MW01201485

Surgery of the Knee

Surgery *of the* Knee

Volume 2

Third Edition

John N. Insall, MD
Clinical Professor of Orthopaedic Surgery
Albert Einstein College of Medicine
Bronx, New York
Director, Insall Scott Kelly Institute for Orthopaedics and Sports Medicine
Beth Israel Medical Center
New York, New York

W. Norman Scott, MD
Chairman, Department of Orthopaedic Surgery
Beth Israel Medical Center
New York, New York
Clinical Professor of Orthopaedic Surgery
Albert Einstein College of Medicine
Bronx, New York
Director, Insall Scott Kelly Institute for Orthopaedics and Sports Medicine
Beth Israel Medical Center
New York, New York

Illustrator: Christopher Wikoff, CMI

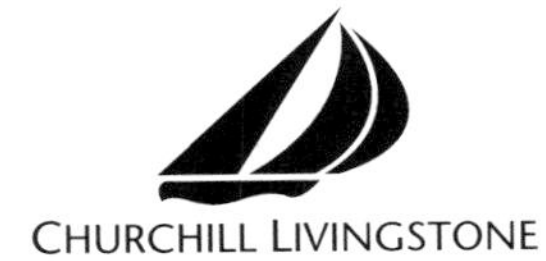

CHURCHILL LIVINGSTONE

A Harcourt Health Sciences Company

New York Edinburgh London Philadelphia San Francisco

CHURCHILL LIVINGSTONE
A Harcourt Health Sciences Company

The Curtis Center
Independence Square West
Philadelphia, Pennsylvania 19106

Library of Congress Cataloging-in-Publication Data

Surgery of the knee / [edited by] John N. Insall, W. Norman Scott; illustrator, Christopher Wikoff.—3rd ed.

p. cm.

Includes bibliographical references and index.

ISBN 0–443–06545–4 (set)

1. Knee—Surgery. I. Insall, John N. II. Scott, W. Norman.
[DNLM: 1. Knee—surgery. 2. Arthroplasty. 3. Knee Injuries—surgery. 4. Ligaments, Articular—injuries. WE 870 S961 2001]

RD561.S87 2001 617.5′82059—dc21 00-024855

Editor-in-Chief, Surgery: Richard H. Lampert
Developmental Editor: Arlene Friday Chappelle
Editor-in-Chief's Assistant: Beth LoGiudice
Copy Editor: Scott Filderman
Production Manager: Frank Polizzano
Illustration Coordinator: Walt Verbitski

SURGERY OF THE KNEE ISBN 0-443-06545-4

Printed in the United States of America.

Last digit is the print number: 9 8 7 6 5 4 3 2 1

➢ Contents

VOLUME 1

SECTION VI

Miscellaneous Conditions and Treatments

49 Inflammatory Arthritis of the Knee

ANDREW G. FRANKS, JR.

GENERAL CONSIDERATIONS

The diagnosis of inflammatory disorders affecting the knee may be facilitated by analysis of the clinical, radiographic, and laboratory studies, with the orthopedist and rheumatologist often combining their diagnostic skills. The classic signs of inflammation (heat, erythema, swelling, and pain) may be variably present in a monoarticular or polyarticular, symmetrical or asymmetrical, or acute or chronic manner, suggesting an array of diagnostic possibilities, involvement of the knee frequently being only part of a more generalized rheumatic disease or systemic illness. The key to successful diagnosis and treatment of nontraumatic acute and chronic inflammatory arthritis of the knee is a systematic approach to the patient that combines thorough history, careful physical examination, and proper use and interpretation of all ancillary studies by the orthopedist and rheumatologist team.

After the history, physical examination, and x-ray films, the initial evaluation of nontraumatic arthritis may include a complete blood count; urinalysis; serum chemistries including liver function, calcium, phosphorous, and uric acid; erythrocyte sedimentation rate; Lyme disease serology; rheumatoid factor; and antinuclear antibodies. If the diagnosis continues to remain unclear, additional blood and radiographic studies as well as synovianalysis, synovial biopsy (Fig. 49.1), and/or arthroscopy may be required.[1] The analysis of synovial fluid (synovianalysis) may be done separately or just prior to irrigation for the arthroscopic evaluation of the inflamed knee, along with direct visualization and a concomitant synovial biopsy. Synovianalysis is more clinically useful than a synovial biopsy alone, with the exception of the granulomatous diseases and amyloidosis.

DIFFERENTIAL DIAGNOSIS

The evolving etiology and prevalence of various inflammatory disorders affecting the knee have recently included Lyme disease, HIV-associated arthritis, and hepatitis C, thereby requiring that the physician maintain a high index of suspicion and not concentrate prematurely on limited diagnostic possibilities. The popularization of fitness and sports has dramatically increased acute injury to the knee, and preexisting or concomitant inflammatory disorders of the knee may be pitfalls in accurate diagnosis and treatment. Also, as a result of advances in health care, an increasing proportion of the population is older; not surprisingly, the prevalence of nontraumatic arthritis of the knee has also grown.

Major advances in our understanding of the pathogenesis of the two most common forms of arthritis, rheumatoid arthritis (RA) and osteoarthritis (OA), have occurred over the past decade (Fig. 49.2). The classic distinction between "inflammatory" and "non-inflammatory" arthritis is rapidly waning. Thus, depending on the underlying pathophysiology, the "inflammation" of RA differs from that of OA and has different therapeutic implications. Knowledge of the pathogenesis of articular damage promises to bring highly specific and effective forms of therapy to decrease the inflammation and articular destruction occurring in these diseases. As more detailed information about the causes of the various forms of arthritis is formulated, more precise treatments directed against the specific etiologies may be developed, and the use of nonspecific anti-inflammatory agents will lessen.

RA is the most prevalent chronic, symmetrical polyarthritis affecting the younger adult population of the United States. The diagnosis of RA is supported by the presence of rheumatoid nodules over extensor surfaces, detection of rheumatoid factor in the serum, x-ray changes of erosion and osteopenia, and synovial fluid inflammatory findings. OA is the most likely cause of progressive pain in the knees aggravated by weight-bearing in the older adult population. It is a heterogeneous group of disorders, each of which leads to varying degress of articular cartilage loss, eburnation of bone, and formation of marginal osteophytes. However, a variety of other conditions can give rise to similar manifestations, and the specific diagnosis requires laboratory data and radiographic and sometimes direct visualization. Lyme disease may cause a monoarticular or polyarticular inflammatory arthritis and may present without a history of tick bite, rash, or constitutional symptoms. Although the diagnosis of Lyme disease is often made clinically, serological blood testing should be used for confirmation of the arthritis, current practice being confirmation of all positive or equivocal enzyme-linked immunosorbent assay results with Western blot analysis.

HIV infection may lead to a wide variety of arthritic syndromes, including variants of Reiter's disease, psoriatic arthritis, and seronegative RA. Therefore, appropriate testing should be performed in those individuals at risk.

Hepatitis C (HCV) infection is transmitted primarily by blood products. As testing was not readily available

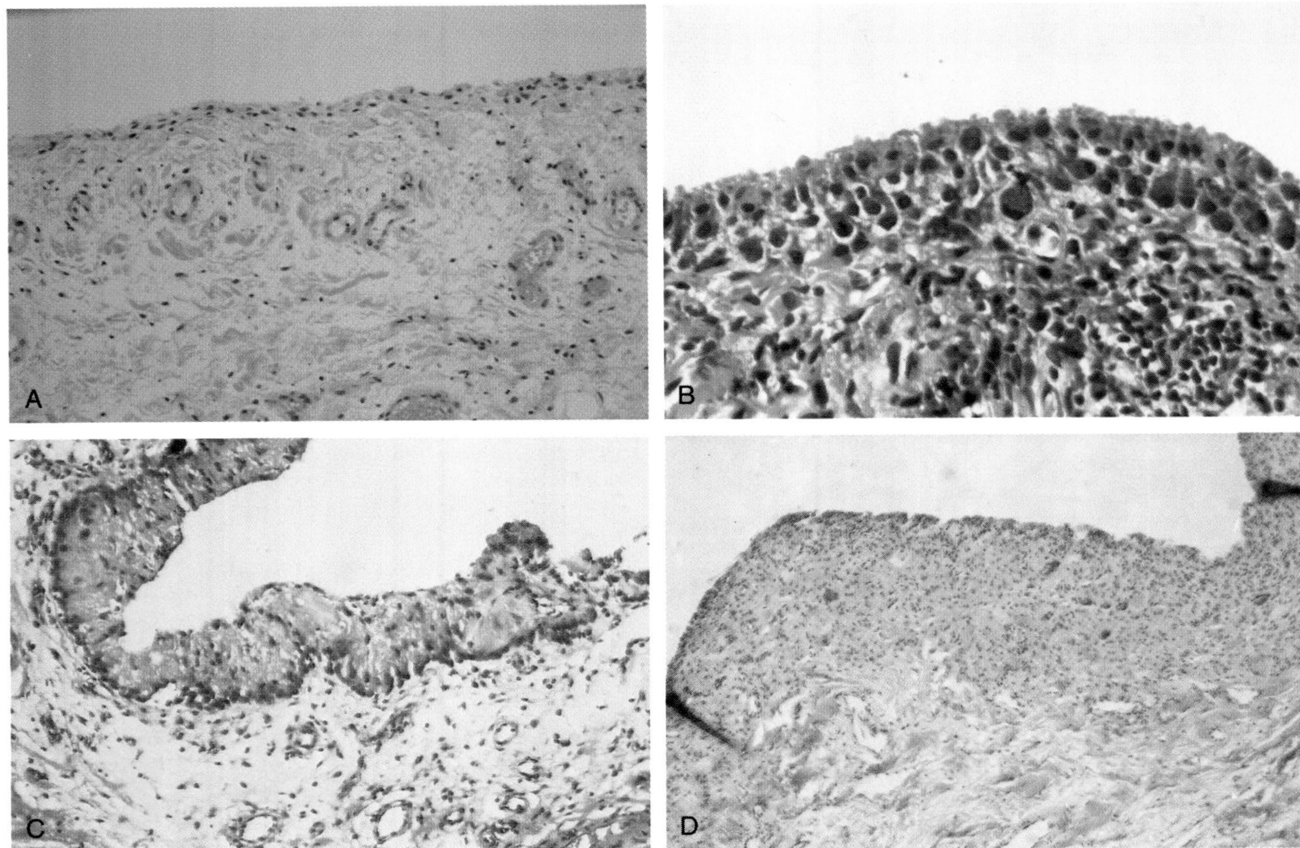

FIGURE 49.1 ➢ *A,* Normal synovium consists of a fine single or double layer of lining "intimal cells" on top of a subintimal zone of vascular and fatty tissue, fibroblasts, and rare histiocytes and mast cells. There is increasing collagen in the vicinity of dense connective tissue structures. *B,* Hyperplastic synovium showing moderate hypertrophy of cells confined to the surface with increasing hyperplasia and hyperplastic cells migrating into the subintimal zone with marked hypertrophy. *C,* Mucinous hyperplasia illustrating secretory potential of synoviocytes. *D,* Superficial zone foreign body giant cell reaction to failed prosthesis. (From Vigorita VJ: The synovium. In Vigorita VJ, Ghelman B: Orthopaedic Pathology. Philadelphia, Lippincott/Williams & Wilkins, 1999.)

until recently, many individuals who have received blood transfusions are also at risk. HCV-infected patients may develop polyarthritis with rheumatoid factors, causing diagnostic confusion with classic RA.[10]

SYNOVIANALYSIS

Synovianalysis may be performed before or with arthroscopy, depending on the clinical setting. Thus, when acute arthritis occurs without a history of trauma, and bacterial infection or crystal-induced arthritis is suspected, synovianalysis performed immediately with a 19 gauge needle (arthrocentesis) may guide initial therapy. Alternately, in those patients with more indolent disease where ancillary studies including radiographs, blood cultures, chemistries, and serologies are unrevealing, synovianalysis may be performed at the time of arthroscopy. Small effusions are best analyzed prior to arthroscopy in order to avoid bleeding caused by the introduction of the arthroscope or dilution with instilled saline and anesthetic. There are two circumstances that require careful exclusion prior to synovianalysis, whether by arthrocentesis or arthroscopy, in order to avoid septic contamination of a sterile joint. Patients with septicemia or with cutaneous or soft-tissue infection mimicking an acute arthritis should not be subjected to arthrocentesis or arthroscopy: direct introduction of the offending organisms into the joint space may occur.[16]

Normal Synovial Fluid

The normal knee joint contains up to 4 mL of synovial fluid with less than 200 white cells per cubic millimeter. In general, small lymphocytes and monocytes predominate with few, if any, polymorphonuclear cells. This fluid is not simply an ultrafiltrate of plasma as are those of serous cavities, because the synovial lining cells (synoviocytes) produce hyaluronate (mucin), a heavy, asymmetrically branched glycosaminoglycan that significantly alters viscosity as well as composition by diminishing water content and interfering with the permeability of large molecules such as fibrinogen, other clotting factors, and globulins. Therefore, normal

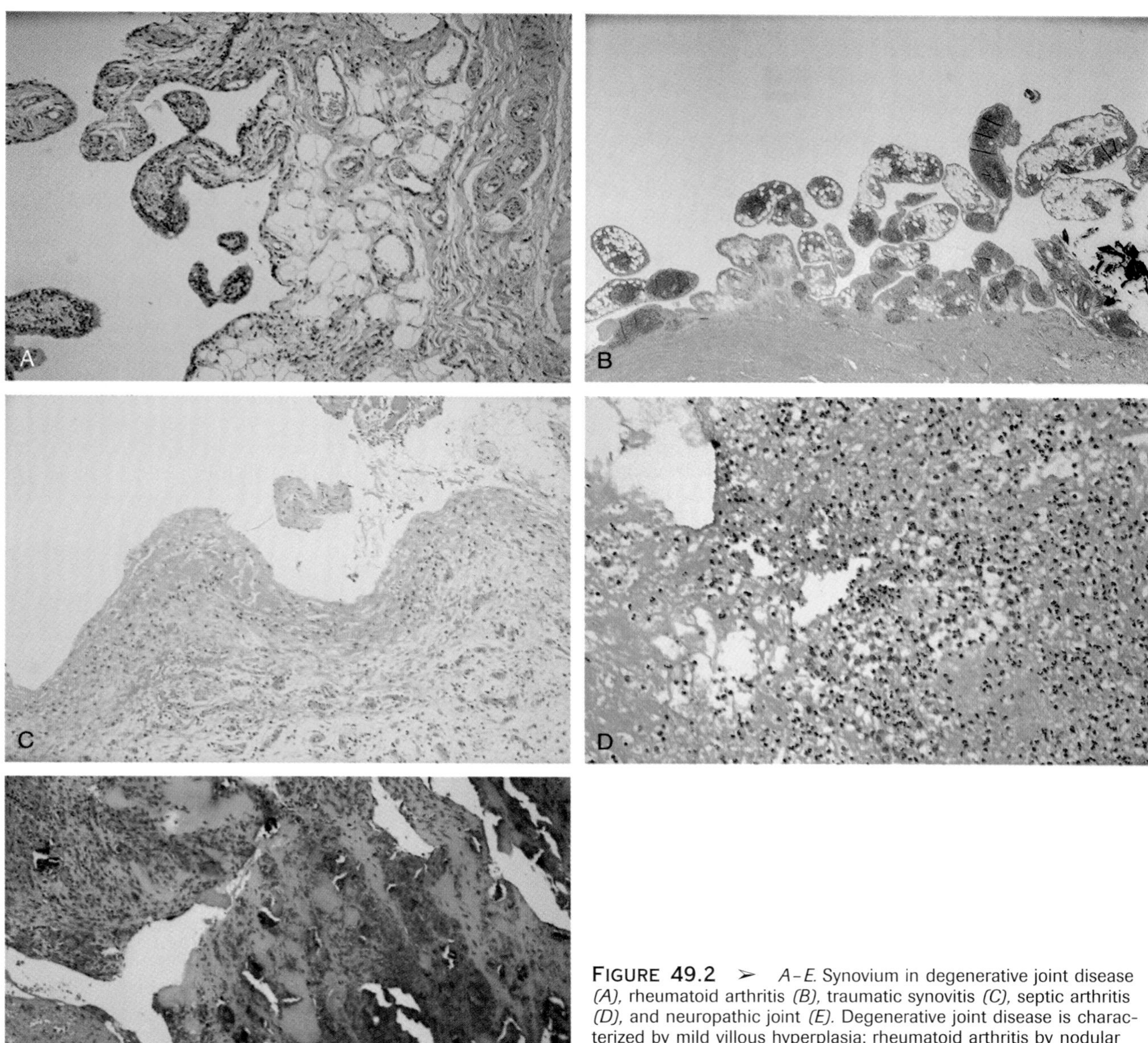

FIGURE 49.2 ➢ *A–E.* Synovium in degenerative joint disease *(A),* rheumatoid arthritis *(B),* traumatic synovitis *(C),* septic arthritis *(D),* and neuropathic joint *(E).* Degenerative joint disease is characterized by mild villous hyperplasia; rheumatoid arthritis by nodular lymphoplasmacytic inflammation; trauma by fibrinous change; septic athritis by leukocytosis; and neuropathic joints by abundant bone and cartilage detritus. (From Vigorita VJ: The synovium. In Vigorita VJ, Ghelman B: Orthopaedic Pathology. Philadelphia, Lippincott/Williams & Wilkins, 1999.)

synovial fluid is of scant volume with few white cells, is highly viscous, does not clot, is transparent, and is colorless or pale yellow (Table 49.1). These features are the basis for correct interpretation of synovianalysis of the abnormal knee joint.[3]

Abnormal Synovial Fluid

Diseases that affect the knee may change the normal characteristics of the synovial fluid in a number of ways, allowing distinctions to be made. Grossly increased volume, decreased viscosity, ability to clot, diminished clarity, and change in color all contribute to the interpretation of synovianalysis. Microscopic analysis for the number and type of cells, as well as presence or absence of crystals, is equally important. The addition of bacteriological, chemical, and immunological tests further enhances the ability to discriminate between the vast number of disorders that may affect the knee. However, the total white cell count and the identification of bacteria or crystals are considered the most important factors in most diagnostic and therapeutic decisions.[20]

Initial descriptions of abnormal joint fluid were simply divided into those that were noninflammatory and those that were inflammatory. The usefulness of this division was eventually increased by the separation of those fluids that were septic and those that were hem-

TABLE 49.1 NORMAL SYNOVIAL FLUID

Volume (Knee)	4 mL
Viscosity (String or mucin clot)	High
Color	Colorless/pale yellow
Clarity	Transparent
Total WBC/mm³	200
Differential WBC:	
PMNs	25%
Lymphocytes	25%
Monocytes	50%
Crystals	None
Protein	2.5 gm/dL
Glucose	90% of blood
Culture	Negative

orrhagic. Therefore, at the present time, four groups of abnormal synovial fluid (Table 49.2) that are clinically useful have been defined. Distinction among these groups is based on synovial fluid volume, viscosity (hyaluronate), clarity, color, cellularity (amount and type), and culture. Further subdivision, particularly within inflammatory noninfectious (group II) synovial fluid, has recently been suggested (Fig. 49.3).

Technique of Synovianalysis

Inadequate or improper technique in performing synovianalysis has been responsible for misinterpretation, sometimes diminishing its importance in assessing joint disease. It is often more informative than performing just a synovial biopsy.[6] Unfortunately, there are more pitfalls in its collection and preparation than with those of other body fluids, and many clinical and hospital laboratories are not thoroughly familiar with the preferred techniques.[12] Therefore, it becomes the responsibility of the physician who performs synovianalysis to become adept in this area, whether performing the tests personally or documenting the correct handling of specimens sent to the laboratory. Although a complete review of specific technique is beyond the scope of this chapter, some general guidelines are suggested below. The reader is referred to detailed descriptions of this subject in the References.

When profuse amounts of extraneous blood are caused by introduction of the needle or arthroscope, the validity of synovianalysis is questionable. However, in situations where smaller numbers of red blood cells may interfere with white cell counts, lysing the red blood cells may be helpful (see below). Once synovial fluid is obtained, approximately 1015 mL is sufficient for complete synovianalysis, although basic studies such as cell count and culture can be obtained on smaller amounts.

The fluid obtained in a sterile syringe should be gently shaken; any needle should be removed from the syringe; and then the fluid should be immediately separated as follows:

1. Sterile tube with sodium heparin (green-topped tubes in many laboratories, if sterile); 3 to 5 mL for stains and cultures, including aerobic, anaerobic, tubercular, and fungal vials, and direct inoculation on chocolate agar for gonococci. Use the same media as for blood cultures. Do not use transport media. Gram's and special stains are best performed on a centrifuged aliquot.
2. Sterile tube with sodium heparin or ethylenediaminetetraacetic acid (EDTA) (green- or purple-topped tubes in many laboratories); 2 to 3 mL for cell counts, differential, cytology, and crystals.
3. Two clean tubes without anticoagulant (plain red-topped tubes in many laboratories); 1 to 2 mL for color, viscosity (string or mucin clot), inclusions, crystals (option from anticoagulated); 1 to 2 mL for total protein, rheumatoid factor, complement, etc.
4. Clean tube with preservative, e.g., oxalate (gray-topped tube in many laboratories); 1 mL for glucose.

Volume

The total volume aspirated may help to determine the severity of the disease process, although it is generally not helpful in distinguishing between the various groups of abnormal fluids. Low volume does not rule out significant disease; rather, the volume of synovial fluid removed on several subsequent synovianalyses is sometimes helpful in determining response to treatment, such as in septic arthritis. Generally more than 4 mL obtained from the knee is considered abnormal.

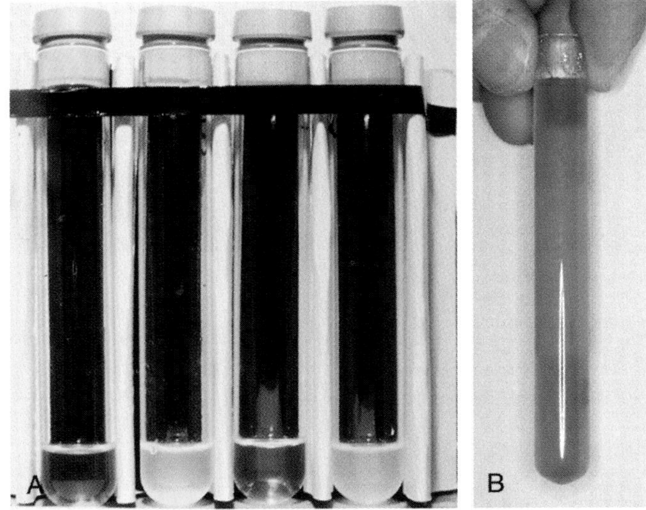

FIGURE 49.3 ➢ *Synovial fluid composite.* Synovial fluid from patients with calcium pyrophosphate crystal deposition (cloudy), normal (clear amber), rheumatoid arthritis (cloudy yellow), and trauma induced (blood stained). Pigmented villonodular synovitis, especially of the diffuse type, can give a bloody or rusty appearance. Septic arthritis yields a turbid yellowish-green. (From Vigorita VJ: The synovium. In Vigorita VJ, Ghelman B: Orthopaedic Pathology. Philadelphia, Lippincott/Williams & Wilkins, 1999.)

TABLE 49.2 CHARACTERISTICS OF ABNORMAL SYNOVIAL FLUID

Group I: Noninflammatory

Volume (knee)	Often >4 mL
Viscosity (string or mucin clot)	High
Color	Straw-colored to yellow
Clarity	Transparent
Total WBC/mm³	200–3000
Differential WBC	
PMNs	<–25%
Lymphocytes	<25%
Monocytes	>50%
Crystals	None
Protein	Usually normal
Glucose	90% of blood
Culture	Negative

Partial List of Associated Conditions

Trauma
Internal derangement
Osteoarthritis
Aseptic necrosis
Osteochondritis dissecans
Osteochondromatosis
Polymyalgia rheumatica
Amyloidosis
Early or resolving inflammation
Acquired immunodeficiency syndrome

Group II: Inflammatory

Volume (knee)	Often >4 mL
Viscosity (string or mucin clot)	Low
Color	Yellow to white
Clarity	Translucent
Total WBC/mm³	2000–75,000
Differential WBC	
PMNs	>50%
Lymphocytes	<25%
Monocytes	25%
Crystals	May be present
Protein	>32.0 g/dL
Glucose	75% of blood or lower
Culture	Negative for bacteria

Partial List of Associated Conditions

a. Often highly inflammatory

Rheumatoid arthritis
Crystal arthritis
Reiter's syndrome
Acute rheumatic fever
Lyme disease

b. Often mildly inflammatory

Psoriatic arthritis
Bowel-related arthritis
Juvenile arthritis
Ankylosing spondylitis
Connective tissue disease
Viral arthritis (including parvovirus)
Tubercular or fungal arthritis

Group III: Septic

Volume (knee)	Usually >4 mL
Viscosity (string or mucin clot)	Low
Color	Variable
Clarity	Opaque
Total WBC/mm³	Usually >100,000
Differential WBC	
PMNs	>75%
Lymphocytes	<10%
Monocytes	<–10%
Crystals	None
Protein	>3.0 g/dL
Glucose	50% of blood or lower
Culture	Positive for bacteria

Partial List of Associated Conditions

Bacterial infections
Tubercular or fungal arthritis (rare)

Group IV: Hemorrhagic

Volume (knee)	Usually >4 mL
Viscosity (string or mucin clot)	Variable
Color	Pink to bloody
Clarity	Variable
Total WBC/mm³	Variable
Differential WBC	
PMNs (%)	Variable
Lymphocytes (%)	Variable
Monocytes (%)	Variable
Crystals	None
Protein	Variable
Glucose	Variable
Culture	Negative

Partial List of Associated Conditions

Trauma (exclude fracture)
Hemorrhagic diatheses:
- Thrombocytopenia
- Anticoagulant therapy
- Hemophilia
- Sickle cell disease
- Malignancy

Neuroarthropathy (Charcot's joint)
Joint prostheses
Tumor:
- Pigmented villonodular synovitis
- Synovial hemangioma

Viscosity

Reduced viscosity results from either the degradation of hyaluronate caused by inflammation or the rapid accumulation of fluid after trauma, which dilutes hyaluronate concentration. Direct measurement of viscosity or hyaluronate is not usually performed; instead, indirect assessment is based on two relatively simple procedures: string test and mucin clot.

When a drop of normal synovial fluid is held between the gloved thumb and index finger, a "string" effect will be noted as the fingers are slowly separated. If viscosity is reduced, separation of the fingers occurs without any bridge of synovial fluid between them. An alternate method is to express fluid one drop at a time from a syringe with the needle removed. Normal synovial fluid droplets form a long string, suggesting honey, whereas low-viscosity fluid appears like water droplets with short tails.

The mucin clot test also correlates with the amount of hyaluronate present and therefore reflects viscosity. When one part normal synovial fluid is added to four parts of 2% acetic acid and shaken, a firm button of clotted hyaluronate protein complex forms at the bottom of the tube after standing for 5 minutes. With degraded hyaluronate from inflammation, no button forms, and the synovial fluid may contain friable shreds of clotted material.

The string test and mucin clot are generally interchangeable in the interpretation of synovial fluid viscosity, with most clinicians performing the former because of its simplicity.[21]

Clarity

The clarity of normal synovial fluid can be reduced by any particulate matter, most commonly increased cellularity, but also by crystals, inclusion bodies, and lipids. The method for detecting loss of clarity generally involves placing black text on a white background, such as newsprint, behind a test tube containing synovial fluid. With a bright light, if the text can be read through the fluid, its clarity is normal (transparent).

Color

The normal synovial fluid is colorless or pale yellow (straw-colored). When blood, not caused by the procedure itself, is found, it generally does not form clots and is evenly distributed throughout the fluid. Inflammatory fluid may appear as deep yellow. Pus may be found, but large numbers of crystals or inflammatory debris may mimic its appearance.

Cell Counts

A grossly bloody fluid may result from the introduction of the needle or arthroscope and is usually evident during the procedure; the blood may be unevenly distributed, often clots, and may decrease as the procedure continues. A hematocrit level from an anticoagulated tube should be obtained on all bloody effusions to determine whether it is blood per se because only moderate amounts of red cells may simulate the appearance of whole blood. If red cells are actually present in the synovial fluid due to the disease process, they are usually evenly distributed, do not clot, and remain consistent throughout the procedure. Because the intra-articular breakdown of these disease-related red cells releases heme, a centrifuged specimen produces xanthochromia. Considered one of the most important aspects of synovianalysis, the total and differential white cell count may be inaccurate if precautions are not observed. It is important that synovial fluid be placed promptly in appropriate anticoagulant and that no clumps of cells are found after gently shaking the tube. If clots remain, this should alert one that the total white cell count may be falsely low. Even if this is correctly done, differences may occur, depending on whether manual or automated counting methods are employed. Manual counts are considered most accurate but have one pitfall: if acetic acid is inadvertently used as the diluent, synovial protein clots will entrap white cells and falsely lower the total count. Therefore, it is imperative that normal saline be used as the diluent. If the effusion is bloody, hypotonic (0.3%) saline should be used to lyse the red cells after a hematocrit is performed. Automated counters are not recommended because of the large number of technical artifacts that may occur.

Crystals

The presence or absence of crystals in synovial fluid is as essential in the evaluation of disorders of the knee as the total cell count and differential, particularly as crystal-induced arthritis may produce inflammation with very high white cell counts overlapping those of septic arthritis. As with the cell count, precautions must be observed in order to obtain an accurate result. Considerable variation in correctly identifying crystals has been documented in clinical and hospital laboratories, and it is strongly recommended that the clinician perform the analysis personally to ensure accuracy, just as the hematologist does with the bone marrow examination.

Collection of the specimen into appropriate tubes is essential for success. As noted above, anticoagulated tubes may be used, but only with sodium heparin or EDTA. If lithium heparin or calcium oxalate is inadvertently used, crystalline artifacts will be produced and cause totally inaccurate results. Although nonanticoagulated specimens may also be used, inaccuracies may be caused by white cells clumps, obscuring identification of crystals. An additional pitfall is the presence of corticosteroid crystals for weeks after their instillation into the joint cavity.

Once the specimen is collected into a tube containing sodium heparin or EDTA, a wet mount should be prepared as soon as possible. This requires placing a drop of synovial fluid on a slide free of dust or scratches, placing a clean cover slip over the drop, and sealing it on all four sides with clear nail polish. Sealing the cover slip avoids the streaming of cells as well as the de novo precipitation of crystals caused by dehydration of the specimen. Assuming the correct collection of the specimen and preparation of the wet mount, the identification of crystals requires use of a compensated, polarized light microscope with a rotating stage. All clinicians who perform synovianalysis should have access to this equipment and be familiar with its use. Without it, significant joint disease will surely be missed. At the present time, four types of pathological crystals may be identified: monosodium urate monohydrate in gout, calcium pyrophosphate dihydrate in pseudogout, calcium oxalate in chronic dialysis arthropathy, and hydroxyapatite in rotator cuff (Milwaukee shoulder) syndrome and erosive osteoarthritis.

The purpose of the compensated, polarized light is twofold. It provides a black background that causes the crystalline material, which is most frequently found intracellularly, to stand out from the cells and other particulate material thus allowing an estimation of size and shape. Also, it provides two optical characteristics of crystals, extinction and elongation (birefringence), which further aids in differentiating the specific type of crystal seen. The reader is referred to the References for detailed discussions on identification of crystals.

Microbiology

The swift identification of septic arthritis of the knee depends on analysis of the synovial fluid. As noted earlier, in patients in whom septicemia or soft-tissue infection is suspected, synovianalysis should be deferred until ancillary data are obtained in order to avoid contaminating a sterile joint.[7]

Once fluid is collected in a sterile tube, aliquots should be placed into both aerobic and anaerobic blood agar vials including tubercular and fungal media, and an additional aliquot should be immediately inoculated onto chocolate agar if gonococcal disease is suspected; Gram's stain for bacteria and special stains for mycobacteria and fungi are best performed on a concentrated (centrifuged) aliquot.

Chemistry and Serology

The total protein of normal synovial fluid is usually about 2 g/dL or approximately 25% that of the blood. If greater than 2.5 g/dL, it is abnormal, with higher levels reflecting the degree of inflammation present. Although fasting specimens are the most accurate, normal synovial fluid glucose is about 90% that of simultaneous blood. With inflammation, the levels of synovial fluid glucose diminish, the lowest levels generally occurring in septic arthritis.

Rheumatoid factor may be found in synovial fluid, even in those patients with negative serum levels. Presumably, this is due to production by the synovial cells themselves; the factor may be found as a nonspecific reaction to many kinds of inflammation. It should not be used as an indicator of RA.

Many other components, such as antinuclear antibodies, DNA, complement, globulins, cryoprecipitates, enzymes, etc., may be found in synovial fluid, but they are of little clinical value at present and are mainly of research interest.

Classification Groups of Abnormal Synovial Fluid

GROUP I (NONINFLAMMATORY)

This includes the noninflammatory synovial fluids typically found in trauma (including internal derangement) and osteoarthritis. Rapid accumulation of high-volume fluid after trauma may dilute the concentration of hyaluronate and reduce the viscosity, thereby causing an abnormal string test or mucin clot. Generally, the white cell counts are low (average 1000 per cubic millimeter) and rarely exceed 3000 cells per cubic millimeter. Grossly bloody synovial fluid (see group IV) may occur after an injury without fracture, although careful exclusion should be performed. Reaccumulation of grossly bloody fluid should suggest other group IV disorders. If OA is suspected clinically but synovianalysis suggests otherwise, evaluation for superimposed crystal arthritis, particularly pseudogout (see group II) or infection (see group III), should be pursued. Advanced OA may produce cartilage fragments and other debris. Worn or damaged prostheses may produce metallic, polymethylmethacrylate, or polyethylene fragments that can sometimes be confused with crystals. Immunodeficiency syndromes, including HIV, may be associated with arthritis, with the synovial fluid sometimes being noninflammatory.

GROUP II (INFLAMMATORY)

Because of the large number of inflammatory disorders included within this broad category, it is useful to divide those that are mildly inflammatory from those that are moderately or severely inflammatory. For mildly inflammatory fluid, this distinction is usually based on the total and differential white cell count, which ranges from 1000 to 5000 per cubic millimeter, less than 30% being polymorphonuclear. Although there is much overlap within group II, disorders such as psoriatic and bowel-related arthritis, lupus, juvenile arthritis, and seronegative arthritis may demonstrate only mild inflammation. Many viral diseases may be associated with joint effusions that produce mild inflammation, generally with large numbers of mononuclear cells. Recent outbreaks of parvovirus infection in adults (after exposure to children with erythema infectiosum caused by the same agent) have been associated with arthritis with mild inflammatory fluid and a predominance of monocytes.[23] Moderate to severe inflammatory fluid is typically found in RA and crystal-induced arthritis, with counts generally ranging from 10,000 to 50,000 per cubic millimeter, more than 50% being polymorphonuclear. Acute rheumatic fever and Reiter's syndrome may also cause high cell counts. Rarely, counts approaching 100,000 cells per cubic millimeter may be found, but infection should be diligently excluded. Lyme arthritis has recently been shown to have varying white cell counts, with a range from 5000 to above 300,000 per cubic millimeter.[4] Cultures from the synovial fluid have not grown the spirochete. Tubercular and fungal infections may have low white cell counts and appear as group II fluid. Also, sarcoma and other malignancies may be found within group II fluid and can be identified by standard cytological analysis.

GROUP III (SEPTIC)

Joint fluid, unlike serum, diminishes the normal phagocytic function of cells and allows uninhibited growth of microbial organisms. Infection must therefore be excluded in any patient with an unexplained arthritis as well as in those patients with other arthritic diseases whose joints remain disparately inflamed. Acute bacterial infection, particularly *Staphylococcus aureus,* produces very high white cell counts, typically 100,000 per cubic millimeter or more, with polymorphonuclear cells constituting at least 90%. However, lower white cell counts are not unusual, particularly in patients treated with antibiotics for any reason prior to synovianalysis. Opportunistic organisms and tubercular or fungal infections may also produce lower white cell counts, with varying amounts of mononuclear and polymorphonuclear cells, and overlap with group II fluids. Gonococcal arthritis may be a difficult diagnosis to establish unless the fluid is plated immediately onto chocolate agar. Disseminated gonococcal infection with arthritis may present with white cell counts below 20,000 per cubic millimeter.

GROUP IV (HEMORRHAGIC)

As little as a 10% admixture of red cells may make a joint fluid look like whole blood, but when the fluid is determined to be truly hemorrhagic (group IV), a number of disorders should be considered. If trauma has occurred, fracture should be excluded. Hemorrhagic diathesis, including hemophilia, sickle cell anemia, thrombocytopenia, and anticoagulant therapy, must be eliminated. Neuroarthropathy (Charcot's joint) may also produce a hemorrhagic fluid. Pigmented villonodular synovitis and synovial hemangioma must be eliminated. In addition, worn or damaged prostheses may cause bleeding within the joint.

Conclusion

Synovianalysis is a critical component in the evaluation of knee joint disease and allows the clinician to make rapid, specific diagnostic and therapeutic decisions. The routine use of synovianalysis can reveal clues to new developments in established disease, such as the superimposition of Lyme arthritis[5] on OA or infection in a rheumatoid knee. If, however, synovianalysis is to remain a valuable tool, it is essential that it be performed precisely.

MEDICAL TREATMENT

Introduction

A significant percentage of all drugs sold in the United States is intended to alleviate musculoskeletal pain and/or inflammation. Nonpharmacological measures, however, are of equal importance in the management of chronic synovitis of the knee. They include patient education, appropriate rest and proper diet, and physical and occupational therapy. Drugs for the treatment of inflammatory arthritis of the knee can be divided into two major categories: nonsteroidal anti-inflammatory drugs (NSAIDs) and disease-modifying antirheumatic drugs (DMARDs). Additionally, adrenocorticosteroids play a role in selected patients.[13] Rapid advances in the biology of inflammation and the recent introduction of novel pharmacological agents have revolutionized the classic treatment algorithms of just a few years ago in both major categories.

Nonsteroidal Anti-Inflammatory Drugs

NSAIDs, including aspirin, have been adequate as the first-line agents for symptomatic control of active disease in most patients with knee synovitis, including OA (primary and secondary) or RA and its variants, but are not considered to have any fundamental effect on the progressive changes that may occur in the joints. NSAIDs describe compounds that owe their pharmacological actions principally to inhibition of the enzyme cyclooxygenase (COX), which is responsible for the conversion of arachidonic acid to prostaglandin and other inflammatory mediators. Unfortunately, side effects are more frequent with NSAIDs than with any other prescription drug. Recently, the discovery of two different COX enzymes, COX-1 and COX-2, has had significant clinical implications: the association of COX-1 inhibition with gastrointestinal side effects including bleeding has led to the rapid development of COX-2-specific compounds, such as MK-966 (Vioxx) and celecoxib (Celebrex). Clinical studies indicate that COX-2-specific inhibition is associated with improved gastrointestinal safety while maintaining therapeutic efficacy and may make many currently available NSAIDs less desirable.[14]

As the therapeutic goal with first-line drugs is symptom relief, guides to efficacy include patient preference, pain relief, relief of stiffness, and functional ability. Often, a sequence of these drugs, in varying doses, must be used on a trial-and-error basis, and it may be advisable to include agents of different classes (Table 49.3) in sequence, possibly increasing the chance of response. Generally a 2- or 3-week trial is sufficient, along with suitable adjustments in dose frequency and strength. Most clinicians choose drugs to be used singly rather than concurrently.

Disease-Modifying Antirheumatic Drugs

The ultimate goal in treatment is to prevent the progression of joint destruction from unremitting synovitis as may occur in RA and related inflammatory disorders. DMARDs have generally been reserved for patients with RA or variants with prolonged, active polyarthritis. These include gold compounds (intramuscular or oral), the antimalarials, sulfasalazine, penicillamine, cytotoxic drugs (particularly azathioprine and methotrexate), and cyclosporine (Neoral). Most recently, leflunomide (Arava) and etanercept (Enbrel) are novel additions in the treatment of RA, opening paths to treatment for which there have been virtually no new medicines developed in years. Etanercept is the first genetically engineered molecule that neutralizes tumor necrosis factor (TNF), a substance produced by the body that plays a role in mounting the immune system's attack against the joints in RA. Etanercept and leflunomide offer the promise of helping those individuals in whom traditional treatments have failed.

Adrenocorticosteroids

Although adrenocorticosteroids are the most potent of the anti-inflammatory agents, the incidence of toxicity

TABLE 49.3 CLASSIFICATION OF SOME NSAIDS

Salicylates:
Aspirin (Acetylated)
Plain, USP
Buffered (Bufferin, Anacin)
Coated (Ecotrin)
Time-release (Bayer Time Release)
Others (Nonacetylated)
Sodium salicylate (Alysine)
Choline magnesium (Trilisate, Arthropan)
Salicylsalicylate (Disalcid)
Diflunisal (Dolobid)
Acetic Acids:
Diclofenac (Voltaren, Arthrotec, Cataflam)
Etodolac (Lodine)
Indomethacin (Indocin)
Sulindac (Clinoril)
Tolmetin (Tolectin)
Propionic Acids:
Ibuprofen (Motrin, Rufen, Advil, etc)
Fenoprofen (Nalfon)
Flurbiprofen (Ansaid)
Oxaprozin (Daypro)
Naproxen (Aleve, Naprosyn, Anaprox, Naprelan)
Ketoprofen (Orudis)
Fenamic Acids:
Mefenamic acid (Ponstel)
Meclofenamic acid (Meclomen)
Naphthyl-Alkalone:
Relafen
Pyrazolones:
Phenylbutazone (Butazolidin)
Oxicams:
Piroxicam (Feldene)
Cox-2 Specific:
MK-966 (Vioxx)
Celecoxib (Celebrex)

associated with systemic administration limits their use in patients with chronic forms of arthritis. Additionally, in acute synovitis of the knee, their use should be restricted until the diagnosis is established with certainty. When major levels of disability are attributable to the knee, intra-articular administration of steroid preparations, as interim adjunctive treatment, may induce periods of improvement that last for several weeks or more. However, injections in individual joints should not be repeated frequently because of the risk of accelerated cartilage destruction.

Individualizing Drug Dosage

The importance of individualizing drug dosage to achieve optimal results is being increasingly recognized. Unfortunately, only the salicylate assays are readily available, and most physicians prescribe the pharmaceutical company's "usual dose" for all other agents. Concentration of drug at receptor sites (the site where a drug is active) relates directly to efficacy and toxicity, and this in turn depends on plasma protein binding (an inactive reservoir of drug) and total daily drug dose. Recently, side effects and toxicity are thought to relate more to concentration of drug rather than to idiosyncratic reactions.

Principles of Adjusting Dose

Most drugs have a narrow therapeutic ratio and do not have clinical assays readily available to determine plasma concentration. Therefore, the physician must adjust the standard or usual dose for each patient. A number of events can alter the optimum plasma concentration for the individual patient, including absorption, protein binding, drug interactions, and biotransformation. Most drugs are prescribed at shorter intervals than their elimination half-life (T1/2) so that with chronic administration accumulation in plasma and tissue occurs until equilibrium is reached. Steady-state levels occur when the amount of drug administered in one dose equals the amount of drug eliminated during that dose interval. Most drugs, including the NSAIDs, are eliminated according to exponential or first-order kinetics whereby a certain percentage of drug is removed independent of dose. They are not significantly influenced by small changes in daily dose, and those with long T1/2s may require weeks to be completely cleared. Some drugs, including the salicylates, demonstrate zero order kinetics whereby a constant amount of drug is removed, and they are therefore considerably dose-dependent. Disproportionately high drug concentrations may be produced by small increases in drug dose.

Clinical Evaluation of Antirheumatic Drugs

The introduction of numerous antirheumatic drugs over the past decade has required more critical appraisal of their usefulness and side effects. Physicians have had to become more sophisticated in the interpretation of clinical trials published in the literature in order to prescribe these drugs correctly. The ability to follow synovial inflammation and cartilage destruction in both RA and OA on a clinical basis has not kept pace with the remarkable advances in understanding the immunological basis for their pathogenesis. Techniques such as computed tomography scans and magnetic resonance imaging have become more sophisticated but obviously do not allow direct visualization and tissue sampling. Rapid technological advances in arthroscopy allow for the performance of diagnostic studies, with synovianalysis and synovial biopsy whenever required, and in the future will provide the necessary follow-up to new treatment protocols.

Aspirin and Salicylates

In addition to their analgesic effect, salicylates are anti-inflammatory. Inhibition of prostaglandin synthesis (acetylated salicylates) and neutrophil function (acetylated and nonacetylated salicylates) appear to be important, although not the only, mechanisms of action. Plain aspirin appears to be as or more effective than its derivatives in both analgesic and anti-inflammatory action.

Clinical Use

Aspirin and salicylates are useful for arthritis of the knee, whether noninflammatory or inflammatory. Dosages of 300 to 600 mg three or four times a day are sufficient for analgesic and mild anti-inflammatory effects. High-dose ("therapeutic") anti-inflammation doses are no longer popular because of the high incidence of gastrointestinal bleeding and other side effects (see below).[19]

USP-formulation plain aspirin is as effective as any, but if not kept dry aspirin will slowly decay to salicylic acid and acetic acid with a vinegary smell. Although not unsafe to use and just as effective when decayed, some patients may tolerate buffered tablets better. Although the small amounts of buffering in commonly sold buffered aspirin may reduce some gastrointestinal side effects, it does not appear to influence the incidence of microbleeding from the stomach.

Aspirin and salicylates should not be used in gout because the effects of salicylate on the serum uric acid (increases) and urinary urate excretion (lowers) can complicate management. The interaction of salicylate with other drugs is extensive but clinically significant in only a few important situations. Thus, although salicylates may compete with or bind to the receptor sites of the other NSAIDs as well as displace them from the plasma protein inactive reservoir, the clinical significance is low or nonexistent. Thus, low-dose aspirin for prevention of heart attack and stroke may be combined with other NSAIDs. Corticosteroids can lower the level of serum salicylate, and when corticosteroids are tapered, a sudden rise in salicylate level may occur. An additive or synergistic effect on gastrointestinal toxicity may also occur. Alcohol may also have this effect on the gastrointestinal tract.

An important interaction of salicylate and other NSAIDs is that with methotrexate, presumably by displacing it from the plasma protein inactive reservoir, thereby raising the amount of drug available to bind the active receptor site, resulting in the increased possibility of bone marrow and liver toxicity. These drugs should be used together cautiously, if at all (see below).

Side Effects and Toxicity of Salicylates

The side effects and toxicity of salicylates, aside from gastrointestinal hemorrhage, are neither chronic nor cumulative and are completely reversible. Tinnitus with a high-pitched ringing, vertigo, dizziness, diminished concentration, and somnolence suggest the need for dose reduction. Aspirin allergy is not uncommon and generally falls into two categories: bronchospasm and urticaria/angioedema. If a patient gives a history of these, it is not unlikely that the patient will also have a similar response to other NSAIDs, which should be used cautiously. The new COX-2–specific NSAIDs may not cross-react in some salicylate-sensitive patients, but this observation requires additional investigation.

The gastrointestinal side effects of acetylated salicylate can be divided into three major categories: symptomatic gastrointestinal distress, microbleeding, and frank gastritis or ulcer with hemorrhage. Nonacetylated salicylates are less troublesome, and some of the newer NSAIDs, especially the COX-2–specific, may greatly reduce gastrointestinal toxicity. Carafate may be more protective than either Tagamet or Zantac when used with salicylates or other NSAIDs. Misoprostol has recently been introduced, and some clinicians use combinations of these agents when the possibility of gastrointestinal intolerance is high and a history of ulcer or hemorrhage is obtained.

The hematological side effects of aspirin include prolongation of the bleeding time and diminished platelet aggregation. This effect can be achieved with as little as one 80-mg tablet per day. In fact, higher doses have no demonstrable increased effect. Presumably, platelet COX is acetylated, and a single tablet inactivates over 90% of this enzyme. This effect takes approximately 5 to 7 days to be eliminated. Sodium salicylate, choline magnesium salicylate, and salicylsalicylate, because of their lack of an acetyl group, have no effect on the enzyme, and some NSAIDs have variable effects (see below).

The hepatic effects of salicylates are usually discovered during routine blood studies and generally consist of elevations of transaminases. Most patients remain asymptomatic, and in this group salicylates may be continued if necessary, although those with extremely high levels or elevation of alkaline phosphatase should be monitored closely for further signs of hepatitis. If nausea, anorexia, or liver tenderness occurs, the dosage should be discontinued.

The effects of aspirin and other NSAIDs on the kidney are numerous and include transient shedding of tubular cells, reduced glomerular filtration and renal blood flow, and alteration of urate excretion. The effect on renal tubules usually occurs during the first week of therapy and gradually disappears, but analgesic nephropathy (chronic interstitial nephritis) should be considered if this occurs later in the course of treatment. Episodic hematuria may also occur, which sometimes leads the physician to search for other causes. The effect on glomerular filtration and renal blood flow is presumably due to aspirin's reduction of renal prostaglandin. Mild proteinuria, edema, and rising BUN/creatinine with alteration of electrolytes may occur. Nonacetylated salicylates have little effect on prostaglandin synthesis and therefore may be more suitable in patients with preexistent renal compromise.

Other Nonsteroidal Anti-Inflammatory Drugs

NSAIDs offer the clinician many alternatives, but without a thorough understanding of their pharmacology, these alternatives can sometimes seem bewildering. Many of these drugs have common properties, such as the potential to bind plasma proteins and the ability to inhibit chemical mediators of inflammation such as prostaglandins and/or leukotrienes.[26] Features such as serum half-life; effects on platelets, liver, or kidney; interaction with other drugs; and dose regimens may make some more suitable than others for the individual patient. Of particular importance, NSAIDs, including the COX-2-specific inhibitors, may significantly reduce the production of renal vasodilatory prostaglandins. All inhibit the enzyme COX, which is involved in the biosynthetic pathway of renal prostaglandin production. Although this effect may be inconsequential on normal kidneys, the presence of preexisting intrinsic renal disease or hyper-reninemic conditions associated with a contracted plasma volume, such as hemorrhage, general anesthesia, salt depletion, diuretic therapy (especially triamterene [Dyazide, Maxzide, Dyrenium]), congestive heart failure, cirrhosis (especially with ascites), or serious infection, may lead to further renal compromise. Specifically, such problems include renal failure due to decreased glomerular filtration, papillary necrosis probably due to medullary ischemia, sodium retention with edema, nephrotic syndrome (which may occur many months after discontinuing NSAIDs), and hyperkalemia and hyponatremia due to suppression of renin production.[22]

Categorizing the various drugs into chemical classes is helpful in organizing changes in therapy. The more commonly available drugs are listed in Table 49.3.

COX-2-Specific Inhibitors

Traditional NSAIDs inhibit COX-1 and COX-2. COX-1 inhibition contributes to its gastrointestinal side effects, whereas COX-2 inhibition contributes to its anti-inflammatory effects. Clinical studies indicate that COX-2-specific inhibition is associated with decreased gastrointestinal side effects including ulcer and bleeding while therapeutic efficacy is maintained.[24]

Effect of Food or Antacids

Many NSAIDs have reduced bioavailability when taken with food or antacids, but clinical variation is common. However, in patients with a high probability of gastrointestinal side effects, many clinicians suggest taking these drugs with meals or antacids during the initial course of treatment.[9] If tolerated, the regimen may then be modified if clinical response is deficient. Switching from aluminum-based to magnesium-based antacids is sometimes helpful. The use of Carafate, 1 g four times a day, may be more protective than Tagamet or Zantac. The introduction of misoprostol for the prevention of upper gastrointestinal bleeding is the reason for its admixture into Arthrotec. Some physicians use these drugs in combination for high-risk patients.

TREATMENT OF SPECIFIC FORMS OF CHRONIC KNEE SYNOVITIS

Osteoarthritis

Aspirin and other NSAIDs, which combine analgesia with anti-inflammation, form the basis for current medical therapy. Pure analgesics, such as acetaminophen and propoxyphene, may be used continuously or intermittently, along with NSAIDs.[2] Narcotic preparations should be limited to the occasional, acute flare of primary OA or the immediate, post-traumatic knee injury. Oral or parenteral corticosteroid treatment should be limited in OA because its benefit is usually short-lived, incremental doses are generally required, and toxicity is high with chronic use. Aspiration as well as joint irrigation of acute or recurrent knee effusion may offer significant relief and may be combined with instillation of corticosteroids or, most recently, hyaluronate (see below). However, intra-articular instillation of corticosteroids, although often helpful with recalcitrant flares, should be used judiciously: the masking of pain may accelerate joint deterioration. Cartilage and subchondral bone may also deteriorate more rapidly with frequent instillation. Pericapsular or ligamentous injections into areas surrounding the joint may be as beneficial but less hazardous. The treatment of OA is rapidly expanding as newer concepts of etiopathogenesis direct attention toward modifying the basic disease processes and many physicians add evolving or experimental forms of therapy such as those below.[18]

Evolving and Experimental Treatment of Osteoarthritis

The treatment of OA is rapidly advancing, and a number of trials have been initiated in an attempt to retard cartilage deterioration.

INTRA-ARTICULAR HYALURONAN DERIVATIVE

The beneficial effects of intra-articular hyaluronan derivative on knee pain in selected patients with OA has been documented, and the derivative is currently available for this purpose. It is best combined with continuous NSAID treatment. However, its effects on the course of the disease, if any, remain to be elucidated.[15]

TETRACYCLINES

Tetracyclines have a variety of anti-inflammatory effects that are mediated by mechanisms independent of their antimicrobial activity. They appear to be potent inhibitors of matrix metalloproteinases, a group of proteolytic enzymes including collagenases, which can degrade articular extracellular matrix, thus causing destruction of articular cartilage. Minocycline and doxycycline are currently under investigation.

GLUCOSAMINE AND CHONDROITIN SULFATE

Modulation of cartilage constituents has been suggested by the combined use of these agents. Glucosamine sulfate is thought to slow cartilage breakdown, possibly by stimulating cartilage to synthesize glycosaminoglycans and proteoglycans and by the inhibition of proteolytic enzymes that damage articular cartilage. Chondroitin sulfate is the predominant glycosaminoglycan found in articular cartilage.[25]

COLCHICINE

The basis for the use of colchicine in inflammatory synovitis that is refractory to NSAIDs is that the majority of patients have evidence of calcium pyrophosphate dihydrate crystals (pseudogout). In addition, colchicine has inhibitory effects on neutrophil chemotaxis.[17]

FISH OIL

Polyunsaturated fatty acids derived from marine sources (fish oil), including eicosapentaenoic acid, have recently been promoted for the treatment of both OA and RA. They appear to have mild anti-inflammatory activity through reduction in arachidonic acid, the precursor of prostaglandin, thus exerting a mild NSAID-like effect.

ANTIMALARIALS

Both chloroquine (Aralen) and hydroxychloroquine (Plaquenil) have been shown to have a salutary healing effect on cartilage, mediated by stabilization of lysosomal membranes and inhibition of cartilage proteases. Their clinical usefulness in OA remains to be determined. These agents are currently used mostly in RA because of their anti-inflammatory and remittive effects.

Rheumatoid Arthritis

RA usually follows one of three patterns: (1) monocyclical, (2) intermittent, and (3) unremitting. About 20% of patients have a monocyclical course, in which all signs and symptoms of RA resolve within 2 years of onset. About 60% develop an intermittent course, with unpredictable flares and remissions as well as variable joint involvement. Most patients in these two groups do fairly well with NSAIDs. However, the remaining 20% develop an unremitting and progressive polyarthritis, which calls for the use of DMARDs. This group may be recognized by any or all of the following: continuous inflammation in all the major joints affected, despite the administration of a succession of NSAIDs; progressive hip or knee involvement; constantly elevated erythrocyte sedimentation rate and/or low-grade anemia, 2 or more hours of morning stiffness, without any benefit from NSAIDs; early afternoon fatigue; frequent extra-articular manifestations; RA latex titers in the thousands; subcutaneous nodules; and progressive deformity on serial radiographs.[11]

DMARDs in Rheumatoid Arthritis

The use of these agents should be reserved for those physicians trained and experienced with their toxicity. They are used for progressively severe RA that has not been controlled by measures such as rest, physical therapy, aspirin and/or NSAIDs, occasional intra-articular steroid injections, or very low-dose parenteral corticosteroids.[27] A brief outline of these drugs follows:

GOLD (ORAL AND INTRAMUSCULAR)

Gold treatment in RA has been extensively studied and its value substantiated, although the mechanism of action remains unknown. Symptomatic improvement may take many months, and patients often require concomitant administration of aspirin or NSAIDs, especially during the initial phase of therapy. Gold therapy may partially or completely correct the blood count, serum albumin, erythrocyte sedimentation rate, hypergammaglobulinemia, and rheumatoid factor. It has also been shown to protect articular cartilage and subchondral bone, thereby possibly diminishing the progressive erosive deformity. Unfortunately, a wide variety of side effects, including stomatitis, rash, diarrhea (primarily oral gold), aplastic anemia (rare), proteinuria, and nephrotic syndrome (rare), occurs in one-third or more of patients, necessitating discontinuing the drug.

Intramuscular gold is available in two forms: gold sodium thiomalate (Myochrysine) and aurothioglucose (Solganal). Both are equally effective, but because of a high incidence of vasomotor (nitritoid) reactions with Myochrysine, including dizziness, sweating, flushing, and syncope, the favored agent is Solganal. Initially, patients are given a test dose of 10 mg. Thereafter, the patient receives 50 mg weekly until a beneficial response is obtained, usually in 3 to 4 months. The intervals between the injections are then increased to 2 weeks and later to 3 or 4 weeks. Results of laboratory studies including complete blood count, platelets, and urine are required before each additional dose.

ANTIMALARIALS

Hydroxychloroquine (Plaquenil) is used more than chloroquine (Aralen) in the United States for the treatment of RA because of a lower incidence of side effects. Plaquenil has a slow onset of action, and patients usually require concomitant administration of NSAIDs to control symptoms. The most dreaded potential toxicity is retinopathy. Fortunately, when the recommended daily dosage is not exceeded and appropriate ophthalmological examinations are performed, progression to loss of visual acuity is rare. A number of other side effects may occur, including headache, rash, alopecia, leucopenia, nausea, and weight loss.

SULFASALAZINE

Sulfasalazine (Azulfidine) has been in widespread use for chronic inflammatory bowel disease for many years. It is metabolized to 5-aminosalicylic acid (mesalamine) and sulfapyridine. Interest in its anti-inflammatory effect in RA and psoriatic arthritis has recently increased, and many physicians use it before resorting to the more traditional DMARDs because of its lower incidence of serious side effects. However, gastrointestinal and hematological side effects, due primarily to the metabolite sulfapyridine, are not uncommon.

PENICILLAMINE (CUPRIMINE, DEPEN)

Penicillamine is a metabolic derivative of penicillin that has been used in the treatment of RA throughout the world. The pattern of improvement is similar to that observed with gold, but its mechanism of action remains unknown. However, there are a number of side effects and toxicities, including rash, aplastic anemia, and nephrotic syndrome. In addition, the drug may induce varied autoimmune syndromes, including myasthenia gravis, lupus erythematosus, and polymyositis. Therefore, its clinical use in the United States has been limited.

AZATHIOPRINE (IMURAN)

Azathioprine (Imuran) is a derivative of 6-mercaptopurine, a cytotoxic agent, and has a slow onset of action, typically 6 months to 1 year. It is used to produce long-term sustained disease suppression rather than to control acute flares, similar to the use of gold and penicillamine. The most frequent serious side effects include leucopenia and thrombocytopenia. In addition, there is an increased risk of neoplasia, particularly leukemia and lymphoma.

METHOTREXATE (RHEUMATREX)

Methotrexate, a cytotoxic folic acid inhibitor, has been used to treat psoriasis, psoriatic arthritis, and RA.[8] Although it does suppress disease activity quickly in a high percentage of patients, there is often a rebound of activity within a few weeks of stopping therapy. Side effects are not uncommon and include vomiting, hair loss, leucopenia, thrombocytopenia, pulmonary and hepatic toxicity, and increased risk of neoplasia. Some physicians have recommended liver biopsy after 2 years of continuous use or a cumulative dose of 1500 mg. The use of NSAIDs, including salicylates, together with methotrexate may potentiate toxicity.

CYCLOSPORINE (NEORAL)

The use of this agent, a transplant drug used to prevent rejection, in a number of autoimmune diseases including RA and psoriatic arthritis has been increasing. Its major toxicity is hypertension and renal insufficiency. Recent studies suggest it has an additive effect when used in combination with low-dose methotrexate.

Newer DMARDs in Rheumatoid Arthritis

LEFLUNOMIDE (ARAVA)

Leflunomide is the first of a new class of immunosuppressive agents that inhibit de novo synthesis of the pyrimidine pathway and arrest the cell cycle at the S phase. It appears to be well tolerated and may be used in combination with NSAIDs and other DMARDs.

ETANERCEPT (ENBREL)

Etanercept is a protein produced by genetic engineering that neutralizes TNF, a substance produced by the body that plays a major role in mounting the immune system's attack against the joints. Patients need to be instructed on how to perform two self-administered subcutaneous injections per week.

A number of other therapies, including anti-TNF monoclonal antibodies such as Remicade, plasmapheresis, leucapheresis, lymphoid or synovial irradiation, and interferon, are also under investigation.

CONCLUSION

A review of the medical treatment of inflammatory arthritis of the knee has been presented. The salicylates and newer NSAIDs including COX-2-specific inhibitors are the drugs of choice for OA as well as the initial treatment for RA and related disorders.[28] DMARDs are of numerous types, and the rationale for their use has been detailed. These agents are utilized in recalcitrant RA and in other forms of chronic inflammatory arthritis.

References

1. Arnold WJ: Office-based arthroscopy. Bull Rheum Dis 41:3, 1992.
2. Bradley JD: Comparison of an antiinflammatory dose of ibuprofen, an analgesic dose of ibuprofen, and acetaminophen in the treatment of patients with osteoarthritis of the knee. N Engl J Med 325:87, 1991.
3. Cohen AS, Brandt KD, Krey PR: Synovial fluid. In Cohen AS, ed: Laboratory Diagnostic Procedures in Rheumatic Disease, 2nd ed. Boston, Little, Brown, 1975, pp 1-62.
4. Culp RW: Lyme arthritis in children: An orthopedic perspective. J Bone Joint Surg Am 69:96, 1987.
5. Evans J: Lyme disease. Curr Opin Rheum 10:339, 1998.
6. Gatter RA: A Practical Handbook of Joint Fluid Analysis. Philadelphia, Lea & Febiger, 1984, pp 1-105.
7. Goldenberg DL, Reed JI: Bacterial arthritis. N Engl J Med 312:764, 1985.
8. Groff GD: Low dose oral methotrexate in rheumatoid arthritis. Semin Arthritis Rheum 12:333, 1983.
9. Griffin MR: Nonsteroidal anti-inflammatory drug use and increased risk for peptic ulcer disease in elderly persons. Ann Intern Med 114:257, 1991.
10. Gumber S, Chopra S: Hepatitis C: A multifaceted disease. Ann Intern Med 123:615, 1995.
11. Harris ED Jr: Rheumatoid arthritis: Pathophysiology and implications for therapy. N Engl J Med 322:1277, 1990.
12. Hasselbacher P: Variation in synovial fluid analysis by hospital laboratories. Arthritis Rheum 30:637, 1987.

13. Kapisinszky N, Keszthelyi B: High-dose methlyprednisolone pulse therapy in patients with rheumatoid arthritis. Ann Rheum Dis 49:567, 1990.
14. Lane NE: Pain management in osteoarthritis: The role of COX-2 inhibitors. J Rheumatol 24:20, 1997.
15. Lohmander LS: Intraarticular hyaluronin injections in the treatment of osteoarthritis of the knee. Ann Rheum Dis 55:424, 1996.
16. McCarty DJ Jr: Synovial fluid. In McCarty DJ Jr, ed: Arthritis and Allied Conditions, 10th ed. Philadelphia, Lea & Febiger, 1985, pp 54-75.
17. Moskowitz RW: Specific drug therapy of experimental osteoarthritis. Semin Arthritis Rheum 11:127, 1981.
18. Moskowitz RW: Osteoarthritis: Diagnosis and Management. Philadelphia, WB Saunders, 1984.
19. Myers SL: Synovial inflammation in patients with early osteoarthritis of the knee. J Rheumatol 17:1662, 1990.
20. Ropes MW, Bauer W: Synovial Fluid Change in Joint Disease. Cambridge, MA, Harvard University Press, 1983, pp 1-150.
21. Schumacher HR: Synovial fluid analysis. In Kelley WN, ed: Textbook of Rheumatology. Philadelphia, WB Saunders, 1981, pp 568-579.
22. Sedor JR, Davidson EW, Dunn MJ: Effects of nonsteroidal antiinflammatory drugs in healthy subjects. Am J Med 81:58, 1986.
23. Semble EL, Agudelo CA, Pegram SP: Human parvovirus B 19 arthropathy in two adults after contact with childhood erythema infectiosum. Am J Med 83:560, 1987.
24. Soll AH: Nonsteroidal antinflammatory drugs and peptic ulcer disease. Ann Intern Med 114:307, 1991.
25. Townheed TE: Glucosamine sulphate in osteoarthritis: A systematic review. J Rheumatol 25:8, 1998.
26. Vane JR: NSAIDs, COX-2 inhibitors, and the gut. Lancet 346: 1105, 1995.
27. Wilder RL: Treatment of the patient with rheumatoid arthritis refractory to standard therapy. JAMA 259:2446, 1988.
28. Ziff M: Rheumatoid arthritis: Its present and future. J Rheumatol 17:127, 1990.

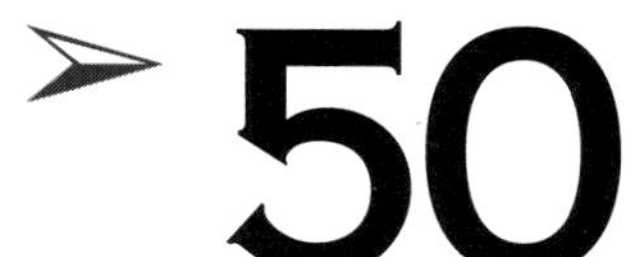

The Synovium: Normal and Pathological Conditions*

VINCENT J. VIGORITA

NORMAL SYNOVIUM: MICROANATOMY AND FUNCTION

Synovium forms when a primitive mesenchymal tissue cavitates, forming a recognizable joint space at approximately 8 weeks of embryonic life (Fig. 50.1).[57] Mature synovium appears pale pink in color and architecturally covers all the surfaces of the joint space, excluding the articular cartilage and most fibrocartilaginous structures. Only in abnormal conditions does the synovium encroach on the surface of articular cartilage, a change classically seen in the reddish "pannus" or inflammatory synovial invasion of the articular cartilage in rheumatoid arthritis.

The synovial membrane, the most superficial layer of the synovium, lines the joint and also forms the linings of tendon sheaths. Parietal and visceral synovium mimic their mesothelial-like counterparts in the thoracic and pericardial cavities. The extensive synovial-like lining cells of tendon sheaths and ligaments explain a host of reactive synovitis and painful clinical tenosynovitis, bursitis, and enthesopathy syndromes. Joint capsule fibrous connective tissue is thought to add to the joint's mechanical strength. The term *joint capsule* refers to the fibrofatty neurovascular tissue that envelopes the nonarticular cartilaginous tissue of the joint space.[43]

In pathological states, synovial-like anatomic structures, not related to a joint space ("synovial metaplasia"),[24] are known to form in a variety of circumstances, including (1) postsurgical states/failed prostheses; (2) failed prostheses, including breast implants[28]; (3) mechanical damage to connective tissue; and (4) experimental settings (injected air or oil in subcutaneous soft tissue[16]).

These structures histologically resemble normal synovium and often have demonstrably similar secretory and phagocytic function.[24]

Normally, the synovium appears smooth and transparent but turns thick, dull, and opaque with pathological change. With hemorrhage, it becomes obviously bloody but in chronic hemarthrosis turns a reddish brown (Fig. 50.2) owing to hemosiderin deposition and the release of iron from red blood cells. In severe bleeding cases, a dark purple color may be noted. The appearance of reddish purple synovium indicates bleeding and may be seen in trauma, bleeding disorders such as hemophilia, and pigmented villonodular synovitis. Whereas in ochronosis (alkaptonuria) the synovium may appear a dull gray, fibrocartilage and articular cartilage will be discolored black. Darkening or blackening may also be seen when there is extensive release of metallic debris. White foci in the synovium usually indicate gout (urate deposition), pseudogout (calcium pyrophosphate crystal deposition), or soft tissue calcifications (deposits caused by trauma or calcinosis syndromes). Cement debris may also lead to pallor.

Microanatomic Structure

The synovium consists of a thin layer of synovial cells or synoviocytes, the intimal layer, above a richly fibrovascular zone, the subintimal layer, that contains arterioles, fat, and other connective tissue cells such as fibroblasts, histiocytes, and occasionally mast cells (Fig. 50.3).[32] The intimal layer of lining cells is usually 1 to 2 cells thick with no discernible differences on light microscopy. The loose connective tissue subintimal zone layer becomes gradually more fibrous at capsular insertions.

The villous appearance of synovium is not necessarily abnormal but rather nonspecific and may be seen in a broad range of conditions (Fig. 50.4). In general, traumatic synovitis and degenerative joint disease (DJD) (osteoarthritis) are attended by edematous change and mild villous hypertrophy. Inflammatory arthritis (classically rheumatoid arthritis) shows a dramatically reddish hyperplastic synovium with fibrinous exudation characterized by abundant tan fibrinous loose bodies, called *rice bodies,* and marked lymphoplasmacytic synovitis. In septic arthritis, leukocytes are seen in tissue. Neuropathic joints and those of rapidly destructive joint processes are characterized by bone and cartilage debris.

Ultrastructure and Function

The intimal zone consists of an admixture of cell types often conveniently classified as those demonstrating macrophage function (synovial A cells) and those more

*Adapted from Vigorita VJ: The synovium. In Vigorita VJ, Ghelman B: Orthopaedic Pathology. Philadelphia, Lippincott/Williams & Wilkins, 1999.

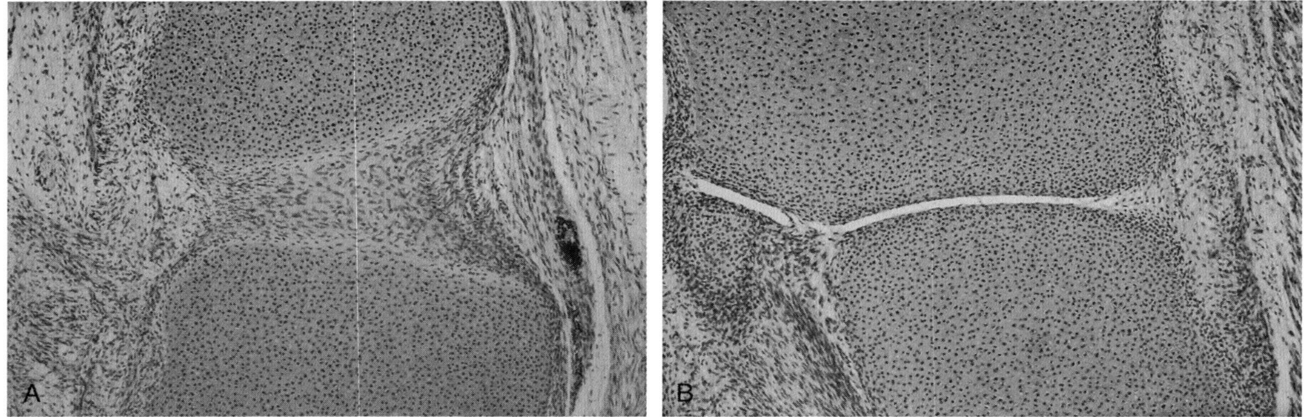

FIGURE 50.1 ➢ Embryonic joint showing evolution of primitive mesenchyma *(A)* into a joint space *(B)* at about 8 weeks of intrauterine life. (From Vigorita VJ: The synovium. In Vigorita VJ, Ghelman B: Orthopaedic Pathology. Philadelphia, Lippincott/Williams & Wilkins, 1999.)

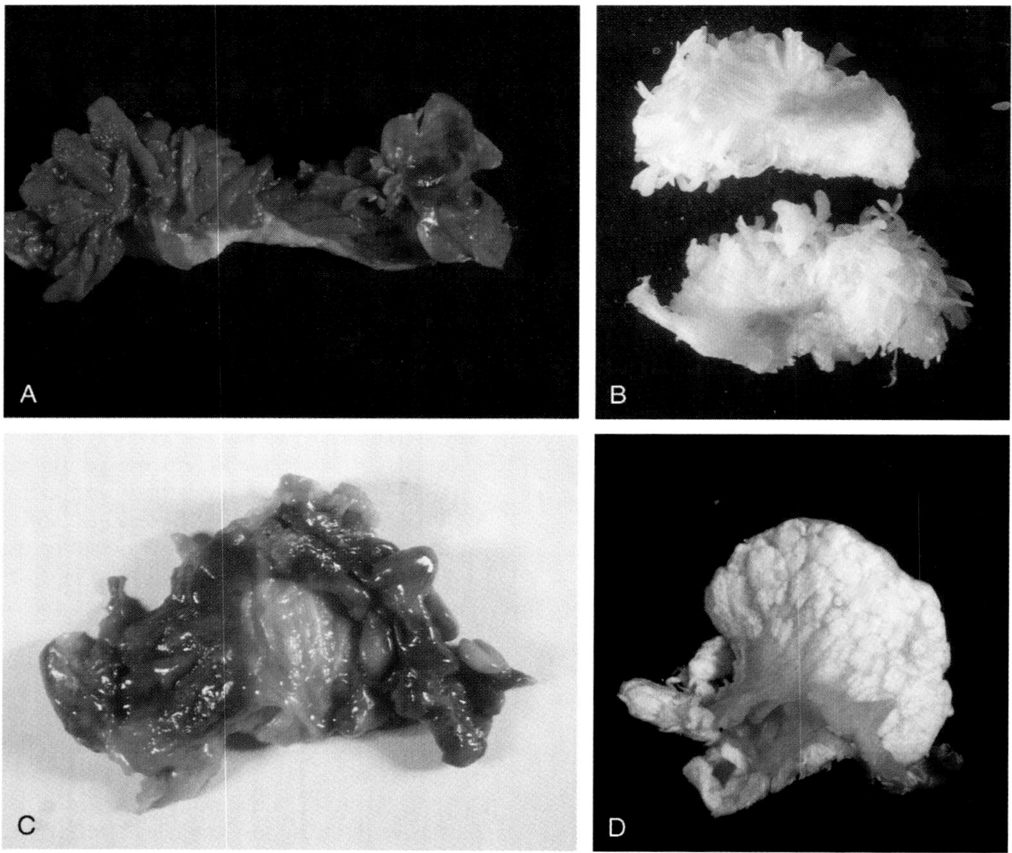

FIGURE 50.2 ➢ Gross appearance of the synovium in pathological states, including bleeding *(A)* and reactions to foreign implant material such as cement and polyethylene *(B)* and metal *(C)*. Bleeding induces a rusty-brown appearance. Implant materials impart a whitening except metal, which induces a darkening or blackening. Crystals such as gout and calcium pyrophosphate deposition can induce a whitening *(D)*. (From Vigorita VJ: The synovium. In Vigorita VJ, Ghelman B: Orthopaedic Pathology. Philadelphia, Lippincott/Williams & Wilkins, 1999.)

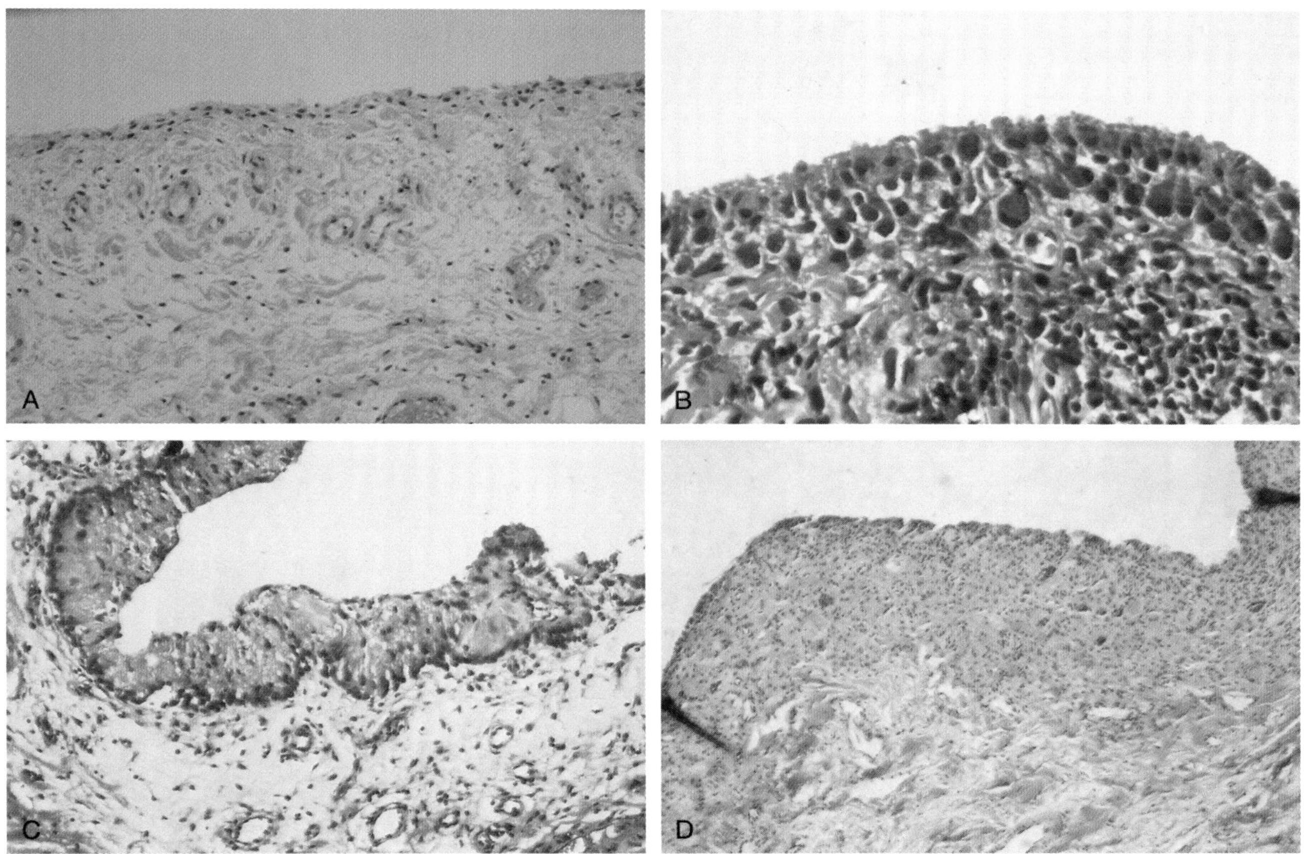

FIGURE 50.3 ➢ *A.* Normal synovium consists of a fine single or double layer of lining "intimal cells" on top of a subintimal zone of vascular and fatty tissue, fibroblasts, and rare histiocytes and mast cells. There is increasing collagen in the vicinity of dense connective tissue structures. *B.* Hyperplastic synovium showing moderate hypertrophy of cells confined to the surface with increasing hyperplasia and hyperplastic cells migrating into the subintimal zone with marked hypertrophy. *C.* Mucinous hyperplasia illustrating secretory potential of synovium. *D.* Superficial zone foreign body giant cell reaction to failed prosthesis. (From Vigorita VJ: The synovium. In Vigorita VJ, Ghelman B: Orthopaedic Pathology. Philadelphia, Lippincott/Williams & Wilkins, 1999.)

synthesizing in function (synovial B cells) (Fig. 50.5). Electron microscopic studies and immunophenotyping studies further characterized these cells.[35] Ultrastructural studies demonstrate abundant mitochondria, Golgi apparatus, vacuoles, lysosomes, phagosomes, vesicles, and surface undulations (characteristics suited to macrophage activity in type A cells) and rough endoplasmic reticulum, free ribosomes, and smoother cytoplasmic profiles (characteristics suited to synthetic activity in type B). As might be expected, synoviocytes may be "intermediate" in nature, featuring organelle functions of both types A and B. Some evidence supports the existence of other cells, such as antigen-type cells (HLA-DR, IA-like).

In fact, the use of special immunological techniques, including monoclonal antibodies, against a range of antigens can confirm that synovial cells consist of many different cell types. Three more or less distinct populations can be defined immunologically.[11]

Arbitrarily designated type 1 for convenience is a group of cells that appear to be related to mononuclear phagocytes based on their expression of antigen and that are consistent with the monocyte macrophage cell lineage. They demonstrate phagocytosis and contain IA antigen and Fc receptors. These cells constitute approximately one-third of the synovial cell population.

A second cell population, type 2, is characterized by nonphagocytic activity and a strong expression of IA antigen with the absence of immunoglobulin (Ig) G Fc receptors and antigens associated with the monocyte lineage, D and T lymphocytes, and fibroblasts. Type 2 cells include the IA antigen-positive dendritic cells. In rheumatoid arthritis a considerable portion of the cells are type 2 cells.

A last cell population, type 3, is characterized by a nonlymphocytic population with characteristics typical of fibroblasts. These are the cells that usually predominate in tissue culture. They lack phagocytic activity and do not express monocyte antigens or IA antigens.

Cell types as defined by immunological studies are consistent with previous morphological observations. Type 1 cells expressing the monocyte macrophage antigens are similar to those historically described as

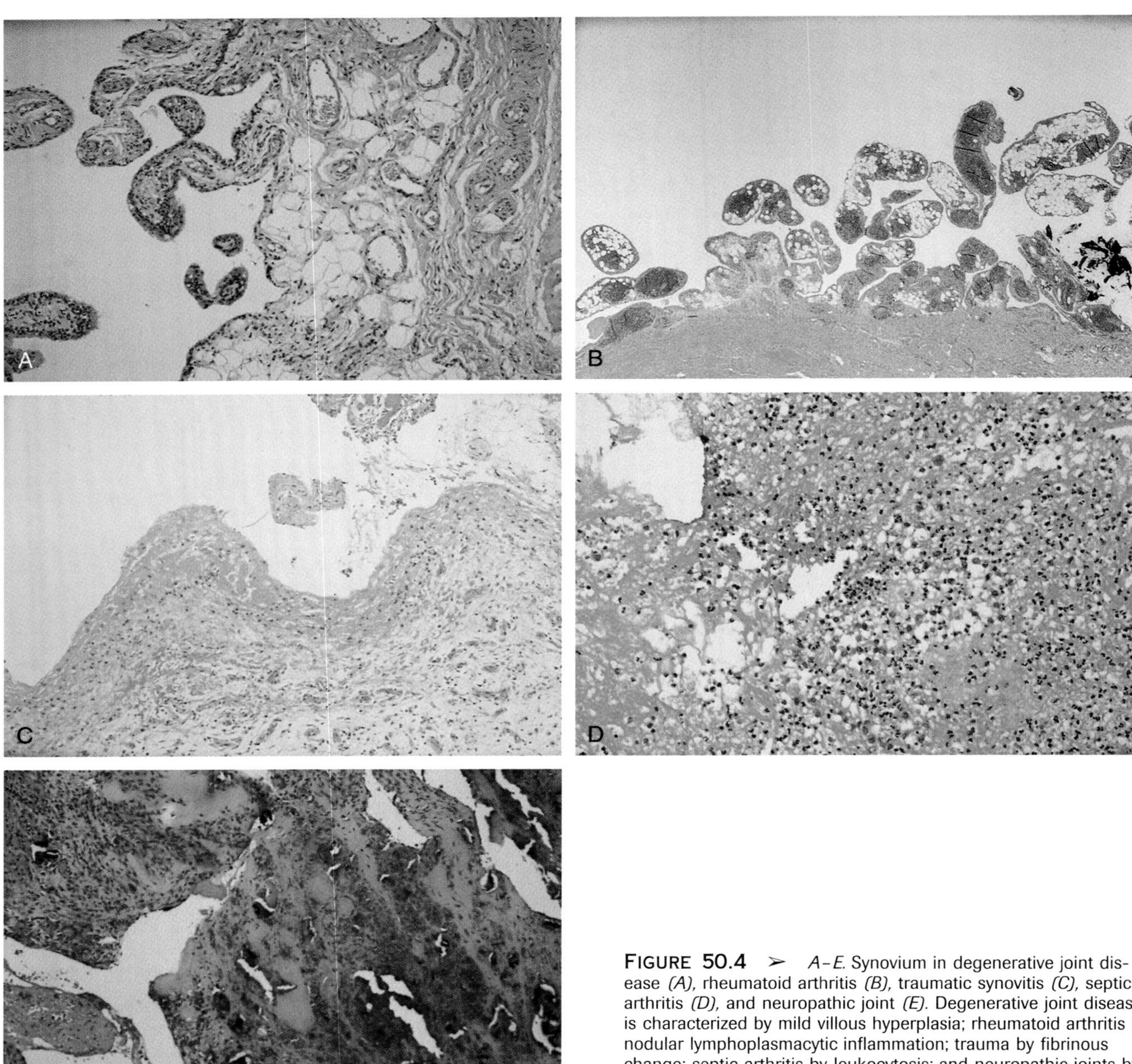

FIGURE 50.4 ➢ *A–E.* Synovium in degenerative joint disease *(A)*, rheumatoid arthritis *(B)*, traumatic synovitis *(C)*, septic arthritis *(D)*, and neuropathic joint *(E)*. Degenerative joint disease is characterized by mild villous hyperplasia; rheumatoid arthritis by nodular lymphoplasmacytic inflammation; trauma by fibrinous change; septic arthritis by leukocytosis; and neuropathic joints by abundant bone and cartilage detritus. (From Vigorita VJ: The synovium. In Vigorita VJ, Ghelman B: Orthopaedic Pathology. Philadelphia, Lippincott/Williams & Wilkins, 1999.)

characterized by phagocytosis type A and type C cells. Type 1 cells are most likely mononuclear phagocytes of bone marrow origin as ascertained by their antigenic marking with monocyte and IA antigen. Modifications in antigen expression suggest that they act more like tissue macrophages in the joint. The historically designated "type B" synovial cell that produces glycosaminoglycans is most likely of the type 3 cell variety, probably mesenchymal in origin. These cells lack IA antigens and most of the differentiated antigens of monocyte macrophage lineage.[11]

The origin of normal synovial lining cells remains controversial, but a dual-cell origin remains plausible with bone marrow derivation for the histocytoid or type A cells and local mesenchymal tissue for fibroblast or type B cells. However, many believe the heterogeneity of synovial cells is more an expression of functional activity resulting from various factors and the cell types are possibly interconvertible.

Although the synovial cells lack desmosomes or tight junctions, characteristic of epithelial tissue, the complexity of this cell structure is evident in the changes seen in various pathological states. Hyperplasia may be limited to a mild increase in intimal cell number, or there may be dramatic change, including large, bizarre cells such as Grimley-Sokoloff giant cells

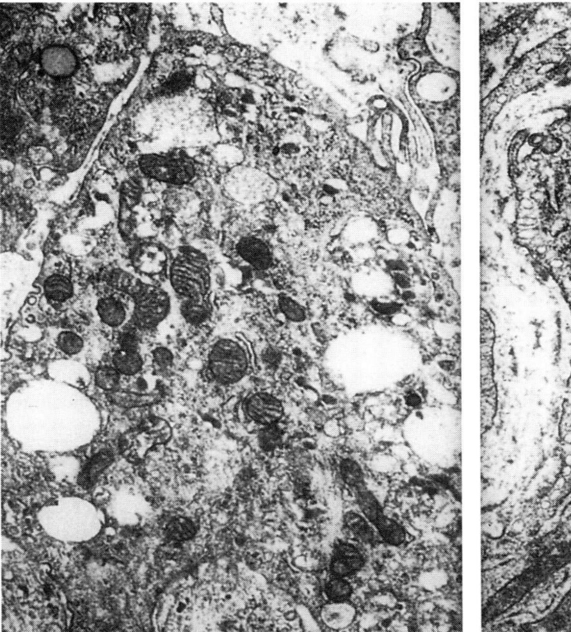
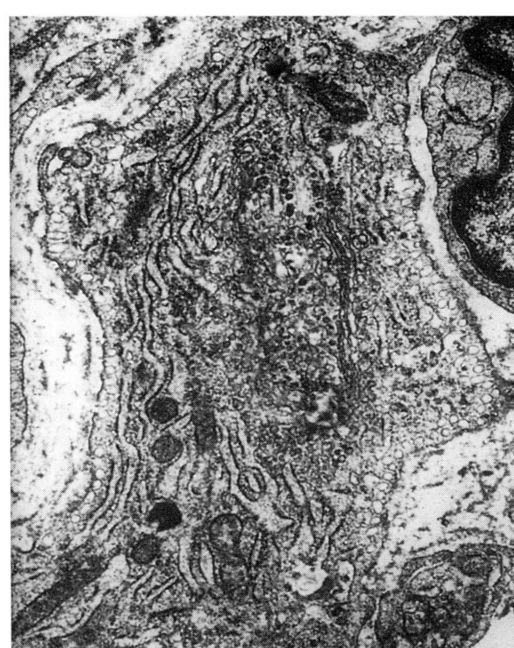

FIGURE 50.5 ➢ Ultrastructure of synovial intimal cells. Type A cells show prominent Golgi cells, vesicles, vacuoles, lysosomes, and mitochondria. Type B cells show abundant rough endoplasmic reticulum. There are no basal lamina separating lining cells from subintimal connective tissue and unless inflamed, rarely cell junctions. (From Vigorita VJ: The synovium. In Vigorita VJ, Ghelman B: Orthopaedic Pathology. Philadelphia, Lippincott/Williams & Wilkins, 1999.)

or even striking mucin-producing cells. In this latter condition (mucinous hypertrophy of the synovium), the copious amount of material secreted testifies to the potential capacity of this membrane (see Fig. 50.3*C*).

Functions of the Synovium

The functions of the synovium are best appreciated by understanding the characteristics of its cellular components and microarchitectural structure. For example, the synovial A cells are suited to phagocytic (or macrophage) activity and ingest native or foreign material, such as hemosiderin in chronic bleeding conditions (hemophilia) or iatrogenically introduced substances (gold in the treatment of rheumatoid arthritis). The phagocytic potential of the synovium is probably best illustrated by the marked foreign body giant cell and histiocytic reaction in some cases of loosened prostheses or in the resorption of bone and cartilage debris in rapidly destructive joint disease or neuropathic joints. Absorption of fluid material by synovial intimal cells is demonstrated ultrastructurally by pinocytotic vesicles and vacuoles. Alternatively, the synovial B cell is suited to synthetic function and most characteristically secretes the hyaluronate protein of synovial fluid, hyaluronate contributing to the lubrication of joint structures. However, more than likely, both type A and type B cells appear to have secretory and phagocytic potential. Other functions in conjunction with the vascular and lymphatic systems of the synovium include the regulation of movement of physiologically important proteins and electrolytes. The lack of a basal lamina and the presence of gaps between synovial cells facilitates interchange between synovial fluid and blood vessels.

SYNOVIAL FLUID

Synovial fluid, a dialysate of plasma, contains small amounts of hyaluronic acid, a copolymer of glucuronic acid and anacetic glycocyamine, a protein complex hyaluronate synthesized by the cells of the synovial membrane. This material gives synovial fluid its high viscosity. In addition, synovial fluid contains cells, mostly mononuclear phagocytes, and neutrophils. Synovial fluid content of glucose, uric acid, and lactate is similar to that in plasma, but there is less total protein. Albumin composes most of the total protein, whereas proteins of higher molecular weight, such as fibrinogen and other globulins, are relatively decreased in comparison to their plasma concentrations.

Arthrocentesis is the procedure whereby the synovial fluid is removed, a procedure that is infrequently complicated by infection. Arthrocentesis may be very helpful in detecting crystal-induced synovitis, such as gout, calcium pyrophosphate crystal deposition disease, and hydroxyapatite crystal deposition disease. Blood, a nonspecific finding, which may be seen in a broad range of conditions, including trauma-induced hemarthrosis and pigmented villonodular synovitis, rheumatoid arthritis, and infection. Collection of synovial fluid in either heparin or liquid ethylenediaminetetraacetic acid (EDTA) will facilitate the identification of crystal deposition disorders. Heparinized tubes should be used for microbial cultures and Gram's stain. For chemical analyses, observation of fresh synovial fluid in a clean test tube may be beneficial be-

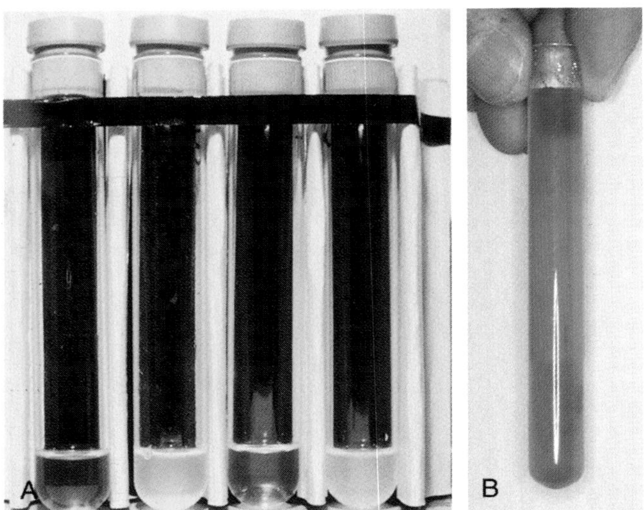

FIGURE 50.6 ➢ Synovial fluid composite. *A*, Synovial fluid from patients with calcium pyrophosphate crystal deposition (cloudy), normal (clear amber), rheumatoid arthritis (cloudy yellow), and trauma induced (blood stained). *B*, Pigmented villonodular synovitis, especially of the diffuse type, can give a bloody or rusty appearance. Septic arthritis yields a turbid yellowish-green. (From Vigorita VJ: The synovium. In Vigorita VJ, Ghelman B: Orthopaedic Pathology. Philadelphia, Lippincott/Williams & Wilkins, 1999.)

cause normal synovial fluid does not clot (low fibrinogen concentration). Subsequent centrifugation can remove cells, fibrin, and other debris for further analysis for lactate, protein, uric acid, glucose, and so on.

Synovial fluid analysis may be grouped for general classification of types of conditions producing synovial fluid (Fig. 50.6 and Table 50.1).[64] Noninflammatory conditions, such as DJD, trauma-induced arthritis, osteochondritis dissecans, and neuropathic arthropathies, or primary synovial metaplastic conditions, such as synovial chondromatosis, are characterized by a yellowish synovial fluid with high viscosity, low leukocyte counts, less than 10 mg/dL of glucose (i.e., below serum level), and low protein. Cultures are negative. This noninflammatory or class I type of synovial fluid group is distinct from the inflammatory or crystal-induced arthropathies, which are characterized by a synovial fluid with low viscosity, a yellow or whitish color, and a variable white count with a greater than 50% neutrophil population. Glucose is usually elevated greater than 25 mg/dL with protein elevation greater than 3 g/dL.

Septic arthritis is usually characterized by a yellowish-green fluid of low viscosity with an elevated leukocyte count with greater than 75% neutrophils. Glucose is usually greater than 25 mg/dL with increased protein levels. A wide range of conditions can induce a hemorrhagic arthropathy, including idiopathic hemosideric synovitis, trauma-induced arthritis, hemophilic arthropathy, and even pigmented villonodular synovitis as a secondary change. This group of synovial disorders are characterized by a reddish-brown color with decreased viscosity and a moderate elevation in white cell count with greater than 25% neutrophils. Glucose is in the normal range, usually 0 to 10 mg below serum level. Protein may be greater than 3 g/dL.

Normal synovial fluid is usually less than 3.5 mL and clear or faintly yellow in color with clear transparency.

TABLE 50.1 CLASSIFICATION OF SYNOVIAL EFFUSIONS

Gross Examination	Gross Synovial Fluid				
	Normal	*Noninflammatory*	*Inflammatory*	*Septic*	*Hemorrhagic*
Volume (mL) (knee)	<3.5	Often >3.5	Often >3.5	Often >3.5	
Viscosity	High	High	Low	Variable	
Color	Colorless to straw	Straw to yellow	Yellow	Variable	
Clarity	Transparent	Transparent	Translucent	Opaque	
Routine laboratory examination					
WBC (mm^3)	<200	200 to 2000	2000 to 75,000	Often >100,000+	
PMN leukocytes (%)	<25%	<25%	>50% often	>75%+	
Culture	Negative	Negative	Negative	Often positive	
Mucin clot	Firm	Firm	Friable	Friable	
Glucose (morning fasting)	Nearly equal to blood	Nearly equal to blood	<50 mg% lower than blood	>50 mg% lower than blood	
		Pathology			
		Osteoarthritis Osteochondromatosis Osteochondritis dissecans Neuroarthropathy	Rheumatoid arthritis Systemic lupus erythematosus Ankylosing spondylitis Gout Chondrocalcinosis (pseudogout)	Bacterial, fungal, and tuberculous infections	Hemorrhagic diatheses Traumatic arthritis Pigmented villonodular synovitis Synovioma

WBC = white blood count; PMN = polymorphonuclear.
Modified from Schumacher HR: Pathologic findings in rheumatoid arthritis. In Schumacher HR, Gall EP (eds): Rheumatoid Arthritis. An Illustrated Guide to Pathology, Diagnosis, and Management. Philadelphia, JB Lippincott, 1988, pp 4.1-4.36.

It has high viscosity as a result of hyaluronic acid and does not clot because of low concentrations of fibrinogen and other clotting factors. In normal synovial fluid, there are fewer than 200 cells/μL with a predominance of mononuclear phagocytes. There is a variable amount of lymphocytes, although both lymphocytes and neutrophils dramatically increase in inflammatory arthropathies.

Eosinophilic synovitis has been described.[67] In 12 cases studied by Tauro,[67] mild elevated eosinophilia in the blood (6%) was associated with normal synovial fluid chemistries but mild leukocytosis consisting of 60% to 90% eosinophils. The differential diagnosis includes suppurative arthritis, including tuberculosis and parasites (endemic filariae noted in the Tauro report) and degenerative and rheumatoid arthritis. Patients responded well to diethylcarbamazine.

Crystal-induced arthropathy can be diagnosed with examination of synovial fluid using polarized light microscopy. Crystals other than gout (urate) and pseudogout (calcium pyrophosphate) may be seen. In chronic noninflammatory disorders, cholesterol crystals may be seen, which are square or rectangular with notched corners. Steroid injections may persist and be detectable as faintly birefringent.

IRON-RELATED CHANGES

Iron in tissue removed during orthopedic or related conditions is usually seen in the form of hemosiderin, typically identified as granular brown pigments in an intracytoplasmic localization. The presence of hemosiderin can be seen in a broad variety of conditions (Table 50.2).[64] Traumatic hemarthrosis is seen in association with soft tissue injuries and fractures, including secondary fractures associated with other pathological states. Iron can be a contributing factor to the pathophysiology of disorders such as hemophilic arthropathy and the transfusional hemosiderosis of thalassemia. Deposition at the mineralization front causing osteoporosis or even osteomalacia can be seen in primary or secondary hemochromatosis. The term "pigmented" in pigmented villonodular synovitis refers to the brown pigmentation caused by coincidental iron deposition in the synovial tissue surrounding the proliferating nodules of the essentially fibrous forming lesion or tumor.

TABLE 50.2 CAUSES OF HEMARTHROSIS

Trauma (with or without fractures)	Anticoagulant therapy
Pigmented villonodular synovitis	Myeloproliferative disease with thrombocytosis
Synovioma and other tumors	Thrombocytopenia
Hemangioma	Scurvy
Charcot's joint or other severe joint destruction	Ruptured aneurysm
Hemophilia or other bleeding disorders	Arteriovenous fistula
Von Willebrand's disease	Idiopathic

Modified from Schumacher HR: Pathologic findings in rheumatoid arthritis. In Schumacher HR, Gall EP (eds): Rheumatoid Arthritis. An Illustrated Guide to Pathology, Diagnosis, and Management. Philadelphia, JB Lippincott, 1988, pp 4.1-4.36.

Yellow color may be seen as a result of the abundant presence of foamy histiocytes.

Incidental hemosiderin deposition seen in association with microscopic or macroscopic hemorrhage is usually of little pathophysiological consequence. However, iron has been linked directly to several important hemosiderin-driven osteoarticular pathologies: trauma-related hemosideric synovitis, hemophilic arthropathy, and the osteoarticular iron osteopathy in hemochromatosis.

The most commonly encountered iron-related injury in orthopedic pathology is that related to hemorrhage into the joint. Considering the rich vascularity of the subintimal layer of the synovium, microscopic bleeds from normal daily use of the joint may be expected. In fact, a few red blood cells are considered normal in joint fluid analysis. Trauma to the knee, however, is often accompanied by significant hemarthrosis, an important association because bleeding—or perhaps more specifically the release of iron from ruptured red blood cells—stimulates clinically significant synovial changes, characterized clinically by pain and swelling.

Acute hemarthrosis of the knee in athletes may result from a wide range of injuries to the meniscus, the cruciate ligaments, fracture of the bone, and even a tear of synovial tissue.[47, 63]

In chronic hemarthrosis, iron will accumulate in the synovium. Histopathological localization includes both the synovial intimal cells and the histiocytic cells of the subintimal zone. Grossly, the synovium may attain a "rusty" appearance (see Fig. 50.3).

Experimental evidence suggests that iron adversely affects synovial function.[48] Chronic hemarthrosis, for example, actually may increase the synthetic function of the otherwise macrophagic synovial type A cell. Hemosideric synovitis without hemophilia is well described clinically.[20] Hemophilia represents this situation in a clinical extreme.[3]

Findings on magnetic resonance imaging (MRI) in iron or hemosiderin accumulation are complex. In general, hemosiderin has a so-called paramagnetic or ferromagnetic property, causing a signal dropout[39] in most cases.

Hemosideric Synovitis

In hemorrhages that occur within the synovium, a highly vascularized tissue, red blood cells eventually disintegrate with phagocytosis occurring by histiocytes. Eventually the hemoglobin is broken down and processed into hemosiderin. It is the hemosiderin that is so characteristically seen as a brown pigmented granular substance in cells of the synovium. Hemosiderin may occur as small minute granules or accumulate into globules up to 25 μm in diameter. The intracellular deposition of hemosiderin is mostly observed in macrophages or histiocytes but may be seen engulfed in various trauma-associated conditions by the hypertrophied synovial lining cells as well. In joints subjected to hemorrhage, hemosiderin may be noted either intracellularly or extracellularly. Cells within different compartments or layers of the synovium may be affected, ranging from the synovial lining cells to the subsynovial proliferating connective tissue cells. The gross appearance of the joint with chronic hemarthrosis is that of a rusty pigmentation, although more acute bleeding may be demonstrable as a blackish-green discoloration.

The response of the human joint to bleeding is clinically denoted by the formation of a hyperplastic vascular synovium within a few days. Examination of the tissue reveals a proliferation of the synovial cells and other subsynovial lining cell connective tissue elements, including often inflammatory cells. Under electron microscope, iron-containing electron-dense particles that are membrane bound, called siderosomes, are noted within the synovial cells and subsynovial macrophages.

Clinically hemosideric synovitis may be due to a wide range of conditions, most notably trauma, particularly chronic trauma leading to chronic hemarthrosis. However, it may also be caused by the use of oral anticoagulant therapies, as a result of breakdown of synovial hemangiomas, or as a secondary phenomenon in conditions such as rheumatoid arthritis, pigmented villonodular synovitis, scurvy, and sickle cell anemia. In fact, the roentgenographic appearances may lead to joint space narrowing, particularly in the hip, and may be confused with other joint destructive ailments. Although most patients with chronic hemarthrosis or with an episode of hemarthrosis recover without any significant sequelae, the potential for joint destruction is present in any patient with bleeding into the joint.

With bleeding into the joint, two pathways may lead to damage. In one mechanism, the red blood cells may break down, causing macrophage activation. The ensuing inflammation may lead to destructive changes in and of itself, as seen, for example, in rheumatoid arthritis. Intracellular hemosiderin precipitates the release of leukocyte- and synovium-derived chondrolytic enzymes.[5] In excessive cases, the iron deposition in organs such as the meniscus may be severe enough to cause mechanical dysfunction and thus degenerative changes. In a second pathway, bleeding may directly lead to synovial proliferation, the release of an uncontrollable cascade of destructive substances such as proteases.

Hemophilia

The adverse effect on synovium in patients with chronic hemorrhage has most extensively been studied in the joint changes of hemophilic arthropathy of the knee.[48] In tissue removed from hemophiliacs, the synovium shows marked villous hypertrophy with extensive hypertrophy and hyperplasia of the synovial lining cells and the subsynovial connective tissue components with abundant intracytoplasmic hemosiderin granule accumulation (Fig. 50.7). In tissue cultures of synovium in hemophilia, pigment-laden fibroblast cells

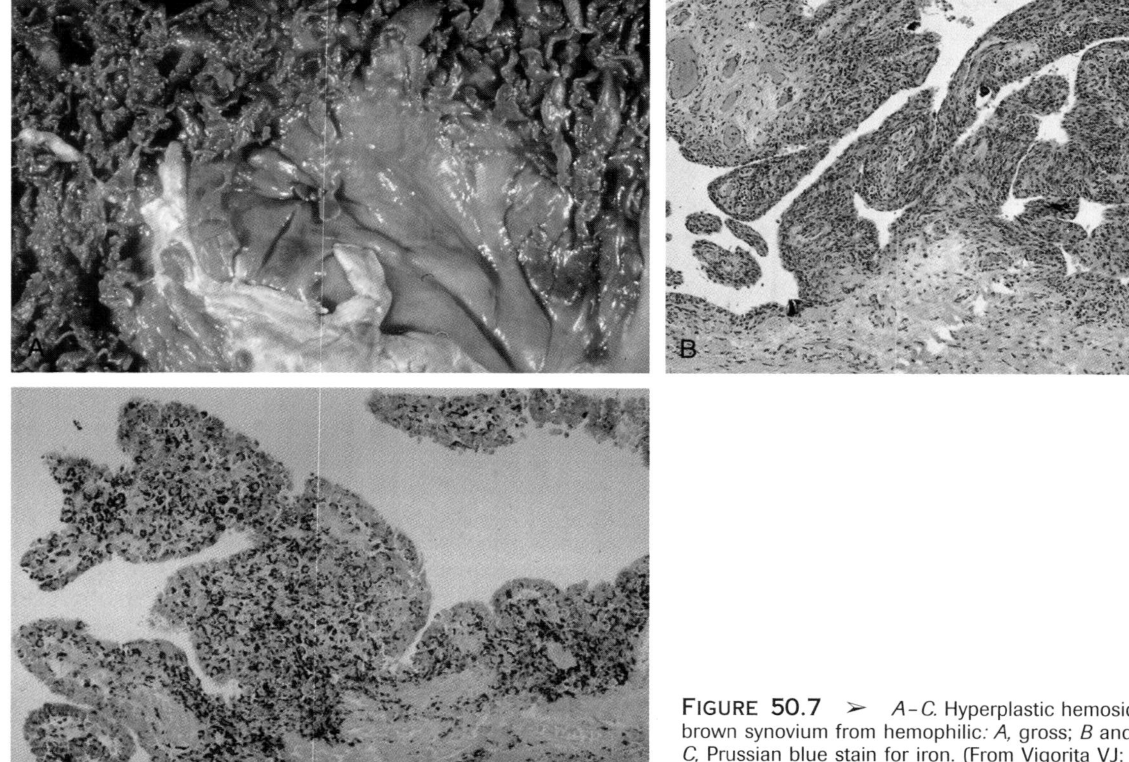

FIGURE 50.7 ➢ *A–C.* Hyperplastic hemosiderin-laden rusty-brown synovium from hemophilic: *A,* gross; *B* and *C,* microscopic; *C,* Prussian blue stain for iron. (From Vigorita VJ: The synovium. In Vigorita VJ, Ghelman B: Orthopaedic Pathology. Philadelphia, Lippincott/Williams & Wilkins, 1999.)

have been shown to proliferate, and explants of the synovial cells have been shown to secrete large amounts of latent collagenase and neutral proteinases establishing the destructive potential of the synovitis in hemophilia. Synovium incited by hemophilia produces enzymes and may do so without coincident inflammation, the latter a significant component to the destructive arthropathy seen in rheumatoid arthritis.

Iron accumulation may, in fact, directly lead to chondrocyte destruction. In experiments aimed at developing a model for pigmented villonodular synovitis, a condition secondary to expanding nodules of proliferative fibroblasts and histiocytes, blood has been experimentally injected into various animal models. The resultant proliferative synovitis is characterized by hyperplasia of fibroblasts, lipid-laden macrophages and giant cells, and extensive hemosiderin accumulation similar to that seen in reactive hemosideric synovitis or hemophilic arthropathy.

Although less visible, iron is known to accumulate in cartilage as well. Extensive hemosiderin deposition leading to grossly visible brown menisci has been observed clinically.[5] In studying hemophilic joints, iron has been localized to superficial chondrocytes, suggesting chondrocytic phagocytic uptake triggering a degradative enzyme release similar to that described in synovial cells. Iron has been histochemically localized to the tidemark in lupus and in hemochromatosis.

Hemophilia A is the most common hereditary coagulation disorder, affecting 20 per 100,000 live male births because of the deficiency, absence, or malfunction of coagulation factor VIII.[60] In normal patients, a very low concentration of factor VIII (0.2 μg/mL plasma) is sufficient for adequate coagulation. Bleeding leading to clinically perceptible illness requires a reduction of at least 75%.

Hemophilia A is a clinically heterogeneous disorder ranging from mild disease (1% to 4% deficiency) to severe disease. Patients with mild or moderate disease may not be recognized unless a significant traumatic event precipitates the observation of abnormal bleeding. Excessive bleeding during surgery may be the first clue. Therapy centers around replacement of factor VIII. Traditionally done with shotgun frozen plasma, cryoprecipitate became available in the 1960s. More recently, purified concentrates have been used. In general, one unit of factor VIII increases plasma activity by 0.024/mL.

Because 0.3 U/mL are usually needed to treat a mild bleeding episode, clinical goals should strive for more than this amount. Therapy has improved morbidity significantly.

Clinically, bleeding is the key, especially into joints. Most commonly involved, in order of frequency, are the knees and elbows, followed by the ankles, shoulders, and hips. Not usually evident in infancy, childhood signs include mild discomfort and joint limitation. Pain and swelling follow. Numerous damaging microhemarthroses have transpired before the initial arousal of clinical suspicion, unfortunately delaying diagnosis.

Roentgenographically, joint space narrowing, loss of articular cartilage, cystic remodeling of bone, and hemophilic pseudotumors characterize the illness. However, strict adherence to maintenance of factor VIII levels to prevent spontaneous hemorrhage has been associated with significantly decreased morbidity and has halted radiographic progression of disease.

Surgical joint reconstruction in hemophiliacs has been attempted to preserve function, but radioactive synoviorthesis and arthroscopic synovectomy have been used.[23]

Intra-articular, intrabursal, and soft tissue bleeding in hemophilia may result in painless masses clinically and roentgenographically mimicking a tumor, called *pseudotumors of hemophilia* (Fig. 50.8). These masses consist of spongy coagula of partially clotted blood encapsulated by thick fibrous membranes. Complications of these so-called hemophilic pseudotumors include muscle and bone damage, infection, and neuropathies. Surgical removal is not without danger. Pseudotumors occur in 1% to 2% of hemophiliacs,[21] mostly in the lower extremity and pelvis. Bleeding in the vicinity of the periosteum has been implicated in the peculiar juxtaosseous changes, among them cyst-like bone changes and large soft tissue masses eroding bone. MRI studies indicate low signal on T1-weighted imaging and high signal on T2-weighted imaging.

Before 1970 hemophilia A was still associated with significant severe disability and even death at a young age. However, median life expectancy has grown significantly throughout the 20th century from 11.4 years to 68 years in carefully monitored populations.[46] However, the transfusion of blood products, including factor VIII concentrates, has led to one of the well-recognized modern complications of hemophilia: transfusion-related AIDS. Life expectancy has now reversed after considerable gains. Large numbers of hemophiliacs developed serologically detectable antibodies to HIV beginning at about 1979. Approximately two-thirds of HIV-positive hemophiliacs have eventually died of AIDS. The risk to the surgeon is minimal if the proper precautions are taken.[29]

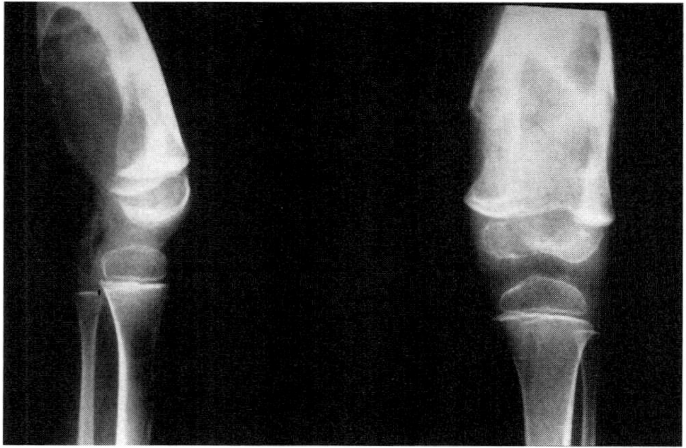

FIGURE 50.8 ➢ Radiograph of hemophilic pseudotumor. (From Vigorita VJ: The synovium. In Vigorita VJ, Ghelman B: Orthopaedic Pathology. Philadelphia, Lippincott/Williams & Wilkins, 1999.)

More recent therapy has used factor VIII concentrates exposed to vigorous virus killing heat treatment or solvent cleaning. Genetically engineered products are now available and are being tested for complications. Expense is a significant consideration.

Hemochromatosis

Much of current knowledge about the effect of iron on tissue comes from studies of hemochromatosis, the systemic disorder in which iron deposition is associated with tissue dysfunction. In general, iron overload has been studied in clinical situations in which there has been hyperplastic refractory anemia, excessive blood transfusions for underlying hematopoietic abnormalities (thalassemia), and hereditary forms of hemochromatosis. In the United States and northern Europe, hereditary hemochromatosis is actually a common cause of iron overload; up to 15% of the population demonstrates the gene in its heterozygous state. The abnormal gene, located on the short arm of chromosome 6, closely linked to the HLAA locus. In hereditary hemochromatosis, there is an increased absorption of dietary iron resulting in excess iron deposition in parenchymal tissues of endocrine organs, liver, and heart; death often results from heart failure or chronic liver disease.

In secondary hemochromatosis, the cause is ineffective erythropoiesis as seen in β-thalassemia and sideroblastic or aplastic anemia for which the treatment is repeated transfusions. Secondary hemochromatosis may also be caused by chronic liver disease, and in certain populations, such as within sub-Saharan Africa, hemochromatosis has been attributed to increased amounts of dietary iron intake such as from large amounts of iron in beer brewed in steel drums. Those at greatest risk probably have a genetic predisposition.[25]

The deposition of iron in bone, particularly at the osteoblast/osteoid interface or at the mineralization front or as hemosiderosis within the hematopoietic cells of the marrow, is a relatively common sequela to both primary and transfusional hemosiderosis. Although the primary organs involved are the heart and the liver with eventual development of cirrhosis and hepatocellular carcinoma and heart failure, endocrine organs are particularly involved. In fact, joint pains in the clinical presentation of arthritis have been noted in 11% of patients carefully clinically analyzed; bone pain is a less frequent cause for presentation.[2]

First recognized in 1964 as a feature of hemochromatosis, arthropathy is now generally believed to be a common clinical symptom. In hemochromatosis, the joint changes may mimic DJD. Less than 50% of patients appear to have clinically osteoarticular problems. The metacarpophalangeal joints and interphalangeal joints are most frequently reported. Wrists, elbows, shoulders, hips, and knees are less frequently affected.[71]

Iron may inhibit the pyrophosphatase activity in cartilage tissue, leading to the precipitation of calcium pyrophosphate crystals, an association between the two which is well recognized.

LEAD SYNOVITIS

The signs and symptoms of lead poisoning are subtle, and recognition of this entity may be difficult. Plumbism is most commonly caused by ingestion of lead-based paint by children; by occupational exposure, such as with painters, lead miners, and workers in battery factories; and by the consumption of contaminated beverages, such as moonshine.[8]

A prototype of lead injury to the joint is the effect of retained bullet fragments.[9] Lead poisoning secondary to retained projectiles is rare but was reported as long ago as the ancient Roman wars (Fig. 50.9). Lead toxicity may cause convulsions, somnolence, mania, delirium tremens, coma, neuritis, nausea, vomiting, abdominal cramps, anorexia, weight loss, renal insufficiency, general malaise, and death. Orthopedic complications include bone cysts, localized arthropathy, pseudarthrosis, and gouty arthritis. Serum levels of lead of as much as 920 μg/dL (44.40 mm/L) have been reported after retention of lead projectiles. The time between injury and onset of symptoms has ranged from 2 days to 40 years, although patients may be asymptomatic for long periods of time.

The location of the projectile in the body is a major factor in the likelihood of the development of lead intoxication. Exposure of lead to acidic synovial fluid results in greater dissolution than does exposure to human serum, water, or soft tissues. A second variable that may affect the duration of the symptomatic period is the surface area of the lead that is exposed to body tissue. Multiple small pellets have a greater surface area than one larger pellet, thus facilitating solubilization. Embedded lead particles usually are not absorbed systemically because they are encapsulated by dense, avascular fibrous tissue, inhibiting their dissolution in body fluids.

The diagnosis of lead intoxication has routinely included analysis of the levels of lead in serum and urine as well as clinical findings.

Studies in which electron microscopy was used suggested that lead is incorporated into cells to a level that causes death of cells, resulting in extracellular deposition of lead. This suggests a need for removing lead fragments from the intra-articular space as soon as possible to avoid localized arthropathy.

The treatment of lead intoxication has consisted primarily of chelation therapy and open techniques for removal of the fragments. Symptomatic lead poisoning can be treated with arthroscopic removal of lead. This technique allows for removal of the fragments, extensive synovectomy, and débridement without the need for an open arthrotomy. Frequently, chelation therapy is given preoperatively to avoid sudden exacerbation of lead intoxication caused by the stress of the operation. Theoretically, lead, which is stored mostly in bone, can be released during stresses such as an operation, fever, immobilization, acidosis, and other conditions, and this would dramatically increase symptoms.

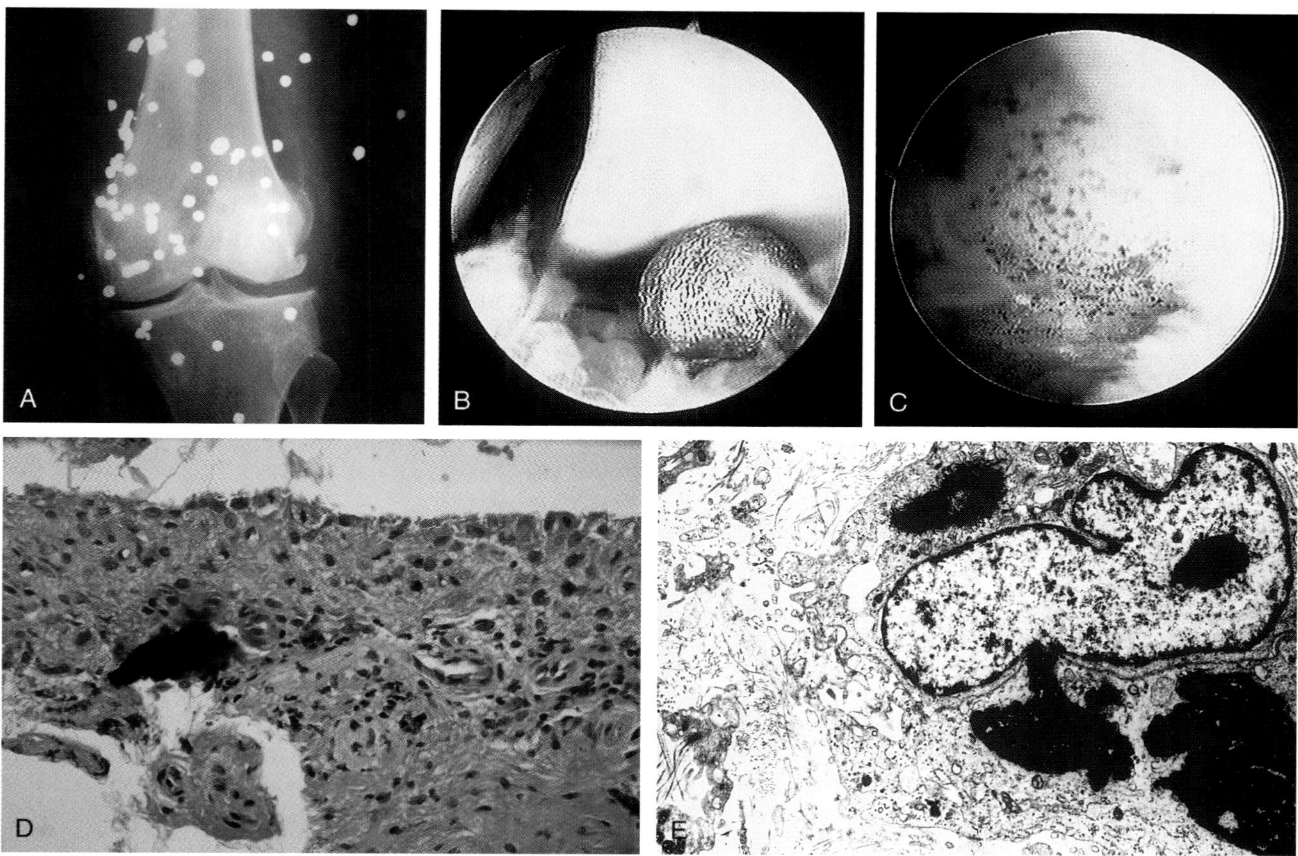

FIGURE 50.9 ➢ Lead synovitis. *A,* Radiograph of the right knee showing multiple lead pellets. *B,* Intraoperative view of the shotgun pellet in the intra-articular space (×10). *C,* Intraoperative view of minute particulate matter engulfing the articular surface of the tibial plateau (×10). *D,* Photomicrograph of hyperplastic and hypertrophied synovial tissue with irregular fragments of foreign material (black). A sparse and patchy chronic inflammation is present (hematoxylin-eosin, ×255). *E,* Transmission electron micrograph of synovial tissue with cytoplasmic electron-dense particulate matter surrounding the nucleus (right) and at the left. The scale marker represents 1 μm (× 9800). (From Vigorita VJ: The synovium. In Vigorita VJ, Ghelman B: Orthopaedic Pathology. Philadelphia, Lippincott/Williams & Wilkins, 1999.)

However, the level of lead might not increase with intervention such as arthroscopy.

Chelation therapy has been given both intravenously and orally. Multiple courses of chelation therapy may be needed to deplete the body stores of lead. It should be combined with operative removal of lead from the intra-articular space, and arthroscopic excision may be an effective way to achieve this goal.

Reported clinical effects of lead on articular structures include extracellular subsynovial lead deposition, synovial hypertrophy and inflammation, and intracellular lead uptake. Radiographic effects reported in animals include synovial lead uptake and arthropathies.

The presence of lead near the joint space can induce microscopic degenerative changes in the joint structures. Lead-implanted knees yield significantly greater degeneration compared with knees with steel, knees undergoing simple arthrotomy, and control knees.

ARTHRITIS

DJD Versus Rheumatoid Arthritis

Although a broad range of disorders may give rise to arthritis, de novo arthritis may be readily classified into two groups: DJD (osteoarthritis)[30] and rheumatoid arthritis.[31] They are distinct etiologically, clinically, roentgenographically, and pathologically (macroscopically and microscopically).

There are significant differences in the primary component of the joint involved. Notwithstanding recent experimental interest in synovial tissue modulation of cartilage destruction by cytokines, such as catabolin (interleukin-1), the synovium in DJD appears, at least initially, to be an innocent bystander, with the brunt of damage initially involving the articular cartilage (fibrillation and eventual denudement) and subsequently the bone (subchondral cyst formation and sclerosis with marginal new bone formation or osteophytosis). Although the synovium may show hyperplasia, this is usually minimal and nonspecific. Synovitis is limited if

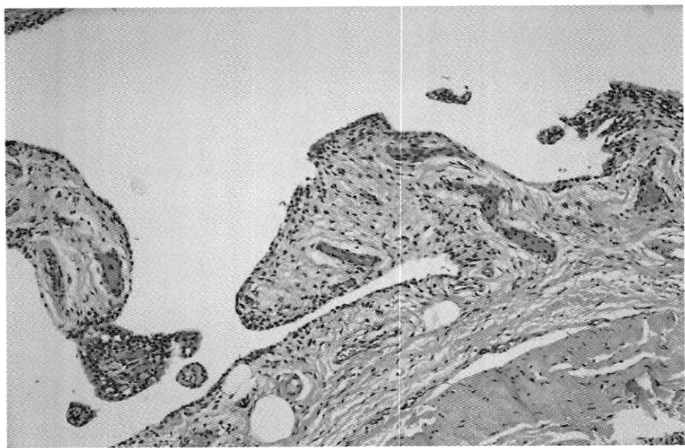

FIGURE 50.10 ➢ Synovium in degenerative joint disease. Villous change with mild hypertrophy and hyperplasia of synovial lining cells.

present at all (Fig. 50.10). Arthroscopic studies revealed that gross signs of inflammation in early DJD, unlike those of rheumatoid arthritis, are limited anatomically to the points of the synovium in close proximity to articular cartilage; the overwhelming remaining synovium is essentially normal.

Rarely does inflammation reach the extent seen in rheumatoid arthritis. In acute rheumatoid arthritis the synovium shows the most significant pathology (Fig. 50.11). Infiltrated by lymphocytes and plasma cells, the synovium becomes hyperplastic and the surface exudes a fibrinous exudate. Changes in the articular cartilage are truly secondary as the pannus, or inflammatory synovium, invades the surface of the joint, causing chondrolysis, eventual cartilage denudement, and, in chronic cases, the appearance of a secondary degenerative phenomenon. However, both chondrolysis and osteoporosis characterize rheumatoid arthritis, thus distinguishing it clearly from DJD.

This distinction is evident in laboratory diagnosis and monitoring. The inflammatory changes in rheumatoid arthritis are discernible in elevated sedimentation rates and positive rheumatoid factors (an elevated immunoglobulin protein, usually IgM, circulating in the serum). There is no equivalent useful laboratory monitor for DJD.

Radiographic changes initially show joint space narrowing and subchondral sclerosis. Eventually, new bone forms at the margins of articular cartilage (osteophytosis), which may give rise to villous synovial hypertrophy and metaplasia leading to chondro-osseous loose bodies.

Variants of DJD include an inflammatory type, characterized by more lymphocytic infiltration and hyperplasia of the synovium, and a rapidly destructive joint process that shows accelerated clinical and roentgenographic joint damage correlated pathologically by ex-

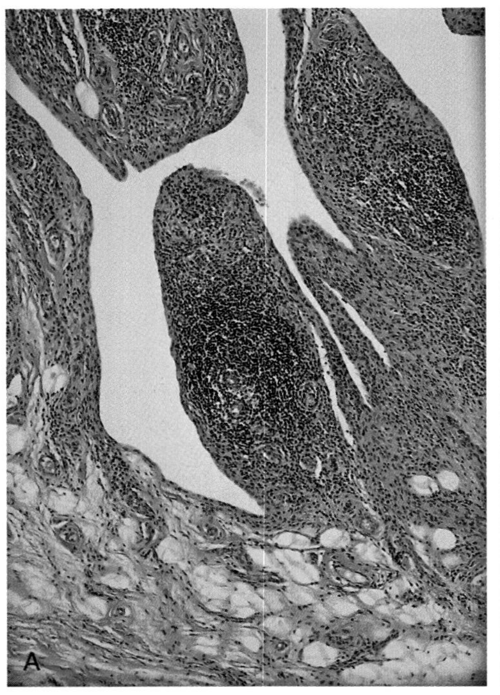

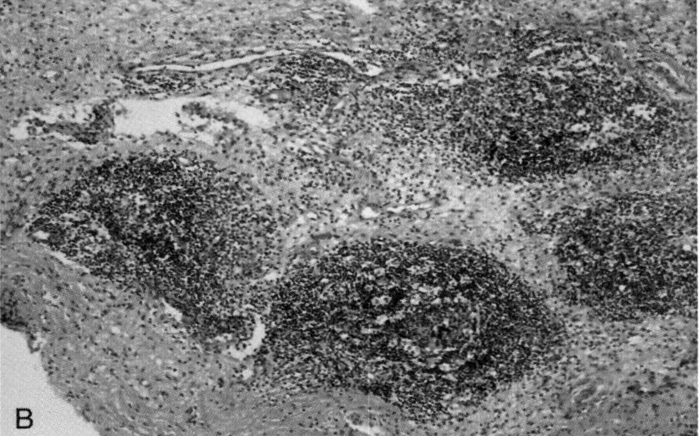

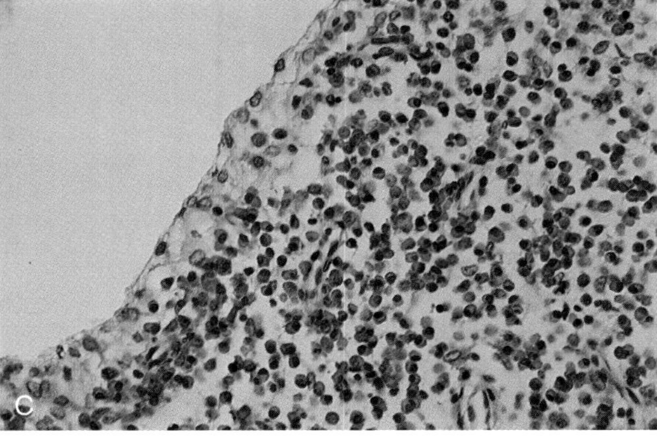

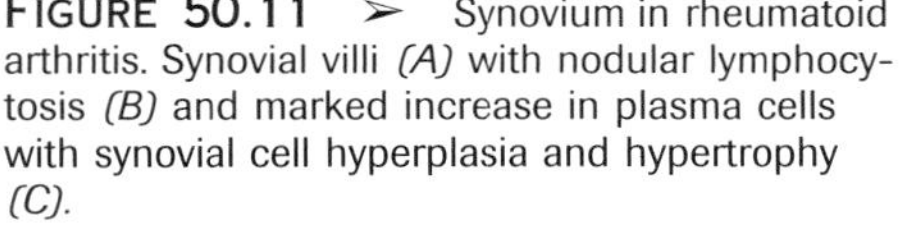

FIGURE 50.11 ➢ Synovium in rheumatoid arthritis. Synovial villi *(A)* with nodular lymphocytosis *(B)* and marked increase in plasma cells with synovial cell hyperplasia and hypertrophy *(C)*.

tensive cartilage and bone debris throughout the joint.[44]

Rheumatoid arthritis is classically a chronic, symmetric, persistent arthritis that may be associated with systemic symptoms and rheumatoid nodules (classically subcutaneous). Its cause remains obscure, but laboratory studies and familial history suggest both immunological and genetic factors in its expression. Most patients with rheumatoid arthritis have a circulating protein in their blood, usually IgM, which is the basis for the "rheumatoid factor test," a nonspecific but often useful serological test in corroborating the clinicopathological diagnosis. Atypical infections may trigger an as yet undetermined genetic predisposition. The presence of rheumatoid factor and elevated sedimentation rates correlates well with the characteristic synovial changes of a hyperemic synovial tissue infiltrated by a pronounced lymphocyte and plasma cell infiltration, often producing a fibrinous exudate. The latter proteinaceous exudation may override the articular bone surfaces of the joint, often creating tan, friable bodies (rice bodies).

Variants

Other disorders have been associated with rheumatoid-like inflammatory joint disease, but these "rheumatoid variants," such as psoriatic arthritis, Reiter's syndrome, and the arthritides associated with colitis, show less inflammatory synovial changes, vary in clinical progression of disease, and usually are not associated with a positive rheumatoid factor.

CRYSTAL-INDUCED SYNOVITIS

Although there are numerous crystals that may deposit in the joint and in the bone proper, two crystals are particularly synoviotropic and associated with clinical articular and osseous pathology and should be specifically contrasted. Gout, resulting from the deposition of sodium urate, and calcium pyrophosphate crystal deposition (pseudogout, chondrocalcinosis) are both frequently encountered crystal deposition disorders presenting with rheumatological or orthopedic complications.[36] In addition, hydroxyapatite crystals may be detected in synovial fluid in association with arthritis and degenerative joint changes. Other crystals, such as oxalosis and cystinosis, are rare and usually associated with kidney-related complications.

Gout

Gout refers to the painful clinical syndrome associated with the precipitation of sodium urate crystals in and around joint surfaces characterized by synovitis and juxta-articular destruction of articular bone. Although gout often presents as a rheumatological or orthopedic syndrome, it is a systemic disorder with the potential deposition of sodium urate crystals and the ensuing inflammatory tophus reaction in virtually any organ in the body with the exception of the brain. Nonetheless, a severe form of hyperuricemia (Lesch-Nyhan syndrome) manifests with severe central nervous system clinical disease.

Gout is far more frequent in males and increases in incidence with age. It usually presents in the adult period. Although there probably are asymptomatic deposits of crystals, more often than not gout is characterized by painful clinical attacks that are usually abrupt in onset involving the small peripheral joints, especially the metatarsal phalangeal joints. The predilection for sodium urate gout crystals to deposit in the peripheral joints of the body suggests that multiple factors may be at work, including factors related to pH and temperature. A gouty attack may last from a half day to several weeks. Although urate levels in the serum are usually elevated (approximately >8.0 mg/dL in men and >6.5 mg/dL in women), this may not necessarily be the case, and well-documented examples of gouty arthritis with large tophus deposits have been associated with normal uric acid levels, at least sporadically. The analysis of synovial fluid in gout cases reflects an inflammatory type of change with leukocytosis and the identification in sediment, in particular of synovial inflamed fluid, of intra- and extracellular needle-shaped crystals that have a characteristic negative birefringence on polarized light microscopy (Fig. 50.12). These morphological changes are useful in differentiating gouty crystals from synovial fluid, contrasting them with other crystals such as those seen in calcium pyrophosphate deposition (CPPD) disorders. A specific and sensitive technique is to use both light microscopy and polarized light microscopy. The addition of a red filter clearly distinguishes the strongly "negative" birefringent crystals. The strongly birefringent crystals parallel to the orientation of the red filter are yellow, and those perpendicular are blue, the so-called eponym "U PAY PEB." "Positive" birefringent crystals of CPPD oriented parallel are blue, and those oriented perpendicular are yellow.

Although there may be a genetic component in a large percentage of gout cases, associated diseases are clearly demonstrable. They include, but are not limited to, diabetes, hypertension, hyperparathyroidism, and hypothyroidism and, in fact, may be precipitated by surgery, including localization around implanted hip prostheses.[4] The association of gout with surgery, particularly repetitive surgeries, is well known. Additional associations or risk factors for gout include lymphoproliferative disorders, particularly polycythemia and diuretic therapy.

Perhaps the most important risk factor in gout is the intake of a high purine-rich diet in patients genetically or otherwise susceptible to the disorder. Here the biochemical understanding of gout is particularly important. Purines and pyrimidines are nitrogen-containing compounds that may coalesce and, with sugars and phosphates, create nucleotides, which form the elements of RNA and DNA. The ability to synthesize purines is universal among living organisms; the final product of purine metabolism is uric acid.

Most gout is seen in adult males. A small group of younger patients, with Lesch-Nyhan syndrome, is of biochemical interest because it pinpoints the defi-

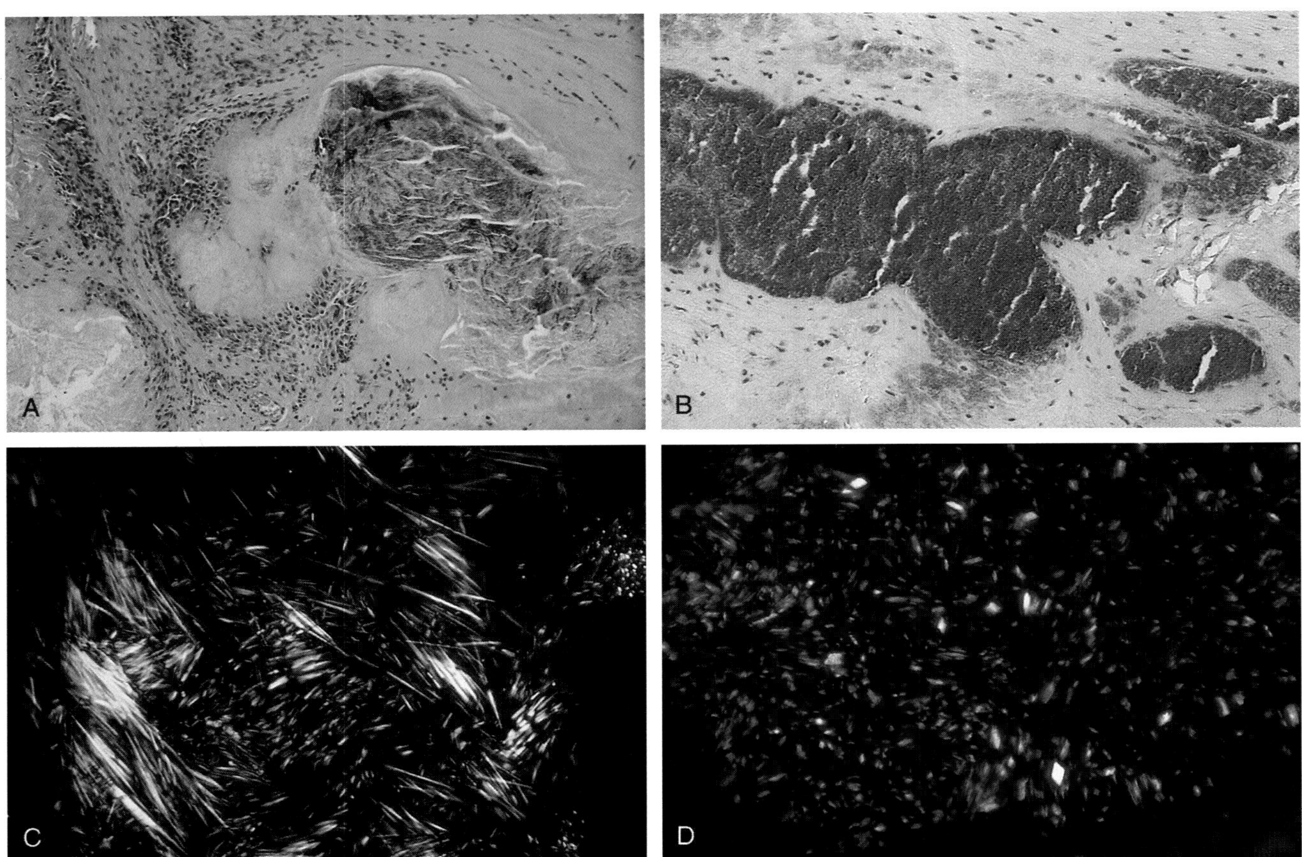

FIGURE 50.12 ➢ Composite: gout versus calcium pyrophosphate crystals. In tissue section, gout *(A)* appears as brown accumulations if not dissolved in routine fixatives (right); otherwise, amorphous whitish spaces remain (left). There is always an associated mononuclear and giant cell inflammation. Calcium pyrophosphate deposition (CPPD) *(B)* appears as purple deposits usually without associated inflammation. On polarized light microscopy, gout crystals appear needle-shaped and brilliantly refractive *(C)*. CPPD is less refractile, and crystals are rhomboid in shape *(D)*.

ciency of the enzyme hypoxanthine-guanine phosphoribisine transferase, pointing to a primary metabolic defect in at least this rare age group with gout.

In other patients, overproduction of uric acid can be linked to high activities of the enzyme phosphoribosyl pyrophosphate (PRPP) synthetase, leading to an increase in the endogenous production of uric acids. These conditions may be associated with genetically transmitted X-linked disorders.

The clinical manifestations of gout have been well described since antiquity. It is clinically characterized by extreme pain around the joints with evident red discoloration of the overlying skin in acute episodes.

Initially, radiographs are unremarkable, with only soft tissue swelling. With progressive attacks and more urate crystal deposition, tophi, which are granulomatous aggregates of crystals, accumulate in the joint tissue, causing discrete radiolucent marginal erosions of the articular bone. Despite significant bone destruction, joint preservation may be well maintained until late in the disease.

Gout may be associated with other crystal deposition disorders, particularly CPPD, or hydroxyapatite deposition. Therefore, its characteristic radiolucent appearance may at times be admixed with radiodensities.

The gross appearance of gout is that of a chalk-white deposit of paste-like consistency (Fig. 50.13). Histologically, it is characterized in synovial fluid by needle-shaped crystals usually within polymorphonuclear leukocytes and in tissue specimens by a characteristic granulomatous inflammatory response. On routine hematoxylin-eosin stain, when crystals have not been dissolved, the crystals have a brown appearance, but sodium urate is particularly soluble in the water component of formalin preparations. Therefore, more often than not the deposition is noted by the characteristic amorphous-looking gray deposits surrounded by a mononuclear and giant cell reaction of varying degrees of severity (see Fig. 50.12). Curiously, as with rheumatoid arthritis, the findings in synovial fluid are characterized by a leukocytosis and in tissue samples by a mononuclear cell population. Crystals from synovial fluid under polarized light are often phagocytosed by inflammatory cells.

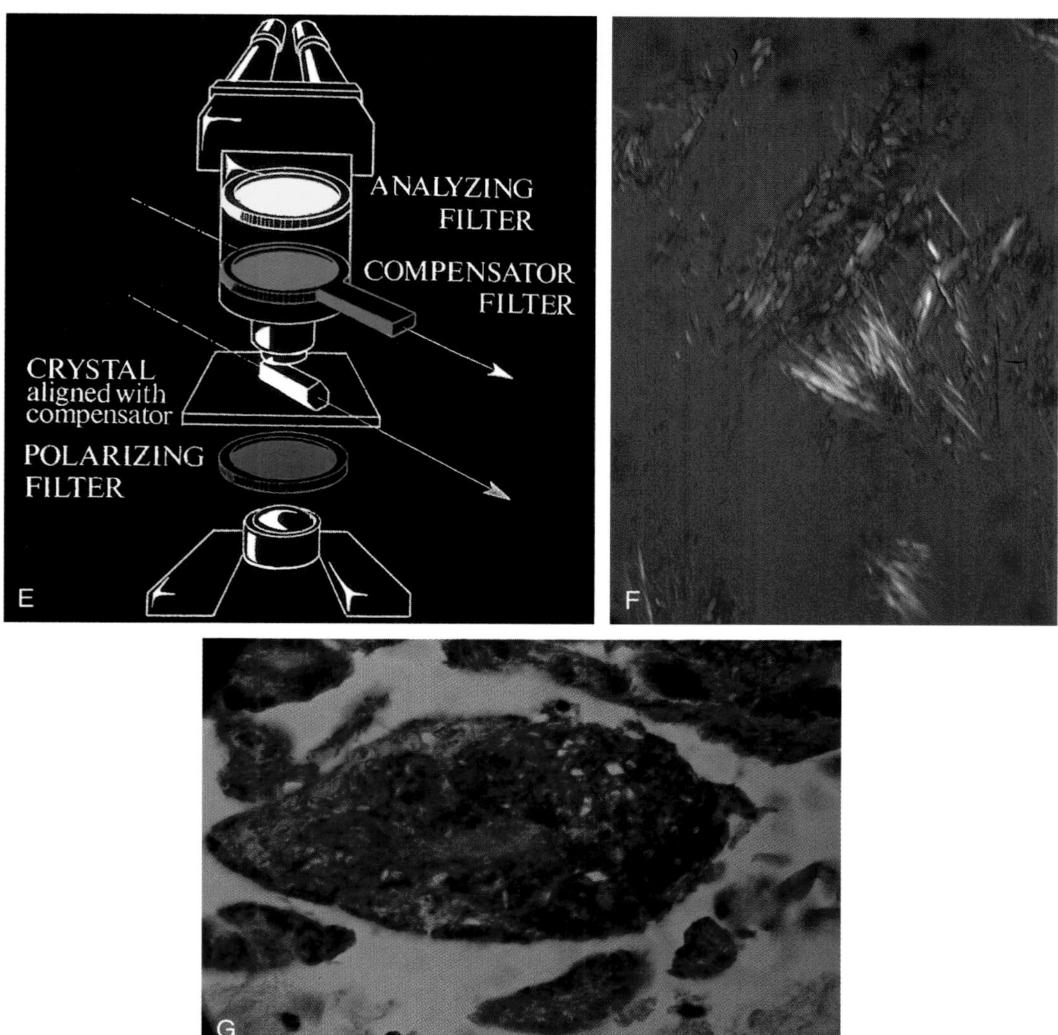

FIGURE 50.12 ➢ *Continued.* On polarized light microscopy with a red compensator filter *(E)*, gout *(U*rate) crystals *(F)* are oriented to the red analyzer filter: *Pa*rallel, *y*ellow; *Pe*rpendicular, *b*lue ("U Pay Peb"). CPPD crystals *(G)* are less oriented but often in the reverse orientation. By convention, the urate orientation of parallel yellow and perpendicular blue is considered negatively birefringent. Conversely, CPPD orientation is positively birefringent. (From Vigorita VJ: The synovium. In Vigorita VJ, Ghelman B: Orthopaedic Pathology. Philadelphia, Lippincott/Williams & Wilkins, 1999.)

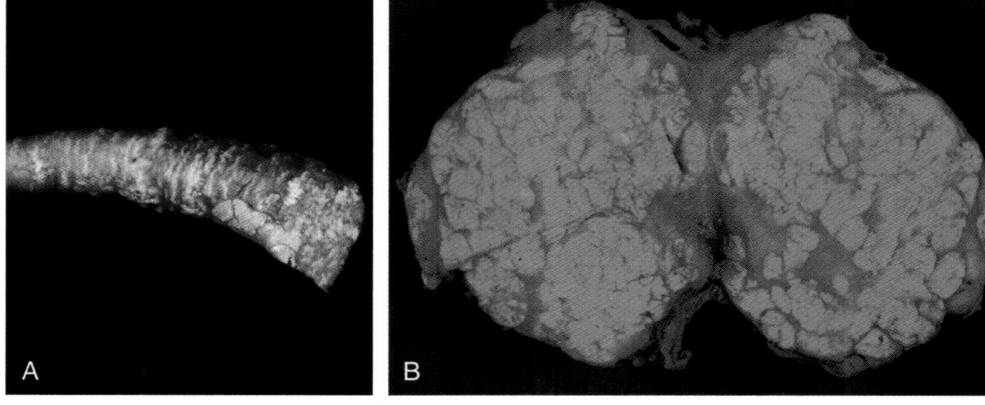

FIGURE 50.13 ➢ Urate crystals seen grossly involving the Achilles tendon *(A)* and synovium *(B)*. The chalk-white deposits have a paste-like consistency. (From Vigorita VJ: The synovium. In Vigorita VJ, Ghelman B: Orthopaedic Pathology. Philadelphia, Lippincott/Williams & Wilkins, 1999.)

TABLE 50.3 SYNOVIOTROPIC CRYSTAL-ASSOCIATED DISORDERS

Variable	Gout	Pseudogout
Crystal	Sodium urate	Calcium pyrophosphates
Radiograph	Early: soft tissue swelling Later: radiolucent erosions around edges of articular cartilage	Fine, radiopaque, linear deposits in the meniscus and articular cartilage
Frequency of occurrence in knee	Common	Very common; increases with age in DJD
Laboratory studies	Elevated serum uric acid	None
Crystal character with polarized light	Needle shaped	Rhomboid
Crystal character with compensated polarized light	Parallel, yellow; perpendicular, blue	Parallel, blue; perpendicular, yellow
Birefringence	Negative	Positive

DJD = degenerative joint disease.
From Vigorita VJ: The synovium. In Vigorita VJ, Ghelman B: Orthopaedic Pathology. Philadelphia, Lippincott/Williams & Wilkins, 1999.

Gout has been associated with osteonecrosis, the mechanism of which is not understood.[13] The clinical differential diagnosis includes septic arthritis.[61]

Finally, the relationship between lead toxicity and gout, first noted by Girrard in 1859 and involving renal dysfunction and hypertension, is also associated with attacks of acute gouty arthritis, or saturnine gout.

Calcium Pyrophosphate Dihydrate Crystal Deposition*

Calcium pyrophosphate dihydrate crystals were first discovered in the early 1960s in the synovial fluid of patients with pseudogout syndrome. It is now well recognized by its roentgenographic appearance: radiodense linear calcifications seen in articular cartilage, fibrocartilage, and soft tissues of the joints. Although CPPD crystal deposition is commonly seen with such diverse conditions as chronic degenerative arthropathy and acute arthritis, it is more common in older people and is seemingly an age-related phenomenon. It can be distinguished clinically, roentgenographically, and pathologically from gout (Table 50.3). By age 80, CPPD crystal formation is seen in at least 25% of Americans. The variation in the reported incidence of CPPD depends on the site and method of detection. For example, in tissue removed at knee replacement for DJD, CPPD crystals are grossly or microscopically seen in nearly 25% of patients. Although preferentially distributed in the meniscus and the layers of the articular cartilage, all tissue, including synovial tissue, may be involved (Fig. 50.14). In this, its most common setting, CPPD is characterized in routine hematoxylin-eosin stain by acellular purplish-gray, granular deposits (see Fig. 50.12).[49] Approximately 50% of the cases reveal positive birefringence on polarized light microscopy with a red analyzer filter. In other cases, crystals may have been cleared by formalin fixation. Inflammation confined to the sites of CPPD may be noted. This localized reaction is seen to a mild degree and usually consists of mononuclear cells. However, inflammatory CPPD, or pseudogout, is associated with considerable inflammation. Occasionally, giant cells may be seen; in fact, the production of loose bodies associated with DJD may also be the site of CPPD deposition. These crystals have also been noted within the confines of other tissue, including cruciate ligaments.

Although the cause of CPPD remains obscure, it appears to be temporally and microscopically related to the degenerative process.[58] Whereas some believe crystals are precipitated in the lacuna margin of dying chondrocytes, CPPD deposition has been linked to the deposition to abnormal hypertrophied chondrocytes.[68] Using special stains, Japanese investigators suggested that the proteoglycans normally inhibiting the normalization are degraded and lost from the extracellular matrix around the chondrocytes, thereby promoting crystal growth.[50] The presence of CPPD in noncartilaginous tissue, like the synovium, may be explained by initial chondrometaplasia.

Probably the most frequent observation of CPPD deposition is that seen in association with DJD, the cause of which is obscure. That DJD may be associated with changes in the inherent structures of the articular cartilage such as collagen and proteoglycan is of interest. Because the cause of CPPD remains unknown, it appears that in some cases tissue differentiation toward cartilage may be a precipitating event or substrate for crystal deposition, a concept supported by noting that calcium pyrophosphate crystals deposit preferentially in fibrocartilage tissue throughout the body. It is possible that modification of the proteoglycan structure, such as that seen in chondrometaplasia and often noted in the vicinity of CPPD deposition, may permit calcification to proceed or perhaps that local activation of certain enzymes such as alkaline phosphatase or inorganic pyrophosphatase leads to inactivation of the calcification inhibitors.

A particularly interesting subpopulation of patients with CPPD are those in whom CPPD deposits take the

* *CPPD* designates the crystal (calcium pyrophosphate) deposition in this disorder. *Pseudogout* refers to the occasional painful occurrence of CPPD-induced arthritis mimicking gout. *Chondrocalcinosis* refers to the fine linear radiopaque densities seen in the joint spaces of involved cases.

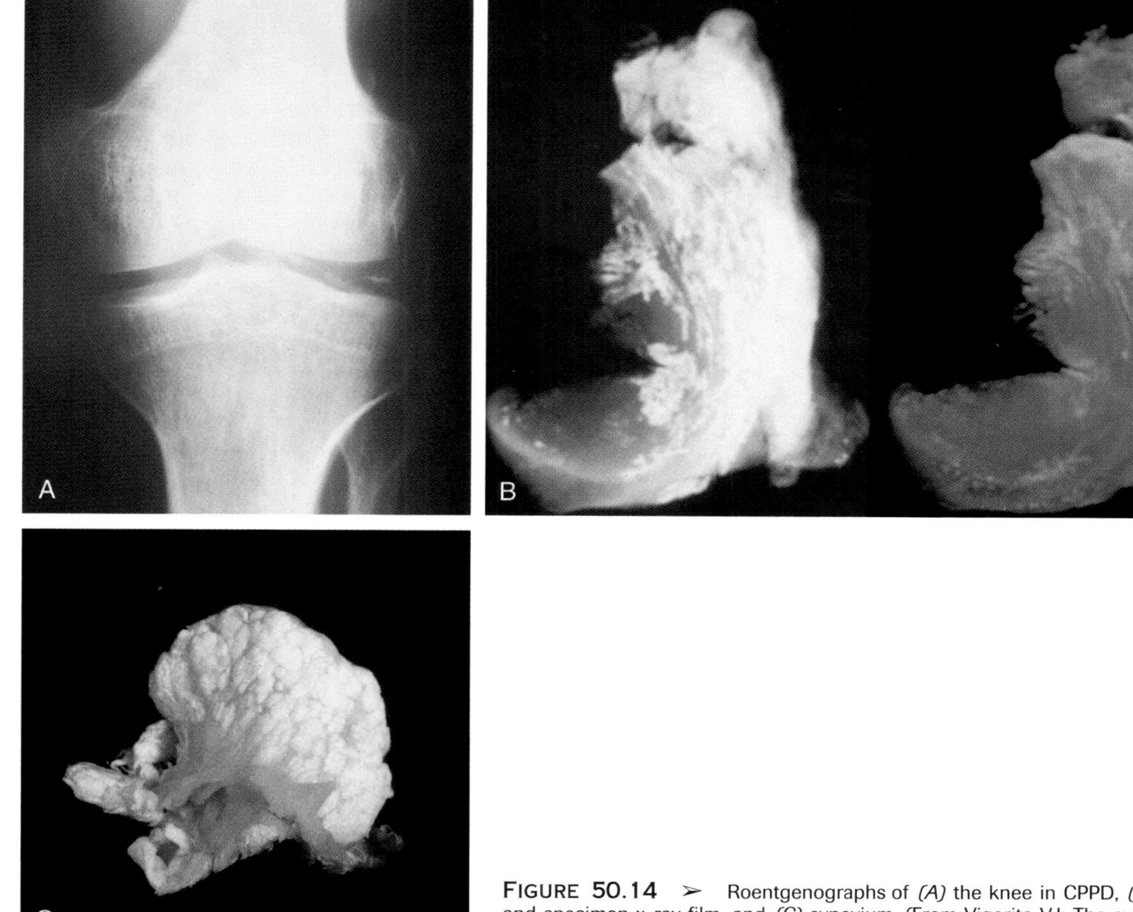

FIGURE 50.14 ➢ Roentgenographs of *(A)* the knee in CPPD, *(B)* meniscus gross and specimen x-ray film, and *(C)* synovium. (From Vigorita VJ: The synovium. In Vigorita VJ, Ghelman B: Orthopaedic Pathology. Philadelphia, Lippincott/Williams & Wilkins, 1999.)

form of bulky tumor-like masses in both articular and para-articular tissues.[65]

Hydroxyapatite Deposition

Hydroxyapatite crystals are the major crystal component of bone, but extraosseous deposition in the soft tissues of the joint space, rotator cuff tendons, and even bursa suggests that precipitation of these crystals may induce an arthropathy in some clinical situations not dissimilar from gout or calcium pyrophosphate crystals. The process may be secondary to traumatic injury to the joint or joint structures, DJD, or a primary crystal-induced arthropathy.

Calcium hydroxyapatite is a basic calcium phosphate, and the calcium hydroxyapatite crystals are characteristically nonbirefringent in contrast to those of gout and pseudogout. Histologically, they are seen as dark-staining clumps usually bluish-purple before decalcification and eosinophilic after decalcification. They are very dissimilar to bone in their staining characteristics, but can be contrasted with bone in that they lack osteocytes within the mineralized matrix. They may be discernible in synovial fluid and have variable morphological appearance. The crystals in tissue removed for clinical symptomatology may be seen in association with a usually sparse mononuclear and giant cell reaction, but, in fact, significant erosive changes of adjacent bone may be noted. Roentgenographically, one observes radiodense calcifications in a wide spectrum of clinical appearances. There may be local deposition in a tumor mass-like fashion or more subtle depositions in periarticular soft tissue. In fact, in association with arthropathies such as DJD, the release of apatite crystals from bone may be a secondary phenomenon in conditions in which crystals are uncovered in synovial fluid analysis. Calcium hydroxyapatite deposition has been described as both monarthric and polyarthric, usually occurring in the later adult years with equal distribution among men and women.

PLICA

Symptomatic synovial plicae are a recognized but rare cause of anterior knee pain.[40] There are at least three generally recognized plicae: suprapatellar, infrapatellar, and mediopatellar. The mediopatellar plica is the synovial fold most often implicated in pathology of the anterior knee. The infrapatellar plica is also known as the ligamentum mucosum.

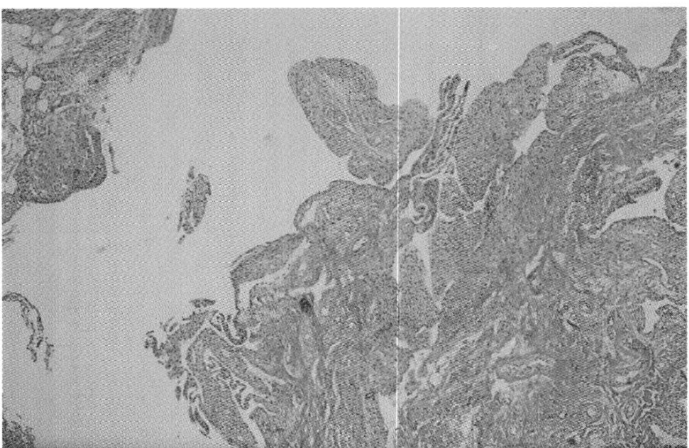

FIGURE 50.15. ➢ Synovial plica histology: bland fibrous membrane lined with rather indistinct synovial-like lining cells. (From Vigorita VJ: The synovium. In Vigorita VJ, Ghelman B: Orthopaedic Pathology. Philadelphia, Lippincott/Williams & Wilkins, 1999.)

Synovial plicae are a common incidental finding at arthroscopy. They are the remnants of incompletely resorbed embryonic septum. Occasionally, a medial plica can become inflamed by impinging on the anterior medial femoral condyle as the knee is flexed. When the condition is chronic, the plica becomes thickened and fibrotic. This is the “medial shelf syndrome.” Conservative therapy consisting of nonsteroidal anti-inflammatory drugs and quadriceps exercises is effective in the majority of cases. Arthroscopic resection is indicated if the plica does not respond to conservative therapy. Histologically, the resected plica is a nondescript fibrotic band covered with either normal or slightly inflamed synovium (Fig. 50.15).

SYNOVIAL DISORDERS

The various components of the synovial subintima explain the source of tumors reported in and around the joint.

- Hemangiomas (arterioles)
- Hemangiopericytoma (the pericyte of the arteriole)
- Fibromas (fibroblast)
- Leiomyomas (smooth muscle of arteriole wall)
- Lipomas, Hoffa’s disease (fat), and lipoma arborescens
- Other: synovial cysts
- Myxomas
- Synovial chondromatosis
- Pigmented villonodular synovitis (PVNS) (fibrohistiocyte)

The cause of the rare malignant tumors arising near joints, called synovial sarcoma and epithelioid sarcoma, is less well known. These latter tumors are highly malignant and are characterized by aggressive and destructive local growth and metastatic potential.

SYNOVIAL TUMORS AND TUMOR-LIKE LESIONS

Synovial Hemangioma

Synovium, the subintimal layer of which is rich in vasculature, may give rise to hemangiomas. They may be described as localized proliferative vascular tissue, which does not preclude their interpretation as a neoplasm, hamartomatous development, or arteriovenous malformation. All three interpretations have their proponents. Hemangiomas may arise from any structure line by synovium and thus have been described as intra-articular and arising from bursal spaces and tendon sheaths.[14]

Synovial hemangioma usually presents as a solitary benign vascular proliferation, most commonly seen in the knee joints of children and adolescents. In one large study, patient age ranged from 9 to 49 years (mean = 25 years).[14] Although the patient may be asymptomatic, there may be swelling, mild pain, or limitation of motion, with the pain and swelling in some instances being of several years’ duration. The knee is the most common location (60%) followed by the elbow (30%), a distribution not unlike that affected by hemophilic hemarthrosis.

Radiological examination reveals a soft tissue density suggesting a mass or synovial effusion.[26] In severe cases, it may cause adjacent bone changes such as periosteal reaction or lucent zones (Fig. 50.16) or phleboliths.

On MRI, synovial hemangiomas have a high signal intensity on T2-weighted images and intermediate signal intensity on T1-weighted images.[26]

Grossly, the knee joint reveals a soft, doughy, brown mass with proliferating villous synovium, frequently mahogany stained by hemosiderin deposition (Fig. 50.17).

Histologically, there is proliferation of vascular channels of various sizes and shapes with surrounding hyperplastic synovium (Fig. 50.18). Patterns described have been cavernous (dilated thin-walled vessels), capillary-size proliferation, and large thick-walled vessels predominating. No mitotic activity is seen. Copious hemosiderin may be seen in patients who have had repeated hemarthrosis. Giant cells, aggregates of inflammatory cells, are not seen. Treatment is surgical excision, after which there are no recurrences.

The differential diagnosis includes chronic hemarthrosis, which is not characterized by nodular tumorous masses of proliferating blood vessels, and pigmented villonodular synovitis, a benign neoplasm of collagen producing fibrohistiocytic growth.

Synovial Lipomatosis (Hoffa’s Disease)

In Hoffa’s disease[37] there is enlargement of the infrapatellar fat pad on either side of the patellar tendon with resulting pain or aching in the anterior compartment of the knee. Pain may be aggravated by physical activity or extension of the knee, with swelling or recurrent effusion, or both, as a consequence.

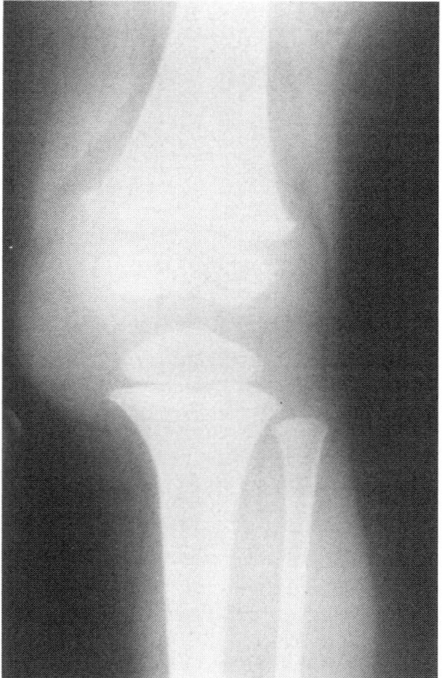
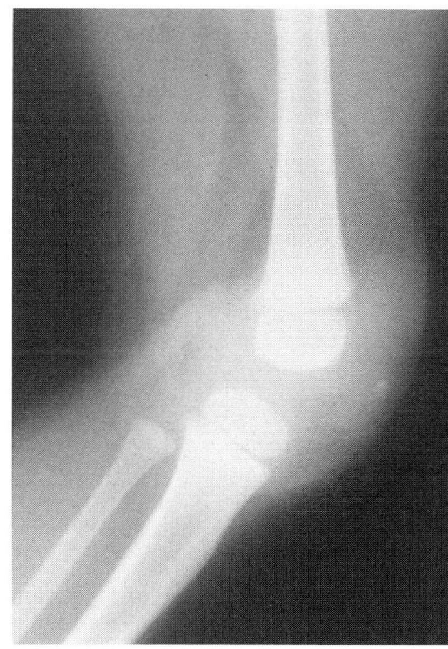

FIGURE 50.16 ➢ Roentgenograph of synovial hemangioma. (From Vigorita VJ: The synovium. In Vigorita VJ, Ghelman B: Orthopaedic Pathology. Philadelphia, Lippincott/Williams & Wilkins, 1999.)

Hoffa's disease may refer to changes in the fat pad caused by trauma. Bleeding in the fat pad is followed at times by fibrosis and calcifications. Fibrosis of the fat pad is best demonstrated on MRI scans. The areas of fibrosis are seen as regions of decreased signal intensity in both T1- and T2-weighted images. Computed tomography (CT) scans may also demonstrate fibrous tissue in the infrapatellar fat pad. Calcifications in the fat pad are well demonstrated by radiographs and should not be confused with intra-articular loose bodies of primary or secondary synovial chondromatosis (Fig. 50.19).

Pathologically, the synovium has a marked papillary proliferative appearance with microscopically evident hyperplasia of the synovial lining cells overlying abundant fat.

Lipoma arborescens refers to intra-articular fatty villonodular proliferations most often found in the knee but also described in other joints such as the wrist, ankle, and hip.[72] Patients usually complain of longstanding, slowly progressive swelling.

Microscopically, there is well-vascularized fat covered by a uniform but thickened synovial cell lining.[27]

Roentgenographically, synovial fat lesions are characterized by extra soft tissue densities on routine x-ray films and MRI signals characteristic of fat with homogeneity.[27]

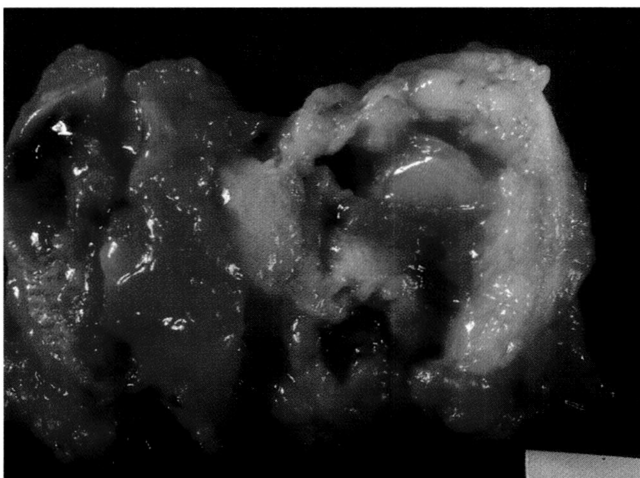

FIGURE 50.17 ➢ Synovial hemangioma: gross appearance showing soft rusty-brown mass. (From Vigorita VJ: The synovium. In Vigorita VJ, Ghelman B: Orthopaedic Pathology. Philadelphia, Lippincott/Williams & Wilkins, 1999.)

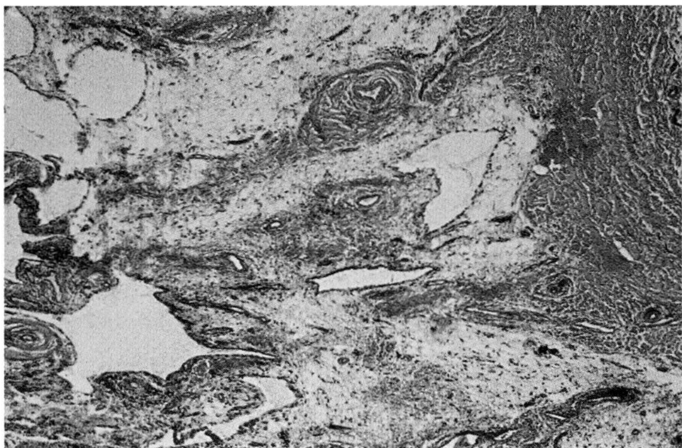

FIGURE 50.18 ➢ Synovial hemangioma. As with hemangiomas in soft tissue, pathology ranges from thick- to thin-walled vessels and may show considerable variation as in arteriovenous malformations. (From Vigorita VJ: The synovium. In Vigorita VJ, Ghelman B: Orthopaedic Pathology. Philadelphia, Lippincott/Williams & Wilkins, 1999.)

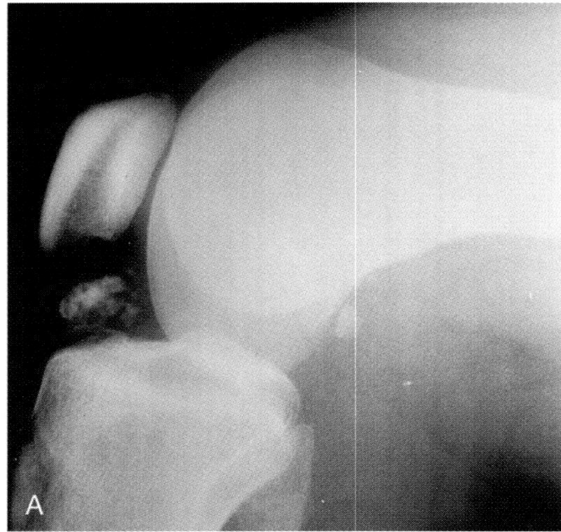

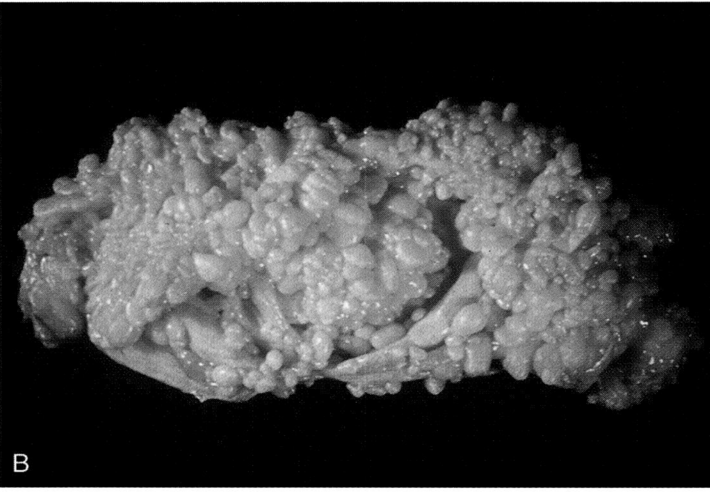

FIGURE 50.19 ➢ *A,* Hoffa's disease: infrapatellar soft tissue (fatty) mass with circumscribed (secondary) calcification. *B,* Hoffa's disease: abundant excess of grossly identifiable fat. (From Vigorita VJ: The synovium. In Vigorita VJ, Ghelman B: Orthopaedic Pathology. Philadelphia, Lippincott/Williams & Wilkins, 1999.)

Juxta-Articular Myoma

The juxta-articular myoma or parameniscal cyst is a type of myxoma or ganglion. Typically, a poorly circumscribed mass that may rapidly enlarge, it is often associated with pain or tenderness and may be symptomatic from weeks to years.[53] They occur more frequently in men and are most typically seen in the knee (shoulder > elbow) and, in particular, in the knee. Many cases have been seen in association with DJD or meniscal tears. Histologically, they are composed of spindle and stellate fibroblasts in an abundant myxoid matrix. A secondary fibroblastic reaction may mimic sarcoma. Most occur in the subcutaneous fat with extension to anatomic components of the joint, including the meniscus, tendons and capsule, and even synovium.

Synovial Cysts

Cysts may be anatomically related to the joints, lined by a synovial membrane and containing synovial fluid.[17] So-called synovial cysts, they are often associated with underlying joint disease such as rheumatoid arthritis or trauma and have been described, or can be expected to develop, in virtually any joint. Those near the knee representing a communication between the gastrocnemius-semimembranous bursa and the knee, "popliteal cysts" are the best described in the literature,[73] but all spaces or potential spaces in communication with a joint are anatomic possibilities.

Synovial cysts may attain a large size and extend far outside the joint in a dissecting fashion. Rupture, mass effects, neuropathies, and vascular compromise are all potential complications. There may be a compensatory function in the development of synovial cysts; some authors believe that synovial cysts help to maintain joint function by decompressing a chronically or acutely effused joint.

Loose Bodies ("Joint Mice")

Loose bodies may occur in any joint, may vary in size and number, and, depending on the cause, consist of a range of normal pathological tissue (Fig. 50.20). They may be asymptomatic or cause pain and interfere mechanically with joint function, causing limited motion, locking, clicking and limping, and even, in extreme cases, subluxation.

Typically consisting of metaplastic cartilage and bone, loose bodies may be formed of fibrin as a result of fibrinous exudation onto the synovial surface in the inflammatory arthritides, particularly rheumatoid arthritis, so-called rice bodies because of their soft, mushy texture and gross appearance. Synovial loose bodies may result from torsion and infarction of nodular pigmented synovitis.

Secondary Chondromatosis

Cartilaginous and osseous loose bodies are the result of DJD, neuropathic joint disease (Charcot's joints), osteochondritis dissecans, meniscal tears, or other trauma. These cartilage segments (with or without underlying bone) may dislodge, fall free into the joint, and continue to grow over prolonged periods of time; the synovial fluid acts as a virtual culture medium (Fig. 50.21).

Grossly, they may be large or small, cartilaginous or osseous, or both, and may or may not show obvious derivation from joint structures such as synovium and fibrocartilage.

Primary Synovial Chondromatosis (Synovial Osteochondromatosis)

The synovium, capable of undergoing metaplasia to cartilage in a broad range of conditions, including trauma and DJD, may produce de novo multiple carti-

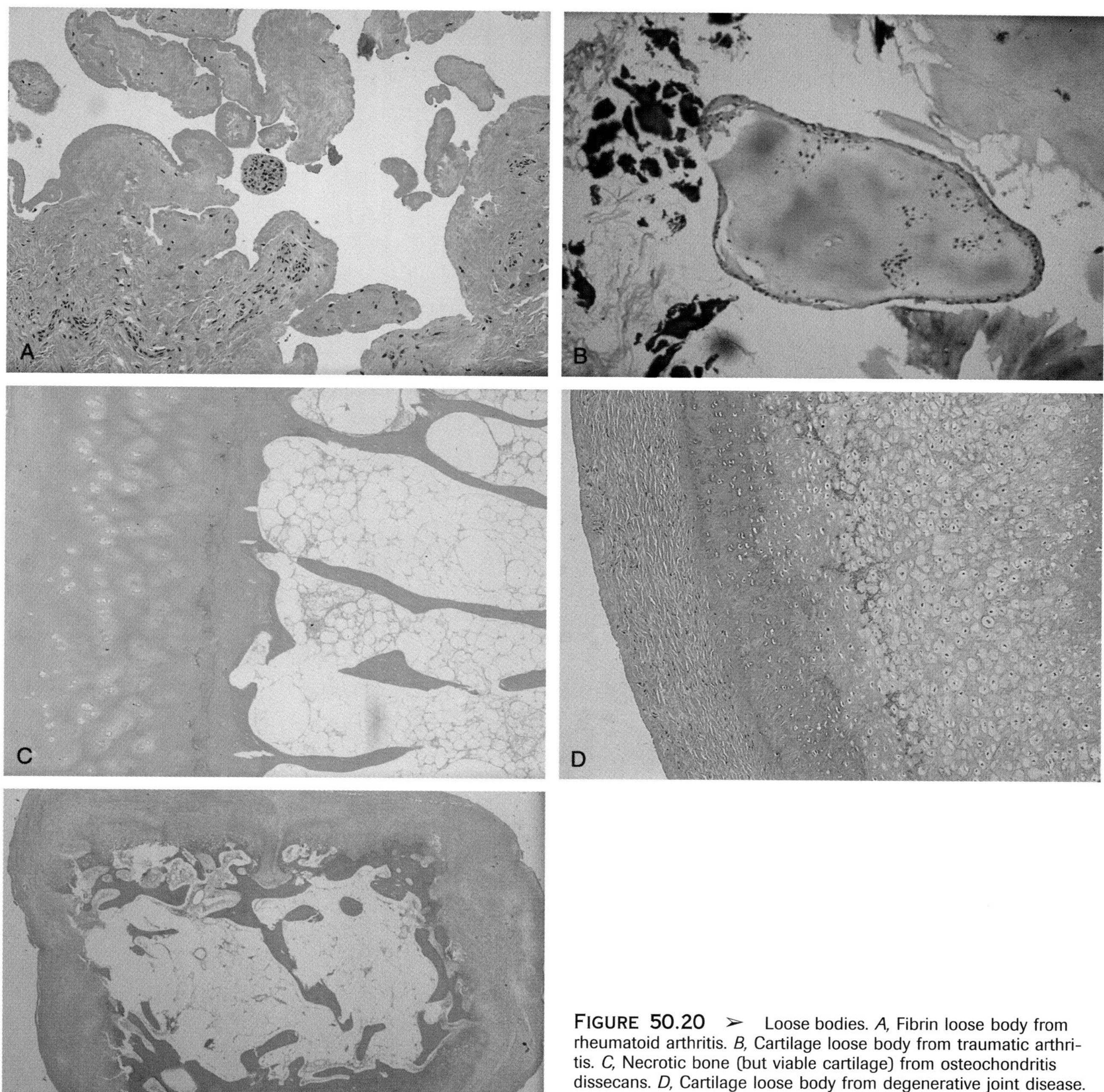

FIGURE 50.20 ➢ Loose bodies. *A,* Fibrin loose body from rheumatoid arthritis. *B,* Cartilage loose body from traumatic arthritis. *C,* Necrotic bone (but viable cartilage) from osteochondritis dissecans. *D,* Cartilage loose body from degenerative joint disease. *E,* Osseous loose body from degenerative joint disease. (From Vigorita VJ: The synovium. In Vigorita VJ, Ghelman B: Orthopaedic Pathology. Philadelphia, Lippincott/Williams & Wilkins, 1999.)

laginous and chondro-osseous loose bodies throughout the joint unrelated to underlying disease. This latter condition, primary synovial chondromatosis (synovial osteochondromatosis), is best characterized as a benign tumorous proliferation. Initially embedded in the synovium, the nodules may dislodge from the synovium and become free loose bodies ranging in number from a few to hundreds.

Synovial chondromatosis is a monarthric condition occurring in the third, fourth, and fifth decades of life, with predilection for the knee, which is involved in more than two-thirds of cases, followed by the elbow, ankle, hip, and shoulder. It is rare in childhood. It is usually associated with swelling and may be associated with pain, limitation of motion, and occasionally clicking or locking. Radiographically, the condition is easily recognized if the cartilaginous bodies have undergone calcification or ossification, which they often do (Fig. 50.22). The numerous radiopaque densities range in size from a millimeter to centimeters, varying considerably in the extent of calcification and size.[15] Arthrography is useful in diagnosing the noncalcified bodies.

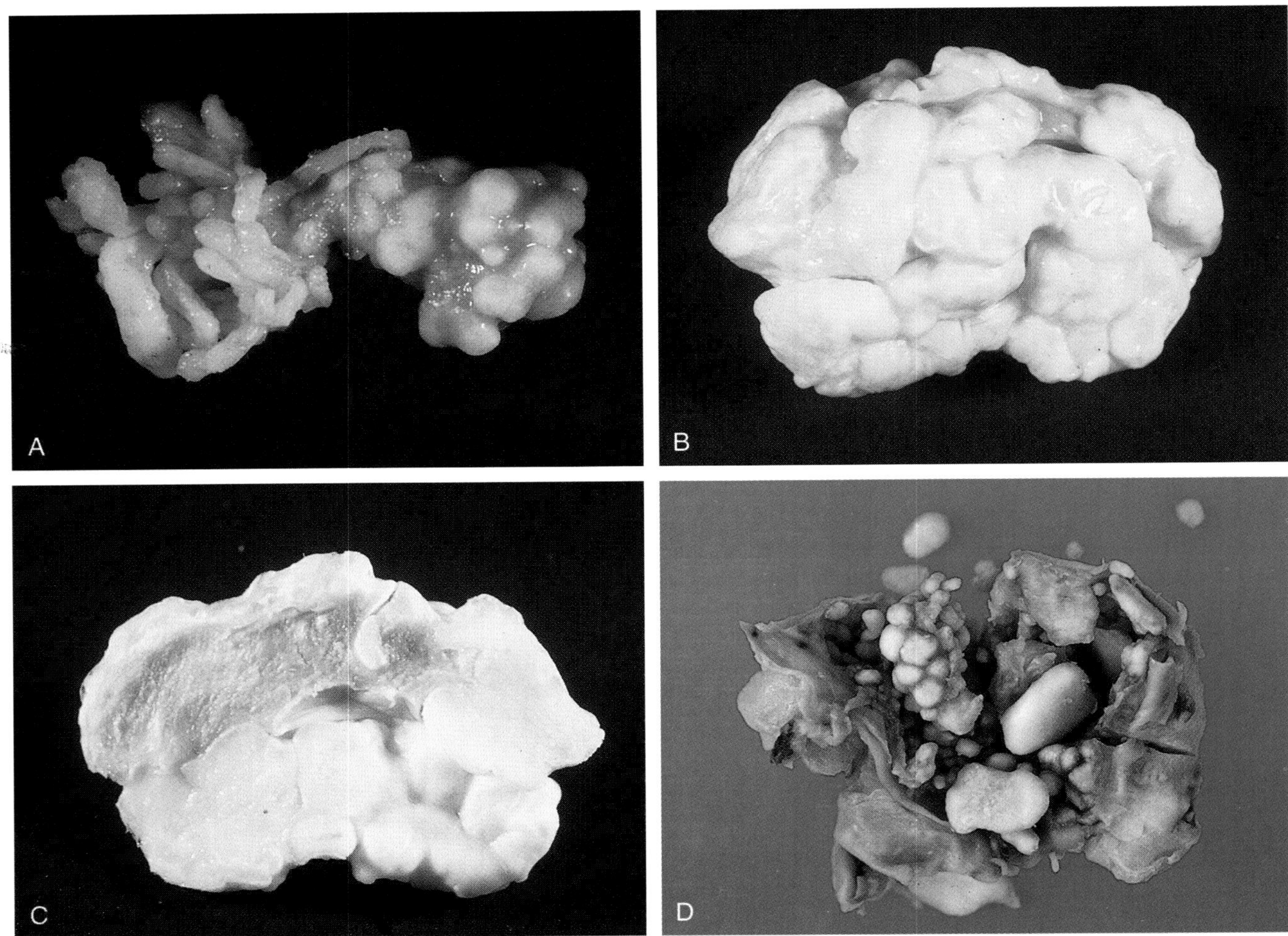

FIGURE 50.21 ➢ Loose bodies (synovial chondromatosis). Gross appearance: small loose body forming from synovial metaplasia *(A)* in contrast to large, free-floating loose body with smooth bosselated cartilaginous surface and bony center (*B, C,* cross-section). *D,* Synovial chondromatosis. Gross appearance: numerous loose bodies of various sizes and shapes fill the joint space. (From Vigorita VJ: The synovium. In Vigorita VJ, Ghelman B: Orthopaedic Pathology. Philadelphia, Lippincott/Williams & Wilkins, 1999.)

Grossly, the synovium shows flake-like bodies, or it may possess an irregular nodular contour. Whitish or translucent bluish-gray nodules, ranging greatly in size and shape, may be more obviously attached on the membrane or floating in the joint space.

Histopathological differences of these bodies supported a distinction between a secondary synovial chondromatosis associated with DJD and a primary synovial chondromatosis not associated with any underlying disorder. The loose bodies in the secondary synovial chondromatosis show more organized cellular growth, often in concentric rings. Progression is orderly with columns of cells usually identifiable. Usually, zones of endochondral ossification are noted. However, transformation between cartilage and bone may be abrupt. In the typical case, orderly zones of transformation from fibrocartilage to hyaline-type cartilage through endochondral ossification to bone may be noted.

In primary synovial chondromatosis, a more disorganized lobular proliferation of cartilage is apparent, resembling the lobular chondroid growth patterns of cartilage neoplasms (Fig. 50.23). There are increased chondrocytes, often crowded and irregular in spatial distribution. Nuclei vary and binucleate cells may be seen. Calcification may be patchy or diffuse. Endochondral ossification, causing confusion with secondary loose bodies, may be noted. Surgical removal of all the nodules is important in preventing recurrence.

If the chondro-osseous bodies are entirely free, loose bodies within the joint, a thorough cleaning of the joint may suffice. However, the disorder may involve chondro-osseous change within the synovial subintimal connective tissue, which may require total synovectomy to prevent recurrence.

Milgram[54] suggested a temporal sequence for synovial chondromatosis beginning with active intrasynovial disease with no loose bodies, followed by transition lesions (intrasynovial and loose) and then purely loose, floating intra-articular bodies. In this scheme, if the last phase could be identified, synovectomy would not be required.

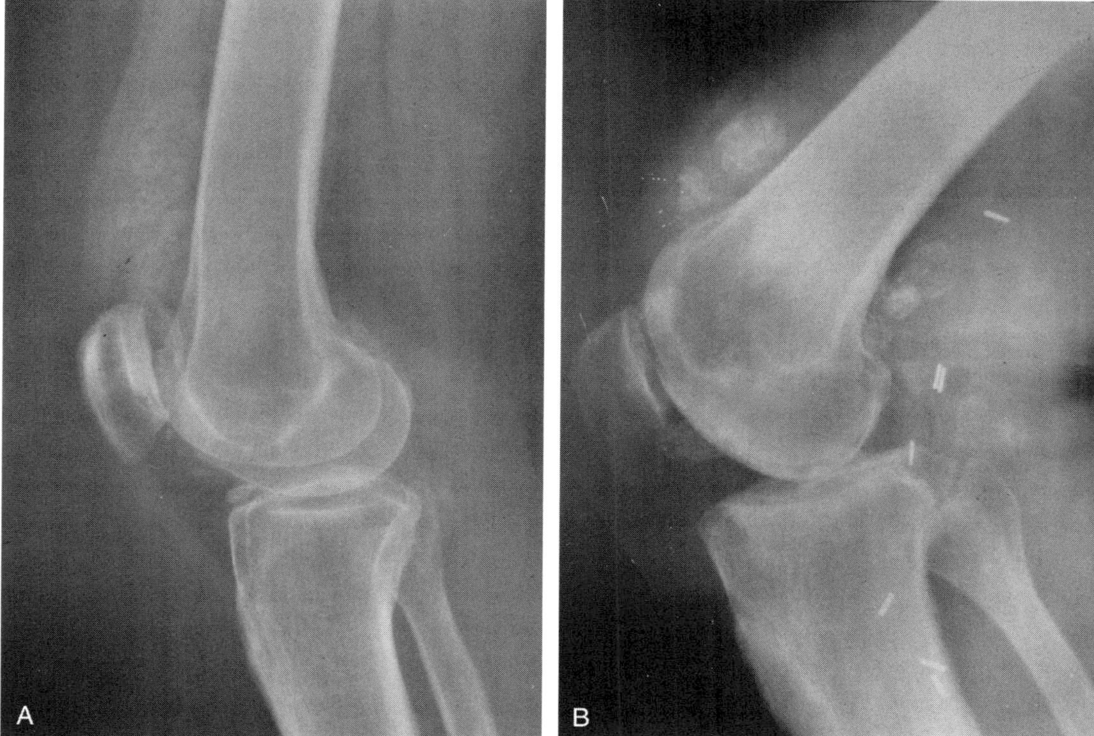

FIGURE 50.22 ➢ *A* and *B,* Synovial chondromatosis of the knee. Lateral radiographs of two different patients demonstrate large areas of calcification projecting inside the joint space, with most of the calcified bodies located in the suprapatellar bursa. Notice that the density, size, and definition of these bodies vary between the patients.

The MRI appearance of synovial chondromatosis depends on the presence of calcium. Areas of calcification will have very low signal intensity. Without calcification, it is a low signal intensity equivalent to muscle on T1-weighted sequences with short repetition times (TR) and short echo times (TE). With T2-weighted sequences (long TR and long TE), the signal intensity will be high, hyaline cartilage being high in water content. Fibrous tissue between the cartilage nodules will give rise to areas of lower signal intensity. A phenomenon similar to synovial chondromatosis may occur within bursae.

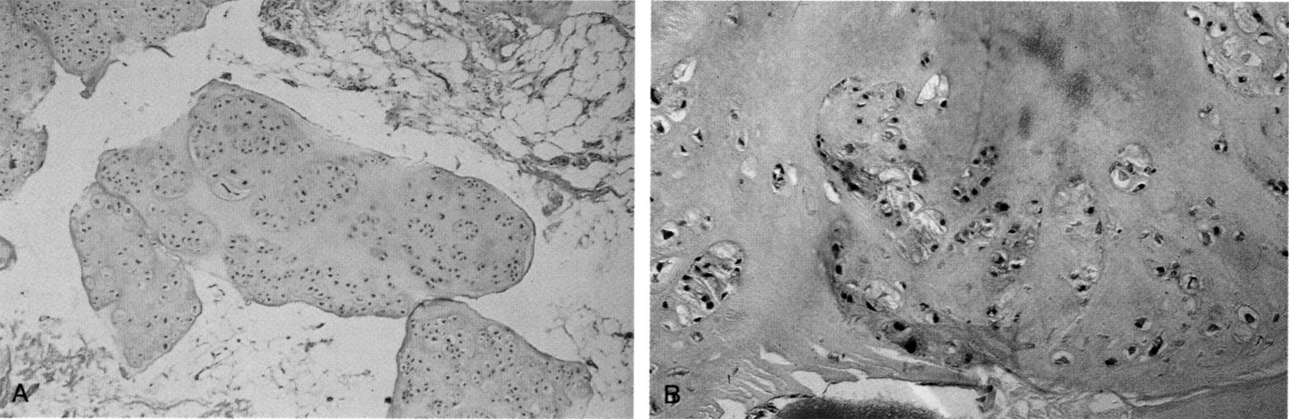

FIGURE 50.23 ➢ *A* and *B,* Primary synovial chondromatosis. Proliferating nodules of cartilage clones are evident, similar to other benign cartilaginous tumors. Atypia and cellularity vary. Calcification and endochondral ossification, when they occur, usually appear less orderly in secondary types. (From Vigorita VJ: The synovium. In Vigorita VJ, Ghelman B: Orthopaedic Pathology. Philadelphia, Lippincott/Williams & Wilkins, 1999.)

Synovial Chondrosarcoma

A malignant tumor arising within the joint is extremely rare.[6] However, chondrosarcomas may arise in the setting of synovial chondromatosis.[33] This condition is suspected when there is evidence of aggressive growth, such as invasion into adjacent extra-articular tissues. Focal areas of atypical and increased cellularity in an otherwise unremarkable case of synovial chondromatosis should not be overdiagnosed. Synovial chondrosarcoma may also arise as a de novo synovial malignancy. The clinical behavior of these neoplasms varies from that of low-grade neoplasm, with a propensity to recur locally, to those that may, in fact, metastasize (primarily to the lungs).

Synovial chondrosarcomas have been reported throughout adult life and have been associated clinically with pain or swelling of usually long-standing duration. The tumor usually involves one joint, the knee more commonly than the hip, elbow, or ankle. Roentgenographically, there is little to distinguish it from synovial chondromatosis except, when present, soft tissue involvement and extensive bone erosion. At operation, cartilaginous lobules extend into the surrounding soft tissue beyond the confines of the joint capsule. Features of chondrosarcoma are seen histologically: marked cellularity, increased cellularity and spindle cells at periphery of lobules, scattered sheets of cells, and myxoid change. Treatment is aggressive surgical removal, resection with reconstruction when possible, and amputation if necessary.

PVNS

PVNS is usually a localized monoarticular, proliferative process that is found in synovial joints and tendon sheaths, most commonly the knee and the tendon sheaths of the digits of the hand (giant cell tumors of tendon sheath [GCTTS]).[59] However, this lesion is also found in the hip, foot, wrist, shoulder, and rarely at other sites. The lesion is rarely polyarthric and does not metastasize, but it may invade bone locally. The localized tenosynovial and diffuse pigmented synovial lesions do not appear to be separate entities, judging from their similar histological characteristics and biological behavior. Tenosynovial nodules in the digits of the hand have been reported to recur in 7% to 45% of patients, and diffuse processes (pigmented villonodular synovitis) of the knee have been reported to recur in as many as 45% of patients.

Clinical presentations depend on the site. In joint lesions, an insidious onset with swelling, stiffness, or discomfort is common. Swelling without trauma and out of proportion to the degree of discomfort is considered typical.[18, 19] The peak incidence of knee lesions is in the third decade.

The joint fluid color is variable, ranging from normal to rusty or brownish-red. The synovium may appear diffusely pigmented or, more commonly, focally pigmented. The pigment is due to both hemosiderin accumulation from microscopic synovial hemorrhage (brown) and aggregations of lipid-laden macrophages (yellow) in the periphery of expanding nodules. Hyperplastic and pigmented changes mimicking those of chronic hemarthrosis in the adjacent synovium are secondary in nature and do not represent the lesion proper.

At least five clinical types of PVNS are identified in the knee[1]: loose body,[2] a localized nodule (pedunculated or embedded in the synovium),[3] aggregates of nodules confined to one compartment,[4] a truly diffuse involvement of the synovium, and synovial PVNS extending into bursa[5] (Fig. 50.24). Localized nodular and nodular aggregate types of PVNS are most common.

Typically, PVNS is monoarticular and is usually observed in early and middle adulthood and rarely at the extreme end of life. Symptoms may be gradual in onset. Clinically, patients may present with discomfort or pain. Swelling, stiffness, locking, and even instability of the knee may occur. Torsion of a pedunculated nodular form of PVNS has been associated with the unusual clinical presentation of acute pain.[38]

The radiological findings are dependent on the anatomy of the involved joint (Figs. 50.25 and 50.26). Articulations with close apposition of the capsule of the joint to the underlying bone, such as the hip, soon develop bone erosions secondary to the abnormal synovial masses. In other joints with greater separation between the capsule and bones, such as the knee where the suprapatellar bursa is placed at a significant distance from the anterior surface of the femur, PVNS usually fails to cause significant bone erosions. The bone erosions are usually well defined, surrounded by minimal or no sclerosis. The erosions are most often located in the bare areas of bone but, at times, can be located in subchondral surfaces. PVNS does not calcify. Often the erosions are located in both sides of a joint but, at times, the condition can be unifocal, causing erosions in only one side of the articular space.

The joint space is usually preserved because articular cartilage generally is not eroded. The hip represents an unusual situation because often these patients can first present with narrowing of the joint space.

The differential diagnosis for PVNS includes any soft tissue mass that causes erosions of adjacent bones such as gout, rheumatoid nodules, tuberculous arthritis, or juxtacortical chondromas. The absence of osteoporosis, joint space narrowing, or calcifications is helpful in making the correct diagnosis of PVNS.

The most common radiographic findings in the knee are soft tissue swelling (see Fig. 50.25). Arthrograms may best demonstrate the nodules as discrete pitting defects. Bone changes are less frequent but may include erosions and degenerative changes. MRI has revealed an isointense or low signal intensity compared with that muscle on T1- and T2-weighted images. However, findings are variable depending on the amount of hemosiderin, lipid, cellularity, and fibrosis. Edema leads to increased T2-weighted images.[66]

The treatment of PVNS is surgical. If an isolated loose body or nodule is confirmed, arthroscopic surgical excision may be attempted. However, the propensity of the lesions to recur (in up to one-third of cases) requires careful examination of the remainder of the

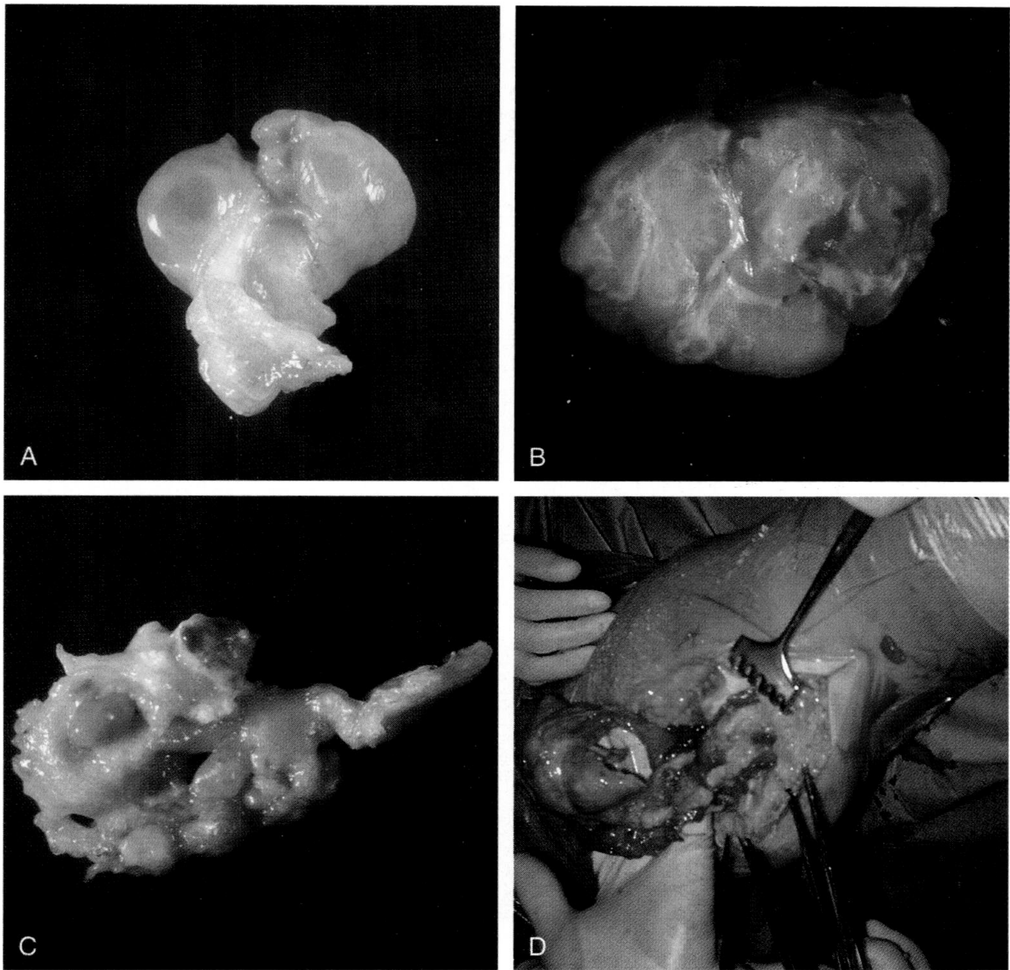

FIGURE 50.24 ➢ Pigmented villonodular synovitis/giant cell tumor of tendon sheath. *A*, Loose body. *B*, Localized nodule (gross appearance, cross-section). *C*, Localized aggregate of multiple nodules. *D*, Diffuse type throughout the joint. (From Vigorita VJ: The synovium. In Vigorita VJ, Ghelman B: Orthopaedic Pathology. Philadelphia, Lippincott/Williams & Wilkins, 1999.)

joint to exclude multiple foci. Smaller nodules may be missed, embedded as they are in the subintimal synovial layers. Recurrences may occur many years after initial treatment.

The diffuse form of PVNS is more problematic and requires total synovectomy. If not removed, PVNS will continue to grow and erode into the articular bone. Bursal PVNS also requires adequate surgical excision and may extend deeply into surrounding soft tissue.

On the basis of ultrastructural and immunohistochemical findings, PVNS/GCTTS can be considered a tumorous proliferation of fibroblasts and histiocytes, i.e., a benign fibrous histiocytoma (Fig. 50.27).[69]

Grossly, the lesions are usually categorized as nodular or villonodular. Solitary nodules or aggregates of confluent nodules are designated nodular, and poorly delineated lesions characterized by plump synovial villi and by small unencapsulated nodules, not necessarily contiguous to one another and often blending into the surrounding tissue, are designated villonodular.

No relationship between duration of symptoms and extent of the fibrosis is evident, indicating that these lesions do not become progressively fibrotic with time. Distinct hyperplasia of the synovial tissue adjacent to the lesion is often present. The giant cells are usually arranged in groups, and there are two types of these cells: one is a truly phagocytic, often densely staining multinucleated cell, and the other is a more inconspicuous cell whose characteristics suggest that it had been formed by fusion of the predominant vesicular, mononuclear, polyhedral stromal cells. Giant cells of the second type are seen commonly in rheumatoid synovitis and may represent multinucleated lining cells of the synovial membrane that are reacting to the proliferating lesions.

Although complete excision of a single nodule or multiple nodules is thought to be essential, total synovectomy may not be necessary. If total synovectomy is not performed, then stiffness, a common postoperative complication of this procedure, may be pre-

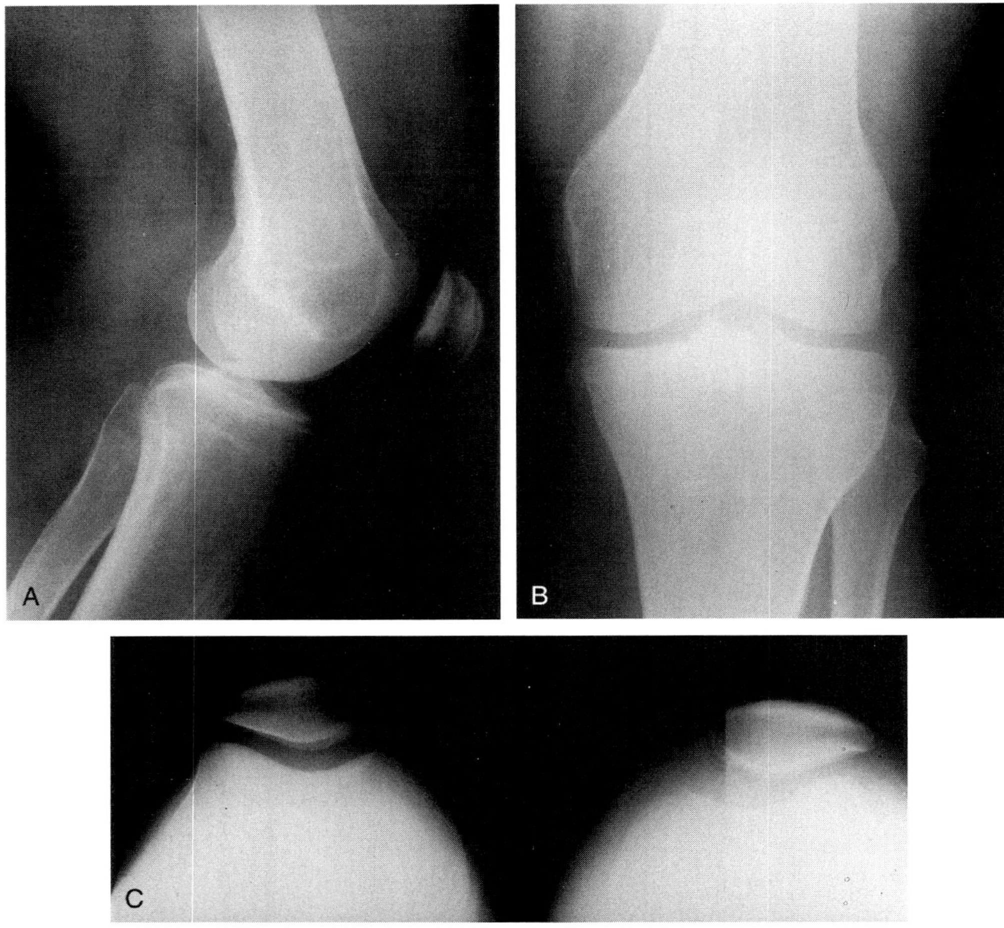

FIGURE 50.25 ➢ Roentgenographs of pigmented villonodular synovitis/giant cell tumor of tendon sheath of the knee. Soft tissue masses as evidence by fullness in posterior compartment *(A)*, fullness of lateral shadows on anteroposterior view *(B)*, and asymmetric shadowing on tunnel view *(C)*. (From Vigorita VJ: The synovium. In Vigorita VJ, Ghelman B: Orthopaedic Pathology. Philadelphia, Lippincott/Williams & Wilkins, 1999.)

vented. Untreated, PVNS may erode and infiltrate surrounding structures, including bone.

Although it has been suggested that pigmented villonodular synovitis is an inflammatory process, its polyclonal proliferation, insignificant degree of inflammation, nodular growth pattern, propensity for recurrence after inadequate removal, and distinct lack of the changes characteristic of the lesion in the adjacent synovial tissue suggest that this is not the case. Inflammatory synovitis, in general, is a diffuse process without nodular changes. The evidence for an inflammatory cause was partially based on the observation that lesions tend to undergo progressive fibrosis. However, there does not seem to be any relationship between the degree of fibrosis and either the duration of symptoms or the size of the lesion. In patients for whom serial biopsies were available or a recurrent lesion was studied, no histological evidence of progressive fibrotic changes is seen. In the overwhelming majority of cases, PVNS appears to be a benign synovial neoplasm with the potential for local recurrence. Because pigmentation of the lesion is secondary to iron deposition and the lesion is usually nodular and rarely shows inflammatory changes, its name is inappropriate.

The differential diagnosis includes both benign and neoplastic conditions. Hemosideric synovitis, as is seen in hemophilia, and the chronic synovitis caused by either rheumatoid arthritis or trauma, do not have a distinct submembranous nodule or nodules composed of proliferating mononuclear and giant cells. Monophasic synovial sarcoma is differentiated by its characteristic increased cellularity, cellular pleomorphism, lack of fibrosis, and high mitotic counts. Other rare lesions such as angioma, hemangiopericytoma, histiocytoma, and fibroma are morphologically homogeneous and, therefore, histologically distinct.

Atypical and malignant variants of PVNS have been described,[70] further substantiating the neoplastic nature of this lesion.

Malignant PVNS has now been described in the knee, ankle, cheek, foot, and thigh.[7] Cases of both primary malignant and transformed benign PVNS are

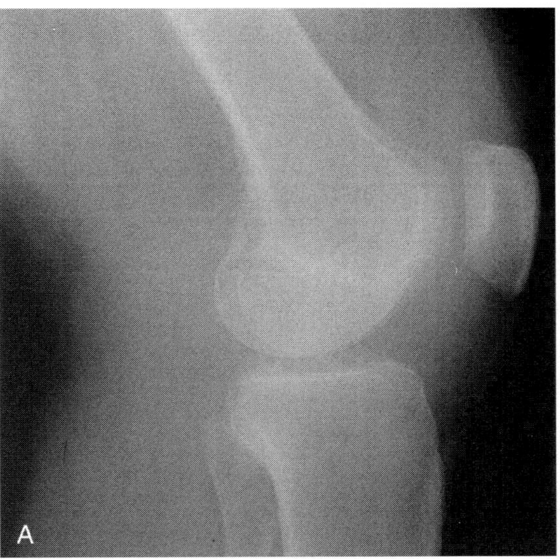

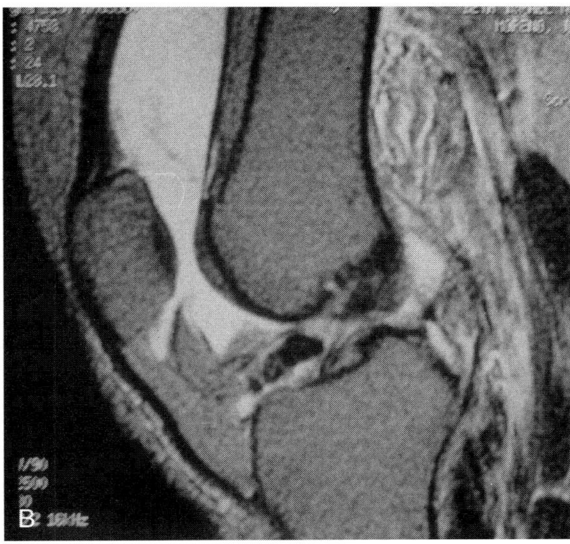

FIGURE 50.26 ➢ Pigmented villonodular synovitis. Lateral radiograph demonstrates fullness of the suprapatellar region resulting from intra-articular effusion. T2-weighted sagittal magnetic resonance image demonstrates areas of signal void anterior to the anterior cruciate ligament and adjacent to the anterior border of the tibial plateau caused by hemosiderin deposition. Notice the large effusion in the suprapatellar bursa.

postulated. Bertoni et al[7] suggested the following features of malignancy:

1. Infiltrative pattern.
2. Large, plump cells with eosinophilic cytoplasm.
3. Large nuclei and prominent nucleoli.
4. Necrotic areas.

Four patients in their series died with metastases (four pulmonary nodes, two inguinal nodes). Patients with malignant PVNS tend to be older with a significant history of local recurrence.

Epithelioid Sarcoma

Epithelioid sarcoma is a malignant soft tissue sarcoma of unknown histogenesis that primarily affects the subcutaneous tissue, fascia, and tendon sheaths of the extremities.[10] It is most commonly seen in the upper extremities as a small, painless, subcutaneous nodule. Because of associated inflammation and even necrotizing granulomatous-like reactions, it may be confused with a benign process. It most often occurs in young males (mean age = 23 years) and tends to recur locally after excision. Progression along tendon sheath and lymphatic pathways has been demonstrated. There is a poor prognosis associated with tumors larger than 3 cm and those that are deeply situated in the soft tissue. Focal necrosis may indicate a worse prognosis.

Although it appears benign, epithelioid sarcoma must be removed at the initial approach. Poor results have been obtained with marginal resection. Wide or radical resection is usually required. Work-up should include radiographs of the involved extremity and chest, MRI to assess local tumor spread, and CT scans of the chest for pulmonary metastases.

Microscopically, cells range from plump spindle cells to rounded or polygonal cells with deep eosinophilic cytoplasm. Resemblance to squamous cells or other epithelial cells has given rise to the name "epithelioid." Characteristic of epithelioid sarcoma is the macroscopic clustering of cells around areas of necrosis in a granulomatous-like fashion.

Varying degrees of fibrosis, cellularity, infiltration, necrosis, and mitotic activity have been described. Immunohistochemically, the lesions are vimentin and keratin positive, a coexpression deemed typical.

Clear Cell Sarcoma

Clear cell sarcomas are rare neoplasms attached to tendons or aponeuroses, often in the foot, ankle, or heel in young adults. The lesions are slow growing and usually painless.

A clear cell sarcoma is composed of a compact mass of polygonal cells, some having a spindle appearance, often with multinucleation. Mitotic activity is scarce. The prognosis for patients with clear cell sarcoma is poor. The lesion has a high recurrence rate, and distant metastases occur within 5 years.

Clear cell sarcoma is now generally believed to originate from the neural crest based on the histochemical demonstration of melanin, ultrastructural demonstration of premelanosomes, and immunohistochemical vimentin and S-100 protein staining.[52]

Alveolar Soft Part Sarcoma

Alveolar soft part sarcoma constitutes less than 1% of soft tissue sarcomas and is characterized histologically by large granular cells dispersed in "alveolus"-like patterns separated by vascular channels.[55] Seen most commonly in women in the second to fourth decade, it is

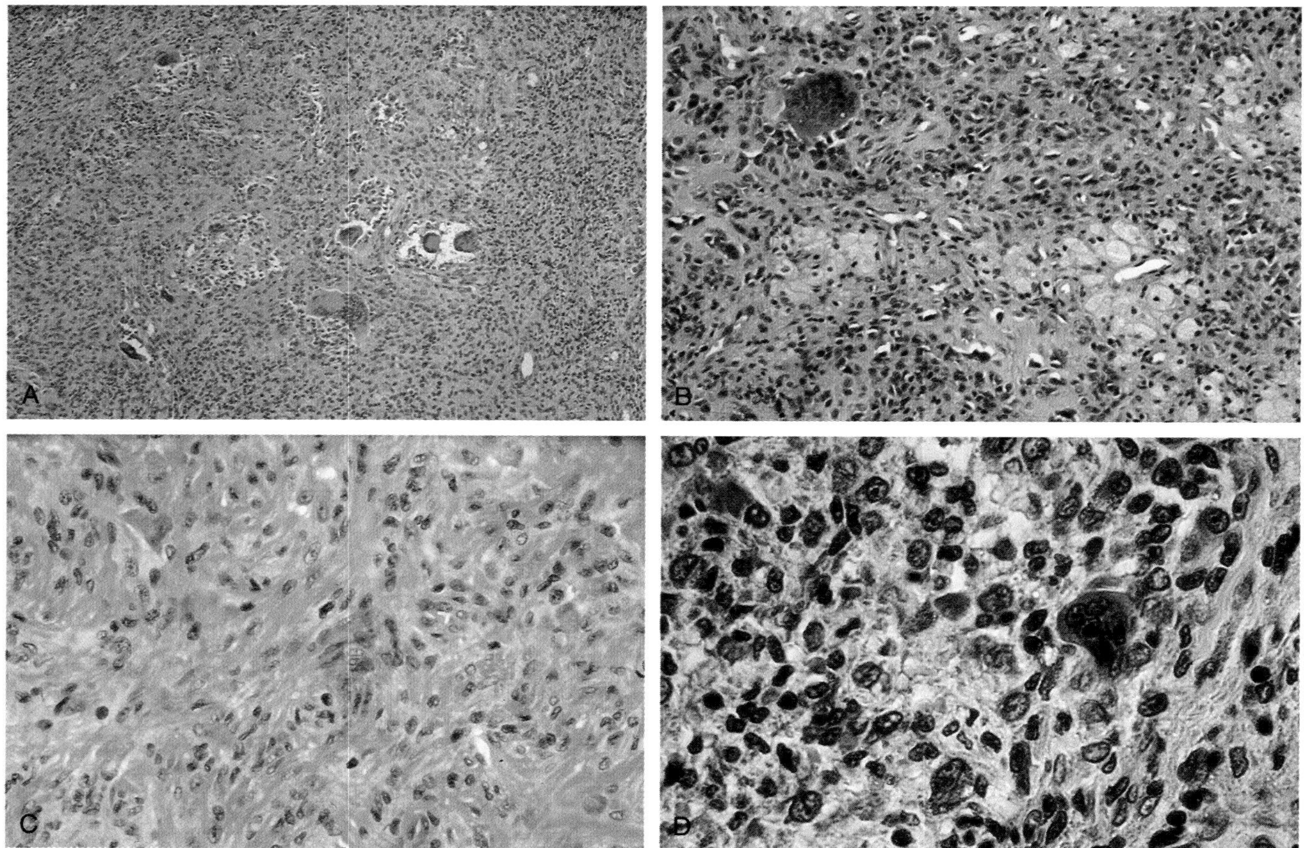

FIGURE 50.27 ➢ Pigmented villonodular synovitis/giant cell tumor of tendon sheath. *A,* Low power reveals sheets of mononuclear cells (fibroblasts and histiocytes) with interspersed giant cells awash in a collagen stroma. *B,* Higher power shows that xanthomatous cells are usually focal in distribution, notably in periphery of lesions; little or no inflammation is evident. *C,* Collagen may predominate in a sea of spindly fibroblasts. *D,* Large multinucleated giant cell whose clear nucleus with prominent dense staining nucleoli is similar to the proliferating surrounding mononuclear cells. (From Vigorita VJ: The synovium. In Vigorita VJ, Ghelman B: Orthopaedic Pathology. Philadelphia, Lippincott/Williams & Wilkins, 1999.)

slow growing but pulsatile, and bruits may be heard. Metastases to the lungs, bones, and brain occur. MRI patterns are high signal intensity relative to muscle on T1-weighted imaging with flow voids. Ten-year disease-free survival is about 50%.

Synovial Sarcoma

Synovial sarcoma is a malignant mesenchymal tumor that usually arises in structures adjacent to the joint, most often in tenosynovium lining anatomic joint structures. It derives its name from the microscopic appearance, which mimics the histological appearance of the embryonic synovium. The anatomic location outside the joint and the occurrence of synovial sarcoma in tissue such as the pleura suggest that the tumor arises from mesenchymal tissue, not synovium.[22] It occurs in close association with tendon sheaths, bursae, and joint capsules and has a propensity to differentiate toward a spindle cell- or fibroblast-like mesodermal cell population as well as an epithelial population, giving it, in its classic presentation, a biphasic microscopic appearance. Intra-articular synovial sarcoma accounts for 10% of cases.[51] It is the fourth most common soft tissue sarcoma, accounting for approximately 10% of all malignant mesenchymal neoplasms. It is most prevalent in patients between the ages of 15 and 35 years, and it characteristically presents as a painful, palpable soft tissue mass.

The radiographic presentation of this malignant tumor is most often that of a soft tissue mass, which in nearly 50% of cases is calcified. The calcifications can be dense, faint, or punctate. The soft tissue mass is usually located close to but outside a joint space. The growth of the tumor eventually results in extension into the adjacent joint and invasion and destruction of the adjacent bones.

Both CT and MRI scans are sensitive technologies in the demonstration of the soft tissue tumor mass that forms synovial sarcoma. The adjacent anatomic structures (muscles, tendons, blood vessels, and nerves) are usually displaced, but at times may be actually invaded by the tumor. The calcifications of synovial sarcoma, if present, are best demonstrated by the CT images. Areas of necrosis may develop, especially in the large synovial sarcomas, resulting in areas of lucency in the CT scans and high intensity signal in the MRI T2-weighted images. The dimensions of the tumor are a significant factor because studies have been published claiming a better prognosis for synovial sarcomas that are smaller than 5 cm in diameter. The more peripheral synovial sarcomas tend to have a better prognosis compared with tumors located more centrally. Approximately 70% of synovial sarcomas occur in the lower extremity.

Histologically, the tumor is diagnosed by the identification of a biphasic cell population (Fig. 50.28). Immunocytochemical and immunohistological staining demonstrated a mesenchymal tissue in one component and epithelial differentiation in the other. Descriptions in the literature of monophasic variants of synovial sarcoma with a predominance of one of these two cell types raised questions about classification.

Monophasic variants tend to occur in distal extremity locations and may carry a poorer prognosis. Prognosis may be related to gross anatomic and histological findings, with a better prognosis in younger patients with tumors smaller than 5 cm, tumors located in the lower extremity with an epithelial gland cellularity greater than 50%, and a mitotic activity of less than 15 mitoses/10 high-power field.[56] Mast cells fewer than 20/high-power field, tumor necrosis, presence of rhabdoid cells, percent glandularity less than 50%, and later stage are possible additional poor prognostic factors.[12, 56] An additional poor prognostic factor is increased staining with antibody to proliferating cell nuclear antigen.

These malignant lesions recur locally and spread by both regional lymph node and pulmonary metastatic routes. Metastases to the lung occur in 75% of patients, to regional lymph nodes in 15%, and to bone in 10%.[41] It is the most common soft tissue sarcoma to metastasize to lymph nodes. Five-year survival rates have been reported to be as low as 21%.

Traditionally, radical surgery or conservative surgery and radiation therapy have been used. A multimodality approach involving surgery, radiotherapy, and combined chemotherapy may improve survival in this highly malignant tumor. In one study of 14 patients with nonmetastasizing synovial sarcoma, encouraging

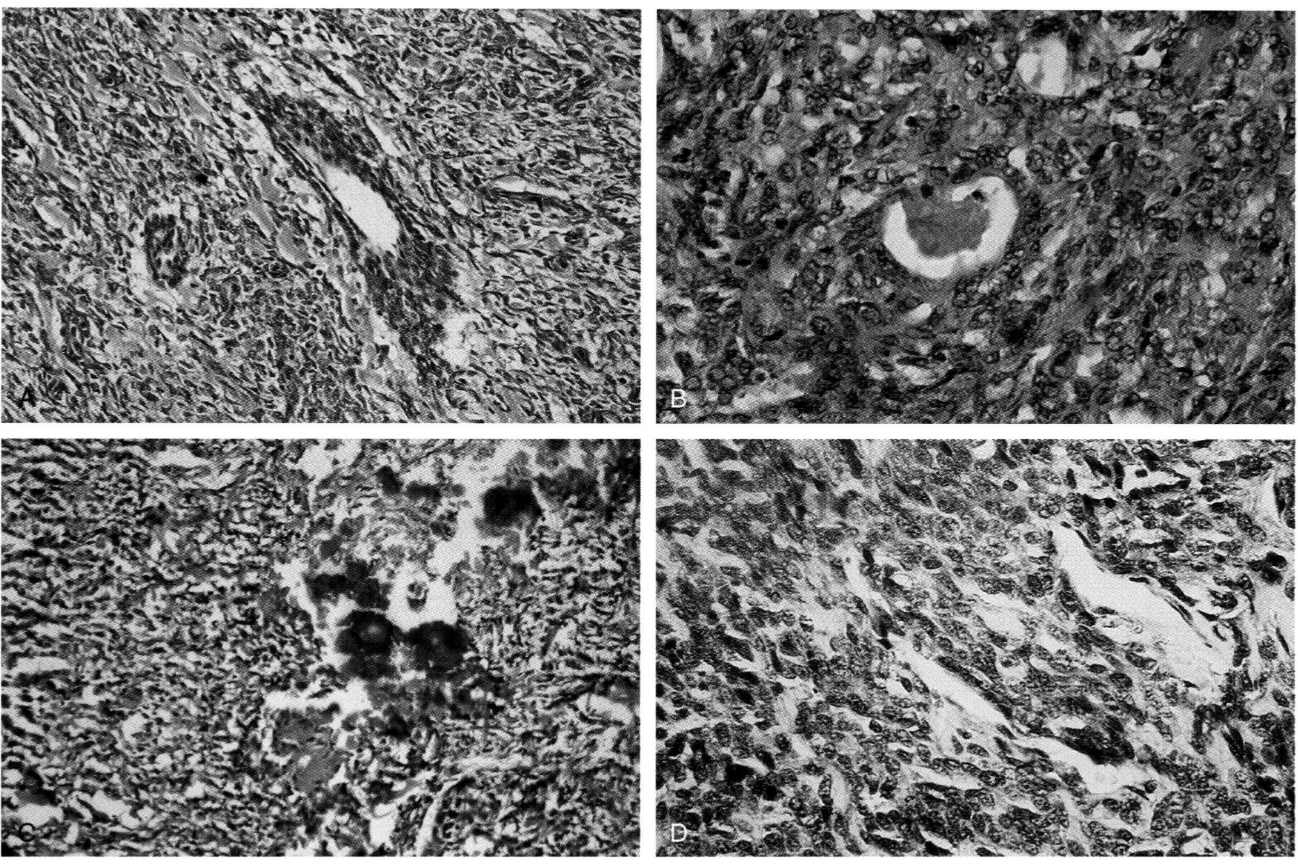

FIGURE 50.28 ➢ Synovial sarcoma. In biphasic synovial sarcoma, gland-like structures are seen in distinction with a spindle-shaped sarcomatous component *(A)*. The epithelial (gland) structures may stand out or blend in with the stroma component *(B)*. Calcification is irregular and may aggregate sufficiently to be seen roentgenographically *(C)*. Monophasic synovial sarcoma is characterized by the typical cleft-like avascular spaces *(D)*. (From Vigorita VJ: The synovium. In Vigorita VJ, Ghelman B: Orthopaedic Pathology. Philadelphia, Lippincott/Williams & Wilkins, 1999.)

results were achieved with intensive chemotherapy (high-dose cisplatin and doxorubicin or high-dose ifosfamide and cisplatin with doxorubicin) and local radiation followed by surgical resection and, in some patients, postoperative chemotherapy.[41] In a similar protocol, event-free survival at 5 years was 75%.[45] Chemotherapy (high-dose ifosfamide) may play a role in metastatic synovial sarcoma.[62]

Characteristic genetic findings include abnormal *bcl-2* proto-oncogene activity.[34]

A characteristic SYT-SSX fusion gene resulting from the chromosome translocation t(X;18)(p11;q11) is detectable in almost all synovial sarcomas and has been reported to be of prognostic significance. Kawai et al[42] found a significant difference between monophasic and biphasic tumors. All biphasic tumors had an SYT-SSX1 fusion transcript. All monophasic tumors had an SYT-SSX2 fusion and had a significantly better metastasis-free survival.[42]

References

1. Abdul-Karim FW, El-Naggar AK, Joyce MJ, et al: Diffuse and localized tenosynovial giant cell tumor and pigmented villonodular synovitis: A clinicopathologic and flow cytometric DNA analysis. Hum Pathol 23:729, 1992.
2. Adams PC, Kertesz AE, Valberg LS: Clinical presentation of hemochromatosis: A changing scene. Am J Med 90:445, 1991.
3. Arnold WD, Hilgartner MW: Hemophilic arthropathy. Current concepts of pathogenesis and management. J Bone Joint Surg Am 59: 287, 1977.
4. Bartles EC: Gout as a complication of surgery. Surg Clin North Am 38:845, 1957.
5. Bennett GL, Leeson MC, Michael A: Extensive hemosiderin deposition in the medial meniscus of a knee. Its possible relationship to degenerative joint disease. Clin Orthop 230:182, 1988.
6. Bertoni F, Unni KK, Beabout JW, et al: Chondrosarcomas of the synovium. Cancer 67:155, 1991.
7. Bertoni F, Unni KK, Beabout JW, et al: Malignant giant cell tumor of the tendon sheaths and joints (malignant pigmented villonodular synovitis). Am J Pathol 21:153, 1997.
8. Bolanos AA, Demizio JP, Vigorita VJ, et al: Lead poisoning from an intra-articular shotgun pellet in the knee treated with arthroscopic extraction and chelation therapy: A case report. J Bone Joint Surg Am 78:422, 1996.
9. Bolanos AA, Vigorita VJ, Meyerson RI, et al: Intra-articular histopathologic changes secondary to local lead intoxication in rabbit knee joints. J Trauma 38:668, 1995.
10. Bos GD, Pritchard DJ, Reiman HM, et al: Epithelioid sarcoma: An analysis of fifty-one cases. J Bone Joint Surg Am 70:862, 1988.
11. Burmester GR, Dimitriu-Bona A, Waters SJ, et al: Identification of three major synovial lining cell populations by monoclonal antibodies directed to Ia antigens and antigens associated with monocytes/macrophages and fibroblasts. Scand J Immunol 17:69, 1983.
12. Cagle LA, Mirra JM, Storm FK, et al: Histologic features relating to prognosis in synovial sarcoma. Cancer 59:1810, 1987.
13. Cooper A, Minutello R, Vigorita VJ, et al: Case report 763. Skeletal Radiol 21:555, 1992.
14. Devaney K, Vinh TN, Sweet DE: Synovial hemangioma: A report of 20 cases with differential diagnostic considerations. Hum Pathol 24:737, 1993.
15. Edeiken J, Edeiken BS, Ayala AG, et al: Giant solitary synovial chondromatosis. Skeletal Radiol 23:23, 1994.
16. Edwards JCW, Sedgwick AD, Willoughby DA: The formation of a structure with the features of synovial lining by subcutaneous injection of air: An in vivo tissue culture system. J Pathol 134: 147, 1981.
17. Fedulla LM, Bonakdarpour A, Moyer RA, et al: Giant synovial cysts. Skeletal Radiol 12:90, 1984.
18. Flandry F, Hughston JC: Current concepts review: Pigmented villonodular synovitis. J Bone Joint Surg Br 69:942, 1987.
19. Flandry F, Hughston JC, McCann SB, et al: Diagnostic features of diffuse pigmented villonodular synovitis of the knee. Clin Orthop 298:212, 1994.
20. France MP, Gupta SK: Nonhemophilic hemosiderotic synovitis of the shoulder. A case report. Clin Orthop 262:132, 1991.
21. Gaary E, Gorlin JB, Jaramillo D: Pseudotumor and arthropathy in the knees of a hemophiliac. Skeletal Radiol 25:85, 1996.
22. Gaertner E, Zeren EH, Fleming MV, et al: Biphasic synovial sarcomas arising in the pleural cavity. A clinicopathologic study of five cases. Am J Surg Pathol 20:36, 1996.
23. Gilbert MS, Radomisli TE: Therapeutic options in the management of hemophilic synovitis. Clin Orthop 343:88, 1997.
24. Gonzalez JG, Ghiselli RW, Santa Cruz DJ: Synovial metaplasia of the skin. Am J Surg Pathol 11:343, 1987.
25. Gordeux V, Mukiibi J, Hasstedt SJ, et al: Iron overload in Africa. Interaction between a gene and dietary iron content. N Engl J Med 326:95, 1992.
26. Greenspan A, Azouz M, Matthews J, et al: Synovial hemangioma: Imaging features in eight histologically proven cases, review of the literature, and differential diagnosis. Skeletal Radiol 24:583, 1995.
27. Grieten M, Buckwalter KA, Cardinal E, et al: Case report 873. Skeletal Radiol 23:652, 1994.
28. Hameed MR, Erlandson R, Rosen PP: Capsular synovial-like hyperplasia around mammary implants similar to detritic synovitis. A morphologic and immunohistochemical study of 15 cases. Am J Surg Pathol 19:433, 1995.
29. Hamilton JB: Human immunodeficiency virus and the orthopaedic surgeon. Clin Orthop 328:31, 1996.
30. Hammerman D: The biology of osteoarthritis. N Engl J Med 320: 1322, 1989.
31. Harris ED: Rheumatoid arthritis: Pathophysiology and implications for therapy. N Engl J Med 322:1277, 1990.
32. Hasselbacher P: Structure of the synovial membrane. Clin Rheum Dis 7:57, 1981.
33. Hermann G, Klein MJ, Abdelwahab DF, et al: Synovial chondrosarcoma arising in synovial chondromatosis of the right hip. Skeletal Radiol 26:366, 1997.
34. Hirakawa N, Naka T, Yamamoto I, et al: Overexpression of bcl-2 protein in synovial sarcoma: A comparative study of other soft tissue spindle cell sarcomas and an additional analysis by fluorescence in situ hybridization. Hum Pathol 27:1060, 1996.
35. Hirohata K, Morimoto K, Kimura H: Ultrastructure of Bone and Joint Diseases, 2nd ed. Tokyo, Igaku-Shoin, 1981.
36. Ho G Jr, DeNuccio M: Gout and pseudogout in hospitalized patients. Arch Intern Med 153:2787, 1993.
37. Hoffa A: The influence of the adipose tissue with regard to the pathology of the knee joint. JAMA 43:795, 1904.
38. Howie CR, Smith GD, Christie J, et al: Torsion of localized pigmented villonodular synovitis of the knee. J Bone Joint Surg Br 67:654, 1985.
39. Hughes TH, Sartoris DJ, Schweitzer ME, et al: Pigmented villonodular synovitis: MRI characteristics. Skeletal Radiol 24:7, 1995.
40. Johnson DP, Eastwood DM, Witherow PJ: Symptomatic synovial plicae of the knee. J Bone Joint Surg Am 75:1485, 1993.
41. Kampe CE, Rosen G, Eilber F, et al: Synovial sarcoma. A study of intensive chemotherapy in 14 patients with localized disease. Cancer 72:2161, 1993.
42. Kawai A, Woodruff J, Healey JH, et al: SYT-SSX gene fusion as a determinant of morphology and prognosis in synovial sarcoma. N Engl J Med 338:153, 1998.
43. Kleftogiannis F, Handley CJ, Campbell MA: Characterization of extracellular matrix macromolecules from bovine synovial capsule. J Orthop Res 12:365, 1994.
44. Komuya AS, Inoue A, Sasaguri Y, et al: Rapidly destructive arthropathy of the hip. Studies on bone resorption factors in joint with a theory of pathogenesis. Clin Orthop 284:273, 1992.
45. Ladenstein R, Treuner J, Koscielniak E, et al: Synovial sarcoma of childhood and adolescence. Report of the German CWS-81 study. Cancer 71:3647, 1993.
46. Larsson SA: Hemophilia in Sweden. Acta Med Scand Suppl 5:1, 1984.

47. Maffulli N. Binfield PM, King JB, et al: Acute haemarthrosis of the knee in athletes. A prospective study of 106 cases. J Bone Joint Surg Br 75:945, 1993.
48. Mainardi CL, Levine PH, Werb Z, et al: Proliferative synovitis in hemophilia. Biochemical and morphological observations. Arthritis Rheum 21:137, 1978.
49. Markel SF, Hart WR: Arthropathy in calcium pyrophosphate dihydrate crystal deposition disease. Arch Pathol Lab Med 106:529, 1982.
50. Masuda I, Ishikawa K, Usuku G: A histologic and immunohistochemical study of calcium pyrophosphate dihydrate crystal deposition disease. Clin Orthop 263:272, 1991.
51. McKinney CD, Mills SE, Fechner RE: Intraarticular synovial sarcoma. Am J Surg Pathol 16:1017, 1992.
52. Mechtersheimer G, Tilgen W, Klar E, et al: Clear cell sarcoma of tendons and aponeuroses: Case presentation with special reference to immunohistochemical findings. Hum Pathol 20:914, 1989.
53. Meis JM, Enzinger FM: Juxta-articular myxoma: A clinical and pathologic study of 65 cases. Hum Pathol 23:639, 1992.
54. Milgram JW: Synovial osteochondromatosis: A histopathologic study of thirty cases. J Bone Joint Surg Am 59:792, 1977.
55. Nakashima Y, Kotoura Y, Kasakura K, et al: Alveolar soft-part sarcoma. A report of ten cases. Clin Orthop 294:259, 1993.
56. Oda Y, Hashimoto H, Tsuneyoshi M, et al: Survival in synovial sarcoma. A multivariate study of prognostic factors with special emphasis on the comparison between early death and long-term survival. Am J Surg Pathol 17:35, 1993.
57. O'Rahilly R, Gardner E: The embryology of movable joints. In Sokoloff L, ed: The Joints and Synovial Fluid, vol 1. New York, Academic Press, 1978, pp 49-103.
58. Pritzker KPH: Calcium pyrophosphate crystal arthropathy: A biomineralization disorder. Hum Pathol 17:543, 1986.
59. Rao S, Vigorita VJ: Pigmented villonodular synovitis (giant-cell tumor of the tendon sheath and synovial membrane). A review of eighty-one cases. J Bone Joint Surg Am 66:76, 1984.
60. Rodriguez-Merchan EC: Effects of hemophilia on articulations of children and adults. Clin Orthop 338:7, 1996.
61. Rogachefsky RA, Carneiro R, Altman RD, et al: Gout presenting as infectious arthritis. J Bone Joint Surg Am 76:269, 1994.
62. Rosen G, Forscher C, Lowenbraun S, et al: Synovial sarcoma. Uniform response of metastases to high dose ifosfamide. Cancer 73:2506, 1994.
63. Safran MR, Johnston-Jones K, Kabo JM, et al: The effect of experimental hemarthrosis on joint stiffness and synovial histology in a rabbit model. Clin Orthop 303:280, 1994.
64. Schumacher HR: Pathologic findings in rheumatoid arthritis. In Schumacher RH, Gall EP, eds: Rheumatoid Arthritis. An Illustrated Guide to Pathology, Diagnosis, and Management. Philadelphia, JB Lippincott, 1988, pp 4.1-4.36.
65. Sone M, Ehara S, Kashiwagi K, et al: Case report 859. Skeletal Radiol 23:475, 1994.
66. Spritzer CE, Malinka MK, Kressel HY: Magnetic resonance imaging of pigmented villonodular synovitis: a report of 2 cases. Skeletal Radiol 16:316, 1987.
67. Tauro B: Eosinophilic synovitis. A new entity? J Bone Joint Surg Br 77:654, 1995.
68. Vigorita VJ: Arthropathy in calcium pyrophosphate dihydrate crystal deposition disease [correspondence]. Arch Pathol Lab Med 107:275, 1993.
69. Vigorita VJ, Nakata K: Ultrastructural findings in nine cases of pigmented villonodular synovitis. In Proceedings of the 29th Annual Meeting of the Orthopaedic Research Society. Anaheim, CA, Orthopaedic Research Society, 1983, p 190.
70. Vogrincic GS, O'Connell JX, Gilks CB: Giant cell tumor of tendon sheath is a polyclonal cellular proliferation. Hum Pathol 28: 815, 1997.
71. Wardle EN, Patton JT: Bone and joint changes in haemochromatosis. Ann Rheum Dis 28:15, 1969.
72. Weitzman G: Lipoma arborescens of the knee. J Bone Joint Surg Am 47:1030, 1965.
73. Wilson PD, Eyre-Brook AL, Francis JD: A clinical and anatomical study of the semimembranous bursa in relation to popliteal cyst. J Bone Joint Surg Am 20:963, 1938.

51

Hemophilia and Knee Arthropathy

PAUL F. LACHIEWICZ

The most common inherited disorders of blood coagulation are classic hemophilia (hemophilia A, factor VIII deficiency), Christmas disease (hemophilia B, factor IX deficiency), and Willebrand's disease. These three hemophilias account for more than 95% of the congenital disorders of blood coagulation, and features of these disorders require orthopedic evaluation and treatment.

Classic hemophilia or factor VIII deficiency and Christmas disease or factor IX deficiency are transmitted in a sex-linked recessive manner. The two disorders are very similar in clinical appearance and are distinguished only by laboratory tests. Factor VIII and factor IX are both glycoproteins that interact in the intrinsic system of blood coagulation to activate factor X, a central protein in the coagulation cascade (Fig. 51.1). Activated factor IX, factor VIII, calcium, and phospholipid form a complex that activates factor X. Activated factor IX is the enzyme that converts factor X to activated factor X, whereas factor VIII has a regulatory or cofactor role in the reaction, accelerating it 1000 times.

Classic hemophilia is more common than Christmas disease. The incidence of classic hemophilia is approximately 100 per 1 million male births, but milder disease is much more common. Classic hemophilia is caused by a deficiency or abnormality of factor VIII procoagulant activity. These patients have a prolonged partial thromboplastin time. The bleeding time is usually normal or only minimally prolonged. Factor VIII activity levels in normal individuals range from 0.6 to 1.5 U/mL. In patients with classic hemophilia, factor VIII levels are less than 0.5 U/mL.

Hemophilia B (Christmas disease), like classic hemophilia, is an X-linked recessive disease. The incidence of hemophilia B is approximately 20 per 1 million male births, but it is relatively more common in certain countries, such as Switzerland. Hemophilia B is caused by an abnormality in factor IX, one of the vitamin K-dependent factors. The partial thromboplastin time is prolonged, but the prothrombin time and thrombin time are normal. The normal level of factor IX is 1.0 U/mL. In patients with hemophilia B, factor IX levels greater than 0.05 U/mL indicate mild disease, levels of 0.01 to 0.05 U/mL indicate moderate disease, and levels below 0.01 U/mL indicate severe disease.

The exact incidence of Willebrand's disease is unknown, but it is probably as frequent as classic hemophilia. Unlike hemophilias A and B, Willebrand's disease is inherited in an autosomal manner, with the more common varieties being autosomal dominant. Willebrand's factor has an important role in primary hemostasis, probably serving as a carrier for factor VIII and promoting adhesion of platelets to the subendothelium and to other platelets. The diagnosis of Willebrand's disease should be suspected in patients with a prolonged bleeding time, reduced factor VIII activity assay, decreased Willebrand's factor, or decreased Willebrand's-related antigen. Bleeding in Willebrand's disease is usually much less severe than in hemophilia A or B. Massive bleeding into joints occurs only in patients with the most severe form of the disease (type III). However, the orthopedic surgeon should be aware that major surgical procedures or trauma may result in serious bleeding.

In this chapter, hemophilia A and B are described together, with the term "hemophilia" used to indicate both disorders, and the disease is specified A or B when there are important differences.

CLINICAL MANIFESTATIONS OF HEMOPHILIA

Factors VIII and IX Levels

The clinical severity of hemophilia is usually related to the plasma level of factor VIII or factor IX. Cases are usually classified as mild, moderate, or severe, depending on the frequency and severity of bleeding episodes and the amount of trauma that causes the bleeding episodes (Table 51.1). A person with mild hemophilia will bleed rarely, if at all, and usually only after significant trauma or surgery. The factor VIII or IX level is usually greater than 0.05 U/mL, or greater than 5% of normal. With moderate hemophilia, the patient may bleed five or six times per year but may have prolonged periods free of bleeding. These patients usually bleed only with mild trauma. In patients with moderate hemophilia, the factor VIII or factor IX level is between 0.01 to 0.05 U/mL, or 1% to 5% of normal. Patients with severe hemophilia may have two or three bleeding episodes per month and typically bleed spontaneously with minimal trauma or with activities of daily living. The factor VIII or factor IX level is less than 0.01 U/mL, or less than 1%.

Hemarthrosis

Hemarthrosis is the most common and most disabling manifestation of hemophilia, and complications of these bleeding episodes bring the patient to the atten-

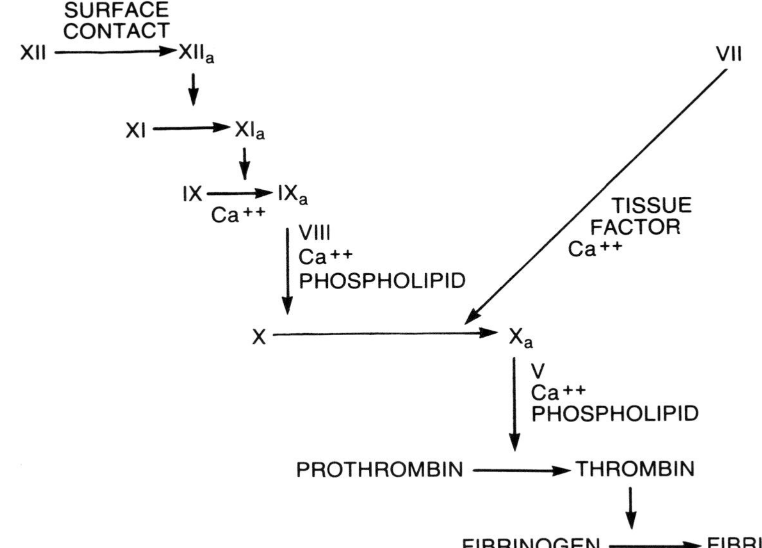

FIGURE 51.1 ➢ The coagulation cascade.

tion of an orthopedist. Although any joint can be involved, the joints most frequently affected, in order of decreasing frequency, are the knees, elbows, ankles, hips, and shoulders. Hemophilic arthropathy of the knee can be classified into three somewhat overlapping clinical groups: acute, subacute, and chronic. Acute hemarthrosis usually begins as a "tingling" sensation in the joint. The prodrome may include stiffness and pain. There is usually not a history of trauma. The hemarthrosis progresses rather rapidly over a few hours. The knee joint becomes swollen, tense, warm, and tender. The overlying skin may be stretched and red. The knee is usually held in flexion, and motion is painful and very restricted. It is not uncommon for the patient to hold the knee in 45 to 75 degrees of flexion. With acute hemarthrosis, pain usually responds rapidly to the administration of appropriate factor concentrates, but resolution of swelling and restriction of motion are related to the amount of blood in the joint. Subacute hemophilic arthropathy, or subacute hemarthrosis, is not as well defined as acute hemarthrosis. It usually develops after two or more joint bleeding episodes. The hemarthrosis persists despite adequate therapy, with thickened palpable synovium and mild to moderate loss of joint motion. Pain is not a prominent feature with subacute arthropathy. Chronic hemophilic arthropathy develops insidiously after subacute joint involvement has been present for a variable period of time (months to years). Most of these patients are young adults with persistent pain in the knee with activity and occasionally at rest. The patient may also have intermittent episodes of acute pain and swelling, related either to synovitis and effusion or to acute bleeding episodes.

TABLE 51.1 **HEMOPHILIA CLINICAL SEVERITY**

Class	Factors VIII and IX Level (% NL)	Bleeding
Mild	>5	Bleeding only with significant trauma or surgery
Moderate	1-5	Occasional spontaneous bleeding; usually bleeding only with mild trauma
Severe	<1	Frequent spontaneous bleeding

NL = normal level.

Muscle Bleeds

Although not directly related to hemarthrosis of the knee, spontaneous bleeding into the muscle compartments of the lower extremity is another feature of severe hemophilia. Aronstam and colleagues[2] described the clinical features, management, and outcome of 178 bleeding episodes into the muscles of the thigh and leg in 37 patients with severe hemophilia. Pain, with motion or at rest, and local tenderness were the presenting symptoms with almost all muscle bleeding episodes. The most frequent sites of bleeding were quadriceps (44%), calf (35%), anterior tibial compartment (7%), thigh adductors (7%), hamstrings (6%), and sartorius (1%). Bleeds into the quadriceps compartment took the longest to resolve, with a mean of 4 days. The first symptom in 66% of muscle bleeds was pain with movement. When the quadriceps were involved, this progressed to pain at rest. There was significant prolongation of recovery time when bleeds of this muscle group were treated more than 2 hours after onset of symptoms. In contrast, bleeds into the calf muscles required fewer transfusions, and there was no prolongation of recovery time when bleeds were treated up to 3 hours after onset of symptoms. Bleeds into the hamstring muscles usually caused restriction of knee motion and occasionally caused restriction of hip motion. Wilson and coworkers[50] suggested that B-mode real-time ultrasound was helpful in the diagnosis of acute muscle and joint bleeding epi-

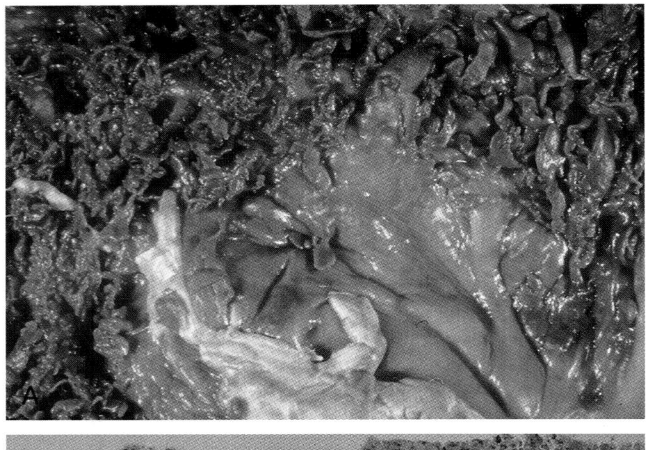

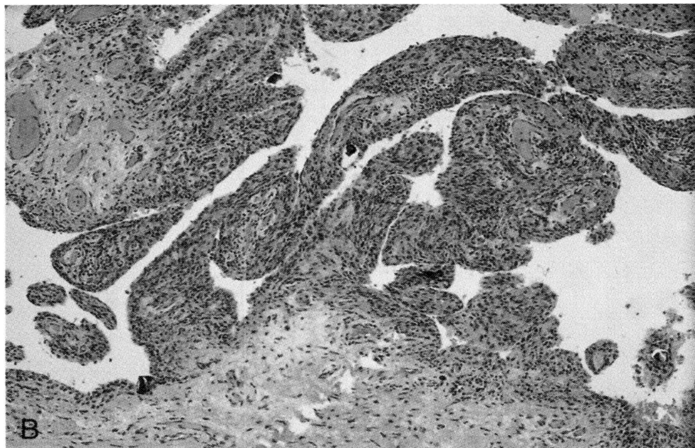

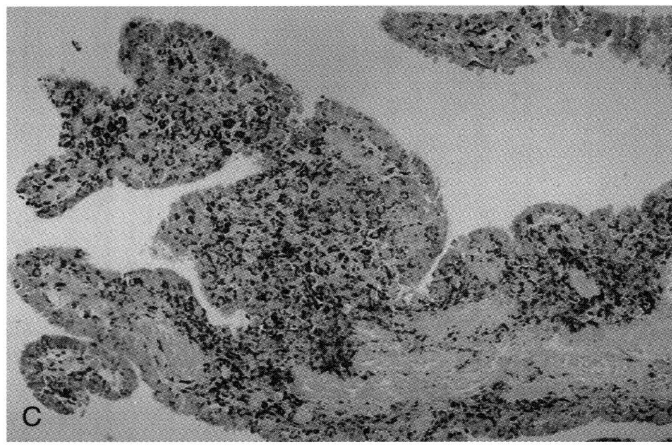

FIGURE 51.2 ➢ *A–C,* Hyperplastic hemosiderin-laden rusty-brown synovium from hemophilic patient: *A,* Gross. *B and C,* Microscopic. *D,* Prussian blue stain for iron. (From Vigorita VJ: The synovium. In Vigorita VJ, Ghelman B: Orthopaedic Pathology. Philadelphia, Lippincott Williams & Wilkins, 1999.)

sodes, especially at the hip and shoulder or when recurrent bleeding was suspected.

PATHOPHYSIOLOGY OF HEMOPHILIC ARTHROPATHY

Hemophilic arthropathy is obviously due to recurrent bleeding into a joint, but the exact mechanism involved in the destructive process is not well understood. The pathophysiology is most likely multifactorial, including general and local physical factors, chemical factors, and inflammatory factors.

The early synovial reaction to intra-articular bleeding is similar to rheumatoid arthritis with synovial hypertrophy, hemosiderin deposition in phagocytic cells, perivascular infiltrates of inflammatory cells, and early fibrosis of the subsynovial layer. There may be marked vascular hyperplasia of the synovium (Figs. 51.2 and 51.3). The hypervascularity and friability of the synovium probably cause an increased tendency to further bleeding, which may become cyclical. A dark red, viscous joint fluid develops with chronic bleeding, and clots form on the synovium. The excess clot formed from chronic hemarthrosis is unlikely to be removed completely by the fibrinolytic system, and organization of the remaining clot leads to the development of fibrous adhesions. Dense intra-articular and subsynovial fibrosis may eventually lead to capsular fibrosis and joint contracture. Increased intra-articular pressure, from hemarthrosis and flexion deformity, may contribute to damage to both synovium and articular cartilage. In the hemophilic knee, nutrition of articular cartilage may be affected by abnormal synovial fluid,

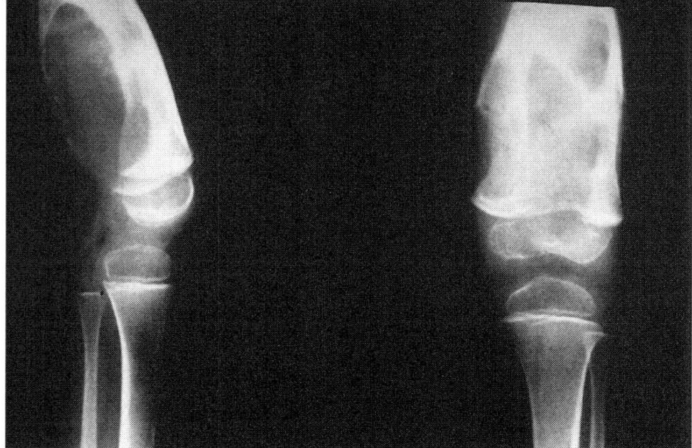

FIGURE 51.3 ➢ Radiograph of hemophilic pseudotumor. (From Vigorita VJ: The synovium. In Vigorita VJ, Ghelman B: Orthopaedic Pathology. Philadelphia, Lippincott Williams & Wilkins, 1999.)

immobilization of the joint, and the presence of fibrous adhesions.

In the later stages of hemophilic arthropathy, articular cartilage lesions, which begin as fibrillation and pitting, progress to erosions. Because little or no bleeding occurs in the subchondral bone, and because pannus formation is limited, destruction of the articular cartilage matrix is probably the result of toxic or chemical factors. It is known that proteolytic enzymes may degrade articular cartilage. Arnold and Hilgartner[1] found that hydrolytic enzymes increased in both hemophilic synovium and joint fluid. High levels of acid phosphatase activity were measured in 56 aspirates from hemophilic joints, and high levels of cathepsin D were measured in 10 specimens of synovial tissue. These enzyme levels were higher than those in patients with rheumatoid arthritis and presumably degraded the extracellular matrix of articular cartilage. Cathepsin D has potent chemotactic activity, and this may play a role in maintaining a chronically inflamed synovium. The role of iron deposition in the pathophysiology of hemophilic arthropathy is not fully established. Stein and Duthie[40] found well-defined cytoplasmic deposits of iron, termed siderosomes, in synovial cells, in subsynovial tissue, and in chondrocytes in the superficial layer of articular cartilage. All cells containing siderosomes showed signs of degeneration. The authors concluded that iron, in the form of cytoplasmic true siderosomes, contributed directly to early degeneration and disintegration of these cells. However, another explanation is that intracellular iron may inhibit the hydrolysis of calcium pyrophosphate and thus permit the precipitation of insoluble calcium pyrophosphate crystals in the articular cartilage matrix, contributing to its deterioration. Roosendaal and colleagues[38] analyzed synovial tissue containing hemosideric deposits from six hemophilic knee joints. Cultures of this tissue had a significantly increased production of interleukin (IL)-1, IL-6, and tumor necrosis factor (TNF) compared with cultures of synovial tissue with a normal appearance. In addition, the supernatant fluids from the cultures showed greater catabolic activity from hemosideritic tissue as determined by the inhibition of the synthesis of articular cartilage matrix. Finally, osteoporosis may develop as a result of disuse and immobilization of the joint. The overgrowth of the epiphyseal plate that is seen in hemophilic children is probably due to the increased blood flow in the capsular and epiphyseal blood vessels, which is part of the reaction to the hemarthrosis.

In summary, the etiology of hemophilic arthropathy is multifactorial. As a result of repeated bleeding episodes, synovial hypertrophy occurs, iron and red cell debris are phagocytized, and hydrolytic enzymes are produced by the proliferating synovium. An inflammatory process develops, cartilage deteriorates, and joint space disappears. The process is completed when subchondral bone is exposed and severe joint fibrosis develops. Elevated intra-articular pressure and immobilization probably play a role in articular cartilage destruction.

RADIOLOGY OF HEMOPHILIC ARTHROPATHY OF THE KNEE

Although the radiographic features of hemophilic arthropathy are not diagnostic, radiographs should be obtained in patients with an acute hemarthrosis and in those presenting with subacute chronic synovitis or a painful joint. In addition, if there is a history of trauma, radiographs should be obtained to exclude a fracture. With knee involvement, there are three minimum radiographs: standing anteroposterior (AP) and lateral views and a tangential view of the patella (either sunrise view or Merchant's view). A "tunnel" view of the knee may occasionally show the femoral intercondylar notch changes sooner than a standard AP view will. Because of the difficulty in evaluating the amount of joint-space narrowing in a knee with a fixed flexion contracture, Johnson and Bobbitt[18] recommended an AP view with the radiographic plate held parallel to the tibial shaft and the beam angled approximately 12 degrees off the perpendicular to the tibia. This may be helpful in determining the true articular cartilage thickness. Magnetic resonance imaging (MRI) of the hemophilic knee may prove helpful in the evaluation of different treatment regimens and when considering patients for synovectomy.[51] In one study of 13 children with severe factor VIII deficiency,[29] MRI findings of one or more target joints caused the investigators to change 40% of the treatment plans based on clinical and plain radiographic data.

In a group of patients with severe hemophilia, before the introduction of factor replacement therapy, Petterson and colleagues[31] showed that radiographic changes are extremely rare before age 3 years, with some changes appearing between 3 and 6 years of age. After age 6 years, almost all patients with severe hemophilia will have radiographic evidence of arthropathy, which progresses until skeletal maturity. Thereafter, arthropathy progresses, but at a much slower pace. There are no reported cases in which the changes have regressed. Arnold and Hilgartner[1] stated that, despite apparently adequate medical treatment for joint bleeding episodes, hemophilic arthropathy continues to progress in many patients with severe disease.

Many radiographic classification systems for hemophilic arthropathy have been proposed since the 1950s, but two systems are in common use. In 1977, Arnold and Hilgartner[1] described a five-stage system for hemophilic arthropathy that attempted to separate the joint changes into stages that have surgical significance (Table 51.2). It is logical, relatively simple, easy to recall, and probably the most commonly used system in the United States. In 1979, Petterson and colleagues[31] described another system that rates eight radiographic changes to grade the arthropathy on a scale of 0 to 13 points. Although this classification system is more difficult to use, it was recommended by the Orthopaedic Advisory Committee at the 1981 meeting of the International Congress of the World Federation

TABLE 51.2 ARNOLD AND HILGARTNER'S RADIOGRAPHIC CLASSIFICATION OF HEMOPHILIC ARTHROPATHY

Stage 0	Normal knee
Stage I	Soft-tissue swelling
Stage II	Soft-tissue swelling, osteopenia, epiphyseal overgrowth, no narrowing of joint space
Stage III	No significant narrowing of joint space, subchondral cysts, osteopenia
Stage IV	Destruction of cartilage and narrowing of joint space
Stage V	End stage, with destruction of joint and gross bony changes

See text for further discussion.
Data from Arnold WD, Hilgartner MW: Hemophilic arthropathy. J Bone Joint Surg Am 59:287, 1977.

of Hemophilia. Greene and colleagues[14] described a modification of the Petterson classification using a four-sign, seven-point system.

The classification system of Arnold and Hilgartner, which separates hemophilic arthropathy into five stages, is outlined in Table 51.2 and discussed below.

Stage 0 is assigned to a normal joint.

In *stage I,* there are no skeletal abnormalities visible on the radiographs, but there is soft-tissue swelling secondary to the hemarthrosis or bleeding into the soft tissues around the joint.

Stage II usually coincides with the clinical stage of subacute hemarthropathy. There is osteopenia, particularly in the epiphyses, and overgrowth of the epiphyses, especially in the knee and elbow. There is no narrowing of the joint space, and there are no bone cysts.

In *stage III,* there is no significant narrowing of the joint space. Subchondral cysts are present. There are changes in the bony contours, with squaring of the patella and femoral condyles, and the femoral intercondylar notch is widened. These changes are probably due to hyperemia and synovitis. Arnold and Hilgartner stated that this is the final stage at which hemophilic arthropathy is reversible by treatment.

Stage IV is characterized by definite narrowing of the joint space that indicates erosion of the articular cartilage. The changes seen in stage III are present and more pronounced stage IV.

Stage V, the final stage, is characterized by complete loss of joint space, with numerous and occasionally large subchondral cysts, extensive enlargement of the epiphyses, and, overall, substantial disorganization of the joint structures. Clinically, in this stage the joint has a fibrous contracture with marked restriction of joint motion, but bleeding episodes may be less frequent. Pathologically, the articular cartilage is absent, with eburnated bone that is discolored with green, brown, or black pigments.

Johnson and Bobbitt[18] studied the relationship of the five stages of the Arnold and Hilgartner classification system with the measured range of motion of the elbow, knee, and ankle joints. In 90 knees of 48 patients with hemophilias A and B, the authors found that the mean arc of motion (flexion minus extension) was about the same, 133 to 134 degrees, in stages 0, I, and II. There was a steady progression of loss of motion with advancing stages, with a mean arc of motion of 120 degrees in stage III, 95 degrees in stage IV, and 47 degrees in stage V. Loss of joint space was the most important radiographic finding related to range of motion.

In the classification system of Petterson and colleagues,[31] eight different radiographic signs are graded to give a cumulative score of 0 to 13 points. A normal joint has a grade of 0. Each of the following signs is allotted one point: osteoporosis, epiphyseal enlargement, and erosion of the joint margin. The remaining five radiographic changes — irregular subchondral surface, incongruity of the joint surfaces, subchondral cyst, narrowing of the joint space, and angular deformity — are assigned 0 points (no changes), 1 point (slight changes), or 2 points (severe changes). Because the categories and point scales are difficult to remember and cumbersome to apply, this system has not been widely used in the United States.

Greene and colleagues[14] devised a simpler radiographic classification system for the knee joint, using only four signs: irregularity of the subchondral surface, joint-space narrowing, erosion of the joint margin, and incongruity of the joint surfaces. In this system, the joint score ranges from 0 to 7 points. The authors compared their newer system with the two previously described classification systems. The newer system and that of Petterson and colleagues were better than that of Arnold and Hilgartner for grading severe arthropathy. With all systems, the range of motion decreased as the arthropathy became more advanced. The utility of the newer system has yet to be tested in a clinical study of medical or surgical treatment of hemophilic arthropathy of the knee.

FACTOR REPLACEMENT THERAPY

The overall management of patients with hemophilia should be supervised by a team of experienced hematologists and orthopedic surgeons. The treatment of hemophilia A consists of factor VIII replacement. In the United States, this has been performed with fresh frozen plasma, a blood bank-prepared cryoprecipitate of fresh plasma, or commercial concentrates of factor VIII. Several different types of commercial concentrate have been developed (Table 51.3).[45] Commercial concentrates are lyophilized, stable at ambient temperatures, and preferred because of their high potency and ease of administration. Heated concentrate is a product prepared from donors screened for human immunodeficiency virus type 1 (HIV1) antibodies and heated at 56° to 68°C during manufacturing to inactivate heat-sensitive viruses (e.g., HIV1). Solvent-detergent-extracted factor VIII concentrate is treated to remove coated viruses, including HIV1 and hepatitis A and B. Monoclonal factor VIII concentrate is an ultrapure product, prepared by using affinity chromatography and viral inactivation steps. Recombinant factor VIII is a synthetic product prepared in Chinese hamster ovary cells. These new techniques and methods for ultrapurification of clotting factors have definitely led to safer and more effective concentrates. No new cases of HIV infection in hemophiliacs have been reported since 1985 except for isolated outbreaks associated with inadequately treated blood products.[26]

Factor VIII may be administered by either intermittent boluses or continuous infusion. Calculation of the dose of factor VIII is performed as follows:

Dose = plasma volume (50% body weight [kg])
(desired factor VIII level (U/mL)
− initial factor VIII level (U/mL)

In patients with severe hemophilia, the initial factor VIII level is less than 0.01 U/mL. Because the half-life of factor VIII in plasma is approximately 12 hours, half the calculated dose should be given every 12 hours.

Hemarthroses and minor muscle bleeds are treated (usually at home) with sufficient concentrate to bring the factor VIII level to 0.50 U/mL (50% of normal). If bleeding continues, the dose is repeated in 12 to 24 hours. Muscle bleeds with neurovascular compromise and retroperitoneal bleeds should be treated for up to 5 to 7 days with doses to bring the factor VIII level to 0.5 to 1.0 U/mL (50% to 100% of normal). In patients with an intracranial hemorrhage and patients undergoing a surgical procedure (synovectomy or total joint arthroplasty), concentrates are given to raise the factor VIII level to 1.0 U/mL (100% of normal) for a variable period of time, and occasionally for as long as 10 to 14 days. Activated prothrombin complex concentrates are used in patients with factor VIII inhibitors and are given in arbitrary doses of 50 to 100 U/kg body weight, rather than in a calculated dose.

The treatment of hemophilia B consists of factor IX replacement using fresh frozen plasma or prothrombin complex concentrates, which are rich in factor IX. Prothrombin complex concentrates (heated) are necessary for serious or persistent bleeding episodes. The dose is calculated with the same formula listed previously for factor VIII replacement. However, because factor IX distribution is approximately twice the plasma volume, it takes twice as much factor IX as factor VIII to achieve a specific level. The half-life of factor IX is 8 to 14 hours. Prothrombin complex concentrates should be given only as intermittent bolus treatment every 12 hours. These concentrates are associated with the risk of hepatitis, are potentially thrombogenic, and may produce a syndrome of disseminated intravascular coagulation. Recombinant factor IX is now available and is being evaluated in clinical studies.[26]

TABLE 51.3 SOURCES OF FACTORS VIII AND IX

Source	Risk of Hepatitis	Risk of HIV	Risk of Hemolysis
Plasma	+	+	(
Cryoprecipitate	+	+	(
Factor VIII Concentrate			
Heated	4+	(	4+
Solvent	−	−	4+
Monoclonal	−	−	−
Recombinant	−	−	−
Factor IX heated	4+	?	−
Activated	4+	−	−

HIV = human immunodeficiency virus.
Symbols: to 4+, degree of increasing risk; (, no risk.
Adapted from White GC: Disorders of blood coagulation. In Stern JH, ed: Internal Medicine. 3rd ed. Boston, Little, Brown, 1990.

Complications of Factor Replacement Therapy

Inhibitors

Inhibitors to factor VIII develop in approximately 15% to 20% of patients treated with factor VIII. These inhibitors are antibodies that have the ability to inactivate factor VIII in coagulation assays and are measured using Bethesda units. There are three distinct clinical groups of patients with inhibitors. In a small number of patients, the level of inhibitor is low (less than 10 Bethesda units). All bleeding episodes in these patients with low-response inhibitors are treated with factor VIII concentrate, but very high doses (up to 4000 units) may be necessary to achieve a satisfactory factor VIII level. In patients with high-response, low-titer inhibitors, the inhibitors remain at low levels until stimulated by administration of factor VIII. This leads to an anamnestic increase in inhibitor level, frequently to very high levels (1000 to 2000 Bethesda units). A third group of patients have inhibitor levels that are high (higher than 20 Bethesda units) and remain high—high-response, high-titer—even without factor VIII administration.

Patients with inhibitors have the same frequency of bleeding episodes as do patients without inhibitors, but those with an inhibitor level above 20 Bethesda units respond poorly, if at all, to treatment with factor VIII concentrates. Patients should be tested for inhibitors before any surgical procedure or when there is a poor response to replacement therapy.

The treatment of serious bleeding episodes in patients with high-response, high-titer inhibitors is very difficult and may include porcine factor VIII, activated prothrombin complex concentrates (factor VIII inhibitor bypassing activity [FEIBA]), or plasmapheresis. The use of factor VIII in patients with high-response, low-titer inhibitors is reserved for life-threatening bleeds. For hemarthroses, treatment with prothrombin complex concentrates is sometimes effective and is less likely to cause an increase in inhibitor level.

Some concern has been raised over the high (25% to 27%) frequency of inhibitor formation during treatment with recombinant factor VIII in previously untreated patients.[26] However, the majority of inhibitors with this product have been low titer, and some inhibitors were transient. Inhibitors to factor IX occur only rarely, in approximately 3% of severely affected patients with hemophilia B, and management is difficult.

Hepatitis

Transfusion-associated hepatitis occurs in a large percentage of hemophiliacs receiving replacement therapy. Although 80% of patients have at least intermittent elevations of liver function test results (transaminases), only about 10% have a history of symptoms. The chronic problems of transfusion-associated hepatitis, including cirrhosis and hypersplenism, occur in a very small number of patients. Both hepatitis B and hepatitis C have been reported as the cause of liver disease in hemophilia. The treatment is supportive, and patients should continue to use appropriate factor VIII concentrates as necessary.

It was hoped that the newer virucidal methods for factor concentrates would eliminate hepatitis from this patient population. However, hepatitis A virus infection was noted in Europe from 1988 to 1992, associated with one particular solvent-detergent factor VIII concentrate.[26] Although hepatitis A transmission may be a rare event, one organization has recommended vaccination of all hemophiliacs older than 2 years who are hepatitis A seronegative. There has been a substantial reduction in (but not a complete elimination of) hepatitis C virus transmission since the new virucidal methods have been used.

Hemolytic Anemia

A hemolytic reaction to infused anti-A or anti-B antibodies may occur in patients with blood groups A, B, or AB who receive a large amount of factor replacement concentrate. Hemolytic anemia has occurred in patients following synovectomy and total knee arthroplasty. Blood typing should obviously be performed before any surgical procedure, and concentrates with low isoagglutinin titers should be used in susceptible patients. Hemolytic anemia, which requires treatment postoperatively, is managed by replacement with washed, packed, type O red blood cells and factor concentrates (monoclonal and recombinant) with low isoagglutinin levels.

Acquired Immunodeficiency Syndrome

A definite association between acquired immunodeficiency syndrome (AIDS) and hemophilia was established by 1984, with a report of 22 cases of AIDS in hemophiliacs.[6] These patients had a complex illness identical in clinical manifestation to the syndrome seen in other groups; 14 had *Pneumocystis carinii* pneumonia, and others had various opportunistic infections. It has been established that the syndrome in hemophiliacs was caused by transmission of HIV1 retrovirus through factor VIII and other factor concentrates that were collected and administered before donor screening and development of heat-treated and other "purified" factor VIII concentrates. Replication of the virus causes disruption of the CD4+ (helper T) lymphocyte, with a variable reduction of the CD4+ lymphocyte count. Patients may later develop opportunistic infections, unusual sarcomas or lymphomas, or multiple or recurrent bacterial infections.

In the hemophilia clinic at the University of North Carolina Hospitals, the overall incidence of seropositive reaction for the HIV1 antibody was 67% in patients with severe factor VIII deficiency, 38% in those with severe factor IX deficiency, and only 9% in those with mild or moderate factor VIII or IX deficiency.[10] None of the patients who had a transfusion with only the newer heat-treated concentrates became seropositive for HIV.

Greene and coworkers[10] reported the results of various orthopedic surgical procedures in hemophiliacs who were seropositive for HIV. In 30 such patients, the preoperative CD4+ lymphocyte count decreased to a mean of 336×10^9 per liter (range, 27 to 708×10^9 per liter). After 26 orthopedic procedures in patients without any previous bacterial infection, only one patient developed a nosocomial infection (forearm cellulitis related to an intravenous catheter). However, in five patients who had unexplained postoperative fever, the preoperative CD4+ lymphocyte count was significantly reduced. In addition, a more rapid progression to AIDS was seen in patients who had a lower preoperative CD4+ lymphocyte count. Therefore, when elective orthopedic surgical procedures in patients with hemophilia are contemplated, the preoperative evaluation should include HIV serological status, CD4+ lymphocyte count, and response to intradermal skin-test antigens. This information may assist in assessing the patient's risk for infection and provide very useful prognostic information. The risk of infection is very minimal with a CD4+ lymphocyte count greater than 400×10^9 per liter.[10] When the CD4+ lymphocyte count is more than 200 but fewer than 400, the risk of infection is probably increased. However, one study found a much higher risk of infection after joint arthroplasty procedures than after nonarthroplasty procedures when the CD4+ lymphocyte count was fewer than 200.[33] Major orthopedic surgical procedures of the knee may be safely performed in patients with hemophilia who are seropositive for HIV if adequate precautions for the patient and for surgical personnel are observed.

TREATMENT OF HEMARTHROSIS

Acute Hemarthrosis: Role of Aspiration

As previously mentioned, a hemophiliac with an acute knee hemarthrosis has a warm, swollen, painful, and tender joint. With the wide availability of factor concentrates and the prevalence of home therapy by a vast majority of hemophiliacs in the United States, aspiration of a knee joint with an acute hemarthrosis will be performed only rarely. However, aspiration of a major hemarthrosis can increase patient comfort and enhance rehabilitation.[34] The removal of the bulk of the hemarthrosis may decrease the risk of progression to chronic synovitis and recurrent hemarthrosis.

A hemophiliac with knee pain and swelling that do not respond rapidly to home or hospital factor replacement therapy should be evaluated for the presence of an inhibitor, and the diagnosis of spontaneous septic arthritis should be considered. Wilkins and Wiedel[49] reported a case of spontaneous pyarthrosis of the knee in an adult hemophiliac. This patient had a low-grade fever, a normal peripheral leukocyte count, and a tender, swollen knee that did not respond to factor VIII replacement therapy. The organism was *Staphylococcus aureus,* and the knee required an open incision and drainage. This author has treated two similar patients with septic arthritis of the knee and the elbow, respectively. A high index of suspicion is required for diagnosis of septic arthritis in a hemophiliac, especially one who is seropositive for HIV1 or who has previously had any manifestions of AIDS. Obviously, before any aspiration, the patient should be checked for an inhibitor and the appropriate factor replacement administered. Immobilization for a short period of time is recommended following a knee aspiration.

Subacute and Chronic Arthropathy

Nonsurgical Management

If a knee fails to respond completely to appropriate factor replacement therapy for an acute hemarthrosis, or if two or more hemarthroses occur in a relatively short period of time, the clinical stage of subacute hemarthrosis or subacute arthropathy usually develops.[35] The knee has a chronic hemarthrosis with palpable synovitis and a slightly restricted range of motion. Subacute hemophilic arthropathy of the knee should be aggressively treated with factor replacement therapy (usually at home) and 2 or 3 weeks of immobilization in a commercially available semiflexible knee splint. If the knee synovitis does not improve, a course of prednisone in doses of 1 to 2 mg/kg body weight is usually given for 5 or 6 days but not longer than 2 weeks. The use of prednisone is probably contraindicated in patients who are seropositive for HIV.

The goals of nonsurgical treatment of subacute hemarthrosis are as follows:

1. To prevent muscle atrophy
2. To preserve a functional range of motion
3. To control repeated hemarthrosis
4. To allow relatively normal function of the knee

Hilgartner and Arnold recommended 6 to 8 weeks of prophylactic replacement therapy combined with active physiotherapy.[1] Specifically, patients are transfused with sufficient factor concentrate at home to raise the plasma level to 20% to 30% of normal three times weekly. After each transfusion and during the following morning, when replacement factor is present, the patient performs an active range-of-motion exercise program under the close supervision of an experienced physical therapist. If range-of-motion exercises are painful, isometric quadriceps exercises alone are recommended.

Greene and Strickler[13] studied the results of a home-modified isokinetic strengthening program in 32 patients with severe hemophilia. The age of the patients ranged from 7 to 51 years, and the stage of arthropathy was stage 0 or normal in 11 knees, stage I in 2 knees, stage III in 13 knees, and stage IV in 27 knees. Measurement of knee extensor and flexor torque, using a Cybex II machine, was performed at the start of the study and at 6 months. The modified isokinetic exercises were performed for 15 minutes every day in the sitting position with the legs hanging freely. Starting with the knees flexed at 90 degrees, the left leg was crossed over the right distal tibia. Simultaneous contracture of the left knee flexors and right knee extensors was begun, and the legs gained full extension over a 5- to 10-second interval. The contralateral maneuver was then performed. The incidence of knee hemarthroses was not increased during the 6 months of exercise. Both knee extensor and knee flexor torque measurements increased in adolescents and adults but not in children younger than 12 years. Thigh circumference increased in more than half the legs. Knees with stage IV arthropathy did not gain as much strength as did knees at other stages. Some of the patients with stage IV knees found that these exercises produced patellar pain. This isokinetic exercise program was recommended for hemophiliacs of all ages with knee arthropathy.

When subacute arthropathy has not been aggressively treated or has progressed, significant knee flexion contractures may develop in association with or even before development of chronic hemophilic arthropathy with joint-space loss (Fig. 51.4). If the knee flexion contracture has been present for only a few months, partial correction may be obtained without surgery. At least four methods have been described for treatment of fixed flexion contractures.

The technique of reversed dynamic slings was developed in Oxford in the 1980s. The advantages of this technique are that quadriceps muscle power is improved and that physiotherapy can be performed during the time of correction. The disadvantage is that it requires hospitalization. The patient's leg is supported by balanced traction in a half-ring Thomas splint with a Pearson knee flexion attachment. Longitudinal skin traction is applied to the calf, but the heel is left free. A padded canvas sling is applied over the distal thigh and is reversed beneath the metal side pieces of the Thomas splint. A traction rope connects the sling to a weight (usually 2.8 kg), and thus a posterior force is applied to the distal part of the anterior aspect of the thigh against the counterpressure of the slings on the posterior surface of the calf. The longitudinal traction and thigh weights are gradually increased over the first 48 hours. The combined forces gradually correct flexion deformity and posterior subluxation of the tibia. When the knee is straight or when no further improvement has occurred for a week, the patient is mobilized with the knee in an open-fronted molded cylinder splint. Factor replacement is not required dur-

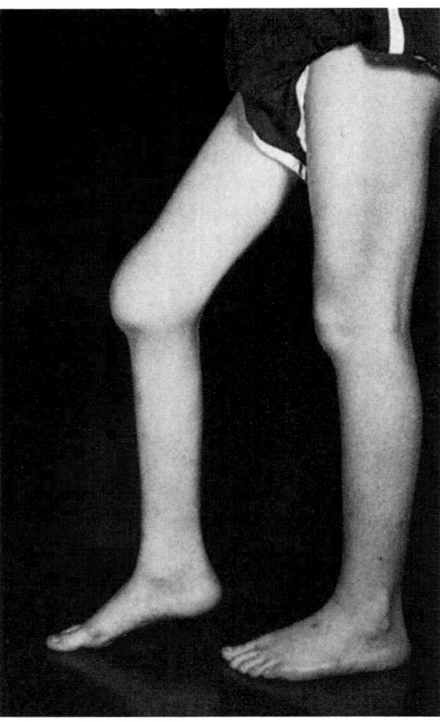

FIGURE 51.4 ➢ Significant knee flexion contracture in an 11-year-old with classic hemophilia.

ing the treatment period. Stein and Dickson[39] compared this technique with serial plaster casts in a prospective study. In patients with reversed dynamic slings, the flexion contracture was reduced by an average of 34 degrees, compared with a reduction of 9 degrees in a serial plaster group.

The extension-desubluxation hinge cast,[3] developed at Orthopedic Hospital in Los Angeles, simultaneously and gradually corrects both subluxation of the tibia on the femur and flexion contracture (Fig. 51.5A, B). An open-front knee cylinder of plaster or thermoplastic material is used. The hinge is adjusted with a wrench daily or twice daily to bring about correction. When the flexion contracture is less than 20 degrees, the cast is removed and a splint applied. Factor replacement may be required during the use of this device.

The knee Dynasplint is an adjustable dynamic splint capable of producing a low-intensity, prolonged-duration force across the knee joint.[21] Two steel struts are placed medially and laterally on the lower extremity and held in place with Velcro closures. An adjustable compression coil spring is contained within the distal calf struts. Two Velcro cuffs and a 4-cm-wide strap act as pressure points, while the posterior thigh cuff and posterior calf cuff prevent rotation of the splint. The splint is initially set at very low tension and is worn for several hours per day. In a study of seven patients with at least a 15-degree flexion contracture, Lang[21] found that four patients gained 5 degrees of extension in an average of 6 months and three patients gained 10 degrees in an average of 9 months. However, three patients had bleeding into the knee during the study.

Greene and colleagues[11] described a protocol using "special Buck's" traction, Quengel casting, and a polypropylene orthosis in patients with high-titer inhibitors and acute and chronic flexion contractures. In their study, nine patients with 15 episodes of chronic knee flexion contractures were treated; four knees had a good result with a contracture of less than 20 degrees at 1 year, but five knees were failures with recurrent contractures. The results of special Buck's traction and bracing were better in patients with acute knee flexion contractures. A good result was obtained in 23 of 25 episodes of acute knee flexion contracture.

Prophylaxis

With the development of newer, safer factor concentrates, interest in routine hemophilia prophylaxis has been revived.[12, 23] Because the main goal is to prevent joint bleeding and hemophilic arthropathy, prophylaxis may be considered optimal management for all persons with severe hemophilia. The most extensive data concerning prophylactic treatment are from Sweden, where prophylaxis was begun in the late 1950s to early 1960s. Nilsson and colleagues[28] reviewed the 25-year experience of prophylaxis for 65 patients with severe hemophilia A. In the youngest group of 21 boys, who started continuous prophylaxis at age 1 to 2 years to prevent factor VIII from falling below 1% of normal, almost no bleeding episodes occurred. The Petterson clinical orthopedic joint score and radiographic scores were zero in all 21 patients. This study and others from international centers have shown that it is now possible to almost completely prevent hemophilic arthropathy by giving effective continuous prophylaxis from an early age and preventing the deficient factor level from falling below 1% of normal.[23, 24, 28] However, in the United States, as in most other countries, economic considerations and cost are the greatest obstacles to implementing this level of routine prophylaxis.

Synovectomy

The rationale for synovectomy of the knee in hemophilia is to prevent or decrease the number of hemarthroses and to prevent or delay the onset of late-stage hemophilic arthropathy. Although the exact mechanism of joint destruction is not fully understood, it is related to the synovial changes caused by bleeding into the joint. One study showed that hemophilic synovial tissue that contained iron deposits had enhanced production of IL-1, IL-6, and TNF (similar to levels found in knee synovium from patients with rheumatoid arthritis).[38] In addition, the fluid from culture of this synovial tissue inhibited the synthesis of articular cartilage matrix. Therefore, the removal of the inflamed and hypervascular synovium should theoretically diminish bleeding and delay or prevent onset of arthritis.

Synovectomy of the knee in hemophilia has been

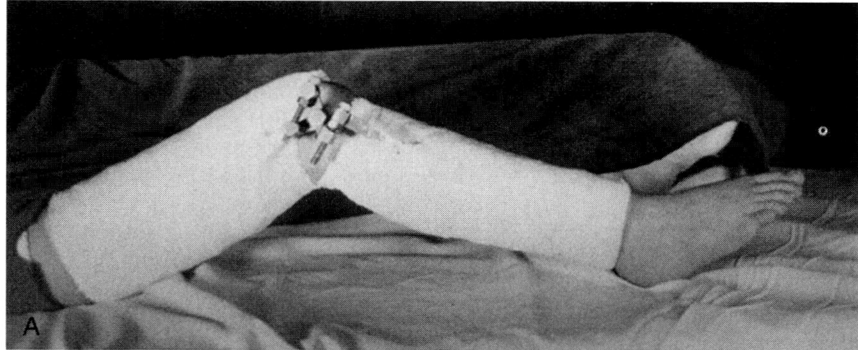

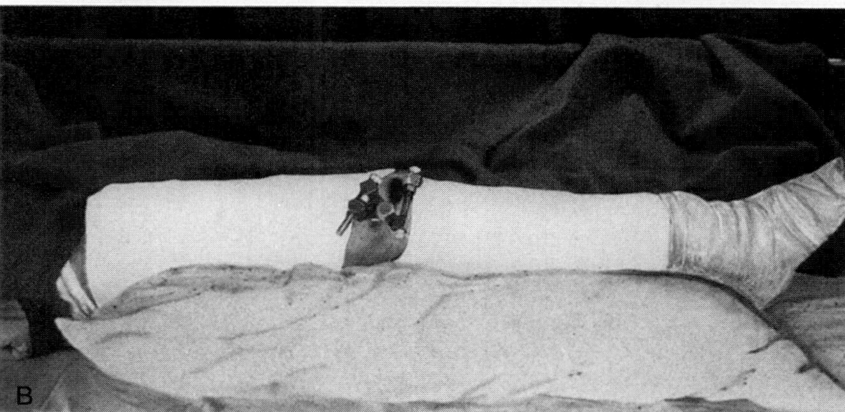

FIGURE 51.5 ➢ *A*, Extension-desubluxation cast on a patient with a 40-degree contracture. *B*, Flexion contracture reduced to 5 degrees after 12 days.

performed as an open surgical procedure, as an arthroscopic procedure, and using radiation from an injectable radionuclide isotope. The indication for synovectomy (by any method) is severe recurrent hemarthroses with persistent synovitis for 3 to 6 months in a patient who has failed to respond to aggressive medical management. Most reports of synovectomy indicate that patients have had one to three bleeds per month for several months despite prophylactic factor replacement, immobilization, and physical therapy. The radiographic stage of arthropathy in the knee to undergo synovectomy should be Arnold and Hilgartner stage I, II, or III—that is, before cartilage space narrowing has occurred. Thus, most patients should be relatively young and have a well-preserved range of motion of the knee.

Open Surgical Synovectomy

Before surgery, a patient who is to undergo a knee synovectomy should have the appropriate factor level measured and should be tested for the presence of a factor inhibitor. A formal "fall-off" study should be performed if a hemophilia A patient's response to factor VIII is not well known. Preoperatively, the appropriate factor concentrate is infused to bring the patient's level to 100%, which is maintained for 48 hours postoperatively. Thereafter, the factor level is maintained at 50% for the first 2 weeks and during periods of aggressive physical therapy. The synovectomy is performed under tourniquet control, and a prophylactic antibiotic (such as cefazolin) is given before tourniquet inflation. A long midline, paramedian, or medial parapatellar incision is made from 7 to 10 cm proximal to the patellar to the medial aspect of the tibial tubercle. This incision permits future reconstructive surgery and allows sufficient exposure for the procedure. The synovium is dissected sharply or with electrocautery from the overlying fibrous capsule. First, the synovium is excised from the suprapatellar region, leaving a thin layer of adipose tissue over the nonarticular surface of the distal femur. Then it is excised from the medial and lateral recesses, from the intercondylar notch, and around the collateral ligaments and menisci. Angled pituitary rongeurs are helpful in removing synovium from the intercondylar region and the posteromedial and posterolateral aspects of the joint. The menisci, cruciate ligaments, and collateral ligaments should be preserved, although minor meniscal tears should be débrided. The tourniquet should be released and the knee packed with moist sponges for several minutes. Thereafter, meticulous hemostasis with electrocautery should be obtained. After hemostasis, the knee is irrigated with saline-antibiotic solution. The wound is closed in layers over suction drains, using nonabsorbable sutures in the quadriceps tendon and capsule and surgical staples in the skin. The lower extremity is then wrapped in a bulky compressive dressing with medial and lateral plaster splints. Although many surgeons recommend initiating continuous passive motion (CPM) immediately, others immobilize the knee for 5 to 7 days following open surgical synovectomy. Thereafter, if the wound is dry and there is no evidence of bleeding, ambulation, CPM, and active assisted range-of-motion exercises are begun, supervised by an experienced physical therapist. It is imperative to monitor the factor level daily and to prohibit motion if the level is inadequate or if the patient senses that bleeding is about to occur. Manipulation is performed between 2 and 3 weeks postoperatively if 90-degree flexion has not been obtained, although this is less likely if CPM devices and aggressive physical therapy are used.

Storti and Ascari[41] first reported the results of open synovectomy in 1969 and described the results in 51 knees at an average follow-up of 3 years. Although the indications for surgery were broad, with their patients receiving much less factor replacement than patients in the United States received, bleeding was eliminated or greatly reduced in 94% of patients. Only 12% of patients were reported to have decreased range of motion. There have been several studies of open synovectomy of the knee.[16, 27, 30, 32] A synthesis of these studies indicates that open surgical synovectomy reliably decreases or eliminates bleeding episodes, but there is usually a concomitant loss of flexion, which may be minimized by aggressive physical therapy and use of a CPM machine. Radiographic progression of arthropathy is probably to be expected. The long-term results of open synovectomy at two European centers have been reported. In Norway, synovectomy (including medial and lateral menisectomy) was performed in nine knees followed up for a mean of 12.6 years (range, 6 to 22 years).[42] Two knees became ankylosed, and total knee arthroplasty was performed or pending in four knees. These authors concluded that although open synovectomy of the knee controls bleeding and pain, the range of motion is decreased and destructive arthropathy is not arrested. In Spain, 27 open synovectomies in patients age 10 to 20 years were followed up for a mean of 15.2 years (range, 12 to 17 years).[36] Two knees had a good result, 10 had a fair result, and 6 had a poor result. Joint function deteriorated and radiographic arthropathy progressed with time.

Arthroscopic Synovectomy

Arthroscopic synovectomy was introduced in 1980 as an alternative to open surgical synovectomy following the success of arthroscopic procedures for other traumatic and degenerative knee conditions.[46] The rationale behind arthroscopic synovectomy of the knee in hemophilia was to provide a similar decrease in bleeding episodes as open synovectomy provides but to avoid the loss of range of motion that occurs in many patients. It was hoped that the morbidity of synovectomy would be decreased and that rehabilitation of the knee would be more rapid.

The preoperative assessment of a patient who is to have an arthroscopic knee synovectomy is identical to that advised for a patient who is to have an open surgical procedure. The arthroscopic synovectomy is performed using general anesthesia and under tourniquet control. The appropriate operative factor level is 100%, and the factor level should be maintained between 70% and 100% for the first 3 to 5 days postoperatively. The factor level is then decreased to 30% to 50% for a variable period of time, depending on the status of the knee and the intensity of physical therapy. Arthroscopic synovectomy of a hemophilic knee is difficult and tedious and is recommended for only an experienced arthroscopist. In one study, arthroscopic synovectomy took an average of 20 minutes longer than open synovectomy took.[36] The technique usually involves five separate portals: anteromedial, anterolateral, medial and lateral suprapatellar, and posteromedial for removal of synovium from the posteromedial aspect of the knee. Motorized large-bore shaving devices are necessary to remove the fibrotic synovium. Copious lavage is recommended before completion of the procedure. A postoperative compression bandage with splints may be applied for 2 to 4 days, or immediate motion may be begun using a CPM device.

Wiedel[46] described the early results of arthroscopic synovectomy in eight patients, mean age 16 years, at follow-up times of 4 to 8 years. Four knees required manipulation — three because of poor knee flexion by 14 days. There was one severe postoperative hemarthrosis that required arthroscopic evacuation. Two knees had recurrent hemarthroses, and both required a second arthroscopic synovectomy with eventual resolution. The range of motion of the knee was improved in three knees and unchanged in three knees. Two knees lost significant flexion — 25 degrees and 40 degrees, respectively. A synthesis of other studies of arthroscopic synovectomy showed that the procedure is certainly feasible but that many knees may still have episodes of recurrent bleeding.[5, 19, 22]

Wiedel[47] described the 10- to 15-year results of nine knees in eight patients (mean age 16 years) who had arthroscopic synovectomy between 1980 and 1985. Two patients required a repeat arthroscopy. At the latest follow-up, some range of motion was lost in four knees, and it was increased or unchanged in five knees. All knees showed progressive radiographic changes, and the greatest change was in those knees with stage II arthropathy at the time of synovectomy. As with open synovectomy, there is no evidence that the arthroscopic technique will prevent progression of arthropathy in these young patients.

Radiation Synovectomy

Radiation synovectomy consists of injection of a radionuclide, in particulate or colloidal form, into the knee to ablate or alter inflamed synovium. Based on experience with this technique for chronic rheumatoid synovitis, investigators have used several isotopes in patients with hemophilia, including ^{198}gold, ^{90}yttrium, ^{165}dysprosium, and ^{32}phosphorus.

The treatment protocol for radiation synovectomy in hemophiliacs consists of factor replacement 1 hour before injection and 12 hours after the injection. After careful sterile preparation and draping, a 22 gauge needle is placed into the knee through a superolateral portal. The position of the needle is confirmed by injection of local anesthetic or by contrast media and radiographs. The radioisotope is injected into the knee, and the system is flushed with local anesthetic. The knee is placed through a range of motion and then placed into a knee immobilizer for 24 hours to decrease leakage. The patient usually remains one night in the hospital and is discharged the following day.

Zuckerman and coworkers[52] treated six knees and one elbow in patients with hemophilia with injections of ^{32}phosphorus. This isotope was chosen because its relatively long half-life (14 days) and relatively low energy would produce a slow and gradual effect that was thought to be desirable. At a very short follow-up time, four patients had decreased pain and effusion and no recurrent hemarthrosis, and three patients were considered to represent partial success, with decreased frequency of hemarthrosis and decreased need for factor replacement. There is concern, however, over possible accumulation of ^{32}phosphorus within bone marrow and possible production of chromosomal aberrations. Since 1984, radiation synovectomy using ^{90}yttrium has been the procedure of choice in hemophilia at the Israel National Hemophilia Center. Heim and coworkers[15] have performed this procedure on 50 joints, including 33 knees. At an average follow-up of 34 months, the incidence of hemarthroses was decreased from one bleed per week to one bleed per month. However, 10% had no response. ^{90}Yttrium radiation synovectomy has also been performed on 40 joints of 20 hemophiliacs in Australia.[4] There were nine knees in this group. The joint bleeding and factor usage were significantly decreased at 6 to 12 months after the procedure. However, elbow joints had a better response than knee joints. Patients who were HIV positive also showed improvement up to 12 months after treatment. These authors concluded that radiation synovectomy was effective and less expensive than surgical synovectomy and was particularly recommended for the HIV-infected patient.[4]

Another study reviewed the long-term results of ^{198}gold radiation synovectomy in 38 knees followed up for a mean of 14 years.[25] The result was good in 8 knees, fair in 23 knees, and poor in 7 knees, using a complex joint score combining pain, bleeding, clinical knee examination, and radiographic changes. Range of motion decreased in 15 knees, and there was gradual radiographic progression in 28 knees.

In the United States, the technique of radiation synovectomy has limited availability and should still be considered investigational.

CHOICE OF PROCEDURE

The most appropriate and effective method of synovectomy for chronic hemophilic synovitis should be individualized. Several factors must be taken into account including age of the patient, expertise of the surgeon, inhibitor status, number of joints involved, amount of synovitis, and availability of agents for radiation synovectomy.[9]

Patients younger than 10 to 12 years may not be able to cooperate with the postoperative physical therapy required after an open procedure. There is concern about chromosomal damage from radiation leakage in this age group. Thus, arthroscopic synovectomy is preferred in younger patients. However, if there is a considerable amount of synovial tissue and the surgeon does not have sufficient expertise with arthroscopic synovectomy, an open synovectomy (without menisectomy) may be preferrable. Because of the risk of bleeding after either surgical procedure, radiation synovectomy is the procedure of choice in patients with an inhibitor. In addition, radiation synovectomy is probably the procedure of choice in patients with multiple joint involvement, HIV positivity, or advanced hepatitis. This limits the exposure and the risks of disease transmission to the surgeon and the operating room staff from contaminated fluids.

Joint Débridement

Débridement of the knee for advanced hemophilic arthropathy has been recommended in two European centers to avoid or delay total knee arthroplasty in young, high-risk patients.[5, 37] In one study, open débridement was performed in 11 knees in 11 patients with a mean age of 29 years (range, 25 to 42 years).[5] With open débridement, synovectomy with removal of meniscal remains and osteophytes was performed with smoothing of articular surfaces. A lateral release of a subluxed patella with proximal or distal realignment was performed in all but one knee. At a mean follow-up of 5.4 years (range, 2 to 11 years), using the Hospital for Special Surgery score, four knees were rated excellent, five good, and two fair. However, all radiographs showed some deterioration. In another study, arthroscopic débridement with or without synovectomy was performed in 20 knees with advanced arthropathy.[37] There was improvement in pain and in ability to extend the knee. However, six knees had severe postoperative bleeding, and there was one infection. There is a very limited role for joint débridement in the treatment of hemophilic arthropathy.

Total Knee Arthroplasty

Following the success of total knee arthroplasties in patients with other arthritic disorders, and considering the availability of factor concentrates, total knee arthroplasty was introduced as an alternative to arthrodesis in patients with chronic hemophilic arthropathy. The principal indication for total knee arthroplasty is severe, disabling pain that is unresponsive to medical treatment. All patients should have an adequate trial of rest, walking supports, and appropriate medication. A poor range of motion or a flexion contracture of the knee alone should not be an indication for the procedure. Ankylosis of the knee, recent sepsis, and prolonged narcotic dependency are contraindications. The presence of a high-titer inhibitor to factor VIII is generally an absolute contraindication, although the procedure has been performed safely in such a patient. An absolute CD4+ lymphocyte count less than 200×10^9

per liter (or 200/mm^3), as mentioned previously,[33] is a relative contraindication to surgery.

Total knee arthroplasty for disabling arthropathy in the hemophiliac is a feasible but technically formidable procedure. It is recommended that total knee arthroplasty be performed only at a center that has physicians experienced in the comprehensive care of hemophiliacs and adequately prepared to manage all possible postoperative complications. The patient should be treated by the orthopedic surgeon in concert with an experienced hematologist. The preoperative hematological evaluation should include a determination of level of factor VIII or IX and level of inhibitor and a survival study of infused appropriate factor concentrate. Serological testing for HIV1, skin testing, and determination of absolute CD4+ lymphocyte count are performed at this author's institution. Radiographic evaluation should include standing AP and lateral views of the knee and a tangential view of the patella. In addition, a standing long-casette hip-knee-ankle film is obtained, because most total knee instrumentation systems include a long intramedullary femoral rod, and the angle of distal femoral resection is selected to reproduce a neutral mechanical axis. The most common deformity in patients with chronic hemophilic arthropathy is a three-plane configuration—that is, a flexion contracture associated with valgus deformity and external rotation of the tibia. However, in one review, 6 of 24 knees had a preoperative varus deformity.[20] Preoperative orthopedic evaluation should include assessment of the deformities, in consideration of intraoperative ligament releases, and evaluation of bone loss, which may require grafting or metallic augmentation blocks or wedges. Preoperative planning, using templates on the lateral radiograph of the knee, is recommended to determine that the procedure can be performed with available, noncustom implants.

Because of the presence of usually severe flexion contractures, as well as valgus or varus deformities, the implant recommended is a cemented, tricompartmental posterior-stabilized prosthesis. Use of less constrained models has had results inferior to use of the total condylar prosthesis or the posterior-stabilized version in the hemophilic knee. Hinged knee arthroplasties are not required and not recommended. A metal-backed tibial component is recommended, both on a theoretical basis and because of a high rate of radiolucent lines and tibial sinkage in one series that used only plain polyethylene tibial components.[7] The patella should be routinely resurfaced with a polyethylene component (Figs. 51.6 and 51.7), unless there has been a previous patellectomy. Cement fixation of all three components is still recommended for the most reliable pain relief and component stability.

Total knee arthroplasty in the hemophilic knee should be performed in an operating room with vertical laminar airflow, and the surgical team should wear closed system "space suits." The procedure is performed under tourniquet control with preoperative cephalosporin antibiotic prophylaxis. The patient should be given appropriate preoperative factor concentrate to achieve a 100% level at the time of surgery. This level is maintained for at least 48 hours postoperatively. A level of 60% of normal is maintained for the next 3 days, and a level of 40% of normal is maintained for 3 more days. The 100% level is obtained if a knee manipulation is to be performed. A level of 20% is maintained for postoperative physical therapy for at least 4 to 6 weeks after the arthroplasty.

A longitudinal midline or paramedian straight skin incision is recommended, followed by a medial arthrotomy. Because of the intra-articular fibrosis and deformities, exposure can be difficult and tedious. On occasion, a "quadriceps snip" or modified Coonse-Adams quadriceps turndown is required for exposure. A synovectomy should be performed following the exposure. Cruciate ligaments are excised and medial or lateral ligament releases are performed, when indicated, before any bone resection. When necessary, it is easier to release the posterior capsule following resections of the distal femur and proximal tibia. Trial components are placed, and the knee should come into full extension intraoperatively. If a flexion contracture remains, the posterior capsule should be released and possibly more distal femur resected. A lateral retinacular release is required in most hemophilic knees to permit proper tracking of the patella and 90 degrees of knee flexion. The tourniquet is deflated before the placement of implants to obtain hemostasis and then reinflated for placement of implants and wound closure. A bulky compressive knee dressing with plaster splints is placed and maintained postoperatively for 3 to 5 days, followed by CPM and active physical therapy. A manipulation under anesthesia is recommended if close to 90 degrees of flexion is not obtained between 2 and 3 weeks after surgery. Pain control after surgery in the hemophiliac is achieved with use of a continuous intravenous morphine solution administered with a "patient-controlled" pump device. Bilateral arthroplasties, if indicated, can be safely performed in one stage with significant reduction in time of hospitalization, amount of factor concentrate replaced, and overall cost.

There are now several well-documented series of total knee arthroplasty in hemophiliacs.[7, 8, 20, 24, 43, 44, 48] The various results must be interpreted with regard to many factors including prosthesis used, presence of patella resurfacing, use of metal-backed tibial components, surgeon's experience, level of factor concentrate, and rating system used (Fig. 51.8).

Figgie and colleagues[7] reviewed 19 knees in 15 patients followed up for a minimum of 5.5 years and an average of 9.5 years. Using the University Hospital Knee Rating Scale, 13 knees had a good or excellent result, whereas 6 knees were failures. The Freeman-Swanson prosthesis was used in 3 knees, the total condylar prosthesis in 12 knees, and the posterior-stabilized prosthesis in 4 knees. The tibial components were all polyethylene, and the patella was not resurfaced in the first 11 knees. Pain relief was excellent in the knees with patella resurfacing, but only the four knees with the posterior-stabilized prosthesis obtained at least 90 degrees of motion. One knee had a deep

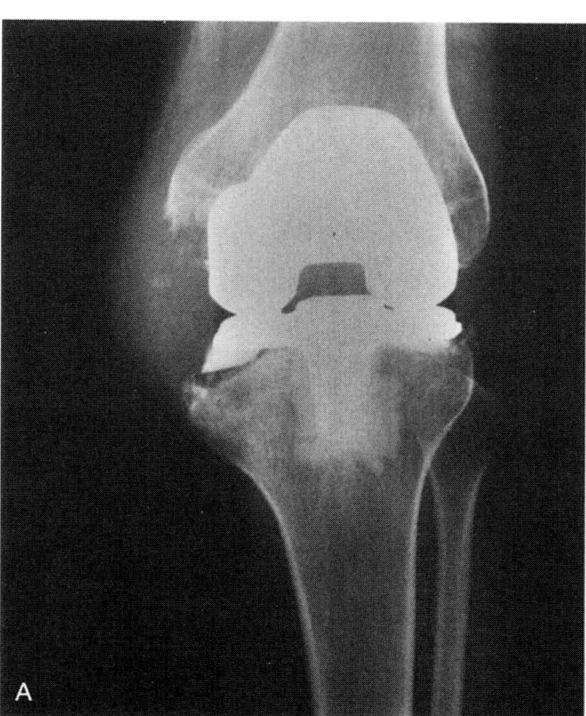

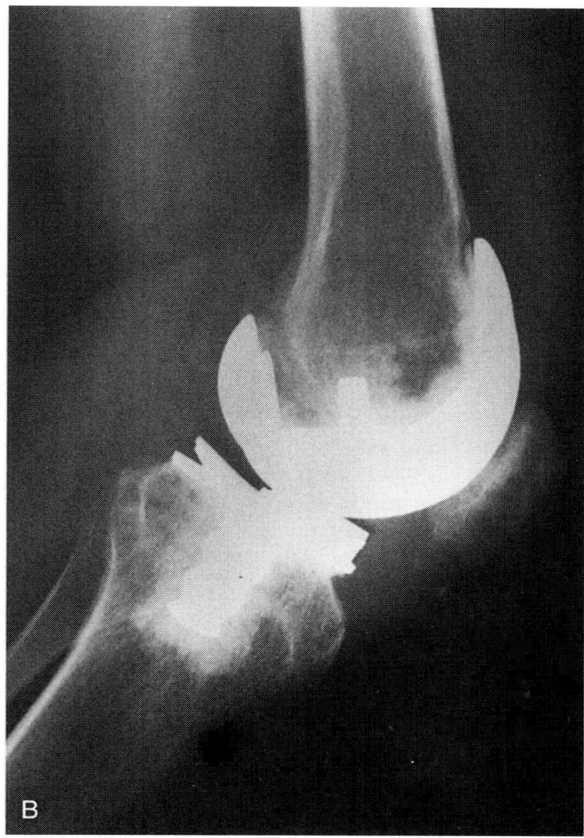

FIGURE 51.6 ➢ *A,* Anteroposterior (AP) radiograph of a 34-year-old man with continued severe pain, recurrent bleeding, and poor motion 6 months after knee arthroplasty. Note the medial soft-tissue swelling. *B,* Lateral radiograph shows that the patella was not resurfaced.

infection that required removal and arthrodesis, and two knees required revision of a loose tibial component. Two knees required additional surgery for patella resurfacing. Complications were frequent in this series and occurred in six of seven knees operated on under only 80% factor coverage. Radiographic review showed progressive tibial radiolucent lines in 13 knees, with subsidence of 3 of these knees.

In a large series from one center, this author and colleagues[20] reviewed 24 total knee arthroplasties performed in 14 patients followed up for a mean of 3.6 years (range, 2 to 9 years). A total condylar prosthesis was used in 17 knees, a posterior-stabilized prosthesis was used in 4 knees, and other prostheses were used in 3 knees. Using the Hospital for Special Surgery Knee Score System, 21 knees had a good or excellent result, with excellent relief of pain and a mean improvement in range of motion of 23 degrees. The mean flexion was 86 degrees, and the mean flexion contracture was 5 degrees in the 21 knees with total condylar or posterior-stabilized prostheses. There were two late infectious complications, requiring implant removal in one knee. There were three other complications: inhibitor development, subcutaneous hematoma, and hemolytic anemia. An incomplete radiolucent line was seen in eight knees at the bone-cement interface of the tibial component. This report describes the most successful results of total knee arthroplasty in hemophilia and probably reflects the surgical and hematological experience of the authors; the most frequent implant was the total condylar prosthesis with patella resurfacing.

Thomason and colleagues[43] reviewed the results of 23 knee arthroplasties in 15 patients followed up for a mean of 7.5 years. Seven patients, all seropositive for HIV, had died at the time of the review. There were two early and two late infections (17%). Although there was good relief of pain, the functional ability of these patients was limited. Two knees had late loosening of the prosthesis, and one was revised. Radiographic review showed migration of only two tibial components.

The largest series was a study of total knee arthroplasties performed at three hemophilia centers.[48] There were 93 knees in 76 patients with a 1- to 14-year follow-up period. The Hospital for Special Surgery Knee Rating System was used and showed a dramatic improvement in pain after surgery. The average arc of motion improved from 57 degrees to 74 degrees. The major concern in this series was the late development of deep infection in 10 knees, usually from a distant source of infection. During the study period, nine pa-

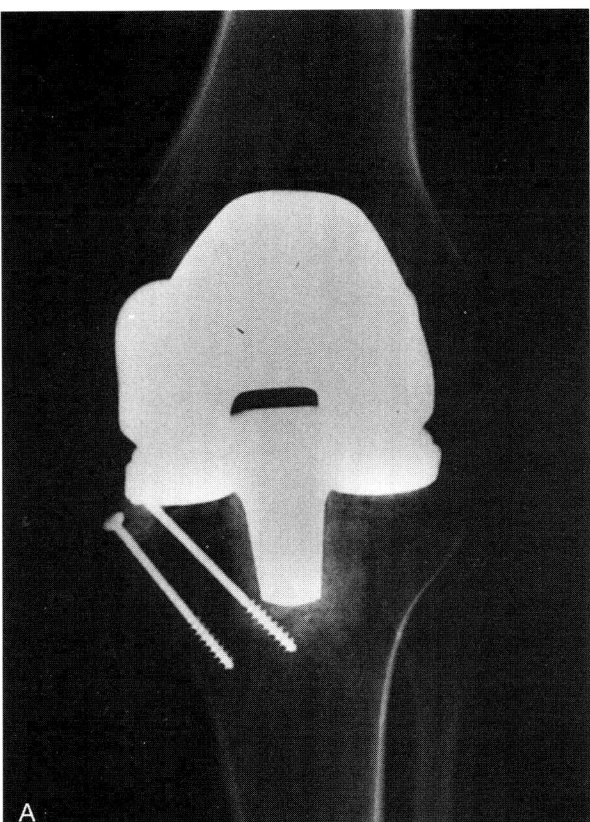

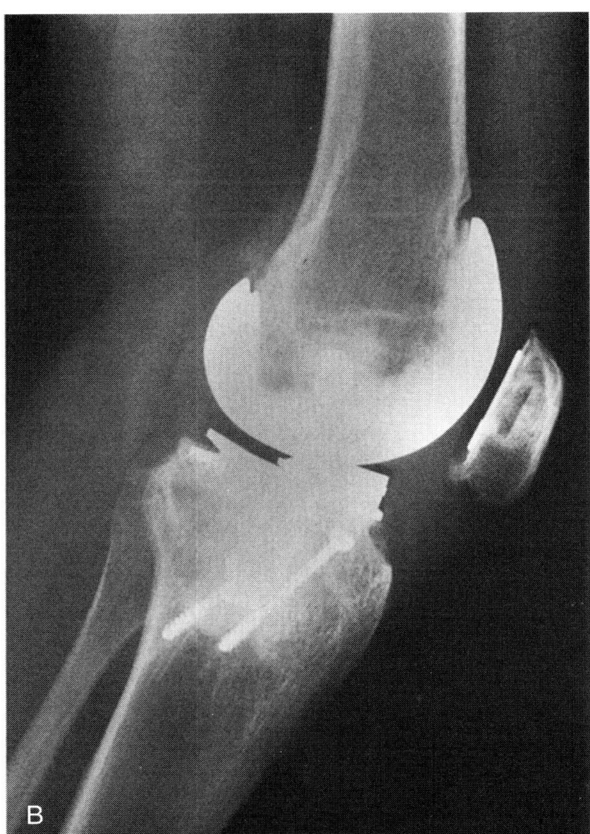

FIGURE 51.7 ➢ *A,* Two-year postoperative anteroposterior (AP) radiograph. The loose medial bone cement was replaced. The components were rigidly fixed. *B,* Two-year postoperative lateral radiograph shows the polyethylene patella prosthesis. Patient had complete relief of pain and 90 degrees of knee flexion. There has been no bleeding since patella replacement.

tients died, and seven of these died from the complication of AIDS. These same surgeons re-reviewed 134 knee arthroplasties in 1992 and documented 14 infections for a late infection rate of 10.4%.[8] The interval between surgery and infection was a mean of 39 months (range, 6 to 108 months). The most common infecting organism was *S. aureus* in seven knees. All patients were HIV positive, with a mean CD4+ count of 202/mm^3 (range, 66 to 449/mm^3). These surgeons now restrict knee arthroplasty to intelligent, cooperative patients who are aware of the risks of surgery and will rapidly treat any infection to prevent hematogenous spread to the knee.

However, Unger and colleagues[44] more recently reported the results of 26 knee arthroplasties in 15 HIV-infected hemophiliacs. The mean patient age was 33 years (range, 25 to 42 years), and all but one of the prostheses were cemented, posterior-stabilized total knee arthroplasties. Half the knees required manipulation to regain motion. All patients were alive at a mean follow-up time of 6.4 years (range, 1 to 9 years). Most importantly, in this group of patients with a mean CD4+ count of 463/mm^3, none of the knee arthroplasties developed an infection and none were revised. Six of the 15 patients received routine zidovudine-azidothymidine (AZT) prophylaxis.

Ragni and colleagues[33] reviewed the prevalence of postoperative infection following orthopedic surgery in HIV-infected hemophiliacs with CD4+ counts of 200/mm^3 or less at 115 hemophilia centers or clinics in the United States. Postoperative infection occurred in 10 (15.1%) of 66 patients who had 74 orthopedic procedures. Nine of the 10 infections involved a total knee arthroplasty, and staphylococcus was the most common organism (60%). These authors determined that the rate of postoperative infection in HIV-positive hemophiliacs with CD4+ counts of 200/mm^3 or less is 10 times higher after total knee arthroplasty than after nonarthroplasty orthopedic procedures.

The use of total knee arthroplasty can be summarized as follows:

1. The procedure can provide excellent relief of pain and can improve motion and function in patients with disabling chronic hemophilic arthropathy.
2. The optimal implant is a cemented posterior-stabilized prosthesis with patella resurfacing.
3. Bleeding complications can be minimized with close hematological supervision.
4. The rate of postoperative infection is higher in HIV positive patients with CD4+ counts of 200/mm^3 or less.

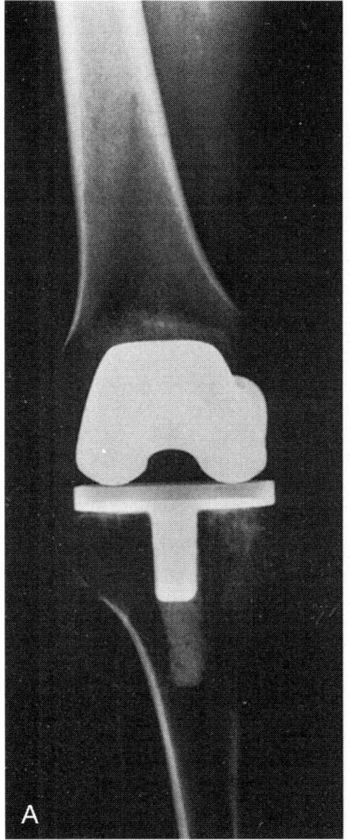

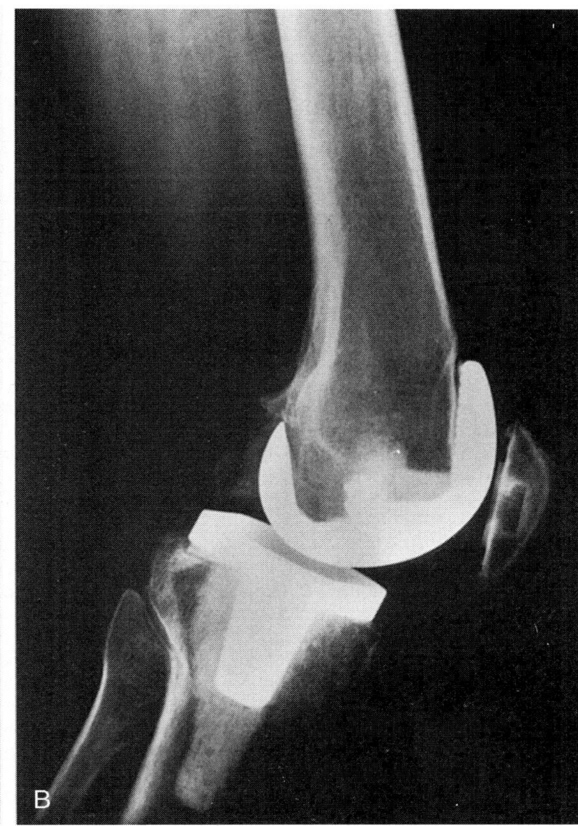

FIGURE 51.8 ➢ Five-year postoperative lateral radiographs of a total condylar prosthesis. There is a small radiolucent line at the anterior femoral cortex.

5. Careful follow-up of these patients is mandatory, with prophylactic antibiotics recommended before dental work and any other invasive procedures.
6. Remote infections must be treated early and aggressively to prevent late hematogeneous infections of the prosthetic knee.
7. The long-term survival of these patients requires an effective treatment for AIDS and its sequelae.

Arthrodesis

The indication for arthrodesis of the knee is disabling pain as a result of stage IV or stage V hemophilic arthropathy in a relatively young patient with unilateral disease who desires to perform strenuous activity. The ipsilateral hip and ankle and the contralateral knee should be relatively normal both clinically and radiographically. The patient should be between the ages of 20 and 40 years. Additional indications are postinfectious arthritis or necessary salvage of an infected total knee arthroplasty. A trial in a long-leg cast may be helpful preoperatively so that the patient realizes the advantages and disadvantages of the procedure.

Houghton and Dickson[17] reported a series of 11 arthrodeses performed over an 11-year period at Oxford. The indication was disabling pain in all cases, and the average preoperative range of motion was only 31 degrees. With their technique of arthrodesis, internal fixation was achieved with crossed 6.5-mm cancellous screws. Postoperatively, the leg was placed in a long-leg cast, which was changed at 2 weeks for suture removal. The cast was continued until there was radiographic evidence of union. In this series, all the arthrodeses united at a mean time of 5.7 months. There were three cases of delayed union, one wound hematoma, and one wound infection. These authors concluded that knee arthrodesis is a successful and definitive procedure in the hemophiliac despite the frequency of complications. At the University of North Carolina Hospitals, three knee arthrodeses, using one or two compression plates, have been performed in young hemophiliacs with high activity demands. All three procedures were successful. Knee arthrodesis will be performed very infrequently in this patient population because of the high incidence of bilateral knee involvement and the presence of other lower-extremity arthritic joints. However, in the young hemophiliac with single knee involvement, poor range of motion, and severe flexion contracture, arthrodesis is still a valuable and reasonable procedure.

References

1. Arnold WD, Hilgartner MW: Hemophilic arthropathy. J Bone Joint Surg Am 59:287, 1977.
2. Aronstam A, Browne RS, Wassef M, et al: The clinical features of early bleeding into the muscles of the lower limb in severe haemophiliacs. J Bone Joint Surg Br 65:19, 1983.

3. Boone D: Extension desubluxation hinge. In Boone D, ed: Comprehensive Management of Hemophilia. Philadelphia, FA Davis, 1976, p 169.
4. Dawson TM, Ryan PRJ, Street AM, et al: Yttrium synovectomy in haemophilic arthropathy. J Rheumatology Br 33:351, 1994.
5. Eickhoff HH, Koch W, Raderschadt G, et al: Arthroscopy for chronic hemophilic synovitis of the knee. Clin Orthop 343:58, 1997.
6. Evatt BL, Ramsey RB, Lawrence DN, et al: The acquired immunodeficiency syndrome in patients with hemophilia. Ann Intern Med 100:499, 1984.
7. Figgie MP, Goldberg VM, Figgie HE III, et al: Total knee arthroplasty for the treatment of chronic hemophilic arthropathy. Clin Orthop 248:98, 1989.
8. Gilbert MS: Hemophilia: The changing role of the orthopedic surgeon in the era of HIV infection. SE Asian J Trop Med Pub Health 24(1):30, 1993.
9. Gilbert MS, Radomisli TE: Therapeutic options in the management of hemophilic synovitis. Clin Orthop 343:88, 1997.
10. Greene WB, DeGnore LT, White GC: Orthopaedic procedures and prognosis in hemophilic patients who are seropositive for human immunodeficiency virus. J Bone Joint Surg Am 72:2, 1990.
11. Greene WB, Howes CL, Mathewson AB: Treatment of knee flexion contractures in hemophiliacs with inhibitors and pre-existent arthropathy. In Gilbert MS, Greene WB, eds: Musculoskeletal Problems in Hemophilia. New York, National Hemophilia Foundation, 1990, p 74.
12. Greene WB, McMillan CW, Warren MW: Prophylactic transfusion for hypertrophic synovitis in children with hemophilia. Clin Orthop 343:19, 1997.
13. Greene WB, Strickler EM: A modified isokinetic strengthening program for patients with severe hemophilia. Dev Med Child Neurol 25:189, 1983.
14. Greene WB, Yankaskas BC, Guilford WB: Roentgenographic classifications of hemophilic arthropathy. J Bone Joint Surg Am 71: 237, 1989.
15. Heim M, Horoszowski H, Lieberman L, et al: Methods and results of radionucleotide synovectomies. In Gilbert MS, Greene WB, eds: Musculoskeletal Problems in Hemophilia. New York, National Hemophilia Foundation, 1990, p 98.
16. Holdredge S, Isaacson J: Open synovectomy of the knee in hemophilia. In Gilbert MS, Greene WB, eds: Musculoskeletal Problems in Hemophilia. New York, National Hemophilia Foundation, 1990, p 87.
17. Houghton GR, Dickson RA: Lower limb arthrodesis in hemophilia. J Bone Joint Surg Br 60:143, 1978.
18. Johnson RP, Bobbitt DP: Five stages of joint disintegration compared with range of motion in hemophilia. Clin Orthop 201:36, 1985.
19. Klein K, Aland C, Kim H, et al: Long term follow-up of arthroscopic synovectomy for chronic hemophilic synovitis. Arthroscopy NY 3(4):231, 1987.
20. Lachiewicz PF, Inglis A, Insall JN, et al: Total knee arthroplasty in hemophilia. J Bone Joint Surg Am 67:1361, 1985.
21. Lang L: Dynasplint for knee flexion contractures. In Gilbert MS, Greene WB, eds: Musculoskeletal Problems in Hemophilia. New York, National Hemophilia Foundation, 1990, p 83.
22. Limbird T, Dennis S: Arthroscope synovectomy and continuous passive motion (CPM) in hemophiliac patients. Arthroscopy NY 3(2):74, 1987.
23. Ljung RCR: Can haemophilic arthropathy be prevented? J Haematol Br 101:215, 1998.
24. Lofqvist T, Nilsson IM, Petersson C: Orthopaedic surgery in hemophilia. 20 years' experience in Sweden. Clin Orthop 332:232, 1996.
25. Merchan ECR, Magallon M, Martin-Villar J, et al: Long term follow up of haemophilic arthropathy treated by Au-198 radiation synovectomy. Int Orthop 17:120, 1993.
26. Moll S, White GC II: Treatment of hemophilias. Curr Op Hematol 2:386, 1995.
27. Montane I, McCollough N, Chun-Yet Lian E: Synovectomy of the knee for hemophilic arthropathy. J Bone Joint Surg Am 68:210, 1986.
28. Nilsson IM, Berntorp E, Löfqvist T, et al: Twenty-five years' experience of prophylactic treatment in severe haemophilia A and B. J Internal Med 232:25, 1992.
29. Nuss R, Kilcoyne RF, Geraghty S, et al: Utility of magnetic resonance imaging for management of hemophilic arthropathy in children. J Pediatr 123:388, 1993.
30. O'Connell FD: Open surgical synovectomy of the knee in hemophilia: A long term follow-up. In Gilbert MS, Greene WB, eds: Musculoskeletal Problems in Hemophilia. New York, National Hemophilia Foundation, 1990, p 91.
31. Petterson H, Ahlberg A, Nilsson IM: A radiographic classification of hemophilic arthropathy. Clin Orthop 149:152, 1980.
32. Post M, Watta G, Telfer M: Synovectomy in hemophilic arthropathy. Clin Orthop 202:139, 1986.
33. Ragni MV, Crossett LS, Herndon JH. Postoperative infection following orthopaedic surgery in human immunodeficiency virus-infected hemophilics with CD4 counts $\leq 200/mm^3$. J Arthroplasty 10:716, 1995.
34. Ribbans WJ, Giangrande P, Beeton K: Conservative treatment of hemarthrosis for prevention of hemophilic synovitis. Clin Orthop 343:12, 1997.
35. Rodriguez-Merchan EC: Pathogenesis, early diagnosis, and prophylaxis for chronic hemophilic synovitis. Clin Orthop 343:6, 1997.
36. Rodriguez-Merchan EC, Galindo E, Ladreda JMM, et al: Surgical synovectomy in haemophilic arthropathy of the knee. Int Orthop 18:38, 1994.
37. Rodriguez-Merchan EC, Magallon M, Galindo E: Joint débridement for haemophilic arthropathy of the knee. Int Orthop 18: 135, 1994.
38. Roosendaal G, Vianen ME, Wenting MJG, et al: Iron deposits and catabolic properties of synovial tissue from patients with haemophilia. J Bone Joint Surg Br 80:540, 1998.
39. Stein H, Dickson RA: Reversed dynamic slings for knee flexion contractures in the hemophiliac. J Bone Joint Surg Am 57:282, 1975.
40. Stein H, Duthie RB: The pathogenesis of chronic haemophilic arthropathy. J Bone Joint Surg Br 63:601, 1989.
41. Storti E, Ascari E: Surgical and chemical synovectomy. Ann NY Acad Sci 240:316, 1975.
42. Teigland JC, Tjonnfjord GE, Evensen SA, et al: Synovectomy for haemophilic arthropathy: 6-21 years of follow-up in 16 patients. J Intern Med 235:239, 1994.
43. Thomason HC III, Wilson FC, Lachiewicz PF, et al: Knee arthroplasty in hemophilic arthropathy. Clin Orthop 360:169, 1999.
44. Unger AS, Kessler CM, Lewis RJ: Total knee arthroplasty in human immunodeficiency virus-infected hemophilics. J Arthroplasty 10:448, 1995.
45. White GC: Disorders of blood coagulation. In Stern JH, ed: Internal Medicine. 3rd ed. Boston, Little, Brown, 1990, p 1048.
46. Wiedel J: Arthroscopic synovectomy for chronic hemophilic synovitis of the knee. Arthroscopy NY 1(3):205, 1985.
47. Wiedel JD: Arthroscopic synovectomy of the knee in hemophilia. Clin Orthop 328:46, 1996.
48. Wiedel J, Luck J, Gilbert M: Total knee arthroplasty in the patient with hemophilia: Evaluation of the long-term results. In Gilbert MS, Greene WB, eds: Musculoskeletal Problems in Hemophilia. New York, National Hemophilia Foundation, 1990, p 152.
49. Wilkins RM, Wiedel JD: Septic arthritis of the knee in a hemophiliac. J Bone Joint Surg Am 65:267, 1983.
50. Wilson DJ, McLardy-Smith PD, Woodham CH, et al: Diagnonstic ultrasound in haemophilia. J Bone Joint Surg Br 69:103, 1987.
51. Yulish BS, Lieberman JM, Strandjord SE, et al: Hemophilic arthropathy: Assessment with MR imaging. Radiology 164:759, 1987.
52. Zuckerman J, Solomon G, Shortkroff S, et al: Principles of radiation synovectomy. In Gilbert MS, Greene WB, eds: Musculoskeletal Problems in Hemophilia. New York, National Hemophilia Foundation, 1990, p 93.

52

HIV Infection and Its Relationship to Knee Disorders

ALISON SELLECK • HENRY MASUR

INTRODUCTION

When caring for patients infected with human immunodeficiency virus (HIV), orthopedic surgeons need to be familiar with the complex nature of HIV infection to make rational decisions regarding diagnosis and treatment of both HIV-related and HIV-unrelated orthopedic and rheumatic conditions. In addition, they must be knowledgeable about modes of transmission of HIV and universal precautions to protect patients, colleagues, and themselves from exposure. In the event of exposure, they need to be familiar with the risk of transmission associated with certain events as well as the current recommendations for postexposure chemoprophylaxis to make informed decisions regarding prophylaxis treatment. Finally, all health care providers should be familiar with and open to discussing prevention with both HIV-infected and noninfected patients because every encounter with a health care provider can have an impact on patient understanding and behavior.

The Centers for Disease Control and Prevention (CDC) estimates that between 650,000 and 900,000 people are living with HIV infection in the United States.[17] As of June 1999, there have been 711,344 reported cases of acquired immunodeficiency syndrome (AIDS). Of these, 60% have died.[29] Moreover, the estimated annual rate of new infections in this country is approximately 40,000 per year.[18] Although these statistics are striking, there is some encouraging news. In general, HIV-infected individuals in developed countries are living longer than in previous years. The age-adjusted death rate from HIV infection in the United States dropped an estimated 42% from 1996 to 1997.[29] This decline in mortality can be attributed to use of potent combination antiretroviral medications, to establishment of guidelines for the management of antiretroviral therapy, to treatment and prophylaxis of opportunistic infections, to establishment of prevention programs, and to increasing expertise in the care of HIV-infected individuals.

Given that the epidemic continues to spread and that people infected with HIV are living longer, nearly all practicing physicians will encounter patients with HIV in their practice. Natural history studies indicate that HIV-infected individuals often live about 8 to 12 years from the time of initial infection to the time of their first major AIDS manifestation.[1, 90] With the use of potent antiretroviral regimens and prophylaxis for opportunistic infections, many individuals currently infected with HIV are living longer and healthier lives.[41, 52] They are participating in activities for fitness and recreation as well as in competitive high school, college, or professional sports. Furthermore, weight training to build lean muscle mass is considered a standard component of treatment and prevention of wasting syndrome in HIV-infected individuals. Consequently, in addition to HIV-related musculoskeletal conditions, these patients experience trauma and degenerative processes just like their uninfected counterparts. Thus, careful evaluation and familiarity with the complex nature of HIV infection will help ensure accurate assessment and appropriate treatment for HIV-infected individuals presenting with orthopedic and rheumatic conditions.

HIV VIROLOGY

HIV-1, HIV-2, human T-cell lymphotropic virus-I (HTLV-I), and HTLV-II are the four known human retroviruses. HIV-1 is by far the most important retrovirus of humans currently known and has been established as the causative agent of AIDS. Retroviruses are a group of RNA viruses that produce reverse transcriptase, an enzyme that converts viral RNA to proviral DNA. This proviral DNA is then integrated into the chromosomal DNA of the host cell.

The hallmark of HIV disease is a profound immunodeficiency resulting primarily from a progressive quantitative and qualitative deficiency of helper T lymphocytes. This subset of helper T cells is defined by the presence of the CD4+ molecule on its surface. Monocytes, macrophages, and follicular dendritic cells express the CD4+ molecule on their surface as well. This CD4+ molecule, together with a coreceptor, serves as the primary receptor for HIV. Although a number of both direct and indirect mechanisms that contribute to CD4+ T lymphocyte depletion and dysfunction have been identified in vitro, a full understanding of the manner in which HIV infection results in a progressive decline in CD4+ lymphocyte counts and immune function remains unclear.

HIV infection is persistent and associated with an extended period during which the usual clinical features of the disease are not apparent. Infection stimulates an immune response to HIV, which initially appears to hinder viral replication but fails to eradicate the virus.[47, 62, 69] Although current potent combination antiretroviral therapy has been shown to slow the decline of immune function,[52] nearly all infected individuals will ultimately experience a progressive deterioration of immune function, resulting in susceptibility to HIV-related complications and opportunistic infections.[53, 64]

CLINICAL MANIFESTATIONS OF HIV

The clinical manifestations of HIV infection include (1) an acute syndrome associated with primary infection, (2) a prolonged asymptomatic state, and (3) a period of profound immunosuppression during which clinical manifestations occur. Natural history studies of HIV infection in individuals not receiving antiretroviral therapy or *Pneumocystis carinii* pneumonia prophylaxis indicate that the average time from initial infection to an AIDS-defining diagnosis is about 10 years and that the time from an AIDS-defining diagnosis to death is about 1 year, although significant variation exists.[1, 90] However, patients receiving potent antiretroviral combinations and aggressive prophylaxis and treatment of opportunistic infections are living longer.[41, 52]

With few exceptions, the level of CD4+ T cells in the blood decreases gradually and progressively in HIV-infected individuals. The rate of CD4+ T cell count decline and the absolute viral burden have been shown to correlate with the time to development of clinical manifestations.[86] Patients often remain asymptomatic during this progressive decline. Active viral replication and progressive immunological impairment occur throughout the course of HIV infection in most patients, even during the clinically latent stage.[91] CD4+ T cell dysfunction has been demonstrated in patients early in the course of infection, even when the CD4+ T cell count is in the low-normal range. Most AIDS-defining opportunistic infections and malignancies occur in the advanced stage of disease. Neurological disease, including peripheral neuropathy, and Kaposi's sarcoma, on the other hand, have been associated with a varied degree of immunodeficiency.

Three basic mechanisms are thought to underlie the production of disease in HIV infection: depletion and functional impairment of CD4+ T lymphocytes, resulting in susceptibility to opportunistic infections and malignancies; development of immune complex–mediated events such as glomerulonephritis or thrombocytopenia; and damage to specific organs such as the heart, brain, peripheral nerves, and lungs because of direct or indirect retroviral effects. The time frame in which these events unfold and the precise disease manifestation in an individual are highly variable, impossible to predict, and presumably the result of a complex interaction between viral factors and host defense mechanisms. Viral factors include size of the inoculum, strain-specific virulence, and viral replicative accuracy and efficiency. Host factors that may predispose to disease progression, such as age at the time of infection, route of transmission, sex, ethnicity, and coinfection with other infectious agents, are less well defined and remain to be conclusively determined for all patient groups.

Primary HIV Infection

It is estimated that 50% to 70% of individuals infected with HIV experience an acute clinical syndrome approximately 3 to 6 weeks after acquisition of infection. The syndrome is usually similar to acute infectious mononucleosis.[48, 75, 107] Clinical manifestations may include generalized symptoms, such as fever, fatigue, malaise, pharyngitis, headache, photophobia, arthralgias, myalgias, anorexia, nausea, vomiting, and diarrhea, and neurological complications such as meningitis, encephalitis, peripheral neuropathy, and myelopathy. Findings may include a morbilliform rash, mucocutaneous ulcerations, thrush, generalized lymphadenopathy, hepatosplenomegaly, elevated transaminases, and leukopenia with atypical lymphocytes. The severity and constellation of manifestations vary. The illness is self-limited with resolution of symptoms within days to weeks. Seroconversion documented by enzyme-linked immunosorbent screening assay (ELISA) and verified by Western blot analysis occurs within 3 to 12 weeks following acquisition of HIV in 99% of exposed persons.[68, 75] Well-documented cases of seroconversion more than 12 weeks after infection are extremely rare.

The clinical manifestations of acute HIV syndrome coincide with a rapid rise in the plasma level of viral RNA and p24 antigen, widespread dissemination of virus, and drop in the CD4+ count.[57] The associated immunodeficiency at this stage results from both reduced numbers and functional impairment of CD4+ T cells and can be accompanied by opportunistic infections. An immune response subsequently develops, leading to decrease in the plasma level of viral RNA, increase in the CD4+ count, and gradual resolution of symptoms. In most patients, the CD4+ count remains mildly depressed for a period of time before progressively declining. In some patients, the CD4+ count returns to normal range, though some qualitative dysfunction remains. A small percentage of patients manifest a fulminant immunological and clinical deterioration after primary infection and may die within 1 to 2 years of acquiring HIV. However, in the majority of patients, primary infection is followed by a prolonged period of clinical latency.

Asymptomatic Infection

The asymptomatic stage of HIV infection is referred to as clinical latency. Active viral replication continues during this asymptomatic period. Although viral loads in many patients, particularly those on potent antiretroviral combinations, may be determined to be below the level of detection in the blood using currently available tests, it has been shown that the virus is still replicating in other reservoirs such as lymphoid tissue.[91]

The rate of disease progression is directly correlated

with HIV RNA levels. A patient with high levels of HIV RNA will progress to symptomatic disease faster than will a patient with low levels of HIV RNA.[13] Although the length of time from initial infection to development of clinical disease varies greatly, the median time is approximately 10 years in the absence of antiretroviral therapy or *P. carinii* pneumonia prophylaxis. Multiple studies have shown that progression to AIDS, frequency of opportunistic infections, and survival correlate directly with CD4+ counts.[14, 23, 82, 93, 104]

The term "long-term survivor" refers to an untreated individual who remains alive for 10 to 15 years after initial infection. A long-term nonprogressor is an individual who has been infected with HIV for 10 or more years, whose CD4+ counts have remained in the normal range despite lack of antiretroviral therapy, and who generally has a low viral burden.

Early Symptomatic Disease, AIDS, and Opportunistic Infections

Once the CD4+ cell count falls below 500, patients often begin to develop signs and symptoms of clinical illness. Common clinical features of early symptomatic disease include vulvovaginal and oropharyngeal candidiasis (thrush), oral hairy leukoplakia, persistent generalized lymphadenopathy, reactivation herpes zoster (shingles), recurrent herpes simplex, aphthous ulcers, molluscum contagiosum, condyloma acuminatum, and thrombocytopenia. Individuals may also experience constitutional symptoms such as persistent fever to 38.5°C or diarrhea lasting more than 1 month. The occurrence of these events in an otherwise asymptomatic individual should prompt consideration of underlying HIV infection.

Opportunistic infections are generally encountered when the CD4+ T cell count declines below 200. Many of the organisms that cause opportunistic infections, such as *P. carinii, Mycobacterium avium* complex (MAC), and cytomegalovirus (CMV), are ubiquitous in nature and do not ordinarily cause disease in the absence of a compromised immune system. Opportunistic infections can also be caused by common bacterial and mycobacterial pathogens. Opportunistic infections are the leading cause of morbidity and mortality in HIV-infected individuals. With the development of more effective management of HIV and more aggressive treatment and prophylaxis of opportunistic infections, the clinical spectrum of disease caused by opportunistic organisms will continue to change.

The median time from the onset of severe immunosuppression (CD4+ count <200) to an AIDS-defining diagnosis (by 1987 criteria) is 12 to 18 months in persons not receiving antiretroviral therapy.[30] Studies have shown that in patients receiving monotherapy with zidovudine (AZT), this time frame was delayed by 9 to 10 months.[63] The onset from severe immunosupression to an AIDS-defining illness in individuals on highly potent antiretroviral combinations has been further delayed to more than 24 months.[52]

In 1993, the CDC revised the AIDS Surveillance Case Definition to include all HIV-infected individuals with a CD4+ cell count of fewer than 200. In addition, recurrent bacterial pneumonia, invasive cervical cancer, and pulmonary tuberculosis were added to the 1987 list of AIDS-defining illness (Table 52.1). The major AIDS-defining diagnosis and the major identifiable cause of death in patients with AIDS is *P. carinii* pneumonia. The risk of infection with *P. carinii* is inversely correlated with CD4+ T cell counts. *P. carinii* pneumonia is most frequently encountered in patients with CD4+ cell counts of fewer than 200 and in those who have had a previous episode of *P. carinii* pneumonia. *P. carinii* pneumonia prophylaxis is recommended in any HIV-infected individual who has experienced a previous episode of *P. carinii* pneumonia or has a CD4+ T cell count of fewer than 200/μL, oral candidiasis, or unexplained fevers for more than 2 weeks.[21]

The most common opportunistic bacterial infection encountered in HIV-infected persons is disseminated mycobacterial infection, particularly with MAC. Infection with MAC is a late complication of HIV infection and is usually seen when CD4+ T cell counts drop below 100/μL. Other common opportunistic infections encountered in advanced stages of HIV infection include toxoplasmosis, CMV retinitis and colitis, *M. tuberculosis,* and superficial and systemic fungal infections.

TRANSMISSION OF HIV

HIV is transmitted between humans by the exchange of body fluids. There are three principle routes: sexual contact, parenteral inoculation, and vertical transmission from an infected mother to her child. Body fluids identified as potentially significant sources of HIV exposure include blood, semen (including pre-ejaculatory fluid), vaginal secretions, breast milk, cerebrospinal fluid, synovial fluid, pleural fluid, peritoneal fluid, pericardial fluid, amniotic fluid, and any body fluid containing blood.[42, 83] Those body fluids considered to represent minimal risk for transmission of HIV include feces, nasal secretions, sputum, saliva, sweat, tears, urine, and vomitus, unless contaminated with visible blood. The quantity of virus isolated from a fluid varies by site and stage of HIV infection. Viral burden in blood and other fluids is highest during acute infection before seroconversion,[62, 69] and in the late stages of HIV disease.[2] HIV has not been shown to be transmitted by casual contact or by insect vectors such as mosquitoes.

Sexual Transmission

Throughout the world, the predominant mode of HIV transmission is through sexual contact. Historically, homosexual contact has accounted for the preponderance of sexual transmission in developed countries. In developing countries, most sexual transmission of HIV is through heterosexual contact. In the United States, aggressive educational programs targeting high-risk behavior in homosexual men has resulted in an increase in "safer sex" practices and a decline in the incidence

TABLE 52.1 REVISED CLASSIFICATION SYSTEM FOR HIV INFECTION AND EXPANDED AIDS SURVEILLANCE CASE DEFINITION FOR ADOLESCENTS AND ADULTS*

	Clinical Categories		
CD4+ T cell Categories	*(A) Asymptomatic, Acute (Primary) HIV or PGL†*	*(B) Symptomatic, Not (A) or (C) Conditions§*	*(C) AIDS-Indicator Conditions¶*
(1) ≥500/μL	A1	B1	C1
(2) 200–4999/μL	A2	B2	C2
(3) <200/μL AIDS-indicator T cell count	A3	B3	C3

* The shaded cells illustrate the expanded AIDS surveillance case definition. Persons with AIDS-indicator conditions (Category C) as well as those with CD4+ T lymphocyte counts <200/μL (Categories A3 or B3) will be reportable as AIDS cases in the United States and Territories, effective January 1, 1993.
† PGL = persistent generalized lymphadenopathy. Clinical Category A includes acute (primary) HIV infection.
§ See text for discussion.
¶ See Appendix B.

Clinical Categories

The clinical categoires of HIV infection are defined as follows:

Category A

Category A consists of one or more of the conditions listed below in an adolescent or adult (≥13 years) with documented HIV infection. Conditions listed in Categories B and C must not have occurred.

- Asymptomatic HIV infection
- Persistent generalized lymphadenopathy
- Acute (primary) HIV infection with accompanying illness or history of acute HIV infection

Category B

Category B consists of symptomatic conditions in an HIV-infected adolescent or adult that are not included among conditions listed in clinical Category C and that meet at least one of the following criteria: (a) the conditions are attributed to HIV infection or are indicative of a defect in cell-mediated immunity; or (b) the conditions are considered by physicians to have a clinical course or to require management that is complicated by HIV infection. **Examples** of conditions in clinical Category B include, **but are not limited to, the following:**

- Bacillary angiomatosis
- Candidiasis, oropharyngeal (thrush)
- Candidiasis, vulvovaginal; persistent, frequent, or poorly responsive to therapy
- Cervical dysplasia (moderate or severe)/cervical carcinoma in situ
- Consitutional symptoms, such as fever (38.5°C) or diarrhea lasting >1 month
- Hairy leukoplakia, oral
- Herpes zoster (shingles), involving at least two distinct episodes or more than one dermatome
- Idiopathic thrombocytopenic purpura
- Listeriosis
- Pelvic inflammatory disease, particularly if complicated by tubo-ovarian abscess
- Peripheral neuropathy

For classification purposes, Category B conditions take precedence over those in Category A. For example, someone previously treated for oral or persistent vaginal candidiasis (and who has not developed a Category C disease) who is now asymptomatic should be classified in clinical Category B.

Category C

Category C includes the clinical conditions listed in the AIDS surveillance case definition (Appendix B). For classification purposes, once a Category C condition has occurred, the person will remain in Category C.

Appendix B. Conditions Included in the 1993 AIDS Surveillance Case Definition

- Candidiasis of bronchi, trachea, or lungs
- Candidiasis, esophageal
- Cervical cancer, invasive*
- Coccidioidomycosis, disseminated or extrapulmonary
- Cryptococcosis, extrapulmonary
- Cryptosporidiosis, chronic intestinal (>1 month's duration)
- Cytomegalovirus disease (other than liver, spleen, or nodes)
- Cytomegalovirus retinitis (with loss or vision)
- Encephalopathy, HIV related
- Herpes simplex: chronic ulcer(s) (>1 month's duration), or bronchitis, pneumonitis, esophagitis
- Histoplasmosis, disseminated or extrapulmonary
- Isosporiasis, chronic intestinal (>1 month's duration)
- Kaposi's sarcoma
- Lymphoma, Burkitt's (or equivalent term)
- Lymphoma, immunoblastic (or equivalent term)
- Lymphoma, primary, of brain
- *Mycobacterium avium* complex or *M. kansasii,* disseminated or extrapulmonary
- *M. tuberculosis,* any site (pulmonary* or extrapulmonary)
- *Mycobacterium,* other species or unidentified species, disseminated or extrapulmonary
- *Pneumocystis carinii* pneumonia
- Pneumonia, recurrent*
- Progressive multifocal leukoencephalopathy
- *Salmonella* septicemia, recurrent
- Toxoplasmosis of brain
- Wasting syndrome due to HIV

* Added in the 1993 expansion of the AIDS surveillance case definition.
AIDS = acquired immunodeficiency syndrome; HIV = human immunodeficiency virus.
From MMWR 41(RR17).

of new cases in this group. On the other hand, the incidence of new cases of AIDS contracted through heterosexual contact is increasing in the United States, particularly among women, African Americans, and teens and young adults.[29]

Regardless of the mode of sexual contact, it is evident that both behavioral and biological factors contribute to the transmission of HIV infection.[26] Transmission of HIV is strongly associated with receptive anal intercourse. Even when intact, the thin, fragile rectal mucosa offers little protection against infection from deposited semen. Moreover, anal intercourse as well as other sexual practices involving the rectum, such as "fisting" and insertion of objects, traumatizes the rectal mucosa, thereby increasing the likelihood of infection during receptive anal intercourse.

HIV can be transmitted to either partner through vaginal intercourse. There is an estimated 20-fold greater chance of transmission of HIV from a man to a woman than from a woman to a man though vaginal intercourse. This is thought to be due in part to the prolonged exposure to infected seminal fluid of the vaginal, cervical, and endometrial mucosa. Transmission of HIV is also closely associated with genital ulceration. Important cofactors in the transmission of HIV include infection with herpes simplex virus, *Treponema pallidum* (syphilis), and *Haemophilus ducreyi* (chancroid).[26, 72] Similarly, genital inflammatory conditions such as cervicitis, urethritis, and epididymitis associated with gonorrhea and chlamydia have been linked with transmission of HIV. Although oral sex appears to be a less efficient mode of transmission of HIV, it is a misperception that oral sex is a form of "safe sex." HIV transmission has been reported as resulting solely from receptive fellatio and insertive cunnilingus. The risk appears to be increased by the presence of oral ulcerations and gum bleeding.

Alcohol consumption and drug use have been associated with the transmission of HIV as well. The disinhibition and poor judgment that accompany alcohol and drug use often lead to unsafe sexual behavior. Other important risk factors for infection include number of sexual contacts, sex with a prostitute, being a prostitute, being a sex partner of an infected person, being a sex partner of an intravenous drug user, and having a history of other sexually transmitted diseases, particularly ulcerative genital disease.[72]

Parenteral Transmission and Intravenous Drug Use

HIV infection in intravenous drug users is highly prevalent throughout the world. Risk factors for HIV infection in intravenous drug users include frequency of injection, number of persons with whom needles are shared, anonymous sharing of needles and other paraphernalia, cocaine use, and use of injection drugs in geographic locations with a high prevalence of HIV infection, such as inner-city areas.[44] This population appears to be functioning as the primary reservoir for the rapid spread of HIV infection into the heterosexual population throughout the world.[28, 29, 36, 79, 94]

Although the risk of infection is highest with direct sharing of needles, the sharing of drug paraphernalia, such as syringes, water, "spoons" and "cookers" used to dissolve drugs in water and to heat drug solutions, and "cottons" (small pieces of cotton or cigarette filters used to filter out particles that could block the needle), can also increase the risk of transmission. Street sellers of syringes and needles often repackage them and sell them as "sterile." Needle or syringe sharing for any use, including skin popping and injecting anabolic steroids, can put one at risk for HIV and other blood-borne infections, such as hepatitis B and C.

Parenteral Transmission and Blood Products

Transmission of HIV infection by blood product transfusion was a major problem in the United States from the late 1970s until 1985, when a serological test for HIV was developed. Unfortunately, the use of pooled clotting factor had already resulted in widespread infection among hemophiliacs. In general, persons with factor VIII deficiency (hemophilia A) have greater factor requirements than do persons with factor IX deficiency (hemophilia B, Christmas disease) and hence have a higher prevalence of HIV infection.[43]

In the United States and in most developed countries, the risk of transmission of HIV infection by transfused blood and blood products is extremely small. From data obtained in the early 1990s, it has been estimated that routine screening fails to detect HIV infection in 1 per 450,000 to 660,000 blood donations.[76] Measures such as testing donated blood for HIV, syphilis, and hepatitis B and C, as well as excluding high-risk donors based on self-reported risk factors, account for this small risk. The majority of false negatives are attributed to donation during the "window period" when the donor is infectious but before HIV antibodies are detectable. In 1995, the U.S. Food and Drug Administration (FDA) recommended that all donated blood and plasma also be screened for HIV-1 p24 antigen. Consequently, the risk of transmission from a single donation of blood is thought to be even smaller than previously estimated. Although p24 antigen testing is very specific, it has failed to detect infection in a few cases in which HIV polymerase chain reaction (PCR) testing was positive. It is anticipated that molecular testing of donated blood will further decrease the risk of transmission. Currently, donated blood is screened for both HIV-1 and HIV-2 antibodies. There have been no reported cases of transmission of HIV-2 (via donated blood) in the United States to date.

Transmission rates in hemophiliacs have been further reduced by the heat treatment of blood products and the development of recombinant factor. Similarly, because the virus is either inactivated or removed during processing, hyperimmune gamma globulin, hepatitis B immune globulin, plasma-derived hepatitis B vaccine, and Rh_0 immune globulin have not been associated with HIV transmission. Nonetheless, in many developing countries, blood transfusions remain an important source of ongoing transmission because of lack of serological screening as a result of economic and technical constraints.

Occupational Transmission of HIV

Parenteral transmission of HIV has emerged as a major concern for health care workers. All well-verified cases of occupationally acquired HIV infection have involved exposure to blood, bloody body fluids, or HIV viral cultures. The majority of exposures resulted from needlestick injuries or cuts. Results of several large studies suggest that the risk of transmission from an infected source with the usual needlestick injury (hollow-bore needle, in contrast to a solid-bore suture needle) approximates 1 per 300 or 0.3%.[65] A retrospective case-control study of occupational HIV infection reported that an increased risk of seroconversion following percutaneous exposure to HIV-infected blood is associated with exposures involving a deep injury; a relatively large quantity of blood, such as with a device visibly contaminated with the patient's blood; or a procedure with a needle placed directly in a vein or artery.[16] In addition, an increased risk of seroconversion is associated with exposures to blood from patients with high viral loads. Presumably, this increased risk is due to the higher titer of HIV in the blood as well as to the presence of more virulent strains of virus. On the other hand, a decreased risk of seroconversion was associated with AZT postexposure prophylaxis.[16] In simulated needlesticks, the use of gloves appears to decrease the amount of blood transferred.[80] Finally, a temporal relationship between implementation of universal precautions and decrease in percutaneous and nonparenteral exposures has been shown.[9, 55]

Although seroconversion has been noted after mucocutaneous exposure to infected blood, the efficiency of transmission by mucocutaneous exposure is substantially less than that with percutaneous needle injury. The risk of seroconversion after mucous membrane exposure has been estimated to be 0.09%.[29] The few documented mucocutaneous exposures involved transmission through mucous membranes or abraded skin. There have been no documented transmissions through intact skin.[59, 65] Factors that might be associated with mucocutaneous transmission of HIV include exposure to an unusually large volume of blood, prolonged contact, and potential portal of entry.[59]

As of June 1998, 54 cases of occupationally acquired HIV infection in health care workers in the United States have been confirmed.[19, 29] An additional 133 health care workers have been classified as having possible occupationally acquired HIV. In these cases, the health care workers have a history of occupational exposure to blood, other body fluids, or HIV-infected laboratory material and report no other identifiable risk factors for HIV infection but do not have documentation of a negative HIV test result before the exposure. Of the 54 confirmed cases, nurses and laboratory technicians are highly represented, and all transmissions involve blood or bloody body fluid except for three involving laboratory workers exposed to HIV viral cultures. Of these 54 confirmed cases, 46 are associated with percutaneous exposures, 5 with mucous membrane exposures, and 2 with both percutaneous and mucous membrane exposures. In one case, the route of exposure is unknown. The source specimen was blood in 49 cases, bloody pleural fluid in 1 case, unspecified fluid in 1 case, and concentrated virus stocks in 3 cases.

Thus far, there have been no confirmed cases of occupationally acquired HIV infection in surgeons or in any personnel after percutaneous exposure with a suture needle. In an anonymous seroprevalence survey of 3420 orthopedic surgeons, 39% of respondents reported percutaneous exposure to patient blood, usually involving a suture needle. Seventy-five percent of these respondents practiced in an area with a relatively high prevalence of HIV infection. 0.8% reported one or more injuries from a sharp object from an HIV-infected patient during the previous year. 3.2% reported a percutaneous injury at some point during their career from a patient known to have HIV infection or AIDS. No cases of occupational infection were identified.[108] However, considerable underreporting of occupational percutaneous injury exists.

Orthopedic procedures, in general, have been shown to have a relatively low percutaneous injury rate compared with other surgical subspecialty procedures. In one observational study, total knee replacement and open reduction with internal fixation of the hip were shown to have percutaneous exposure rates of 8% and 7%, respectively. All other orthopedic procedures were shown to have a combined percutaneous exposure rate of 2%.[109] The incidence of skin and mucous membrane contact with blood has been estimated to be 16.7 contacts per 100 orthopedic procedures.[108] Hand contact has been most closely associated with the duration of the procedure, whereas body contact has been associated with the estimated blood loss.[110]

Universal precautions recommended by the CDC to protect health care workers from contact with potentially infected body fluids emphasize barrier techniques to prevent skin and mucous membrane exposure from contacting blood and other body fluids.[22, 32] The major criticism of barrier precautions is that they often fail to prevent injuries with sharp instruments (e.g., needlestick punctures, cuts), which are the source of more than 80% of confirmed cases of occupationally acquired HIV infection.[43] Nonetheless, as noted above, the use of gloves appears to decrease the amount of blood transferred in simulated needlesticks, while the implementation of universal precautions has been temporally related to a decrease in the frequency of needlesticks.[9, 80] In 1992, the U.S. Occupational Safety and Health Administration (OSHA) established mandatory regulations requiring national standards for the prevention of occupational exposure to hepatitis B and HIV. These include guidelines for disposal of sharp instruments such as not recapping needles and using designated boxes. A review of the circumstances of reported exposures suggests that the risks of transmission could have been decreased or prevented if universal precautions and OSHA guidelines had been followed. This observation is supported by Tokars et al in their observational study of percutaneous injuries during surgery, in which injuries often occurred when fingers were used instead of instruments to hold tissue or suture needles during suturing or when instruments were being handled by a coworker.[109]

Although exposure to HIV is a significant concern for health care workers, exposure to other pathogens such as hepatitis B and C, *M. tuberculosis,* and, less commonly, HTLV-I and HTLV-II should also be considered. In fact, the risk of hepatitis B and C infection after percutaneous injury ranges from 2% to 40% and from 3% to 10%, respectively, compared with 0.3% for HIV.[59] It has been projected that of the approximately 1000 health care workers infected with hepatitis B in 1994, 22 will die as a result of infection.[101] Consequently, it is advisable for all health care workers to be vaccinated for hepatitis B. Moreover, hepatitis C, the most common chronic blood-borne infection in the United States, results in chronic infection in 75% to 85% of infected individuals.[34] There is no vaccine available for hepatitis C.

In addition to protecting health care workers from HIV and other blood-borne pathogens, universal precautions protect patients from infected health care personnel, especially those performing invasive procedures. Few controversies involving HIV infection have generated as much media or public-sector commentary as the highly publicized incident of HIV transmission from a Florida dentist to at least six of his patients.[39, 40, 45] Documentation that the dentist was the source of infection was based on the lack of alternative substantive risk factors in several of his patients, the fact that all patients underwent multiple procedures, including extractions following the onset of the dentist's symptomatic disease, and the genetic analysis of HIV strains. Although it is evident that the dentist was the source of infection in these patients, the mechanism of transmission remains unclear.

More recently, Lot et al reported a case of probable transmission of HIV from an orthopedic surgeon to a patient in France.[78] After the surgeon was diagnosed with HIV in 1995, serological tests were obtained from 983 patients of the infected surgeon. One patient tested positive. This patient, a 67-year-old woman, had no other identifiable risks for HIV exposure. She tested negative for HIV before placement of a total hip prosthesis with bone graft. She subsequently underwent hip aspiration and removal of the prosthesis by the same surgeon. She received two units of packed red blood cells after the third procedure. However, the donor of the bone graft and both units of blood have tested negative for HIV infection. The patient had no reported sexual exposure to HIV. In addition, the surgeon reported a high frequency of intraoperative injury. Molecular analysis indicated that the viral sequences obtained from the surgeon and patient are closely related.[11] Although the patient did undergo noninvasive teeth whitening in Indonesia, where HIV infection is prevalent, and the mechanism and date of transmission could not be established with certainty, it appears as if the most likely source of infection was the surgeon.[60]

As of January 1995, retrospective investigations of 22,759 patients of HIV-infected health care workers in the United States failed to identify a single case of provider-to-patient transmission of HIV aside from the Florida dental cases.[96] Moreover, as of 1998, investigations of HIV-infected individuals with no identifiable risk reported to the CDC failed to establish any additional cases of nosocomial HIV transmission.[27] It has been estimated that the average risk of HIV transmission from a surgeon to a patient because of percutaneous injury during an invasive procedure is 2.4 to 24 per million.[10] All numerical estimates of risk are hypothetical. Thus, although rare, the risk of provider-to-patient transmission of HIV during invasive procedures does exist.

Consequently, in 1996, the CDC issued updated guidelines for the prevention of transmission of HIV and hepatitis B by health care workers who perform exposure-prone invasive procedures.[33] In general, these guidelines advocate use of universal precautions, voluntary testing for HIV and hepatitis B and hepatitis C of health care workers who perform exposure-prone procedures, and counseling of infected workers who perform exposure-prone procedures (by an expert review panel). The responsibility for developing and implementing such guidelines has been delegated to the state level. The net effect of these recommendations has been intensification of the ongoing medical, legal, and political debate of this emotionally charged issue.

Transmission Issues in Surgery

Given their prolonged and repeated exposure to potentially large volumes of blood, surgeons' concern about possible occupational acquisition of HIV infection is understandable. However, studies have documented that nurses, followed by house staff and operating room nurses and technicians, are at greatest risk for occupational sharp instrument injuries,[84] the type of injury most likely to be associated with transmission of HIV infection. Factors that may influence the risk of HIV transmission during surgery include skill and training level of the surgeon, surgical procedure being performed, volume and duration of blood exposure during the procedure, number of procedures performed, and conditions under which the procedure is performed — that is, emergent versus elective.[7] Procedures undertaken to reduce the risk of exposure to HIV and other blood-borne pathogens include restriction of operating room personnel, double-gloving, use of protective eyewear and appropriate garment shields, and minimizing sharp instrument use.[7, 95]

Although HIV-1 has been demonstrated to remain viable in the cool vapors and aerosols produced by several common surgical power instruments, the significance of this exposure as a potential risk for transmission of HIV infection to surgeons during procedures is unknown.[73] Interestingly, no infectious HIV was detected in aerosols generated by electrocautery or with manual wound irrigation syringe. Serological surveys of orthopedic surgeons have not yet identified any infected physicians who appear to have acquired HIV infection through occupational exposure.[7] It is conceivable that in the future surgeons will be identified who have been infected with HIV as a consequence of the practice of their profession. However, based on current knowledge of infection rates and inefficiency of HIV transmission, such an event is likely to be a rare occurrence.

HIV infection of bone is well documented,[13, 85, 97] and reports of transmission of HIV infection in bone-transplantation recipients[37, 102] highlight the concern that every precaution be taken to avoid this devastating complication. The primary safeguards against potential transmission of HIV by bone allograft are screening and testing of patients.[77] The freezing step in bone tissue banking probably results in further reduction of the risk of transmission.[13, 102] Techniques designed to minimize requirements for blood transfusions during operative procedures include intraoperative autologous transfusion[12] and postoperative blood salvage,[103] both of which may serve to further minimize the risk of parenteral HIV transmission.

Transmission and Sports

There have been no documented cases to date of HIV transmission during participation in athletic activities. The risk of transmission during sports participation is estimated to be extremely low and would be expected to occur only after direct body contact, presumably of mucous membranes or open skin, with blood. There is no risk of HIV transmission through sports activities where bleeding does not occur.[17] Transmission of both HIV and hepatitis B and C can occur by sharing razors, toothbrushes, and needles used to administer anabolic steroids.

In their joint position statement on HIV and other blood-borne pathogens in sports, the American Medical Society for Sports Medicine and the American Academy of Sports Medicine maintain that sports medicine practitioners should play a role in the education of infected and uninfected athletes, their families, and the sports community regarding disease transmission and prevention.[4] Athletes should be advised that it is their responsibility to report wounds and injuries in a timely manner. If an athlete is bleeding, his or her participation should be interrupted. After the wound stops bleeding and has been antiseptically cleaned and securely bandaged, participation may be resumed. Universal precautions and basic principles of hygiene should be observed. In addition, the position statement asserts that sports medicine practitioners should be knowledgeable about management issues of HIV-infected athletes and should maintain the confidentiality of HIV-infected athletes.

Vertical Transmission

Although HIV infection can be transmitted from an infected mother to her fetus throughout pregnancy, most transmissions occur at or near delivery. AZT alone and nevirapine alone have been shown to significantly reduce the rate of perinatal transmission.[46] Consequently, all pregnant women should be tested for HIV infection. In addition, all HIV-infected women should be counseled about the risks and benefits of antiretroviral therapy for both the mother and the infant.[35]

TESTING

Individuals who should undergo HIV testing include (1) persons with current or past sexually transmitted disease; (2) those in known high-risk groups (intravenous drug users, gay and bisexual men, hemophiliacs, regular sexual partners of persons in these categories and of persons with known HIV infection); (3) those in lower-risk categories (prostitutes, persons who received blood products from 1977 to May 1985, and heterosexual persons with at least one sex partner in the past 12 months or noncompliance with condom use in the past 6 months); (4) those who consider themselves at risk or who request the test; (5) pregnant women; (6) those with active tuberculosis; (7) those with occupational exposures (both recipient and source); (8) those patients age 15 to 54 years admitted to hospitals where the seroprevalence exceeds 1% or AIDS case rates exceed 1 per 1,000 discharges; (9) health care workers who perform exposure-prone invasive procedures, depending on institutional policies; (10) blood, semen, and organ donors; and (11) those patients with clinical or laboratory findings suggestive of HIV.[8]

The diagnosis of HIV infection is based on antibodies to the virus detected by an ELISA and confirmed by Western blot. Criteria for a positive HIV test are a positive ELISA result followed by a positive Western blot result. A positive Western blot result requires the identification of antibodies to two of the following viral proteins: p24, gp 41, gp 120/160. The accuracy of HIV serology is excellent, with a reported sensitivity of 99.3% and a specificity of 99.7%.[38]

Antibody to HIV usually appears 3 to 12 weeks after primary infection but may take as long as 6 months to appear. False-negative results occur most frequently in recently infected persons before seroconversion. The newer, more sensitive antibody tests reduce the typical window period to 3 to 4 weeks. False-negative test results have also been reported in individuals with agammaglobulinemia, in individuals infected with strains showing little genetic homology with HIV-1, and in those who remain persistently seronegative because of an "atypical host response." The most common cause of false-positive test results is vaccination with experimental HIV-1 vaccines.[8]

Indeterminate results may occur in an HIV-infected individual who either is in the process of seroconversion or has advanced HIV infection with decreased titers of antibodies. Indeterminate results have also been reported in uninfected individuals who have cross-reacting alloantibodies from pregnancy, blood transfusions, or organ transplantation; in individuals who have autoantibodies as seen with collagen-vascular disease, autoimmune diseases, and malignancy; or in recipients of experimental HIV-1 vaccines. An individual infected with HIV-2 may have a positive or indeterminate result on Western blot for HIV-1. Repeat testing at 3 and 6 months is generally advocated for individuals with indeterminate test results.

Additional methods for establishing HIV infection include HIV p24 antigen testing, HIV DNA and RNA PCR, and viral culture of peripheral blood mononuclear cells. None of these tests is considered superior to the routine serology noted above. They may be useful in individuals with indeterminate tests, for virological monitoring in therapeutic trials, and for HIV detection when routine serological tests are likely to be misleading. Quantitative HIV RNA (viral load) is also useful for predicting progression and for therapeutic monitoring. In fact, it has been shown that HIV RNA levels are the most important measure of therapeutic response.[86] Viral burden testing does not test immune function, nor does it detect viral burden in compartments other than blood (lymph nodes, central nervous system, genital secretions). CD4+ cell count testing, on the other hand, determines immunocompetence and serves as an independent predictor of prognosis. The viral load should be obtained only at times of clinical stability and with the same laboratory and technology.

Informed consent is an important issue with regard to HIV testing. It is required by law in most states and recommended in all other states. HIV testing has the potential to significantly affect an individual's life. A person who tests positive must cope with the diagnosis of an incurable disease. He or she may experience depression, anxiety, and isolation, as well as changing family and personal relationships. Furthermore, a person may face discrimination from insurance carriers, health care workers, employers, and coworkers. Consequently, both pretest and posttest counseling for all individuals receiving HIV testing should be provided. Almost universally, documented patient consent is required before HIV testing. However, some states permit testing of the source without consent in cases of occupational exposures of health care workers. In addition, testing of all blood, bone marrow, semen, and organ donors is mandatory.

TREATMENT OF HIV

Management of Antiretroviral Drugs

The explosion of information regarding HIV, the increasing number of antiretroviral medications, the development of resistance patterns to these medications, and the long-term survival of many patients with HIV have led to increasing complexity in the treatment of HIV-infected individuals. This complexity has necessitated the formalization of guidelines for management of antiretroviral agents, management and prophylaxis of opportunistic infections, and management of occupational exposure to HIV and recommendations for postexposure prophylaxis.[1, 17, 18, 29] These guidelines are prepared by a panel of leading experts in the field of HIV care and the U.S. Department of Health and Human Services. They are frequently updated and readily available.[90] Antiretroviral therapies are medically complex and are associated with a significant number of side effects and drug interactions, which can complicate both physician management and patient adherence. Although the guidelines recommend that management of HIV-infected individuals be supervised by a physician experienced in HIV care, nearly all physicians will participate in the care of HIV-infected individuals at some time and thus should be familiar with the principles set forth by the guidelines.

There are no formal guidelines for the preoperative evaluation of HIV-infected patients. In general, consultation with a clinician experienced in the care of HIV-infected individuals is appropriate. In addition to potential opportunistic infections, patients with HIV infection are predisposed to a variety of organ-system deficiencies. Thrombocytopenia, anemia, and leukopenia because of bone marrow suppression from antiretroviral medications or infiltration by opportunistic pathogens or HIV, or because of an autoimmune phenomenon, are common. Renal insufficiency from HIV nephropathy, drug toxicity, and various other etiologies is frequently encountered. Patients infected with HIV often have elevated liver enzymes because of medications or chronic infection with hepatitis B or C. Adrenal insufficiency in HIV infection is well documented. Moreover, HIV-infected individuals may be predisposed to premature coronary artery disease and dilated cardiomyopathy as a result of antiretroviral medications and HIV itself.[41, 52] Finally, protease inhibitors, a common class of antiretroviral medications, have been associated with glucose intolerance and diabetes, as well as dyslipidemia.

In addition, a fair number of both well-documented and theoretical drug interactions have been reported with protease inhibitors, a common class of antiretroviral medication. Dosing adjustments may be required. Medications that should be avoided or used with caution in patients taking protease inhibitors include, but are not limited to, some benzodiazepines; the antihistamines astemizole and terfenadine; the analgesics meperidine, piroxicam, and propoxyphene; the antidepressant bupropion; the motility agent cisapride; and ergot alkaloids. Some reasonable alternatives include temazepam, lorazepam, loratadine, oxycodone, aspirin, acetaminophen, and ibuprofen.

Management of Occupational Exposure to HIV and Recommendations for Postexposure Prophylaxis

Many experts suggest that all health care workers consider the pros and cons of postexposure prophylaxis before an occupational exposure occurs so that they may be better prepared to take immediate action and

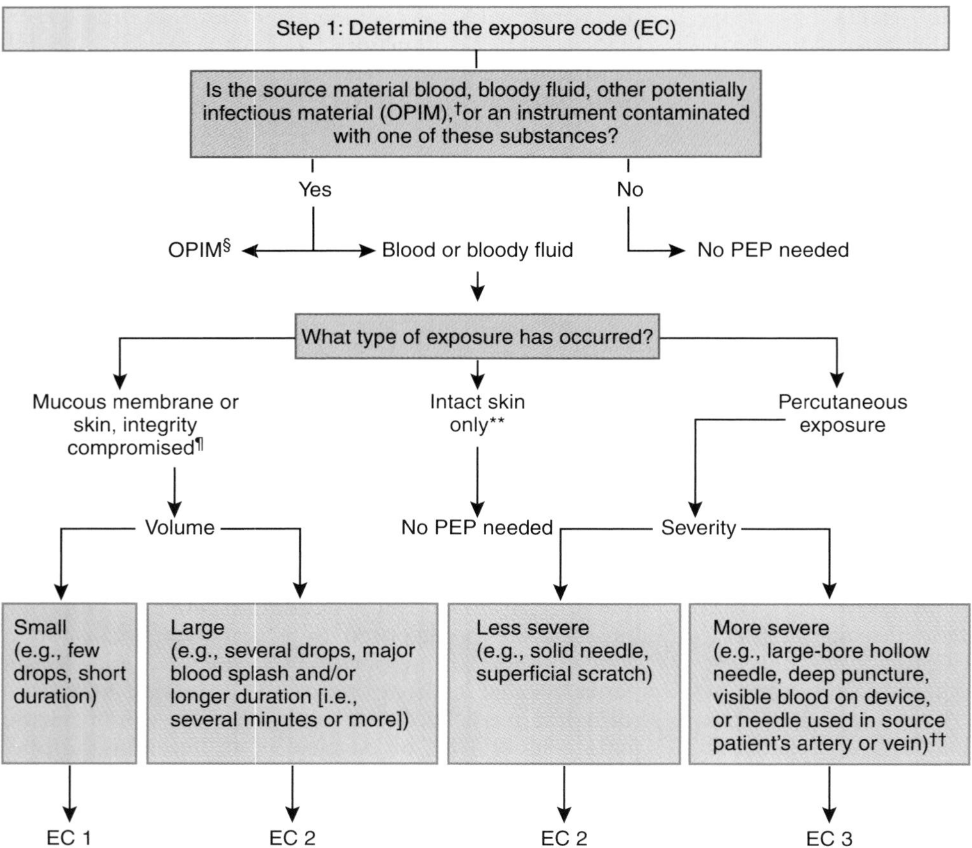

This algorithm is intended to guide initial decisions about PEP and should be used in conjunction with other guidance provided in this report.

† Semen or vaginal secretions; cerebrospinal, synovial, pleural, peritoneal, pericardial, or amniotic fluids; or tissue.

§ Exposures to OPIM must be evaluated on a case-by-case basis. In general, these body substances are considered a low risk for transmission in health-care settings. Any unprotected contact to concentrated HIV in a research laboratory or production facility is considered an occupational exposure that requires clinical evaluation to determine the need for PEP.

¶ Skin integrity is considered compromised if there is evidence of chapped skin, dermatitis, abrasion, or open wound.

** Contact with intact skin is not normally considered a risk for HIV transmission. However, if the exposure was to blood, and the circumstance suggests a higher volume exposure (e.g., an extensive area of skin was exposed or there was prolonged contact with blood), the risk for HIV transmission should be considered.

†† The combination of these severity factors (e.g., large-bore hollow needle *and* deep puncture) contributes to an elevated risk for transmission if the source person is HIV-positive.

FIGURE 52.1 ➢ Determining the need for human immunodeficiency virus (HIV) postexposure prophylaxis (PEP) after an occupational exposure. (From Centers for Disease Control and Prevention: Public Health Service guidelines for the management of health care worker exposures to HIV and recommendations for postexposure prophylaxis. MMWR 47[RR7]:14–15, 1998.)

to cope with the anxiety of decision making and the uncertainty of outcome. All known and suspected exposures should be reported, regardless of how small the perceived risk, because collective data continues to provide much of our understanding regarding transmission risk.

The Public Health Service recommendations[31] for postexposure prophylaxis are based on an algorithm that stratifies the risk of transmission based on the type and degree of exposure as well as the likelihood of infectivity of the source (Fig. 52.1). The first action after any exposure is to wash the skin with soap and water or flush mucous membranes with water immediately. The next action is prompt reporting of the exposure. If antiretroviral therapy is indeed indicated, it should be initiated within hours of exposure.

Step 1 of the algorithm is to determine the Exposure Code (EC). The EC is determined by the source material, the type of exposure, and the severity of exposure. Exposure to source material that is blood or bloody fluid or to instruments contaminated with these substances requires further consideration of risk. Exposure to other potentially infectious materials such as semen; vaginal secretions; and cerebrospinal, synovial, pleural, peritoneal, pericardial, and amniotic fluids is determined on a case-by-case basis. In general, these body fluids are considered to have a low risk for transmission.

The type of exposure is classified as (1) intact skin only, (2) mucous membrane or skin with compromised integrity (chapped skin, dermatitis, abrasion, or open wound), or (3) percutaneous exposure. Expo-

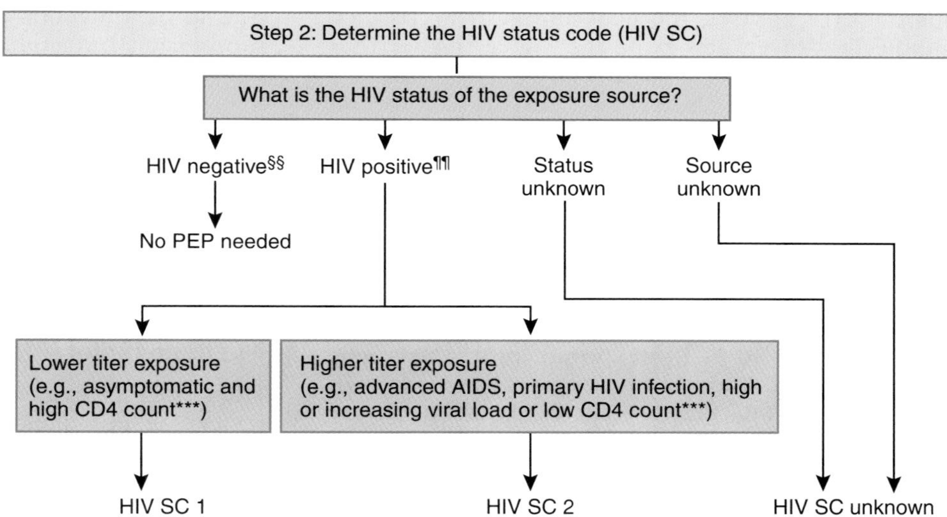

§§ A source is considered negative for HIV infection if there is laboratory documentation of a negative HIV antibody, HIV polymerase chain reaction (PCR), or HIV p24 antigen test result from a specimen collected at or near the time of exposure and there is no clinical evidence of recent retroviral-like illness.

¶¶ A source is considered infected with HIV (HIV positive) if there has been a positive laboratory result for HIV antibody, HIV PCR, or HIV p24 antigen or physician-diagnosed AIDS.

*** Examples are used as surrogates to estimate HIV titer in an exposure source for purposes of considering PEP regimens and do not reflect all clinical situations that may be observed. Although a high HIV titer (HIV SC 2) in an exposure source has been associated with an increased risk for transmission, the possibility of transmission from a source with low HIV titer also must be considered.

Step 3: Determine the PEP recommendation

EC	HIV SC	PEP recommendation
1	1	**PEP may not be warranted.** Exposure type does not pose a known risk for HIV transmission. Whether the risk for drug toxicity outweighs the benefit of PEP should be decided by the exposed HCW and treating clinician.
1	1	**Consider basic regimen.**§§§ Exposure type poses a negligible risk for HIV transmission. A high HIV titer in the source may justify consideration of PEP. Whether the risk for drug toxicity outweighs the benefit of PEP should be decided by the exposed HCW and treating clinician.
2	1	**Recommend basic regimen.** Most HIV exposures are in this category; no increased risk for HIV transmission has been observed but use of PEP is appropriate.
2	2	**Recommend expanded regimen.**††† Exposure type represents an increased HIV transmission risk.
3	1 or 2	**Recommend expanded regimen.** Exposure type represents an increased HIV transmission risk.
Unknown		If the source or, in the case of an unknown source, the setting where the exposure occurred suggests a possible risk for HIV exposure and the EC is 2 or 3, consider PEP basic regimen.

§§§ Basic regimen is four weeks of zidovudine, 600 mg per day in two or three divided doses, *and* lamivudine, 150 mg twice daily.

††† Expanded regimen is the basic regimen plus *either* indinavir, 800 mg every 8 hours, *or* nelfinavir, 750 mg three times a day.

FIGURE 52.1 ➢ *Continued*

sure to intact skin is not normally considered a risk for HIV transmission, and thus postexposure prophylaxis is not recommended. However, if the exposure entails a large volume of blood with an extensive area of intact skin or prolonged contact, the risk of HIV should be considered. On the other hand, if the exposure occurs via mucous membranes or skin with compromised integrity, then the volume of exposure should be determined. A small exposure entails a few drops or a short duration of contact and is classified as EC 1. A large exposure entails several drops, a major splash, or prolonged contact and is classified as EC 2. Percutaneous exposures are classified by severity. Penetration with a solid needle and a superficial scratch are considered less severe and are classified as EC 2. Deep puncture or penetration with a hollow needle, a needle used in a source artery or vein, or a needle with visible blood on the device is considered more severe exposure and is classified as EC 3.

Step 2 of the algorithm is to determine the HIV Status Code (SC). The initial classification scheme requires determination of the HIV status of the exposure source. A source is considered to be HIV negative if there is documentation of a negative HIV antibody, HIV PCR, or HIV p24 antigen test result from a specimen collected at or near the time of exposure and if there is no clinical evidence of an acute or recent retroviral-like illness.

If the source is determined to be HIV negative, no postexposure prophylaxis is recommended. If the source is HIV positive, the exposure is then classified as either a "lower titer exposure" or a "higher titer exposure." An individual who has asymptomatic HIV infection and a high CD4+ cell count (and a low viral load) can be considered a lower titer exposure and thus classified as HIV SC 1. An individual with advanced AIDS, primary HIV infection, a high or increasing viral load, or a low CD4+ count should be considered a higher titer exposure and thus classified as SC 2. Situations in which the HIV status of the source is unknown or the source itself is unknown are classified as SC Unknown.

For EC 1 and SC 1, postexposure prophylaxis may not be warranted because drug toxicity may outweigh the risk of HIV transmission. For EC 1 and SC 2, the exposure poses negligible risk. Thus, the consideration of AZT and 3TC prophylaxis is recommended (Table 52.2). Although no increased risk of transmission has been observed in the category of EC 2 and SC 1, most exposures occur in this category, and thus AZT and 3TC prophylaxis is recommended. Finally, for categories EC 2 and SC 2 or EC 3 (regardless of SC), AZT, 3TC, and indinavir or nelfinavir are indicated because an increased risk of transmission has been observed.

The guidelines recommend that health care workers exposed to HIV undergo serological testing at baseline, 6 weeks, 3 months, 6 months, and possibly 1 year after exposure. In addition, exposed health care workers should practice safer sex or abstain from sex until serology is negative 6 months after exposure. Moreover, they should seek medical evaluation for any acute illness that develops during the follow-up period, which may indicate the development of acute HIV infection.

HIV INFECTION AND MUSCULOSKELETAL DISEASE

Nearly 75% of HIV-infected individuals report musculoskeletal symptoms.[74] Infectious, inflammatory, and neoplastic processes are all represented in the spectrum of rheumatic manifestations of HIV disease. The frequency and type of processes clinically manifested appear to be a function of the patient's level of immunosuppression and primary risk factor for HIV infection. Infectious and neoplastic complications are frequently seen in patients with late-stage infection[70, 100] who commonly, although not exclusively, have intravenous drug use as their risk factor for HIV infection.[88] In contrast, reactive rheumatological processes can occur in persons with early or late symptomatic disease[89, 98] and are reported more consistently in patients with HIV infection acquired through homosexual activity.[15]

Musculoskeletal Infections

From their retrospective cohort study and literature review of musculoskeletal infections in patients with HIV disease, Vassilopoulos et al estimated the incidence to be 0.3% to 3.5%.[112] Septic arthritis, osteomyelitis, pyomyositis, avascular necrosis, and bursitis are the most common orthopedic infectious complications seen in patients with HIV infection.[70, 88, 89, 112] Infection occurs with conventional or atypical bacteria, fungi, or other opportunistic organisms. Diagnosis depends on isolation of the infecting organism from synovial fluid, bone, muscle, or blood. Despite the low incidence, HIV-infected individuals with musculoskeletal infections experience significant morbidity and mortality.[112]

In addition, a resurgence of tuberculosis has paralleled the emergence of the HIV epidemic. *M. tuberculosis* has been associated with increased frequency in infectious musculoskeletal disorders in HIV-infected patients. Although classic Pott's disease still occurs, tuberculosis appears to be a very aggressive disease, associated with frequent dissemination, multidrug resistance, and high mortality in patients with HIV infection. Consequently, orthopedic surgeons must be aware that pulmonary disease may coexist and must take appropriate respiratory isolation precautions to prevent the spread of infection to other patients and health care workers.

Septic arthritis is usually monoarticular, with the knee[70] and hip[88] most commonly involved. Unusual sites of joint infection, including sternoclavicular and sacroiliac joints and intervertebral discs, have been de-

TABLE 52.2 BASIC AND EXPANDED POSTEXPOSURE PROPHYLAXIS REGIMENS*

Regimen Category	Application	Drug Regimen
Basic	Occupational HIV exposures for which there is a recognized transmission risk (see Fig. 52.1)	4 weeks (28 days) of both zidovudine 600 mg every day in divided doses (i.e., 300 mg twice a day, 200 mg three times a day, or 100 mg every 4 hours) **and** lamivudine 150 mg twice a day.
Expanded	Occupational HIV exposures that pose an increased risk for transmission (e.g., larger volume of blood and/or higher virus titer in blood) (see Fig. 52.1).	Basic regimen plus **either** indinavir 800 mg every 8 hours **or** nelfinavir 750 mg three times a day.*

* Indinavir should be taken on an empty stomach (i.e., without food or with a light meal) and with increased fluid consumption (i.e., drinking six 8-oz. glasses of water throughout the day); nelfinavir should be taken with meals.

HIV = human immunodeficiency virus.

From Centers for Disease Control and Prevention: Public Health Service recommendations for management of health care worker exposures to HIV and recommendations for postexposure prophylaxis. MMWR 47(RR7):21, 1998.

scribed in intravenous drug users.[74] Infection of the joint occurs via hematogenous spread or direct extension from an adjacent soft-tissue or bone infection. Polyarticular involvement is usually seen in the setting of disseminated disease.

Staphylococcus aureus and *Candida albicans* are the most frequently isolated pathogens.[70, 88, 89] In addition to a variety of conventional bacterial organisms, several uncommon organisms have been isolated as well. These include fungi, *M. tuberculosis,* and atypical mycobacterium.[99] Clinically, septic arthritis caused by *S. aureus* presents similarly in both seropositive and seronegative patients. Erythema, effusion, and tenderness are usually noted on examination. Although atypical organisms such as fungi and mycobacteria often result in a chronic infectious arthritis in seronegative individuals, an acute or subacute infectious arthritic process may ensue in seropositive patients.[74]

Although effusion is often present, synovial fluid cultures may frequently be negative, despite the presence of organisms on Gram's stain, wet mount, or acid-fast bacillus smears.[70] Blood cultures may be helpful in definitively establishing a microbiological diagnosis, although discordant blood and joint culture results have been reported.[49, 81] Synovial biopsies may be necessary to isolate fungi and mycobacteria from joints. Imaging studies, such as serial radiograms and or radionuclide bone scans, should be performed in patients with septic arthritis to eliminate the possibility of coexistent osteomyelitis.[74] In addition, septic bursitis caused by *S. aureus* has been reported in a number of patients with HIV infection.[112]

Although the relationship between HIV risk factors and incidence of septic arthritis has yet to be clearly defined, it appears as if septic arthritis occurs more frequently in patients with intravenous drug use and hemophilia as risk factors.[88, 89] The degree of immunosuppression does not appear to be a contributing factor for infection with pathogens commonly introduced via needles. However, infection with opportunistic pathogens tends to occur in patients with more advanced HIV disease and CD4+ cell counts of fewer than 100. One study revealed a median CD4+ count of 241 in a group of seropositive patients with septic arthritis.[112]

The most commonly isolated pathogens in osteomyelitis are *S. aureus* and atypical mycobacterium species.[112] Hirsch et al reported that the rate of infections because of atypical mycobacteria and *M. tuberculosis* was 676-fold and 35-fold higher, respectively, in HIV-infected patients compared with the general population.[67] Generally, fungal osteomyelitis is uncommon, but when it does occur it is hematogenously spread and thus often occurs in more than one bone.[100]

In patients with osteomyelitis, bone biopsy is usually required to establish the diagnosis. In addition, osteomyelitis is associated with a high mortality rate in HIV-positive patients, likely because of their immunocompromised state. Osteomyelitis is more frequently seen in advanced HIV disease with a median CD4+ count documented in one study at 41.[112]

Bacillary angiomatosis associated with disseminated cat-scratch bacillus has also been reported.[6, 66, 111] This clinical syndrome is characterized by subcutaneous nodules and osteolytic lesions that are typically culture negative on biopsy and aspirate. Electron microscopy and histopathological examination of the vascular soft tissue may verify the presence of cat-scratch bacillus.

Once primarily seen in tropical climates, pyomyositis appears to be associated with advanced HIV infection in temperate climates. By far the most common organism identified in HIV-infected individuals is *S. aureus*.[50, 112] Other organisms reported include streptococcal and salmonella species as well as *Toxoplasma gondii, Cryptococcus neoformans, M. avium* complex, and microsporidia.[74, 112]

Inflammatory Conditions of the Joints

Inflammatory musculoskeletal complications, particularly arthritis, arthralgia, and myalgia, are common in HIV infection.[15] Arthralgias are the most common musculoskeletal manifestations seen during the course of HIV infection[89] and can be present in approximately 35% to 40% of patients.[54, 98] Three primary types of arthritis have been described in association with HIV infection: reactive arthritis (Reiter's syndrome), psoriatic arthritis, and HIV-associated arthritis.

Arthrocentesis is necessary in HIV-infected patients with subacute and chronic arthritis before attributing such arthritides to a noninfectious cause. As discussed above, synovial biopsies are sometimes necessary for isolation of fungi and mycobacteria.[74] Identification of such organisms is particularly important for both initiating appropriate therapy and avoiding the inappropriate use of immunosuppressive agents (e.g., methotrexate) in patients who are already immunocompromised.

Arthralgias are the most common musculoskeletal manifestation seen during the course of HIV infection[89] and can be present in approximately 35% to 40% of patients.[54, 98] Diffuse arthralgias may be seen in the setting of acute primary infection as well as at other times during the course of the HIV infection. The large joints, such as the knee, shoulder, and elbow, are most commonly involved. Symptoms are usually of moderate intensity and intermittent but, rarely, can be extremely severe and debilitating. Often the clinical examination is without evidence of inflammatory signs.[3] Simple analgesics are usually adequate for treatment of the arthralgias in HIV-infected individuals.

Reiter's syndrome is reported as a common rheumatological syndrome in HIV infection, although the true association with HIV infection remains unclear. The presentation is similar to idiopathic Reiter's syndrome, with asymmetric oligoarthritis of the large joints (knees, shoulders, and ankles). Enthesopathies of the Achilles' tendon, plantar fascia, and anterior and posterior tibial tendons are common. Patients may present with gait disturbances secondary to these enthesopathies combined with multidigit dactylitis of the toes.[74]

The classic triad of arthritis, urethritis, and conjunctivitis is seen in a much smaller proportion of patients. Urethritis has been found in 59% of HIV-infected individuals with Reiter's syndrome, conjunctivitis in 47%, keratoderma blennorrhagicum in 25%, and circinate balanitis in 29%.[74] Organisms such as *Salmonella typhimurium, Shigella flexneri, Campylobacter fetus, Ureaplasma urealyticum,* and *Yersinia* species have been found in less than one third of HIV-infected patients with reactive arthritis. However, an antecedent culture-negative diarrheal illness often precedes the onset of Reiter's syndrome and reactive arthritis in HIV-infected patients.[74] In a patient with a Reiter's-like arthritis but lacking the other defining features, it may be more appropriate to classify the patient as having nonspecific reactive arthritis.

The signs and symptoms of Reiter's syndrome can occur before the onset of clinical immunodeficiency. Given the possible association of Reiter's syndrome with HIV infection, patients presenting to a physician with Reiter's syndrome or reactive arthritis should be questioned about HIV risk factors. Both noninfected and HIV-infected Caucasion North American patients with Reiter's syndrome have high human leukocyte antigen (HLA)-B27 seropositivity. In contrast, in a cohort of 13 African-American patients with Reiter's syndrome and HIV infection, no HLA-B27 seropositivity was found. This finding may reflect the low prevalence of HLA-B27 in African-American people in general.[74]

HIV-associated arthritis is an oligoarthritis that primarily involves the knees and ankles. It is characterized by brief episodes of debilitating pain. The peak intensity occurs within 1 to 4 weeks and often remits within 6 weeks to 6 months. Intense pain may necessitate the use of narcotics, nonsteroidal anti-inflammatory drugs (NSAIDs), and intra-articular corticosteroids. Arthrocentesis reveals fluid that is noninflammatory. Synovial biopsy reveals a chronic mononuclear infiltrate. Antecedent infections, mucocutaneous lesions, and ophthalmological and urogenital features commonly seen with Reiter's syndrome and psoriatic arthritis are not associated with these patients. Rheumatological markers (HLA-B27, rheumatoid factor, antinuclear antibodies) and bacterial and viral cultures are negative in these patients as well. The pathophysiology is unknown; however, a direct viral infection, an immune-complex deposition in the joint, and a form of reactive arthritis have been proposed as possible mechanisms.[3, 74]

Psoriasis and psoriatic arthritis are reported more frequently in HIV-infected individuals than in the general population. Psoriatic arthritis may precede, occur concomitantly, or follow the clinical onset of AIDS. It is frequently an asymmetric, polyarticular disease that can be accompanied by enthesopathy and dactylitis. The clinical course is variable, ranging from mild to rapidly progressive and deforming.[50] Psoriatic arthritis may occur alone or in conjunction with psoriatic skin lesions. Various types of psoriatic skin lesions, including vulgaris, guttate, sebopsoriasis, pustular, and exfoliative erythroderma forms have been described in both HIV-positive and HIV-negative individuals.

Painful articular syndrome involves the acute onset of painful arthralgias in up to three joints. The physical examination is not suggestive of synovitis. The pain usually resolves within 24 hours. Narcotics may be required because NSAIDs often do not adequately control the pain. This syndrome appears to be unique to HIV-infected patients. Avascular necrosis has been reported in HIV-infected patients and should be considered in the differential diagnosis.[74, 106] Other considerations include infections with parvovirus B19 and hepatitis C.

Peripheral sensory neuropathy is common in HIV-infected individuals. HIV-related axonal degeneration or nerve destruction because of the antiretroviral agents d4T and ddI are the most common causes. Peripheral neuropathy may lead to gait disturbance with subsequent mechanical derangement of weight-bearing joints over time.

Patients with these lesions often have a history of corticosteroid use and substantial exercise. These lesions do not appear to be related to coagulopathies or lipid abnormalities. The knee has not been reported to be involved, yet, by avascular necrosis.

Avascular Necrosis

An increasing number of reports describe avascular necrosis involving one or both hips. Other bones can be affected. The cause of this condition is not known nor is the natural history clear. One cross-sectional study found that 4.5% of HIV-infected patients who deny symptoms have lesions involving one or both hips. At least some of these patients develop substantial pain and ultimately undergo hip replacement.

Neoplastic Complications

Kaposi's sarcoma, the most common neoplasm reported in adults with HIV infection, can be present at any stage of HIV disease. Sites of involvement include skin and viscera as well as bone and muscle. Lesions may be asymptomatic or painful. Computed tomography (CT) scan may reveal osteolytic bone lesions that may be associated with periosteal reaction and an overlying soft-tissue mass.[105] Bone scans and plain films may be negative. Early bone changes may be best detected with magnetic resonance imaging (MRI). Muscle involvement may be seen on MRI as well.

Non-Hodgkin's lymphoma (NHL), the second most common tumor found in adults with AIDS, is the most common tumor found in children with AIDS. The central nervous system and the gastrointestinal tract are the most common sites of involvement, although bone and muscle involvement is fairly common as well. Patients with bone involvement may present with pain and pathological fractures, whereas patients with muscle involvement may complain of painful swelling, which may mimic pyomyositis or thrombophlebitis. Plain films and CT of bone lesions may reveal osteolytic lesions with cortical destruction, sclerosis, indistinct transition zone, periosteal reaction, pathological fractures, and an associated soft-tissue mass.[105]

Although NHL and Kaposi's sarcoma are well described in patients with HIV infection, reports of the occurrence of malignant plasma cell tumors are relatively uncommon.[61, 87] Historically, multiple myeloma and extramedullary plasmacytomas are diseases associated with an older population and are extraordinarily rare in young persons. Their detection in young adults with HIV infection suggests that these tumors may represent another complication of HIV disease.

Loss of Bone Density

Patients with HIV disease have been reported to develop premature osteoporosis. The cause is unclear. Osteopenia has been reported to be associated with lipodystrophy and protease inhibitors.[113, 114] The consequences of this osteoporosis and the utility of therapy are being studied. Pathological fractures have not yet been reported.

SUMMARY

Virtually all physicians, including orthopedic surgeons, will encounter individuals with HIV infection in their practice of medicine. Orthopedic surgeons need to be familiar with the risks of acquiring HIV from needlesticks, other surgical accidents, and blood transfusions as well as the principles of risk reduction to ensure the safety of both patients and the entire health care team. Moreover, individuals infected with HIV are living longer, healthier, and more active lives. Consequently, orthopedists need to be aware of the possibility that their patients may have orthopedic complications not only because of HIV, but also independent of HIV infection. Thus, individuals with HIV infection deserve the same careful diagnostic and therapeutic management as uninfected patients. Finally, nearly all practicing physicians will encounter patients who are at risk for acquiring HIV infection, likely to be HIV infected, or already diagnosed with HIV infection but not receiving adequate care. In such situations, frank discussion about prevention of transmission and testing as well as referral to an HIV specialist, when indicated, may contribute to the overall health of the individual as well as to efforts to stem the tides of the HIV epidemic.

References

1. Alcabes P: Incubation period of human immunodeficiency virus. Epidemiol Rev 15:303, 1993.
2. Allain JP: Long term evaluation of HIV antigen and antibodies to p24 and gp41 in patients with hemophilia: Potential clinical importance. N Engl J Med 317:1114, 1987.
3. Alpiner N: Rehabilitation in joint and connective tissue diseases. 1. Systemic diseases. Arch Phys Med Rehab 76(5):S32, 1995.
4. American Medical Society for Sports Medicine and the American Academy of Sports Medicine: Human immunodeficiency virus (HIV) and other blood-borne pathogens in sports. Joint position statement. Am J Sports Med 26(4):510, 1995.
5. Barbaro G: Incidence of dilated cardiomyopathy and detection of HIV in myocardial cells of HIV-positive patients. N Engl J Med 339:1093, 1998.
6. Baron AL: Osteolytic lesions and bacillary angiomatosis in HIV infection: Radiologic differentiation from AIDS-related Kaposi sarcoma. Radiology 177:77, 1990.
7. Bartlett JG: HIV infection and surgeons. Curr Probl Surg 29: 197, 1992.
8. Bartlett JG: Medical Management of HIV Infection. Baltimore, MD, Johns Hopkins University Department of Infectious Disease, 1998.
9. Beekmann SE: Temporal association between implementation of universal precautions and a sustained, progressive decrease in percutaneous exposures to blood. Clin Inf Dis 18:562, 1994.
10. Bell DM: Preventing bloodborne pathogen transmission from health-care workers to patients. The CDC perspective. Surg Clin North Am 75(6):1189, 1995.
11. Blanchard A: Molecular evidence for nosocomial transmission of human immunodeficiency virus from a surgeon to one of his patients. J Virol 72:4537, 1998.
12. Bovill DF, Norris TR: The efficacy of intraoperative autologous transfusion in major shoulder surgery. Clin Orthop 240:137, 1989.
13. Buck BE: Human immunodeficiency virus cultured from bone. Implications for transplantation. Clin Orthop 240:249, 1990.
14. Burcham J: CD4 percent is the best predictor of development of AIDS in cohort of HIV-infected homosexual men. AIDS 5: 365, 1991.
15. Buskila D, Gladman D: Musculoskeletal manifestations of infection with human immunodeficiency virus. Rev Infect Dis 12: 223, 1990.
16. Cardo DM et al: A case-control study of HIV seroconversion in health care workers after percutaneous exposure. N Engl J Med 337:1485, 1997.
17. Centers for Disease Control and Prevention. HIV/AIDS Surveillance Report 11(1):1, 1999.
18. Centers for Disease Control and Prevention and National Center for HIV, STD, TB Prevention: CDC Update: Combating complacency in HIV prevention. http://www.cdc.gov/nchstp/hiv_aids/pubs/facts/combat.htm. Updated July 1998.
19. Centers for Disease Control and Prevention and National Center for HIV, STD, TB Prevention: Preventing occupational HIV transmission to health care workers. http://www.gov/nchstp/hiv_aids. Updated October 1998.
20. Centers for Disease Control and Prevention National AIDS Clearinghouse: (1-800-458-5231; http://www.cdcnac.org).
21. Centers for Disease Control and Prevention: 1999 USPHS/IDSA guidelines for the prevention of opportunistic infections in persons infected with human immunodeficiency virus. http://www.hivatis.org.
22. Centers for Disease Control and Prevention: Guidelines for prevention of transmission of human immunodeficiency virus and hepatitis B virus to health-care and public safety workers. MMWR 38(S6):3, 1989.
23. Centers for Disease Control and Prevention: Guidelines for prophylaxis against *Pneumocystis carinii* pneumonia for persons infected with HIV. MMWR 38(Suppl 6):S1, 1989.
24. Centers for Disease Control and Prevention: Guidelines for the use of antiretroviral agents in HIV-infected adults and adolescents. http://www.hivatis.org.
25. Management of possible sexual, injecting drug use, or other nonoccupational exposure to HIV, including considerations related to antiretroviral therapy. http://www.hivatis.org.
26. Centers for Disease Control and Prevention: HIV prevention through early detection and treatment of other sexually transmitted diseases—United States and recommendations of the Advisory Committee for HIV and STD Prevention. MMWR 47(RR12):1, 1998.
27. Centers for Disease Control and Prevention: HIV/AIDS surveillance report. 9:21, 1998.
28. Centers for Disease Control and Prevention. Basic statistics—cumulative cases. http://www.cdc.gov/hiv/stats/cumulati.htm.
29. Centers for Disease Control and Prevention. Current trends in preliminary analysis: HIV serosurvey of orthopedic surgeons, 1991. MMWR 40:309, 1991.
30. Centers for Disease Control and Prevention: Projections of the number of persons diagnosed with AIDS and the number of immunosuppressed HIV-infected persons, United States, 1992–1994. MMWR 41(RR18), 1992.
31. Centers for Disease Control and Prevention: Public Health Service guidelines for the management of health care worker ex-

posures to HIV and recommendations for post-exposure prophylaxis. MMWR 47(RR7):1, 1998.
32. Centers for Disease Control and Prevention: Recommendations for prevention of HIV transmission in health-care settings. MMWR 36(S2), 1987.
33. Centers for Disease Control and Prevention: U.S. Public Health Service recommendations for management of health care worker exposures to HIV and recommendations for post-exposure prophylaxis. MMWR 47(RR7):1, 1998.
34. Centers for Disease Control and Prevention: Recommendations for prevention and control of hepatitis C virus infection and HCV-related chronic disease. 47(RR19):1, 1998.
35. Centers for Disease Control and Prevention: U.S. Public Health Service Task Force recommendations for the use of antiretroviral drugs in pregnant women infected with HIV-1 for maternal health and for reducing perinatal HIV-1 transmission in the United States. http://www.hivatis.org.
36. Centers for Disease Control and Prevention: The HIV/AIDS epidemic: The first ten years. MMWR 40:357, 1991.
37. Centers for Disease Control and Prevention: Transmission of HIV through bone transplantation: Case report and public health recommendations. MMWR 37:587, 1988.
38. Centers for Disease Control and Prevention: Update: Serologic testing for HIV-1 antibody—United States, 1988 and 1989. MMWR 39:380, 1990.
39. Centers for Disease Control and Prevention: Update: Transmission of HIV infection during an invasive dental procedure—Florida. MMWR 40:21, 1991.
40. Centers for Disease Control and Prevention: Update: Transmission of HIV infection during an invasive dental procedure—Florida. MMWR 40:377, 1991.
41. Centers for Disease Control and Prevention: Update: trends in AIDS incidence, deaths, and prevalence—United States, 1996. MMWR 46:155, 1997.
42. Centers for Disease Control and Prevention: Update: Universal precautions for prevention of transmission of human immunodeficiency virus, hepatitis B virus, and other blood borne pathogens in healthcare settings. MMWR 37:377, 1988.
43. Chaisson RE: Epidemiology of human immunodeficiency virus and acquired immunodeficiency syndrome: In Gorabach SL, ed: Infectious Diseases. Philadelphia, WB Saunders, 1992, p 912.
44. Chin J: Global estimates of AIDS cases and HIV infection. AIDS 4(S1):S277, 1990.
45. Ciesielski C et al: Transmission of human immunodeficiency virus in a dental practice. Ann Intern Med 116:798, 1992.
46. Connor EM et al. Reduction of maternal-infant transmission of human immunodeficiency virus type-1 with zidovudine treatment. N Engl J Med 331:1173, 1994.
47. Coombs RW et al: Plasma viremia in human immunodeficiency virus infection. N Engl J Med 321:1626, 1989.
48. Cooper DA et al: Acute AIDS retrovirus infection. Definition of a clinical illness associated with seroconversion. Lancet 1:537, 1985.
49. Crawford EJ, Baird PR: An orthopaedic presentation of AIDS: Brief report. J Bone Joint Surg Br 69:672, 1987.
50. Cuellar ML: HIV infection-associated inflammatory musculoskeletal disorders. Rheum Dis Clin North Am 24(2):403, 1998.
51. Denning DW: Acute myelopathy associated with primary infection with human immunodeficiency virus. Br Med J 294:143, 1987.
52. Detels R: Effectiveness of potent anti-retroviral therapy on time to AIDS and death in men with known HIV infection duration. JAMA 280:1497, 1998.
53. Enger C: Survival from early, intermediate and late stages of HIV infection. JAMA 275:1329, 1996.
54. Espinoza LR: There is an association between human immunodeficiency virus infection and spondyloarthropathies. Rheum Dis Clin North Am 18:257, 1992.
55. Fahey BJ: Frequency of non-parenteral occupational exposures to blood and body fluids before and after universal precautions training. Am J Med 90:145, 1991.
56. Farthing C, Gazzard B: Acute illnesses associated with HTLV-III seroconversion [letter]. Lancet 1:935, 1985.
57. Fauci AS: Immunopathogenic mechanisms of HIV infection. Ann Intern Med 124:654, 1996.
58. Fox R: Clinical manifestations of acute infection with human immunodeficiency virus in a cohort of gay men. AIDS 1:35, 1987.
59. Gerberding JL: Management of occupational exposures to blood-borne viruses. N Engl J Med 332:444, 1995.
60. Gerberding, JL: Editorial. Provider-to-patient HIV transmission: How to keep it exceedingly rare. Ann Intern Med 130:64, 1999.
61. Gold JE: Malignant plasma cell tumors in human immunodeficiency virus-infected patients. Cancer 66:363, 1990.
62. Goudsmit J: Expression of human immunodeficiency virus antigen in serum and cerebral spinal fluid during acute and chronic infection. Lancet 2:177, 1986.
63. Graham NMH: Effect of zidovudine and PCP prophylaxis on progression of HIV-1 infection to AIDS. Lancet 338:265, 1991.
64. Haynes BF: Toward an understanding of the correlates of protective immunity to HIV infection. Science 271:325, 1996.
65. Henderson DK: Risk for occupational transmission of human immunodeficiency virus type 1 associated with clinical exposures. A prospective evaluation. Ann Intern Med 113:740, 1990.
66. Herts BR: Soft tissue and osseous lesions caused by bacillary angiomatosis: Unusual manifestations of cat-scratch fever in patients with AIDS. AJR Am J Roentgeneol 157:1249, 1991.
67. Hirsch R: Human immunodeficiency virus-associated atypical mycobacterial skeletal infections. Semin Arthritis Rheum 25: 347, 1996.
68. Ho DD: Primary human T-lymphotrophic virus type III infection. Ann Intern Med 103:880, 1985.
69. Ho DD: Quantitation of human immunodeficiency virus type 1 in the blood of infected persons. N Engl J Med 321:1621, 1989.
70. Hughes RA: Septic bone, joint and muscle lesions associated with human immunodeficiency virus infection. Br J Rheumatol 31:381, 1992.
71. Ippolito G: The risk of occupational human immunodeficiency virus infection in health care workers: Italian multicenter study. Arch Intern Med 153:1451, 1993.
72. Johnson AM, Laga M: Heterosexual transmission of HIV. AIDS 2(S1):S49, 1988.
73. Johnson GK, Robinson WS: Human immunodeficiency virus in the vapors of surgical power instruments. J Med Virol 33:47, 1991.
74. Kaye, BR: Rheumatologic manifestations of HIV infections. Clin Rev Allergy Immunol 14(4):385, 1996.
75. Kessler HA: Diagnosis of human immunodeficiency virus infection in seronegative homosexuals presenting with an acute viral syndrome. JAMA 258:1196, 1987.
76. Lackritz EM: Estimated risk of transmission of the human immunodeficiency virus by screened blood in the United States. N Engl J Med 333:1721, 1995.
77. LaPrarie AJ, Gross M: A simplified protocol for banking bone transplantation from surgical donors requiring a 90-day quarantine and an HIV-1 antibody test. Can J Surg 34:41, 1991.
78. Lot F: Probable transmission of HIV from an orthopedic surgeon to a patient in France. Ann Intern Med 130:1, 1999.
79. Mann JM: AIDS—the second decade: A global perspective. J Infect Dis 165:245, 1992.
80. Mast ST: Efficacy of gloves in reducing blood volumes transferred during simulated needlestick injury. J Infect Dis 168: 1589, 1993.
81. Masters DL, Lentino JR: Cervical osteomyelitis related Nocardia asteroides. J Infect Dis 149:824, 1984.
82. Masur H: CD4 counts as predictors of opportunistic pneumonias in human immunodeficiency virus infection. Ann Intern Med 111:223, 1989.
83. Matava MJ: Serial quantification of human immunodeficiency virus in an arthroscopic effluent. Case report. Arthroscopy 13(6):739, 1997.
84. McCormick RD: Epidemiology of hospital sharps injuries: A 14-year prospective study in the pre-AIDS and AIDS eras. Am J Med 91:S301, 1991.
85. Mellert W: Infection of human fibroblasts and osteoblast-like cells with HIV-1. AIDS 4:527, 1990.
86. Mellors JW: Plasma viral load and CD4+ lymphocytes as prognostic markers of HIV-1 infection. Ann Intern Med 126:946, 1997.
87. Meyers SA: Kaposi sarcoma involving bone: CT demonstration in a patient with AIDS. J Comput Assist Tomogr 14:161, 1990.

88. Munoz FS: Osteoarticular infection associated with the human immunodeficiency virus. Clin Exp Rheumatol 9:489, 1991.
89. Munoz FS: Rheumatic manifestations in 556 patients with human immunodeficiency virus infection. Semin Arthritis Rheum 21:30, 1991.
90. Niu MT: Primary human immunodeficiency virus type I infection: Review of pathogenesis and early treatment intervention in human and animal retrovirus infections. JID 168:1490, 1993.
91. Pantaleo G: HIV infection is active and progressive in lymphoid tissue during the clinically latent stage of disease. Nature 362: 355, 1993.
92. Paton P: Coronary artery lesions and human immunodeficiency virus infection. Res Virol 144:225, 1993.
93. Polis MA, Masur H: Predicting the progression to AIDS. Am J Med 89:701, 1990.
94. Quinn TC: The epidemiology of AIDS: A decade of experience. Curr Clin Top Infect Dis 11:61, 1991.
95. Raahave D, Bremmelgaard A: New operative technique to reduce surgeons' risk of HIV infection. J Hosp Infect 18(Suppl A):S177, 1991.
96. Robert LM: Investigations of patients of health care workers infected with HIV. The Centers for Disease Control and Prevention database. Ann Intern Med 122:653, 1995.
97. Roder W: HIV infection in human bone. J Bone Joint Surg Br 74:179, 1992.
98. Rowe IF: Arthritis in the acquired immunodeficiency syndrome and other viral infections. Curr Opin Rheumatol 3:621, 1991.
99. Rowe IF: HIV- and AIDS-related musculoskeletal problems. Curr Opin Rheumatol 2:642, 1990.
100. Sabbagh M: Bone manifestations associated with the acquired immunodeficiency syndrome. Ann Med Interne (Paris) 143:50, 1992.
101. Shapiro CN: Occupational risk of infection with hepatitis B and hepatitis C virus. Surg Clin North Am 75(6):1047, 1995.
102. Simonds RJ: Transmission of human immunodeficiency virus type 1 from a seronegative organ and tissue donor. N Engl J Med 326:726, 1992.
103. Slagis SV: Postoperative blood salvage in total hip and knee arthroplasty. A randomized controlled trial. J Bone Joint Surg Am 73:591, 1991.
104. Taylor JM: CD4 percentage, CD4 number, and CD4:CD8 ratio in HIV infection: Which to choose and how to use. J AIDS 2: 114, 1989.
105. Tehranzadeh J: The spectrum of osteoarticular and soft tissue changes in patients with human immunodeficiency (HIV) infection. Crit Rev Diagn Imag 37(4):305, 1996.
106. Timpone J: Avascular Necrosis in HIV+ Patients a Potential Link to Protease Inhibitors. Abstract 680. Sixth Conference on Retroviruses and Opportunistic Infections, January 31 - February 4, 1999.
107. Tindall B: Characterization of the acute clinical illness associated with human immunodeficiency virus infection. Arch Intern Med 148:945, 1988.
108. Tokars JI: A survey of occupational blood contact and HIV infection among orthopedic surgeons. JAMA 268:489, 1992.
109. Tokars JI: Percutaneous injuries during surgical procedures. JAMA 267:2899, 1992.
110. Tokars JI: Surveillance of HIV infection and zidovudine use among health care workers after occupational exposure to HIV-infected blood. Ann Intern Med 118:913, 1993.
111. Van der Wouw PA: Disseminated cat-scratch disease in a patient with AIDS. AIDS 3:751, 1989.
112. Vassilopoulos D: Musculoskeletal infections in patients with human immunodeficiency virus infection. Medicine 76:284, 1997.
113. Tebas P: Accelerated bone mineral loss in HIV-infected patients receiving patient antiretroviral therapy. Abstract 207. 7th Conference on Retrovirus and Opportunistic Infections. January 30, 2000.
114. Hoy J: Osteopenia in a randomized, multicenter study of protease inhibitor (PI) substitution in patients with the lipodystrophy syndrome and well-controlled HIV viremia. Abstract 208. 7th Conference on Retrovirus and Opportunisitic Infections. January 30, 2000.

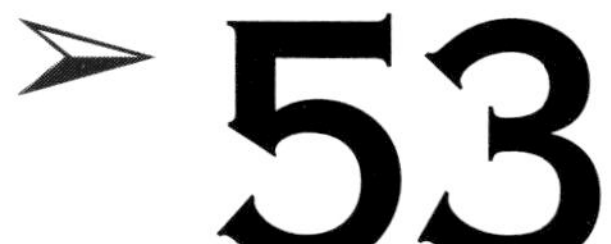

Complex Regional Pain Syndromes, Types I (Reflex Sympathetic Dystrophy) and II (Causalgia)

BRADLEY S. GALER

Although in the past decade there has been an increased awareness and academic interest among pain specialists with regard to the syndrome classically referred to as *reflex sympathetic dystrophy* (RSD), little new knowledge has been gained about its pathophysiology. However, much that was taught in the past about RSD has been questioned, if not discarded, as medical folklore not based in scientific fact.

In 1993, an expert panel of the International Association for the Study of Pain (IASP) recommended that the terms *reflex sympathetic dystrophy* and *causalgia* be replaced with *complex regional pain syndrome* (CRPS) type I and type II, respectively, with well-defined clinical diagnostic criteria (see later discussion). This new taxonomy has been accepted by most pain specialists, but other physicians, such as orthopedic surgeons, have yet to be educated about these important changes. One aim of this chapter is to familiarize the orthopedic physician with this new nomenclature.

CRPS (RSD) most commonly occurs in a distal extremity (i.e., the foot or hand), although CRPS by definition can be present in any bodily area covered by skin. Symptoms and signs of CRPS can and do occur in the knee. However, no reports or studies have been published to date using the new diagnostic criteria of CRPS with knee involvement. Thus, this chapter's recommendations are made based on prior RSD of the knee literature (which is scarce), the pain medicine field's consensus with regard to CRPS, and my personal experience with CRPS of the knee and other body parts. (For more complete and up-to-date information on CRPS, the reader is referred to Galer et al.[22])

CRPS DIAGNOSTIC CRITERIA

> Many medical disorders have no clear single diagnostic "gold standard" (e.g., known measurable etiological process or laboratory test result) that unequivocally indicates the presence or absence of the disorder. Most disease states reflect a spectrum of associated signs and symptoms. Often no prototypic signs and symptoms define the presentation of a given disorder across all cases. Thus, development of standardized, reliable diagnostic criteria and decision rules to identify disorders is the only way to allow adequate generalizability for appropriate treatment selection and identification of reproducible research samples. Medicine continually attempts to classify symptoms and signs into distinct categories with the goal of achieving standardized diagnostic criteria and hence leading to improved understanding of symptom/sign pathophysiology and eventually to improved treatment.[19]

Unlike many other disorders in orthopedic medicine, the problem with many chronic pain disorders, including CRPS/RSD, is that no laboratory testing can identify or confirm the diagnosis. Thus, physicians must develop, study, and agree on clinical diagnostic criteria to identify disease entities, which, it is hoped, lead to improved therapeutic outcomes. Currently, the pain medicine field is actively refining the clinical criteria of this disorder.

Why Was RSD Renamed CRPS?

Over the past decade or so, confusion arose as to the diagnostic criteria for RSD. No single diagnostic criterion was widely accepted by clinicians and researchers worldwide. Diagnostic criteria differed among different specialists. This lack of consensus retarded progress regarding this disorder's pathophysiology and made interpretation of clinical trials difficult.

In 1993, a consensus group of pain medicine experts (a Special Consensus Workshop of the IASP) gathered with the defined task of re-evaluating the clinical syndromes of RSD and causalgia.[49] This group agreed to dismantle the terms RSD and causalgia. Besides the lack of diagnostic criteria for RSD, the experts agreed that (1) much medical folklore exists with reference to RSD and causalgia, which reflected early anecdotal physician personal experiences rather than scientific clinical study, (2) many patients do not demonstrate the classically described dystrophic signs, such as atrophy and changes in skin, nails, and hair, and (3) many, if not most, patients with this disorder do not report significant relief with a sympathetic blockade.

CRPS CRITERIA

The diagnostic criteria for CRPS as defined in 1993 were accepted by the IASP Classification Committee and published in 1994[35] (Table 53.1). Importantly, as with all clinically based criteria, it is understood that these published criteria should and must evolve based on the results of scientifically performed validation studies.

Unlike prior criteria of RSD and causalgia, the diagnostic criteria for CRPS are purely clinical (i.e., there is no need for laboratory testing or a positive response to sympathetic block). All that is needed is a history, pain, and symptom description and physical signs that fulfill the diagnostic criteria.

CRPS is divided into two subtypes based on the type of injury that apparently initiated the disorder: type I follows a soft tissue injury, akin to RSD, whereas type II follows a well-defined nerve injury, akin to causalgia. Both types I and II are otherwise identical, with the same diagnostic symptoms and signs. However, it may not always be possible to identify whether a patient's CRPS followed injury to nerve, soft tissue, or both, which may be the case in CRPS of the knee. No published studies have assessed the CRPS diagnostic criteria with symptoms and signs in the knee. I have used the CRPS criteria successfully in patients with unexplained knee pain.

For most knee pain patients who meet the IASP diagnostic criteria for CRPS, it is unclear whether it is type I (i.e., associated with soft tissue injury) or type II (i.e., associated with a nerve injury) or perhaps a combination of both types I and II. (For prognostic and therapeutic issues, it appears that type I and type II behave similarly; thus, the division may only be an academic point.) A retrospective study reported that 35 of 35 (100%) RSD patients examined "had clinical evidence of insult to the inferior branch of the saphenous nerve."[39] Yet I have cared for patients with knee CRPS in whom such nerve injury has not been apparent.

TABLE 53.1 COMPLEX REGIONAL PAIN SYNDROME (CRPS) DIAGNOSTIC CRITERIA

CRPS Type I

1. The presence of an initiating noxious event or a cause of immobilization.
2. Continuing pain, allodynia, or hyperalgesia with which the pain is disproportionate to any inciting event.
3. Evidence at some time of edema, changes in skin blood flow (skin color changes, skin temperature changes >1.1°C difference from the homologous body part), or abnormal sudomotor activity in the region of pain.
4. This diagnosis is excluded by the existence of conditions that would otherwise account for the degree of pain and dysfunction.

CRPS Type II

1. The presence of continuing pain, allodynia, or hyperalgesia after a nerve injury, not necessarily limited to the distribution of the injured nerve.
2. Evidence at some time of edema, changes in skin blood flow (skin color changes, skin temperature changes >1.1°C), or abnormal sudomotor activity in the region of pain.
3. This diagnosis is excluded by the existence of conditions that would otherwise account for the degree of pain and dysfunction.

Adapted from Merskey H, Bogduk N: Classification of Chronic Pain. Seattle, IASP Press, 1994.

SYMPATHETICALLY MAINTAINED PAIN

Sympathetically maintained pain (SMP) is defined as pain that is maintained by sympathetic efferent innervation or by circulating catecholamines.[49] Thus, SMP is a pain mechanism and not a clinical diagnosis. The term SMP should only be used in clinical practice to describe a patient's report of pain relief after a sympatholytic procedure; that is, if a patient reports good pain relief after a sympathetic block, then that patient can be said to have SMP. If a patient does not report significant pain reduction with a sympathetic block, then she or he may be said to have sympathetically independent pain (SIP).

SMP is a pain mechanism, whereas CRPS is a clinical diagnosis. Thus, the term SMP cannot be used interchangeably with CRPS. By definition, SMP cannot be defined by the presence of dysautonomic symptoms and signs, such as skin color changes, skin temperature changes, and sudomotor abnormalities. Patients with CRPS may or may not have SMP. Other pain patients who do not have CRPS may or may not have SMP. In fact, it is currently believed that the majority of CRPS patients do not have SMP but instead have SIP. Moreover, response to sympathetic block may be partial; therefore, a CRPS patient may have components of both SMP and SIP.

EPIDEMIOLOGY

To date, no well-designed prospective studies have assessed the epidemiology of this disorder, whether using old RSD/causalgia criteria or the new CRPS criteria in the general nonmilitary population. Several studies assessed some basic demographic information regarding RSD, but these suffer from selection bias because they mostly reflect patients seen in a tertiary care setting.

RSD patients seen in a Netherlands tertiary referral surgical clinic were reported as having a median age of 41 years (range 4 to 84 years) and a mean duration of RSD of 405 days.[54] A tertiary university-based pain center in the United States found that their patients had a mean age of 41.8 years (range - 18 to 71 years), a mean age at injury of 37.7 years (range 14 to 64 years), and a mean duration of CRPS symptoms before pain center evaluation of 30 months (range 2 to 168 months).[2] Both studies found a female preponderance:

a 3:1 ratio[54] in the Netherlands population and a 2.3:1 ratio in U.S. pain clinic patients.[2] Most patients had CRPS involving a single limb, with a fairly equal involvement of the upper versus lower extremities.[2, 53]

Overall in the RSD patient population, one study reported that 65% of their patients' RSD developed in association with trauma, most commonly a fracture, 19% with an "operation," 2% with an "inflammatory process," and 4% "after various other precipitants, such as injection or intravenous infusion."[54] The U.S. chronic pain clinic study found the following inciting events: 29% strain or sprain, 24% postsurgical, and 11% contusion/crush injury.[2] Both studies identified patients with no known precipitating cause, ranging from 10% to 23%.[2, 54]

No studies assessed epidemiological factors using the CRPS criteria with knee involvement. However, several studies reported on the development of RSD after orthopedic procedures. A large prospective study involving "21 experienced arthroscopists" assessed complications associated with arthroscopic surgery of the knee and other joints.[46] (Importantly, the data from this study should be interpreted cautiously; they may be biased because data collection was by monthly questionnaires completed by the performing surgeon and not the patient.) This study assessed a total of 10,262 procedures, of which 8741 (85%) were performed in the knee, and reported that 173 (1.68%) complications occurred, of which 2.9% were RSD. A similar retrospective study of 2640 arthroscopic procedures on the knee found a total of 216 complications (8.2%), of which 126 were categorized as major, including RSD.[45] This study also found a higher rate of RSD in patients with an industrial injury. Yet another study noted that arthroscopic procedures were the most common precipitating event for the development of RSD in the knee.[37] A case review reported that 23 of 36 patients with RSD "primarily affecting the knee" had injuries or operation on the patellofemoral joint as a trigger.[29] Thus, based on the current literature, there is a small but definite risk for the development of RSD/CRPS associated with knee surgery, most notably arthroscopy.

CRPS PATHOPHYSIOLOGY

The pathophysiology of CRPS is not known. It is not known why, after a soft tissue injury, only a minority of people experience CRPS. It is not known why traumatic incidents in the same person, such as a minor ankle sprain, can result repeatedly in self-limited traumas that resolve and another seemingly similar incident can result in CRPS. Even with CRPS type II, it is not known why, with the same nerve injury, one person experiences no chronic pain, another has severe neuropathic pain, and yet another experiences CRPS.

Most authorities hypothesize that CRPS most likely develops from abnormalities throughout the neuraxis, including peripheral nervous system, central nervous system, and autonomic nervous system.[22] Also, the involvement of regional myofascial dysfunction (i.e., focal dysfunctional, spastic muscle) may also play an important role in CRPS.[42] The degree to which each system is involved probably varies among patients. Furthermore, psychological factors, ongoing stress, and disuse of the involved body part have a direct impact on the entire nervous system and musculoskeletal system.

Thus, most likely one single pathophysiological process is not responsible for the development and maintenance of CRPS. Rather, CRPS is likely a heterogeneous disorder with several different underlying pathophysiological mechanisms that result in similar clinical symptoms and signs (Table 53.2). Perhaps the different patterns of symptoms and signs observed

TABLE 53.2 POSTULATED PATHOPHYSIOLOGICAL MECHANISMS

Mechanism	Description
Aberrant healing	Exaggerated and persistent inflammatory response is present. Local release of substance P, CGRP, bradykinin, leukotrienes, histamine, prostaglandins, and serotonin into the damaged tissues may result in vasodilation and increased vascular permeability.[31]
Disuse	Physiological changes associated with not using a body part are present, including swelling (dependent edema), cold (decreased blood flow), and trophic changes (decreased blood flow). Immobilizing a rodent limb with casting for several weeks results in significant allodynia (pain caused by non-noxious stimulation) and changes within the dorsal horn similar to those caused by peripheral nerve injury.[34, 52] After uncomplicated orthopedic surgery and casting, a study demonstrated that a majority of patients postoperatively experience CRPS symptoms and signs, these resolve with time and physical therapy.[9]
Myofascial	Tight spastic muscles may be primarily or secondarily involved in the symptoms in some CRPS patients. On examination, up to 61% of CRPS patients had evidence of trigger points in the proximal musculature that reproduced CRPS signs and symptoms when palpated.[42]
Peripheral somatic nerve	In CRPS type II, as with any other peripheral neuropathic pain, it is presumed that abnormal ectopic impulses develop at the site of injury and adjacent to the dorsal root ganglia. In CRPS type I, abnormal somatic nerve function may be present even if EMG/NCV are normal; EMG/NCV only measure large fiber function and cannot test small fiber function. In addition, they do not assess neurotransmitter/neuropeptide alerations within the PNS.
Spinal cord	Abnormal impulses from peripheral nerve result in abnormal sensitivity of dorsal horn neurons.
Brain	All pain is ultimately perceived in the brain. Autonomic nervous system has a CNS component that, when stimulated, results in peripheral dysautonomic signs. Alterations in the thalamus have been shown in PET scanning of CRPS patients.[3]

CGRP = calcitonin gene-related peptide; CRPS = complex regional pain syndrome; EMG = electromyogram; NCV = nerve conduction velocity; PET = positron emission tomography; PNS = peripheral nervous system.

among CRPS patients may be reflective of the different underlying pathophysiologies.

NEW THOUGHTS REGARDING THE SYMPATHETIC NERVOUS SYSTEM AND CRPS/RSD

The classic teaching of RSD has been that the major underlying cause is a disturbance in the sympathetic nervous system.[7, 8] This belief emanated from physicians' clinical experience that patients with RSD reported pain relief with sympathetic nerve block. In addition, it was believed that the only viable explanation for the unusual and prominent vasomotor changes associated with this disorder, such as the focal skin color and temperature changes, was considered an abnormal sympathetic tone in the involved limb; hence, the term *dysautonomic signs* was coined to describe these abnormalities.

However, it must be realized that prior diagnostic criteria required patients to have reported good pain relief after a sympathetic blockade in order to be diagnosed with RSD. Thus, by definition, all RSD patients responded to sympathetic block or they did not have RSD.

Moreover, clinical data suggested that the involvement of the sympathetic nervous system in CRPS (and RSD) may not be responsible for the symptoms and signs associated with this disorder. Studies questioned the mechanism of action in which sympathetic blocks produce pain relief. For instance, results from several studies suggested nonsympathetic involvement: (1) after selective sympathetic blockade, such as lumbar sympathetic block, there is a clinically significant systemic absorption of local anesthetic, which can result in clinically relevant activity in other regions of the nervous system besides the sympathetic nervous system[4, 56]; (2) after selective sympathetic blockade, there has been documented spillage of local anesthetic onto adjacent nonsympathetic nerve fibers[27]; (3) the degree of pain relief obtained from sympathetic blockade does not correlate with the degree of sympathetic dysfunction[13, 41]; (4) time of onset and duration of pain relief do not correlate with the timing of sympathetic block[17, 41]; and (5) the CRPS-affected limbs' catecholamine concentration does not correlate with pain relief after sympathetic blockade.[15]

ARE THERE RISK FACTORS FOR CRPS?

Many factors have been postulated to be risk factors that may predispose individuals to CRPS/RSD, including extensive immobilization (and disuse), cigarette smoking, genetic predisposition, and psychological factors.[9, 28, 33, 38] However, none of these factors have been scientifically proven to actually increase the risk for CRPS. In fact, psychological factors, such as patient personality and the presence of comorbid psychiatric disorders, have been shown not to have any relevance with regard to predisposing patients to CRPS/RSD.[12, 32] Yet some intriguing data suggest that physiological or psychological stress at the time of an injury may predispose persons to CRPS.[16, 22, 36]

CRPS TREATMENT

No treatment, whether procedural or medical, can cure CRPS. No treatment has been shown in a large controlled study to alleviate the pain and other symptoms in a majority of CRPS sufferers. Unfortunately, the overall clinical experience with all medical and procedural treatments is poor. (Several excellent detailed treatment reviews have been published and are recommended reading.[22, 30, 51]) However, many CRPS/RSD patients do experience significant symptomatic relief and improved functional status when participating in a multidisciplinary therapeutic regimen, including, but not limited to, medical interventions, active physiotherapeutic modalities, and stress management training. In fact, this multidisciplinary approach is the therapeutic gold standard currently recommended.[22, 48]

Multidisciplinary Treatment

The primary goal of multidisciplinary management is to improve functional restoration of the CRPS body region through long-term, quota-based physical/occupational therapy. The physician's role is to provide pain and symptom relief via medication or procedures and to manage the overall treatment team. The psychologist's role is to identify co-morbid psychiatric conditions, such as depression, post-traumatic stress disorder, and anxiety disorder. Psychological treatment approaches include cognitive-behavioral techniques and supportive psychotherapy, with the goal of teaching the patient pain-coping skills. The physiotherapist's role, probably the key interventionalist and therapeutic provider, is to organize and manage the daily rehabilitative treatment of the patient. It is imperative that all medical providers are experienced in the care of CRPS patients and work closely as a cohesive team, with frequent team meetings to address patient progress. Multidisciplinary management of CRPS can be painstakingly slow (for both patient and providers), taking several months to a year or even longer. The key is slow, gradual, yet persistent documented functional improvement.[22]

Recommended Medical Therapies

Anesthetic Techniques

SYMPATHETIC BLOCKADE

As discussed, the earlier teaching of necessitating a series of sympathetic blocks has been discarded. This dramatic change in recommendations is based on worldwide experience that (1) a majority of patients do not respond to sympathetic blockade and (2) if a patient does not respond to one block (that was performed well), then proceeding with more blocks is not warranted.

Yet every CRPS patient should receive at least one well-performed sympathetic block because, for a minority of patients, the response will be dramatic. Knee CRPS patients should obtain a lumbar sympathetic block from an experienced pain anesthesiologist. If a patient does have SMP, then significant pain and symptom relief is observed. Importantly, when such a patient is encountered, it is imperative that active physical therapy be performed immediately while the patient is afforded relief from the block.

Intravenous Lidocaine Infusion and Oral Mexiletine

It is well established that an intravenous lidocaine infusion (5 mg/kg body weight infused over 30 minutes into a *nonpainful* limb) will result in significant pain relief for a majority of neuropathic pain patients.[21] Although not well studied in CRPS, the clinical experience of pain specialists is that many CRPS patients do obtain relief from this procedure. However, the vast majority of patients who do report relief with systemic lidocaine infusion experience only transient pain relief, on the order of several hours. Many pain centers use an intravenous lidocaine infusion as a predictive test to assess whether a patient should then be prescribed the oral analogue of lidocaine, mexiletine.[20]

Injections into the Knee

No literature exists assessing the efficacy and safety of direct injection of substances into the knee for the treatment of knee CRPS/RSD. As with surgery performed on a CRPS-affected body part, injections into a knee with CRPS run the risk of exacerbating the condition. Although it has not been studied, an interesting therapy that perhaps has some theoretical grounding is intra-articular opioid injection. Such treatment requires future study.

ORAL MEDICATION

As with other chronic pain conditions, oral medication is prescribed using a trial-and-error method with subsequent drug trials. The key is to aggressively titrate each drug prescribed at least weekly until the patient reports substantial pain relief or intolerable side effects (with the exception of corticosteroids). It is also very important to titrate one drug at a time and discontinue a drug if intolerable side effects are reported.

CORTICOSTEROIDS

In several very small uncontrolled case series, pulse doses of corticosteroids (60-80 mg/day) for 2 to 12 weeks have been reported to be beneficial in RSD patients.[10] All of these patients were treated within weeks to several months of symptom onset, and none reported long-term follow-up data. Clinical experience with corticosteroids in CRPS patients who have had symptoms for more than 6 months is poor. Chronic steroid treatment should not be prescribed.

GABAPENTIN

Although there are no controlled studies published assessing gabapentin for the treatment of CRPS, most pain specialists use gabapentin as their first-line agent for CRPS. In my experience, at least one-third of CRPS patients report noticeable pain and symptom relief and tolerable side effects from gabapentin. The drug dosage must be titrated at least weekly to a maximum of 6000 mg/day; the average successful dose is approximately 3600 mg, although some patients need a smaller dose and some need a larger dose.

ORAL SYMPATHOLYTIC AGENTS

Although case series have reported benefit from prazosin,[1] phenoxybenzamine,[23] and terazosin,[50] the clinical experience for these agents is poor, with significant side effects and rarely significant pain relief.

CLONIDINE

A small uncontrolled study reported that several RSD patients with SMP observed relief of allodynia (skin sensitivity) under the application site of a transdermal clonidine patch.[11] Clinical experience has been poor with all systemic versions of clonidine because of significant systemic side effects. On the horizon, however, is a new formulation of topical clonidine gel with only local peripheral activity and minimal systemic activity, which has been shown in an open-label pilot study to relieve pain and allodynia in some CRPS patients.[14]

TOPICAL LIDOCAINE PATCH

A topical lidocaine patch that has Food and Drug Administration-approved indication for postherpetic neuralgia (shingles) has been used with some success to help treat the pain of CRPS, although controlled trials have not been performed.[18] This novel drug alleviates pain and allodynia in postherpetic neuralgia by a local anesthetic effect without any systemic activity.[43]

TRICYCLIC ANTIDEPRESSANTS

Unlike their use for the treatment of other neuropathic pains, tricyclic antidepressants for CRPS have a poor clinical experience. However, as in many other chronic pain states, these drugs are often prescribed to improve sleep.

CALCIUM CHANNEL BLOCKERS AND β-BLOCKERS

Although several case reports have been published claiming pain relief from calcium channel blockers,[40] the clinical experience is poor for these agents. A placebo-controlled trial failed to show efficacy for the β-blocker propranolol.[44] Thus, these agents have fallen out of favor for the treatment of CRPS.

CALCITONIN

A newer agent, calcitonin, has some controlled evidence suggesting efficacy in RSD[6, 24] when prescribed within 8 weeks of injury. However, the clinical experience using intranasal calcitonin for the treatment of CRPS has been disappointing.

OPIOIDS

Most chronic pain experts believe that some patients with CRPS will experience significant pain relief with minimal side effects from opioids, allowing for improved functional compliance with an active physiotherapy program. However, as with most drugs in this condition, only a minority of CRPS patients report dramatic relief and no side effects. When prescribing opioids as the primary medication, a long-acting opioid, such as methadone or sustained-release formulations of morphine and oxycodone, should be prescribed using time-contingent dosing (i.e., around-the-clock and not as needed). The dose should be titrated as described earlier, as with any other oral agent.

Implantable Spinal Devices

Spinal cord stimulation and intrathecal opioid pumps have been proposed for the treatment of many types of chronic pain, including CRPS. No controlled clinical studies have been published regarding their usage in CRPS, although case series of successful implantation have been published.[5, 25, 26] Many pain experts report a gradual diminution of efficacy, even in those patients with initial symptomatic relief. Intrathecal opioid and spinal cord stimulation should be reserved for CRPS patients in whom more conservative approaches have failed.[47]

SURGICAL SYMPATHECTOMY

Surgical sympathectomy should be considered only in those knee CRPS patients who consistently report significant pain and symptom relief after lumbar sympathetic blockade, yet whose duration of relief is transient. However, even in patients who reliably experience relief with each local anesthetic sympathetic ganglion block, extended pain relief after surgical ablation of the sympathetic fibers is not guaranteed. In fact, patients may report no relief at all or may even complain of a worsening of their underlying CRPS after the surgical procedure. The response rate reported in the literature for surgical sympathectomy varies from 12% to 97%, depending on the series and follow-up time.[55] In addition, postsympathectomy syndrome is a common complication of lumbar sympathectomy, characterized by pain in the anterior thigh.

PHYSIOTHERAPY

Even though most authorities currently agree that an active physiotherapy program is probably the most crucial therapeutic piece to treating CRPS, no studies have been published assessing different techniques. Although many therapists use "passive" modalities, such as warm and cold baths, ultrasonography, and electrical stimulation, the "active" modalities are more important, such as stretching, strengthening, and aerobic conditioning.

The goal of an active program is to restore range of motion, strength, and motor control as well as build functional tolerance to activities such as standing, sitting, and walking. To attain these goals, appropriate dosing of exercise is critical such that, for each individual activity or specific exercise, a baseline is first established (i.e., the amount of exercise that causes the patient to feel increased pain, muscle weakness, or fatigue). During each subsequent session (or every week), the number of repetitions and times are increased by 5% to 10%. This formula allows the individual to begin exercising at a level that is well within a reasonable level of exercise tolerance and then progress at a gentle, reasonable rate. Patients are instructed to perform exactly that number of repetitions, not more or less, regardless of pain. The implementation of quota-based exercise dosing helps the individual increase functional physical ability while decreasing the oscillation cycles of activity tolerance inherent to pain-contingent dosing of activity.[22]

An important technique in treating the allodynia associated with CRPS is "desensitization." Desensitization is a progressive technique to gradually habituate the patient to non-noxious stimuli. Thus, the patient progresses through a sequence of materials from very soft, light textures to extremely course, irritating surfaces, which are rubbed directly against the affected skin region. Gradually, the affected limb habituates to increasingly irritating textures, until the patient can easily tolerate the touch of clothing, bed sheets, towels, and so on during normal activities of daily living. (For a more detailed discussion on specific physiotherapy programs for CRPS, the reader is referred to Galer et al.[22])

CONCLUSION

Much still needs to be learned about CRPS. Yet patients who suffer from this unusual and poorly understood condition can obtain both symptomatic relief and improved function with therapies that are currently available. Of primary therapeutic importance is that the CRPS patient be treated by a knowledgeable multidisciplinary pain team using medical, psychological, and physiotherapeutic modalities.

References

1. Abram SE, Lightfoot RW: Treatment of long-standing causalgia with prazosin. Reg Anesth 6:79, 1981.
2. Allen G, Galer BS, Schwartz L: Epidemiological review of 134 patients with complex regional pain syndrome evaluated at a chronic pain clinic. Pain 80:539, 1999.
3. Apkarian AV: Primary somatosensory cortex and pain. Pain Forum 5:188, 1996.
4. Backonja M, Gombar K: Serum lidocaine levels following stellate ganglion sympathetic blocks and intravenous lidocaine injection. J Pain Symptom Manage 7:2, 1992.

5. Barolet G, Schartzman R, Woo R: Epidural spinal cord stimulation in the management of reflex sympathetic dystrophy. Stereotact Funct Neurosurg 53:29, 1989.
6. Bickerstaff DR, Kanis JA: The use of nasal calcitonin in the treatment of post-traumatic algodystrophy. Br J Rheumatol 30: 291, 1991.
7. Bonica JJ: The Management of Pain. Philadelphia, Lea & Febiger, 1953.
8. Bonica JJ: The Management of Pain. Philadelphia, Lea & Febiger, 1990.
9. Butler SH, Galer BS, Bernirshka S: Disuse as a cause of signs and symptoms of CRPS-I [abstract]. In Proceedings of the 8th World Congress on Pain. Seattle, IASP Press, 1996, p 401.
10. Christensen K, Jensen EM, Noer I: The reflex sympathetic dystrophy syndrome response to treatment with systemic corticosteroids. Acta Chir Scand 148:653, 1982.
11. Davis KD, Treede RD, Raja SN, et al: Topical application of clonidine relieves hyperalgesia in patients with sympathetically maintained pain. Pain 47:309, 1991.
12. DeGood DE, Cundiff GW, Adams LE, et al: A psychosocial and behavioral comparison of RSD, low back pain, and headache patients. Pain 54:317, 1993.
13. Dellemijn PJI, Fields HL, Allen RR, et al: The interpretation of pain relief and sensory changes following sympathetic block. Brain 17:1475, 1994.
14. Devers A, Galer BS: Topically applied clonidine gel relieves neuropathic pain: Results of open-label pilot studies. Presented at the 17th Annual Scientific Meeting of the American Pain Society, 1998, p 124.
15. Drummond PD, Fincj PM, Smythe GA: Reflex sympathetic dystrophy: The significance of differing plasma catecholamine concentrations in affected and unaffected limbs. Brain 114:2025, 1991.
16. Ecker A: Norepinephrine in reflex sympathetic dystrophy: An hypothesis. Clin J Pain 5:313, 1989.
17. Galer BS: Preliminary report: Peak pain relief is delayed and duration of relief is extended following intravenous phentolamine infusion. Reg Anesth 20:444, 1995.
18. Devers A, Galer BS: Topical lidocaine patch relieves a variety of neuropathic pain conditions: An open label experience. Clin J Pain, in press.
19. Galer BS, Bruehl S, Harden RN: IASP diagnostic criteria for complex regional pain syndrome: A preliminary empirical validation study. Clin J Pain 14:48, 1998.
20. Galer BS, Harle, J, Rowbotham MC: Response to intravenous lidocaine infusion predicts subsequent response to oral mexiletine: A prospective study. J Pain Symptom Manage 12:161, 1996.
21. Galer BS, Miller KV, Rowbotham MC: Response to intravenous lidocaine infusion differs based on clinical diagnosis and site of nervous system injury. Neurology 43:1233, 1993.
22. Galer BS, Schwartz L, Allan R: Complex regional pain syndromes-type I/RSD and type II/CRPS. In Loeser JDL, ed: Bonica's Management of Pain. Philadelphia, Williams & Wilkins, 2000.
23. Ghostine SY, Comair YG, Turner DM, et al: Phenoxybenzamine in the treatment of causalgia. Report of 40 cases. J Neurosurg 60:1263, 1984.
24. Gobelet C, Meier JL, Schaffner W, et al: Calcitonin and reflex sympathetic dystrophy syndrome. Clin Rheum 5:382, 1986.
25. Gobelet C, Waldburger M, Meier JL: The effect of adding calcitonin to physical treatment of reflex sympathetic dystrophy. Pain 48:171, 1992.
26. Goodman R, Brisman R: Treatment of lower extremity reflex sympathetic dystrophy with continuous intrathecal morphine infusion. Appl Neurophysiol 50:425, 1987.
27. Hogan QH, Erickson SJ, Haddox JD, et al: The spread of solutions during stellate ganglion block. Reg Anesth 17:78, 1992.
28. Howard SA, Hawthorne KB, Jackson WT: Reflex sympathetic dystrophy and cigarette smoking. J Hand Surg Am 13:470, 1988.
29. Katz MM, Hungerford DS: Reflex sympathetic dystrophy affecting the knee. J Bone Joint Surg Br 69:797, 1987.
30. Kingery WS: A critical review of controlled clinical trials for peripheral neuropathic pain and complex regional pain syndromes. Pain 73:123, 1997.
31. Levine JD, Fields HL, Basbaum AL: Peptides and the primary afferent nociceptor. J Neurosci 13:2273, 1993.
32. Lynch ME: Psychological aspects of reflex sympathetic dystrophy: A review of the adult and paediatric literature. Pain 49:337, 1992.
33. Mailis A, Wade J: Profile of caucasian women with possible genetic predisposition to reflex sympathetic dystrophy: A pilot study. Clin J Pain 10:210, 1994.
34. Maves TJ, Smith B: Pain behaviors and sensory alterations following immobilization of the rat hindpaw [abstract]. In Proceedings of the 8th World Congress on Pain. Seattle, IASP Press, 1996, p 118.
35. Merskey H, Bogduk N: Classification of Chronic Pain. Seattle, IASP Press, 1994.
36. Nathan PW: Pain and the sympathetic nervous system. J Auton Nerv Syst 7:363, 1983.
37. O'Brien SJ, Ngeow J, Gibne MA, et al: Reflex sympathetic dystrophy of the knee. Causes, diagnosis, and treatment. Am J Sports Med 23:655, 1995.
38. Pawelka S, Fialka V, Ernst E: Reflex sympathetic dystrophy and cigarette smoking. J Hand Surg Am 18:168, 1993.
39. Poehling GG, Pollock FE, Koman LA: Reflex sympathetic dystrophy of the knee after sensory nerve injury. Arthroscopy 4:31, 1988.
40. Prough DS, McLeskey CH, Poehling GG, et al: Efficacy of oral nifedipine in the treatment of reflex sympathetic dystrophy. Anesthesiology 62:769, 1985.
41. Raja SR: Nerve blocks in the evaluation of chronic pain: A plea for caution in their use and interpretation. Anesthesiology 86:4, 1997.
42. Rashiq S, Galer BS: Myofascial dysfunction in complex regional pain syndrome: A retrospective prevalence study. Clin J Pain 15: 151, 1999.
43. Rowbotham MC, Davies PJ, Verkempinck CM, et al: Lidocaine patch: Double-blind controlled study of a new treatment method for postherpetic neuralgia. Pain 65:39, 1996.
44. Scadding JW, Wall PD, Parry W, et al: Clinical trial of propranolol in post-traumatic neuralgia. Pain 14:283, 1982.
45. Sherman OH, Fox JM, Snyder SJ, Del Pizzo W, et al: Arthroscopy—"No problem surgery." An analysis of complications in two thousand six hunderd and forty cases. J Bone Joint Surg Am 68:256, 1986.
46. Small NC: Complications in arthroscopic surgery performed by experienced arthroscopists. Arthroscopy 4:215, 1988.
47. Stangl JA, Loeser JD: Intraspinal opioid infusion therapy in the treatment of chronic nonmalignant pain. Current Rev Pain 1: 353, 1997.
48. Stanton-Hicks M, Baron R, Boas R: Consensus report—Complex regional syndromes: Guidelines for therapy. Clin J Pain 14:155, 1998.
49. Stanton-Hicks M, Janig W, Hassenbusch S, et al: Reflex sympathetic dystrophy: Changing concepts and taxonomy. Pain 63: 127, 1995.
50. Stevens DS, Robins VF, Price HM: Treatment of sympathetically maintained pain with terazosin. Reg Anesth 18:318, 1993.
51. Tanelian DT: Reflex sympathetic dystrophy: A reevaluation of the literature. Pain Forum 5:247, 1996.
52. Ushida T, Willis WD: Effect of contracture-induced pain in rat: Electrophysiological and behavioral study [abstract]. In Proceedings of the 8th World Congress on Pain. Seattle, IASP Press, 1996, p 6.
53. Veldman PH, Goris RJ. Multiple reflex sympathetic dystrophy. Which patients are at risk for developing a recurrence of reflex sympathetic dystrophy in the same or another limb. Pain 64:463, 1996.
54. Veldman PH, Reynen HM, Arntz IE, et al: Signs and symptoms of reflex sympathetic dystrophy: Prospective study of 829 patients. Lancet 342:1012, 1993.
55. White JC, Sweet WH: Pain and the Neurosurgeon. Springfield, IL, Charles C Thomas, 1969.
56. Wulf H, Gleim M, Schele HA: Plasma concentrations of bupivacaine after lumbar sympathetic block. Anesth Analg 79:918, 1994.

54 Anesthesia

VIRGINIA D. WADE

INTRODUCTION

The practice of anesthesia has undergone dramatic change in recent years, raising the so-called standard of care, that is, the level of care physicians of similar training and experience practice under similar circumstances.[20] New pharmaceutical agents, monitoring equipment, and invasive monitoring techniques have contributed to an increasingly complex specialty, taking the practice to a higher level of care, thus affording patients greater safety and a smooth anesthetic course. Selection of appropriate anesthetic agents and techniques is guided by analyses of critical incidents and outcome studies. This chapter focuses on the most recent advances in anesthesia and the selection of appropriate anesthetic agents and techniques for the management of patients undergoing knee surgery.

PRACTICE STANDARDS IN ANESTHESIA

In 1985 the anesthesia departments of the Harvard-affiliated hospitals adopted standards for patient monitoring during anesthesia.[23] This marked the first attempt in the history of anesthesia practice to standardize anesthesia care. The Harvard standards were then used to formulate the national guidelines set forth by the American Society of Anesthesiologists (ASA) in 1986, and amended in 1998.[3] These two important publications were drafted in order to reduce anesthesia-related morbidity and mortality. The result has been a significant reduction in malpractice claims, leading to a reduction in anesthesia malpractice premiums in many states. Failure to adhere to the current practice standards not only deprives the patient of a safe anesthetic, but has resulted in allegations of negligent misconduct.[20]

The success of the national guidelines for patient monitoring has prompted the ASA to develop practice guidelines for a variety of anesthesia care issues. The purpose of these guidelines is to enhance the quality and efficiency of care, including cost-effective utilization of services, increased patient satisfaction, avoidance of cancellations and delays, and a reduction in perioperative morbidity. Based on the analyses of current literature, the expert opinions of several task force members have been compiled in a series of reports titled Practice Guidelines. Topics include preanesthesia assessment, anesthetic monitoring, postanesthesia care, preoperative fasting, latex allergy, acute and chronic pain management, blood component therapy, and pulmonary artery catheterization. These guidelines are now available to the practitioner and the public on the Internet website of the ASA (http://www.asahq.org).

Basic Standards for Preanesthesia Care

Preoperative evaluation is required for all patients receiving more than nonsupplemental local anesthesia. An anesthesiologist is responsible for determining the medical status of the patient and formulating a plan of anesthesia care. The development of the plan is based on the review of the medical records, including the history and physical examination, the preoperative interview and consultation, and preoperative testing. It is the responsibility of the anesthesiologist to inform the patient of the anesthesia plan and to document this plan in the medical record.

Monitoring Standards

The contention that nearly all anesthetic mishaps are preventable through safety monitoring has been the subject of several articles. Eichhorn and associates[23] have reviewed the records of more than 1 million patients who received general anesthesia over a 12-year period. There were only 11 major accidents solely attributable to anesthesia. Seven of the 11 cases were due to hypoventilation. Epidemiological studies have indicated that the use of respiratory monitors does reduce the incidence of anesthesia-related morbidity and mortality.[12, 15, 23, 47, 65]

Monitoring practices must satisfy the requirements that oxygenation (oxygen), ventilation (carbon dioxide), circulation, and temperature be continually monitored by an anesthesiologist. Routine monitoring of the anesthetized patient now includes the application of an automated blood pressure cuff, a continuous electrocardiogram (EKG), core temperature measurement, and the use of at least one respiratory monitor for all cases, regardless of the type of anesthesia administered.[3, 12, 23, 65] Two respiratory monitors, the pulse oximeter and end-tidal CO_2 monitor, have virtually eliminated the accidental undetected esophageal intubation that has often resulted in anesthesia-related morbidity and mortality.[23] During regional anesthesia or local anesthesia with sedation, adequate oxygenation is confirmed by the use of a pulse oximeter, accompanied by clinical observation of ventilation by the anesthesiologist. When an endotracheal tube or laryngeal airway is inserted, its position must be verified by an end-tidal CO_2 monitor.[3]

Pulse Oximetry

The pulse oximeter is a noninvasive and easy-to-use device that has revolutionized anesthesia practice since its introduction in 1983. Oxygen saturation of hemoglobin is accurately measured by reflecting light through a pulsating vascular bed, most commonly the fingertip, producing a waveform and a measurable difference in the absorption of light between reduced and oxygenated hemoglobin. The calculated difference is converted to a percent saturation using Beer's law. The pulse oximeter is recommended for all cases, including general, regional, and local anesthesia with sedation.[3, 23, 48]

Capnography

The culprit in many costly verdicts and settlements has been the failure to adequately oxygenate the anesthetized patient. End-tidal CO_2 monitoring continuously evaluates the adequacy of exhaled carbon dioxide gas, affording a timely diagnosis of accidental esophageal intubation, as well as a variety of other conditions in which suboptimal ventilation requires immediate intervention (bronchospasm, pulmonary embolism, kinked endotracheal tube, anesthesia circuit disconnect). The end-tidal CO_2 monitor is required for all cases of general anesthesia when an endotracheal tube or laryngeal airway is inserted.[3]

Temperature

Perioperative monitoring of temperature is required when clinically significant changes in temperature are anticipated. Perioperative maintenance of normothermia has been shown to reduce the incidence of morbid cardiac events. In a randomized clinical trial involving 300 patients with cardiac risk factors or documented coronary artery disease, patients were assessed in a double-blind fashion to measure the relative risk of a morbid cardiac event (unstable angina, ischemia, cardiac arrest, or myocardial infarction) in the presence of temperature changes. The results showed that hypothermia, defined as a core temperature of 36.7°C or lower, was an independent indicator of morbid cardiac events. When normothermia was maintained by thermal treatment, there was a 55% reduction in risk of a cardiac event.[28]

Invasive Monitoring

The appropriate indications for pulmonary artery catheter monitoring have been debated for more than a decade. The Swan-Ganz catheter was originally introduced in 1978 to measure pulmonary capillary wedge pressure (PCWP). Its ability to measure pressure changes in the pulmonary artery serves as an indicator of myocardial ischemia, based on the observation that an ischemic myocardium results in hypokinesis in the left ventricle, translating into an increase in left-heart and pulmonary artery (PA) pressures. Early detection of ischemia was then postulated to affect therapy and outcome. However, several studies have failed to demonstrate a change in patient outcome associated with its use. A randomized controlled trial involving 146 patients found no difference in therapy or outcome in patients who were monitored by PA catheters compared with central venous catheter-monitored patients.[52] Another prospective, randomized trial[8] has demonstrated that catheterization of patients 12 hours before elective lower-limb revascularization did not produce better outcome than placement 3 hours before surgery. If PA catheters were used preoperatively to optimize cardiac status, patients were less likely to experience intraoperative cardiac events such as tachycardia, hypotension, and arrhythmias, but there was no difference in perioperative morbidity and mortality, thus minimizing the indications for its use. Furthermore, the risk of catheter-related sepsis and other complications appears to increase significantly if the catheter remains beyond 72 hours.[4] Therefore, at present there is insufficient evidence to support the use of early preoperative Swan-Ganz catheter monitoring (e.g., the night before surgery) in patients who are scheduled for elective surgery.[52]

The measurement of PCWP as an indicator of ischemia has been studied by others. Mangano has demonstrated that acute increases in PCWP are indicative of ischemia, but the absence of elevated PCWP does not ensure the absence of ischemia.[36, 37] One large observational study by Rao and colleagues[55] remains the leading research paper in the debate over the relationship between PCWP and patient outcome. In this study, 733 high-risk patients with previous myocardial infarction who underwent noncardiac surgery were monitored with Swan-Ganz catheters in the perioperative period. The PCWP exceeded 25 mm Hg in 29 patients, and 28% of the patients with elevated PCWP developed a myocardial infarction during the postoperative period, versus less than 1% of those without elevated pressures. This study suggests that there is a relationship between intraoperative cardiac dysfunction and outcome. Rao concluded that the use of PA catheters lowered reinfarction rates and mortality rates when compared with unmonitored patients.

Following an extensive review of the literature, a task force of the ASA has developed recommendations for use of the Swan-Ganz catheter in the perioperative period.[52] Upon its review of the literature, the task force has recommended that the decision to use a PA catheter should be based on the hemodynamic risk of the individual rather than on the type of procedure planned. They further state that pulmonary catheterization is inappropriate as a routine practice, acceptable only in selected patients undergoing procedures associated with complications from hemodynamic changes (e.g., cardiac surgery, aortic reconstruction), or for patients who are entering surgery with advanced cardiopulmonary disease.[52] The risk of a serious complication using a PA catheter is on the order of .1% to .5%, including infection, arrhythmia, thromboembolic phenomena, and fatal PA rupture.

ANESTHETIC CONSIDERATIONS FOR CRUCIATE LIGAMENT RECONSTRUCTION

General Versus Regional Anesthesia

The techniques applicable to arthroscopic cruciate ligament reconstruction are regional (spinal or epidural) and general anesthesia. It is the experience of the author that general anesthesia still holds an advantage over regional anesthesia for cruciate ligament reconstruction. The choice takes into consideration the preferences of both the patient and the surgeon, the potential risks and benefits of the type of anesthetic for the proposed surgery, the patient's health status, and overall patient satisfaction. General anesthesia also satisfies the requirements of a busy operating room setting, providing maximum efficiency in the operating room and shortened recovery room stays. General anesthesia has the advantage of being easier to perform, with rapid onset and recovery. A survey conducted by Shevde and Panagopoulos[58] reported that 69% of 800 patients surveyed preferred general anesthesia when given the choice, whereas 22% expressed a preference for local anesthesia to avoid the effects of general anesthesia. Only 9% were willing to elect regional anesthesia. The study also pointed out that patients' highest concern preoperatively was the anesthesiologist's experience and qualifications. A similar study by Erikksson and associates[26] evaluated the efficacy of local versus general anesthesia for knee surgery. The authors reported that of their patients who received either local, spinal, or general anesthesia, general anesthesia had the highest acceptance rate (97%).

Routine intra-articular injection of a combined solution of the local anesthetic bupivacaine and small amounts of opiates has allowed for early passive motion and mobilization following a general anesthetic. Anti-inflammatory medications, such as parenteral ketorolac (Toradol), and oral analgesics have proved satisfactory for the majority of patients, with intravenous narcotics reserved for only the difficult pain management patient.

General Anesthetic Agents

Propofol

Propofol (Diprivan) continues to be hailed as the single most important pharmacological agent for the induction and maintenance of general anesthesia. It is believed to be responsible for an increase in overall patient satisfaction. Propofol is chemically related to phenol, and analogous to the barbiturates, it produces dose-dependent central nervous system depression and loss of consciousness. Propofol has an elimination half-life of 55 minutes, in contrast to pentothal's elimination time of 5 to 12 hours. This distinct advantage over the barbiturates allows for rapid recovery from general anesthesia with little or no hangover effect. Recent studies have compared propofol anesthesia to the more conventional thiopental-inhalation anesthetic.[21, 49] The times to awakening and clear-headedness were significantly earlier in the propofol-N_2O group,[1, 21] and the incidence of postoperative nausea and vomiting was significantly less.[21, 39]

Opioids

Opioids is an inclusive term that applies to all drugs that bind to morphine receptors. The newer synthetic opioids fentanyl, sufentanil, and alfentanil, are highly potent, short-acting intravenous agents that provide excellent analgesia with minimal side effects. Because opioids are not complete anesthetics, they are used in combination with other drugs such as propofol, benzodiazepines, inhaled anesthetics, and muscle relaxants. When coupled with the sedative-hypnotic propofol, opioids produce excellent anesthesia and analgesia within minutes, followed by rapid recovery.

Inhalation Agents

The role of inhalation anesthetics is changing, with a reduction in their use for the majority of general anesthetics. Replacing the inhalation agents are intravenous drugs, which produce stable hemodynamics and more rapid recovery. The inhaled anesthetics of greatest importance are the weakly potent gas nitrous oxide and the volatile anesthetics isoflurane and sevoflurane. The effects of volatile inhaled agents include respiratory depression and muscle relaxation. They are responsible for dose-dependent decreases in blood pressure by virtue of their vasodilating effects. By the same mechanism, they produce increases in cerebral blood flow. Nitrous oxide alone produces a mild increase in vascular resistance, but when used in combination with opioids and volatile anesthetics, it decreases blood pressure and cardiac output. Myocardial depression produced by volatile anesthetics may be enhanced by the concomitant use of beta blockers and calcium channel blockers, used frequently in the treatment of hypertension.

Local Anesthetics

At the present time, patients who undergo anterior cruciate ligament reconstruction in many institutions are treated as inpatients, but improved management of postoperative pain may soon allow for satisfactory same day discharge. Routine use of intra-articular local anesthetic has allowed patients to enter the recovery room with a significant reduction in pain.[14, 26, 42, 43] Early studies on the use of bupivacaine in weak concentration (.25%) demonstrated its ineffectiveness in controlling pain postoperatively.[38] More recently, Smith and co-workers[60] assessed the efficacy of a volume of 30 mL of .5% bupivacaine (150 mg) for postoperative analgesia following general anesthesia in a randomized, double-blind protocol. Patients who received bupivacaine had significantly fewer opioid requirements and improved mobility, and were discharged from the recovery room an average of 30 minutes earlier than the placebo group. A study at the Cleveland Clinic Foundation in Ohio has demonstrated that the use of a bupivacaine-morphine combination for intra-articular injection produces the best postoperative analgesia[66] when compared with bupivacaine alone. This study confirms previous reports of the beneficial effects of small doses of opiates in local anesthetic solutions.

The most important consideration in the use of local anesthetics is the potential for systemic toxicity. Meinig and associates[41] conducted an important study to assess plasma concentrations of bupivacaine with epinephrine; 1:200,000 (.5% = 5 mg/mL; 30 mL = 150 mg) was used in this study, and venous plasma samples were analyzed by the highly sensitive method of gas chromatography and mass spectrometry. Peak absorption of bupivacaine following intra-articular injection of 30 mL occurred 20 minutes postinjection, with a mean plasma level that was one-third to one-fifth the level reported to produce toxicity. The maximum recommended doses of local anesthetics are listed in Table 54.1.[73]

Complications of General Anesthesia

Improved patient monitoring and new pharmacological agents have contributed to lowering the incidence of complications related solely to anesthesia. Eichhorn and associates[23] at the Harvard-affiliated hospitals reviewed the records over more than 1 million healthy patients who received anesthesia and found 11 major accidents solely attributable to anesthesia (.1 in 10,000), with 5 deaths and 4 permanent neurological injuries. The conclusion is that general anesthesia in the otherwise healthy patient is safe. Less serious complications, including dental injury, bronchospasm, laryngospasm, pharyngitis, tracheitis, and glottic edema are either preventable or easily treated. Aspiration of gastric contents is largely preventable, with adherence to some basic guidelines.

Factors that influence the incidence of complications of general anesthesia include disease states such as asthma, hypertension, diabetes, morbid obesity, rheumatoid arthritis, coronary artery disease, and advanced age. In all cases, routine medications should be continued up to the time of surgery. In most cases, the anesthetic plan for knee surgery in these patients favors the use of regional anesthesia to avoid airway difficulties such as bronchospasm in asthmatics, cervical spine manipulation in rheumatoid patients, and the significant risk of aspiration in the morbidly obese and those patients with a history of gastroesophageal reflux. Patients with coronary artery disease or advanced age also benefit from the use of regional anesthesia because of the favorable hemodynamics seen under regional blockade.[18, 69, 74, 75]

Guidelines for Preoperative Fasting

Pulmonary aspiration is regarded as one of the more serious complications of general anesthesia. Guidelines for preoperative fasting, recently revised by the ASA, are now available to assist the practitioner in decision-making, to avoid the risk of aspiration and the complications of pneumonia and sepsis, and to avoid delays and cancellations. Recommendations are for healthy patients with no predisposing factors to pulmonary aspiration, before procedures requiring general anesthesia, regional anesthesia, or sedation-analgesia (monitored anesthesia care). The guidelines focus on preoperative fasting and the use of pharmacological agents commonly employed to reduce gastric fluid acidity and volume. Revised guidelines are summarized in Table 54.2,[51] and include withholding clear fluids for 2 to 4 hours, full liquids or a "light" meal, defined as toast and a clear liquid, for 6 hours, and a full meal for 8 hours or more. The routine use of gastrointestinal stimulants, gastric acid blockers, antacids, and antiemetics to reduce the risks of pulmonary aspiration in patients who have no apparent risk is not recommended. Patients at risk for aspiration include the morbidly obese and those with hiatal hernia, gastroesophageal reflux disease, and diabetes. The anesthetic management of these patients requires different airway management techniques to reduce the risk of aspiration, and the recommendations for preoperative fasting do not necessarily apply.

TABLE 54.1 Recommended Doses of Local Anesthetic Agents

		Plain Solutions		Epinephrine-Containing Solutions	
Agent	*Concentration %*	*Maximum Adult Dose (mg)*	*Maximum Dose (mg/kg)*	*Maximum Adult Dose (mg)*	*Maximum Dose (mg/kg)*
Short duration					
Procaine	1-2	800	11	1000	14
Chloroprocaine					
Moderate duration					
Lidocaine	.5-1	300	4	500	7
Mepivacaine	.5-1	300	4	500	7
Prilocaine	.5-1	500	7	600	8
Long duration					
Bupivacaine	.25-.5	175	2.5	225	3

From White PF: Outpatient Anesthesia. New York, Churchill Livingstone, 1990, p 264. Used by permission.

TABLE 54.2 SUMMARY OF FASTING RECOMMENDATIONS TO REDUCE THE RISK OF PULMONARY ASPIRATION*

Ingested Material	Minimum Fasting Period†
Clear liquids‡	2 h
Breast milk	4 h
Infant formula	6 h
Non-human milk§	6 h
Light meal¶	6 h

* These recommendations apply to healthy patients who are undergoing elective procedures. They are not intended for women in labor. Following the guidelines does not guarantee that a complete gastric emptying has occurred.

† The fasting periods noted above apply to all ages.

‡ Examples of clear liquids include water, fruit juices without pulp, carbonated beverages, clear tea, and black coffee.

§ Since non-human milk is similar to solids in gastric emptying time, the amount ingested must be considered when determining an appropriate fasting period.

¶ A light meal typically consists of toast and clear liquids. Meals that include fried or fatty foods or meat may prolong gastric emptying time. Both the amount and type of foods ingested must be considered when determining an appropriate fasting period.

ANESTHETIC CONSIDERATIONS FOR TOTAL KNEE ARTHROPLASTY

Knee pain due to severe degenerative arthritis is no longer considered to be an inevitable part of aging. Total knee arthroplasty (TKA) has been performed successfully for more than 25 years, and studies indicate that the newly designed prostheses relieve pain in more than 95% of patients and restore adequate range of motion to enable the resumption of activities of daily living. TKA is being performed on nearly 150,000 Americans annually, and with the aging of American society the trend is obvious. Patients presenting for TKA require special attention in the perioperative period, and the evolving standard of care in anesthesia for TKA clearly favors the use of regional anesthesia, with few exceptions.

Preoperative Assessment

Patients who present for TKA range from the young with rheumatoid arthritis to the elderly with osteoarthritis. In all cases, the evaluation begins with a thorough history, physical examination, and routine laboratory tests. In patients with preexisting disease, medical records should be procured to determine the presence or absence of recent change in medical status. The medical consultant should be called upon to decide whether additional testing is warranted. Depending on the results of tests, it may be necessary to institute medical therapy to optimize the patient's medical condition prior to elective surgery. There is no doubt that a well-conducted preoperative evaluation is essential to the delivery of a safe and successful anesthetic.

Preoperative Autologous Donation

Approximately 12 million units of red blood cells (RBCs) are transfused each year in the United States,[51] many of which are administered to surgical patients. Preoperative autologous donation has become routine practice for the majority of patients undergoing elective TKA. When appropriate, preoperative autologous blood donation, intraoperative and postoperative blood recovery, acute normovolemic hemodilution, and measures to decrease blood loss (deliberate hypotension and pharmacological agents) have proved to be beneficial in reducing the risk of allogeneic blood transfusion. The indications for transfusion of autologous RBCs may be more liberal than for allogeneic RBCs because of the lower (but still significant) risks associated with the former.

Autologous blood has a shelf life of 35 to 42 days, depending on the type of anticoagulant used. In most cases, one to two units of autologous blood are donated for unilateral total knee replacement, and two to three units for bilateral knee arthroplasty, in the 1 to 2 weeks before surgery. Following a protocol of cementing all prostheses, intraoperative tourniquet deflation and hemostasis, and closed drainage with reinfusion, replacement of blood initially occurs in the form of reinfused blood recovered from the surgical drain, followed by infusion of autologous blood. At the Beth Israel Hospital North Division, on an annual basis approximately 350 patients donate autologous blood for elective orthopedic procedures. In 1998 alone, 367 units of autologous blood were wasted on expiration. This represents approximately 50% of the total number of units donated. For this reason, patients are now routinely managed with preoperative donation of 1 unit for unilateral TKA, and 2 units for bilateral TKA. Patients with infected knee prostheses for removal and reimplant procedures are unable to donate autologous blood or benefit from reinfusion techniques. Patients with preexisting anemia are also unsuitable for autologous blood donation. Erythropoietin therapy has been shown to decrease the allogeneic blood requirements of these patients.[28] Routine use of erythropoietin for 10 days before surgery in doses of 300 U/kg has significantly reduced requirements for transfusion (Fig. 54.1).[27, 56]

Guidelines for Blood Component Therapy

The proposed benefit of RBC transfusion is an increase in oxygen-carrying capacity. In healthy subjects, tissue oxygenation is maintained at hematocrit values as low as 18% to 25%.[62] A mild to moderate blood loss (15% to 30% of total blood volume) is usually tolerated because of compensatory increases in cardiac output, provided normovolemia is achieved by crystalloid therapy. There are conditions under which compensatory mechanisms may be altered, thus making symptoms of anemia unreliable in the decision-making process. This is especially true for the elderly, patients with left ventricular dysfunction, and patients on beta blockers or calcium channel blockers. Changes in vital signs are also masked by anesthetics. It is important to note that intraoperative myocardial ischemia is associated with tachycardia in only 26% of patients, and with changes in blood pressure in only 10% of patients.[62]

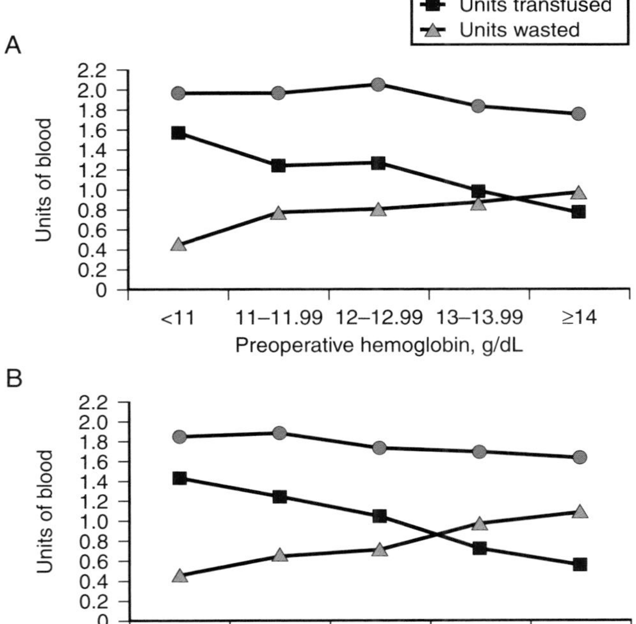

FIGURE 54.1 ➢ Units of autologous blood donated, transfused, and discarded (wasted) in total hip arthroplasty *(A)* and TKA patients *(B)* stratified by preoperative hemoglobin. (Redrawn from Sculco TP, Galliana J: Blood management experience: Relationship between autologous blood donation and transfusion in orthopedic surgery. Orthopedics 22 Suppl:s133, 1999.)

The ASA has developed recommendations for blood component therapy. After extensive review of the literature, a task force has concluded that the use of a single hemoglobin "trigger" for all patients is not recommended; that transfusion of RBCs is rarely indicated when the hemoglobin concentration is greater than 10 g/dL and is almost always indicated when it is less than 6 g/dL, especially when the anemia is acute; the determination of whether intermediate hemoglobin concentrations (6 to 10 g/dL) justify or require RBC transfusion should be based on the patient's risk for complications of inadequate oxygenation.[62]

Surgical patients with evidence of altered coagulation usually require platelet transfusion if the platelet count is less than 50 × 1,000,000,000/1 and rarely require therapy if it is greater than 100 × 1,000,000,000/1.[51] The ASA task force further states that prophylactic platelet transfusion is ineffective when thrombocytopenia is due to increased platelet destruction. Fresh-frozen plasma is indicated for urgent reversal of warfarin therapy, correction of known coagulation factor deficiencies for which specific concentrates are unavailable, and correction of microvascular bleeding when prothrombin and partial thromboplastin times are greater than 1.5 times normal. It is contraindicated for volume expansion. Cryoprecipitate should be considered for patients with von Willebrand's disease unresponsive to desmopressin, bleeding patients with von Willebrand's disease, and bleeding patients with fibrinogen levels below 80 to 100 mg/dL. The task force recommends careful adherence to proper indications for blood component therapy to reduce the risks of transfusion.[51]

Assessment of the High-Risk Patient

Perioperative Cardiac Morbidity

Perioperative cardiac morbidity is the leading cause of death following surgery and anesthesia.[36] One in four Americans is affected by cardiovascular disease, and the prevalence increases with age. Since TKA is performed predominantly in elderly patients, a large prevalence of underlying cardiovascular disease is expected.

The evaluation of cardiac disease is difficult in patients who are debilitated by arthritis. Very often the history of exertional chest pain, still regarded as one of the most sensitive indicators of coronary artery disease, is absent. Furthermore, about half of all patients suffering from angina have a normal resting EKG,[61] and an exercise test may not be feasible. Patients who give a history of chest pain or previous myocardial infarction (MI) may be assumed to have atherosclerotic heart disease. For patients in whom cardiac disease is known, or is highly suspected, the decision about whether to obtain noninvasive echocardiogram and stress testing should be based on the potential to modify perioperative care.

Nuclear scans are routinely used to identify the presence of ischemic heart disease. In those patients who are unable to exercise, the radionuclide technique using thallium-labeled dipyridamole (Persantine) produces results similar to those seen with exercise.[10, 22, 61] This imaging technique is both sensitive (80%) and specific (89% to 100%) for detection of coronary stenosis.[10, 22] The value of coronary revascularization before noncardiac surgery has not been studied in a randomized prospective manner, but several cohort studies have suggested that patients who undergo coronary artery bypass grafting have decreased risk during subsequent surgery.[36, 37]

The incidence of perioperative ischemia in patients with diagnosed coronary artery disease is approximately 40% in various studies. The most recent data suggest that the incidence of ischemia is greatest in the postoperative period. Marsch and associates[38] have conducted a study of unselected patients for lower-limb arthroplasty under regional anesthesia, to determine the prevalence of myocardial ischemia. Ninety-nine episodes occurred in 16 patients (31%), and 56% of the ischemic episodes were clinically silent. Thirteen episodes occurred in the preoperative period, one intraoperatively, and 85 postoperatively. Thus the greatest risk for ischemia occurred in the postoperative period.

Various epidemiological studies of patients with a history of MI who undergo anesthesia for noncardiac surgery have been reported.[46, 53, 59] The results are strikingly similar. Most studies confirm that perioperative reinfarction rate is in the range of 30% to 40% in the first 6 months after a previous MI. Those patients who had an MI more than 6 months prior to surgery have a reinfarction rate of 5% to 8%, whereas those without a previous history of MI have an overall risk of .1% to .7%. Thus the more recent the MI, the more likely is reinfarction. Another major prognostic indicator of adverse outcome in anesthesia, along with MI, is the presence of congestive heart failure.[30] Identification of patients with left ventricular dysfunction and decreased reserve allows for preoperative optimization of cardiac function with therapeutic intervention. Insertion of a Swan-Ganz catheter for perioperative fluid management may be indicated, but is no substitute for preoperative therapeutic management.[52]

Rheumatoid Arthritis

A smaller subset of high-risk patients who present for TKA arthroplasty are those suffering from rheumatoid arthritis. The knee is involved in nearly 60% of patients with rheumatoid arthritis, and the majority of these patients have bilateral joint involvement. Pain is the primary indication for surgery. Anesthetic considerations for the patient with rheumatoid arthritis are many, due to the systemic nature of the disease. Frequently there is multiple symmetric joint involvement, as well as pulmonary, cardiovascular, and hematologic manifestations. Rheumatoid lung is the term used to describe the restrictive pattern of lung disease that occurs secondary to fibrosis, and cardiac involvement may progress to congestive heart failure in advanced cases. Cervical spine arthritis is present in many patients with rheumatoid arthritis, causing severe pain and neurological symptoms, including paresthesias and even paresis. Cervical vertebral erosion and subluxation may occur, particuarly at the atlantoaxial joint. Great care must be exercised in positioning the rheumatoid patient, especially during tracheal intubation. Plain films of the cervical spine are recommended to assess the degree of subluxation in flexion and extension, but are not necessarily diagnostic of spinal cord compression. Magnetic resonance imaging is now employed to demonstrate pannus formation, which frequently compromises the spinal canal and cannot be detected by plain films.[47] Involvement of the cricoarytenoid and temporomandibular joints is also common in rheumatoid patients, making airway management difficult. In view of the potential airway problems, regional anesthesia has become the preferred technique for knee surgery in rheumatoid patients.

Morbid Obesity

Another group of patients frequently encountered in anesthesia for TKA are those who are morbidly obese, defined as weighing more than twice ideal body weight. Osteoarthritis is more common in the obese population, as are diabetes, hiatal hernia, thromboembolism formation, and cardiovascular disease. Massive obesity is often accompanied by a syndrome comprising hypersomnolence and episodes of sleep apnea, respiratory hypoxemia and hypoventilation, increased cardiac output, and congestive heart failure. If a history of hypersomnolence is obtained, the patient may be suffering from hypoxemia, decreased cardiac reserve, or both. Preoperative evaluation of left-ventricular function is indicated in the evaluation of these patients, as well as evaluation of baseline arterial blood gases.

Morbidly obese patients are known to be at risk for pulmonary aspiration and rapid deterioration of oxygenation in the presence of anesthetics. The use of regional anesthesia is preferred for lower extremity surgery in obese patients. An overly anxious patient may require sedation sufficient to produce a sleep-like state. Oxygen desaturation and hypoventilation are expected under sedation, and may require the use of an endotracheal tube under a combined general and regional technique. In this way, hemodynamic stability and thromboprophylaxis are provided by regional anesthesia, with controlled ventilation and adequate oxygenation. Insertion of a Swan-Ganz catheter may be required to guide fluid replacement in the perioperative period.

REGIONAL ANESTHESIA FOR TKA

Spinal and epidural block, commonly referred to as regional anesthesia, are similar in their ability to produce selective anesthesia to the lower extremity, with the advantage of muscle relaxation (Table 54.3). Both techniques have enjoyed renewed popularity among patients undergoing TKA. Patient bias has limited the use of regional anesthesia in the past, although a well-conducted preoperative discussion often proves effective in dispelling the fear of being awake, being able to feel pain, or the commonly feared adverse outcome of permanent neurological injury. A large body of clinical research now exists to support the use of regional anesthesia for TKA. Information from several recent outcome studies may soon lead to the acceptance of regional anesthesia as the standard of care for all patients undergoing TKA, with few exceptions.

Advantages of Regional Anesthesia

Thromboprophylaxis

Major orthopedic procedures are associated with a high risk of thromboembolic complications. Information obtained from many recent studies indicates that regional anesthesia significantly reduces the incidence of deep-vein thrombosis and pulmonary thromboembolism. Modig and associates[44, 45] in Sweden have demonstrated a significant decrease in proximal deep-vein thrombosis formation when comparing epidural to general anesthesia for TKA (Table 54.4).

Sharrock et al[57] at The Hospital for Special Surgery retrospectively reviewed the incidence of deep-vein

TABLE 54.3 KNEE SURGERY

Block	L1	L2	L3	L4	L5	S1	S2
Spinal							
Hyperbaric	✓✓	✓✓	✓✓	✓✓	✓✓	✓✓	✓✓
Isobaric	✓	✓	✓	✓	✓	✓	✓
Epidural							
Lumbar	✓	✓	✓✓	✓✓✓	✓✓	✓✓	✓
Caudal		✓	✓	✓✓	✓✓	✓✓	✓✓
Peripheral nerve							
Sciatic nerve				✓	✓	✓	✓
Femoral nerve		✓	✓	✓			
Obturator nerve	✓	✓	✓	✓	✓	✓	✓
Lateral femoral cutaneous nerve		✓	✓				
Efficacy							
1. Hyperbaric spinal							
2. Isobaric spinal							
3. Lumbar epidural							
4. Sciatic-femoral-obturator nerve block							
5. Caudal epidural							

From Raj P: Clinical Practice of Regional Anesthesia. New York, Churchill Livingstone, 1991, p 248.
Note: Supine position precludes hypobaric spinal.

thrombosis in a large series of patients who had received general anesthesia for TKA, and then compared them with a similar group who received epidural anesthesia. Postoperative deep-vein thrombosis, known to occur to 40% to 80% of patients following TKA, was seen in 48% of 277 patients who had regional anesthesia, compared with an incidence of 64% ($p < .001$) of 264 patients who had received general anesthesia. In patients who underwent bilateral TKA, deep-vein thrombosis developed in 80% of the patients who had general anesthesia, versus 65% of the patients who had epidural anesthesia ($p < .05$). Postulated mechanisms for the apparent prophylaxis include improved blood flow to the lower extremities, and local anesthetic interaction with various blood elements, resulting in decreased coagulation and cell adhesiveness.[11] The results of this study and others suggest that the use of epidural anesthesia is beneficial for thromboprophylaxis in knee replacement surgery.

Hemodynamic Stability

The preferred use of regional anesthesia for TKA is supported by numerous reports of the favorable hemodynamics produced by regional blockade. Valli and Rosenberg[69] reported that prolonged use of a thigh tourniquet produced marked hypertensive responses (more than 30% of control values) in patients under general anesthesia, and no rise in blood pressure in patients under regional anesthesia. This finding translates into a reduction in left-ventricular strain and a decrease in blood loss. Damask and colleagues[18] used invasive monitoring to demonstrate the physiological effects of epidural anesthesia on hemodynamic response. They found a significant reduction in myocardial oxygen demand as measured by reductions of oxygen consumption. Explanations of the cardiovascular benefits of regional anesthesia include more stable hemodynamics due to afferent blockade, decreased sympathetic tone, and decreased ventricular preload and afterload, with fewer episodes of myocardial ischemia. A number of studies in patients with known cardiac disease have compared the effects of general versus regional anesthesia on the incidence of perioperative infarction, dysrhythmias, and congestive heart failure. The results are conflicting; however, one study has demonstrated a significant benefit from the combined use of epidural anesthesia and postoperative epidural analgesia. Yeager and associates[74] conducted a randomized trial to evaluate the relationship between anesthetic techniques and

TABLE 54.4 DISTRIBUTION AND LOCATION OF DEEP-VEIN THROMBOSIS (DVT) AND FREQUENCY OF PULMONARY EMBOLISM (PE) IN TWO GROUPS OF PATIENTS

Anesthetic Technique	Patients (n)	DVT (Thigh Veins) n (%)	DVT (Thigh and Calf Veins) n (%)	PE n (%)
"Continuous" epidural anesthesia	48	8 (17)	21 (44)	5 (10)
General anesthesia: ketobemidone postoperatively	46	30 (65)	38 (83)	15 (33)
Significance		$p < .001$	$p < .001$	$p < .01$

From Modig J, et al: Reg Anesth 1986.

postoperative morbidity in high-risk surgical patients. They found that critically ill patients who received general anesthesia had an overall complication rate that was "strikingly higher" than a similar group who received epidural anesthesia. Complications included congestive heart failure, MI, cardiac arrhythmias, and respiratory failure. The cost of hospitalization was higher in the general anesthesia group, and the investigators terminated the study because of the significant differences in morbidity between the two groups.

Physiology of Regional Blockade

Local anesthetic injected into the lumbar, intrathecal, or epidural space produces a conduction block of sensory and motor nervous transmission, as well as blockade of the thoracolumbar sympathetic outflow tracts. A small dose of intraspinal local anesthetic acts directly on the spinal cord, whereas the major site of action of local anesthetic in the epidural space is at the nerve roots and the dorsal root ganglia beyond the point of meningeal covering (Fig. 54.2). A much larger dose of local anesthetic is necessary to achieve a satisfactory epidural block. Inadvertent injection of a large dose of local anesthetic into the cerebrospinal fluid (CSF) during the performance of an epidural may result in total spinal anesthesia and cardiovascular collapse.

The proper use of regional anesthesia for TKA requires a thorough understanding of the effects of conduction blockade. The most important physiological response to regional anesthesia involves the denervation of arteriolar and venous smooth muscle, with reductions in preload, afterload, and cardiac output. Alterations in these parameters may be accentuated in hypovolemic patients, resulting in dramatic reductions in blood pressure. Prehydration of patients who present for TKA is of paramount importance, since most patients have donated autologous blood within the preoperative period. Patients who have a documented history of cardiovascular disease may benefit from the use of invasive monitoring to optimize fluid status prior to surgery.

In order to adequately anesthetize the knee joint, a minimum sensory level of T10 is required to ensure sensory and motor blockade (Figs. 54.3 and 54.4). When establishing a regional block, the level of sympathetic block extends about two spinal segments below the sensory level.[64] High sympathetic thoracic blockade (T1 - T4) involves the cardiothoracic sympathetics, with unopposed vagal activity causing bradycardia or even cardiac arrest. Prompt treatment of bradycardia with atropine and beta-adrenergic vasopressors is indicated in high regional blockade.

Local Anesthetic Agents

The mechanism of action of local anesthetic agents has been elucidated. Transmission of nervous stimuli along a nerve cell axon occurs due to increased permeability of the nerve cell membrane to sodium. The presence of local anesthetic blocks the rapid influx of sodium that must occur for transmission to take place.[62] Small sensory fibers are the most readily blocked, requiring about half the local anesthetic concentration necessary to produce skeletal muscle relaxation (Table 54.5).[64] Higher levels of local anesthetics result in stabilization of all excitable membranes, including central nervous system (CNS) and cardiac mus-

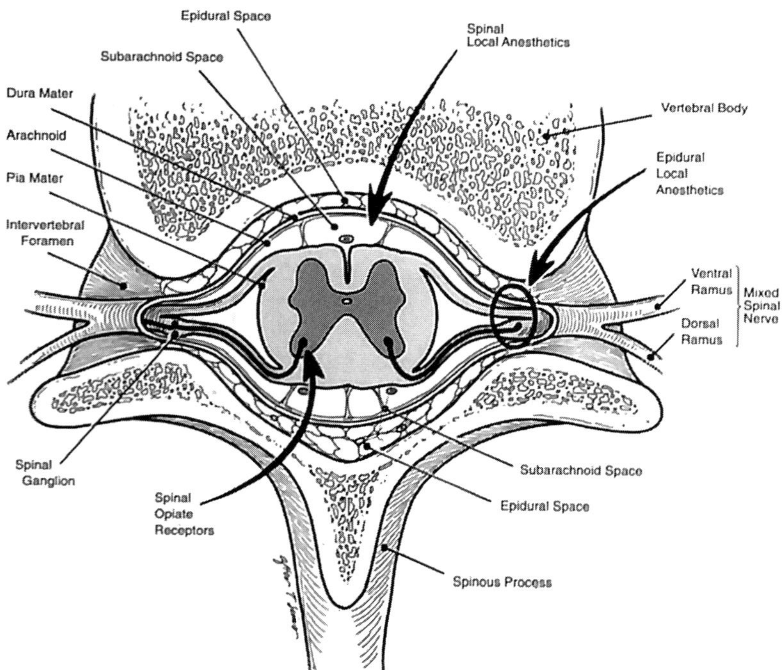

FIGURE 54.2 ➢ Cross-sectional view of the vertebral column shows site of action of local anesthetics and opiates. (From Scott WN: The Knee, vol 1. St. Louis, Mosby-Year Book, 1994, p 307.)

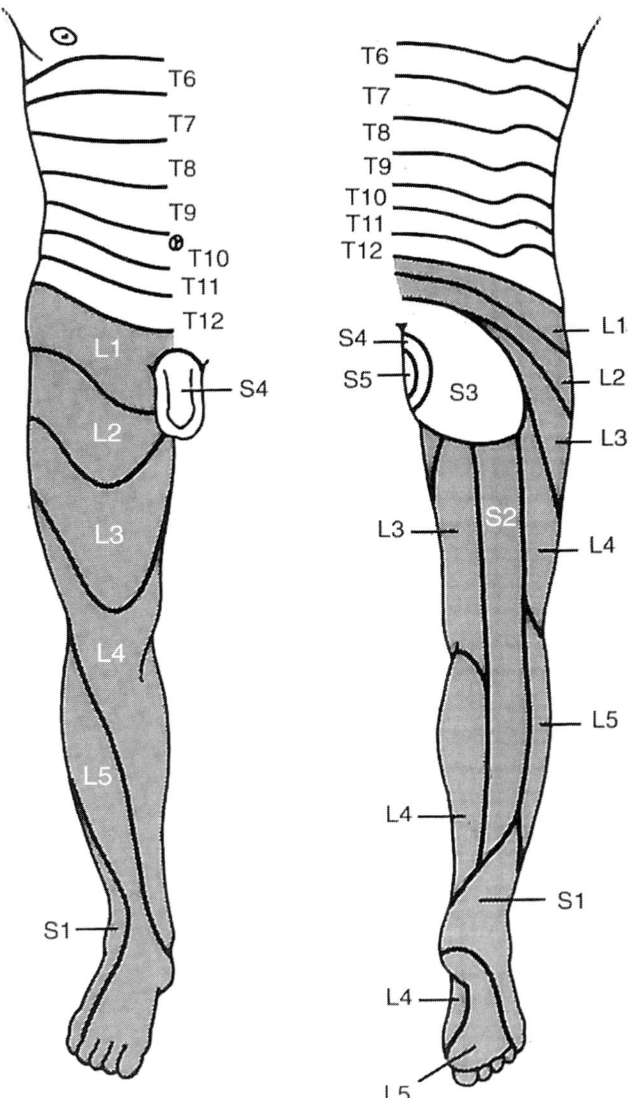

FIGURE 54.3 ➢ For surgery of knee region, L1-S2 dermatomes must be anesthetized. (From Scott WN: The Knee, vol 1. St. Louis, Mosby-Year Book, 1994, p 308.)

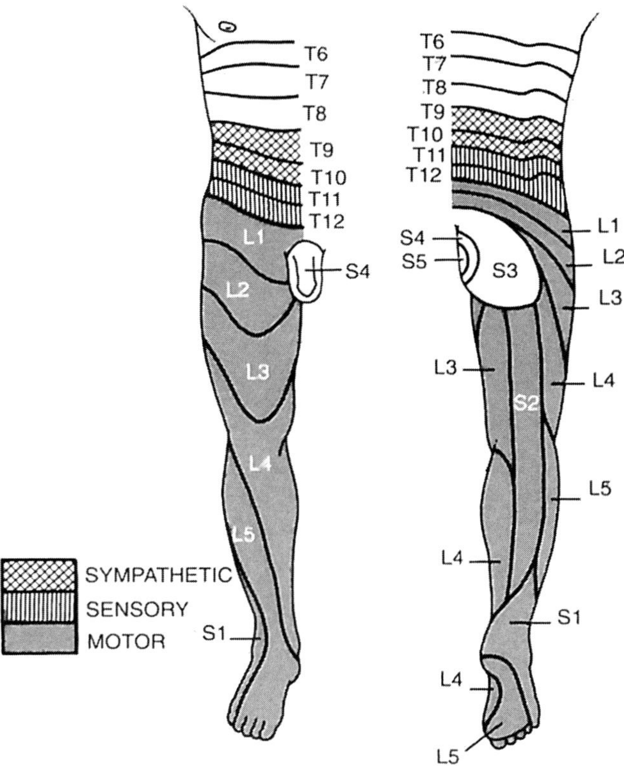

FIGURE 54.4 ➢ Zones of differential blockade. Sympathetic blockade averages two dermatomes above sensory level. Motor blockade averages two dermatomes below sensory level. (From Scott WN: The Knee, vol 1. St. Louis, Mosby-Year Book, 1994, p 308.)

cle membranes. The two most important areas of concern in the use of local anesthetics are their duration of action and their relative toxicities.

Local anesthetics are divided into two main groups according to their chemical structure and metabolism. The ester group is rapidly broken down by the plasma enzyme pseudocholinesterase. The advantage of this type of metabolism is the virtual elimination of systemic toxicity following accidental intravascular injection. Chloroprocaine (Nesacaine) is the only ester-type local anesthetic used in epidural anesthesia, and pro-

TABLE 54.5 Relative Size and Susceptibility to Blockade by Local Anesthetics of Types of Nerve Fibers

Fiber Type	Myelin	Diameter (μm)	Sensitivity to Block	Function
Type A				
Alpha	Yes	12-20	+	Proprioception, motor
Beta	Yes	5-12	++	Proprioception, motor
Gamma	Yes	3-6	++	Muscle tone
Delta	Yes	2-5	+++	Pain, temperature, touch
Type B	Yes	<3	++++	Preganglionic autonomic
Type C	No	.3-1.2	++++	Pain and postganglionic autonomic

From Miller RD, Stoelting RK: Basics of Anesthesia. New York, Churchill Livingstone, 1984. Used by permission.
++++ = extremely sensitive; +++ = very sensitive; ++ = moderately sensitive; + = slightly sensitive.

caine (Tetracaine) is the ester-linked local agent commonly used for spinal anesthesia. Early case reports of permanent neurological deficit following inadvertent spinal injection of chloroprocaine have been investigated and found to be linked to the preservative bisulfite.[29] Newer preparations of Nesacaine are preservative-free, and are now considered safe for use in epidural anesthesia.

The amide group of local anesthetics includes lidocaine (Xylocaine) and bupivacaine (Marcaine). These agents are metabolized in the liver, and the main concern with their use is the potential for systemic toxicity. The use of additives such as epinephrine, in a dilution of 1:200,000, is safe and effective in reducing the rate of systemic absorption to match the rate of metabolism. Vasoconstrictors are also useful in prolonging the duration of action of anesthetics by about 50%, presumably by the same mechanism of reduced absorption.

Local Anesthetic Toxicity

Local anesthetic toxicity involves the CNS and the cardiovascular system. The CNS is more sensitive to the effects of high plasma concentration of local anesthetics than the cardiovascular system. Early manifestations of CNS toxicity include restlessness, tremors, visual and auditory disturbances, and progressive agitation. These symptoms eventually give way to frank seizure activity and finally CNS depression. Treatment of CNS toxicity includes prompt airway management and the use of diazepam.[19]

Higher plasma levels of local anesthetics produce hypotension, slowing of cardiac conduction, bradycardia, and in severe cases, cardiac arrest. The long-acting amide local anesthetic bupivacaine (Marcaine) has been associated with a greater risk of cardiac toxicity than other local anesthetics.[2, 64] Several case reports of cardiac arrest following intravascular injection of small amounts of Marcaine have led to the conclusion that a narrow safety margin exists in the development of toxicity. It is now recognized that bupivacaine is a highly lipid-soluble local anesthetic that avidly binds to cardiac smooth muscle cells, blocking sodium channels in a slowly reversible manner, and may result in cardiac arrest.[2, 13, 33] The treatment of bupivacaine-induced cardiovascular collapse should be aggressive and sustained. Controlled ventilation with 100% oxygen, correction of acidosis, closed chest massage, and cardioversion are first-line measures. Resuscitation with bretylium has been found useful in the treatment of this refractory cardiac arrest.[33]

SERIOUS COMPLICATIONS RELATED TO REGIONAL ANESTHESIA

Headache

A postspinal headache is the most common complication of regional anesthesia, now minimized by the use of finer gauge spinal needles, but still a serious complication of epidural anesthesia with accidental dural puncture by a large bore epidural needle. Mild forms of headache are treated with aggressive fluid management and bed rest, since the headache is posture dependent. If severe headache continues beyond 48 hours, an autologous blood patch is used to seal off the persistent leak of CSF. Case reports of cerebral hematoma following spinal headache indicate prompt management in severe cases.[71]

Infection

Meningitis, adhesive arachnoiditis, and epidural abscess are rare complications of regional anesthesia that usually appear later in the postoperative period. The majority of cases reported are the result of endogenous local or systemic infection. Treatment includes antibiotics and, in the case of abscess, surgical drainage.

Intravascular Injection of Local Anesthesia

The epidural space is filled with fat and the epidural plexus of veins, as well as the peripheral nerves. Inadvertent intravascular injection of local anesthetic may occur in an attempted epidural, leading to local anesthetic toxicity. Prevention of inadvertent intravascular injection once again involves the simple use of a test dose to detect early signs of toxicity, such as circumoral numbness or tinnitus.

Total Spinal Anesthesia

Accidental dural puncture in an attempted epidural anesthetic may result in a large volume of local anesthetic reaching the CSF. Because the total volume of local anesthetic for spinal block is approximately one-twentieth that used to achieve epidural anesthesia, the result of undetected dural puncture is high or total spinal block. Treatment includes immediate cardiopulmonary resuscitation with controlled ventilation, fluids, atropine for bradycardia or arrest, and vasopressors. Prevention of this complication involves the careful use of small test doses of local anesthetic prior to administration of the full volume into the epidural space.

Seizures

Seizures occurring during placement of a regional anesthetic are the result of elevated blood levels of local anesthetic. The risk of developing toxic blood levels of local anesthetics is virtually nonexistent in spinal anesthesia, where small amounts of local anesthetics are used. The use of higher volumes of locally placed anesthetics increases the risk of elevated blood levels. For this reason, an epidural poses a small risk of toxicity, estimated in the series by Auroy and co-workers[6] to be 1.3 in 10,000 epidural anesthetics, compared with 0 in 10,000 for spinal anesthesia.

Epidural Hematoma

Prior to the introduction of low-molecular-weight heparin to the United States in 1993, epidural or spinal hematoma after regional anesthesia was considered rare.[72] From 1993 to 1998, the US Food and Drug Administration has received reports of 43 cases of spinal or epidural hematoma associated with the use of the low-molecular-weight heparin enoxaparin (Lovenox) in patients undergoing spinal or epidural anesthesia. Thirty-six of the 42 patients who developed spinal or epidural hematoma while receiving Lovenox did so for the prevention of deep-vein thrombosis associated with surgery (knee or hip replacement). Symptoms of spinal cord compression began on the average of 2 to 3 days after enoxaparin therapy had begun. Emergency laminectomy was performed in 28 patients, with permanent paraplegia occurring in 16 patients. Nearly all 16 patients had a continuous epidural catheter technique, and developed symptoms within a few hours after catheter removal.[32] It is estimated that the frequency of spinal hematoma among patients receiving enoxaparin is between 1 in 1,000 and 1 in 10,000. The frequency of this grave complication in the absence of anticoagulant therapy is reported to be on the order of 1 in 100,000. An important factor contributing to the higher frequency of spinal hematoma seen in the United States is the use of higher doses of Lovenox, averaging 30 mg twice daily, as compared with 40 mg once daily used for many years in Europe. The development of severe back pain accompanied by rapid onset of neurological symptoms signals the possibility of an epidural hematoma. Treatment requires surgical drainage to decompress the spinal cord.

Neurological Injury

Neurological sequelae following regional anesthesia are rare. The various forms of neurological injury are radiculopathy, cauda equina syndrome, and paraplegia. Individual case reports of rare events include postoperative radiculopathy associated with difficult needle placement in spinal anesthesia, cauda equina syndrome after spinal anesthesia, and epidural hematoma with spinal cord compression following epidural anesthesia. The most comprehensive multicenter review of complications related to regional anesthesia has emerged from France, in a remarkable effort on the part of 735 anesthesiologists.[6] The anesthesiologists were avid practitioners of regional anesthesia, averaging more than 30 cases of regional anesthesia per month. The number of consecutive regional anesthetics performed over a 5-month period was more than 100,000, including 40,000 spinal anesthetics, 30,000 epidural anesthetics, 20,000 peripheral nerve blocks, and 11,000 intravenous regional anesthetics. The serious complications they reported are summarized in Table 54.6, and include radicular deficit, cauda equina syndrome, paraplegia, seizures, and cardiac arrest. Reports of 98 severe complications were received, of which 89 were attributable to anesthesia.

The French study reported 34 neurological injuries in 100,000 consecutive patients. Injuries were considered permanent after 3 months (5 of 34). All injuries presented within 48 hours after surgery. There was a higher incidence of neurological injury after spinal anesthesia (6 per 10,000 cases) than after the epidural. In total, there were 19 cases of radiculopathy following spinal anesthesia and 5 cases following epidural anesthesia. Two-thirds of the 34 patients with neurological deficits had either a paresthesia or pain at the time of needle placement or injection. Thirteen of 34 neurological complications were not associated with pain, paresthesias, or technical problems, and 12 of the 13 occurred after spinal anesthesia. Seventy-five percent of these patients had received hyperbaric lidocaine, 5%, in a dose of 75 mg or greater. Cauda equina syndrome occurred in five patients, all of whom received spinal anesthesia with hyperbaric bupivacaine or lidocaine. Two of the patients suffered permanent radiculopathy or cauda equina syndrome. There was one reported case of paraplegia following an uneventful epidural anesthetic combined with general anesthesia, during which surgery the patient suffered hypovolemic hypotension. The cause of paraplegia was pre-

TABLE 54.6 CLASSIFICATION OF COMPLICATIONS

	Reported	No Detail	Unrelated to Regional Anesthesia	Completely or Partially Related to Regional Anesthesia
Cardiac arrest	33	0	1	32
Radicular deficit	34	0	6	28
Seizures	24	1	0	23
Cauda equina syndrome	6	0	1	5
Paraplegia	1	0	0	1
Total	98	1	8	89
Death related to the event	7	0	0	7

* Circulatory arrest (n = 1): sudden onset of diffuse erythema and Quincke's edema immediately after intravenous injection of metoclopramide and midazolam during spinal anesthesia for cesarean section. Radicular deficit (n = 1): postoperative diagnosis of multiple sclerosis associated with upper extremity neurological deficit after an uneventful epidural anesthesia. Radicular deficit (n = 1): patient suffering from a preoperative advanced polyradiculoneuritis. Radicular deficit (n = 2): psychiatric patients complaining of variable postoperative neurological symptoms after spinal anesthesia. Radicular deficit (n = 2): sciatic pain occurring 13 and 15 days after spinal anesthesia. Cauda equina syndrome (n = 1): isolated sexual impotence without any associated objective clinical sign.

Auroy Y, Narchi P, Messiah A, et al: Serious complications related to regional anesthesia: Results of a prospective survey in France. Anesthesiology 87:479, 1997.

sumed to be anterior spinal artery hypoperfusion. There were no case reports of spinal or epidural hematoma, a result of compliance with recommendations of a French consensus to avoid regional anesthesia in patients who are taking anticoagulants preoperatively. This study from France confirms that regional anesthesia is safe in experienced hands, with the risk of death being .7 in 10,000 cases, and the risk of permanent neurological injury .5 in 10,000.

Cardiac Arrest

The incidence of cardiac arrest and neurological injury related to regional anesthesia is very low, but both were more than three standard deviations greater after spinal anesthesia than after other regional anesthetics.[6] Auroy and colleagues reported 32 cardiac arrests in more than 100,000 regional anesthetics, 26 of which occurred during spinal anesthesia (6.4 ± 1.2 per 10,000 patients), and 3 during epidural anesthesia (1 ± .4 per 10,000 patients). The incidence of cardiac arrest with spinal anesthesia was significantly greater than with epidural anesthesia ($p < .05$, Table 54.7). Seven of the 32 cardiac arrests were fatal, and 6 of the 7 fatalities occurred during spinal anesthesia, the seventh resulting from an MI during a peripheral nerve block. Sedation was not given, nor was cyanosis observed before any of the cardiac arrests. All cardiac arrests were preceded by bradycardia. All three cases of cardiac arrest during epidural anesthesia were reversible, and all three cases of cardiac arrest reported at the time of cementing of total hip prostheses were fatal. Variables that were statistically significant in assessing the risk of death after cardiac arrest were age and physical status, the time between onset of block and occurrence of cardiac arrest, and the operative procedure. The average age of nonsurvivors was 82 ± 7, with higher-risk patients (preexisting disease) at greater risk for nonsurvival. The time between the onset of block and occurrence of cardiac arrest was significantly greater in nonsurvivors than among survivors (42 ± 19 minutes versus 17 ± 16 minutes). The average blood loss in patients suffering cardiac arrest was 700 mL for nine cardiac arrest patients, four of whom were nonsurvivors. Total hip arthroplasty (THA) was more frequently the type of surgery associated with nonsurvival (5 of 6 THA patients were among nonsurvivors compared with 2 of 20 in non-THA surgeries; $p < .05$). The survival rate of patients suffering a cardiac arrest during spinal anesthesia is surprisingly low, considering that the patients were being monitored and attended by a trained anesthesiologist at the time of arrest.

A widely quoted study by Caplan and associates[12] has been compared to the French survey of Auroy. Caplan and associates conducted a closed claims analysis of major anesthetic mishaps involving regional anesthesia. The study was aimed at identifying any trend or pattern of management that might have led to the otherwise unexplained cardiac arrests. Spanning an 8-year interval, 14 cases of unexplained cardiac arrest occurred in young (35 ± 15 years), healthy patients who had received spinal anesthesia. Two patterns emerged from the study. The first was the use of

TABLE 54.7 Number and Incidence of Severe Complications Related to Regional Anesthesia

	Type of Anesthesia				
Critical Serious Event	*Spinal (40,640)*	*Epidural (30,413)*	*Peripheral Nerve Blocks (21,278)*	*Intravenous Regional (11,229)*	*Total (103,730)*
Cardiac	26	3	3	0	32
	(6.4)	(1)*	(1.4)†		(3.1)
	(3.9–8.9)	(.2–2.9)	(.3–4.1)	(0–3.3)	(2–4.1)
Death	6	0	1	0	7
	(1.5)		(.5)		(.9)
	(.3–2.7)	(0–1.2)	(0–2.6)	(0–3.3)	(.2–1.2)
Seizures	0	4	16	3	23
		(1.3)	(7.5)‡	(2.7)	(2.2)
	(0–.9)	(.4–3.4)	(3.9–11.2)	(.5–7.8)	(1.3–3.1)
Neurological injury	24	6	4	0	34
	(5.9)	(2)*	(1.9)‡	(2.7)§	(3.3)
	(3.5–8.3)	(.4–3.6)	(.5–4.8)	(.5–7.8)	(2.2–4.4)
Radiculopathy	19	5	4	0	28
	(4.7)	(1.6)*	(1.9)		(2.7)
	(2.6–6.8)	(.5–3.8)	(.5–4.8)	(0–3.3)	(1.7–3.7)
Cauda equina syndrome	5	0	0	0	5
	(1.2)				(.5)
	(.1–2.3)	(0–1.2)	(0–1.7)	(0–3.3)	(.2–1.1)
Paraplegia	0	1	0	0	3
		(.3)			(.1)
	(0–.9)	(0–1.8)	(0–1.7)	(0–3.3)	(0–0.5)

Values are, in order, the number, the incidence/10,000, and the 95% confidence interval.
* Epidural vs spinal ($p < .05$).
† Peripheral nerve blocks vs spinal ($p < .05$).
‡ Peripheral nerve blocks vs epidural ($p < .05$).
§ Intravenous regional vs epidural and spinal ($p < .05$).
Auroy Y, Narchi P, Messiah A, et al: Serious complications related to regional anesthesia: Results of a prospective survey in France. Anesthesiology 87:479, 1997.

sedation sufficient to produce a sleep-like state in which there was no spontaneous verbalization on the part of the patient. In these cases, the first sign of cardiac arrest was cyanosis, suggesting that respiratory embarrassment predisposed the patient to cardiac arrest. The second pattern to emerge was the poor neurological outcome in these otherwise young and healthy patients. All but 1 of 14 cases were unable to resume self-care, despite prompt attention at the time of arrest. Six patients died, eight survived the initial treatment, and only four regained consciousness. The neurological outcome in these patients was worse than the Seattle experience for out-of-hospital cardiac arrests in patients with underlying coronary artery disease. Explanations for the poor outcome following cardiac arrest under spinal anesthesia include sympathetic blockade resulting in peripheral pooling of blood volume, decreased cerebral and coronary perfusion, as well as a decreased response to beta-adrenergic stimulants used in resuscitation. Recommendations based on this study include vigilance when using sedatives in regional anesthesia, routine use of oximetry to detect early respiratory depression, and use of a full resuscitating dose of epinephrine to overcome sympathetic blockade.[12]

CONTRAINDICATIONS TO REGIONAL ANESTHESIA

Contraindications to regional anesthesia are few. Allergic reactions to local anesthetics are exceedingly rare, and historical reports often indict additives such as epinephrine or a toxic reaction. Infection, either systemic or at the site of intended injection, is a contraindication to the use of regional anesthesia. Deformities of the lumbosacral spine and previous laminectomy are not considered to be contraindications to the use of regional anesthesia, although they may make performance of the block more difficult.[53] Coagulopathies and blood dyscrasias must be corrected prior to any attempt at regional anesthesia to avoid the risk of spinal hematoma.

Anticoagulants and Regional Anesthesia

The guidelines for use of regional anesthesia and low-molecular-weight heparin have been revised following a series of case reports of spinal hematoma following epidural anesthesia in the presence of enoxaparin (Lovenox).[32] It is recommended that patients who receive low-molecular-weight heparin postoperatively should receive their first dose no earlier than 24 hours postoperatively, and that the epidural catheter may remain overnight, as long as the catheter is removed 2 hours prior to initiation of enoxaparin. Patients already on preoperative low-molecular-weight heparin have altered coagulation, and in the case of surgery, should not have an epidural catheter technique. If regional anesthesia is the preferred technique, a single-shot spinal may be performed only for patients who received their last dose 24 hours prior to surgery. In the event of administration of low-molecular-weight heparin in the presence of an epidural catheter, removal of the catheter should be delayed for at least 10 to 12 hours after the last dose of enoxaparin, and subsequent dosing should not occur for at least 2 hours after catheter removal.[32]

Antiplatelet drugs such as aspirin and nonsteroidal anti-inflammatory agents, by themselves, have not been found to present significant risk for developing a spinal hematoma in patients having spinal or epidural anesthesia.[25] In cases of chronic use of oral anticoagulants such as warfarin (Coumadin), the anticoagulant must be stopped prior to regional anesthesia, and prothrombin time normalized. Low-dose heparin, also frequently used in orthopedic patients for prophylaxis against venous thromboembolism, does not contraindicate the use of spinal or epidural anesthesia, unless there is concomitant use of other anticoagulants.[26] When full therapeutic anticoagulation with heparin is indicated, heparin administration should be timed 1 hour from the placement of the needle and/or catheter, and the catheter should remain in place for 2 to 4 hours after the last heparin dose.[32]

CONCLUSION

Experience in performing anesthetics varies among practitioners, with some anesthesiologists in academic environments supervising less experienced individuals. The approach to teaching and reinforcing vigilance as a preventive measure cannot be overemphasized. Complications of anesthesia occur in experienced hands nonetheless. In support of the continued effort to improve patient safety, the ASA has created practice standards to be adhered to nationwide. Much of this information has been published and is now available on the World Wide Web.

Medical Information on the Internet

The ability to communicate information globally and almost instantaneously via a loosely connected network of computers has made the Internet a popular resource for its nearly 100 million daily users.[54] Within the Internet, information is disseminated simply by using some abbreviated text, or hypertext (http), referred to as an Internet address. For example, the current practice standards in anesthesia may be located by accessing the Internet and typing in the address http://www.asahq.org. Another source of medical information is the database known as Pub Med (www.ncbi.nlm.nih.gov/pubmed/), for the location of medical publications and medically related research articles. Websites that provide information to the orthopedic community include the American Academy of Orthopaedic Surgeons (http://www.aaos.org) and Orthopaedic Web Links (OWL) (http://www.orthogate.org/owl/orthpat.html); patient education for orthopedic-related topics include the OrthoGate at http://www.orthogate.org/ and the WebMD (http://www.webmd.com). The proliferation of published medical material on the Internet has led to some skepticism and concern as to its reliability. The ease of tracking information should encourage medical professionals worldwide to develop a strategy for accessing information on the Internet.

References

1. Adam HK, Briggs LP, Bahar M, et al: Pharmacokinetic evaluation of ICI 35868 in man: Single induction doses with different rates of injection. Br J Anaesth 55:97, 1983.
2. Albright GA: Cardiac arrest following regional anesthesia with etidocaine or bupivacaine. Anesthesiology 51:285, 1979.
3. American Society of Anesthesiologists Task Force: Standards for basic intraoperative monitoring. American Society of Anesthesiologists Newsletter. Approved by the House of Delegates, Oct 25, 1985.
4. Applefeld JJ, Caruthers TE, Reno DJ, et al: Assessment of the sterility of long-term cardiac catheterization using thermodilution Swan-Ganz catheter. Chest 74:377, 1978.
5. Arens JF: A practice parameter overview. Anesthesiology 78:229, 1993.
6. Auroy Y, Narchi P, Messiah A, et al: Serious complications related to regional anesthesia: Results of a prospective survey in France. Anesthesiology 87:479, 1997.
7. Bergqvist D, Lindblad B, Matzsch T: Risk of combining low-molecular-weight heparin for thromboprophylaxis and epidural or spinal anesthesia. Semin Thromb Hemost 19:147, 1993.
8. Berlauk JF, Abrams JH, Gilmour IJ, et al: Preoperative optimization of cardiovascular hemodynamics improves outcome in peripheral vascular surgery: A prospective, randomized clinical trial. Ann Surg 214:289, 1991.
9. Bierbaum BE, Galanta JO, Rubash HE, et al: Prediction of red cell transfusion in orthopedic surgery. Paper presented at the 65th Annual Meeting of the American Academy of Orthopaedic Surgeons, March 19, 1998, New Orleans, LA. Paper 380.
10. Boucher CA, et al: Determination of cardiac risk by dipyridamole-thallium imaging before peripheral vascular surgery. N Engl J Med 312:389, 1985.
11. Bromage PR: Continuous epidural analgesia and thromboembolism prophylaxis. In Bromage PR, ed: Epidural Analgesia. Philadelphia, WB Saunders, 1978, pp 240–257.
12. Caplan RA, et al: Unexplained cardiac arrest during spinal anesthesia. Anesthesiology 68:5, 1988.
13. Chinwa SS, Macleod A, Day B: Intraarticular bupivacaine (Marcaine) after arthroscopic meniscectomy: A randomized double-blind controlled study. Arthroscopy 5:33, 1989.
14. Clarkson CW, Hondeghem LM: Mechanism for bupivacaine depression of cardiac conduction: Fast block of sodium channels during the action potential with slow recovery from block during diastole. Anesthesiology 62:396, 1985.
15. Cooper JB, et al: Effects of informational feedback and pulse oximetry on the incidence of anesthesia complications. Anesthesiology 70:199, 1987.
16. Covino BG, Lambert DH: Efficacy in comparison to general anesthesia. In Raj PP, ed: Clinical Practice of Regional Anesthesia. New York, Churchill Livingstone, 1991, pp 173–185.
17. Crews JC, Clark RB: Effect of alkalinization on the pH of local anesthetic solutions. Anesth Analg 66:1203, 1987.
18. Damask MC, Weissman C, Todd G: General versus epidural anesthesia for femoral-popliteal bypass surgery. J Clin Anesth 2:71–75, 1990.
19. DeJong RH, Heavner JE: Diazepam prevents and aborts lidocaine convulsions in monkeys. Anesthesiology 41:226, 1974.
20. Dornette WHL: The standard of care. In Dornette WHL, ed: Legal Issues in Anesthesia Practice. Philadelphia, FA Davis, 1991, pp 24–38.
21. Doze NA, Shafer A, White PF: Recovery characteristics following propofol anesthesia: A comparison with thiopental-isoflurane. Anesthesiology 67:398, 1987.
22. Eagle KA, et al: Dipyridamole-thallium scanning in patients undergoing vascular surgery. JAMA 257:2185, 1987.
23. Eichhorn JH, et al: Standards for patient monitoring during anesthesia at Harvard Medical School. JAMA 256:1017, 1986.
24. Eichhorn JH: Prevention of intraoperative anesthesia accidents and related severe injury through safety monitoring. Anesthesiology 70:572, 1989.
25. Enneking FK, Benson HT: Oral anticoagulants and regional anesthesia: A perspective. Reg Anesth Pain Med 23(6 Suppl 2):140, 1998.
26. Erikksson E, et al: Knee arthroscopy with local anesthesia in ambulatory patients: Methods, results and patient compliance. Orthopedics 9:186, 1986.
27. Faris PM, Spence RK, Larholt KM, et al: The predictive power of baseline hemoglobin for transfusion risk in surgery patients. Orthopedics 1999:22 Suppl.
28. Frank SM, Flusher LA, Breslow MJ: Anesthesiology and critical care medicine. Johns Hopkins department of critical care medicine. JAMA 277:1127, 1997.
29. Gerancher J: Cauda equina syndrome following a single spinal administration of 5% hyperbaric lidocaine through a 25-gauge Whitaker needle. Anesthesiology 87:687, 1997.
30. Goldman L: Cardiac risks and complications of noncardiac surgery. Ann Intern Med 98:504, 1983.
31. Guidelines for preoperative fasting and the use of pharmacologic agents to reduce the risk of pulmonary aspiration: Application to healthy patients undergoing elective procedures. A Report by the American Society of Anesthesiologists Task Force. Copyright 1999 Anesthesiology http://www.asahq.org.
32. Horlocker TT, Heit JA: Low-molecular-weight heparin: Biochemistry, pharmacology, perioperative prophylaxis regimens, and guidelines for regional anesthetic management. Anesth Analg 85: 874, 1997.
33. Kasten GW, Martin ST: Bupivacaine cardiovascular toxicity: Comparison of treatment with bretylium and lidocaine. Anesth Analg 64:911, 1985.
34. Liu SS, Mulroy MF: Neuroaxial anesthesia and analgesia in the presence of standard heparin. Reg Anesth Pain Med 23(6 Suppl 2):157, 1998.
35. Lumpkin MM: FDA public health advisory. Anesthesiology 88: 27A, 1998.
36. Mangano DT, et al: Association of perioperative myocardial ischemia with cardiac morbidity in men undergoing noncardiac surgery. N Engl J Med 323:1781, 1990.
37. Mangano DT: Perioperative cardiac morbidity. Anesthesiology 72:153, 1990.
38. Marsch SCU, et al: Perioperative myocardial ischemia in patients undergoing elective hip arthroplasty during lumbar regional anesthesia. Anesthesiology 76:518, 1992.
39. Martin RC, et al: Diagnostic and operative arthroscopy of the knee under local anesthesia with parenteral medication. Am J Sports Med 17:436, 1989.
40. McCollum JSC, Milligan KR, Dundee JW: The antiemetic action of propofol. Anaesthesia 43:239, 1988.
41. Meinig RP, et al: Plasma bupivacaine levels following single dose intraarticular instillation for arthroscopy. Am J Sports Med 16: 295, 1988.
42. Milligan KA, et al: Intraarticular bupivacaine for pain relief in day case patients. Anaesthesia 43:563, 1988.
43. Mitchell RWD, Smith G: The control of postoperative pain. Br J Anaesth 63:147, 1989.
44. Modig J, et al: Thromboembolism after total hip replacement: Role of epidural and general anesthesia. Anesth Analg 62:174, 1983.
45. Modig J, Maripuu E, Sahlstedt B: Thromboembolism following total hip replacement. A prospective investigation of 94 patients with emphasis on the efficacy of lumbar epidural anesthesia in prophylaxis. Reg Anesth 11:72, 1986.
46. Moffitt EA, et al: Myocardial infarction after general anesthesia. JAMA 199:318, 1972.
47. Murakami DM, Bassett LW, Seeger LL: Advances in imaging in rheumatoid arthritis. Clin Orthop 265:83, 1991.
48. Orkin FK: Practice standards: The Midas touch or the emperor's new clothes? Anesthesiology 70:567, 1989.
49. Philip BK: Local anesthesia and sedation techniques. In White PF, ed: Outpatient Anesthesia. New York, Churchill Livingstone, 1990, p 264.
50. Plosker H, et al: A comparison of Diprivan and thiamylal sodium for the induction and maintenance of outpatient anesthesia. Anesthesiology 63:366, 1985.
51. Practice Guidelines for Blood Component Therapy: A report by

the American Society of Anesthesiologists Task Force on blood component therapy. Anesthesiology 84:732, 1996.
52. Practice guidelines for pulmonary artery catheterization. A report by the American Society of Anesthesiologists Task Force. Anesthesiology 78:380, 1993.
53. Raj PP, et al: Rationale and choice for surgical procedures. In Raj PP, ed: Clinical Practice of Regional Anesthesia. New York, Churchill Livingstone, 1990.
54. Rampil IJ: Medical information on the Internet. Anesthesiology 89:1223, 1998.
55. Rao TK, Jacobs KH, El Etr AA: Reinfarction following anesthesia in patients with myocardial infarction. Anesthesiology 59:499, 1983.
56. Sculco TP, Galliana J: Blood management experience: Relationship between autologous blood donation and transfusion in orthopedic surgery. Orthopedics 22 Suppl: 1999.
57. Sharrock NE, et al: Effects of epidural anesthesia on deep vein thrombosis after total knee arthroscopy. J Bone Joint Surg Am 73:502, 1991.
58. Shevde K, Panagopoulos G: A survey of 800 patients' knowledge, attitudes, and concerns regarding anesthesia. Anesth Analg 73:190, 1991.
59. Shoemaker WC, Appel PL, Kram HB, et al: Prospective trial of supranormal values of survivors as therapeutic goals in high-risk surgical patients. Chest 94:1176, 1988.
60. Smith I, et al: Effects of local anesthesia on recovery after outpatient arthroscopy. Anesth Analg 73:536, 1991.
61. Steen PA, Tinker JH, Tarhan S: Myocardial reinfarction after anesthesia and surgery. JAMA 239:256, 1976.
62. Stehling LC: Practice guidelines for blood component therapy. Park Ridge, IL, American Society of Anesthesiologists. Anesthesiology 82:1971, 1995.
63. Steingart R, Scheuer J: Assessment of myocardial ischemia. In Hurst JW, Schlant RL, eds: The Heart, the Arteries, and Veins. New York, McGraw-Hill, 1990, pp 351-368.
64. Stoelting RK, Miller RD: Basics of Anesthesia. New York, Churchill Livingstone, 1984, p 83.
65. Stoelting RK: Pharmacology and Physiology in Anesthetic Practice. Philadelphia, JB Lippincott, 1987, pp 148-168.
66. Tezlaff J: Bupivacaine-morphine combination best for ACL repair. Am J Sports Med 26:524, 1998.
67. Tinker JH, et al: Role of monitoring devices in prevention of anesthetic mishaps. A closed claims analysis. Anesthesiology 71: 541, 1989.
68. Ummey WF, Rowlingson JC: Do antiplatelet agents contribute to the development of perioperative spinal hematoma? Reg Anesth Pain Med 23(6 Suppl 2):146, 1998.
69. Valli H, Rosenberg PH: Effects of three anesthesia methods on hemodynamic responses connected with the use of thigh tourniquet in orthopedic patients. Acta Anesthesiol Scand 29:142, 1985.
70. Way WL, Trevor AJ: Pharmacology of intravenous nonnarcotic anesthetics. In Miller RD, ed: Anesthesia, 2nd ed. New York, Churchill Livingstone, 1986, pp 779-883.
71. Wedel DJ, Mulroy MF: Hemiparesis following dural puncture. Anesthesiology 59:475, 1983.
72. Weitz JI: Low-molecular-weight heparins. N Engl J Med 337:688, 1997.
73. White PF, ed: Outpatient Anesthesia. New York, Churchill Livingstone, 1990, p 264.
74. Yeager MP, et al: Epidural anesthesia and analgesia in high-risk surgical patients. Anesthesiology 66:729, 1987.
75. Yeager MP: Outcome of pain management. Anesth Clin North Am 7:241, 1989.

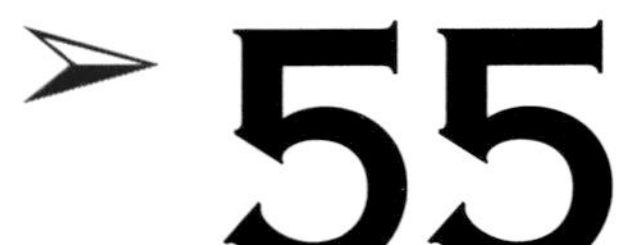

Anesthetic Considerations in Knee Surgery: The Ambulatory Patient

SUNDAR KOPPOLU • SOMUSANDARAM THIAGARAJAH

Sixty percent of all surgical procedures are now done in the United States on an ambulatory basis, and it is expected that in the next few years this rate will increase to 65% to 70%. Although ophthalmology cases make up the bulk of ambulatory surgical procedures (27%), orthopedic ambulatory surgery cases comprise 6%.[1]

ADVANTAGES OF AMBULATORY SURGERY

The advantages of performing surgery on an ambulatory basis are substantial, among them

1. Economic: financial incentive to reduce hospital costs up to 40% to 80% depending on the facility and surgical procedure
2. Less disruption of personal life, especially for children
3. Reduced risk of hospital infection
4. Convenience for the patient and the surgeon
5. No need for 24-hour service; helps in expanding community medical care

Whereas in the past only physical status class I and II patients (Table 55.1) received ambulatory surgery care, now more and more class III and IV patients are being seen.

Geriatric and higher risk patients (physical status classes III and IV) may be considered acceptable candidates for outpatient surgery if their systemic disease is well controlled and their medical condition is optimized. Excluded as acceptable candidates are medically unstable patients and those with inadequate postoperative home care, including pain management. Implementation of inappropriate procedures based on the patient's general condition and age leads to unnecessary hospital admission.

CONTRAINDICATIONS TO AMBULATORY SURGERY

Contraindications of ambulatory surgery are as follows:

1. Premature infants younger than 50 weeks' gestational age.
2. Infants with apneic episodes.
3. Respiratory distress syndrome.
4. Bronchopulmonary dysplasia.
5. Family history of sudden infant death syndrome.
6. History of malignant hyperpyrexia.
7. Morbid obesity.
8. Acute substance abuse.
9. Patient on monoamine inhibitors.
10. Severe bronchospastic disease.
11. Social factors, including patient refusal of escort on discharge home and lack of responsible adult at home.

The ambulatory surgical center can be free standing with or without hospital affiliation, office based, or hospital based but at a different location than the main operating room area. Wherever the ambulatory surgical center is located, it must meet Joint Commission on the Accreditation of Healthcare Organizations standards.

TABLE 55.1 AMERICAN SOCIETY OF ANESTHESIOLOGISTS PHYSICAL STATUS CLASSIFICATION

Class	Description
1	A healthy patient Example: inguinal hernia in an otherwise healthy patient
2	A patient with mild systemic disease Examples: chronic bronchitis; moderate obesity; diet-controlled diabetes mellitus; old myocardial infarction; mild hypertension
3	A patient with severe systemic disease that is not incapacitating Examples: coronary artery disease with angina; insulin-dependent diabetes mellitus; morbid obesity; moderate to severe
4	A patient with incapacitating systemic disease that is a constant threat to life Examples: organic heart disease with marked cardiac insufficiency, unstable angina, intractable arrhythmia; advanced pulmonary, renal, hepatic, or endocrine insufficiency
5	A moribund patient not expected to survive for 24 hours with or without operation Example: ruptured abdominal aneurysm with profound shock
Emergency (E)	The suffix E is used to denote the presumed poorer physical status of any patient in one of these categories who undergoes emergency surgery (e.g., 2E)

TABLE 55.2 INFILTRATION ANESTHESIA FOR AMBULATORY SURGERY PATIENTS

Agent	Concentration (%)	Plain Solutions			Epinephrine-Containing Solutions		
		Max. Adult Dose (mg)	*Max. Dose (mg/kg)*	*Duration (min)*	*Max. Adult Dose (mg)*	*Max. Dose (mg/kg)*	*Duration (min)*
Short Duration							
Procaine	1-2	800	11	15-30	1000	14	30-90
Chloroprocaine							
Moderate Duration							
Lidocaine	0.5-1	300	4	30-60	500	7	120-360
Mepivacaine	0.5-1	300	4	45-90	500	7	120-360
Bupivacaine	0.25	200	4	60-120			

PREOPERATIVE SCREENING

Surgeons' evaluation is very important in determining whether a particular procedure can be performed on an ambulatory basis. Proper help at home after the procedure and pain management should be taken into consideration.

There is no substitute for a good patient history and physical examination. The minimal laboratory requirement at Beth Israel Medical Center (New York) includes a complete blood count dated within 1 year, chest x-ray film, and electrocardiogram for patients older than 50 years. If warranted by the patient's medical condition, further evaluation may be necessary. The American College of Obstetrics and Gynecology (ACOG) does not require mandatory testing for pregnancy in all females of childbearing age, but it does recommend testing if there is any question after a thorough history or in the event of suggestive signs and symptoms. It is also very important to elicit a history of motion sickness. These patients are prone to experience nausea and vomiting after certain procedures such as laparoscopy and eye muscle surgery. Women early in their menstrual cycle tend to experience more nausea after anesthesia.

PREMEDICATION

When patients are capable, they are now allowed to walk to the operating room, which makes them feel that they can walk in and walk out after the procedure. Occasionally, a few patients require diazepam (Valium) for sedation preoperatively. Too much sedation, however, will prolong the recovery.

Some patients are more prone to regurgitation and aspiration under anesthesia:

1. Obese patients.
2. Diabetic patients.
3. Patients with a history of hiatal hernia.
4. Pregnant patients.

DIFFERENT ANESTHESIA TECHNIQUES

Anesthesia for surgery of the knee in ambulatory patients can be provided by the following techniques:

1. Local anesthesia into the knee and skin infiltration for incision sites either with systemic sedation or with no sedation.
2. Regional anesthesia (either spinal or epidural and intravenous Bier block).
3. General anesthesia.

The choice of anesthesia depends on the patient's general medical condition and willingness to receive regional anesthesia and type of surgery.

The maximum amount of local anesthesia agents that can be used is given in Tables 55.2 and 55.3.

KETOROLAC TROMETHAMINE (TORADOL)

Early discharge from the hospital in a safe and comfortable state is the goal of ambulatory surgery patient management. Problems in the immediate postoperative period that can impede this goal are nausea, vomiting, somnolence, urinary retention, and, most important, pain at the surgical site. Pain relief is commonly

TABLE 55.3 MAJOR NERVE BLOCKS FOR AMBULATORY SURGERY PATIENTS

Agent	Usual Concentration (%)	Plain Solutions				Epinephrine-Containing Solutions			
		Usual Adult Volume	*Max. Adult Dose (mg)*	*Usual Onset (min)*	*Usual Duration (min)*	*Usual Adult Volume*	*Max. Adult Dose (mg)*	*Usual Onset (min)*	*Usual Duration (min)*
Chloroprocaine	2-3	25-40	800	10-20	30-50	30-60	1000	10-20	60-120
Lidocaine	1-1.5	20-30	300	10-20	60-90	30-50	500	10-20	120-140
Mepivacaine	1-1.5	20-30	300	10-20	60-120	30-50	500	10-20	180-300
Bupivacaine	0.5	20-25	300	20	60-120				

achieved with narcotics, but at the expense of exacerbating other adverse effects. Ketorolac is a nonsteroidal anti-inflammatory drug (NSAID) with attractive properties. It has approximately one-half the analgesic properties of morphine[5] and, therefore, can be used as an alternative or adjunct to narcotics. It blocks the enzyme cyclooxygenase and prevents conversion of arachidonic acid to the precursors of prostaglandins and thus the formation of pain-producing prostaglandins. The analgesic properties of ketorolac are comparable to those of fentanyl, meperidine (Demerol), ibuprofen, piroxicam, indomethacin, and diclofenac.[3, 7, 8] The adverse effects of narcotics — somnolence, respiratory depression, depression of gastrointestinal (GI) motility, nausea, vomiting, and urinary retention — are nonexistent with ketorolac.[6] In mild to moderate surgical pain, ketorolac is useful as a single agent. However, when pain is severe, it is used as an adjunct to narcotics. It has clinically significant opioid-sparing effects, thereby limiting the side effects of narcotics. Other interesting features of ketorolac are the absence of psychomotor and addictive effects. Irritation at the injection site is absent with ketorolac.[8]

Compared with fentanyl, ketorolac has a slow onset of action. Therefore, to be effective in the immediate postoperative period, it should be administered early, preferably preoperatively, especially if the surgery is of short duration.[4, 12] The action begins in 10 minutes, peaks at 40 to 60 minutes, and lasts 6 hours. Also, the initial dosage should be adequate: for adults, 60 mg followed by 30 mg every 4 to 6 hours. Clearance is reduced in the elderly. The drug can be given either intravenously or intramuscularly; however, the route that is superior is not yet known. Sporadic articles in the literature describe the use of ketorolac intra-articularly in patients undergoing knee arthroscopic surgery.[10]

Ketorolac is not without side effects. Like all NSAIDs, ketorolac can cause GI bleeding, hematological abnormalities, and kidney dysfunction. Ketorolac inhibits platelet aggregation by reversible inhibition of prostaglandin synthetase and is of no clinical significance. However, there are claims that platelet dysfunction worsens with spinal anesthesia.[11] In one case report, hemiparesis developed in a patient as a result of a spinal hematoma after spinal anesthesia, which was established after multiple attempts. This patient was being treated concurrently with ketorolac.[2] Because it is highly protein bound, it could displace drugs like warfarin (Coumadin) and potentiate bleeding. The incidence of GI bleeding is estimated at less than 0.3% and usually occurs when the drug is used for more than 30 days.

Ketorolac should be avoided in patients with congestive heart failure, hypovolemia, and cirrhosis. In these patients, the renin-angiotensin system is activated and releases the vasoactive substances that cause renal artery vasoconstriction. Prostaglandins in these patients negate the renal artery vasoconstriction and prevent renal dysfunction. Ketorolac, if given, will block prostaglandin formation, renal artery vasoconstriction will continue unabated, and renal dysfunction may ensue.[9] Therefore, ketorolac should be avoided in these patients.

INTRA-ARTICULAR ANESTHETICS FOR KNEE SURGERY

Ambulatory patients experience excruciating pain after surgery of the cruciate ligaments or menisci. Early mobilization and physiotherapy of the joint in the postoperative period further worsen the pain to intolerable levels. The chemicals released from surgically traumatized tissues sensitize the peripheral nociceptors and cause pain. Adequate pain management is, therefore, an integral step for a successful surgical outcome.

Parenteral narcotics were used in the past to control pain. However, narcotics cause somnolence, emesis, and urinary retention and increase time until discharge. To overcome these adverse effects, intra-articular injections of local anesthetics instead of parenteral narcotics were attempted. Bupivacaine, because of its long duration of action, was injected intra-articularly at the end of surgery.[19]

The literature is replete with information on intra-articular medications. Local anesthetics, narcotics, clonidine, and nonsteroidal analgesics have been tried.[13] One study evaluated the effect of intra-articular injection of morphine, 1 mg, Demerol, 10 mg or fentanyl, 10 μg, and concluded that Demerol was the most effective of the three in producing analgesia.[17] The effect of intra-articular ketorolac is equivocal; some claim it is equally effective as morphine or bupivacaine, whereas others refute its efficacy.[14, 15] Alkalinizing prilocaine for intra-articular injection did not improve pain relief.[16] Increasing the dose of intra-articular morphine from 1 mg to 3 mg had no beneficial effect.

In one study, a combination of 20 mL of 0.25% bupivacaine and 1 mg of morphine injected intra-articularly 20 minutes before a surgical incision was made provided very effective analgesia. The postoperative analgesia was <2 on a 1- to 10-cm visual analog scale and lasted for 6 hours[18].

Oral analgesics are usually adequate for diagnostic arthroscopic examination.

SELECTION OF ANESTHETICS

General Anesthesia

Arthroscopic surgery of the knee in ambulatory patients may be performed for diagnostic or therapeutic purposes. Therapeutic arthroscopy may be performed for evacuation of hemarthrosis, removal of a loose body, or repair of a torn cruciate ligament or a fractured meniscus.

General anesthesia is the most common anesthetic technique for ambulatory arthroscopic surgery and is preferred by patients and surgeons. General anesthesia can be administered intravenously or via inhalation, but a balanced technique combining both seems to be more popular. Short-acting and quickly cleared anesthetics have appeared on the market. The anesthetic management of these ambulatory patients is challenging. The anesthesiologist should aim to provide a pain-free, nonemetic, and quick recovering postoperative period.

Preparation

The analgesic component can be achieved with NSAIDs for mild to moderate pain. Severe pain can be treated with ketorolac or other NSAIDs with modest doses of narcotics. Some patients may experience nausea and vomiting with narcotic analgesics. The emetic side effects of narcotics can be minimized by decreasing the dose and combining them with NSAIDs. Ketorolac is the commonly used NSAID for these patients.[35] Ideally, pain control should begin early, preferably pre- or intraoperatively.

Preemptive analgesia is another method of minimizing postoperative pain.[26] If the sensory innervation of the surgical site is blocked before the surgical incision is made the analgesic requirement during the postoperative period is significantly less. Sensory blockade can be achieved with spinal or epidural anesthesia or by direct infiltration of the operative site.

Antiemetics

Postoperative nausea and vomiting (PONV) are major problems, although the exact reason is not clear. The use of intraoperative fentanyl or morphine causes a higher incidence of emesis.[29, 34] Nitrous oxide, preoperative dehydration, motion sickness, middle ear disease, and timing early in the menstrual cycle are other implicated factors. Some types of surgery are predisposed to PONV. Use of droperidol, metoclopramide, or ondansetron and avoidance of intraoperative use of nitrous oxide are some measures to minimize postoperative emesis. Ondansetron is a 5-HT_3 serotonin receptor antagonist that is very effective against PONV, and its effect is dose related. An adequate dose of droperidol is claimed to be more effective than ondansetron.[23] Droperidol, metoclopramide, and ondansetron can cause extrapyramidal symptoms and require benzodiazepine to control them.[33] Droperidol causes agitation and feelings of impending doom if given to unpremedicated patients and can be avoided if given after the patient is anesthetized. Tropisetron and granisetron have been added to the antiemetic pharmacology.[20, 24] (Table 55.4).

Selection of Anesthesia

Selecting anesthesia to shorten the recovery phase is another aspect of patient management. Propofol, sevoflurane, desflurane, and remifentanil have been added to the armamentarium of anesthetics for quick, pain-free, nonemetic emergence. Skill and experience of the anesthesiologist, rather than the agents itself, are major determinants of such an emergence from anesthesia.

INDUCING AGENTS

Of the inducing agents, propofol is ideal because of its quick clearance and antiemetic effect. Thiopental sodium (Pentothal) has been used for many years and is inexpensive. However, large and repeated doses must be avoided to shorten postoperative recovery. Etomidate is useful in cardiovascular-compromised patients. Pain at the injection site, nausea, vomiting, and myoclonal symptoms are limiting factors.

Maintenance of Anesthesia

INHALATIONAL AGENTS

The most commonly used inhalational agents are halothane, enflurane, and isoflurane. As mentioned, however, desflurane and sevoflurane have been added to the group. In choosing an ideal volatile agent for ambulatory surgery, the anesthesiologist must select one known for its quick induction and recovery, adequate potency, minimal adverse effects, and lack of metabolites. In comparing the available agents for quick induction and recovery, one should examine the physical property blood/gas solubility (partition coefficient). The lower the blood/gas solubility, the quicker are induction and emergence. The volatile agents, in ascending order of blood/gas solubility, are desflurane, nitrous oxide, sevoflurane, isoflurane, enflurane, and halothane (Table 55.5). Emergence is slowest with halothane.

The potency of an inhalational agent is determined by its minimal alveolar concentration (MAC). In order of potency, the old group—halothane, isoflurane, and enflurane—have greater potency than sevoflurane, which closely follows. Desflurane ranks much lower. In selecting an agent with high potency and low blood gas solubility, sevoflurane ranks first, closely followed by isoflurane. Desflurane has a low partition coefficient, making it attractive for quick induction and emergence. However, the pungent smell of desflurane is irritating to the airways and is liable to cause coughing and laryngospasm during induction and emergence. Also, it has a low boiling point (23°C) and high saturated vapor pressure, making it difficult to store and dispense in normal vaporizers. Other notable features are the higher incidence of postoperative nausea

TABLE 55.4 ANTIEMETICS FOR AMBULATORY SURGERY PATIENTS

Variable	Ondansetron	Tropisetron	Granisetron	Droperidol
Dose (mg)	4–8	2–5	2.5	0.6–1.25
Half-life (hours)	3.5	8–12	3–4	4–6

TABLE 55.5 **PHYSICAL PROPERTIES OF VOLATILE ANESTHETIC AGENTS**

Variable	Halothane	Enflurane	Isoflurane	Desflurane	Sevoflurane
Blood/gas solubility	2.3	1.9	1.4	0.42	0.6
MAC	0.75	1.68	1.15	6–7	2
Boiling point	50.2	56.5	48.5	23.5	58.5
Saturated vapor pressure	243.3	172	240	664	160

MAC = minimal alveolar concentration.

and vomiting compared with propofol, its low potency (MAC 6), and tachycardia associated with its use.

Sevoflurane is nonirritating to the airways and odorless and is, therefore, an ideal anesthetic agent for induction in both children and adults. Sevoflurane is claimed to be equally good as propofol in adults.[36] Sevoflurane has significantly more muscle relaxant properties than the other volatile agents. It potentiates the muscle relaxants and even provides relaxation of its own, adequate for tracheal intubation. However, the instability of sevoflurane, especially with soda lime, is worrisome although not clinically significant. Adverse effects of its metabolites have not been demonstrated as yet. In hypoxic states in animals, sevoflurane has produced histological hepatotoxic features similar to those of isoflurane.

INTRAVENOUS AGENTS

Remifentanil is an ultra-short-acting opioid that equilibrates with the brain in 1.3 minutes and has an elimination half-life of 6 to 11 minutes. It is an ester that rapidly undergoes degradation by the plasma and tissue-nonspecific esterases. Pseudocholinesterase does not affect the metabolism of remifentanil. Generally, a bolus dose of 1 μg/kg followed by an infusion of 0.25 to 1 μg/kg/min is used to maintain analgesia. Like all narcotics, remifentanil causes bradycardia, hypotension, chest wall rigidity, and postoperative nausea and vomiting. However, a bolus dose alone may cause these side effects, particularly muscle rigidity and respiratory depression. Therefore, it should not be used unless treatment for these side effects is readily accessible. Histamine release is claimed to be absent with remifentanil. It seems to be ideally suited for intraoperatively painful procedures with minimal postoperative pain. Because of its short half-life, for those procedures with lingering postoperative pain, supplemental analgesics are needed.[22, 25]

Fentanyl, alfentanil, and sufentanil are the other three opioids available. Fentanyl is commonly used. Sufentanil is five to 10 times stronger than fentanyl and provides effective postoperative analgesia with less drowsiness and nausea than the other narcotics. However, dose and surgery must be carefully selected[30, 32] (Table 55.6).

Use of propofol to maintain anesthesia is also very common. After the initial induction bolus dose of 2 to 2.5 mg/kg, anesthesia is maintained with an infusion of 200 μg/kg/min and then gradually tapered and titrated to 100 to 150 μg/kg/min. Propofol can be combined with nitrous oxide and amnesic agents such as midazolam. It results in a quicker recovery with a clear sensorium and emesis-free postoperative period.[28]

MUSCLE RELAXANTS

In selecting a muscle relaxant, Savarese[31] recommended the use of short and intermediate-acting drugs, particularly if extubation is planned at the end of surgery as done in ambulatory patients.[31] Postoperative train-of-four ratio >90% is required to prevent postoperative pulmonary complications and is more easily achieved with short- and intermediate-acting drugs rather than long-acting relaxants.[27] Continuous infusion, rather than bolus administration, of these relaxants to achieve intraoperative paralysis is claimed to produce predictable relaxation, easy reversibility, and cost savings.

Succinylcholine is a short-acting drug ideal for tracheal intubation. However, postoperative myalgia, one of its adverse effects, is worse in ambulating patients.[21]

TABLE 55.6 **DOSE REGIMENS FOR INTRAVENOUS ANESTHETICS**

Drug	Loading Dose (μg/kg)	Maintenance Infusion (μg/kg/min)	Recovery Time (min)	Potency in Comparison to Morphine
Alfentanil	10–30	0.5–2	15–30	10–20 times
Fentanyl	2–4	0.02–0.08	45–60	100 times
Sufentanil	0.25–0.75	0.005–0.01	15–30	500–1000 times
Remifentanil	1.0	0.25–1.0	Immediate	?
Propofol	1000–2500	120–200	5–10	—

TABLE 55.7 **MUSCLE RELAXANTS**

Drug	ED95 (mg/kg)	Intubation (mg/kg)	Duration TOF 70%		Infusion Rate (μg/kg/min)	Recovery Slope 5%–59% Twitch (min)
Mivacurium	0.08	0.2-0.25	25-30 min	Histamine	3-8	13-16
Cisatracurium	0.05	0.1-0.2	60-90 min	—	1-2	30-35
Rocuronium	0.3	0.6-1.2	45-120 min	Mild vagolytic	6-12	30-60

ED95 = effective dose at 95%; TOF = train-of-four ratio.

Also, an occasional patient (1:3000) may manifest prolonged apnea after administration of succinylcholine because of a lack or deficiency of pseudocholinesterase. Skill in the use of other drugs instead of succinylcholine for tracheal intubation is, therefore, an advantage. Rocuronium has fast onset of action and is used for tracheal intubation (Table 55.7). If the surgery is short, mivacurium can be used. Mivacurium has a slow onset, but when primed and topped up before laryngoscopy, its action can be hastened.[31]

LARYNGEAL MASK AIRWAY (LMA) AND CUFFED OROPHARYNGEAL AIRWAY (COPA)

In selected patients, laryngeal mask airway (LMA) or cuffed oropharyngeal airway (COPA) can be used, thus avoiding tracheal intubation or mask ventilation and their related adverse effects. Also, muscle relaxants and deeper planes of anesthesia can be avoided with LMA or COPA. As opposed to tracheal intubation, with LMA or COPA there is a quick and smooth emergence as well as fewer effects of anesthetics, resulting in a more pleasant outcome for patients.

The anesthetic management of these ambulatory patients is challenging. A multifaceted approach is needed to achieve a comfortable, alert, and pain-free patient in the immediate postoperative period:

1. Antiemetics should be administered early, particularly in susceptible patients.
2. Consider providing preemptive analgesia before the surgical incision is made.
3. Select the least invasive but appropriate type of modality for airway management (LMA, COPA, mask, or an endotracheal tube).
4. Provide analgesia for the postoperative period with a non-narcotic, epidural, spinal, intra-articular injection, or nerve block.
5. Select an ideal anesthetic and, if necessary, a muscle relaxant, and carefully tailor the doses.

POSTOPERATIVE COURSE

In general, the incidence of nausea and vomiting is less after regional anesthesia than general anesthesia. The recovery time depends on the anesthetic agents used. Because of the availability of short-acting anesthetic agents and their antiemetic properties, patients are able to be discharged home within 2 hours after general anesthesia.

DISCHARGE CRITERIA

The following criteria should be considered before the patient is discharged home:

1. Vital signs must be stable for more than 1 hour.
2. The patient must have no evidence of respiratory depression.
3. The patient must also be
   a. Oriented to place and time.
   b. Able to ingest oral fluids without nausea and vomiting.
   c. Able to void.
   d. Able to walk without assistance.
4. The patient must have
   a. Minimal nausea and vomiting.
   b. No excessive pain.
   c. No bleeding.

Patients who received high doses of local anesthetics can have impaired psychomotor skills in the postoperative period.

References

1. Society for Ambulatory Anesthesia: Outpatient surgery information. http://www.sambahq.org.
2. Gerancher JC, Waterer R, Middleton J: Transient paraparesis after postdural puncture spinal hematoma in a patient receiving ketorolac Anesthesiology. 86:490-494, 1997.
3. Lysak SZ, Anderson PT, Carithers RA, et al: Postoperative effects of fentanyl, ketorolac, and piroxicam as analgesics for outpatient laparoscopic procedures. Obstet Gynecol 83(2):270-275, 1994.
4. McLaughlin ME: The intraoperative administration of ketorolac tromethamine in evaluating length of stay in a same day surgery unit. AANA J 62(5):433-436, 1994.
5. McQuire DA, Sanders K, Hendricks SD: Comparison of ketorolac and opioid analgesics in postoperative ACL reconstruction outpatient pain control. Arthroscopy 9(6):653-661, 1993.
6. Mendel HG, Guarnieri KM, Sundt LM, et al: The effects of ketorolac and fentanyl on postoperative vomiting analgesic requirements in children undergoing strabismus surgery. Anesth Analg 80(6):1129-1133, 1995.
7. Morley-Forster P, Newton PT, Cook MJ: Ketorolac and indomethacin are equally efficacious for relief of minor postoperative pain. Can J Anesth 40(12):1126-1130, 1993.
8. Morrow BC, Bunting H, Milligan KR: A comparison of diclofenac and ketorolac for postoperative analgesia following day-case arthroscopy of the knee joint. Anaesthesia 48(7):585-587, 1993.
9. Murrell GC, Leake T, Hughes PJ: A comparison of the efficacy of ketorolac and indomethacin for postoperative analgesia following laparoscopic surgery in day patients. Anaesth Intensive Care 24(2):237-240, 1996.
10. Reuben SS, Connelly NR: Postoperative analgesia for outpatient arthroscopic knee surgery with intraarticular bupivacaine and ketorolac. Anesth Analg 80(6):1154-1157, 1995.

11. Thwaites B, Nigus D, Bouska G, et al: Intravenous ketorolac tromethamine worsens platelet function during knee arthroscopy under spinal anesthesia. Anesth Analg 82:1176-1181, 1996.
12. Twersky RS, Lebovits A, Williams C, et al: Ketorolac versus fentanyl for postoperative pain management in outpatients. Clin J Pain 11(2): 127-133, 1995.
13. Niemi L, Pitkanen M, Tuominen M, et al: Intraarticular morphine for pain relief after knee arthroscopy performed under regional anesthesia. Acta Anaesthesiol Scand 38:402-405, 1994.
14. Reuben SS, Connelly NR: Postarthroscopic meniscus repair analgesia with intraarticular ketorolac or morphine. Anesth Analg 82: 1036-1039, 1996.
15. Reuben SS, Connelly NR: Postoperative analgesia for outpatient arthroscopic knee surgery with intraarticular bupivacaine and ketorolac. Anesth Analg 80(6) 1154-1157, 1995.
16. Richmond CE: Alkalinization of local anaesthetic for intra-articular instillation during arthroscopy. Br J Anaesth 73:190-193, 1994.
17. Soderlund A, Westman L, Ersmark H, et al: Analgesia following arthroscopy—A comparison of intra-articular morphine, pethidine and fentanyl. Acta Anaesthesiol Scand 41:6-11, 1997.
18. Tezlaff JE: Intra-articular saline, bupivacaine, or bupivacaine plus morphine for post-op pain relief. Am J Sports Med 26:524-529, 1998.
19. Tierney GS, Wright RW, Smith JP, et al: Anterior cruciate ligament reconstruction as an outpatient procedure. Am J Sports Med 23:755-756, 1995.
20. Chan MTV, Chui PT, Ho WS, et al: Single dose tropisetron for preventing postoperative nausea and vomiting after breast surgery. Anesth Analg 87:931-935, 1998.
21. Churchill-Davidson HC: Suxamethonium chloride and muscle pain. BMJ 74:75, 1954.
22. Fortier J, Chung F, Moote C, et al: Remifentanil vs alfentanil for ambulatory surgery using preoperative naproxen Na for pain management. Anesthesiology 87:A15, 1997.
23. Fortney J, Graczyk S, Creed M, et al: Comparison of ondansetron and droperidol as prophylactic antiemetic therapy for elective outpatient surgical procedures. Anesthesiology 87:A21, 1997.
24. Fujii Y, Toyooka H, Tanaka H: Prevention of postoperative nausea and vomiting with a combination of granisetron and droperidol. Anesth Analg 86:613-616, 1998.
25. Glass PSA, Hardman D, Kamiyama Y, et al: Preliminary pharmacokinetics and pharmacodynamics of an ultra short acting opioid: Remifentanil. Anesth Analg 77:1031-1040, 1993.
26. Kissin I: Preemptive analgesia. Anesthesiology 84:1015-1019. 1996.
27. Kopman AF, Yee PS, Neuman GG: Relationship of train-of-four fade to clinical signs and symptoms of residual paralysis in awake volunteers. Anesthesiology 86:765, 1997.
28. Korttila K, Ostman P, Faure E, et al: Randomized comparison of recovery after propofol-nitrous oxide versus thiopentone-isoflurane-nitrous oxide anesthesia in patients undergoing ambulatory surgery. Acta Anaesthesiol Scand 34:400-403, 1990.
29. Mendel HG, Guarnieri KM, Sundt LM, et al: The effects of ketorolac and fentanyl on postoperative vomiting and analgesic requirements in children undergoing strabismus surgery. Anesth Analg 80:1129-1133, 1995.
30. Phitayakoran P, Melnick BM, Vicinie AF: Comparison of continuous sufentanil and fentanyl infusions for outpatient anaesthesia. Can J Anaesth 34:242-245, 1987.
31. Saverese J: Some considerations on the new muscle relaxants. In IARS Review Course Lectures. IARS, 1998.
32. Shafer SL, Varvel JR: Pharmacokinetics, pharmacodynamics, and rational opioid selection. Anesthesiology 74:53-63, 1991.
33. Tolan MM, Fuhrman TM, Tsueda K: Perioperative extrapyramidal reactions associated with ondansetron. Anesthesiology 90:340-341, 1998.
34. Weinstein MS, Nicolson SC, Schreiner MS: A single dose of morphine sulphate increases the incidence of vomiting after outpatient inguinal surgery in children. Anesthesiology 81:572-577, 1994.
35. Yee JO, Koshiver JE, Allbon C, et al: Comparison of intramuscular ketorolac tromethamine and morphine sulphate for analgesia of pain after major surgery. Pharmacotherapy 6:253, 1986.
36. Zarate E, Song D, White PF: Use of sevoflurane as an alternative to propofol for induction of anesthesia in outpatients undergoing laparoscopic cholecystectomy. Anesthesiology 87: A1, 1997.

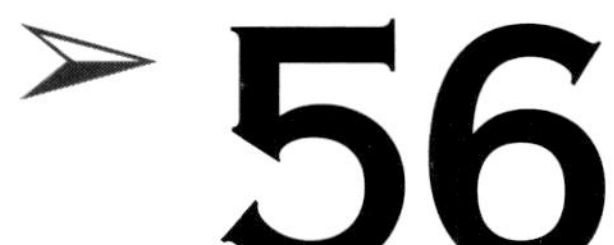

Anesthetic Considerations in Knee Surgery—Choice of Anesthesia and the Relationship to DVT

NIGEL E. SHARROCK

The risk of deep vein thrombosis (DVT) following knee surgery depends on the type of surgery performed, patient characteristics, the form of thromboprophylaxis, and the type of anesthesia. The risk of DVT following knee arthroscopy is approximately 3%,[4] and it is questionable whether the type of anesthesia influences this rate. The patients at risk of developing DVT following reconstructive knee surgery include those over 40 years of age,[22] those having sustained lower limb fracture about the knee, and those undergoing total knee arthroplasty (TKA) or high tibial osteotomy. The studies demonstrating an effect of anesthesia on DVT have been performed in patients undergoing TKA, but the observations probably also apply to high tibial osteotomy. With fractures, the thrombogenic stimulus is already activated, and it is unknown whether anesthetic practice can modify this process. For these reasons, this chapter will discuss in detail the influence of anesthesia on DVT with TKA.

RATE OF DVT: EPIDURAL VERSUS GENERAL ANESTHESIA

A number of studies have assessed the effect of anesthesia on DVT rate following TKA.[8, 11, 19, 26] In a randomized trial of epidural anesthesia and general anesthesia (GA) in 48 patients, a significantly lower rate of DVT was noted in the epidural group (59% GA vs 18% epidural anesthesia).[8] In a further trial, the overall DVT rate was similar, but the proximal DVT rate was lower with epidural anesthesia.[11] In a large retrospective series of 541 patients undergoing TKA between 1984 and 1988, the DVT rate was 64.3% for GA and 48% for epidural anesthesia ($p < .0001$).[19] The rates for unilateral TKA were 56% and 42%, respectively ($p < 0.01$).[19] The rate of proximal DVT (popliteal or thigh) was 7% with GA and 3% with epidural anesthesia.[19] In a subsequent randomized trial of epidural anesthesia versus GA for unilateral TKA in 178 patients at the same institution, the rate was 48% for GA and 40% for epidural anesthesia.[26] In both studies, all patients had ascending venography to assess DVT. These four studies demonstrate that epidural anesthesia confers a benefit in reducing overall DVT rate by at least 20% and may reduce the rate of proximal DVT even further. However, by itself, epidural anesthesia is insufficient DVT prophylaxis.

Role of Epidural Analgesia

It has been assumed that extending the epidural analgesia postoperatively would enhance the intraoperative benefit of epidural anesthesia on DVT formation.[1, 14] However, this has not been demonstrated and may not be the case.[20] Epidural analgesia infusion with 0.125% bupivacaine and fentanyl 5 μg/mL does not increase femoral venous blood flow following surgery,[9] so it is unlikely to influence DVT formation by reducing stasis. On the other hand, foot flexion/extension exercises markedly increase femoral venous blood flow during epidural analgesia.[9, 25] An alert, cooperative patient comfortable with epidural analgesia may be able to enhance lower extremity blood flow by being able to perform these exercises. In these regards, it has been demonstrated that epidural anesthesia and analgesia enhance rehabilitation following TKA.[21, 26] Factors that facilitate early ambulation may indirectly prevent propagation of DVT or enhance clot lysis.

RISK OF PULMONARY EMBOLISM

In the retrospective study previously cited, the rate of positive lung scan was 9% with GA and 6% with epidural.[19] In the randomized trial, the rate was 12% with GA and 9% with epidural anesthesia.[26] The lung scan data is inconclusive, but in a retrospective study of death following total hip and knee arthroplasty, the rate of death from pulmonary embolism (PE) was reduced six-fold with epidural anesthesia as compared with GA.[16] The overall death rate for unilateral TKA was reduced from 0.44% to 0.07% ($p = 0.01$).[16] These data attest to the outcome benefit of epidural anesthesia rather than GA for TKA.

MECHANISM OF DVT

Recent studies have demonstrated that thrombi form primarily during rather than following TKA. Parmet et al[15] aspirated fresh thrombi from the femoral vein following release of a tourniquet during TKA. Echogenic shower of emboli, both small and moderately large, can be seen following release of a tourniquet during TKA. Markers of thrombosis increase significantly during TKA, and the increase is most marked following release of the tourniquet.[17, 18] Finally, Maynard et al[10] demonstrated that 70% of the patients who developed DVT had venographic evidence of thrombi within hours of the end of surgery.

Thrombi may extend or lyze following surgery, and most treatment is focused on the postoperative period. However, the ultimate success in preventing DVT has to be directed at preventing DVT during surgery. In this regard, administration of heparin during surgery can suppress fibrin formation.[17] Unfortunately, this regime does not prevent DVT formation.[23]

Whether the beneficial effect of epidural anesthesia occurs during or immediately following surgery is unknown.[18] In a study of markers of thrombosis, there were no differences between epidural anesthesia or GA with TKA performed under tourniquet.[18] Fibrinolytic mechanisms were likewise not influenced by the type of anesthesia.[18] These data suggest that the effect of epidural anesthesia may be in the immediate postoperative period rather than during surgery with the tourniquet inflated. A possible mechanism whereby epidural anesthesia may decrease DVT rate is by enhancing lower extremity blood flow.[1, 3] A period of enhanced "deep venous washout" could reduce the thrombogenic load in the vein. This is, of course, speculation. TKA is a profound thrombogenic stimulus, and studies are needed to better understand this process so that rational means of preventing it can be developed.

SPINAL COMPARED TO EPIDURAL ANESTHESIA

No comparison trials of spinal versus either GA or epidural anesthesia are available in relation to DVT after TKA. However, both epidural and spinal anesthesia prevent DVT after total hip arthroplasty when compared with GA,[2, 13] so it is likely that spinal anesthesia also confers a benefit over GA for TKA. The physiological effects of spinal anesthesia are similar to those of epidural anesthesia. The one disadvantage of spinal anesthesia is the inability to provide optimal postoperative analgesia. As stated earlier, it is possible that by augmenting rehabilitation and early ambulation, epidural analgesia may retard extension of existing thrombi.

Interrelationship of Low-Molecular-Weight Heparin and Epidural Analgesia

Concerns over the concurrent use of low-molecular-weight heparin (LMWH) and epidural anesthesia have existed for some time.[12] The recent Food and Drug Administration advisory has highlighted the concern and focused on two issues.[5] First, epidural anesthesia should not be performed on a patient who has had an injection of LMWH within 12 hours. Second, it is risky to use LMWH in patients with an epidural catheter in place. It is, however, safe to use LMWH following surgery in a patient who had epidural or spinal anesthesia, but the catheter must be withdrawn before administering LMWH.

There has been much discussion about the dose of LMWH administration and the timing of LMWH injections in relation to inserting or withdrawing the epidural catheter.[7] In addition, there appears to be an apparent difference in the U.S. when compared with the European experience.[7] The problem, however, remains: there is a risk of epidural hematoma and permanent paraplegia when LMWH is administered concurrently with epidural analgesia. Timing the withdrawal of the catheter in relationship to LMWH injections is wishful thinking as catheters may pull out spontaneously. Reducing dosage may help, but one is still dealing with patient outliers and interpatient responses to heparin vary markedly.

I believe that a prudent approach is to use epidural anesthesia and postoperative epidural analgesia without LMWH and reserve the use of LMWH to patients who receive general anesthesia or spinal or epidural for surgery alone.

Interrelationship of Epidural and Other Modalities of DVT Prophylaxis

Epidural anesthesia is associated with an overall DVT rate of 40% to 50%. However, a subset analysis of patients undergoing TKA at the author's hospital from 1986 to 1990 demonstrated some interesting facts. First, one surgeon had a DVT rate of 58%, whereas two other surgeons had a combined rate of 35% ($p < .0001$).[20] Furthermore, the rates for both surgeons decreased during this period.[20] This suggested that other modifiable factors might influence DVT rate with epidural anesthesia. Of note in this study was that 24 hours of epidural analgesia did not reduce DVT rate.

Subsequently, two studies have demonstrated that pneumatic compression devices can lower DVT rate in conjunction with epidural anesthesia. Haas et al[6] and Westrich and Sculco,[24] using thigh-high or foot pumps, respectively, have shown that DVT rates of 25% to 30% can be achieved by using epidural anesthesia, aspirin 650 mg daily, and pneumatic compression. These devices are usually only used for 2 or 3 days, because once patients begin to ambulate, compliance is poor.

Nevertheless, this multimodal approach using epidural anesthesia, postoperative epidural analgesia, aspirin, pneumatic compression, and early rehabilitation provides rates of DVT comparable to those with LMWH. The one advantage of this approach is the better analgesia and reduced risk of wound bleeding.

CONCLUSION

Epidural anesthesia reduces the rate of DVT following TKA. By itself, it is insufficient prophylaxis. By combining the benefit of epidural anesthesia and analgesia, pneumatic compression devices, aspirin, and early ambulation, effective thromboprophylaxis can be achieved with minimal risk of bleeding. LMWH should not be used in conjunction with epidural analgesia. Further studies are needed to identify factors contributing to thrombogenesis during and following TKA to provide a rational basis for further prophylaxis.

References

1. Dalldorf PG, Perkins FM, Totterman S, et al: Deep venous thrombosis following total hip arthroplasty: Effects of prolonged postoperative epidural anesthesia. J Arthroplasty 9:61, 1994.
2. Davis FM, Laurenson VG, Gillespie WJ, et al: Deep vein thrombosis after total hip replacement. J Bone Joint Surg Br 71:181, 1989.
3. Davis FM, Laurenson VG, Gillespie WJ, et al: Leg blood flow during total hip replacement under spinal or general 4. Durica S, Raskob G, Johnson C, et al: Incidence of deep-vein thrombosis after arthroscopic knee surgery [abstract]. Thromb Haemost 183, 1997.
4. Durica S, Raskob G, Johnson C, et al: Incidence of deep-vein thrombosis after arthroscopic knee surgery [abstract]. Thromb Haemost 183, 1997.
5. FDA Public Health Advisory: Reports of epidural or spinal hematomas with the concurrent use of low molecular weight heparin and spinal/epidural anesthesia or spinal puncture. U.S. Department of Health and Human Resources, 1997.
6. Haas SB, Insall JN, Scuderi GR, et al: Pneumatic sequential-compression boots compared with aspirin prophylaxis of deep-vein thrombosis after total knee arthroplasty. J Bone Joint Surg Am 72:27, 1990.
7. Horlocker TT, Wedel DJ: Neuraxial block and low-molecular-weight heparin: Balancing perioperative analgesia and thromboprophylaxis. Regional Anesth Pain Manage 23:164, 1998.
8. Jørgensen LN, Lind B, Hauch O, et al: Thrombin-antithrombin III-complex and fibrin degradation products in plasma: Surgery and postoperative deep venous thrombosis. Thromb Res 59:69, 1990.
9. Markel DC, Urquhart B, Derkowska I, et al: Effect of epidural analgesia on venous blood flow after hip arthroplasty. Clin Orthop 334:168, 1997.
10. Maynard MJ, Sculco TP, Ghelman B: Progression and regression of deep vein thrombosis after total knee arthroplasty. Clin Orthop 273:125, 1991.
11. Mitchell D, Friedman RJ, Baker JD III, et al: Prevention of thromboembolic disease following total knee arthroplasty. Clin Orthop 269:109, 1991.
12. Modig J: Spinal or epidural anaesthesia with low molecular weight heparin for thromboprophylaxis requires careful postoperative neurological observation. Acta Anaesthesiol Scand 36: 603, 1992.
13. Modig J, Borg T, Karlström G, et al: Thromboembolism after total hip replacement: Role of epidural and general anesthesia. Anesth Analg 62:174, 1983.
14. Modig J, Maripuu E, Sahlstedt B: Thromboembolism following total hip replacement: A prospective investigation of 94 patients with emphasis on the efficacy of lumbar epidural anesthesia in prophylaxis. Reg Anesth 11:72, 1986.
15. Parmet JL, Berman AT, Horrow JC, et al: Thromboembolism coincident with tourniquet deflation during total knee arthroplasty. Lancet 341:1057, 1993.
16. Sharrock NE, Cazan MG, Hargett MJL, et al: Changes in mortality after total hip and knee arthroplasty over a ten-year period. Anesth Analg 80:242, 1995.
17. Sharrock NE, Go G, Sculco TP, et al: Changes in circulatory indices of thrombosis and fibrinolysis during total knee arthroplasty performed under tourniquet. J Arthroplasty 10:523, 1995.
18. Sharrock NE, Go G, Williams-Russo P, et al: Comparison of extradural and general anaesthesia on the fibrinolytic response to total knee arthroplasty. Br J Anaesth 79:29, 1997.
19. Sharrock NE, Haas SB, Hargett MJ, et al: Effects of epidural anesthesia on the incidence of deep-vein thrombosis after total knee arthroplasty. J Bone Joint Surg Am 73:502, 1991.
20. Sharrock NE, Hargett MJ, Urquhart B, et al: Factors affecting deep vein thrombosis rate following total knee arthroplasty under epidural anesthesia. J Arthroplasty 8:133, 1993.
21. Singelyn FJ, Deyaert M, Joris D, et al: Effects of intravenous patient-controlled analgesia with morphine, continuous epidural analgesia, and continuous three-in-one block on postoperative pain and knee rehabilitation after unilateral total knee arthroplasty. Anesth Analg 87:88, 1998.
22. Stringer MD, Steadman CA, Hedges AR, et al: Deep vein thrombosis after elective knee surgery: An incidence study in 312 patients. J Bone Joint Surg Br 71:492, 1989.
23. Westrich G: Thromboembolic disease prophylaxis in total knee arthroplasty using intraoperative heparin and postoperative pneumatic plantar compression. J Arthroplasty, in press.
24. Westrich GH, Sculco TP: Prophylaxis against deep venous thrombosis after total knee arthroplasty: Pneumatic plantar compression and aspirin compared with aspirin alone. J Bone Joint Surg Am 78:826, 1996.
25. Westrich GH, Specht LM, Sharrock NE, et al: Venous haemodynamics after total knee arthroplasty: Evaluation of active dorsal to plantar flexion and several mechanical compression devices. J Bone Joint Surg Br 80:1057, 1998.
26. Williams-Russo P, Sharrock NE, Haas SB, et al: Randomized trial of epidural versus general anesthesia: Outcomes after primary total knee replacement. Clin Orthop 331:199, 1996.

57 Pain Management in Knee Surgery

DERMOT R. FITZGIBBON • LAURA LEWIS MANTELL • PAUL S. TUMBER

INTRODUCTION

Pain occurring from surgery to the knee is variable in intensity. Surgical procedures may produce minimal trauma with relatively little noxious stimulation, or procedures such as extensive open reconstruction may result in prolonged periods of intense pain and slow rehabilitation. The challenge for the clinician involved in the care of these patients is to provide adequate pain management for variable nociceptive-producing surgeries in both inpatient and outpatient populations. This chapter provides guidelines in these areas. It includes discussion of the problems associated with undertreatment of surgical pain, discussion of general principles of management, and separate discussions of pain management for the commonly performed surgical procedures of knee arthroscopy-meniscectomy, anterior cruciate ligament (ACL) reconstruction, and total knee arthroplasty (TKA). General guidelines on the use of oral analgesics are also discussed.

OVERVIEW

Treatment Imperative

Advantages to aggressive pain management include accelerated rehabilitation, earlier hospital discharge, and improved patient satisfaction.[36, 64, 120] However, for years it has been recognized that the management of postoperative pain has been inadequate and problematic despite advances in pain management.[65, 74, 82] Reasons for the undertreatment of postoperative pain include inadequate assessment of the intensity of pain, lack of information or knowledge regarding currently available options for treating surgical pain, inadequate information on effective dose ranges and duration of action of opioids, and unfounded fears of causing respiratory depression and addiction. Acute pain management guidelines have been published by a variety of professional bodies, such as the American Society of Anesthesiologists,[6] the U.S. Department of Health and Human Services, the Agency for Health Care Policy and Research,[1] the American Pain Society,[5] the International Association for the Study of Pain,[95] and the Royal College of Surgeons of England and the College of Anaesthetists,[24] in an effort to address these issues. Results of studies examining the incidence of addiction arising from treatment of postsurgical pain with opioids do not support a rational basis for this fear. Accordingly, for both physiological and humanitarian reasons, prescribers' fear of patient addiction must not be allowed to deter adequate opioid dosing.[81, 90, 92]

Untreated or poorly treated postoperative pain results in adverse physiological and psychological effects. All surgical procedures are followed by pain, which may amplify endocrine metabolic responses, autonomic reflexes, nausea, and muscle spasm, and thereby delay restoration of function. Not surprisingly, postoperative pain can be a major source of fear and anxiety in patients.[89] Insomnia may accompany inadequately controlled pain with further detriment to recovery. Effective management of postoperative pain can attenuate these responses.[19, 58-61, 89]

Given these facts, the mandate to manage postoperative pain aggressively is incontrovertible. The first step toward meeting that responsibility, for both the surgical team and its supporting institution, is to affirm the obligation to deliver the best pain relief that can safely be provided. A dedicated acute pain service assists the surgeon and the patient by expanding the range of analgesic options and by providing highly individualized daily postoperative care. Once integrated into standard care, acute pain management dramatically improves the postoperative experience for both surgeon and patient.

Patient Assessment

The most common cause of unrelieved pain in a hospital setting is failure of the medical staff to routinely assess pain and pain relief.[28, 77] Often, patients will not report pain unless asked about it. Those who have difficulty communicating, such as very young children and cognitively impaired patients, are at greatest risk for unrelieved pain.

Patient self-report should always be the primary source of information for the measurement of symptoms. Observer ratings of symptom severity correlate poorly with patient ratings. Discrepancies are most pronounced in patients reporting severe pain.[40] Although some objective signs can be monitored, the information gathered must only complement patient self-reporting. An assessment of pain intensity should include an evaluation of not only present pain intensity but also pain at its least and worst. The most commonly used tools for pain assessment are the Visual Analogue Scale, the Numeric Rating Scale, and the Verbal Descriptor Scale. In clinical settings, they approach equivalency.[49] It should be noted that when pain severity is rated at the midpoint or higher on numeric rating scales, patients report interference with daily function disproportionately greater than when pain severity is rated below the midpoint.[23, 122, 123]

Patient-Specific Care

Following thorough assessment, the key to optimizing pain relief is individualizing care. Studies have demonstrated that the range of blood concentrations varies fourfold to fivefold between patients having received the same dose of an opioid analgesic.[8] Moreover, the range in dose requirements varies 8- to 10-fold for patients having undergone the same surgical procedure. The most important determinant of dose requirement is age, not weight.[71] Doses should be increased until the desired effect is reached or until side effects intervene. Safe dosing requires knowledge about patient history with pain and analgesics, about systemic disease and the medications used to treat it, and about renal function. Intersubject variability is the rule, so rigid protocols enlisting one drug cannot hope to address all patients' needs. Changing opioids in the face of disturbing side effects is appropriate because patients respond differently to different opioids.[75]

Treatment Modalities

The nature of the surgical procedure and whether or not the patient is discharged after surgery influence the treatment of postoperative pain. It is well known that surgical procedures vary in the degree of pain produced. Treatment options are listed in Table 57.1. Treatment strategies for patients discharged the day of surgery must include use of techniques or medications that will facilitate early discharge and that will not significantly impair function after discharge. The most effective methods of controlling pain after knee surgery for patients who remain in the hospital include epidural and nerve-blocking techniques, intravenous patient-controlled analgesia (PCA), and oral analgesics. Although commonly used, intramuscular injections should be avoided (see "Injections").

Epidural Analgesia

Epidural opioids have been used since the 1980s for the relief of pain.[26, 125] Epidural opioid delivery offers analgesia superior to that delivered by parenteral or oral routes.[33, 34, 109] The administration of epidural opioids seems to attenuate the neurohumoral stress response and may thereby enhance the immune status of postoperative patients,[11] a distinct advantage because pain may diminish the immune response of surgical patients by contributing to the surgical stress response.[101]

Nerve Blocks

Femoral nerve blocks result in superior pain relief compared with conventional intramuscular injections.[32] Singelyn et al showed that these blocks produce pain relief equal to that of epidural analgesia with even fewer side effects.[109]

Patient-Controlled Analgesia

PCA increased in popularity in the 1980s and, where available, has largely supplanted the use of injections for the treatment of postoperative pain. Advantages include individualization of therapy[29] and better pain relief compared with conventional therapy (injections) with less sedation.[12, 62] Additionally, patients report a preference for and satisfaction with PCA over injections.[14, 113]

Injections

Injections are painful, produce wide fluctuations in drug absorption, and take 30 to 60 minutes to reach peak effect. Consequently, patients receiving intramuscular injections frequently experience inadequate pain control with a significant incidence of side effects.

Oral Analgesics

Excellent pain relief can be achieved with oral analgesics, assuming adequate gastrointestinal absorption. Al-

TABLE 57.1 TREATMENT OPTIONS FOR THE MANAGEMENT OF INPATIENT AND OUTPATIENT PAIN AFTER KNEE SURGERY

Inpatient	Outpatient
Oral Analgesia	Oral Analgesia
Opioid ± nonopioid	Opioid ± nonopioid
Parenteral Analgesia	Intra-Articular Injection (also for some inpatients)
IM opioids—administered PRN	Local anesthetic ± opioids
IV opioids—PRN; PCA ± CI	Ketorolac
IM/IV ketorolac (Toradol)	Glucocorticoids
Neuraxial Analgesia	Parenteral Analgesia
Epidural catheter (opioid ± local anesthesia)	IM/IV ketorolac (before discharge)
Intrathecal (single dose; opioid)	IV opioids (minimal)
Peripheral Nerve Blocks	Peripheral Nerve Blocks
Single injection (femoral, sciatic, psoas)	Single injection (femoral nerve)
Continuous infusion (femoral nerve)	

CI = continuous infusion; IM = intramuscular; IV = intravenous; PCA = patient-controlled analgesia; PRN = as needed.

though oral analgesics were once believed to be useful only for mild pain, excellent analgesia can be achieved with oral opioid analgesics provided adequate doses at appropriate intervals are prescribed. Their utility is limited in the postoperative patient experiencing severe *incident* pain—pain related to movement—because of the time lag to pain relief. (See "Oral Medications" for the management of postoperative pain.)

Side Effects of Opioids

Opioid-related side effects include nausea, sedation, constipation, pruritus, urinary retention, dysphoria, and respiratory depression. It is important to recognize that respiratory rate depression from opioids is a late event and is usually preceded by ventilatory depression and sedation. It is, therefore, exceedingly important that levels of sedation be monitored frequently. Because opioids frequently cause side effects such as itching, nausea, and vomiting, it is important to anticipate and appropriately treat these side effects to ensure delivery of effective pain management. Opioid administration may contribute to orthostatic hypotension as the result of arterial and venous vasodilatation. Significant decreases in blood pressure do not generally occur unless the patient has coexistent hypovolemia. True allergies to opioids are rare, and anaphylaxis following the administration of any opioid by any route is extremely rare.[20] Although seemingly daunting, severe respiratory depression or respiratory arrest from opioids is rare but nevertheless requires appropriate dosing and careful patient monitoring to avoid this potentially lethal complication.[96]

Special Considerations

Elderly Patients

The effects of opioids on elderly patients may be unpredictable. Altered pharmacokinetics compared with younger patients may in part explain this. Elderly patients have reduced glomerular filtration rates, which may allow active opioid metabolites such as normeperidine and morphine-6-glucuronide to accumulate and cause cognitive impairment. The elderly patient may also experience a higher peak effect and a longer duration of effect, in part because of prolonged elimination from plasma.[53, 54]

Meperidine

Because meperidine (Demerol) is so widely prescribed, a warning about its potential danger is warranted. Meperidine is metabolized to normeperidine, a toxic metabolite, and has a long elimination half-life of 15 to 20 hours. Normeperidine is excreted by the kidneys and can easily accumulate in patients with renal insufficiency and even in patients with normally functioning kidneys. Symptoms of normeperidine toxicity include dysphoria, irritability, hyperreflexia, and generalized seizures. These can occur while patients are receiving standard clinical doses. Meperidine should not be prescribed for more than 48 hours, and no more than 600 to 1000 mg should be given over the first 24 hours.

POSTOPERATIVE PAIN MANAGEMENT FOR KNEE ARTHROSCOPY AND MENISCECTOMY

Outpatient care is preferable for the majority of patients undergoing arthroscopic examination or surgery of the knee. In addition to the clear economic benefits of outpatient surgery, many patients prefer it. Weale et al[126] reported on the acceptability and safety of arthroscopic knee surgery in outpatients and in patients admitted overnight. Although pain after hospital discharge was similar in both groups, outpatient management was preferred by 90% of outpatients and by 64% of those admitted overnight. Pain after arthroscopic surgery is a significant factor in delaying patient discharge.[18] A variety of agents and techniques are advocated for successful pain management after arthroscopic knee surgery (Table 57.2). Each of these modalities (alone or in combination) will be discussed.

Diverse medications have been given by intra-articular injection, either alone or in combination, at the conclusion of arthroscopic knee surgery. Beneficial effects have been reported with all these agents, but in analyzing these claims it is important to remember some basic principles for evaluating the efficacy of analgesic agents. Claims of beneficial effects occurring with a particular agent or technique need to be interpreted cautiously because studies that are not randomized or properly blinded may result in overestimation of treatment effect.[104] Classic analgesic trial design includes both active and placebo control. This is to ensure that if no difference is found between test analgesic and placebo, the correct interpretation of a negative result can be made if the standard (active control) analgesic gives a significant difference from that of placebo. In addition, variability in the extent of the arthroscopic procedure is one of the confounding factors that may influence postoperative pain, and this may be more difficult to control than in studies of other surgeries. Many other factors are often not reported in any significant detail, such as specific pathology and its extent, type and extent of surgery, inten-

TABLE 57.2 MODALITIES USED FOR MANAGEMENT OF PAIN FOLLOWING ARTHROSCOPIC KNEE SURGERY

Physical	Medication
Cryotherapy	*Systemic:*
	Opioids (PO/IM/IV)
	NSAIDs (PO/IM/IV)
	Intra-articular:
	Local anesthetics
	Opioids
	Ketorolac
	Glucocorticoids

IM = intramuscular; IV = intravenous; NSAIDs = nonsteroidal anti-inflammatory drugs; PO = orally.

sity and duration of pain experienced before surgery, and outcome of surgery (e.g., whether or not the pathology was corrected).

Intra-articular local anesthetics are often used in the management and prevention of pain after arthroscopic knee surgery. Although most studies demonstrate benefit from intra-articular local anesthetic administration,[2, 22, 39, 42, 93, 111] the effect appears to be short lived (less than 6 hours)[48, 63, 98] and does not influence convalescence significantly.[39] Indeed, the main benefit from intra-articular local anesthetics is improved pain control in the early postoperative period, thus facilitating early discharge from the hospital.

Intra-articular injections of opioids (and ketorolac, discussed later) have possible advantages over systemic injections, including enhanced efficacy and reduced systemic side effects. Local opioid receptors have been isolated in inflamed synovial tissue, and intra-articular opioids have been shown to produce potent antinociceptive effects by interacting with them.[117] The presence of inflammation in peripheral tissues has been postulated as a prerequisite for the satisfactory analgesic effects of locally administered opioids.[115-117] Research has been undertaken regarding the efficacy of low-dose intra-articular morphine (0.5 to 5 mg) in mediating peripheral analgesia. The minimum dose tested (0.5 mg) did not show any analgesic effect.[114] In supportive studies, intra-articular morphine at doses of 1 to 5 mg produced significant pain relief with a variable onset time of 0 to 3 hours after administration and a variable duration of 24 to 48 hours.[55] Two studies compared the effect of different doses of morphine.[43, 66] No dose response was detected either between 1 and 3 mg or between 2 and 5 mg morphine. Although studies have revealed effective pain relief for up to 48 hours from the administration of single doses of intra-articular morphine,[2, 27, 114] this effect and duration are controversial because other studies have not demonstrated any significant clinical effect.[42, 93] Furthermore, the effects of intra-articular morphine on overall convalescence remain to be evaluated.

The combination of intra-articular morphine and bupivacaine may enhance pain relief within the first 24 hours,[55] but some authors dispute this.[52] Heine et al[43] assessed the long-term effect of intra-articular morphine and bupivacaine by measuring pain at rest, pain on standing, and ability to walk for 7 days after intra-articular injection of bupivacaine and bupivacaine-morphine at the end of arthroscopic knee surgery. Patients who received the bupivacaine-morphine combination had significantly lower pain scores at rest (12 hours and on day 1), on standing (12 hours and on day 1), and on walking (12 hours) and a significantly lower oral analgesic requirement for 3 days after surgery. Indeed, most later studies published on successful pain management following arthroscopic surgery for the first 24 hours appear to favor the combination of intra-articular morphine and bupivacaine.

Nonsteroidal anti-inflammatory drugs (NSAIDs), administered by various routes, have also proven useful in relieving pain after arthroscopy,[88, 110] probably from their ability to mediate pain and inflammation at the surgical site. Systemic ketorolac (intravenous [IV] or intramuscular [IM]) is commonly used to manage post-arthroscopic knee pain. Early postoperative pain scores were similar when either systemic ketorolac or intra-articular bupivacaine was administered after arthroscopic knee surgery.[110] Reuben et al[98] have shown that intra-articular ketorolac with bupivacaine results in a significant improvement in pain relief (as measured by decreased patient discomfort, increased time to first analgesic request, and decreased need for postoperative analgesics for the first 24 hours after surgery) compared with either agent individually. Intra-articular ketorolac and intra-articular morphine provided equally effective pain relief, but their combination failed to demonstrate any further benefit.[99] However, there are concerns about the effects of NSAIDs on cartilage, even when given parenterally.[16] Different NSAIDs have different effects on cartilage metabolism, with some having marked catabolic effects.[38] Cook et al[25] caution against the widespread and routine use of intra-articular NSAIDs until their safety and efficacy can be established.

The effectiveness of intra-articular glucocorticoids after arthrosopic knee surgery has been studied by several authors.[94, 124] Wang et al[124] demonstrated that intra-articular triamcinolone reduced pain intensity for 24 hours after arthroscopic knee surgery. Rasmussen et al[94] contrasted the effects of intra-articular bupivacaine-morphine-methylprednisolone (BMP) versus bupivacaine-morphine (BM) or saline on postmeniscectomy pain, mobilization, and convalescence in a double-blind randomized study of 60 patients undergoing arthroscopic meniscectomy. Patients received 40 mL saline, 30 mL bupivacaine (5 mg/mL) + 10 mL morphine (0.4 mg/mL), or 30 mL bupivacaine (5 mg/mL) + 10 mL morphine (0.4 mg/mL) + 1 mL methylprednisolone (40 mg/mL). BM significantly reduced pain, time of immobilization, and duration of convalescence. The addition of methylprednisolone further reduced pain, use of additional analgesics, joint swelling, and convalescence; improved muscle function; and prevented the inflammatory response to surgery. Pain scores during leg lift, flexion to 90 degrees, and walking stairs were significantly less in the BMP group compared with the other two groups and between the BM group and the saline group (Fig. 57.1). The number of days using crutches until being pain free and returning to work were reduced in the BMP group compared with the other two groups ($p \leq 0.05$), but recovery was also enhanced in the BM group compared with the saline group (Fig. 57.2). At day 10, there was a significant difference in joint effusion between the saline and BMP groups. The beneficial effect of glucocorticoids may be through an anti-inflammatory effect on inflamed tissue,[41] but, in addition, there may be a direct inhibitory effect on transmission in nociceptive C fibers.[50] However, further large-scale studies are required to assess the safety of using glucocorticoids for this type of surgery.

Oral opioids or NSAIDs, or both, are routinely used for pain control after arthroscopic surgery. The use of combination opioid-nonopioid analgesics on a short-

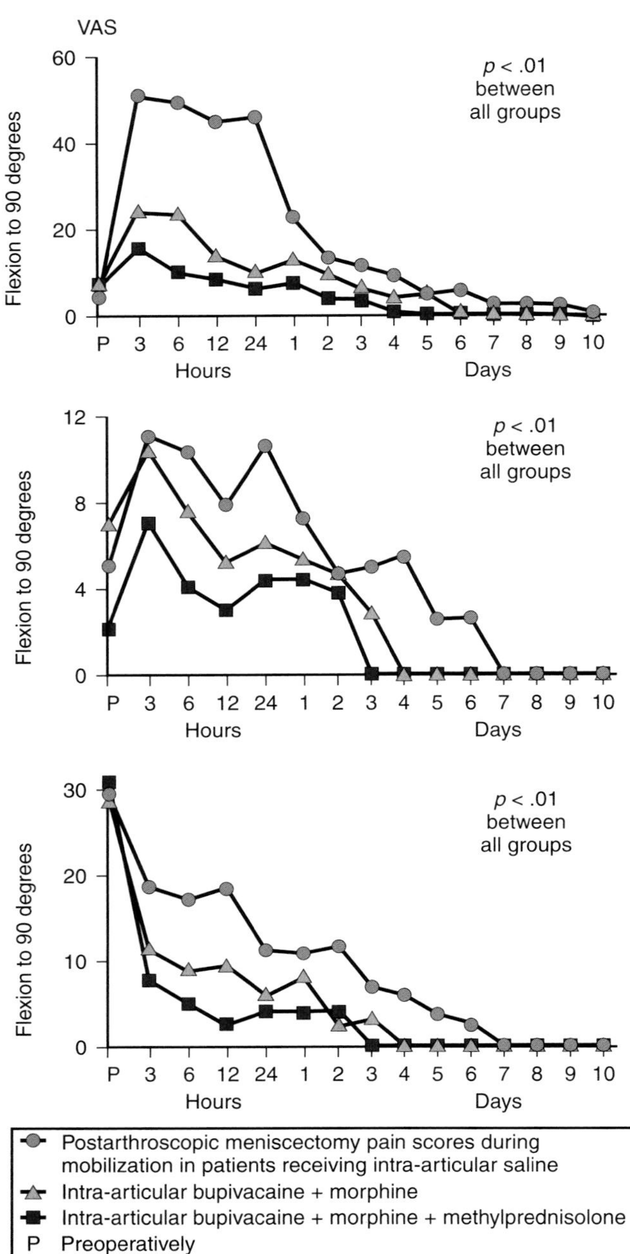

FIGURE 57.1 ➢ Postarthroscopic meniscectomy pain scores during mobilization in patients receiving intra-articular saline (●..●), intra-articular bupivacaine + morphine (●--●), or intra-articular bupivacaine + morphine + methylprednisolone (●-●) (median values). P = preoperatively. (Redrawn from Rasmussen S, Larsen AS, Thomsen ST, et al: Intra-articular glucocorticoid, bupivacaine and morphine reduces pain, inflammatory response and convalescence after arthroscopic meniscectomy. Pain 78[2]:132, 1998.)

term, as-needed basis is probably sufficient for the majority of patients undergoing diagnostic arthroscopy. However, patients experiencing constant pain after surgical arthroscopy would benefit from scheduled, time-contingent opioids, as discussed later. The use of scheduled NSAIDs is also likely to be of benefit in these patients. Pedersen et al[88] demonstrated the beneficial effects of scheduled 10-day use of naproxen in patients following arthroscopic knee surgery. Patients taking naproxen were able to return to work significantly sooner than were those who did not receive naproxen (median of 10 days versus 30 days, respectively).

The direct application of cold (cryotherapy) to trau-

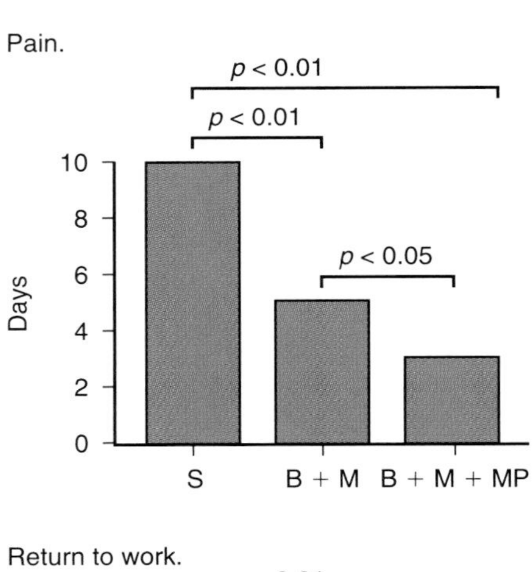

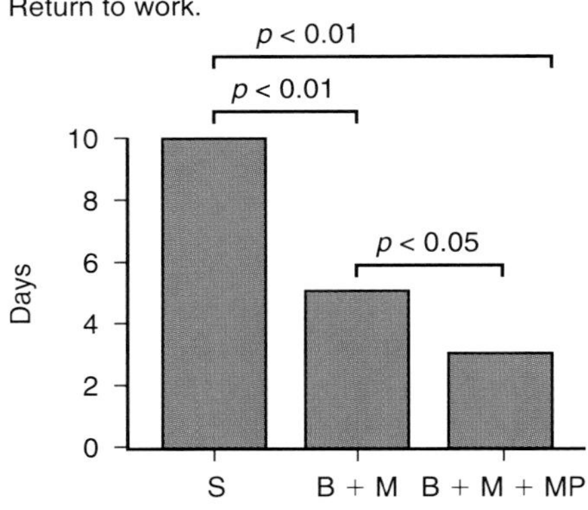

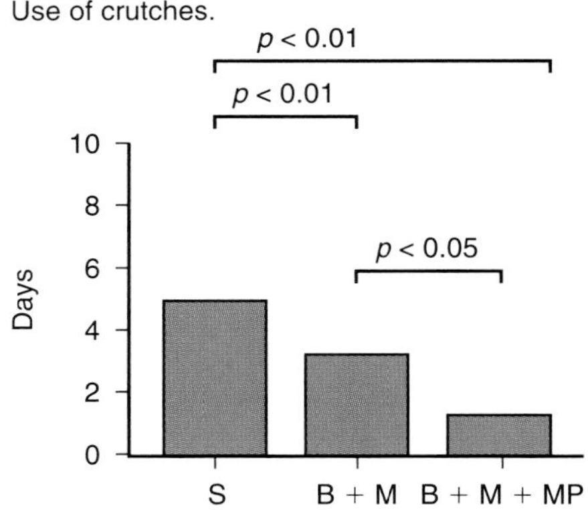

FIGURE 57.2 ➢ Time to being pain free, returning to work, and using crutches following arthroscopic meniscectomy with intra-articular saline (S), bupivacaine + morphine (B + M) or bupivacaine + morphine + methylprednisolone (B + M + MP) (median values). (Redrawn from Rasmussen S, Larsen AS, Thomsen ST, et al: Intra-articular glucocorticoid, bupivacaine and morphine reduces pain, inflammatory response and convalescence after arthroscopic meniscectomy. Pain 78[2]:133, 1998.)

matized tissue has long been known to provide beneficial effects. Although the exact mechanism for its action is not completely understood, cryotherapy is used to decrease edema, limit inflammation, decrease hematoma formation, and decrease pain.[79] A number of methods have been used to provide cold pressure dressings, including ice and elastic bandages. Commercial devices that provide continuous application of a combined cooling and compression system, such as the Cryo/Cuff (Cryo/Cuff, Aircast Inc., Summit, NJ), have also been developed to provide similar beneficial effects. Whitelaw et al[128] demonstrated that the Cryo/Cuff is a useful adjunct in the rehabilitation of knee arthroscopy patients.

Although patients recover more rapidly from arthroscopic meniscectomy than from open meniscectomy, arthroscopic surgery is often followed by weeks of pain and disability. Patients typically return to work within 1 to 2 weeks, even when pain and swelling are brought under control, and full recovery may require 6 weeks.[30, 118] Effective pain management, which facilitates rehabilitation,[88] needs to continue throughout recovery until pain subsides.

POSTOPERATIVE PAIN MANAGEMENT FOR ARTHROSCOPIC ACL REPAIR

Arthroscopic ACL repair is more painful than arthroscopic non-ACL knee surgery. Although pain intensity may be equally high in both groups on postoperative days 1 and 2, ACL patients typically use significantly more opioids and have higher pain scores in the first week after surgery than do non-ACL patients.[129] Brown et al[17] examined the intensity and duration of pain after arthroscopically assisted ACL reconstruction during the first 5 postoperative days. During surgery, ketorolac was given intravenously and bupivacaine was injected into the joint space and the graft donor site. After surgery, all patients received scheduled doses of oral acetaminophen and ketorolac and oxycodone as required. Pain intensity at rest and with activity was highest on the second postoperative day. Oxycodone consumption also peaked on the second postoperative day. Eighty-nine percent of patients reported overall pain intensity as mild or moderate. Five-day cumulative mean pain scores for patients unable to perform straight leg raises were higher than for those able to successfully perform them, suggesting that pain may inhibit function and, therefore, early rehabilitation.

Poor control of postoperative pain is a common reason for delay in discharge after ACL reconstruction. Outpatient ACL reconstructive surgery is possible in the cooperative, motivated patient and is associated with significant cost savings and no apparent increase in the complication rate.[7, 56, 100] After ambulatory ACL surgery, a multimodal approach for pain control is useful and includes the use of perioperative NSAIDs and intra-articular bupivacaine, postoperative cryotherapy with an external cooling system, and effective oral analgesia. Aronwitz and Kleinbart[7] demonstrated the multimodal approach, with intra-articular bupivacaine-morphine, parenteral ketorolac (both intraoperative and before discharge), an external cooling system, and oral analgesics after discharge providing good pain relief with minimal morbidity.

McGuire et al demonstrated that ketorolac provided pain control as good as, or in some cases, better than parenteral opioid therapy.[78] Hoher et al[45] demonstrated short-term (first postoperative day only) benefit from intra-articular bupivacaine. Joshi et al[51] demonstrated that intra-articular morphine significantly reduced pain scores and systemic analgesic use during the first 24 hours after ACL repair. However, Reuben et al,[100] using a multimodal analgesic approach, failed to demonstrate any benefit from intra-articular morphine in this setting. Femoral nerve block (single injection or continuous infusion) is a safe and effective form of pain control after inpatient ACL repair.[31, 86, 119] Single-injection femoral nerve block may provide effective pain relief for up to 29 hours after injection.[31] However, the safety and efficacy of this block have not been reported extensively for outpatient ACL repair. A number of studies demonstrate beneficial pain-relieving effects lasting 24 to 48 hours with intra-articular morphine-bupivacaine,[15, 57] with further beneficial effects if combined with an external cooling system.[15] Continuous-flow cold therapy is safe and effective for outpatient ACL reconstruction and reduces pain medication requirements.[10]

Outpatient ACL reconstruction is not an option for every patient, especially those with demonstrated preoperative opioid tolerance, those who have had difficulty with pain control after previous surgical procedures, and those who have difficulty following pain control instructions. Most inpatients are hospitalized for relatively short periods of 24 to 48 hours. Although previously popular for inpatient pain management after ACL repair, epidural opioids and local anesthetics are probably unnecessary and may delay early hospital discharge.[67, 68, 112] A multimodal approach to pain control appears optimal and facilitates early discharge. Popp et al[91] demonstrated that parenteral ketorolac and oral oxycodone provided comparable pain relief with fewer undesirable side effects than PCA morphine.

POSTOPERATIVE PAIN MANAGEMENT FOR TKA

Postoperative pain after TKA is a major concern. Sixty percent of TKA patients experience severe pain, and 30% experience moderate pain.[13] After open knee surgery, pain can be associated with severe reflex spasms of the quadriceps muscle, causing further pain and impaired muscle function. Severe and uncontrolled pain hinders early intense physical therapy, the most influential factor for good postoperative knee rehabilitation.[102, 107] To further complicate pain management options, patients undergoing TKA are often elderly, and thus the ramifications of inadequate pain relief may include increased risk of deep venous thrombosis, coronary ischemic events, blood loss from the opera-

TABLE 57.3 NONOPIOID ANALGESICS FOR THE TREATMENT OF ACUTE PAIN*

Agent	Oral Dose (mg)	Interval (hr)	Maximum Daily Dose (mg)	Comments
		Salicylates		
Aspirin	500–1000	4–6	6000	Prolonged platelet effect. Discontinue 5–7 days before surgery.
Choline magnesium trisalicylate	1000–1500	12	4000	No antiplatelet effect
Acetaminophen	500–1000	4–6	4000	Hepatotoxic with sustained high dose (>4 g/day)
		NSAIDS		
Diclofenac (Voltaren)	50–100	6–12	200	All NSAIDs
Etodolac (Lodine)	200	6–8	1200	Reversible decrease in platelet aggregation (24 hr)
Ibuprofen (motrin)	400	4–6	3200	
Indomethacin (Indocin)	25	8–12	150	Can produce GI effects
Ketoprofen (Orudis)	50	6–8	300	Can cause renal insufficiency
Mefenamic acid (Ponstel)	500 initial; 250 subsequent	6	1000	
Naproxen (Naprosyn)	500	12	1250	
Piroxicam (Feldene)	10	12	40	
Sulindac (Clinoril)	150	12	400	
Tolmetin (Tolectin)	400	8	2000	

* Trade names for individual drugs are listed in parentheses.
GI = gastrointestinal; NSAIDs = nonsteroidal anti-inflammatory drugs.

tive knee, and a significant increase in the duration of hospitalization required for adequate rehabilitation.

Few studies have assessed the influence of the postoperative analgesic technique on knee rehabilitation after TKA. Most published data report on the effectiveness of a particular technique on reducing postoperative pain intensity only. Options for pain control after TKA include parenteral opioids (IM or, more commonly, IV via PCA), parenteral ketorolac, locoregional analgesia (single injection or repeated injections with catheters), and epidural analgesia (opioids or opioids combined with local anesthetics). In choosing the best pain management technique, patient-related factors (e.g., patient preference) and the institutional commitment to pain management are factors for consideration. The optimal use of any analgesic technique requires knowledge, skill, experience, and attentiveness to individual patient responses. A well-planned and organized pain service is essential to ensure optimal comfort and safety using sophisticated treatment options.

Since its inception into clinical practice, PCA with intravenous opioids has become a widely used technique for pain control after most major surgeries. Compared with IM administration, IV opioids administered by PCA provide superior pain relief and patient comfort for patients undergoing TKA.[113] The use of a patient-controlled feature often enhances patient satisfaction because of the sense of control conferred.[21, 108] Pain after TKA may be inadequately treated with PCA in some patients. After TKA, visual analog pain scale scores range from 40 to 80 (out of 100) during the immediate postoperative period and slowly decline by the first postoperative day with opioids.[35, 44, 106] In spite of advances in technology and the introduction of more complex and safer programmable delivery techniques, the potential of PCA is still limited by variability in analgesic requirements and occurrence of undesirable side effects.[70] The addition of ketorolac, if not contraindicated, improves pain relief after TKA, but pain control during the immediate postoperative period remains difficult.[35, 37]

Peripheral nerve blocks are useful analgesic adjuncts for the immediate postoperative period after TKA even when added to IV PCA opioids plus NSAIDs, probably by prevention of quadriceps muscle spasm. Combined sciatic and femoral nerve blocks with bupivacaine can significantly reduce systemic analgesic requirements for the first 24 hours after TKA.[4] Allen et al[3] showed that a single-injection femoral nerve block with bupivacaine provided significant pain reduction until the second postoperative day after TKA. Postoperative single-shot femoral nerve blocks can decrease pain from the surgical incision and block reflexive quadriceps muscle spasm. Furthermore, a number of studies have advocated the use of continuous femoral nerve blockade with bupivacaine, citing equivalent pain relief to epidural analgesia but a lower incidence of side effects.[32, 103, 106, 109] However, additional block of the sciatic nerve may be necessary to ensure pain relief during the active rehabilitation phase.[73]

Epidural analgesia has become one of the most important techniques for providing effective pain relief after TKA. Preoperative placement of an epidural catheter allows for continuous pain control both intraoperatively and postoperatively for extended periods. The benefits of epidural analgesia (decreased pain, improved range of motion, improved ambulation, and reduced fatigue) may have the most impact on patient outcome when combined with protocols emphasizing early mobilization and early rehabilitation.[72, 83] Compared with parenteral opioid treatment, epidural analgesia is associated with more rapid achievement of all postoperative rehabilitative goals and, in some studies, shorter hospital stay.[72, 87, 130] Opioids (usually morphine or fentanyl) or local anesthetic agents (bupivacaine or ropivacaine), or both, are commonly administered by the epidural route. Epidural morphine provides superior analgesia compared with the IV route.[69, 80, 127] However, although epidural morphine provides excellent overall pain relief after TKA, relief may be inconsistent, particularly when movement is required, and a high incidence of side effects such as nausea, vomiting, urinary retention, and pruritus may be experienced.[9] Combining local anesthetics with opioids will enhance analgesic efficacy in this situation.[72, 84, 121] In addition, epidural local anesthetics will reduce the incidence of painful quadriceps muscle spasms.[109] However, local anesthetics may produce undesirable side effects including hypotension, sensory and motor block, and urinary retention. Careful selection of the lowest effective concentration of local anesthetic with monitoring of effect is required. Studies suggest some possible advantages to using ropivacaine instead of bupivacaine.[84] Ideally, epidural analgesia should be continued until the patient is ambulating without pain and tolerating oral analgesics.

The high incidence of deep vein thrombosis (DVT) after total knee replacement surgery, even in patients who receive DVT prophylaxis, is well documented.[105] The use of low-molecular-weight heparins (LMWHs) has increased in popularity as a pharmacological method of DVT prophylaxis. The U.S. Food and Drug Administration (FDA) issued a public health advisory calling attention to reports of patients who developed spinal or epidural hematomas after having spinal or epidural anesthesia administered while LMWHs were administered. The FDA advises practitioners to carefully weigh potential risks versus benefits before initiating neuraxial intervention in patients receiving or scheduled to receive anticoagulation therapy. Placement of epidural catheters should be delayed for 12 hours after the last LMWH dose. Subsequent LMWH dosing should be delayed for at least 1 hour after needle or epidural catheter placement. Removal of epidural catheters postoperatively should be delayed for at least 12 hours after a dose of LMWH. Subsequent dosing should not occur for at least 1 hour after catheter removal.[46]

ORAL MEDICATIONS FOR THE MANAGEMENT OF POSTOPERATIVE PAIN

The role of oral analgesics, both opioid and nonopioid, deserves special consideration because almost all postoperative orthopedic patients will be treated with oral medications either immediately after surgery or later in the postoperative course.

Nonopioid Analgesics

Nonopioid analgesics are useful either alone for the management of mild to moderate pain or in combination with opioids for more severe pain. Nonopioids include the salicylates, acetaminophen, and NSAIDs. Patients may experience variable degrees of pain relief from a particular drug, and familiarity with several different NSAIDs will enable the clinician to best respond to patient needs. Commonly used drugs and dosing guidelines are listed in Table 57.3. Optimal use of these drugs requires an understanding of their clinical pharmacology, including dosing guidelines and potential adverse effects.

The primary benefit of nonopioids in the perioperative period is enhancement of pain relief provided by opioids and avoidance of opioid-related problems such as sedation and constipation. NSAIDs also provide useful anti-inflammatory and antipyretic effects. Unfortunately, nonopioid analgesics are not devoid of problems. All drugs in this class demonstrate a ceiling effect to effective pain relief. Doses should be no higher than necessary for clinical effect because the incidence of major adverse effects is dose related.[76] NSAIDs may precipitate acute renal insufficiency in susceptible patients (e.g., if dehydrated, elderly, diabetic, septic, or having preexisting heart, renal, or liver disease). NSAIDs may also cause gastric ulceration and bleeding in some patients (especially if there is a history of peptic ulceration, corticosteroid use, or anticoagulants). Many NSAIDs will reversibly inhibit platelet function for a period of 24 to 48 hours (aspirin effects last 1 week), and, therefore, caution is indicated when thrombocytopenia or coagulopathies are present.

Most NSAIDs used in the United States are administered by the oral or rectal route. The FDA approved ketorolac tromethamine for parenteral use in 1990, and it is still the only one of its kind available in the United States. Several studies have demonstrated that regular postoperative administration of ketorolac can reduce the requirement for morphine by approximately 30% to 40% in patients requiring major orthopedic procedures such as TKA.[35, 37] The use of ketorolac either parenterally or orally is limited to 5 days because of an increased incidence of drug-related side effects if use of the drug is extended beyond this period. Therefore, it is most effectively used in the immediate postoperative period, and patients should be switched to a different NSAID once an oral regimen is tolerated. Dosing guidelines for ketorolac are listed in Table 57.4.

Opioids

Prescribe opioids on a scheduled basis to optimize pain control and minimize peak and trough blood levels typically seen with as-needed regimens, especially in the early postoperative period when pain is likely to be most intense. For a scheduled regimen, patients are instructed to take opioids around the clock (typically every 3 to 4 hours) with an allotment for breakthrough dosing as required. Compared with scheduled regimens, an as-needed regimen, particularly if used for patients with moderate to severe pain, may result in patients requiring more analgesics as they attempt to "catch up" to their pain, thus exposing them to a higher incidence of side effects such as dysphoria, sedation, and nausea.

It is common clinical practice to initiate opioid ther-

TABLE 57.4 DOSING GUIDELINES FOR PARENTERAL KETOROLAC: SINGLE AND MULTIPLE DOSING GUIDELINES

Patient Group	Single Dose, IM	Single Dose, IV	Repeated Dose, IM/IV	Maximum Daily Dose
Age <65 yr, no risk factors	60 mg	30 mg	30 mg every 6 hr	120 mg/d (max 5 days)
Age >65 yr, weight <50 kg, history of renal impairment	30 mg	15 mg	15 mg every 6 hr	60 mg/d (max 5 days)

IM = intramuscular; IV = intravenous.

apy with a combination product, usually one in which aspirin or acetaminophen is combined with codeine, oxycodone, hydrocodone, or propoxyphene. Opioids may also be combined with NSAIDs for postoperative pain management (Table 57.5). These agents are relatively cheap, simple to use, and usually efficacious in the management of mild to moderate postoperative pain such as after arthroscopic knee surgery. However, daily doses of these combination products are limited by the nonopioid component, and care should be exercised to avoid nonopioid-related toxicity.

Patients who fail to obtain adequate pain relief at maximal doses of opioid-nonopioid combinations should be switched to an opioid-only preparation. Moderate to severe pain requires dosing with short-acting oral opioids every 3 to 4 hours. Patients who require frequent dosing may benefit from the addition of a sustained-release opioid. The sustained-release form of oxycodone (OxyContin) is conveniently dosed at 12-hour intervals and provides steady plasma levels during this period.[97] Factors influencing the selection of opioids include physician preference and patient prior experience. Provided an adequate dose is prescribed, these drugs are equianalgesic and usually differ only in side effect profiles (Table 57.6). The occurrence of side effects with a particular drug is generally unpredictable and related to individual patient exposure and prior experience. Patients who have been appropriately titrated with a particular opioid but experience dose-limiting side effects may benefit from trials with different opioids to minimize side effects.

The agonist-antagonist opioids (pentazocine, butorphanol, and nalbuphine) and the partial agonists (buprenorphine) are not recommended for routine use for moderate to severe pain. These drugs exhibit a ceiling effect for pain relief and, if combined with other opioids, may further reduce the effectiveness of opioids and precipitate an opioid withdrawal reaction.[47] In addition, pentazocine can cause confusion and hallucinations, further limiting its use.[85]

Management of the opioid substance abuser is a difficult but increasingly common clinical problem. The use of opioids for pain control raises several treatment questions including how to treat pain in patients who have a high tolerance to opioids, how to mitigate this population's drug-seeking and potentially manipulative behavior, how to deal with patients who may have unreliable medical histories, and how to deal with patients who do not comply with treatment recommendations.

Clinicians should distinguish between the temporal characteristics of the abuse behaviors. Three scenarios may be encountered: the recovering addict who has not used drugs for years, the recovering addict in a

TABLE 57.5 RECOMMENDED STARTING DOSES AND INTERVALS FOR COMMONLY USED ORAL OPIOIDS*

Opioid	Starting Dose/Interval	Example: *Trade Name*	Example: *Components*
Codeine (cd)	30-60 mg q 3-4 hr	Tylenol #2	cd 15; apap 300
		Tylenol #3	cd 30; apap 300
		Tylenol #4	cd 60; apap 300
Oxycodone (od)	5-10 mg q 3-4 hr	Percocet	od 5; apap 325
		Percodan	od 4.5; asa 325
		Roxicodone	od 5
		Roxicet	od 5; apap 325
		Tylox	od 5; apap 500
Hydrocodone (hd)	5-10 mg q 3-4 hr	Lorcet	hd 10; apap 650
		Lortab	hd (2.5, 7.5, 10); apap 500
		Norco	hd 10; apap 325
		Vicodin	hd 5; apap 500
		Vicodin ES	hd 7.5; apap 750
		Vicoprofen	hd 7.5; ibu 200
Hydromorphone (hm)	2-4 mg q 3-4 hr	Dilaudid	hm 1, 2, 4, 8
Meperidine	50-150 mg q 3 hr (max 800 mg per day, not recommended for oral use)	Demerol	Meperidine 50, 100
Propoxyphene (px)	65 mg q 3-4 hr (max 390 mg per day)	Darvon	px 65
		Wygesic	px 65; apap 650

* Dosage strengths of each component are listed in milligrams.
apap = acetaminophen; asa = aspirin; ibu = ibuprofen.

TABLE 57.6 EQUIANALGESIC DOSES OF OPIOID ANALGESICS AND EXPECTED DURATION OF ACTION*

	Dose (mg) Equianalgesic to 10 mg IM Morphine			
Drug	*IM*	*PO*	*Half-Life (hr)*	*Duration of Action (hr)*
Codeine	130	200	2-3	2-4
Dihydrocodeine	-	200	2-3	2-4
Oxycodone	-	20	2-3	2-4
Hydrocodone	-	20	2-3	2-4
Propoxyphene	-	65	2-3	2-4
Morphine	10	60 (single dose) 30 (repeated dose)	2-3	3-4
Hydromorphone	1.5	7.5	2-3	2-4
Methadone*	10	10	15-190	4-8
Meperidine	75	300	2-3	3-4

* Repeated doses of methadone result in drug accumulation. Doses may need to be adjusted after 3 days.
IM = intramuscular; PO = orally.

methadone maintenance program, and the addict who is currently abusing illicit or prescription drugs or both. For example, a distant history of substance abuse might predispose the patient to reemergence of substance-abuse behaviors with the stress of surgery and postoperative pain but may not require treatment approaches different from those appropriate for non-addicted patients. Individualized care should be provided in dealing with each scenario, and relevant pharmacological principles of opioid use should be followed. For example, likelihood of preexisting opioid tolerance should be recognized because high doses of opioids may be required, and treatment with an opioid agonist-antagonist should not be started because these agents may precipitate withdrawal in this setting. Consultation with a pain service or addiction specialist is advised for clinicians who do not commonly encounter or manage these patients.

CONCLUSION

Prolonged pain and disability characterize recovery from surgical procedures of the knee. Variable degrees of postoperative pain intensity, the need for early ambulation and rehabilitation, and the increasing frequency of outpatient surgical procedures pose challenges to the clinician caring for the postoperative needs of these patient. Effective pain management can further the goals of the orthopedic surgeon for his or her patients. Strategies for management include careful assessment of pain and its impact on function, use of appropriate and effective intra-articular pain-relieving medications, selection of modern pain management techniques, and correct use of oral analgesics. Consultation with appropriate specialists is recommended for patients whose pain does not respond to the above measures.

References

1. Agency for Health Care Policy and Research: Acute Pain Management: Operative or Medical Procedures and Trauma: Clinical Practice Guideline. Rockville, MD, Author, 1992.
2. Allen GC, St. Amand MA, Lui AC, et al: Postarthroscopy analgesia with intraarticular bupivacaine/morphine. A randomized clinical trial. Anesthesiology 79(3):475, 1993.
3. Allen HW, Liu SS, Ware PD, et al: Peripheral nerve blocks improve analgesia after total knee replacement surgery. Anesth Analg 87(1):93, 1998.
4. Allen JG, Denny NM, Oakman N: Postoperative analgesia following total knee arthroplasty: A study comparing spinal anesthesia and combined sciatic femoral 3-in-1 block. Reg Anesth Pain Med 23(2):142, 1998.
5. American Pain Society Quality of Care Committee: Quality improvement guidelines for the treatment of acute pain and cancer pain. JAMA 274(23):1874, 1995.
6. American Society of Anesthesiologists, Task Force on Pain Management: Practice guidelines for acute pain management in the perioperative setting. Anesthesiology 82(4):1071, 1995.
7. Aronowitz ER, Kleinbart FA: Outpatient ACL reconstruction using intraoperative local analgesia and oral postoperative pain medication. Orthopedics 21(7):781, 1998.
8. Austin KL, Stapleton JV, Mather LE: Multiple intramuscular injections: A major source of variability in analgesic response to meperidine. Pain 8(1):47, 1980.
9. Baker MW, Tullos HS, Bryan WJ, et al: The use of epidural morphine in patients undergoing total knee arthroplasty. J Arthroplasty 4(2):157, 1989.
10. Barber FA, McGuire DA, Click S: Continuous-flow cold therapy for outpatient anterior cruciate ligament reconstruction. Arthroscopy 14(2):130, 1998.
11. Bauer M, Rensing H, Ziegenfuss T: Anesthesia and perioperative immune function. Anaesthesist 47(7):538, 1998.
12. Boldt J, Thaler E, Lehmann A, et al: Pain management in cardiac surgery patients: Comparison between standard therapy and patient-controlled analgesia regimen. J Cardiothorac Vasc Anesth 12(6):654, 1998.
13. Bonica JJ: Postoperative pain. In Bonica JJ, Loeser JD, Chapman CR, et al, eds: The Management of Pain, 2nd ed., vol. 1. Philadelphia, Lea & Febiger, 1990, p 461.
14. Boulanger A, Choiniere M, Roy D, et al: Comparison between patient-controlled analgesia and intramuscular meperidine after thoracotomy. Can J Anaesth 40(5):409, 1993.
15. Brandsson S, Rydgren B, Hedner T, et al: Postoperative analgesic effects of an external cooling system and intra-articular bupivacaine/morphine after arthroscopic cruciate ligament surgery. Knee Surg Sports Traumatol Arthrosc 4(4):200, 1996.
16. Brandt KD, Slowman-Kovacs S: Nonsteroidal antiinflammatory drugs in treatment of osteoarthritis. Clin Orthop 213:84, 1986.
17. Brown DW, Curry CM, Ruterbories LM, et al: Evaluation of pain after arthroscopically assisted anterior cruciate ligament reconstruction. Am J Sports Med 25(2):182, 1997.
18. Cardosa M, Rudkin GE, Osborne GA: Outcome from day-case knee arthroscopy in a major teaching hospital. Arthroscopy 10(6):624, 1994.
19. Carpenter RL: Optimizing postoperative pain management. Am Fam Physician 56(3):835, 1997.
20. Chaney MA: Side effects of intrathecal and epidural opioids. Can J Anaesth 42(10):891, 1995.
21. Chapman CR: Psychological aspects of postoperative pain control. Acta Anaesthesiol Belg 43(1):41, 1992.

22. Chirwa SS, MacLeod BA, Day B: Intraarticular bupivacaine (Marcaine) after arthroscopic meniscectomy: A randomized double-blind controlled study. Arthroscopy 5(1):33, 1989.
23. Cleeland CS: Effects of attitudes on cancer pain control. In Straton Hill JC, Fields WS, eds: Drug Treatment of Cancer Pain in a Drug Oriented Society. New York, Raven Press, 1989.
24. Commission of the Provision of Surgical Services: Report of the Working Party on Pain after Surgery: The Royal College of Surgeons of England and the College of Anaesthetists. London, The Royal College of Surgeons, 1990.
25. Cook TM, Nolan JP, Tuckey JP: Postarthroscopic meniscus repair analgesia with intraarticular ketorolac or morphine [letter]. Anesth Analg 84(2):466, 1997.
26. Cousins MJ, Mather LE: Intrathecal and epidural administration of opioids. Anesthesiology 61(3):276, 1984.
27. Dalsgaard J, Felsby S, Juelsgaard P, et al: Low-dose intra-articular morphine analgesia in day case knee arthroscopy: A randomized double-blinded prospective study. Pain 56(2):151, 1994.
28. Donovan M, Dillon P, McGuire L: Incidence and characteristics of pain in a sample of medical-surgical inpatients. Pain 30(1): 69, 1987.
29. Dubois M: Patient-controlled analgesia for acute pain. Clin J Pain 5(Suppl 1):S8, 1989.
30. Durand A, Richards CL, Malouin F: Strength recovery and muscle activation of the knee extensor and flexor muscles after arthroscopic meniscectomy. A pilot study. Clin Orthop 262: 210, 1991.
31. Edkin BS, Spindler KP, Flanagan JF: Femoral nerve block as an alternative to parenteral narcotics for pain control after anterior cruciate ligament reconstruction. Arthroscopy 11(4):404, 1995.
32. Edwards ND, Wright EM: Continuous low-dose 3-in-1 nerve blockade for postoperative pain relief after total knee replacement. Anesth Analg 75(2):265, 1992.
33. Egan KJ, Ready LB: Patient satisfaction with intravenous PCA or epidural morphine. Can J Anaesth 41(1):6, 1994.
34. Eriksson-Mjoberg M, Svensson JO, Almkvist O, et al: Extradural morphine gives better pain relief than patient-controlled i.v. morphine after hysterectomy. Br J Anaesth 78(1):10, 1997.
35. Etches RC, Warriner CB, Badner N, et al: Continuous intravenous administration of ketorolac reduces pain and morphine consumption after total hip or knee arthroplasty. Anesth Analg 81(6):1175, 1995.
36. Fisher DA, Trimble S, Clapp B, et al: Effect of a patient management system on outcomes of total hip and knee arthroplasty. Clin Orthop 345:155, 1997.
37. Fragen RJ, Stulberg SD, Wixson R, et al: Effect of ketorolac tromethamine on bleeding and on requirements for analgesia after total knee arthroplasty. J Bone Joint Surg Am 77(7):998, 1995.
38. Fujii K, Tajiri K, Kajiwara T, et al: Effects of NSAID on collagen and proteoglycan synthesis of cultured chondrocytes. J Rheumatol Suppl 18:28, 1989.
39. Geutjens G, Hambidge JE: Analgesic effects of intraarticular bupivacaine after day-case arthroscopy. Arthroscopy 10(3):299, 1994.
40. Grossman SA, Sheidler VR, Swedeen K, et al: Correlation of patient and caregiver ratings of cancer pain. J Pain Symptom Manage 6(2):53, 1991.
41. Hargreaves KM, Costello A: Glucocorticoids suppress levels of immunoreactive bradykinin in inflamed tissue as evaluated by microdialysis probes. Clin Pharmacol Ther 48(2):168, 1990.
42. Heard SO, Edwards WT, Ferrari D, et al: Analgesic effect of intraarticular bupivacaine or morphine after arthroscopic knee surgery: A randomized, prospective, double-blind study. Anesth Analg 74(6):822, 1992.
43. Heine MF, Tillet ED, Tsueda K, et al: Intra-articular morphine after arthroscopic knee operation. Br J Anaesth 73(3):413, 1994.
44. Hirst GC, Lang SA, Dust WN, et al: Femoral nerve block. Single injection versus continuous infusion for total knee arthroplasty. Reg Anesth 21(4):292, 1996.
45. Hoher J, Kersten D, Bouillon B, et al: Local and intra-articular infiltration of bupivacaine before surgery: Effect on postoperative pain after anterior cruciate ligament reconstruction. Arthroscopy 13(2):210, 1997.
46. Horlocker TT, Wedel DJ: Neuraxial block and low-molecular-weight heparin: Balancing perioperative analgesia and thromboprophylaxis. Reg Anesth Pain Med 23(6 Suppl 2):164, 1998.
47. Hoskin PJ, Hanks GW: Opioid agonist-antagonist drugs in acute and chronic pain states. Drugs 41(3):326, 1991.
48. Jaureguito JW, Wilcox JF, Cohn SJ, et al: A comparison of intraarticular morphine and bupivacaine for pain control after outpatient knee arthroscopy. A prospective, randomized, double-blinded study. Am J Sports Med 23(3):350, 1995.
49. Jensen MP, Karoly P, Braver S: The measurement of clinical pain intensity: A comparison of six methods. Pain 27(1):117, 1986.
50. Johansson A, Hao J, Sjolund B: Local corticosteroid application blocks transmission in normal nociceptive C-fibres. Acta Anaesthesiol Scand 34(5): 335, 1990.
51. Joshi GP, McCarroll SM, McSwiney M, et al: Effects of intraarticular morphine on analgesic requirements after anterior cruciate ligament repair. Reg Anesth 18(4):254, 1993.
52. Joshi GP, McCarroll SM, O'Brien TM, et al: Intraarticular analgesia following knee arthroscopy. Anesth Analg 76(2):333, 1993.
53. Kaiko RF: Basics of opioid analgesic pharmacodynamics. J Pain Symptom Manage 1(2):103, 1986.
54. Kaiko RF, Wallenstein SL, Rogers AG, et al: Narcotics in the elderly. Med Clin North Am 66(5):1079, 1982.
55. Kalso E, Tramer MR, Carroll D, et al: Pain relief from intra-articular morphine after knee surgery: A qualitative systematic review. Pain 71(2):127, 1997.
56. Kao JT, Giangarra CE, Singer G, et al: A comparison of outpatient and inpatient anterior cruciate ligament reconstruction surgery. Arthroscopy 11(2):151, 1995.
57. Karlsson J, Rydgren B, Eriksson B, et al: Postoperative analgesic effects of intra-articular bupivacaine and morphine after arthroscopic cruciate ligament surgery. Knee Surg Sports Traumatol Arthrosc 3(1):55, 1995.
58. Kehlet H: The stress response to surgery: Release mechanisms and the modifying effect of pain relief. Acta Chir Scand Suppl 550:22, 1989.
59. Kehlet H: The surgical stress response: Should it be prevented? Can J Surg 34(6):565, 1991.
60. Kehlet H: Effect of pain relief on the surgical stress response. Reg Anesth 21(6 Suppl):35, 1996.
61. Kehlet H: Multimodal approach to control postoperative pathophysiology and rehabilitation. Br J Anaesth 78(5):606, 1997.
62. Kenady DE, Wilson JF, Schwartz RW, et al: A randomized comparison of patient-controlled versus standard analgesic requirements in patients undergoing cholecystectomy. Surg Gynecol Obstet 174(3):216, 1992.
63. Khoury GF, Chen AC, Garland DE, et al: Intraarticular morphine, bupivacaine, and morphine/bupivacaine for pain control after knee videoarthroscopy. Anesthesiology 77(2):263, 1992.
64. Klein EA, Grass JA, Calabrese DA, et al: Maintaining quality of care and patient satisfaction with radical prostatectomy in the era of cost containment. Urology 48(2):269, 1996.
65. Kuhn S, Cooke K, Collins M, et al: Perceptions of pain relief after surgery. BMJ 300(6741):1687, 1990.
66. Laurent SC, Nolan JP, Pozo JL, et al: Addition of morphine to intra-articular bupivacaine does not improve analgesia after day-case arthroscopy. Br J Anaesth 72(2):170, 1994.
67. Loper KA, Ready LB: Epidural morphine after anterior cruciate ligament repair: A comparison with patient-controlled intravenous morphine. Anesth Analg 68(3):350, 1989.
68. Loper KA, Ready LB, Downey M, et al: Epidural and intravenous fentanyl infusions are clinically equivalent after knee surgery. Anesth Analg 70(1):72, 1990.
69. Loper KA, Ready LB, Nessly M, et al: Epidural morphine provides greater pain relief than patient-controlled intravenous morphine following cholecystectomy. Anesth Analg 69(6):826, 1989.
70. Love DR, Owen H, Ilsley AH, et al: A comparison of variable-dose patient-controlled analgesia with fixed-dose patient-controlled analgesia. Anesth Analg 83(5):1060, 1996.
71. Macintyre PE, Jarvis DA: Age is the best predictor of postoperative morphine requirements. Pain 64(2):357, 1996.
72. Mahoney OM, Noble PC, Davidson J, et al: The effect of continuous epidural analgesia on postoperative pain, rehabilitation,

and duration of hospitalization in total knee arthroplasty. Clin Orthop 260:30, 1990.
73. Mansour NY, Bennetts FE: An observational study of combined continuous lumbar plexus and single-shot sciatic nerve blocks for post-knee surgery analgesia. Reg Anesth 21(4):287, 1996.
74. Marks RM, Sachar EJ: Undertreatment of medical inpatients with narcotic analgesics. Ann Intern Med 78(2):173, 1973.
75. Mather LE: Opioids: A pharmacologist's delight! Clin Exp Pharmacol Physiol 22(11):833, 1995.
76. Matzke GR: Nonrenal toxicities of acetaminophen, aspirin, and nonsteroidal anti-inflammatory agents. Am J Kidney Dis 28:S63, 1996.
77. Max MB: Improving outcomes of analgesic treatment: Is education enough? Ann Intern Med 113(11):885, 1990.
78. McGuire DA, Sanders K, Hendricks SD: Comparison of ketorolac and opioid analgesics in postoperative ACL reconstruction outpatient pain control. Arthroscopy 9(6):653, 1993.
79. McMaster WC, Liddle S: Cryotherapy influence on posttraumatic limb edema. Clin Orthop 150:283, 1980.
80. McQueen DA, Kelly HK, Wright TF: A comparison of epidural and non-epidural anesthesia and analgesia in total hip or knee arthroplasty patients. Orthopedics 15(2):169, 1992.
81. Medina JL, Diamond S: Drug dependency in patients with chronic headaches. Headache 17(1):12, 1977.
82. Melzack R, Abbott FV, Zackon W, et al: Pain on a surgical ward: A survey of the duration and intensity of pain and the effectiveness of medication. Pain 29(1):67, 1987.
83. Moiniche S, Hjortso NC, Hansen BL, et al: The effect of balanced analgesia on early convalescence after major orthopaedic surgery. Acta Anaesthesiol Scand 38(4):328, 1994.
84. Muldoon T, Milligan K, Quinn P, et al: Comparison between extradural infusion of ropivacaine or bupivacaine for the prevention of postoperative pain after total knee arthroplasty. Br J Anaesth 80(5):680, 1998.
85. Musacchio JM: The psychotomimetic effects of opiates and the sigma receptor. Neuropsychopharmacology 3(3):191, 1990.
86. Nakamura SJ, Conte-Hernandez A, Galloway MT: The efficacy of regional anesthesia for outpatient anterior cruciate ligament reconstruction. Arthroscopy 13(6):699, 1997.
87. Pati AB, Perme DC, Trail M, et al: Rehabilitation parameters in total knee replacement patients undergoing epidural vs. conventional analgesia. J Orthop Sports Phys Ther 19(2):88, 1994.
88. Pedersen P, Nielsen KD, Jensen PE: The efficacy of Na-naproxen after diagnostic and therapeutic arthroscopy of the knee joint. Arthroscopy 9(2):170, 1993.
89. Perry F, Parker RK, White PF, et al: Role of psychological factors in postoperative pain control and recovery with patient-controlled analgesia. Clin J Pain 10(1):57, 1994.
90. Perry S, Heidrich G: Management of pain during debridement: A survey of U.S. burn units. Pain 13(3):267, 1982.
91. Popp JE, Sanko WA, Sinha AK, et al: A comparison of ketorolac tromethamine/oxycodone versus patient-controlled analgesia with morphine in anterior cruciate ligament reconstruction patients. Arthroscopy 14(8):816, 1998.
92. Porter J, Jick H: Addiction rare in patients treated with narcotics [letter]. N Engl J Med 302(2):123, 1980.
93. Raja SN, Dickstein RE, Johnson CA: Comparison of postoperative analgesic effects of intraarticular bupivacaine and morphine following arthroscopic knee surgery. Anesthesiology 77(6):1143, 1992.
94. Rasmussen S, Larsen AS, Thomsen ST, et al: Intra-articular glucocorticoid, bupivacaine and morphine reduces pain, inflammatory response and convalescence after arthroscopic meniscectomy. Pain 78(2):131, 1998.
95. Ready LB, Edwards WT: Management of Acute Pain: A Practical Guide. Seattle, WA, IASP Publications, 1992.
96. Ready LB, Loper KA, Nessly M, et al: Postoperative epidural morphine is safe on surgical wards. Anesthesiology 75(3):452, 1991.
97. Reder RF, Oshlack B, Miotto JB, et al: Steady-state bioavailability of controlled-release oxycodone in normal subjects. Clin Ther 18(1):95, 1996.
98. Reuben SS, Connelly NR: Postoperative analgesia for outpatient arthroscopic knee surgery with intraarticular bupivacaine and ketorolac. Anesth Analg 80(6):1154, 1995.
99. Reuben SS, Connelly NR: Postarthroscopic meniscus repair analgesia with intraarticular ketorolac or morphine. Anesth Analg 82(5):1036, 1996.
100. Reuben SS, Steinberg RB, Cohen MA, et al: Intraarticular morphine in the multimodal analgesic management of postoperative pain after ambulatory anterior cruciate ligament repair. Anesth Analg 86(2):374, 1998.
101. Rutberg H, Hakanson E, Anderberg B, et al: Effects of the extradural administration of morphine, or bupivacaine, on the endocrine response to upper abdominal surgery. Br J Anaesth 56(3):233, 1984.
102. Ryu J, Saito S, Yamamoto K, et al: Factors influencing the postoperative range of motion in total knee arthroplasty. Bull Hosp Jt Dis 53(3):35, 1993.
103. Schultz P, Anker-Moller E, Dahl JB, et al: Postoperative pain treatment after open knee surgery: Continuous lumbar plexus block with bupivacaine versus epidural morphine. Reg Anesth 16(1):34, 1991.
104. Schulz KF, Chalmers I, Hayes RJ, et al: Empirical evidence of bias. Dimensions of methodological quality associated with estimates of treatment effects in controlled trials. JAMA 273(5): 408, 1995.
105. Sculco TP: Establishing a universal protocol for deep vein thrombosis following orthopedic surgery: Total knee arthroplasty. Orthopedics 19(Suppl):6, 1996.
106. Serpell MG, Millar FA, Thomson MF: Comparison of lumbar plexus block versus conventional opioid analgesia after total knee replacement. Anaesthesia 46(4):275, 1991.
107. Shoji H, Solomonow M, Yoshino S, et al: Factors affecting postoperative flexion in total knee arthroplasty. Orthopedics 13(6):643, 1990.
108. Sinatra RS: Current methods of controlling post-operative pain. Yale J Biol Med 64(4):351, 1991.
109. Singelyn FJ, Deyaert M, Joris D, et al: Effects of intravenous patient-controlled analgesia with morphine, continuous epidural analgesia, and continuous three-in-one block on postoperative pain and knee rehabilitation after unilateral total knee arthroplasty. Anesth Analg 87(1):88, 1998.
110. Smith I, Shively RA, White PF: Effects of ketorolac and bupivacaine on recovery after outpatient arthroscopy. Anesth Analg 75(2):208, 1992.
111. Smith I, Van Hemelrijck J, White PF, et al: Effects of local anesthesia on recovery after outpatient arthroscopy. Anesth Analg 73(5):536, 1991.
112. Solheim E, Strand T: Postoperative pain after anterior cruciate ligament reconstruction using a transligamentous approach. Am J Sports Med 21(4):507, 1993.
113. Spetzler B, Anderson L: Patient-controlled analgesia in the total joint arthroplasty patient. Clin Orthop 215:122, 1987.
114. Stein C, Comisel K, Haimerl E, et al: Analgesic effect of intraarticular morphine after arthroscopic knee surgery. N Engl J Med 325(16):1123, 1991.
115. Stein C, Gramsch C, Herz A: Intrinsic mechanisms of antinociception in inflammation: local opioid receptors and beta-endorphin. J Neurosci 10(4):1292, 1990.
116. Stein C, Hassan AH, Przewlocki R, et al: Opioids from immunocytes interact with receptors on sensory nerves to inhibit nociception in inflammation. Proc Natl Acad Sci 87(15):5935, 1990.
117. Stein C, Millan MJ, Shippenberg TS, et al: Peripheral opioid receptors mediating antinociception in inflammation. Evidence for involvement of mu, delta and kappa receptors. J Pharmacol Exp Ther 248(3):1269, 1989.
118. St-Pierre DM: Rehabilitation following arthroscopic meniscectomy. Sports Med 20(5):338, 1995.
119. Tetzlaff JE, Andrish J, O'Hara J Jr, et al: Effectiveness of bupivacaine administered via femoral nerve catheter for pain control after anterior cruciate ligament repair. J Clin Anesth 9(7):542, 1997.
120. Tighe SQ, Bie JA, Nelson RA, et al: The acute pain service: Effective or expensive care? Anaesthesia 53(4):397, 1998.
121. Turner G, Blake D, Buckland M, et al: Continuous extradural infusion of ropivacaine for prevention of postoperative pain after major orthopaedic surgery. Br J Anaesth 76(5):606, 1996.
122. Wallenstein SL: Measurement of pain and analgesia in cancer patients. Cancer 53(10 Suppl):2260, 1984.
123. Wallenstein SL, Heidrich GD, Kaiko R, et al: Clinical evaluation

of mild analgesics: The measurement of clinical pain. Br J Clin Pharmacol 10(Suppl 2):319, 1980.
124. Wang JJ, Ho ST, Lee SC, et al: Intraarticular triamcinolone acetonide for pain control after arthroscopic knee surgery. Anesth Analg 87(5):1113, 1998.
125. Wang JK, Nauss LA, Thomas JE: Pain relief by intrathecally applied morphine in man. Anesthesiology 50(2):149, 1979.
126. Weale AE, Ackroyd CE, Mani GV, et al: Day-case or short-stay admission for arthroscopic knee surgery: A randomised controlled trial. Ann R Coll Surg Engl 80(2):146, 1998.
127. Weller R, Rosenblum M, Conard P, et al: Comparison of epidural and patient-controlled intravenous morphine following joint replacement surgery. Can J Anaesth 38(5):582, 1991.
128. Whitelaw GP, DeMuth KA, Demos HA, et al: The use of the Cryo/Cuff versus ice and elastic wrap in the postoperative care of knee arthroscopy patients. Am J Knee Surg 8(1):28, 1995.
129. Williams JS Jr, Wexler G, Novak PJ, et al: A prospective study of pain and analgesic use in outpatient endoscopic anterior cruciate ligament reconstruction. Arthroscopy 14(6):613, 1998.
130. Williams-Russo P, Sharrock NE, Haas SB, et al: Randomized trial of epidural versus general anesthesia: Outcomes after primary total knee replacement. Clin Orthop 331:199, 1996.

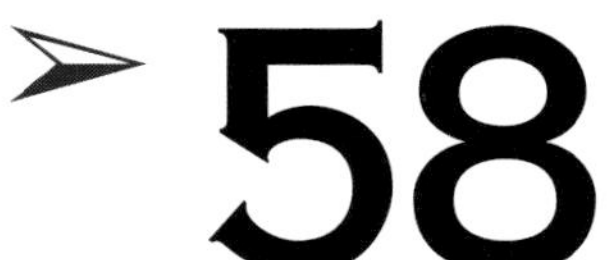

Gene Therapy in Treatment of Knee Disorders

JOHNNY HUARD • VLADIMIR MARTINEK • FREDDIE H. FU

The treatment of knee disorders has improved since the 1970s as a consequence of new minimally invasive operative techniques, novel instruments, modern rehabilitation, medications, and increasing knowledge about the biomechanics of the knee joint.

Despite this progress, there are still deficits in the therapy of injuries originating from a limited healing capacity in most tissues of the musculoskeletal system. Ligaments, tendons, menisci, and articular cartilage are tissues with low blood supply and a reduced cell turnover. For this reason, the healing process is prolonged and often results in the formation of an inferior scar or a tissue defect.

Various cytokines, or growth factors, have been identified as substances capable of modifying the healing process in tissues.[1] Growth factors are small peptides that can be synthesized both by the resident cells at the injury site (e.g., fibroblasts, endothelial cells, mesenchymal stem cells) and by the infiltrating reparatory or inflammatory cells (e.g., platelets, macrophages, monocytes). They are capable of stimulating cell proliferation, migration, and differentiation as well as the matrix synthesis in different tissues (Table 58.1)[2] The gene encoding for most of the growth factors has been determined and, using recombinant DNA technology, these proteins can be produced in large quantity for the purpose of treatment.[3]

TABLE 58.1 EFFECT OF GROWTH FACTORS IN TISSUES OF THE MUSCULOSKELETAL SYSTEM

	Hyaline Cartilage	Meniscus	Ligament Tendon	Bone
IGF-1	+	+/−	+/−	+
bFGF	+	+	+/−	+
NGF		−	−	
aFGF		−	+/−	
PDGF AA		−	+/−	
PDGF AB		+	+/−	
PDGF BB			+	
EGF	+	+	+	
TGF-α		+	−	
TGF-β	+	+/−	+/−	+
BMP-2	+	+		+
HGF		+	+	
CDMP (1 to 3)	+			

+ = positive effect; − = no or negative effect; aFGF = acidic fibroblast growth factor; bFGF = basic fibroblast growth factor; BMP-2 = bone morphogenetic protein-2; CDMP = cartilage-derived morphogenetic proteins; EGF = endothelial growth factor; HGF = hepatocyte growth factor; IGF-1 = insulin-like growth factor 1; NGF = nerve growth factor; PDGF = platelet-derived growth factor; TGF-α = transforming growth factor-α; TGF-β = transforming growth factor-β.

Although the direct injection of these human recombinant proteins has some beneficial effect on the healing process,[4] very high dosages and repeated injections are often required because of the relatively short biological half-life. Another major limitation of using these human recombinant growth factor proteins to promote healing is their delivery to the injured site.[4] In fact, the use of various strategies, including polymers, pumps, and heparin, has been investigated to achieve sustained persistence of these proteins. Although these approaches have been capable of improving the local persistence of the growth factor proteins, the results remain limited. Among the different methods developed for local administration of growth factors, gene therapy based on the use of various gene transfer techniques has proved the most promising.[5]

GENE THERAPY

Definition

Gene therapy is a technique relying on the alteration of the cellular genetic information. Originally, gene therapy was conceived for the manipulation of germline cells for the treatment of inheritable genetic disorders, but this method is greatly limited by the inefficient technology and considerable ethical concerns. Meanwhile, gene manipulation of somatic cells has been widely achieved for many tissues.[5] Gene therapy can be applied to orthopedics using the transfer of defined genes encoding for growth factors, cytokines, and antibiotics into the target tissue. Thus, therapeutic substances can be highly and persistently produced directly at the site of injuries by the local cells, with concentrations of encoded therapeutic substances capable of improving the healing process.

Vectors

For gene expression, the transferred DNA material has to enter the nucleus, where it either integrates into the chromosomes of the host cells or remains separated from the host DNA in the form of an episome. After transcription, the generated mRNA is transported

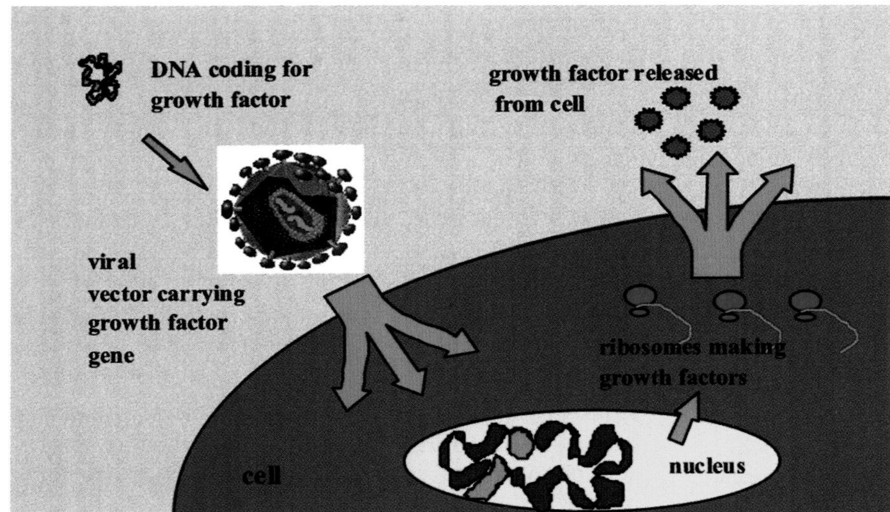

FIGURE 58.1 ➢ Gene transfer using a viral vector.

outside the nucleus and serves as a matrix for the production of proteins (e.g., growth factors) in the ribosomes (Fig. 58.1). The transduced cells by the vector can consequently express the growth factors and cytokines of interest and become a reservoir of secreting molecules capable of improving the healing process.

Viral and nonviral vectors can be used for delivery of genetic material into cells (Table 58.2). The nonviral gene transfer systems are usually easier to produce and have a significantly lower cell toxicity and immunogenicity than the viral vectors, but the overall use of the nonviral systems has been hindered by the low transfection efficiencies despite using large amounts of DNA. Different approaches are being investigated to improve nonviral gene transfer (e.g., the use of necrotic agents to increase the permeability of the nonviral vectors and the development of liposomes), but their success remains limited.

Currently, viral gene vectors present a more efficient method.[4] Before a virus is used in gene therapy, all genes encoding for pathogenic proteins must be deleted and replaced by the gene of interest. In fact, many years of basic research were required to characterize and remove the pathogenic genes from the viral genomes. The native ability of the virus to enter (infect) the cell and express its own genetic material within the infected cell could then be utilized. The most commonly used viruses in gene therapy currently are adenovirus, retrovirus, adeno-associated virus, and herpes simplex virus. Although viral vectors display a high efficiency of transfer to many cell types, their cytotoxicity (herpes simplex virus), immunogenicity (adenovirus), and inability to transduce postmitotic cells (retrovirus) have limited their general application for gene therapy purposes (see Table 58.2). Consequently, new viral vectors with reduced cytotoxicity and immunogenicity are under development.[3]

TABLE 58.2 COMMON VECTORS USED FOR GENE DELIVERY INTO CELLS

Gene Delivery	Vectors	Specifications
Nonviral	Liposomes DNA gene gun DNA-protein complex Naked DNA	Low efficiency of gene delivery Low immunogenicity Easy to produce
Viral	Adenovirus	Infects mitotic/postmitotic cells Low cytotoxicity Immune rejection problems
	Retrovirus	Low toxicity/immunogenicity Infects mitotically active cells only Low gene insert capacity
	Adeno-associated virus	Low toxicity/immunogenicity High persistence of gene transfer Low gene insert capacity
	Herpes simplex virus	Large insert capacity Infects mitotic/postmitotic cells Immune rejection problems

Strategies

Various gene delivery strategies, such as direct and systemic, can be used to achieve gene transfer to the knee and the musculoskeletal system. The systemic delivery of the viral vectors consists of injecting the vector in the bloodstream, resulting in the dissemination of the vector to the target tissues. This approach offers a major advantage when the target tissue is difficult to reach by direct injection. Moreover, systemic delivery often displays better distribution of the vectors within the targeted tissues because direct injection of the vectors often results in a localized expression at the injected site. The major disadvantages of this technology are the high number of vectors required and the lack of specificity of expression, because the majority of the vectors are disseminated in the lung and the liver. Furthermore, the lack of blood supply makes this approach inappropriate for some knee injuries and disorders (meniscus and cartilage).

Two basic strategies for direct gene therapy to the musculoskeletal system have been extensively investigated.[4] Either the vectors are directly injected in the host tissues (in vivo) or the cells of the injured tissue are removed, genetically altered (transduced/transfected) in vitro, and directly re-injected in the tissues (ex vivo). The direct, in vivo method is technically simpler, but the ex vivo gene delivery offers more safety because the gene manipulation takes place under controlled conditions outside the body (Fig. 58.2). Furthermore, the ex vivo approach leads to the delivery of growth factors and cytokines as well as endogenous cells capable of responding to the stimuli and participating in the healing process. Approaches based on tissue engineering, which aim at using cells from different tissues (mesenchymal stem cells, muscle-derived cells, dermal fibroblasts) to deliver genes, may bring additional opportunities to improve the healing process of various tissues of the musculoskeletal system. Selecting the appropriate procedure depends on various factors such as the division rate of the target cells, pathophysiology of the disorder, availability of cells from the injured tissues, and type of vector used.

Limitations

For the treatment of knee disorders, the major concern with gene therapy is safety. Although gene therapy may be a "last chance" treatment option in cases of malignancies or severe genetic disorders (e.g., Duchenne's muscular dystrophy, Gaucher's disease, cystic fibrosis), the risk of many side effects and potential consequences of gene therapy may be unacceptable in elective orthopedics. Virus vectors integrating into the genome of the cells pose the danger of insertional mutagenesis.[6] Possible abnormal regulation of cell growth, toxicity due to chronic overexpression of the growth factor protein, and development of a malignancy are theoretically conceivable, although cases have never been reported. Vectors that do not integrate into the native DNA avoid these risks but remain greatly limited by the lack of persistent expressions of the desired genes in the target tissues. The loss of expression of the transferred gene over a few weeks is a frequent and not fully understood phenomenon, especially for adenoviral vectors. However, a temporary and self-limiting gene expression could be useful in the treatment of musculoskeletal injuries, for which only transient high levels of growth factors are necessary to promote the healing response.

GENE THERAPY IN TREATMENT OF KNEE DISORDERS

Arthritis

Arthritis is a common disorder of the knee joint with different causes. Gene therapy is suggested to deliver therapeutic recombinant proteins relevant to the noninflammatory, inflammatory, infectious, and hemorrhagic origins of the diseased knee joint.[4] With ex vivo and in vivo methods, genes have been successfully introduced locally to the synovial tissue of the animal knee joints.[7–17]

One of the promising therapeutic approaches in gene therapy is the transfer of the interleukin-1 receptor antagonist protein (IRAP) into the inflammatory knee joint.[8, 11–13] Interleukin-1 (IL-1) is a cytokine highly expressed in inflammatory knee disorders, especially in rheumatoid arthritis and osteoarthritis.[18] It is thought that IL-1 is the leading proinflammatory cytokine responsible for inducing protease synthesis and cartilage catabolism. Synovial cells mediated ex vivo transfer of IRAP using a retrovirus and led to a significant increase of this receptor antagonist in the joint[8] and to an anti-inflammatory effect in the rabbit knee joint.

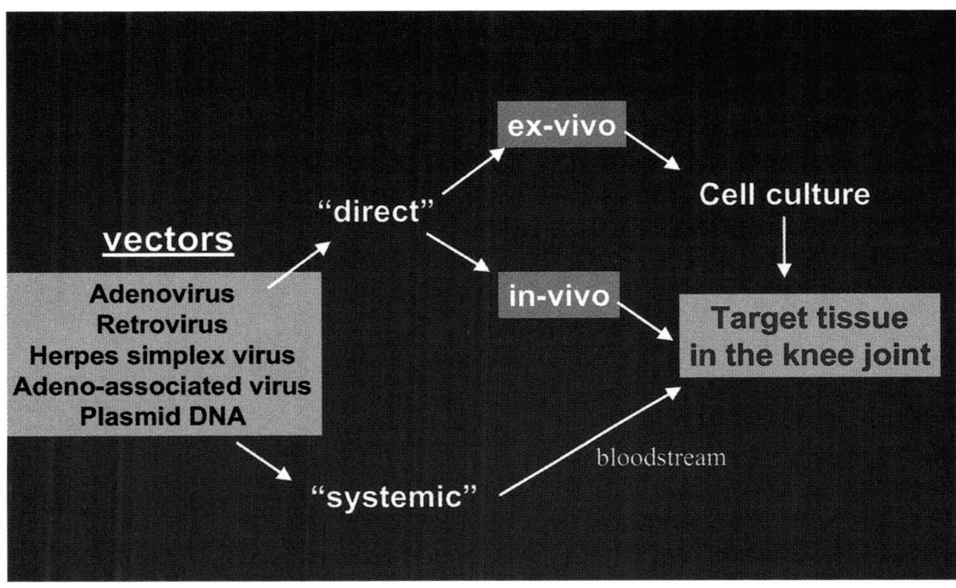

FIGURE 58.2 ➢ Gene delivery strategies into the joint.

Among the other anti-inflammatory cytokines, IL-10 has received growing attention for its anti-inflammatory properties and independent effects on T-cell reactivity.[18] Local delivery of replication-defective adenovirus expressing IL-10 significantly reduced the inflammation in experimentally induced arthritis in rabbits.[14] Interestingly, the anti-inflammatory effect was achieved not only in the injected knee joints but in the contralateral knees that received, as control, an adenovirus carrying a marker gene as well as in distal joints. Similar systemic therapeutic effects of adenovirus-carrying IL-10 were demonstrated in murine collagen-induced arthritis.[19]

Success in animal studies led to the approval of the first human clinical trial of gene therapy for a nonlethal disease.[4] In this trial, the human IRAP gene was delivered by an ex vivo method using synovial cells to the metacarpophalangeal joints of postmenopausal women suffering from rheumatoid arthritis. The goal of the first trials was to test the safety of the approach; although the experiment is still ongoing, no adverse reaction associated with the applied gene therapy has been noted.[18]

The treatment of osteoarthritis may require different gene therapy approaches.[4] However, ex vivo gene transfer based on the use of transduced chondrocytes encoding genes for growth factors to inhibit the breakdown of cells or to enhance synthesis of the matrix is under investigation.[20, 21]

Cartilage Lesion

Damage to articular cartilage in the knee joint leads to premature osteoarthritis and may cause a considerable decrease in quality of life and enormous long-term health care costs.[22] Articular cartilage in adults does not possess blood supply, lymphatic drainage, or neural elements; furthermore, the chondrocytes are sheltered from the nutritional synovial fluid and reparative recognition by their large extracellular matrix. For these reasons, the regeneration of damaged articular cartilage is very limited.[23]

The common operative techniques for therapy of injured articular cartilage are subchondral drilling or microfracture, transplantation of autologous or allogeneic chondrocytes, autogenous or allogeneic osteochondral transplantation, and the use of scaffolds.[24] Despite some promising clinical results,[25] new strategies are required to obtain consistently good long-term results. Growth factors, including bone morphogenetic protein-2 (BMP-2), basic fibroblast growth factor (bFGF), transforming growth factor-β (TGF-β), endothelial growth factor (EGF), insulin-like growth factor-1 (IGF-1), and cartilage-derived morphogenetic proteins (CDMP), have been identified in vitro and in vivo with positive effects on chondrocytes and cartilage healing[26–30] (see Table 58.1). Several gene therapy techniques are currently being investigated for treatment of cartilage defects, but the most efficient way to solve this sophisticated problem has not yet been established.[20, 31] However, a therapeutic effect of gene therapy on cartilage tissue in vivo was demonstrated in rabbit intervertebral discs using an adenovirus-mediated transfer of human TGF-β_1.[32] This study demonstrated transfer of TGF-β_1 to rabbit nucleus pulposus cells in vivo, resulting in increased TGF-β_1 levels and proteoglycan synthesis. It has also been shown that ex vivo transduced periosteal cells using BMP-7 can affect healing of the articular cartilage in rabbits in vivo.[33]

ACL Rupture

The anterior cruciate ligament (ACL) is the second most frequently injured knee ligament, with over 100,000 estimated ACL ruptures each year in the United States.[34] The ACL has a low healing capacity.[35] To restore the normal knee function after complete ACL rupture, surgical reconstruction using autograft or allograft tendons is required.[36, 37] These treatments are both linked to disadvantages (i.e., additional injury through harvesting of the autograft,[38] transmission of infectious diseases [hepatitis B, HIV], and immunorejection of the allografts[39]). For ACL replacement with autologous material, both the bone-patella tendon-bone graft (BPTB) and the hamstring tendon graft represent the standard choice.[36] Although ACL replacement surgery has been significantly improved in recent years, the challenge to improve and accelerate the healing after ACL reconstruction remains.

Because of a ligamentization process, which can take up to 3 years,[40] the transplanted graft undergoes a period of weakness. For this reason, rehabilitation after ACL reconstruction remains slow: Even with professional athletes, the recommendation is to refrain from competitive sports for 6 months.

Several studies have shown a positive effect of growth factors (platelet-derived growth factor AB [PDGF-AB], IGF-1, EGF, bFGF, TGF-β) on the ACL fibroblast metabolism[2, 41–45] (see Table 58.1). The data suggest that these specific growth factors improve the healing of the ACL or the ligamentization of the ACL graft. Gene therapy that addresses these issues is promising as a delivery system to the ligaments.[46] The first feasibility studies have demonstrated the ability of the ligaments to be transduced with viral vectors expressing marker genes in vivo.[47, 48] Although no transfer of a therapeutic gene was achieved in the ACL in vivo, a positive effect of therapeutic genes on healing of the patella ligament was demonstrated using nonviral vector-mediated gene transfer of PDGF-B and hepatocyte growth factor/scatter factor.[49, 50]

Using the autologous semitendinosus and/or gracilis tendon for ACL reconstruction, surgeons also face some problems resulting from the tendon-to-bone healing in the femoral and tibial tunnel, which seems to be inferior to the bone-to-bone fixation of the BPTB graft. The delivery of BMP-2 and many other growth factors at the insertion site may solve this problem and improve the healing of the tendon in the bone tunnel.[51]

Meniscus Lesion

Meniscal tears due to twisting or compression forces are common sports injuries. Several repair techniques,

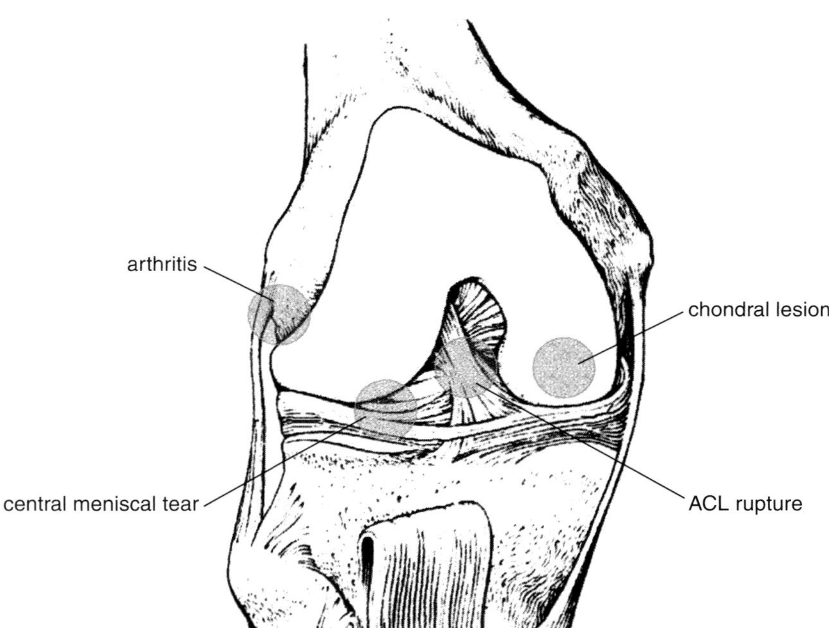

FIGURE 58.3 ➢ Aims of gene therapy in treatment of knee disorders.

including sutures, arrows, and staples, have been developed to preserve the menisci,[52] but only tears in the vascularized peripheral third of the meniscus can heal.[53] Meniscal lesions in the avascular central part do not heal and present an unsolved clinical problem because even partial resection of the meniscus leads over time to cartilage damage and osteoarthritis.[54] Experimental studies have shown that the healing process in the central part of the meniscus might be promoted by some chemotactic or mitogenic stimuli delivered by fibrin clot, synovial tissue, or growth factors (TGF-α, TGF-β, bFGF, EGF, PDGF-AB, HGF)[41, 55–61] (see Table 58.1). The goals of gene therapy for meniscal healing would be to (1) transduce cells located at the central meniscal tears directly with vectors or indirectly with autologous cells expressing growth factor genes to stimulate cell proliferation and matrix synthesis in meniscal fibroblasts and (2) to reach efficient healing. The first gene therapy approach for meniscal healing in vivo was achieved using retroviral vector expressing TGF-β_1 gene in rabbits.[58]

After a complete loss of the meniscus due to an extended injury or to repeated resections, most patients experience rapid impairment of knee function. Without treatment, osteoarthritis develops in most patients in 5 to 10 years.[62] Treatment after meniscal de-

TABLE 58.3 THERAPEUTIC GENE DELIVERY IN TISSUES OF THE MUSCULOSKELETAL SYSTEM

Authors/Year	Tissue	Strategy	Vector
Nakamura et al, 1998[49]	Tendon	In vivo	HVJ liposome PDGF-B
Natsuume et al, 1998[66]		In vivo	HVJ-liposome HGF/SF
Goto et al, 1999[58]	Meniscus	Ex vivo	retro TGF-β_1
Powell et al, 1999[67]	Muscle	Ex vivo	retro rhGH/xeno myoblasts
Lieberman et al, 1997[68]	Bone	Ex vivo	retro BMP-2/stromal cells
Lieberman et al, 1997[68]		In vivo	ad BMP-2
Lou et al, 1999[69]		In vivo	ad BMP-2
Baltzer et al, 1999[70]		In vivo	ad BMP-2, ad TGF-β
Nishida et al, 1999[32]	Cartilage	In vivo	ad TGF-β_1
Grande et al, 1999[33]		Ex vivo	retro BMP-7/periosteal cells
Pelletier et al, 1999[13]	Joint	In vivo	plasmid DNA IR-1 RA
Ghivizzani et al, 1998[10]		In vivo	ad IL-1 recept, ad TNF-α recept
Otani et al, 1996[11]		Ex vivo	retro IRAP
Bandara et al, 1993[8]		Ex vivo	retro IRAP/synoviocytes
Hung et al, 1994[12]		Ex vivo	retro IRAP/synoviocytes
Pelletier et al, 1999[13]		In vivo	plasmid DNA IL-1 RA
Lechman et al, 1999[14]		In vivo	ad IL-10, ad lacZ
Bakker et al, 1999[15]		In vivo	ad TGF-β
Ikeda et al, 1998[16]		In vivo	ad lacZ, ad TFG-β_1
Apparailly et al, 1998[19]	Systemic	Systemic	ad IL-10

pletion is limited. In order to find a therapeutic solution, meniscal transplantation with allograft has been performed.[36] Clinical studies on this issue are rare and cite failure rates up to 60% after less than 2 years.[63, 64] Experimental studies show slow immune rejection problems taking part in the transplanted meniscal allografts.[65] The pretreatment of meniscus allografts with viral vectors expressing growth factors, which could lead to the acceleration of graft healing, restructuring, and limitation of immune rejection by delivering immunosuppressive substances, may further improve the success of meniscal allograft transplantation.

FUTURE DIRECTIONS

Although gene therapy is not yet established as an approved therapeutic technique, the potential is great for the treatment of knee disorders (Fig. 58.3). Until recently, only a few therapeutic gene therapy techniques had been shown to be effective in human joints.[4] At the experimental level, many studies have proved the feasibility of gene delivery into different tissues of the musculoskeletal system (Table 58.3). Beyond this stage, initial experimental studies demonstrated positive effects of transduced genes (especially BMP-2, IGF-1, TGF-β) in vivo. The main obstacle today seems to be the availability of vectors carrying effective genes, but many laboratories working on the engineering of these vectors have made great progress.[3] In general, gene therapy will potentially help us to develop efficient therapies for tissues with low healing capacity (cartilage, meniscus, ligament) and for other disorders such as osseous nonunion or arthritis.

REFERENCES

1. Trippel SB: Growth factors as therapeutic agents. Instr Course Lect 46:473, 1997.
2. Schmidt CC, Georgescu HI, Kwoh CK, et al: Effect of growth factors on the proliferation of fibroblasts from the medial collateral and anterior cruciate ligaments. J Orthop Res 13:184, 1995.
3. Robbins PD, Ghivizzani SC: Viral vectors for gene therapy. Pharmacol Ther 80:35, 1998.
4. Evans CH, Robbins PD: Possible orthopedic applications of gene therapy. J Bone Joint Surg Am 77:1103, 1995.
5. Mulligan RC: The basic science of gene therapy. Science 260: 926, 1993.
6. Crystal RG: Transfer of genes to humans: Early lessons and obstacles to success. Science 270:404, 1995.
7. Nita I, Ghivizzani SC, Galea-Lauri J, et al: Direct gene delivery to synovium: An evaluation of potential vectors in vitro and in vivo. Arthritis Rheum 39:820, 1996.
8. Bandara G, Mueller GM, Galea-Lauri J, et al: Intraarticular expression of biologically active interleukin 1-receptor-antagonist protein by ex vivo gene transfer. Proc Natl Acad Sci U S A 90: 10764, 1993.
9. Roessler BJ, Allen ED, Wilson JM, et al: Adenoviral-mediated gene transfer to rabbit synovium in vivo. J Clin Invest 92:1085, 1993.
10. Ghivizzani SC, Lechman ER, Kang R, et al: Direct adenovirus-mediated gene transfer of interleukin 1 and tumor necrosis factor alpha soluble receptors to rabbit knees with experimental arthritis has local and distal anti-arthritic effects. Proc Natl Acad Sci U S A 95:4613, 1998.
11. Otani K, Nita I, Macaulay W, et al: Suppression of antigen-induced arthritis in rabbits by ex vivo gene therapy. J Immunol 156:3558, 1996.
12. Hung GL, Galea-Lauri J, Mueller GM, et al: Suppression of intra-articular responses to interleukin-1 by transfer of the interleukin-1 receptor antagonist gene to synovium. Gene Ther 1:64, 1994.
13. Pelletier JP, Fernandes JC, Tardif G, et al: Direct in vivo transfer of the IL-IRA gene in osteoarthritic rabbit knee joints: Prevention of the disease progression. Oral presentation at the 45th Annual Meeting, ORS, February 1, 1999, Anaheim, CA.
14. Lechman ER, Ghivizzani SC, Mi Z, et al: In vivo delivery of viral IL-10 by replication-defective adenovirus ameliorates disease pathology in a rabbit antigen-induced arthritis model. Poster presentation at the 45th Annual Meeting, ORS, February 1, 1999, Anaheim, CA.
15. Bakker AC, Beuningen H, Van Lent P, et al: Adenovector-mediated gene transfer of active TGF beta 1 in the murine knee joint induced fibrosis and osteophyte formation. Poster presentation at the 45th Annual Meeting, ORS, February 1, 1999, Anaheim, CA.
16. Ikeda T, Kubo T, Arai Y, et al: Adenovirus mediated gene delivery to the joints of guinea pigs. J Rheumatol 25:1666, 1998.
17. Day CS, Kasemkijwattana C, Menetrey J, et al: Myoblast-mediated gene transfer to the joint. J Orthop Res 15:894, 1997.
18. Evans CH, Ghivizzani SC, Kang R, et al: Gene therapy for rheumatic diseases. Arthritis Rheum 42:1, 1999.
19. Apparailly F, Verwaerde C, Jacquet C, et al: Adenovirus-mediated transfer of viral IL-10 gene inhibits murine collagen-induced arthritis. J Immunol 160:5213, 1998.
20. Kang R, Marui T, Ghivizzani SC, et al: Ex vivo gene transfer to chondrocytes in full-thickness articular cartilage defects: A feasibility study. Osteoarthritis Cartilage 5:139, 1997.
21. Arai Y, Kubo T, Kobayashi K, et al: Adenovirus vector-mediated gene transduction to chondrocytes: In vitro evaluation of therapeutic efficacy of transforming growth factor-beta 1 and heat shock protein 70 gene transduction. J Rheumatol 24:1787, 1997.
22. O'Driscoll SW: The healing and regeneration of articular cartilage. J Bone Joint Surg Am 80:1795, 1998.
23. Shapiro F, Koide S, Glimcher MJ: Cell origin and differentiation in the repair of full-thickness defects of articular cartilage. J Bone Joint Surg Am 75:532, 1993.
24. O'Driscoll SW, Keeley FW, Salter RB: The chondrogenic potential of free autogenous periosteal grafts for biological resurfacing of major full-thickness defects in joint surfaces under the influence of continuous passive motion: An experimental investigation in the rabbit. J Bone Joint Surg Am 68:1017, 1986.
25. Minas T, Peterson L: Advanced techniques in autologous chondrocyte transplantation. Clin Sports Med 18:13, 1999.
26. Hunziker EB, Rosenberg LC: Repair of partial-thickness defects in articular cartilage: Cell recruitment from the synovial membrane. J Bone Joint Surg Am 78:721, 1996.
27. Cuevas P, Burgos J, Baird A: Basic fibroblast growth factor (FGF) promotes cartilage repair in vivo. Biochem Biophys Res Commun 156:611, 1988.
28. Arai Y, Kubo T, Kobayashi K, et al: Adenovirus vector-mediated gene transduction to chondrocytes: In vitro evaluation of therapeutic efficacy of transforming growth factor-beta 1 and heat shock protein 70 gene transduction. J Rheumatol 24:1787, 1997.
29. Sellers RS, Peluso D, Morris EA: The effect of recombinant human bone morphogenetic protein-2 (rhBMP-2) on the healing of full-thickness defects of articular cartilage. J Bone Joint Surg Am 79:1452, 1997.
30. Erlacher L, Ng CK, Ullrich R, et al: Presence of cartilage-derived morphogenetic proteins in articular cartilage and enhancement of matrix replacement in vitro. Arthritis Rheum 41:263, 1998.
31. Stone KR, Steadman JR, Rodkey WG, et al: Regeneration of meniscal cartilage with use of a collagen scaffold: Analysis of preliminary data. J Bone Joint Surg Am 79:1770, 1997.
32. Nishida K, Kang R, Suh JK, et al: Adenovirus mediated transfer of human TGF-beta 1 encoding gene to the rabbit intervertebral disc in vivo. Oral presentation at the 45th Annual Meeting, ORS, February 1, 1999, Anaheim, CA.
33. Grande DA, Mason J, Paulino C, et al: Gene enhanced tissue engineering for repair of osteochondral defects. Oral presentation at the 45th Annual Meeting, ORS, February 1, 1999, Anaheim, CA.

34. Miyasaka KC, Daniel DM, Hirschman P: The incidence of knee ligament injuries in the general population. Am J Knee Surg 4:3, 1991.
35. Hawkins RJ, Misamore GW, Merritt TR: Followup of the acute nonoperated isolated anterior cruciate ligament tear. Am J Sports Med 14:205, 1986.
36. Siegel MG, Roberts CS: Meniscal allografts. Clin Sports Med 12: 59, 1993.
37. O'Donoghue DH, Frank GR, Jeter GL, et al: Repair and reconstruction of the anterior cruciate ligament in dogs: Factors influencing long-term results. J Bone Joint Surg Am 53:710, 1971.
38. Aglietti P, Buzzi R, D'Andria S, et al: Patellofemoral problems after intraarticular anterior cruciate ligament reconstruction. Clin Orthop 188:195, 1993.
39. Marks PH, Cameron M, Fu FH: [Reconstruction of the cruciate ligaments with allogeneic transplants: Techniques, results and perspectives]. Orthopade 22:386, 1993.
40. Rougraff B, Shelbourne KD, Gerth PK, et al: Arthroscopic and histologic analysis of human patellar tendon autografts used for anterior cruciate ligament reconstruction. Am J Sports Med 21: 277, 1993.
41. Spindler KP, Mayes CE, Miller RR, et al: Regional mitogenic response of the meniscus to platelet-derived growth factor (PDGF-AB). J Orthop Res 13:201, 1995.
42. Marui T, Niyibizi C, Georgescu HI, et al: Effect of growth factors on matrix synthesis by ligament fibroblasts. J Orthop Res 15:18, 1997.
43. Scherping SCJ, Schmidt CC, Georgescu HI, et al: Effect of growth factors on the proliferation of ligament fibroblasts from skeletally mature rabbits. Connect Tissue Res 36:1, 1997.
44. DesRosiers EA, Yahia L, Rivard CH: Proliferative and matrix synthesis response of canine anterior cruciate ligament fibroblasts submitted to combined growth factors. J Orthop Res 14:200, 1996.
45. Scherping SCJ, Schmidt CC, Georgescu HI, et al: Effect of growth factors on the proliferation of ligament fibroblasts from skeletally mature rabbits. Connect Tissue Res 36:1, 1997.
46. Menetrey J, Kasemkijwattana C, Day CS, et al: Direct, fibroblast and myoblast mediated gene transfer to the anterior cruciate ligament. J Tissue Engineering 5:435, 1999.
47. Gerich TG, Lobenhoffer HP, Fu FH, et al: Virally mediated gene transfer in the patellar tendon: An experimental study in rabbits. Unfallchirurg 100:354, 1997.
48. Hildebrand KA, Deie M, Allen CR, et al: Early expression of marker genes in the rabbit medial collateral and anterior cruciate ligaments: The use of different viral vectors and the effects of injury. J Orthop Res 17:37, 1999.
49. Nakamura N, Shino K, Natsuume T, et al: Early biological effect of in vivo gene transfer of platelet-derived growth factor (PDGF)-B into healing patellar ligament. Gene Ther 5:1165, 1998.
50. Natsuume T, Nakamura N, Shino K, et al: In vivo introduction of hepatocyte growth factor/scatter factor (HGF/SF) into healing patellar ligament. Oral presentation at the 44th Annual Meeting, ORS, March 16, 1999, New Orleans, LA.
51. Gerich TG, Kang R, Fu FH, et al: Gene transfer to the patellar tendon. Knee Surg Sports Traumatol Arthrosc 5:118, 1997.
52. DeHaven KE: Meniscus repair. Am J Sports Med 27:242, 1999.
53. Arnoczky SP, Warren RF: The microvasculature of the meniscus and its response to injury: An experimental study in the dog. Am J Sports Med 11:131, 1983.
54. Bolano LE, Grana WA: Isolated arthroscopic partial meniscectomy: Functional radiographic evaluation at five years. Am J Sports Med 21:432, 1993.
55. Arnoczky SP, Warren RF, Spivak JM: Meniscal repair using an exogenous fibrin clot: An experimental study in dogs. J Bone Joint Surg Am 70:1209, 1988.
56. Webber RJ, Zitaglio T, Hough AJJ: Serum-free culture of rabbit meniscal fibrochondrocytes: Proliferative response. J Orthop Res 6:13, 1988.
57. Hashimoto J, Kurosaka M, Yoshiya S, et al: Meniscal repair using fibrin sealant and endothelial cell growth factor: An experimental study in dogs. Am J Sports Med 20:537, 1992.
58. Goto H, Shuler FD, Niyibizi C, et al: Gene transfer to meniscal lesion: TGF-ß1 gene retrovirally transduced into meniscal fibrochondrocytes upregulates matrix synthesis. Oral presentation at the ISAKOS Congress, May 29–June 2, 1999, Washington, DC.
59. Attia B, Bhargava MM, Dolan M, et al: Effect of cytokines on proliferation and migration of bovine meniscal cells. Poster presentation at the 43rd Annual Meeting, ORS, February 9, 1999, San Francisco, CA.
60. Shirakura K, Niijima M, Kobuna Y, et al: Free synovium promotes meniscal healing: Synovium, muscle and synthetic mesh compared in dogs. Acta Orthop Scand 68:51, 1997.
61. Kasemkijwattana C, Menetrey J, Goto H, et al: The use of growth factors, gene therapy and tissue engineering to improve meniscal healing. Poster presentation at the 45th Annual Meeting, ORS, February 1, 1999, Anaheim, CA.
62. Jorgensen U, Sonne-Holm S, Lauridsen F, et al: Long-term follow-up of meniscectomy in athletes: A prospective longitudinal study. J Bone Joint Surg Br 69:80, 1987.
63. de Boer HH, Koudstaal J: Failed meniscus transplantation: A report of three cases. Clin Orthop 306:155, 1994.
64. Noyes FR: A histological study of failed human meniscal allografts. Oral presentation at Speciality Day, Arthroscopy Association of North America, February 19, 1995, Orlando, FL.
65. Seneviratne AM, Suzuki K, Warren RF, et al: The basic biology of meniscus allograft transplantation in humans. Poster presentation at the 45th Annual Meeting, ORS, February 1, 1999, Anaheim, CA.
66. Natsuume T, Nakamura N, Shino K, et al: In vivo introduction of hepatocyte growth factor/scatter factor (HGF/SF) into healing patellar ligament. Oral presentation at the 44th Annual Meeting, ORS, March 16, 1998, New Orleans, LA.
67. Powell C, Shansky J, Del Tatto M, et al: Tissue-engineered human bioartificial muscles expressing a foreign recombinant protein for gene therapy. Hum Gene Ther 10:565, 1999.
68. Lieberman JR, Le LQ, Wu L: Regional gene therapy with a BMP-2 producing stromal cell line induces heterotopic and orthotopic bone formation in rodents. J Orthop Res 16:330, 1998.
69. Lou J, Xu F, Merkel K, et al: Gene therapy: Adenovirus-mediated human bone morphogenetic protein-2 gene transfer induces mesenchymal progenitor cell proliferation and differentiation in vitro and bone formation in vivo. J Orthop Res 17:43, 1999.
70. Baltzer AWA, Evans CH, Whalen JD, et al: Bone healing induced by adenoviral based gene therapy with BMP-2 and TGF beta. Poster presentation at the 45th Annual Meeting, ORS, February 1, 1999, Anaheim, CA.

SECTION VII

Plastic Surgery

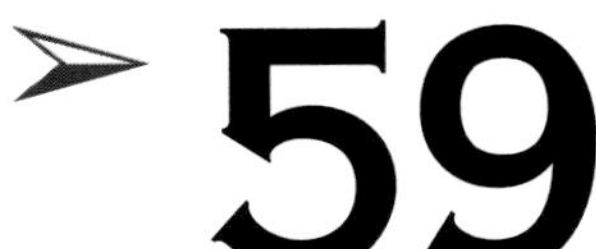

Soft-Tissue Considerations About the Knee: Prevention and Treatment of Problems

FRED D. CUSHNER • SUSAN CRAIG SCOTT • W. NORMAN SCOTT

INTRODUCTION

Paramount to a successful total knee arthroplasty (TKA) is appropriate wound healing. Failure to obtain appropriate healing not only thwarts the goals of early mobilization and rapid rehabilitation, but also can lead to complications such as prosthesis infection, need for further reconstructive surgical procedures, prolonged hospitalizations, and failed expectations from the patient and physician. This chapter will focus on the prevention, early recognition, and treatment options.

VASCULAR ANATOMY

The blood supply of the anterior soft tissue to the knee is made up of perforating arteries from numerous vessels[1–5] (Fig. 59.1). Studies have been undertaken to evaluate this blood supply, which consists of six main arteries that make up an extraosseous parapatellar anastomotic ring.[1–5] These vessels would include the medial and lateral superior genicular vessels, medial and lateral inferior genicular vessels, and a supreme genicular and anterior tibial recurrent artery. There is also a branch of the profunda femoris that adds to this anastomotic ring. The origin of the superior and inferior vessels is the popliteal artery. These branches supply the skin soft tissue envelope in the immediate proximity to the joint including the local skin. Should interruption of these vessels occur in the presence of local ischemic conditions, potential anastomotic communications may occur.[6]

In addition to the above intrinsic vessels, there are three additional extrinsic vessels. The first are branches from the profunda femoris. These branches not only supply the rectus femoris, vastus intermedius, and vastus lateralis but also send, via the dermal plexus, perforating branches to the superior region of the inferior skin.

The second extrinsic vessel is the supreme genicular vessel. This is a branch of the superficial femoral artery that travels through the adductor canal before dividing into two branches; the musculoarticular branch as well as the saphenous artery. It is the musculoarticular branch that runs medially in the vastus medialis, later to supply the medial aspect of the joint as well as the medial and superior aspect of overlying skin. The saphenous artery branch travels inferiorly and goes inferior to the sartorius tendon. This vessel ends in a terminal vessel that supplies the skin just below the medial tibial plateau.

A third extrinsic vessel is a recurrent branch of the anterior tibial artery. This is a branch of the popliteal artery that eventually joins the lateral inferior genicular artery and supplies the skin overlying and lateral to the patellar ligament.

It therefore can be seen that this vasculature is a plentiful random blood supply that, in most cases, can tolerate a single incision. Unfortunately, not all incisions for total knee arthroplasty (TKA) are primary or free of previous incisions or compromised local conditions. An understanding of this vascular anatomy is needed, as well as the risk factors noted below, to help avoid compromise of the overlying skin.

PREVENTION OF WOUND PROBLEMS

The blood supply to the anterior skin is a random plentiful blood supply that exists under most circumstances without compromise. Most knees without previous surgery can tolerate a single midline incision such as performed for TKA. Unfortunately, the fact is that it can jeopardize a patient's normal healing. Recognition of a compromised skin tissue envelope before surgery can aid in the detection of healing problems before they occur. Prevention of wound problems can be divided into the diagnosis of systemic factors as well as local knee factors that could lead to skin compromise at the time of the indicated TKA.

Patient Systemic Factors

It is standard to perform a thorough medical history as well as a physical examination prior to performing a TKA. While often this is done at the time of preadmission testing with emphasis placed on pulmonary and cardiac status, the patient must also be assessed for wound healing potential.

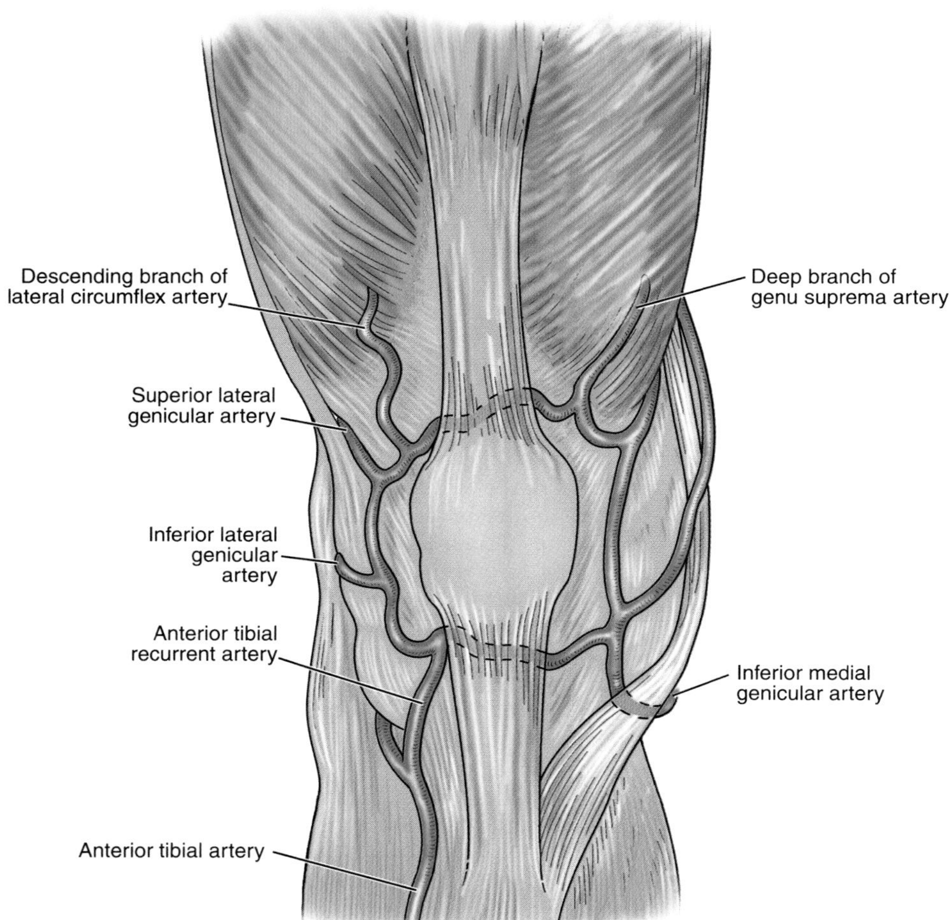

FIGURE 59.1 ➢ Blood supply.

Vascular status is a factor that may play a role in postoperative wound healing. While preoperative x-ray films easily show a varus or valgus deformity, careful review may also demonstrate calcified popliteal vessels and signs of arterial sclerosis despite palpable pulses. A vascular surgery consult may be necessary to decide if vascular reconstruction is necessary and to determine if changes in the normal TKA protocol are needed. For example, in some instances it may be deemed necessary to perform the TKA without the use of a tourniquet, whereas in patients with a previous vascular reconstruction, intravenous heparin may be needed intraoperatively to help keep the graft patent and free of thrombus. The heparin can be reversed intraoperatively before tourniquet deflation.

Aside from vascular status, other systemic factors must be addressed. Anemia has long been thought to play a role in wound healing[7, 8] with patients with a hematocrit less than 35% thought to be in jeopardy for a wound healing failure.[9] Anemia may play a role through a decreased oxygen tension at the wound edges.[10, 11] A nutritional component may also exist especially in cases in which a deficiency causes anemia to be present. Hypovolemia may also be associated with anemia and may be another factor to consider, but not all authors agree.[9] Heughan concluded that anemia is well tolerated in an otherwise healthy individual and that a mild or moderate anemia in these healthy patients would not have impaired oxygen delivery to their wounds. This author did not think that preoperative transfusions to aid in wound healing were necessary.[9] This does not mean that anemia should be ignored; treatable causes of anemia such as deficiency anemia should be addressed.

It is now protocol for our patients to receive a complete blood cell count prior to booking their TKA. As indicated in more detail in other chapters of this text, anemia is addressed and erythropoietin supplementation is initiated before surgery. The goal is to avoid disease transmission associated with allogeneic transfusions and the immunosuppression effect.

The nutritional status of the patient may also play a role in wound healing. In the severe nutritional deficiency states, protein is still necessary to aid in proper healing. Decreased albumin levels ($<$3.5 g/dL) as well as total leucocyte count ($<$1500) may make a patient more prone to wound failure.[12, 13] Although it is unlikely that a patient will present with severe nutritional deficiency at the time of the TKA, even more mild forms should be corrected prior to this elective procedure.

Obesity is another nutritional factor that may play a role in placing a patient more at risk for wound healing difficulty.[14, 15] Technically, exposure is more difficult in a markedly obese patient. The thickness of the outermost tissue layer as well as physical limitations on flexion of the limb may lead to more vigorous skin retraction that could lead to soft-tissue devascularization. Wong and colleagues[16] found a direct relationship between obesity and poor wound healing, whereas other studies have shown delayed healing and an increase in wound drainage postoperatively.[14] This does not mean that total knee arthroplasty should not be performed in an obese patient. Two studies performed in our institution that address the TKA and the obese patient are as follows: Stein and Insall found a higher incidence of patellofemoral pain (30% versus 14%) for obese patients but no difference in wound complications was noted.[17] A 10-year follow-up on this same series of patients was performed, and once again there was no increased revision rate or wound difficulties noted.[18] Since controlling obesity prior to surgery is extremely difficult, perhaps emphasis should be placed on meticulous surgical technique, adequate exposure, and proper skin handling. The use of heavy-toothed forceps, crushing clamps, or excessive retraction should be avoided. This helps to not push borderline but viable skin to compromise. Continuous retraction should not be performed, and the sustained crushing effect of retractors should be avoided. Continued retraction can increase local edema and compromise blood flow.

One potentially correctable systemic factor is cigarette smoking. Aside from its pulmonary effects, cigarette smoking can play a role in wound healing. By having a direct inhibitory effect on the microcirculation of the dermis, skin circulation can be compromised.[19, 20, 21] This occurs via the vasoconstrictor effect of nicotine as well as its byproduct cotinine.[2] Cotinine has a long half-life in a patient's body fat; therefore, cessation of smoking must be undertaken at least 3 weeks before surgery to eliminate its vasoconstrictor effects.[19, 20, 21]

Some medical illnesses may also play a role in wound healing. These may be difficult to separate because numerous patients may have several of these conditions. For example, a patient may have diabetes as well as obesity, but in separating wound healing factors and wound healing problems, these patients might be multifactorial.

Diabetes has long been thought to be associated with delays in wound healing. Wong and associates[16] demonstrated a delay in wound healing in the diabetic patient with increase in wound separation, erythema, and/or swelling noted. It has been postulated that delayed collagen synthesis and delayed wound tensile strength may play a role in the phenomenon. The mechanism may also be multifactorial because both small and large vessels may show signs of peripheral vascular disease.

Wilson and coworkers[14] looked at risk factors for infection following TKA, and diabetes was noted to not be a significant risk factor in this group.

Rheumatoid arthritis patients may be at more risk for wound healing problems.[22] This effect may also be multifactorial, with anemia, nutritional status, and steroid use as possible factors. Wong and associates[16] found a 30% increase in wound complication in rheumatoid arthritis patients compared with an osteoarthritic group. Garner and associates[23] did not have similar results, with no delays in healing noted. It may be the corticosteroids used to treat the rheumatoid arthritis that is the most important factor in wound healing problems in rheumatoid arthritic patients. Wilson showed increased infection rates with a rheumatoid arthritic patient but only in those treated with corticosteroids.[14] It is our experience that rheumatoid arthritic patients may have atrophic skin, and caution should be used when placing adherent drapes as well as in removing them.

This leads to one last factor, systemic medications. As mentioned, the use of corticosteroids may interfere with the healing process at several points in the healing cycle.[2, 22, 24] A decrease in fibroblast proliferation as well as a reduction of collagen clearance from the healing wound may be noted with corticosteroid use.[25, 26] Garner and coworkers looked at the role of long-term steroid use (more than 3 years), and a higher rate of infection and wound healing delay was noted with steroid use.[23] Since often it is not possible to eliminate corticosteroids from the therapeutic treatment of rheumatoid arthritis, the surgeon should be aware of their usage and appropriate skin care should be followed.

Other factors have been postulated to play a role in the occurrence of wound healing delays. Although age, gender, nonsteroidal anti-inflammatory drug usage, and surgical blood loss have been evaluated, no direct relationship has been noted between these factors and delayed wound healing.

Local Factors

Just as systemic patient conditions may play a role in wound healing, so may local factors present at the operative site. Local factors include not only previously placed skin incisions but also factors such as the degree of deformity, rotational component of the deformity, skin adherence, or previous skin trauma such as burns (Fig. 59.2). Previously placed skin incisions may be present from a high tibial osteotomy as well as open medial or lateral meniscectomies, open fracture management, or newer cartilage transplantation procedures. Numerous studies have shown an increase of wound healing difficulties in these knees with numerous incisions.[2, 27] Problems can arise from an avascular skin bridge between the new and previous incision, but may also be related to decreased subcutaneous tissue with its decrease in elasticity secondary to skin adherence. The treatment of skin with a compromised local environment will be discussed in other areas of this chapter.

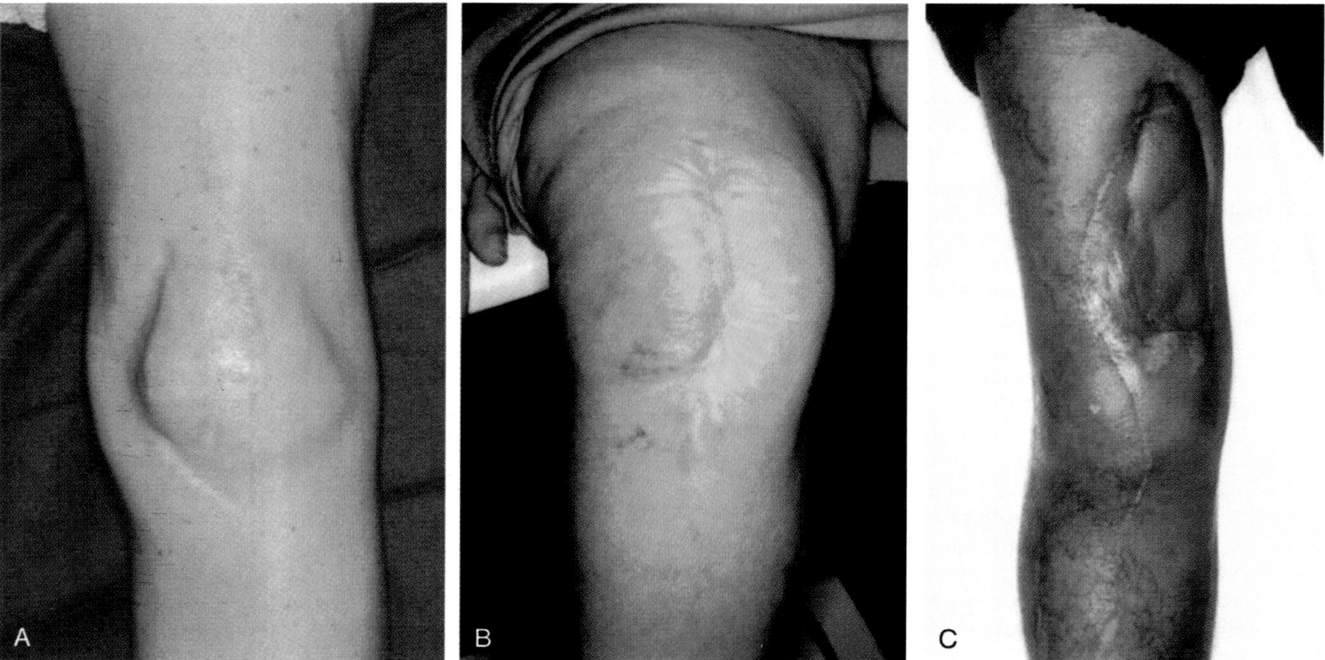

FIGURE 59.2 ➢ Local factors that may play a role in wound healing: numerous previous incisions, adherent skin, previous trauma such as burns.

Surgical Technique Factors

Although systemic as well as local factors may be identified prior to surgery, often little can be done to correct these conditions. However, surgical technique can be modified to enhance wound healing potential and aid in the prevention of wound healing problems. Starting with the knee approach, an adequate skin incision should be chosen. This enhances exposure and aids in avoidance of excessive skin retraction. Care should be taken in the handling of the skin edges and in preservation of the subcutaneous fascial layer. Large flaps are not necessary and should be avoided. Ideally, no lateral flap is needed, but occasionally adhesions can be encountered in the subcutaneous layer with valgus deformities that may require a surgical release. Therefore, should a flap be necessary, it should be as minimal and as deep as possible to preserve the blood supply to this dermal plexus.

Lateral release rate is important because numerous studies have shown that the patients receiving a lateral retinacular release show a decrease in skin oxygen tension at the healing wound edges, resulting in increased risk of wound complications.[10] Although proper component position, patella thickness, and component rotation may decrease the lateral release rate, a lateral release may still be necessary. By preserving the superior genicular vessel, some of these skin healing problems may be avoided.[10]

An understanding of the vascular anatomy shows that the lateral retinacular release with its standard medial parapatellar approach will transect with the medial and lateral genicular vessels, including both the superior and inferior branches. Johnson and Eastwood[10] noted a decrease in skin oxygen tension when a lateral release was performed. The rate of superficial drainage and infection rates was also increased in those patients undergoing a lateral release. If a lateral flap is necessary, a large flap should be avoided. We prefer an all-inside approach with minimal flap to help seal the postoperative hemarthrosis into the joint itself. A large lateral flap in conjunction with a lateral release may allow the postoperative hematoma to travel to the subcutaneous level, leading to pressure on the skin from the hematoma as well as prolonged drainage.

With no previous incision, the midline approach is used; a correct skin incision is paramount to preventing wound-healing difficulties. Johnson and associates[28, 29] evaluated skin oxygen tension for a variety of incisions and concluded that a medial side circulation predominance did exist within the cutaneous circulation. Therefore, the lateral wound edges showed lower oxygen tension initially as well as during the immediate postoperative period. By postoperative day 8, the preoperative levels were noted to return to normal. This is just another reason why large lateral flaps should be avoided. With previous placed skin incisions, the initial incision becomes more difficult, but these incisions may not always be avoided. If avoidance is not possible, an attempt is made to incorporate the new incision within the old. Transverse incisions can be crossed in most instances at 90-degree angles with little or no threat of local skin compromise.[30, 31, 32] A wide scar with minimal subcutaneous tissue may be at risk because this may disrupt the underlying dermal plexus.[30] Treatment includes avoiding these areas or using tissue expanders as discussed below. The distance between the skin incisions may also put the knee at risk.[33] If a skin bridge is less than 2.5 cm, once again, tissue expanders should be considered. All closure sutures are not equal, with 20% more reaction noted when the subcuticular layer was closed with polydioxane rather than polyglycolic suture material.[34]

Surgical integrity of the medial retinaculum must be maintained during the postoperative period. Flexion of the knee after closure of the retinaculum is a quick way to evaluate suture integrity. Should sutures break under direct visualization, they can be replaced prior to closure of the more superficial layers. Loss of retinaculum integrity may play a role in the prevention of postoperative hematoma. It should be noted that absorbable sutures become significantly weaker during the first week following surgery. For example, Monocryl (Ethicon, Somerville, NJ) retains only 60% to 70% of its original strength at 7 days whereas coated Vicryl suture (Ethicon, Somerville, NJ) retains 75% of its original strength at 14 days postoperatively. Newer sutures such as Panacryl suture (Ethicon, Inc. Somerville, NJ) maintain 80% of their original strength up to 3 months following the procedure[35] (Fig. 59.3).

If closure is difficult at the time of surgery, new skin closure systems are available (Suiz-Closure, Zimmer, Warsaw, IN) that stretch the skin, increasing its elasticity for an easier closure (Fig. 59.4).

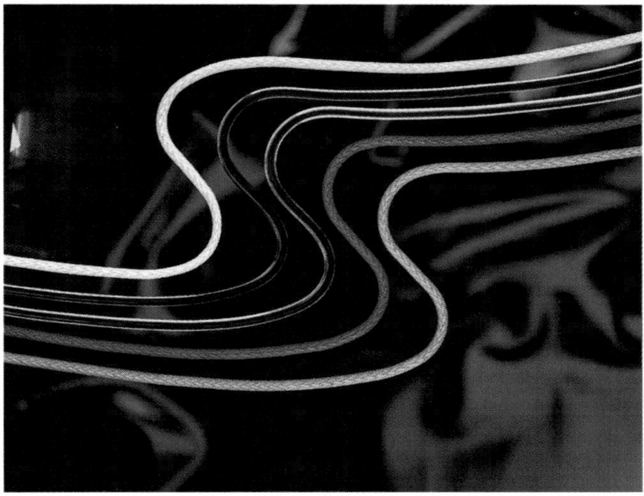

FIGURE 59.3 ➢ Sutures vary in design, absorption, and strength at postoperative intervals.

Postoperative Factors

Discussion of the prevention of wound healing problems would not be complete without addressing postoperative factors. Avoidance of hemarthrosis is thought to be very important in decreasing wound healing problems. A large hematoma can serve as a culture medium for infection, but local skin compromise may occur from pressure on the subcutaneous tissue. At our institution, a tourniquet deflation is performed

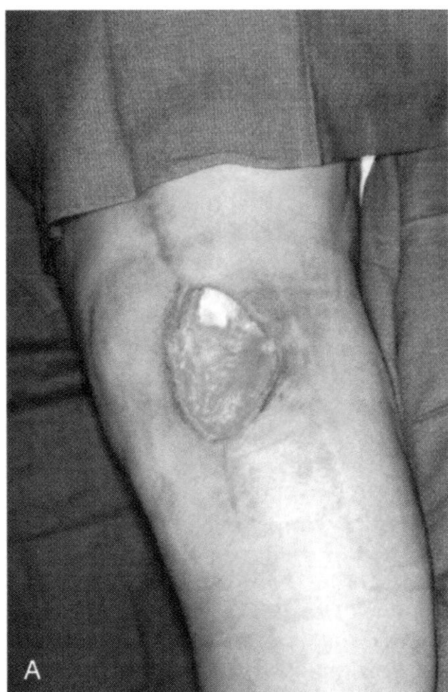

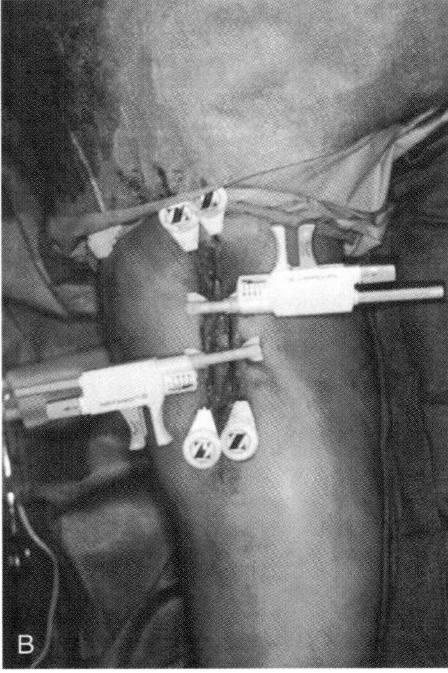

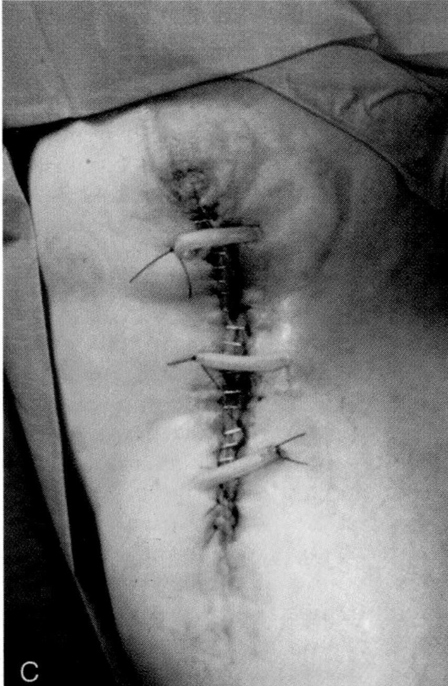

FIGURE 59.4 ➢ A defect closed with the aid of a skin stretching system. *A,* The defect. *B,* Clamps in place. *C,* The wound at closure.

prior to closure. This is done to visualize and cauterize perforating arteries that may lead to the hemarthrosis formation. This is not a universal finding—other authors have concluded that intraoperative tourniquet deflation leads to increased bleeding compared with tourniquet deflation at the close of the case.[36] Abdel-Salem and Byres formed a prospective randomized study where no tourniquet was used.[37] Other authors concluded that despite a higher blood loss over the control group, the no-tourniquet group showed less postoperative pain and fewer infections.[37]

Regarding postoperative hemarthrosis, another controversy is use of postoperative drains. Holt and coworkers examined blood loss and wound problems in drained and undrained knees, noting 40% of the undrained knees and 0% of the drained knees required dressing reinforcement.[38] It should be noted that the undrained knees also had a higher incidence of ecchymosis. These authors concluded that drains are effective in preventing the accumulation of blood in the surrounding soft tissues. Not all authors agree with these conclusions; Crevoisier and colleagues[39] concluded that there is no advantage of closed suction drain usage. They examined 32 patients and divided them into a drained and undrained group and found no difference between the two cohorts. This was a small study, probably of insufficient size, to draw a definitive conclusion on a risk of wound infections because it occurs in less than 1% of cases. Ovadin and associates[40] evaluated 58 knees that were also divided into the drained and undrained group. Although there was little difference in the rate of infection, there was more serous drainage in the undrained group. Therefore, at our institution we use postoperative drains, not only for hemarthrosis avoidance but also reinfusion benefits. With the use of reinfusion drains, the allogenic transfusion rate has been reduced to approximately 2% for the unicompartmental knee. Drains were removed on the first postoperative day as prophylaxis antibiotics ended. Drinkwater and coworkers has shown a decrease in bacterial colonization when drains are removed during this 24-hour period.[41]

Some concern has been raised over bleeding complications with postoperative deep venous thrombosis prophylaxis. It should be noted that bleeding complications have been noted with placebo as well as low-molecular-weight heparin and warfarin usage. Stulberg and associates[42] evaluated 638 total knee arthroplasties and noticed a wound complication rate of 18.1%, with 10.6% having culture-negative drainage. Increased bleeding has also been noted with low-molecular-weight heparin, with bleeding complications of 2% to 5% noted in the literature.[43, 44, 45] It should be noted that bleeding problems are multifactorial and perhaps some wound complications could be avoided with careful hemostasis, proper dosing of agents, and meticulous closure.

Continued passive motion (CPM) has been advocated as a method to increase knee range of motion following TKA, and its usage is common at many institutions. Johnson showed a decrease in skin oxygen tension when the CPM past 40 degrees was used during the first three days following the procedure.[46] This is not universal in that Yashar[47] found no increased wound problems with the accelerated flexion program. In these patients, 70 to 100 degrees was used immediately in the recovery room and no increased wound problems were present. Although immediate CPM is used commonly without difficulty, patients with compromised skin circulation or compromised local environment perhaps would benefit from a slower rehabilitation protocol compared with those who are not at risk.

It can be seen that wound complications can be prevented or decreased by understanding the vascularity that exists to the anterior skin envelope. Recognition of systemic, local, surgical, and postoperative factors may lead to the prevention of wound-healing problems.

TREATMENT

Obviously the best form of treatment is the prevention of wound problems before they occur. In the preceding discussions, the systemic factors, local factors, and postoperative protocols may all play a role in wound healing. If prevention fails, the surgeon is left with treating the wound complication while still attempting preservation of the prosthesis with acceptable range of motion and function. Treatment is, therefore, dependent on the type of wound complication: serous drainage, tense hematoma, superficial soft-tissue necrosis, and full-thickness necrosis. Of course, these complications can occur with and without the presence of infection (other chapters of this text are dedicated to the discussion of infection). Obviously when dealing with wound compromise, infection must be ruled out as well as prevented from developing through local wound care and aggressive, but correct, antibiotic usage.

Prevention

Because not all factors can be corrected before surgery and not even the best of surgeons can erase the effect of previously placed incisions, suspect knees can be treated preoperatively with a tissue expander technique. Gold and colleagues reported on the first 10 patients using this technique at our institution.[48] This study gradually expanded the skin envelope over an average of 64.5 days, and all wounds healed without incident. To date more than 30 knees have been treated pre-TKA with tissue expansion. This has become our method of choice when a knee shows evidence of local soft-tissue compromise. We use soft-tissue expansion when it is believed that the quality and viability of soft tissue are compromised. This may be secondary to previously placed numerous incisions or secondary to trauma that caused increased adherence of the skin to the tibial plateau below. Granted, these criteria for using soft-tissue expanders may be subjective, but any patient with adherent immobile skin or numerous previously placed incisions is considered a candidate for this procedure. Severe angular deformities with a rotational deformity are also candidates for this procedure. This is necessary since on correction of increased angular deformities, insufficient skin coverage, once appropriate alignment is maintained, may occur. We have been quite happy with the use of tissue expanders and no longer use the "sham" incision. This was employed in the past for those patients with increased risk of wound necrosis. A plain incision was made and performed to the depth of the subcutaneous tissue. Skin flaps were elevated and the wound was closed in a standard fashion. The wound was then observed for its healing potential: If it healed without incident, a TKA could be performed with greater confidence. If the wound failed, local measures were used to obtain healing without the added pressures of an exposed prosthesis. This is mentioned for historical review, and due to the success of tissue expansion, we no longer advocate this technique.

TECHNIQUE OF TISSUE EXPANSION

Tissue expanders are placed in the operating room under local anesthesia. We currently use a mixture of Xylocaine (.05%) and 1:1,000,000 epinephrine. Approximately 300 mL is injected into the subcutaneous space. This is continued until the subcutaneous tissue blanches. A small incision is then made in line with a planned TKA. We typically use two 200-mL expanders, which are placed 90 degrees to each other. Placement of the tissue expanders can be adjusted to accommodate the local skin conditions. A subcutaneous pocket is then created and the tissue expander balloon is inserted. Once in place, the patient is admitted for 24 hours and the knee immobilized for 1 week. After 1 week gradual expansion is begun and an average of 10% of the expander volume is inserted weekly. Capillary refill, less than 5 seconds, and patient comfort are monitored. The expander volume to be injected can be increased if tolerated by the patient. At the time of revision, we prefer to wait 2 weeks from the last expander injections. These expanders are easily removed at the time of surgery through the planned arthrotomy incision. It is our experience that skin is plentiful following tissue expanders usage and, although trimming of excess skin is possible, it is often not needed (Fig. 59.5). We currently recommend subcutaneous drains to be placed to decrease hematoma formation in the previously expanded pocket. Once the skin has been expanded, a choice of using the old incision or creating a new one exists. When possible the incision deemed most adequate is used. We have found that the tissue expanders enhance the vascularity of the flap safely around the old incision to be utilized. If the prior incision is not adequate, then a new longitudinal incision can be chosen. If when fin-

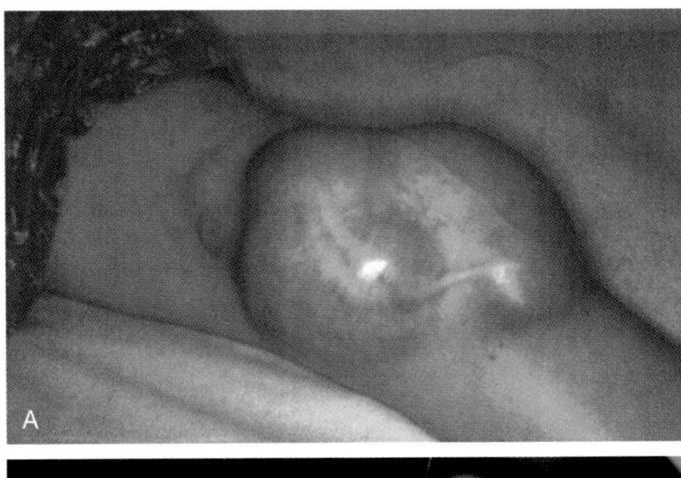

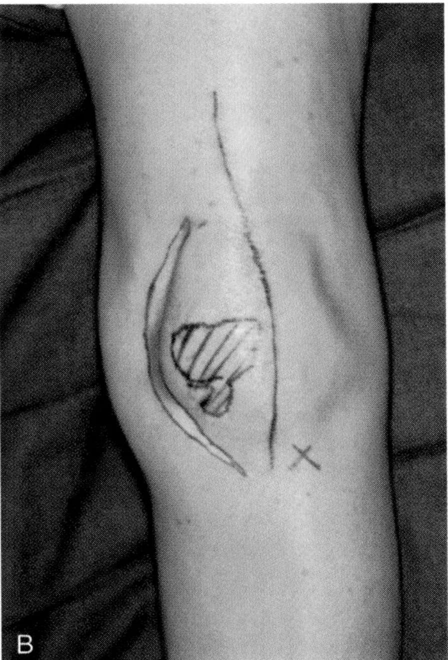

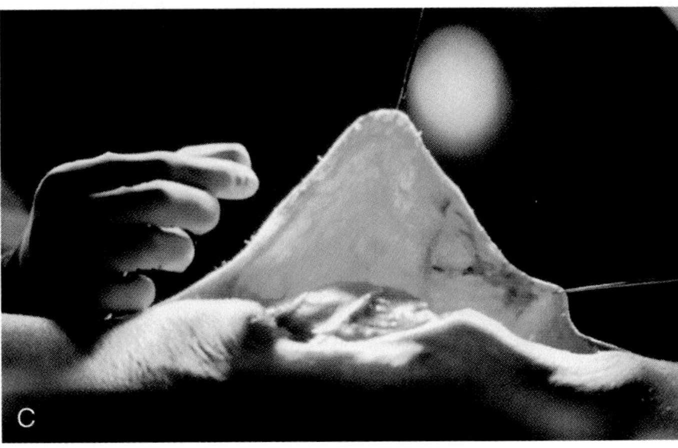

FIGURE 59.5 ➢ Preoperative use of tissue expanders. *A*, Knee with numerous previous incisions. *B*, Tissue expanders in place. *C*, Abundant skin available at time of TKA.

ished, excess skin is present, the skin bridge between the prior incision and the new incision can be excised and the remaining skin edges reapproximated. We have found that this is often not necessary.

This technique has been successful before the TKA; case reports of success are seen in revision TKA,[49, 50] and infected TKA revision is reported. By allowing primary closure without tension, this technique allows for the ability to perform standard rehabilitation protocols as well as immediate postoperative range of motion. More important, more invasive procedures can be avoided. Others have found the technique useful in wound difficulties. Riederman and Noyes[51] described the use of the tissue expanders in five patients with severe patellofemoral arthrosis. In these patients, tissue expanders were used before a McKay osteotomy because of previously placed incisions, and no complications over the wounds were noted.

While potential complications such as hematoma, infection, prosthesis exposure, and prosthesis failure do exist, with this technique they can be limited. Benefits include allowing primary closure without tension as well as immediate range of motion and ability to use CPM. Following the use of tissue expanders, standard rehabilitation protocol is followed and reconstructive procedures such as flap coverage are avoided.

Prolonged Serous Drainage

Prolonged serous drainage can occur after TKA. The question that remains for all surgeons is when to explore this wound. Often other factors such as excessive erythema or purulence may lead to wound exploration, but when these are not present the wounds can initially be observed. The cause of this prolonged drainage may be secondary to a large hematoma, and if drainage is not resolved in 5 to 7 days, surgical evaluation may become necessary. Hematoma may adversely affect the wound as any increasing soft-tissue

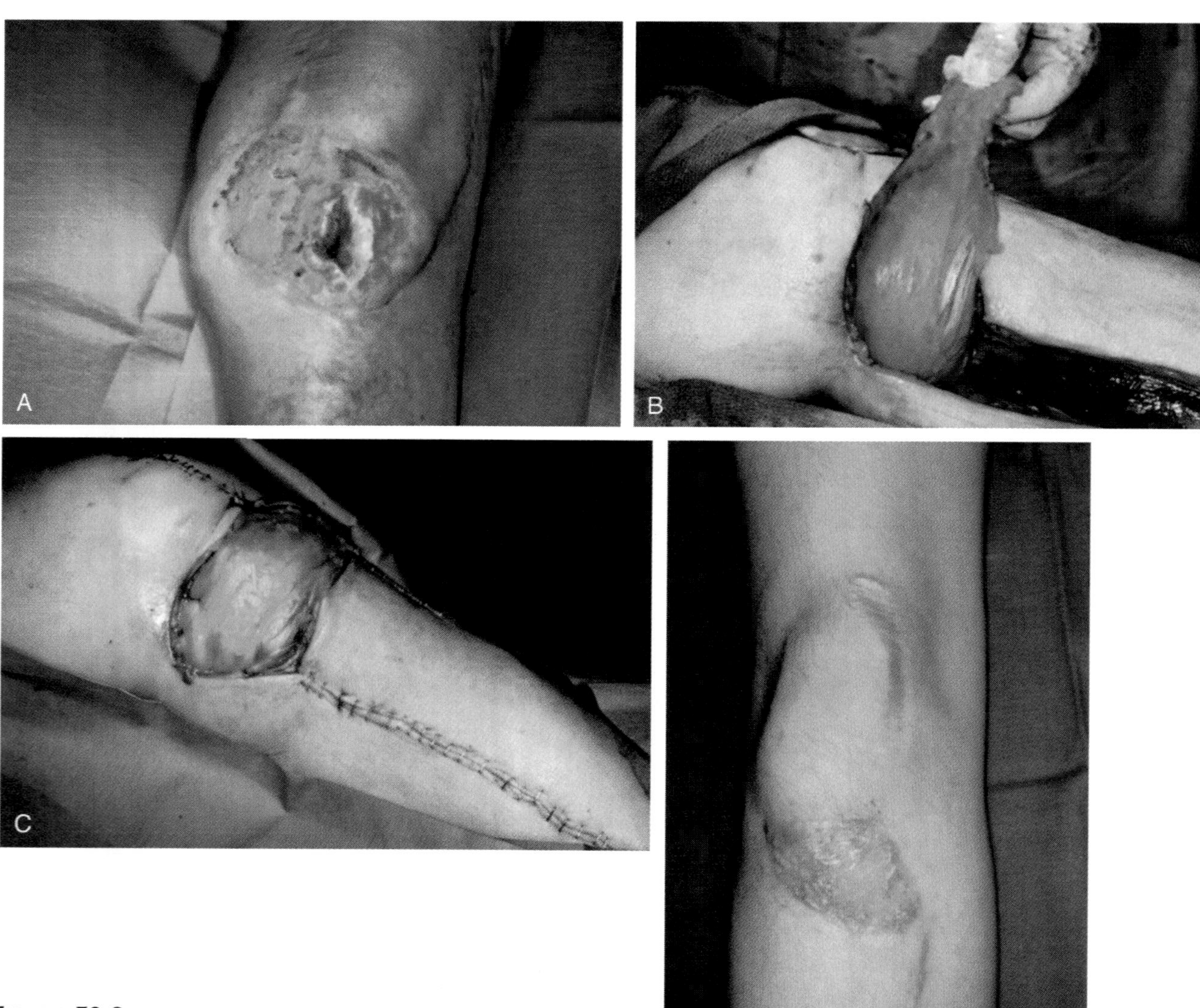

FIGURE 59.6 ➢ Use of gastrocnemius flap. *A*, Anterior eschar with exposed prosthesis. *B*, The flap is rotated to provide coverage. *C*, Flap in place. *D*, The healed flap.

tension can. The toxic breakdown of hemoglobin may also play a role in wound healing difficulties. While prolonged drainage occurs, physical therapy and CPM may be limited. It should be noted that not all prolonged drainage is noninfected; 17% to 50% of chronically draining wounds show later evidence of infection.[52, 53, 54] It is for this reason that not all authors agree with this observation of prolonged draining wounds. Weiss and Krackow[52] reported on early intervention with eight draining TKAs and concluded that early intervention may prevent a deep-tissue prosthetic infection.

Deep Tissue Hematoma

Although a tense hematoma that is not draining can occur, once again, initial observation can be performed. With any signs of local skin compromise, increased pain, or limited range of motion, surgical exploration can be performed. CPM and physical therapy may be limited during this period. The patient's pain and limited range of motion may lead to earlier drainage of the hematoma, so normal postoperative protocol may be followed.

Superficial Soft-Tissue Necrosis

Superficial infections can be classified as wound lesions that do not penetrate to the level of the prosthesis and bone. This category is general and will include the benign stitch abscess that improves with suture débridement and dressing changes and the superficial soft-tissue infection secondary to cellulitis. A superficial infection should be treated aggressively, with cultures changed prior to the initiation of antibiotics for a presumed organism. With the presence of superficial soft-tissue necrosis, CPM and physical therapy should be discontinued. Clinically it is difficult to separate a superficial from a deep necrosis, and surgical exploration may be necessary to evaluate for deep penetration.

Despite aggressive treatment, superficial infection may lead to skin necrosis. While initially necrosis less than 3 cm can be treated with local wound débridement under anesthesia and immobilization,[55] it is important that at the time of débridement, all dead tissue will be removed. If under surgical exploration the infection is noted to be superficial, then local wound débridement techniques may be adequate. If the prosthesis becomes exposed during débridement, the necrosis is judged to be no longer superficial, and treatment for a major skin necrosis is required.

Treatment of a superficial necrosis begins with local wound care. This can be through local débridement, observation, and appropriate antibiotic coverage.[2] During this period, when skin viability is plentiful, the wound can be found to declare itself. With no evidence of infection, tissue débridement can wait until the eschar separates. During this period the wound may be contracting. With contraction, the side of the wound coverage may decrease. Small wounds may be allowed to heal by secondary intention. The benefits of healing by secondary intention include avoidance of another surgical procedure as well as the ability to continue with range of motion. During secondary intention, both active and passive range of motion can be continued.

Skin grafting is indicated when the time for the untreated healing is longer than the healing of a routine skin grafting and the postoperative 5 to 7 days that accompany it. Skin graft viability requires penetration of vascular buds to the underlying wound bed; therefore, proper immobilization is needed. For the skin graft to heal, infection must also be controlled. The wounds should be followed closely and viability assessed.

A third option for the treatment of superficial necrosis is a local fasciocutaneous flap. Hallock[56] describes six patients in whom extratensial soft-tissue coverage was performed with this technique. The diagnosis of infection must be ruled out for this technique to work if infection cannot be noted.

Full-Thickness, Soft-Tissue Necrosis

Full-thickness, soft-tissue necrosis is the most serious of wound problems. This includes deep penetration of soft tissue and exposure of the bone and joint below. Coverage options involve major surgical reconstructions, and overall result of the TKA is therefore compromised. Options include advancement of local tissue or the transfer of distant tissue in the form of a free flap.[57, 58] Unfortunately, due to the complex nature of this problem, the prosthesis is often removed to treat the soft-tissue difficulties. Early plastic surgery intervention cannot be emphasized enough.[59]

Salvage with a gastrocnemius flap is well described in the orthopedic and the plastic surgery literature.[60, 61, 62, 63] Usually the medial head of the gastrocnemius muscle is used because of its wide arc of motion. It can be detached distally from its insertion on the Achilles tendon and rotated proximally. The lateral gastrocnemius can also be used especially for lateral wound difficulties. It is the medial gastrocnemius that is used for defects around the patella and tibial tubercle. These flaps can be utilized for necrosis in approximately two-thirds of the tibia, whereas the distal one-third tibial lesions require free flap coverage (Fig. 59.6).

For most knees in which gastrocnemius flaps are not adequate, such as large defects with an exposed prosthesis, coverage can be accomplished with a free-tissue transfer to the latissimus dorsi muscle, rectus abdominis muscle, or a scapular free flap. All these methods have been described and are reliable to obtain coverage.[2] Gerwin and coworkers[57] treated 12 patients with exposed prostheses with a medial gastrocnemius flap, and 92% healing was achieved.[57] A similar experience was noted by Markovich with muscle flap coverage.[50] Markovich and associates described the result of five latissimus dorsi free flaps, six medial gastrocnemius flaps, and two rectus abdomini free flaps with 100% wound revascularization noted.[58] Prosthesis retention was achieved in 83% of the cases. It is no surprise that the worst results were noted when flaps were used to treat an infected prosthesis.

More recently, Nahabedian and associates describe their 10-year results of 35 complex TKA wounds with aggressive wound management as an 83% prosthesis salvage rate and a 97% limb salvage rate.[64] The importance of early plastic surgery consultation, aggressive débridement, and early coverage cannot be overemphasized.

CONCLUSION

Wound problems are not always avoidable with TKA. Despite meticulous surgical technique, closure, and postoperative care, wound failure can occur. Early recognition is of utmost importance. The key is to identify those patients at risk of systemic, local, or surgical factors and to prevent local wound healing difficulties before they occur. When they do occur, aggressive early treatment is needed, and despite the occurrence of significant wound problems, both prosthesis retention and an acceptable long-term function can be achieved.

References

1. Scapinelli R: Studies on the vasculature of the human knee. Acta Anat 70:305, 1968.
2. Craig SM: Soft Tissue Considerations in the Failed Total Knee Arthroplasty. In Scott WN, ed: The Knee. St. Louis, Mosby-Yearbook, 1994, vol. 2, pp 1279-1295.
3. Abbott LC, Carpenter WF: Surgical approaches to the knee joint. J Bone Joint Surg 227:277, 1945.
4. Bjorkstrom S, Goldie IF: A study of the arterial supply of the patellae in the normal state, in chondromalacia, chondromalaica patellae and in osteonecrosis. Acta Orthop Scand 51:63, 1980.
5. Waisbrod H, Treiman N: Intra-osseous venography in patellofemoral disorders: A preliminary report. J Bone Joint Surg Br 62:454, 1980.
6. Taylor GI, Palmer JH: The vascular territories (angiosomes) of the body: Experimental study and clinical applications. Br J Plast Surg 40:113, 1987.
7. Arey LB: Wound Healing. Physiol. Rev. 16: 327, 1966
8. Glenn F, Moore SW: The Disruption of Abdominal Wounds. Surg. Gynec. Obstet. 72: 1041, 1941
9. Heughan C, Chir B, Grislis G, et al: The effect of anemia on wound healing. Ann Surg 179:163, 1974.
10. Johnson DD, Eastwood DM: Lateral patellar release in knee arthroplasty: Effect on wound healing. J Arthroplasty 7 (Supp):407, 1992.
11. Archauer BM, Black KS, Litke DK: Transcutaneous pO_2 in flaps: A new method of surgical prediction. Plast Reconst Surg 65:738, 1980.
12. Ecker ML, Lotke PA: Postoperative care of the total knee patient. Orthop Clin North Am 20:55, 1989.
13. Dickhaut SC, DeLee JL, Pase CP: Nutritional statistics. Importance in predicting wound healing after amputation. J Bone Joint Surg Am 66:71, 1984.
14. Wilson MG, Kelley K, Thornhill TS: Infection as a complication of total knee replacement arthroplasty: Risk factors and treatment in sixty-seven cases. J Bone Joint Surg Am 72:878, 1990.
15. Cruse PJ, Foord R: A five-year prospective study or 23,649 surgical wounds. Arch Surg 107:206, 1973.
16. Wong R, Lotke P, Ecker M: Factors influencing wound healing after total knee arthroplasty. Orthop Trans 10:497, 1986.
17. Stein SH, Insall JN: Total knee arthroplasty in obese patients. J Bone Joint Surg Am 72:1400, 1990.
18. Griffin FM, Scuderi GR, Insall JN, et al: Total knee arthroplasty in patients who were obese with 10 years follow-up. CORR 356: 28, 1998.
19. Benowitz NL, Jacob P III: Daily intake of nicotine during cigarette smoking. Clin Pharmacol Ther 35:494, 1984.
20. Benowitz NL, Kuyt F, Jacob P: Influence of nicotine on cardiovascular and hormonal effects of cigarette smoking. Clin Pharmacol Ther 36:74, 1984.
21. Benowitz NL: Cotinine disposition and effects. Clin Pharmacol Ther 34:664, 1983.
22. Klein NE, Cox LU: Wound problems in total knee arthroplasty. In Fu FH, Harner CD, Vince KG, et al, eds: Knee Surgery. Baltimore, Williams & Wilkins, 2nd vol 1994, pp 1539-1552.
23. Garner RW, Mowot AG, Hazleman BL: Wound healing after operations on patients with rheumatoid arthritis. J Bone Joint Surg Br 55:134, 1973.
24. Green JP: Steroid therapy and wound healing in surgical patients. BJ Surg 52:523, 1965.
25. Wahl LM: Hormonal resolution of macrophage collagenase activity. Biochem Biophys Res Commun 74:838, 1977.
26. Werb Z: Biochemical actions of glucocorticoids on macrophages in culture. J Exp Med 147:1695, 1978.
27. Grogan TJ, Dores F, Rolling J, et al: Deep sepsis following total knee arthroplasty. J Bone Joint Surg Am 687:226, 1986.
28. Johnson DD: Midline or parapatellar incision for knee arthroplasty. A comparative study of wound viability. J Bone Joint Surg Br 70:656, 1988.
29. Johnson DD, Houshton TA, Redford P: Anterior midline or medial parapatellar incision for arthroplasty of the knee. A comparative study. J Bone Joint Surg Br 68:812, 1986.
30. Dennis PA: Wound complications in total knee arthroplasty. Inst Course Lecture 46:165, 1997.
31. Ecker ML, Lotke PA: Wound healing complications. In Rand JA, ed: Total Knee Arthroplasty. New York, Raven Press, 1993, pp 403-407.
32. Windsor RE, Insall JN, Vince KE: Technical consideration of total knee arthroplasty after proximal tibial osteotomy. J Bone Joint Surg Am 70:547, 1988.
33. Rosenberg AG: Surgical technique of posterior cruciate sacrificing and preserving total knee arthroplasty. In Rand, JA, ed: Total Knee Arthroplasty. New York, Lippincott-Raven, 1993, p 115.
34. Casha JN: Suture reaction following skin closure with subcuticular polydionanone in total knee arthroplasty. J Arthrop 11:859, 1996.
35. Ethicon Wound Closure Manual, 1994 Ethicon, Inc. a Johnson & Johnson Co., Somerville, NJ. Product Information pp 126-131; Panacryl Suture Package Insert 389175.
36. Faralli VJ, Lotke PA, Orenstein E: Blood loss after total knee replacement: Effects of early motion. Presented at 55th annual meeting of AAOS, New Orleans, Feb. 1998.
37. Abdel-Salem, Byres KS: Effects of tourniquet during total knee arthroplasty. A prospective randomized study. J Bone Joint Surg Br 77:250, 1995.
38. Holt BT, Parks NL, Ensh GA, et al: Comparison of closed reduction drainage and no drainage after primary total knee arthroplasty. Orthopaedics 20:1121, 1997.
39. Crevoisier XM, Reber P, Noesberger B: Is suction drainage necessary after total knee joint arthroplasty? A prospective study. Arch Orthop Trauma Surg 117:121, 1998.
40. Ovadin D, Luger E, Bickels J, et al: Efficacy of closed wound drainage after total joint arthroplasty. A prospective randomized study. J. Arthroplasty 12:317, 1997.
41. Drinkwater CJ, Neil MJ: Optimal timing of wound drain removal following total joint arthroplasty. J Arthroplasty 10:185, 1995.
42. Stulberg BN, Insall JN, Williams GW, et al: Deep vein thrombosis following total knee replacement. J Bone Joint Surg Am 2:194, 1984.
43. Levine MN, Gent M, Hirsh J, et al: Ardeparin (low molecular weight heparin) vs. graduated compression stockings for the prevention of venous thromboembolism. A randomized trial in patients undergoing knee surgery. Arch Inter Med 156:851, 1996.
44. Leclerc JR, Geerts WN, DesJardins L, et al: Prevention of venous thromboembolism (WTE) after knee arthroplasty—A randomized double-blind trial comparing a low molecular-weight heparin fragment (enoxaparin) to warfarin. Blood 84:246a, 1992.
45. Spiro TE, Fitzgerald RH, Trowbridge AA, et al: Enoxaparin—A low molecular weight heparin and warfarin for the prevention

of venous thomboembolic disease after elective knee replacement surgery. Blood 84:246a, 1994.
46. Johnson DD: The effect of continuous passive motion on wound healing and joint mobility after total knee arthroplasty. J Bone Joint Surg Am 78:421, 1990.
47. Yashar AA: Continuous passive motion with accelerated flexion after total knee arthroplasty. Clin Orthop 345:38, 1997.
48. Gold DA, Scott SC, Scott WN: Soft tissue expansion prior to arthroplasty in the multiply operated knee—A new method of preventing catastrophic skin problems. J Arthroplasty 11:512, 1996.
49. Santore RF, Kaufman D, Robbins AJ, et al: Tissue expansion prior to revision total knee arthroplasty. J Arthroplasty 12:475, 1997.
50. Namba RS, Diao E: Tissue expansion for staged reimplantation of infected total knee arthroplasty. J Arthrop 12:471, 1997.
51. Riederman R, Noyes FR: Soft tissue skin expansion of contracted tissues prior to knee surgery. Am J Knee Surg 4:195, 1991.
52. Weiss AP, Krackow KA: Perisistent wound drainage after primary total knee arthroplasty. J Arthroplasty 8:285, 1993.
53. Bergstrom S, Krutson K, Lidgren L: Treatment of infected knee arthroplasty. Clin Orthop 245:173, 1989.
54. Insall J, Aglietti P: A five to seven-year follow-up of unicondylar arthroplasty. J Bone Joint Surg Am 62:1329, 1980.
55. Sculco TP: Local wound complications after total knee arthroplasty. In Ranawat C, ed: Total Condylar Knee Arthroplasty: Technique, Results and Complications. New York, Springer-Verlag, 1985, pp 194-196.
56. Hallock GG: Salvage of total knee arthroplasty with local fasciocutaneous flaps. J Bone Joint Surg Br 72:1236, 1990.
57. Gerwin M, Rothaus KU, Windsor RE, et al: Gastrocnemius muscle flap coverage of exposed or infected knee prosthesis. Clin Orthop 286:64, 1993.
58. Markovich G, Door LD, Klein NE, et al: Muscle flaps in knee arthroplasty. Clin Orthop 321:122, 1995.
59. Bergstrom S, Carlsson A, Relander M, et al: Treatment of the exposed knee prosthesis. Acta Orthop Scand 58:662, 1987.
60. Eckhardt JJ, Lesavoy MA, Dubrow TJ, et al: Exposed endo-prosthesis. Clin Orthop 251:220, 1990.
61. Hemphill CS, Ebert FR, Muench AG: The medial gastrocnemius muscle flap in the treatment of wound complications following total knee arthroplasty. Orthopaedics 15:477, 1992.
62. Peled IJ, Franki U, Wexler MR: Salvage of exposed knee prosthesis by gastrocnemius myocutaneous flap coverage. Orthopedics 6:1320, 1983.
63. Salibian AH, Sanford HA: Salvage of an infected total knee prosthesis with medial and lateral gastrocnemius muscle flaps. J Bone Joint Surg Am 6:681, 1983.
64. Nahabedian ML, Orlando JL, Delanois RE, et al: Salvage procedures for complex soft tissue defects of the knee. CORR 356: 119, 1998.

SECTION VIII

Fractures About the Knee

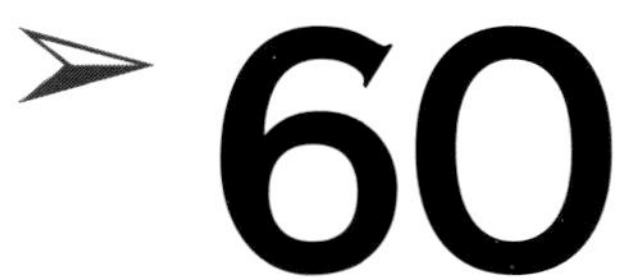

Supracondylar and Distal Femur Fractures

ANTHONY T. SORKIN • DAVID L. HELFET

RELEVANT ANATOMY

Bone

The distal femur traditionally refers to the lower third of the bone. Description of this anatomic area in the literature varies from the distal 7.6 to 15 cm of the femur.[1–4] The supracondylar (metaphyseal) area of the distal femur provides a unique transition between the cylindrical shape of the shaft (diaphysis) and the rhomboidal shape of the intracondylar (epiphyseal) area. It is in the supracondylar area that the distal femur flares, especially medially, to provide a stable platform for the articular condyles. The two condyles are separated anteriorly by a small, articular, longitudinal depression (trochlea) that articulates with the two facets of the patella. The femoral condyles are separated posteriorly by the intercondylar notch. The larger medial condyle has a readily identifiable tubercle on its medial surface for insertion of the adductor magnus.

The orientation and relationship of the shaft of the femur relative to the articular surface are important when considering management of fractures of the distal femur. In the coronal plane, the shaft of the femur is set at a valgus angle of 6 to 9 degrees to the plane of the articular surface[3, 5] and aligned slightly over the lateral condyle. In the sagittal plane, the shaft is aligned over the anterior portion of the articular surface, leaving the posterior portion of the condyles extended posteriorly to act as runners in their articulation with the tibial plateaus. In addition, on the transverse or axial plane, the posterior portions of both condyles are wider than they are anteriorly. A transverse cut through the condyles demonstrates a trapezoidal shape with up to a 25% decrease in width from posterior to anterior.[3]

Muscle

The four muscles that make up a majority of the anterior thigh are collectively known as the quadriceps femoris. The four "heads" consist of the vastus lateralis, the vastus intermedius (deepest), the vastus medialis, and the rectus femoris (most superficial). The anterior or extensor compartment is separated from the posterior compartment by both the medial and the lateral intermuscular septa. These fascial expansions are important landmarks used during various surgical approaches to the distal femur. The posterior compartment consists of three large fusiform muscles called the hamstrings: the semimembranosus, semitendinosus, and biceps femoris. Together they form the rudimentary medial (semimembranosus, semitendinosus) and lateral (biceps femoris) boundaries of the popliteal fossa.

The powerful muscles of the distal thigh produce characteristic deformities after both supracondylar and intracondylar fractures. The combination of the quadriceps femoris anteriorly and the hamstring and gastrocnemius muscles posteriorly tend to lead to shortening and consequent sagittal plane deformity. If an intracondylar fracture is present, additional significant rotational deformities occur.

Vascular Supply

Of surgical importance on the medial side of the distal thigh is the superficial femoral artery, which is the continuation of the external iliac artery. The artery travels between the anterior and medial compartments through the adductor canal with the femoral vein and saphenous nerve. The femoral artery and vein then pass through a small opening in the adductor magnus (approximately 10 cm proximal to the knee joint) into the popliteal fossa.

The femoral artery, renamed the popliteal artery once it enters the popliteal fossa, then gives off several branches as it passes posterior to the knee joint, including the superior and inferior branches of the medial and lateral geniculate arteries. Interestingly, although the lateral femoral condyle is supplied by both the superior and the inferior lateral geniculate arteries via a persistent anastomotic link, there is not a similar watershed supplying the medial femoral condyle.[9] In fact, the medial femoral condyle relies almost exclusively on branches of the superior medial geniculate artery as they pass just anterior to the medial epicondyle.[9] It is imperative, therefore, that these structures be identified and protected in any medial approaches to the distal femur.

Alignment

There are two important axes to consider concerning the overall alignment of the distal femur. The anatomic axis, as mentioned previously, is measured at the intersection of a longitudinal mid-diaphyseal line and the knee joint axis (transcondylar line). The anatomic axis subtends the knee joint axis at an angle of 6 to 9 degrees from the vertical.[3, 5, 10] The mechanical, or weightbearing, axis is measured at the intersection of a line extending from the center of the femoral head to the center of the knee joint axis and the transcondylar line. This angle measured at the lateral aspect of the distal femur averages 87 degrees, or 3 degrees from the vertical.[3, 5, 10] These angles are averages based on cadaveric studies, and it is important to confirm the measurements from the contralateral extremity, when available, before planning intervention.

EPIDEMIOLOGY

Incidence

Supracondylar and distal femur fractures account for 4% to 7% of all femur fractures.[6, 7, 11] When fractures of the hip are excluded, fractures of the distal femur occur in 31% of the remaining femur fractures.[8] Given the advances in safety technology as well as the increasing longevity of the population, the incidence of these injuries will certainly rise.

There are two major patient populations in which fractures of the distal femur occur: young persons (consequent to high-energy trauma) and the elderly (after low-energy injuries).[2, 6, 11–13]

In the younger group, the fractures are often open and comminuted. They usually result from a high-energy blow on the anterolateral aspect of the flexed knee or from a direct blow on the lateral aspect of the extended knee. A majority of these injuries occur from vehicular accidents (especially motorcycles), but some occur as a result of industrial accidents or falls.[2, 13–15] Most of these patients are less than 35 years of age, and there is a male predominance.[3]

In the older group, the mechanism commonly involves a much lower energy of impact, such as falling from a standing position onto a flexed knee. In a study of patients 65 years or older from Minnesota, two thirds of the fractures caused by the lower-energy trauma were preceded by either a previous age-related fracture (hip, wrist) or by radiographic evidence of osteopenia.[8] In that study, the older group showed a definite predominance of females.[8] Although supracondylar comminution often is equivalent in both groups, younger patients have a higher incidence of more significant intra-articular injury as well as segmental and more proximal shaft comminution.[16]

Associated Injuries

Fractures of the distal femur, especially those involving younger patients sustaining a higher-energy mechanism of injury, are frequently associated with other concomitant skeletal, thoracic, and visceral injuries. This discussion deals only with injuries associated with distal femur fractures that involve the ipsilateral extremity.

The most common mechanism for distal femur fracture is a direct blow on the flexed knee. The position of the leg and hip at time of impact determines the presence of other major injuries, including ipsilateral acetabular fractures, hip dislocations, and femoral neck or shaft fractures. Careful evaluation of these polytraumatized patients is required to ensure that appropriate preoperative planning allows fixation of all the injuries in concert and with prioritization.

Fractures of the distal femur may be associated with various soft-tissue injuries of the knee joint. Ligamentous injuries to the knee in association with supracondylar femoral fractures occur in about 20% of cases.[22] These injuries may be difficult to diagnose prior to stabilization of the femur. They may require careful physical examination after treatment of the femur fracture as well as stress radiographs or magnetic resonance imaging to confirm the diagnosis.

As discussed previously, the femoral and popliteal arteries are close to the femur in both the adductor canal and popliteal fossa. Displaced and high-energy fractures place the artery at significant risk for injury, not only because of its proximity to the fracture but also because of its lack of mobility due to its tethering proximally by the adductor canal and distally by the soleus canal.[17] The popliteal artery is at risk for injury in up to 40% of patients who sustain significant, concomitant ligamentous injuries to the ipsilateral knee (such as a posterior dislocation).[18–21] If there is evidence of a diminished pulse or ischemia of the ipsilateral extremity in the setting of a distal femur fracture, immediate surgical exploration or angiography is mandatory.

Distal femur fractures, especially those involving a higher-energy mechanism of injury in a sagittally directed force, may be associated with a fracture of either tibial plateau or tibial shaft. This injury complex, or "floating knee" syndrome, has a 5% to 39% incidence of knee ligament injury[23, 24] and a 31% incidence of compartment syndrome involving either the thigh or lower leg.[25] The associated tibia fractures are commonly open and highly comminuted.[23, 25, 26]

Classification

Neer and associates[27] devised one of the early classification schemes for supracondylar-intercondylar femur fractures (Fig. 60.1). The system divided fractures of the distal femur into three distinct categories:

I. Minimal displacement.
II. Displacement of the condyles relative to the shaft.
III. Concomitant supracondylar or shaft comminution.

Although simple to apply, the Neer classification system did not accurately portend prognosis and therefore is no longer commonly used.

Seinsheimer[1] published a more intricate scheme in 1980 (Fig. 60.2). Fractures of the distal femur were divided into four basic groups:

I. Nondisplaced fractures—any fracture with less than 2-mm displacement of fractured fragments.
II. Fractures involving only the distal metaphysis, without extension into the intercondylar region.
   A Two-part fractures.

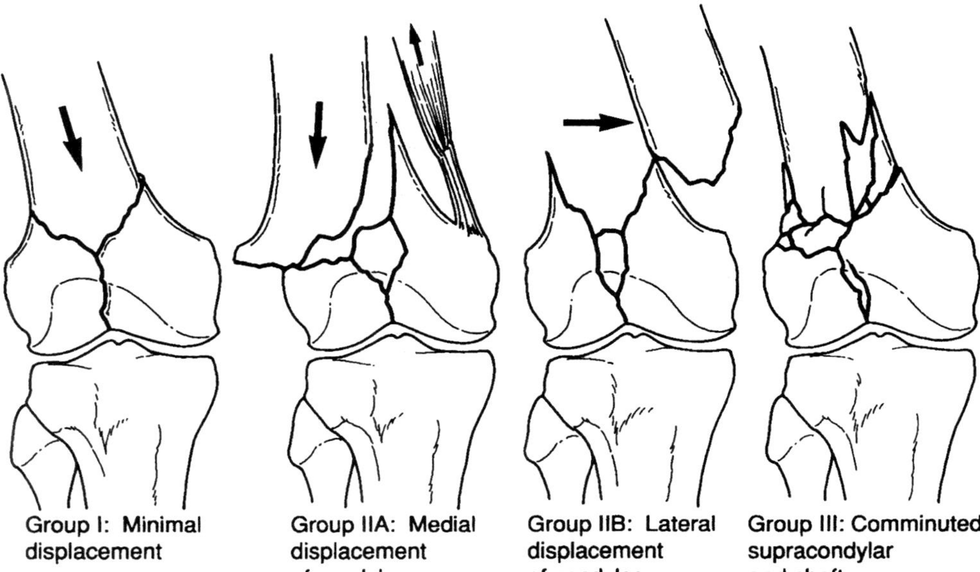

FIGURE 60.1 ➢ The Neer classification.

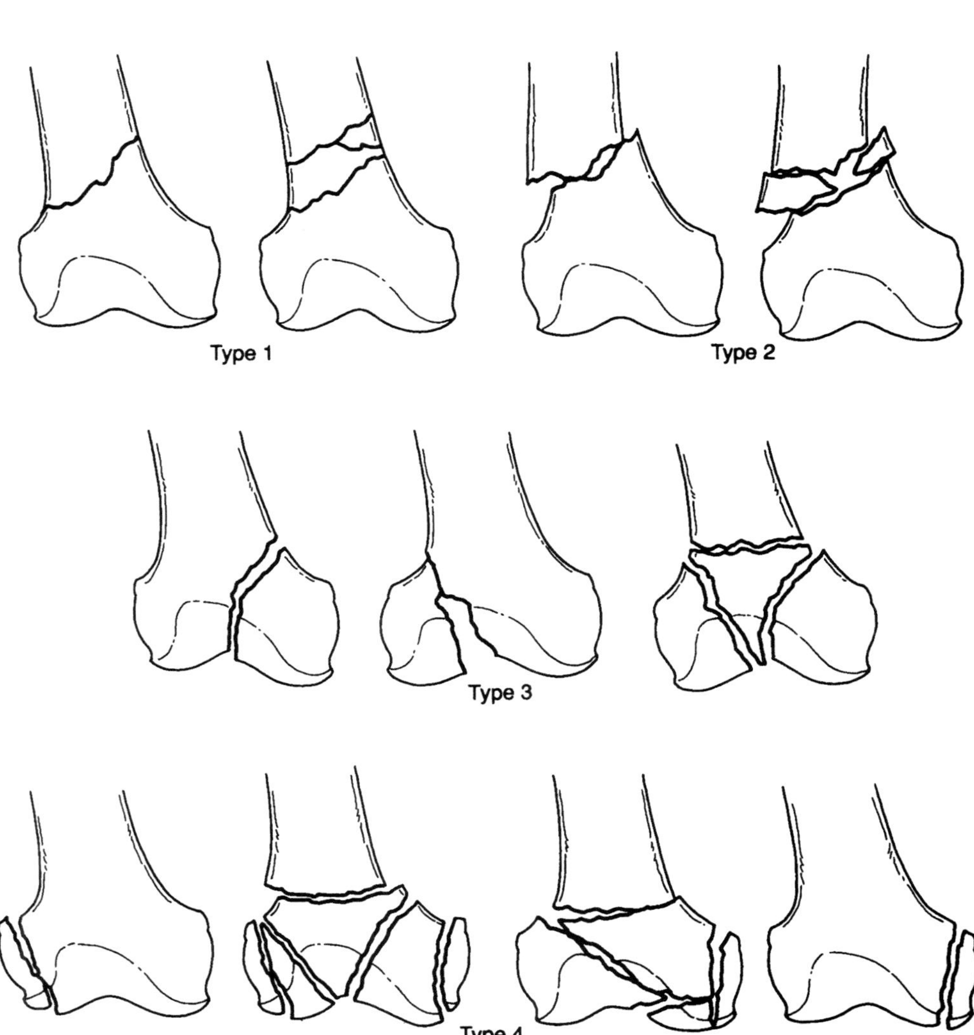

FIGURE 60.2 ➢ The Seinsheimer classification.

B. Comminuted fractures.

III. Fractures involving the intercondylar notch in which one or both condyles are separate fragments.
   A. Medial condyle is the separate fragment; the lateral condyle remains in continuity with the shaft.
   B. Lateral condyle is the separate fragment; the medial condyle remains in continuity with the shaft.
   C. Both condyles are separated from each other as well as from the shaft.

IV. Fractures involving the articular surface of the condyles.
   A. Fracture through the medial condyle with at least two fragments.
   B. Fracture through the lateral condyle with at least two fragments.
   C. Complex and more highly comminuted fractures extending into one condyle and the intercondylar notch, both condyles, or all three; this pattern commonly involves a metaphyseal fracture.

Seinsheimer[1] was able to identify several epidemiological patterns of injury as a result of this fracture classification scheme. Patients with type I, nondisplaced fractures, or type II, two-part supracondylar fractures, were older and had a history of pathological osteoporosis prior to injury. Patients diagnosed with a type IV injury with significant articular comminution, however, were substantially younger. In addition, the fractures with more comminution were found to be the result of higher-energy trauma and therefore had a predictably worse outcome.

More recently, the Swiss AO/ASIF Group developed a standard classification scheme for fractures that is widely accepted in the trauma community (Fig. 60.3). Müller and associates[28] in 1991 updated the AO classification system and divided fractures of the distal femur into three main groups: type A, extra-articular; type B, unicondylar; and type C, bicondylar. The main groups are then subdivided:

A. Extra-articular fractures.
   A1. Simple.
   A2. Two-part supracondylar.
   A3. Comminuted supracondylar.

B. Unicondylar fractures.
   B1. Lateral condyle, sagittal plane.
   B2. Medial condyle, sagittal plane.
   B3. Lateral or medial condyle, coronal plane.

C. Bicondylar fractures.
   C1. Noncomminuted, supracondylar with intercondylar extension ("T" or "Y").
   C2. Comminuted supracondylar with intercondylar extension ("T" or "Y").
   C3. Comminuted supracondylar with comminuted intercondylar involvement.

The AO/ASIF classification system also provides for an additional level of specificity to further describe the orientation or position of the primary fracture line or fragment, but for the purposes of this review that discussion will be omitted. The scheme as it relates to the distal femur has proved to be a reliable predictor of injury severity, mechanism of injury, and prognosis. In progressing from A to C, the severity of the fracture and the energy of the trauma increase as the prognosis for a good result decreases. The same is true for the 1 to 3 subdivisions. A patient with a C3 fracture, therefore, sustained a higher-energy injury and has a worse prognosis than a similar patient with a B1 fracture.

DIAGNOSIS

History and Physical Examination

One of the vital steps in the treatment of a patient with a distal femur fracture is taking a thorough history and performing a careful physical examination. Even in the setting of a low-energy, isolated injury, following standard ACLS/ATLS guidelines should be routine and provides experience when dealing with a polytraumatized patient.

The entire lower extremity should be scrutinized from the pelvis to the foot in search of associated skeletal and soft-tissue injuries. Diminished or absent pulses should be documented immediately with a bedside Doppler instrument and then evaluated either with urgent surgical exploration or angiography. Equally as important in terms of the limb is careful documentation of the neurological status of the affected extremity. The sciatic nerve and its subsequent divisions are close to the popliteal artery in the popliteal fossa and are therefore subject to similar traumatic injuries. Although documented neurological injuries from isolated supracondylar femur fractures are not common,[54] neurological status is an important prognostic indicator of limb viability.

As in all traumatic injuries to an extremity, one must remain alert to the possibility of compartment syndrome. If the diagnosis by physical examination is in question in a tense thigh, compartment pressures must be documented using any number of available methods. Finally, traumatic open and contaminated wounds to the lower extremity are usually easily diagnosed, and their treatment is rather straightforward. Because many distal femur fractures result from a direct blow, all deep abrasions and lacerations should be aggressively evaluated for communication with the fracture or the knee joint.

Radiographic Examination

Radiographic examination of a fracture of the distal femur and supracondylar region requires two 90-degree orthogonal views. Anteroposterior (AP) and lateral plain radiographs are standard. Although screening AP radiographs occasionally are used to confirm the presence of a skeletal injury, the most qualitative information for the purposes of classification and treatment are gained from traction radiographs. Oblique views of the knee may facilitate diagnosis of fracture extension into the articular surface. Computed tomography

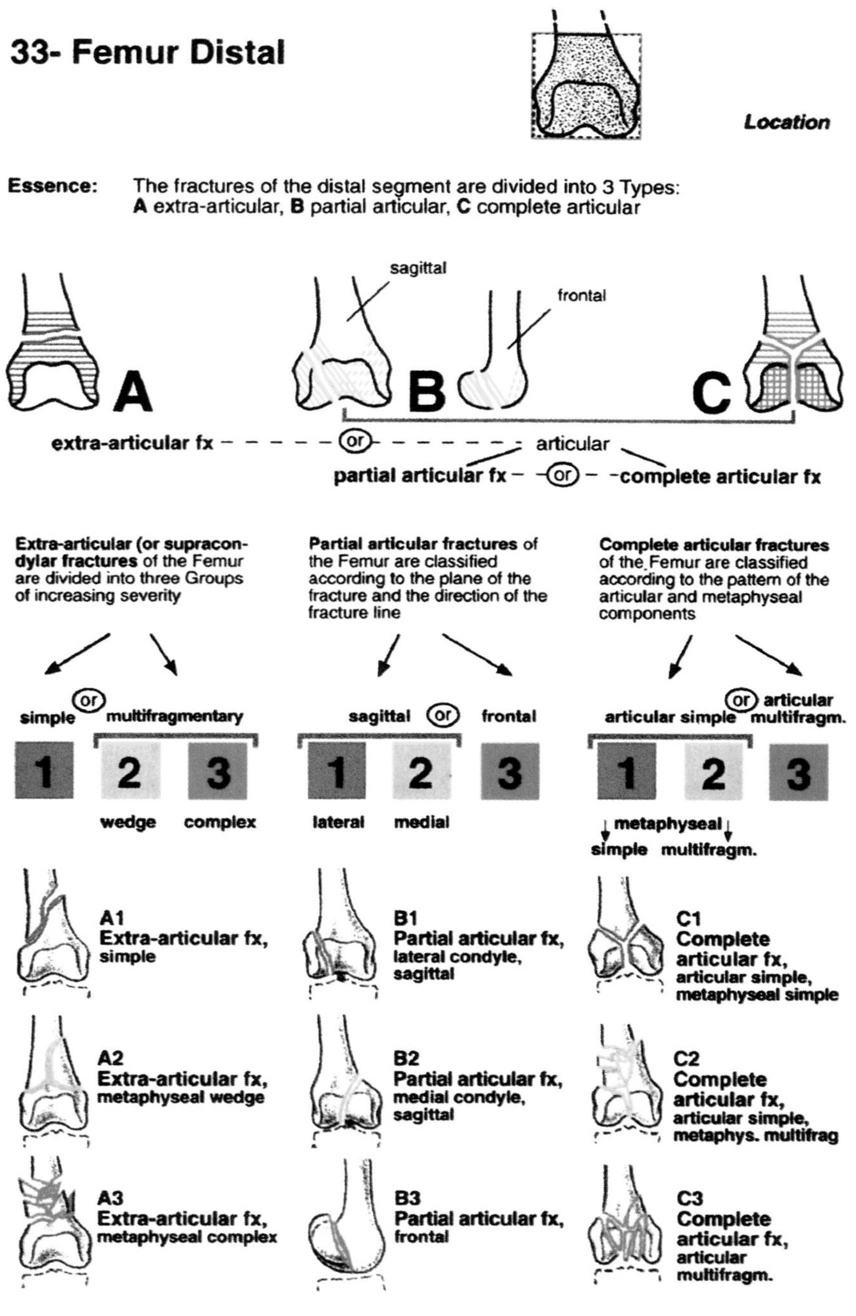

FIGURE 60.3 ➢ The AO/ASIF classification. (From Müller ME, Nazarian S, Koch P, Schatzker J: The Comprehensive Classification of Fractures of Long Bones. Bern, M.E. Müller Foundation, 1995.)

may be a useful adjunct to delineate the extent of supracondylar comminution and articular involvement. Although previous studies have concentrated on the area of segmental, ipsilateral involvement of the femur,[30, 31] the same principle of precise identification of coronal and sagittal plane articular involvement for the purpose of preoperative planning may be applied to an isolated distal femur fracture.

The importance of complete radiographic evaluation of the entire femur, from the ipsilateral pelvis to the knee, cannot be overstated when a skeletal injury to the femur has been identified at any level. Butler and associates,[30] in a review of 684 femoral shaft fractures, identified a 3% incidence of ipsilateral supracondylar or intracondylar involvement. Full radiographic examination of the knee might also reveal involvement of the tibial plateaus that would affect fixation planning.

In the setting of significant comminution, comparison radiographs of the unaffected, contralateral femur from the pelvis to the knee may provide useful information for reconstruction. They provide a template not only to assess the patient's normal valgus alignment of the distal femur but to guide the overall axial alignment of the limb.

Distal femur fractures associated with frank dislocation or the ligamentous equivalent should undergo immediate angiographic evaluation or surgical exploration because of the reported 40% incidence of arterial injuries associated with knee dislocations.[18–21] Identification of ligamentous injury in the acute setting is quite difficult and limited because of the instability of the extremity from the fracture and issues of pain control. Ligamentous instability noted in the operating room after skeletal fixation of a comminuted, high-energy injury, however, should receive thorough and immediate attention to rule out the presence of a partial vascular injury or intimal flap. As mentioned previously, absent or diminished pulses associated with a distal femur fracture when compared with the unaffected extremity should be aggressively managed with immediate angiography or surgical exploration.

MANAGEMENT

Conservative Nonoperative Management

Prior to the modern era of internal fixation and the subsequent wave of enthusiasm for intramedullary fixation, femur fractures were treated with traction and bracing. Several different techniques for the application of traction were developed in the early part of the 20th century that employed either a single proximal tibial pin or a combination of a tibial pin with a second, supracondylar pin.[32–38, 43] After an appropriate period of immobilization, usually 3 to 5 months, progressive weightbearing was initiated with the use of braces or calipers.[39]

Maintaining alignment and reduction of distal femur fractures by conservative measures, however, soon became recognized as an entity separate from fractures of the shaft of the femur. In 1921, Trethowan[39] commented that when traction devices "prove insufficient for correct reposition, there should be no hesitation in cutting down and transfixing the fragments with long screws or autogenous bone pegs." Other subsequent investigators, concurring with the difficulty of maintaining adequate reduction of this subset of femur fractures as well as the late complications of prolonged bedrest and knee-joint stiffness,[36, 40] advocated open reduction.[41]

More contemporary investigators, however, continue to advocate the conservative management of these difficult fractures,[42, 44, 45] especially in the subset of patients who present biological or mechanical challenges to treatment by open methods. These patients include the elderly with significant osteopenia or comminution and paraplegics or other nonambulatory patients. In the 1970s, investigators such as Connolly and associates[47, 48] and Mays and Neufeld[46] made advances in the closed treatment of distal femur fractures that allowed earlier motion and less prolonged recumbency. Nonetheless, conservatively managed distal femur fractures were not free from complications such as shortening, angular/rotational deformity, and post-traumatic arthritis from joint incongruity and associated limitation of motion.[11] Nonoperative management of displaced distal femur fractures should be reserved only for patients who have a special circumstance that either obviates the need or contraindicates the necessity for surgical intervention.

Operative Management

Open Reduction, Internal Fixation

One of the earliest comments on internal fixation of distal femur fractures is found in *Orthopaedic Surgery of Injuries,* edited by Sir Robert Jones and published in 1921.[39] Several authors in the 1940s and 1950s did report on the use of internal fixation with Blount blade plates but without overwhelming success.[49–51] Obtaining consistently good results with internal fixation was so difficult that, in the 1960s, two separate groups published landmark papers once again advocating the conservative treatment of distal femur fractures.

Stewart and associates[12] found only 54% good or excellent results with open treatment of distal femur fractures while achieving 67% good or excellent results with those treated with closed methods. The poorer outcome in the group undergoing surgery was due to infection, inadequate surgical technique, and insufficient fixation. In 1967, Neer and associates[27] published their experience treating 110 supracondylar femur fractures over a 24-year period and proposed the classification system outlined previously. Again, the operative group demonstrated considerably less success (52% satisfactory) compared with the conservative group (90% satisfactory). However, the criteria accepted for a satisfactory outcome in this study would not be acceptable today; in addition, inadequate technique and insufficient fixation once again plagued the operative group. In fact, many of the patients in the operative group underwent prolonged immobilization due to the tenuous nature of the fixation, thereby negating the benefits of internal fixation.

In 1958, the Swiss AO Group was formed to advance fracture care by restoring full function to the affected limb while avoiding the complications of conservative management and prolonged immobilization.[28] They recommended certain principles of fracture treatment that remain today as the mainstays of fracture management: anatomic reduction of the fracture fragments, preservation of the blood supply, stable internal fixation, and early mobilization. They stressed repeatedly that the goal of fracture treatment must include not only union of the skeletal injury but also full recovery of limb function with maintenance of soft-tissue integrity.[28]

Wenzl and associates[52] were the first to report on a series of distal femur fractures treated with the AO principles. They reported 73.5% good or excellent results with 112 patients, which was far better than any other published data up to that time and included much more stringent criteria for outcome determination than any previous study. Schatzker and associates[53] reported similar results using the same AO principles after treating 32 of 71 supracondylar femur fractures with open reduction, internal fixation (ORIF). Although they achieved 75% good or excellent results compared with 32% in the conservative group, they still cautioned against the use of internal fixation for all patients, especially in elderly patients with severe osteoporosis or those with nondisplaced fractures.

Schatzker and Lambert[54] later reported on an additional series of 35 supracondylar femur fractures treated with ORIF. Of the 17 cases treated with AO principles, they achieved over 70% good and excellent results. When the same implants were used but the AO principles were not followed, however, they only achieved 21% good or excellent results. Of the cases in the latter group, they noted several consistent problems that led to their poor outcome: incomplete reduction, lack of interfragmentary compression, failure to use autogenous graft to fill areas of comminution or medial bone loss, ineffective use of cement to supplement osteoporotic bone, and inappropriate use of the angled blade plate. Given that failure in this particular cohort was related more to overwhelming osteopenia and not technical error, Schatzker and Lambert[54] recommended closed reduction and cast bracing as an alternative to surgery for this particular group of elderly patients. Schatzker,[55] upon later revisiting the issue of fixation in the osteoporotic distal femur, stated that if the supracondylar segment contained less than 2 to 3 cm of comminution, the fragments should be pushed out of the way and the extremity shortened in the process of fixation. This process "not only enhances axial stability, facilitates fixation and union, but it also allows one to use the fragments as bone graft."[55]

During the next 15 years, 72% to 92% good or excellent results[56–61] were reported in the literature by investigators utilizing AO principles of ORIF in the treatment of distal femur fractures. Of interest, both Healy and associates[60] and Siliski and associates[61] found that increasing age did not seem to adversely affect surgical outcome or functional result.

In their prospective, randomized study of operative intervention (Dynamic Condylar Screw [DCS], Synthes, Paoli, PA) versus conservative, nonoperative management of displaced, intra-articular fractures of the distal femur in an elderly cohort, Butt and associates[62] reported similar results. Patients in the surgical group achieved 53% good or excellent results; those in the nonoperative group achieved only 31%. Patients in the nonoperative group also had considerably longer hospital stays as well as a much higher incidence of serious complications, including deep venous thrombosis, pressure sores, urinary infections, respiratory infections, and malunion or nonunion.[62] This was the first prospective study demonstrating that operative intervention in the elderly population utilizing AO principles had results that far surpassed those realized in treating these injuries conservatively.

Several other investigators have had similar results using the DCS device as an alternative to other traditional forms of ORIF such as the blade plate or condylar buttress plate, especially in the elderly.[2, 7, 63–66] Giles and associates[2] reported that the lag screw provided compression across the fractured intracondylar surface that proved beneficial in maintaining reduction and allowing early motion in the elderly population with osteoporotic bone.

Following the principles of indirect reduction championed by Mast and associates,[67] some investigators have attempted to apply biological fixation and minimal soft-tissue stripping techniques to the basic tenets of the AO method. Ostrum and Geel[68] reported 86.6% good or excellent results using indirect reduction techniques with various forms of ORIF. The group, however, relied on the less-stringent Neer rating system (a satisfactory result requires only 70 degrees of flexion) for its outcome scoring. Bolhofner and associates[69] found 84% good or excellent results in their series of 57 patients with supracondylar femur fractures treated with open, indirect reduction and internal fixation. To assess outcome, the authors used the modified Schatzker scale, which requires at least 100 degrees of flexion, less than 10 degrees of flexion contracture, and less than 5 degrees of varus malalignment to achieve a good or excellent result.

Although the condylar buttress plate has been used successfully to treat distal femur fractures, especially those with intercondylar comminution,[68, 69] the use of this implant in the setting of significant supracondylar medial comminution has potential problems. The lack of a rigid interface between the screws and the plate can lead to collapse and varus malalignment. This device, although not as strong as either the DCS or the blade plate, does provide for multiple 6.5-mm lag screws to be placed across intracondylar comminution, however. Koval and associates[83] addressed the lack of rigidity of the condylar buttress plate by comparing it in a cadaveric biomechanical study with a blade plate and a modified condylar buttress plate with four distal "locked" screw holes. The locked buttress plate demonstrated significantly greater fixation stability and equal rigidity to torsion and lateral bending than either of the two other plates.

Acknowledging that complex fractures associated with significant medial comminution can lead to varus malalignment, Sanders and associates[70] proposed double-plating of the distal femur. They achieved union in all patients. The medial buttress plate may be placed through a second formal incision or a percutaneous technique. Matelic and associates[84] have also reported a technique to augment medial stability in seven patients with nonunion by introducing a medial endosteal plate through the nonunion that is transfixed with screws from the lateral plate.

Other attempts at achieving union by means of ORIF of distal femur fractures have led some investigators to use alternative implants. Using the principle that less-rigid fixation provides for more robust and expedient formation of callus,[71, 72] Pemberton and associates[73] reported a series of 22 patients treated with a carbon-fiber plate used in conjunction with AO 4.5-mm and 6.5-mm cancellous screws. Of the 19 patients (average age, 80 years) who survived 12 months, 89% demonstrated radiographic union by 5 months. There were no implant failures or infections. The authors did note that their range of motion was less than the acceptable range for a younger cohort of patients, but these authors thought that it was a permissible trade-off to achieve nearly 90% union in this difficult treatment group.

Intramedullary Nail Fixation

During the late 1970s, alternatives to the technically demanding surgical principles of the AO Group were relentlessly pursued. In 1977, Zickel and associates[74] introduced the supracondylar Zickel device for the treatment of distal femur fractures. The device consisted of tapered rods introduced into the medullary canal through both the medial and the lateral condyles and secured distally with transcondylar screws. Although early results revealed 82% good or excellent results, four patients with significant intra-articular involvement required adjunctive fixation and more than 50% underwent prolonged postoperative immobilization. Zickel and associates[75] subsequently published a report on a series of 67 patients in which the union rate was near 100%, but again they reported that more than 50% of patients with intra-articular involvement had less than 90 degrees of motion. Shelbourne and Brueckmann[76] reported on the use of Rush rod fixation for fractures of the distal femur. The authors stressed that adjunctive cerclage wiring of metaphyseal segments with minimal soft-tissue stripping would be required for comminuted supracondylar fractures.

As early as 1940, Kuntsher[77] was recommending the use of antegrade intramedullary nails for the treatment of femur fractures. Several authors have applied the technique of antegrade nailing for the treatment of distal femur fractures in hopes of limiting the complications of ORIF while obtaining comparable rates of union. Specifically, closed intramedullary nailing leads to indirect reduction with no soft-tissue stripping or interruption of the fracture hematoma at the fracture site.[78, 79] Both Leung and associates[15] and Butler and associates[30] reported excellent results treating most types of supracondylar femur fractures with antegrade nails. The technique, however, is not effective for type B and most C3 fracture patterns.

In fractures with intracondylar involvement, distal percutaneous screw fixation or limited ORIF must be performed prior to antegrade nailing. The authors also warned that fractures with intra-articular involvement require restricted weightbearing because of limitations of the implant rigidity in the distal femur, which is quite different from the typical antegrade nailing rehabilitation protocol. With this limitation, Leung and associates[15] found 97% union and 95% good or excellent results.

Tornetta and Tiburzi[81] found no antegrade intramedullary nail hardware failures, excellent motion, and no nonunions in a series 38 patients with distal femur fractures secondary to gunshot wounds. The major complication they noted in their younger population was a 50% incidence of valgus malalignment in the six patients in whom nailing was performed in the lateral position. In 1998, in a series of 20 fractures, Dominguez and associates[80] found no fair or poor outcomes and only one nonunion (treated successfully with nail exchange). All patients had full extension and at least 100 degrees of flexion, giving the study group an average HSS score of 87 (excellent). Unfortunately, this study was limited by the large drop-out rate of the patient cohort (4 patients died, 11 were lost to follow-up).

During the early 1990s, there was a groundswell of enthusiasm for the use of retrograde intramedullary devices. One of the early devices was the GSH (Green, Seligson, Henry) supracondylar intramedullary nail. Henry and associates[82] thought that the intramedullary position of the nail provided a biomechanical advantage over plates and screws by decreasing the lever arm to the axis of deformation. They also postulated that the medial parapatellar approach would offer direct visualization of the joint surface.

After mechanical testing of the retrograde nail versus the DCS in synthetic bones, Firoozbaksh and associates[85] reported that the bending stiffness in varus and flexion was not significantly different in the two constructs. Although the plate was notably stiffer in lateral bending and torsion, the most common modes of failure for the implants in vivo occurred in varus and flexion—therefore, both devices were found to be biomechanically adequate in the treatment of distal femur fractures. Koval and associates[86] found similar results in an osteoporotic cadaver model, comparing the DCS with both an antegrade nail and a short retrograde nail. However, they recommended that the plate be used when maximum stiffness of the construct is desired. The antegrade nail demonstrated the least amount of stiffness to lateral bending and torsion at the level of the distal femoral osteotomy site. David and associates[87] reported similar results.

Ito and associates[88] compared the blade plate with the GSH nail and a new AO supracondylar femoral nail that utilizes a spiral blade. Again, the nails were found to be as stiff in AP bending but inferior in torsion and varus during axial load when compared with the plate. Finally, Voor and associates[89] performed fatigue testing on composite femurs instrumented with either a twelve-hole or a five-hole intramedullary supracondylar nail. They demonstrated no failures of the five-hole design of either the 11-mm or the 12-mm diameter, suggesting that for optimal fixation, a nail with fewer holes and therefore fewer stress-risers should be selected.

The literature shows mixed results with the use of the GSH device. Lucas and associates,[90] in their series of 25 type A and C fractures, demonstrated union of all injuries (although 4 of the 19 type C fractures required bone grafting). Danziger and associates[91] found 94% good or excellent results with only one nonunion in their series of 16 patients, which included 10 C2 and 3 C3 fractures. In their initial experience with 41 fractures, however, Iannacone and associates[92] reported four nonunions, five delayed unions, and four stress fatigue fractures with the GSH device. The nail failures all involved the 11-mm nail with 6.4-mm locking screws. The latter part of the study included 14 nails after modification to 12-mm and 13-mm diameters with 5.0-mm locking screws. None of these devices failed.

Janzing and associates[93] reported on a consecutive series of 24 elderly patients treated with the GSH device and found that all injuries healed with 89% good or excellent results using the Neer scoring system. The authors mentioned several frustrations with the device and instrumentation, including poor purchase of the distal locking screws in osteoporotic bone and difficulties with the targeting device for the proximal screws.

External Fixation

Several reports have commented on the use of external fixation for the treatment of distal femur fractures.[94, 95] Marsh and associates[96] reported on a diverse series of 13 patients treated with a monolateral fixator. Five of the fractures were open, and five required vascular repair. Twelve of the fractures healed with an average of just over 4 months in the fixator. The one nonunion also represented the only infection; after further surgical intervention, this patient went on to experience union. The authors found 77% good results using the Iowa Knee Score. In their review of the use of hybrid external fixation in periarticular fractures of the lower extremity, Hutson and Zych[97] included 19 distal femur fractures as part of their patient cohort. After an average of 6 months in the fixator, they found one nonunion, two pin tract infections requiring IV antibiotics, one episode of septic arthritis requiring arthrotomy and débridement, and one episode of deep infection within the fracture zone.

Primary Total Knee Arthroplasty

Although many in the field of fracture fixation consider the procedure radical, treating supracondylar femur fractures in carefully selected patients with a primary total knee arthroplasty has been supported in the literature.[99] In 1992, Bell and associates[98] reported on a cohort of 13 elderly patients (average age, 84 years) with comminuted distal femur fractures (10 of 13 fractures were classified as Müller type C). Twelve of the patients were able to bear weight as tolerated immediately after the surgery and were mobile by the fourth postoperative day. They found that 11 of the patients returned to their premorbid level of functioning within 12 weeks of injury. Although the follow-up was limited to a minimum of 6 months, they reported no infections or loosening of the components. Certainly, advances concerning the biomechanics of hinged total knee arthroplasties will bring wider acceptance of this treatment in the elderly, highly comminuted and osteoporotic patient population.

Adjunctive Use of Bone Cement

Benum[100] originally described the use of bone cement as an adjunct to fixation of extra-articular distal femur fractures in the elderly in the late 1970s. Of the study group, 86% tolerated early mobilization and went on to heal uneventfully. Younger and associates[101] reported on a refinement of Benum's technique and found 79% satisfactory to excellent results in 17 distal femur fractures, several of which included an intercondylar component. Their technique involves fixation of the distal fragment with a DCS implant, followed by application of cement in its "doughy" state into the medullary canal of the distal femur, taking care to avoid applying cement to the fracture surfaces. The cancellous bone is removed from the proximal shaft and saved. The proximal shaft is then filled with cement to the level of the plate. The fracture is reduced, and the proximal screw holes are drilled through the matured "cement" canal. The cancellous bone is then used as graft around the fracture site. This method offers the advantage of more stable fixation in compromised bone but requires meticulous technique and is time-consuming.

Bone Grafting

Several investigators have advocated the use of autologous bone grafting at time of fracture stabilization for distal femur fractures.[2, 3, 11, 54, 59] In most cases the application of bone graft is reserved for comminuted fractures in severely osteoporotic patients, younger patients after a high-energy injury, and patients who lack adequate medial "column" stability after fixation. Delayed or secondary bone grafting has also been recommended for open fractures and those that have undergone significant soft-tissue stripping and devascularization. In these cases, the time delay to the bone graft procedure depends on the viability of the surrounding soft-tissue envelope. Frequently, a delay of 6 weeks is suggested from the time of soft-tissue coverage to the secondary bone grafting procedure. The bone graft is meant to help preserve the local biological milieu and the integrity of the implant to tip the balance in the "race between fracture healing and plate breakage."[11]

Ostrum and Geel,[68] concurring with previous authors that the bone graft procedure may not be necessary and is not without morbidity,[101] reported on a series of 30 fractures of the distal femur treated with indirect reduction and lateral plating without the use of primary bone grafting. They found 86% excellent to satisfactory results and suggest that bone grafting be reserved only for severely open injuries with markedly devascularized fragments or extreme osteoporosis. In 1996, Bolhofner and associates[69] prospectively reported on a series of 57 fractures of the distal femur treated with indirect reduction and without bone grafting with 84% good and excellent results.

SURGICAL APPROACHES

There are several different surgical approaches to the distal femur that vary according to the type of fracture and method of fixation. A radiolucent operating room table should be used for the reduction and the application of retrograde nails, plates and screws, external fixators, and total knee arthroplasties. An antegrade femoral nail may be inserted with the patient supine on a standard table with bump under the ipsilateral buttock, in the lateral position on a standard table, or supine on a fracture table. The affected extremity should be draped free except when a fracture table will be used. A tourniquet should be used in all cases with open reduction, but it should be applied after draping and in a sterile fashion so that the surgical field is not compromised. All open wounds should be closed over a drain. Perioperative antibiotics are standard. Prior to preparing and draping the extremity, adequate AP and lateral accessibility of the fracture site with the image intensifier should be verified.

Posterolateral Approach to the Distal Femur

A longitudinal incision is made along the lateral aspect of the distal thigh, extending from the proximal extension of the fracture distally to the lateral femoral epicondyle. The incision is then gently curved anteriorly and medially to a point midway between the tibial tubercle and the inferior pole of the patella. The anterior portion of the iliotibial band may be detached and reflected posteriorly or split along its anterior third in line with its fibers. The vastus lateralis fascia is then split longitudinally, and the muscle fibers are bluntly dissected from the anterior surface of the lateral intermuscular septum. Care must be taken to identify and ligate the perforating branches of the profunda femoris artery.

The dissection may be extended distally with a lateral parapatellar arthrotomy. The patella may be subluxated medially to provide exposure of the intercondylar notch and trochlea. This is the standard approach for ORIF of the distal femur. Visualization of the medial condyle and reduction of some comminuted intra-articular fractures may be challenging with this approach. Releasing the lateral meniscus at the anterior horn just lateral to the intermeniscal ligament attachment may significantly improve visualization. The meniscus is repaired with two 4-0 proline sutures prior to closure.

The anterolateral approach to the distal femur is similar, except the incision should be placed slightly more anterior and the plane of deep dissection is between the vastus lateralis and the rectus femoris. Several extensile exposures from the lateral approach have been suggested, including a tibial tubercle osteotomy.[57, 59]

Anterior and Anteromedial Approach

The anterior approach is familiar to most surgeons and is most commonly used for total knee arthroplasty. The incision is longitudinal along the anterior surface of the distal thigh, extending across the knee joint and terminating along the medial surface of the tibial tubercle. A standard medial parapatellar arthrotomy is performed, and the dissection is carried proximally between the vastus medialis and the rectus femoris. This approach is useful for medial condyle fractures but is not recommended for comminuted supracondylar fractures.

Starr and associates[142] described a variation of the anterior approach. After the anterior incision is made, a lateral parapatellar arthrotomy is performed distally. The dissection is carried proximally by identification of the fibers of the vastus lateralis muscle and blunt teasing of the fibers medially while the iliotibial band is retracted laterally. Proximal dissection is continued by blunt dissection of the fibers of the vastus lateralis from the lateral intermuscular septum, similar to the lateral approach. Again, care must be taken to ligate the perforating arterial branches arising from the intermuscular septum. The patella is retracted medially, and Homann or Bennett retractors are placed to expose the entire anterior and anterolateral distal femur. This approach offers excellent visualization of the joint surface and allows easy access to the starting point for fixed angle devices. The anterior incision is advantageous versus the lateral J incision because it does not compromise future arthroplasty or reconstructive exposure.

COMPLICATIONS

Infection

The most significant early complication of operative treatment of distal femur fractures is infection. Although the infection rate was previously reported to be as high as 20%,[12, 27] contemporary refinements in surgical technique and patient selection have dropped it to 7% or less.[2, 58, 60, 65, 68, 69] Factors that contribute to the risk of early infection include high-energy traumatic injury with significant stripping or devascularization of the bony fragments, open fractures, extensive or prolonged surgical dissection, and inadequate skeletal stabilization.[3]

To combat the risk of infection, the surgical approach should be performed with meticulous, sharp dissection; flaps should be held without self-retaining retractors whenever possible; and perioperative parenteral antibiotics should be administered. Several investigators[68, 69] have championed the techniques of Mast and associates,[67] including their tenets of indirect reduction and biological, stable fixation. Drains should be applied to all surgical wounds after careful hemostasis has been achieved. It is important that the reduction and fixation achieved in the operating room allow early active and active-assisted range of motion in the immediate perioperative period.

Open fractures of the distal femur should undergo initial, immediate débridement independent of and prior to attempts at surgical stabilization. The wound should be left open and serially débrided until clinical assessment suggests that closure has become favorable. Ostermann and associates[120] reported a statistically significant decrease in the incidence of acute infection in Gustilo IIIB/IIIC fractures and chronic osteomyelitis in Gustilo II/IIIB fractures with the application of antibiotic PMMA beads (aminoglycoside) during the initial débridement of limb fractures. Although no prospective study currently justifies the application of this technique in the setting of open distal femur fractures, it may play a role in further reducing the incidence of infection and late reconstruction. The application of acute antibiotic beads or a bead pouch in severely open injury may also reduce the total number of trips to the operating room for serial débridements and therefore have economic implications as well.

In the unfortunate circumstance of an acute postoperative infection, the wound should undergo aggressive and repeated débridements in the operating room. Again, antibiotic beads may be applied. The wound may be closed over beads and a drain; in the absence of beads, the extra-articular component should be left open for delayed primary or secondary intention closure. After diagnosis of an acute, deep infection, parenteral antibiotics should be continued on an outpatient basis for a total of 6 weeks. The key to prevention of this complication is to maintain a high index of suspicion throughout the perioperative period.

Nonunion

Nonunion of fractures of the distal femur has been reported with both nonoperative and operative management of these injuries. The incidence of nonunion after conservative management has been reported to be as high as 22%.[1, 12, 45, 47, 139] The incidence of nonunion after open reduction and internal fixation in the early literature ranged from 10% to 19%.[12, 27] A review of the contemporary literature, however, reveals a much more acceptable rate of nonunion, ranging from 0% to 4%.[2, 7, 54, 58–60, 65, 140] Nonunions of the distal femur occur most frequently in the supracondylar region, rarely in the intracondylar extension of the fracture.[3] Factors that commonly predispose to nonunion after a supracondylar femur fracture include (1) significant bone loss, (2) high-energy injuries, especially those associated with open contamination and periosteal stripping, (3) fractures treated with inadequate fixation, (4) lack of application of autogenous bone graft during the index procedure, and (5) wound infection.[3]

Management of nonunion of a supracondylar femur fracture can be extremely difficult. The most effective management technique is adequate prophylaxis, including stable internal fixation and early joint motion. Nonunion of the supracondylar region frequently leads to joint stiffness, followed by the development of a pseudoarthrosis at the nonunion site providing juxta-articular motion. Helfet and Lorich[3] advised the use of a reamed intramedullary device for the treatment of a nonunion in this area if there is adequate room distally for cross-lock fixation. With more distal pathology, a fixed-angle device such as the blade plate provides the most stable fixation.

Whenever ORIF is used for a nonunion in the supracondylar region, autogenous bone graft should be harvested and generously applied after decortication or petaling of the surrounding bone. The addition of lag screws and compression of the nonunion via an articulating tension device significantly increases the stability of the construct. In all cases, aggressive arthrolysis and mobilization of the knee joint are essential to diminish the forces on the supracondylar fixation. If there is not enough bone distally to accept an ORIF implant, salvage with a total knee arthroplasty in older patients or with a long, transarticular intramedullary nail in younger patients.[141]

Malunion

Malunion after supracondylar femur fracture is a significant problem, especially with conservative management. The modes of failure include axial malalignment, shortening, and malrotation. If an appropriate and acceptable reduction of these injuries cannot be maintained by conservative means, early surgical intervention should be considered. Neer and associates[27] reported a 5% incidence of malunion (15 degrees angulation and/or 2 cm displacement) after conservative management.

Malunion may also result from operative treatment of these complex injuries. Varus malalignment has been reported after ORIF in the setting of significant supracondylar comminution, especially on the medial side.[27, 58, 70] To avoid this complication, medial bone grafting and the addition of a medial plate have been advocated.[70] Sagittal plane deformities (flexion, extension) may also occur after ORIF of a small distal fragment. Adequate preoperative radiographs, planning, and application of the appropriate implant diminish the occurrence of these complications.

Malrotation and valgus angulation are common complications after intramedullary fixation of a supracondylar femur fracture, especially if the procedure is performed in a retrograde manner on a radiolucent table. Vigilance during insertion and cross-locking of the device is the main prophylaxis for this form of malunion.

Complete evaluation of an established malunion of the distal femur includes plain long leg standing radiographs and a computed tomographic scanogram for length and rotation. Full appreciation of both the clinical and radiographic deformity requires that the examination be performed with the patella facing directly anterior. Radiographs of the contralateral, unaffected side may be necessary to assess a patient's native limb alignment.

Failure of Fixation

Loss of fixation of a supracondylar femur fracture can occur regardless of the type of surgical intervention. Factors that may lead to this complication include (1) significant supracondylar comminution, (2) elderly patient population with marked osteopenia, (3) low transcondylar and intercondylar fractures in which adequate fixation stability is difficult to achieve, (4) poor patient compliance with rehabilitation protocols, and (5) infection.[3] Postoperative mobilization is preferred, including active and active-assisted range of motion. If the fixation stability of the fracture is judged to be inadequate or poor in the operating room, serious consideration should be given to an adjunctive procedure such as bone grafting, supplemental bone cement, or medial plating. If adequate fixation is still not achieved, motion exercises should be delayed and the immobilized extremity should be monitored closely for failure. If the hardware does fail, the type of the injury and the fixation failure should be considered when contemplating revision versus continued observation.

Infection must be considered whenever fixation fails, especially when it is diagnosed late. Prior to intervention, appropriate preoperative work-up includes a leukocyte count with manual differential, erythrocyte sedimentation rate, C-reactive protein, and aspiration for culture and Gram's stain. If an infection is suspected or diagnosed, a staged reconstructive procedure is indicated.

Decreased Knee Motion

Poor motion after periarticular fractures is a common complication, and the distal femur is not an exception. As with other complications noted after a supracondylar femur fracture, prophylaxis is the most effective treatment. Early motion after stable internal fixation, especially in the setting of intracondylar extension, is vital to avoid late stiffness and contracture. The etiology of poor postoperative motion is varied: (1) malreduction of the articular surface, (2) intra-articular hardware, (3) joint adhesions, (4) capsular or ligamentous scarring, (5) extra-articular muscle contracture, and (6) post-traumatic arthritis.[3]

After determining the cause of the poor motion, appropriate steps may be taken to address the problem directly. If malreduction of the articular surface is suspected, the risks and realistic gains of hardware revision should be considered and discussed with the patient. All intra-articular hardware should be removed. Joint adhesions can be treated with aggressive physical therapy followed by manipulation under anesthesia for recalcitrant cases. Joint stiffness secondary to capsular contracture may be addressed at the time of manipulation with surgical release. Quadriceps and hamstring muscle contractures should be identified and treated at the time of manipulation as well.

Quadriceps adhesions and contracture are common after ORIF and frequently require release from the anterior aspect of the femur. Hamstring contractures may be effectively treated with careful percutaneous release along its distal, tendinous portion, both medially and laterally. Post-traumatic arthritis is common after high-energy injuries and should be treated with nonsteroidal anti-inflammatory agents as well as physical therapy. Arthroscopy may be required to evaluate the joint surface and débride post-traumatic and degenerative pathology within the knee. In severe cases, realignment osteotomy, arthrodesis, or arthroplasty may be considered as a salvage procedure.

SUPRACONDYLAR FEMUR FRACTURE IPSILATERAL TO A TOTAL KNEE ARTHROPLASTY

A supracondylar femur fracture proximal to a total knee arthroplasty (TKA) presents several additional challenges compared with the injuries discussed to this point. Historical review of the literature demonstrates the wide variety of treatment options.[65, 102–110] In his review article of the literature from the 1980s, Ayers[111] commented that there seemed to be near-equal good and excellent results for both surgical (69%) and nonsurgical treatment (68%). These findings are similar to those reported by Chen and associates.[121] With the increasing prevalence of this injury complex as well as with further refinements in both surgical technique and implants, the indications for either surgical or nonsurgical treatment should become more clearly delineated.

Epidemiology

The incidence of supracondylar femur fractures ipsilateral to a TKA ranges from 0.3% to 2.5%.[102, 103, 106, 109, 111–113, 117] Predisposing factors to this injury include chronic immunosuppressive or steroid therapy, neurological disorders, rheumatoid arthritis, malalignment, and revision arthroplasty associated with distal femoral bone loss.[103, 110, 126] Arthrofibrosis[103] (leading to a stress fracture in the metaphysis) and polyethylene wear debris[114] have also been implicated in the etiology of supracondylar periprosthetic femur fractures. Although it was originally thought that notching of the anterior cortex was a significant predisposing factor for fracture,[102, 103] Ritter and associates[108] found only one fracture in a review of 180 patients undergoing TKA who had anterior femoral notching. The authors, however, concede that anterior femoral notching may play a more prominent etiological role in the setting of marked osteoporosis.

Liu and associates[115] have reported preliminary data suggesting that the bone mineral density in the supracondylar area of patients 1 year after TKA is 10% to 13% lower than in age-matched controls. After the first year, the bone mineral density equilibrates. Although the authors speculate about the cause of this phenomenon, further study is required to elucidate its significance in the development of a distal femur fracture. The most common mechanism of injury in this older age group is minor trauma, such as a fall from a standing position on a flexed knee.[109, 113, 116]

Classification

Several investigators have adapted the Neer classification system for distal femur fractures to apply in this periprosthetic setting.[27, 104, 106] Within this three-part classification scheme, a type I fracture is minimally (less than 5 mm of translation and 5 degrees of angulation) or not displaced. A type II fracture describes either medial (type IIA) or lateral (type IIB) displacement of the shaft relative to the distal segment. Type III fractures demonstrate significant supracondylar comminution. To further simplify the classification of these injuries, many investigators[3, 110, 121] have combined Neer type II and III fractures into a single group, yielding a classification scheme with either type I fractures (minimally or not displaced) and type II fractures (displaced or comminuted). More recently, Rorabeck and associates[126] further modified the classification of these injuries with the addition of a type III fracture, which includes displaced or nondisplaced fractures associated with a loose femoral component.

Management

Conservative Nonoperative Management

Conservative management of supracondylar periprosthetic fractures, including closed reduction, traction, casting, and/or cast-bracing, was recommended for most of these injuries when they first were being reported in the literature.[104–107, 110, 124] The rates of malunion and nonunion in comminuted fractures, however, were unacceptably high in two of the larger series.[103, 106] In more recent years, the pendulum has swung toward operative treatment of displaced or comminuted injuries with the increased availability of various "specialized" implants and experience in dealing with this complex problem. Conservative management of supracondylar periprosthetic fractures, therefore, is currently recommended for nondisplaced or minimally displaced fractures in which adequate alignment of the injured segment may be easily maintained with closed reduction and immobilization.[118, 119, 125] Typical treatment includes closed reduction (if necessary) followed by either traction or cast immobilization for 2 to 4 weeks.[111, 117] Gentle range-of-motion exercises in a hinged cast or brace are then initiated while the non-weightbearing activity restriction is continued until there is radiographic evidence of healing.

In their meta-analysis of the treatment of these injuries, Chen and associates[121] reported that 35 of 47 patients (74%) experienced a satisfactory outcome with casting alone and 43 of 71 patients (67%) experienced a satisfactory outcome with traction and casting. The poorer results with traction and casting likely reflect the fact that patients who required traction had displaced fractures.

Operative Management

The indications for open management of a supracondylar periprosthetic femur fracture include low-energy injuries that do not maintain adequate alignment with closed techniques, fractures with a significant amount of associated comminution, open fractures, fractures associated with a loose femoral component, and fractures in patients who would not otherwise effectively tolerate traction and bracing because of medical or physical constraints.

OPEN REDUCTION, INTERNAL FIXATION

After finding unacceptable rates of nonunion and malunion with conservative treatment of these injuries, several investigators[103, 111, 122, 123] advocated immediate open reduction and rigid internal fixation for displaced supracondylar periprosthetic femur fractures. Many different devices are available for ORIF, including fixed-angle periarticular plates, cobra plates, buttress plates, blade plates, and condylar screws. The plate-screw option usually requires that the distal fragment have at least one intact cortex (either medial or lateral) of sufficient density to accept fixation.

Although the condylar screw is the least technically demanding of the devices to implant, the lag screw is bulky and requires the removal of valuable bone during the reaming process. The buttress plates are also relatively easy to apply but offer inferior fixation and should be reserved for salvage procedures. The fixed-angle blade plate provides excellent fixation in periprosthetic fractures because the blade can be juxtaposed to the lugs of the femoral component or along the back of the intercondylar box of a posterior stabilized component. Even in osteoporotic bone, the 95-degree angled blade plate dictates a mild valgus angle to the comminuted fracture site in the setting of a stable femoral arthroplasty component. If stable fixation cannot be achieved intraoperatively, augmentation of the fixation is required. Some investigators[118] have advocated augmentation via a small window on the lateral cortex of the lateral femoral condyle, through which the metaphysis may be packed or injected with autograft, allograft, or bone cement. Zehntner and Ganz[135] described augmentation of screw holes through the osteoporotic bone of the distal segment with bone cement injected through a syringe.

Healy and associates[118] reported on a group of 20 supracondylar periprosthetic femur fractures treated with open reduction and stable internal fixation. Fifteen of these patients also underwent primary bone grafting. The authors found 90% union (two patients required repeat ORIF) and return of the average Knee Society score to its premorbid level. Zehntner and Ganz[135] found satisfactory results with the use of condylar buttress plates in a cohort of six patients, all of whom returned to their premorbid level of ambulation. Moran and associates,[125] while advocating the use of ORIF for displaced periprosthetic femur fractures, reported only 67% satisfactory results in their cohort of 15 patients and acknowledged the significant rate of complications with this technique. Chen and associates[121] reported 65% satisfactory outcome in their analysis of 52 patients in the literature. Not all investigators have reported equally satisfactory results.[104, 107, 133]

FRACTURE REDUCTION AND TECHNIQUES FOR STABILIZATION

As discussed previously, fractures of the distal femur present with a wide range of injury severity, including supracondylar comminution and possible articular involvement. Treating physicians, therefore, must have a multiplicity of surgical techniques at their disposal to treat these complicated injuries.

95-DEGREE CONDYLAR BLADE PLATE

Either an anterior or a lateral approach may be employed with the 95-degree blade plate. The incision for the anterior approach, however, is usually longer than anticipated, depending on the volume of the quadriceps mechanism. Care should be taken to limit perios-

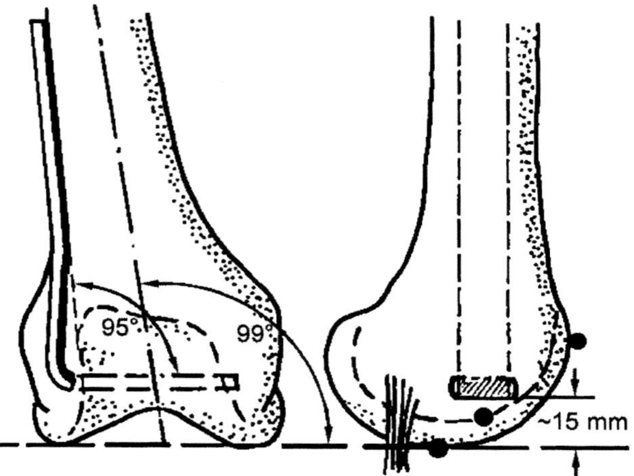

FIGURE 60.4 ➢ Insertion site for the 95-degree Condylar Blade Plate is 1.5 to 2 mm cephalad from the inferior articular surface in the coronal plane and in the middle third of the anterior half of the width of the lateral femoral condyle in the sagittal plane.

teal stripping of the lateral aspect of the distal femur. Homann retractors should be used to aid in exposure rather than wider, blunt instruments such as Bennett retractors.

The first step in treating a periarticular fracture of the distal femur is anatomic reduction of the articular surface. Provisional 2-mm K-wires should be placed laterally to medially to hold the reduction. Placement of intercondylar lag screws should be delayed until the insertion site for the blade plate has been planned.

The length of the blade and side plate are determined through preoperative planning. Insertion site for the blade plate is 1.5 to 2 mm cephalad from the inferior articular surface in the coronal plane and in the middle third of the anterior half of the width of the lateral femoral condyle in the sagittal plane (Fig. 60.4). The insertion point must be determined exactly so that an anatomic reduction of the supracondylar portion of the fracture can be maintained when the side plate is reduced to the femoral shaft. Once determined, the insertion site should be marked with cautery. Several intercondylar, 6.5-mm, partially threaded, cancellous lag screws then can be placed from the lateral to medial aspects. The screws should be inserted just cephalad to the blade-plate insertion site. Although the medial cortex can be violated with the drill, care should be taken to ensure that the screws remain unicortical. Medial cortex penetration with a 6.5-mm lag screw may contribute to long-term pain and disability with knee motion. Occasionally, a 16-mm threaded 6.5-mm screw is required instead of a 32-mm screw to keep all of the threads across the fracture site. To ensure that the screws are directed outside of the path of the blade plate, the seating chisel may be placed first as outlined later.

Once the condyles are anatomically reduced and internally fixed, the distal portion of the femur must be reduced and attached to the femoral shaft (Fig. 60.5). This is accomplished with meticulous insertion of the blade plate into the distal femur. Two temporary 2-mm K-wires are placed as guides for insertion of the seating chisel for the 95-degree condylar blade plate. K-wire No. 1 is inserted across the knee joint parallel to the inferior aspect of the medial and lateral condyles. K-wire No. 2 is inserted anteriorly across the patellofemoral joint, sloping from anterior to posterior and parallel to the condyles in the coronal plane. The definitive or "summation" K-wire No. 3 is inserted approximately 1 cm cephalad to the inferior aspect of the articular surface, just inferior to the area marked with cautery for the insertion of the seating chisel. This final K-wire No. 3, which is placed parallel to K-wire No. 1 in the coronal plane and parallel to K-wire No. 2 in the axial plane, acts as the definitive guide for the placement of the seating chisel. In fractures without supracondylar comminution, the position of the summation wire can also be verified with the condylar guide (represents a mirror image of the blade plate). The provisional K-wires No. 1 and No. 2 should be removed before the seating chisel is tapped into position.

In young patients with dense trabecular cancellous bone, attempting to pass the seating chisel without predrilling the condylar blade plate tract may lead to loss of reduction or additional comminution at the insertion site. Predrilling is easily accomplished using three 4.5-mm drill bits and the appropriate three-hole guide. The guide is placed along the distal femur against the summation K-wire No. 3. The three drill bits are then passed across the distal femur parallel in all planes to summation K-wire No. 3.

Starting with the middle hole, intraoperative fluoroscopy is used to verify the parallel position of the drill holes to the summation K-wire. It is vital to accurately assess the sagittal (flexion/extension) alignment of the guide against the distal femur prior to creating the drill holes and passing the seating chisel. Although a few degrees of correction can be used to adjust the blade during insertion, sagittal plane malalignment is one of the more common mistakes during the application of this device. The window in the lateral cortex is then expanded with the router in the three drill holes. To seat the "axilla" of the blade plate fully against the bone, it is often necessary to remove a 0.5- to 1.0-cm strip of bone underlying the most caudad portion of the side plate with an osteotome.

The seating chisel is assembled with the seating chisel guide. This allows greater control of the sagittal plane alignment as the chisel is passed across the condyles. It may be helpful to take the long slap hammer and place it perpendicularly over the guide. This maneuver allows the surgeon some mechanical advantage in holding and controlling rotation during chisel insertion. It may also be helpful to insert the chisel under fluoroscopic guidance, especially for the inexperienced surgeon. The seating chisel is inserted to a predetermined depth. It should be appreciated that the distal femur is a trapezoid, with a 25-degree angle on the medial side from the posterior to anterior aspects. Again, care must be taken not to penetrate the medial cortex with the seating chisel. On an AP radiograph,

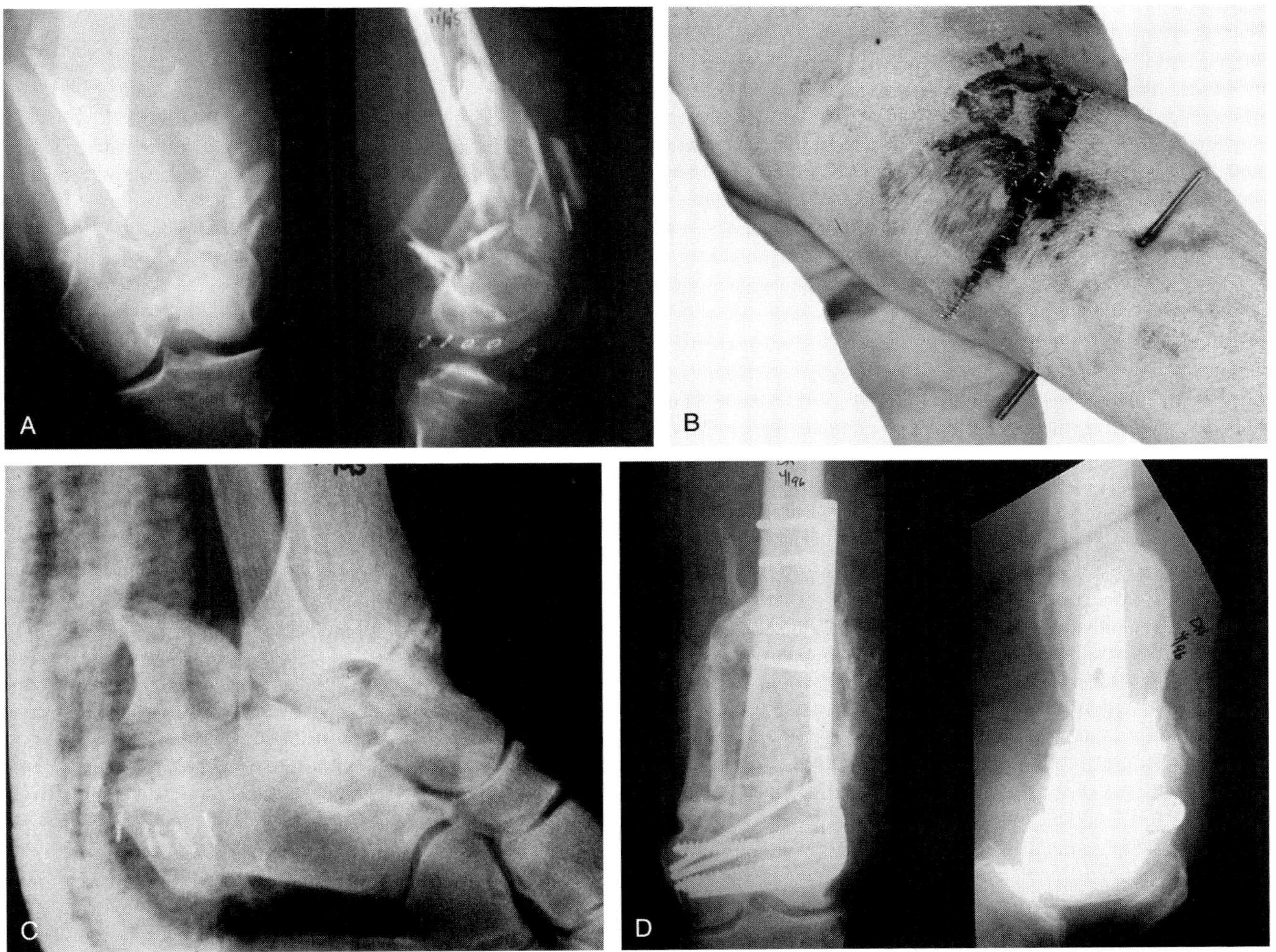

FIGURE 60.5 ➢ A 75-year-old female was a restrained passenger in a high-speed motor vehicle accident and sustained an open left femur fracture and a right open talus fracture dislocation. Ten days after initial irrigation and débridement and traction for the left open femur, she was transferred for definitive care. She underwent ORIF using a 95-degree blade plate with lag-screw placement and removal of the talus and primary fusion of the tibia to the calcaneus. *A,* Anteroposterior and lateral radiographs showing an AO C2 supracondylar distal femur fracture. *B,* Clinical preoperative photograph at 10 days post injury showing the previously open wound and traction pin. *C,* Lateral radiograph of the right ankle demonstrating a posterior fracture dislocation of the talus. *D,* Anteroposterior and lateral radiographs 5 months after ORIF with placement of a 95-degree blade plate demonstrating bone healing/union.

the chisel appears "too short" because of the underlying shadow of the wider posterior medial femoral condyle. The 95-degree condylar blade plate is then inserted along the prepared tract in the femoral condyles and impacted to lie flush with the lateral cortex.

Prior to reduction of the supracondylar portion of the injury, the distal femoral fixation is further augmented by insertion of one or two fully threaded 6.5-mm screws through the most distal aspect of the plate. This not only enhances the rotational stability of the condylar fragment but prevents lateral excursion of the blade during application of axial compression. The distal portion of the femur, now securely attached to the blade plate, is then reduced to the femoral shaft and held in position with one or two Verbrugge clamps. In fractures without significant comminution, axial compression can be achieved with the articulated tension device; occasionally, in cases without bone loss and after an anatomic reduction, additional compression may be applied by loading screws through the dynamic compression plate. In fractures with comminution or bone loss, the viable fragments with soft-tissue attachments may be keyed into position after appropriate ligamentotaxis has been applied. Whenever possible, lag screws across the supracondylar portion of the fracture should be inserted through the plate.

The 95-degree condylar blade plate is indicated for most supracondylar and bicondylar distal femur fractures. Distal fixation is achieved by the contact of the broad surface of the blade and the addition of the distal cancellous lag screws through the plate into the condyles. In very low transcondylar fractures, especially in elderly patients, distal fixation with the condylar blade plate may be inadequate and alternate methods are indicated. If there is significant comminution of the condyles or of the intercondylar area, adequate fixation of the distal femur with this device may not be possible.

DYNAMIC CONDYLAR SCREW AND SIDE PLATE

The design of the DCS and side plate is similar to that of the 95-degree condylar blade plate, except that the blade is replaced with a 95-degree cannulated compression screw. The condylar compression screw is generally easier to insert into the condyles than the 95-degree condylar blade plate for the following reasons:

- It is a cannulated screw system inserted over a guide wire. Most surgeons are already familiar with this type of system, which is frequently used to fix intertrochanteric fractures.
- Because a power-driven triple reamer is used over the guide wire for the compression screw, the intercondylar tract for the screw is precut and eliminates the complications associated with hammering the chisel across the condyles.
- The system eliminates the need for meticulous sagittal-plane control when the compression screw is inserted across the condyles because of the free rotation of the side plate around the screw.

The operative technique for insertion of the DCS is similar to that for the 95-degree condylar blade plate except in the technique for insertion of the compression screw (Fig. 60.6). Provisional K-wires No. 1 and No. 2 are inserted. The starting point for the DCS, however, is approximately 2 cm cephalad to the articular surface and at the junction of the anterior and middle thirds of the sagittal width of the lateral femoral condyle. This is just proximal to the cephaloposterior edge of the window for insertion of the blade plate.

In this system, the "summation" wire becomes the definitive guide for the cannulated screw system. The 230-mm guide wire with a threaded tip is inserted into the premarked area along the lateral cortex parallel to both provisional K-wires. The condylar compression screw angle guide may be helpful in the absence of significant comminution. The guide wire should be inserted until it is felt to just penetrate the medial cortex. Again, even with fluoroscopy, determining the medial edge of the distal femur in the AP plane can be deceiving given the trapezoidal shape of the condyles. A reverse-calibrated measuring device is placed over the guide wire to allow direct measurement of the length. The triple reamer is then set for 10 mm less than the measured length to avoid penetration of the medial cortex. A cannulated screw of correct length is then inserted over the wire (Fig. 60.7). In elderly patients with osteoporotic bone, a condylar screw 5 mm longer than the measured length may be chosen in an attempt to gain better fixation. The appropriate length side plate is then placed over the compression screw (Fig. 60.8). The remainder of the technique is similar to that described for the 95-degree condylar blade plate (Figs. 60.9 and 60.10).

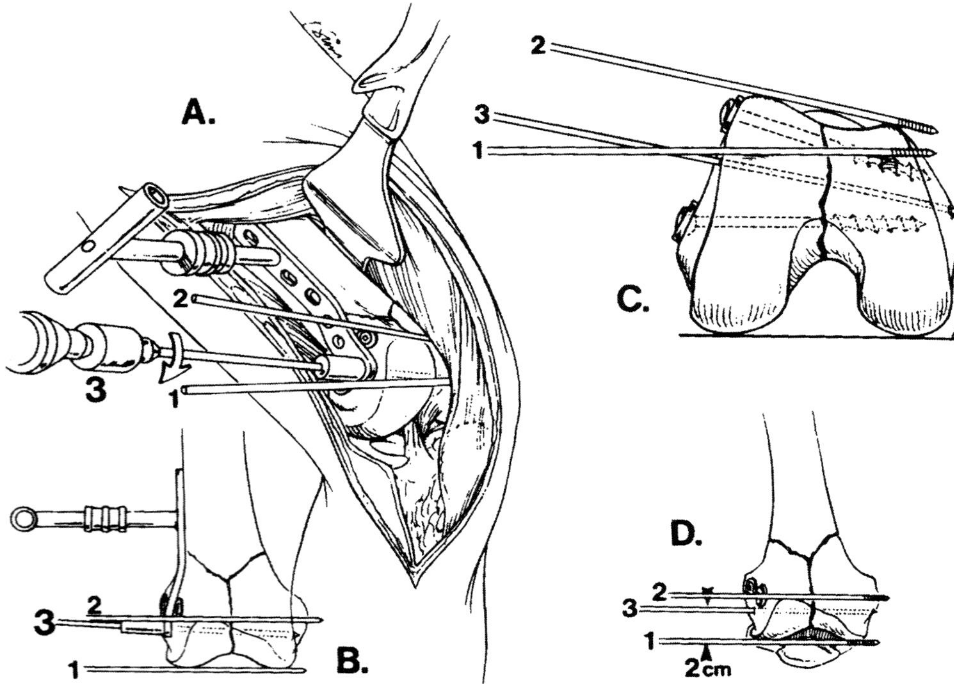

FIGURE 60.6 ➢ The condylar screw system. Placement of the three directional guide wires (1, 2, and 3, respectively). *A,* The first wire is parallel to the joint axis. *B,* The second wire shows the inclination of the patellofemoral joint and slopes down from the lateral to medial aspects. *C,* The third wire is parallel to both the first and second wires and serves as the definitive guide for the triple reamer and large condylar screw. *D,* The point of entry for the third wire should be about 2 cm from the joint and in line with the femoral shaft. (From Miza RD: Supracondylar and articular fractures of the restricted distal femur. In Chapman MW, ed: Operative Orthopaedics. Philadelphia, Lippincott, 1988.)

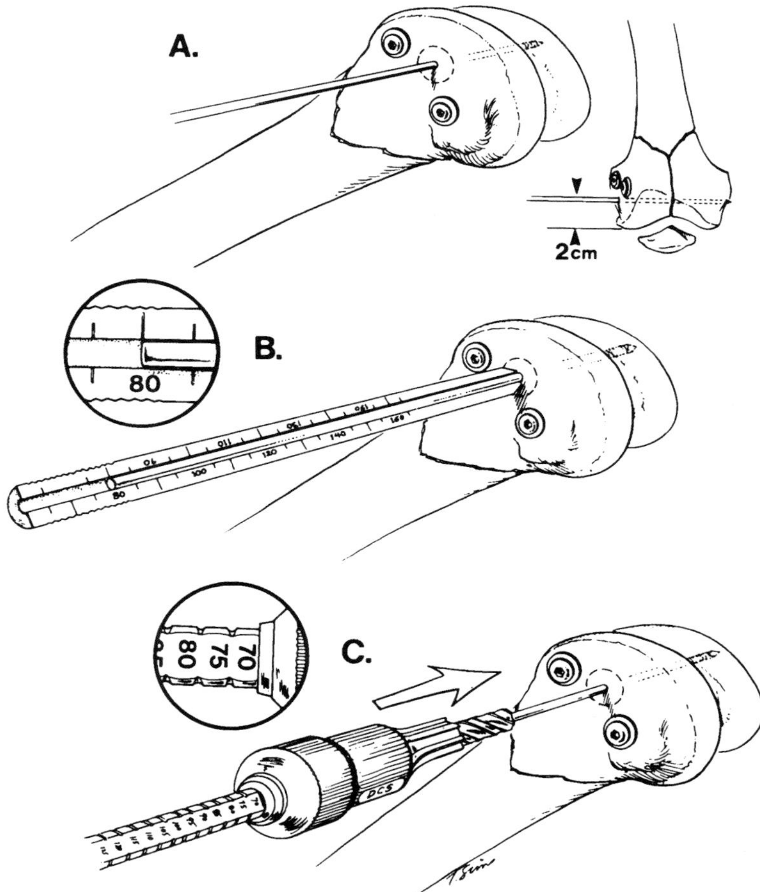

FIGURE 60.7 ➢ Preparation of the tunnel for placement of the condylar screw. *A,* The point of entry for the condylar lag screw should be about 2 cm from the knee joint and in line with the middle of the femoral shaft or slightly anterior. The third wire should be parallel with the knee joint axis, and the tip should just penetrate the medial cortex. *B,* Reverse calibration on the measuring device allows direct measurement of the guide pin depth if a standard 9-inch or 230-mm wire is used. *C,* The depth setting on the triple reamer should be approximately 10 mm less than the measurement from the direct measuring device. The triple reamer is cannulated and can be slipped over the guide wire. (From Miza RD: Supracondylar and articular fractures of the restricted distal femur. In Chapman MW, ed: Operative Orthopaedics. Philadelphia, Lippincott, 1988.)

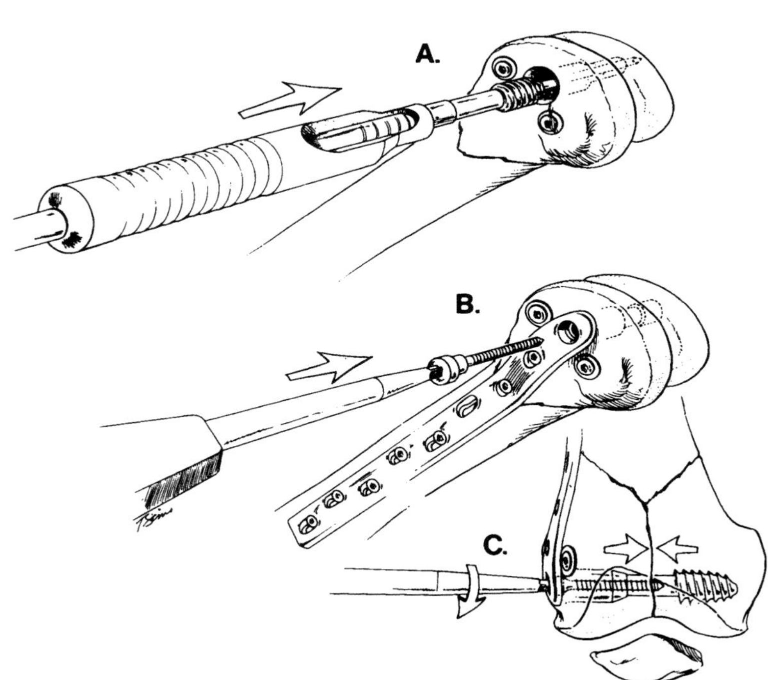

FIGURE 60.8 ➢ Placement of the condylar compression screw plate. *A,* The cannulated condylar screw is slipped over the guide wire and inserted into the reamed hole. *B,* The compressing screw is inserted. *C,* The compressing screw is tightened, resulting in interfragmentary compression between the split condyles. (From Miza RD: Supracondylar and articular fractures of the restricted distal femur. In Chapman MW, ed: Operative Orthopaedics. Philadelphia, Lippincott, 1988.)

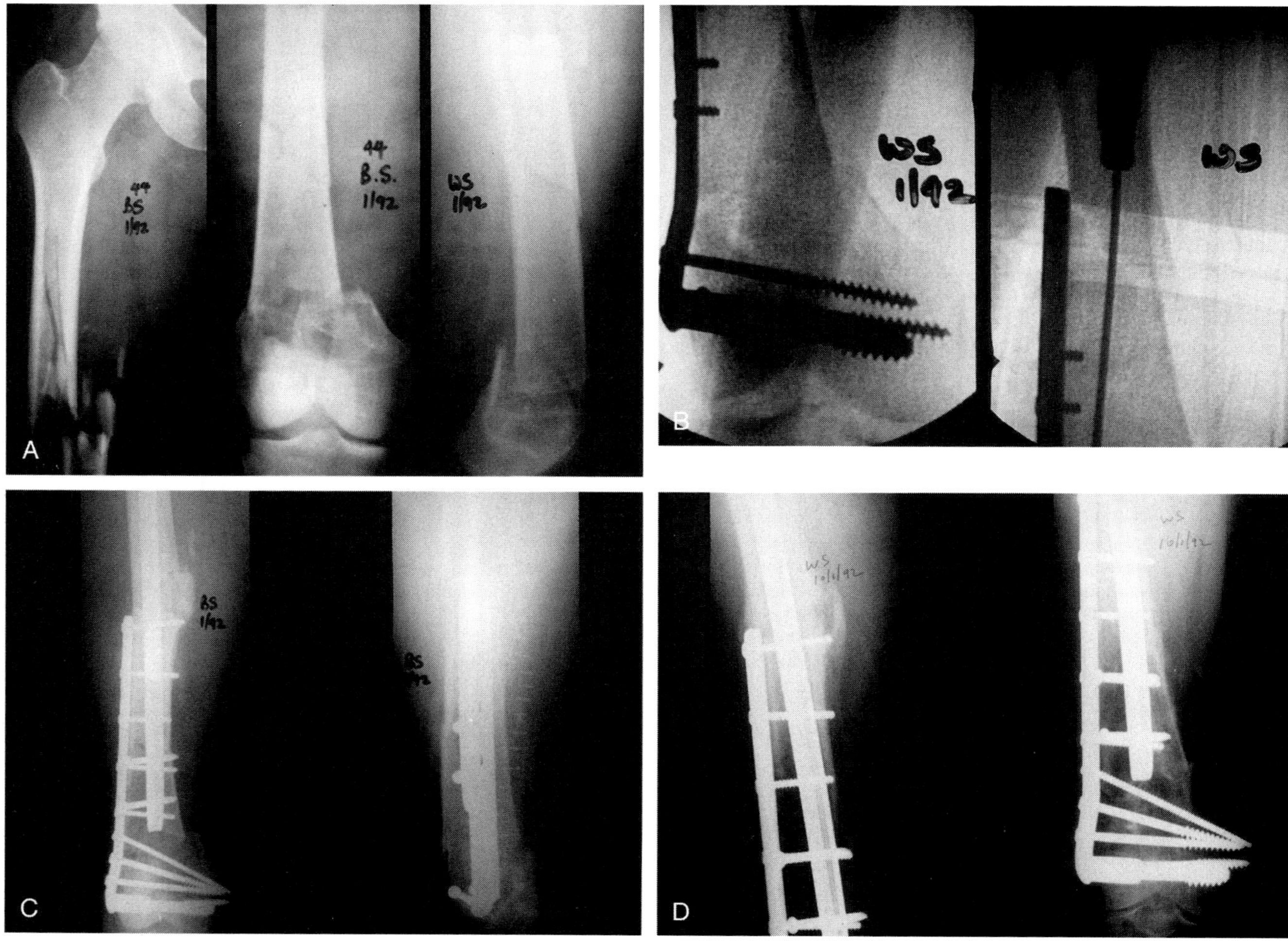

FIGURE 60.9 ➢ A 44-year-old male was involved in a motor vehicle accident and suffered closed ipsilateral segmental fractures of the femoral shaft and a supracondylar/intercondylar fracture of the distal femur. He subsequently underwent ORIF of the supracondylar/intracondylar fracture of the distal femur with a Dynamic Condylar Screw (DCS) and antegrade intramedullary locked nailing for the segmental fracture of the femoral shaft. *A,* Anteroposterior and lateral radiographs showing an AO 32 C3.1 fracture of the femoral shaft and AO 33 C2.1 supracondylar distal femur fracture. *B,* Perioperative fluoroscopic image showing placement of the DCS and plate and guide wire for the antegrade intramedullary nail. *C,* Postoperative anteroposterior and lateral radiographs showing satisfactory reduction and stabilization of the femoral diaphysis and distal femur. *D,* Anteroposterior radiographs taken 9 months after ORIF demonstrating bone healing/union.

CONDYLAR BUTTRESS PLATE

The condylar buttress plate was designed to allow multiple lag screw fixation of complex condylar fractures. It consists of a broad compression side plate and a bifurcated, precontoured distal portion to fit the lateral surface of the lateral femoral condyle. Because they are precontoured, the plates are "side-specific" and each set should have plates for both the right and left sides. Although up to six lag screws can be inserted through the plate into the distal femur, it is not a fixed-angle device and therefore is susceptible to axial malalignment. It should only be used when the fracture morphology does not allow the use of either the 95-degree condylar blade plate or the DCS and side plate. Its primary indications are as follows:

- Low transcondylar fractures or comminuted fractures of the lateral or medial condyles in which stable fixation with a fixed-angle device is perceived to be inadequate.
- Coronal or very comminuted articular fractures in which screw fixation of the condyles precludes the use of a fixed-angle device.

The condylar buttress plate should be a part of the armamentarium available for fixation of all distal femur fractures should intraoperative complications preclude the use of another device. One of the more common initial complications with the condylar buttress plate is relative valgus axial malalignment from applying lag screws through the plate without some plate pre-bend. Frequently, a radiograph of the contra-

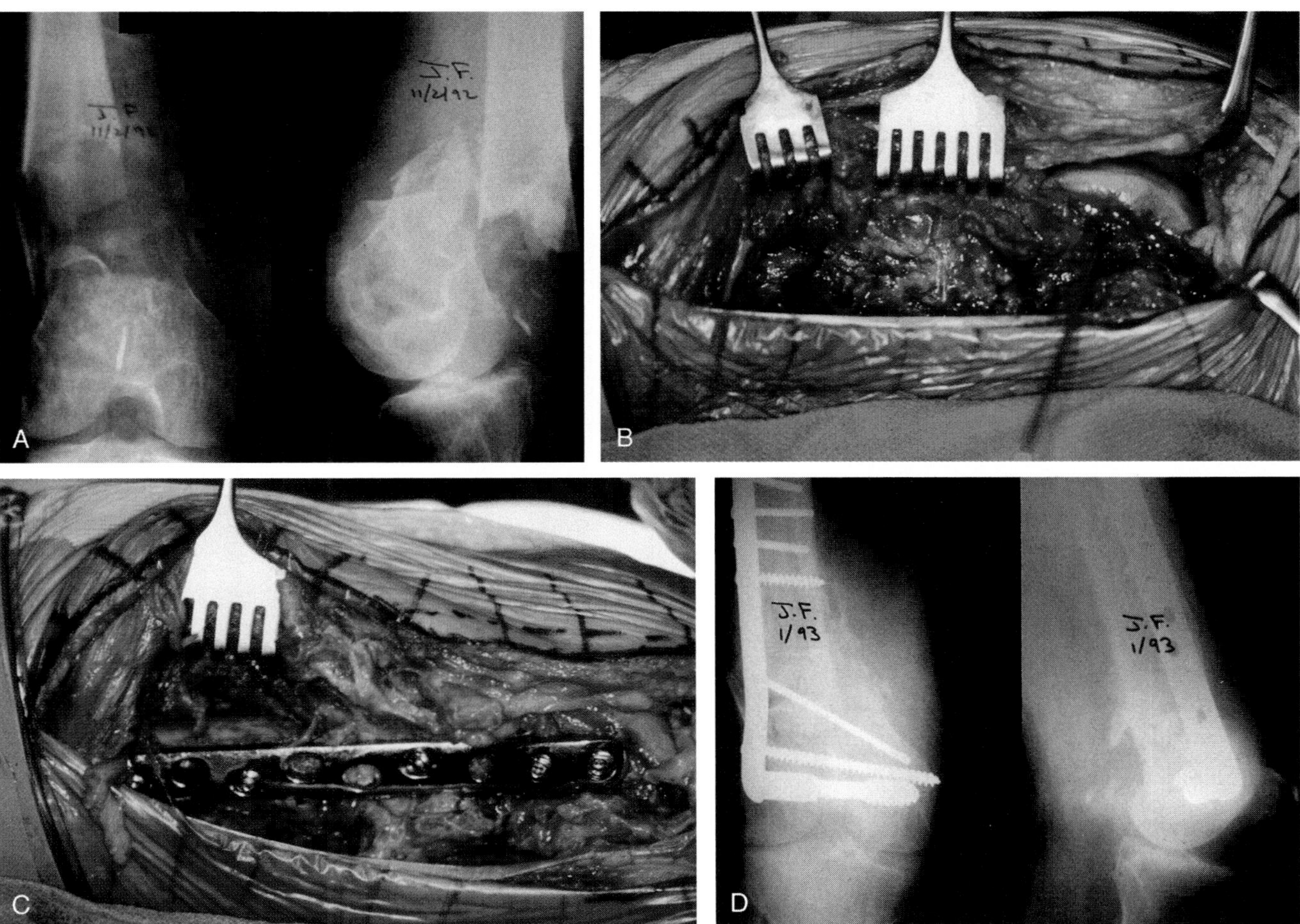

FIGURE 60.10 ➢ An 82-year-old male pedestrian was struck by an automobile while crossing an intersection. He sustained a closed right supracondylar femur fracture. He was placed in tibial traction and then transferred for definitive care. He underwent ORIF and placement of a Dynamic Condylar Screw (DCS). *A,* Anteroposterior and lateral radiographs showing an AO 33 A3 supracondylar distal femur fracture. *B,* Intraoperative photograph showing placement of the 230-mm guide wire with a threaded tip into the premarked area along the lateral cortex parallel to both provisional K-wires for DCS insertion. *C,* Intraoperative photograph showing the inserted DCS and side plate. *D,* Anteroposterior and lateral radiographs taken 5 months after ORIF with DCS demonstrating bone healing/union.

lateral distal femur provides some clues as to the patient's normal axial alignment. Even though the plates are precontoured, they usually require some pre-bend to approximate the patient's anatomy (Fig. 60.11).

Because the condylar buttress plate is not a fixed-angle device, it does not resist axial loading as well as other devices and therefore may lead to relative late varus malalignment. Several vendors manufacture a hybrid plate that allows multiple lag-screw fixation distally with screws that also thread into the plate. This essentially adds to the axial stability of the construct by providing the plate with "fixed-angle screws." These devices are new, and extensive clinical and biomechanical testing is pending.

ANTEGRADE INTRAMEDULLARY NAIL FIXATION

As discussed previously, some authors have advocated the treatment of distal femur fractures with reamed antegrade nailing.[15, 30] The technique involves open anatomic reduction and fixation of the periarticular fractures followed by closed, reamed antegrade nailing of the femur. This technique has been shown to be a viable treatment option for some type A and occasional C1/C2 fractures.[15]

Although specific techniques vary, in general patients should be placed supine on a radiolucent table. Any intra-articular fracture extension should be reduced and fixed with 6.5-mm lag screws through an

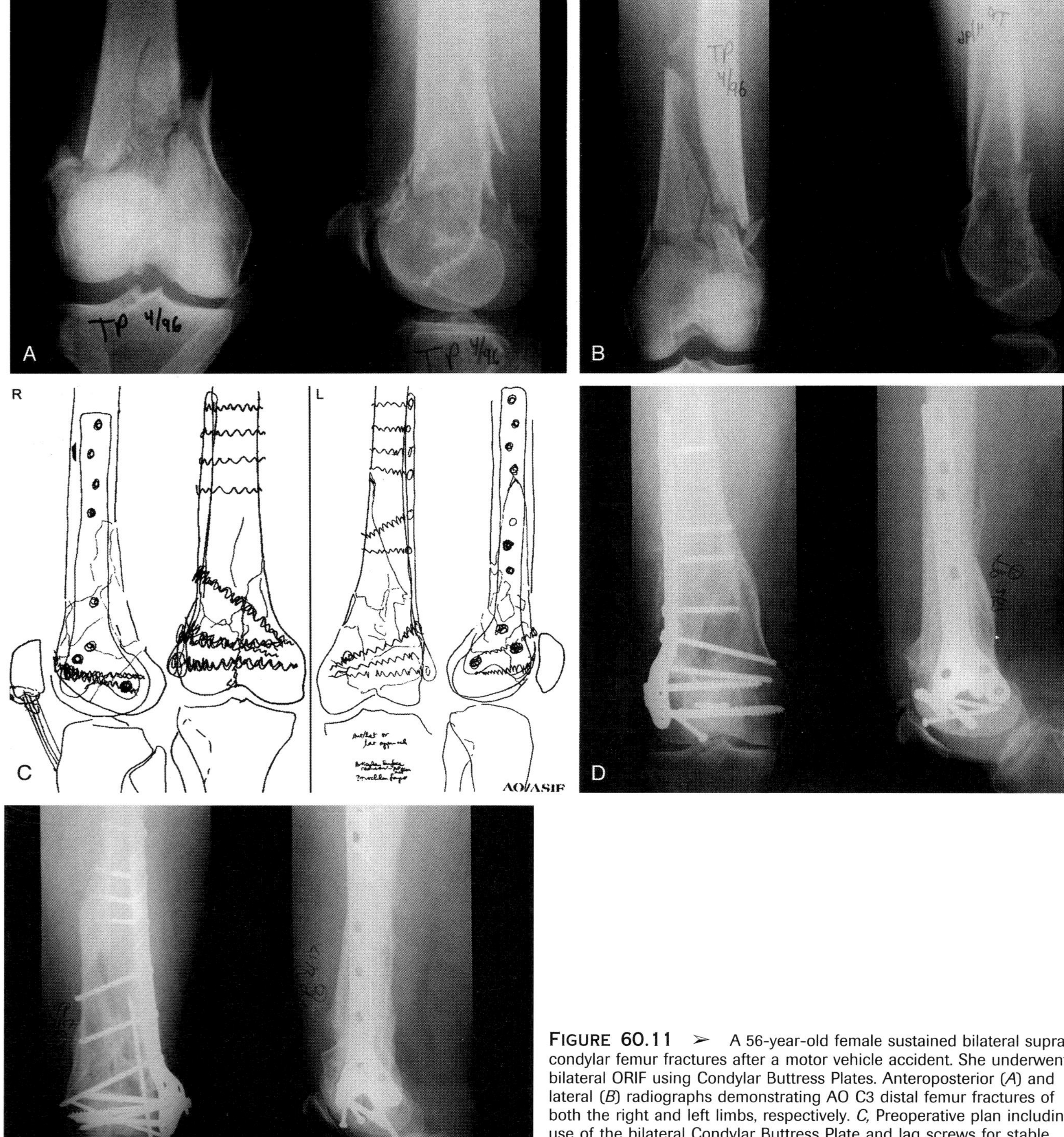

FIGURE 60.11 ➢ A 56-year-old female sustained bilateral supracondylar femur fractures after a motor vehicle accident. She underwent bilateral ORIF using Condylar Buttress Plates. Anteroposterior (*A*) and lateral (*B*) radiographs demonstrating AO C3 distal femur fractures of both the right and left limbs, respectively. *C*, Preoperative plan including use of the bilateral Condylar Buttress Plate and lag screws for stable fixation. Anteroposterior (*D*) and lateral (*E*) radiographs taken 1 year after ORIF demonstrate union/bone healing.

adequate anterior arthrotomy. The entire joint surface should be visualized to aid in obtaining anatomic reduction. The arthrotomy is then closed over a suction drain and the leg is re-prepared for the closed nailing. Depending on the experience of the surgeon, the nailing may be performed with the patient supine on a fracture table with skeletal traction or on a radiolucent table without traction. This procedure is much more technically demanding than a standard antegrade femoral nail because meticulous attention must be paid to the length of the device as well as the axial and rotational alignment of the reduction. This is especially

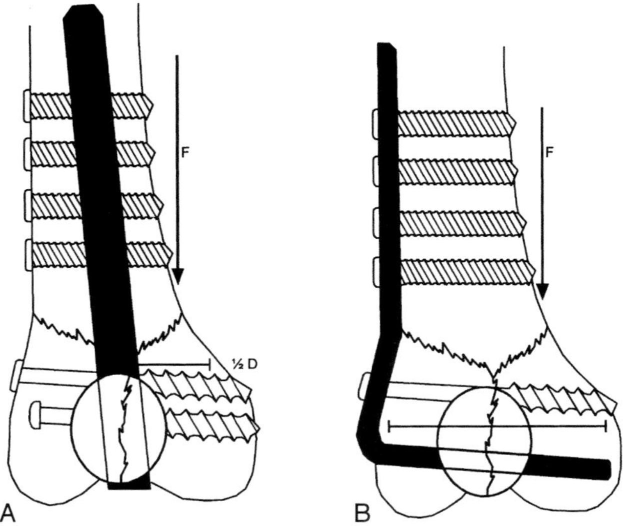

FIGURE 60.12 ➢ Supracondylar type A fracture reduced and stabilized with (*A*) a retrograde nail and (*B*) a 95-degree blade plate. The forces (F) are better distributed along the axis of the bone in the intramedullary nail than with the 95-degree blade plate. D = diameter.

important when the nail is inserted with the patient in the lateral position because of the tendency of the leg to fall into excessive external rotation and valgus.

RETROGRADE INTRAMEDULLARY NAIL FIXATION

Several groups have reported on the use of the GSH nail for the treatment of distal femur fractures with varying levels of success.[90–93] The GSH nail is fully cannulated and is produced with several different lengths to accommodate various injury patterns. The distal locking holes are quite caudad on the nail and therefore may stretch the indications for use of this device to include low transcondylar fractures (Figs. 60.12 and 60.13).

The patient should be placed supine on a radiolucent table with a bump under the knee. For patients with intra-articular extension of their fracture, a standard arthrotomy (as opposed to a "percutaneous" incision advocated by some) should be performed so that anatomic reduction of the articular surface can be visualized. Again, the condyles should be internally stabilized with several 6.5-mm lag screws. Care must be taken not to interfere with the intercondylar starting point or the course of the nail when inserting the lag screws. A curved awl or twist drill is used to create the starting point, found just anterior to the insertion of the posterior cruciate ligament. On a true lateral radiograph of the distal femur, the starting point is found at the junction of Blumensat's line and a line extended from the posterior cortex of the femur. The appropriate length nail is then passed over a guide wire across the manually reduced fracture. The cross-locking in the GSH system is accomplished both proximally and distally through an aiming device. It is important to bury the tip of the nail below the articular surface. This should be verified on a true lateral radiograph by ensuring that the nail is cephalad to Blumensat's line.

Several variations of the GSH nail have been produced that include more numerous length options as well as AP proximal locking. This allows the retrograde nail to be inserted past the isthmus and subtrochanteric area where stress-risers from the cross-locks might be less of a concern. The Distal Femoral Nail (Synthes, Paoli, PA) has, in addition, an end cap that locks the most distal cross-lock into position, creating a fixed angle between the nail and the cross-lock. Clinical trials with this new generation of intramedullary devices are ongoing.

INTRAMEDULLARY NAIL FIXATION

Treatment of supracondylar periprosthetic femur fractures with retrograde intramedullary devices is gaining popularity.[119, 127–131] The retrograde nails allow an opportunity to gain fixation of poor-quality, osteoporotic bone without the risks and complications of a large incision and dissection. A caveat to the use of these devices is that they require careful preoperative planning and knowledge of the brand and type of indwelling femoral component. Most of the manufacturers are currently producing components that are compatible with these devices. In some of the older models, however, the intercondylar distance or notch opening may be limiting.[119]

An intercondylar distance of at least 12 mm is required for application of most of the retrograde intramedullary devices on the market. If the brand of the component cannot be determined from standard AP and lateral radiographs, a notch view should be attempted. In addition, posterior stabilized components usually have a box distal cut that articulates with the constrained tibial component. Only a few of these systems currently have an opening in the box that would accommodate a retrograde device (IB II, Zimmer, Warsaw, IN). Retrograde nails may not be used if the femoral component has an intramedullary stem. It is incumbent on the surgeon to verify the identity of the components prior to surgery. If this is not possible, alternative methods of fixation should be tentatively planned and provided for during the surgery.

Jabczenski and Crawford[130] reported on four patients that all healed with no complications. Rolston and associates[119] similarly found excellent results in their limited study of four patients treated with a retrograde femoral nail. They reported that the retrograde nail had several advantages over the plate-screw option, including decreased operative time, more rigid fixation, and access to the fracture without exposing the fracture hematoma or stripping of the fragment periosteum. McLaren and associates[137] reported good results in their series of seven patients. In all of the patients, healing eventually occurred. Four of the patients demonstrated return of their premorbid motion; the remaining three sustained losses of knee flexion of 10 to 20 degrees. Several other investigators have re-

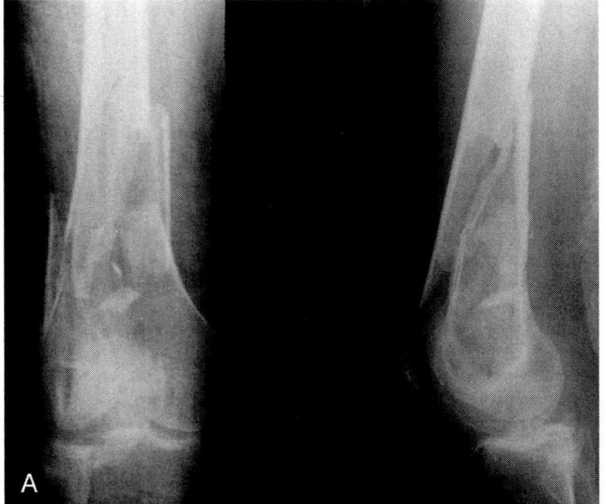

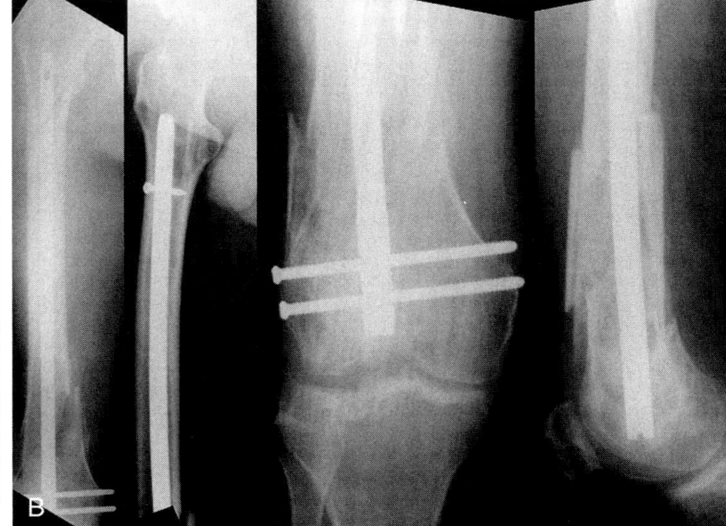

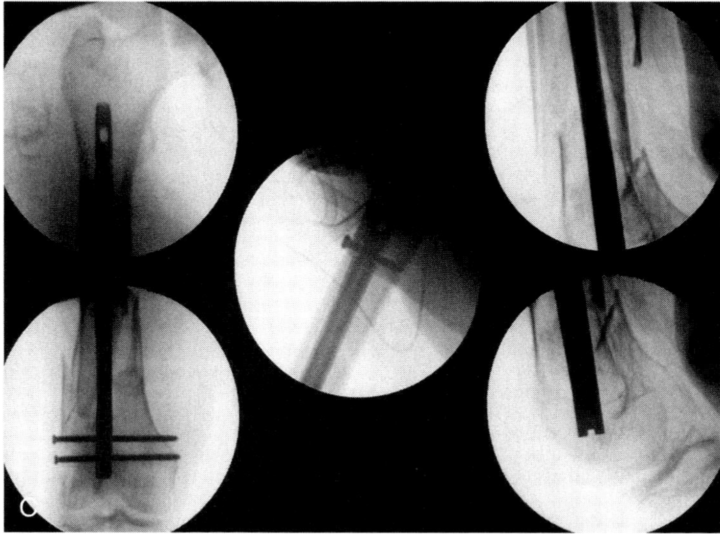

FIGURE 60.13 ➢ A 65-year-old diabetic presented to the emergency department after a fall. He complained of leg pain and denied other injuries. He was previously fully ambulatory with excellent knee motion. ORIF was performed using a retrograde locked intramedullary nail. *A,* Anteroposterior and lateral radiographs demonstrating an AO C2 right intra-articular distal femur fracture. *B,* Intraoperative anteroposterior and lateral fluoroscopic views showing insertion of a retrograde intramedullary nail with good reduction of the articular condyles and restoration of length, alignment, and rotation of the shaft. *C,* Anteroposterior and lateral radiographs taken 3 months after ORIF demonstrating progressive bone healing.

ported satisfactory results with treatment of these complex injuries with supracondylar retrograde nails.[131, 136]

REVISION TOTAL KNEE ARTHROPLASTY

There are several options for the treatment of type III fractures and select type II fractures with severely comminuted and osteoporotic bone. If the femoral component is loose, it may be revised at the time of fracture fixation or in a delayed fashion after fracture union has been achieved.[138] Revision of the femoral component should include a long-stemmed, uncemented femoral component; a linked tumor-like prosthesis; or an allograft/component composite. Every attempt should be made to retain and use a stable tibial component. Although early revision of the femoral component with a long-stemmed prosthesis or distal femoral replacement (allograft or component) is effective, Engh and Ammeen[138] have suggested that there are advantages to attempting fracture fixation initially and delaying the revision procedure. First, revision of prosthesis adjacent to a healed supracondylar fracture is technically much less demanding. Second, by allowing at least some of the comminution to consolidate and heal, it is more likely that a standard revision component rather than a large custom or tumor prosthesis will suffice.

The stem or stem extension should be inserted without cement into the medullary canal of the femur and be long enough to allow tight diaphyseal contact. Engh and Ammeen[138] recommend a stem that is at least 150 mm in length to gain purchase in the distal aspect of the isthmus. A custom, long-stemmed component can be modified with the addition of screw holes for proximal cross-locking. The distal femoral replacement prostheses, allograft/component composites, and tumor prostheses are all applied using standard cement technique. Care must be taken to properly align the femoral component perpendicular to the axis of the tibial component prior to stabilization. To obtain correct alignment, the femur is flexed to 90 degrees and the trochlear portion of the femoral component is aligned to the longitudinal axis of the tibia. In order to maintain the appropriate level of the joint-line, intercalated segments of allograft may be placed between the proximal segment and the component.[138]

It is difficult to compare the results of various reports in the literature using these techniques because of the rarity of the injury and the wide variety of implants available. Chen and associates[121] found 92% satisfactory outcomes in 11 patients. Cordiero and associates[133] reported on five patients treated with a custom-made stemmed revision component who went on to heal without complication. In their meta-analysis of treatment of these injuries, McLaren and associates[137] found that 24 of 25 patients treated with a long-stemmed femoral component had a satisfactory outcome. Kraay and associates[134] reported on the use of large, distal femoral allografts in conjunction with stemmed femoral components in a semi-constrained knee system. They found satisfactory results in all patients with limited early outcome due to the death of three patients prior to the 2-year follow-up.

Complications

A significant number of complications are reported whether these injuries are managed conservatively or operatively. The three complications most commonly reported are infection, malunion, and nonunion. In their review of the literature, Chen and associates[121] found a 30% complication rate in both the conservatively managed group (33 of 199 cases) and the operative group (23 of 77 cases).

As anticipated, the incidence of infection was statistically higher in the operative group (n = 6) than in the conservative group (n = 1).[121] In the conservatively managed group, the incidences of malunion and nonunion were 9% and 11%, respectively. The incidences of malunion and nonunion in the operative group were 4.5% and 8%, respectively. These rates compared favorably in the two groups, and the differences were not statistically different.[121] Other complications in conservatively managed patients include poor knee motion,[125] deep venous thrombosis, and contralateral below-knee amputation from heel-slough in a diabetic patient.[121] Additional surgical complications include poor knee motion, proximal migration,[138] amputation, and death.[121] Since the time of the study performed by Chen and associates,[121] the percentage of these cases treated operatively is increasing because of the increasing prevalence of the injury and recent technological advancements in implants.

References

1. Seinsheimer F III: Fractures of the distal femur. Clin Orthop 153:169, 1980.
2. Giles JB, DeLee JC, Heckman J, et al: Supracondylar-intercondylar fractures of the femur treated with a supracondylar plate and lag screw. J Bone Joint Surg Am 64:864, 1982.
3. Helfet DL, Lorich DG: Fractures of the distal femur. In Browner BD, Jupiter JB, Levine AM, Trafton PG, eds: Skeletal Trauma, 2nd ed, vol 2. Philadelphia, WB Saunders, 1997, p 2033.
4. Newman JH: Supracondylar fractures of the femur: Injury. Br J Acc Surg 21:280, 1990.
5. Paley D, Herzenberg JE, Tetsworth K, et al: Deformity planning for frontal and sagittal plane corrective osteotomies. Orthop Clin North Am 25(3):426, 1994.
6. Kolmert L, Wulff K: Epidemiology and treatment of distal femoral fractures in adults. Acta Orthop Scand 53:957, 1982.
7. Regazzoni P, Leutenegger A, Ruedi T, et al: Erste Erfahrungen mit der dynamischen Kondylenschraube bei distalen Femurfrakturen. Helv Chir Acta 53:61, 1986.
8. Arneson TJ, Melton LJ, Lewallen DG, et al: Epidemiology of diaphyseal and distal femoral fractures in Rochester, Minnesota, 1965–1984. Clin Orthop 234:188, 1988.
9. Reddy AS, Frederick RW: Evaluation of the interosseous and extraosseous blood supply to the distal femoral condyles. Am J Sports Med 26(3):415, 1998.
10. Yoshoika Y, Siu D, Cooke DV: The anatomy and functional axes of the femur. J Bone Joint Surg Am 69:873, 1987.
11. Mize RD: Treatment options for fractures of the distal femur. Instr Course Lect 43:109, 1994.
12. Stewart MJ, Sisk TD, Wallace SL: Fractures of the distal third of the femur: A comparison of methods of treatment. J Bone Joint Surg Am 48:784, 1966.
13. Yang RS, Liu HG, Liu TK: Supracondylar fractures of the femur. J Trauma 30:315, 1990.
14. Mize RD: Surgical management of complex fractures of the distal femur. Clin Orthop 240:77, 1989.
15. Leung KS, Shen WY, So WS, et al: Interlocking intramedullary nailing for supracondylar and intercondylar fractures of the distal part of the femur. J Bone Joint Surg Am 73:332, 1991.
16. Schatzker J, Tile M: The Rationale of Operative Fracture Care. New York, Springer-Verlag, 1987.
17. Aglietti P, Buzzi R: Fractures of the femoral condyles. In Insall JN, Windsor RE, Scott WN, et al, eds: Surgery of the Knee, 2nd ed, vol 2. New York, Churchill Livingstone, 1993, p 983.
18. Green NE, Allen FL: Vascular injuries associated with dislocation of the knee. J Bone Joint Surg Am 59:236, 1977.
19. Kennedy JC: Complete dislocation of the knee joint. J Bone Joint Surg Am 45:889, 1963.
20. Meyers MH, Moore TM, Harvey JP: Traumatic dislocation of the knee joint. J Bone Joint Surg Am 68:430, 1975.
21. Sisto DJ, Warren RF: Complete knee dislocation. Clin Orthop 198:94, 1985.
22. Walling AK, Seradge H, Spiegel PG: Injuries to the knee ligaments with fractures of the femur. J Bone Joint Surg Am 64:1324, 1982.
23. Schiedts D, Mukisi M, Bouger D, et al: [Ipsilateral fractures of the femoral and tibial diaphyses]. Rev Chir Orthop Reparatrice Appar Mot 82(6):535, 1996.
24. van Raay JJ, Raaymakers EL, Dupree HW: Knee ligament injuries combined with ipsilateral tibial and femoral diaphyseal fractures: The "floating knee." Arch Orthop Trauma Surg 110(2):75, 1991.
25. Volk CP, Zwalley J, Ruth JT, Brumback RJ: Floating knee injuries and compartment syndrome. Abstract presented at 1997 OTA Meeting.
26. Gregory P, DiCicco J, Karpik K, et al: Ipsilateral fractures of the femur and tibia: Treatment with retrograde femoral nailing and unreamed tibial nailing. J Orthop Trauma 10(5):309, 1996.
27. Neer CS, Grantham SA, Shelton ML: Supracondylar fracture of the adult femur. J Bone Joint Surg Am 49:591, 1967.
28. Müller ME, Allgower M, Schnieder R, et al: Manual of Internal Fixation, 3rd ed. New York, Springer-Verlag, 1991.
30. Butler MS, Brumback RJ, Ellison TS, et al: Interlocking intramedullary nailing for ipsilateral fractures of the femoral shaft and distal part of the femur. J Bone Joint Surg Am 73(10):1492, 1991.
31. Yang KH, Han DY, Park HW, et al: Fracture of the ipsilateral neck of the femur in shaft nailing: The role of CT in diagnosis. J Bone Joint Surg Br 80(4):673, 1998.
32. Hampton OP: Wounds of the Extremities in Military Surgery. St. Louis, CV Mosby, 1951.
33. Kirshner M: Ueber Nagelextension. Beitr Klin Chir 64:266, 1909.
34. Mahorner HR, Bradburn M: Fractures of the femur: Report of 308 cases. Surg Gynecol Obstet 56:1066, 1933.

35. Modlin J: Double skeletal traction in battle fractures of the lower femur. Bull U S Army Med Dept 4:119, 1945.
36. Steinman FR: Eine neue Extensionmethode in der Frakturenbehandlung. Zentralbl Chir 34:398, 1907.
37. Wiggins HE: Vertical traction in open fractures of the femur. U S Armed Forces Med J 4:1633, 1953.
38. Magnuson PB, Stack JK: Fractures. Philadelphia, JB Lippincott, 1949.
39. Trethowan WH: Simple fractures of the upper and lower limbs. In Jones, Sir Robert, ed: Orthopaedic Surgery of Injuries, vol 1. London, Oxford University Press, 1921, p 57.
40. Tees JD: Fracture at the lower end of the femur. Am J Surg 38: 656, 1937.
41. Kennedy Col. RH: Fractures that require open reduction. In Thomson JE, ed: The American Academy of Orthopaedic Surgeons Presents Lectures on Reconstruction Surgery. Michigan, Edwards Brothers. 1944, p 465.
42. Smillie IS: Injuries to the Knee Joint, 4th ed. Baltimore, Williams & Wilkins, 1971, p 246.
43. Bohler L: The Treatment of Fractures, 4th ed. Bristol, England, Wright, 1935.
44. Charnley J: The Closed Treatment of Common Fractures, 3rd ed. Edinburgh, E&S Livingstone, 1961.
45. Mooney V, Nickel VL, Harvey JP, et al: Cast-brace treatment for fractures of the distal part of the femur: A prospective controlled study of one hundred and fifty patients. J Bone Joint Surg Am 52:1563, 1970.
46. Mays J, Neufeld AJ: Skeletal traction methods. Clin Orthop 102: 144, 1974.
47. Connolly JF, Dehne E, Lafollette B: Closed reduction and early cast-brace ambulation in the treatment of femoral fractures: II. Results in 143 fractures. J Bone Joint Surg Am 55:1581, 1973.
48. Connolly JF, King P: Closed reduction and early cast-brace ambulation in the treatment of femoral fractures: I. An in vivo quantitative analysis of immobilization in skeletal traction and a cast-brace. J Bone Joint Surg Am 55:1559, 1973.
49. Altenberg AR, Shorkey RL: Blade-plate fixation in nonunion and in complicated fractures of the supracondylar region of the femur. J Bone Joint Surg Am 31:312, 1949.
50. Unmansky AL: Blade-plate internal fixation for fracture of the distal end of the femur. Bull Hosp Jt Dis 9:18, 1948.
51. White EH, Russin LA: Supracondylar fractures of the femur treated by internal fixation with immediate knee motion. Am J Surg 22:801, 1956.
52. Wenzl H, Casey PA, Herbert P, et al: Die Operative Behandlung der Distalen Femurfraktur. AO Bull December, 1970.
53. Schatzker J, Horne G, Waddell J: The Toronto experience with the supracondylar fracture of the femur, 1966–1972. Injury 6: 113, 1975.
54. Schatzker J, Lambert DC: Supracondylar fractures of the distal femur. Clin Orthop 138:77, 1979.
55. Schatzker J: Fractures of the distal femur revisited. Clin Orthop 347:43, 1998.
56. Slatis P, Ryoppy S, Huttinen V: AO osteosynthesis of fractures of the distal third of the femur. Acta Orthop Scand 42:162, 1971.
57. Olerud S: Operative treatment of supracondylar-condylar fractures of the femur: Technique and results in fifteen cases. J Bone Joint Surg Am 54:1015, 1972.
58. Chiron HS, Casey P: Fractures of the distal third of the femur treated by internal fixation. Clin Orthop 100:160, 1974.
59. Mize RD, Bucholz RW, Grogan DP: Surgical treatment of displaced, comminuted fractures of the distal end of the femur. J Bone Joint Surg Am 64:871, 1982.
60. Healy WL, Brooker AF: Distal femoral fractures: Comparison of open and closed methods of treatment. Clin Orthop 174:166, 1983.
61. Siliski JM, Mahring M, Hofer HP: Supracondylar-intercondylar fractures of the femur: Treatment by internal fixation. J Bone Joint Surg Am 71:95, 1989.
62. Butt MS, Krikler SR, Ali MS: Displaced fractures of the distal femur in elderly patients. J Bone Joint Surg Am 77:110, 1995.
63. Hall MF: Two-plane fixation of acute supracondylar and intracondylar fractures of the femur. South Med J 71:1474, 1978.
64. Prichett JW: Supracondylar fractures of the femur. Clin Orthop 184:173, 1984.
65. Sanders R, Regazzoni P, Reudi T: Treatment of supracondylar-intra-articular fractures of the femur using the dynamic condylar screw. J Orthop Trauma 3:214, 1989.
66. Shewring DJ, Meggitt BF: Fractures of the distal femur treated with the AO dynamic condylar screw. J Bone Joint Surg Am 74:122, 1992.
67. Mast J, Jakob R, Ganz R: Planning and Reduction Techniques in Fracture Surgery. New York, Springer-Verlag, 1989.
68. Ostrum RF, Geel C: Indirect reduction and internal fixation of supracondylar femur fractures without bone graft. J Orthop Trauma 9(4):278, 1995.
69. Bolhofner BR, Carmen B, Clifford P: The results of open reduction and internal fixation of distal femur fractures using a biologic (indirect) reduction technique. J Orthop Trauma 10(6): 372, 1996.
70. Sanders RW, Swiontkowski M, Rosen H, et al: Complex fractures and malunions of the distal femur: Results of treatment with double plates. J Bone Joint Surg Am 73:341, 1991.
71. McKibbon B: The biology of fracture healing in long bones. J Bone Joint Surg Br 60:150, 1978.
72. Tayton K, Johnson-Nurse C, McKibbon B, et al: The use of semi-rigid carbon-fibre-reinforced plastic plates for fixation of human fractures: Results of preliminary trials. J Bone Joint Surg Br 64:105, 1982.
73. Pemberton DJ, Evans PD, Grant A, et al: Fractures of the distal femur in the elderly treated with a carbon fibre supracondylar plate. Injury 25:317, 1994.
74. Zickel RE, Fietti VG, Lawsing JF, et al: A new intramedullary fixation device for the distal third of the femur. Clin Orthop 125:185, 1977.
75. Zickel RE, Hobeika P, Robbins DS: Zickel Supracondylar Nails for fractures of the distal end of the femur. Clin Orthop 212: 79, 1986.
76. Shelbourne KD, Brueckmann FR: Rush-pin fixation of supracondylar and intercondylar fractures of the femur. J Bone Joint Surg Am 64:161, 1982.
77. Kuntsher G: Practice of Intramedullary Nailing. Translated by Rinne HH. Springfield, IL, Charles C Thomas, 1967.
78. O'Sullivan ME, Chao EY, Kelly PJ: Current concepts review: The effects of fixation of fracture healing. J Bone Joint Surg Am 71:306, 1989.
79. Rand JA, An KN, Chao EY, et al: A comparison of the effect of open intramedullary nailing and compression-plate fixation on fracture-site blood flow and fracture union. J Bone Joint Surg Am 63:427, 1981.
80. Dominguez I, Moro Rodriguez E, De Pedro Moro JA, et al: Antegrade nailing for fractures of the distal femur. Clin Orthop 350:74, 1998.
81. Tornetta P, Tiburzi D: Anterograde interlocked nailing of distal femoral fractures after gunshot wounds. J Orthop Trauma 8(3): 220, 1994.
82. Henry S, Trager S, Green S, et al: Management of supracondylar fractures of the femur with the GSH Supracondylar Nail. Contemp Orthop 22:631, 1991.
83. Koval KJ, Hoehl JJ, Kummer FJ, et al: Distal femoral fixation: A biomechanical comparison of the standard condylar buttress plate, a locked buttress plate, and the 95-degree blade plate. J Orthop Trauma 11(7):521, 1997.
84. Matelic TM, Monroe MT, Mast JW: The use of endosteal substitution in the treatment of recalcitrant nonunions of the femur: Report of seven cases. J Orthop Trauma 10:1, 1996.
85. Firoozbaksh K, Behzadi K, DeCoster TA, et al: Mechanics of retrograde nail versus plate fixation for supracondylar femur fractures. J Orthop Trauma 9:152, 1995.
86. Koval KJ, Kummer FJ, Bharam S, et al: Distal femoral fixation: A laboratory comparison of the 95° plate, antegrade and retrograde inserted reamed intramedullary nails. J Orthop Trauma 10:378, 1996.
87. David SM, Harrow ME, Peindl RD, et al: Comparative biomechanical analysis of supracondylar femur fracture fixation: Locked intramedullary nail versus 95-degree angled plate. J Orthop Trauma 11:344, 1997.
88. Ito K, Grass R, Zwipp H: Internal fixation of supracondylar femoral fractures: Comparative biomechanical performance of the 95-degree blade plate and retrograde nails. J Orthop Trauma 12:259, 1998.

89. Voor MJ, Verst DA, Mladsi SW, et al: Fatigue properties of a twelve-hole versus a five-hole intramedullary supracondylar nail. J Orthop Trauma 11:98, 1997.
90. Lucas SE, Seligson D, Henry SL: Intramedullary supracondylar nailing of femoral fractures: A preliminary report of the GSH supracondylar nail. Clin Orthop 296:200, 1993.
91. Danziger M, Caucci D, Zechner SB, et al: Treatment of intercondylar and supracondylar distal femur fractures using the GSH supracondylar nail. Am J Orthop 8:684, 1995.
92. Iannacone WM, Bennett FS, DeLong WG, et al: Initial experience with the treatment of supracondylar femoral fractures using the supracondylar intramedullary nail: A preliminary report. J Orthop Trauma 8(4):322, 1994.
93. Janzing HM, Stockman B, Van Damme G, et al: The retrograde intramedullary nail: Prospective experience in patients older than sixty-five years. J Orthop Trauma 12(5):330, 1998.
94. Noer HH, Cristensen N: Distale Femur Frakturer behandelt met extern Fiksation med Orthofix. Ugeskr Laeger 155:2699, 1993.
95. Ronen G, Michaelson M, Waisbrod H: External fixation in war injuries. Injury 6:94, 1976.
96. Marsh JL, Jansen H, Yoong HK, et al: Supracondylar fractures of the femur treated by external fixation. J Orthop Trauma 11(6): 405, 1997.
97. Hutson JJ, Zych GA: Infections in periarticular fractures of the lower extremity treated with tensioned wire hybrid fixators. J Orthop Trauma 12(3):214, 1998.
98. Bell KM, Johnstone AJ, Court-Brown CM, et al: Primary knee arthroplasty for distal femoral fractures in elderly patients. J Bone Joint Surg Br 74:400, 1992.
99. Wolfgang GL: Primary total knee arthroplasty for intercondylar fracture of the femur in a rheumatoid arthritic patient. Clin Orthop 171:80, 1982.
100. Benum P: The use of bone cement as an adjunct to internal fixation of supracondylar fractures of osteoporotic femurs. Acta Orthop Scand 48:52, 1977.
101. Younger EM, Chapman MW: Morbidity at bone graft donor sites. J Orthop Trauma 3:192, 1989.
102. Aaron RK, Scott R: Supracondylar fracture of the femur after total knee arthroplasty. Clin Orthop 219:136, 1987.
103. Culp RW, Schmidt RG, Hanks G, et al: Supracondylar fracture of the femur following prosthetic knee arthroplasty. Clin Orthop 222:212, 1987.
104. Figgie MP, Goldberg VM, Figgie HE, et al: The results of treatment of supracondylar fracture above total knee arthroplasty. J Arthroplasty 5:267, 1990.
105. Hirsh DM, Bhalla S, Roffman M: Supracondylar fracture of the femur following total knee replacement: Report of 4 cases. J Bone Joint Surg Am 63:162, 1981.
106. Merkel KD, Johnson EW: Supracondylar fracture of the femur after total knee arthroplasty. J Bone Joint Surg Am 68:29, 1986.
107. Nielson BF, Petersen VS, Vanmarken JE: Fracture of the femur after knee arthroplasty. Acta Orthop Scand 59:155, 1988.
108. Ritter MA, Faris PM, Keating EM: Anterior femoral notching and ipsilateral supracondylar femur fracture in total knee arthroplasty. J Arthroplasty 3:185, 1988.
109. Sisto DJ, Lachiewicz PF, Insall JN: Treatment of supracondylar fractures following prosthetic arthroplasty of the knee. Clin Orthop 196:265, 1985.
110. DiGioia AM, Rubash HE: Periprosthetic fractures of the femur after total knee arthroplasty: A literature review and treatment algorithm. Clin Orthop 271:135, 1991.
111. Ayers DC: Supracondylar fracture of the distal femur proximal to a total knee replacement. Instr Course Lect 47:197, 1997.
112. Delport PH, Van Audekerke R, Martens M, et al: Conservative treatment of ipsilateral supracondylar femoral fracture after total knee arthroplasty. J Trauma 24:846, 1984.
113. Huo MH, Sculco TP: Complications in primary total knee arthroplasty. Orthop Rev 19:781, 1990.
114. Rand JA: Supracondylar fracture of the femur associated with polyethylene wear after total knee arthroplasty. J Bone Joint Surg Am 76:1389, 1994.
115. Liu TK, Yang RS, Chieng PU, et al: Periprosthetic bone mineral density of the distal femur after total knee arthroplasty. Int Orthop 19:346, 1995.
116. Smith WJ, Martin SL, Mabrey JD: Use of a supracondylar nail for treatment of a supracondylar fracture of the femur following total knee arthroplasty. J Arthroplasty 11:210, 1995.
117. Sochart DH, Hardinge K: Nonsurgical management of supracondylar fracture above total knee arthroplasty. J Arthroplasty 12: 830, 1997.
118. Healy WL, Siliski JM, Incavo SJ: Operative treatment of distal femur fractures proximal to total knee replacements. J Bone Joint Surg Am 75:27, 1993.
119. Rolston LR, Christ DJ, Halpern A, et al: Treatment of supracondylar fractures of the femur proximal to a total knee arthroplasty. 77:924, 1995.
120. Ostermann PA, Seligson D, Henry SL: Local antibiotic therapy for severe open fractures: A review of 1085 consecutive cases. J Bone Joint Surg Br 77:93, 1995.
121. Chen F, Mont MA, Bachner RS: Management of ipsilateral supracondylar femur fractures following total knee arthroplasty. J Arthroplasty 9(5):521, 1994.
122. Bogoch E, Hastings D, Gross A, et al: Supracondylar fractures of the femur adjacent to resurfacing and MacIntosh arthroplasties of the knee in patients with rheumatoid arthritis. Clin Orthop 229:213, 1988.
123. Garnavos C, Rafiq M, Henry AP: Treatment of femoral fracture above a knee prosthesis: 18 cases followed 0.5–14 years. Acta Orthop Scand 65:610, 1994.
124. Cain PR, Rubash HE, Wissinger HA, et al: Periprosthetic femoral fractures following total knee arthroplasty. Clin Orthop 208: 205, 1986.
125. Moran MC, Brick GW, Sledge CB, et al: Supracondylar femoral fracture following total knee arthroplasty. Clin Orthop 324:196, 1996.
126. Rorabeck CH, Angliss RD, Lewis PL: Fractures of the femur, tibia, and patella after total knee arthroplasty: Decision making and principles of management. Instr Course Lect 47:449, 1998.
127. Hanks GA, Mathews HH, Routson GW, et al: Supracondylar fracture of the femur following total knee arthroplasty. J Arthroplasty 4:289, 1989.
128. Smith WJ, Martin SL, Mabrey JD: Use of a supracondylar nail for treatment of a supracondylar fracture of the femur following total knee arthroplasty. J Arthroplasty 11:210, 1996.
129. Ritter MA, Keating EM, Faris PM, et al: Rush rod fixation of supracondylar fractures above total knee arthroplasties. J Arthroplasty 10:213, 1995.
130. Jabczenski FF, Crawford M: Retrograde intramedullary nailing of supracondylar femur fractures above total knee arthroplasty. J Arthroplasty 10:95, 1995.
131. Murrell GA, Nunley JA: Interlocked supracondylar intramedullary nails for supracondylar fractures after total knee arthroplasty: A new treatment method. J Arthroplasty 10:37, 1995.
132. Oxborrow NJ, Stone MH: A new method of treatment for periprosthetic supracondylar fractures of the femur for prostheses with a stemmed femoral component. J Arthroplasty 12:596, 1997.
133. Cordiero EN, Costa RC, Carazzato JG, et al: Periprosthetic fractures in patients with total knee arthroplasties. Clin Orthop 252:182, 1990.
134. Kraay MJ, Goldberg VM, Figgie MP, et al: Distal femoral replacement with allograft/prosthetic reconstruction for treatment of supracondylar fractures in patients with total knee arthroplasty. J Arthroplasty 7:7, 1992.
135. Zehntner MK, Ganz R: Internal fixation of supracondylar fractures after condylar total knee arthroplasty. Clin Orthop 293:219, 1993.
136. Henry SL: Management of supracondylar fractures proximal to total knee arthroplasty with the GSH supracondylar nail. Contemp Orthop 31:231, 1995.
137. McLaren AC, Dupont JA, Schroeber DC: Open reduction internal fixation of supracondylar fractures above total knee arthroplasties using the supracondylar rod. Clin Orthop 302:194, 1994.
138. Engh GA, Ammeen DJ: Periprosthetic fractures adjacent to total knee implants: Treatment and clinical results. Instr Course Lect 47:437, 1998.
139. Borgen D, Sprague BL: Treatment of distal femoral fractures with early weight bearing. Clin Orthop 111:156, 1975.
140. Zickel RE: Nonunions of fractures of the proximal and distal

thirds of the shaft of the femur. Instr Course Lect 37:173, 1988.

141. Beall MS, Nebel E, Baily R: Transarticular fixation in the treatment of nonunion of supracondylar fractures of the femur: A salvage procedure. J Bone Joint Surg Am 61:1018, 1979.

142. Starr AJ, Jones AL, Reinert CM: The "Swashbuckler:" A modified anterior approach for fractures of the distal femur. J Orthop Trauma 13:138, 1999.

143. Aglietti P, Buzzi R: Fractures of the femoral condyles. In Insall JN, Windsor RE, Kelly MA, et al, eds: Surgery of the Knee. New York: Churchill Livingstone, 1993, p 983.

61 Tibial Plateau Fractures

WALTER W. VIRKUS • DAVID L. HELFET

ANATOMY

The tibial plateau forms the articular portion of the proximal tibia and articulates with the condyles of the distal femur to form the knee joint. The surface of the tibial plateau slopes posteriorly and inferiorly 10 to 15 degrees in the coronal plane. In the sagittal plane, the plateau lies at nearly a right angle to the axis of the tibial shaft, forming an angle of 3 degrees of varus. This varus is a result of the lateral plateau being higher than the medial plateau. Additionally, the lateral plateau is smaller and convex, whereas the medial plateau is larger and concave. This is helpful when trying to identify the respective plateaus on a lateral radiograph or fluoroscopic image.

The height of the lateral plateau compared with the medial plateau must be considered when placing screws across the joint line so that screws placed from the lateral side do not enter the medial joint. The slight varus alignment of the proximal tibia results in slightly eccentric load distribution across the tibial plateau. In a normally aligned lower extremity, the medial plateau bears more weight than the lateral plateau.[60] This asymmetric weightbearing contributes to increased medial subarticular bone formation and results in the medial plateau being stronger and denser. This may contribute to a lower incidence of medial plateau fractures. When medial fractures occur, they usually involve a higher level of energy, often resulting in associated ligament, nerve, or other soft-tissue injury.

Between the plateaus lies a nonarticular area, which contains the anterior and posterior tibial spines. The anterior spine is larger and more medial and lies just posterior to the insertion of the anterior cruciate ligament (ACL). The posterior spine is much smaller and more lateral and is only a small portion of the insertion of the posterior cruciate ligament. The area of the tibial spines is often comminuted in high-energy fractures involving the tibial plateau, and it is important to restore both the position of the spines and the width of the nonarticular area of the plateau.

The medial and lateral menisci are semilunar, triangular-shaped fibrocartilages that rest between the femoral condyles and the tibial plateaus. They are known to serve an important function in load sharing along with the articular cartilage.[80] The peripheral third of the menisci is vascular, and tears in this area have reparative ability. The inner third is avascular, and these tears have no healing potential. The middle third of the meniscus constitutes the "gray zone."

The lateral meniscus is larger and covers a larger percentage of the lateral plateau than the medial meniscus on the medial plateau. The menisci are connected to each other anteriorly by the intermeniscal ligament. They are attached to the rim of the respective tibial plateaus by the meniscotibial or coronary ligaments. Finally, the anterior attachment of the lateral meniscus is slightly posterior to that of the medial meniscus. These anatomic nuances of the menisci are important to remember during attempts to restore these structures when they are damaged.

The stability of the knee is maintained by its ligamentous restraints. The medial and lateral collateral ligaments are the primary stabilizers to valgus and varus stress respectively. The ACL is the primary restraint to anterior translation of the tibia; the posterior cruciate prevents posterior translation. In injuries to the lateral plateau, the lateral ligament complex usually remains intact, but the medial collateral ligament is often disrupted. In injuries to the medial plateau, the lateral ligaments are almost always disrupted. The ACL, and less commonly the posterior cruciate ligament, can undergo intersubstance stretch, frank rupture, or avulsion of their insertions, more commonly with higher-energy injuries.

MECHANISM OF INJURY

Tibial plateau fractures result from one of three mechanisms of injury: axial load, side loading, or a combination. The actual fracture is caused by the femoral condyle being driven into the tibial plateau. Historically, these occurred by bumper strikes, but currently the more common mechanisms include motor vehicle accidents and falls.[10, 53, 65] Side loading tends to cause injury to an isolated plateau, lateral for valgus loads and medial for varus loads.[47] The valgus mechanical axis of the lower extremity, as well as the susceptibility of the leg to a medially directed blow, partially explains the higher incidence of lateral fractures. The protection afforded by the contralateral leg may explain the low incidence of medial plateau fractures. Axial load tends to produce injury to both sides of the plateau.

In addition to the direction of the force applied to the knee, the resultant fracture depends on the energy involved in the injury, the position of the knee upon impact, and the structural strength of the involved bone, which is related to the age of the patient.[47] Of these factors, the strength of the bone probably plays the largest role in the resulting fracture pattern. Young patients with stiffer bone generally get split or wedge fractures as a result of the shear force imparted by the bone's ability to withstand compression. In older patients, the bone is less able to withstand compression, resulting in depression fractures of the plateau. In slightly younger patients, the interplay of these mechanisms results in a combination split and depression fracture. Patient age also plays a role in associated injuries. Younger patients have a higher incidence of ligamentous injuries, most likely related to the increased energy required to cause bony injury, compared with the older population, wherein ligament injury is less common.

Plateau injuries can occur with minimal energy, as with falls with a valgus load in the elderly, or with very high energy, as with bumper strikes or falls from a height. The energy imparted to the plateau largely determines the amount of comminution and displacement of the resultant fracture. Higher-energy injuries also lead to an increased soft-tissue injury and the possibility of compartment syndrome.[83]

CLASSIFICATION

A classification system is most useful if it is easy to apply and remember, describes a logical progression of injury severity, and has prognostic ability. A number of classifications have been used for tibial plateau fractures.

Rasmussen[63] proposed one of the early classifications for tibial plateau fractures. He first divided the injuries into the plateau that was injured — the lateral plateau, the medial plateau, or both. He then subdivided them into the particular fracture pattern, either split, split-compression, or pure compression. This resulted in a classification system that is fairly easy to use, has a logical progression of severity, and is somewhat prognostic.

Hohl et al[35] used a modification of a system described by Hohl and Moore[88] for fractures and fracture-dislocations of the tibial plateau. The authors described seven fracture types. Type I was minimally displaced. Types II and III were local compression and split-compression, respectively. Type IV was a total condylar fracture, which basically involved a fracture line that went through the tibial eminence, avoiding the articular surface, and resulted in a free-floating plateau. Type V was a split fracture. Type VI was a rim avulsion or compression fracture, which occurred peripherally and could only occur with associated ligament disruption. Type VII fractures were called bicondylar fractures, and these were severe injuries with damage to both plateaus as well as to the nonarticular area between the plateaus. One problem with this classification is that there is no differentiation between injuries to the medial and lateral plateaus. A second problem is that there is no progression of severity — for example, split fractures appear after total condylar fractures — and therefore the system has no prognostic use.

The Association for the Study of Internal Fixation presented a classification for tibial plateau fractures that is part of a classification system for all fractures of the skeletal system[61] (Fig. 61.1). This classification has been adopted by the Orthopaedic Trauma Association. General categories in the system are divided into nonarticular metaphyseal fractures, partial articular fractures, and complete articular fractures. Fractures are also assigned a number, from 1 to 3, that corresponds to the amount of comminution. Overall, this classification is comprehensive and excellent for investigational purposes.

The classification proposed by Schatzker is the classification currently used by most North American surgeons[70, 83] (Fig. 61.2). In this classification, as the fracture type increases, the treatment is more difficult and the prognosis is poorer. In summary, types I to III are low-energy injuries occurring in progressively older patients and types IV to VI are injuries involving increasingly higher energy, resulting in more comminution and soft-tissue injury.

Type I injuries occur in young patients with strong bone and are a split or wedge fracture of the lateral plateau. The size of the split fragment varies. There is a high incidence of meniscal tears in this injury, and the meniscus may even be trapped in the fracture. Type II fractures occur in an older population and consist of a lateral split fragment but also describe an articular depression injury just medial to the split. Type III injuries occur in the elderly and are a pure depression injury.

The magnitude and area of the depression varies. Type IV injuries are fractures of the medial plateau. These are divided into type IVA fractures, which are split fractures, and type IVB fractures, which are depression injuries of the medial plateau. The fracture line in the medial split fractures often crosses over the midline and exits lateral to the tibial spine. The type IVA injuries typically involve lateral collateral and ACL injuries, and many consider them to constitute a fracture/dislocation of the knee. Type V fractures are split fractures of both plateaus, often called bicondylar fractures. In these fractures, a portion of intact metaphysis is still attached to the tibial shaft, which distinguishes them from type VI fractures. Type VI injuries describe a variety of articular injury patterns, but the fracture extends distally, resulting in a dissociation of the entire metaphysis and epiphysis from the tibial shaft. These are high-energy injuries, often with severe comminution and soft-tissue injury.

CLINICAL EVALUATION

A fracture of the tibial plateau should be in the differential diagnosis of any injury of the knee. A history of axial load or side force to the knee should raise suspicion further. Once the fracture is suspected, thorough evaluation of the patient and extremity involved is vital to a successful treatment outcome. When the fractured plateau is part of a constellation of injuries in a polytraumatized patient, it must be placed in its proper perspective. Standard trauma resuscitative protocols and ATLS must be adhered to in these patients. Airway, breathing, and circulation concurrent with a primary injury survey must precede any evaluation of extremity injuries. Initial radiographic studies, including lateral cervical spine, pelvis, and chest radiographs, should also precede radiographic evaluation of the extremities.

When appropriate, evaluation of the knee should be

41- Tibia/Fibula Proximal

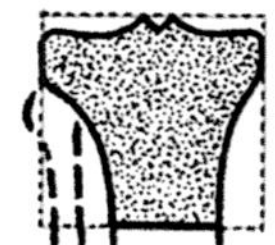

Location

Essence: The fractures of the distal segment are divided into 3 Types:
A extra-articular, **B** partial articular, **C** complete articular

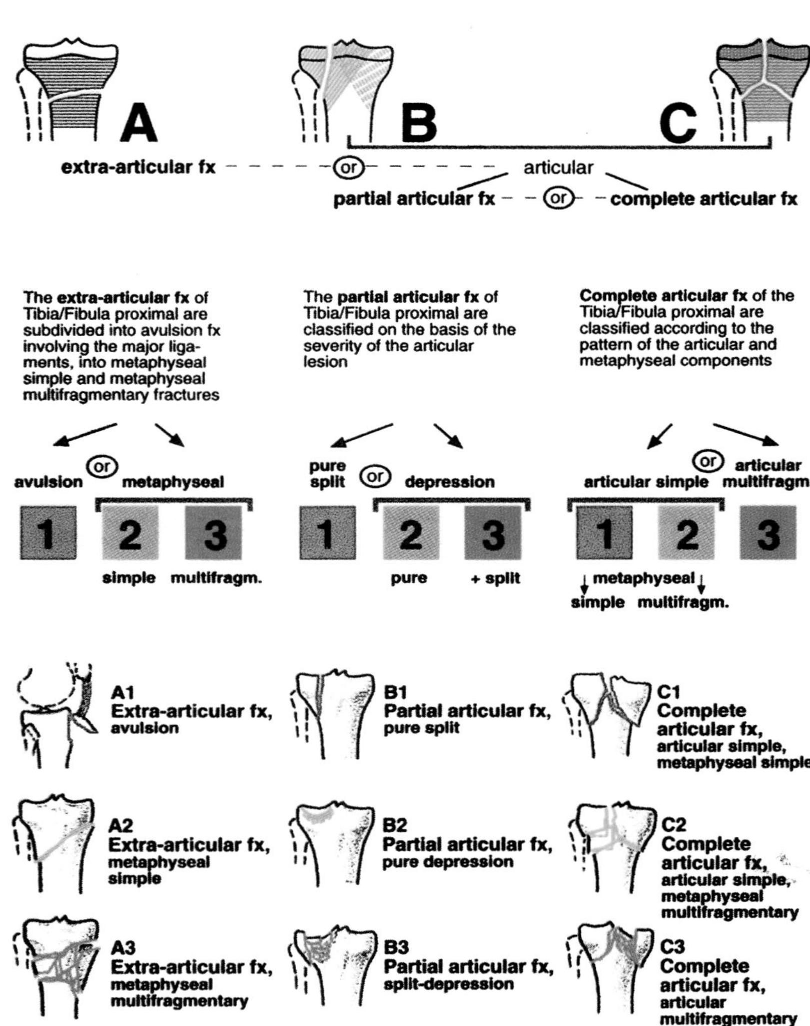

FIGURE 61.1 ➢ The AO/ASIF Classification. (From Müller ME, Nazarian S, Koch P, Schatzker J: The Comprehensive Classification of Fractures of Long Bones. Bern, M.E. Müller Foundation, 1995.)

included in a comprehensive evaluation of the involved extremity; in fact, the entire skeletal system should be included when indicated. Visual examination of the knee often reveals an effusion, although if the knee capsule has been torn, the hemarthrosis will decompress into the surrounding soft tissue. If the effusion is tense, aspiration of the acute hemarthrosis usually increases the patient's comfort level. Careful inspection should look for open wounds over fracture lines. Abrasions, contusions, and blisters should be noted because they may affect the approach to fixation. Ligamentous examination, unless performed with anesthesia, is often too painful for the patient to tolerate, and it is difficult to determine whether instability is due to joint depression or ligamentous laxity. Suspicion for ligament injuries should be high, especially in younger patients with type IV, V, and VI injuries.

Careful neurological and vascular examination must be documented. Popliteal artery injury is rare but is catastrophic if missed. If pulses are not equal upon palpation, Doppler examination with ankle-brachial indices should be performed. A ratio of 0.9 or less suggests arterial injury, and in this case arteriography should be performed.[56] Neurological injury, usually in the form of a peroneal nerve injury, is not uncommon, especially in medial plateau fractures.[70] Careful motor and sensory evaluation of all the lower leg nerves is mandatory.

Finally, a careful evaluation for compartment syndrome must be performed. The usual signs of tense

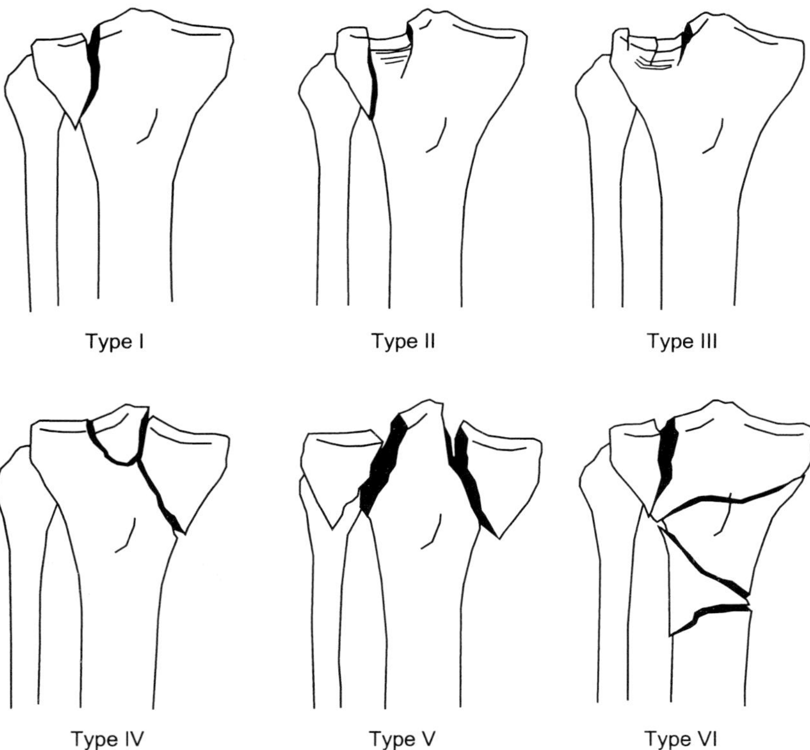

FIGURE 61.2 ➢ The Schatzker classification.

compartments, pain with passive extension of the toes or ankle, and increasing numbness or cyanosis should be assessed in all tibial plateau fractures, but especially type V and VI fractures.[3] Compartment syndrome can occur even after the first 24 hours; we have seen a number of cases involving delayed presentation after transfer from the primary institution. If any question of compartment syndrome exists, the compartment pressures should be measured and fasciotomy performed if pressures are elevated.

IMAGING STUDIES

Radiographs

Plain orthogonal radiographs are the mainstay of radiographic evaluation of tibial plateau fractures (Fig. 61.3). They should be centered on the knee joint, and if possible the anteroposterior (AP) view should be angled 10 degrees in a craniocaudal direction to approximate the posterior slope of the plateau. The AP view should be inspected for fracture lines extending

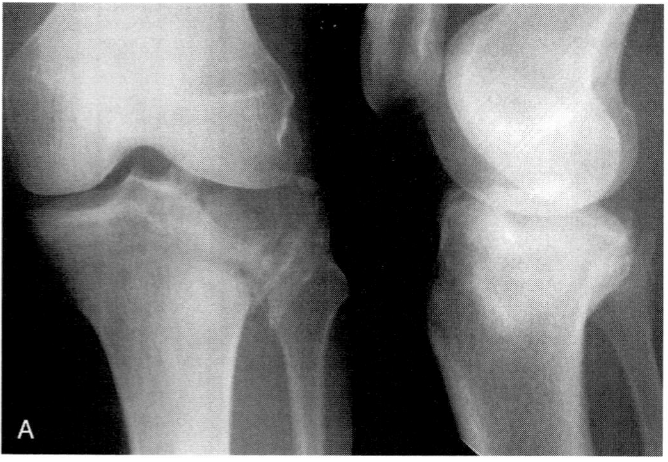

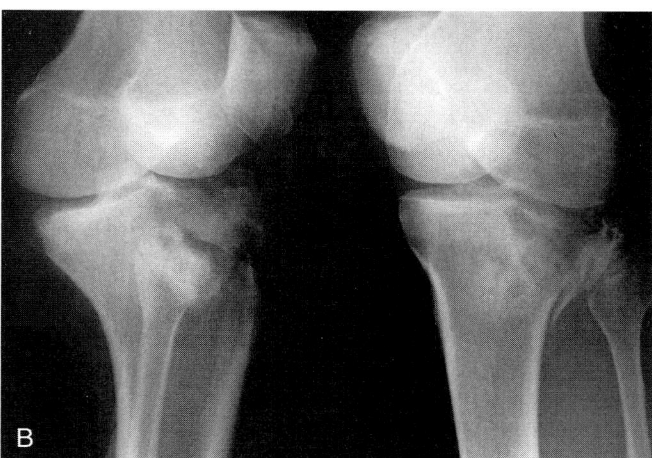

FIGURE 61.3 ➢ *A*, AP and lateral radiographs of a Schatzker type II tibial plateau fracture. *B*, Corresponding oblique radiographs.

into the joint, for widening of the plateau in relation to the femoral condyles, and for avulsion fractures of the collateral ligaments or the ACL insertion. The lateral view often shows a depressed fragment if each plateau is carefully analyzed individually. It is useful to remember that on the lateral view, the lateral plateau appears convex and the medial plateau appears concave. The lateral view often shows a coronal split or widening, indicating a posterior or posteromedial fragment.

Supplementary radiographs include oblique views and stress views. Oblique views should be obtained in almost all cases of suspected tibial plateau fractures. They will often show a significant injury when the AP and lateral radiographs look fairly unremarkable. When the injury is obvious on the AP and lateral radiographs, however, the obliques rarely add significant information unless computed tomography (CT) is not possible.

Stress views are labor-intensive, can be very uncomfortable for the patient unless performed with anesthesia, and rarely add to treatment decision-making. Historically, they were used to help assess the stability of the knee, which often was the determining factor between operative and nonoperative treatment.[63] Presently, the determination for surgical treatment is based more often on fracture displacement; therefore, stress views are less useful unless ligamentous instability cannot be differentiated from fracture instability. They can serve a purpose in eliciting whether manipulation and ligamentotaxis will enable fragments to be reduced closed, allowing percutaneous or closed treatment techniques to be used.

Computed Tomography

For all but the most basic fractures, CT, usually with sagittal and coronal reconstructions, is the study of choice when additional information about the fracture pattern is desirable (Fig. 61.4). Chan et al demonstrated that information from CT scans significantly changed both the fracture classification and the surgical plan compared with plain radiographs alone.[14] For the most part, CT has replaced standard tomography for detailed evaluation of these injuries. Standard tomography is time consuming, exposes the patient to a large amount of radiation, and is more difficult to interpret than modern CT techniques. CT can also be done through a plaster splint or cast, which makes it more comfortable for the patient and more convenient for the surgeon.

Modern techniques, such as spiral CT, allow a detailed study to be completed in minutes, and modern software can format 2-D and 3-D reconstructions with remarkable resolution. CT offers excellent bony detail, although it is not very helpful in evaluating soft-tissue injuries. CT axial views are helpful in delineating the direction of the major fracture lines and can precisely identify the location of any depressed fragments. It also enables the surgeon to identify fracture lines and depressions not appreciated on plain radiographs. Coronal and sagittal reconstructions quantitatively delineate the amount of depression of fracture fragments as well as showing any malalignment in these planes.

Magnetic Resonance Imaging

Magnetic resonance technology is progressing rapidly. Magnetic resonance imaging (MRI) has the unique ability to assess soft-tissue injuries in the knee with great accuracy. Unfortunately, MRI is less useful in delineating bony anatomy, and even soft-tissue pathology can be difficult to assess in the traumatized knee in which edema and hematoma are present and the anatomy is severely distorted. Studies in which MRI was performed on tibial plateau fractures showed associated soft-tissue injuries in 45% or more of patients.[37, 50] A study being performed jointly with our institution showed that at least 8 mm of lateral displacement, or at least 4 mm of depression, resulted in a 95% incidence of lateral meniscal injury.[86]

Some surgeons think that because of the high incidence of ligamentous and meniscal injuries, MRI is a more useful adjunctive study than CT. In the single published study comparing CT with MRI for evaluation of tibial plateau fractures, MRI was found to be equal or better than CT in determining fracture configuration in 86% of cases.[50] At present, however, most surgeons are more comfortable reading CT scans. CT remains the radiological study of choice to fully evaluate the pathoanatomy, as well as to plan the surgery, of tibial plateau fractures in most institutions treating large numbers of these injuries.

Angiography

Angiography is indicated when the vascularity of the lower leg is in question. Although uncommon, it is possible for fracture fragments or the initial injury displacement to damage the popliteal artery or the trifurcation. In cases of absent distal pulses, an ankle-brachial index should be obtained: a ratio below 0.9 should prompt angiographic examination.[56] In cases of obvious leg ischemia, angiography may be helpful in localizing the injured area but should not delay vascular exploration and subsequent revascularization.

METHODS AND RESULTS OF TREATMENT

A variety of treatment options are available depending on the type of injury and the preferences and abilities of the treating surgeon. One must be careful in referring to various treatments as "conservative" or "operative." In many cases, what is historically considered conservative treatment may have complications that are worse than operative treatments.

That being said, there is certainly a role for nonoperative treatment in some tibial plateau fractures. Historically, nearly all tibial plateau fractures received nonoperative treatment with traction or casting,

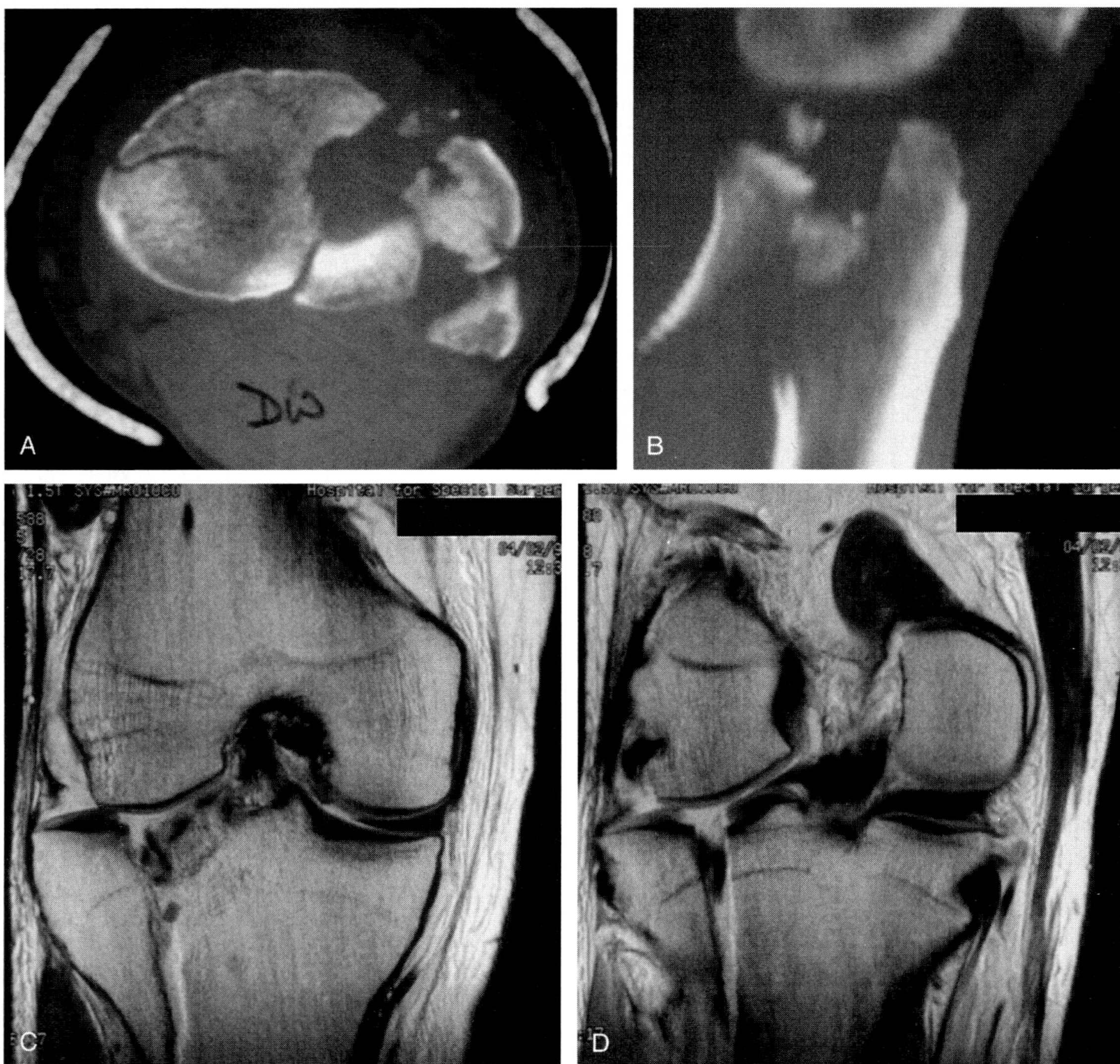

FIGURE 61.4 ➢ CT and MRI. *A*, Axial CT of a 38-year-old male with a Schatzker type II tibial plateau fracture. Sagittal and coronal fracture lines are easily visible. *B*, Corresponding sagittal reconstruction showing the depressed fragment. *C*, Coronal MRI of a 31-year-old male with a Schatzker type II tibial plateau fracture. The depression is visible just lateral to the tibial spine. *D*, Same patient as in *C*, showing articular cartilage fragments and lateral meniscus within the split fracture.

mostly because of the poor results with early internal fixation techniques.[4, 15, 23, 59, 62, 74, 77] Multiple studies showed that more complex fractures did not do well with nonoperative treatment.[10, 18, 23, 70, 79] Gradually, increasing evidence showed that early motion and restoration of alignment were key elements in obtaining a good result.[4, 34, 36, 70]

Now, improved techniques of internal fixation, a better understanding of the importance of preserving soft-tissue and local vascularity, and recognition of the need for early motion and aggressive physiotherapy have lead to improved results in operative treatment of these fractures. Regardless of the treatment method, the goals of treatment are the same—namely, to maximize joint congruity and maintain alignment of the leg.

Traction and Casting

Although traction or casting was a mainstay of nonoperative treatment in the past, their indications in present times are few.[4, 23, 65] Skeletal traction with range-of-motion exercises is used when medical comorbidities or other injuries present too great a risk for operative treatment, when soft-tissue injury prevents internal or external fixation, or when significant comminution exists, preventing adequate reduction and fixation.[83] It is important that the patient receives passive motion and, if possible, performs active motion exercises of the knee to prevent stiffness. Acceptable results have been shown in patients treated with this method.[4, 44, 65]

Casting has been used historically for immobilization

of these injuries but now is rarely if ever indicated in the treatment of tibial plateau fractures.[16, 23, 65] Casting for the 6 to 8 weeks that is needed to heal to the point of partial stability leads to severe stiffness in any articular fracture.[30, 34, 70] In the knee, this stiffness can be particularly refractory because the knee joint is composed of two articulations, the patellofemoral and the femorotibial. Casting has largely been replaced by various bracing techniques that allow early knee motion.

Bracing

In fractures of the tibial plateau that are minimally or non-displaced, treatment with a brace is preferred to casting. Bracing is also used in patients with poor health who are not good surgical candidates. An off-the-shelf rehabilitation-type brace can be applied to most patients and comfortably locked in a mild degree of flexion for a period of 1 to 2 weeks. The patient can be mobilized in a non-weightbearing manner with this treatment regimen. Then, 1 or 2 weeks after the injury, the brace can be unlocked and motion exercises and physiotherapy can begin to prevent joint stiffness. Although rarely needed, the metal braces can be bent to preferentially load either the medial or the lateral plateau, protecting the injured side. Bracing is often used in conjunction with minimal internal fixation, which holds the benefits of improved joint reduction and stability as well as minimizing operative complications.

Good historical as well as recent results have been obtained with cast bracing either alone or as an adjunctive treatment.[12, 18, 20, 24, 68, 72, 85] Duwelius and Connolly[24] reported on 73 fractures treated with closed reduction and cast bracing. Twelve of these patients had minimal fixation with screws or pins, based on instability in extension. They reported 89% good and excellent results at 5 years of follow-up, despite poor radiographic results in many cases. The complication rate was 12%. Brown and Sprague[12] treated 30 patients with a cast brace and weightbearing as tolerated. Follow-up was only 9 months, but the patients had excellent motion, no loss of position, and minimal pain. Scotland and Wardlaw treated patients in a brace and allowed them to bear weight as tolerated.[72] In 29 patients, 7 treated with limited internal fixation, only 1 had a bad result with cast-brace treatment.

Criteria for good and excellent results were less stringent in the past than is the case currently. In most grading systems, any motion over 90 degrees was considered acceptable, as was moderate pain after activity. It is difficult to compare older results to newer ones because of the variety of outcome measures used. The patients in Brown and Sprague's study underwent long-term review by DeCoster et al.[18] At an average of 11 years of follow-up, only 61% had good results. The average Iowa Knee Score was 71, compared with 94 in age-matched controls. Sixty-six percent of patients had no or only mild radiographic arthrosis. The authors concluded that cast-brace treatment of minimally displaced fractures yielded good results, but the results were much more unpredictable in bicondylar fractures.

Percutaneous Fixation

Percutaneous screws and, more rarely, plate fixation are useful treatment modalities for many tibial plateau fractures. Percutaneous screws can be used in conjunction with limited open or percutaneous reduction techniques for displaced fractures (see Fig. 61.8C). Percutaneous plates can be useful when compromised soft tissues make standard open plating less desirable or when a second plate is needed opposite the main plate.

Percutaneous screws of any size can be used, but cannulated 7.0-mm or 7.3-mm screws are the most common and are typically used in the epiphyseal area of the plateau. Washers are generally used to prevent the screws from advancing into the softer cancellous bone in this area. Smaller 4.5-mm or 3.5-mm screws can be used, allowing more directional freedom and a larger number to be placed, especially in the immediate subchondral region.

Percutaneous screws should be placed under fluoroscopic guidance to prevent penetration of the chondral surface. In displaced fractures, fluoroscopy can also be used in conjunction with bone-reduction clamps or spiked pushers placed though small stab incisions to obtain reduction of displaced fragments. The ideal example is the mildly displaced split-type fracture, which can be reduced and held with a "King-Tong" or pointed pelvic reduction clamp and fixed with two percutaneous 7.0-mm screws with washers. Percutaneous screws can also be placed subchondrally to buttress a joint depression that has been elevated through a metaphyseal window.

Results of percutaneous fixation have been good in general, although most studies group this technique with other types of fixation. Keogh et al[48] presented early results of fractures fixed with percutaneous screws. They found no residual deformity and only one loss of reduction, occurring in an unreliable patient with a Schatzker type V injury. Satisfactory results were noted in 11 patients, with 1 fair and 1 poor result. Duwelius et al[25] reported a group of patients with various types of internal fixation, a majority of which were percutaneous screws. Overall, their results were good, although patients with C3 injuries had poorer results. Koval et al[52] presented a group of 18 patients treated with indirect closed reduction and percutaneous screw fixation. They were able to achieve anatomic reduction in 72% and found no loss of reduction and no residual deformities. Overall results were excellent in 33%, good in 56%, and fair in 11% of cases. They concluded that anatomic reduction could be obtained in split-type fractures but that depressions were poorly reduced by this technique. Scheerlinck et al[71] reported the follow-up of 38 of 52 patients treated with percutaneous fixation. Ten of these patients had external fixation as either the sole fixation or as supplemental fixation. Arthroscopy and fluoroscopy facilitated assessment of reduction in all

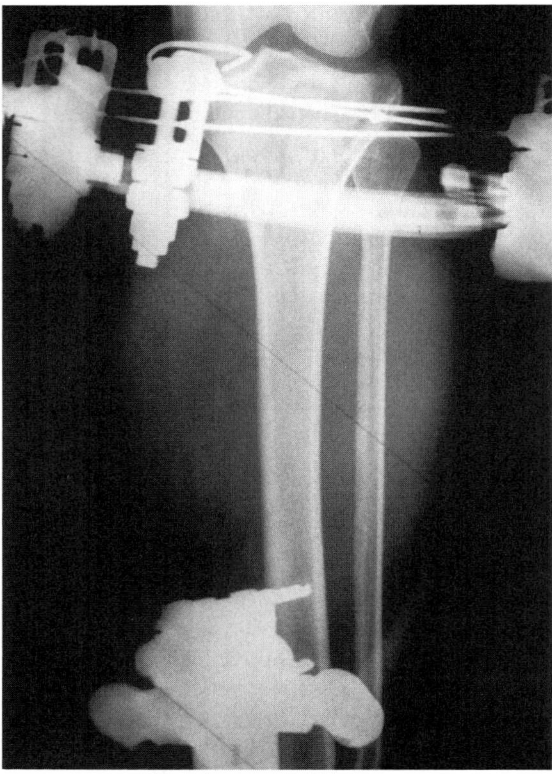

FIGURE 61.5 ➢ Schatzker type V tibial plateau fracture reconstructed using a hybrid external fixator. Compression across the fracture lines is obtained via the tensioned olive wires.

cases. Thirty-five of 38 patients had excellent or good results according to the HSS knee score at an average of 5 years of follow-up. Again, results were not as good in C-type injuries.

Percutaneous plating is a relatively new technique wherein plates are advanced through small stab incisions made proximal or distal to the fracture line and screws are placed through separate small incisions over the plate holes. These plates are usually smaller-caliber malleable plates that contour to the bone upon placement of screws. We use them commonly as a medial buttress for bicondylar fractures or fractures with metaphyseal-diaphyseal dissociation when a larger, more stable plate is being used on the lateral side. This allows dual side fixation without complete stripping of the soft tissue off the proximal tibia, thus avoiding a large devascularized bone or soft-tissue segment ("dead-bone sandwich") that will delay healing and increase the risk of infection.

External Fixation

External fixation is a modular fixation modality that has many applications in the management of tibial plateau fractures. External fixators can use half-pins, thin wires, or both (Fig. 61.5). There are many commercial brands of each, and most perform adequately. The main differences between fixators are the ease of construction, freedom of manipulation, and cost. The indications for an external fixator in tibial plateau fractures can be divided into three: temporary stabilization, adjunct stabilization, and definitive fixation.

An external fixator can be used as temporary fixation in tibial plateau fractures that are open, in patients too unstable to undergo definitive internal fixation, or in patients with compartment syndrome or excessive swelling that prevents immediate internal fixation. In these cases, an external fixator that spans the knee can be applied quickly and distraction can be applied across the knee to restore length, rotation, and proper alignment in the coronal and sagittal planes. This allows open wounds to be managed with dressing changes or other appropriate treatments and provides relative stability to the fracture fragments, minimizing pain and soft-tissue irritation.

Half-pins, usually 5 mm in diameter, can be placed anteromedially into the tibial shaft and either anteriorly or laterally into the femoral shaft. We prefer lateral femoral shaft pins because they are much less damaging to the quadriceps and therefore cause less skin and muscle irritation. Lateral femoral pins are also less painful, have a lower incidence of drainage and infection, and allow faster return of knee motion once they are removed. If internal plate fixation may eventually be used for definitive fixation, ensure that the tibial external fixator half-pins are placed sufficiently distal so that the subsequent open incision will not be contaminated by the previously placed fixator pins. Meticulous pin care is essential to allow later conversion to internal fixation when the patient's soft tissue and overall condition permit.

External fixation can also be used as definitive treatment for tibial plateau fractures. This may be indicated when the soft-tissue envelope is unlikely to be amenable to open fixation even after a delay. Some have recommended external fixation alone because they think that acceptable results can be obtained in these fractures irrespective of the soft-tissue injury, without the inherent risks of open reduction and internal fixation.[81, 84] Most external fixation methods are amenable to use as definitive fixation, including half-pin uniplanar and multiplanar frames, thin-wire ring fixators, and so-called hybrid fixators. Each frame configuration has its advantages and disadvantages, and much is determined by individual surgeon preference. Thin-wire fixators have the advantage of being able to apply some compression across fracture fragments by use of olive or beaded guide wires placed in opposing directions across fracture planes. Gaudinez et al reported on the use of a hybrid fixator in type V and VI tibial plateau fractures.[29] They treated 16 patients, 10 of whom had open injuries. The average time to union was 19 weeks. They found no deep infections and no malalignment, and range of motion averaged 85 degrees. Four patients had superficial pin tract infections, and 15 of 16 had degenerative changes on radiographs at 1 year of follow-up.

In most cases in which external fixators are used as definitive fixation, they are used in conjunction with percutaneous screw or limited internal fixation of the articular surface.[22, 57, 75, 82, 84] In these circumstances, the fixator serves as a buttress of the articular surface to the tibial shaft, substituting for an internally placed buttress plate. This function can be achieved with thin-wire, half-pin, or hybrid fixators. Thin-wire or hybrid fixators are usually technically easier in these cases because the thin wires are easier to direct around the periarticular lag screws. An external fixator can also be used to provide medial support after lateral plate fixation of bicondylar fractures. In these circumstances, a simple two-pin low-profile fixator can serve as an alternative to medial plating when it is thought that the lateral fixation alone is unable to adequately stabilize and prevent varus collapse of the medial side.[11]

The results of external fixation supplementing limited or percutaneous internal fixation have been promising. Unfortunately, almost all are plagued by pin tract problems, long healing times, and difficulty in maintaining tibial alignment. It must be remembered that most of these studies have been performed in the most severe, difficult to treat fractures, and the learning curve is still being mastered. Marsh et al[57] presented their results using limited internal fixation and a uniplanar external fixator. They had 21 fractures, of which 7 were open. Articular reductions were achieved percutaneously, through an open wound, or via open reduction. At an average of 3 years of follow-up, all fractures had healed in an average of 12 weeks. The average Iowa Knee Score was 87. Three patients had tibial malalignment, seven needed antibiotics for pin tract infections, and two needed arthrotomy for septic arthritis.

Stamer et al[75] treated 23 Schatzker type VI fractures with a hybrid fixator and limited open reduction, internal fixation (ORIF), or percutaneous screws. Their average healing time was 4.4 months. They incurred three deep infections (all in patients who underwent limited ORIF), one varus malunion, and one pin tract infection. According to their grading scale, they had 13 excellent results, 3 good, 1 fair, and 6 poor. They thought that most of the poor results were related to concomitant injuries.

Weiner et al[84] treated 50 fractures with hybrid ring fixators. Articular reduction was obtained closed in 15 patients and open in 30. They had 38% superficial pin tract infections, 4% nonunions, and 4% malunions. The mean HSS knee score was 90, and the grade of radiographic reduction was good or excellent in 82%.

Dendrinos[22] reported on 24 patients treated with percutaneous or open fixation supplemented with an Ilizarov circular fixator. Average time to union was 14 weeks. They had no deep infections, but they did have two malunions, and seven patients had less than 110 degrees of motion at 3-year follow-up.

Watson and Coufal also used an Ilizarov fixator with limited open fixation.[82] In a population of 14 high-energy Schatzker type I and II fractures, they were able to achieve union in 4.5 months, with 12 good and excellent results. They had five minor pin infections and one superficial skin slough.

With extremely unstable fracture patterns wherein

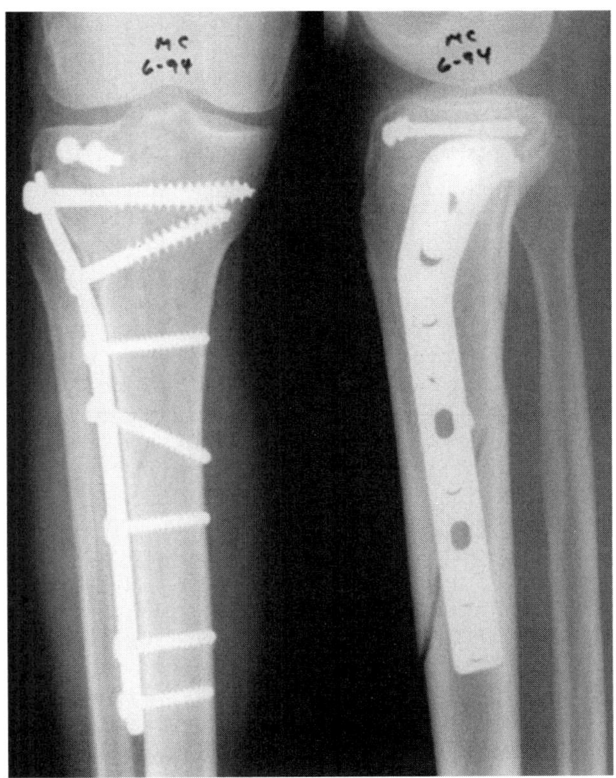

FIGURE 61.6 ➢ Schatzker type VI tibial plateau fracture reconstructed with open reduction, internal fixation (ORIF) using a lateral tibial head plate.

stable internal fixation will be difficult to obtain, or with tenuous soft-tissue status, a spanning fixator can be placed (or left on if previously applied) to add temporary stability until early bone or soft-tissue healing occurs. The spanning fixator provides more reliable stability than a brace or cast and avoids the soft-tissue problems inherent to these methods of support. If the spanning fixator is left on for only a short time, knee motion can be recovered with physiotherapy or, in severe cases, closed manipulation.

Open Reduction, Internal Fixation

A change in philosophy regarding articular fractures, in conjunction with advances in plate design, reduction techniques, and soft-tissue preservation—all pioneered by the AO/ASIF—have dramatically improved the results obtainable using ORIF for these injuries. When performed with correct technique in the proper setting, with an anatomic reduction of the articular surface, formal ORIF of the tibial plateau to the shaft of the tibia allows stable fixation sufficient to allow primary bone healing while aggressive early joint motion is encouraged (Fig. 61.6). More recently, the trend has been toward less bulky, lower-profile implants that are less damaging to the surrounding soft tissues yet still provide sturdy fixation. A variety of plate shapes and sizes are available; the choice of implant must be based on the fracture configuration and soft-tissue envelope.

Typically, buttress plates function to support a bone graft used to elevate a joint depression or to prevent distal migration of a split fragment. Preshaped L- and T-shaped plates have long been available for this purpose, but straight plates can also be molded to the proximal tibia for this use. Smaller T- and L-shaped plates have become available, and the lower profile of these implants may limit injury to the soft tissue. A buttress plate is suggested when a metaphyseal window is made to facilitate elevation of a depressed joint fragment; however, the need for a plate to buttress a large split fragment is controversial.[51] Large, sturdier, hockey stick-shaped plates are available for use in fracture patterns wherein the metaphysis is dissociated from the tibial shaft. Although no particular implant or fixation method is amenable to all fractures of a particular type, the general goals and principles of ORIF should be maintained: (1) anatomic articular reconstruction, (2) preservation of soft tissue and bone viability (i.e., minimal additional soft-tissue disruption), (3) stable fixation sufficient to allow immediate motion, and (4) maintenance of alignment, length, and rotation.

It is difficult to analyze and compare the literature concerning ORIF of tibial plateau fractures. In recent decades, numerous classification and outcome scores have been used by a variety of authors. Furthermore, many studies grouped the results of operatively and nonoperatively treated fractures together. Finally, many studies reported results on both low-energy and high-energy injuries together, leading to the problem of comparing "apples and oranges."

Schatzker et al[70] were among the first surgeons using modern techniques of ORIF to recommend this approach for plateau fractures. They treated 40 patients with ORIF, using various techniques depending on the fracture type. The results were graded as acceptable in 78% of the operatively treated group compared with 58% in the nonoperatively treated group. They thought that most of the failures in the operative group were the result of inadequate reductions, errors in technique, or concomitant ligament injuries. In patients who were treated with the combination of ORIF with a buttress plate, bone graft, and early motion, outcomes were satisfactory in 88%. There was only one wound infection. They concluded that all but minimally displaced stable fractures should undergo operative treatment. However, they cautioned that "results of poor open reduction are far worse than the results of poor nonoperative treatment."

Waddell et al[79] presented 69 patients treated operatively. They had 62% satisfactory results and only two superficial infections. They recommended ORIF in cases with more than 1 cm of displacement, cases of valgus instability, and young patients. More recently, Tscherne and Lobenhoffer[78] reported the results of 190 patients, 144 treated operatively. These included a large percentage of high-energy injuries. These patients had mean Lysholm Knee Scores of 78 for isolated plateau injuries. More complex fracture dislocation injuries had mean scores of 69. Complications included deep infections in 4% and malalignment in 4%. Lachiewicz and Funcik[53] had good or excellent results in 40 of 43 patients treated with ORIF. At only 2.7 years of follow-up, however, 23% of patients had some degree of radiographic arthrosis.

Clearly, an anatomic reduction and stable fixation would be the natural choice for any articular fracture, including the tibial plateau, if this could be reliably accomplished without complications, especially infection and soft-tissue slough. It is the soft-tissue status and the ability to accomplish such ORIF without causing significant compromise of the soft tissue and the resulting blood supply to the bone that determine whether ORIF is possible.

TREATMENT DECISION-MAKING

Indications for Surgery

The indication for operative versus nonoperative treatment of tibial plateau fractures remains controversial, with only general principles available to guide treatment decisions. Although minimally displaced or nondisplaced fractures routinely do well with nonoperative treatment, higher-energy, comminuted injuries have been shown to do poorly with nonsurgical treatment.[10, 18, 70, 79] Objective criteria such as knee instability or amount of joint depression have been used to assist in the treatment decision.[63, 70, 79] The amount of joint depression that can be accepted is not agreed on, and these criteria have often been altered as perceived improvements in fixation techniques have evolved. Historically, 10 mm or less of depression was thought to be tolerated by the joint; however, this has been challenged.[70, 79] Depressions from 4 to 10 mm have been suggested as limits for nonoperative treatment.[4, 18, 34, 39, 54, 59, 70]

The ultimate treatment decision must be based on many factors, including the fracture pattern, the soft-tissue condition, additional injuries, and the experience of the surgeon. This involves a characterization of the "personality" of the injury. An assessment of the energy of the injury and the status of the soft tissue of the injured leg are paramount in the treatment decision. Open treatment through severely traumatized soft tissue is most predictive of infection and soft-tissue slough and must be avoided. Other factors that must be considered in the decision-making process include the patient's overall health, occupation, and expected compliance, as well as the ability of the treating surgeon to obtain an acceptable reduction and stable fixation.

Absolute indications for operative treatment are rare but include open fractures and fractures with an associated arterial injury. The general relative indications for operative treatment include displaced split or depressed fractures leading to joint instability, bicondylar fractures, fractures associated with a fracture of the ipsilateral tibial shaft or distal femur, fracture/dislocations, displaced medial plateau fractures, and pathological fractures.

Timing of Surgery

If operative treatment of a fracture is preferable, the timing of surgery must be considered. ORIF is not advisable in the acute postinjury period if there is already excessive bruising, swelling, or blistering in the area of the operative field. If ORIF is going to be performed, it should be delayed until the swelling has resolved and hematoma-filled fracture blisters have ruptured and dried. In general, the "wrinkle test" is a good indicator that acute swelling is sufficiently decreased to proceed with open approaches.

Controversy exists as to whether incisions can be safely made through clear serous blisters, but this should probably be avoided if at all possible. The fracture should be stabilized in the interim with either a soft, padded, long-leg splint or a spanning external fixator. These fractures occur in metaphyseal bone, and callus formation will be present as early as 2 weeks after injury. After 3 to 4 weeks, fracture lines may be sufficiently obscured as to make anatomic reduction extremely difficult. If it is unlikely that the soft-tissue envelope will present a friendly environment for ORIF within 2 or 3 weeks of the injury, percutaneous techniques or nonoperative treatment should be considered.

Preoperative Planning

Presurgical planning is a vital part of the operative treatment of tibial plateau fractures.[58] A surgical tactic forces the surgeon to fully study and understand the fracture configuration and potential problems that may arise. This helps ensure that all needed imaging studies and implants are obtained. It is often useful to have radiographs of the contralateral proximal tibia for templating purposes. Axial CT views can help identify individual fracture fragments and the ideal placement and direction of lag screws. The need for supplemental approaches can also be suggested by these images. In bicondylar fractures, it is useful to identify the side to be reconstructed first, usually the less-comminuted side. Preoperative planning also allows the surgeon to determine the ideal approach, patient position, and need for bone grafting. In addition, the final preoperative drawing of the reduction and surgical montage provides a template of the ideal result (i.e., for critical self-evaluation and quality control).

Approaches

The direct lateral approach is preferable for injuries of lateral plateau. A midline incision can be used for lateral injuries but involves considerable soft-tissue dissection. If the lateral approach is used and medial fixation is considered necessary, this can be performed percutaneously or through a second small medial incision. In such cases, maintain a skin bridge of at least 8 cm. In the direct lateral approach, a straight or hockey-stick incision is made anterolaterally from just proximal to the joint line to just distal to the tibial tubercle, ending about 1 cm lateral to the tibial crest. The incision is extended down through the iliotibial band proximally and the fascia of the anterior compartment distally. The tibialis anterior muscle is elevated supraperiosteally off the proximal tibia to the level of the capsule. The capsule is incised in line with the incision, with care being taken not to cut the lateral meniscus. By incising the capsule proximally and distally first, one can extend the incision toward the meniscus while directly looking at the meniscus from above and below.

Visualization of the plateau can usually be obtained by flexing the knee and exerting a gentle varus stress to the leg, thereby opening the lateral compartment of the knee. If there is a split fracture of the plateau, the lateral meniscus is usually no longer attached to the rim of the lateral plateau, and the lateral plateau fragment can be opened up using its posterior soft tissue as a hinge. If the lateral meniscus remains attached to the rim of the lateral plateau, a submeniscal incision can be performed by transecting the meniscotibial ligament and allowing the meniscus to be elevated so that the surface of the plateau can be inspected. Some surgeons prefer to cut the anterior horn of the lateral meniscus near its insertion to the intermeniscal ligament and then repair it during the closure.[46, 62]

Often there is a tear of the lateral meniscus, and this should be assessed. If there is a peripheral tear, it should be repaired; this can be easily accomplished by placing sutures through the torn peripheral edge of the meniscus under direct vision and tying the sutures over the capsule after it is repaired during the closure. Placing these sutures during the approach allows the surgeon to use them to retract the meniscus for visualization during the reduction (see Fig. 61.9C). A tear of the inner third of the meniscus should probably be débrided to prevent symptoms resulting from an unstable meniscal fragment. As much meniscus as possible should be retained, and meniscectomy should never be routinely performed for visualization in tibial plateau fractures.

After the fracture is reduced and stabilized, the meniscal sutures are passed through the capsule, the capsule is repaired, and the sutures are tied. The iliotibial band is repaired. The fascia of the anterior compartment should generally be left open. If any concern about residual swelling and compartment syndrome exists during closure, the anterior compartment fascia should be fully released. In isolated low-energy fractures in which there is minimal swelling, the fascia can be closed, which has the advantage of preventing a later cosmetically displeasing bulge of the tibialis anterior muscle.

The midline approach is favored by some, usually for bicondylar fractures, because it can give good exposure to both the lateral and medial plateaus. Additionally, the midline approach uses the same skin incision as is used for total knee arthroplasty, so future salvage arthroplasty will not be made more difficult by lateral or medial skin incisions. Some authors further enhance this approach by either making a Z-cut of the patellar tendon or performing a tibial tubercle osteotomy.[27, 69] The disadvantage of the midline approach is that to reduce and fix both condyles from this approach, a significant amount of soft-tissue dissection is required, resulting in devascularized fracture fragments and a potential "dead-bone" sandwich, which delays fracture healing and increases the potential for skin slough and infection (Fig. 61.7). The current trend favors a lateral incision and performing a separate limited medial incision as necessary.

Occasionally, there is a posteromedial coronal fracture fragment, in addition to the lateral plateau injury, which cannot be reduced from the standard lateral or even midline incision. In these circumstances, one can make an additional posteromedial incision and gain access to the fragment in the interval between the medial head of the gastrocnemius muscle and the semitendinosus tendon. This allows good visualization of the reduction, as well as room to place a posterior to anterior lag screw or a small buttress plate.[6, 17, 32]

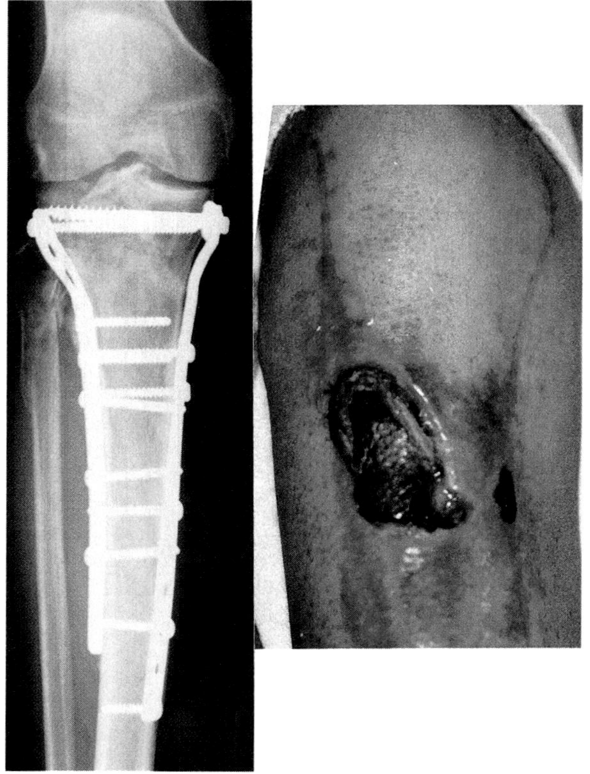

FIGURE 61.7 ➢ Schatzker type VI tibial plateau fracture in a 42-year-old man involved in a motor vehicle crash. Reconstruction was performed with ORIF using two large plates applied through separate incisions with a narrow skin bridge, resulting in a "dead-bone sandwich" and a necrosed skin flap. Osteomyelitis was avoided by expeditious irrigation and débridement and soft-tissue coverage with a rotational flap.

Assessing Reduction

The ability to assess the reduction prior to placing fixation is paramount in the operative treatment of tibial plateau fractures. There are three methods of assessing the intraoperative reduction: fluoroscopically, arthroscopically, and via direct visualization. Intraoperative fluoroscopy can be useful in assessing the reduction in both open and percutaneous treatment of tibial plateau fractures. Intraoperative use of the C-arm allows multiple views and projections to be obtained, which can accurately show the position of the fracture fragments and any implants. Fluoroscopy should not be used as the final assessment of joint congruity, however, because a number of studies have shown that seemingly congruent joint reductions on fluoroscopy have step-offs when standard radiographs are obtained.[52] Similarly, fluoroscopy can be misleading in the determination of overall tibial alignment because it is impossible to get the entire tibia on one fluoroscopic image.

Spot views of the proximal tibia tend to suggest more varus than is present and seen if the entire tibia is imaged on one radiographic plate. It is suggested that plain AP and lateral radiographs centered on the joint line, as well as separate full-length AP and lateral tibia radiographs, be obtained for the final evaluation of the tibial plateau articular reduction and alignment prior to leaving the operating room.

When the joint depression consists of many fragments or other factors limit fluoroscopic evaluation of the joint reduction, arthroscopy can be used to confirm adequate joint reduction. The use of percutaneous fixation with arthroscopic visualization allows joint restoration without a formal open reduction. Disadvantages of this technique include difficulty in visualization, added equipment for the operating room staff to manage, and case reports of compartment syndrome due to extravasation of the arthroscopy fluid.[5] The potential for compartment syndrome has led to the recommendation that a pump not be used if the arthroscope is used.

Proponents of the arthroscopic technique tout its ability to visualize the articular reduction without an open approach or mobilizing of the menisci, to assess and treat other intra-articular pathology, and to facilitate rehabilitation by minimizing iatrogenic soft-tissue injury. Detractors of the arthroscopic technique of visualization of acute tibial plateau fractures point out a number of disadvantages. First, many surgeons think that for injuries in the lateral compartment, the meniscus covers such a significant portion of the plateau that much of the fracture displacement, especially fractures near the rim, will occur under the meniscus, which can be difficult to visualize with the arthroscope. Second, some surgeons think that simple split fractures can be adequately assessed using fluoroscopy and that fractures that would be better assessed by arthroscopy—namely, fractures with a depressed component—require a buttress plate for stable fixation. Placement of a buttress plate obviously necessitates an open approach, in which case the articular reduction can be assessed by direct visualization. Third, many think that arthroscopy does not provide enough improvement in their ability to assess articular reduction over fluoroscopy to warrant the risk of compartment syndrome or the added equipment demands inherent to arthroscopy.

Early results have been good in patients in whom arthroscopy was used for visualization of the articular reduction. Holzach et al reported the results of 15 lateral plateau fractures reduced under arthroscopic guidance.[38] All had bone grafting, and 10 had internal fixation. Twelve of 15 were found to have anatomic reduction according to radiographic evaluation, and 14 of 15 had excellent results at 3 years of follow-up. Dwyer and Bobic[26] reported on seven patients treated with the use of an arthroscope. Six of seven had internal fixation. All seven had good results. Bernfeld et al reported on nine patients with an average of 10 months of follow-up.[8] All had good or excellent reductions, and eight of nine had good or excellent clinical results. In the only direct comparison of arthroscopic versus open reduction, Fowble et al[28] reported on 23 patients, 12 treated with arthroscopic reduction and percutaneous fixation, 11 treated with ORIF. They found 100% anatomic reduction in the arthroscopic group compared with 55% in the ORIF group. Long-term outcomes were not measured, but at 6 months of follow-up, the arthroscopic group had better range of motion. There was one deep infection in the ORIF group.

Associated Injuries

Treatment of associated soft-tissue injuries remains controversial. The high incidence of ligament and meniscal injuries has been previously identified, but with improved imaging techniques such as MRI, this incidence appears to be even higher than was previously recognized.[37, 50, 86] The treatment of associated meniscal disorders is generally accepted. Central tears without the potential for healing should be débrided, leaving as much intact rim as possible. Peripheral tears and capsular detachments should be repaired. Under no circumstances should the meniscus be removed to facilitate visualization of the plateau.

Treatment of associated ligamentous injuries remains unclear. Good results have been obtained in patients in whom obvious collateral ligament disruptions were not repaired, and it is well established that isolated medial collateral tears heal with nonoperative treatment.[43] Some authors, however, have reported improved results after repairing associated collateral ligament injuries.[21] Currently, most surgeons treating large numbers of these injuries repair a collateral ligament only if there is a bony avulsion or if it can be done without additional soft-tissue dissection, which is rare.

Cruciate ligament injuries are more straightforward. Many high-energy type V and VI injuries have a bony avulsion of the ACL insertion, and these should be repaired. This can still result in some anterior laxity, however, because of actual intraligamentous stretch at the time of injury before bony avulsion. Acute substance ruptures of the ACL are not improved by direct repair and should be left alone initially. ACL reconstruction is not indicated at the time of fracture treatment and can be performed as needed after both fracture healing and rehabilitation are complete.

Treatment Recommendations

Type I

Split fractures of the lateral condyle usually occur in a young population, and an anatomic reduction of the articular surface must be the goal. Fortunately, these fracture fragments are typically fairly large, with minimal comminution. These fractures are often amenable to closed reduction and percutaneous screw fixation (Fig. 61.8). A varus stress often reduces the split component by virtue of its capsular attachments, or a femoral distractor can be used. Occasionally, the lateral meniscus may be impacted into the fracture site, preventing closed reduction. Fine adjustments of the reduction and temporary fixation can be obtained with a "King Tong" pelvic clamp or pointed bone clamp placed around the bone through small lateral and medial stab incisions. Two large 7.0-mm or 7.3-mm cannulated screws, or 6.5-mm noncannulated, partially threaded lag screws with washers, can then be placed under fluoroscopic guidance. If preoperative CT was obtained, the fracture line can be identified on the axial views, allowing the screws to be directed to cross the fracture line as near to perpendicular as possible. In general, there is no benefit to having screws coming from both lateral to medial and medial to lateral in unicondylar fractures. As to the number of screws and need for buttress plating, a study by Koval et al showed that there was no significant difference between two side-by-side lag screws, two lag screws and a third screw and washer at the fracture line functioning as a small buttress plate, and a formal L-buttress plate with lag screws placed through the plate.[51] This applies to normal bone, however; in osteoporotic bone, a buttress plate should be employed.

Type II

Reduction of type II fractures is facilitated by the split component of the fracture. This typically allows the lateral portion of the plateau to be hinged open, permitting the depressed portion of the fracture to be elevated under direct vision. Also, the distal fracture line of the split fragment is usually readily visible on the tibia, often with edges that can be keyed into place anatomically. This shows the correct lateral height that must be obtained as the depressed fragment is elevated. The lateral-most portion of the intact medial plateau or tibial spine is usually visible, which can also be used to ensure correct elevation. Care must be taken to identify the intact medial portion of the joint, with the understanding that the lateral portion of the anterior spine is often depressed and only intact medially. If the main depressed portion of the plateau is elevated to an incompletely elevated anterior spine, a step-off persists between the depression fragment and the split fragment.

Type II fractures are best approached laterally, as described previously (Fig. 61.9). After the lateral split fragment is reflected laterally, the entire depressed fragment is identified. The depressed fragments are

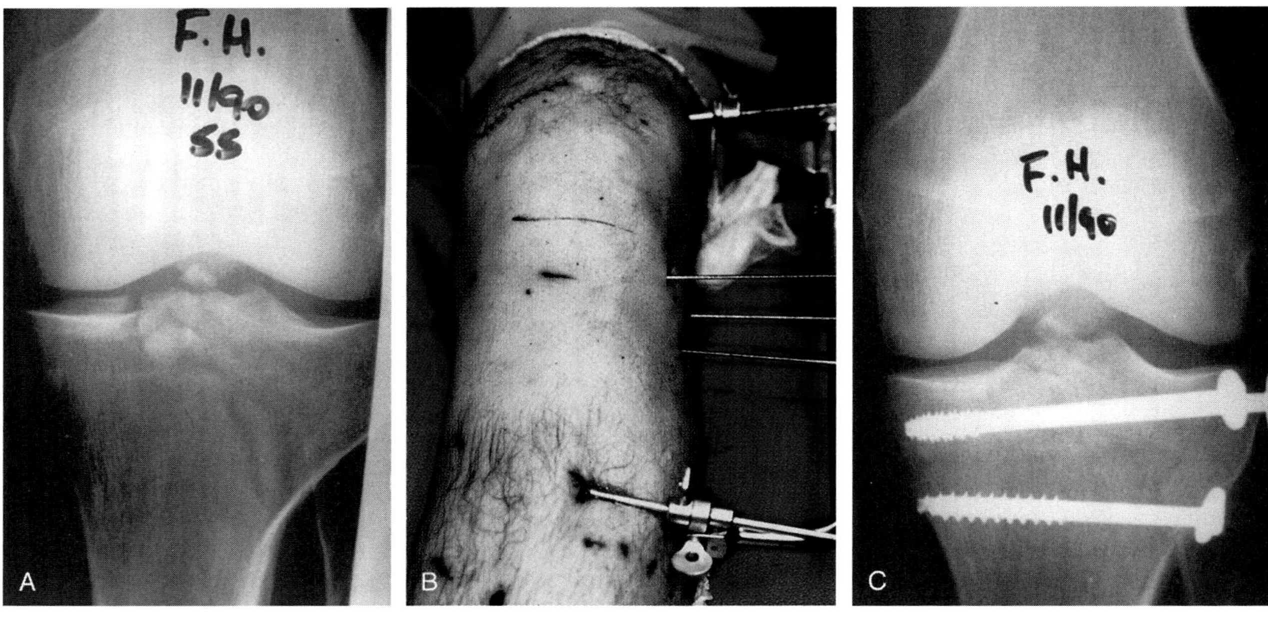

FIGURE 61.8 ➢ Schatzker type I tibial plateau fracture in a 30-year-old male who fell from a ladder. *A*, Preoperative anteroposterior radiograph. *B*, Intraoperative picture showing femoral distractor being used to obtain indirect reduction, with guide wires for the cannulated screws in place. *C*, Postoperative anteroposterior radiograph showing anatomic reduction of the tibial plateau.

partially elevated en masse with a flat, wide elevator. At this point it is generally recommended that bone graft be placed under the depressed articular fragments and the articular depression be elevated indirectly by elevation of the bone graft and subchondral bone. We have started achieving this with a unicortical or bicortical rectangle of iliac crest bone graft, as opposed to the pure cancellous graft we used previously. We find that the articular fragments elevate more easily as well as more evenly by indirect elevation through the cortical piece of bone. This cortical bone block is cut from the iliac crest to a size to fill the remaining subchondral defect as completely as possible. The remaining gaps can be filled with cancellous bone graft. Allograft and porous hydroxyapatite have also been used for grafting defects with good results.[13, 78] New bone graft substitutes are appearing in the marketplace rapidly, and their utility in these injuries must be assessed individually. The lateral split fragment is rotated closed, and its anatomic reduction can be assessed by observing its distal and anterior fracture lines. The plateau can also be partially visualized by elevating the meniscus. A K-wire is then placed for provisional fixation. At this point, the C-arm can be used to radiographically assess the articular reduction. The plate is affixed to the metaphysis by placing a screw in the sliding hole so that fine proximal-distal adjustments can be made. After final adjustments are made, a lag screw is placed through one of the proximal holes. This can be a 4.5-mm screw placed after overdrilling the lateral cortex or a partially threaded 6.5-mm screw. This is followed by a second lag screw and the distal plate screws. Final radiographs are obtained, followed by meniscal repair if necessary and closure as described previously.

Type III

Type III fractures have an intact lateral plateau rim with depressed articular fragments. Direct elevation of these depressed articular fragments is required for reduction. This is usually accomplished by making a window in the metaphyseal bone under the depression. The depression is elevated and the resulting defect filled with bone graft. A buttress plate is used as in type II fractures, with careful subchondral placement of the screws required to prevent settling of the articular surface.

Alternatively, type III injuries can be reduced under arthroscopic guidance (Fig. 61.10). Under tourniquet, the arthroscope is inserted into the knee and hematoma and fracture debris are removed. An intra-articular arthroscopic inspection for associated injuries is carried out. After identification of the depressed fragment, a guide wire is placed percutaneously into the metaphysis and advanced until it is observed entering the depressed fragment intra-articularly. A large cannulated drill is carefully advanced to the subchondral level. Bone graft is placed into this tunnel and elevated until the depressed portion of the articular surface is brought to the proper height. After the tunnel is completely packed with bone graft, screws are placed across the joint in the subchondral bone to prevent collapse of the elevated joint surface.

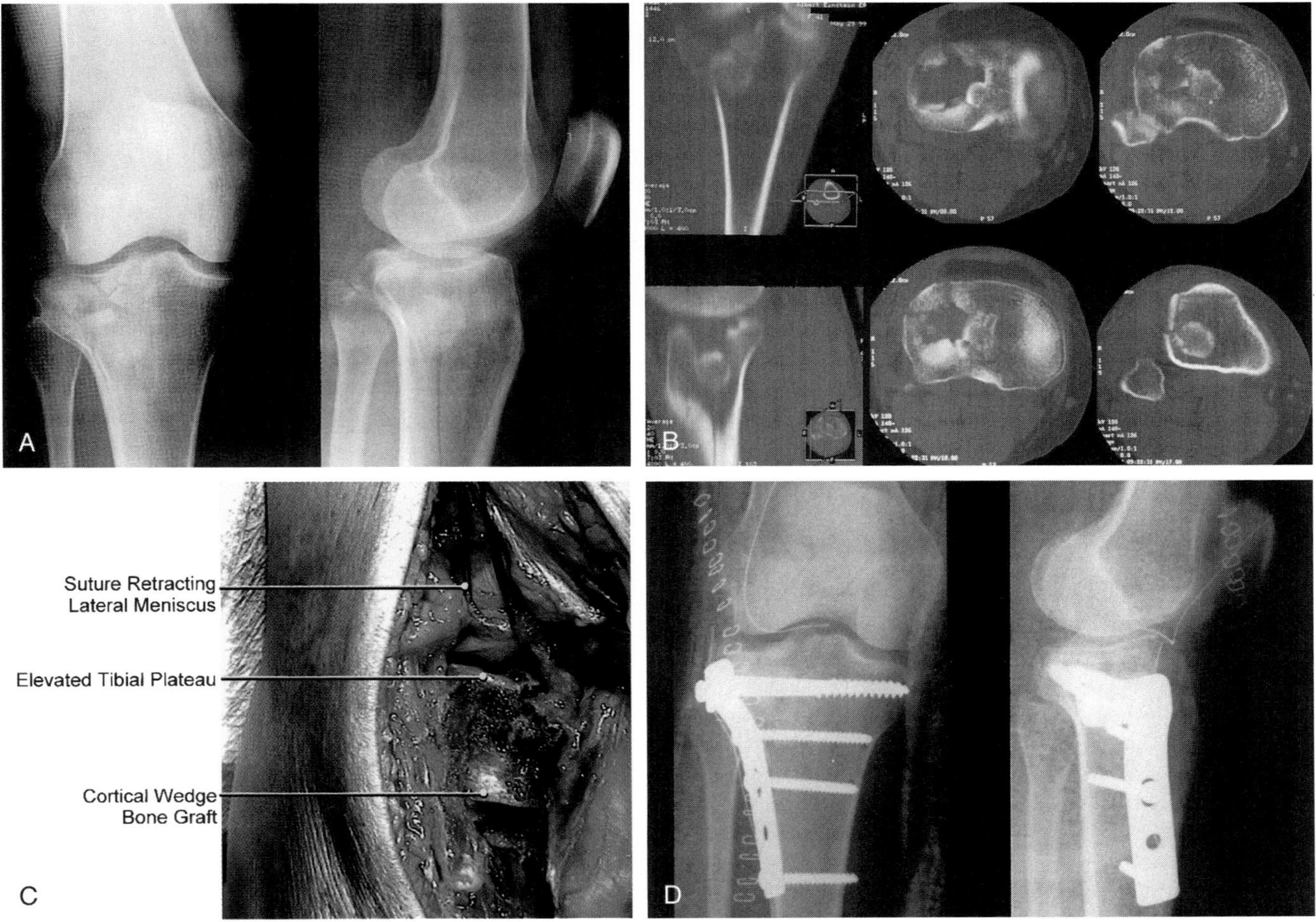

FIGURE 61.9 ➢ A Schatzker type II tibial plateau fracture in a 35-year-old female involved in a motor vehicle crash. *A*, Preoperative anteroposterior and lateral radiographs. *B*, Preoperative CT scan showing the split as well as a large depression fragment. *C*, Intraoperative picture showing indirect elevation of the depression fragment en masse using an iliac crest bone block. *D*, Postoperative anteroposterior and lateral radiographs showing reduction and stabilization of the tibial plateau fracture.

Type IV

Type IV fractures can look deceivingly simple, but they are not the equivalent of a lateral plateau fracture occurring on the medial side. Unlike the lateral side where the plateau fractures off the leg, the leg is usually fractured off the medial plateau in type IV fractures. The medial plateau actually represents the intact stable fragment. There is usually complete disruption of the lateral ligaments and stabilizing soft tissues as well as ACL and posterior cruciate ligament injuries. Many classify this injury as a fracture/dislocation. This is important to understand when treatment decisions are being formulated because the entire lower leg will be acting as a long lever arm on the fixation placed medially. Complicating the articular reconstruction is the fact that the fracture line often crosses through to the lateral side or even enters the joint medially and laterally, leaving the spines as a free fragment or fragments. If a tibial head plate is used on the medial side, the plate made for the contralateral leg must be used because the plate is essentially placed backward.

Type V

Type V fractures are difficult because, although a portion of the metaphysis may remain attached to the tibial shaft, there is often no intact cartilage on this remaining metaphyseal spike. This makes it difficult to determine how much to elevate the bicondylar articular surfaces. These fractures also typically have quite a bit of comminution in the area of the tibial spines, leading to a tendency to overcompress the plateau (i.e., making the plateau too narrow compared with the distal femur). Furthermore, there is often a need to place fixation medially or posteromedially.

Fixation of these fractures can be undertaken through either a lateral approach or a midline approach. We prefer the lateral approach, knowing that a medial or posteromedial approach may be necessary

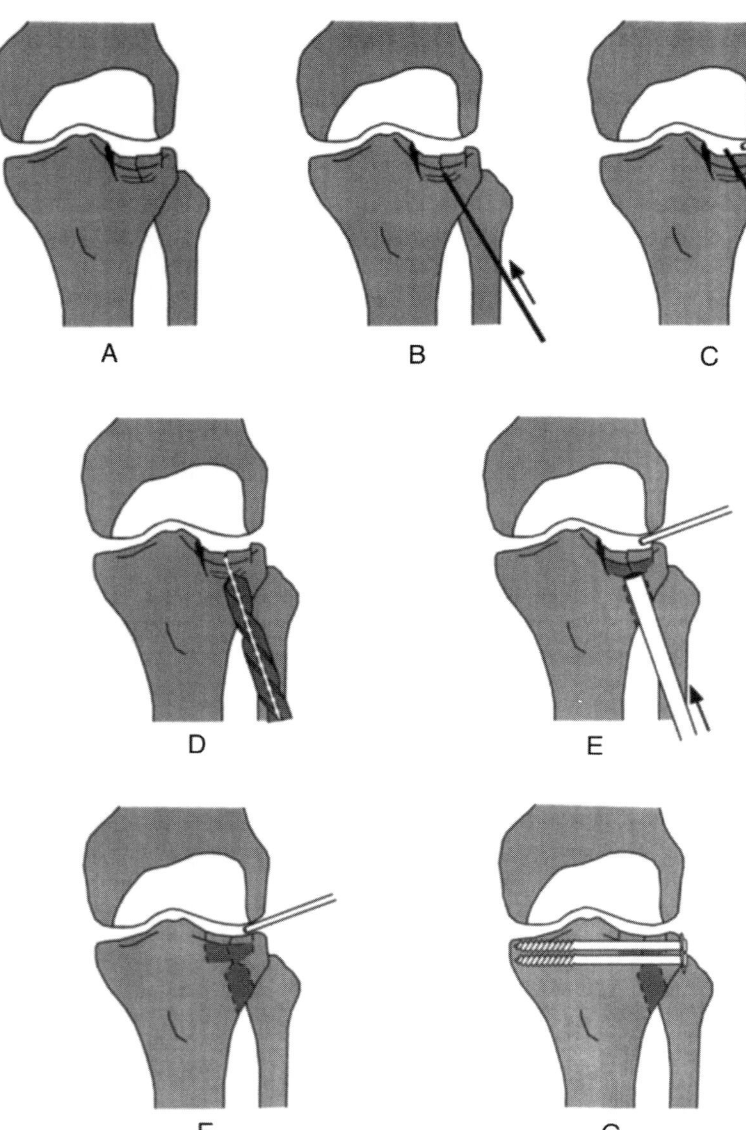

FIGURE 61.10 ➢ Technique for reduction and arthroscopic assessment of reduction in a Schatzker type III tibial plateau fracture. *A*, Preoperative anteroposterior view showing articular depression. *B*, Guide wire being passed through the metaphyseal cortex into the depressed fragment. *C*, Penetration of the fragment is confirmed by arthroscopic visualization of the wire entering the joint through the depression. *D*, A cannulated drill is passed over the wire until it is just under the depressed fragment. Fluoroscopy aids in determining the depth of the drill. *E*, Bone graft is placed into the drilled channel, and the articular surface is elevated indirectly. *F*, Reduction is confirmed by visualization through the arthroscope. *G*, Two or three 3.5-mm screws are placed across the joint surface. These screws must be placed immediately under the chondral surface to prevent collapse of the elevated surface.

secondarily. It is important to fully identify the distal and anterior extent of the lateral plateau fragment because the keying of this fragment will define the height for restoring the remainder of the joint. If the lateral plateau fragment is comminuted and anatomic reduction is unlikely to be obtainable initially, one should consider beginning the reconstruction with anatomic reduction of the medial side. When comminution exists in the area of the tibial spines, it is often prudent to simply reduce each plateau directly by its respective fracture lines along the metaphysis, then place screws across the plateau in a nonlag fashion to stabilize the articular surface but prevent overcompression. The femoral distractor can be a useful tool in obtaining reduction. One or even two distractors can be placed on either or both sides of the knee to counteract the tendency toward shortening.[58] Parallel Schanz pins placed near the epicondyles of the distal femur and midshaft in the tibia enable the femoral distractor to distract in the line of the joint, minimizing translational effects.

Typically, a buttress plate or lateral tibial head plate is used laterally, with a flattened semitubular or reconstruction plate used medially, depending on the inherent stability. Occasionally, the medial plate can be placed percutaneously if a near-anatomic reduction can be obtained with closed reduction techniques (Fig. 61.11C, D). This is accomplished by making a small incision proximal or distal to the fracture line and using an elevator to create a supraperiosteal tunnel under the soft tissue.

A plate is bent to the approximate curvature of the medial metaphysis and slid through the previously created tunnel. The plate can usually be a short four- or five-hole plate. The screws are placed through small stab incisions. If indirect reduction is not obtainable, the medial plate can be applied by making a small incision directly medial and using minimal soft-tissue

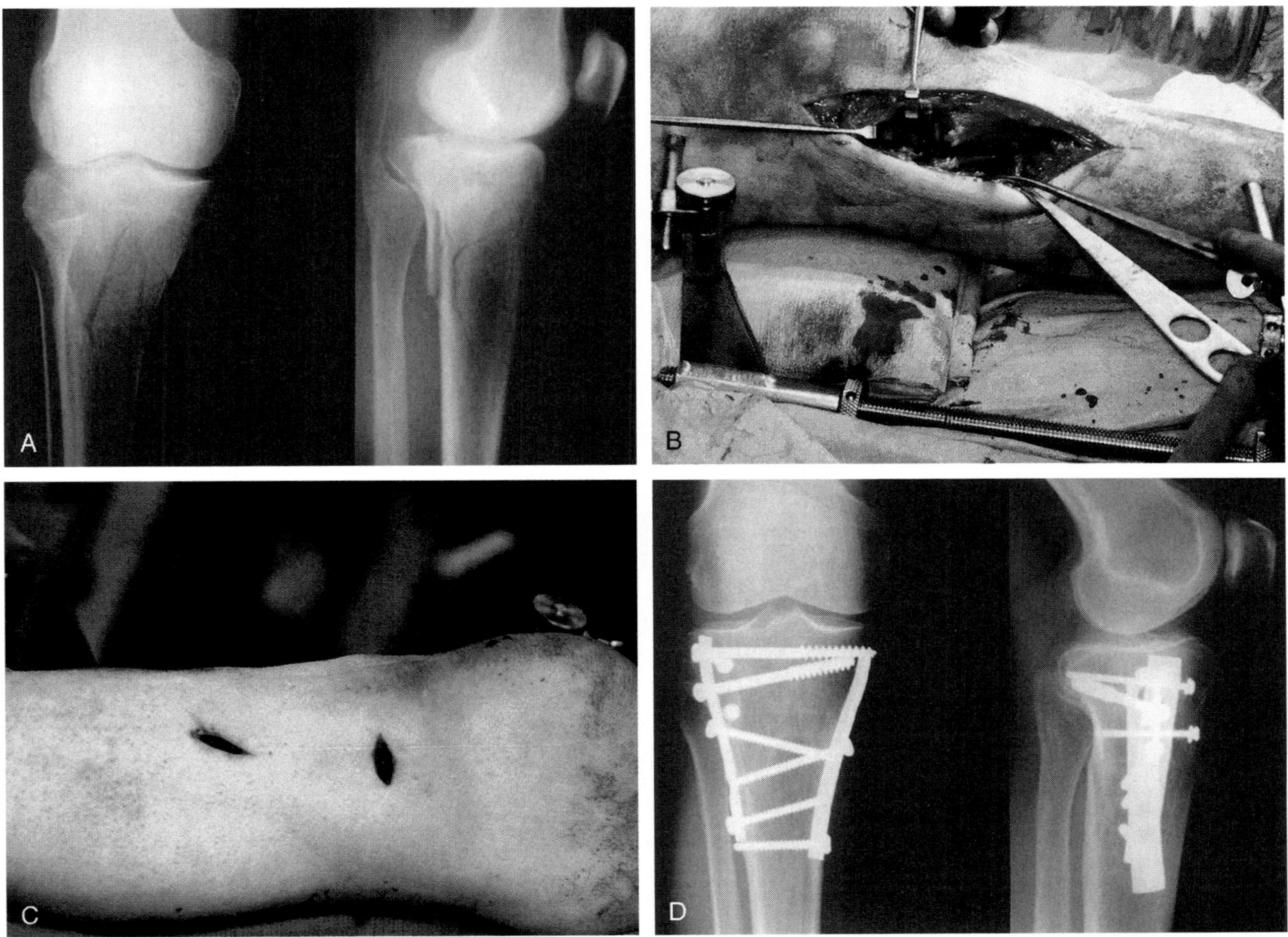

FIGURE 61.11 ➢ Schatzker type VI tibial plateau fracture in a 48-year-old male involved in a motor vehicle crash. *A*, Preoperative AP and lateral radiographs showing complete dissociation of the tibial plateau from the tibial shaft. *B*, Intraoperative picture showing a laterally placed femoral distractor placed for ligamentotaxis and varus load to allow elevation of the articular fragments. Soft-tissue stripping is minimized by a direct lateral approach. *C*, Intraoperative picture showing the incisions used for application of a percutaneous medial buttress plate. *D*, Postoperative radiographs showing anatomic reduction of the articular surface and a healed tibial shaft.

dissection; the fracture can be reduced under direct vision and the plate applied. Alternatively, a simple two-pin medial fixator can be used as a buttress, with one Schanz pin placed in the tibial shaft distally and one Schanz pin in the medial plateau proximally, connected by a simple bar (Fig. 61.12C). Bone grafting should be performed if comminution exists either at the metaphyseal fracture lines or in the area of the spines, or prophylactically if extensive soft-tissue stripping was needed for hardware placement.

Type VI

Type VI fractures are the most difficult fractures to treat. First, there is a complete dissociation of the articular surface from the tibial shaft, leaving no stable base upon which to reconstruct the plateau. Second, these are usually high-energy injuries, often with severe soft-tissue injuries and significant comminution. One must carefully consider the soft tissue in these injuries when choosing a treatment plan. A significant delay before ORIF, or alternative methods such as limited internal fixation with external fixation, may be necessary.

Ideally, fixation of type VI fractures proceeds by an anatomic reconstruction of the lateral and medial plateaus, followed by attachment of the reconstructed plateaus and metaphysis to the tibial shaft (see Fig. 61.11). This is difficult if there is comminution in the area of the tibial spines because it makes assessment of both joint width and height very difficult. Also, an anterior fragment with the tibial tubercle is often displaced and requires an anterior-to-posterior lag screw to prevent displacement. As in type V fractures, a lateral approach, with a supplemental medial approach as needed, is used. Fully threaded screws may be necessary across the joint to avoid overcompression. Bone graft in the region of the tibial spines may also be

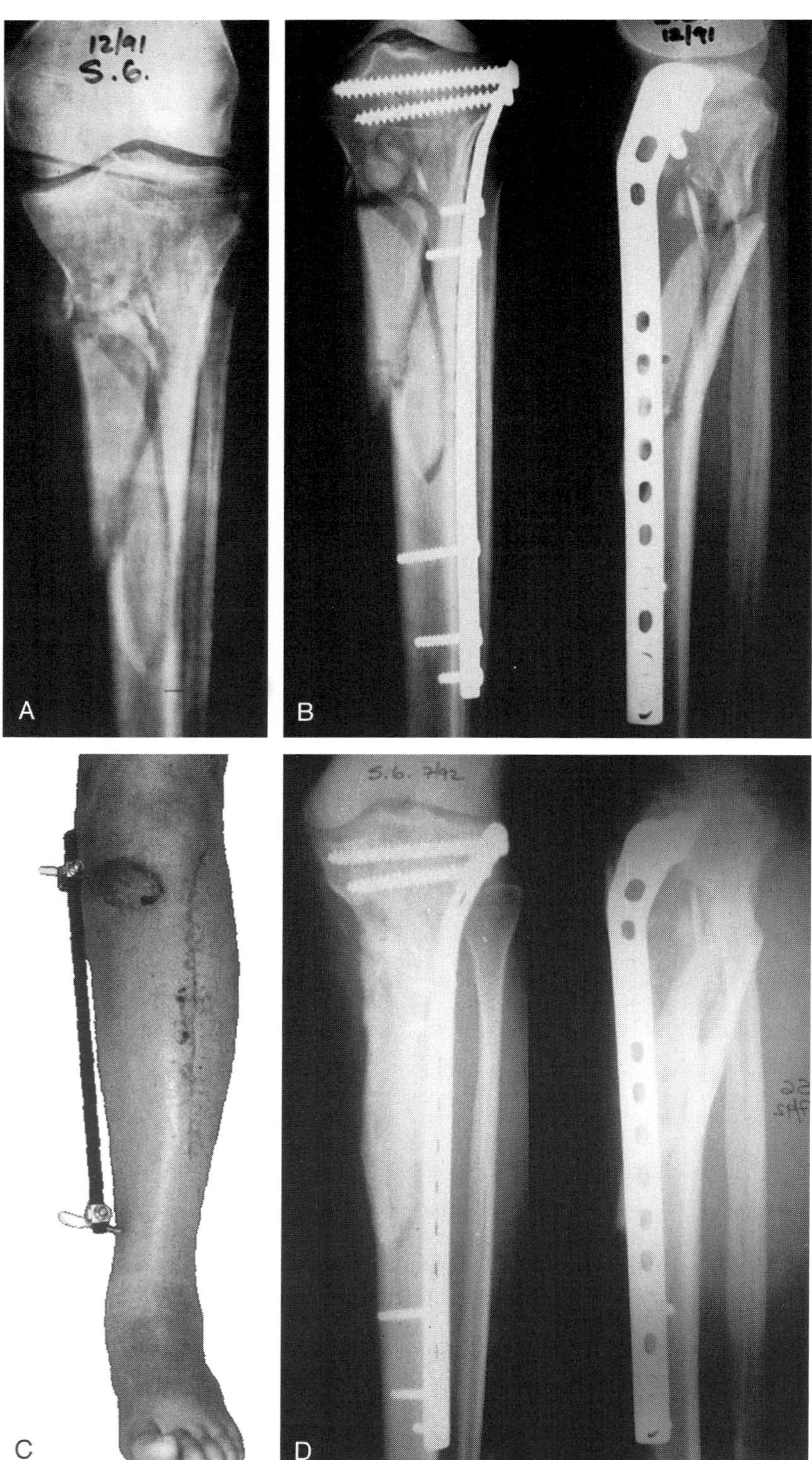

FIGURE 61.12 ➢ Schatzker type VI tibial plateau fracture in a 34-year-old female involved in a motor vehicle crash. There was a grade II open wound on the medial side. *A*, Preoperative anteroposterior radiograph showing comminution of the tibial shaft and a small minimally displaced fracture line extending into the joint near the tibial spine. *B*, Intraoperative anteroposterior and lateral radiographs after lateral plate fixation. Medial fixation was thought to be a poor option because of the presence of an open wound. *C*, Clinical photograph showing a simple two-pin medial fixator applied to buttress the medial side of the plateau and shaft. A medial gastrocnemius flap was rotated to provide soft-tissue coverage for the open medial wound. *D*, Anteroposterior and lateral radiographs showing bone union with no malalignment.

necessary. Once two crossing screws are placed and the articular surface is stable, it can be attached to the tibial shaft, usually with a tibial head buttress plate. The smaller buttress plates are not usually sturdy enough to tolerate the forces generated by the long lever arm of the leg in these fractures.

In a majority of cases, supplemental fixation is necessary on the medial side (see Fig. 61.12). If there is a posteromedial fragment, it can be reduced under direct vision via a posteromedial approach. Fixation of this fragment is obtained with a small one-third or semitubular plate placed as an antiglide plate, with a lag screw placed from posterior to anterior through one of the top plate holes (Fig. 61.13).

Open Fractures and Fractures With Compromised Soft Tissue

Open injuries and fractures with severely compromised soft tissues present a significant treatment dilemma. Thorough, emergent irrigation and débridement is necessary to minimize the chance of delayed bony infection or even septic arthritis, but one must simultaneously consider future reconstruction. Incisions used to extend open wounds for débridement should anticipate incisions that may be needed for ORIF. Likewise, incisions for release of compartment syndrome should be given similar consideration. In these circumstances, placing the lateral incision for compartment release slightly more anterior than usual generally allows release of both the anterior and the lateral compartments but still allows good access to the anterolateral tibial metaphysis if subsequent plating is required. An attempt should be made to avoid extending the compartment releases into the fracture lines, thereby creating an open fracture.

The timing of hardware placement in open tibial plateau fractures is controversial. When the wound is minimally contaminated and débridement is good, some advocate acute joint reconstruction with lag screws and buttressing with a plate, a thin-wire fixator, or a spanning external fixator.[7, 75, 82, 84] If the wound is severely contaminated, the joint should be spanned with an external fixator, with joint reconstruction taking place when a clean wound is obtained after subsequent débridements. When a fasciotomy is necessary, expedient coverage of the soft tissue is paramount. Attempts should be made to close the skin within 72 hours; if skin closure is not possible, split-thickness skin grafting should be performed. If skin on only one side of the fasciotomy can be closed, it is preferable to close the lateral side and skin graft the medial side, thus providing better coverage for a subsequent lateral ORIF.

Often in tibial plateau fractures with severe soft-tissue injuries or compartment syndrome, fixation is best obtained with limited internal fixation of the articular surface and external fixation. Thin-wire fixation with a hybrid-type fixator is our preference in these circumstances (Fig. 61.14). Attempting fluoroscopy-assisted closed reduction, but resorting to minimal arthrotomy and open reduction if necessary, the articular surface is reduced. Temporary fixation is obtained with K-wires. Lag screw fixation is achieved with cannulated, partially threaded screws. Using the C-arm to guide wire placement, a smooth thin wire is placed just distal and parallel to the joint line in the coronal plane. The wires should be at least 14 mm distal to the joint line to prevent penetration of the capsular reflection.[19, 41, 64] Capsular penetration by the pins can lead to drainage of synovial fluid, an increased incidence of bone and soft-tissue infection, and septic arthritis if the pin becomes superficially infected during the treatment course.[76, 87]

A second wire, with an olive or bead, is placed posterolaterally to anteromedially. Some prefer to place this wire into the fibular and across the proximal tibiofibular joint. There is a low incidence of com-

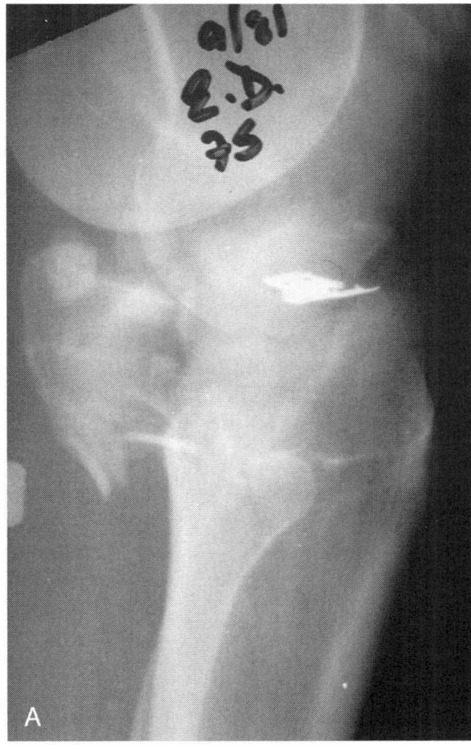

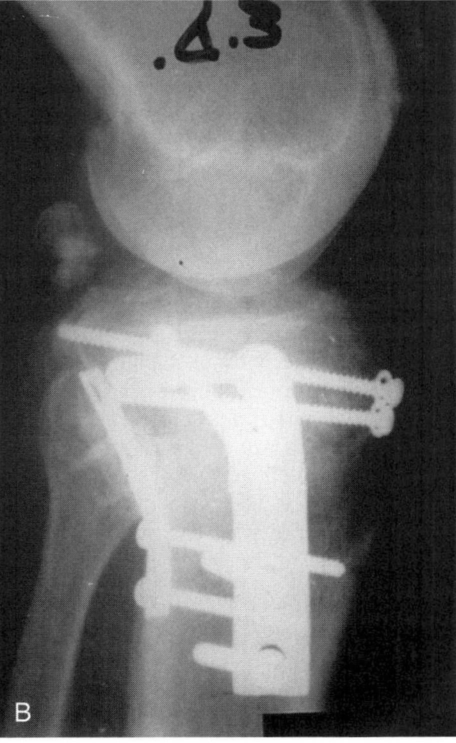

FIGURE 61.13 ➢ A 75-year-old diabetic who was a pedestrian struck by a motor vehicle. *A*, Lateral radiograph showing a displaced posteromedial fragment. *B*, Postoperative lateral radiograph showing the fragment reduced with a one-third tubular antiglide plate placed through a direct posteromedial approach.

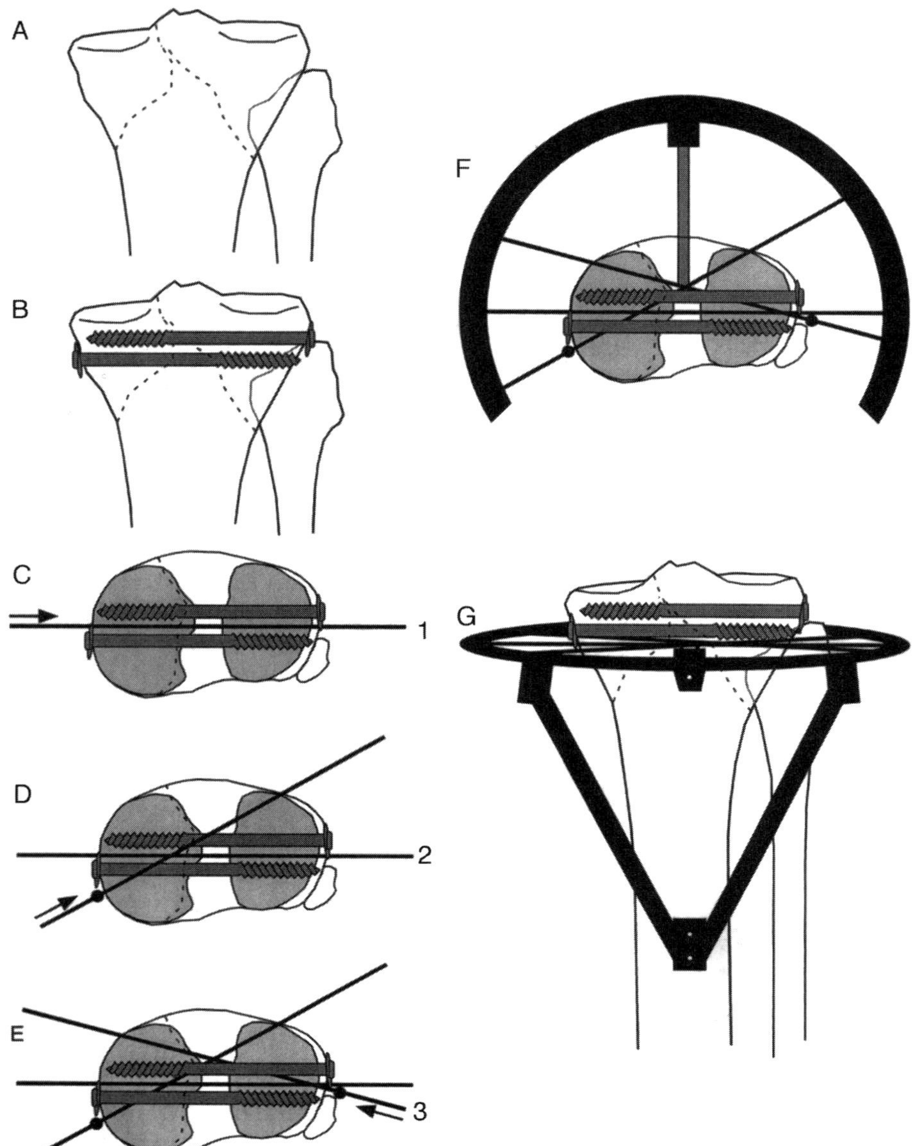

FIGURE 61.14 ➢ Technique for reduction and fixation of a Schatzker type V tibial plateau fracture using cannulated screws and a hybrid external fixator. *A,* Reduction is obtained via open or closed methods and held with a reduction clamp. *B,* Cannulated screws are placed to hold the articular reduction. *C,* Smooth guide wire for the external fixator is placed in the coronal plane, at least 14 mm distal to the joint line. *D,* The second wire, with a bead or olive, is passed posteromedially to anterolaterally. *E,* A third wire, also beaded, is passed posterolaterally to anteromedially. *F,* Wires are appropriately tensioned and fixed to the ring. An optional half-pin can be placed from the anterior to posterior aspects and attached to the ring for increased stability. *G,* Half-pins are placed into the tibial shaft, and the distal pins are connected to the ring with the appropriate clamps and bars.

munication of this joint with the femorotibial joint, which could further increase the risk of septic arthritis if the wire became superficially infected. We therefore prefer to place the wire just anterior to the fibula and have it exit medially as close to the patellar tendon as possible without violating it or the pes tendons.

The final wire, again a beaded wire, is placed posteromedially to anterolaterally. By having the wire exit near the patellar tendon, the maximum angle is produced between the two crossing wires, which maximizes the stability of the wire fixation. A ring is fixed to the wires by the appropriate connectors. A distance of approximately two fingerbreadths should be maintained between the skin and the ring throughout the circumference of the ring, and the ring should be positioned to allow as much knee flexion as possible before the ring impinges on the posterior thigh.

The wires must be tensioned. The initial smooth wire is usually tensioned first. The beaded wires must be tensioned from the proper direction so that the bead will be pulled against the cortex of the metaphysis. The ring is now well fixed to the proximal tibia, and attention is directed to the tibial shaft segment. Two or three 4.5-mm half-pins are placed bicortically into the distal third of the tibial shaft, anteriorly to posteriorly. The appropriate pin clamp is affixed to the pins, and the clamp is attached to the ring with the appropriate clamps and bars. Fluoroscopy and plain radiographs are used to adjust the tibial alignment as discussed previously.

The use of pins placed into the foot is controversial. In cases of severe proximal soft-tissue injury and swelling, the foot should be immobilized to rest the proximal muscles that control the foot and allow leg swelling to diminish. This can be done with either a resting foot splint that is attached to the external fixator with straps or by placing small pins into the first metatarsal and connecting these pins to the fixator. Some think that by placing pins into the foot, it is easier to prevent an equinus contracture, which tends to develop while the patient is minimally mobile.

Elderly Patients

Fractures of the tibial plateau in the elderly population are common, likely because of weaker osteoporotic bone and an increased propensity for falls. Fractures in this elderly group are likely to continue to increase as the aging population continues to grow. Tibial plateau fractures in older patients are typically low-energy type II or III fractures, although a high-energy injury in any age group leads to type V and VI fractures, as typically occur in younger patients. Fracture treatment in the elderly is more difficult because of their inability to tolerate the immobility associated with conservative treatment and their osteoporotic bone, which makes obtaining stable internal fixation difficult. Osteoporosis, however, is not a contraindication to internal fixation.[70]

Good results have been reported for treatment of tibial plateau fractures in the elderly. Biyani et al reported on a group of 32 patients with a mean age of 71.7 years, all of whom underwent standard ORIF.[9] They had 72% good or excellent results clinically and 69% good or excellent results radiographically. There was no association between radiographic and clinical results. There were no infectious complications, but one patient did lose reduction postoperatively. Levy et al also had good results with operative treatment of tibial plateau fractures in the elderly population.[55] They performed an 11-year follow-up of 19 patients, all at least 65 years old at the time of injury. There were good or excellent results in 79% but four (20%) superficial infections.

Postoperative Care

Postoperatively, the patient's management is determined by the stability of the fixation and the soft-tissue integrity. Ideally, motion of the knee should begin immediately, if the fracture is well fixed and the soft tissue is not compromised. Continuous passive motion is an excellent method of early joint mobilization,[67] but care must be exercised if the soft tissues are tenuous. Studies have shown that the oxygen tension in the anterior skin about the knee decreases with flexion above 40 degrees.[45] If significant swelling or a closure under tension exists, it is prudent to place the entire leg in a soft, bulky, mildly compressive dressing in 10 degrees of flexion, stabilized with plaster splints for 48 to 72 hours. If the wound appears less tenuous at this time, it can be placed into a rehabilitation-type brace, and continuous passive motion can be started. If the soft tissues are not a concern, it is acceptable to place a soft dressing on the wound and begin passive motion immediately with a long-leg brace in place. Continuous epidural anesthesia in the postoperative period may facilitate motion by controlling pain, but the patient must be monitored for compartment syndrome for at least 48 hours after surgery.[42] Closed-suction drains and prophylactic antibiotics are typically maintained for 24 to 48 hours. Patients are typically light partial weightbearing for 6 to 12 weeks, although some studies have reported that early weightbearing does not lead to loss of reduction.[72]

Diligent care must also be taken to prevent an equinus contracture of the foot in all patients, but especially those treated with either internal or external fixation. External fixators should be maintained for 10 to 12 weeks if the pins allow. Draining pins may be managed with oral antibiotics for 7 to 10 days, but if there is no improvement the pins must be removed or exchanged. At the time of planned fixator removal, it is prudent to disconnect the ring from the shaft pins and stress the fracture under fluoroscopy to ensure solid healing, before removing pins and wires.

COMPLICATIONS

Infection

Infection can be a devastating complication of tibial plateau fracture management because of its intra-articular location. Other than open fractures, most deep infections in tibial plateau fractures result from insufficient attention to the soft-tissue envelope. Open fixation in a leg with severe swelling or blisters, wide exposures with extensive periosteal stripping, two incisions with too narrow a skin bridge, and overly aggressive early range of motion all increase the chances of wound breakdown and subsequent infection. Superficial wound problems in the early postoperative period should be treated aggressively with antibiotics, and there should be a low threshold for repeat irrigation and débridement. Any deep infection should be similarly treated, and the knee joint should be opened and irrigated to prevent unappreciated septic arthritis from causing permanent damage to the articular cartilage.

Early in the postoperative period, implants that are stable may be retained but should be aggressively irrigated and undergo mechanical débridement. Unstable implants and implants in a late infection should be removed. If the plateau is unstable after implant removal, a spanning external fixator should be placed to maintain relative stability. Antibiotic beads, either under a closed soft-tissue envelope or as a bead pouch, can be useful to deliver local antibiotic while awaiting final closure. Rotational or free flaps are often needed to obtain closure in many cases with deep infection.

Stiffness

Arthrofibrosis and resulting stiffness is common after tibial plateau fractures, particularly in more severe injuries. Prevention is the best treatment, but this depends on adequate, stable fixation allowing aggressive mobilization. When fixation is tenuous, the fracture must be protected by limiting motion; stiffness is more common in these cases. When stiffness occurs, it should be treated with motion exercises in physiotherapy. Often in severe injuries, a 5- to 10-degree flexion contracture results, but flexion of at least 120 degrees should be obtainable. If the range of motion is not improving with physiotherapy and the fracture is healed, closed manipulation under anesthesia can be performed. This is ideally performed under epidural block wherein the epidural catheter can be left in place postoperatively, and inpatient CPM can continue for 2 to 3 days. Manipulation can be performed in conjunction with arthroscopic lysis of adhesions in some cases. An aggressive outpatient therapy program is vital after any of these treatments.

Arthrosis

Post-traumatic arthrosis occurs in some tibial plateau injuries despite attempts at or even successful anatomic joint reconstruction. The articular cartilage damage occurring at the time of injury, the bony comminution common to these injuries, and the associated soft-tissue injuries all predispose the joint to arthrosis. Honkonen[40] reported that 44% of his patients had arthrosis at an average of 7.6 years of follow-up. When the meniscus had been totally removed, this percentage rose to 74%. He found that normal or slight valgus alignment and an intact meniscus led to the best prognosis. However, in contradistinction to his findings, it is important to appreciate that numerous other studies have shown no correlation between radiographic arthrosis and clinical symptoms.[4, 24, 52, 65]

Salvage for post-traumatic arthrosis depends on the age of the patient, the status of the individual plateaus, the alignment, and the bone stock of the leg. Osteotomy is a good option for patients who have some residual malalignment or who have one plateau with better cartilage coverage than the other.

Osteotomy should be of the tibia if the tibia has residual malalignment, or of the distal femur if the tibia is properly aligned and a more varus alignment of the knee is preferred. Arthrodesis is the treatment of choice in younger patients with poor articular coverage of both plateaus, although they are almost always reluctant to agree to this procedure. In older patients, or patients who refuse arthrodesis, total knee arthroplasty (TKA) is a good option. TKA can be considerably more difficult in these cases because of previous incisions, retained hardware, malalignment, or lack of bone stock. Roffi and Merritt[66] reported the follow-up of 13 patients who underwent TKA after a tibial plateau fracture. The success rate was only 61% at only 1 year. Newer techniques involving tibial osteochondral allografts have been performed with mixed results.[33] These techniques may provide another option for treatment of young patients with unicondylar degeneration in the future, but they must still be considered experimental at this time.

Malalignment

Malalignment of the knee can result from tibial plateau fractures if care is not taken during treatment, whether operative or nonoperative (Fig. 61.15). Type V and VI fractures are the most likely to lead to malalignment, although this can occur in unicondylar fractures if the plateau is not anatomically elevated. Normally, the mechanical axis of the leg crosses through the knee between the tibial spines. If the plateau is not restored anatomically, the axis will shift either medially or laterally and the respective compartment of the knee will be overstressed. In general, slight valgus alignment is better tolerated than varus alignment. Malalignment can also exist in the sagittal plane, with resultant excessive or minimized posterior tibial slope. This alters the loading of the articular surfaces as well as the flexion and extension range of the knee joint.

Excessive coronal or sagittal plane alignment can be treated with osteotomy, correction of deformity, and ORIF. This is best undertaken after the fractures and soft tissues have all healed. Preoperative planning is vital for these procedures to help ensure adequate final alignment. Focusing on only the knee must be avoided. The overall alignment of the leg must be

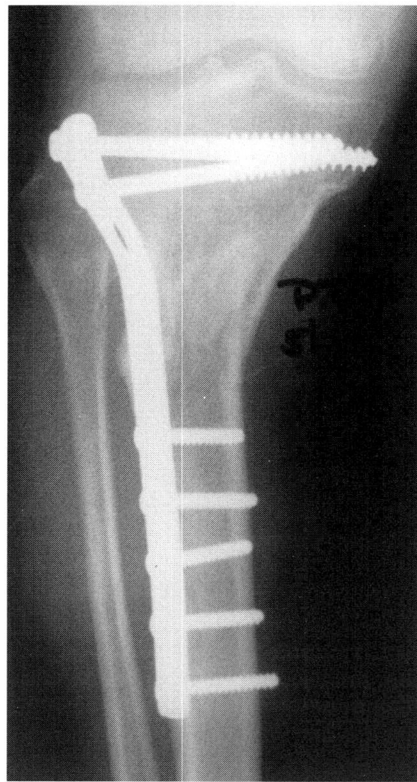

FIGURE 61.15 ➢ Radiograph of a 51-year-old male who suffered a Schatzker type VI tibial plateau fracture while skiing. Residual varus malalignment of the proximal tibia resulted after ORIF, likely because of insufficient support of the medial side. This led to medial knee pain, likely the result of overloading of the medial compartment of the knee.

considered to avoid joint alterations proximally and distally.

Loss of Fixation and Nonunion

Significant loss of fixation is rare if stable fixation is obtained initially, although small amounts of settling can occur, usually of elevated depression fragments. If stable fixation is not obtainable at the initial operation, the postoperative mobilization regimen should be altered to protect against excessive stress to suboptimal fixation. Fixation that fails in the early postoperative period should be revised if significant malalignment or joint incongruity results and the soft tissue is amenable.

Nonunions in tibial plateau fractures are rare and usually occur in the metaphysis after high-energy injuries.[49] The potential for nonunion or delayed union can often be identified at the time of initial injury, and bone grafting should be performed primarily in these cases. If healing is delayed in the postoperative course, early bone grafting should be performed.

Thromboembolic Disease

The problem of deep venous thrombosis (DVT) and pulmonary embolism in the trauma patient in general, and the lower-extremity trauma patient in particular, is well known.[31] Abelseth et al[1] reported an overall incidence of DVT of 28% in patients with fractures distal to the hip but an alarming 43% for patients with tibial plateau fractures. All trauma patients, including those with tibial plateau fractures, are at high risk for proximal DVT and subsequent pulmonary embolism. Care must be taken, however, not to overdo anticoagulation because a deep hematoma could lead to skin slough and infection. If more than a few days transpire between injury and fixation, a Doppler study of the lower extremities may be indicated to identify thrombi that may become dislodged during the reconstruction procedure. If thrombi are present, a vena caval filter may be indicated.

CONCLUSIONS

Tibial plateau fractures are severe injuries to a joint that bears significant load with daily activities. Treatment can be and often is complicated by a variety of patient and injury factors other than the bony injury. In some situations, the surgeon must realize that the severity of the injury prevents an anatomic reconstruction of the limb and that attempts at such can be more detrimental to both patient and limb than accepting a lesser result initially. Unfortunately, absolute objective treatment criteria and methods are not in place, largely because of the wide spectrum of injury severity.

Some treatment principles have evolved to guide the care of these significant lower-extremity injuries. Immobilization for any extended length of time greatly diminishes the chances for a good clinical result, particularly after operative treatment. Joint instability or large residual articular depressions lead to a suboptimal result. Open approaches through a swollen, traumatized soft-tissue envelope often lead to draining incisions, skin slough, and infection, and if large fragments of bone are devascularized (dead-bone sandwich), osteomyelitis may develop. If even a partial reduction can be obtained and motion can be maintained, good clinical results are possible even if radiographic results are suboptimal. Finally, every effort must be made to preserve meniscal and articular cartilage to minimize long-term degeneration of the joint.

Fortunately, advances in imaging, implants, and surgical techniques aid in the treatment of all injuries, including those of the tibial plateau. Future advances in indirect or minimally invasive reduction techniques; smaller, stronger implants; and advances in fixation devices should enable better results while limiting the potential for complications and poorer outcomes.

REFERENCES

1. Abelseth G, Buckley RE, Pineo GE, et al: Incidence of deep-vein thrombosis in patients with fractures of the lower extremity distal to the hip. J Orthop Trauma 10:230, 1996.
2. Aglietti P, Buzzi R: Fractures of the femoral condyles. In Insall JN, Windsor RE, Kelly MA, eds: Surgery of the Knee, 2nd ed, vol 2. New York, Churchill Livingstone, 1993, p 983.
3. Andrews JR, Tedder JL, Godbout BP: Bicondylar tibial plateau fracture complicated by compartment syndrome. Orthop Rev 21: 317, 1992.
4. Apley AG: Fractures of the lateral tibial condyle treated by skeletal traction and early mobilization. J Bone Joint Surg Br 38:699, 1956.
5. Belanger M, Fadale P: Compartment syndrome of the leg after arthroscopic examination of a tibial plateau fracture: Case report and review of the literature. Arthroscopy 13:646, 1997.
6. Bendayan J, Noblin JD, Freeland AE: Posteromedial second incision to reduce and stabilize a displaced posterior fragment that can occur in Schatzker type V bicondylar tibial plateau fractures. Orthopedics 19:903, 1996.
7. Benirschke SK: Immediate internal fixation of open, complex tibial plateau fractures: Treatment by a standard protocol. J Orthop Trauma 6:78, 1992.
8. Bernfeld B, Kligman M, Roffman M: Arthroscopic assistance for unselected tibial plateau fractures. Arthroscopy 12:598, 1996.
9. Biyani A, Reddy NS, Chaudhury J, et al: The results of surgical management of displaced tibial plateau fractures in the elderly. Injury 26:291, 1995.
10. Blokker CP: Tibial plateau fractures. Clin Orthop 182:193, 1984.
11. Bolhofner BR: Indirect reduction and composite fixation of extraarticular proximal tibial fractures. Clin Orthop 315:75, 1995.
12. Brown GA, Sprague BL: Cast brace treatment of plateau and bicondylar fractures of the proximal tibia. Clin Orthop 119:184, 1976.
13. Bucholz RW: Interporous hydroxyapatite as a bone graft substitute in tibial plateau fractures. Clin Orthop 240:53, 1989.
14. Chan PS, Klimkiewicz JJ, Luchetti WT, et al: Impact of CT scan on treatment plan and fracture classification of tibial plateau fractures. J Orthop Trauma 11:484, 1997.
15. Charnley J: The Closed Treatment of Common Fractures, 3rd ed. Baltimore, Williams & Wilkins, 1961.
16. Chuinard EG: Fractures of the condyles of the tibia. Clin Orthop 37:115, 1964.
17. De Boeck H, Opdecam P: Posteromedial tibial plateau fractures: Operative treatment by posterior approach. Clin Orthop 320: 125, 1995.
18. DeCoster TA, Nepola JV, el-Khoury GY: Cast brace treatment of proximal tibia fractures: A ten-year follow-up study. Clin Orthop 321:196, 1988.
19. DeCoster TA, Crawford MK, Kraut MAS: Safe extracapsular

placement of proximal tibia transfixation pins. J Orthop Trauma 13:236, 1999.
20. Delamarter RB, Hohl M: The cast brace and tibial plateau fractures. Clin Orthop 242:26, 1989.
21. Delamarter RB, Hohl M, Hopp E Jr: Ligament injuries associated with tibial plateau fractures. Clin Orthop 250:226, 1990.
22. Dendrinos GK: Treatment of high energy tibial plateau fractures by the Ilizarov circular fixator. J Bone Joint Surg Br 78:710, 1996.
23. Drennan DB, Locher FG, Maylahn DJ: Fractures of the tibial plateau: Treatment by closed reduction and spica cast. J Bone Joint Surg Am 61:989, 1979.
24. Duwelius PJ, Connolly JF: Closed reduction of tibial plateau fractures: A comparison of functional and radiographic results. Clin Orthop 230:116, 1988.
25. Duwelius PJ, Rangitsch MR, Colville MR, et al: Treatment of tibial plateau fractures by limited internal fixation. Clin Orthop 339:47, 1997.
26. Dwyer KA, Bobic VR: Arthroscopic management of tibial plateau fractures. Injury 23:261, 1992.
27. Fernandez DL: Anterior approach to the knee with osteotomy of the tibial tubercle for bicondylar tibial fractures. J Bone Joint Surg Am 70:208, 1988.
28. Fowble CD, Zimmer JW, Schepsis AA: The role of arthroscopy in the assessment and treatment of tibial plateau fractures. Arthroscopy 9:584, 1993.
29. Gaudinez RF, Mallik AR, Szporn M: Hybrid external fixation of comminuted tibial plateau fractures. Clin Orthop 328:203, 1996.
30. Gausewitz S, Hohl M: The significance of early motion in the treatment of tibial plateau fractures. Clin Orthop 202:135, 1986.
31. Geerts WH, Code KI, Jay RM, et al: A prospective study of venous thromboembolism after major trauma. N Engl J Med 331: 1601, 1994.
32. Georgiadis GM: Combined anterior and posterior approaches for complex tibial plateau fractures. J Bone Joint Surg Br 76:285, 1994.
33. Ghazavi MT, Pritzker KP, Davis AM, et al: Fresh osteochondral allografts for post-traumatic osteochondral defects of the knee. J Bone Joint Surg Br 79:1008, 1999.
34. Hohl M: Tibial condyle fractures. J Bone Joint Surg Am 49:1455, 1967.
35. Hohl M, Johnson EE, Wiss DS: Fractures of the proximal tibia and fibula. In Rockwood and Green's Fractures in Adults, 2nd ed. Philadelphia, JB Lippincott, 1991, p 1725.
36. Hohl M, Luck JV: Fractures of the tibial condyle. J Bone Joint Surg Am 38:1001, 1956.
37. Holt MD, Williams LA, Dent CM: MRI in the management of tibial plateau fractures. Injury 26:595, 1995.
38. Holzach P, Matter P, Minter J: Arthroscopically assisted treatment of lateral tibial plateau fractures in skiers: Use of a cannulated reduction system. J Orthop Trauma 8:273, 1994.
39. Honkonen SE: Indications for surgical treatment of tibial condyle fractures. Clin Orthop 302:199, 1994.
40. Honkonen SE: Degenerative arthritis after tibial plateau fractures. J Orthop Trauma 9:273, 1995.
41. Hyman J, Moore T: Anatomy of the distal knee joint and pyarthrosis following external fixation. J Orthop Trauma 13:241, 1999.
42. Iaquinto JM, Pienkowski D, Thornsberry R, et al: Increased neurologic complications associated with postoperative epidural analgesia after tibial fracture fixation. Am J Orthop 26:604, 1997.
43. Indelicato PA: Nonoperative treatment of complete tears of the medial collateral ligament of the knee. J Bone Joint Surg Am 65: 323, 1983.
44. Jensen DB, Rude C, Duus B, Bjerg-Nielsen A: Tibial plateau fractures: A comparison of conservative and surgical treatment. J Bone Joint Surg Br 72:49, 1990.
45. Johnson DP: The effect of continuous passive motion on wound-healing and joint mobility after knee arthroplasty. J Bone Joint Surg Am 72:421, 1990.
46. Karas EH, Weiner LS, Yang EC: The use of an anterior incision of the meniscus for exposure of tibial plateau fractures requiring open reduction and internal fixation. J Orthop Trauma 10:243, 1996.
47. Kennedy J, Bailey W: Experimental tibial plateau fractures. J Bone Joint Surg Am 50:1522, 1968.
48. Keogh P, Kelly C, Cashman WF, et al: Percutaneous screw fixation of tibial plateau fractures. Injury 23:387, 1992.
49. King GJ, Schatzker J: Nonunion of a complex tibial plateau fracture. J Orthop Trauma 5:209, 1991.
50. Kode L, Lieberman JM, Motta AO, et al: Evaluation of tibial plateau fractures: Efficacy of MR imaging compared with CT. AJR Am J Roentgenol 163:141, 1994.
51. Koval KJ, Polatsch D, Kummer FJ, et al: Split fractures of the lateral tibial plateau: Evaluation of three fixation methods. J Orthop Trauma 10:304, 1996.
52. Koval KJ, Sanders RW, Borrelli JD Jr, et al: Indirect reduction and percutaneous screw fixation of displaced tibial plateau fractures. J Orthop Trauma 6:340, 1992.
53. Lachiewicz PF, Funcik T: Factors influencing the results of open reduction and internal fixation of tibial plateau fractures. Clin Orthop 259:210, 1990.
54. Lansinger O, Bergman B, Korner L, Andersson GBJ: Tibial condylar fractures: A twenty year follow-up. J Bone Joint Surg Am 68: 13, 1986.
55. Levy O, Salai M, Ganel A, et al: The operative results of tibial plateau fractures in older patients: A long-term follow-up and review. Bull Hosp Joint Dis 53:15, 1993.
56. Lynch K, Johansen K: Can Doppler pressure measurement replace "exclusion" arteriography in the diagnosis of occult extremity arterial trauma? Ann Surg 214:737, 1991.
57. Marsh JL, Smith ST, Do TT: External fixation and limited internal fixation for complex fractures of the tibial plateau. J Bone Joint Surg Am 77:661, 1995.
58. Mast JW, Ganz R, Jakob RP: Planning and Reduction Technique in Fracture Surgery. New York, Springer-Verlag, 1989, p 1.
59. Moore TM, Patzakis MJ, Harvey JP: Tibial plateau fractures: Definition, demographics, treatment rationale, and long-term results of closed traction management or operative reduction. J Orthop Trauma 1:97, 1987.
60. Morrison JB: The mechanics of the knee joint in relation to normal walking. J Biomech 3:51, 1970.
61. Müller ME, Nazarian S, Koch P, et al: The Comprehensive Classification of Fractures of Long Bones. Berlin, Springer-Verlag, 1990.
62. Perry CR, Evans LG, Rice S, et al: A new surgical approach to fractures of the lateral tibial plateau. J Bone Joint Surg Am 66: 1236, 1984.
63. Rasmussen PS: Tibial condylar fractures: Impairment of knee joint stability as an indication for surgical treatment. J Bone Joint Surg Am 55:1331, 1973.
64. Reid JS, Vanslyke M, Moulton MJR, et al: Safe placement of proximal tibial transfixation wires with respect to intracapsular penetration: Orthopaedic Trauma Association meeting. Orthop Trans 1995.
65. Roberts JM: Fractures of the condyles of the tibia: An anatomical and clinical end-result study of one hundred cases. J Bone Joint Surg Am 50:1505, 1998.
66. Roffi RP, Merritt PO: Total knee replacement after fractures about the knee. Orthop Rev 19:614, 1990.
67. Salter RB, Simmonds DF, Malcolm BW, et al: The biological effect of continuous passive motion on the healing of full-thickness defects in articular cartilage: An experimental investigation in the rabbit. J Bone Joint Surg Am 62:1232, 1980.
68. Sarmiento A, Kinman PB, Latta LL: Fracture of the proximal tibia and tibial condyles: A clinical and laboratory comparative study. Clin Orthop 145:136, 1979.
69. Schatzker J: Fractures of the tibial plateau. In The Rationale of Operative Fracture Care. Springer-Verlag, 1987, p 279.
70. Schatzker J, McBroom R, Bruce D: The tibial plateau fracture: The Toronto experience 1968–1975. Clin Orthop 138:94, 1979.
71. Scheerlinck T, Ng CS, Handelberg F, et al: Medium-term results of percutaneous, arthroscopically-assisted osteosynthesis of fractures of the tibial plateau. J Bone Joint Surg Br 80:959, 1998.
72. Scotland T, Wardlaw D: The use of cast-bracing as treatment for fractures of the tibial plateau. J Bone Joint Surg Br 63:575, 1981.
73. Segal D, Mallik AR, Wetzler MJ, et al: Early weight bearing of lateral tibial plateau fractures. Clin Orthop 294:232, 1993.
74. Slee GC: Fractures of the tibial condyles. J Bone Joint Surg Br 37:427, 1955.
75. Stamer DT, Schenk R, Staggers B, et al: Bicondylar tibial plateau

fractures treated with a hybrid ring external fixator: A preliminary study. J Orthop Trauma 8:455, 1994.
76. Stevens MA, De Coster TA, Garcia F, et al: Septic knee from Ilizarov transfixation tibial pin. Iowa Orthop J 1995;15:217, 1995.
77. Stokel EA, Sadasivan KK: Tibial plateau fractures: Standardized evaluation of operative results. Orthopedics 14:263, 1991.
78. Tscherne H, Lobenhoffer P: Tibial plateau fractures: Management and expected results. Clin Orthop 292:87, 1993.
79. Waddell JP, Johnston DWC, Neidre A: Fractures of the tibial plateau: A review of ninety-five patients and comparison of treatment methods. J Trauma 21:376, 1981.
80. Walker PS, Erkman MJ: The role of the menisci in force transmission across the knee. Clin Orthop 109:184, 1975.
81. Watson JT: High-energy fractures of the tibial plateau. Orthop Clin North Am 25:723, 1994.
82. Watson JT, Coufal C: Treatment of complex lateral plateau fractures using Ilizarov techniques. Clin Orthop 353:97, 1998.
83. Watson JT, Schatzker J: Tibial plateau fractures. In Browner B, Jupiter J, Levine AM, et al, eds: Skeletal Trauma, 2nd ed, vol 2. Philadelphia, WB Saunders, 1998, p 2143.
84. Weiner LS, Kelley M, Yang E, et al: The use of combination internal fixation and hybrid external fixation in severe proximal tibia fractures. J Orthop Trauma 9:244, 1995.
85. Weissman SL, Herold ZH: Fractures of the tibial plateau. Clin Orthop 33:194, 1964.
86. Yacoubian SV, Nevins RT, Sallis JG, et al: Evaluation of soft tissue injuries in high energy tibial plateau fractures by MRI. 1999 (unpublished).
87. Yang EC, Weiner L, Strauss E, et al: Metaphyseal dissociation fractures of the proximal tibia: An analysis of treatment and complications. Am J Orthop 24:695, 1995.
88. Moore T: Fracture dislocation of the knee. Clin Orthop 156:128, 1981.

62 Fractures of the Patella

THOMAS E. BROWN • DAVID R. DIDUCH

INTRODUCTION

Fractures of the patella are relatively common injuries, representing approximately 1% of all skeletal fractures.[10] The patella is prone to injury by virtue of its anterior location, the large forces generated through it, and the minimal amount of overlying soft tissue protecting it from direct trauma. Despite its relatively small size in relation to the distal femur and proximal tibia, functional impairment following suboptimally treated fractures may be significant, resulting in joint stiffness, quadriceps weakness, painful post-traumatic arthritis, or a combination of all three. Because of the range of injuries to the patella, treatment options vary considerably. Yet, the goals of treatment remain constant and are of paramount importance: restoring the functional integrity of the extensor mechanism and maintaining or restoring the articular surface of the patella.

ANATOMY OF PATELLA AND EXTENSOR MECHANISM

The patella is the largest sesamoid bone and has a "rounded triangle" shape, with its most distal aspect anteroinferiorly termed the apex and its proximal portion termed the basis.[10]

The articular surface of the patella is composed of seven facets, divided by several bony ridges (Fig. 62.1). A large vertical ridge separates the lateral and medial facets, and a smaller vertical ridge medially defines the odd facet, a small narrow strip of articular surface. Two additional horizontal ridges create superior, intermediate, and inferior facets.[55]

Variance in the size and shape of the patellar facets was characterized and classified by Wiberg[87] into three main types:

- Type I: The medial and lateral facets are both concave and roughly equal in size.
- Type II: The medial, concave facet is smaller than the lateral.
- Type III: The medial facet is smaller than the lateral but is convex-shaped.

Baumgartl[6] further characterized the patellar facets into three additional types: type II-III, a small, flat medial facet; type IV, a very small, steeply sloped medial facet with medial ridge present; and type V (Jaegerhut patella), no medial facet or vertical ridge. These classification schemes essentially describe the relative constancy of the lateral facet with varying degrees of medial patellar facet dysplasia.

One particularly important point regarding the bony architecture of the patella is that the proximal three-fourths of the patella is covered with a thick articular cartilage, and the distal one-fourth (the distal pole) is entirely extra-articular. This anatomic peculiarity becomes clinically important when treating certain types of patellar fractures.[24]

The extensor mechanism, of which the patella is an integral component, consists of the quadriceps mechanism, the patellar retinaculum, and the patellar tendon. The quadriceps consists of four separate muscles: the rectus femoris, the vastus medialis, the vastus lateralis, and the vastus intermedius. The tendons of these four muscles blend distally into a complex insertion into the patella[55] (Fig. 62.2).

The rectus femoris muscle occupies the most central and superficial position in the quadriceps.[2] Its muscle fibers run somewhat medially in relation to the shaft of the femur, forming an angle between the two of 7 to 10 degrees.[44]

The vastus medialis consists of two parts. A more proximal portion, the vastus medialis longus, attaches to the patella at an angle between 15 and 18 degrees. The more distal portion, the vastus medialis obliquus, attaches to the patella at an angle between 50 and 55 degrees.[44] The oblique orientation of the muscle fibers and short tendonous attachment of the vastus medialis contribute to the importance of the vastus medialis as a dynamic stabilizing force for patellar tracking.

The vastus lateralis attaches to the patella more proximally than the vastus medialis, at a more vertical angle of approximately 30 degrees. Its most medial fibers insert into the superolateral aspect of the patella, and the lateral fibers traverse past the patella, contributing to the lateral retinaculum and fusing with the iliotibial tract.[44]

The vastus intermedius lies deep to the other three muscles, with most of its fibers attaching directly into the superior aspect of the patella.

The fascia lata over the anterior aspect of the knee combines with the aponeurosis of both the vastus medialis and vastus lateralis to form the retinaculum, which inserts directly on either side of the proximal tibia. Thickenings of the capsule, which connect the medial and lateral edges of the patella to their corresponding epicondyles, are termed the patellofemoral ligaments, which complete the retinaculum. The patellar retinaculum performs two important functions: stabilization of the patella and, along with the iliotibial band, secondary knee extensors.[10, 55]

The patellar tendon, a stout, flat structure measuring approximately 5 cm in length, is formed primarily by continuation of central fibers of the rectus femoris and inserts into the tibial tubercle. Blending with the patel-

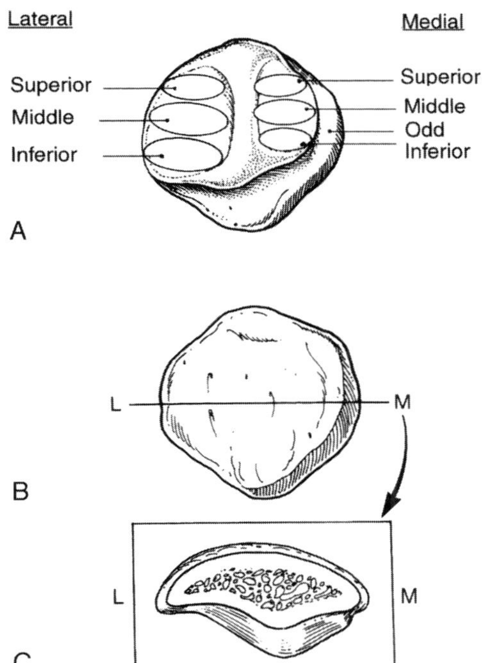

FIGURE 62.1 ➢ *A* illustrates the seven patellar facets. *B* illustrates the anterior surface. *C* illustrates the cross-section of a Wiberg II patella. (From Scuderi G: The Patella. New York, Springer Verlag, 1995.)

lar tendon on either side are fascial expansions of the iliotibial band and patellar retinaculum.

The arterial blood supply to the patella is derived mainly from the peripatellar plexus, which receives contributions from six separate arteries (Fig. 62.3). This plexus helps preserve the vascularity of fracture fragments even in comminuted patellar fractures (Fig. 62.4). The supreme geniculate artery branches from the superficial femoral artery at the level of the adductor canal. There are four geniculate arteries originating from the popliteal artery. The superolateral geniculate is the most superior of the four and joins the peripatellar plexus at its most superior point. The superomedial geniculate artery branches from the popliteal artery just above the joint line and enters the plexus at the midpoint of the patella on the medial side. The inferolateral geniculate arises from the popliteal artery just below the joint line and courses anteriorly adjacent to the lateral meniscus. It proceeds superiorly to join the plexus. The inferomedial geniculate is the most inferior of the four vessels originating from the popliteal artery. It courses anteriorly 2 cm below the joint line and then proceeds superiorly to join the plexus. The final branch contributing to the peripatellar plexus is the recurrent anterior tibial artery, which is a branch of the anterior tibial artery at the point where the vessel penetrates the interosseous membrane 1 cm below the proximal tibiofibular joint. It then courses superiorly to join the plexus.[68] Despite the symmetric appearance of the peripatellar plexus, Scapinelli[67] demonstrated that the functional blood supply to the patella is from the distal to the proximal aspect.[70]

Biomechanics of the Extensor Mechanism

The patella has three functions: increase the strength of the quadriceps, act as a protective shield for the femoral condyles and, less importantly, when absent changes the cosmetic appearance of the knee.[79] The most important function is its mechanical role in increasing the strength of the extensor mechanism. The patella, by virtue of its thickness, displaces the tendon away from the center of rotation of the knee, thereby increasing its moment arm, which increases the force of knee extension by as much as 50%, dependent on the angle of the knee (Fig. 62.5). Numerous clinical studies have documented up to a 50% decrease in isokinetic strength following patellectomy.[21, 22, 53, 78, 84]

During initial extension from a fully flexed position, the patella serves as a mechanical link between the quadriceps and the patellar tendon. This link allows for torque generated from the quadriceps to be transferred to the tibia. The torque generated is considerable, ranging from four up to eight times body weight in athletes.[35] As extension progresses to 135 degrees, the patella engages the intercondylar notch. At this angle, the patellar-contact surface of the femur is occupied by both the patella and the quadriceps tendon proximally. As extension progresses, the contact area

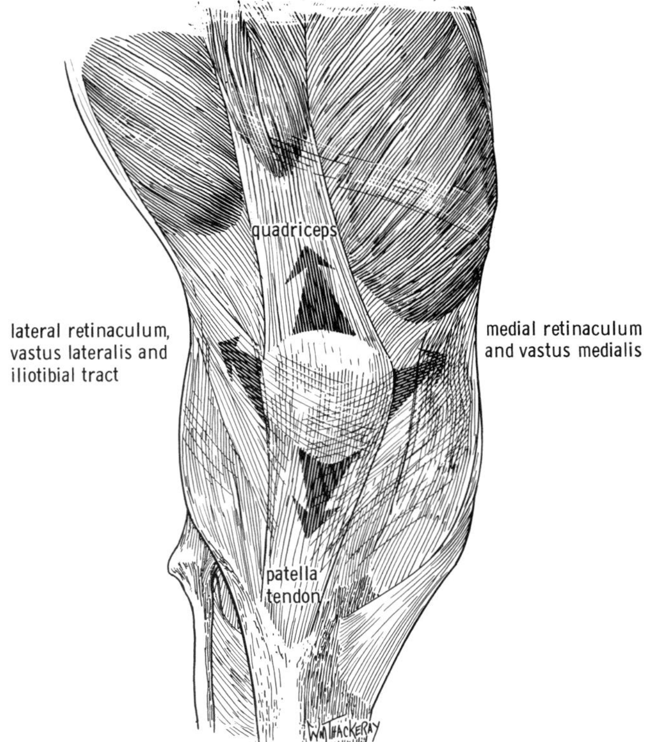

FIGURE 62.2 ➢ The patella is anchored and stabilized to the knee by four structures in a cruciform fashion: the patellar tendon inferiorly, the quadriceps tendon superiorly, and the retinacular medially and laterally.

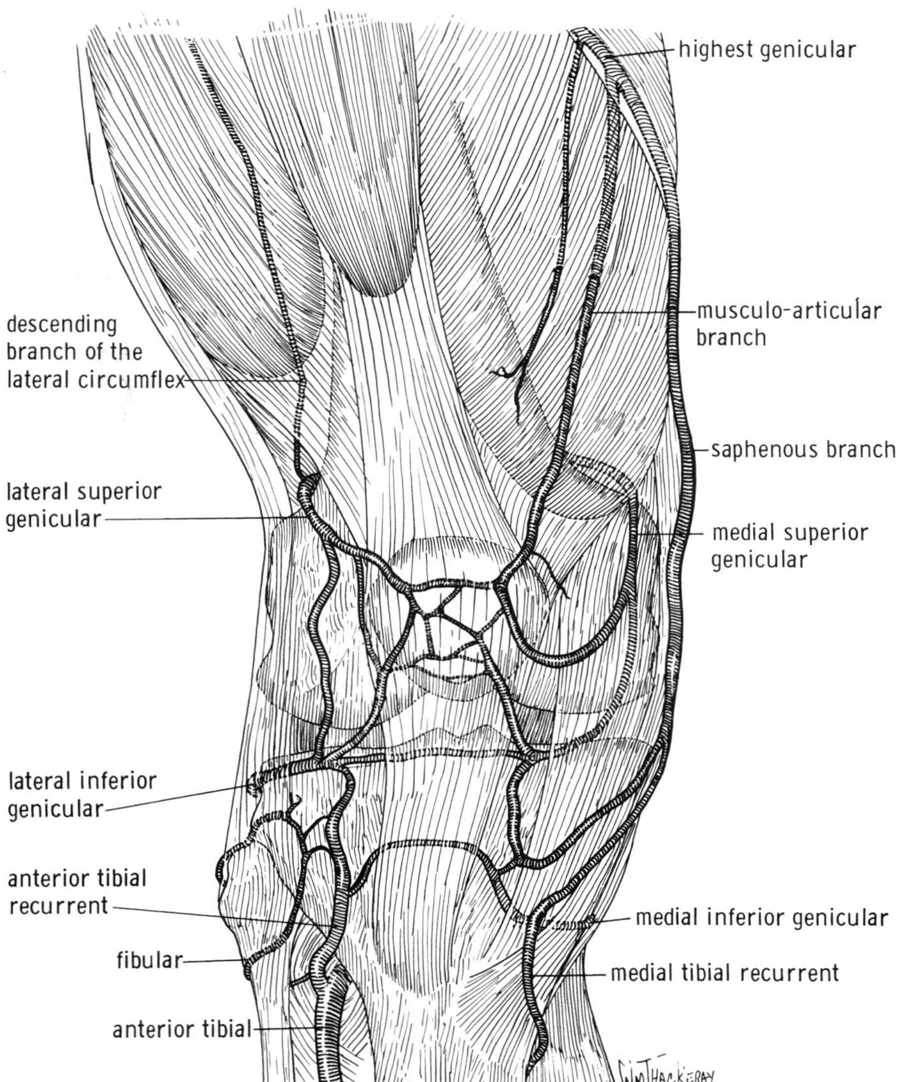

FIGURE 62.3 ➢ Anastomosis at the front of the knee formed by genicular branches from the popliteal artery and descending branches, which connect the femoral artery proximally with the popliteal and anterior tibeal arteries distally.

of the quadriceps tendon on the femur decreases progressively until at 45 degrees, the patella is the only portion of the extensor mechanism to contact the femur. It is during the terminal portion of extension when the increased moment arm of the patella becomes important, because it requires twice as much torque to extend the knee the final 15 degrees than it does to extend it from a maximally flexed position up to 15 degrees.[44]

Because of the high torque generated by the extensor mechanism and the convex configuration of the patella, compressive forces on the patella are quite high, ranging from 3.3 times body weight with stair-climbing up to 7.6 times body weight while squatting.[47] Although patellofemoral forces are generally less than tibiofemoral forces with weightbearing and knee motion, because of the smaller contact areas of the patellofemoral joint, it has been estimated that the contact stresses on the patellofemoral joint are higher than on any other major weightbearing joint.[17]

The contact area between the patella and femur changes in location and extent during range of motion. The patella centers within the trochlear groove at around 20 degrees of flexion. As flexion continues, the contact area on the patella, a horizontal band across both condyles, moves proximally and reaches a maximum at 90 degrees of flexion. Beyond 90 degrees, the contact area separates into two discrete areas of contact on the patellar facets.[3, 32] As the contact area moves proximally on the patella, the contact area on the trochlea moves more distally with increasing flexion (Fig. 62.6).

MECHANISM OF INJURY

Fractures of the patella may be direct, indirect, or a combination. Direct injuries involve a blow to the anterior knee and may be either low-energy, as sustained from a fall, or high-energy, as from a motor vehicle accident. Indirect trauma occurs with a violent contraction of the quadriceps with the knee bent, which literally pulls the patella apart and concomitantly dis-

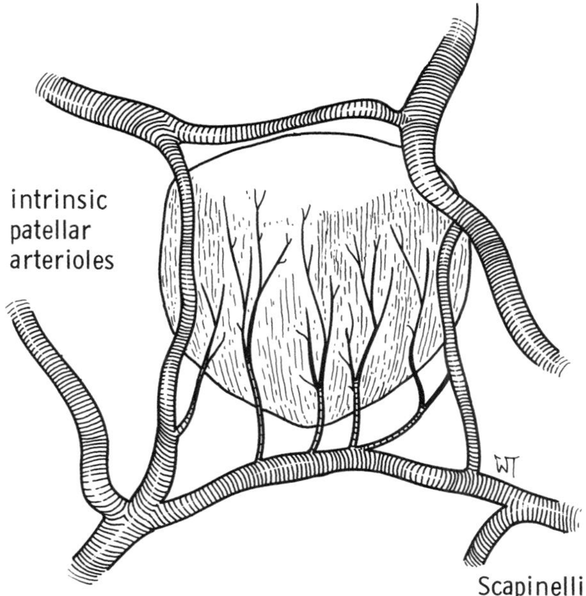

FIGURE 62.4 ➢ Vascular circle around the patella, which, according to Scapinelli,[62] supplies the patella by nutrient arteries that enter predominantly at the inferior pole. The genicular arteries and their branches lie in the most superficial layer of the deep fascia.

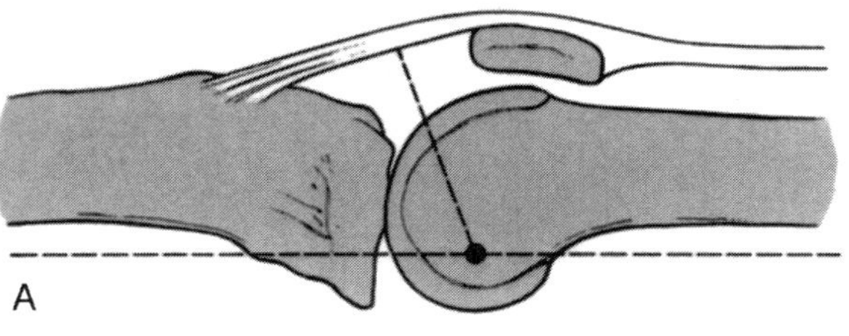

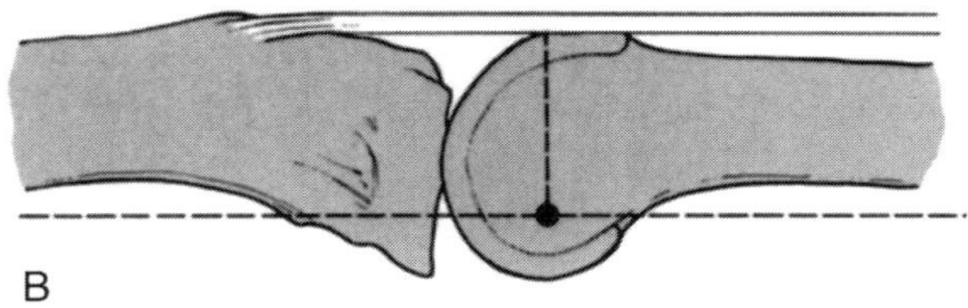

FIGURE 62.5 ➢ In *A,* the patella increases the effective moment arm. In *B,* after patellectomy, the moment arm is decreased, diminishing extensor force. (From Sanders R: Patella fractures and extensor mechanism injuries. In Browner B, ed: Skeletal Trauma. Philadelphia, W.B. Saunders, 1992.)

rupts the patellar retinacular portion of the extensor mechanism. Previous classification systems for fractures of the patella were based on the mechanism of injury, with transverse fractures the result of indirect trauma and comminuted fractures the result of direct injury.[85] It is now evident that some types of patella fractures can be caused by either mechanism, and other factors, such as the patient age, degree of knee flexion, the extent of osteoporosis, and the energy absorbed by the patella, can influence the sustained fracture pattern. In many instances, it is difficult to reconstruct the events leading to injury, and most likely it is a combination of direct forces, muscle contraction, and joint collapse that results in fracture.[1]

Diagnosis

Historical information obtained from the patient usually includes a direct blow to the anterior knee, a fall from a height, or a near fall with strong contraction of the quadriceps on a loaded, flexed knee. The onset of anterior pain, acute effusion of the knee, and inability or limited ability to walk following the fall are also important clinical indicators of injury to the extensor mechanism. Other important information that should

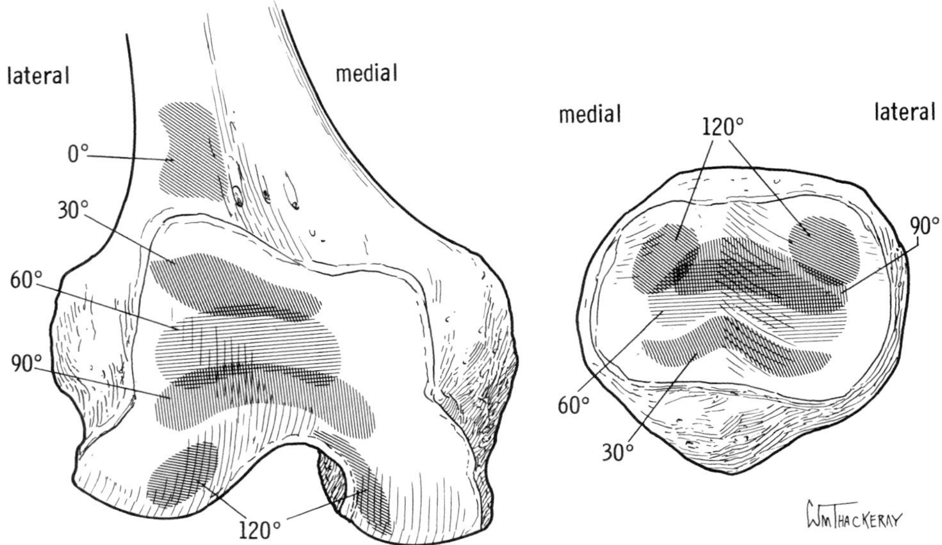

FIGURE 62.6 ➢ Patellofemoral contact zones. (From Aglietti P, Insall JN, Walker PS, et al: A new patella prosthesis. Clin Orthop 107:175, 1975.)

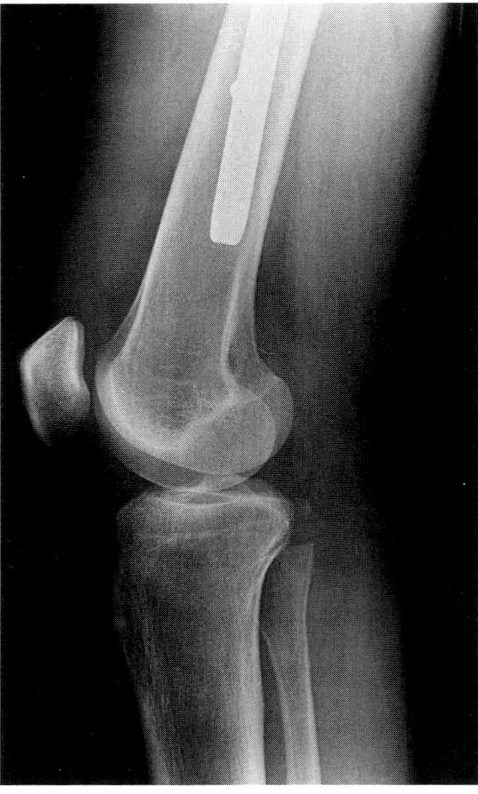

FIGURE 62.7 ➢ Lateral radiograph of a previously undiagnosed patella fracture in a multiply-injured patient.

be obtained includes the presence of pain at other sites, especially if the accident involved a high-energy mechanism such as a motor vehicle.

Physical examination should include inspection of the skin for abrasions, contusions, or lacerations. If there is any question whether a laceration is an open fracture or communicates with the knee joint, sterile aspiration of the knee followed by the infusion of saline with methylene blue dye and local anesthetic will quickly determine joint or bone contamination if infused fluid exits from the wound. Additionally, local anesthetic in the knee may facilitate a more complete examination. The knee should be palpated gently for determination of any skeletal defects, size of effusion, or any ligamentous instability. If the history or examination raises suspicion for other orthopedic injuries, especially with the ipsilateral limb, these should be examined as well. Competence of the extensor mechanism should be tested by determining the patient's ability to perform a straight-leg raise or extend the partially flexed knee against gravity.

Plain radiography is usually all that is required to confirm an injury to the patella or extensor mechanism. On occasion, more subtle injuries such as osteochondral fractures or partial extensor mechanism disruption will require more speciaized studies such as computed tomography or magnetic resonance imaging. Appropriate standard plain radiographic views include an adequate anteroposterior (AP) and lateral view of the knee and tangential view of the patellofemoral joint. The AP view should be performed on a 14-inch × 17-inch cassette to evaluate the distal femur and proximal tibia for concomitant injuries. The AP view should be evaluated for the position of the patella in the midline within the femoral sulcus and the patellar height in relation to its distal pole and the profile of the femoral condyles.

Occasionally, a bipartite or tripartite patella can be mistaken for a fracture.[48] This normal variant is caused by separate ossification centers of the patella that fail to fuse. It is usually located on the superolateral aspect of the patella, is usually bilateral, and requires no treatment. It is not associated with focal bony tenderness or compromise of extensor mechanism function. Comparative x-ray films of the contralateral knee may be obtained to confirm the diagnosis.

The lateral view of the knee will clearly define a transverse or comminuted patellar fracture. Other, more subtle, information can be obtained with less obvious injuries or fracture patterns. The lateral view should include a good profile of the tibial tubercle to detect an avulsion from this site. Additionally, the position of the patella and its relationship to the femur should be observed. The most reliable indicator of the height of the patella is the Insall-Salvati ratio, which compares the length of the patella with the length the patellar tendon. A normal ratio is 1.02 (±0.13); a ratio of less than 1.0 may indicate a patellar tendon rup-

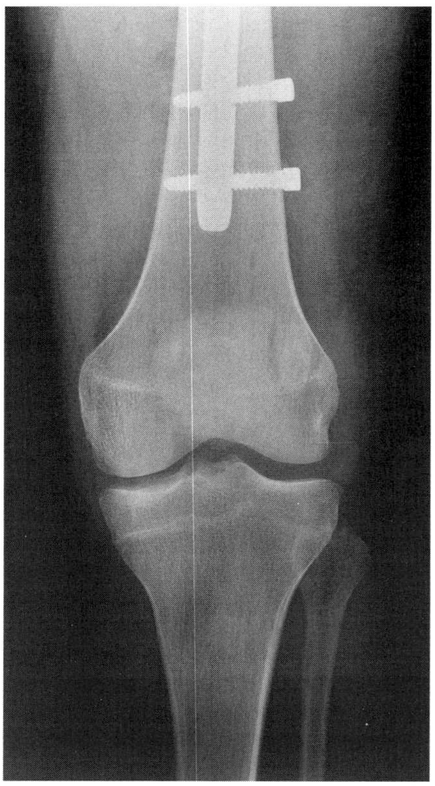

FIGURE 62.8 ➢ Anteroposterior radiograph of this same patient more clearly identifies the patella fracture.

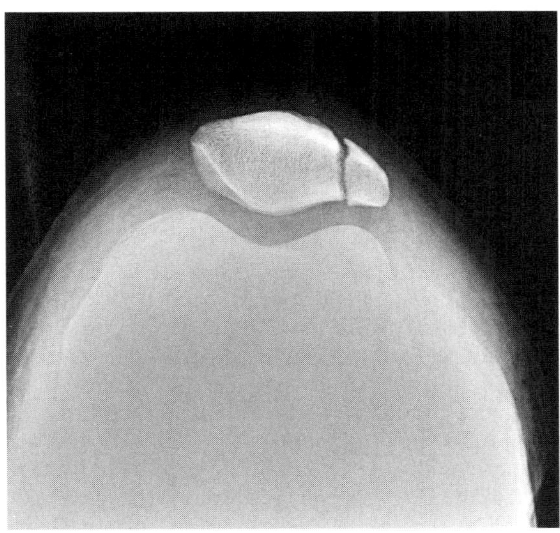

FIGURE 62.9 ➢ Merchant's view clearly demonstrates the displaced longitudinal fracture.

ture.[18, 39] The relation of the distal pole of the patella to the distal physeal scar remnant (Blumensaat's line) can also be compared to look for extensor mechanism disruption.[56]

The tangential view of the patellofemoral joint is helpful in identifying osteochondral fractures as well as marginal or vertical fractures that may not be readily apparent on the AP or the lateral views of the knee (Figs. 62.7 to 62.11). The Merchant view is the most practical view in the trauma evaluation because of the lack of participation required by the patient and the supine passive positioning of the limb at 45 degrees of flexion.[49]

PATELLA FRACTURE CLASSIFICATION

Patella fractures can be classified by the degree of displacement, fracture pattern, the proposed mechanism of injury, or by a combination of two or more of these descriptors. With the wide variability in patella fracture patterns, no single classification system has been effective in stratifying fracture patterns and their respective outcomes.[8, 10, 69] Because of this difficulty, most authors have reported long-term results according to the type of treatment as opposed to the type of fracture.[8, 10, 11, 19, 45, 50, 69, 81]

Displaced patella fractures are defined as those fractures with greater than 3 mm between fracture fragments and/or an articular incongruity of greater than 2 mm.[8, 10, 48, 69] Because of the articular step-off, these fractures are usually treated operatively.

Classification by mechanism of injury is based on a direct blow, such as from a fall or motor vehicle accident, or by an indirect mechanism that occurs with violent quadriceps contraction on a loaded flexed knee. As stated previously, the mechanism of injury may not be readily determined, and varied fracture patterns may occur with the same injury mechanism.[79]

Fracture classification by the configuration of the fracture line(s) provides the most useful information to the surgeon, especially when this includes characterization of the degree of displacement associated with the fracture pattern. Described fracture patterns of the patella include transverse, vertical, stellate (comminuted), apical or marginal, and osteochondral. In addition, sleeve fractures with a large portion of the distal fragment being articular cartilage can occur in skeletally immature patients (Fig. 62.12).

Nonoperative Treatment

Successful nonoperative treatment of patella fractures depends most of all on the relative lack of displacement or separation between fragments, lack of articular incongruity, and the integrity of the extensor mechanism. Longitudinal fractures are best suited for nonoperative management, as the pull of the intact extensor mechanism is parallel to the fracture, thereby helping prevent displacement (Fig. 62.13). Nonoperative treatment should provide good-to-excellent results in more than 90% of patella fractures.[10] Relative indications for nonoperative treatment include the elderly low-demand patient with significant osteopenia, making rigid fixation impossible, and patients for whom general or regional anesthesia is contraindicated because of preexisting medical conditions.

Nonoperative treatment consists of the application of a well-padded cylinder cast in near full-extension for

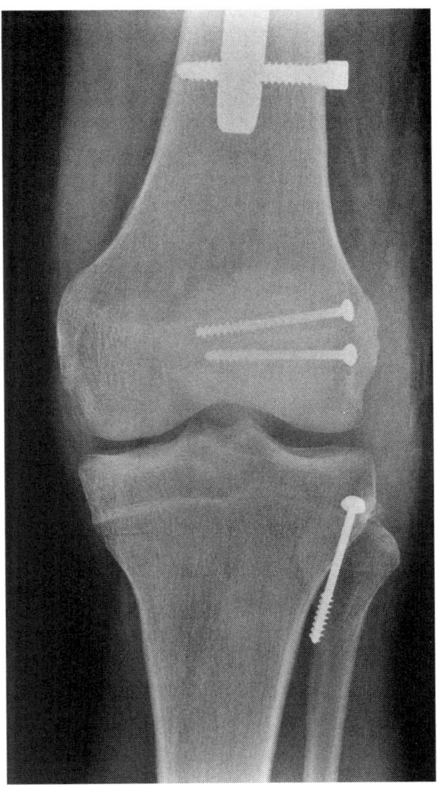

FIGURE 62.10 ➢ Postoperative radiograph of the patella repaired with cancellous screws.

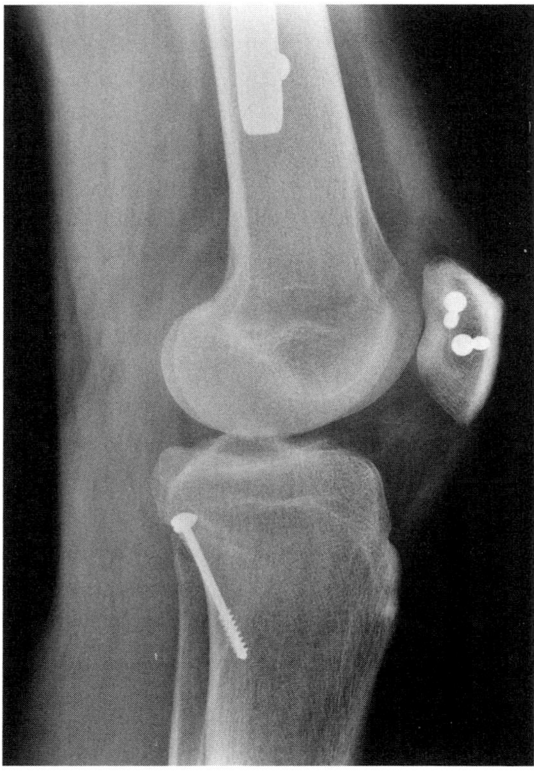

FIGURE 62.11 ➢ Lateral postoperative radiograph of screw fixation.

4 to 6 weeks, with weightbearing to tolerance for longitudinal fractures and partial weightbearing for nondisplaced transverse fractures. Patients are encouraged to perform straight-leg raises in the cast to maintain some quadriceps muscle strength. If patient reliability and compliance are not a concern, a hinged knee brace locked in extension may be substituted for the cylinder cast. Extension is maintained until fracture consolidation is evident on radiographs, at which time gentle, active range of motion exercises may be implemented.

Operative Treatment

Operative treatment for patella fractures is indicated for displacement between fragments of 3 mm or more or for articular incongruity or step-off of greater than 2 mm.[24] Goals of surgical treatment are to obtain an accurate reduction of the fracture and provide rigid fixation or repair so as to allow for early range of motion of the knee.

Surgical techniques can be divided into three main categories: internal fixation, partial patellectomy with reattachment of the extensor mechanism to the remaining patella, and total patellectomy. On occasion, it is possible to combine internal fixation with partial patellectomy techniques in order to preserve more patellar bone within the extensor mechanism.

Surgical exposure, preferably under tourniquet control, can be performed through either a transverse or vertical skin incision. We prefer the more utilitarian vertical incision, which provides excellent exposure for any of the surgical techniques employed, and it can be utilized later with little concern for soft-tissue problems should additional surgical procedures to the knee be necessary.[82] In the event of an open patella fracture, the laceration should be incorporated into the skin incision if possible. Following adequate exposure of the fracture, the joint should be evaluated for articular damage to the patella and femur. Additionally, the retinacular and proximal and distal soft-tissue attachments to the patella should be assessed before selecting the definitive surgical repair technique. Small comminuted bone fragments, especially those with no soft-tissue attachment, should be removed before attempted reduction. During reduction, the articular surface must be accessible for palpation and direct visualization in order to assess the quality of reduction. Additional exposure may be necessary by extending the arthrotomy vertically through a preexisting retinacular tear. Intraoperative radiographs may be required to assess the articular reduction.

Internal Fixation

A variety of techniques have been described to stabilize displaced patella fractures: wires in a cerclage or tension band configuration, screw fixation, and a combination of these methods. Of historic interest, initial wiring techniques employed circumferential cerclage of the patella, followed by cast treatment in extension for 4 to 6 weeks.[4, 10, 46, 68] Magnuson[46] and Payr[52] advocated the use of a wire passed through two vertical, longitudinal drill holes. Anderson suggested the use of equatorial circumferential wiring.[4] The early wiring techniques were less than optimal for treatment of these fractures because of the inability to start early motion postoperatively, lack of compression at the articular surface, and the risk of displacement if tensile forces were placed on the construct. Others have advocated screw fixation for transverse or longitudinal fractures.[25, 63, 73]

The Association for the Study of Internal Fixation (ASIF) has popularized the technique of tension band cerclage of the patella, with or without the addition of longitudinal Kirschner wires. This method is ideal for transverse patellar fractures, as it allows for immediate range of motion postoperatively. Two stainless steel 18-gauge wires (1.2 mm) are placed anteriorly through the quadriceps and patellar tendons, with one placed in a figure-of-eight fashion, the other in a cerclage configuration (Figs. 62.14 and 62.15). Tightening of the wires over-reduces the transverse fracture, but when the knee is flexed, the pressure of the femoral condyles against the patella transforms the tension into interfragmentary compression. Two twisting sites for the wires have been shown to provide greater compression.[64] This method can be augmented with two parallel 2-mm Kirschner wires placed longitudinally

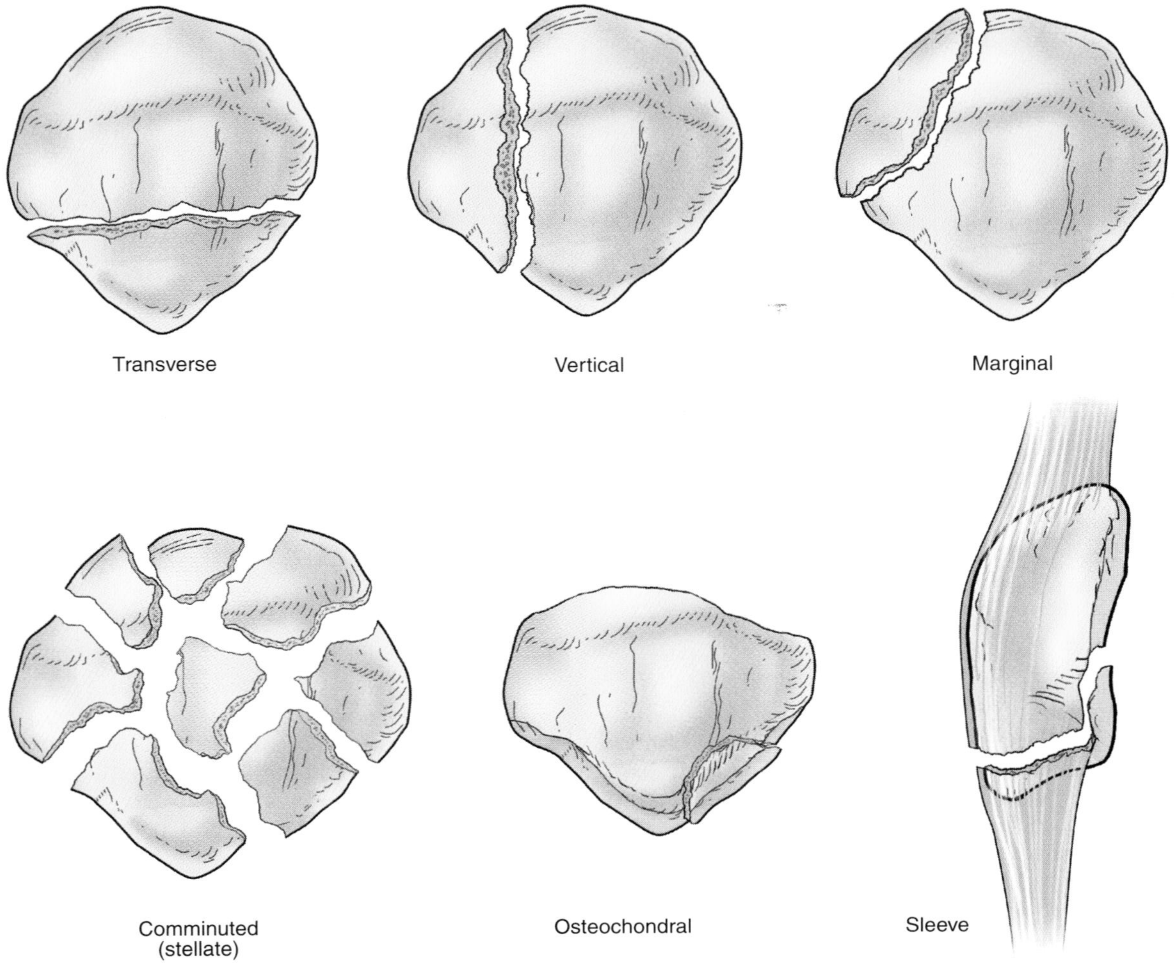

Transverse

Vertical

Marginal

Comminuted (stellate)

Osteochondral

Sleeve

FIGURE 62.12 ➢ Classification of patella fractures based on fracture configuration. (Redrawn from Cramer K, Moed B: Patellar fractures: Contemporary approach to treatment. JAAOS 5:323, 1997.)

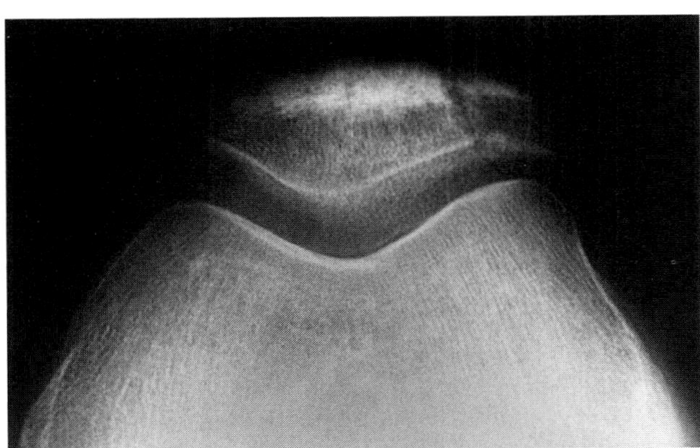

FIGURE 62.13 ➢ Merchant's view demonstrates maintenance of articular congruity following closed treatment for this longitudinal patella fracture.

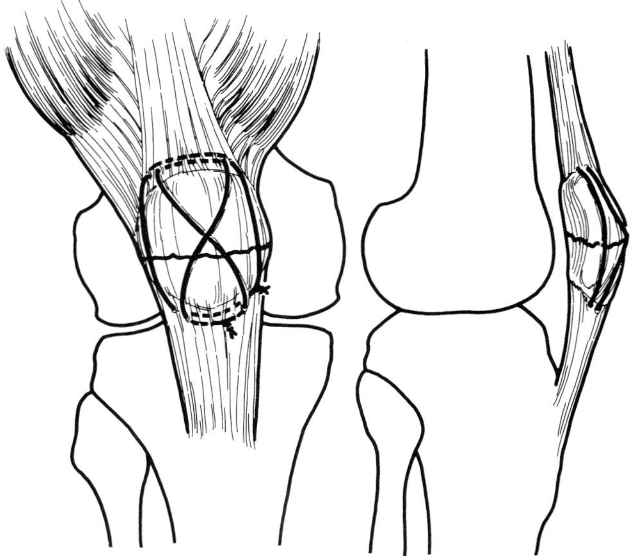

FIGURE 62.14 ➢ Tension cerclage of patellar fractures.

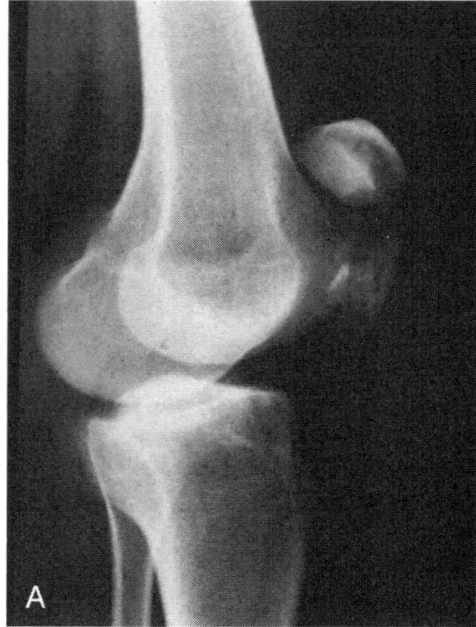

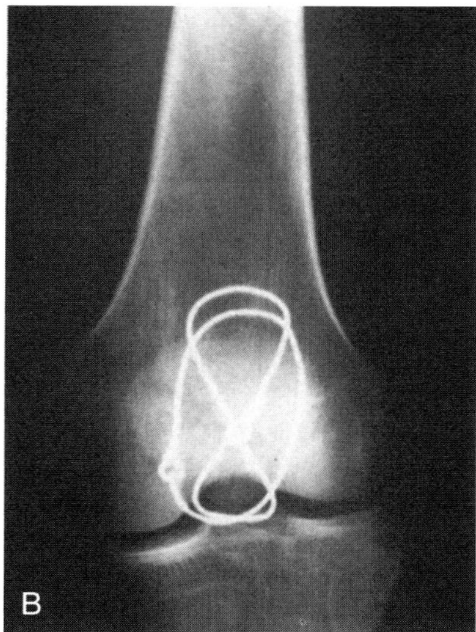

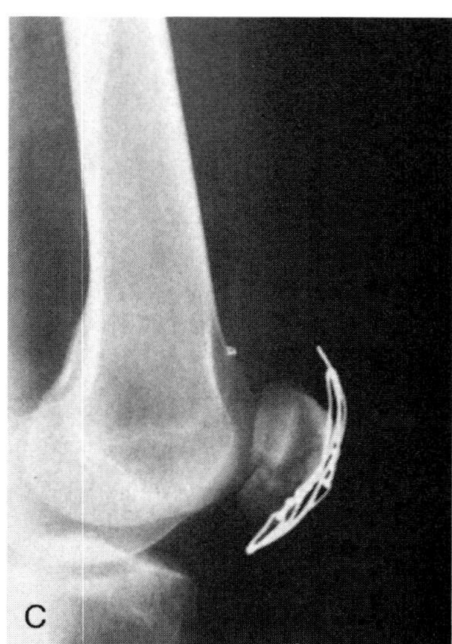

FIGURE 62.15 ➢ *A*, Transverse fracture of the patella with some distal fragment comminution. *B* and *C*, Treated with tension band cerclage with two wires; after 1 month, the fracture shows good healing, with a little step on the articular surface.

through the patella, which helps prevent tilting of the distal fragment (Figs. 62.16 and 62.17). This same technique has been employed with comminuted patella fractures. A variation of the tension band technique, according to Lotke and Ecker,[45] is to utilize a tension band construct with the wire placed through longitudinal drill holes in the patella (Fig. 62.18). In order to minimize the risk of subsequent hardware irritation, No. 5 nonabsorbable polyester sutures may be substituted for the stainless steel wires used in tension banding the patella (Fig. 62.19). Sutures alone are more prone to failure than wires and may require cast immobilization. The use of nonabsorbable suture in a cerclage fashion may be used for internal fixation of the sleeve fracture of the patella seen most often in the pediatric population (Fig. 62.20).[77]

Cannulated screws with a tension band wire placed through the screws have also been reported to provide excellent fracture fixation. This technique is very similar to the ASIF tension band technique, with 3.5-mm cannulated screws being substituted for the Kirschner wires. Care must be taken to avoid protruding the threads of the screws beyond the far cortex, which may lead to early wire failure[17] (Fig. 62.21).

Internal fixation with 3.5-mm- to 4.5-mm-diameter screws may also be used for fixation of patella fractures. In simple transverse or displaced longitudinal fractures in patients with good bone stock, two parallel screws placed across the fracture utilizing lag technique may be all that is required (Fig. 62.22). Additionally, screw fixation or additional Kirschner wires may be used to convert more comminuted fracture patterns into those that are amenable to tension band fixation[24] (Fig. 62.23). A comminuted central portion of the patella, unamenable to fixation, may be removed and the remaining fragments fixed with screw fixation (Fig. 62.24).

The knee is mobilized early, with no cast needed. The knee is kept in 20 to 25 degrees of flexion, with flexion allowed to about 70 degrees using a hinged knee brace. No extension is permitted beyond 20 degrees for the first 3 weeks, and partial weightbearing is allowed for the first 4 weeks. Cast immobilization is reserved only for those fractures where adequate fixation was not achieved.

A biomechanical study comparing the strength of four different fixation techniques (circumferential wiring, tension band wiring, modified tension band over K-wires, and the Lotke and Ecker technique) with simulated transverse fractures and retinacular disruption identified the circumferential wiring method as providing the weakest fixation, with up to 20 mm of displacement with tension stress. The tension band wiring method showed improved stability, with only 2.5 mm of displacement. The addition of Kirschner wires to modify the tension band technique further improved fracture stability. Surprisingly, the technique of Lotke and Ecker showed fracture stability similar to the modified tension band method, with less than 1 mm of maximum displacement at the fracture site.[15] It was concluded that the combination of transosseous fixation and tension band principles offered the best results. More recently, Carpenter et al[17] compared modified tension band technique with the tension band technique incorporated into cannulated screws and screws alone in a simulated leg-extension model. Their results demonstrated that the anterior tension band with incorporated cannulated screws failed at higher loads than screws alone or the standard modified tension band. Additionally, the modified tension band allowed more fracture displacement under tension stress than the other two methods.

Clinical results published to date following internal fixation have reported the best results with tension

Text continued on page 1304

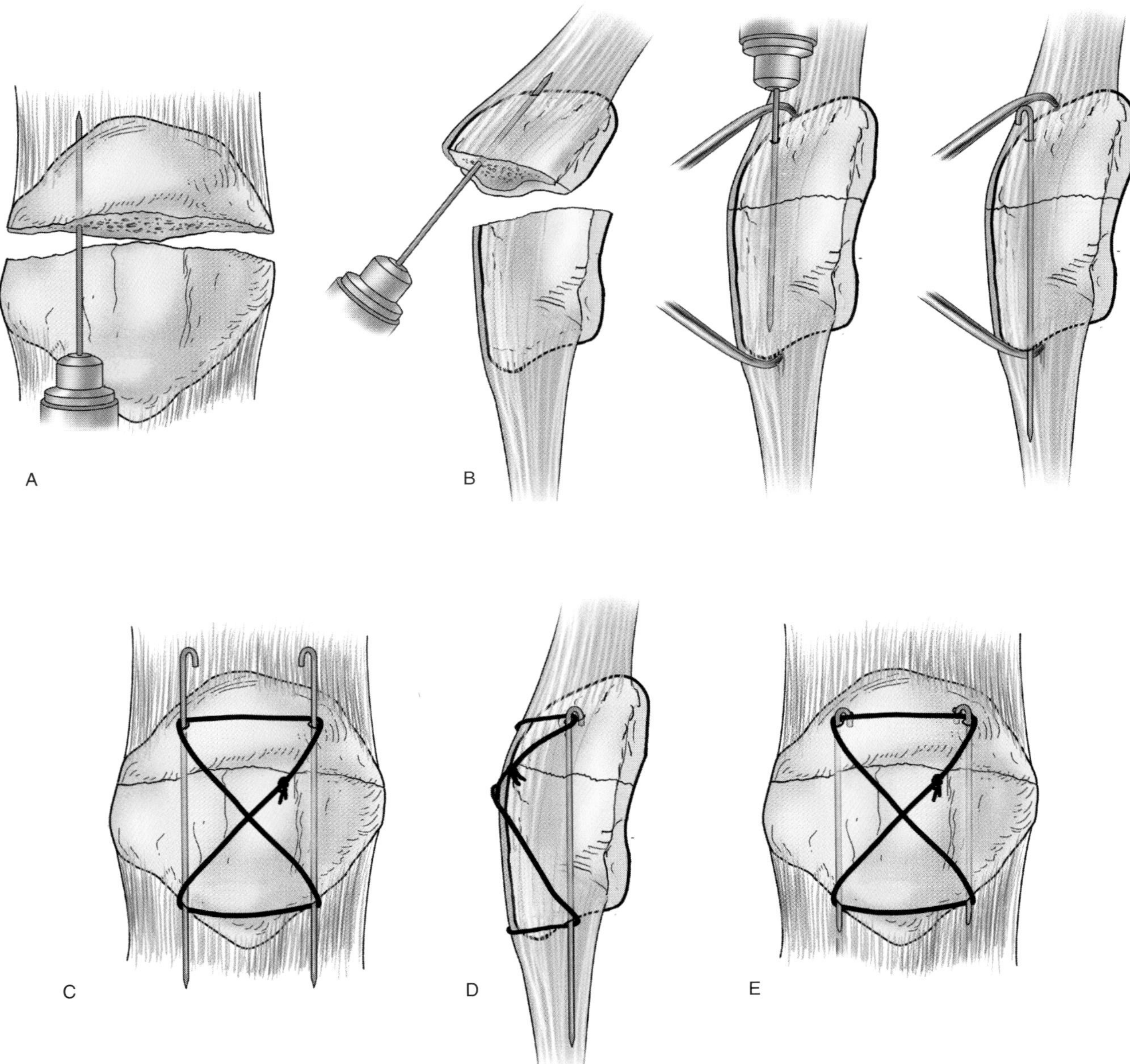

FIGURE 62.16 ➢ The tension band technique for patella fractures. *A,* Kirschner wires are placed retrograde from distal to proximal to the fracture's edge of the proximal fragment. *B,* The fracture is reduced and held with bone clamps while the Kirschner wires are advanced distally across the fracture site. *C,* A figure-of-eight tension band wire is passed around the Kirschner wires and tightened. *D,* The Kirschner wires are countersunk proximally, and excess wire is removed distally. (Redrawn from Scuderi G: The Patella. New York, Springer Verlag, 1995.)

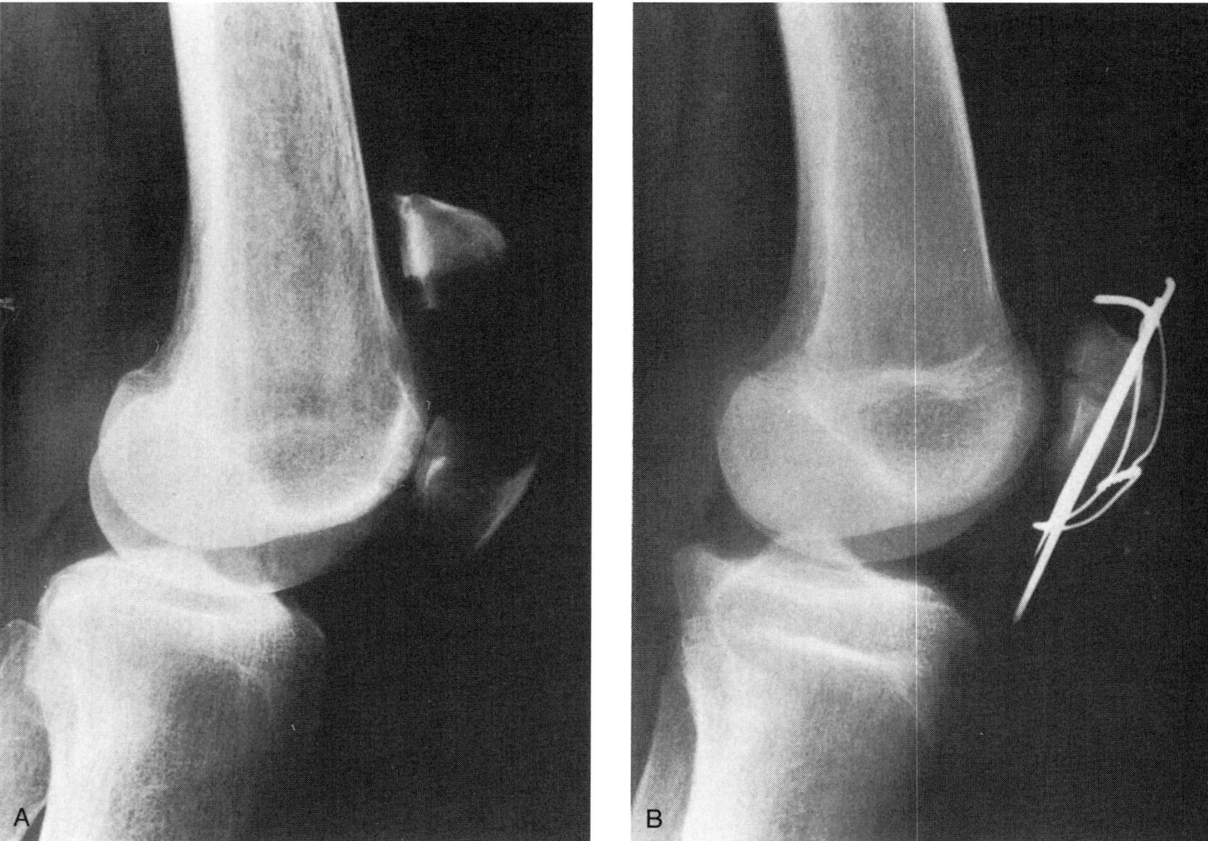

FIGURE 62.17 ➢ *A*, Transverse fracture of the patella. *B*, Treated with modified tension cerclage. The K-pins were too long and had to be removed at 3 months after secure healing of the fracture. (From Aglietti P, Scarfi G. Trattamento chirurgico delle fratture di rotula. Arch Putti 30:301, 1980.)

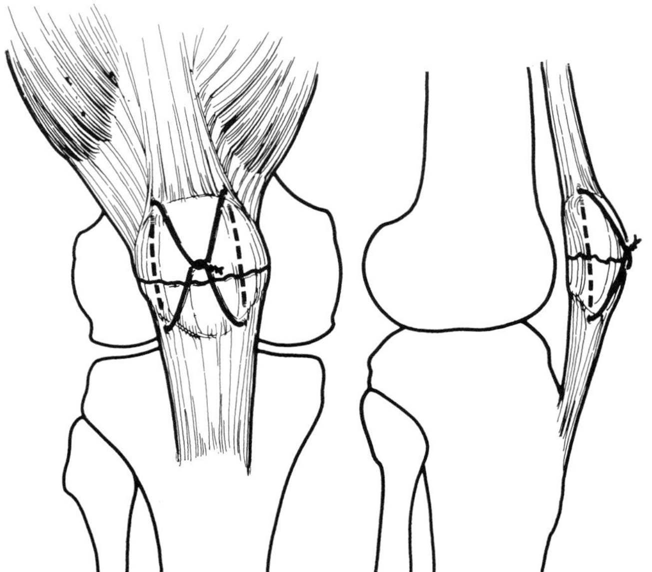

FIGURE 62.18 ➢ Internal fixation of a transverse fracture of the patella according to the method of Lotke and Ecker.

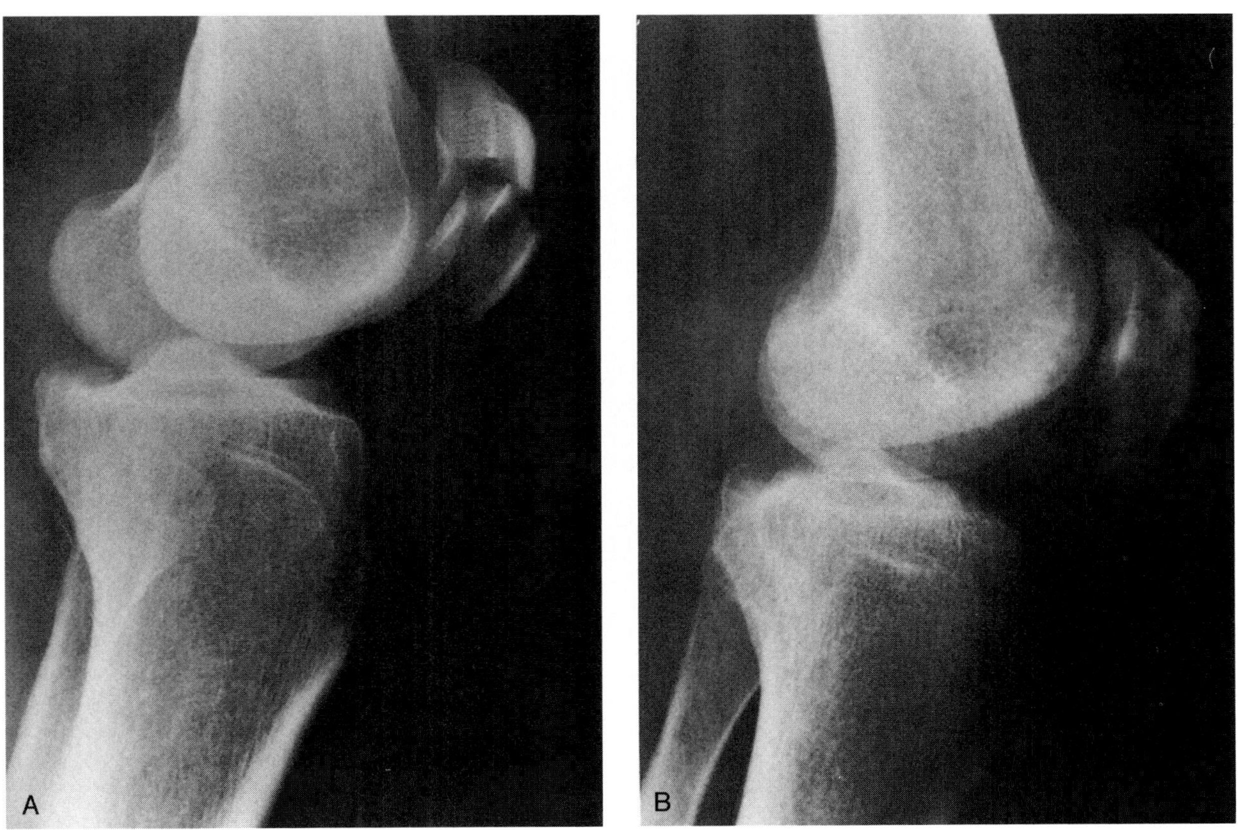

FIGURE 62.19 ➢ *A,* Transverse patella fracture treated with traditional circumferential cerclage with suture fixation. *B,* Good result after 6 weeks of cast immobilization.

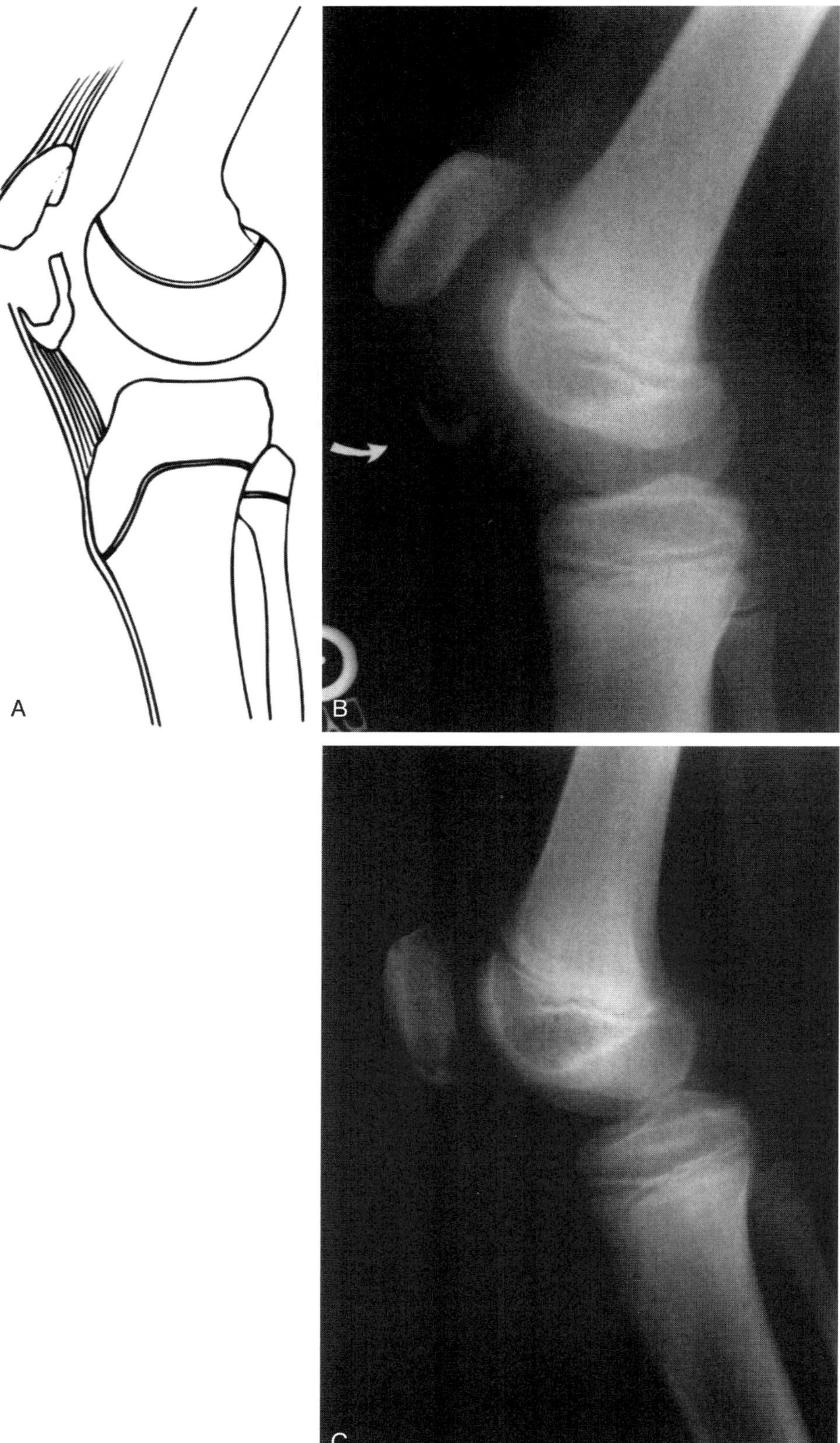

FIGURE 62.20 ➢ *A,* Sleeve fracture of the patella. *B,* The cartilage on the distal fragment is not seen in this projection, but the fracture fragment is evident. *C,* The healed fracture following open reduction and internal fixation. (From Sponseller P, Beaty J: Fractures and dislocations about the knee. In Rockwood C, Wilkins K, Beaty J, eds: Fractures in Children, 4th ed. Philadelphia, Lippincott-Raven, 1996, p 1287.)

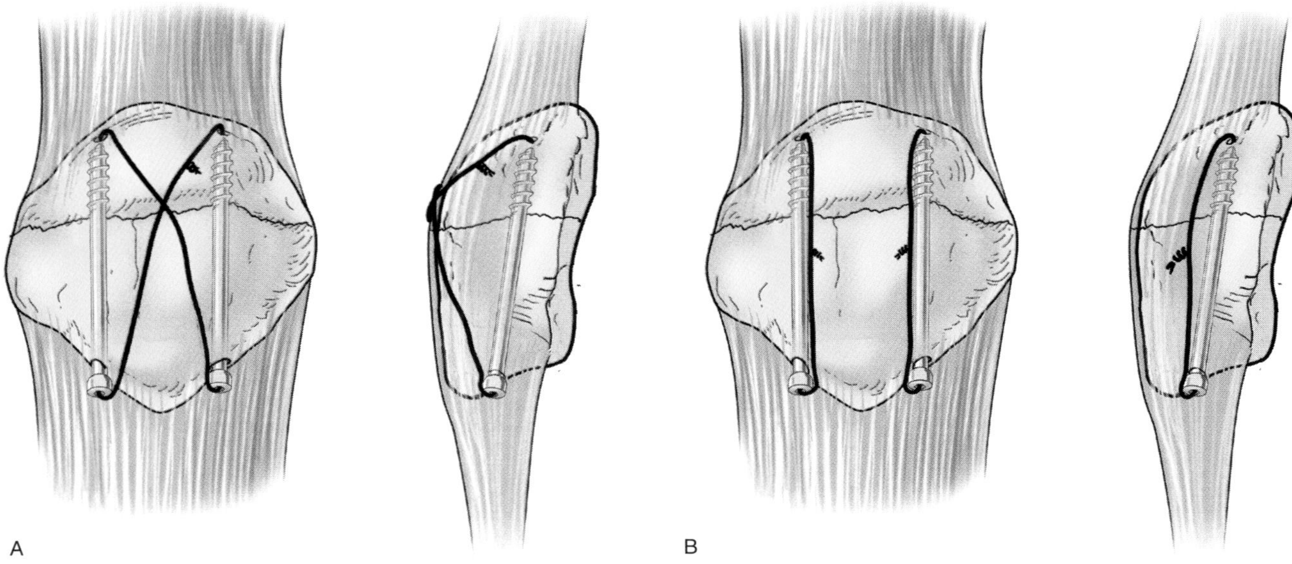

FIGURE 62.21 ➢ *A,* Cannulated screws augmented with a figure-of-eight tension band anteriorly. Note that the threads of the screw do not cross the fracture site. *B,* The separate tension bands are applied vertically. (Redrawn from Cramer K, Moed B: Patellar fractures: Contemporary approach to treatment. JAAOS 5:323, 1997.)

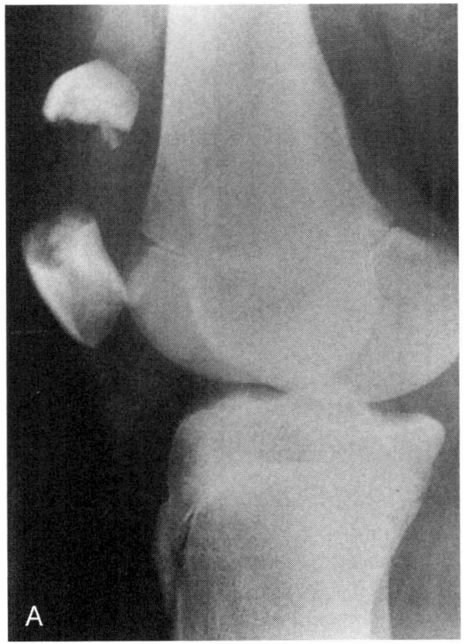

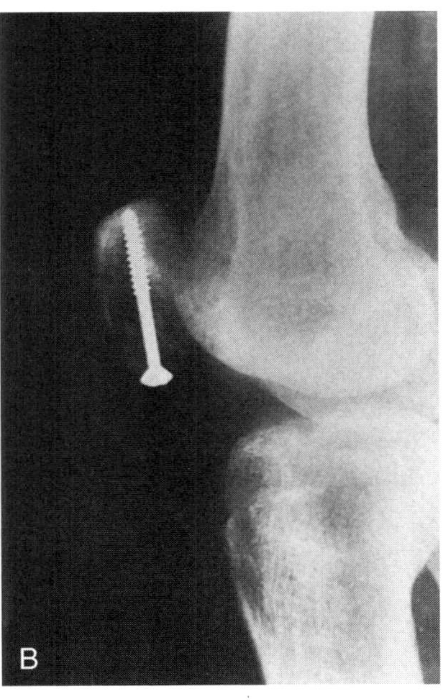

FIGURE 62.22 ➢ *A,* Transverse fracture of the upper third of the patella. *B,* Treated with a screw; showing good result at 1 year. (From Aglietti P, Scarfi G: Trattamento chirurgico delle fratture di rotula. Arch Putti 30:301, 1980.)

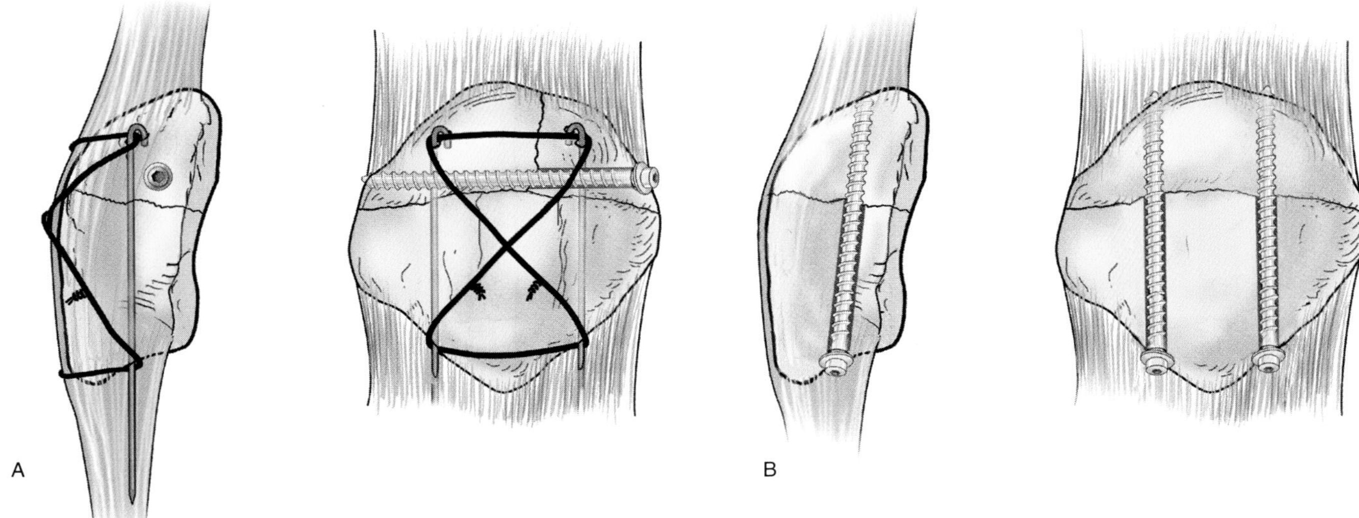

FIGURE 62.23 ➢ *A,* The transverse screw converts this comminuted fracture into a simple transverse fracture. *B,* Lag screws without tension band augmentation. (Redrawn from Cramer K, Moed B: Patella fractures: Contemporary approach to treatment. JAAOS 5:323, 1997.)

band wiring, with 86% of patients reporting excellent or good results.[8, 9, 42] Bostman et al[9] reported significantly better results with the modified tension band technique compared with circumferential wiring, partial patellectomy, or screw fixation. The data regarding the results of surgical treatment should be interpreted with caution; most surgical results have been reported by the method of surgical treatment rather than by the actual type of fracture treated.[8, 10, 11, 19, 45, 50, 81]

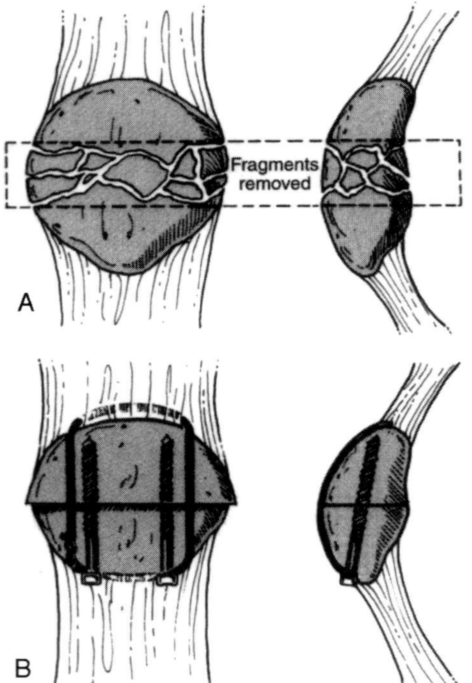

FIGURE 62.24 ➢ *A,* The comminuted fragments are removed, and the fracture surfaces are cut evenly, with subsequent reduction and fixation with screws plus wire cerclage in *B.* (From Scuderi G: The Patella. New York, Springer Verlag, 1995.)

Our preferred treatment for the majority of fractures amenable to internal fixation is the use of the modified tension band over Kirschner wires or through cannulated screws, with an additional circumferential wire or suture for more comminuted fractures.

Partial Patellectomy

Partial patellectomy is indicated when the amount of patellar comminution prevents secure fixation of all fracture fragments. Retention of as much congruous articular surface is desirable; therefore, internal fixation of larger fragments with screw or Kirschner-wire fixation may help minimize the amount of bone lost with partial patellectomy and extensor mechanism repair.[24]

Following adequate exposure, unsalvageable comminuted fragments are removed while preserving as much soft tissue as possible. Longitudinal drill holes are placed through the remaining patella to serve as tunnels for the tendon sutures. It is imperative that the holes be placed near the articular surface so that the patella does not tilt abnormally. A tendon-grasping, locking, nonabsorbable, suture is placed through the tendon, passed through the bone tunnels, and tied over the bony bridge. An overlapping repair of the retinacular tears is then performed (Figs. 62.25 and 62.26). If protection of the repair is deemed necessary for immediate postoperative motion, the repair may be protected by a cable or wire passed through the tibial tubercle distally and just proximal to the superior patella.[54] Postoperatively, partial weightbearing in full extension is allowed, with range-of-motion exercises dependent on the security of the repair and/or the use

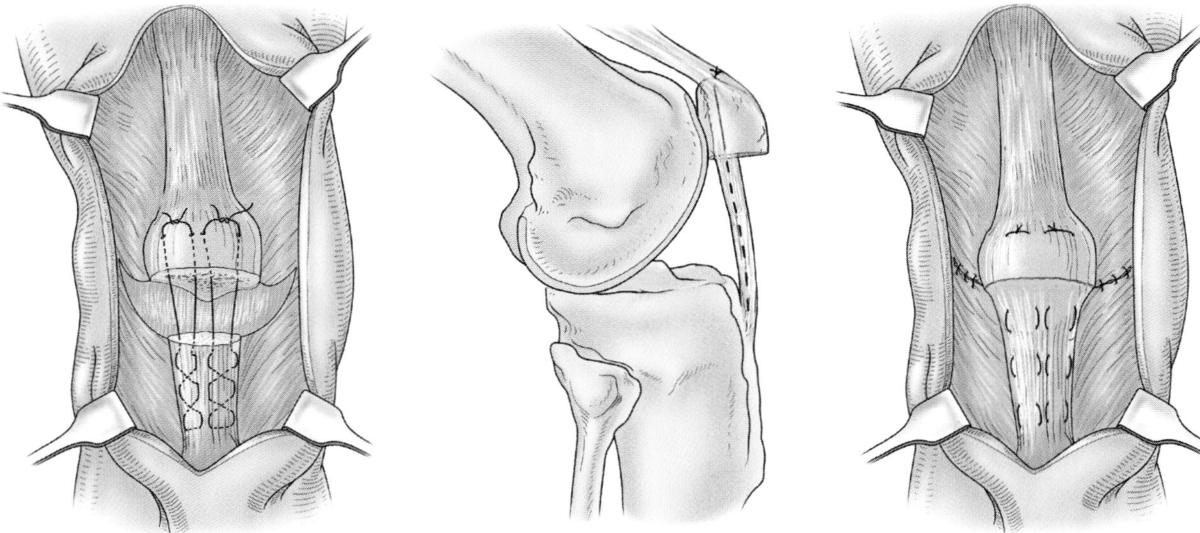

FIGURE 62.25 ➢ Technique of partial patellectomy. Note the placement of the patellar tendon at the articular surface of the remaining patella. (Redrawn from Cramer K, Moed B: Patellar fractures: Contemporary approach to treatment. JAAOS 5:323, 1997.)

of a load-sharing wire or cable. Extension splinting for ambulation is continued for 4 to 6 weeks, at which time aggressive quadriceps strengthening may commence.

Clinical results following partial patellectomy are favorable, with studies reporting good or excellent results in 78% to 86% of patients.[8-10, 60] Other reports have demonstrated comparable results between partial patellectomy and internal fixation.[9, 10, 51] Bostrom[10] reported on a group of patients with a transverse patellar fracture with inferior pole comminution. Of these, 88% treated with partial patellectomy had good-to-excellent results, compared with 74% treated with internal fixation. Given this information, partial patellectomy should be considered if adequate internal fixation of a comminuted fracture cannot be achieved. Most reports involving partial patellectomy involve predominantly distal pole fractures that to a large extent, are extra-articular.[8, 51, 60] Results for proximal pole excision and tendon repair have not been reported to date.

Total Patellectomy

Total patellectomy is rarely required and should be reserved for those instances in which the comminu-

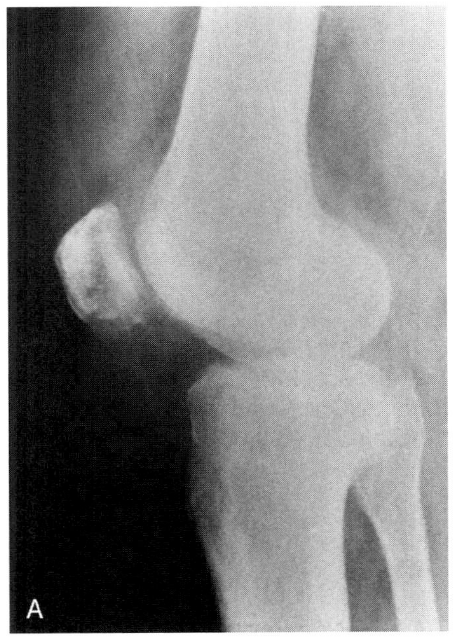

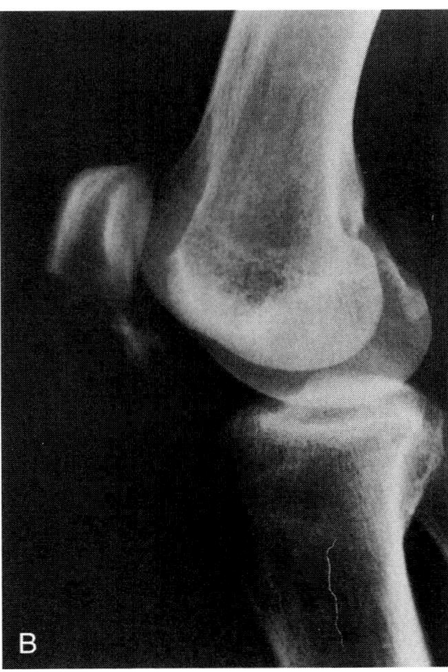

FIGURE 62.26 ➢ *A,* Distal patellar fracture of the apex. *B,* Treated with partial patellectomy. Good result at 1 year. (From Aglietti P, Scarfi G: Trattamento chirurgico delle fratture di rotula. Arch Putti 30:301, 1980.)

tion is so extensive that it is impossible to retain any congruous fragments for articulation with the femur. Function postpatellectomy is usually compromised, and for that reason it should be considered a salvage operation when no other surgical alternatives exist. The point at which bone retention is futile and total patellectomy is indicated has not been determined. Saltzman et al[60] was unable to show a correlation between the clinical outcome and the size of the retained fragment of patella. Pandey et al[51] believed that retention of even a small fragment of bone may provide a biomechanical advantage over total patellectomy.

If a complete patellectomy is necessary, it is important to restore the normal tension within the extensor mechanism following repair to minimize the loss of the biomechanical advantage generated by the patella. The extensor mechanism is effectively lengthened by patellectomy; therefore, some form of tissue imbrication is necessary to avoid a significant extensor lag.[61] Following the resection of all loose bone fragments, with retention of as much soft tissue as possible, repair of the extensor mechanism can be performed with multiple tendon-grasping, nonabsorbable sutures. The retinacular disruption should also be repaired to restore the appropriate extensor mechanism tension. It is important that 80 to 90 degrees of flexion be possible on the operating table without placing undue tension on the repair. In the event that inadequate soft tissue is available for a primary repair or for soft-tissue augmentation, it may be necessary to perform an inverted V-plasty of the quadriceps tendon to fill the defect.[71] Postoperatively, the leg is kept in extension for 2 to 3 weeks to allow for adequate soft-tissue healing. Following this period of immobilization, an extensive and lengthy (up to 2 years) rehabilitation program is initiated.

If soft tissues permit, our preferred method for total patellectomy is that described by Compere et al[23] (Fig. 62.27), which maintains the continuity and tubularizes the extensor mechanism following patellar excision. Frequently, ossification will occur within the tubularized patella tendon, creating a "pseudo patella" that will enhance the mechanical advantage of the extensor mechanism.

Results following a complete patellectomy have generally been inferior compared with those for partial patellectomy or internal fixation. Prior to the advent of tension band fixation, poor reconstructive methods and results (usually a simple cerclage wire) may have justified total excision of the patella.[14, 26] Numerous studies have reported poor outcomes following total patellectomy when compared with those following partial excision or internal fixation. Sutton et al[78] compared total patellectomy with partial patellectomy in terms of quadriceps strength and functional ability. Their results revealed a 49% reduction in extensor mechanism strength with total excision. Functionally, after total excision, patients lacked the ability to support their weight on the affected leg with stair climbing. Long-term follow-ups on patellectomy patients have also demonstrated less than optimal results. Einola et al[29] reported on 28 patients monitored for an average of 7.5 years post excision, with only 6 patients having a good result. A common finding was persistent quadriceps atrophy, along with pain and weakness in the knee with activity. Scott[65] reported similar long-term results, with only 4 of 71 patients satisfied with their result. More than half of these patients experienced weakness, and 90% experienced pain with activity. Atrophy of the quadriceps was a consistent finding. Sorensen[75] thought that attempt to salvage some patella was usually indicated, given the poor functional outcome of patients following total excision. Patients complained of pain and giving way of the affected knee with running and stair climbing. Additionally, no patients regained full quadriceps strength following patellectomy.

COMPLICATIONS

Loss of Knee Motion

Decreased range of motion following patellar fracture treatment is probably the most common complication encountered. The motion lost is usually in the terminal degrees of flexion and is well tolerated by most pa-

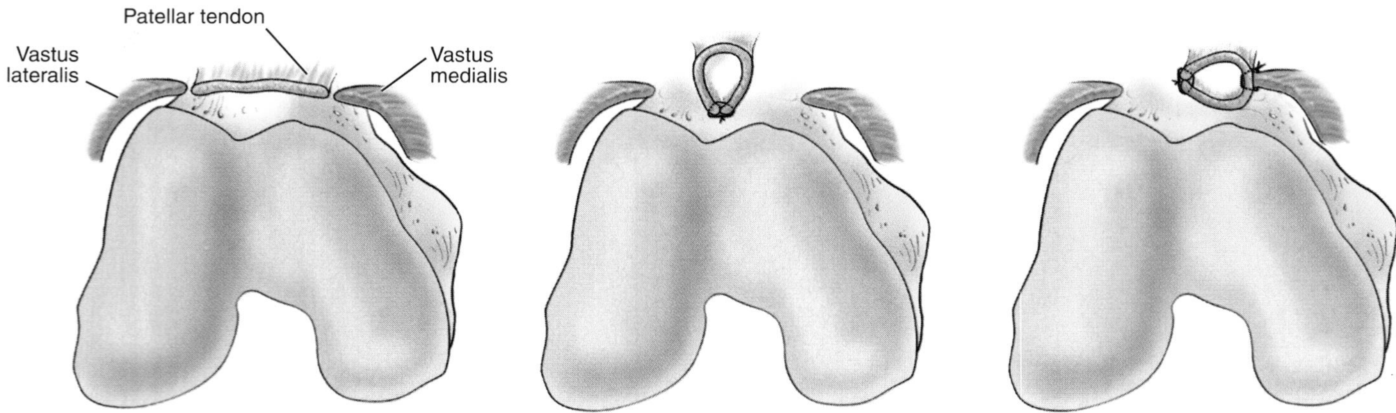

FIGURE 62.27 ➢ Compere's technique for patellectomy (see text). Ossification will occur within the tube.

tients.[24] With the advent of tension band techniques, early range of motion is permitted, which usually results in a functional range of motion after fracture healing. In the event that some symptomatic stiffness results following fracture healing, an intense physical therapy program may help improve the functional range of motion. In rare instances, a manipulation of the knee under anesthesia with or without arthroscopic lysis of adhesions may be required if a prolonged therapy program fails to yield beneficial results. We try to determine the need for further intervention at 3 months postoperatively. The indications and timing for these interventions are not clearly delineated in the literature.

Infection

Infection rates following operative treatment of patella fractures have ranged from 3% to 10%.[8, 36, 74] Because of their superficial location, patella fractures are often accompanied by varying degrees of soft-tissue injury, ranging from superficial abrasions to frank, open fractures. For open fractures, internal fixation should accompany emergent débridement and irrigation to reduce further soft-tissue damage and minimize the risk for infection. For closed injuries, some consideration can be given to postponing definitive fracture fixation until the soft tissues have had a chance to heal. Regardless of the timing of the definitive fracture fixation, careful handling of the soft tissue is mandatory to minimize the risk of infection. Superficial postoperative infections may be managed by a brief period of immobilization and antibiotic therapy until the infection resolves. Deep infection requires more aggressive treatment, including serial open débridements and irrigation, with definitive wound closure withheld until the wound is clean. If the fracture has not yet healed, internal fixation devices should be retained if possible. Once fracture healing has occurred and persistent infection is present, hardware removal in addition to débridement and irrigation should be performed.

Loss of Reduction

Reports of loss of operative reduction or the loss of internal fixation of patella fractures have ranged from none to 20% in the literature[8, 36, 74]. Many factors may contribute to this complication, including inadequate fixation, extensive comminution, patient noncompliance with activity and weightbearing restrictions, and early mobilization for constructs not amenable to early motion.[42, 74] If the resulting displacement or incongruity is minimal, a period of immobilization may be attempted to salvage the operation and allow the fracture to heal. If, on the other hand, the loss of reduction is too great or the extensor mechanism has been compromised, reoperation is indicated.

Delayed Union and Nonunion

With the advent of new surgical fixation methods, delayed union and nonunion have become extremely uncommon. Carpenter et al[17] reported a nonunion rate of less than 1% following operative reduction and fixation. If a delayed union is diagnosed, a period of immobilization may allow the fracture to consolidate. If a fracture fails to unite following a period of immobilization, consideration should be given to a repeated attempt at rigid fixation with autogenous bone-grafting. Weber and Cech[86] reported on their operative revision of patellar nonunions, with subsequent 100% union using standard fixation techniques.

For neglected nonunions with wide separation between the fragments, an attempt should be made at reconstructing the extensor mechanism. If the nonunion is longstanding, it may be necessary to perform a quadricepsplasty to mobilize a shortened, contracted quadriceps tendon prior to fracture fixation.[34]

Osteoarthrosis

Degeneration of the patellofemoral joint following patella fracture has several causes. Some are a direct result of the injury, and others are iatrogenic. First, articular damage may occur at the time of injury, and despite successful restoration of the articular surface, post-traumatic arthrosis may develop. Second, exuberant callous formation following apparent successful treatment (operative or nonoperative) of a comminuted patella fracture may also lead to patellofemoral joint degeneration.[61] Third, inadequate restoration of the articular surface has been defined as a source of subsequent joint degeneration. Fourth, improper placement and repair of the patellar tendon on the patellar remnant following a partial patellectomy has been shown to lead to patellofemoral arthritis.[28] Long-term follow-up studies of patients after patella fracture have demonstrated an increased incidence of radiographic degeneration when compared with the uninvolved knee.[34, 75]

Hardware Irritation

Although irritation of the soft tissues by underlying hardware is not a true complication of treatment, it occurs often enough to warrant mentioning, and patients should be counseled preoperatively of the possible need for hardware removal after fracture healing. Two studies[36, 74] have quoted an incidence of 15% of soft-tissue irritation from retained hardware, necessitating removal. Hardware removal should be done on an elective basis after complete fracture healing and restoration of knee motion.

PATELLA FRACTURES IN TOTAL KNEE ARTHROPLASTY

Fracture of the patella occurs infrequently following total knee replacement. However, it is probably the most frequently occurring periprosthetic fracture about the knee.[61] Reported incidence of patella fractures following patellar resurfacing has ranged from 0.33% to as high as 6.3% in one series.[16, 33]

A multitude of risk factors for patella fracture following total knee arthroplasty have been compiled in the literature, and these have been categorized into patient-related factors, implant design factors, and surgical technique factors[43] (Table 62.1).

Excessive body weight and an increased activity level have been associated with an increased incidence of patellar fracture.[27, 37, 80] Excessive postoperative flexion has also been associated with patella fractures in some series,[2, 37] and others have found no relationship between range of motion and fracture.[72] Osteoporotic bone secondary to rheumatoid arthritis and long-term steroid use have also been identified as risk factors for fracture.[66] Although little can be done surgically to alter these patient-related risk factors for fracture, knowledge of their presence should alert the surgeon to avoid further compromising the success of patellar resurfacing by means of careful surgical technique and implant selection decisions.

The design of the component can also influence the risk of patella fracture. Patellar buttons with a central peg are believed to result in more frequent fractures, especially if there is perforation of the anterior cortex of the patella.[12, 16, 66] The type of fixation used for the patella has also been implicated, with some authors believing that the use of cementless pegs increases the incidence of fracture, others believing that the thermal effects of polymerizing bone cement may increase the risk of patellar fracture.[20] Patellar components that are designed to be inset within the periphery of the patella have also been associated with so-called "rim" fractures of the peripheral portion of the patella.[43] Insall[37] believes that excessive knee motion and increased activity postoperatively places patients at risk for patella fracture, but this in effect is a testament to the success of the total knee arthroplasty.

TABLE 62.1 RISK FACTORS FOR PATELLA FRACTURE

Patient factors
- Osteoporosis
- Rheumatoid arthritis
- Male sex
- Overactivity
- Excessive knee motion

Implant factors
- Patellar replacement/nonreplacement
- Central peg
- Cementless implants
- PCL-substituting prosthesis
- Inset design
- Polyethylene osteolysis

Technical factors
- Excessive resection
- Inadequate resection
- Anterior patella perforation
- Revision surgery
- Cement usage
- Malalignment
- Patella subluxation/dislocation
- Patella blood supply disruption

The goal of patellar resurfacing is to recreate the original dimensions of the patella after prosthetic replacement. Any deviation from this technique increases the risk for patellar fracture. Excessive bone resection may predispose the thin bone to fracture by virtue of its inability to withstand the physiological strains placed on it. This also applies to asymmetric resurfacing, with the thin portion at risk for failure.[59, 66, 80] Conversely, inadequate bone resection may thicken the patellofemoral joint excessively, which may lead to patellar fracture through increased contact forces.[5, 13, 80] If the appropriate femoral and tibial rotation is not achieved, maltracking of the patella may occur, which will increase the forces on the patellofemoral joint, potentially leading to subluxation and/or fracture.[30, 72] Additionally, anterior placement of the femur may increase the forces across the patellofemoral joint, potentially leading to fracture.

The other iatrogenic risk factor for patella fracture is circulatory embarrassment to the patella as a result of the surgical exposure and correction of patellofemoral maltracking due to a lateral retinacular release. Avascular necrosis of the patella has been reported following ligation of the superior lateral geniculate artery, especially when associated with a medial arthrotomy.[12, 20, 40, 67] However, other authors have disputed this claim.[38, 57, 58] Despite the controversy, it is recommended that an attempt should be made to spare the superior lateral geniculate artery during lateral release if at all possible, understanding that good patellofemoral tracking should take precedence over conservation of this vessel. It is difficult to stratify the many risk factors associated with periprosthetic patella fractures in terms of their relative contribution to this complication. Figgie et al,[30] in their review of 36 patella fractures after condylar total knee arthroplasty, concluded that the most serious contributing factor to patella fracture was the overall alignment of the prosthesis. Malalignment also had a major impact on the severity of the fracture and on the prognosis following treatment for the patella fracture.

Classification of periprosthetic patellar fractures has also been confusing, with many systems having been developed to help guide treatment and predict prognosis. Fractures may be classified by mechanism of injury, such as direct or indirect, or stress fractures, with no identifiable injury. Insall[38] divided patella fractures by configuration of the fracture: horizontal, vertical, and comminuted. He also categorized periprosthetic fractures into traumatic injuries, which were often displaced (Fig. 62.28) and required operative intervention, and fatigue fractures (Figs. 62.29 and 62.30), which are best treated with a period of decreased motion or activity until asymptomatic. Perhaps the most useful classification system in terms of guiding treatment is that described by Goldberg et al,[31] which attempts to account for patellar fracture pattern and any concomitant extensor mechanism pathology (Fig. 62.31).

Type I fractures are marginal fractures with no extension into the implant-bone interface and have no exten-

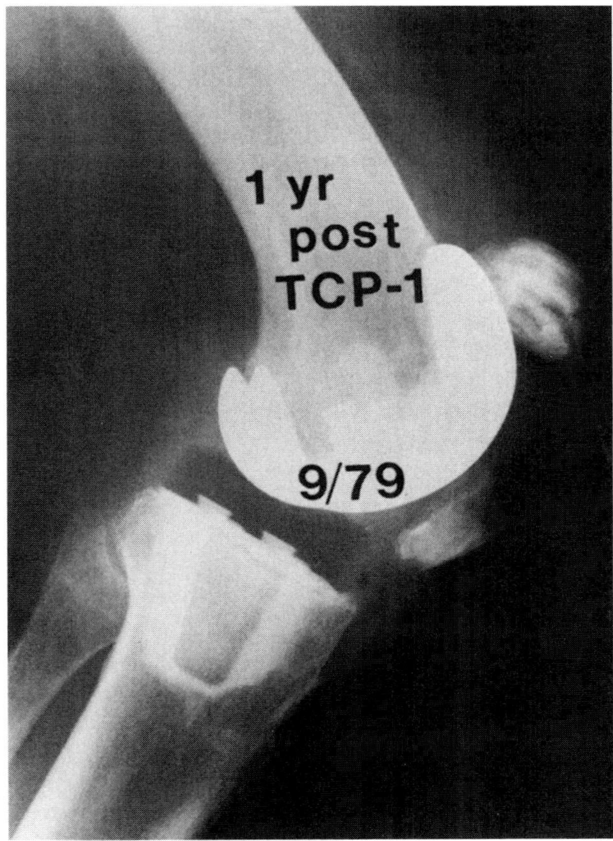

FIGURE 62.28 ➢ Post-traumatic vertical fracture of the patella, requiring open reduction.

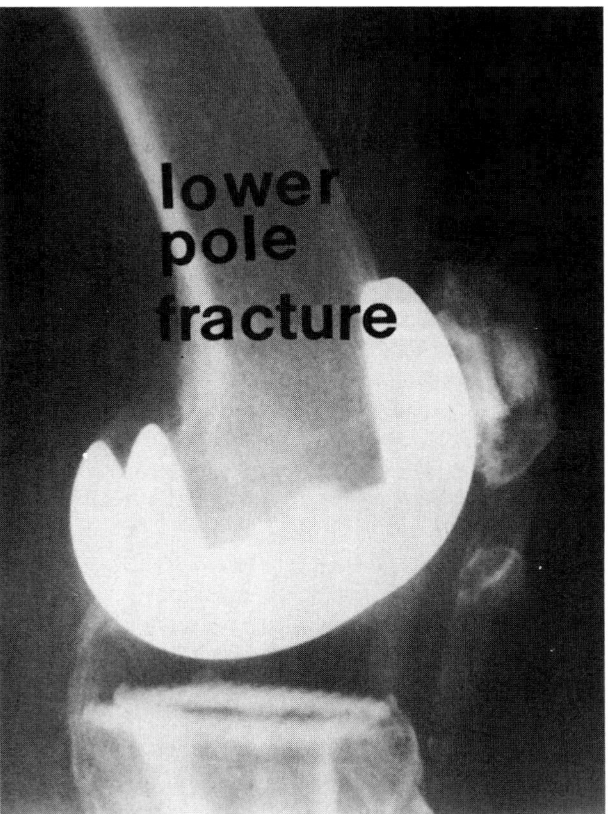

FIGURE 62.29 ➢ Vertical fatigue fracture of the patella. In contradistinction to the traumatic fractures, this type usually heals spontaneously, as occurred in this case.

sor mechanism injury. Type II fractures are characterized by either disruption of the extensor mechanism, or disruption of the implant-bone interface. Type III injuries involve the inferior pole of the patella with subtype III-A having patellar tendon disruption and subtype III-B having an intact patellar tendon. Type IV fractures are those associated with patellofemoral dislocation.

Management of periprosthetic patellar fractures must be guided by a number of factors, and it is important to evaluate all components of the arthroplasty in order to optimize treatment results. As Figgie et al[30] concluded in their review, the overall alignment of the arthrolpasty is critical, and failure to address this may compromise the results of periprosthetic patella fracture treatment.

Treatment

Patella fractures after total knee arthroplasty can often be treated nonoperatively, if no significant displacement or extensor lag exists. Fractures that are marginal and have no extension into the bone-implant interface or disruption of the extensor mechanism (type I) can be successfully treated by a period of bracing or casting until fracture consolidation occurs (see Fig. 62.24). Even comminuted fractures with little displacement with an intact prosthesis and extensor mechanism can be treated without surgical intervention. If component loosening has occurred, it may be prudent to allow the fracture to consolidate before attempting component revision, as opposed to attempting both in the acute setting.[76] Grossly loose or free-floating implants

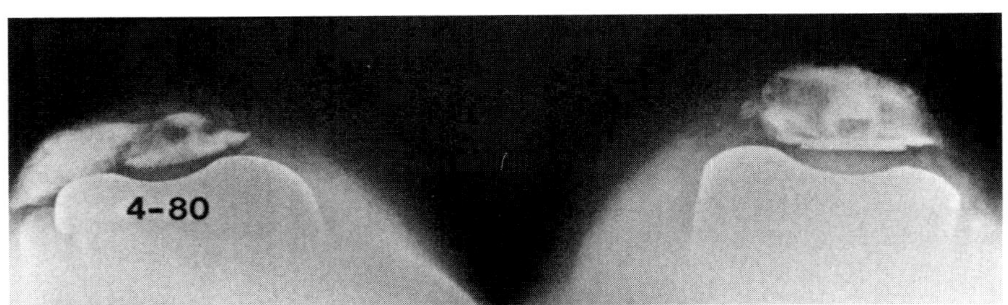

FIGURE 62.30 ➢ Horizontal fatigue fracture of the patella.

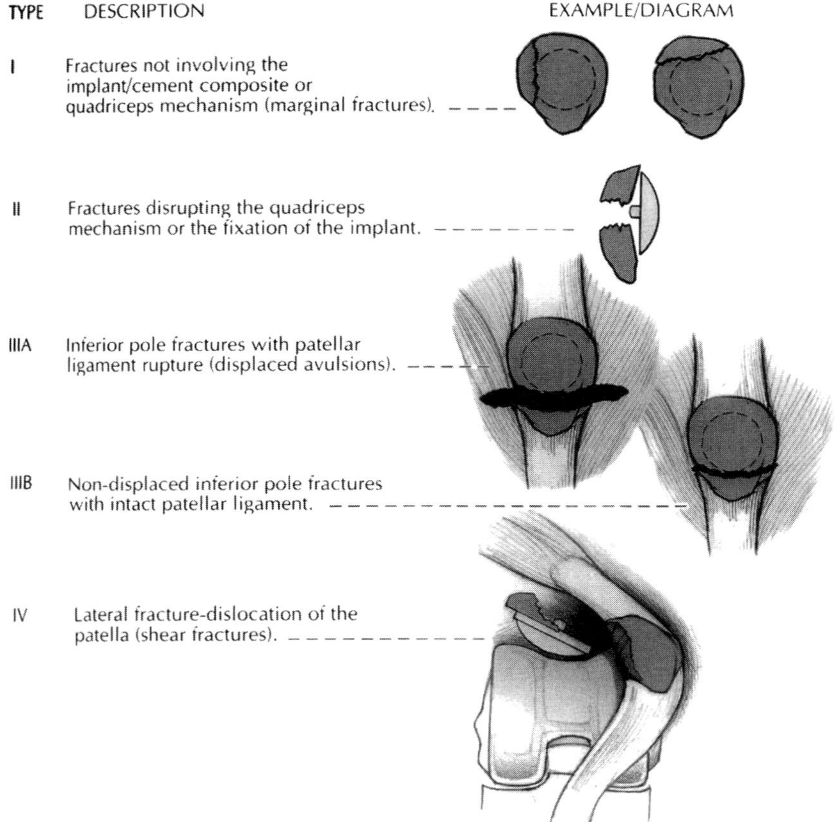

FIGURE 62.31 ➢ Goldberg[31] classification of patella fractures following total knee arthroplasty. (From Kolessar D, Rand J: Extensor mechanism problems following total knee arthroplasty. In Morrey B, ed: Reconstructive Surgery of the Joints, 2nd ed. New York, Churchill Livingstone, 1996.)

may require removal to prevent further damage to the joint or extensor mechanism. Fractures that involve disruption of the extensor mechanism (types II and IIIB) mandate surgical repair to minimize the functional disability of a permanent extensor lag. Patellar fractures with significant displacement should also be treated with open reduction and internal fixation.[3, 13, 31, 33] Standard tension band wiring with supplemental Kirschner wires or screws is not always possible, owing to osteopenic bone, poor capacity to heal, and the presence of a patellar component, so that cerclage wiring may be the only surgical option. Because of the compromised fixation, early postoperative motion may not be possible.[83] If surgical repair of a patella fracture is not possible, and resurfacing of the patellar remnant is not technically feasible, a patelloplasty (partial patellectomy without resurfacing) is much more preferable than a total patellectomy. Conserving a portion of the patella helps maintain the biomechanical advantage of the extensor mechanism and also minimizes the risk of tendon rupture and total knee arthroplasty instability sometimes seen after total patellectomy.[7, 83]

In summary, for patella fractures following total knee arthroplasty, most of these injuries do well without surgery, despite an unusual radiographic appearance. Operative treatment may be more detrimental than conservative management.

References

1. Aglietti P, Buzzi B: Fractures of the patella. In Insall J, ed: Surgery of the Knee, 2nd ed. New York, Churchill Livingstone, 1993.
2. Aglietti P, Buzzi B, Gaudanzi A: Patellofemoral functional results and complications with the posterior stabilized total condylar prosthesis. J Arthroplasty 3:17, 1988.
3. Aglietti P, Insall J, Walker P, et al: A new patellar prosthesis. Clin Orthop 180:158, 1981.
4. Anderson L: Fractures. In Crenshaw DI, ed: Campbell's Operative Orthopaedics, 5th ed. St. Louis, Mosby, 1971.
5. Barnes C, Scott R: Patellofemoral complications of total knee replacement. Instr Course Lect, AAOS, 42:304, 1993.
6. Baumgartl F: Das Kniegelenk. Berlin, Springer Verlag, 1964.
7. Bayne O, Cameron H: Total knee arthroplasty following patellectomy. Clin Orthop 186:112, 1984.
8. Bostman O, Kivilvoto O, Nirhama J: Comminuted displaced fractures of the patella. Injury 13:196, 1981.
9. Bostman O, Kivilvoto O, Santavirta S, et al: Fractures of the patella treated by operation. Arch Orthop Trauma Surg 102:78, 1983.
10. Bostrom A: Fracture of the patella: A study of 422 patellar fractures. Acta Orthop Scand 143:1, 1972.
11. Bostrom A: Longitudinal fractures of the patella. Rec Surg Traumatol 14:136, 1974.
12. Brick G, Scott R: Blood supply to the patella: Significance in total knee arthroplasty. J Arthroplasty 4:75, 1989.
13. Brick G, Scott R: The patellofemoral component of total knee arthroplasty. Clin Orthop 231:163, 1988.
14. Brooke J: The treatment of fractured patella by excision: A study of morphology and function. Br J Surg 24:733, 1936.
15. Buzzi R, Aglietti P: Fratture transversali di rotulz: Valutazione

spereimentale del metodo di fissazione intema di Lotke e Ecker. Arch Putti 37:283, 1989.
16. Cameron H, Fedorkow D: The patella in total knee arthroplasty. Clin Orthop 165:197, 1982.
17. Carpenter J, Kasman R, Matthews L: Patella fractures. Instr Course Lect, AAOS, 43:97, 1994.
18. Carson W, James S, Larson R, et al: Patellofemoral disorders: II—Radiographic examination. Clin Orthop 185:178, 1984.
19. Chiroff R: A new technique for the treatment of comminuted transverse fractures of the patella. Surg Gynecol Obstet 79:909, 1977.
20. Clayton M, Thirupathi R: Patellar complications after total condylar arthroplasty. Clin Orthop 170:152, 1982.
21. Coffer H: Mechanical function of the patella. J Bone Joint Surg Am 53:1551, 1971.
22. Coffer H: Patellobiomechanics. Clin Orthop 144:51, 1979.
23. Compere C, Hill J, Lewinnek G, et al: A new method of patellectomy for patellofemoral arthritis. J Bone Joint Surg Am 61:714, 1979.
24. Cramer K, Moed B: Patellar fractures: Contemporary approach to treatment. JAAOS 5:323, 1997.
25. De Palma AF: Diseases of the Knee. Philadelphia, JB Lippincott, 1954.
26. Dobbie R, Ryerson S: The treatment of fractured patella by excision. Am J Surg 55:339, 1942.
27. Dupont J, Baker S: Complications of patellofemoral resurfacing in total knee arthroplasty. Orthop Trans 6:369, 1982.
28. Duthie H, Hutchinson J:The results of partial and total excision of the patella. J Bone Joint Surg, Br 40:75, 1958.
29. Einola S, Aho A, Kallio P: Patellectomy after fracture. Acta Orthop Scand 47:441, 1976.
30. Figgie H, Goldberg V, Figgie M, et al: The effect of alignment on fractures of the patella after condylar total knee arthroplasty. J Bone Joint Surg Am 71:1031, 1989.
31. Goldberg V, Figgie H, Inglis A, et al: Patella fracture type and prognosis in condylar total knee arthroplasty. Clin Orthop 236: 115, 1988.
32. Goodfellow J, Hungerford D, Woods C: Patellofemoral joint mechanics and pathology of chondromalacia-patella. J Bone Joint Surg Br 59:291, 1976.
33. Grace J, Sim F: Fracture of the patella after total knee arthroplasty. Clin Orthop 230:168, 1988.
34. Hesketh K: Experiences with the Thompson quadriceps-plasty. J Bone Joint Surg Br 45:491, 1963.
35. Huberti H, Hayes W, Stone J, et al: Force ratios in the quadriceps tendon and ligamentum patella. J Orthop Res 2:49, 1984.
36. Hung L, Chan K, Chow Y, et al: Fractured patella: Operative treatment using the tension band principle. Injury 16:343, 1985.
37. Insall J, Dethmers D: Revision of total knee arthroplasty. Clin Orthop 170:123, 1982.
38. Insall J, Haas S: Complications of Total Knee Arthroplasty. In Insall J, ed: Surgery of the Knee, 2nd ed. New York, Churchill Livingstone, 1993.
39. Insall J, Goldberg V, Salvati E: Recurrent dislocation of the high riding patella. Clin Orthop 88:67, 1972.
40. Kayler D, Lyttle D: Surgical interruption of patellar blood supply by total knee arthroplasty. Clin Orthop 229:221, 1988.
41. Kolessar D, Rand J: Extensor mechanism problems following total knee arthroplasty. In Morrey B, ed: Reconstructive Surgery of the Joints, 2nd ed. New York, Churchill Lavingstone, 1996.
42. Levack B, Flannagan J, Hobbs S: Results of surgical treatment of patella fractures. J Bone and Joint Br 67:416, 1985.
43. Lewis P, Rorabeck C: Periprosthetic fractures. In Engh G, ed: Revision Total Knee Arthroplasty. Philadelphia, Williams & Wilkins, 1997.
44. Lieb F, Perry J: Quadriceps function. J Bone and Joint Am 50: 1535, 1968.
45. Lotke P, Ecker M: Transverse fractures of the patella. Clin Orthop 158:180, 1981.
46. Magnuson P: Fractures, 2nd ed. Philadelphia, JB. Lippincott, 1933.
47. Matthews L, Sanstegard D, Henke J: Load-bearing characteristics of the patellofemoral joint. Acta Orthop Scand 48:511, 1977.
48. McMaster P: Fractures of the patella. Clin Orthop 4:24, 1953.
49. Merchant A, Mercer R, Jacobsen R, et al: Roentgenographic analysis of patellofemoral congruence. J Bone and Joint Am 56:1391, 1974.
50. Nummi J: Operative treatment of patella fractures. Acta Orthop Scand 42:437, 1971.
51. Pandey A, Pandey S, Pandey P: Results of partial patellectomy. Acta Orthop Traum Surg 110:246, 1991.
52. Payr E: Zur operativen Behandlung der Kniegelenksteife nach langdauernder Ruhigstellung. Zentralbl Chir 44:809, 1917.
53. Peeples R, Margo M: Function after patelectomy. Clin Orthop 132:180, 1978.
54. Perry C, McCarthy J, Kain C, et al: Patellar fixation protected with a load-sharing cable: A mechanical and clinical study. J Orthop Trauma 2:234, 1988.
55. Reider B, Marshall J, Kostin B, et al: The anterior aspect of the knee joint. J Bone Joint Surg Am 63:351, 1981.
56. Resneck D, Niwayama G: Disorders of Bone and Joint Disorders, 2nd ed. Philadelphia, W.B. Saunders, 1988.
57. Ritter M, Campbell E: Postoperative patellar complications with or without lateral release during total knee arthroplasty. Clin Orthop 219:163, 1987.
58. Ritter M, Keating E, Faris P: Clinical roentgenographic and scintographic results after interruption of the superior lateral genicular artery during total knee arthroplasty. Clin Orthop 248:145, 1989.
59. Reuben J, McDonald C, Woodward P, et al: Effect of patella thickness on patella strain following total knee arthroplasty. J Arthroplasty 6:251, 1991.
60. Saltzman C, Goulet J, McClellan R, et al: Results of treatment of displaced patella fractures by partial patellectomy. J Bone Joint Surg Am 72:1279, 1990.
61. Sanders R: Patella fractures and extensor mechanism injuries. In Browner B, ed: Skeletal Trauma, Philadelphia, W. B. Saunders, 1992.
62. Scapinelli R: Blood supply of the human patella. J Bone Joint Surg Br 3:563, 1967.
63. Schatzker J, Tile M: The Rationale of Operative Fracture Care. New York, Springer Verlag, 1987.
64. Schauwecker R: The Practice of Osteosynthesis. Stuttgart, Georg Thieme, 1974.
65. Scott J: Fractures of the patella. J Bone Joint Surg Br 31:76, 1949.
66. Scott R: Duopatellar total knee replacement: The Brigham experience. Orthop Clin North Am 13:89, 1982.
67. Scucki G, Scharf S, Meltzer L, et al: The relationship of lateral release to patella viability in total knee arthroplasty. J Arthroplasty 2:209, 1987.
68. Scuderi G: The Patella, New York, Springer-Verlag, 1995.
69. Seligo W: Fractures of the patella. Recons Surg Traumatol 12: 1281, 1971.
70. Shim S, Leung G: Blood supply of the knee joint: A microangiographic study in children and adults. Clin Orthop 208:119, 1986.
71. Shorbe H, Dobson C: Patellectomy. J Bone Joint Surg Am 40: 1281, 1958.
72. Sirrison A, Noble J, Harding K: Complications of the Altenborough knee replacement. J Bone Joint Surg Br 68:100, 1986.
73. Smillie IS: Injuries of the Knee Joint, 4th ed. Edinburgh, Churchill Livingstone, 1970.
74. Smith S, Cramer K, Kargus D, et al: Early complications in the operative treatment of patella fractures. J Orthop Trauma 11: 183, 1997.
75. Sorensen K: The later prognosis after fracture of the patella. Acta Orthop Scand 47:441, 1976.
76. Spitzer A, Vince K: Patella considerations in total knee replacement. In Scuderi G, ed: The Patella, New York, Springer Verlag, 1995.
77. Sponseller P, Beaty J: Fractures and dislocations about the knee. In Rockwood C, Wilkins K, Beaty J, eds: Fractures in Children, 4th ed. Philadelphia, J.B. Lippincott, 1996. p 1287,
78. Sutton F, Thompson C, Lipke J, et al: The effect of patellectomy on knee function. J Bone Joint Am 58:537, 1976.
79. Templeman D: Fractures of the patella. In Fractures and Dislocations. St. Louis, Mosby, 1993.

80. Thompson F, Hood R, Insall J: Patella fractures in total knee arthroplasty. Orthop Trans 5:490, 1981.
81. Thompson J: Comminuted fractures of the patella. J Bone Joint Surg Am 1935; 17:431, 1935.
82. Vince K, Cameron H: Total knee arthroplasty following patellectomy. Clin Orthop 186:112, 1984.
83. Vince K, McPherson E: The patella in total knee arthroplasty. Orthop Clin North Am 23:675, 1992.
84. Watkins M, Harris B, Wender S: Effect of patellectomy on the function of the quadriceps and hamstrings. J Bone Joint Surg Am 65:390, 1983.
85. Watson-Jones R: Fractures and Joint Injuries. Baltimore, Williams & Wilkins, 1952.
86. Weber B, Cech O: Pseudarthrosis. New York, Grune and Stratton, 1976.
87. Wiberg G: Roentgenographic and anatomic studies of the patellofemoral joint. Acta Orthop Scand 12:319, 1941.

63 Periprosthetic Fractures

ROBERT E. BOOTH, JR. • DAVID G. NAZARIAN

The second millennium marks a human life expectancy more than double that of the first while simultaneously creating an ever-expanding population of patients with total knee arthroplasties (TKA) that are nonetheless expected to endure for unanticipated intervals in increasingly frail hosts.

Conventional wisdom would suggest that patients with a successful TKA are at no greater risk for traumatic fracture than their unoperated cohorts. However, when periprosthetic fractures do occur, there is no question that the biological and sociological conditions that precipitated the injury in the first place only serve to compound the difficulty of its reconstruction. The typical patient suffers polyarticular arthritis, general debilitation, neurological dysfunction, multiple systemic illnesses, and a constitutional intolerance of bed rest and restricted ambulation. Their osseous skeleton is almost definitionally osteopenic, frustrating traditional methods of stabilization and fixation. The competing surgical principles of proscribed activity to facilitate fracture healing must be balanced against early motion to preclude joint stiffness. Worse, the deficiencies of the index arthroplasty — often invisible in the myopia of the responsible surgeon — require coincidental revision not only to effect a successful articulation but also to decompress the healing fracture and promote osteosynthesis.

As a general rule, therefore, periprosthetic fractures demand more aggressive and more innovative concepts and techniques of reconstruction, which are the essential focus of the ensuing discussion.

INTRAOPERATIVE FRACTURES

Intraoperative fractures about a total knee prosthesis are reportedly rare, but the true incidence is unknown as most go unnoticed by the operating surgeon.[13] Small cortical infractions are occasionally seen in immediate postoperative films, but they rarely progress to pathological significance. This is partly because of the protected weightbearing status that many arthroplasties require. Additionally, these periprosthetic fissures are protected and partially stabilized by the very prosthetic components that occasioned them.

On the femoral side of an arthroplasty, the most common intraoperative fractures are vertically oriented and involve the metaphyseal junction of the femoral condyle and shaft. They are frequently sustained by the periosteal hinge, and many require no further stabilization if the collaterals are intact and properly tensioned. The most common cause for these fractures is aggressive impaction of the femoral component. Indeed, sufficient force is often generated that even more proximal fractures of the hip[16] have been described. The intercondylar fractures, however, are most common in posterior stabilized knee designs, in which the asymmetric impaction of the intercondylar prosthetic box may disrupt the femoral cortical integrity. Lombardi[27] described a series of these injuries, most of which went on to uncomplicated union. Potential avoidance of this rare fracture remains one of the few good reasons for preferring a cruciate-retaining to a cruciate-substituting design. If the surgeon is anxious about the stability of such a fracture, the addition of an intramedullary rod to the femoral prosthesis provides excellent stabilization. Screws and other external fixation devices are usually excessive and difficult to apply to the osteopenic periprosthetic bone.

With the advent of intramedullary and posterior-referencing instrumentation systems — as opposed to the earlier anterior-referencing designs — the incidence of femoral notching is not insignificant. This, in a sense, constitutes an iatrogenic fracture as well, as even a 3-mm disruption of the distal femoral cortical bone reduces the integrity of that area by 28%. Although the direct relationship of anterior notches or "blends" to supracondylar fractures is still debatable, most surgeons feel it prudent to protect a substantial anterior defect with an intramedullary femoral stem extension.

Femoral intramedullary roddings are not without their own complications. As the length of the femoral intramedullary device approaches 150 mm or more, the impact of the narrow femoral isthmus and anterior femoral bowing makes the standard straight intramedullary rods at risk to create a cortical disruption or fracture, usually on the anterolateral femoral surface. Once again, many of these fractures are not identified at the time of surgery because they are obscured by the proximal soft tissues. If such a rodding fracture does occur, the conventional wisdom suggests that it is appropriate to bypass the defect by a distance equivalent to 2½ femoral canal diameters.

As a general rule, all such periprosthetic fractures are best stabilized without intramedullary cementation, because the pressurization of the cement will penetrate the fracture defects, retarding osteosynthesis or sequestrating isolated fragments.

Intraoperative tibial periprosthetic fractures are even less common, particularly in primary knee arthroplasty. The uniform anatomy and high compressive strength of the proximal tibial metaphysis — at least for the first 15 mm — means that even the most vigorous prosthetic impaction is unlikely to induce a fracture (Fig. 63.1). In cruciate-retaining total knee designs, the appropriate tibial stem is commonly placed more anteriorly in the sagittal plane to accommodate the poste-

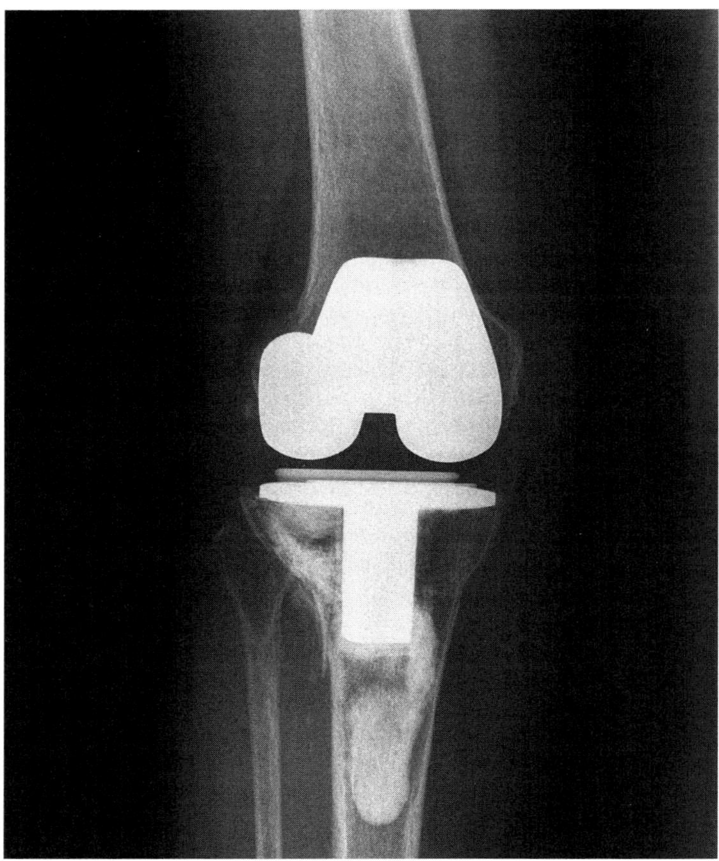

FIGURE 63.1 ➢ Intraoperative lateral tibial metaphyseal fracture from impaction of tibial component.

rior cruciate bone block and ligament. Cruciate-substituting knees have been shown to have better results with slightly posteriorly oriented stems, which creates the potential for posterior cortical disruptions at the time of instrumentation or implantation. Although this hazard may well be worth the risk because of the unsurpassed results of cemented cruciate-substituting tibial trays, one must be careful not to penetrate the posterior tibial cortex during surgery. Should this occur, these lesions do not require a stem extension to bypass the defect, but care must be taken to prevent cement extrusion into the posterior neurovascular structures.

Tibial intramedullary stems can, once again, create potential problems of their own. The center of the tibial metaphysis is not precisely the center of the knee, which is located several millimeters laterally in the coronal plane. Thus, the act of reaming a tibial intramedullary canal longitudinally to avoid fracture may cause medial overhang of the tibial tray unless an offset stem can be employed. Most tibial shaft violations therefore occur on the anteromedial cortex. Because of the stabilizing effect of the fibula, minor tibial fractures are even more intrinsically stable than their femoral counterparts, are generally loaded vertically in their posture of maximum strength, and therefore rarely need additional stabilization or protection.

Intraoperative patellar fractures are extremely rare in primary TKA, although a congenital bipartite patella or the fibrous union of a prior patellar fracture may create similar challenges. One option in this setting is simply not to resurface the patella. Most physicians are not intimidated by this prospect and would prefer to proceed with patellar resurfacing with good result.

Intraoperative periprosthetic fractures are unquestionably more common in the revision setting, where it is frequently observed that the knees' soft tissues have become stiff and the hard tissues have become soft. As a consequence of this biological reversal, one occasionally sees avulsion fractures on the convex or tension sides of the articulation. Thus, separation of the cortical shell of the medial femoral condyle or even the tibial tuberosity at the time of exposure or prosthetic reimplantation can occur. The tibial tuberosity *must* be reattached and secured, using either staples, screws, or intraosseous anchors. Unfortunately, the limb usually must be restricted in its flexion postoperatively. On the other hand, the more common medial femoral condylar avulsion, as long as it remains attached proximally by a periosteal sleeve, is intrinsically stable and may require no supplemental fixation. Metallic fixation devices work poorly anyway in this stress-shielded osteopenic bone, and a better choice may be to correct the overall limb alignment closer to neutral to protect these structures from excessive tension.

POSTOPERATIVE PERIPROSTHETIC FRACTURES

Femoral Fractures

The femoral component of any TKA surrounds and protects the distal femur while at the same time inducing stress shielding and a radical transition in the modulus of elasticity at the junction of the femoral diaphysis and metaphysis. Thus, it is not surprising that the most common and most problematic postoperative periprosthetic fracture is in the supracondylar area. Most of the patients who sustain these injuries are elderly, infirm, and poorly muscled. Some studies have suggested a high incidence of neurological abnormalities as well.[7]

Supracondylar fractures are defined, by general agreement, as those occurring within 15 cm of the joint line. There exists, in fact, a biological "no man's land" between 4 and 15 cm from the end of the femur. Fractures that occur at the level of or distal to the transepicondylar axis — such as are seen with failed unicompartmental or Geomedic designs — can be treated by a fairly simple revision technology, although often requiring distal femoral augmentation to replace lost bone. Conversely, fractures occurring more than 15 cm from the joint are in the area of the femoral diaphysis, where better bone quality and a tubular anatomic geometry allow a wide variety of intramedullary and extramedullary fixation techniques to be successful. It is in the intervening area that the greatest challenges are found. Indeed, as a general rule, the greater the distance from the articulation, the easier the fracture is to treat. All periprosthetic fractures present the unique dilemma of balancing the competing principles of immobilization of the fracture until healing occurs versus maintaining joint motion to preclude stiffness.

If untreated or undertreated, supracondylar femoral fractures will all adopt the same deformity, whether or not malunion occurs. The typical posture of the fracture is in adduction, flexion, and internal rotation of the distal component, largely as a response to the dominant muscle forces about the knee. Should a malunion occur, its impact is determined not only by the degree of the deformity but also the distance of the deformity from the joint. For example, a 5-degree varus malunion at a distance 7 cm from the joint line will produce less malalignment than a 5-degree deformity 15 cm from the joint line. Deformities that occur in the plane of action of the joint, in this case sagittal flexion and extension, are less troublesome than those that occur out of the plane of motion of the joint.

Before initiating treatment of any supracondylar fracture, it is advisable for the surgeon to consider four issues operative in the creation of the fracture. First, how severe was the trauma that produced the injury? Fractures that occur with minimal provocation are generally associated with severe osteopenia, and more aggressive stabilization techniques may be required than were originally imagined.

Second, how severe is the bony comminution about the fracture site? Another principle of supracondylar fracture management is that they are always worse under direct vision in the operating room than they appeared on preoperative x-ray films. Thus, any significant amount of comminution may require intercalary or onlay bone grafting, about which more will be said later, but whose availability should be investigated before surgery (Fig. 63.2).

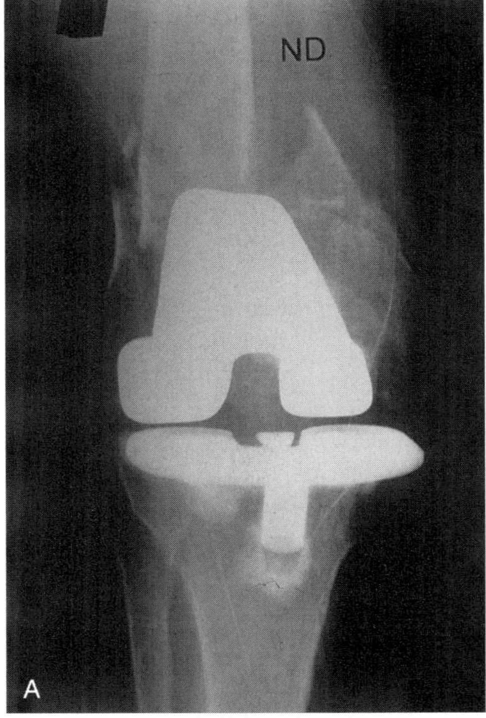

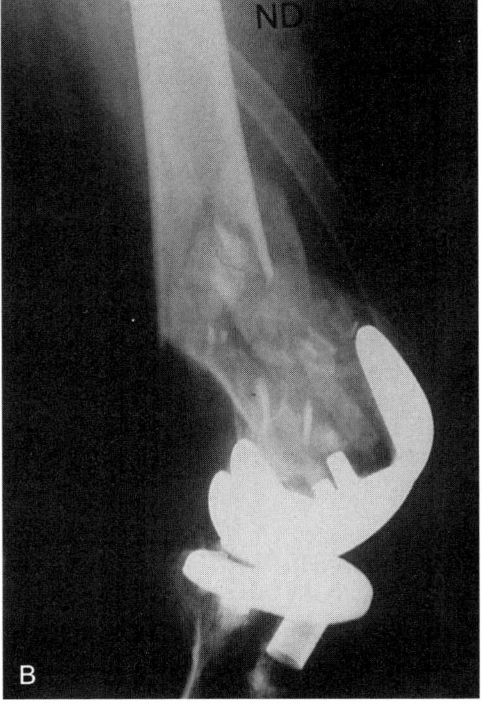

FIGURE 63.2 ➢ Supracondylar fracture with comminution too severe for open surgical treatment.

Third, how successful was the primary TKA before the fracture occurred? Most supracondylar fractures, in the authors' experience, are associated with a stiff or unstable total joint, a condition that undoubtedly contributed to the occurrence of the fracture or its nonunion/malunion. In these situations it is inadequate and inappropriate simply to repair the fracture alone. Obviously, the probability of fracture healing will be reduced by an unsatisfactory adjacent arthroplasty, and even a successful osteosynthesis will leave the limb unimproved from its prefracture condition. Thus in this situation the surgeon should optimally consider simultaneous revision of the failed TKA and internal fixation of the supracondylar fracture.

Last, it is important for the surgeon to make some determination about the stability of the prosthetic components themselves — their status before the injury as well as whether the implants have been loosened by the injury. This is often very difficult to accomplish once the fracture has occurred, yet the surgeon must be prepared to replace or revise components that are found to be loose at the time of surgery. The success of nonoperative treatment of supracondylar fractures will be compromised by loose components, although this condition is often not apparent. However, if one or more of the components has become loose, then conservative or nonoperative treatment of the fracture is usually inappropriate.

Although a host of biological and sociological factors ultimately affect the therapeutic choice for a supracondylar periprosthetic fracture, the two most crucial issues remain the "character" of the fracture itself and the quality of the antecedent arthroplasty. Although several classification systems have been proposed to codify this decision process, perhaps the most useful is that proposed by Lewis and Rorabeck.[26]

Type I: Prosthesis intact — undisplaced fracture.

Type II: Prosthesis intact — displaced fracture.

Type III: Failed prosthesis — displaced or undisplaced fracture.

Whereas the first two categories speak for themselves, the third deserves detailed consideration. Prostheses that are loose, failing for mechanical or biological reasons, unstable, the result of prior unsuccessful attempts at stabilization, or — as is most common in the authors' experience — excessively stiff and lacking in range of motion, are probably best served by simultaneous revisional arthroplasty and fracture stabilization. The economic imperatives of millennial medical care may additionally dictate more aggressive interventional therapies, as the economic costs of extended conservative therapy and sequential surgeries may be prohibitive.

TYPE I: UNDISPLACED SUPRACONDYLAR FRACTURES

Undisplaced supracondylar fractures about an entirely normal prosthesis are fortunately quite uncommon. Should they occur, however, the optimal treatment is either a cast or preferably a cast-brace with an initial period of immobilization followed by range-of-motion exercise. Intense scrutiny is requisite during the healing period, as these fractures notoriously slip into the typical attitude of flexion, adduction, and internal rotation with little provocation. Intervention is appropriate at the earliest sign of deformity, and internal fixation is necessary at that point. To be successful in the conservative mode, both extreme patient compliance with bracing and protected weightbearing as well as compulsive physician scrutiny on at least a weekly basis are required.

Frequently, conservative therapy is not an option for other reasons. Obesity often renders casting or cast-bracing ineffective. Protected weightbearing can be difficult in the elderly or infirm or those with compromised upper extremities. Even such issues as the unavailability of transportation to the patient for frequent physician visits may influence the treatment option toward surgical stabilization.

Although several authors[5, 31, 32] have reported small series of type I fractures treated conservatively, their focus has been on the rate of healing, which was high, but not on the postoperative range of motion and the ultimate quality of the arthroplasty. Contemporary standards for a successful TKA are high, as are patient expectations. The early range of motion necessitated to prevent arthrofibrosis requires great attention and compulsive scrutiny during the healing period.

If surgical stabilization is needed, for any of a variety of reasons, there are several technical options. The Richards DCS screw, the AO blade plate, and the Zickel supracondylar rod have all been variously employed, but with no literary substantiation in type I fractures. DCS screws and blade plates have limited applicability, largely determined by the internal geometry of the femoral prosthesis, which may prevent their appropriate positioning. Conventional wisdom suggests that the stress shielding of a femoral prosthesis will create sufficient periarticular osteopenia that the screws in particular should penetrate the medial femoral cortex to have any hope of secure purchase.

Zickel's supracondylar rods are less substantial, usually employing a 90-degree lateral intramedullary rod and a 75-degree medial intramedullary rod. If successful, they have the virtue of early joint mobility, particularly when coupled with a supplementary cast-brace.

Rush rods have also been described as providing satisfactory stabilization of supracondylar periprosthetic fractures. (Fig. 63.3). They are minimally invasive and extremely inexpensive, not inconsiderable virtues today. Ritter and associates have reported a series of 22 patients treated with Rush rods, all of whom healed within 4 months.[36] The patients averaged 108 degrees of knee flexion. Two instances of valgus malalignment occurred, but the authors attributed this to technical errors. An additional attraction of the Rush rod approach is that its minimally invasive nature provides the least opportunity for iatrogenic displacement of the fracture during surgical stabilization.

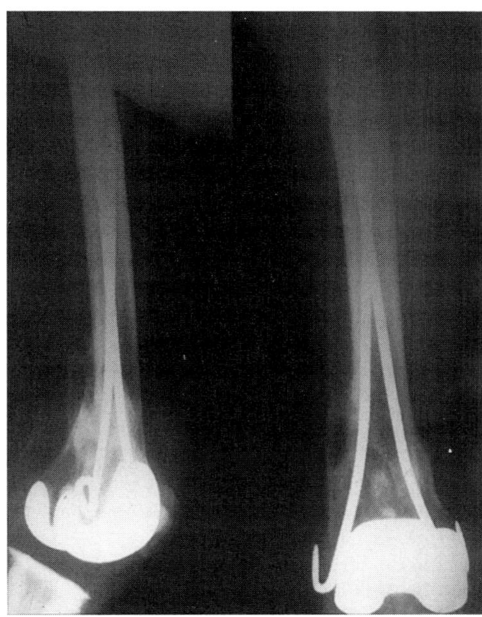

FIGURE 63.3 ➢ Rush rod stabilization of undisplaced supracondylar fracture.

TYPE II: DISPLACED SUPRACONDYLAR FRACTURES

It is recommended that all displaced supracondylar periprosthetic fractures be treated operatively, as the incidence of progressive displacement, nonunion, and malunion is extremely high. Attempts at closed reduction of these fractures may be transiently successful, but recurrent deformity is almost uniformly observed. As previously discussed, the deforming muscular forces about the knee tend to drive the distal component of the fracture into varus, adduction, and internal rotation. These vectors must be sufficiently resisted not only to prevent recurrent deformity but also to allow for early joint motion.

External fixators are frequently advocated and occasionally employed in the treatment of displaced supracondylar fractures. The periprosthetic osteopenia renders small pins ineffective, and the prospect of a pin tract infection so close to an arthroplasty would make external fixation relatively contraindicated for these fractures. Only one reported series[31] endorses this concept, reporting early activity and no nonunions, with an average range of motion of 101 degrees.

A variety of plate-and-screw techniques have been described for these fractures, and each has its own merits. Traditionally, the blade plate has been popular, although it is technically difficult and occasionally limited by the internal geometry of the femoral component.

Moran and coworkers[32] included nine blade plate fixations in their series of 15 supracondylar fractures. Fully one-third of their cases failed, however, with shortening and nonunion and malunion as a result.

Other authors have had similar difficulties with plate-and-screw fixation. Cordeiro and colleagues described three patients, all of whom developed a varus malunion.[6] Figgie and associates reported a 50% incidence of nonunion in their series of 10 fractures,[11] and Nielsen and coworkers had 100% failure in three cases with high infectious complications.[34]

On the other hand, Zehntner and Ganz had uniform success in a series of six patients, although all required either bone graft or methylmethacrylate supplementa-

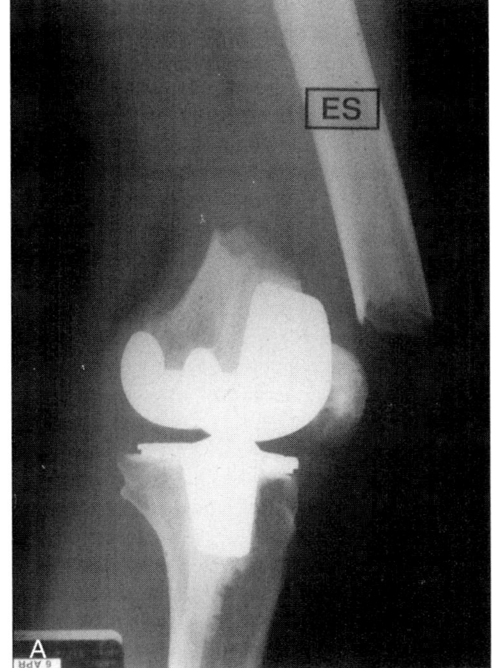

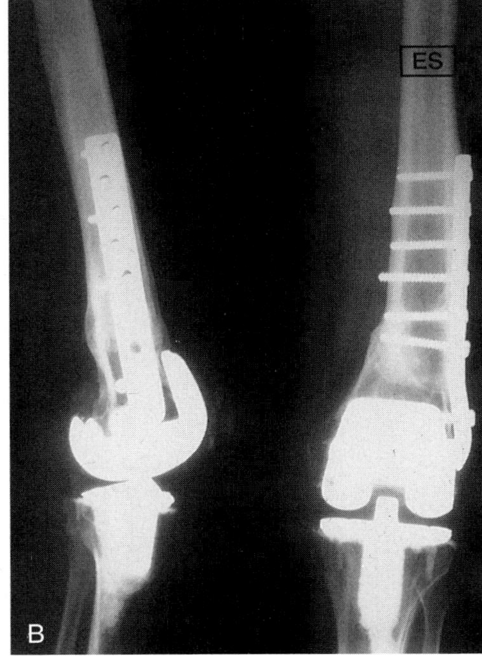

FIGURE 63.4 ➢ Displaced supracondylar fracture treated with plate and screw with mild malunion.

tion of the metallic fixation.[40] Finally, Healy and colleagues had success in 18 of 20 fractures treated with blade plates, condylar screws, or buttress plates.[17] Two patients required reoperation, and supplemental bone grafting was necessary in 15 of the 22 fractures. Nonetheless, all patients returned to their prefracture functional level, as defined by Knee Society scoring (Fig. 63.4).

Perhaps the most frustrating aspect of plate-and-screw stabilization attempts is that even technically perfect surgical efforts can deteriorate with the passage of time, into nonunions and malunions. Many physicians, even in the face of an adequate osteosynthesis, would protect the limb with an external cast-brace for 3 to 6 months. As with the conservative treatment of type I fractures, meticulous management and frequent observation of the fracture are required.

The newest and most attractive technique for stabilization of supracondylar periprosthetic fractures involves the use of the Supracondylar Intramedullary Nail (Smith & Nephew Richards). In concept, this is a minimally invasive procedure that, while technically demanding and radiographically dependent, requires only a small arthrotomy and relatively little disruption of the fracture hematoma and periosteum[19] (Fig. 63.5).

The rods are available in diameters from 11 to 13 mm, but an accurate knowledge of the patient's knee prosthesis is necessary to determine candidacy for this procedure.

Only femoral components with an open intercondylar notch are appropriate, and the intercondylar diameters of most prostheses are readily available (Table 63.1).

If the prosthetic intercondylar diameter is truly unknown or unavailable, radiographs can occasionally approximate this distance or the surgeon should be prepared to modify the femoral component with a Midas Rex bur to accommodate the rod. The latter technique is not generally recommended.

It should be noted that obese thighs are severely problematic, as the extramedullary guide for transfixing screws may simply not fit. Severe comminution of the femoral bone proximal to the prosthesis may produce shortening and rotation, deformities that should be corrected before final placement of the stabilizing screws. This is technically quite difficult and requires significant surgical judgment. In cases of severe com-

TABLE 63.1 INTERCONDYLAR DISTANCES OF COMMONLY USED TOTAL CONDYLAR KNEE IMPLANTS*

Implant	Intercondylar Distance (mm)
Miller-Galante (Zimmer, Warsaw, IN)	12
Insall-Burstein (Zimmer, Warsaw, IN)	14–19
Biomet (Warsaw, IN)	22
Intermedics (Austin, TX)	18
AMK (DePuy, Warsaw, IN)	14–17
Osteonics (Allendale, NJ)	19
PFC (Johnson & Johnson, New Brunswick, NJ)	20
Kirschner wires (Timonium, MD)	20
Genesis (Smith & Nephew Richards, Memphis, TN)	20
Duracon (Howmedica, Rutherford, NJ)	12–16

* Reproduced, with modification, from Jabczenski FF, Crawford M: Retrograde intramedullary nailing of supracondylar femur fractures above total knee arthroplasty. A preliminary report of four cases. J Arthroplasty 10:100, 1995.[22]

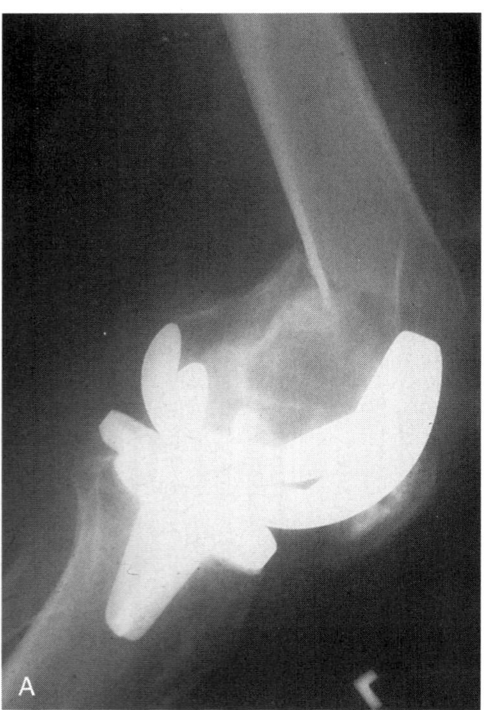

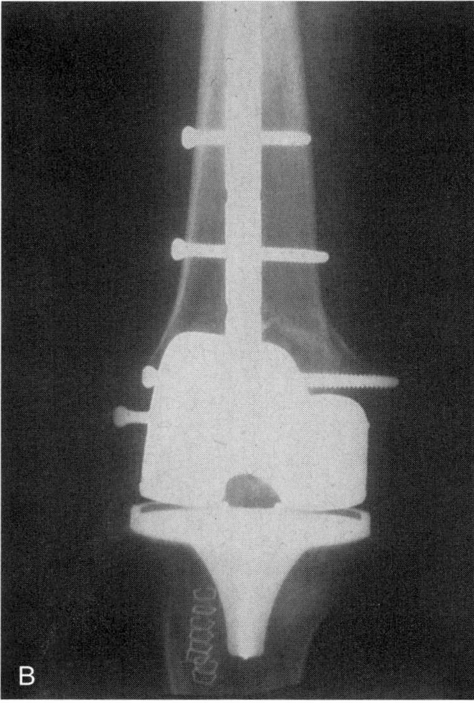

FIGURE 63.5 ➢ Displaced supracondylar fracture treated with supracondylar intramedullary nail.

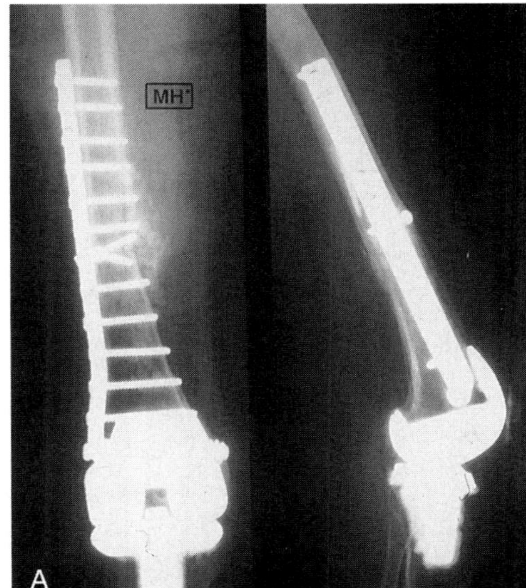

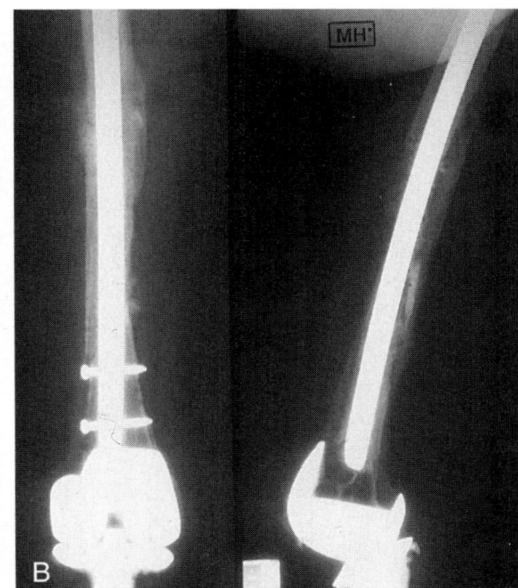

FIGURE 63.6 ➢ Femoral nonunion treated with antegrade intramedullary nail.

minution, proximal bone grafting should be considered, and copious amounts of graft material may be necessary to fill the distal femoral metaphysis. These techniques are well described in several publications, notably Henry and Booth.[19]

Several small series substantiate this technique. Rolston et al,[37] McLaren et al,[28] Jabczenski and Crawford,[22] Murrell and Nunley,[33] and Engh and Ammeen[9] have all reported very satisfactory outcomes. Most have contemplated or employed bone graft material or methylmethacrylate to stabilize the fracture. Although the predictable complications of nonunion, arthrofibrosis, infection, femoral shortening, and intrusion of the rod into the joint can occur, supracondylar intramedullary rods appear to be the optimal fixation technique at present for type II fractures (Fig. 63.6).

TYPE III: SUPRACONDYLAR FRACTURES WITH FAILED ARTHROPLASTY

A supracondylar femoral fracture is very frequently associated with a failed TKA. Indeed, this may be the most common scenario, because knees that are unstable or stiff predispose the patient to falls and other minor traumas that produce the fracture. If the quality of the arthroplasty is not known before the fracture, this factor may be difficult to quantify in the postfracture evaluation. In the authors' experience, the majority of supracondylar periprosthetic fractures referred for care have preexisting malalignment, instability from soft tissue imbalance or polyethylene wear, or stiffness from oversized components or tight posterior cruciate ligaments. These maloccurrences not only precipitate a fracture but also will compromise its treatment. For example, a cruciate-retaining TKA with an excessively tight posterior cruciate ligament (PCL) and thus limited flexion is more likely to fracture and is at higher risk for nonunion because of the increased stresses across the fracture site during the time of healing. The operative surgeon must be prepared to address *all these issues* in order to achieve a satisfactory result.

Two alternative treatment approaches are available. In the first, one may choose to treat the fracture alone, ignoring the prosthetic deficiencies and achieving solid femoral healing, after which a secondary revisional arthroplasty can be performed. This option is particularly attractive in instances of severely comminuted bone, the possibility of periprosthetic infection, and inadequate surgical materials or experience. The penalty for this option, obviously, is postoperative stiffness, which may be difficult to reverse, even with a subsequent revisional arthroplasty. On the other hand, any suspicion of infection can be defined, custom or special prosthetic devices can be prepared, and less constrained components are generally employed, thus potentially enhancing the longevity of the revisional arthroplasty.

The second option is the simultaneous revision of the failed arthroplasty and stabilization of the fractured femur. The advantage of this approach is a single procedure, early mobilization of the patient with significantly reduced morbidity and expense, and a lower incidence of arthrofibrosis. On the other hand, absolute stabilization of the fracture must be achieved intraoperatively, often at the expense of cemented intramedullary stems and constrained components. The surgery is exponentially more difficult than a simple revisional arthroplasty, usually requiring supplemental prosthetic and biological materials not commonly found other than in major joint replacement centers (Fig. 63.7).

The revision of a malunited supracondylar fracture is not without challenges of its own. The typical attitude of flexion, adduction, and internal rotation of the femoral component will frequently require a supracondylar osteotomy in the area of the prior fracture (Fig. 63.8). Many techniques have been described for this including butt cuts, step cuts, and oblique biplanar

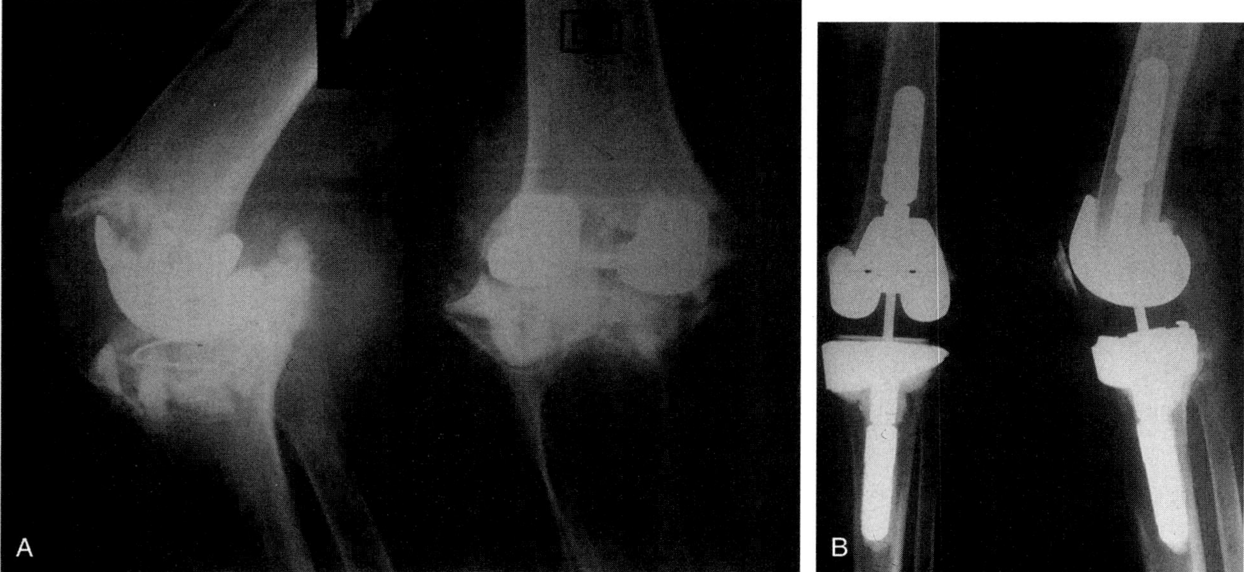

FIGURE 63.7 ➢ Low supracondylar fracture with failed arthroplasty, treated with revisional arthroplasty using substantial augmentations.

cuts. The last are the authors' preference because they have several distinct advantages. First, the obliquity of the distal femoral osteotomy will allow, depending on its degree, variable correction of both sagittal alignment and the flexion deformity (Fig. 63.9). That is, the more oblique the osteotomy, the more the rotated distal fragment will come up out of flexion and into proper coronal alignment. This osteotomy also produces a broader bone surface for healing, rotational stability without the supplemental use of plates or screws, and a very pleasing radiographic appearance on the anteroposterior x-ray film. Butt cuts and step cuts, although technically easier, do not share these virtues and should be avoided (Fig. 63.10).

In approaching these procedures, a long midline extensile approach is most helpful, exposing both the arthroplasty and the fracture. In general it is best to deal with the fracture first, such that its extent and requirements be known early in the case so that bone graft material can be thawed and prepared for use. Once the fracture has been identified and exposed, one can remove the failed total knee, taking greatest

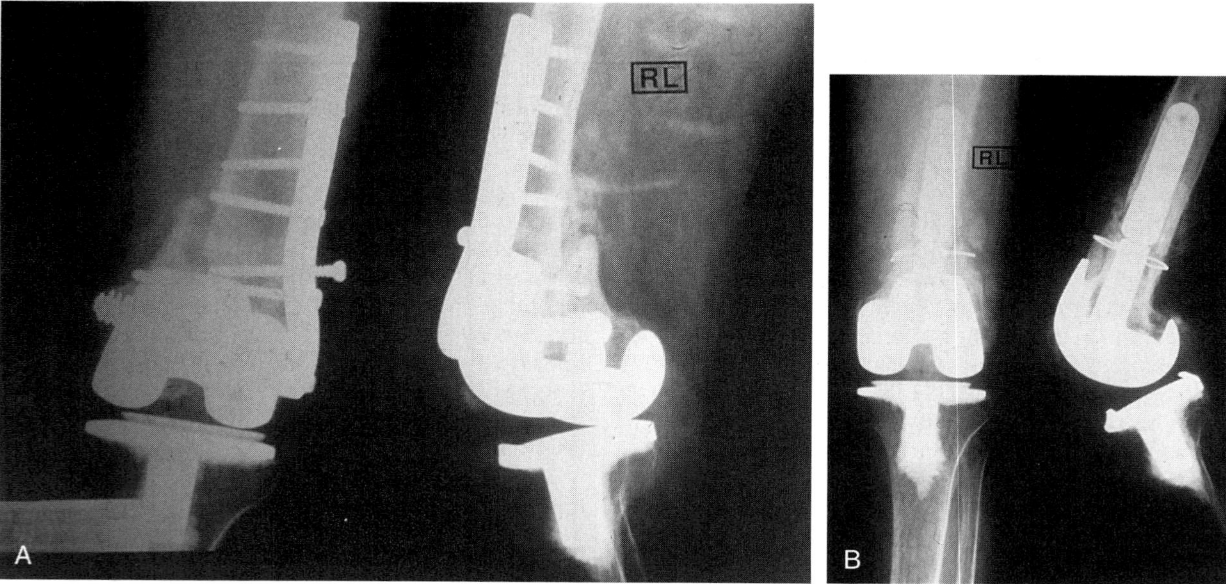

FIGURE 63.8 ➢ Nonunion of supracondylar fracture with stiff TKA, treated with femoral revisional arthroplasty and intramedullary stems.

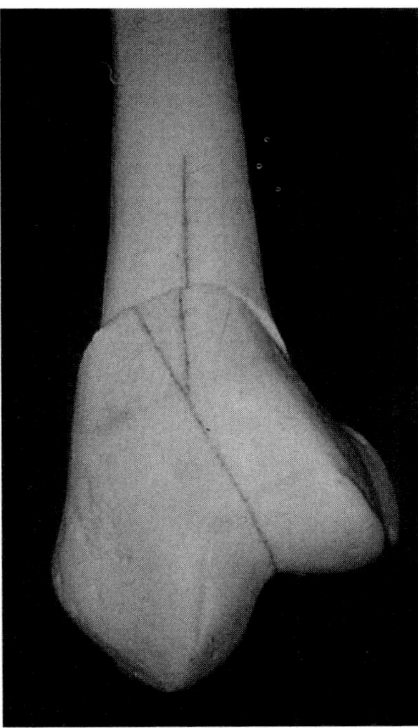

FIGURE 63.9 ➢ Oblique supracondylar femoral osteotomy showing potential angle of corrected alignment.

care with the femoral component so that an intercondylar infraction is not added to the existing supracondylar fracture. Should that unfortunate event occur, all is not lost, as the femoral condyles with their attendant collateral ligaments can be preserved and cemented to the femoral prosthesis at the time of reconstruction. Nonetheless, this complication significantly increases the technical difficulty of the procedure and is best avoided.

As previously observed, the severity of the fracture and its degree of comminution routinely exceed the radiographic appearance. One must thus be prepared to use an intercalary graft to restore the bony anatomy of the femoral metaphysis. This allows the preservation of limb length, the restoration of rotational alignment, and the appropriate substrate onto which comminuted host bone fragments or supplemental allograft can be secured. If allograft is not available, a large proximal femoral defect may result, radically increasing the chances of nonunion or malunion above the total knee. Long intramedullary stems may be necessary, and the cementation of these stems should be done advisedly but enthusiastically if it is necessary for stability at the time of the reduction. As a general rule, unless alignment, rotation, and stability are achieved at surgery, the construct will ultimately fail.

The results of simultaneous revisional arthroplasty and fracture stabilization have been reported several times. The largest series by McLaren and colleagues,[28] found a satisfactory result in 24 of 25 knees. Seven patients reported by Kraay and associates[23] required cemented fixation of the stems, semiconstrained prostheses, and significant bone graft material. Although the osseous results were satisfactory, two of the seven patients had sufficient instability to require chronic bracing. Cordeiro and coworkers[6] described five fractures treated with custom long-stemmed components, all of which healed with good result. Suffice it to say that these results were achieved despite heroic procedures requiring extensive experience and abundant resources.

POSTOPERATIVE PERIPROSTHETIC TIBIAL FRACTURES

True tibial periprosthetic fractures are actually quite rare, possibly because of the fairly standard use of an intramedullary stem, the supplemental support against

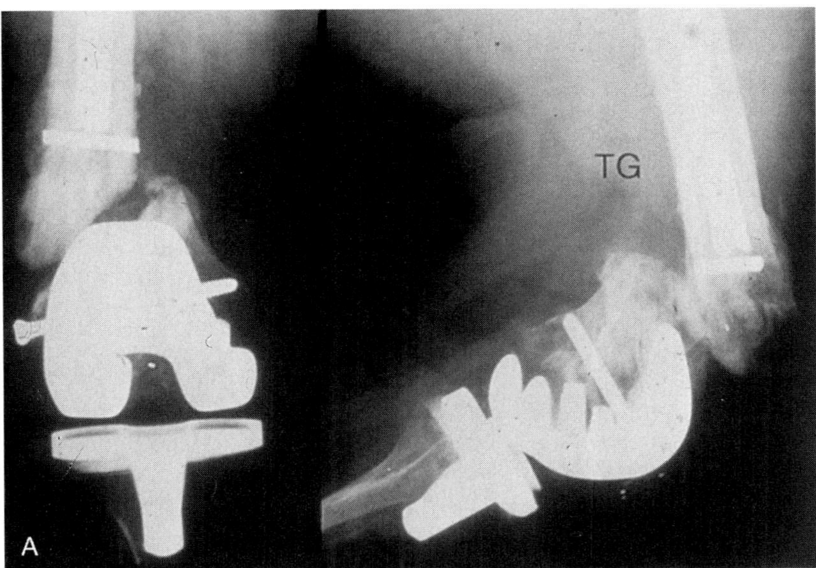

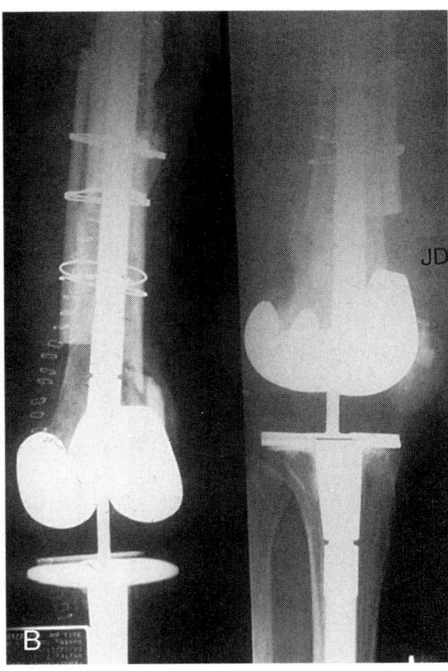

FIGURE 63.10 ➢ Supracondylar nonunion treated with oblique osteotomy, revisional arthroplasty, and bone graft supplementation.

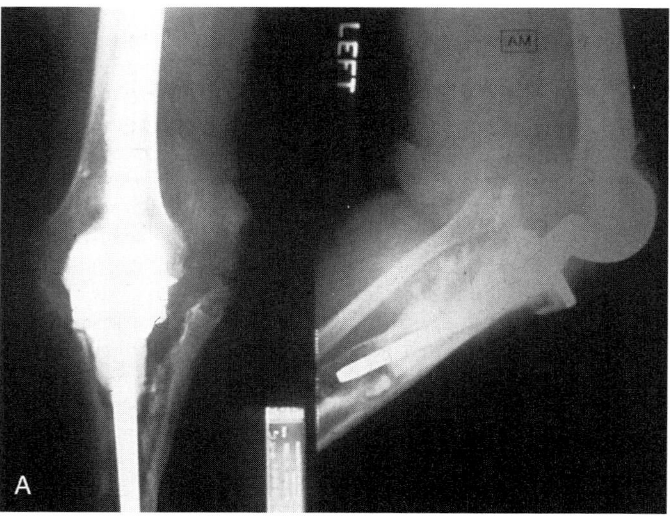

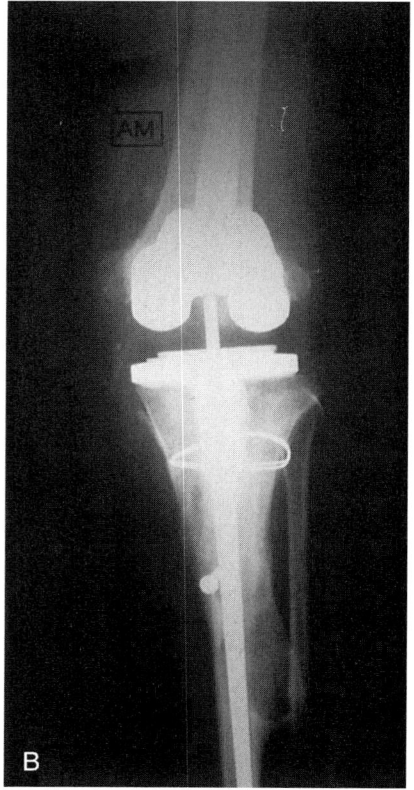

FIGURE 63.11 ➢ Comminuted tibial periprosthetic fracture around a hinged prosthesis, treated with massive bone allograft and intramedullary stems.

torque and shear provided by the intact fibula, or the fact that most loads visited upon the tibia are compressive in nature and not as exaggerated by periprosthetic stress shielding as is the femur. For whatever reason, few orthopedic surgeons have been forced to confront a periprosthetic tibial fracture (Fig. 63.11).

The definitive review of tibial periprosthetic fractures was reported by Felix and associates,[10] in which they reviewed 102 fractures after TKA. Eighty-three

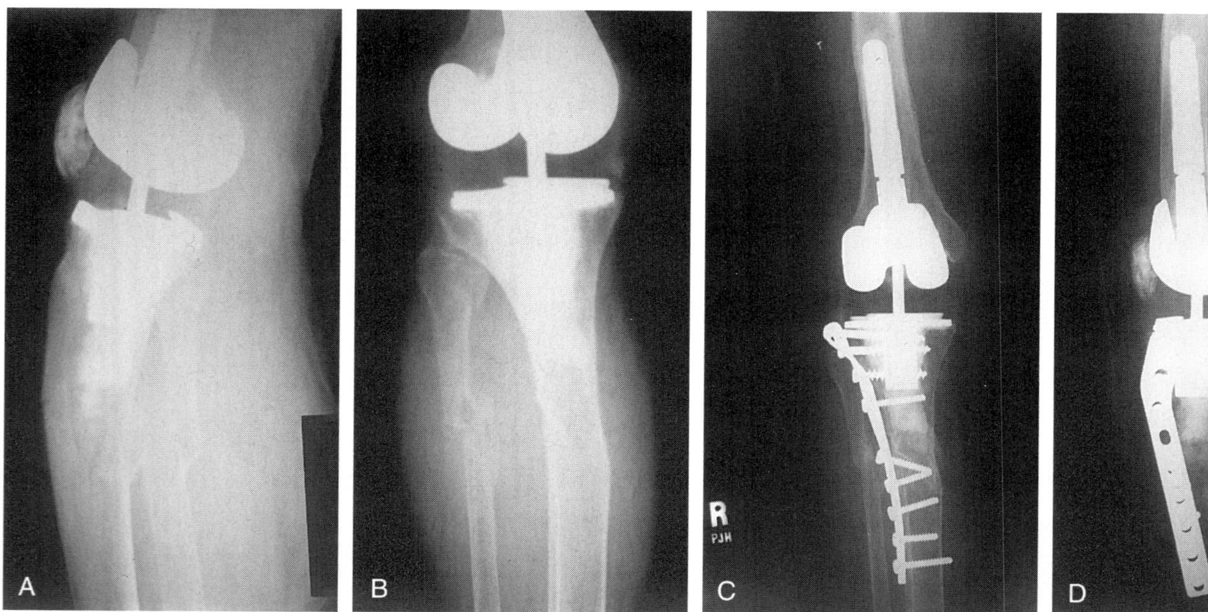

FIGURE 63.12 ➢ Tibia-fibula fracture below tibial prosthesis, treated with open reduction and internal fixation.

were postoperative, and their classification system is helpful from a conceptual if not therapeutic viewpoint. Type I fractures occurred at the tibial plateau and were largely the result of varus malalignment. This is similar to a previous series of 15 fractures reported by Rand and Coventry in 1980.[35] The tibial component is frequently loose, and revision of the arthroplasty is required with supplemental reconstruction of the medial femoral bone. This category largely represents stress fractures secondary to malalignment, and the advent of intramedullary instrumentation systems has radically reduced the incidence of this problem.

Type II fractures, which occurred around the prosthetic stem, were largely traumatic in origin; because of prosthetic loosening, they required revisional surgery with extended stem stabilization. In all, 22 patients were identified with this injury, and the results of surgical correction were generally excellent.

Type III fractures occurring distal to the tip of the intramedullary stem were largely traumatic in origin, but were not necessarily associated with loosening of the tibial prosthesis. These fractures were treated variously with casting or open reduction and internal fixation, again with excellent results. Only 17 patients sustained this injury in the Mayo Clinic experience (Fig. 63.12A, D).

Type IV fractures involved the tibial tuberosity and were extremely rare, with only two examples being identified. The stability of the prosthesis was not jeopardized, and standard fracture treatment techniques provided excellent results.

POSTOPERATIVE PERIPROSTHETIC PATELLAR FRACTURES

Periprosthetic patellar fractures are also quite infrequent, and their true incidence is obscured by the fact that most are asymptomatic. The principal factors responsible for their occurrence are diminished vascularity and increased stress after an arthroplasty. The arthrotomy necessary for any TKA necessarily diminishes the vascular supply to the extensor mechanism. Additional maneuvers such as fat pad excision, lateral retinacular release, and quadriceps snip or turndown further compound this problem, leading to a susceptibility to fracture and to avascular necrosis of the patellar bone. Some reduction in patellar sensation is also produced by resurfacing, and attempts at full denervation to diminish potential anterior knee pain are probably unwise.

The bone resection necessary for placement of patellar prosthesis also compromises bone strength. Excessive resection — generally considered below 15 mm of residual bone — clearly predisposes to patellar fragility and fracture.[39] Interestingly, insufficient bone resection is also problematic, as it creates an "overstuffed joint" wherein increased patellar or femoral component thickness produces excessive stresses frequently leading to proximal or distal avulsion fractures. Component malalignment (particularly inadequate external rotation of the femoral component) produces transverse stresses that may lead to similar fractures. Excessive weight is also a consideration, as the quadriceps is known to generate as much as eight times body weight to effect rising from a seated position or descending stairs. Thus, patellar resurfacing in the morbidly obese may require judicious consideration.

The majority of postoperative periprosthetic patellar fractures are indeed asymptomatic; some are accompanied by rupture or dysfunction of the extensor mechanism and are quite apparent to the patient. Pain, swelling, and a hemarthrosis may ensue. Many of these incidents occur, as one might expect, with stair climbing and rising from a seated position. Interestingly, while direct falls onto the resurfaced patella can produce fractures, these are the least common mechanism of all.

The majority of periprosthetic patellar fractures should be treated conservatively with restricted motion and observation, as most will heal with minimal if any loss of function. As with other periprosthetic fractures, two issues determine the potential need for operative treatment: the stability of the patellar prosthesis and the integrity of the extensor mechanism. Obviously, if the patellar button is loose or displaced, operative intervention is highly likely. It should be noted, however, that many patellar buttons are loose and asymptomatic, covered by a "patellar meniscus" of fibrous tissue that maintains them in their place. It is thus displacement more than radiographic loosening of the patellar button that would dictate operative intervention.

The integrity of the extensor mechanism is also a concern; Hozack and colleagues[21] have shown that the results of conservative or surgical repairs are compromised when the patient presents with an extensor lag. In most instances it is preferable to place the patient in a restricted motion brace for at least 6 weeks, with gentle range of motion thereafter. Although the mild extensor lag may persist, the continuity of the extensor mechanism may be sufficient to avoid surgery.

Vertical fractures clearly are at less risk to displace than transverse fractures, which have the potential for late extensor dysfunction. The transverse fractures are often easily treated surgically with standard tension-banding techniques. Avulsion of the superior or inferior pole of the patella may produce a patella baja or patella alta, and reconstitution of the extensor — with or without resection of the avulsed fragment — will be required. These cases should be approached with some trepidation, however, as the repairs are often more difficult than imagined. Occasionally one encounters avascular necrosis of the patella at surgery, and a patellectomy may be necessary. This, of course, compromises extensor strength significantly, as well as the anteroposterior stability of the arthroplasty.

Supplementation of an extensor repair should also be considered. Cadambi and Engh have popularized the semitendinosus graft[4] with a supplemental cerclage wire from the patella to the tibial tubercle. The authors' preference is to use a long strip of fascia lata, resected with a tendon stripper from the lateral thigh, and left intact at its insertion into Gerdy's tubercle. The proximal tail of the tendon is woven through the extensor mechanism and secured to the medial tibial metaphysis, providing a very strong supplement to the primary extensor repair.

Some element of diminished vascularity is responsible in almost all patellar fractures and extensor disruptions. More aggressive surgeries to correct this problem may only devascularize the extensor further. Very occasionally, an entire extensor allograft may be necessary to reconstitute limb extension. This technique has been described in detail by Booth and Nazarian,[2] with good results in 36 of 38 patients.

Despite all the ingenious attempts at reconstruction of a periprosthetic patellar fracture, the results have generally been dismal. Four articles from the same year show Goldberg and colleagues[14] reporting poor surgical results in 13 of 19 knees; Grace and Sim[15] had failures in 3 of 8 procedures; Hozack and associates[21] had only 1 of 7 patients with an extensor lag with a good result after surgery; and Brick and Scott[3] had failures of fixation in 3 of 4 surgically treated fractures. Clearly, there is a great deal of room for improvement in the management of all periprosthetic fractures.

References

1. Barker LG, Ryan WG, Paul AS, et al: Zickel supracondylar nail to treat supracondylar fracture of the femur in patients with total knee replacements. Internat J Orthop Trauma 3:183, 1993.
2. Booth RE Jr, Nazarian DG, Paczkoskie V, et al: Extensor mechanism allografts in total knee arthroplasty. Accepted by Clin Orthop for publication in 1999.
3. Brick, GW, Scott RD: The patellofemoral component of total knee arthroplasty. Clin Orthop 231:163, 1988.
4. Cadambi A, Engh GA: Use of a semitendinosus tendon autogenous graft for rupture of the patellar ligament after total knee arthroplasty. A report of seven cases. J Bone Joint Surg Am 74: 974, 1992.
5. Chen F, Mont MA, Bachner RS: Management of ipsilateral supracondylar femur fractures following total knee arthroplasty. J Arthroplasty 9:521, 1994.
6. Cordeiro EN, Costa RC, Carazzato JG, et al: Periprosthetic fractures in patients with total knee arthroplasties. Clin Orthop 252: 182, 1990.
7. Culp RW, Schmidt RG, Hanks G, et al: Supracondylar fracture of the femur following prosthetic knee arthroplasty. Clin Orthop 222:212, 1987.
8. Emerson RH Jr, Head WC, Malinin TI: Reconstruction of patellar tendon rupture after total knee arthroplasty with an extensor mechanism allograft. Clin Orthop 260:154, 1990.
9. Engh GA, Ammeen DJ: Periprosthetic fractures adjacent to total knee implants. J Bone Joint Surg Am 79:1100, 1997.
10. Felix NA, Stuart MJ, Hanssen AD: Periprosthetic fractures of the tibia associated with total knee arthroplasty. Clin Orthop 345: 113, 1997.
11. Figgie HE III, Goldberg VM, Figgie MP, et al: The effect of alignment of the implant on fractures of the patella after condylar total knee arthroplasty. J Bone Joint Surg Am 71:1031, 1989.
12. Figgie MP, Goldberg VM, Figgie HE III, et al: The results of treatment of supracondylar fracture above total knee arthroplasty. J Arthroplasty 5:267, 1990.
13. Fipp G: Stress fractures of the femoral neck following total knee arthroplasty. J Arthroplasty 3:347, 1988.
14. Goldberg VM, Figgie HE III, Inglis AE, et al: Patellar fracture type and prognosis in condylar total knee arthroplasty. Clin Orthop 236:115, 1988.
15. Grace JN, Sim FH: Fracture of the patella after total knee arthroplasty. Clin Orthop 230:168, 1988.
16. Hardy DC, Delince PE, Yasik E, et al: Stress fracture of the hip. An unusual complication of total knee arthroplasty. Clin Orthop 281:140, 1992.
17. Healy WL, Siliski JM, Incavo SJ: Operative treatment of distal femoral fractures proximal to total knee replacements. J Bone Joint Surg Am 75:27, 1993.
18. Henry SL: Management of supracondylar fractures proximal to total knee arthroplasty with the GSH supracondylar nail. Contemp Orthop 31:231, 1995.
19. Henry SL, Booth RE Jr: Management of supracondylar fractures above total knee prostheses. Tech Orthop 9:243, 1994.
20. Howes JP, Sakka SA, Riley TBH: A modified prosthesis with an interlocking nail stem for the treatment of supracondylar femoral fractures after total knee replacement: A report of three cases. Orthopedics. Internat ed 3:303, 1995.
21. Hozack WJ, Goll SR, Lotke PA, et al: The treatment of patellar fractures after total knee arthroplasty. Clin Orthop 236:123, 1988.
22. Jabczenski FF, Crawford M: Retrograde intramedullary nailing of supracondylar femur fractures above total knee arthroplasty. A preliminary report of four cases. J Arthroplasty 10:95, 1995.
23. Kraay MJ, Goldberg VM, Figgie MP, et al: Distal femoral replacement with allograft/prosthetic reconstruction for treatment of supracondylar fractures in patients with total knee arthroplasty. J Arthroplasty 7:7, 1992.
24. Krackow KA, Thomas SC, Jones LC: A new stitch for ligament-tendon fixation. Brief note. J Bone Joint Surg Am 68:764, 1986.
25. Le Blanc JM: Patellar complications in total knee arthroplasty. A literature review. Orthop Rev 18:296, 1989.
26. Lewis PL, Rorabeck CH: Periprosthetic fractures. In Engh GA, Rorabeck CH, eds: Revision Total Knee Arthroplasty. Baltimore, Williams & Wilkins, 1997, pp. 275–295.
27. Lombardi AV Jr, Mallory TH, Waterman RA, et al: Intercondylar distal femoral fracture. An unreported complication of posterior-stabilized total knee arthroplasty. J Arthroplasty 10:643, 1995.
28. McLaren AC, Dupont JA, Schroeber DC: Open reduction internal fixation of supracondylar fractures above total knee arthroplasties using the intramedullary supracondylar rod. Clin Orthop 302:94, 1994.
29. Madsen F, Kjersgaard-Andersen P, Juhl M, et al: A custom-made prosthesis for the treatment of supracondylar femoral fractures after total knee arthroplasty: Report of four cases. J Orthop Trauma 3:333, 1989.
30. Maniar RN, Umlas ME, Rodriguez JA, et al: Supracondylar femoral fracture above a PFC posterior cruciate–substituting total knee arthroplasty treated with supracondylar nailing. A unique technical problem. J Arthroplasty 11:637, 1996.
31. Merkel KD, Johnson EW Jr: Supracondylar fracture of the femur after total knee arthroplasty. J Bone Joint Surg Am 68:29, 1986.
32. Moran MC, Brick GW, Sledge CB, et al: Supracondylar femoral fracture following total knee arthroplasty. Clin Orthop 324:196, 1996.
33. Murrell GA, Nunley JA: Interlocked supracondylar intramedullary nails for supracondylar fractures after total knee arthroplasty. A new treatment method. J Arthroplasty 10:37, 1995.
34. Nielsen BF, Petersen VS, Varmarken JE: Fracture of the femur after knee arthroplasty. Acta Orthop Scand 59:155, 1988.
35. Rand JA, Coventry MB: Stress fractures after total knee arthroplasty. J Bone Joint Surg Am 62:226, 1980.
36. Ritter MA, Keating EM, Farris PM, et al: Rush rod fixation of supracondylar fractures above total knee arthroplasties. J Arthroplasty 10:213, 1995.
37. Rolston LR, Christ DJ, Halpern A, et al: Treatment of supracondylar fractures of the femur proximal to a total knee arthroplasty. A report of four cases. J Bone Joint Surg Am 77:924, 1995.
38. Rosenfield AL, McQueen D: Zickel supracondylar fixation device and Dall-Miles cables for supracondylar fractures of the femur following total knee arthroplasty. Tech Orthop 6:86, 1991.
39. Scott RD, Turoff N, Ewald FC: Stress fracture of the patella following duopatellar total knee arthroplasty with patellar resurfacing. Clin Orthop 170:147, 1982.
40. Zehntner MK, Ganz R: Internal fixation of supracondylar fractures after condylar total knee arthroplasty. Clin Orthop 293: 219, 1993.

SECTION IX

The Pediatric Knee

64

Normal Growth and Development in the Skeletally Immature Knee

J. CRAIG MORRISON • GREGORY A. MENCIO

INTRODUCTION

More attention has been given to the development of the human knee than to any other joint. The size, complex nature, and clinical importance of the knee joint have made the knee the subject of intense interest. Although the literature is extensive, it is admittedly incomplete. In this chapter, we will attempt to summarize the literature pertaining to the development of the knee. The purpose is to outline its normal growth and development. Where applicable, we will discuss how deviations from normal lead to the development of clinically relevant anomalies and how aspects of normal development can sometimes mimic the pathologic conditions we strive to identify and treat. (Chapter 1 provides a more in-depth survey of the embryology of the knee. However, because of the gradual nature of growth and development of the skeletally immature knee and the lack of a definite demarcation in development between the prenatal period and birth, a brief discussion of embryological anatomy is also included here.)

Embryologically, all synovial joints are formed in a similar manner (Fig. 64.1). After the limb buds appear, chondrification of primitive mesenchymal cells (the blastema) begins in the regions of future bones, stopping short of the areas corresponding to the future joints. In these sites, a homogenous interzone of blastema persists, from which the synovium, joint capsule, menisci, and intra-articular ligaments eventually develop. The major step in synovial joint formation is cavitation of the interzone. In the knee, three separate cavities form initially and, as the process proceeds, up to six cavities eventually develop. The cavities include the suprapatellar, medial and lateral meniscofemoral, and medial and lateral meniscotibial, which coalesce to create a joint similar in structure and appearance to that of the adult knee, and the tibiofibular joint, which remains separate (Fig. 64.2).

After birth, the knee changes more in size than shape. The epiphyses ossify the menisci, the ligaments mature, and the knee gradually becomes more recognizable on radiographs. Angular alignment changes from varus to valgus.[12, 29] At a gross and microscopic level, form evolves to allow optimal function in the changing biomechanical environment of the growing child.

THE TIBIOFEMORAL ANGLE

Changes in the angular alignment of the knee are undoubtedly the most visually obvious in the developing limb. Angular malalignment between the femur and tibia (bowlegs and knock-knees) is a common source of parental concern and of office visits to the orthopedist. The development of the tibiofemoral angle in children is well defined.[12, 29] Working knowledge of this natural history is essential in order to differentiate normal anatomy and variations from pathological malalignment.

The alignment of the lower limbs normally progresses from a maximal amount of varus angulation at birth to valgus in early childhood (Fig. 64.3). On average, the tibiofemoral angle measures about 16 degrees varus at birth, gradually straightens by about 18 months to 2 years of age, and reaches maximum valgus by age 4 years. Females tend to have slightly more genu valgum than males (about 2 degrees). As growth continues, the valgus alignment slowly decreases to more closely approximate the physiological valgus of adulthood by 7 to 9 years of age. In adolescence there is little further change, although after 14 years of age boys show a gradual but significant decrease in valgus compared with girls. By age 16 years, valgus angulation averages about 4 degrees in males compared with about 5 degrees in females.

Clinically, it is useful to follow the angular alignment of the limbs at different stages of development by measuring the intercondylar (IC) and intermalleolar (IM) distances.[12] The distance between the femoral condyles (IC distance), as measured in the supine position with the medial malleoli just touching, can be used to quantify changes in varus alignment. At 6 months of age, the mean IC distance is about 2.6 cm and should decrease to 0 cm by age 2 years, reflecting normal development. After the onset of valgus, the distance between the medial malleoli, or the IM distance, can be used to follow changes in angular alignment of the limb. Normally, the IM distance is at a maximum of 3.5 cm (± 2.0 cm) by age 3 to 4 years. Measurements within 2 standard deviations of the mean are considered normal; therefore, IM distances as high as 8 cm may reflect normal variation in children up to the age of 11 years.[4, 12, 29, 32]

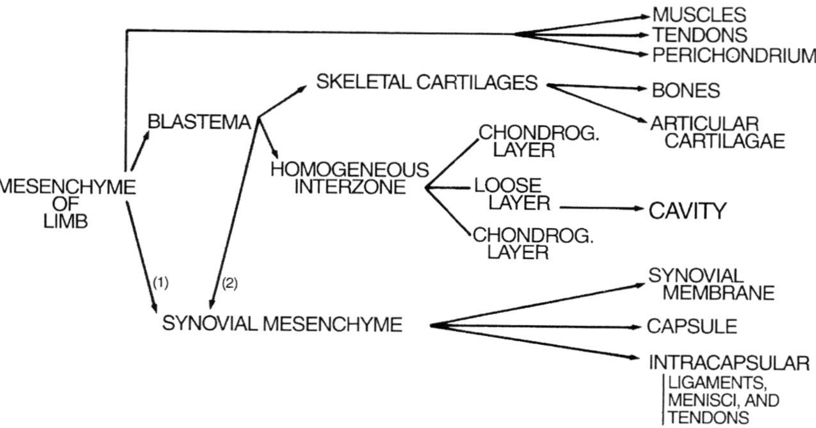

FIGURE 64.1 ➢ Flow diagram showing the stages in the embryological development of a synovial joint. (From O'Rahilly R, Gardner E: The embryology of movable joints. In Sokoloff L, ed: The Joints and Synovial Fluid, vol 1. New York, Academic Press, Inc. 1978, p 77.)

THE DISTAL FEMUR

The epiphysis of the distal femur forms from a single ossific nucleus. It is the first epiphysis to ossify and the last to fuse. Ossification of the distal femoral epiphysis is evident in the prenatal period between 32 and 40 weeks of gestation. This process, like that of all secondary ossification, begins with the appearance of well-defined cartilage canals early in fetal development. These canals form from mesenchymal cells that penetrate the avascular cartilaginous anlage. The mesenchymal cells eventually line these canals and differentiate into vascular elements forming distinct arterioles, capillaries, and veins. Shortly after this differentiation, the chondrocytes in the central epiphysis hypertrophy, mitotic activity increases, and ossification commences. Presumably, these vascular networks supply a source of osteoblastic precursor cells that contribute to the initiation of this process. As ossification expands, the canals lose their organization, fill with fibrous tissue elements, and become incorporated into the ossific nucleus.[2]

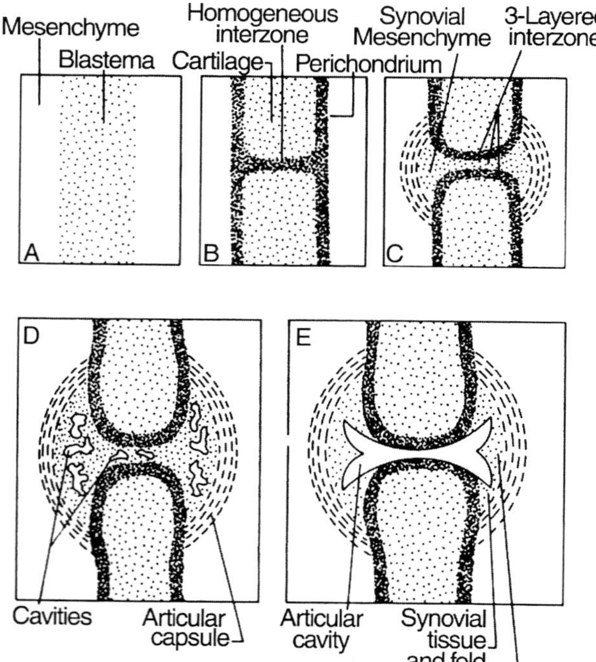

FIGURE 64.2 ➢ Stages in the embryological development of the knee joint. Chondrification of primitive mesenchymal cells (blastema) stops short of the area corresponding to the site of the future joint *(A, B)*. Development of a homogeneous interzone and synovial mesenchyme from which the joint cavity and soft-tissue elements (synovium, joint capsule, menisci, and intra-articular ligaments) are formed *(C)*. Cavitation of the interzone into compartments (suprapatellar, medial and lateral meniscofemoral, medial and lateral meniscotibial), which eventually coalesce to form the knee joint *(D,E)*. (From O'Rahilly R, Gardner E: The embryology of movable joints. In Sokoloff L, ed: The Joints and Synovial Fluid, vol 1. New York, Academic Press, Inc., 1978, p 77.)

The distal femoral epiphysis is the largest epiphysis in the body and, during development, grows more rapidly than any other. Variations in the pattern of ossification exist and can be erroneously interpreted as evidence of disease. Therefore, it is important to have some knowledge of the normal existence of irregularities in the developing epiphysis. Caffey et al[3] delineated some of these variants in their review of 147 radiographs of normal knees in children between the ages of 3 and 13 years. Caffey and colleagues divided the variants into three groups. Group I showed roughening of the epiphyseal margins, with occasional separate foci of calcification. In group II there were larger localized marginal irregularities that appeared as indentations. Group III was similar to group II except that there was an isolated bone island lying in the marginal indentation (Fig. 64.4).

An explanation for these radiographic irregularities can be extrapolated from an understanding of the epiphyseal ossification process. In a rapidly growing epiphysis, the zones of proliferating cartilage and provisional calcification are deeper than in a slowly growing epiphysis. During the rapid-growth phase, the process of cartilage proliferation and provisional calcification does not proceed in the usual orderly fashion, resulting in a deep zone within the epiphysis in which spotty mineralization occurs. Foci of provisional calcification can appear beyond the image of the main calcified mass of the primary ossific nucleus,

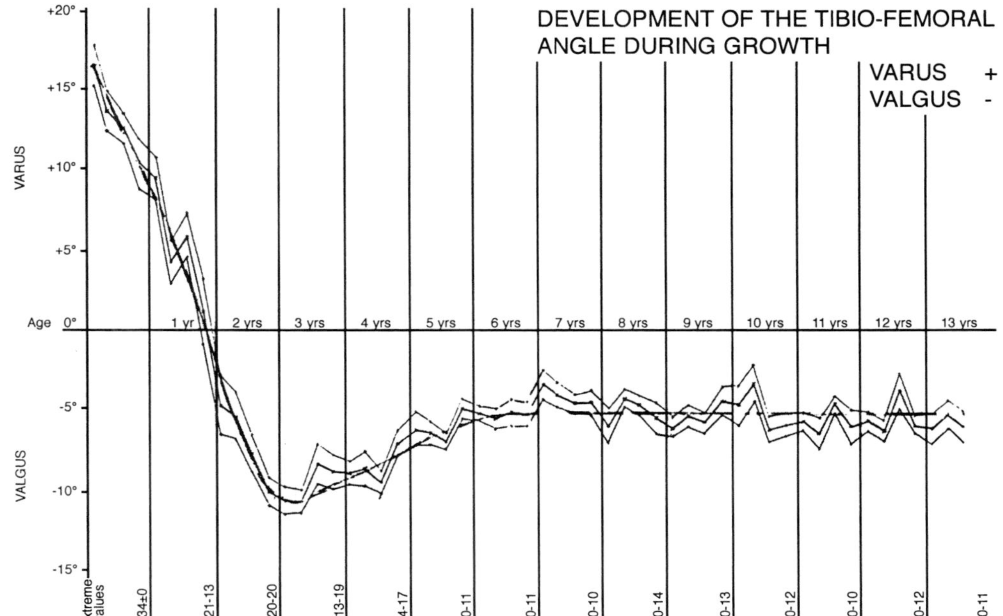

FIGURE 64.3 ➢ Graph illustrating the development of the tibiofemoral angle during growth, based on measurement from 1480 examinations of 979 children. The jagged lines represent the mean value and standard deviation at any given age and the smooth line the general trend. Note the progression from maximal varus at birth to maximal valgus by about 3 to 4 years and resolution to physiological valgus of adulthood by 7 to 9 years of age. (From Salenius P, Vankka E: The development of the tibiofemoral angle in children. J Bone Joint Surg Am 57:260, 1975.)

giving rise to the radiographic appearance seen in group I variants (see Fig. 64.4A). As the ossification process proceeds, osteoblasts invade and replace the partially calcified cartilage in the periphery with trabecular bone, and a regular outline again appears.[3]

In group II variation, provisional calcification is relatively retarded in a focal area, producing a radiolucent defect (see Fig. 64.4B). Within this defect, a focus of calcification can develop apart from the main epiphysis, giving rise to the appearance typical of group III variants (see Fig. 64.4B). The irregularities characteristic of groups II and III mimic the radiographic appear-

FIGURE 64.4 ➢ Normal variations in the ossification patterns of the distal femoral epiphysis. Variation occurs when the normal process of calcification cannot keep pace with the rate of cartilage proliferation during periods of growth. Group 1 variation *(A, arrowhead)* is characterized by roughening of the epiphyseal margins and scattered foci of calcification. Group II *(B, solid arrow)* variation is characterized by a more focal radiolucent defect, reflecting a more focal retardation in the process of provisional calcification. In group III variation *(B, open arrow)*, a central island of ossification develops within the radiolucent area and may develop apart from the main epiphysis.

ance of osteochondritis dissecans and are usually present bilaterally. With increasing age, all of these irregularities steadily decrease from prevalences as high as 90% at age 4 years to less than 20% by age 12 years. Nonetheless, it is conceivable that during the periods of growth acceleration, a transition from smooth to irregular outline may be repeated.[3, 26]

In addition to rapid growth, the distal femur also provides an abundance of growth. Seventy percent of the growth of the femur and 37% of the growth of the lower extremity come from the distal femoral physis. Thus, it contributes more to longitudinal growth than any other physis. The rate of growth is estimated to be approximately 0.9 cm/y. It slows considerably at skeletal-age 13 years in females and 15 years in males. The timing of complete closure is variable and may occur as late as the 3rd decade.

Orientation of this physis is horizontal, but it is not at all smooth. It undulates markedly from side to side as well as front to back. The convex processes of the metaphysis interdigitate with their respective cup-shaped counterparts in the epiphysis, creating a topographic configuration that is inherently stable to shear and torsional forces. The size of this physis and its complex topography explain the frequency of partial or complete growth arrest following traumatic separation. First, significant force is required to cause separation of this growth plate. Second, damage to the germinal cells of the physis may occur as the interdigitations displace and grind against each other at the moment of injury or during attempted reduction maneuvers. Finally, the complex configuration of the physis makes anatomic reduction difficult to achieve.[1]

THE PATELLA AND PATELLOFEMORAL ARTICULATION

The condensation of cells that ultimately form the patella develops in the 7th week of gestation and is located deep to the patellar tendon rather than embedded in it.[10] These cells form an expanding mass of unossified cartilage that is morphologically similar to the final shape of the mature patella. Ossification commences between 4 and 6 years of age, begins centrally and, like the distal femur, may be marked by irregular, granular margins (Fig. 64.5A). The process is often multifocal, and as many as six irregular centers may be seen. These coalesce quickly to form a single, rapidly enlarging, ossific nucleus. However, a distinct separation may persist between the superior and inferior portions of the ossification center, which may be mistaken for a fracture (Fig. 64.5B).[14]

A bipartite patella is another variant that may be mistaken for a fracture. Although a single case of a bipartite patella has been reported following trauma in a previously normal knee, this condition most likely represents a developmental anomaly. It is characterized by the presence of an accessory ossification cen-

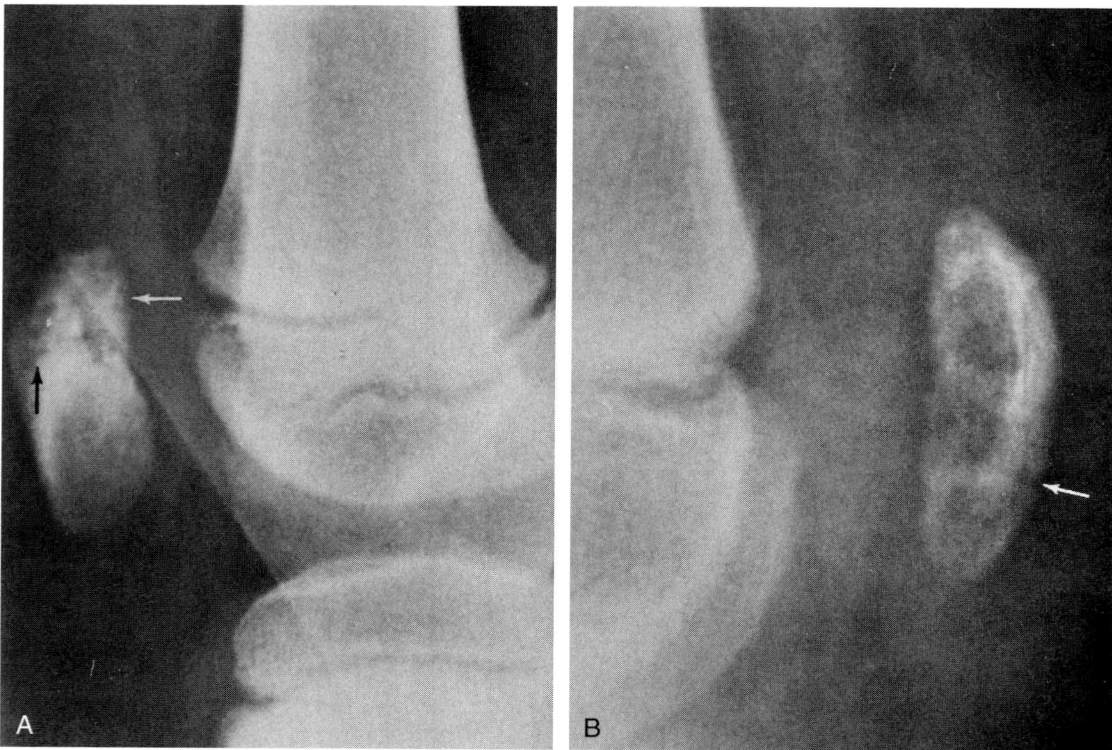

FIGURE 64.5 ➢ Variations in the pattern of ossification of the patella. Ossification characterized by irregular, granular margins *(A)*. Persistent separation between ossification centers mimicking fracture *(B)*. (From Keats TE, ed: An Atlas of Normal Roentgen Variants That May Simulate Disease. Chicago, Yearbook Medical Publishers, 1973, p 197.)

ter in the superolateral part of the patella that is never incorporated into the primary nucleus.[24] There is cartilaginous and articular congruity between the fragments despite the appearance of osseous incongruity. A separate ossification center at the inferior pole of the patella is not believed to exist as a normal variant. In the absence of acute disruption of the extensor mechanism, bony fragmentation in this area usually represents a chronic overuse syndrome known as Sinding-Larsen-Johansson (the patellar equivalent of Osgood-Schlatter disease).[22]

By the 2nd decade of life, the ossific expansion of the patella slows significantly, allowing the formation of a well-defined subchondral plate at the chondro-osseous margins. This peripheral maturation gives the patella a smooth appearance except at the superolateral region, which often remains irregular until adolescence (or persists as a bipartite patella). The trabecular bone also changes with age, responding to the biomechanical demands of an enlarging quadriceps muscle mass and longer moment arm. The trabeculae progressively thicken and orient longitudinally as seen on the lateral radiograph.[22, 28]

Normally, the medial and lateral articular surfaces of the patella are equal and subtend equivalent angles in all stages of development. However, the radiographic appearance does not accurately reflect the actual articular contours of the patella until after 10 to 12 years of age.[22] In a similar manner, the osseous angle of the femoral sulcus does not truly reflect its cartilaginous model until adolescence. Although the early radiographic appearance suggests otherwise, the patellofemoral articulation has been demonstrated by ultrasound to be well formed and congruent even in the neonate.[19] Thus, the actual depth of the femoral sulcus does not change. Instead, the changing radiographic appearance of the sulcus actually reflects the osseous maturation of the existing cartilaginous model of the distal femur. Accompanying this change is a progressive thinning of cartilage lining the medial and lateral facets so that by adolescence the thickest cartilage lies in the deepest part of the sulcus. A shallow sulcus angle (normal, 145 degrees), either the result of congenital dysplasia or the consequence of maltracking with gradual plastic deformation, is thought to play a role in the development of patellar instability. Radiographic measurements have been described to assess the sulcus angle; however, the developmental chronology of the patellofemoral articulation precludes using these parameters until adolescence.[9, 15] On the other hand, ultrasound may allow detection of abnormalities in the earlier stages of growth.

The morphological development of a child's patella also explains the low incidence and differing presentation of patellar fractures in comparison to adults. The osseous portion of the patella is cushioned by a surrounding layer of thick cartilage, making direct trauma a rare mechanism of injury.[28] However, the transitional chondro-osseous composition of the peripheral margin of the patella, which is weaker than the attached soft tissues, makes avulsion of the superior, inferior, or medial poles a much more common mechanism of fracture. In these injuries, the bulk of the avulsed fragment is usually cartilaginous, and radiographs typically underrepresent the true extent of skeletal involvement, often showing only a tiny bone fragment despite the clinical presentation of pain, joint effusion, and extensor mechanism disruption.[11] For the same reasons, osteochondral fractures of the patella or either femoral condyle following acute dislocation of the patella can be missed or underestimated, making the presence of a sizable loose body or significant intra-articular incongruity.

THE PROXIMAL TIBIA

At birth, the proximal tibial epiphysis consists entirely of a cartilaginous anlage that is very similar morphologically to its shape at the time of skeletal maturity. The height of the epiphysis is greater on the lateral than on the medial side. In skeletally immature cadavers, even the normal posterior slope of the articular surface has been shown to be present in this early stage of development.[23] The physis is transverse, and its interface with the proximal metaphysis is smooth.

The ossific nucleus appears radiographically as early as 2 months of age and is well established by 3 months of age. Ossification begins as a centrally located sphere slightly closer to the metaphyseal than to the articular surface.[23, 28] Over the next 5 to 6 years, the ossification center enlarges peripherally, taking on a more elliptical shape. This rapid expansion often results in irregular chondro-osseous margins and the appearance of accessory peripheral ossicles, which may be mistaken for trauma or musculoskeletal sepsis (i.e., septic arthritis or subacute osteomyelitis).

At 6 to 7 years of age, the rapid peripheral expansion of the ossific nucleus slows. This stage of development is characterized radiographically by smooth epiphyseal borders. All accessory ossific granules have coalesced with the central ossific nucleus, and the margins of the ellipse stabilize at a point 1 to 3 mm from the metaphyseal rim. In early adolescence, the margins again expand to become even with the periphery of the metaphysis.[23]

The intercondylar eminence develops concomitantly with the proximal epiphysis. By 2 years of age, there is a central extension of the cartilaginous epiphysis corresponding to the site of development of the tibial spines. Ossification of this structure is visible above the level of the tibial articular surface as a single radiopaque entity by 5 to 6 years of age. The spines continue to mature, and by age 10 they appear as distinct anterior (medial) and posterior (lateral) structures of varying size. Rarely, the eminence may be tripartite.[23] The eminence serves as the site of attachment of the cruciate ligaments and is not covered by articular cartilage after chondro-osseous maturation is complete.[18]

Fractures of the tibial spines are most likely to occur in late childhood and early adolescence when these rapidly growing, but incompletely ossified, structures are more susceptible to tensile stress than the attached cruciate ligaments. Failure occurs by osteochondral avulsion rather than by ligamentous disruption. Fracture of the anterior spine by the anterior cruciate ligament is the more common injury, but isolated avulsion of the posterior spine (by the posterior cruciate ligament) may also occur.[28] In radiographic studies of the developing proximal tibia, the relatively short spines in the earliest stages of ossification (7 to 10 years of age) were not always appreciated with standard anteroposterior views.[23] The downward, posterior slope of the articular surface of the proximal tibia also contributes to the difficulty imaging the spines on this view. For these reasons, lateral and/or oblique radiographs may be necessary to visualize a fracture of the tibial eminence in the younger child.

The proximal tibial physis remains relatively smooth and transverse during the early growth and development of the knee. Its epiphyseal side is slightly convex, and its metaphyseal side is slightly concave. During to first 2 years of life, a central undulation develops anteriorly at the site of the future tibial tuberosity. By age 5 or 6 years, multiple smaller undulations begin to appear in the physis and can be appreciated in gross sections. These continue to grow in number and size so that they are readily visible radiographically by ages 9 or 10 years. Physiological epiphyseodesis begins in early adolescence. It begins centrally and proceeds peripherally. The physis thins, and the subchondral bone on the epiphyseal and metaphyseal side thickens. After closure, the thickened subchondral remnants persist for several years as a "ghost" or physeal "scar," which eventually remodels so that it is no longer visible in the adult.[23]

The ossification of the tibial tubercle is highly variable, occurring between the ages of 8 and 12 years in girls and 9 and 14 years in boys. Until this time, the undulation in the anterior aspect of the proximal tibial epiphysis and a slight indention in the anterior metaphysis are the only radiographic suggestion of the tibial tuberosity. However, the tibial tubercle does exist as a discrete cartilaginous structure by the 15th week of fetal development. At birth it is well developed but lies proximal to its adult location. During postnatal development it "migrates" distally to its adult position below the level of the horizontal physis.[22]

Several months after birth, a vertically oriented extension of the proximal physis extends beneath the cartilaginous tubercle. Initially, the tuberosity is composed of fibrocartilage. Secondary ossification of the fibrocartilaginous tuberosity occurs during a period in the maturation process referred to as the apophyseal phase. The process begins at the distal pole of the tuberosity and proceeds proximally toward the horizontal epiphysis until the two centers abut. An intervening cartilaginous bridge separates the two ossification centers until about age 15 years, when they coalesce. In the final stage of tubercle maturation, the physis closes (Fig. 64.6).[8] The process of closure of this vertically oriented physis occurs in a proximal-to-distal direction between ages 13 to 15 years in females and 15 to 19 years in males. The histologic composition of the physis changes concomitantly as it ossifies, from fibrocartilage to columnar physeal cartilage in a proximal-to-distal direction except for the very tip of the tuberosity that remains as fibrocartilage.[22]

During most of development, the patellar tendon inserts into the more distal aspect of the tuberosity. It is postulated that the fibrocartilaginous nature of the immature physis is well suited to resist the tensile stresses imparted through the patellar tendon. As the secondary ossification center of the tuberosity matures, changes in the anatomy of the tubercle and extensor mechanism and in the histological structure of the distal epiphyseal cartilage predispose this region to a repetitive stress injury known as Osgood-Schlatter disease.

Cells in the region of the secondary ossification cen-

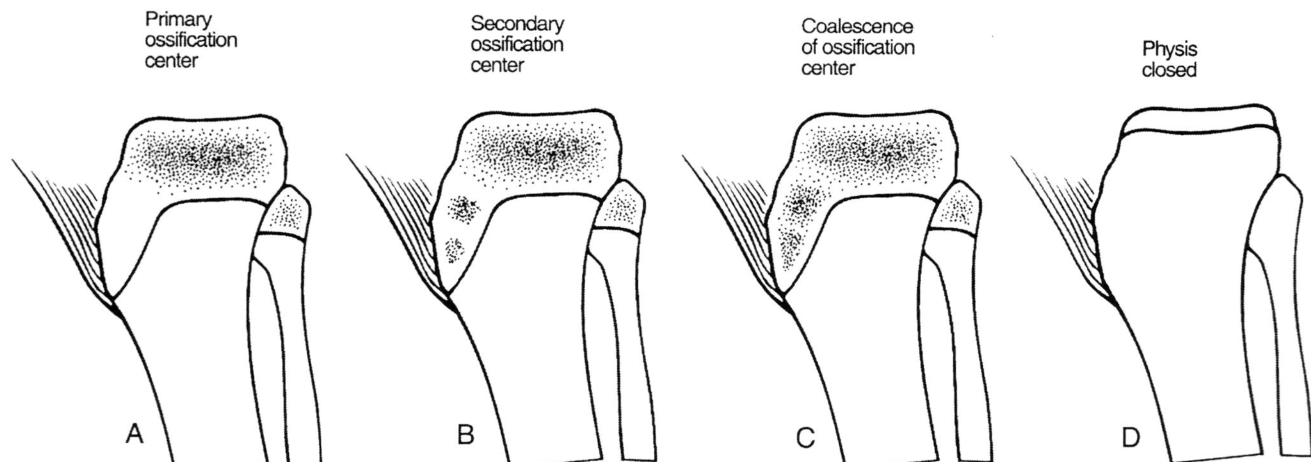

FIGURE 64.6 ➢ Ossification of the tibial tubercle. The tibial tubercle is present as a discrete fibrocartilaginous structure at birth *(A)*. Appearance of the secondary ossification centers occurs during the apophyseal stage (ages 8 to 12 years for girls, 9 to 14 years for boys) *(B)*. Coalescence of the ossification centers is complete by about age 15 years *(C)*. Physeal closure occurs in a proximal-to-distal direction *(D)*. (From Rockwood CA, ed: Fractures in Children, 3rd ed. Philadelphia, JB Lippincott Co., 1991, p 1208.)

ter hypertrophy, and as ossification of the tubercle proceeds, fibrocartilage that is relatively resistant to tensile forces is replaced by bone. Both the hypertrophic cells in the preossification stage of development and the bone in the early phases of ossification are much more susceptible to repetitive tensile stresses than their precursor. Coincidentally, the patellar tendon gradually develops a more extensive proximal insertion on the anterior surface of the tuberosity that results in dissipation of the tensile stresses to the histologically susceptible area of the physis. The typical injury resulting from repetitive stress to the tibial tuberosity is a separation of the immature chondro-osseous structures in the anterior aspect of the tubercle; the deeper layers of the apophysis and the cartilage of the underlying physis remain intact. If the process occurs in the preossification phase of development of the physis, or if the avulsed fragments are completely cartilaginous, symptoms will precede radiographic evidence of the diagnosis. However, with normal maturation, the avulsed fragments continue to grow and ossify and eventually become visible as separate bony fragments. Typically, the tissue between the avulsed bony fragments and the underlying tuberosity also ossifies, creating the appearance of "overgrowth" of the tubercle at skeletal maturity. Alternatively, the avulsed segment may persist as a fibrocartilaginous pseudarthrosis or a separate ossicle embedded within the patellar tendon.[22]

Traumatic avulsion of the tibial tuberosity occurs most commonly during the period of physiological epiphysiodesis of the composite proximal tibial ossification center, which exists as a continuous physis following coalescence of the two secondary ossification centers.[28] Closure of the proximal (horizontal) tibial physis begins centrally and proceeds in a centrifugal pattern. Closure of the vertical physis under the tuberosity follows in a proximal-to-distal direction. As opposed to the repetitive stress mechanism associated with Osgood-Schlatter disease, fractures of the tuberosity are typically caused by a single major stress generated by the extensor mechanism. Initial failure of the physis typically occurs distally and then extends proximally owing to the sequence of physiological epiphysiodesis of the proximal tibia.[22]

PROXIMAL TIBIOFIBULAR JOINT

The proximal fibular epiphysis is unossified at birth. Like the proximal tibia, the physis is initially transverse and smooth but develops undulations. The physis is situated 5 to 10 mm distal to the tibial physis throughout development. Appearance of the secondary ossification center is quite variable, ranging from as early as 2 years of age to as late as 4 years. The ossification process begins just above the physis and extends proximally. The styloid remains cartilaginous until late in skeletal maturation. Physeal closure occurs at about 15 years in males and 14 years in females.[23]

The proximal tibiofibular joint begins to form at about 12 weeks of fetal age and develops in a manner typical of other synovial joints. Narrow cavities appear between the lateral aspect of the tibial epiphysis and the medial aspect of the fibular epiphysis. Development of synovial tissue and formation of articular cartilage and a fibrous capsule then ensues. The fully developed articulation is present at birth as a plane joint between the lateral tibial condyle and the head of the fibula. Communication between the proximal tibiofibular joint and the knee is present in about 10% of knees. As the knee develops, the joint expands volumetrically but does not change its morphological contours. It becomes evident radiographically as the tibial and fibular epiphyses ossify.

The inclination of the proximal tibiofibular articulation is highly variable among normal subjects. Two basic anatomic types have been described (Fig. 64.7). The first is a more horizontal articulation, with less than 20 degrees of inclination, that is positioned under and behind a projection of the lateral edge of the tibial epiphysis. This configuration provides anterior stability and prevents significant forward displacement of the fibula. The second type has a more oblique orientation, with more than 20 degrees of inclination but ranging up to 80 degrees. The amount of articular cartilage decreases as the obliquity of the joint increases. Because of the steeper inclination and diminished surface area, this type of articulation tends to

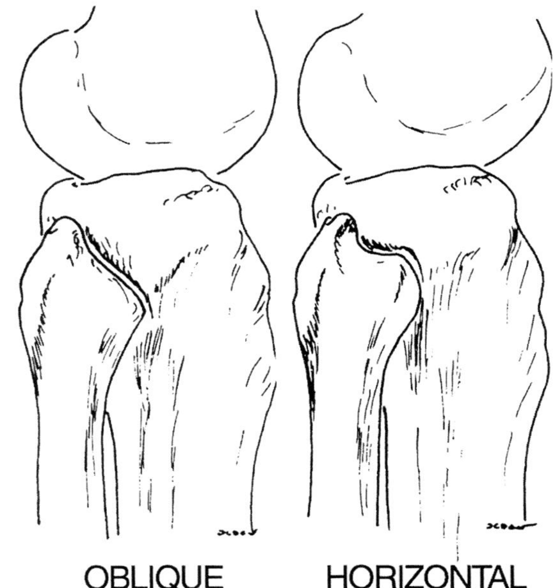

FIGURE 64.7 ➢ Anatomy of the proximal tibiofibular joint. The more horizontal articulation (right) typically has less than 20 degrees of inclination and is positioned under and behind a projection of the lateral edge of the tibial epiphysis. This configuration provides anterior stability and prevents significant forward displacement of the fibula. The more oblique articulation (left) is inclined more than 20 degrees, ranging up to 80 degrees. The steeper orientation and diminished surface area make this type of articulation inherently less stable and more prone to disruption. (From Ogden JA: The anatomy and function of the proximal tibiofibular joint. Clin Orthop 101:187, 1974.)

have less rotatory mobility and is the variant that is more frequently associated with disruption.[21, 23, 27]

This joint functions to dissipate torsional stresses transmitted from the ankle and lateral bending moments applied to the tibia and to absorb tensile loads generated by weightbearing. The major stabilizer of the proximal tibiofibular joint is the lateral collateral ligament, which inserts into the perichondrium of the fibular epiphysis. With the knee in extension, the ligament is taught and holds the fibula in its normal position. As the knee flexes the ligament relaxes, allowing a variable degree of anteroposterior translation of the proximal fibula. Symptomatic subluxation of this articulation is a common problem in children with generalized ligamentous laxity and is most often seen in preadolescent females. Fortunately, the problem is usually a self-limited one that resolves as the elasticity of the soft tissues begins to diminish during the process of physiological maturation.[21]

THE DEVELOPMENT OF SYNOVIAL PLICAE

Synovial mesenchyme forms in the peripheral portion of the interzone in the developing embryo. In time, this mesenchyme is vascularized and invaded by macrophages. It becomes looser in appearance as joint cavitation begins.[25] It is believed that the knee joint is originally composed of medial and lateral femuromeniscal compartments and a suprapatellar compartment. These three compartments are partitioned by septa of synovium. Through cellular apoptosis, these septa normally undergo progressive involution to lead to the formation of a single joint space.[6] Plicae are believed to be the result of incomplete dissolution of these septa.

The more common infrapatellar (ligamentum mucosum) and suprapatellar plicae are regarded as remnants of the septa, dividing the femuromeniscal compartments and the suprapatellar bursa, respectively. The ligamentum mucosum is usually not relevant clinically. Occasionally, a suprapatellar plica persists as a complete septum, in which case it most often presents as a symptomatic, suprapatellar mass.[26] Lateral and mediopatellar plicae are much less common but are more often pathological than the supra- and infrapatellar variants. They are thought to be remnants of involuting mesenchymal synovium rather than residual septa. Medial plicae are estimated to be roughly 30 times more common than lateral plicae. The higher incidence of medial plicae is thought to be related to the more lateral position of the patella during development. It is postulated that a greater bulk of mesenchymal tissue is present in the wider medial interval between the patella and femur and that involution of this tissue is more apt to be incomplete than on the lateral side where less tissue is present. Medial plicae have been identified in up to 35% of cadaveric fetuses and adults, suggesting that they may represent normal developmental variants.[20] Pathological conditions are estimated to be present in about 10% of mediopatellar plicae.[7]

MENISCUS

Differentiation of synovial mesenchyme into rudimentary meniscal structures begins during week 8 of gestation. Organization proceeds rapidly, and the structures are distinguished clearly by weeks 9 to 10.[16] Initially, growth of the menisci is more rapid than that of the corresponding tibial plateaus. By 28 weeks, the rate of growth of the tibial plateau relative to the meniscus equalizes and remains fairly constant through the remainder of fetal and postnatal development. Although the surface area of both menisci is about equal, the lateral meniscus covers a greater percentage of its plateau than does the medial meniscus at all ages.

Much speculation has been made as to the origination of the discoid meniscus. Smillie[30] attributed this anomaly to failure of resorption of the central portion of the meniscus during embryological development. Kaplan[13] and, more recently, Clark and Ogden[5] disputed this theory. In their studies of the embryological and postnatal development of the menisci in humans, they were unable to identify a discoid-shaped structure at any stage of normal development. Clark and Ogden found several knees in perinatal specimens with small or absent coronary ligaments but normal lateral menisci. Based on their observations, they postulated a developmental etiology of this anomaly in which failure of formation of the posterior meniscotibial (coronary) ligaments leaves only the meniscofemoral (Wrisberg's and Humphry's) ligaments as posterior stabilizers. The ensuing hypermobility leads to the eventual hypertrophic and discoid changes in the meniscus seen clinically.

Histologically, the prenatal menisci are highly cellular and well vascularized. Following birth, the structure of the menisci gradually changes in response to the evolving biomechanical environment of the knee. The general makeup becomes less cellular and, as the nucleus-to-cytoplasm ratio decreases, the architecture of the extracellular collagen becomes more organized. Bundles of collagen orient themselves in a predominantly circumferential fashion, with crossing radial fibers located mainly at the articular surfaces. As the menisci increase in size with the growth of the distal femur and proximal tibia, they also change in shape to accommodate the changing areas of contact between the femoral and tibial articulations. Most of the substantial architectural refinements are evident by the age of 3 years, reflecting an adaptation to the progressive weightbearing function of the knee associated with upright posture and bipedal gait.

The vascularity of the menisci also changes during postnatal development. At birth, blood vessels can be identified throughout the entire meniscus. By 9 months, they predominate in the peripheral one-third, although they can still be found centrally, perfusing the inner margin of the meniscus. This pattern of sparse central vascularity persists into the preadolescent years, after which the central third becomes essentially avascular. This age-related difference in meniscal vascularity has been used to support a more aggressive approach to repair torn menisci in children, regardless of the zone of injury or pattern of tear.[5]

THE LIGAMENTS

The organization of the ligaments of the knee is complete at birth. Meridia-Velasco[17] performed a cadaveric study of human embryo and fetal knees and found that the patellar tendon is the first ligament to form. The posterior cruciate ligament develops next, followed by the anterior. Both structures arise from the articular interzone. The lateral (fibular) collateral ligament forms next. It lies outside of and is separate from the joint capsule. In contrast, the medial collateral ligament begins as a condensation of the joint capsule and maintains this relationship throughout the maturation sequence. It is the last of the four major ligaments to form. Both of the collateral ligaments take origin from the respective medial and lateral aspects of the distal femoral epiphysis. The fibular collateral ligament inserts primarily into the proximal fibular epiphysis but also has some attachment to the proximal tibial epiphysis and, to a lesser extent, the proximal tibial metaphysis. The medial collateral ligament has a major attachment to the proximal tibial metaphysis, under the pes anserinus, but also has significant attachments to the epiphysis.[23]

There have been no longitudinal studies of ligamentous development in the knee after birth. However, it is a fact that ligamentous injuries in the skeletally immature are less common than in adults. Generalized ligamentous laxity is thought to be a protective factor in the preadolescent age group. In older children, there is a predisposition to major epiphyseal injury, based on observations of the failure patterns of the tibial tuberosity, tibial eminence, and periarticular physes.[22, 28] Anatomically, the major ligaments attach primarily to epiphyseal structures. The simple explanation for the observed patterns of failure in the distal femur and proximal tibia is that the maturing chondroepiphyseal structures (physes and perichondrium of the epiphyses) are weaker than the attached ligaments and thus more susceptible to tensile stresses. However, the interplay among many anatomic and biomechanical factors, including the general configuration of the epiphyses, the angular alignment and moments about the knee, and muscular attachments, are probably as important in determining the failure modes.

SUMMARY

Embryologically, the knee develops in a manner similar to that of other synovial joints. The joint-cavity and soft-tissue elements (synovium, joint capsule, menisci, and ligaments) develop from a homogeneous interzone and synovial mesenchyme in the center of the developing limb bud. The interzone cavitates into compartments (suprapatellar, medial, and lateral meniscofemoral and medial and lateral meniscotibial) that eventually coalesce to form the knee joint before birth. After birth, the knee changes more in size than in shape.

Changes in the angular alignment of the knee are visually the most obvious. The development of the tibiofemoral angle—from maximal varus alignment at birth to physiological valgus by age 7 to 9 years—has been well defined and provides a basis for evaluating angular malalignment of the limbs in children. Variations in the ossification patterns of the patella and distal femur epiphysis may occur when the normal process of calcification cannot keep pace with the rate of cartilage proliferation, particularly during periods of rapid skeletal growth. The radiographic appearance of these normal variants may be mistaken for pathological conditions of the chondroepiphyses if one is not aware of their existence and origins.

The literature regarding development of the soft-tissue structures about the knee is relatively sparse. The menisci begin to differentiate from synovial mesenchyme in the 1st trimester. After birth, structural adaptation occurs rapidly at both a gross and histological level in response to weightbearing. By age 3 years, most of the substantial architectural changes are evident. In similar fashion, organization of the ligaments of the knee is complete at birth. All of the ligaments have firm attachments into portions of the epiphyses about the knee.

The characteristics of the soft tissues and the transitional composition of the chondro-osseous structures in large part determine the typical injury patterns about the knee at various stages of development. Incompletely ossified structures are more susceptible to tensile stress than are the soft-tissue elements that attach to them. Thus, failure is more likely to occur by osteochondral avulsion or epiphyseal separation than by ligamentous disruption. The exact stage of development of the structures and pattern of loading ultimately determine the specific type of injury.

References

1. Brashear H Jr: Epiphyseal fractures. J Bone Joint Surg Am 41(6): 1055, 1959.
2. Burkus J, Ganey T, Ogden J: Development of the cartilage canals and the secondary center of ossification in the distal chondroepiphysis of the prenatal human femur. Yale J Biol Med 66(3):193, 1993.
3. Caffey J, Madell S, Royer C, et al: Ossification of the distal femoral epiphysis. J Bone Joint Surg Am 40(3):647, 1958.
4. Cahuzac J, Vardon D, Sales de Gauzy J: Development of the clinical tibiofemoral angle in normal adolescents: A study of 427 normal subjects from 10 to 16 years of age. J Bone Joint Surg Br 77(5):729, 1995.
5. Clark C, Ogden J: Development of the menisci of the human knee joint: Morphologic changes and their potential role in childhood meniscal injury. J Bone Joint Surg Br 65(4):538, 1983.
6. Deutsch A, Resnick D, Dalinka M, et al: Synovial plicae of the knee. Radiology 141(3):627, 1981.
7. Dupont J: Synovial plicae of the knee: Controversies and review. Clin Sports Med 16(1):87, 1997.
8. Ehrenborg G: The Osgood-Schlatter lesion: A clinical and experimental study. Acta Chir Scand (suppl) 288:1, 1962.
9. Fulkerson J: Patellofemoral pain disorders: Evaluation and management. J Am Acad Orthop Surg 2:124, 1994.
10. Gardner E, O'Rahilly R: The early development of the knee joint in staged human embryos. J Anat 102(2):289, 1968.
11. Grogan D, Carey T, Leffers D, Ogden J: Avulsion fractures of the patella. J Pediatr Orthop 10(6):721, 1990.
12. Heath C, Staheli L: Normal limits of knee angle in white children: Genu varum and genu valgum. J Pediatr Orthop 13(2):259, 1993.
13. Kaplan E: Discoid lateral meniscus of the knee. J Bone Joint Surg Am 39(1):77, 1957.

14. Keats T, ed: An Atlas of Normal Roentgen Variants That May Simulate Disease. Chicago: Yearbook Medical Publishers, 1973.
15. Merchant A, Mercer R, Jacobsen R, et al: Roentgenographic analysis of patellofemoral congruence. J Bone Joint Surg Am 56(7): 1391, 1974.
16. Meridia-Velasco J, Sanchez-Montesinos I: Development of the human knee joint. Anat Rec 248(2):269, 1997.
17. Meridia-Velasco J, Sanchez-Montesinos I: Development of the human knee joint ligaments. Anat Rec 248(2):259, 1997.
18. Meyers M, McKeever F: Fracture of the intercondylar eminence of the tibia. J Bone Joint Surg Am 41(2):209, 1959.
19. Nietosvaara Y: The femoral sulcus in children: An ultrasonographic study. J Bone Joint Surg Br 76(5):807, 1994.
20. Ogata S, Uhthoff H: The development of the synovial plicae in human knee joints: An embryologic study. Arthroscopy 6(4):315, 1990.
21. Ogden J: Anatomy and function of the proximal tibiofibular joint. Clin Orthop 101(1):186, 1974.
22. Ogden J. Radiology of postnatal skeletal development: Patella and tibial tuberosity. Skeletal Radiol 11:246, 1984.
23. Ogden J: Radiology of postnatal skeletal development: Proximal tibia and fibula. Skeletal Radiol 11:169, 1984.
24. Ogden J, McCarthy S, Jokl P: The painful bipartite patella. J Pediatr Orthop 2(3):263, 1982.
25. O'Rahilly R, Gardner E: The embryology of movable joints. In Sokoloff L, ed: The Joints and Synovial Fluid. New York, Academic Press, Inc., 1978, p 491.
26. Pipkin G: Knee injuries: The role of suprapatellar plica and suprapatellar bursa in simulation internal derangements. Clin Orthop 74:161, 1971.
27. Resnick D, Newell J, Guerra J, et al: Proximal tibiofibular joint: Anatomic-pathologic-radiographic correlation. Am J Roentgenol 131:133, 1978.
28. Rockwood C, Kaye W, King R, eds: Fractures in Children, 3rd ed. Philadelphia, J.B. Lippincott Co., 1991.
29. Salenius P, Vankka E: The development of the tibiofemoral angle in children. J Bone Joint Surg Am 57(2):259, 1975.
30. Smillie I: The congenital discoid meniscus. J Bone Joint Surg Br 30(4):671, 1948.
31. Sontag L, Pyle S: Variations in the calcification pattern in epiphyses: Their nature and significance. Am J Roentgenol 45:50, 1941.
32. White GR, Mencio GA: Genu valgum in children: Diagnostic and therapeutic alternatives. J Am Acad Orthop Surg 3:275, 1995.

65 Congenital Deformities of the Knee

William C. Warner, Jr. • S. Terry Canale • James H. Beaty

CONGENITAL DISLOCATION AND SUBLUXATION OF THE KNEE

Congenital dislocation (recurvatum) of the knee is rare, with a reported incidence ranging from 0.017 to 0.7 occurrences per 1000 births. Some authors have estimated that congenital hip dislocation is from 40 to 80 times more common than congenital dislocation of the knee.[5, 10, 11, 14] Congenital knee dislocation is two to three times more frequent in females than in males, the right and left knees are equally affected, and about a third of patients have bilateral dislocations.

The cause of congenital knee dislocation is unknown, although several theories have been proposed. Birth trauma was an early suggestion, but studies by Katz, Gorgano, and Soper[11] showed that, in a fetus, the distal femoral epiphysis displaces before the knee dislocates. Fetal molding was suggested by Shattock,[19] who postulated that the feet become locked beneath the mandible or beneath the axilla, causing hyperextension of the knee. Although breech presentation is more common in patients with congenital knee dislocations, this is not the cause in most patients. Katz et al[11] reported that hypoplasia and attenuation of the anterior cruciate ligament (ACL) were the cause of congenital knee dislocation and that this condition was a genetic trait or was induced in the developing embryo before 9 weeks' gestation. In dissections of fetal knees of less than 28 weeks' gestation, the authors found the cruciate ligaments to be the principal structure preventing anterior dislocation of the knee. However, Curtis and Fisher[5] believed the changes in the cruciate ligaments to be secondary to, rather than a cause of, knee dislocation in infants. Middleton[13] theorized that congenital knee dislocation resulted from quadriceps contracture, but, again, it is not known whether quadriceps contacture is a cause or a result of the dislocation. Ferris and Aichroth[7] suggested that intrauterine ischemia similar to a compartmental syndrome might cause quadriceps contracture that results in knee dislocation.

In some patients, heredity appears to be a factor. McFarlane[12] reported on three children with congenital knee dislocations, all of whom had the same mother but three different, normal fathers. Provenzano,[16] in a review of 200 patients with congenital knee dislocations, found 7 patients with positive family histories. These familial occurrences may represent Larsen's syndrome with congenital knee dislocation.

Congenital knee dislocation occurs in association with other skeletal anomalies in 82% to 88% of patients,[5, 10, 11] most frequently with congenital dislocation of the hip (45%) (Fig. 65.1), congenital deformities of the feet (31%), and congenital dislocation of the elbow (10%). Other reported associated anomalies include cleft palate and cleft lip, spina bifida, hydrocephalus, Down syndrome, cryptorchidism, angiomata, facial paralysis, and imperforate anus. Syndromes such as arthrogryposis and Larsen's syndrome are also associated with congenital dislocation of the knee.

Classification

The term congenital dislocation of the knee includes a spectrum of conditions that are usually classified according to the severity of the deformity (Fig. 65.2). Grade I is congenital hyperextension of the knee, with minimal or no subluxation of the tibia on the femur. The knee is in 15 to 20 degrees of hyperextension and can be passively manipulated into 45 to 90 degrees of flexion. Grade II is congenital subluxation of the knee, in which the epiphysis of the tibia is displaced forward on the anterior aspect of the femoral condyles, with some contact remaining between the tibial and femoral articular surfaces. The knee is held in 25 to 45 degrees of hyperextension and can be flexed only to a neutral position. Grade III is congenital dislocation of the knee in which the upper tibial epiphysis is totally displaced in front of the femoral condyles with no contact between the articular surfaces.

Carlson and O'Connor[4] also identified three types of patients with congenital knee dislocations: those with an isolated dislocation, those with multiple dislocations, and those with known syndromes. Ferris and Jackson[8] described four children with six "congenital snapping knees," in whom anterior subluxation of the tibia on the femur occurred with knee extension and spontaneously reduced with knee flexion. These children had no marked recurvatum deformity, and knee flexion was not restricted by quadriceps fibrosis. All four children, however, had other major clinical anomalies and ACL insufficiency. The most obvious clinical sign was an audible and palpable "clunk" that accompanied both subluxation and reduction. Curtis and Fisher[6] described 10 knees in five children with a similar condition they called "heritable congenital tibiofemoral subluxation."

Adapted from Warner WC Jr, Canale ST, Beaty JH: Congenital Deformities of the Knee. In Scott WN: The Knee, vol 1. St. Louis, Mosby-Year Book, 1994, pp 209-227.

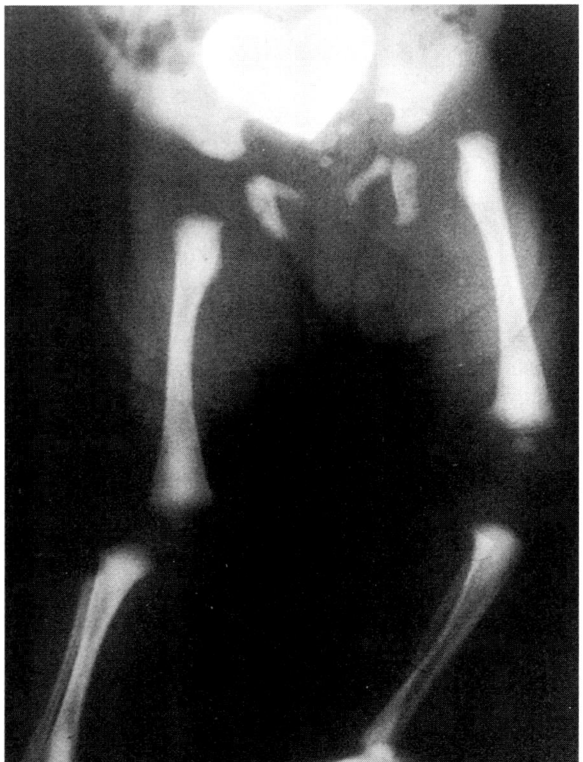

FIGURE 65.1 ➢ Radiograph of patient with congenital dislocation of right knee and left hip. (From Scott WN: The Knee, vol 1. St. Louis, Mosby-Year Book, 1994, p 210.)

Clinical Examination

The hyperextension of the knee is distinctive, and the diagnosis can be easily made by visual inspection (Fig. 65.3). Knee flexion is limited, and the knee can be extended farther than its hyperextended position. Lateral radiographs demonstrate either partial displacement (subluxation) or complete dislocation of the tibia on the femur, with the tibial plateau sloped posteriorly (Fig. 65.4). Anteroposterior views show associated lateral and rotary subluxation and valgus deformity of the knee. The ossification centers of the proximal tibia and distal femur are usually hypoplastic or occasionally absent.

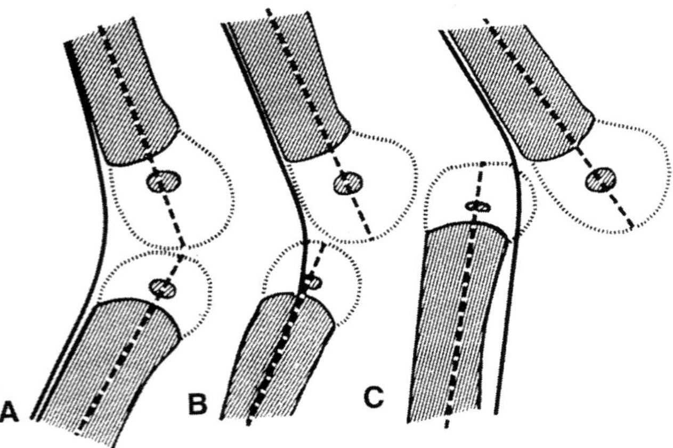

FIGURE 65.2 ➢ Grades of congenital hyperextension, subluxation, and dislocation of the knee. *A,* Hyperextension. *B,* Subluxation. *C,* Dislocation. (From Curtis BH, Fisher RL: Congenital hyperextension with anterior subluxation of the knee: Surgical treatment and long-term observations. J Bone Joint Surg Am 51:225, 1964.)

Pathological Findings

The pathology varies with the severity of the deformity, but contractures of the quadriceps mechanism and the anterior capsule are constants.[2] In a true dislocation, the tibia is anterior to the femoral condyles. Lateral and rotary subluxation and valgus deformity may be caused by contractures of the iliotibial band and the lateral intermuscular septum. Curtis and Fisher[5] observed that the vastus lateralis and the lateral structures about the knee tend to be more involved. They also found that the suprapatellar pouch was obliterated in more severely involved knees and that in more than half their patients, the patella was dislocated laterally. In severe anterior dislocations, the collateral ligaments coursed anteriorly from their femoral attachments and the hamstring muscles subluxed anteriorly to function as extensors of the knee in the deformed position. The popliteal vessels and nerves were normal. Austwick and Dandy[1] found that the posterior cruciate ligament was short and tight, and Katz et al[11]

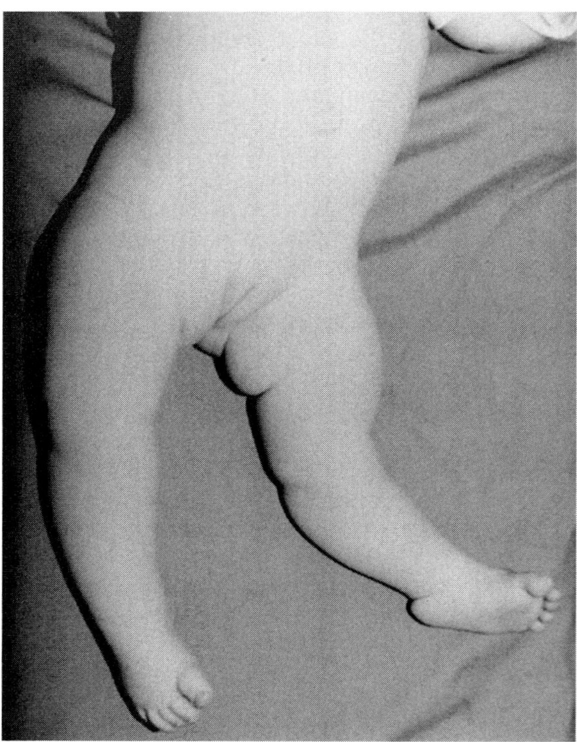

FIGURE 65.3 ➢ Clinical appearance of congenital dislocation of the knee *(left)*. (From Scott WN: The Knee, vol 1. St. Louis, Mosby-Year Book, 1994, p 212.)

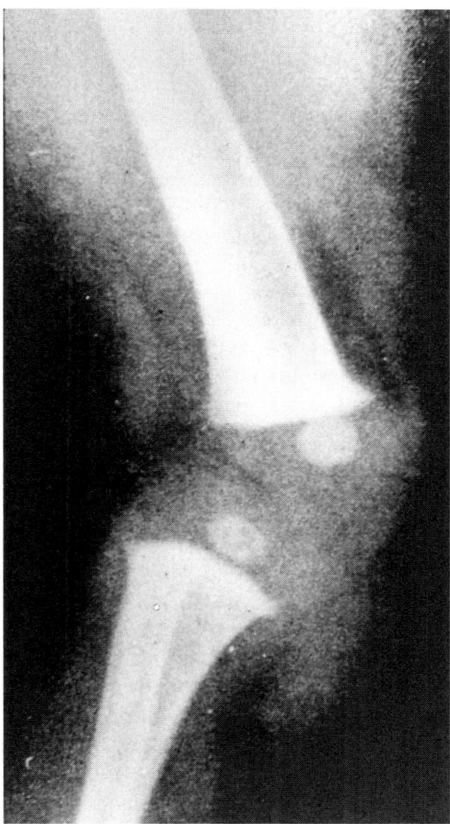

FIGURE 65.4 ➢ Lateral radiograph of patient with complete dislocation of tibia on femur. (From Scott WN: The Knee, vol 1. St. Louis, Mosby–Year Book, 1994, p 212.)

found that the ACL was hypoplastic or absent and that the tibial plateau sloped posteriorly.

Treatment

The treatment of congenital hyperextension and subluxation of the knee depends on the severity of the deformity and the age at which treatment is begun. In newborns with mild or moderate hyperextension or subluxation, serial manipulation and casting should begin as soon as possible, although Haga et al[9] recommended observation for the first month based on six patients who had spontaneous reduction with minimal treatment. The knee is manipulated and casted every 2 weeks in as much flexion as can be easily obtained. Forceful casting in flexion has been cited as a cause of posterior sloping of the tibial plateau. After 90 degrees of flexion are obtained by casting, the knee can be maintained in flexion in a Pavlik harness, as described by Nogi and MacEwen.[14] Lateral subluxation of the knee is a contraindication to the use of a Pavlik harness because the harness will aggravate the lateral subluxation.

If the subluxation or dislocation cannot be reduced by serial manipulation, surgery is usually necessary.[16] Skin and skeletal traction have been used to reduce the dislocation and to obtain 45 degrees of knee flexion before a casting program is begun. Most often, however, open reduction and quadricepsplasty are required. Surgery should be done before the infant begins to try to walk, preferably at about 6 months. Several procedures have been described for the treatment of congenital knee dislocation, but all involve lengthening of the quadriceps mechanism and release of the anterior capsule. The technique described by Curtis and Fisher[6] is most commonly used. This involves anterior exposure of the knee joint, V-Y lengthening of the quadriceps tendon (Fig. 65.5), transverse release of the anterior capsule, and release of any intra-articular adhesions. Any significant contracture of the iliotibial band is also released. Bell, Atkins, and Sharrard[2] recommended a distal quadriceps muscle slide procedure if adequate flexion cannot be obtained (Fig. 65.6). After release of contracted structures, the collateral ligaments and displaced hamstring tendons are returned to their proper positions. Katz et al[11] recommended reconstruction of the ACL with a slip of patellar tendon, whereas Tachdjian used the semitendinosus tendon for cruciate ligament reconstruction. If the ACL is lax, its tibial insertion can be moved at the time of reduction. Roy and Crawford[18] described a percutaneous quadriceps lengthening technique in which a small stab incision is made one to two patellar lengths superior to the patella in the midline (Fig. 65.7). The fascia overlying the rectus portion of the quadriceps is released through this incision. Medial and lateral stab incisions are then made at the superior

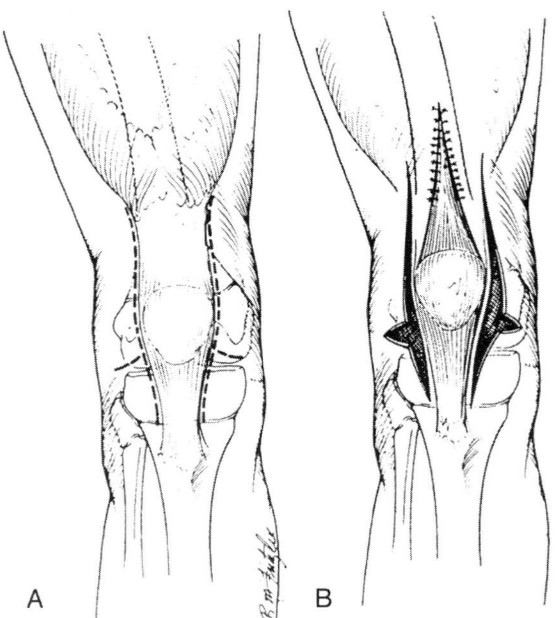

FIGURE 65.5 ➢ Curtis and Fisher technique for congenital dislocation of the knee. *A,* Lines of incision to release anterior capsule medially and laterally, as well as medial and lateral retinacula of quadriceps mechanism. *B,* Correction after soft-tissue release and lengthening of rectus femoris muscle. (From Canale ST, Beaty JH, eds: Operative Pediatric Orthopaedics. St. Louis, Mosby–Year Book, 1991, p 127.)

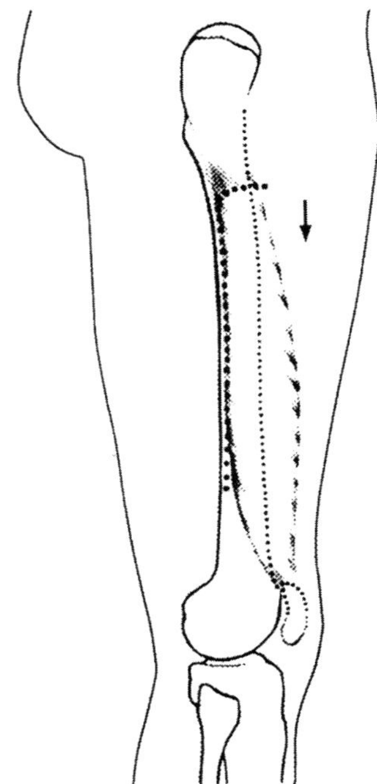

FIGURE 65.6 ➢ Lateral approach required to perform quadriceps muscle slide procedure. (Redrawn from Bell MJ, Atkins RM, Sharrard WJW: Irreducible congenital dislocation of the knee: Aetiology and management. J Bone Joint Surg Br 69:403, 1987.)

border of the patella for release of the medial and lateral quadriceps and the retinaculum. In older children, full flexion may not be obtained and a femoral or tibial osteotomy may be necessary. In adults who have developed disabling arthritis, arthrodesis is recommended.

CONGENITAL ABSENCE OF THE ANTERIOR CRUCIATE LIGAMENT

Congenital absence of the ACL is rare. Although this condition was initially described in association with congenital knee dislocation, it is not known if the absence of the ACL is primary or secondary, and several authors have reported absence of the ACL as a distinct, solitary entity.[20, 22] It has also been reported in association with congenital short femur,[20, 23] congenital absence of the menisci,[28] congenital ring meniscus,[21, 25] and thrombocytopenic absent radius syndrome.[26, 29]

Absence of the ACL may or may not cause symptoms. Thomas et al[27] reported that half of their patients were asymptomatic. Of those who had symptoms, most reported giving way of the knee at least once a week. All the patients except one, however, were active with little restriction on their daily activities. Physical examination usually reveals a positive anterior drawer test and at least a grade 3 Lachman sign. Radiological evidence of hypoplasia of one or both tibial spines is suggestive of congenital ligament deficiency. The intercondylar notch is V-shaped or shallow, and the lateral femoral condyle may be hypoplastic.

It is not known if the natural history of congenital absence of the ACL is the same as traumatic absence. In patients with tibial or femoral dysplasia, the diagnosis is important because subluxation or dislocation of the knee has been reported after femoral lengthening when the ACL is absent.[24] Before femoral lengthening is done, radiographs should be carefully scrutinized for any evidence of absence of the ACL.

Because most patients with congenital absence of the ACL are asymptomatic or have only mild symptoms and because the natural history is unknown, treatment at present usually consists of observation or bracing for symptomatic patients.

CONGENITAL DISLOCATION OF THE PATELLA

The congenitally dislocated patella is dislocated laterally and cannot be reduced by closed manipulation. The condition may be unilateral or bilateral, and a familial tendency has been reported. Mumford[38] reported on a patient who had six maternal relatives with congenital patellar dislocations. The condition has also been reported in association with other abnormalities, including arthrogryposis and Down syndrome.[37] Stanisavljevic et al[39] suggested that the primary pathology in this condition is failure of the medial rotation of the myotome that contains the quadriceps musculature. This medial rotation usually occurs during the first trimester of gestation.

The patella is dislocated on the lateral side of the lateral femoral condyle and is hypoplastic and misshapen; the lateral femoral condyle is flattened anteri-

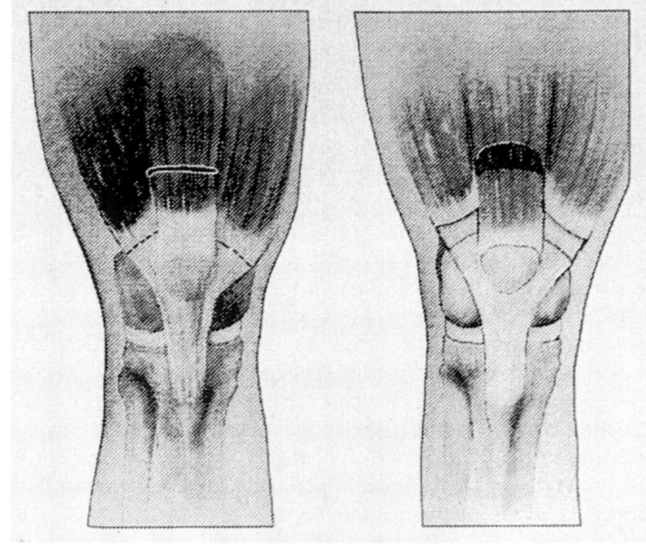

FIGURE 65.7 ➢ Percutaneous quadriceps recession technique. (From Roy DR, Crawford AH: Percutaneous quadriceps recession: A technique for management of congenital hyperextension deformity of the knee in the neonate. J Pediatr Orthop 9:717, 1989.)

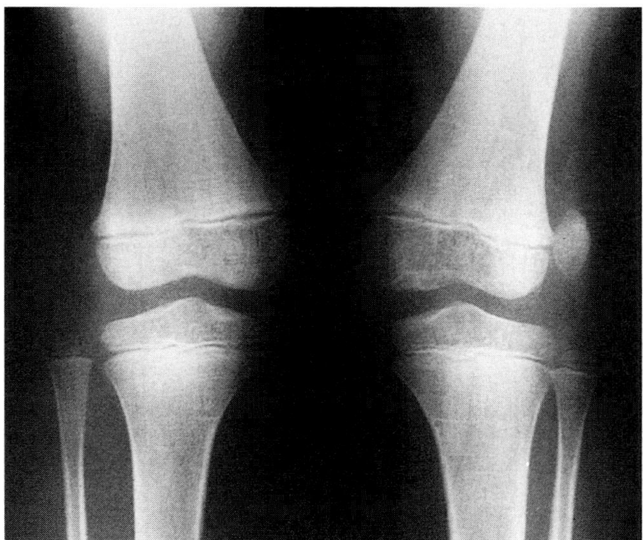

FIGURE 65.8 ➢ Untreated congenital dislocation of patella in a 5-year-old child; note fixed position of patella on lateral aspect of lateral femoral condyle. (From Scott WN: The Knee, vol 1. St. Louis, Mosby-Year Book, 1994, p 215.)

orly.[33] The vastus lateralis muscle may be absent, and the iliotibial band may be attached to the patella.[34] Varying degrees of genu valgum are present, and the tibia tends to externally rotate and subluxate laterally. With the patella dislocated, the quadriceps flexes the knee and externally rotates the tibia.

Because the patella is small at birth and is not ossified until age 2 to 3 years, the diagnosis often is overlooked.[39, 42] Congenital patellar dislocation should be suspected in an infant with fixed flexion deformity of the knee and excessive lateral rotation of the tibia. Usually, the knee cannot be actively extended from a flexed position because of the altered pull of the quadriceps muscles. The femoral condyles can be palpated, and the patella can be located above the fibular head. Radiographs are usually not helpful until age 3 to 5 years because of the lack of patellar ossification. Before this age, lateral radiographs show a loss of the normal quadriceps soft-tissue shadow. Walker, Rang, and Daneman[41] reported the use of ultrasonography to determine the position of the patella and to help in early diagnosis.

When the patella remains dislocated, walking is often delayed and difficult because of the loss of active knee extension. Secondary articular and bony changes occur in the patella, lateral femoral condyle, and intercondylar notch (Fig. 65.8). The valgus stress stretches

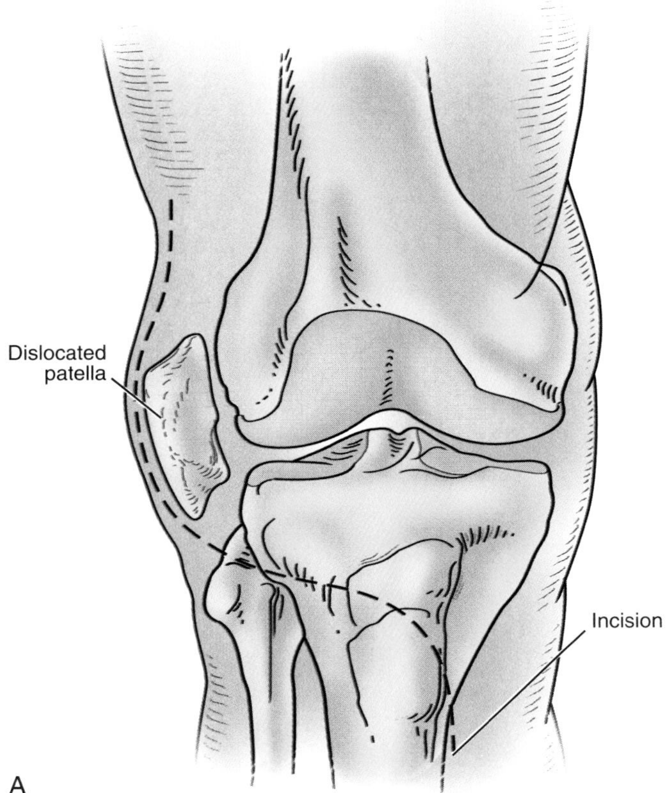

FIGURE 65.9 ➢ Medial transfer of the patellar tendon for congenital patellar dislocation. *A,* Skin incision.

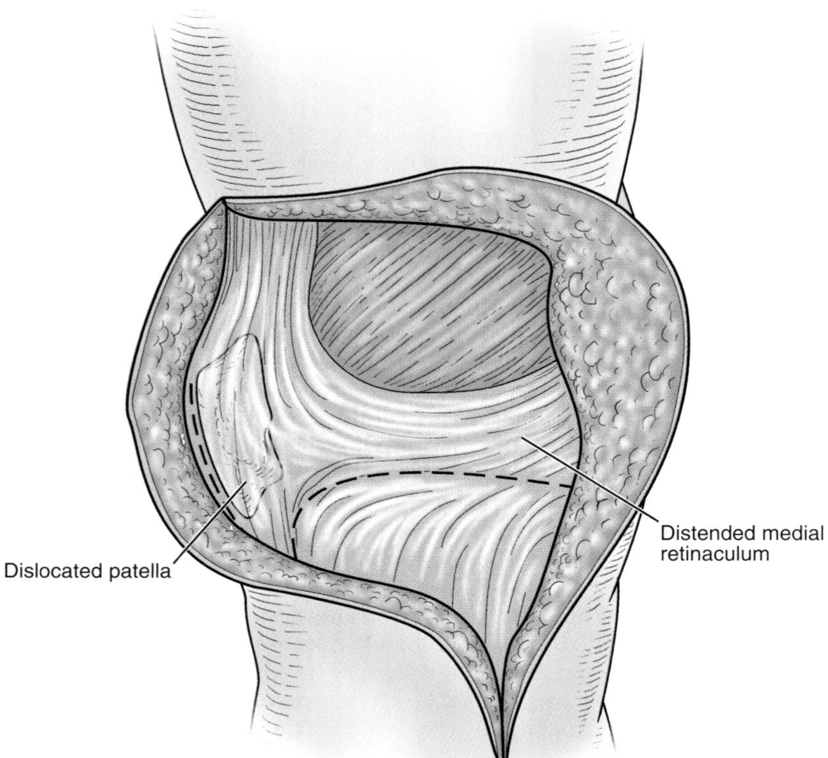

FIGURE 65.9 ➢ *Continued B,* Detachment of skin with fat layer from patellar retinacula and adjacent structures.

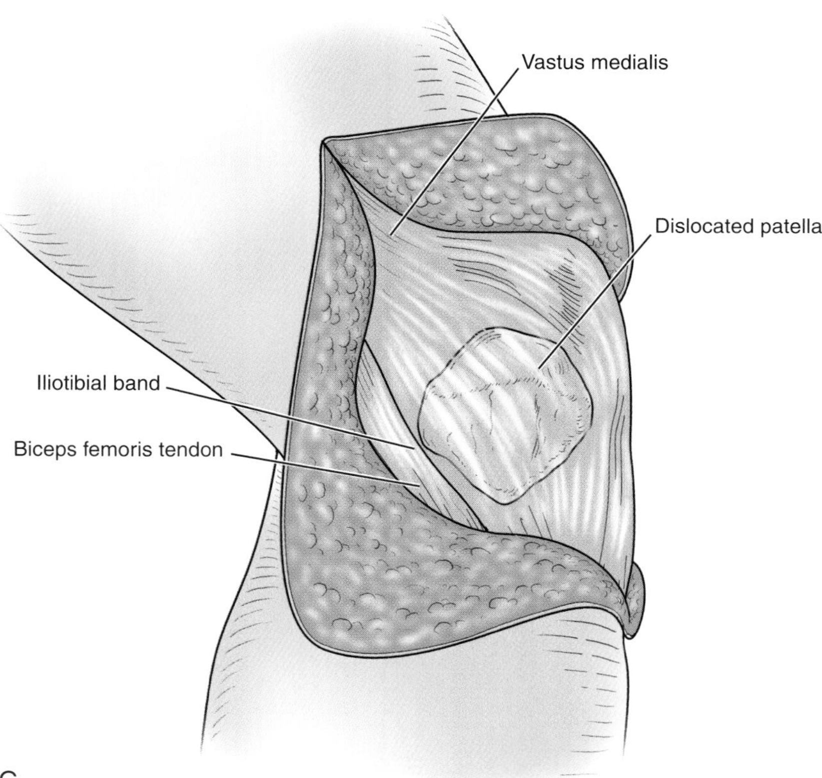

FIGURE 65.9 ➢ *Continued C,* Oblique division of tight iliotibial band and biceps femoris.

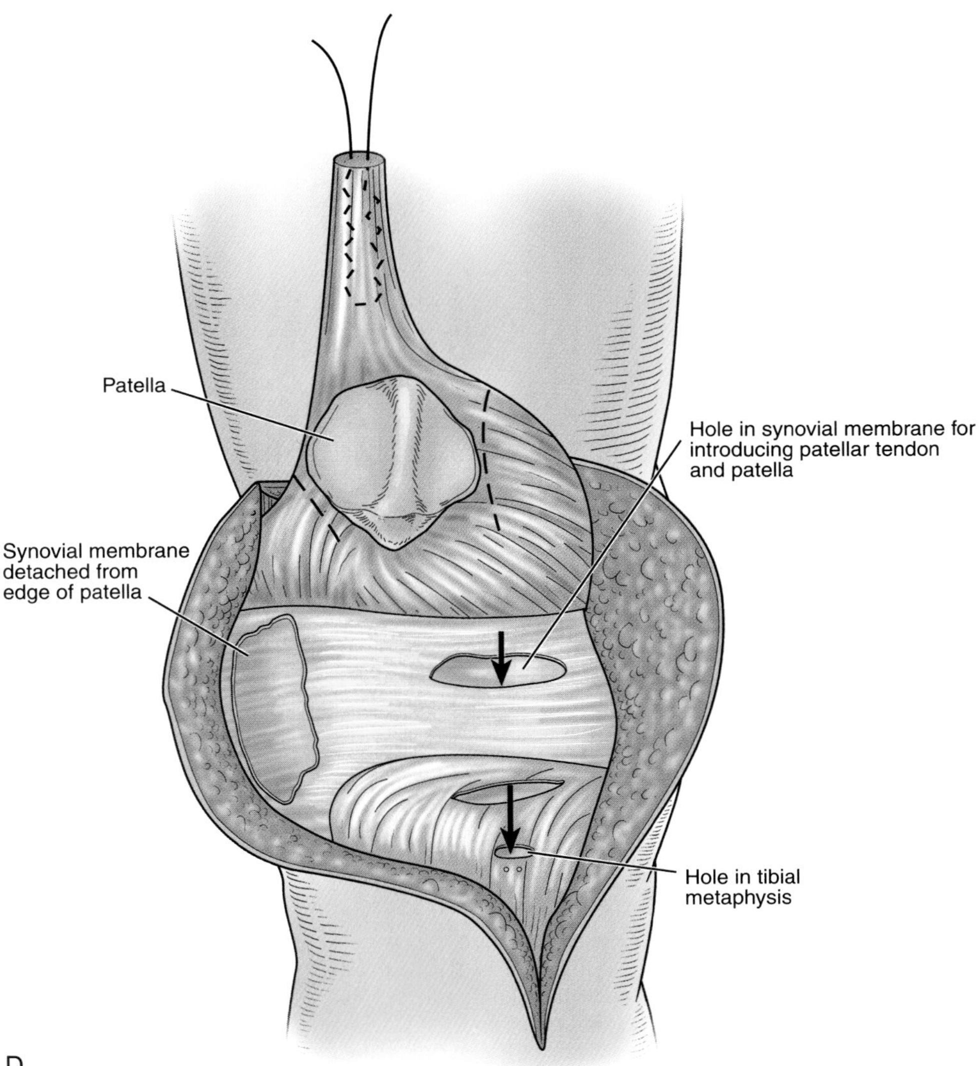

FIGURE 65.9 ➢ *Continued D,* Patella and tendon passed through opening in synovial membrane; tendon passed out through opening in capsule. Patella remains in closed synovial cavity. Tendon is buried in hole in metaphysis.

the medial collateral ligament, and the capsule on the medial and anteromedial aspects of the joint becomes hypertrophic.[32, 35, 40]

Closed reduction is impossible, and the deformity can be corrected only by surgery.[39] Because the severity of the deformity is directly related to the length of time it remains uncorrected, surgery should be performed as soon as the diagnosis is made. Stanisavljevic et al.[39] described rotation of the muscle mass, the patella, and the lateral half of the tendon to correct malrotation of the quadriceps muscle. Others have used extensive lateral releases combined with medial imbrication of the vastus lateralis muscle for realignment of the patella[31] and, if necessary, for tenodesis of the semitendinosus tendon.[30] More recently, Langenskiöld and Ritsilä[36] reported good results after mobilization of the patella and medial transfer of the patellar tendon. A hole in the synovial membrane is made to accept the patella in its new position. The iliotibial band and biceps femoris tendon should be lengthened at the same time (Fig. 65.9). Moving the patellar tendon insertion must be done carefully to prevent growth arrest of the tibial tubercle and iatrogenic recurvatum deformity. In general, results after treatment of congenital dislocation of the patella are not as good as those after traumatic recurrent dislocation because of recurrence and decreased range of motion.

NAIL-PATELLA SYNDROME

Nail-patella syndrome (hereditary onycho-osteodysplasia) is a rare dysplasia with four characteristic findings: dysplasia of the fingernails, hypoplasia or absence of the patella, radial head dislocations, and iliac horns.[43-49] Nephropathy accompanied by mild proteinuria is also a common manifestation of this syndrome. Other skeletal deformities such as foot abnormalities, most commonly a clubfoot deformity[46]; shoulder girdle

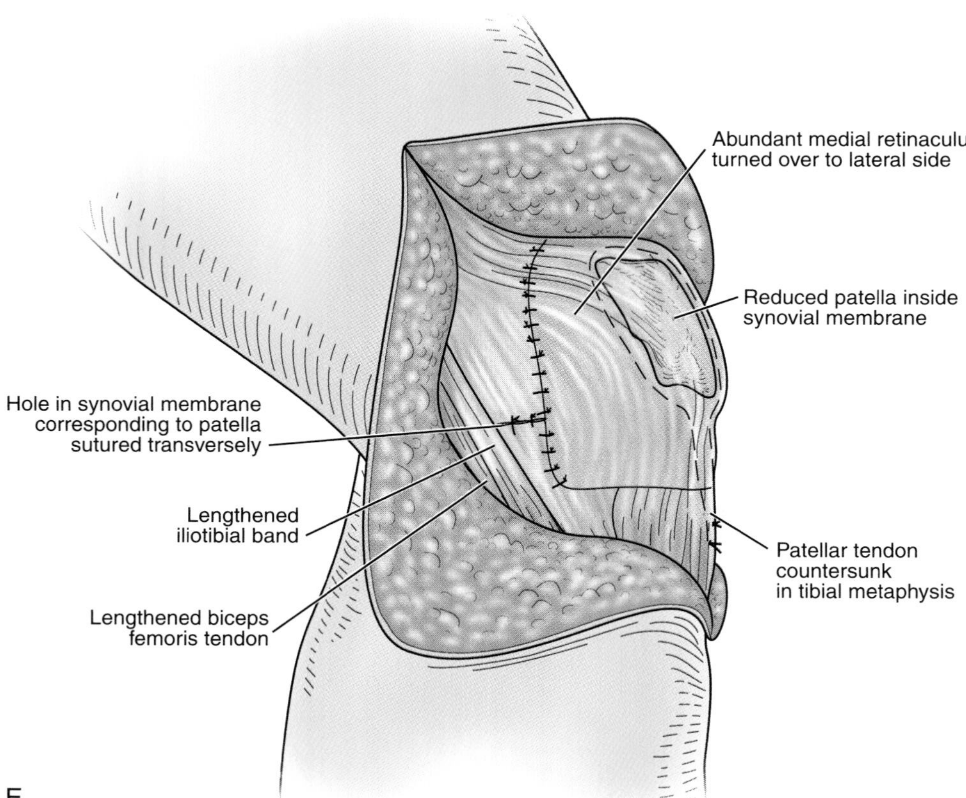

FIGURE 65.9 ➢ *Continued E,* Medial retinaculum with part of vastus lateralis turned over to lateral side and sutured to synovial membrane. (Redrawn from Langenskiöld A, Ritsilä V: Congenital dislocation of the patella and its operative treatment. J Pediatr Orthop 12: 315, 1992.)

dysplasia[47]; and clavicular horns[49] have been reported. The reported incidence of this condition in the United States is 4.5 per 1 million. The inheritance pattern is autosomal dominant with linkage to the ABO blood group locus. Involved family members have the same blood group type, but no specific blood group has a higher rate of carrying the syndrome. The fingernails are either hypoplastic or absent, but the toenails are usually not involved. Involved fingernails have splitting, spooning, and ridging, with lesser degrees of changes in the fingernails on the ulnar side of the hand. The thumbnails are always involved. Iliac horns, considered pathognomonic of the disease, are bilateral, smooth, bony outgrowths from the posterior ilium. They cause no symptoms, have no effect on gait, and need no treatment.

The patella is either hypoplastic or absent and may be abnormally shaped and unstable. Contracture of the quadriceps muscles and atrophy of the vastus medialis are common. Hypoplasia of the femoral condyles and an intercondylar synovial septum also have been reported,[48] as have late degenerative changes of the knee joint. Guidera et al[46] reported the best surgical results with combined proximal and distal patellar realignments, quadricepsplasties for extension contractures, and full posterior and capsular releases for flexion deformities. Femoral osteotomies were required in some patients for residual deformities.

BIPARTITE PATELLA

The patella may arise from two or more centers of ossification. If a separate center of ossification does not fuse with the main body of the patella, it is attached to the patella by fibrocartilaginous tissue, resulting in bipartite patella.[56, 61] Most ossicles are superolateral, but lateral, medial, and inferior lesions have been reported. Saupe[62] classified bipartite patella based on the position of the accessory ossification center (Fig. 65.10): type I, at the inferior pole (5%); type II, at the lateral margin (20%); and type II, at the superolateral pole (75%). Bipartite patella is bilateral in about 40% of patients, is usually asymptomatic, and is often a coincidental finding on radiographs obtained for some other reason.[51, 53] Pain in the superolateral pole of the patella is usually caused by an overuse syndrome, such as chondromalacia, rather than by bipartite patella.[50, 52, 55] Occasionally, excessive lateral tension from the vastus lateralis results in hypermobility of the bipartite patella.[57, 58, 60] To demonstrate this hypermobility, Ishikawa[57] described the "squatting position test," in which a skyline view of patella is obtained with the patient in a squatting position. This view showed a wider separation of the accessory fragment than did non-weightbearing skyline views. Occasionally, a superolateral lesion can be mistaken for an acute patellar fracture. Ogden et al[61] and Needoff[59]

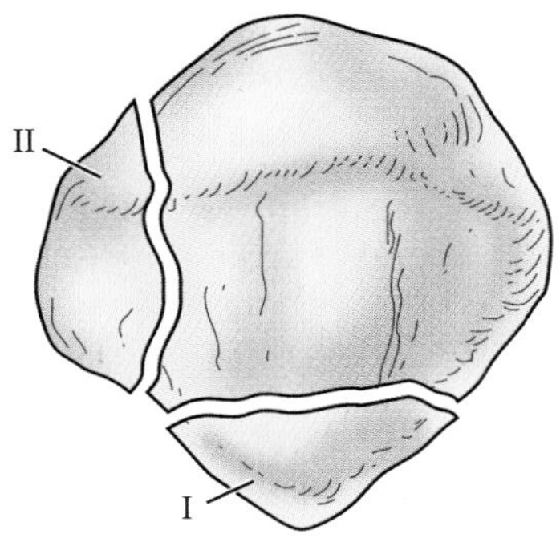

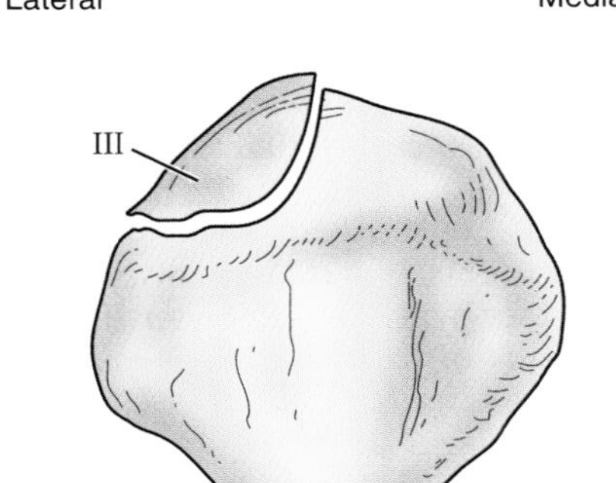

FIGURE 65.10 ➢ Saupe classification of bipartite patella. (Redrawn from Bourne MH, Bianco AJ Jr: Bipartite patella in the adolescent: Results of surgical excision. J Pediatr Orthop 10:69, 1990.)

suggested that bone scanning may be helpful in making the diagnosis of a fracture of the superolateral pole of the patella.

Restriction of competitive activity, use of nonsteroidal anti-inflammatories, and a program of short-arc exercises generally allow resolution of symptoms. Repetitive microtrauma may fracture the synchondrosis and produce pain;[54, 61] this usually resolves with 3 weeks of knee immobilization. If symptoms persist after nonoperative treatment, surgery may be indicated. Surgery for bipartite patella includes (1) excision of the accessory fragment, (2) lateral retinacular release, (3) subperiosteal release of vastus lateralis described by Ogata,[60] and (4) open reduction and internal fixation with bone grafting of the fragment. Excision of a bipartite patella is rarely indicated, except for persistent pain in older adolescents and young adults who have not responded to conservative treatment and who wish to continue competitive sports. Bourne and Bianco[50] reported marked improvement in 15 of 16 patients with symptomatic bipartite patella after surgical excision of the fragment. Ishikawa et al[57] reported good results after excision in all nine of their patients. Mori et al[58] reported that 15 of 16 bipartite patellae united 8 months after lateral retinacular release. This supports the theory that sustained lateral traction acting on the bipartite patella causes pain. Open reduction and grafting are rarely indicated.

DISCOID MENISCUS

As the name suggests, a discoid meniscus is disc shaped rather than semilunar, as normal menisci are. This abnormality has been reported to occur in 1.4% to 15.5% of the population. Ikeuchi[77] reported a 16.6% incidence in Japanese people. The medial or lateral meniscus may be discoid, but most often the lateral meniscus is abnormal. Involvement is often bilateral, and there is no sex predilection. Dashefsky[68] reported a familial incidence of discoid lateral meniscus, and Gebhart and Rosenthal[74] described identical twins with bilateral lateral discoid menisci.

The two most widely accepted etiologies for discoid meniscus are those proposed by Smillie[84] and Kaplan.[78] Smillie suggested that discoid meniscus resulted from an arrest at varying stages of embryological meniscal development. He divided discoid lateral meniscus into three forms: primitive, intermediate, and infantile. Kaplan, however, found no cartilaginous disc representing the meniscus at any stage of human embryological development nor in any comparative anatomic dissections. He believed that the meniscus formed normally but that, instead of its normal attachments to the posterior tibial plateau, it was attached to the lateral suface of the medial femoral condyle by the meniscofemoral ligament (Wrisberg's ligament). Because of the abnormal attachment, knee extension pulls the lateral meniscus into the intercondylar area. According to Kaplan, constant medial-lateral motion and irritation of the lateral meniscus transforms an intially normal, semilunar meniscus into a thick, fibrocartilaginous mass, or discoid meniscus.

Watanabe et al[90] classified discoid meniscus into three types based on arthroscopic findings: Wrisberg's ligament, complete, and incomplete. The Wrisberg's-ligament type has no attachment to the tibial plateau posteriorly, and its only posterior attachment is through the lateral meniscofemoral ligament, resulting in a hypermobile lateral meniscus. The complete type has intact attachments and is not hypermobile. The incomplete type differs from the complete type only in size.

A discoid meniscus is from 0.5 to 1.3 cm thick, is oval or almost circular in shape, and is a solid mass of fibrocartilage. Cystic degeneration with central cavities is common. Histological examination shows ridges in the meniscus and mucoid degeneration, indicating that the menisci are subjected to increased wear.

Discoid menisci are often asymptomatic. Dickhaut and DeLee[70] found that complete discoid menisci were usually asymptomatic and that Wrisberg's-ligament types were symptomatic. Symptoms usually occur by the sixth to eighth year of life, most often with snapping or clicking in the knee and a sensation of giving way or catching. Examination elicits a palpable "clunk" during the last 15 to 20 degrees of extension of the flexed knee. A fullness can be detected along the lateral joint line. Joint effusion and thigh atrophy may also be present.

Plain radiographs show widening of the lateral joint space compared with the other side. Flattening of the lateral femoral condyle and cupping of the lateral aspect of the tibial plateau are also suggestive of discoid meniscus. Magnetic resonance imaging (MRI) is the diagnostic method of choice (Fig. 65.11).[65, 66, 75, 83, 85] Silverman[83] reported that three or more adjacent MRI cuts with meniscal heights of more than 5 mm are indicative of a discoid meniscus. MRI also has the advantage of being able to demonstrate intrasubstance pathology that may not extend to the surface and may not be seen by arthroscopy.[65, 75, 85]

In children, conservative management of discoid mensicus is recommended because of the well-documented occurrence of degenerative knee joint changes after meniscectomy.[79, 80, 91] A short period of immobilization is followed by restriction of activities and progressive quadriceps-strengthening exercises. If the knee frequently locks or if function is significantly impaired, surgery is indicated. The type of surgery depends on the type of lesion identified at surgery. Good results have been reported after saucerization and partial meniscectomy of asymptomatic, stable lesions,[71, 72] but hypermobile, Wrisberg's-ligament-type partial meniscectomy results in an unstable meniscal rim. In Wrisberg's-ligament type, in which the posterior ligamentous attachments are not intact, treatment may include peripheral repair of the discoid meniscus and partial meniscectomy or total meniscectomy. Dickhaut and DeLee[70] and Aichroth et al[53] recommended total meniscectomy for symptomatic, Wrisberg's-ligament-type lesions, despite the fact that degenerative changes will occur, because the snapping and occasional locking of the knee caused by an unstable meniscal rim are functionally disabling. Washington et al,[89] however, reported only minimal degenerative changes in eight patients 17 years after total menisectomy for a discoid meniscus. Sugawara et al[87] found that of nine knees requiring repeat arthroscopic surgery, seven had lateral discoid menisci treated with partial meniscectomy. Although none had meniscal tears at the time of initial surgery, five had horizontal tears at the second procedure. The authors recommended observation for asymptomatic discoid menisci with no tears and subtotal or total meniscectomy for symptomatic menisci or those with tears. Fujikawa et al[73] recommended partial meniscectomy only when the discoid meniscus is not thick, severely degenerated, or hypermobile. Several reports in the literature indicate that better results are obtained with arthroscopic meniscectomy than with open meniscectomy.[64, 67, 69, 76, 88] Rosenberg et al[82] reported peripheral reattachment of a Wrisberg's-ligament-type discoid meniscus after central partial meniscectomy. At second-look arthroscopy 12 months later, healing was evident. The efficacy of this procedure has not been documented by other authors.

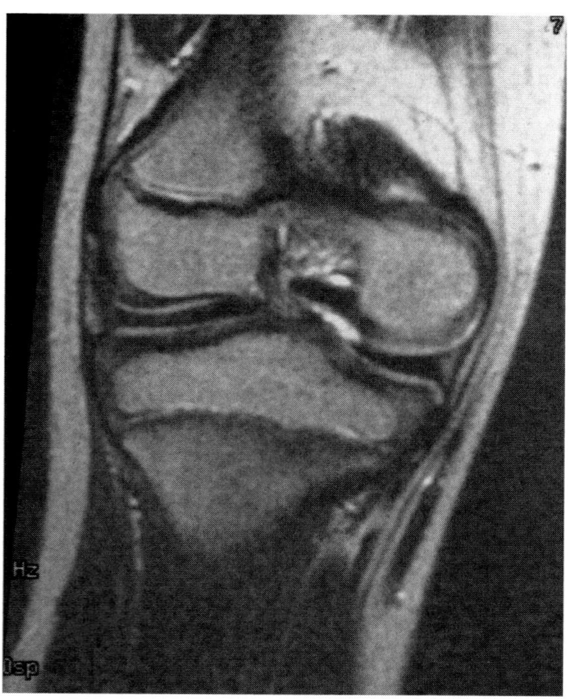

FIGURE 65.11 ➢ Magnetic resonance image of knee with discoid meniscus showing increased thickness of meniscus.

POPLITEAL CYSTS

Popliteal cysts usually arise between the semimembranosus and gastrocnemius tendons and represent an enlargement of the bursa between these two muscles. Popliteal cysts are usually unilateral, occur between the ages of 2 and 14 years, and are more common in males than in females.[92, 93] The lesion is usually distal to the popliteal crease and is prominent with the knee hyperextended. MRI[95] and ultrasonography[98] have been reported for evaluation of popliteal cysts. Most popliteal cysts in children are isolated bursal sac formations and are not related to pathology in the knee joint; they are rarely symptomatic. Treatment is conservative, and surgery is usually not indicated for popliteal cysts in children.[94, 97] Most cysts resolve spontaneously within 1 to 2 years. Dinham[94] found that 73% of untreated and 24% of recurrent cysts resolved within 5 years. He also found that more than half of cysts surgically removed recurred. Excision is indicated only for persistent, symptomatic lesions.

GENU VARUM AND GENU VALGUM

The angular alignment of the lower extremities normally varies with age. Bowlegs (genu varum) and knock knees (genu valgum) are common problems for which parents seek orthopedic advice. Most bowlegs and knock knees in children represent normal physiological development and correct spontaneously with age. Normal physiological causes must be differentiated from pathological causes of genu varum and genu valgum;[100, 102] to treat the physiological causes is overtreatment, and not to treat the pathological causes is undertreatment. Generally, the terms bowlegs and knock knees denote physiological conditions, and the terms genu varum and genu valgum indicate pathological conditions.

In newborns, mild to moderate medial bowing of the lower limbs is normal and persists until the age of 2 to 3 years, when knock knees begin to develop. Knock knees spontaneously correct between the ages of 4 and 10 years. In their study of the natural history of angular development of the lower extremity, Salenius and Vankka[107] measured the tibiofemoral angle in 1480 normal children and found that it was similar in girls and boys (Fig. 65.12). Between birth and 1 year, the tibiofemoral angle was 15 degrees of varus; this gradually corrected to neutral by 1.5 years. During the second and third years of life, the tibiofemoral angle increased to an average of 12 degrees of valgus, and by 7 years this valgus alignment gradually corrected to that of normal adulthood (8 degrees valgus in females and 7 degrees valgus in males).

Clinical measurements of the distance between the medial malleoli for knock knees and the distance between the femoral condyles for bowlegs have been used for evaluating progression of angular deformities, but these measurements are not accurate or reproducible.

Physiological Bowlegs

As determined by Salenius and Vankaa,[107] bowlegs are normal from birth to 1.5 years. Internal tibial torsion usually accentuates the bowleg deformity. The bowing is symmetric and bilateral and is present in both the femur and the tibia. Unilateral bowing or acute angulation indicates the possiblity of a pathological cause for the deformity. Differential diagnoses include Blount's disease; metabolic bone disease (rickets), asymmetric growth arrest caused by trauma, infection, tumor, bone dysplasia, and congenital longitudinal deficiency of the tibia with relative overgrowth of the fibula. In physiological bowing, lateral thrust of the tibia is not present as it is in Blount's disease. Radiographs show medial tilting of both knee and ankle joints (Fig. 65.13). The tibia is angulated medially at the junction of the proximal and middle thirds, and the femur is angulated medially at the distal third.

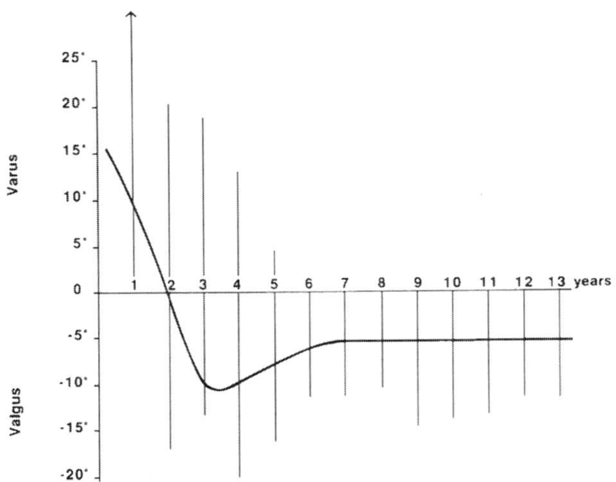

FIGURE 65.12 ➢ Femoral-tibial angle by age group in normal children. Vertical lines show range of normal for subject in study population. (From Salenius P, Vankka E: The development of the tibiofemoral angle in children. J Bone Joint Surg Am 57:259, 1975.)

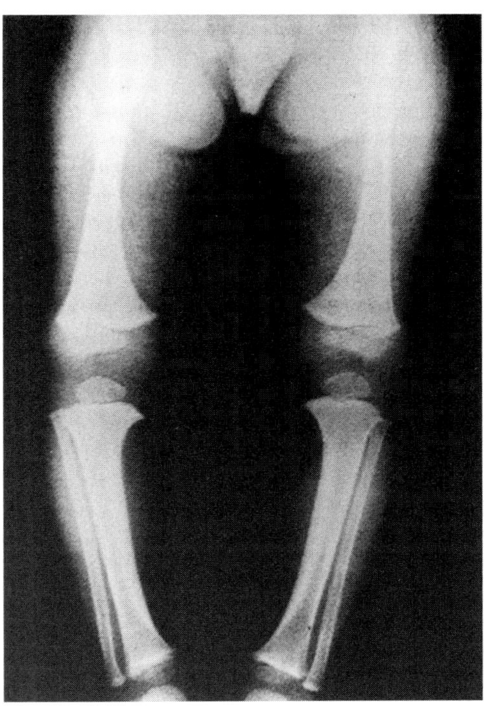

FIGURE 65.13 ➢ Radiograph of patient with physiological bowing shows symmetric bowing of femur and tibia. (From Scott WN: The Knee, vol 1. St. Louis, Mosby-Year Book, 1994, p. 218.)

The medial cortices of the tibia and the femur are thickened and sclerosed. Robertson[106] found that in children younger than 2 years, both the proximal and the distal ends of the tibia were frequently bowed and both ends remodeled at the same rate whether the tibia was braced or not.

Children with physiological bowlegs should be evaluated at 6-month intervals, and their parents should be reassured. Use of night splints (Denis Browne splint), wearing of corrective shoes, and active and passive exercises have been advocated, but these have produced no change in the appearence of the extremities other than that expected from normal growth and development.

Physiological Knock Knees

Physiological knock knees normally occur between the ages of 3 and 5 years and cause the cosmetic problems of flatfoot and awkward gait. Pain in the calf and the anterior aspect of the thigh may also be present. Knock knees correct without treatment in approximately 95% of children. Shoe modifications and bracing have not been proven effective in correcting physiological knock knees. For those few children in whom the deformity persists, surgical correction may be indicated. Howorth[103] recommended surgical correction if the genu valgum persists after age 10 years and if the intermalleolar distance measures more than 7.5 to 10 cm with the medial femoral condyles touching.

Medial femoral or tibial physeal arrest or varus tibial or femoral osteotomy can be used for correction of the valgus deformity. Howorth,[103] Herring and Kling,[102] and Zuege et al[108] recommended physeal stapling for correction of genu valgum. Stapling of the distal femoral epiphysis and the proximal tibial physis will correct genu valgum if sufficient growth remains, but correction is unpredictable because of a "rebound" increase in growth after staple removal. Zeuge et al[108] suggested allowing for 5 degrees of rebound growth after staple removal, of which 1 to 2 degrees are corrected after closure of the physis. Stapling should be done after age 11 years in girls and after age 12 years in boys. The staples should not be left in place for more than a year because longitudinal growth may not resume after removal if they are left in place longer. To effectively stop the growth of the medial physis, the staple prongs must be placed parallel to the physis. The amount of correction can be predicted mathematically using the transverse area of the physis, the length of the leg distal to the physis, and the amount of growth that will occur on the unarrested side of the plate based on skeletal age. Medial distal femoral or proximal tibial hemiepiphysiodesis, singularly or in combination, can also be used for correction of genu valgum. Bowen et al[99] developed a chart based on the Green-Anderson chart for predicting correction obtainable by medial epiphysiodesis. This chart is useful as a general guideline, but it is not exact. Patients must be followed up closely to prevent overcorrection. As a general rule, after tibial hemiepiphysiodesis, 5 degrees of angular correction can be expected for each year of remaining growth, and after femoral hemiepiphysiodesis, 7 degrees of correction can be expected for each year of remaining growth. Varus osteotomy has the advantage of completely correcting the genu valgum deformity at the time of surgery; however, this is a much more complicated procedure with a greater risk of complications, such as peroneal nerve palsy and compartmental syndrome.

BLOUNT'S DISEASE

Blount's disease is a developmental condition that affects the medial side of the proximal tibial epiphysis and causes a varus deformity of the tibia. Although its exact incidence is unknown, Smith[159] found only 37 children with Blount's disease among 5000 children with bowlegs, an incidence of less than 1%. Two distinct forms of the disease are manifested at different ages. Infantile Blount's disease affects children between ages 1 and 3 years, and the adolescent form affects children older than 8 years.

The infantile form is usually bilateral (60% to 80%), progressive, and associated with internal tibial torsion. This form must be differentiated from physiological bowlegs. In Blount's disease, the varus deformity becomes progressively severe, whereas physiological bowlegs tend to resolve with growth. In Blount's disease, the tibia alone is angulated; in physiological bowing, both the tibia and the femur are angulated. The exact cause of infantile Blount's disease is unknown. The most widely accepted theory is that early ambulation and obesity accentuate normal infantile physiological genu varum in suspectible individuals.[109, 114, 120, 123, 131, 139, 141, 142, 147, 155] Early walking when physiological genu varum is at its peak has been thought to cause Blount's disease because the weight-bearing force is transmitted across the medial tibiofemoral component, slowing the growth of the medial tibial physis, according to the Heuter-Volkman principle that increased pressure on a physis inhibits growth. Cook et al[120] developed a biomechanical model that demonstrated sufficient force to retard physeal growth in a 2-year-old child with 20 degrees of varus. They predicted that only 10 degrees of varus were necessary to retard growth in a 5-year-old child of normal weight. A combination of developmental and hereditary factors is the most likely cause.

The adolescent form of Blount's disease is less common and is less often associated with internal tibial torsion.[135, 148, 162] Adolescent Blount's disease has been attributed to residual genu varum from childhood, compounded by obesity and the accelerated growth rate of adolescence that results in progression of the varus deformity.[110, 122, 161, 163] Other proposed etiologies are occult trauma,[144] infection,[144] and formation of a bony bar.[112] Carter et al[118] demonstrated that the histopathology of the tibial physis in late-onset tibia vara is essentially the same as that in slipped, capital femoral epiphysis.

Pathological changes, described by Blount[113] and Langenskiöld,[143] include irregular cartilage columns, scattered areas of hypertrophic chondrocytes, hypocellular fibrocartilage, and delayed and irregular ossification of the metaphysis, physis, and epiphysis.

Clinically, Blount's disease produces abrupt angulation of the proximal tibia because of growth disturbance of the posteromedial portion of the proximal tibia. A lateral thrust of the tibia can be felt during ambulation. Internal tibial torsion is present.[157] The knee is stable in extension, but in 10 to 20 degrees of flexion, some medial-lateral instability is present.

Langenskiöld[143] classified the radiographic changes caused by Blount's disease into six stages based on the characteristic medial metaphyseal fragmentation, depression, and beaking that progress with age (Fig. 65.14). The initial stage of infantile Blount's disease and that of extreme physiological bowlegs are difficult to differentiate. Caffey[116] suggested that the main differential radiographic finding in a child in whom tibia vara is developing is a sharp angulation of the medial cortex of the proximal tibial metaphysis, in contrast to the lateral cortex, which remains nearly straight. Levine and Drennan[146] described the use of the metaphyseal-diaphyseal angle to predict which children will progress from physiological bowlegs to Blount's disease (Fig. 65.15). On an anteroposterior radiograph, this angle is formed by the intersection of a line drawn through the widest portion of the proximal tibial metaphysis (between the medial and lateral me-

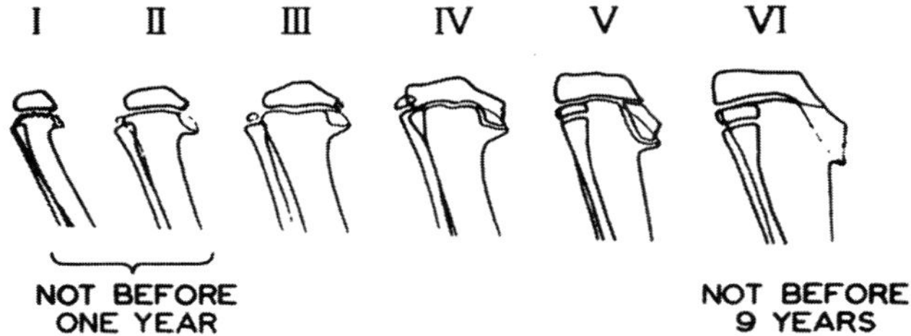

FIGURE 65.14 ➢ Langenskiöld classification of radiographic changes in Blount's disease. Stages show progressively increasing deformity of proximal tibia. In stage V, physis is angulated 90 degrees, and in stage VI, physis is fused. (Redrawn from Langenskiöld A, Riskä EB: Tibia vara (osteochondrosis deformans tibiae): A survey of 71 cases. J Bone Joint Surg Am 46:1405, 1964.)

taphyseal beaks) and a line drawn perpendicular to the longitudinal axis of the tibial metaphysis. Levine and Drennan[146] found that tibia vara progressed and Blount's disease developed in 96% of patients whose metaphyseal-diaphyseal angles measured more than 11 degrees. Tibia vara did not progress and Blount's disease did not develop in 80% of patients in whom the metaphyseal-diaphyseal angles measured less than 11 degrees. This measurement is not totally reliable[133] and can vary if the radiograph is made with any external or internal rotation of the lower extremity. Henderson et al[136] found an interobserver variability of ±4.6 degrees in measurements of the metaphyseal-diaphyseal angle, and they recommended that this difference be considered in comparing a patient's angle with the criterion of 11 degrees. Foreman and Robertson,[128] however, found the measurement reliable and easily obtainable. Feldman and Schoenecker[126] found that when the metaphyseal-diaphyseal angle was 16 degrees or more, the risk of a false-positive error decreased to less than 5%. Based on these findings, they recommended initiating treatment for early infantile tibia vara only if the metaphyseal-diaphyseal angle was 16 degrees or more.

O'Neill and MacEwen[149] examined roentgenograms of 39 knees in children younger than 30 months who had bowlegs. They found a poorer prognosis in those children in whom the fibula was longer than the tibia and in those who had more acute proximal tibial angulation than distal femoral angulation. The authors emphasized the importance of comparing the degree of bowing with the normal developmental pattern and noted that a significant deviation suggested a poor prognosis for spontaneous resolution of the deformity.

Arthrography outlines the tibial plateau and may show the hypertrophied, nonossified cartilage that is not visible on plain roentgenograms.[121, 137]

Treatment of Blount's disease depends on the age of the child and the severity of the varus deformity. Some children younger than 3 years with stage I or stage II involvement may improve without treatment or can be treated in an ambulatory orthosis that produces a valgus stress at the proximal tibia.[114, 155] Daytime ambulatory bracing has been shown to be effective in correcting tibia vara in children younger than 3 years with Langenskiöld stage I or stage II involvement and a metaphyseal diaphyseal angle of more than 16 degrees.[153, 154, 164] Loder and Johnson,[147] however, found bracing to be effective in only approximately 50% of patients, even in young children, and recommended that bracing be used only as a trial in young children.

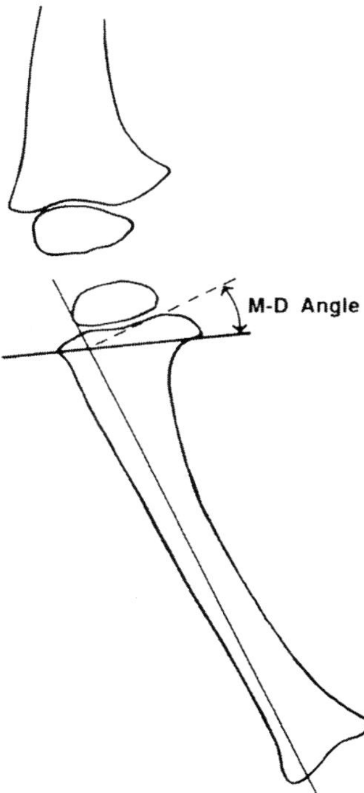

FIGURE 65.15 ➢ Metaphyseal-diaphyseal angle described by Levine and Drennan. Values greater than 11 degrees are consistent with Blount's disease. (Redrawn from Levine AM, Drennan JC: Physiological bowing and tibia vara: The metaphyseal-diaphyseal angle in the measurement of bowleg deformities. J Bone Joint Surg Am 64: 1158, 1982.)

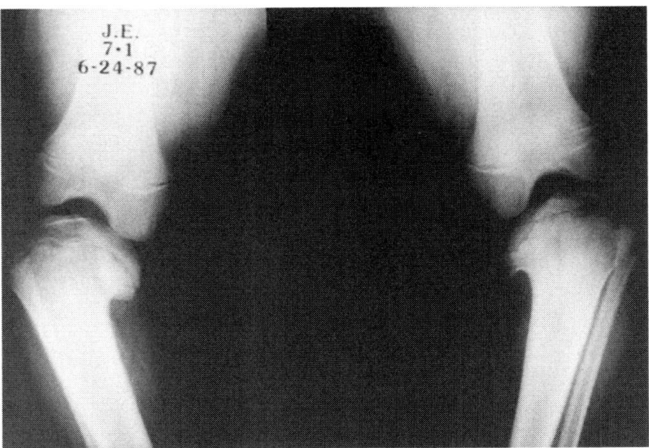

FIGURE 65.16 ➢ Radiograph of 7-year-old child with infantile Blount's disease. (From Scott WN: The Knee, vol 1. St Louis, Mosby-Year Book, 1994, p. 221.)

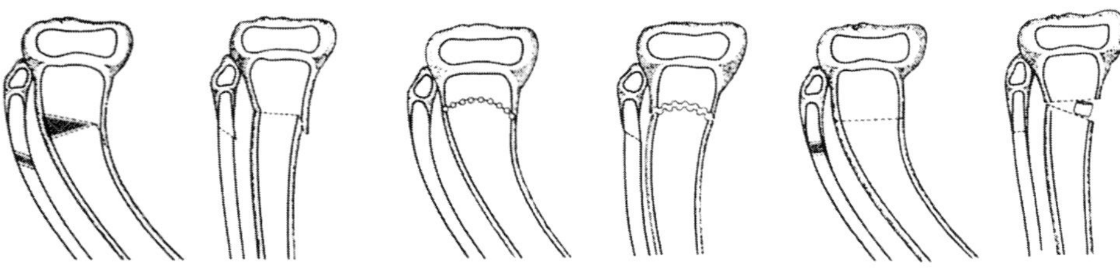

FIGURE 65.17 ➢ Types of osteotomies for correction of deformity in Blount's disease: Closing wedge osteotomy. Crescent-shaped osteotomy. Opening wedge osteotomy. (Modified from Canale ST, Beaty JH, eds: Operative Pediatric Orthopaedics. St. Louis, Mosby-Year Book, 1991.)

Early surgical treatment is the mainstay of treatment in children between the ages of 3 and 5 years because at this age, the diagnosis of Blount's disease is established, its natural history is known to be progressive, and recurrence after surgery is less likely than when the child is older than 5 years. Surgical correction should be considered for children older than 3 years with Langenskiöld stage II involvement and for all children with stage III or greater involvement.[127, 137, 155] Schoenecker et al,[155] Beaty et al,[111] and Doyle[125] reported better results if the osteotomy was performed before age 5 years; after this age, recurrence of the varus deformity requiring repeat correction was much more likely. Schoenecker et al[155] found that postoperative correction to within −5 or +5 degrees of neutral in children younger than 5 years predictably produced satisfactory results. Loder and Johnston[147] reported that single tibial osteotomy produced good results in 85% of patients younger than 4 years, whereas multiple osteotomies were required in children 4 to 8 years old.

The most difficult treatment decisions are in children between the ages of 5 and 10 years with untreated or recurrent infantile Blount's disease (Fig. 65.16). In these children, so much deformity is present and so much damage has been done to the physis that recurrence of the deformity is likely. Treatment options include multiple tibial osteotomies, elevation of the tibial plateau, and osteotomy combined with epiphysiodesis followed by a limb length equalization procedure.[132, 156] In children older than 10 years with residual deformity of infantile Blount's disease, three-level epiphyseal-metaphyseal osteotomy is indicated.

Several techniques have been described for tibial valgus osteotomies, including closing and opening wedge osteotomies and a crescent-shaped osteotomy[117, 145, 150] (Fig. 65.17) Rab[152] described an oblique osteotomy that corrected internal tibial torsion as well as the varus deformity (Fig. 65.18). In children older than 9 years with Langenskiöld stage V or VI involvement, bony bar resection[112] or epiphysiodesis of the lateral tibial and fibular epiphyses may be indicated in addition to the valgus osteotomy. Physeal bar resection alone has been reported to be effective when premature closure of the physis is evident, but significant angular deformity cannot be corrected by resection alone. Epiphysiodesis should be performed between 9 years of age and skeletal maturity. In unilateral deformity, epiphysiodesis of the uninvolved leg may be in-

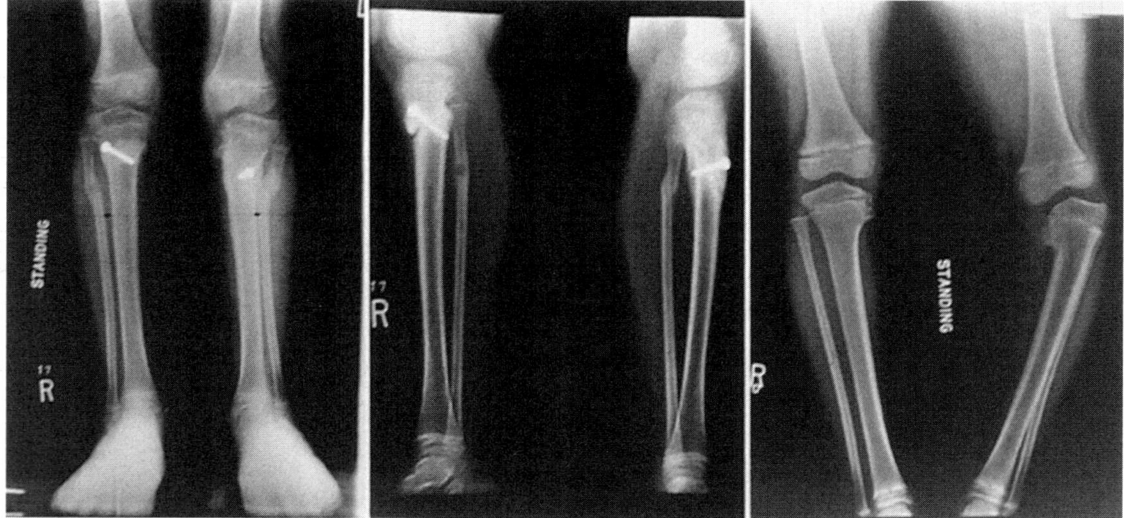

FIGURE 65.18 ➢ *A*, Preoperative radiograph of child with Blount's disease. *B*, Immediately after Rab-type osteotomy for correction of varus deformity. *C*, Six weeks after osteotomy. (From Scott WN: The Knee, vol. 1. St. Louis, Mosby-Year Book, 1994, p 222.)

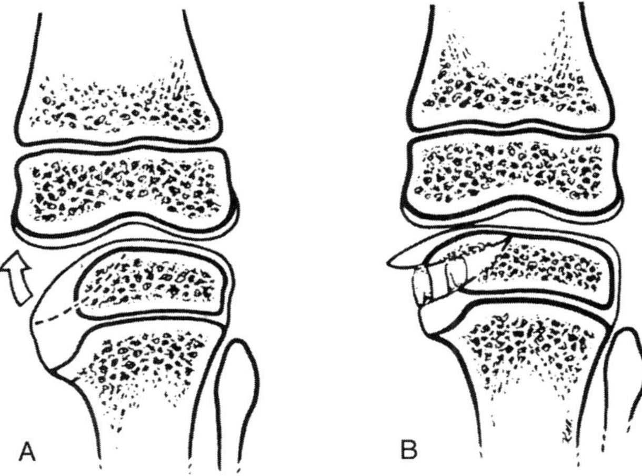

FIGURE 65.19 ➢ Epiphyseal-metaphyseal osteotomy. *A*, Curved osteotomy of epiphysis. *B*, Elevation of tibial condyle. (From Siffert RS: Intraepiphyseal osteotomy for progressive tibia vara: Case report and rationale for management. J Pediatr Orthop 2:81, 1982.)

dicated to prevent leg-length discrepancy. Osteotomy or epiphyseal distraction with external fixation has been reported for correction of the deformity, especially in obese patients.[119, 124, 130, 131, 151]

The prognosis of adolescent Blount's disease is better than that of the infantile form.[161] The deformity progresses more slowly, and recurrence is uncommon. Treatment has traditionally consisted of proximal tibial osteotomy, but Henderson et al[134] instead recommended lateral tibial hemiepiphysiodesis for patients with open proximal tibial physes because of the high incidence of complications and malalignment after tibial osteotomy. According to the authors, lateral tibial hemiepiphysiodesis does not interfere with later osteotomy, if necessary, and may actually make the osteotomy technically easier by decreasing the amount of correction that is required. The authors reserve tibial osteotomy as initial treatment for patients with severe deformities and closed or nearly closed proximal tibial physes.

For significant sloping deformity, Ingram,[138] Siffert,[158] and others[160] described an epiphyseal-metaphyseal osteotomy (Fig. 65.19) to restore knee articular anatomy to nearly normal and to prevent posterior subluxation with knee flexion. This procedure is indicated only in children older than 9 years with Langenskiöld stage V or VI involvement, severe sloping deformity, or premature closure of the medial physis (Fig. 65.20).

Kline et al[140] and Schoenecker et al[156] emphasized the importance of femoral varus deformity in older children with severe Blount's disease. In six adolescent patients, Kline et al[140] found that from 34% to 75% of the net genu varum deformity was contributed by the femur, whereas in eight patients with infantile disease, all genu varum deformity was in the tibiae. Schoenecker et al[156] recommended tibial osteotomy combined with elevation of the medial tibial plateau and epiphysiodesis of the lateral proximal tibial and proximal fibular epiphyses to restore as much anatomic configuration as possible.

FOCAL FIBROCARTILAGINOUS DYSPLASIA

Focal fibrocartilaginous dysplasia is a rare cause of varus deformity of the knee in children.[165-173] The lesion occurs in the proximal and medial tibial metaphysis, usually in children 1 to 2 years old.[165] The etiology is unknown. Abnormal development of fibrocartilage at the site of the insertion of the pes anserinus tendon has been proposed as a possible cause.[166] Genu varum is localized distal to the physis, as opposed to Blount's

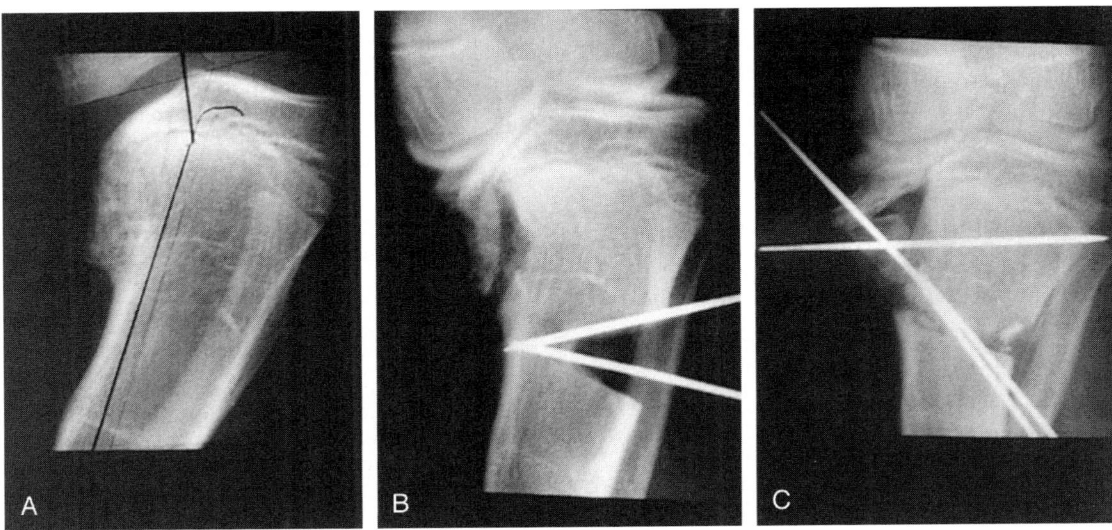

FIGURE 65.20 ➢ Epiphyseal-metaphyseal osteotomy. *A*, Preoperative deformity. *B and C*, Intraoperative radiographs. (From Scott WN: The Knee, vol 1. St. Louis, Mosby-Year Book, 1994, p 223.)

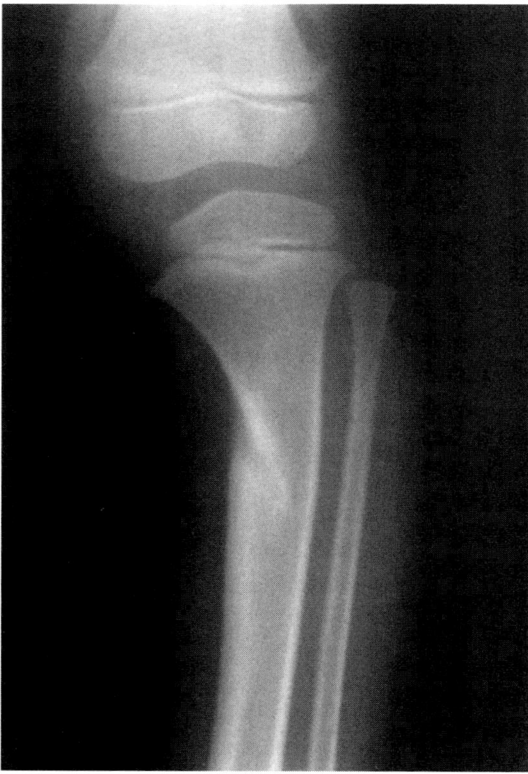

FIGURE 65.21 ➢ Varus deformity of proximal tibia secondary to focal fibrocartilaginous dysplasia.

disease, in which the varus angulation is located at the level of the physis. A radiolucent cortical defect with surrounding sclerosis is visible on plain radiographs (Fig. 65.21). Biopsies of this lesion consist of dense fibrous tissue. Initially, the varus deformity increases and then spontaneously resolves.[166] Because of this tendency for spontaneous correction, observation is the recommended treatment of this lesion. Surgery is recommended only in patients who show no signs of spontaneous correction of the deformity.

References

Congenital Dislocation and Subluxation of the Knee

1. Austwick DH, Dandy DJ: Early operation for congenital subluxation of the knee. J Pediatr Orthop 3:85, 1983.
2. Bell MJ, Atkins RM, Sharrard WJW: Irreducible congenital dislocation of the knee: Aetiology and management. J Bone Joint Surg Br 69:403, 1987.
3. Bensahel H, Dal Monte A, Hjelmstedt A, et al: Congenital dislocation of the knee. J Pediatr Orthop 9:174, 1989.
4. Carlson DH, O'Connor J: Congenital dislocation of the knee. Am J Roentgenol 127:465, 1976.
5. Curtis BH, Fisher RL: Congenital hyperextension with anterior subluxation of the knee: Surgical treatment and long-term observations. J Bone Joint Surg Am 51:255, 1964.
6. Curtis BH, Fisher RL: Heritable congenital tibiofemoral suluxation: Clinical features and surgical treatment. J Bone Joint Surg Am 52:1104, 1970.
7. Ferris B, Aichroth P: The treatment of congenital knee dislocation: A review of nineteen knees. Clin Orthop 216:136, 1987.
8. Ferris BD, Jackson AM: Congenital snapping knee: Habitual anterior subluxation of the tibia in extension. J Bone Joint Surg Br 72:453, 1990.
9. Haga N, Nakamura S, Sakaguchi R, et al: Congenital dislocation of the knee reduced spontaneously or with minimal treatment. J Pediatr Orthop 17:59, 1997.
10. Johnson E, Audell R, Oppenheim WL: Congenital dislocation of the knee. J Pediatr Orthop 7:194, 1987.
11. Katz MP, Grogono BJ, Soper KC: The etiology and treatment of congenital dislocation of the knee. J Bone Joint Surg Br 49:112, 1967.
12. McFarlane AL: A report on four cases of congenital genu recurvatum occurring in one family. Br J Surg 34:388, 1947.
13. Middleton DS: The pathology of genu recurvatum. Br J Surg 22: 696, 1935.
14. Neibauer JJ, King DE: Congenital dislocation of the knee. J Bone Joint Surg Am 42:207, 1960.
15. Nogi J, MacEwen GD: Congenital dislocation of the knee. J Pediatr Orthop 2:509, 1982.
16. Provenzano F: Congenital dislocation of the knee. N Eng J Med 236:360, 1947.
17. Roach JW, Richards BS: Instructional case: Congenital dislocation of the knee. J Pediatr Orthop 8:226, 1988.
18. Roy DR, Crawford AH: Percutaneous quadriceps recession: A technique for management of congenital hyperextension deformity of the knee in the neonate. J Pediatr Orthop 9:717, 1989.
19. Shattock SG: Genu recurvatum in a foetus at term. Trans Pathol Soc Lond 42:280, 1891.

Congenital Absence of the Anterior Cruciate Ligament

20. Barrett GR, Tomasin JD: Bilateral congenital absence of the anterior cruciate ligament. Orthopedics 11:431, 1988.
21. Basmajian JV: A ring-shaped medial semi-lunar cartilage. J Bone Joint Surg Br 34:638, 1952.
22. Johansson E, Aparisi T: Congenital absence of the cruciate ligaments: A case report and review of the literature. Clin Orthop 162:108, 1982.
23. Johansson E, Aparisi T: Missing cruciate ligament in congenital short femur. J Bone Joint Surg Am 65:1109, 1983.
24. Kaelin A, Hulin PH, Carlioz H: Congenital aplasia of the cruciate ligaments: A report of six cases. J Bone Joint Surg Br 68: 827, 1986.
25. Noble J: Congenital absence of the anterior cruciate ligament associated with a ring meniscus: Report of a case. J Bone Joint Surg Am 57:1165, 1975.
26. Schoenecker PL et al: Dysplasia of the knee joint in association with the thrombocytopenia absent radius syndrome. Orthop Trans 5:404, 1981.
27. Thomas NP, Jackson AM, Aichroth PM: Congenital absence of the anterior cruciate ligament: A common component of knee dysplasia. J Bone Joint Surg Br 67:572, 1985.
28. Tolo VT: Congenital absence of the menisci and cruciate ligaments of the knee: A case report. J Bone Joint Surg Am 63: 1022, 1981.
29. Torode IP, Gillespie R: Anteroposterior instability of the knee: A sign of congenital limb deficiency. J Pediatr Orthop 3:467, 1983.

Congenital Dislocation of the Patella

30. Baker RH et al: The semitendinosus tenodesis for recurrent dislocation of the patella. J Bone Joint Surg Br 54:103, 1972.
31. Gao GX, Lee EH, Bose K: Surgical management of congenital and habitual dislocation of the patella. J Pediatr Orthop 10:255, 1990.
32. Green JP, Waugh W: Congenital lateral dislocation of the patella. J Bone Joint Surg Br 50:285, 1968.
33. Gunn DR: Contracture of the quadriceps muscle: A discussion

on the etiology and relationship to recurrent dislocation of the patella. J Bone Joint Surg Br 46:492, 1964.
34. Jeffreys TE: Recurrent dislocation of the patella due to abnormal attachment of the ilio-tibial tract. J Bone Joint Surg Br 45: 740, 1963.
35. Jones RDS, Fisher RL, Curtis BH: Congenital dislocation of the patella. Clin Orthop 119:177, 1976.
36. Langenskiöld AL, Ritsilä V: Congenital dislocation of the patella and its operative treatment. J Pediatr Orthop 12:315, 1992.
37. McCall RE, Lessenberry HB: Bilateral congenital dislocation of the patella. J Pediatr Orthop 7:100, 1987.
38. Mumford EB: Congenital dislocation of the patella: Case report with a history of four generations. J Bone Joint Surg 29:1083, 1947.
39. Stanisavljevic S, Zemenick G, Miller D: Congenital, irreducible, permanent lateral dislocation of the patella. Clin Orthop 116: 190, 1976.
40. Støren H: Congenital complete dislocation of patella causing serious disability in childhood: The operative treatment. Acta Orthop Scand 36:301, 1965.
41. Walker J, Rang M, Daneman A: Ultrasonography of the unossified patella in young children. J Pediatr Orthop 11:100, 1991.
42. Zeier FG, Dissanayke C: Congenital dislocation of the patella. Clin Orthop 148:140, 1980.

Nail-Patella Syndrome

43. Beals RK, Eckhardt AL: Hereditary onycho-osteodysplasia (nail-patella) syndrome: A report of nine kindreds. J Bone Joint Surg Am 51:505, 1969.
44. Duncan JG, Souter WA: Hereditary onycho-osteodysplasia. The nail patella syndrome. J Bone Joint Surg Br 45:242, 1964.
45. Garces MA et al: Hereditary onchyo-osteo-dysplasia (HOOD syndrome): A report of two cases. Skeletal Radiol 8:55, 1982.
46. Guidera KJ et al: Nail patella syndrome: a review of 44 orthopaedic patients. J Pediatr Orthop 11:737, 1991.
47. Loomer RL: Shoulder girdle dysplasia associated with nail patella syndrome: A case report and literature review. Clin Orthop 238:112, 1989.
48. Yakish SD, Fu FH: Long-term follow-up of the treatment of a family with nail-patella syndrome. J Pediatr Orthop 3:360, 1983.
49. Yarali HN, Erden GA, Karaarslan F, et al: Clavicular horn: Another bony projection in nail-patella syndrome. Pediatr Radiol 25:549, 1995.

Bipartite Patella

50. Bourne MH, Bianco AJ Jr: Bipartite patella in the adolescent: Results of surgical excision. J Pediatr Orthop 10:69, 1990.
51. Carter SR: Traumatic separation of a bipartite patella. Injury 20: 244, 1989.
52. Casscells SW: Chondromalacia of the patella. J Pediatr Orthop 2:560, 1982.
53. DeLee JC, Dickhaut SC: The discoid lateral meniscus syndrome. J Bone Joint Surg Am 64:1068, 1982.
54. Green WT Jr: Painful bipartite patella: A report of three cases. Clin Orthop 110:197, 1975.
55. Halpern AA, Hewitt O: Painful medial bipartite patellae. Clin Orthop 134: 180, 1978.
56. Insall J: Current concepts review: Patellar pain. J Bone Joint Surg Am 64:147, 1982.
57. Ishikawa H, Sakurai A, Hirata S, et al: Painful bipartite patella in young athletes: The diagnostic value of skyline views taken in squatting position and the results of surgical excision. Clin Orthop Rel Res 305:223, 1994.
58. Mori Y, Okumo H, Iketani H, et al: Efficacy of lateral retinacular release for painful bipartite patella. Am J Sports Med 23:13, 1995.
59. Needoff M: Like father, like son: A tale of two patellae. J Orthop Trauma 4:163, 1990.
60. Ogata K: Painful bipartite patella: A new approach to operative treatment. J Bone Joint Surg Am 76:573, 1994.
61. Ogden JA, McCarthy SM, Joke P: The painful bipartite patella. J Pediatr Orthop 2:263, 1982.
62. Singer KM, Henry J: Knee problems in children and adolescents. Clin Sport Med 4:385, 1985.

Discoid Meniscus

63. Aichroth PM, Patel DV, Marx CL: Congenital discoid lateral meniscus in children: A follow-up study and evolution of management. J Bone Joint Surg Br 73:932, 1991.
64. Albertsson M, Gillquist J: Discoid lateral meniscus: A report of 29 cases. Arthroscopy 4:211, 1988.
65. Auge W II, Kaeding CC: Case report: Bilateral discoid medial menisci with extensive intrasubstance cleavage tears: MRI and arthroscopic correlation. Arthroscopy 10:313, 1994.
66. Barnes CL, McCarthy RE, VanderSchildden JL, et al: Discoid lateral meniscus in a young child: Case report and review of the literature. J Pediatr Orthop 8:707, 1987.
67. Bellier G, Dupont JY, Larrain M, et al: Lateral discoid menisci in children. Arthroscopy 5:52, 1989.
68. Dashefsky JH: Discoid lateral meniscus in three members of a family: Case reports. J Bone Joint Surg Am 53:1208, 1971.
69. Dickason JM, Del Pizzo W, Blazina ME, et al: A series of ten discoid medial menisci. Clin Orthop 168:76, 1982.
70. Dickhaut SC, DeLee JC: The discoid lateral-meniscus syndrome. J Bone Joint Surg Am 64:1068, 1982.
71. Dimakopoulos P, Patel D: Partial excision of discoid meniscus: Arthroscopic operation of 10 patients. Acta Orthop Scand 61: 40, 1990.
72. Fritschy D, Gonseth D: Discoid lateral meniscus. Inter Orthop (SICOT) 15:145, 1991.
73. Fujikawa K, Iseki F, Mikura Y: Partial resection of the discoid meniscus in the child's knee. J Bone Joint Surg Br 63:391, 1981.
74. Gebhardt MC, Rosenthal RK: Bilateral discoid meniscus in identical twins. J Bone Joint Surg Am 61:1110, 1979.
75. Hamada M, Shino K, Kawano K, et al: Usefulness of magnetic resonance imaging for detecting intrasubstance tears and/or degeneration of lateral discoid meniscus. Arthroscopy 10:645, 1994.
76. Hayashi LK, Yamaga H, Ida K, et al: Arthroscopic meniscectomy for discoid lateral meniscus in children. J Bone Joint Surg Am 70:1495, 1988.
77. Ikeuchi H: Arthroscopic treatment of the discoid lateral meniscus: Technique and long-term results. Clin Orthop 167:19, 1982.
78. Kaplan EB: Discoid lateral meniscus of the knee joint: nature, mechanism, and operative treatment. J Bone Joint Surg Am 39: 77, 1957.
79. Manzione M, Pizzutillo PD, Peoples AB, et al: Meniscectomy in children: A long-term follow-up study. Am J Sports Med 11:111, 1983.
80. Medlar RC, Mandiberg JJ, Lyne ED: Meniscectomies in children: Report of long-term results (mean, 8.3 years) of 26 children. Am J Sports Med 8:87, 1980.
81. Pellacci F, Montanari G, Prosperi P, et al: Lateral discoid meniscus: Treatment and results. Arthroscopy 8:526, 1992.
82. Rosenberg TD et al: Discoid lateral meniscus: Case report of arthroscopic attachment of a symptomatic Wrisberg-ligament type. Arthroscopy 3:277, 1987.
83. Silverman JM, Mink JH, Deutsch AL: Discoid menisci of the knee: MR imaging appearance. Radiology 173:351, 1989.
84. Smillie IS: The congenital discoid meniscus. J Bone Joint Surg Br 30:671, 1948.
85. Stark JE, Siegel MJ, Weinberger E, et al: Discoid menisci in children: MR features. J Comp Assist Tomog 19:608, 1995.
86. Stern A, Hallel T: Medial discoid meniscus with cyst formation in a child. J Pediatr Orthop 8:471, 1988.
87. Sugawara O, Miyatsu M, Yamashita I, et al: Problems with repeated arthroscopic surgery in the discoid meniscus. Arthroscopy 7:68, 1991.
88. Vandermeer RD, Cunningham FK: Arthroscopic treatment of the discoid lateral meniscus: Results of long-term follow-up. Arthroscopy 5:101, 1989.

89. Washington ER, Root L, Liener UC: Discoid lateral meniscus in children: Long-term follow-up after excision. J Bone Joint Surg Am 77:1357, 1995.
90. Watanabe M, Takeda S, Ikeuchi H: Atlas of Arthroscopy. 3rd ed. Berlin, Springer, 1979.
91. Zaman M, Leonard MA: Meniscectomy in children: Results in 59 knees. Injury 12:425, 1981.

Popliteal Cysts

92. Baker ND: Evaluation of popliteal cysts. Rheum Dis Clin North Am 17:803, 1991.
93. Baker WM: On the formation of synovial cysts in the leg in connection with disease of the knee joint. St Bart Hosp Rep 13:245, 1877.
94. Dinhamn JM: Popliteal cysts in children: The case against surgery. J Bone Joint Surg Br 57:69, 1975.
95. Fielding JR, Franklin PD, Kustan J: Popliteal cysts: A reassessment using magnetic resonance imaging. Skeletal Radiol 20: 433, 1991.
96. Hughston JC, Baker CL, Mello W: Popliteal cyst: A surgical approach. Orthopedics 14:147, 1991.
97. Massari L et al: Diagnosis and treatment of popliteal cysts. Chir Organi Mov 75:245, 1990.
98. Szer IS et al: Ultrasonography in the study of prevalence and clinical evolution of popliteal cysts in children with knee effusions. J Rheumatol 19:458, 1992.

Bowlegs and Knock Knees

99. Bowen JR et al: Partial epiphysiodesis at the knee to correct angular deformity. Clin Orthop 198:184, 1985.
100. Davids JR et al: Angular deformity of the lower extremity in children with renal osteodystrophy. J Pediatr Orthop 12:291, 1992.
101. Engel GM, Staheli LT: The natural history of torsion and other factors influencing gait in childhood. Clin Orthop 99:12, 1974.
102. Herring JA, Kling TF Jr: Genu valgus: An instructional case. J Pediatr Orthop 5:236, 1985.
103. Howorth B: Knock knees. Clin Orthop 77:233, 1971.
104. Jackson SW, Cozen L: Genu valgus as a complication of proximal tibial metaphyseal fractures in children. J Bone Joint Surg Am 53:1571, 1971.
105. McDade W: Bow legs and knock knees. Pediatr Clin North Am 24:825, 1977.
106. Robertson WW Jr: Distal tibial deformity in bowlegs. J Pediatr Orthop 7:324, 1987.
107. Salenius P, Vankka E: The development of the tibiofemoral angle in children. J Bone Joint Surg Am 57:259, 1975.
108. Zeuge RC, Kempken TC, Blount WP: Epiphyseal stapling for angular deformities of the knee. J Bone Joint Surg Am 61:320, 1979.

Blount's Disease

109. Arkin AM, Katz JF: The effects of pressure on epiphyseal growth: The mechanism of plasticity of growing. J Bone Joint Surg Am 38:1056, 1956.
110. Bathfield CA, Beighton PH: Blount disease: A review of etiological factors in 110 patients. Clin Orthop 135:29, 1978.
111. Beaty JH, Coscia MF, Holt M: Blount's Disease. Paper presented at the Southern Orthopaedic Association, Edinburgh, Scotland, September 1988.
112. Beck CL et al: Physeal bridge resection in infantile Blount disease. J Pediatr Orthop 7:161, 1987.
113. Blount WP: Tibia vara, osteochondrosis deformans tibiae. J Bone Joint Surg 19:1, 1937.
114. Blount WP: Tibia vara, osteochondrosis deformans tibiae. Curr Pract Orthop Surg 3:141, 1966.
115. Bradway JK, Klassen RA, Peterson HA: Blount disease: A review of the English literature. J Pediatr Orthop 7:472, 1987.
116. Caffey JP: Pediatric X-Ray Diagnosis. 7th ed. Chicago, Year Book Medical Publishers, 1978.
117. Canale ST, Harper MC: Biotrigonometric analysis and practical applications of osteotomies of the tibia in children. AAOS Instr Course Lect 30:85, 1981.
118. Carter JR et al: Late-onset tibia vara: A histopathologic analysis. A comparative evaluation with infantile tibia vara and slipped capital femoral epiphysis. J Pediatr Orthop 8:187, 1988.
119. Coogan PG, Fox JA, Fitch RD: Treatment of adolescent Blount disease with the circular external fixation device and distraction osteogenesis. J Pediatr Orthop 16:450, 1996.
120. Cook SD et al: A biomechanical analysis of the etiology of tibia vara. J Pediatr Orthop 3:449, 1983.
121. Dalinka MK et al: Arthrography in Blount's disease. Radiology 113:161, 1974.
122. Davids JR, Huskamp M, Bagley AM: A dynamic biomechanical analysis of the etiology of adolescent tibia vara. J Pediatr Orthop 16:461, 1996.
123. Deitz WH, Gross WL, Kirkpatrick JA: Blount's disease (tibia vara): Another skeletal disorder associated with childhood obesity. J Pediatr 101:735, 1982.
124. De Pablos J, Alfaro J, Barrious C: Treatment of adolescent Blount disease by asymmetric physeal distraction. J Pediatr Orthop 17:54, 1997.
125. Doyle BS, Volk AG, Smith CF: Infantile Blount disease: Long-term follow-up of surgically treated patients at skeletal maturity. J Pediatr Orthop 16:469, 1996.
126. Feldman MD, Schoenecker PL: Use of the metaphyseal-diaphyseal angle in the evaluation of bowed legs. J Bone Joint Surg Am 76:1752, 1994.
127. Ferriter P, Shapira F: Infantile tibia vara: Factors affecting outcome following proximal tibial osteotomy. J Pediatr Orthop 7:1, 1987.
128. Foreman KA, Robertson WW Jr: Radiographic measurement of infantile tibia vara. J Pediatr Orthp 5:452, 1985.
129. Ganel A, Heim M, Farine I: Asymmetric epiphyseal distraction in the treatment of Blount's disease. Orthop Rev 15:237, 1986.
130. Gaudinez R, Adar U: Use of Orthofix T-Garache fixator in late-onset tibia vara. J Pediatr Orthop 16:455, 1996.
131. Golding JSR, MacNeil-Smith JDG: Observations on the etiology of tibia vara. J Bone Joint Surg Br 45:320, 1963.
132. Gregosiewicz A et al: Double-elevating osteotomy of tibiae in the treatment of severe cases of Blount's disease. J Pediatr Orthop 9:178, 1989.
133. Hägglund G, Ingvarsson T, Ramgren B, et al: Metaphyseal-diaphyseal angle in Blount's disease: A 30-year follow-up of 13 unoperated children. Acta Orthop Scand 68:167, 1997.
134. Henderson RC, Kemp GJ, Greene WB: Adolescent tibia vara: Alternatives for operative treatment. J Bone Joint Surg Am 74: 342, 1992.
135. Henderson RC, Kemp J, Hayes PRL: Prevalence of late-onset tibia vara. J Pediatr Orthop 13:255, 1993.
136. Henderson RC et al: Variability in radiographic measurement of bowleg deformities in children. J Pediatr Orthop 10:491, 1990.
137. Hofmann A, Jones RE, Herring JA: Blount's disease after skeletal maturity. J Bone Joint Surg Am 64:1004, 1982.
138. Ingram AJ: Personal communication, 1984.
139. Kessel L: Annotations on the etiology and treatment of tibia vara. J Bone Joint Surg Br 52:93, 1970.
140. Kline SC, Bostrum M, Griffin PP: Femoral varus: An important component in late-onset Blount's disease. J Pediatr Orthop 12: 197, 1992.
141. Kling TF Jr: Tibia vara: A mechanical problem. Orthop Trans 5: 138, 1981.
142. Langenskiöld A: Tibia vara: A critical review. Clin Orthop 246: 195, 1989.
143. Langenskiöld A: Tibia vara: Osteochondrosis deformas tibiae: Blount's disease. Clin Orthop 158:77, 1981.
144. Langenskiöld A, Riska EB: Tibia vara (osteochondrosis deformans tibiae): A survey of 71 cases. J Bone Joint Surg Am 46: 1405, 1964.
145. Laurencin CT, Ferriter PJ, Millis MB: Oblique proximal tibial osteotomy for the correction of tibia vara in the young. Clin Orthop Rel Res 327:218, 1996.
146. Levine AM, Drennan JC: Physiological bowing and tibia vara: The metaphyseal-diaphyseal angle in the measurement of bowleg deformities. J Bone Joint Surg Am 64:1158, 1982.

147. Loder RT, Johnston CE II: Infantile tibia vara. J Pediatr Orthop 7:639, 1987.
148. Loder RT, Schaffer JJ, Bardenstein MB: Late-onset tibia vara. J Pediatr Orthop 11:162, 1991.
149. O'Neill DA, MacEwen GD: Early roentgenographic evaluation of bowlegged children. J Pediatr Orthop 2:547, 1982.
150. Martin SD, Moran MC, Martin TL, et al: Proximal tibial osteotomy with compression plate fixation for tibia vara. J Pediatr Orthop 14:619, 1994.
151. Price CT, Scott DS, Greenberg DA: Dynamic axial external fixation in the surgical treatment of tibia vara. J Pediatr Orthop 15: 236, 1995.
152. Rab GT: Oblique tibial osteotomy for Blount's disease (tibia vara). J Pediatr Orthop 8:715, 1988.
153. Raney EM, Topoleski TA, Yaghoubian R, et al: Orthotic treatment of infantile tibia vara. J Pediatr Orthop 18:670, 1998.
154. Richards BS, Katz DE, Sims JB: Effectiveness of brace treatment in early infantile Blount's disease. J Pediatr Orthop 18:374, 1998.
155. Schoenecker PL et al: Blount's disease: A retrospective review and recommendations for treatment. J Pediatr Orthop 5:181, 1985.
156. Schoenecker PL et al.: Elevation of the medial plateau of the tibia in the treatment of Blount disease. J Bone Joint Surg Am 74:351, 1992.
157. Siffert RS, Katz JR: The intra-articular deformity in osteochondrosis deformans tibiae. J Bone Joint Surg Am 52:800, 1970.
158. Siffert RS: Intraepiphyseal osteotomy for progressive tibia vara: Case report and rationale for management. J Pediatr Orthop 2: 81, 1982.
159. Smith JF: Current concepts review: Tibia vara (Blount's disease). J Bone Joint Surg Am 64:630, 1982.
160. Støren H: Operative elevation of the medial tibial joint surface in Blount's disease: One case observed for 18 years after operation. Acta Orthop Scand 40:788, 1969.
161. Thompson GF, Carter JR: Late-onset tibia vara (Blount's disease): Current concepts. Clin Orthop 255:24, 1990.
162. Thompson GH, Carter JR, Smith CW: Late onset tibia vara: A comparative analysis. J Pediatr Orthop 4:185, 1984.
163. Wenger DR, Mickelson M, Maynard JA: The evolution and histopathology of adolescent tibia vara. J Pediatr Orthop 4:78, 1984.
164. Zionts LE, Shean CJ: Brace treatment of early infantile tibia vara. J Pediatr Orthop 18:102, 1998.

Focal Fibrocartilaginous Dysplasia

165. Albiñana J, Cuervo M, Certucha JA, et al: Five additional cases of local fibrocartilaginous dysplasia. J Pediatr Orthop Part B 6: 52, 1997.
166. Bell SN, Campbell PE, Cole WG, et al: Tibia vara caused by focal fibrocartilaginous dysplasia: three case reports. J Bone Joint Surg Br 67:780, 1985.
167. Bradish CF, Davies SJM, Malone M: Tibia vara due to focal fibrocartilaginous dysplasia: The natural history. J Bone Joint Surg Br 70:106, 1988.
168. Cockshott WP, Martin R, Friedman L, et al: Focal fibrocartilaginous dysplasia and tibia vara: A case report. Skeletal Radiol 23: 333, 1994.
169. Husien AMA, Kale VR: Case report: Tibia vara caused by focal fibrocartilaginous dysplasia. Clin Radiol 40:104, 1989.
170. Kariya Y, Taniguichi K, Yagisawa H, et al: Focal fibrocartilaginous dysplasia: Consideration of healing process. J Pediatr Orthop 11:545, 1991.
171. Meyer JS, Davidson RS, Hubbard AM, et al: MRI of focal fibrocartilaginous dysplasia. J Pediatr Orthop 13:304, 1993.
172. Olney BW, Cole WG, Menelaus MB: Three additional cases of focal fibrocartilaginous dysplasia causing tibia vara. J Pediatr Orthop 10: 405, 1990.
173. Zayer M: Tibia vara in focal fibrocartilaginous dysplasia: A report of two cases. Acta Orthop Scand 63:353, 1992.

66 The Pediatric Knee—Evaluation and Treatment

MININDER S. KOCHER • LYLE J. MICHELI

KNEE EVALUATION IN THE PEDIATRIC PATIENT

Knee injuries in children and adolescents are unique to the growing body and specific to the demands of the involved sport or activity. The musculoskeletal system of the skeletally immature patient differs from that of the adult in significant ways. Bone of children and adolescents is more susceptible to injury, including unique patterns such as plastic deformation. Fractures in children heal more quickly than in adults. Most fractures in children are able to be treated closed, and those requiring operative fixation often need less rigid constructs than fractures in adults need. Children have a greater potential to remodel after bony injury owing to their thicker periosteum and ongoing growth potential. Ligaments in children tend to have greater laxity and, in general, are stronger than the physis, thus predisposing to physeal injury. The physis is unique to the growing skeleton, and sequelae of physeal injury include growth arrest and angular deformity. The growing skeleton may induce muscle imbalance and stiffness across joints, predisposing to injury, particularly during periods of rapid growth. The developing knee has a larger cartilage component than the adult knee has, with physeal cartilage of the distal femur and proximal tibia, apophyseal cartilage of the patella and tibial tubercle, and articular cartilage of the distal femoral and proximal tibial epiphyses. The susceptibility of this growing cartilage to injury allows for unique injuries including osteochondritis, osteochondrosis, apophysitis, and osteochondral injury.[125, 367, 371]

History and Physical Examination

The diagnosis of knee pain in children can be difficult because children are poor historians and the symptoms they describe are frequently vague and generalized. Children younger than age 6 or 7 years are usually unable to reliably localize pain. Thus, their manifestation of a knee disorder may be only a limp or a refusal to walk.

Knee pain is a common presenting complaint. The differential diagnoses of knee pain in the skeletally immature patient are numerous and differ substantially from adult knee pain (Table 66.1). Consideration should always be given to referred pain from hip disorders (particularly slipped capital femoral epiphysis), tumors, and systemic illnesses (such as hemophilia, Reiter's syndrome, and juvenile rheumatoid arthritis [JRA]).[21, 170, 211, 321, 324, 367]

The history should include onset of symptoms (duration, acute versus chronic, acute injury versus insidious injury), location and character of pain, mechanical symptoms, instability, bilaterality, relation of symptoms to activity, previous history of symptoms, involvement of other joints, systemic symptoms, other medical problems, family history of musculoskeletal problems, growth history, developmental history, and activity or competitive level. The parents' concerns should always be elicited and addressed. In addition to physical examination of the knee, assessment should be made of gait, height, appropriate developmental milestones, physical maturity, hip examination, rotational and mechanical alignment of lower extremities, spinal deformity, presence of masses, and overall fitness level. A screening test for constitutional joint looseness should be performed using the maneuvers listed in Table 66.2. The child is considered hypermobile if he or she can perform three of the five maneuvers listed. A simple screening test has recently been described that allows grading of relative laxity. Loose-jointed children may be more prone to injury.[31, 125]

Imaging should be used to supplement a careful history and thorough physical examination. X-ray films

TABLE 66.1 DIFFERENTIAL DIAGNOSIS OF KNEE PAIN IN CHILDREN AND ADOLESCENTS

Acute fracture (distal femur, proximal tibia, patella, tibial spine)
Stress fracture
Physeal injury
Osteochondritis dissecans
Osgood-Schlatter disease
Sinding-Larsen-Johansson disease
Ligament injury (ACL, PCL, MCL, LCL)
Meniscal injury
Discoid meniscus
Patellofemoral pain
Patellofemoral subluxation/dislocation
Plica
Patellar tendinitis
Prepatellar bursitis
Pes anserinus bursitis
Osteomyelitis
Septic arthritis
Juvenile rheumatoid arthritis
Tumor
Hemophilia
Referred pain from hip disease

ACL = anterior cruciate ligament; LCL = lateral collateral ligament; MCL = medial collateral ligament; PCL = posterior cruciate ligament.

TABLE 66.2 SIGNS OF LIGAMENT HYPERMOBILITY

Ability to touch floor with palms with knees straight
Ability to extend the metacarpophalangeal (MCP) joint of the little finger more than 90 degrees
Ability to abduct the thumb so it touches the forearm
Hyperextension of elbow more than 10 degrees
Hyperextension of knee more than 10 degrees

should be obtained first, particularly for unilateral knee pain. Roentgenographic comparison views of the opposite knee are often helpful in assessing unusual-appearing ossification centers or apophyses. X-ray films of the ipsilateral hip are indicated if the history or examination cannot refer the abnormality to the knee or if there are findings on hip examination. An anteroposterior (AP) x-ray film of the left wrist can be used to determine skeletal age. Standard knee x-ray films include AP and lateral views. Additional views may be beneficial, such as notch views for evaluating osteochondritis dissecans (OCD) or tibial spine avulsion, tangential views of the patellofemoral joint (Merchant's skyline) to assess patellofemoral dysplasia or subluxation, and stress views to consider physeal or collateral ligament injury. In addition, full-length 3-in AP lower-extremity films may be used to assess alignment, and scanograms may be used to assess leg-length discrepancy. Bone scans can aid in the assessment of OCD or in the localization of osteomyelitis or tumor. Magnetic resonance imaging (MRI) is useful in evaluating the physis and osteomyelitis. It is also frequently used to evaluate intra-articular pathology. MRI is often helpful in evaluating complete anterior cruciate ligament (ACL) injuries and the extent of OCD lesions; however, the accuracy of MRI of the knee in younger patients may be more limited than in adults, particularly for discoid menisci, meniscal tears, and partial ligament injuries.[103, 178, 184, 332, 395] In addition, recent studies have found the presence of signal changes within the menisci of asymptomatic children or children with menisci found to be normal at arthroscopy.[168, 178, 346]

Hemarthrosis

The most common causes of acute hemarthrosis in children are patellar dislocation, ACL injury, and osteochondral fracture. In children who underwent arthroscopy to evaluate acute hemarthrosis, Vahasarja and coworkers found 35% patellar dislocation and 23% ligament injuries in 138 children, Stanitski and colleagues found ACL tears in 47% of preadolescents and 65% of adolescents and meniscal tears in 47% of preadolescents and 45% of adolescents, Kloeppel-Wirth et al found 26% ACL injury and 23% patellar dislocation in 35 children, and Eiskjaer and coworkers found 45% ACL injury and 28% patellar dislocation in 40 pediatric patients.[93, 182, 334, 356] Thus, arthroscopy should be considered in children with acute hemarthrosis because of the high incidence of significant lesions. In particular, arthroscopy may be useful in the diagnosis and management of osteochondral fracture, which is relatively common after patellar dislocation and was radiographically silent in 5 of 14 patients in Matelic's series and 14 of 19 patients in Vahasarja's series.[220, 356, 357]

Hemophilia should be considered in any child presenting with hemarthrosis with a minimal history of trauma. The knee is the second most common bleeding site after the elbow. Treatment of hemophilia consists of factor VIII replacement to >25% for intramuscular bleeds, >50% for intra-articular bleeds, and 100% postoperatively. Arthroscopic synovectomy in the child or adolescent with a boggy synovium has been shown to decrease the number of bleeding episodes and reduce pain, but it may cause a loss of motion in some patients. Pigmented villonodular synovitis should also be included in the differential diagnosis of hemarthrosis in the adolescent.[21, 61, 120]

Arthroscopy in Children

Knee arthroscopy in children and adolescents is safe, yields high diagnostic accuracy, and allows treatment of a variety of intra-articular conditions.[17, 133, 214, 355, 357, 394]

In adolescents and older children, a standard 5-mm arthroscope may be used as in adults; however, a smaller 2.7-mm arthroscope provides more effective and gentler examination in smaller knees of younger children. General anesthesia is usually required in children because they are often unable to safely comply with sedation or regional anesthesia. Arthroscopy in children is safe. In a series of 202 arthroscopies in the knees of children age 5 to 18 years, there were no complications, and the procedure was found to be easier than in adults owing to children's more compliant joints.

Arthroscopy for diagnosis is frequently performed in children. Correlation of arthroscopic findings and preoperative diagnosis varies from 18% to 78.5% in the literature with most reports at approximately 50% correlation, with poorer diagnostic accuracy in younger children and for meniscal lesions.[17, 37, 92, 93, 132, 133, 141, 165, 247, 332, 344, 355, 356, 357] Because of the often poor accuracy of clinical diagnosis, arthroscopy offers substantial diagnostic benefit, and additional unsuspected lesions are not uncommonly found.

Arthroscopy also has substantial therapeutic benefit in children and adolescents, such as the management of ACL tears, meniscal tears, discoid menisci, tibial spine fracture fixation, septic arthritis, OCD, osteochondral fracture, patellofemoral maltracking, and plicae.[17, 37, 92, 93, 132, 133, 141, 165, 214, 247, 330–332, 344, 355–357, 394]

PATELLOFEMORAL DYSPLASIA

Patellofemoral dysplasia includes a spectrum of disorders involving malalignment of the patella within the femoral trochlea, resulting in patellar instability or anterior knee pain, or both. Merchant classified the spectrum of patellofemoral dysplasias into four groups according to severity: lateral patellar compression syndrome, chronic subluxating patella, recurrent dislocating patella, and chronic dislocating patella.[229] Reider and colleagues noted a correlation between the severity of lower-extremity malalignment and the severity of patellofemoral dysplasia symptoms.[286] Patellofemoral dysfunction is the most common cause of chronic knee pain in the child and the adolescent. Asymptomatic forms of patellofemoral dysplasia may predispose the child to symptoms only after traumatic or repetitive insult.

Anterior knee pain and patellofemoral instability can be chronic, frustrating entities for both the patient and the clinician; however, they can be treated successfully through an understanding of risk factors and patellofemoral biomechanics, a careful physical examination and accurate diagnosis, and a rational treatment plan.[107, 112, 232, 233, 237, 314, 333, 347, 389]

Etiology, Biomechanics, and Risk Factors

Patellofemoral dysplasia may have genetic or developmental etiology. It is common in genetic and connective tissue disorders with increased joint laxity. Some children with patellofemoral dysplasia give a history of antecedent trauma, such as direct blows, resulting in acute patellar subluxation or dislocation. More commonly, symptoms begin after the repetitive microtrauma of sports training, especially during the adolescent growth spurt.[232, 333, 347, 389]

Rapid growth in adolescents results in increased tension in the muscle-tendon units, which are stretched to accommodate longer bones. The thicker and less compliant vastus lateralis and iliotibial band exert a relatively unbalanced, laterally directed force. The resultant changes in patellar tracking may contribute to the onset of anterior pain and instability. The risk factors for patellofemoral dysplasia are usually multifactorial (Table 66.3).[3, 4, 59, 112, 125, 149, 232, 233, 237, 321, 330, 333]

Patellofemoral dysfunction, particularly chondromalacia and lateral patellar compression syndrome, may result from overuse injury to a knee predisposed to dysfunction because of patellofemoral dysplasia. Chondromalacia and anterior knee pain are activity related.

TABLE 66.3 FACTORS ASSOCIATED WITH PATELLOFEMORAL MALALIGNMENT

1. Q (quadriceps) angle greater than 15 degrees
2. Lateral patellar tilt
3. Patella alta
4. Vastus lateralis contracture
5. Medial retinaculum laxity
6. Previous medial arthrotomy
7. Genu recurvatum
8. Genu valgum
9. Generalized ligamentous laxity
10. Lateral femoral condyle hypoplasia
11. Shallow trochlear groove
12. Pronated and planus feet
13. Vastus medialis atrophy/hypoplasia
14. Femoral anteversion/external tibial torsion

Certain activities, such as jumping, place high demands on the patellofemoral joint, whereas other activities, such as running, may result in cumulative repetitive microtrauma. The prevalence of chondromalacia is related to activity level in children.[338] In addition, comparisons between large groups of children with anterior knee pain and those without pain have found differences in activity level, not lower extremity alignment or joint mobility, to correlate with the presence of pain.[95]

Reaction forces across the patellofemoral joint approximate one half of body weight with level walking, 3 to 4 times body weight with stair climbing, and nearly 10 times body weight with jumping activities or extension against resistance.[52] Therefore, even slight changes in congruity may increase areas of pressure beyond physiological limits. The rectus femoris, vastus lateralis, and vastus intermedius pull the patella along the long axis of the femur, which is approximately 7 degrees from vertical (anatomic valgus) in older children. The resultant force on the patella from the quadriceps proximally and the patellar tendon distally is directed laterally and balanced by the medial pull of the oblique fibers of the vastus medialis. Static stabilizers include the patellar retinaculum and the medial and lateral patellofemoral ligaments.

Patella alta can contribute to patellofemoral dysplasia. Proximal migration of the patella correlates with femoral growth rate, indicating that patella alta in some cases is acquired during the growth spurt rather than inherited. Girls have a slightly greater correlation between femoral growth rate and incidence of patella alta.[236] The size of a high patellae is also frequently smaller than normal.[324] Distal transposition of patella alta will likely increase patellofemoral pressure, thus worsening pain and accelerating the development of degenerative changes. Treatment should be directed toward the tight lateral retinaculum and lateral subluxation, if present.

Clinical Features

Patients with anterior knee pain typically complain of poorly localized pain about the patellofemoral joint, which is often correlated with activity or positioning. The pain is usually of a dull, achy nature without mechanical symptoms. The pain may worsen with jumping and climbing activities or may be present with prolonged sitting. Patients with patellofemoral instability may complain of frank dislocation or subtle subluxation, depending on the magnitude of instability. In addition, they often complain of giving way. It is important to evaluate mechanism of injury, acuity, previous treatment, and status of the contralateral knee.

In addition to examination of the patellofemoral joint, the physical examination should include gait evaluation, lower-extremity alignment, Q angle, hip examination, foot examination, knee stability, generalized ligamentous laxity, and knee range of motion.[12] Flexibility and strength of the quadriceps (particularly the vastus medialis obliquus) and hamstrings should be assessed.[164] The presence of patella alta, patella baja, Osgood-Schlatter disease, or Sinding-Larsen-Johansson disease should be ascertained. Examination of the patellofemoral joint should include an assessment of patellar glide and patellar tilt. Limited medial displacement and limited tilt should alert the clinician to the possibility of tight retinacular structures. Tracking of the patella should be observed as the patient slowly extends the knee. Lateral displacement of the patella as the knee approaches full extension is described as "J tracking." Pain may be present on resisted extension, compression of the patellofemoral joint, or palpation of the patella. Crepitus may be present on active or passive range of motion. Patients with instability may have a positive apprehension test with a laterally directed force.[333, 347, 389]

Radiographic Evaluation

Routine four-view radiographic images of the knee (AP, lateral, tunnel, and skyline views) should be obtained in the pediatric patient with unilateral symptoms, significant initial symptoms, or symptoms unresponsive to management. Osteochondral fracture of the patella may be appreciated on x-rays; however, a substantial number of chondral or osteochondral fractures are undetected by plain radiography. In any pediatric patient with patellar dislocation, osteochondral fracture should be considered because the rate of associated osteochondral fracture of the patella or lateral femoral condyle may be as high as 40% in some series.[123, 256, 333, 352] A multitude of radiographic measurements of the patellofemoral relationship exist including assessments of patellofemoral dysplasia, congruence, tilt, subluxation, and patellar height.[3] In the skeletally immature knee, patellar height can be determined using the ratio of the distance between the center of the patella and the midpoint of the tibial epiphyseal line to the distance between the midpoints of the distal femoral and proximal tibial epiphyseal lines (Fig. 66.1).[186] Computed tomography (CT) may be of additional benefit in assessing the extent of patella tilt or subluxation.[128, 328] MRI can be used to evaluate OCD of the patella. Sonography may be useful to assess the patella and extensor mechanism in young patients with limited ossification.[239, 364] These imaging assessments of the patellofemoral joint are limited, however, because they represent static images (often non-weightbearing) of a dynamic dysfunction. In addition, radiographic ratios may be unreliable and are age dependent in the skeletally immature knee, related to stage of ossification and maturation.[3, 186, 365]

Chondromalacia

Chondromalacia patellae is a pathological diagnosis resulting from patellofemoral dysfunction. It is not a clinical diagnosis, and efforts should be focused on identifying more precise etiologies of anterior knee pain such as patellofemoral dysplasia, patellar instability, osteochondral fracture, OCD, pathological plica, patellar

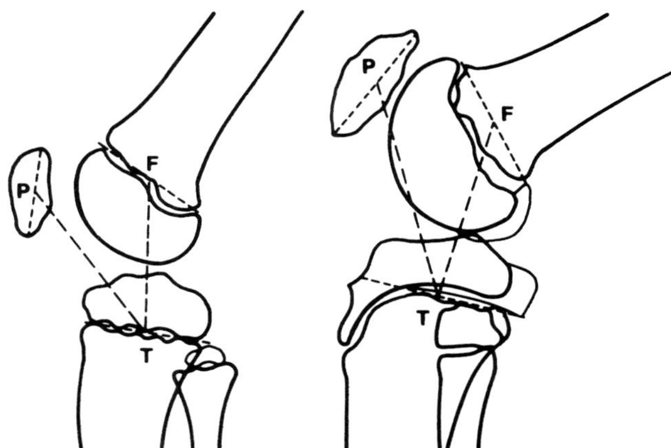

FIGURE 66.1 ➢ Epiphyseal line midpoint method for measurement of patellar height. The average PT:FT ratio is 1.31 ± 0.09 in full extension and decreases to 0.99 ± 0.06 at 90 degrees of flexion. P = patella, F = femur, T = tibia. (From Koshino T, Sugimoto K: J Pediatr Orthop 92:216, 1989.)

tendinitis, Sinding-Larsen-Johansson disease, Osgood-Schlatter disease, and bipartite patella.[333, 347, 389]

Insall described four stages of chondromalacia: stage I is softening of the cartilage from edema, stage II is fissuring with softened areas, stage III is breakdown of the articular cartilage (fasciculation), and stage IV refers to osteoarthritis with erosive changes and exposure of articular bone.[95, 149] Based on autopsy studies in children, grade I and II lesions can appear on the medial and central patellar segments in healthy, normal children.[245] Fissuring appears to be due to matrix destruction from mechanical stresses.[245] Some authors have noted that in younger children, fissuring of the cartilage appears early, unlike in adults, where softening is the usual initial cartilage change.[63] It is controversial whether chondromalacia in children is the precursor to patellofemoral arthritis in the adult.

In younger children, only the medial facet may exhibit softening, and an effusion is uncommon. In children age 13 to 16 years, effusion can occur and there may be fissuring of the central ridge with occasional erosion. In older patients (18 to 20 years) with a longer duration of symptoms, fissuring becomes more common, with erosions also seen. With age, the lateral facet becomes involved and erosions become more extensive, leading to the appearance of osteoarthritis.[245]

Metaplasia of chondrocytes has been observed in lesions of the central ridge of the patella in adolescents, suggesting the ability of cartilage to repair itself by cellular multiplication.[245] The subchondral layer may also possess regenerative capabilities in children. Softening, fibrillation, and fissuring in children with patellofemoral dysplasia can repair to a smooth surface if the causal mechanical factors are corrected. High-grade chondropathy associated with patellofemoral dysplasia is uncommon in children with open physes. With skeletal maturation, advanced chondromalacia and arthritis are seen more frequently.

The cause of pain associated with chondromalacia is poorly understood because articular cartilage is aneural. Theories include increased intraosseous pressure, stimulation of pain receptors in peripatellar soft tissues, and synovitis secondary to cartilage breakdown. There is often a poor correlation between the intensity of pain and the degree of chondromalacia. However, pain seems to correlate with subchondral bone injury.[147, 149]

Lateral Patellar Compression Syndrome

Lateral patellar compression syndrome (LPCS) is the mildest form of patellofemoral dysplasia. The pathogenesis of LPCS is loss of the dynamic equilibrium of the patella in the trochlea, leading to narrowing of the joint space from lateral compression and subsequent irritation and fragmentation of the cartilage from repetitive motion.[333, 347, 389]

Symptoms usually include insidious onset of vague, poorly localized pain over the anterior aspect of the knee. Pain typically worsens with stair climbing, prolonged sitting with the knee flexed, and playing sports, particularly jumping sports. Locking, crepitus, giving way, and swelling may be present at more advanced stages. On examination, there is usually no evidence of overt patellar malalignment, but a lateral tilt of the patella may be observed. With quadriceps contraction in full extension, lateral subluxation of the patella may be observed and pain may be elicited. A tight iliotibial band or lateral retinaculum may or may not be present. Roentgenographic evidence of lateral tilting may be found on the skyline view. CT axial views of the patella at 30, 60, and 90 degrees of flexion may show narrowing of the lateral patellofemoral joint with or without lateral subluxation.

Treatment of LPCS should initially be nonoperative. Exercises should be prescribed to stretch the iliotibial band and mobilize the patella. Medial quadriceps strengthening should be done by straight-leg raising against increasing amounts of resistance of thigh flexion in semi-Fowler's position. These exercises allow for quadriceps contraction without painful patellofemoral movement. We refer to these as static progressive resistive exercises. The straight-leg lifting should be done regularly, increasing resistance by 1 to 2 lb weekly if it does not result in significant pain or quadriceps lag. The goal in adolescents is 10 static quadriceps lifts of 10 to 12 lb. Ability to lift 12 lb for three sets of 10 repetitions has resulted in resolution of symptoms in 91% of patients in these authors' clinic. In a young adult, the goal may go up to sets of 25 lb. Short-arc (less than 40 degrees) exercises may benefit the tracking mechanism but should be avoided if they are painful. Swimming is an ideal exercise because it maintains muscle tone while minimizing patellofemoral compressive forces. Children should be encouraged to refrain from activities that produce high patellofemoral compressive forces such as running, jumping, climbing, squatting, and other long-arc knee extension or hyperflexion activities. Oral anti-inflammatory drugs and icing may be useful in decreasing pain, but in our experience, they are not often helpful over the long term in children.[233, 311, 330, 333, 347, 389]

Although the scientific basis remains conjectural, neoprene elastic braces with a patella cutout (Palumbo brace) may give physical or psychological comfort. They may be helpful in allowing an earlier return to sports. Theoretically, they help contain the maltracking of the patella by distributing the force of the quadriceps around the circumference of the knee and by providing bolsters to mechanically discourage subluxation. Also, braces may improve proprioceptive sensation. In addition, patellar taping, using the technique of McConnell, can be taught to the patient. Foot orthotics may also be of some use for minor lower-extremity malalignments.[200, 225, 233, 311, 330]

Many series have reported success rates over 75% in rendering patients asymptomatic with return to full athletic activity using nonoperative care. Supervised physical therapy for up to 6 months may sometimes be necessary. If symptoms recur, return to physical therapy usually results in resolution. If no relief of symptoms occurs after 3 to 6 months, one must search further for the cause of the problem, which is usually malalignment, and surgical correction may be required.[112, 232, 301, 321, 330, 333, 337, 347, 389]

If there is no patellar laxity, we use the lateral release as our first choice of operative therapy because it has a low morbidity and does not alter the extensor mechanism or preclude later reconstructions if required. The lateral release may help relieve pain by decreasing the lateral compression force, resulting in patellar tilt, or by relieving pressure on the tight lateral peripatellar structures. The procedure may be performed arthroscopically with visualization of patellar tilt, grading of chondromalacia, evaluation of other intra-articular pathology, and assessment of maltracking before and after release. Successful results range widely, from 33% to 77%, owing to patient selection or to variation in technique. Unsuccessful results are associated with significant malalignment, high Q angle, ligamentous laxity, genu valgum or recurvatum, high body weight, persistent lateral maltracking, and female sex. Medial patellar subluxation as a complication of lateral release has been reported. There is little correlation between results and extent of chondromalacia, roentgenographic findings, and patella height.[4, 25, 112, 145, 149, 237, 330, 337, 389]

We perform open realignment if nonoperative treatment and lateral release fail and if anatomic malalignment exists. Options for open realignment include combinations of lateral release, medial reefing and vastus medialis advancement, and medialization of the patellar tendon (Fig. 66.2). Some series report more than 75% good or excellent results with these procedures after 2 to 10 years. Satisfactory results correlate with normalization of patellar alignment on Merchant's view.[112, 149, 232, 347, 389]

Tibial tubercle realignment procedures in children with open physes are contraindicated because of the possibility of arrest of the tibial tubercle apophysis with resultant hyperextension deformity. The Roux-Goldthwait (patellar tendon lateral hemitransfer) or

Galeazzi-Baker (semitendinosis tenodesis) procedures (see Fig. 66.2) can be used to improve distal alignment in children who fail lateral release and medial reefing with vastus medialis advancement without comprising the physis. We prefer the latter procedure, which involves a proximal quadricepsplasty and lateral release with the semitendinosis used for tenodesis to the patella, resulting in a medially directed distal force without insult to the apophysis.[25, 29, 64, 105, 130, 196, 232, 305]

Older children with a Q angle of greater than 25 degrees and closed physes (or less than 1 cm of remaining growth) can have a tibial tubercle osteotomy of the Elmslie-Trillat type or Fulkerson type, medially or anteromedially transferring the tubercle along with a proximal quadricepsplasty and lateral release.[232, 333, 347, 389]

Chronic Subluxating Patella

The next stage in the continuum of patellofemoral dysplasias is the chronic subluxating patella. Pain beneath the patella is more severe. In addition, swelling, clicks, and giving way may be present. Instability permits the patella to be subluxed out of the intercondylar groove. The patella then snaps back into place rather than going on to complete dislocation. It is more apt to occur during quadriceps contraction with the knee flexed, the foot fixed to the ground, and the tibia laterally rotated. Patellofemoral tenderness, crepitus, apprehension, effusion, and quadriceps atrophy may be evident on examination. Dynamically, lateral deviation of the patella may be observed with excessive patellar glide. Roentgenographically, the patella often rides laterally in the trochlear groove with abnormal congruence.

Management of the chronic subluxating patella should begin with nonoperative measures as discussed for LPCS. The number and extent of subluxation may decrease with age. Nonoperative measures are less successful than LPCS. For patients who fail nonoperative management, surgical options follow those outlined for LPCS. Chondromalacia may be more advanced. Osteochondral fracture of the patella or lateral femoral condyle can occur with significant patellar subluxation.[130, 149, 232, 333, 347, 389]

Recurrent Patellar Dislocation

In recurrent patellar dislocation, the patella repeatedly frankly dislocates laterally with certain stresses and then usually spontaneously reduces with extension or further flexion. This disorder can begin as young as age 5 years but usually does not present until adolescence or young adulthood. The tendency to redislocate is greater if the primary dislocation occurs when the patient is younger than 20 years.[20, 155]

Normally, the patella first strikes the lateral condyle with flexion and then moves medially into the sulcus. If the lateral condyle is hypoplastic or if other predisposing factors exist (see Table 66.3), the patella will dislocate laterally with flexion. Dislocation is more likely with high patellae when the tibia is slightly flexed and externally rotated on the abducted femur with tension from the contracting quadriceps. The dislocation can occur when the patient twists while standing or changes direction while running. Recurrent patellar dislocation can also commence if a traumatic episode is superimposed on a biomechanically predisposed child with LPCS or patellar subluxation. Familial and congenital forms of recurrent patellar dislocation have been described. Predisposing congenital anomalies include a hypoplastic lateral femoral condyle, hypoplastic patella (nail-patella syndrome), and a tight iliotibial band and vastus lateralis (arthrogryposis multiplex congenita). Patellar instability associated with conditions characterized by ligamentous laxity, such as Down syndrome or Ehlers-Danlos syndrome, present a significant challenge.[101, 228, 232, 238, 333, 347, 389]

Osteochondral fractures and chondromalacia of the lateral condyle or medial patellar facet occur as the patella either dislocates or relocates back in the trochlear groove. The incidence of osteochondral fracture with patellar dislocation approximates 40% in some series.[123, 256, 333, 352] Resultant loose bodies can cause recurrent locking and effusions.

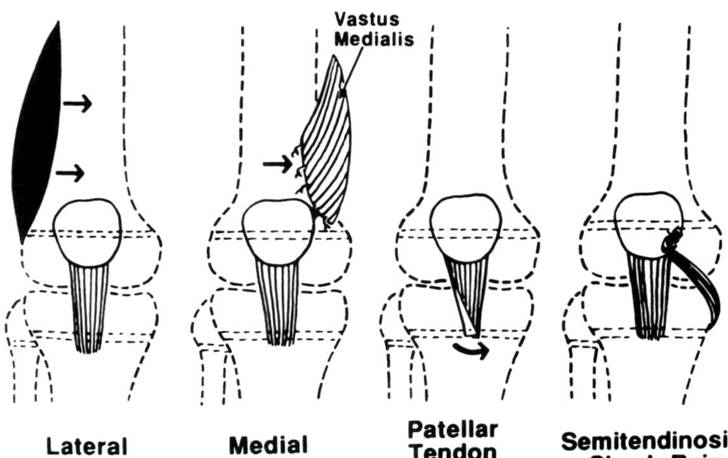

FIGURE 66.2 ➢ Patellofemoral realignment operations in the skeletally immature. (From Staheli LT: The lower limb. In: Morrissy RT, ed: Lovell and Winters' Pediatric Orthopaedics, 3rd ed. Philadelphia, Lippincott, 1990.)

The patient complains of multiple episodes of frank dislocation, often with spontaneous relocation. When examining a knee with a dislocated patella, the knee remains flexed, the patella is visible laterally, and there is a concavity anteriorly over the trochlear groove. The patella can be relocated by lifting the foot to straighten the knee, reducing quadriceps tension. Sometimes gentle pressure over the lateral aspect of the patella is necessary. When examining the knee with a relocated patella, there is often excessive lateral glide, a positive apprehension test result, effusion, vastus medialis atrophy, and pain with patellofemoral compression. Medial tenderness indicates medial retinacular and possibly vastus medialis tear.

After the first dislocation, and if no signs of loose fragments are present, the knee should be immobilized after reduction for 4 weeks followed by static progressive resistive exercises and lateral stretching. Surgery is usually required in children or adolescents with recurrent dislocations. An arthroscopic lateral release can be initially attempted if hypermobility is not present. Success may be limited, especially in cases of recurrent dislocation; however, the associated morbidity is minimal and does not preclude future open realignment. Open realignment options include combinations of lateral release, medial reefing, vastus medialis advancement, patellar tendon hemitransfer, semitendinosis tenodesis, and tibial tubercle transfer in older patients. In addition, transfer of the medial third of the patellar tendon to the deep medial collateral ligament (MCL) has been described.[43, 108]

Chronic Patellar Dislocation

Chronic patellar dislocation, also called habitual dislocation, is rare and is the most severe form of patellofemoral dysplasia. The patella laterally dislocates with each knee flexion and reduces with each extension, as opposed to recurrent dislocating patella, which involves intermittent dislocation. The primary abnormality is tightness of the vastus lateralis and its fascia, the vastus intermedius, and the iliotibial band. The tibia may also be subluxated laterally on the femur as a result of lateral tightness.[101, 232, 333, 347, 389]

A congenital form exists resulting from malposition of the entire extensor mechanism on the femur. These are usually irreducible or, if reducible, unstable. The cause is probably failure of internal rotation of the myotome, which contains the quadriceps femoris and patella in utero. Children with congenital habitual dislocation may have other genetic derangements such as Down syndrome. An acquired form of habitual dislocation has been reported as a result of infantile quadriceps fibrosis. The acquired form has also been termed obligatory dislocation because infants are unable to flex the knee without first dislocating the patella.[329, 378]

The patient may complain of a clicking or clunking sensation with each flexion and extension of the knee. Over time, the knee becomes painful and the child keeps the knee continuously flexed with the patella dislocated laterally, eventually developing a flexion contracture. The diagnosis is confirmed by visualization and palpation of the laterally displaced patella and by roentgenogram. With severe contractures of the vastus lateralis, the patella may be permanently dislocated. In newborns, the knee may not extend. Ultrasound is useful in locating the unossified patella.[239]

Early surgical intervention is recommended before associated abnormalities such as flexion contracture, genu valgum, maldevelopment of the patellofemoral joint, and external rotation of the tibia become severe, rendering treatment more difficult. Release of the lateral retinaculum and iliotibial band should be performed. The vastus lateralis should be mobilized from the lateral intermuscular septum, patella, and central slip of the quadriceps. The vastus medialis should be transferred distally and laterally. Fibrotic bands in the vastus lateralis or intermedius should be excised. Subperiosteal dissection of the entire quadriceps off the femur with complete medial displacement may be necessary. In older children, the patellar tendon may require transfer. Occasionally, the patella adheres to the periosteum and perichondrium over the lateral condyle, and great care must be used to free the patella without injury to its articular surface. Treatment of associated flexion contractures from a chronically dislocated patella requires surgical release because traction and serial casting have been unsuccessful.[232, 329, 333, 347, 389]

OVERUSE INJURIES

Overuse injuries are caused by chronic, repetitive microtrauma, usually related to sports, causing submaximal insults to local tissues that result in pain. Common sites of overuse injuries in the athletic child are the knee, elbow, shoulder, and spine. The frequency of overuse injuries in children has been increasing because of increased participation in sports and high competitive levels of many youth sports. Year-round training at high-intensity levels and highly repetitive levels results in repetitive microtrauma to the growing musculoskeletal system, which causes overuse injuries. In the skeletally immature athlete, the physes, chondroepiphyses, apophyses, and regions of ligamentous insertion are particularly vulnerable to repetitive microtrauma.

The most frequent risk factor for overuse injury is training error. Improper technique or too-rapid increase in training intensity or duration results in repetitive injuries to the developing skeleton that are above the normal reparative threshold. Training error also includes improper technique from poor coaching and supervision. Contributing to training error are the often high demands placed on the youth athlete by her or his parents or coaches, who treat her or him as a little professional athlete instead of as a child.

Muscle-tendon imbalance is another risk factor for overuse injury. Growth decreases flexibility as muscle-tendon units elongate, especially during growth spurts. In addition, although strength increases with growth, increased strength may not be uniform. Anatomic malalignment is also a risk factor for overuse injuries. Femoral anteversion, leg-length discrepancy, foot pronation, tibial torsion, patella alta, and increased lumbar lordosis may all contribute to abnormal stresses with repetitive activities. Other factors to consider when assessing a patient with overuse injury include poor equipment (especially shoes), playing surface, nutritional factors, psychological factors, systemic illnesses, and poor conditioning.[213, 265]

Overuse injury may manifest clinically as pain, stress fracture, osteochondral injury, articular cartilage wear, subluxation, growth disturbance, or exertional compartmental syndrome. In addition, overuse may predispose to acute injuries. The evaluation of a child suspected of having an overuse injury should include assessment of the aforementioned risk factors. Treatment first consists of relative rest and conservative measures aimed at correcting risk factors. Return to full activity should be slow and progressive. The "10% per week" rule for increasing the duration and intensity of training is helpful. In addition, an upper limit of cumulative exercise dose should be empirically determined.

Osgood-Schlatter Disease

Osgood-Schlatter disease (OSD), or tibial osteochondrosis, is the most common traction apophysitis and overuse injury in the knee of adolescent athletes. The condition develops from repetitive microtrauma to the tibial tubercle at the time of formation of the secondary ossification center. Symptoms typically occur at the onset of the growth spurt in adolescent boys, usually ages 13 to 14 (range 10 to 15 years). The condition is activity related with higher prevalence rates in active children and in participants of jumping sports such as basketball or volleyball. As the participation of girls in sports has increased, so has their incidence of OSD, typically occurring at ages 10 and 11 years (the skeletal maturity equivalent of 13- to 14-year-old boys), with a range of 8 to 13 years. Girls are often involved in gymnastics, soccer, and other jumping sports.[190]

The tibial tubercle progresses through four radiographic and histological stages of development: cartilaginous, apophyseal, epiphyseal, and bony incorporation into the adult tibia. OSD is caused by multiple submaximal avulsion fractures of the patellar tendon insertion on the tibial tubercle apophysis. The fractures result from repetitive traction microtrauma from the stress of an unbalanced, tightened extensor mechanism that is capable of generating great forces, particularly during eccentric contraction. There do not appear to be abnormalities of skeletal maturation or histological physeal abnormalities in patients with OSD. Some children with OSD develop bony ossicles in the tendon that may result in late symptoms. Vigorous jumping rarely leads to complete displacement of the apophysis.[189, 241, 263, 388]

Symptoms include the insidious onset of a low-grade ache associated with activity that is localized to the area of the tibial tubercle. The pain is aggravated by acceleration and deceleration forces as well as by direct blows. Bilaterality is seen in approximately 20% to 35% of cases, although it is not unusual to see bilateral tubercle enlargement with unilateral symptoms. The patient or the parents may be concerned about tumor, given the size of tubercle enlargement in some cases. On examination, there is tenderness and sometimes swelling over the tubercle and adjacent patellar tendon, often with a bony or cartilaginous prominence. Pain is reproduced with resisted extension from a flexed position. Occasional associated findings are tight quadriceps with decreased flexibility and patellar maltracking.

Roentgenographic evaluation is done to rule out other processes. X-ray films may demonstrate a simple bony prominence of the tubercle with fragmentation of the ossific nucleus or a free bony fragment proximal to the tubercle in the patellar tendon. Comparison views of the contralateral knee may be helpful in differentiating nonpathological multicentric ossification. A consistent x-ray finding in OSD is more than 4 mm of soft-tissue swelling over the tibial anterior articular surface, seen best with low-energy (50 to 60 kV) lateral xeroradiographs. Ultrasound is also effective in demonstrating tubercle fragmentation and edematous thickening of the patellar tendon insertion, infrapatellar fat pad and bursa, and subcutaneous tissue. MRI can elucidate patellar tendon thickening and chronic tendon tears.[81, 140, 185, 194, 308]

Exercises should be instituted to restore strength and flexibility to the extensor mechanism because OSD is often associated with a tight quadriceps that becomes weaker with the onset of pain. Because dynamic quadriceps exercises are painful, static progressive resistive exercises should be performed with the goal of eventually lifting 12 to 15 lb, as for LPCS. Quadriceps stretching should also be performed.[202, 233]

Activity should be limited, with 2 to 3 weeks of relative rest. Patients should avoid sports requiring running, jumping, or kneeling until all symptoms resolve, but cross-training with bicycling and swimming should be encouraged. If walking is uncomfortable, a protective crutch gait with a knee immobilizer can be used while the patient initiates the stretching and strengthening program. Frequently, as much as a 3-month layoff from the offending sport may be required. Knee pads or braces that leave the patella open, preventing direct mechanical impact to the tubercle, may allow the child to continue to play with reduced pain. If symptoms are severe, a cylinder cast for 2 to 4 weeks with crutch ambulation can be used. Casting is rarely recommended, however, because it can make a tight, weak quadriceps mechanism even tighter and weaker. Corticosteroid injection is contraindicated because the cause is not inflammatory and steroid injection can result in skin thinning and weakening of the tendon. Oral anti-inflammatory drugs may be of benefit. Icing after activity can help alleviate acute symptoms. Symptoms may recur with resumption of sports, requiring a repeat cycle of rest, strengthening, stretching, and activity modification. However, the process is usually self-limited, stopping when growth stops and the tibial tubercle apophysis matures and fuses. Patients are more likely to have chronic symptoms after maturity if initial radiographs show fragmentation of the apophysis. A bony prominence at the tubercle that is susceptible to tenderness from direct blows or kneeling may be a residuum of OSD in the adult. ACL reconstruction can be performed in adults with residual OSD using the central third patellar tendon graft without compromising knee function.[189, 223]

Surgical excision may be necessary for patients who fail nonoperative management and who have free ossific nuclei over the tubercle or within the patellar tendon. Excision before skeletal maturity may be complicated by residual bony prominences, decreased range of motion, and recurvatum deformity. Other procedures described include drilling of the tuberosity, placement of bone plugs, tuberosity debulking, and linear osteotomy with complete excision of the tibial tuberosity. Success rates are improved in the older child near skeletal maturity.[189, 241, 353]

Sinding-Larsen-Johansson Syndrome

Sinding-Larsen-Johansson syndrome (SLJS) or patellar osteochondrosis, is an overuse traction apophysitis or avulsion resulting from dynamic stress and microtrauma at the proximal patellar tendon insertion onto the inferior patellar pole. SLJS is a condition similar to OSD, except that it occurs at the opposite end of the patellar tendon and is analogous to jumper's knee in the skeletally mature athlete. Histological analysis demonstrates pathological changes in the tendon tissue adjacent to the tendon-bone junction. Adjacent patellar fragments are usually nonpathological accessory ossification centers. Rarely, a displaced fracture of the distal patellar pole may result. The condition is most common in adolescent boys age 9 to 13 years.[81, 109, 226, 354]

The presentation and history are similar to that of OSD, but the pain is at the distal pole of the patella. Many patients report a history of a single episode of macrotrauma, such as a fall that significantly worsens symptomotology. Pain typically occurs with running, jumping, or climbing of stairs. On examination, there is tenderness over the distal pole of the patella and adjacent patellar tendon insertion. Frequently, the quadriceps will be tight but relatively weak.

Lateral roentgenograms may be normal or show elongation of the distal patellar pole or small avulsion ossicle. Fragmentation at the distal pole may represent a more severe injury as the tendon fibers and periosteum avulse and undergo subsequent necrosis and calcification. Fragmentation may also represent a patellar sleeve fracture or nonpathological multicentric centers of ossification, found in 2% to 5% of normal adolescents. A roentgenogram of the opposite knee is helpful for differentiation. Ultrasonography will also demonstrate fragmentation of the distal pole and patellar tendon thickening.

Treatment of this syndrome is similar to that of OSD, including relative rest, cross-training, and quadriceps strengthening and stretching. Symptoms are usually self-limited. If symptoms are severe, immobilization can be used to attain some healing before beginning muscle rehabilitation. Patients who fail nonoperative management with persistent symptoms that limit function may be surgical candidates for ossicle excision.[81, 109, 226, 354]

Breaststroker's Knee

Pain at the medial aspect of the knee is frequently encountered in breaststroke swimmers. Pain initially occurs during the final thrust of the whipkick and progresses to being symptomatic with other athletic and nonathletic activities. The site of knee pain is related to the particular whipkick technique, as analyzed by underwater movies. In particular, increased hip abduction angles at kick initiation and limited hip internal rotation may predispose to medial knee injury. Tibial collateral ligament pain is associated with forceful adduction of the legs with the knees extended. Patellofemoral symptoms are associated with rapid extension of the knee with the legs abducted, the tibia externally rotated, and the feet dorsiflexed. The patella is pulled proximally and medially, causing the medial facet to abut the intercondylar ridge. In addition, there may be an increased incidence of symptomatic synovial plicae and medial synovitis. In patients using the whipkick for more than 8 years, early patellofemoral osteoarthritis can develop.[175, 296, 297, 342, 362]

On examination, there is tenderness at the medial patellar facet, medial femoral intercondylar ridge, and tibial collateral ligament. Treatment consists of warming up, icing, and ultrasound. Patients should train occasionally using other types of kicks and have 2 months of total rest from swimming per year. Errors in whipkick technique should be corrected.[175, 296, 297, 342, 362]

Synovial Plicae

The embryonic knee is partitioned into suprapatellar, medial, and lateral compartments by synovial septa. Thus, synovial plicae and synovial shelves are normal embryological remnants. Medial suprapatellar synovial plicae are most common and are frequently bilateral. The medial plica attaches medially at the undersurface of the quadriceps tendon and extends distally around the patella and over the medial femoral condyle to insert into the fat pad. Most plicae are asymptomatic and are seen as incidental findings at arthroscopy. Occasionally, following acute or chronic trauma, particularly in the adolescent athlete participating in running or jumping sports, synovial plicae become inflamed and undergo progressive fibrosis and thickening. Plicae are commonly seen in the adolescent knee but are unusual in the infantile or juvenile knee. It is hypothesized that plicae become prominent with the adolescent growth spurt as the extensor mechanism elongates and tightens. This pulls the patella proximally and laterally, increasing tension on the medial synovium, resulting in shelf formation.[50, 79, 240, 251, 276, 280, 360, 371]

Patients usually complain of medial parapatellar pain and sometimes experience snapping. Symptomatic plicae often present as an overuse syndrome with activity-related pain; however, some patients give a history of acute injury. Symptoms can mimic a meniscal or chondral lesion. A snapping sensation can be felt on flexion-extension of the knee, particularly with the leg internally rotated. In addition, the plica may be palpable over the medial femoral condyle or posterior to the medial edge of the inferior patellar pole. When inflamed, the palpable plica is tender locally and can become painful on impingement on the medial femoral condyle or entrapment in the patellofemoral joint. Plain radiograms are usually normal. MRI can detect plicae but, in practice, is more useful to rule out other intra-articular lesions as the cause of knee pain.[50, 240, 253, 276, 280, 360]

Symptoms are often relieved by a supervised program of relative rest, progressive resistance exercises, patellar mobilization, and stretching of the hamstrings, gastrocnemius, and quadriceps.[13] Intraplical steroid and local anesthetic injection has been used; however, we discourage this in children and adolescents.[296] Arthroscopic plica resection may be necessary for recalcitrant cases. Good results are generally obtained with careful identification of pathological plica syndrome and with isolated lesions.[85, 104, 159, 179, 251, 259] Care should be taken to excise the plica shelf while leaving the medial synovial and retinacular wall. Indiscriminate resection of normal plica should be discouraged. A pathological plica can be identified by an appropriate history and confirmatory physical examination along with arthroscopic findings of a thickened, fibrotic plica with concomitant articular erosion. Lateral patellar subluxation may contribute to the pathoetiology of symptomatic medial plicae resulting from tension and impingement on the medial femoral condyle or in the patellofemoral joint. Therefore, careful assessment of patellar tracking should be done with the anticipation of possible lateral release in addition to plica resection should there be evidence of lateral patellar subluxation.[231b]

Chondromalacia Fabellae

The fabella, or "little bean," is a sesamoid bone about 2.0 × 2.5 cm within the lateral head of the gastrocnemius that articulates with the posterior aspect of the lateral femoral condyle. The incidence of the fabella in the normal population is approximately 10% to 15%, and it is bilateral in more than one half of cases.[372, 373]

Chondromalacia fabellae, or fabella syndrome, is unique to adolescents age 15 to 17 years. Because the patients are almost always athletic and usually have no history of trauma, the cause is presumably overuse. Pain is believed to be a result of roughened articular cartilage and synovial irritation, suggesting abnormal wear. Pain can also be due to fracture or irritation of the peroneal nerve by local compression. The symptomatic fabella can be either bony or cartilaginous precursor. The patient complains of intermittent sharp pain localized to the posterolateral aspect of the knee. Symptoms are exacerbated with gastrocnemius contraction when the knee is loaded in full extension, as in ballet dancers. On examination, the fabella is often palpable, and pain is reproduced on compressing the fabella against the femoral condyle. Radiograms demonstrate the bony fabella or suggest a cartilaginous fabella.

Nonoperative management consists of splinting or casting, temporary restriction of activities, and analgesics. Steroid injection may be beneficial in the older patient. Patients with persistent symptoms are candidates for surgical excision. Enucleation usually results in relief of symptoms and minimal morbidity.[372, 373]

Patellar Stress Fracture

Patellar stress fractures should be suspected with insidious onset of activity-related patellar pain in a child with overuse risk factors, the most significant of which is training error in running and jumping sports placing high demands on the extensor mechanism. Stress fractures result from a failure of normal bone homeostasis because of excessive demands of repetitive microtrauma or overuse with inadequate time for healing. The resultant microfractures then summate into a clinical stress fracture. Usually the stress fractures are transverse, indicating a longitudinal load.[87, 234, 265, 304]

On examination, there is focal tenderness, swelling, quadriceps atrophy, and loss of full flexion. Early roentgenograms are normal or equivocal and may not be positive for 6 to 8 weeks. Technetium bone scan or MRI allows early diagnosis. The patient should eliminate or modify the etiological activity and predisposing factors, thus breaking the cycle to allow healing. Some authors recommend immobilization for 6 to 8 weeks in extension followed by extensive rehabilitation. These authors encourage cross-training activities and weightbearing within the limits of pain. Full activity should then be resumed gradually.

Bipartite Patellae

Normally, the cartilaginous anlage of the patella forms from one center of ossification. In bipartite patellae, an accessory center of ossification forms a separate ossicle that is attached to the body of the patella by a fibrous or cartilaginous junction. The main body of the patella begins ossification at age 3 to 4 years, whereas the accessory center usually appears later, between age 8 to 12 years. The most common site of accessory ossification is the superolateral corner (75%), followed by the lateral margin (20%) and the inferior pole (5%) (Fig. 66.3). The prevalence of multipartite patellae is between 1% to 5% in the general population, and approximately 50% are bilateral. Boys are involved more frequently than are girls.[94, 262, 370]

Multipartite patellae are usually asymptomatic radiographic findings. Symptoms may occur at the patella-accessory ossicle junction because of acute trauma or repetitive microtrauma. The presenting complaint is often pain on the superolateral pole or lateral border of the patella during or following vigorous exercise or an acute blow. Some patients present with swelling or catching of the knee. Patients are usually adolescent males, although adults may develop symptomatic bipartite patellae. Acute flexion or forceful quadriceps contraction worsens the pain. The patella is often enlarged, and there is often a prominence on the superolateral or lateral margin of the patella that is tender to palpation in symptomatic cases. Radiographs demonstrate the accessory ossification center. It may be difficult to distinguish between an inferior pole bipartite patella and a patellar sleeve fracture or Sinding-Larsen-Johansson disease. Films of the contralateral knee may be beneficial. Skyline views in a squatting position may demonstrate separation at the ossicle-patella junction.[151] It is important to rule out other causes of pain such as patellofemoral dysplasia because bipartite patellae are usually asymptomatic.

Treatment depends on chronicity of symptoms. Acute, macrotraumatic injuries are usually treated with immobilization for 3 to 4 weeks, providing the fragment is not displaced. Duration of immobilization is determined clinically as the radiolucent line between the accessory center and the body of the patella persists. Displaced ossicles of sufficient size are treated as fracture-separations with open reduction and internal fixation. Chronic, microtraumatic injuries are treated by brief immobilization, relative rest, activity modificaton, short-arc exercises, and stretching. Symptomatic nonunion may occur because of poor chondro-osseous healing. If symptoms persist, fragment excision usually produces excellent results.[44, 150, 151] In addition, lateral retinacular release and detachment of the vastus lateralis insertion into the painful fragment have been used with good results to treat painful bipartite patellae.[246, 260]

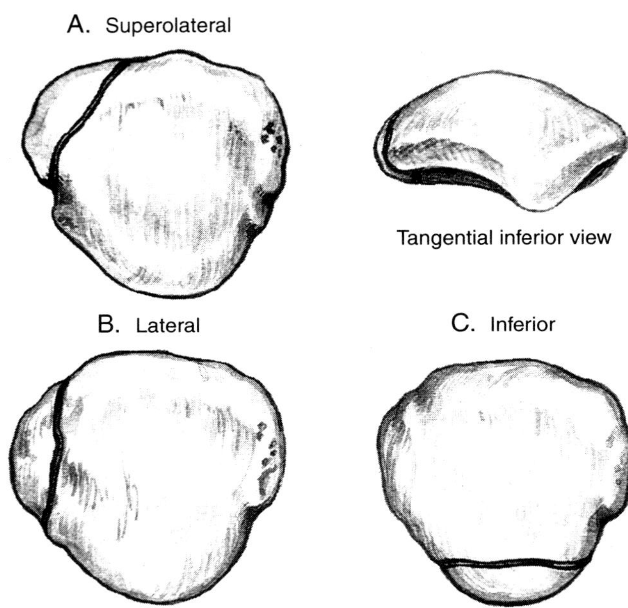

FIGURE 66.3 ➢ Anatomic sites of accessory ossification centers of the patella. *A*, Superolateral pole. *B*, Lateral. *C*, Inferior. (From Tachdjian MO: Clinical Pediatric Orthopedics: The Art of Diagnosis and Principles of Management. Stamford, Appleton & Lange, 1997.)

ACUTE KNEE TRAUMA

Acute Patellar Dislocation

Acute patellar dislocations usually occur as a result of a direct blow but may occur with a valgus, external rotation force. Dislocation is lateral. Many patients with acute dislocation have predisposing patellofemoral dysplasia. Osteochondral fractures of the lateral femoral trochlea, medial patellar facet, or both are being increasingly recognized and may occur in as many as 40% of patellar dislocations in some series.[123, 256, 296, 333, 352] The diagnosis of the acutely dislocated patella is straightforward, with the patella prominent on the lateral aspect of the knee. The medial retinaculum and patellofemoral ligaments are torn. Many patients spontaneously reduce after dislocation, and in these cases the diagnosis is inferential. The child may have sensed that the patella popped out and that there was deformity. There is often a large hemarthrosis with tenderness of the torn medial retinaculum. The examiner should check for malalignment, patellofemoral dysplasia, and vastus medialis atrophy. MRI is unreliable in detecting osteochondral fractures.[232, 347, 389]

Treatment of acute patellar dislocations consists of 2 to 3 weeks of immobilization followed by progressive rehabilitation of the quadriceps and hamstrings. Results are good, particularly in those with normal realignment. Recurrence rates vary from 17% to 44% depending on the presence of associated extensor malalignment. For patients with significant trauma or those with mechanical symptoms, arthroscopy can be useful in identifying and treating associated osteochondral fractures. In addition, reconstruction of the vastus medialis gap and an associated lateral release may be beneficial. For patients with recurrence associated with significant malalignment, proximal or distal realignment procedures may be necessary.[232, 347, 389]

Patellar Fracture

Patellar fractures in skeletally immature patients are unusual, accounting for 1% of all patellar fractures.[261] However, they can occur in the pediatric athlete as a result of a direct blow or indirectly from forced quadriceps contraction against a fixed, flexed knee. Adolescent patellar fractures secondary to direct blows are often stellate, whereas patellar fractures in the younger child are usually transvere. Patellar fractures must be differentiated from bipartite patellae in which the accessory ossicle usually involves the superolateral portion of the body of the patella. The diagnosis of patella fracture is usually made by pain over the patella and weakness with extensor lag. With displaced fractures, there is a gap and often inability to actively extend the knee. Minimally displaced fractures may be difficult to identify radiographically because of the incomplete ossification of the patella. The fracture is often best visualized on the lateral view. Nondisplaced fractures are treated with immobilization in extension. Displaced fractures involving a substantial fragment are treated with open reduction and internal fixation. Excision of fracture fragments in a comminuted fracture is performed only as a last resort because of poor results of partial patellectomy in children.[35, 73, 122, 217, 285]

Patellar sleeve fractures are rare, acute injuries that are unique to children and occur most commonly at the inferior pole of the patella. Predisposing factors are rapid growth, peripheral chondro-osseous transformation, increased stress of competitive sports, and patellofemoral instability, making the older child and adolescent most susceptible.[136] The patella in the newborn is composed entirely of cartilage and begins to ossify at age 4 to 6 years. The process begins as a multifocal, centrally located ossification that develops a constantly remodeling chondro-osseous transformation around the entire periphery. The peripheral bone, therefore, is the least mature and the most susceptible to fractures. The sleeve fracture is most commonly due to avulsion of the patellar tendon from the distal pole, with a small fragment of bone and a variable portion of the patellar articular cartilage. The cause is a sudden forceful knee contraction while the knee is flexed; it most commonly occurs in jumpers. Medial avulsion fractures can occur following lateral patellar dislocations. Superior pole sleeve avulsions have also been reported.[40, 109, 123, 142, 387]

With patellar sleeve fracture, there is hemarthrosis and lack of extension. A gap will be palpable below the patella at the site of the avulsion. Roentgenograms reveal an effusion and patella alta. The fragment of avulsed bone is not always detectable because it may be largely cartilaginous and have minimal osseous composition. MRI can prove useful in delineating the extent of cartilaginous injury and displacement. Arthroscopic examination should be considered to confirm the status of the articular cartilage. If there is displacement of the articular surface, open reduction and internal fixation with tension band wiring and Kirschner wires are recommended. Alternatively, repair of the patellar tendon to the inferior patellar pole with heavy, nonabsorbable sutures may be performed. Nondisplaced fractures are treated with long-leg or cylinder cast immobilization.[30, 40, 109, 123, 142, 387]

Tibial Tubercle Fracture

The tibial tubercle forms at 13 weeks of gestation as a cartilaginous extension of the proximal tibial epiphysis. It develops as a secondary center of ossification at approximately 8 years of age, coalescing with the proximal tuberosity and epiphysis at approximately 12 years of age. The tubercle-epiphysis bony unit then fuses with the tibial metaphysis at age 15 to 17, starting posteriorly and proximally, with the area deep to the tuberosity fusing last. The physis of the tibial tuberosity is unique because it does not have the histological structure of other growth plates. The zones of proliferation and hypertrophy are replaced by fibrocartilage that dissipates the high tensile forces generated by the extensor mechanism more effectively than do hyaline cartilage growth plates.

Avulsion fractures of the tibial tubercle occur in adolescents between 13 and 16 years of age—close to the end of growth. Children with OSD are predisposed to tubercle fracture.[263, 264, 384] The injury usually occurs during jumping, particularly in basketball, because of a strong contraction of the quadriceps against a fixed, flexed leg. The injury occurs in adolescents undergoing physiological epiphyseodesis, similar to Tillaux's fracture of the ankle. Patients complain of pain at the tibial tubercle. On examination, there is often tenderness at the tubercle with pain and weakness of knee extension. Radiograms, particularly the lateral view, demonstrate the fracture, and comparison views of the contralateral knee may be necessary to differentiate the fracture from an open physis.[65, 131, 263, 264]

Three types of fractures have been classified (Watson-Jones classification) based on the degree of involvement of the proximal tibial epiphysis (Fig. 66.4): type I is a fracture involving only the tibial tubercle; type II is a fracture that occurs after the coalescence of the tuberosity ossification center to the metaphysis, resulting in a fracture that splits the epiphysis of the tuberosity from the epiphysis of the proximal tibia; and type III is a fracture that involves the proximal tibial epiphysis and extends into the articular surface. In type III fractures, the growth plate beneath the tubercle is separated, and the fracture tracks through the anterior proximal tibial physis.[382] Because the posterior physis has closed in the typical age group, the fracture then tracks proximally through the epiphysis and into the joint.

Nondisplaced fractures can be treated nonoperatively with the knee immobilized in extension in a cast. With displacement, open reduction and internal fixation should be performed. Displaced type III fractures must have anatomic reduction to restore the integrity of the articular surface. Screws are usually used for fixation with protection in a long-leg cast for 5 to 7 weeks postoperatively. Isometric quadriceps exercises can be begun in the cast after pain resolves, and range-of-motion exercises with quadriceps strengthening are initiated after cast removal.[290, 291, 382]

Compartmental syndrome has been reported as a complication of type III fracture.[325, 382] Recurvatum deformity is rare even with screw fixation across the physis because the demographic age group is usually undergoing physiological epiphyseodesis. Recurvatum may occur, however, in patients younger than 11 years, with substantial growth remaining. Temporary fixation with smooth wires should be used in these cases. Malunion can result in extensor lag or post-traumatic arthritis if there is significant articular incongruity. Articular injuries, particularly meniscal tears, may occur in association with tibial tuberosity fractures, most commonly type III fractures.[382] Leg-length discrepancies can also occur in type III fractures.[382]

Distal Femoral Physeal Fracture

Distal femoral physeal fractures account for less than 1% of all pediatric fractures, 1% to 5% of all physeal fractures, and 15% of lower-extremity physeal fractures.[261, 325] At the turn of the century, this injury most commonly resulted from violent hyperextension of the leg as a result of the leg being caught in the spokes of

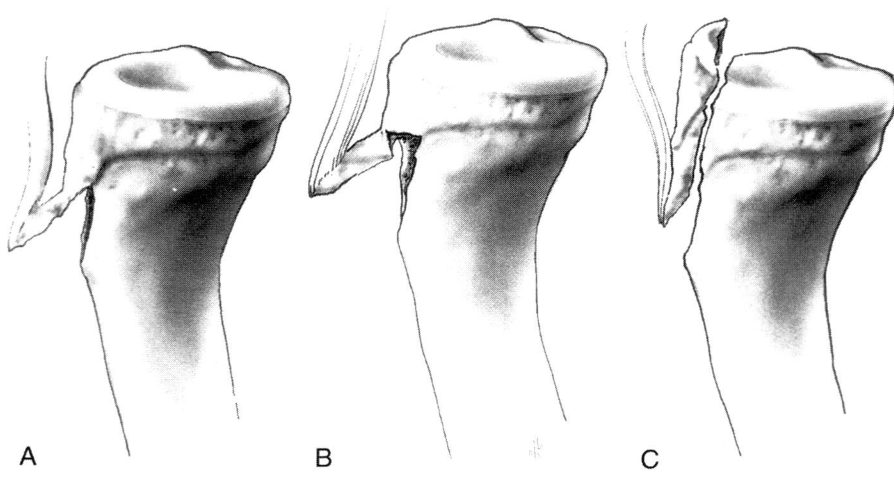

FIGURE 66.4 ➢ Classification of tibial tuberosity fractures. *A,* Type I fracture through the secondary ossification center of the tibial tubercle. *B,* Type II fracture at the junction of the tibial tubercle and proximal tibial ossification centers. *C,* Type III intra-articular fracture through the proximal tibial epiphysis. (From Devito DP: Management of fractures and their complications. In: Morrissy RT, Weinstein S, eds: Lovell and Winters' Pediatric Orthopaedics, 4th ed. Philadelphia, Lippincott, 1996.)

a wagon wheel, often resulting in vascular injury, infection, amputation, or death. Today, the most common mechanisms of injury are sports and motor vehicle accidents. Although amputation and death are now uncommon results of this type of injury, sequelae of angular deformity and leg-length discrepancy are not uncommon.

The secondary center of ossification of the distal femur appears during the ninth fetal week and is the only epiphyseal ossification center present at full-term birth. The distal femoral physis is the largest and fastest growing in the body. It contributes 70% of the growth of the femur and 37% of the growth of the lower extremity. It grows at an average rate of ⅜ in or 9 mm per year, slowing at a mean skeletal age of 13 years in girls and 15 years in boys. The distal femoral physis is extra-articular. The joint capsule, medial collateral ligament, lateral collateral ligament, and cruciate ligaments all originate from the distal femoral epiphysis (Fig. 66.5). Thus, the physis is vulnerable to forces

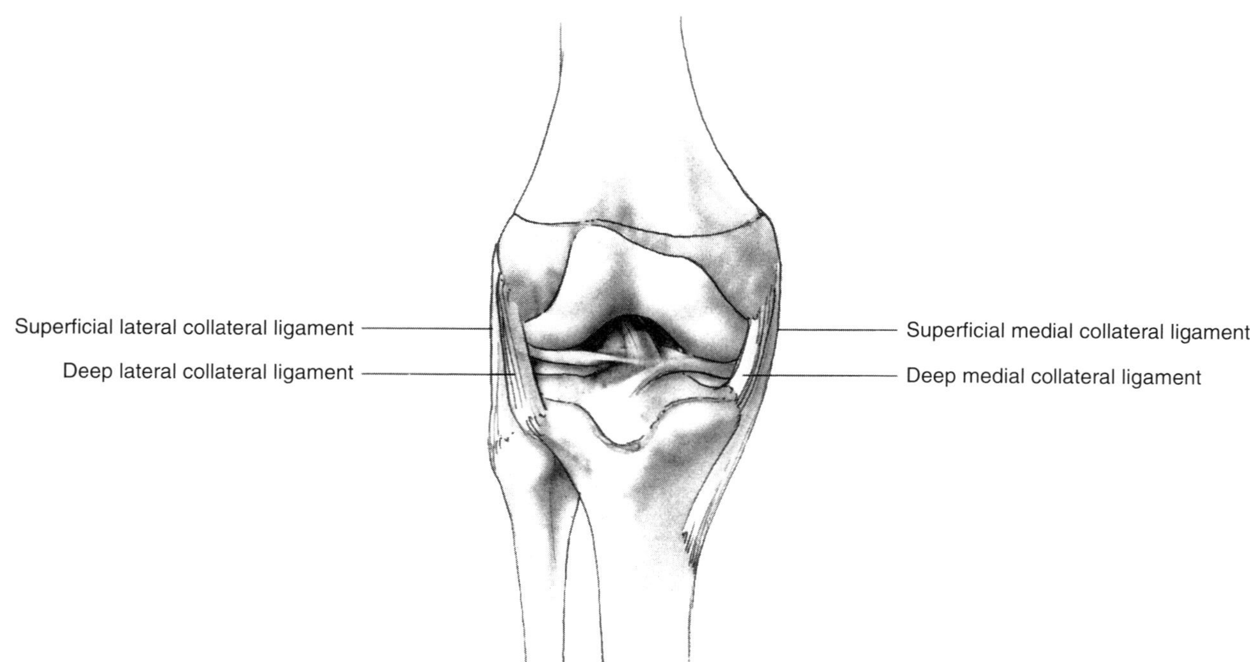

FIGURE 66.5 ➢ The collateral ligaments of the knee insert distal to both the distal femoral and proximal tibial epiphyses. Thus, stress to the knee will more often result in distal femoral physeal injury than in collateral ligament sprain. (From Busch MT: Sports medicine. In: Morrissy RT, Weinstein SL, eds: Lovell and Winters' Pediatric Orthopaedics, 4th ed. Philadelphia, Lippincott, 1996.)

applied to the distal femur. With valgus forces, physeal injury is more common than medial collateral injury in the skeletally immature. Similarly, with varus forces, physeal injury is more common than lateral collateral ligament injury. Distal femoral physeal fracture is much more common than proximal tibial physeal injury because the proximal tibial physis is protected by the spanning medial collateral ligament, lateral collateral ligament, patellar tendon, and gastrocnemius muscles. The medial heads of the gastrocnemius and the plantaris muscles do originate proximal to the distal femoral physis and thus provide some limited stability. The popliteal artery lies in close proximity to the distal metaphysis of the femur and is tethered by the geniculate arterial branches. Hyperextension fracture-separations with anterior displacement of the distal femoral epiphysis place the popliteal artery at risk of injury. Also, the peroneal nerve is at risk of injury with varus angulation of a distal femoral physeal fracture.

Many distal femoral physeal fractures occur during the growth spurt of early adolescence as the femoral and tibial moment arms increase, the muscle forces increase, the distal femoral physis undergoes relative weakening, the ligaments undergo relative strengthening, and the participation in competitive sports increases. The patient usually presents with pain after an acute, often violent, injury. Examination of the knee can be difficult because of extreme pain. The neurovascular status of the lower extremity must be carefully examined. Palpation along the damaged physis reveals tenderness. With displacement, there may be obvious deformity. Radiographs are usually sufficient to demonstrate the fracture pattern in displaced fractures and may be sufficient to demonstrate the fracture pattern in Salter-Harris II to IV injuries. Nondisplaced Salter-Harris I fractures may have normal x-rays initially and demonstrate periosteal healing bone in 2 weeks. Stress radiographs in the sedated patient may demonstrate the physeal injury but may cause further trauma to the growth plate. CT scans are sometimes necessary to determine the amount of displacement as in assessing joint congruity in Salter-Harris III fractures. MRI may allow greater accuracy in classifying physeal injury and may also allow assessment of the extent of physeal injury and physeal arrest (Fig. 66.6).[73, 118, 157, 261]

Distal femoral physeal fractures are classified based on the Salter-Harris classification. Salter-Harris I fractures occur at all ages. Child abuse should be ruled

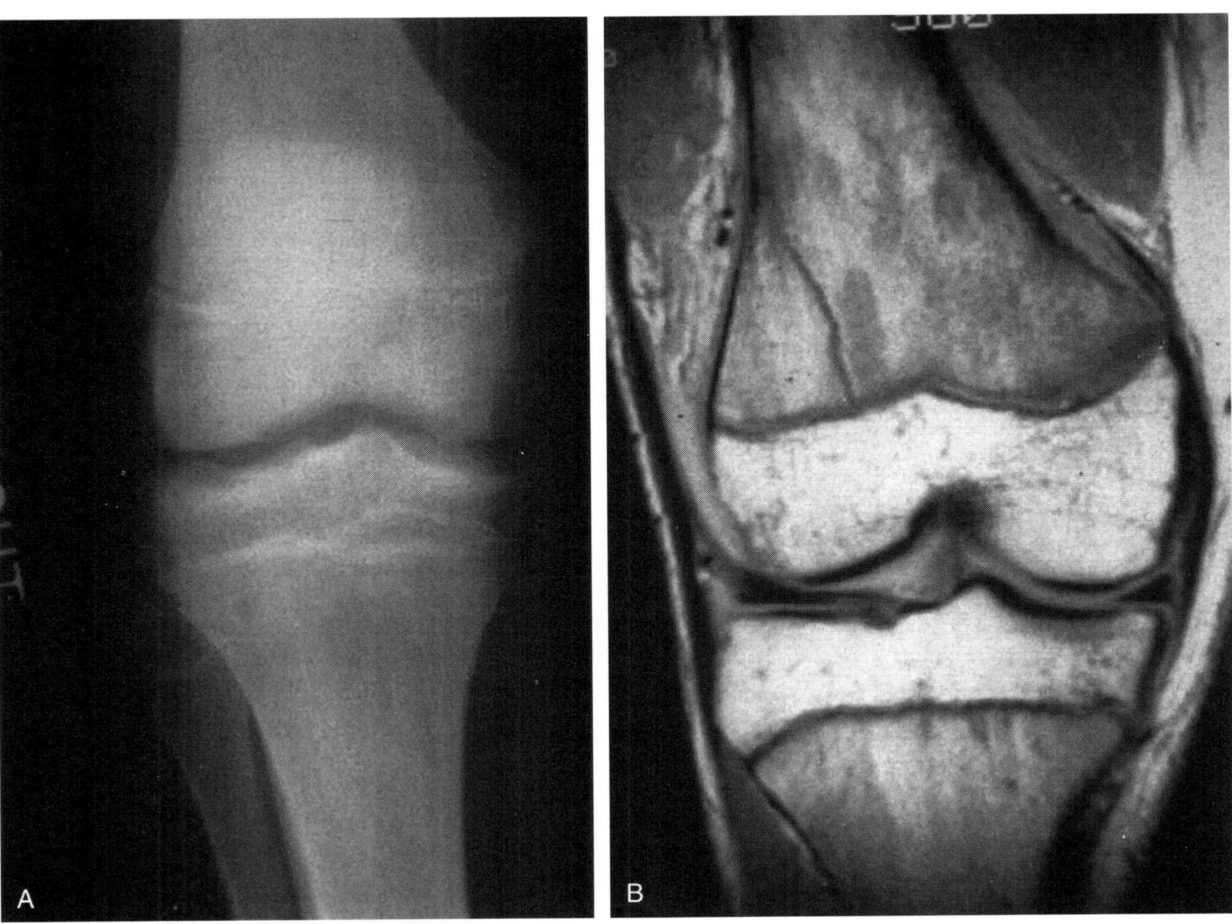

FIGURE 66.6 ➢ *A*, Apparently normal plain x-ray of a 14-year-old boy after a hockey injury. *B*, MRI reveals a nondisplaced Salter-Harris II fracture. (From Scott WN: The Knee, vol. 1. St. Louis, Mosby-Year Book, 1994, p 244.)

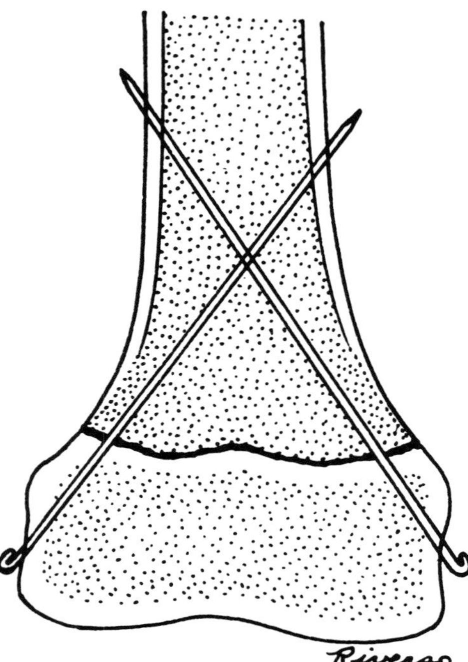

FIGURE 66.7 ➢ Fixation technique for Salter-Harris I or II distal femoral physeal fractures using crossed smooth wires. (From Canale ST: Fractures and dislocations. In Canale ST, Beaty JH, eds: Operative Pediatric Orthopaedics. St. Louis, Mosby–Year Book, 1991, pp 837-1032.)

out in children younger than 1 year with this injury. Salter-Harris II fractures are most common. Coronal displacement is usually to the side of the attached metaphyseal fragment, the Thurston-Holland fragment. The portion of physis associated with the Thurston-Holland fragment is usually spared from arrest. Salter-Harris III fractures propagate through the physis and exit the epiphysis into the joint. The most common location of articular exit is the intercondylar notch. A significant hemarthrosis is usually associated with this injury. Salter-Harris IV injuries are uncommon. Involvement of both the metaphysis and the epiphysis can result in significant joint and physeal incongruity. Salter-Harris V injuries involve crushing of the physis and are usually diagnosed in retrospect.

Nondisplaced fractures are treated closed, with a single-leg hip spica cast until early healing at 2 to 3 weeks, followed by long-leg casting. Long-leg casting may be used initially in thin patients with quite stable fractures. Displaced Salter-Harris I and II fractures are treated with gentle reduction under general anesthesia. Angulation in the plane of motion is better tolerated than is varus-valgus angulation. Acceptable angulation includes up to 20 to 30 degrees of flexion-extension in the frontal plane, 5 to 6 degrees of varus-valgus in the coronal plane, and no rotational malalignment. The intact periosteum and Thurston-Holland fragment can be used to aid reduction. Fractures with anterior displacement of the epiphysis are most easily reduced with the patient prone. Fractures that are stable after reduction may be treated closed; however, most significantly displaced fractures are unstable and thus require internal fixation. For Salter-Harris II fractures with a sufficiently large Thurston-Holland fragment, horizontal screws through the metaphyseal fragment across the metaphysis to engage the far cortex are used. For Salter-Harris I fractures and Salter-Harris II fractures with a small metaphyseal fragment, smooth Kirschner wires are introduced through each femoral condyle, cross each other proximal to the reduced growth plate, and penetrate the opposite cortex (Fig. 66.7). Displaced Salter-Harris III and IV fractures require an anatomic reduction for articular and physeal integrity and are usually treated with open reduction and internal fixation with screws parallel to the physis, followed by long-leg casting (Fig. 66.8). Ideally, the internal fixation should avoid crossing the physis to prevent further risk of growth arrest. Fractures of the distal femoral physis usually heal in 4 to 6 weeks. Cast immobilization is maintained during this time, and smooth pins are removed at the time of radiographic healing.[60, 118, 234, 291, 325]

Complications are not infrequently associated with distal femoral physeal fractures. Major vascular injury is uncommon, occurring in approximately 2% of displaced fractures. Injury to the popliteal artery can occur with anterior displacement of the epiphysis because it remains tethered by the geniculate arterial branches, resulting in transection, intimal tear, or spasm. Fractures associated with a nonperfused leg should undergo arteriogram and vascular exploration in the operating room. The fracture should be stabilized to prevent further vascular injury and to allow for a stable vascular repair. Progressive angular deformity can occur after distal femoral physeal fracture because of a peripheral physeal arrest, and leg-length discrepancy can occur because of a central arrest. The incidence of angular deformity ranges from 5% to 30%, and the incidence of leg-length discrepancy varies from 7% to 40% in various series (Table 66.4). Growth arrests may occur with all fracture types and are seen not infrequently even after Salter-Harris I or II injuries. Parents should be warned about the high risk of growth arrest after distal femoral physeal fracture and the need for careful follow-up. Even with anatomic reduction, the risk of growth disturbance may correlate more closely with amount of initial displacement instead of fracture type. Poor prognostic factors for growth arrest include greater than 50% initial displacement, inadequate reduction, younger age, and crushing injuries. Bar excision can be attempted when there is less than 50% of the physis involved and there is significant growth (>2 cm) remaining. Other options include completion epiphyseodesis of the involved side; shoe lift (<2 cm); epiphyseodesis of the contralateral side (2 to 5 cm discrepancy); lengthening procedures (>5 cm discrepancy); shortening procedures (<5 cm and skeletal maturity); and osteotomies, partial epiphyseodesis, or Ilizarov correction for angular deformity. Knee ligament instability after distal femoral physeal fracture is increasingly recognized with rates between 25% and 45% in various series.[11, 28, 38, 74, 76, 91, 117, 169, 199, 210, 288, 339]

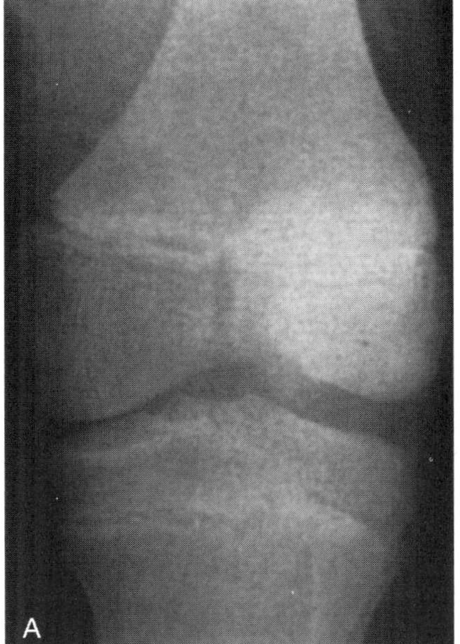

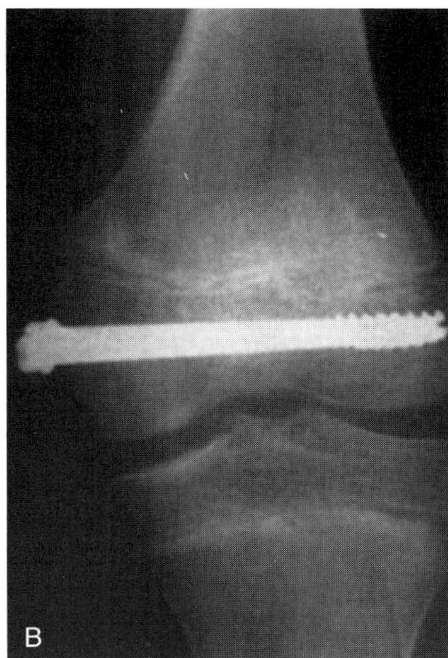

FIGURE 66.8 ➢ *A,* Anteroposterior roentgenogram of Salter-Harris III fracture of the distal femur. *B,* Fixation with two horizontal cancellous compression screws extending across the epiphyseal fragment parallel to the physis, restoring the articular surface. (From Beaty JH, Roberts JM: Fractures and dislocations of the knee. In Rockwood CA, Wilkins KE, King RE, eds: Fractures in Children, 3rd ed. Philadelphia, JB Lippincott, 1991, pp 1165–1270.)

Proximal Tibial Physeal Fracture

The proximal tibial epiphyseal ossification center appears between the first and third postnatal months. It enlarges peripherally in an irregular fashion. The ossification does not reach the tibial eminence until late childhood. The ossification center of the proximal fibula appears at approximately 3 years of age. The proximal tibial physis accounts for approximately 25% of the growth of the leg, or ¼ in per year. The cruciate ligaments and knee joint capsule insert onto the proximal tibial epiphysis. The proximal tibial physis is well protected laterally by the fibula and the lateral collateral ligament inserting on the fibula, medially by the superficial medial collateral ligament inserting on the proximal tibial metaphysis, anteriorly by the tibial tuberosity and the patellar tendon inserting on the tuberosity, and posteriorly by the gastrocnemius and the hamstrings tendons. The distal portion of the popliteal artery lies close to the posterior aspect of the upper tibia and is anchored to the posterior knee capsule by septae and the geniculate arteries.

Because of its protected position, injuries to the proximal tibial physis are rare, accounting for less than 1% of all physeal injuries and 0.5% of all pediatric fractures.[261, 325] Two thirds of proximal tibial physeal fractures are Salter-Harris I or II fractures. Type III and IV fractures are usually the result of severe trauma and are uncommon. Most patients present after high-energy acute trauma with pain localized to the proximal tibia. Deformity may be present with displacement. A thorough neurovascular examination is essential. Radiograms are usually sufficient to delineate the fracture pattern.

Nondisplaced fractures are treated closed with a long-leg cast until healing, which usually occurs at 4 to 6 weeks. Most displaced Salter-Harris I or II fractures of the proximal tibia can be reduced under general anesthesia with gentle longitudinal traction. If stable, the patient is placed in a long-leg cast. The patient should have frequent neurovascular examinations after the reduction. Unstable fractures should be pinned with smooth Kirschner wires to maintain reduction. If anatomic reduction of Salter-Harris type III or IV fractures cannot be obtained closed, open reduction and internal fixation are essential to reestablish articular and physeal congruity. The fixation should be parallel to the physis without violating it, if possible. Undisplaced proximal tibial fractures can be unstable; therefore, they require frequent follow-up to identify displacement.[9, 10, 53, 57, 60, 73, 111, 281, 290, 291, 312, 325]

Vascular injury is the most serious complication associated with displaced proximal tibial physeal fractures. The popliteal artery is intimately associated with

TABLE 66.4 COMPLICATIONS AFTER DISTAL FEMORAL PHYSEAL FRACTURE

Series	Incidence	
Angular Deformity		
Aitken & Magill[11]	1/15	7%
Lombardo & Harvey[210]	11/34	32%
Stephens et al[339]	4/20	20%
Roberts[291]	9/50	18%
Sponseller & Beaty[325]	1/21	5%
Leg-Length Discrepancy		
Aitken & Magill[11]	1/15	7%
Lombardo & Harvey[210]	13/34	38%
Stephens et al[339]	8/20	40%
Roberts[291]	11/50	22%
Sponseller and Beaty[325]	3/21	14%
Ligament Instability		
Aitken & Magill[11]	4/9	44%
Lombardo & Harvey[210]	8/34	24%
Stephens et al[339]	5/20	25%
Bertin & Goble[38]	7/16	44%

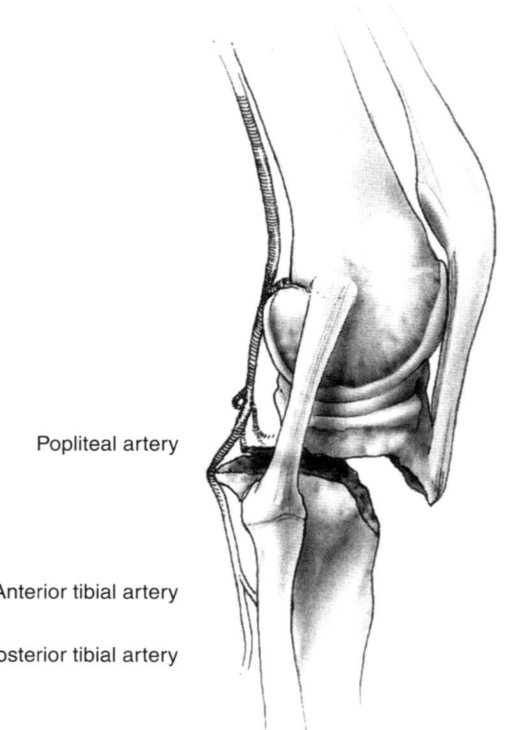

FIGURE 66.9 ➢ Proximal tibial physeal fracture. Injury to the popliteal artery can occur with posterior displacement of the distal tibial segment. (From Devito DP: Management of fractures and their complications. In: Morrissy RT, Weinstein SI, eds: Lovell and Winters' Pediatric Orthopaedics, 4th ed. Philadelphia, Lippincott, 1996.)

the posterior aspect of the proximal tibia (Fig. 66.9). With anterior displacement of the proximal tibial epiphysis, the upper end of the tibial metaphysis may injure the popliteal artery, which is tethered in this region by the geniculate branches. In addition, angular deformity and leg-length discrepancy can occur after fracture as in distal femoral physeal fractures. Associated ligamentous injury, particularly tibial ACL avulsions, can also be seen. A Salter-Harris type III medial fracture has been described with a superficial medial collateral ligament tear and a lateral type IV fracture.[9, 10, 53, 57, 60, 73, 111, 281, 290, 291, 312, 325]

OSTEOCHONDRITIS DISSECANS

OCD is a nonacute derangement involving necrosis of subchondral bone. The sites of OCD are, in decreasing order, knee, ankle, elbow, and hip. The knee is by far the most common location, and 10% of cases are bilateral and symmetric. The incidence of OCD of the knee has been reported as 4% of all knee radiographs and as 18 per 100,000 females and 29 per 100,000 males.[8, 204] Most commonly, OCD appears during the second decade of life but has been documented in children as young as 4 years and in adults up to age 50 years. The incidence of juvenile OCD seems to be increasing, females seem to be involved more frequently, and the mean age of juvenile OCD patients seems to be decreasing from approximately 13 years to around 11 years. This may be due to increased participation in competitive youth sports by younger children. The frequency in males is two to three times that of females. The most common location is the lateral aspect of the medial femoral condyle (70%) (Fig. 66.10). OCD also occurs in the lateral femoral condyle (20%), usually the posterior weightbearing region, and in the patella (10%), usually the distal half.[54, 66]

The cause of OCD is unknown. OCD most likely represents the result of cumulative stress to subchondral bone, resulting in subchondral stress fractures. Other causes or contributing factors include microvascular alterations, acute macrotrauma (osteochondral fracture), osteonecrosis, endocrinopathy, ligamentous laxity, osteochondrosis, and familial predisposition. Most patients do not report a single traumatic event. However, most patients with OCD are active and athletic, with exposure to sports at a young age being a risk factor. This suggests a cause of cumulative injury from repetitive microtrauma. The target tissue in OCD is the subchondral bone, rather than the articular cartilage. Stress fractures may provoke vascular compromise, resulting in the finding of a variably viable bone nucleus covered with intact articular cartilage. Pathologically, OCD appears as dead, avascular bone under normal cartilage. Early or developing OCD is seen as an expanding concentric lesion in an otherwise normal epiphysis. Later, the lesion may separate from the femoral condyle and become free in the joint.[54, 66, 96, 248, 249, 272]

Two distinct forms exist: juvenile OCD and adult OCD. The distinguishing feature is that juvenile OCD occurs in patients with an open epiphyseal plate. Once established, adult OCD has a significantly poorer prognosis than does juvenile OCD. Adult OCD can arise de novo in the skeletally mature knee; however, the majority of young adults with OCD have symptoms dating back to skeletal immaturity and thus most likely represent juvenile OCD that did not heal.[54]

Symptoms are nonspecific. As aforementioned, there is usually a chronic history without an acute event, often dating back to an age of skeletal immaturity. Initially, the patient complains of vague, activity-related knee pain and swelling. The pain may progress to activities of daily living. In later stages, the patient may complain of mechanical symptoms and instability because of loose bodies or unstable OCD flaps. On examination, there may be palpable tenderness over the femoral condyle or an effusion. A consistent finding is thigh atrophy. Pain can sometimes be elicited with internal rotation of the leg and gradual extension of the knee. At 25 to 30 degrees of flexion, the tibial spine impinges on the lateral aspect of the medial femoral condyle producing pain (Wilson's sign). The patient may, therefore, ambulate with the leg externally rotated to avoid impingement. Roentgenograms are usually diagnostic, showing craterlike areas of rarefaction in subchondral bone. There may be associated loose bodies or sequestra. The lesion is often more visible and more extensive on the notch view as opposed to the AP view. Patellar OCD is often best ap-

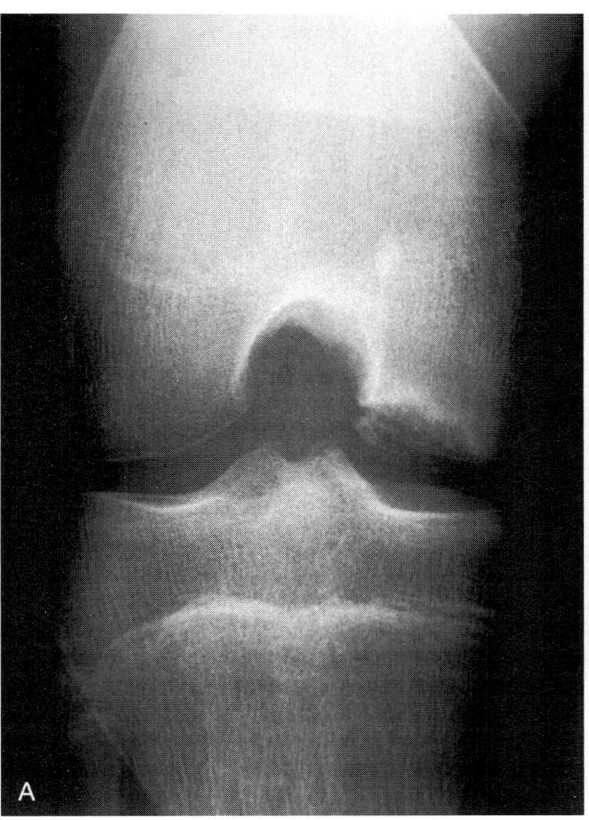

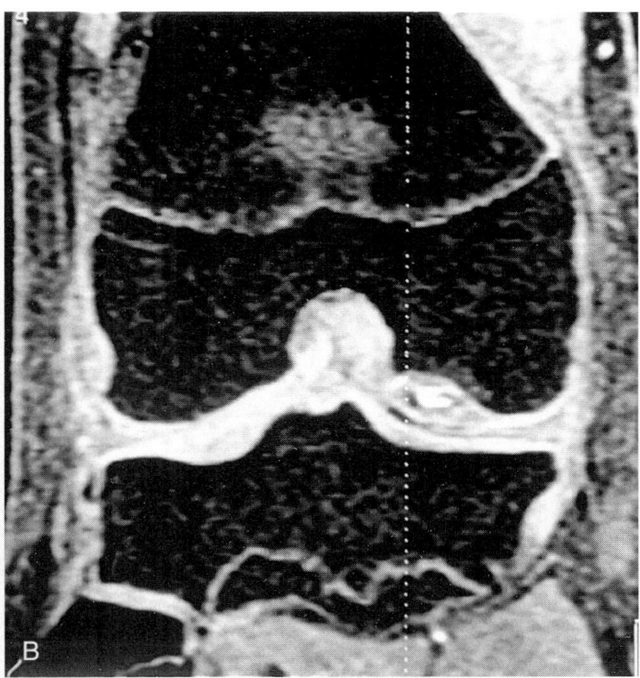

FIGURE 66.10 ➢ Osteochondritis dissecans. *A*, AP (notch view) radiograph demonstrating involvement of the medial femoral condyle. *B*, Corresponding MRI view.

preciated on the skyline view. X-rays may be temporally insensitive to changes in OCD activity, often lagging behind symptoms and not providing evidence of metabolic activity. MRI is specific and sensitive for early detection of OCD. In addition, it often aids in assessing the condition of the articular cartilage (magnetic resonance arthrograms especially) and the healing response. Bone scans have been used to follow metabolic activity associated with the OCD lesion. They may be helpful in assessing the extent of involvement and the healing potential, thus guiding treatment. Periodic scanning at 4-month intervals has been advocated to follow the progression of disease and response to treatment. Quantitative bone scans and computerized blood flow analysis may provide more reliable prognostic information.[55, 56, 66, 86, 119, 206, 230, 271]

OCD has been classified on the basis of plain x-ray and bone scan findings related to activity of the femoral condyles and the adjacent tibial plateau (Fig. 66.11). Stage 0 has a normal radiographic and scintigraphic appearance with clinical symptoms. Stage 1 has normal scintigraphy with a radiographically visible defect. Stage 2 has increased scintigraphic uptake in the radiographically visible lesion. Stage 1 and 2 OCD may be asymptomatic. Stage 3 has increased scintigraphic uptake in both the lesion and the femoral condyle. Stage 4 also has increased uptake in the adjacent tibial plateau. Stage 3 and 4 lesions are always symptomatic.[54–56, 206]

The goal of treatment in OCD is to alleviate pain, prevent further injury, aid in healing of the lesion, and maintain a smooth congruent joint surface to avoid early development of degenerative arthritis. The natural history of OCD allows for healing, particularly in juvenile lesions. There is a definite role for initial nonoperative management of juvenile OCD, consisting of relative rest and cessation of the offending activity. As in fracture healing, crutches may be initially necessary if there is pain with ambulation. Immobilization is controversial, with some advocating casting with limited weightbearing to protect the cartilage from its loss of mechanical support because of the subchondral injury. Others discourage immobilization because of its detrimental effect on articular cartilage. These authors have had good results with treating OCD with fracture principles, especially in prepubescents, using casting and limiting weightbearing for 6 to 8 weeks. When the patient is symptom free, weightbearing as tolerated is allowed. Follow-up is every 6 to 8 weeks until clinical, radiographic, and scintigraphic evaluation reveal healing. Healing is assumed when the patient is symptom free, clinical examination is normal, radiographs show no further progression, and scintigram shows a decrease in activity to uptake in the lesion only. It may take 10 months to reach this point of healing. Competitive sports are prohibited during this time. As healing continues, conditioning with nonimpact sports, such as swimming, bicycling, and strength training, are added, provided the child remains asymptomatic. Compliance may be difficult for some patients and their families because restriction from competitive athletic participation may be prolonged. However, the excel-

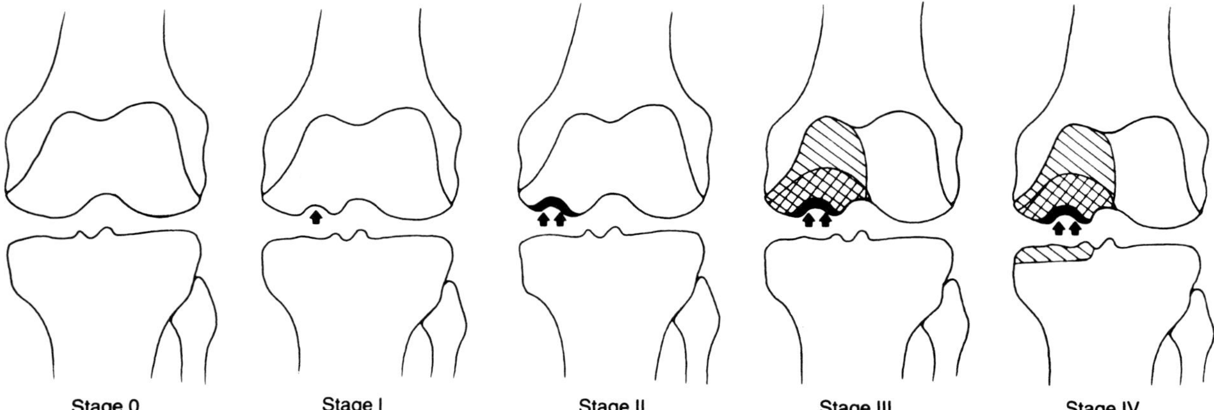

FIGURE 66.11 ➢ Classification of juvenile osteochondritis dissecans on the basis of the radiographic and scintigraphic appearance. Stage 0 is a normal radiographic and scintigraphic appearance. In stage 1, a defect on the femoral condyle is visible radiographically but not scintigraphically. In stage 2, the scintigram shows increased uptake in the lesion. In stage 3, the increased isotope uptake is seen in both the lesion and the femoral condyle. In stage 4, there is also increased uptake in the tibial plateau. (From Cahill BR: Osteochondritis dissecans of the knee. J Am Acad Orthop Surg 3:237, 1995. Copyright 1995 American Academy of Orthopaedic Surgeons.)

lent long-term results of successful nonoperative treatment, particularly in the skeletally immature patient, should be emphasized. Nonoperative management will allow resolution of most intact stable lesions before physeal closure.[54, 66, 146, 197, 320]

Operative treatment is indicated for large lesions, detachment or instability of the OCD fragment, persistence of symptoms or worsening of symptoms despite nonoperative management, and skeletal maturity because healing from nonoperative measures is less likely. Loose or unstable fragments are treated with repair. Internal fixation of the fragment can be accomplished arthroscopically with bone pegs, smooth wires, biodegradable pins, cannulated screws, fibrin sealant, and articular screws. Postoperatively after drilling or fragment reattachment, the leg is immobilized for 2 to 4 weeks and protected from weightbearing for 8 to 12 weeks. Poor results are predictable from removal of a substantial fragment in a weightbearing area. Removal of a loose or unstable fragment from a non-weightbearing area is acceptable. If the lesion has been loose or unstable for months, restoring the joint surface arthroscopically is technically prohibitive, requiring arthrotomy. Partially detached and loose juvenile OCD fragments tend to grow, while the crater of the lesion retains its original dimensions. Thus, there is frequently size mismatch for chronic lesions, necessitating open management consisting of trimming, curetting of the femoral defect, drilling, and internal fixation. Grafting may be necessary to fill subchondral defects or to enhance healing. Stable lesions with intact articular cartilage at arthroscopy can be treated with transarticular drilling.[126b] If the lesion is stable and there is sufficient metabolic activity (such as a stage 3 bone scan), drilling of the subchondral bone alone may suffice to initiate healing. For stable lesions with metabolic activity confined to the lesion alone (stage 2 bone scan), additional bone grafting may be beneficial to induce healing. Overall, good results can be obtained in most patients, with poor results more likely in older patients and in those with chronic lesions or larger lesions. For the rare instances where there is no alternative to removal of a juvenile OCD lesion in a weightbearing location, a fresh or fresh-frozen osteochondral allograft should be considered. Autologous chondrocyte implantation holds promise for OCD lesions because good short-term results have been obtained in the management of focal articular cartilage defects of the femoral condyles; however, the long-term function of the repair cartilage remains to be proven.[5, 14, 46, 49, 54, 66, 146, 191, 197, 198, 203, 215]

MENISCAL INJURIES

Originating from the differentiation of mesenchymal tissue within the limb bud, the meniscus becomes defined by the eighth fetal week. By the 14th week, the meniscus has established its adult relationship. At no point in its development is the meniscus discoid.[167] During embryological development and even at birth, the vascular supply of the meniscus enters from the periphery and extends throughout the entire width. At birth, the meniscus is densely cellular with spindle-shaped and polygonal fibrochondrocytes. After birth, there is a progressive decrease in vascularity that occurs from the inner to the outer region, a progressive decrease in cellularity, and an increase in collagen content.[67] By the ninth month post partum, the inner third is avascular, and by age 10 to 11 years, the meniscus becomes similar to that of the adult, with blood vessels primarily in the peripheral third adjacent to the coronary ligaments. The meniscus grows commensurate with the growth of the tibial plateaus and femoral condyle. Around age 3 years, as the child assumes the upright position more frequently, collagen fibers become more abundant and their orientation changes to a more highly organized circumferential pattern. Radially oriented fibers develop on the tibial and femoral surfaces of the meniscus to resist longitudinal splitting.

Meniscal Tears

The true incidence of meniscal tears in children is unknown, but they are very unusual in children younger than 10 years unless associated with a discoid meniscus. The biomechanical and vascular environment may be responsible for the low incidence in children. As the child approaches adolescence, the incidence of meniscal tears increases significantly.[82] Children and adolescents have different tear patterns than adults have. The majority are bucket-handle tears and complete longitudinal tears with a significant portion of the meniscus peripherally detached.[17, 177, 334] Some series have found lateral meniscus tears to outnumber medial meniscus tears in children and adolescents, whereas others have found medial tears to be more common.[17, 138, 177, 289, 334]

The most frequent mechanism of injury involves the weightbearing position with a moderate degree of flexion while sustaining a bending or twisting force. However, some children with meniscus tears present without a specific history of trauma. Symptoms are usually nonspecific. Acutely, there may be a catching sensation with a rapid hemarthrosis. There may be medial or lateral pain, which is usually activity-related. Mechanical symptoms of catching and locking may be present. Joint line tenderness may be present. Provocative tests, such as McMurray's maneuver or Apley's grind test, may have positive results. Range of motion may be limited, and there is often quadriceps atrophy. Plain radiographs may be useful to rule out other disorders that may mimic a meniscal tear, such as osteochondral fracture, OCD, or a loose body. MRI is often helpful to evaluate the extent of meniscal tears and other intra-articular lesions. However, MRI can yield false-positive results for meniscal tear because of changing meniscal hydration and cellularity in the developing knee.[103, 184, 332, 346, 361, 395] In diagnosing a meniscal tear by MRI, care should be taken to note signal change that extends to the surface in children and adolescents.

Because of the greater vascularity of the younger meniscus, its reparative ability is greater than in the adult. If the patient has a full range of motion without locking, nonoperative therapy can be used.[374] At arthroscopy, stable peripheral tears measuring less than 10 mm in length, which are less than 3 mm manually displaceable, and small radial tears measuring less than 3 mm may be left alone to heal. Fenestration, trephination, rasping, or débriding the tear edges may enhance healing. Many meniscal tears in children may be reparable, particularly bucket-handle tears and unstable or large peripheral tears. Repair techniques are similar to those used in adults: inside-out techniques, outside-in techniques, and all-inside techniques. In knees with both a reparable meniscus tear and an ACL tear, ACL reconstruction should be performed in addition to meniscus repair to provide a stable environment for healing.[116] With increased recognition of the biomechanical importance of the meniscus and the sequelae of degenerative arthritis associated with complete meniscectomy, meniscus excision today is rarely total. Complete meniscectomy in children predictably leads to early degenerative changes.[1, 78, 218, 227, 322, 358, 386, 391] The long-term outcome of arthroscopic partial meniscectomy in young patients is still unknown. The biomechanical effect of partial meniscectomy is highly variable depending on amount removed, location, articular geometry, and associated lesions. Results for meniscal repair in children and adolescents appear more favorable than for adults; however, the long-term results are not known.

Meniscal Cysts

Cysts associated with meniscal tears occur in adolescents as well as in adults. They are most often found with lateral meniscal tears and with horizontal cleavage tears. Pain and swelling are the usual complaints. The pain is activity related and is located about the joint line. There may not be mechanical symptoms. The cyst may not be apparent with the patient supine and the knee extended. Knee flexion with comparison with the contralateral uninvolved knee often demonstrates the cyst. The cyst may extrude over the proximal tibia or about the distal iliotibial band laterally.

Aspiration and corticosteroid injection have been used to treat meniscal cysts in adults, with variable success. However, we tend to avoid corticosteroid injection in young patients. Excision of the meniscal tear may result in resolution of the meniscal cyst. However, in children and adolescents, the cyst may persist. Thus, open ligation and excision of the cyst along with arthroscopic débridement of the meniscal tear usually result in resolution of the cyst and the symptoms.[299]

Discoid Meniscus

The true incidence of discoid menisci in children is unknown because many cases are asymptomatic, but it has been estimated at 3% to 5% of the American population and higher (approximately 15%) in the Asian population.[103, 163] Bilaterality occurs in approximately 25% of cases. In terms of the etiology of discoid menisci, it was thought that they might represent an embryological failure of resorption of the central portion of the meniscus during development.[319] However, it has been shown that in humans and in many other species, there is no stage of embryological development in which the meniscus is discoid.[167] It has been further hypothesized that because of increased mobility, discoid changes occur to compensate for instability of the meniscus during development.[67, 101, 167]

Discoid menisci occur almost always laterally, although medial discoid menisci have been documented.[22] Discoid menisci are classified based on their morphology and on the presence of the coronary (meniscotibial) ligaments (Fig. 66.12).[366] Type I menisci are completely discoid, generally extending across the entire lateral tibial plateau. Type II menisci are incom-

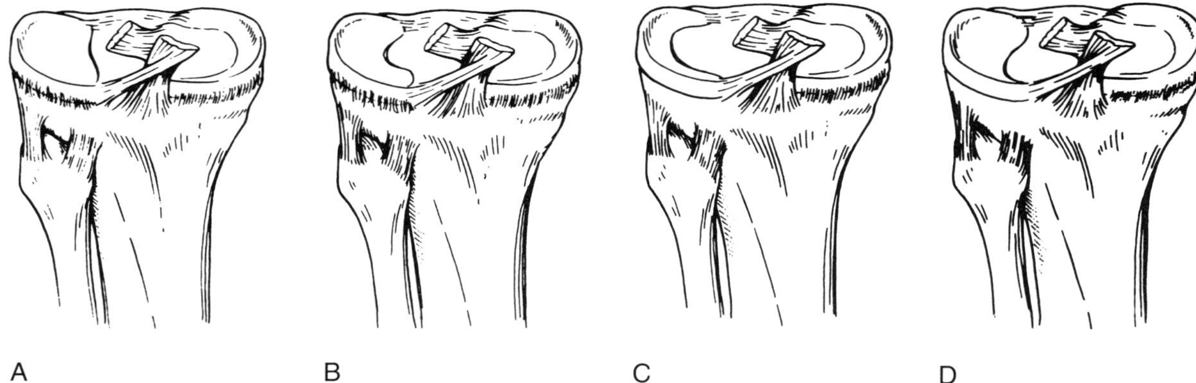

FIGURE 66.12 ➢ Posterior views of lateral discoid menisci. *A*, Type I complete discoid meniscus. *B*, Type II incomplete discoid meniscus. *C*, Type III Wrisberg's variant with normal shape. *D*, Type III Wrisberg's variant with discoid shape. (From Jordan MR: Lateral meniscal variants. J Am Acad Orthop Surg 4:191, 1996. Copyright 1996 American Academy of Orthopaedic Surgeons.)

plete. The central portion of the meniscus extends across the lateral tibial plateau farther than normal, but not completely. Type III menisci, Wrisberg's type, lack coronary ligament meniscotibial attachment at the posterior horn, resulting in instability of the posterior horn, which is secured only by the meniscofemoral ligaments. Type III menisci may be normally shaped or discoid shaped.

Discoid menisci usually present in the young patient as a snapping knee. There is often a dramatic snapping or popping with knee motion that produces minimal or momentary pain. There is a history of frequent catching and locking. On examination, the clunking can be reproduced with McMurray's maneuvers. The knee seems to momentarily subluxate. In the older child and adolescent, the presenting symptoms are usually those of a meniscal tear and not of instability: pain, swelling, and mechanical symptoms.[27, 88, 163, 383] On plain radiographs, few patients have the classic findings of widening of the lateral joint, squaring of the lateral femoral condyle, and cupping of the tibial plateau (Fig. 66.13). MRI may demonstrate discoid menisci on coronal sections in which the transverse meniscal diameter will be greater than 15 mm, or 20% of the tibial width (see Fig. 66.13).[316] However, although MRI is extremely specific for discoid meniscus, it is not very sensitive, with a high rate of false-negative interpretations.[184]

Discoid menisci are more prone to mechanical stress because they are thicker, are more poorly vascularized, and, in some cases, have a loose posterior or anterior attachment.[67] For type I and II discoid menisci, the most common tear pattern is longitudinal, with horizontal tears also occurring. For type III menisci, there may be complex degenerative tears or no tear at all.

No treatment is required for the asymptomatic discoid meniscus discovered incidentally. For the symptomatic patient with type I or II discoid meniscus, arthroscopic saucerization is performed by débridement of the central portion with contouring of the remaining rim to a 6-mm rim for type I menisci and an 8-mm rim for type II menisci. Wider widths are prone to retear. Frequently, a peripheral indentation made by the femoral condyle can be identified in the meniscus, which can be used as a convenient marker for the limits of saucerization. Type III discoid menisci have traditionally been treated with total meniscectomy. However, because of the risk of developing early degenerative changes after total meniscectomy, attachment of the unstable rim to the capsule is preferred although technically challenging.[8, 34, 134, 278, 294, 340, 359, 368]

KNEE LIGAMENT INJURIES

Injury patterns in the skeletally immature knee are dependent on the stage of musculoskeletal development. Young children tend to sustain fractures, particularly metaphyseal fractures and buckle fractures. In older children, between ages 7 and 11 years, both physeal and ligament injuries may occur. Physeal injuries predominate during the adolescent growth spurt when the physis is relatively weakest. During late adolescence, as physes fuse, ligament injury is more common, as in adults.[321, 343] Ligaments may undergo a relative reduction in strength and laxity as children approach adulthood, for both males and females.[31, 63]

Knee ligament injuries can occur in association with other fractures or can occur as isolated ligamentous or bony avulsion injuries. Knee ligament instability after distal femoral physeal fracture is increasingly recognized, with rates between 25% and 45% in various series.[11, 38, 210, 339] Ligament injuries occur with all Salter-Harris types, although type III fractures may be especially at risk because they frequently exit intra-articularly at the intercondylar notch. ACL injuries are most common. Similarly, knee ligament injuries can occur in association with proximal tibial physeal fractures, particularly Salter-Harris III fractures. MCL injuries are most common.

On physical examination for collateral ligament injuries in children, particular attention should be paid to determining the site of injury: physis, midsubstance ligament, or ligament insertion. Varus-valgus and ante-

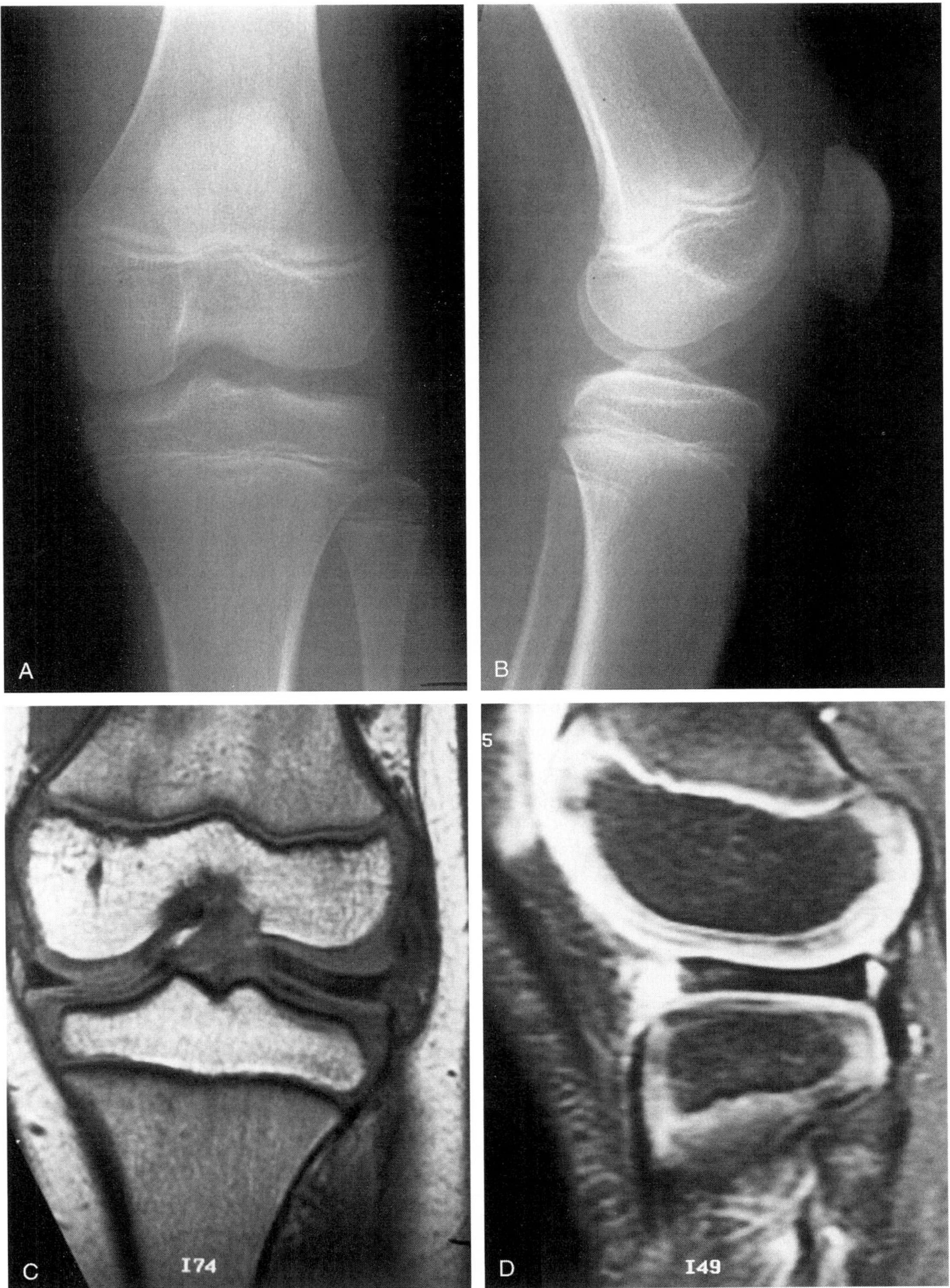

FIGURE 66.13 ➢ Imaging of lateral discoid meniscus. *A*, AP radiograph demonstrating lateral compartment widening and squaring of the lateral femoral condyle and lateral tibial plateau. *B*, Lateral radiograph demonstrating flattening of lateral femoral condyle. *C*, Coronal and *D*, Sagittal MRI images demonstrating lateral discoid meniscus.

rior-posterior laxity should always be compared with the uninvolved side because of the nonpathological laxity present in many children at various stages of development. For cruciate ligament injuries, Lachman, drawer, and pivot-shift tests should be performed as in adults. Grading of laxity is important because partial ligament injuries are common in children. Examination may be difficult in the younger child because of patient apprehension and pain. If the diagnosis is in doubt, arthroscopy or MRI should be performed. Although MRI is sensitive for complete tears, it has poor sensitivity for partial tears.[184]

Anterior Cruciate Ligament Injury

The type of ACL injury in the skeletally immature patient, either tibial spine avulsion or midsubstance tear, depends on the loading conditions and the stage of maturity of the knee. Avulsion fractures predominate in conditions of lower loads over a longer loading period, whereas midsubstance tears occur more commonly in conditions of larger loads over a shorter loading period. Avulsion fractures predominate in children and prepubescents, whereas midsubstance tears occur more commonly in later adolescence and skeletal maturity. However, midsubstance tears have been reported in children as young as 4 years, and tibial spine avulsion fractures are seen in adults.[257, 303, 345]

Tibial Spine Fracture

The tibial eminence refers to the region of anterior tibial plateau between the anterior horns of the medial and lateral menisci. The ACL attaches to the fossa anterior to the medial tibial spine. Some ACL fibers pass beneath the transverse meniscal ligament, blending with the anterior horn of the lateral meniscus. The tibial ACL attachment is wider and shorter than the femoral attachment. With sufficient stress to the ACL in the skeletally immature child, an avulsion can occur through the relatively weaker cancellous bone beneath its insertion in the tibial subchondral plate.

The most common mechanism of tibial eminence fracture is forced valgus and external rotation of the tibia, although tibial spine avulsion fractures can also occur from hyperflexion, hyperextension, or tibial internal rotation. Classically, pediatric tibial spine fractures occur from bicycling accidents, although they are also seen with pedestrian–motor vehicle accidents or sports trauma.[32, 135, 231, 244, 252, 268, 287, 379, 392]

Meyers and McKeever, and later Zaricznyj, classified tibial spine avulsions into four types (Fig. 66.14): type I is minimally displaced, type II occurs when the fragment is hinged but still attached, type III is complete displacement of the fragment, and type IV is comminution of the fragment.[231, 392] Type III is more common in children who are older than 11 years.

On physical examination, there is often a hemarthrosis and limited motion. Sagittal plane laxity is often present, but the contralateral knee should be assessed for physiological laxity. Associated MCL injury should be evaluated. Roentgenograms typically demonstrate the fracture, seen best on the lateral and tunnel views.

For nondisplaced or minimally (type I or II) displaced fractures, treatment is in a long-leg cast for 6 to 8 weeks. Some authors recommend immobilization in full extension or hyperextension to allow the femoral condyle to compress the fragment toward its fracture bed. Ultimately, the optimal position for maintenance of reduction should be confirmed by imaging or direct arthroscopic observation. We have often found this position to be flexed 15 to 30 degrees to relax the posterolateral ACL bundle. In cast, the child may perform partial weightbearing after 72 hours.

For hinged or displaced fractures (types II to IV) (Fig. 66.15) or for any fracture with a positive Lachman sign, we favor reduction under arthroscopic control. It is frequently necessary to remove clots and

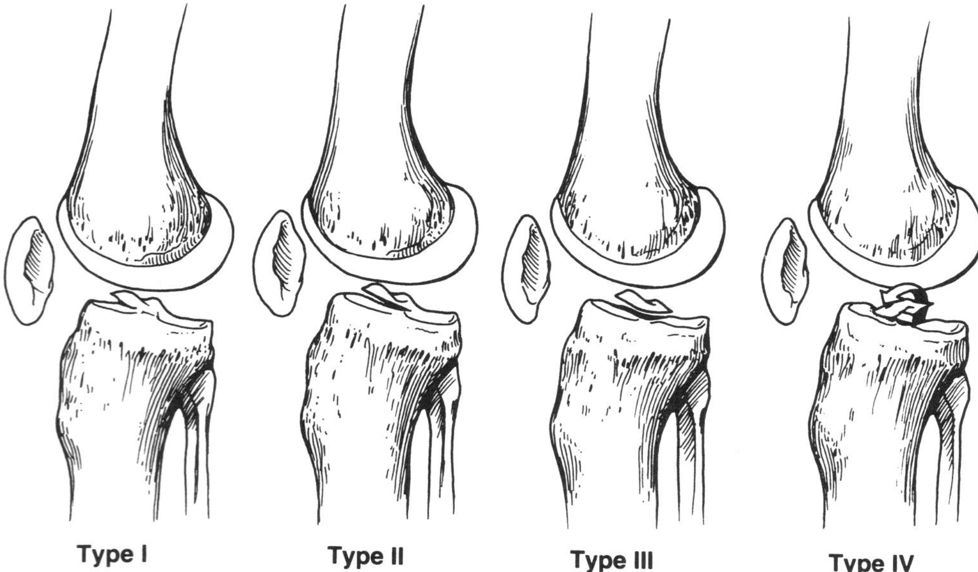

FIGURE 66.14 ➢ Tibial spine fractures. Type I fracture is minimally displaced, Type II fracture is hinged, Type III fracture is completely displaced, and Type IV fracture is completely displaced and rotated. (From Stanitski CL: Anterior cruciate ligament injury in the skeletally immature patient: Diagnosis and treatment. J Am Acad Orthop Surg 3:146, 1995.)

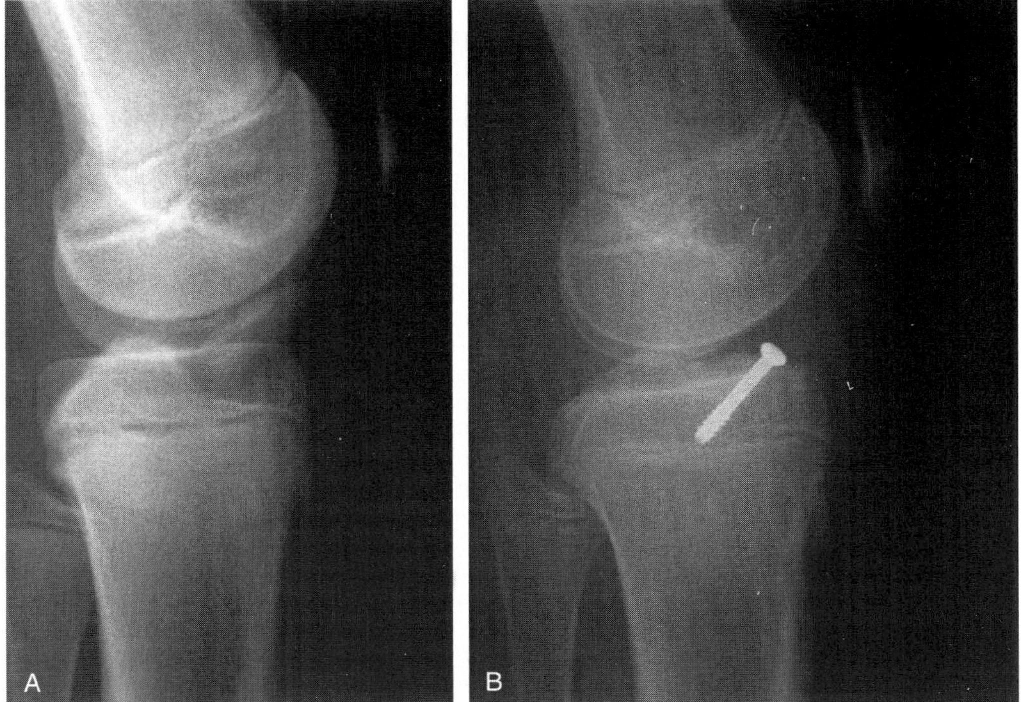

FIGURE 66.15 ➢ Tibial spine fracture. *A,* Lateral radiograph demonstrating a displaced, type III tibial eminence fracture. *B,* Postoperative lateral radiograph after arthroscopic reduction and fixation with a cannulated epiphyseal screw.

debris from the bed and to remove intervening meniscus or articular cartilage to get a satisfactory reduction. After reduction, fixation may not be necessary if extension maintains proper position; however, fixation is often needed to maintain reduction in displaced fractures. Fixation can usually be done arthroscopically or with a small arthrotomy. If the bony fragment is too small for pin or cannulated screw fixation, sutures can be used. Several large, strong sutures are passed into the avulsion site and weaved through the ACL using a suture punch. The sutures are then brought out of the proximal tibial epiphysis anteriorly with a suture passer and tied. The leg is then immobilized at 30 degrees for 6 weeks. Alternatively, the fragment can be sutured to the anterior horn of the medial or lateral meniscus over the front lip of the fragment. If the fragment is large enough, pins can be inserted retrograde through the proximal tibial epiphysis into the reduced tibial spine fragment. A second procedure to remove the pins after healing is usually required. Intra-articular fixation with 3.5-mm cannulated screws provides strong fragment fixation; however, care must be taken to remain intraepiphyseal, to avoid damage to the proximal tibial physis. Again, a second procedure is usually required to remove the screw.[32, 135, 231, 244, 252, 268, 287, 379, 392]

The overall prognosis is good to excellent if satisfactory reduction is achieved and maintained while healing.[32, 124, 135, 231, 244, 252, 268, 287, 379, 392] Most series have found residual laxity after open or closed treatment for all fracture types up to 6 mm greater than the unaffected side, and worse with higher fracture types, pedestrian-motor vehicle accident trauma, or associated ligament tears.[32] This increased laxity may be a result of greater spine height from increased local blood supply, functionally lengthening the ACL, or a result of associated injury to the ACL itself. Some suggest countersinking the fragment or partially plicating the ACL to precompensate for the observed increased laxity.[124] However, in fractures that are appropriately reduced, this increased laxity is rarely symptomatic or functionally limiting in most series. Another complication that is not uncommon after tibial spine fracture, even after anatomic reduction, is loss of extension. This is thought to be due to the local increase in blood supply during healing, which leads to spine enlargement, causing a mechanical block to extension. Notchplasty can be performed if the patient is near skeletal maturity, to regain extension.

Midsubstance Tears

Midsubstance ACL injury in skeletally immature patients has received increasing attention.[16, 18, 41, 116, 156, 171, 205, 207, 208, 222, 224, 242, 254, 274, 282, 331, 343, 369, 376, 381] Although the true incidence and prevalence of ACL injuries in the skeletally immature patient is unknown, these injuries appear to be increasingly common. This may be due to a combination of factors including increased participation in sports, increased competitive levels at younger ages, decreased level of conditioning, increased awareness of injuries in children and adolescents, and increased awareness of knee ligament injuries with arthroscopy and MRI.

In the child or adolescent with acute knee hemarthrosis, ACL injury is not uncommon. ACL injury has been reported in 26% to 65% of pediatric knees with acute hemarthroses in various series.[93, 182, 334, 356] ACL injuries in children and adolescents frequently have associated MCL or meniscal injuries. The preoperative clinical diagnosis often correlates poorly with arthroscopic findings of acute knee injuries in children, with agreement rates of 18% to 78.5% in the literature with most reports at approximately 50% agreement.[17, 37, 93, 132, 133, 141, 165, 247, 332, 344, 355, 356] Furthermore, MRI is particularly insensitive for partial ACL injuries.[184] Thus, a potential ACL injury should always be considered in the skeletally immature knee with an acute hemarthrosis.

The natural history of ACL injuries in the skeletally immature knee depends on the extent of injury. Unlike in adults, a large proportion of midsubstance tears in skeletally immature patients are partial ACL tears. Partial ACL injuries with intact secondary restraints appear to have a good prognosis. In a review of 35 young adults with arthroscopically proven partial ACL tears at an average follow-up of 41 months, Buckley et al found that 86% were minimally symptomatic and that 40% had returned to preinjury performance level after a program of protected early weightbearing, range-of-motion, and strengthening exercises.[51] Angel and Hall studied 27 children (average age, 14.5 years) with arthroscopically documented ACL injuries at a mean follow-up of 51 months after injury who were treated with physical therapy, no bracing, and no limitations. Twelve of 18 children with partial tears were satisfied with their outcome, whereas only 2 of 7 with complete tears were satisfied.[18] Others have also found poor results of complete ACL tears in children and adolescents. Graf and coworkers reported poor results at 15 months with new meniscal tears and episodes of instability in seven of eight skeletally immature patients who did not undergo ACL reconstruction or activity limitations.[116] Similarly, Mizuta et al found that in 18 skeletally immature patients followed up an average of 51 months after complete ACL tear, all had symptoms, only 1 had returned to preinjury sports level, 6 developed secondary meniscal tears, and radiographic changes were found in 11 patients.[242] Janarv and colleagues found that 16 of 23 skeletally immature patients treated with rehabilitation eventually needed reconstruction. The patients who did not require reconstruction were younger and less active.[156] McCarroll and colleagues found better results for surgical management of complete ACL injuries in prepubescent and junior high school patients. Of 16 prepubescent patients treated conservatively, 9 ceased sports participation, 4 sustained at least one reinjury, and only 3 were able to return to sports. Of 24 patients treated surgically, 22 returned to sports.[222] In a group of 73 junior high school athletes with midsubstance tears, every child treated nonoperatively reported instability, and 94% developed a meniscal tear. Ninety-two percent of patients treated surgically returned to sports.[224] Pressman and coworkers also found more stable and functional knees in children with a complete tear of the ACL who underwent reconstruction.[282]

We use nonoperative management for patients with partial ACL injuries and for prepubescent patients with complete tears. For patients with partial ligament injuries, physical therapy and activity modification are used. If laxity is increased, these authors recommend 12 weeks of protective bracing to assist in healing, then supplemental bracing during cutting sports for 2 years. Reconstruction is performed for those who fail nonoperative treatment. Prepubescent children with complete ACL tears are treated nonoperatively initially, provided there is not an associated meniscal tear requiring repair or multiple ligament injury. These children are treated with a rehabilitation program, protection with a customized brace, and activity modification until they are closer to skeletal maturity. Although the prognosis for successful nonoperative management alone may be limited in these young patients, many are protected until further skeletal maturity, thus allowing a more reliable surgical reconstruction. Patients who develop recurrent instability, giving way, or meniscal tears are then candidates for surgical reconstruction.

Surgical management of ACL tears in skeletally immature knees includes extra-articular reconstructions and intra-articular reconstructions that are nontransphyseal, partially transphyseal, or completely transphyseal.[331] As in adults, direct repair of the torn ACL is usually ineffective because of rapid inflammation and degeneration, along with ligament attenuation.[83, 331] Purely extra-articular reconstructions have also yielded unpredictable results in the adolescent knee.[77, 195, 254, 331]

Physeal sparing reconstructions are, in general, performed in prepubescents or Tanner stage 1 patients who have substantial growth remaining and have failed nonoperative management. We use a combined extra-articular and nontransphyseal intra-articular reconstruction using the iliotibial band (Fig. 66.16). A portion of the iliotibial band is taken as a graft with its insertion maintained distally. A "notchplasty" is performed that stays well below the distal femoral physis and creates a groove at the over-the-top position for the graft. A trough is created at the anterior-superior aspect of the proximal tibial epiphysis using a rasp. The graft courses from Gerdy's tubercle, proximally around the lateral femoral condyle, through the posterior capsule, around the over-the-top position, through the notch, and out the trough and is sutured to the periosteum in a metaphyseal trough medial to the tibial tubercle. The graft is also sutured proximally to the lateral intermuscular septum at the superior aspect of the lateral femoral condyle. By maintaining the iliotibial band insertion at Gerdy's tubercle and coursing it proximally around the lateral femoral condyle, an extra-articular reconstructive component is added to assist in anterolateral stability.[235b] Other nontransphyseal reconstruction techniques include using a portion of the patellar tendon, as described by DeLee and Bergfeld, or hamstrings tendons, as described by Brief, which are kept attached distally, passed over the anterior tibia and under the intermeniscal ligament, and fixed in the over-the-top position to the lateral femoral condyle metaphysis, avoiding the physis.[48, 84] The advantage of the nontransphyseal reconstructions is that they avoid the physis; however, the disadvantages are the lack of isometry and the tendency to elongate, thus providing partial stability. In Brief's series, eight of nine patients were satisfied, but all required bracing and some precautions.[48] Parker et al performed a similar procedure using hamstrings tendons in six skeletally immature patients, with the addition of a femoral metaphyseal groove to augment the over-the-top position and a direct repair of the ACL.[274] At follow-up averaging 32 months, four of five patients had returned to preinjury level of sports participation with excellent objective testing and no evidence of growth disturbance.

Partial transphyseal reconstructions are, in general, used in adolescents who have growth remaining (greater than 1 cm of growth or Tanner 2 stage) and who have instability or further injury after nonoperative management. Partial transphyseal techniques involve using hamstring or patellar tendon grafts brought in continuity through a drill hole in the central tibial physis and placed in the over-the-top femoral position or through the lateral distal femoral epiphysis. Lipscomb and Anderson used semitendinosis and gracilis tendon grafts fed through 0.25-in drill holes that crossed the center of the proximal tibial physis and then out the lateral femoral condylar epiphysis without crossing the distal physis. Supplementation was performed with Losee procedure using the iliotibial band. Results were good to excellent in 23 of the 24 children, age 12 to 15 years, after an average of 35 months. No growth abnormalities developed associated with drilling across the tibial physis.[205] Fowler also had excellent results, with full return to preoperative activities in 29 patients younger than 14 years who were reconstructed with hamstrings graft with intact distal insertion or quadriceps tendon graft placed through the central tibial physis and fixed in the over-the-top position. There were no angular deformities or leg-length discrepancies even in young children with more than 5 cm of expected growth remaining.[207, 208, 331] The lack of growth disturbance with soft-tissue grafting across open physes has been confirmed in animal models but is likely very dependent on the size of physeal violation.[129, 216, 327, 376] Andrews and colleagues used allograft tissue, 7-mm fascia lata or Achilles tendon grafts, through a tibial transphyseal tunnel and fixed in the over-the-top femoral position in eight patients ranging from age 10 to 15 years.[16] At an average 58-month follow-up, six patients had excellent results, one patient had a flexion contracture, and one graft reruptured 4 years postoperatively. Bisson et al reported two graft ruptures in nine skeletally immature patients treated with semitendinosis and gracilis tendon grafts through a tibial tunnel and fixed in the over-the-top position. There were no

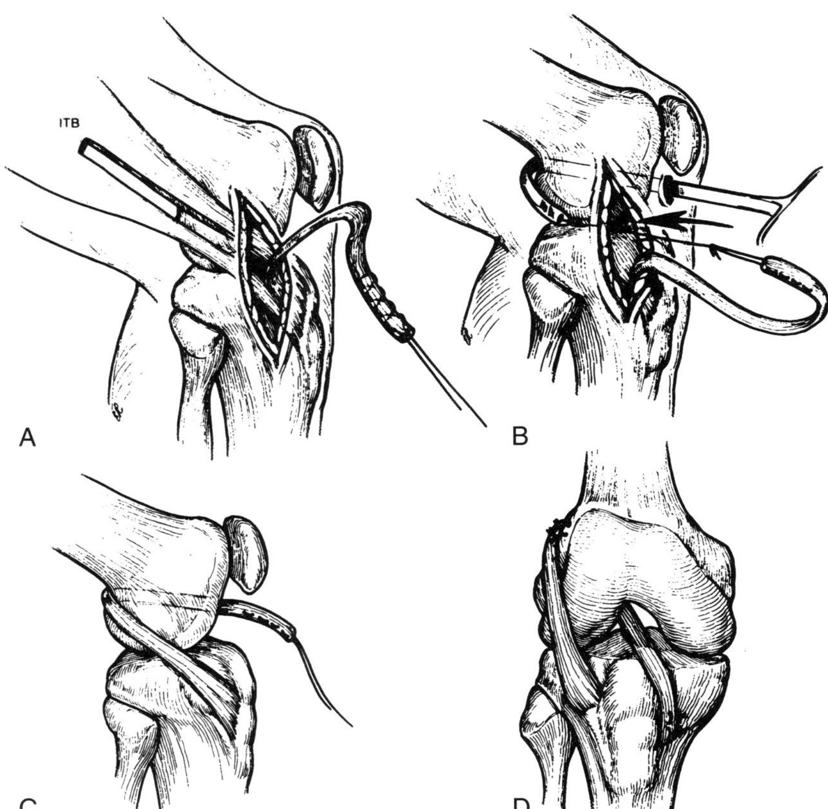

FIGURE 66.16 ➢ Combined extra-articular and nontransphyseal intra-articular ACL reconstruction. *A*, Harvesting of iliotibial band graft. *B*, Curved passer reaches through notch and around lateral femoral condyle to retrieve graft. *C*, Passage of graft around lateral condyle and over-the-top position, and through notchplasty. *D*, Graft sutured to periosteum medial to the tibial tubercle and sutured proximally at the superior aspect of the lateral femoral condyle.

growth disturbances, and the remaining seven patients had excellent results.[41]

Complete transphyseal reconstructions are, in general, used in older adolescents approaching skeletal maturity (less than 1 cm of growth remaining; bone age 13 years for males and 14 years for females, or Tanner stage 3) who have failed nonoperative management or who have a poor prognosis for successful nonoperative management given their activity level and the presence of a complete tear. Complete transphyseal techniques involve using a hamstrings or bone-patellar tendon-bone graft through standard tibial and femoral tunnels that violate the physis. McCarroll et al reported on 58 skeletally immature patients who were followed up at an average of 4.3 years after arthroscopically proven complete ACL tear.[224] The 20 more mature (Tanner 3) patients underwent initial ACL reconstruction, and the 38 less mature (Tanner 1 or 2) patients were managed nonoperatively. Twenty-seven of these 38 patients treated nonoperatively developed symptomatic meniscal tears, and all were eventually treated with ACL reconstruction when closer to skeletal maturity. ACL reconstruction was performed with patellar tendon grafts placed through femoral and tibial transphyseal tunnels. Ninety percent of patients returned to preinjury level of sports, and no growth disturbances were detected.

Posterior Cruciate Ligament Injury

Posterior cruciate ligment (PCL) injuries are much less common in children and adolescents. In the skeletally immature knee, PCL injuries involve avulsions from the femoral or tibial insertions, with femoral avulsion predominating.[106, 114, 152, 173, 221, 295, 300, 343, 351, 390] Isolated PCL injuries are extremely rare. Hyperextension appears to be the most common mechanism of injury clinically. In adult cadaver experiments, hyperextension consistently avulsed the tibial attachment of the PCL, whereas femoral avulsion was difficult to reproduce but occurred in the knee flexed 45 degrees with a posterior force applied to the tibia.[173] In the skeletally immature knee, however, the chondro-osseous junction of the femoral origin of the PCL may be the weakest link.

The PCL-deficient pediatric knee is often symptomatic with instability and variable amounts of pain. On examination, there may be posterior sag and increased posterior displacement with the posterior drawer test. External rotation through the knee should be examined in 30 degrees of flexion to rule out associated posterolateral corner injury. Concomitant injury to the MCL, lateral collateral ligament, posterolateral corner, ACL, meniscus (especially posterior horn injuries), and physis may occur with PCL injury. Radiographs may not demonstrate the avulsion if it is nondisplaced or primarily cartilaginous. Examination under anesthesia, stress radiographs, MRI, and arthroscopy have all been used to further evaluate the injury (Fig. 66.17).

Nonoperative management of nondisplaced fractures in a long-leg cast usually results in good functional results despite some persistent laxity.[106] However, for avulsion fractures with displacement or significant laxity, nonoperative management has yielded poorer results than has surgical repair.[114, 221, 300, 343, 351] In addition, results from early surgical repair seem to be

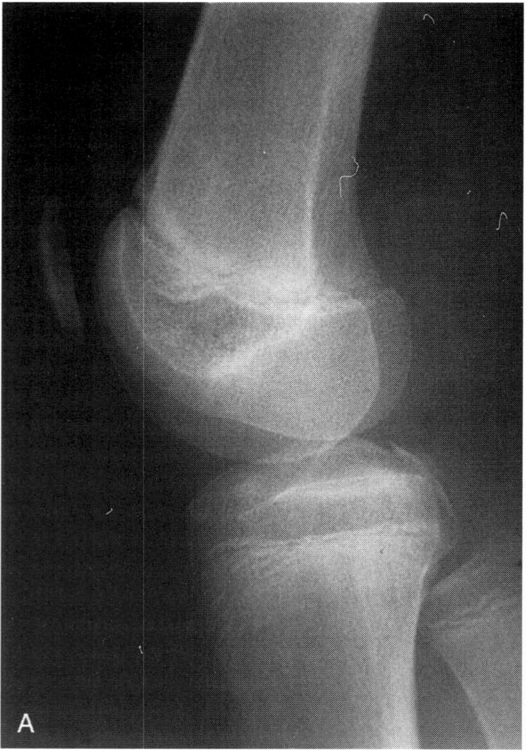

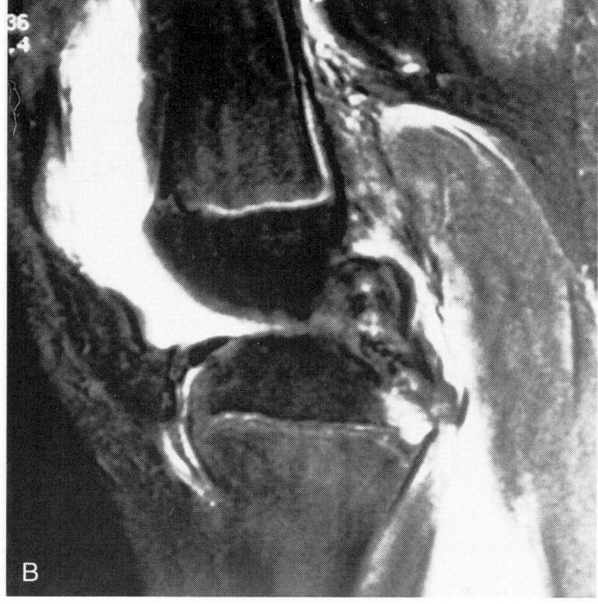

FIGURE 66.17 ➢ PCL avulsion. *A*, Lateral radiograph demonstrating avulsion of the tibial insertion of the PCL. *B*, Corresponding MRI view.

better than those from late repair.[114, 351] Direct repair of the avulsed fragment has been performed posteriorly by both open and arthroscopic techniques, avoiding the physis with fixation.

Medial Collateral Ligament Injury

The MCL originates distal to the distal femoral physis and inserts distal to the proximal tibial physis (see Fig. 66.5). Thus, distal femoral physeal fractures are more common and isolated MCL tears are unusual in children and early adolescents, although this injury has been reported in children as young as 4 years.[337] MCL injuries do occur more frequently, however, in the older adolescent approaching skeletal maturity and can occur in association with ACL midsubstance tears, tibial spine avulsion fractures, distal femoral Salter-Harris type III physeal fractures, PCL injuries, and meniscal tears.

The usual mechanism of MCL injury involves a valgus force to the knee. On examination, localization of the region of injury should be performed by eliciting tenderness over the femoral insertion, midsubstance, or tibial insertion. Laxity of the uninvolved MCL should be tested. Stress radiograms, examination under anesthesia, and MRI can be used to differentiate from distal femoral Salter-Harris I physeal injury. MRI or arthroscopy can be useful to further evaluate associated intra-articular injuries.

Nonoperative management of isolated MCL injuries has yielded good results, similar to those for adults.[148, 162, 243, 343] For grade I and II injuries, we use a short period of immobilization followed by use of a hinged brace and early range-of-motion exercises. For grade III injuries, we use a hinged brace locked at 20 to 30 degrees until acute symptoms subside, usually in 10 to 14 days. Range-of-motion exercise is then initiated followed by progressive strengthening, beginning with straight-leg raises. Bracing is continued for a total of 4 to 6 weeks. For grade III avulsions from the adductor tubercle, we use a long leg cast flexed to 60 degrees with 15 degrees of internal rotation for 4 to 6 weeks.

For grossly unstable midsubstance or distal grade III tears with stress roentgenograms showing more than 8 mm of opening than the normal stressed side, operative repair may be indicated because the ligament can become incarcerated in the joint. Some authors recommend open repair for combined MCL-Salter-Harris type III proximal tibia fractures or MCL-ACL injuries. Fixation of the ligament should be to the epiphysis and not to the physis or metaphysis to avoid physeal damage or compressive forces that may hinder growth. Midsubstance tears can be repaired directly with sutures.

Lateral Collateral Ligament Injury

Lateral collateral ligament injuries are rare in children. Diagnosis is by physical examination and roentgenographic stress tests to rule out the more common distal femoral physeal fracture. The sites of disruption are, in decreasing order, fibular head, femoral insertion, and midsubstance. A flake of bone from the lateral tibial plateau can be seen on films if there is an associated lateral capsular avulsion. Concomitant ACL injury, more common in adolescents than in younger children, is suggested by anterolateral instability.[174] MRI can be used to evaluate internal derangement such as ACL or meniscal tears that may require arthroscopic management. Surgical repair should be considered in adolescents with complete disruption and marked varus or posterolateral instability.

Knee Ligament Hypermobility Syndrome

Hypermobility can lead to joint pain and swelling, primarily during childhood and adolescence. Symptoms usually accompany activity and resolve with rest. Carter and Wilkinson proposed five tests (see Table 66.2) to aid in the detection of hypermobility; a joint is considered hypermobile if at least three of the five maneuvers listed can be performed.[52] Joint laxity is age dependent but is usually similar for boys and girls. Almost 50% of toddlers and preschoolers are hypermobile by the aforementioned criteria, falling to 5% by age 6 years and remaining constant until early adulthood.[52] Similarly, instrumented measures of knee laxity usually demonstrate increased laxity in childhood that decreases in adolescence and is similar for boys and girls. In most children, hypermobility is idiopathic, and probably represents one end in a spectrum of physiological characteristics, like intoeing. However, joint hyperlaxity can be partly inherited as an autosomal dominant trait or may be part of connective tissue abnormalities seen in Down, Marfan's, and Ehlers-Danlos syndromes.

Except for patellofemoral instability, children with hypermobility are not predisposed to ligament injury any more than is the general population.[336] Treatment consists primarily of muscle strengthening for joint stability with orthotic use, such as foot orthotics for hyperpronation or patella-stabilizing knee sleeves for patellar instability. Surgical procedures may be necessary for recurrent patellar dislocation.

CONGENITAL KNEE DISLOCATION

Congenital knee dislocation is a very rare (1.7 per 100,000 births) congenital deformity characterized by varying degrees of hyperextension and recurvatum of the knees. It may occur as an isolated disorder or in association with dislocated hips, clubfoot, myelodysplasia, Larsen's syndrome, or arthrogryposis.[6, 23, 36, 68, 75, 98, 101, 102, 121, 126, 143, 153, 154, 160, 201, 212, 250, 258, 275, 292, 298, 310, 315]

Patients often have a history of breech presentation. It is important to examine the entire child to rule out associated abnormalities. About half of patients with congenital knee subluxation-dislocation have associated hip dislocation, and about 10% have elbow dislocation. Foot deformities, such as clubfoot or calcaneus foot, occur in approximately one third of patients. The patient may have features suggestive of a syndrome such as Down, Ehlers-Danlos, arthrogryposis multiplex congenita, or Larsen's syndrome. Other associated anomalies include imperforate anus, cryptorchidism, spina bifida, hydrocephalus, cleft palate, facial paralysis, and camptodactyly.

Leveuf and Pais classified three grades of knee dislocation, which represent a spectrum of severity of involvement (Fig. 66.18).[201] In grade I, there is recurvatum but minimal anterior translation of the tibia. The knee can be passively flexed beyond neutral to 45 to 60 degrees but bounces back to 10 to 20 degrees of hyperextension. In grade II, there is anterior subluxation of the tibia. The knee can be passively flexed only to neutral and is postured in 20 to 40 degrees of hyperextension. In grade III, there is complete anterior dislocation of the tibia with limited flexion.

Physical examination findings vary with the grade of involvement. The femoral condyles may be prominent posteriorly, and there may be a transverse crease in the front of the knee. Flexion is limited to varying extents with a tendency to bounce back into hyperextension after passive flexion. The hyperextension deformity is associated with varying degrees of genu valgum and iliotibial band contracture. In more severe cases, the hamstrings, particularly the medial hamstrings, are displaced anteriorly, acting as knee extensors. The quadriceps is contracted, and the patellar tendon is shortened to a varying degree. The patella may be hypoplastic, and the cruciate ligaments may be absent. In severe cases, there is abundant fibrous tissue proliferation and adhesions in the suprapatellar pouch that tether the extensor mechanism.[6, 23, 36, 68, 75, 98, 101, 102, 121, 126, 143, 153, 154, 160, 201, 212, 250, 258, 275, 292, 298, 310, 315]

AP and true lateral radiographs are taken for evaluation. In infants, the ossification centers of the distal femur and proximal tibia may be delayed. Normally, the distal femoral secondary center of ossification is present at birth. Determining the articular relationship and differentiating between varying degrees of hyperextension (type I), subluxation (type II), and dislocation (type III) can be difficult on radiography given the inability to image the cartilaginous epiphyses and articular surfaces. Ultrasound has proven useful in depicting the cartilaginous relationship of the distal femur and proximal tibia in infants.[275] In addition to assessing the articular relationship, MRI can provide additional information about the menisci, the cruciate ligaments, the suprapatellar pouch, and the extensor mechanism. MRI in this age group, however, requires sedation.

Management depends on the severity of deformity. In general, the knee should be treated before the hip in limbs containing both problems. Grade I knees are managed by serial splinting of the knee into progressive flexion following gentle passive manipulation. Once 90 degrees of knee flexion can be obtained, usually after approximately 6 weeks of serial casting, a Pavlik harness can be used for dynamic retention of knee flexion, or a bivalve cast can be used at night with stretching during the day. Grade II knees are managed by serial cast application followed by dynamic splinting. Ultrasound can be used to confirm reduction. Resistant extension contracture or failure of reduction is treated with quadriceps lengthening. Alternatively, traction has been used. Grade III knees require major open reduction, usually between 3 and 6 months of age. Procedures vary but involve quadriceps release and lengthening, transverse anterior capsular release, and hamstring tendon relocation for stabilization. Postoperatively, a cast is worn for 3 weeks, followed by bivalved night casting with manipulation during the day.[6, 23, 36, 68, 75, 98, 101, 102, 121, 126, 143, 153, 154, 160, 201, 212, 250, 258, 275, 292, 298, 310, 315]

FLEXION AND EXTENSION CONTRACTURES

Flexion Contracture

Knee flexion contractures of up to 20 degrees can be normal in healthy newborns and resolve during the first 6 months of life.[33] Pathological flexion contractures can occur in association with multiple disorders including congenital patellar dislocations, poliomyelitis, JRA, myelodysplasia, arthrogryposis multiplex congen-

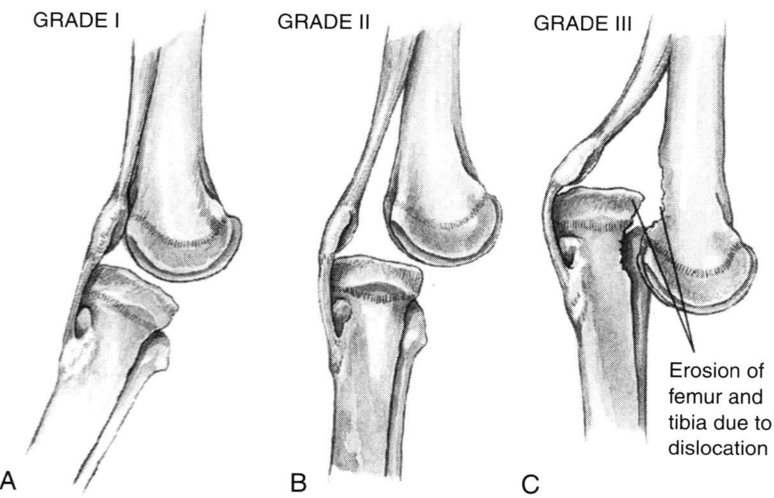

FIGURE 66.18 ➢ Congenital knee dislocation. *A,* Grade I—Minimal anterior translation of the tibia, knee hyperextension usually between 10 and 20 degrees, and passive knee flexion beyond neutral to 45 to 60 degrees of flexion. *B,* Grade II—Anterior subluxation of the tibia, knee hyperextension of 20 to 40 degrees, and passive knee flexion to neutral. *C,* Complete anterior dislocation of the tibia. (From Tachdjian MO: Clinical Pediatric Orthopedics: The Art of Diagnosis and Principles of Management. Stamford, Appleton & Lange, 1997.)

ita, pterygium syndromes, multiple hereditary exostoses, hemarthrosis (bleeding disorders), inflammatory lesions of the synovium (JRA, pigmented villonodular synovitis), internal derangement of the knee, spasticity related to cerebral palsy, spinal cord tumor, or tethered cord.[127, 143, 273, 302] In cerebral palsy, the flexion contracture may be due to muscle imbalance involving tight hamstrings, ankle equinous, or a hip flexion contracture, because the knee must be flexed to hold the body's center of gravity directly over its base.[39] In children with myelomeningocele, the cause may be spastic hamstring or gastrocnemius muscles or simply lack of motion aggravated by early wheelchair use.[2, 385]

With severe contractures, the tibia is posteriorly subluxated. With long-standing deformities, the posterior aspect of the femoral condyles becomes flattened and the tibia develops a forward slope, making maintenance of joint congruity difficult. Mild bony abnormalities are not believed to be a significant etiological factor in flexion deformities and are more likely a result of the altered weightbearing statics. In children with high spinal lesions, flexion contractures can be prevented by early splinting and physical therapy. In children with spasticity, such as cerebral palsy patients, night splinting may be of some benefit.[15]

The advantages of correction can be obtained only if the patient has potential and desire to walk with crutches, sufficient intelligence, and no significant upper extremity weakness or spasticity. Spinal segmental function to L3 is prerequisite for functional ambulation in most cases.[2, 385] If these conditions are not met, the flexion deformity may be left uncorrected unless it interferes with sitting or hygiene. In correcting flexion deformities, one must produce a stable joint so that it can bear weight. Usually correction to less than 20 degrees is required. If the tibia is posteriorly subluxated, it must be reduced during correction. Concomitant hip flexion contractures of greater than 30 degrees should generally be corrected before the knee deformity. However, if the knee contracture is greater than 45 degrees and worse than the hip contracture, then the knee should be treated first.

Deformities of up to 15 degrees can usually be corrected by physical therapy or serial casting. If there is no sensation, as in myelomeningocele, correction by casting and traction are hazardous and surgical correction is recommended.[2, 385] There are four basic procedures available; the first two will work only if quadriceps strength is at least grade 3 out of 5: (1) hamstring tendon division or elongation; (2) hamstring tendon transplantation to the distal femur; (3) if the quadriceps is paralyzed as confirmed by electrical stimulation, transplantation of the hamstring tendon to the patella; and (4) supracondylar femoral osteotomy.

Recommended surgical treatment for most flexion contractures of 15 to 30 degrees is posterior capsulotomy and flexor release. The procedure involves dissection of all tendons crossing the popliteal fossa including the hamstrings and gastrocnemius. The PCL is divided if full extension is still not attainable. After the releases, the knee should not be straightened immediately because of the risk to contracted neurovascular structures. Gradual straightening must be developed over a 6- to 12-week period using traction, serial casting, or both. If a flexion deformity recurs after one correction, hamstring tendon transfer to the distal femur or patella (if the quadriceps is paralyzed) should be considered. Supracondylar femoral osteotomies are usually reserved for patients older than 16 years with contractures of more than 30 to 45 degrees, or after failed flexor release. Osteotomy is usually successful but only if combined with transplantation of the hamstring tendon to the femur or patella.

Extension Contracture

The most common cause of extension contractures in children is infantile quadriceps fibrosis as a result of multiple intramuscular injections in the thigh.[309] Other causes include myelomeningocele, Larsen's syndrome, arthrogryposis multiplex congenita, poliomyelitis, and congenital recurrent patellar dislocation.[19, 39, 298, 302, 323] Extension contractures can also occur after distal femur fractures as a result of fibrous hematoma and ischemia in the overlying quadriceps. Patella alta commonly accompanies extension contractures.

Knees that do not bend may aid in walking initially, but as the child grows it becomes increasingly difficult to sit, use a wheelchair, and get in and out of a car. Flexion to at least 90 degrees is necessary to reduce the lever arm to prevent fractures and to allow the child to sit comfortably. In some societies, further flexion is necessary to allow kneeling.

In myelomeningocele, children with a lesion below L3 will likely be able to ambulate with assistance. In children with lesions above L3 with muscle imbalance or flail limbs, the goal is to allow comfortable sitting. Serial casting is frequently effective in arthrogryposis multiplex congenita and other causes of extension contractures and should be attempted before surgery. Extension contractures caused by myelomeningocele, however, do not usually respond to nonoperative therapy.[19, 39]

In children with infantile quadriceps fibrosis, physical therapy is usually unsuccessful, so surgical therapy should be performed early. Open quadricepsplasty usually involves V-Y advancement of the central slip of quadriceps tendon, release of the iliotibial band, and transverse division of the anterior joint capsule.[75] The knee is then immobilized in 45 degrees of flexion, which is eventually increased to 90 degrees. Percutaneous quadriceps resection has been shown to be just as effective as open procedures, making it the preferred initial technique in many cases.[298] Stab incisions are made at the superior border of the patella to release the medial and lateral quadriceps and retinaculum. Children who previously had good quadriceps function are able to maintain active extension. A proximal approach has also been developed to avoid the complications of V-Y plasty such as extension lag, hemarthrosis, and conspicuous scarring.[309] The basis of the procedure is that the fibrous area involves usually the vastus lateralis and frequently the vastus intermedius. A vertical incision is made over the greater trochanter, and the vastus lateralis origin is exposed and detached from the trochanteric line and the lateral intermuscular septum. As the lateralis retracts, the intermedius is exposed and likewise released. The patient is then splinted in maximum flexion for 3 to 4 weeks. In neglected cases of extension contracture, condylar flattening can develop, making attainment of full flexion impossible with soft-tissue procedures alone. Supracondylar flexion femoral osteotomy can restore useful flexion in these instances.

ANGULATORY DEFORMITIES

Genu varum and genu valgum in children are most commonly physiological. Normally, children are in approximately 15 degrees of varus angulation at birth, which resolves to neutral by age 18 months, develops to 10 degrees of valgus angulation by ages 3 to 6 years, and finally plateaus to 5 to 6 degrees of valgus angulation by age 7 years.[176, 180, 181, 270, 313]

The differential diagnosis of genu varum (Table 66.5) includes physiological genu varum, tibia vara (proximal metaphyseal beaking), rickets (low serum phosphorus), post-traumatic deformities (history of trauma), metaphyseal chondroplasia or other skeletal dysplasias (short stature with multiple metaphyseal deformities), and postinfectious deformities. Pathological genu varum is most commonly a result of tibia vara, also referred to as Blount's disease. Pathological genu valgum (Table 66.6) should be suspected if the valgus angulation is severe (greater than 4 in between the medial malleoli) or asymmetric or if the child has a history of trauma or infection or has associated dysplastic features (e.g., scoliosis, short stature). The most common cause of pathological genu valgum is fracture, resulting in distal femoral or proximal tibial physeal stimulation or arrest. Less common causes include JRA, poliomyelitis, fluorosis, long periods of immobilization, chronic infections, storage diseases, rickets, and various dysplasias. Genu valgum can be accentuated by anteversion, internal rotation of the femur, external tibial torsion, obesity, and ligamentous laxity.[72, 209, 255, 269, 284, 349]

For physiological angulatory deformities, no treatment is necessary. For pathological deformities, the indications for surgery are pain and significant functional or cosmetic deformity. Prophylactic treatment for angulation of more than 10 degrees may be necessary to prevent articular overload and future degenerative arthritis. Treatment of post-traumatic angulatory deformities and tibia vara will be discussed separately. Surgical options include osteotomies and partial epiphyseodeses. Osteotomies can be performed with external fixation (Ilizarov, Orthofix) or with internal fixation. Opening wedge osteotomies provide length, whereas closing wedge osteotomies shorten. Osteotomies provide maximum correction when closest to the deformity; however, in children with significant growth remaining, periarticular osteotomies are precluded by the physis.[183] Partial epiphyseodesis will correct angular deformities depending on the amount of growth remaining.[45] Partial epiphyseodesis can be performed with percutaneous drilling, Phemister technique's or with staples. Resection of bony bridges may be performed for patients with partial arrests and significant remaining growth.[169]

TABLE 66.5 CAUSES OF GENU VARUM

Apparent genu varum
Physiological genu varum
Congenital familial tibia vara
Tibia vara (Blount's disease)
Asymmetric growth arrest of medial distal femur or proximal tibia because of infection, fracture, or tumor
Rickets
Skeletal dysplasia (achondroplasia, metaphyseal dysplasia)
Congenital longitudinal deficiency of the tibia with relative fibular overgrowth
Lead or fluoride intoxication

TABLE 66.6 CAUSES OF GENU VALGUM

1. Physiological genu valgum
2. Post-traumatic overgrowth
3. Longitudinal deficiency of the fibula
4. Iliotibial band contracture
5. Asymmetric growth arrest of lateral distal femoral or proximal tibial physis because of infection, fracture, or tumor
6. Arthritis
7. Skeletal dysplasia (Morquio's syndrome, Ollier's disease, hereditary multiple osteocartilaginous exostoses, multiple epiphyseal dysplasia)
8. Osteogenesis imperfecta
9. Metabolic bone disease or renal osteodystrophy

Post-Traumatic Deformities

Post-traumatic angulatory deformities about the knee are usually valgus deformities. Valgus deviation occurs in 1% of fractures of the proximal tibial metaphysis in children, most commonly in those younger than 5 years. Roentgenograms may show oblique Harris' growth arrest lines indicating asymmetric physeal closure. An average tibial overgrowth of 1 cm often accompanies post-traumatic valgus deformities. The growth is thought to be a result of stimulation and increased activity of the medial physis. It can also occur from lateral physeal arrest.

Post-traumatic valgus deformity progresses during fracture healing for up to 18 months with an average time to maximal deformity of 12 months. Gradual resolution then usually occurs with complete correction in most cases by 28 to 52 months. The amount of correction is greater in the child with more growth remaining.[24, 26, 90, 317, 393]

Immediate treatment is usually not necessary for post-traumatic genu valgum owing to the high frequency of spontaneous resolution. Parents should be reassured and the child should be followed up. If spontaneous improvement is insufficient by early adolescence or if functional problems result, surgical treatment may be necessary. Correction can be accomplished by osteotomy or partial epiphyseodesis. Resection of a physeal bridge may be indicated if there is a peripheral arrest with significant growth remaining.

Tibia Vara (Blount's Disease)

Three forms of tibia vara, or Blount's disease, have been described (Table 66.7). The infantile form is the most common, with an onset at age 1 to 3 years; the juvenile form has an onset at age 4 to 10 years, and the adolescent form has an onset at age 11 years or older. The differences in the three groups include age of onset, amount of remaining growth, and magnitude of medial compressive forces. Therefore, the infantile form has potential for the greatest deformity and the adolescent type for the least. Some authors group the juvenile and adolescent forms together into the "late-onset" type because of their similar roentgenographic features, which differ from those of the infantile group. Langenskiöld radiographically classified the progressive stages of tibia vara with age (Fig. 66.19).[47, 71, 97, 100, 137, 161, 193, 209, 219, 267, 283, 306, 349, 375]

Familial cases have been reported for both the infantile and the late-onset varieties. Both forms occur three times more frequently in males, and most of the children are obese. In the infantile and juvenile forms, bilaterality is seen in 50% to 80% of cases, whereas bilaterality is seen in only 20% of the adolescent form. In the infantile variety, the chief complaint is the deformity, whereas in the late-onset type, the complaint is pain with activity or long-term standing. The pathogenesis of tibia vara involves growth retardation of the posteromedial aspect of the proximal tibial physis and epiphysis because of abnormal weightbearing stress and medial compressive forces on varus knees.[71, 375] Weightbearing and walking are requisites for the development of tibia vara. The predisposed child is an obese African-American child with significant physiological tibia vara who walked at an early age and stretched his lateral knee ligaments. Asymmetric pressure and repetitive microtrauma result medially, causing chondrocyte injury and matrix necrosis of the posteromedial physis. Medial growth is suppressed, and ultimately an osseous bridge forms, producing a permanent and progressive varus deformity.

TABLE 66.7 INFANTILE VERSUS LATE-ONSET BLOUNT'S DISEASE

Characteristic	Infantile	Late-Onset
Race	Black	Black
Sex	Male	Male
Weight	Obese	Obese
Bilaterality	75%	20% (adolescent), 50% (juvenile)
Varus angulation	24 degrees	15 degrees
Palpable medial metaphyseal beak	Prominent	Absent
Internal tibial torsion	Present	Mild
Leg-length discrepancy	Present	Mild
X-ray medial metaphyseal beak	Marked	Mild
Chief complaint	Deformity	Pain
Progression	Marked	Mild

Infantile Tibia Vara

Signs of tibia vara should be looked for in toddlers with genu varum after age 24 months. Signs include asymmetric bowing, progressive deformity, or lack of spontaneous resolution. The disorder progresses most rapidly between 3 and 6 years of age. Affected children may have an apparent lateral thrust to the knee during the stance phase caused by varus instability. A prominent medial tibial metaphyseal beak is palpable. Children with infantile tibia vara may display the following roentgenographic features: sharp varus angulation of the metaphysis, a widened and irregular physeal line medially, a medially sloped and irregularly ossified epiphysis, and prominent beaking and fragmentation of the medial tibial metaphysis. Roentgenographic changes have not been reported before age 18 months and are rare before age 2 years. The diagnosis is made by a metaphyseal-diaphyseal angle of greater than 11 degrees after age 2 years.[97]

Treatment should begin as soon as the diagnosis is confirmed because earlier treatment has a better prognosis.[137, 306] There is little indication for simply observing roentgenographically confirmed infantile tibia vara. In children diagnosed before age 3 years, a full hip-knee-ankle-foot orthosis should be worn at least 23 hours per day. Valgus correction should be increased every 2 months until roentgenograms demonstrate absolute valgus alignment. The child is then weaned off the orthosis over several months. Resolution of the metaphyseal beak lesion should begin before discontinuing the brace completely. Bracing is successful in at least 50% of cases. If bracing is not successful after 1 year, corrective osteotomy should be performed. If the diagnosis is made after age 3 years, corrective proximal tibial metaphyseal osteotomy is recommended to correct to 5 degrees of valgus angulation while the child is supine on the operating table. If the medial physis is too disrupted with a partial arrest, resection of the bar may be indicated if there is greater than 2 years of growth remaining. Osteotomy may be required and may need to be repeated with growth and recurrent deformity.[100]

Late-Onset Tibia Vara

The late-onset form has a more ossified proximal medial tibial epiphysis that is less vulnerable to deformity and is more slowly progressive. Frequently in adolescent tibia vara, there is precedent mild trauma or repetitive stress. The deformity can range from 5 to 45 degrees in the juvenile form and from 10 to 20 degrees in the adolescent form. The proximal medial tibial metaphyseal beak is only slightly palpable, in contrast to the more prominent beak of the infantile group.

Late-onset tibia vara requires surgery if there is significant functional impairment or pain, or if sufficient

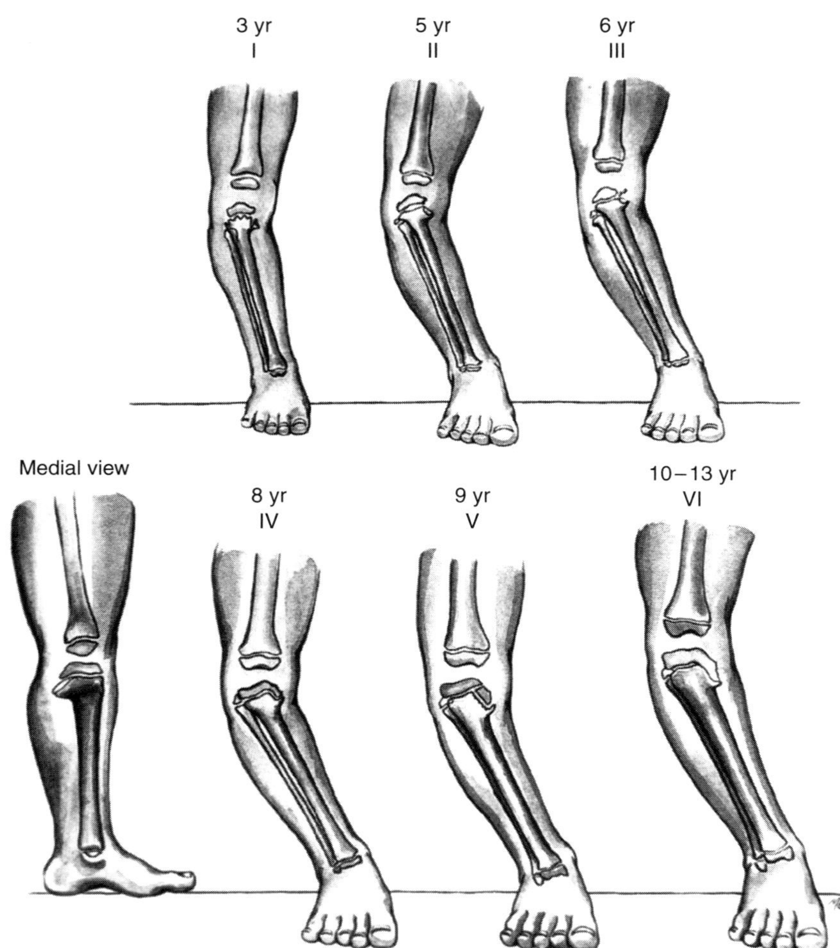

FIGURE 66.19 ➢ Langenskiöld's classification of progressive stages of Blount's disease. (From Tachdjian MO: Clinical Pediatric Orthopedics: The Art of Diagnosis and Principles of Management. Stamford, Appleton & Lange, 1997.)

deformity is present to predispose to degenerative arthritis. Physeal bony bar resection and proximal tibial metaphyseal valgus osteotomies should be performed to correct to at least neutral. Osteotomies can be stabilized with internal or external fixation. Epiphyseodesis of the lateral tibia and fibula is another option in children older than 9 years and before skeletal maturity.

Juvenile-onset-type tibia vara has the worst prognosis, with 25% to 50% recurrence of deformity after surgical correction. If deformity recurs, indicating significant physeal damage, physeal bridge resection with placement of an interposition graft may be necessary.[47, 71, 97, 100, 137, 161, 193, 209, 219, 267, 283, 306, 349, 375]

TABLE 66.8 NEOPLASMS ABOUT THE KNEE

Lesion	Number
Benign bone	101
Osteochondroma	27
Nonossifying fibroma	23
Chondroblastoma	11
Osteoid osteoma	9
Malignant bone	59
Osteosarcoma	48
Ewing's sarcoma	8
Benign soft tissue	18
Desmoid	4
Lipoma	3
Malignant soft tissue	13
Synovial sarcoma	5
Neurofibrosarcoma	5
Other	8

NEOPLASMS ABOUT THE KNEE

Bone tumors in children often arise from the metaphyses of the proximal tibia or distal femur and result in knee pain. Gebhardt and colleagues reviewed 199 tumors about the knee in children age 1 to 18 years; the diagnoses are shown in Table 66.8.[110]

Tumors about the knee usually present with pain. There may be symptoms mimicking intra-articular derangements. Night pain or systemic symptoms may be present. Family history and history of fever, chills, weight loss, chronicity of symptoms, and relief of pain with medicines should be sought. Laboratory analysis should include erythrocyte sedimentation rate, complete blood count (infection, leukemia), and calcium and phosphorus (metabolic bone disease) and alkaline phosphatase (higher in osteosarcoma, lymphoma, or Ewing's sarcoma) levels. Radiographs of the involved region should be obtained. If malignancy is suspected, the appropriate staging workup should be instituted including chest film, bone scan, CT, and MRI.

After staging and a preliminary diagnosis, an incisional biopsy using the most direct route with a longitudinal incision is the procedure of choice. The biopsy incision should take into account the potential resection margins and, in general, should be performed by the individual who will be performing the resection and reconstruction. Samples should always be sent for both pathology and microbiology.

Osteochondroma

Osteochondroma, or benign solitary osteocartilaginous exostosis, is probably the most common tumor about the knee. The lesion can appear at any age, usually before age 20 years, and enlarges especially during the adolescent growth spurt into the third decade. It is usually an asymptomatic incidental finding. Roentgenograms show a sessile or pedunculated outgrowth from the distal femoral or proximal tibial metaphyseal cortex, usually projecting away from the joint. The marrow of the outgrowth communicates with that of the bone, distinguishing it from periosteal osteosarcoma. The lesion is topped by a cartilaginous cap. Removal is not necessary unless it becomes symptomatic by nerve irritation, bursitis, or pressure. Malignant degeneration is extraordinarily rare.[110, 279, 326]

Fibrous Cortical Defect and Nonossifying Fibroma

Fibrous cortical defect (FCD) and nonossifying fibroma (NOF) are extremely common and have the same histological features, differing only in location. FCD refers to the lesion when confined to the cortex, whereas NOF involves the medullary canal. Both are most common in the metaphyses of long bones and are most frequent about the knee. These lesions are often incidental findings and are probably not neoplasms but represent defects in the growth plate, or fibrous periosteum, or represent local disturbances of ossification. Both are self-limiting and frequently disappear near skeletal maturity. On rare occasion, pathological fracture can occur through an NOF lesion in a load-bearing region.[110, 113, 326]

Roentgenograms show well-demarcated, round, or oval metaphyseal lytic, usually septated, lesions with a sclerotic border. The lesions are frequently multiple and symmetric. No treatment is necessary unless the lesion is greater than 50% of the diameter of the bone, rendering it susceptible to pathological fractures. Treatment is then curettage and bone graft.

Chondroblastoma

Chondroblastoma is a benign epiphyseal tumor in the skeletally immature patient. The patient will have constant, inflammatory-type pain. Roentgenograms show a round-to-oval lytic lesion with punctate calcifications confined to the epiphysis. Treatment is curettage and bone graft. Local recurrence is seen.[110, 326]

Osteoid Osteoma

Osteoid osteoma is a benign osteoblastic lesion that can occur in the distal femoral epiphysis, intra-articularly, or at Gerdy's tubercle. Signs and symptoms include a sharp, gnawing pain relieved by aspirin, local tenderness, effusion, and leg-length inequality. Osteoid osteoma of the hip commonly presents as knee pain. Roentgenograms show a lucent nidus less than 1 cm in diameter surrounded by bony sclerosis in the cortex, periosteum, or medullary cavity. Treatment is excision of the nidus.[110, 235, 326, 350]

Osteosarcoma

Fifty percent of all osteosarcomas occur about the knee because of the rapid growth at the distal femur and proximal tibia. Osteosarcoma often presents as the spontaneous onset of pain or pain after minor trauma that does not go away. The pain becomes severe and constant and is worse at night. A mass may be palpable. Roentgenograms may show a poorly marginated, infiltrative lytic lesion with a soft-tissue mass. MRI evaluates the extent of the lesion. Chest CT should be performed to rule out metastases. Treatment consists of adjuvant chemotherapy, wide resection, and limb salvage when possible using allograft tissue or prosthetic reconstruction. Another reconstructive option is rotationplasty.[58, 115, 187, 188]

Popliteal Cyst

The popliteal cyst is the most common soft-tissue lesion about the knee in children. It is twice as common in males as in females and can be found in children age 2 to 14 years. The incidence decreases after age 9 years. It is usually asymptomatic and of insidious onset. The cysts are often noted by parents and may enlarge or diminish. The common site is medial, originating in the gastrocnemius-semimembranosis bursa immediately distal to the popliteal crease. Unlike those in adults, popliteal cysts in children rarely communicate with the knee joint and are not usually related to intra-articular lesions.

The cyst is best observed with the child prone and the knee extended. It is smooth and firm and occurs under or adjacent to the medial head of the gastrocnemius. No treatment is required if the lesion is asymptomatic and no intra-articular lesion is present. If left untreated, the majority will disappear spontaneously after 1 to 2 years. Aspiration and cortisone injection are usually unsuccessful and not recommended. If surgical excision is performed, a high recurrence rate of up to 40% is seen. Surgery should be restricted to those whose disability restricts activity.[89, 110, 326]

KNEE INFECTIONS

Septic Arthritis

In neonates (younger than 6 months), the most common joint affected by sepsis is the hip, followed by the shoulder and then the knee. Some authors believe males are more susceptible to septic arthritis, with as much as a threefold higher incidence. Forty-one percent of neonates have concurrent infections elsewhere, the most common being *Escherichia coli* gastroenteritis. In the neonate, the most consistent sign is reduced movement of the affected limb. Less consistent findings are lethargy, irritability, and failure to gain weight. Fever is often present, and erythrocyte sedimentation rate and white blood cell count are usually elevated but can be normal. Roentgenograms show evidence of bone and joint infection only when it is well established. The diagnosis is established by aspiration and culture of joint fluid with an elevated joint white blood cell count. Common organisms in this age group include *Staphylococcus aureus, E. coli,* and group B streptococci. *Haemophilus influenzae* is being seen with less frequency since vaccination has become routine. Treatment is aspiration or arthroscopic irrigation and intravenous antibiotics followed by oral antibiotics based on the sensitivity of the culture.

Older children with septic knees are generally febrile and acutely ill and usually present with pain, swelling, decreased range of motion, and refusal to bear weight. The pathogenesis is usually hematogenous spread to the synovium from another source, or from direct innoculation via a penetrating wound. The child may have an antecedent or concomitant infection such as otitis media or an upper respiratory infection. Pyogenic arthritis may also arise from adjacent osteomyelitis. The most common organisms in this age group are *S. aureus,* followed by group A streptococci and *H. influenzae.* The child usually has a fever and a high white blood cell count and erythrocyte sedimentation rate, but both can be normal. Roentgenograms may show osteopenia as a result of adjacent inflammation in long-standing cases. Bone scan or MRI may be helpful to evaluate osteomyelitis. The diagnosis is established by a joint aspirate, which should be sent for culture and sensitivity, and by white blood cell count. Blood cultures should be obtained because up to 50% of cases have negative joint fluid cultures. Arthroscopic drainage and irrigation should be performed, followed by a course of intravenous antibiotics, which are switched to oral antibiotics after a variable time period. Loculations should be débrided and drains left in for 2 to 3 days. Motion is encouraged. Multiple needle aspirations for treatment of septic arthritis of the knee have been used but may not remove all loculations and debris. Arthroscopic treatment has been shown to be as effective as open arthrotomy but with much lower morbidity. Patients should be closely followed for sequelae of growth arrest, leg-length discrepancy, angular deformity, and osteonecrosis.[59, 144, 158, 266, 277, 318, 341, 348, 363]

Osteomyelitis

Osteomyelitis of the distal femur and proximal tibia is not uncommon given the large amount of growth in this region. The principle etiology involves hematogenous spread, which occurs as a result of bacterial translocation from the low-flow capillary loops of the juxtaphyseal metaphysis. Patients often present with pain, fever, and limp or inability to walk. Erythrocyte sedimentation rate and white blood cell counts are usually elevated. Radiographic changes depend on the chronicity of the process and may initially show periosteal elevation with subtle lucency to an involucrum and sequestrum in late stages. Bone scan or MRI can be used to further delineate the location and extent of the involved process. Aspiration at the area of maximal bony tenderness is essential in obtaining cultures to guide treatment and to rule out abscess. Treatment consists of a course of intravenous antibiotics followed by oral antibiotics. Surgical débridement may be necessary for an abscess or for failure to improve clinically with antibiotics. Sequelae include deformity, leg-length discrepancy, septic arthritis, physeal arrest, osteonecrosis, and establishment of chronic osteomyelitis.[192]

Lyme Arthritis

Lyme disease is caused by the spirochete *Borrelia burgdorferi,* which is carried by the deer tick. Lyme arthritis should be considered in any child with brief, intermittent attacks of joint pain and swelling and a history of a rash or fever with possible exposure to the carrier.

The presenting complaint is pain and swelling, usually in the knee. There may be a history of a circular erythematous migratory rash, headaches, and malaise. On examination, there is diffuse swelling of the knee joint with warmth. There may be associated neurological or cardiac abnormalities. The diagnosis is made by demonstration of elevated titers of immunoglobulin (Ig) M and IgG antibodies against the spirochete. Treatment consists of antibiotics such as penicillin or tetracycline.[80, 335, 380]

JUVENILE RHEUMATOID ARTHRITIS

JRA most commonly involves the knee, followed by the ankle and the elbow. Symptoms often begin at an early age and involve swelling, warmth, pain, decreased range of motion, and impaired ambulation. JRA is often a diagnosis of exclusion, whose diagnostic criteria are listed in Table 66.9. Multiple joints may be involved (polyarticular = 5 or more, pauciarticular = 4 or less). Rheumatoid factor may be positive, and the erythrocyte sedimentation rate and white blood cell count are usually elevated. Aspiration of the knee yields nonpurulent fluid with an elevated white blood cell count.[139, 172, 307]

Children with the polyarticular form seem to have a poorer prognosis with respect to destructive and reactive changes and development of rheumatoid arthri-

TABLE 66.9 DIAGNOSTIC CRITERIA FOR CLASSIFICATION OF JUVENILE RHEUMATOID ARTHRITIS

1. Onset before age 16 years
2. Arthritis in one or more joints defined as swelling or effusion or the presence of two or more of the following signs: limitation of range of motion, tenderness or pain on motion, and increased heat
3. Duration of disease of 6 weeks to 3 months
4. Type of onset of disease during the first 4 to 6 months classified as
   a. Polyarthritis—five or more joints
   b. Oligoarthritis—four joints or fewer
   c. Systemic disease
      1. Arthritis
      2. Intermittent fever
      3. Rheumatoid rash
      4. Visceral disease (hepatosplenomegaly, lymphadenopathy)
5. Exclusion of other disease

tis.[42] The pauciarticular form is often self-limiting. Abnormalities resulting from JRA include genu valgum, posterior tibial subluxation, lateral compartment bone loss, and patellar subluxation. Leg-length discrepancy can also occur with lengthening of the involved leg in younger children and shortening of the involved leg from premature physeal closure in older children and adolescents.[172, 377]

The first line of treatment in JRA is medical therapy using nonsteroidal anti-inflammatory drugs. The next line of therapy involves slow-acting remittent drugs, such as gold, followed by cytotoxic agents, such as methotrexate, and then finally corticosteroids. Surgery is indicated if nonoperative management fails. In selected patients with persistent chronic synovitis, arthroscopic synovectomy will give temporary relief. Physical therapy with active and passive range-of-motion exercises with night splinting can prevent flexion contractures. Total knee replacement is an option for patients who have reached skeletal maturity and who have end-stage destruction with substantial disability.[284]

References

1. Abdon P, Turner MS, Pettersson H, et al: A long-term follow-up study of total meniscectomy in children. Clin Orthop 257:166, 1990.
2. Abraham E, Verinder DGR, Sharrard WJW: The treatment of flexion contracture of the knee in myelomeningocele. J Bone Joint Surg Br 59:433, 1977.
3. Aglietti P, Insall JN, Cerulli G: Patellar pain and incongruence. I: Measurements of incongruence. Clin Orthop 176:217, 1983.
4. Aglietti P, Pisaneschi A, Buzzi R, et al: Arthroscopic lateral release for patellar pain or instability. Arthroscopy 5:176, 1989.
5. Aglietti P, Buzzi R, Bassi PB, et al: Arthroscopic drilling in juvenile osteochondritis dissecans of the medial femoral condyle. Athroscopy 10:286, 1994.
6. Ahmadi B, Shahriaree H, Silver CM: Severe congenital genu recurvatum. Case report. J Bone Joint Surg Am 61:622, 1979.
7. Aichroth P: Osteochondritis dissecans of the knee: A clinical survey. J Bone Joint Surg Br 53:440, 1971.
8. Aichroth PM, Patel DV, Marx CI: Congenital discoid lateral meniscus in children. A follow-up study and evolution of management. J Bone Joint Surg Br 73:932, 1991.
9. Aitken AP: Fractures of the proximal tibial epiphyseal cartilage. Clin Orthop 41:92, 1965.
10. Aitken AP, Ingersoll RE: Fractures of the proximal tibial epiphyseal cartilage. J Bone Joint Surg Am 38:787, 1956.
11. Aitken A, Magill H: Fractures involving the distal femoral epiphyseal cartilage. J Bone Joint Surg Am 36:96, 1952.
12. Al-Rawi Z, Nessan AH: Joint hypermobility in patients with chondromalacia patellae. Br J Rheum 36:1324, 1997.
13. Amatuzzi MM, Fazzi A, Varella MH: Pathologic synovial plica of the knee. Results of conservative treatment. Am J Sports Med 18:466, 1990.
14. Anderson AF, Richards DB, Pagnani MJ, et al: Antegrade drilling for osteochondritis dissecans of the knee. Arthroscopy 13:319, 1997.
15. Anderson JP, Snow B, Dorey FJ, et al: Efficacy of soft splints in reducing severe knee-flexion contractures. Dev Med Child Neurol 30:502, 1988.
16. Andrews M, Noyes FR, Barber-Westin SD: Anterior cruciate ligament allograft reconstruction in the skeletally immature athlete. Am J Sports Med 22:48, 1994.
17. Angel KR, Hall DJ: The role of arthroscopy in children and adolescents. Arthroscopy 5:192, 1989.
18. Angel KR, Hall DJ: Anterior cruciate ligament injury in children and adolescents. Arthroscopy 5:197, 1989.
19. Aprin H, Kilfoyle AM: Extension contracture of the knees in patients with meningomyelocele. Clin Orthop 144:260, 1979.
20. Arnbjornsson A, Egund N, Rydling O: The natural history of recurrent dislocation of the patella: Long-term results of conservative and opeative treatment. J Bone Joint Surg Br 74:140, 1992.
21. Aronstam A, Painter MJ, Eddey JV: Multiple bleeds in haemophilia A. Clin Lab Haematol 1:275, 1979.
22. Auge WK, Kaeing CC: Bilateral discoid medial menisci with extensive intrasubstance cleavage tears. Arthroscopy 10:313, 1994.
23. Austick DH, Dandy DJ: Early operation for congenital subluxation of the knee. J Pediatr Orthop 3:85, 1983.
24. Bahnson D, Lovell W: Genu valgum following fracture of the proximal tibial metaphysis in children. Orthop Trans 4:306, 1980.
25. Baker RH, Carroll N, Dewar FP, et al: The semitendinosus tenodesis for recurrent dislocation of the patella. J Bone Joint Surg Br 54:103, 1972.
26. Baithazar D, Pappas A: Acquired valgus deformity of the tibia in children. J Pediatr Orthop 4:538, 1984.
27. Barnes CL, McCarthy RE, VanderSchilden JL, et al: Discoid lateral meniscus in a young child: Case report and review of the literature. J Pediatr Orthop 8:707, 1988.
28. Bassett FH III, Goldner JL: Fractures involving the distal femoral epiphyseal growth line. South Med J 55:545, 1962.
29. Baski DP: Restoration of dynamic stability of the patella by pes anserinus transposition. A new approach. J Bone Joint Surg Br 63:399, 1981.
30. Bates DG, Hresko MT, Jaramillo D: Patellar sleeve fracture: demonstration with MR imaging. Radiology 193:825, 1994.
31. Baxter MP: Assessment of normal pediatric knee ligament laxity using the Genucom. J Pediatr Orthop 8:546, 1988.
32. Baxter MP, Wiley JJ: Fractures of the tibial spine in children. An evaluation of knee stability. J Bone Joint Surg Br 70:228, 1988.
33. Beaty JH: Congenital anomalies of the lower and upper extremities. In Canale ST, Beaty JH, eds: Operative pediatric orthopaedics. St. Louis, Mosby-Year Book, 1991, pp 73-186.
34. Bellier G, Dupont JY, Larrain M, et al: Lateral discoid menisci in children. Arthroscopy 5:52, 1989.
35. Belman DA, Neviaser RJ: Transverse fracture of the patella in a child. J Trauma 13:917, 1973.
36. Bensahel H, DalMonte A, Hjelmstedt A, et al: Congenital dislocation of the knee. J Pediatr Orthop 9:174, 1989.
37. Bergstrom R, Gillquist, Lysholm J, et al: Arthroscopy of the knee in children. J Pediatr Orthop 4:542, 1984.

38. Bertin K, Goble E: Ligament injuries associated with physeal fractures about the knee. Clin Orthop 177:188, 1983.
39. Birch A: Surgery of the knee in children with spina bifida. Dev Med Child Neurol Supp 8:1, 1976.
40. Bishay M: Sleeve fracture of the upper pole of the patella. J Bone Joint Surg Br 73:339, 1991.
41. Bisson LJ, Wickiewicz T, Levinson M, et al: ACL reconstruction in children with open physes. Orthopedics 21:659, 1998.
42. Blane CE, Ragsdale CG, Herzenberg JE: Predicting outcome at the knee in juvenile rheumatoid arthritis. Clin Exp Rheumatol 8:85, 1990.
43. Bonnard C, et al: Patellar instability in children. Result of transposition of the medial third of patellar tendon. Rev Chir Orthop 76:473, 1990.
44. Bourne MH, Bianco AJ Jr: Bipartite patella in the adolescent: Results of surgical excision. J Pediatr Orthop 10:69, 1990.
45. Bowen JR, Leahey JL, Zhang ZH, et al: Partial epiphysiodesis at the knee to correct angular deformity. Clin Orthop 198:184, 1985.
46. Bradley J, Dandy DJ: Results of drilling osteochondritis dissecans before skeletal maturity. J Bone Joint Surg Br 71:642, 1989.
47. Bradway JK, Klassen RA, Peterson HA: Blount's disease: A review of the English literature. J Pediatr Orthop 7:472, 1987.
48. Brief LB: Anterior cruciate ligament reconstruction without drill holes. Arthroscopy 7:350, 1991.
49. Brittberg M, Lindahl A, Nilsson A, et al: Treatment of deep cartilage defects in the knee with autologous chondrocyte transplantation. N Engl J Med 331:889, 1994.
50. Broom MJ, Fulkerson JP: The plica syndrome: A new perspective. Orthop Clin North Am 17:279, 1986.
51. Buckley SL, Barrack RL, Alexander AH: The natural history of conservatively treated partial anterior cruciate ligament tears. Am J Sports Med 17:221, 1989.
52. Buff HU, Jones LC, Hungerford DS, et al: Experimental determination of forces transmitted across the patellofemoral joint. J Biomech 21:17, 1988.
53. Burkhart SS, Peterson HA: Fractures of the proximal tibial epiphysis. J Bone Joint Surg Am 61:996, 1979.
54. Cahill BR: Osteochondritis dissecans of the knee: Treatment of juvenile and adult forms. J Am Acad Orthop Surg 3:237, 1995.
55. Cahill BR, Berg BC: 99m-Technetium phosphate compound joint scinitigraphy in the management of juvenile osteochondritis dissecans of the femoral condyles. Am J Sports Med 11:329, 1989.
56. Cahill BR: The results of conservative management of juvenile osteochondritis dissecans using joint scintigraphy: A prospective study. Am J Sports Med 17:601, 1989.
57. Caillon F, Rigault P, Padovani JP, et al: Injuries of the upper end of the tibia in children. With the exclusion of fractures of the tibial shaft. Chir Pediatr 31:322, 1990.
58. Cammisa FP Jr: The Van Nes tibia rotationplasty. A functionally viable reconstructive procedure in children who have a tumor of the distal end of the femur. J Bone Joint Surg Am 72:1541, 1990.
59. Canale ST: Sports medicine. In Canale ST, Beaty JH, eds: Operative pediatric orthopaedics. St. Louis, Mosby-Year Book, 1991, pp 777-836.
60. Canale ST: Fractures and dislocations. In Canale ST, Beaty JH, eds: Operative Pediatric Orthopaedics. St. Louis, Mosby-Year Book, 1991, pp 837-1032.
61. Canale ST, Dugdale M, Howard BC: Synovectomy of the knee in young patients with hemophilia. South Med J 81:1480, 1988.
62. Carter C, Wilkinson J: Persistent joint laxity and congenital dislocation of the hip. J Bone Joint Surg Am 46:40, 1964.
63. Cheng JC, Chan P, Hui P: Joint laxity in children. J Pediatr Orthop 11:752, 1991.
64. Chrisman OD, Sook GA, Wilson TC: A long-term prospective study of the Hauser and Roux-Goldthwait procedures for recurrent patellar dislocation. Clin Orthop 144:27, 1979.
65. Christic MJ, Dvonch VM: Tibial tuberosity avulsion fracture in adolescents. J Pediatr Orthop 1:391, 1981.
66. Clanton TO, DeLee JC: Osteochondritis dissecans: History, pathophysiology, and current treatment concepts. Clin Orthop 167:50, 1982.
67. Clark CR, Ogden JA: Development of the menisci of the human knee joint. Morphological changes and their potential role in childhood meniscal injury. J Bone Joint Surg Am 65:538, 1983.
68. Clarren SK, Smith DW: Congenital deformities. Pediatr Clin North Am 24:665, 1977.
69. Colville J: Neonatal septic arthritis. Clinical review of twenty-three patients. J Ir Med Assoc 71:127, 1978.
70. Convery FR, Meyers MH, Akeson WH: Fresh osteochondral allografting of the femoral condyle. Clin Orthop 273:139, 1991.
71. Cook SE, Lavernia CJ, Burke SW, et al: A biomechanical analysis of the etiology of tibia vara. J Pediatr Orthop 3:449, 1983.
72. Cozen L: Knock-knee deformity in children. Congenital and acquired. Clin Orthop 258:191, 1990.
73. Crawford AH: Fractures about the knee in children. Orthop Clin North Am 7:639, 1976.
74. Criswell AR, Hand WL, Butler JE: Abduction injuries of the distal femoral epiphysis. Clin Orthop 115:189, 1976.
75. Curtis B, Fisher A: Heritable congenital tibiofemoral subluxation: Clinical features and surgical treatment. J Bone Joint Surg Am 52:1104, 1970.
76. Czitrom AA, Salter RB, Willis RB: Fractures involving the distal epiphyseal plate of the femur. Int Orthop 4:269, 1981.
77. Dahlstedt L, Dalen N, Jonsson U: Extraarticular repair of the unstable knee. Disappointing 6-year results of the Slocum and Ellison operations. Acta Orthop Scand 9:687, 1988.
78. Dai L, Zhang W, Xu Y: Meniscal injury in children: Long-term results after meniscectomy. Knee Surg, Sports Trauma, Arthroscopy 5:77, 1997.
79. Dandy DJ: Anatomy of the medial suprapatellar plica and medial synovial shelf. Arthroscopy 6:79, 1990.
80. Davidson RS: Orthopaedic complications of Lyme disease in children. Biomed Pharmacol 143:405, 1989.
81. De Flaviiss L, Nessi R, Scaglione P, et al: Ultrasonic diagnosis of Osgood-Schlatter and Sinding-Larsen-Johansson diseases of the knee. Skeletal Radiol 18:193, 1989.
82. DeHaven K, Lintner D: Athletic injuries: Comparison by age, sport, and gender. Am J Sports Med 14:218, 1986.
83. DeLee J, Curtis R: Anterior cruciate ligament insufficiency in children. Clin Orthop 172:112, 1983.
84. DeLee JC: ACL insufficiency in children. In Feagin JA Jr, ed: The Crucial Ligaments. New York, Churchill Livingstone, 1988, pp. 439-447.
85. Denti M, Monteleone M, Berardi A, et al: Medial patellar synovial plica syndrome: The influence of associated pathology on long-term results. Chir Organi Movimento 79:273, 1994.
86. DeSmet AA, Fisher DR, Graf BK, et al: Osteochondritis dissecans of the knee: Value of MR imaging in determining lesion stability and the presence of articular cartilage efects. Am J Roentgen 155:549, 1990.
87. Dickason JM, Fox JM: Fracture of the patella due to over-use syndrome in a child. Am J Sports Med 10:248, 1982.
88. Dickaut S, DeLee J: The discoid lateral-meniscus syndrome. J Bone Joint Surg Am 64:1068, 1982.
89. Dinham JM: Popliteal cysts in children. The case against surgery. J Bone Joint Surg Br 57:69, 1975.
90. Dol Monte A, Manes E, Cammarota V: Post-traumatic genu valgum in children. Ital J Orthop Traumatol 9:5, 1983.
91. Ehrlich MG, Strain RE Jr: Epiphyseal injuries about the knee. Orthop Clin North Am 10:91, 1979.
92. Eiskjaer S, Larsen ST: Arthroscopy of the knee in children. Acta Orthop Scand 58:273, 1987.
93. Eiskjaer S, Larsen ST, Schmidt MB: The significance of hemarthrosis of the knee in children. Arch Orthop Trauma Surg 107: 96, 1988.
94. Echeverria TS, Bersani FA: Acute fracture simulating a symptomatic bipartite patella. Am J Sports Med 8:48, 1980
95. Fairbank HAT: Generalized diseases of the skeleton. Proc R Soc Lond 28:611, 1935.
96. Federico DJ, Lynch K, Jokl P: Osteochondritis dissecans of the knee: A historical review of etiology and treatment. Arthroscopy 6:190, 1990.
97. Feldman MD, Schoeneker PL: Use of the metaphyseal-diaphyseal angle in the evaluation of bowleg. J Bone Joint Surg Am 75:1602, 1993.
98. Ferris B, Aichroth P: The treatment of congenital knee dislocation. Clin Orthop 216:135, 1987.

99. Ferris BD, Jackson AM: Congenital snapping knee. Habitual anterior subluxation of the tibia in extension. J Bone Joint Surg Br 72:453, 1990.
100. Ferriter P, Shapiro F: Infantile tibia vara: Factors affecting outcome following proximal tibial osteotomy. J Pediatr Orthop 7:1, 1987.
101. Ferrone JD Jr: Congenital deformities about the knee. Orthop Clin North Am 7:323, 1976.
102. Finder JA: Congenital hyperextension of the knee. J Bone Joint Surg Br 46:783, 1964.
103. Fischer SP, Fox JM, Del Pizzo W, et al: Accuracy of diagnoses from magnetic resonance imaging of the knee: a multi-center analysis of one thousand and fourteen patients. J Bone Joint Surg Am 73:2, 1991.
104. Flanagan JP, Trakru S, Meyer M, et al: Arthroscopic excision of symptomatic medial plica. A study of 118 knees with 1-14 year follow-up. Acta Orthop Scand 65:408, 1994.
105. Fondren FB, Goldner JL, Bassett FH 3d: Recurrent dislocation of the patella treated by the modified Roux-Goldthwait procedure: A prospective study of forty-seven knees. J Bone Joint Surg Am 67:993, 1985.
106. Frank C, Strother R: Isolated posterior cruciate ligament injury in a child: literature review and a case report. Can J Surg 32: 373, 1989.
107. Fulkerson JP, Shea KP: Disorders of patellofemoral alignment. J Bone Joint Surg Am 72:1424, 1990.
108. Gao GX, Lee EH, Bose K: Surgical management of congenital and habitual dislocation of the patella. J Pediatr Orthop 10:255, 1990.
109. Gardiner JS, McInerney VK, Avella DG, et al: Injuries to the inferior pole of the patella in children. Orthop Rev 19:643, 1990.
110. Gebhardt MC, Ready JE, Mankin HJ: Tumors about the knee in children. Clin Orthop 255:86, 1990.
111. Gill J, Chakrabarti H, Becker S: Fractures of the proximal tibial epiphysis. Injury 14:324, 1983.
112. Goldberg B: Patellofemoral malalignment. Pediatr Ann 26:32, 1997.
113. Gong YR: Fibrous cortical defect. Radiologic analysis of 6 cases. Chin Med J 102:868, 1989.
114. Goodrich A, Ballard A: Posterior cruciate ligament avulsion associated with ipsilateral femur fracture in a 10-year-old child. J Trauma 28:1393, 1988.
115. Gottsauner-Wolf F, Kotz R, Knahr K, et al: Rotationplasty for limb salvage in the treatment of malignant tumors at the knee. J Bone Joint Surge Am 73:1365, 1991.
116. Graf BK, Lange RH, Fujisaki CK, et al: Anterior cruciate ligament tear in skeletally immature patients: Meniscal pathology at presentation and after attempted conservative treatment. Arthroscopy 8:229, 1992.
117. Graham JM, Gross RH: Distal femoral physeal problem fractures. Clin Orthop 255:51, 1990.
118. Grana WA: Physeal fractures about the knee. J Am Acad Orthop Surg 3:63, 1995.
119. Green W, Banks H: Osteochondritis dissecans in children. J Bone Joint Surg Am 35:26, 1953.
120. Gregosiewicz A, Wosko I, Kandzierski G: Intraarticular bleeding in children with hemophilia: The prevention of arthropathy. J Pediatr Orthop 9:182, 1989.
121. Griffin PP: The lower limb. In Lovell WW, Winter RB, eds: Pediatric Orthopaedics, vol 2. Philadelphia, JB Lippincott, 1986.
122. Griswold AS: Fractures of the patella. Clin Orthop 4:44 1954.
123. Grogan DP, Carey TP, Leffers D, et al: Avulsion fractures of the patella. J Pediatr Orthop 10:721, 1990.
124. Gronkvist H, Hirsch G, Johansson L: Fractures of the anterior tibial spine in children. J Pediatr Orthop 4:465, 1984.
125. Grossman RB, Nicholas JA: Common disorders of the knee. Orthop Clin North Am 8:619, 1977.
126. Gugenheim JJ, Rosenthal RK, Simon SR: Knee flexion deformities and genu recurvatum in cerebral palsy: Roentgenographic findings. Dev Med Child Neurol 21:563, 1979.
126b. Guhl JF: Arthroscopic treatment of osteochondritis dissecans. Clin Orthop 167:65, 1982.
127. Guidera KJ, Kortright L, Barber V, et al: Radiographic changes in arthrogrypotic knees. Skeletal Radiol 20:193, 1991.
128. Guzzanti V, Gigante A, DiLazzaro A, et al: Patellofemoral malalignment in adolescents: Computerized tomographic assessment with or without quadriceps contraction. Am J Sports Med 22:50, 1994.
129. Guzzanti V, Falciglia F, Gigante A, et al: The effect of intra-articular ACL reconstruction on the growth plates of rabbits. J Bone Joint Surg Br 76:960, 1994.
130. Hall JE, Micheli LJ, McManama GB Jr: Semitendinosis tenodesis for recurrent subluxation or dislocation of the patella. Clin Orthop 144:31, 1979.
131. Hand WL, Hand CR, Dunn AW: Tibial tuberosity avulsion fracture in adolescents. J Bone Joint Surg Am 53:1579, 1971.
132. Harvell JC Jr, Fu FH, Stanitski CL: Diagnostic arthroscopy of the knee in children and adolescents. Orthopedics 12:1555, 1989.
133. Haus J, Refior HJ: The importance of arthroscopy in sports injuries in children and adolescents. Knee Surg Sports Trauma Arthroscopy 1:34, 1993.
134. Hayashi LK, Yamaga H, Ida K, et al: Arthroscopic meniscectomy for discoid lateral meniscus in children. J Bone Joint Surg Am 70:1495, 1988.
135. Hayes J, Masear V: Avulsion fracture of the tibia eminence associated with severe medial ligamentous injury in an adolescent. Am J Sports Med 12:330, 1984.
136. Heckman JD, Alkire CC: Distal patellar pole fractures: A proposed common mechanism of injury. Am J Sports Med 12:424, 1984.
137. Henderson RC, Kemp GJ, Greene WB: Adolescent tibia vara: Alternatives for operative treatment. J Bone Joint Surg Am 74: 342, 1992.
138. Helfet A: Mechanism of derangement of the medial semilunar cartilage and their management. J Bone Joint Surg Br 41:319, 1959.
139. Herve-Somma CM, Sebag GH, Prieur AM, et al: Juvenile rheumatoid arthritis of the knee: MR evaluation with Gd-DOTA. Radiology 182:93, 1992.
140. Hogh J, Lund B: The sequelae of Osgood-Schlatter's disease in adults. Int Orthop 12:213, 1988
141. Hope PG. Arthroscopy in children. J Royal Soc Med 84:29, 1991.
142. Houghton GR, Ackroyd CE: Sleeve fractures of the patella in children: a report of three cases. J Bone Joint Surg Br 61:165, 1979.
143. Houston CS, Reed MH, Desautels JEL: Separating Larsen syndrome from the "arthrogryposis basket." J Assoc Can Radiol 32: 206, 1981.
144. Howard JB, Highgenboten CL, Nelson JD: Residual effects of septic arthritis in infancy and childhood. JAMA 236:932, 1976.
145. Hughston JC, Deese M: Medial subluxation of the patella as a complication of lateral retinacular release. Am J Sports Med 16: 383, 1988.
146. Hughston JC, Hergenroeder PT, Courtenay BG: Osteochondritis dissecans of the femoral condyles. J Bone Joint Surg Am 66: 1340, 1984.
147. Imai N, Tomatsu T: Cartilage lesions in the knee of adolescents and young adults: Arthroscopic analysis. Arthroscopy 7:198, 1991.
148. Indelicato P: Non-operative treatment of complete tears of the medial collateral ligament of the knee. J Bone Joint Surg Am 65:323, 1983.
149. Insall JN, Aglietti P, Tria AJ Jr: Patellar pain and incongruence. II: Clinical application. Clin Orthop 176:225, 1983.
150. Iossifidis A, Brueton RN: Painful bipartite patella following injury. Injury 26:175, 1995.
151. Ishikawa H, Sakurai A, Hirata S, et al: Painful bipartite patella in young athletes: The diagnostic value of skyline views taken in squatting position and the results of surgical excision. Clin Orthop 305:223, 1994.
152. Itakazu M, Yamane T, Shoen S: Incomplete avulsion of the femoral attachment of the posterior cruciate ligament with an osteochondral fragment in a twelve-year-old boy. Arch Orthop Trauma Surg 110:55, 1990.
153. Iwaya T, Sakaguchi R, Tsuyama N: The treatment of congenital dislocation of the knee with the Pavlik harness. Int Orthop 7: 25, 1983.
154. Jacobsen K, Vopalecky F: Congenital dislocation of the knee. Acta Orthop Scand 56:1, 1985.

155. Jackson AM: Recurrent dislocation of the patella. J Bone Joint Surg Br 74:2, 1992.
156. Janarv PM, Nystrom A, Werner S, et al: Anterior cruciate ligament injuries in skeletally immature patients. J Pediatr Orthop 16:673, 1996.
157. Jaramillo D, Hoffer FA, Shapiro F, et al: MR imaging of fractures of the growth plate. Am J Roentgen 155:1261, 1990.
158. Jerosch J, Hoffstetter I, Schroder M, et al: Septic arthritis: Arthroscopic management with local antibiotic treatment. Acta Orthop Belg 61:126, 1995.
159. Johnson DP, Eastwood DM, Witherow PJ: Symptomatic synovial plicae of the knee. J Bone Joint Surg Am 75:1485, 1993.
160. Johnson E, Audel R, Oppenheim WL: Congenital dislocation of the knee. J Pediatr Orthop 7:194, 1987.
161. Johnston CE: Infantile tibia vara. Clin Orthop 255:13, 1990.
162. Jones R, Henley M, Francis P: Nonoperative management of isolated grade III collateral ligament injury in high school football players. Clin Orthop 213:137, 1986.
163. Jordan MR: Lateral meniscal variants: Evaluation and treatment. J Am Acad Orthop Surg 4:191, 1996.
164. Jozwiak M, Pietrzak S: Patella position versus length of hamstring muscles in children. J Pediatr Orthop 18:268, 1998.
165. Juhl M, Boe S: Arthroscopy in children, with special emphasis on meniscal lesions. Injury 17:171, 1986.
166. Kannus P, Jarvinen M: Knee ligament injuries in adolescents. Eight year follow-up of conservative management. J Bone Joint Surg Br 70:772, 1988.
167. Kaplan EB: Discoid lateral meniscus of the knee joint: Nature, mechanism, and operative treatment. J Bone Joint Surg Am 39:77, 1957.
168. Kaplan PA, Nelson NL, Garvin KL, et al: MR of the knee: The significance of high signal in the meniscus that does not clearly extend to the surface. AJR Am J Roentgenol 156:333, 1991.
169. Kasser JR: Physeal bar resections after growth arrest about the knee. Clin Orthop 255: 68, 1990.
170. Kasser JR: Bone and joint diseases. In Canale ST, Beaty JH, eds: Operative Pediatric Orthopaedics. St. Louis, Mosby-Year Book, 1991, pp 1047-1072.
171. Kellenberger A, von Laer L: Nonosseous lesions of the anterior cruciate ligaments in childhood and adolescence. Prog Pediatr Surg 25:123, 1990.
172. Kelley WN: Textbook of Rheumatology, 3rd ed. Philadelphia, WB Saunders, 1989, pp 1298-1301.
173. Kennedy J, Grainger A: The posterior cruciate ligament. J Trauma 7:367, 1976.
174. Kennedy J, Stewart A, Walker D: Anterolateral rotary instability of the knee joint. An early analysis of the Ellison procedure. J Bone Joint Surg Am 60:1031, 1978.
175. Keskinen K, Eriksson E, Komi P: Breaststroke swimmer's knee. A biomechanical and arthroscopic study. Am J Sports Med 8: 228, 1980.
176. Killam PE: Orthopedic assessment of young children: Developmental variations. Nurse Pract 14:27, 1989.
177. King A: Meniscal lesions in children and adolescents: A review of the pathology and clinical presentation. Injury 15:105, 1983.
178. King SJ, Carty HM, Brady O: Magnetic resonance imaging of knee injuries in children. Ped Radiol 26:287, 1996.
179. Kinnard P, Levesque RY: The plica syndrome: A syndrome of controversy. Clin Orthop 183:141, 1984.
180. Kling TF Jr: Angular deformities of the lower limbs in children. Orthop Clin North Am 18:513, 1987.
181. Kling TF Jr: Angular and torsional deformities of the lower limbs in children. Clin Orthop 176:136, 1983.
182. Kloeppel-Wirth S, Koltai JL, Dittmer H: Significance of arthroscopy in children with knee joint injuries. Eur J Pediatr Surg 2: 169, 1992.
183. Knapp DR, Price CT: Correction of distal femoral deformity. Clin Orthop 255:75, 1990.
184. Kocher MS, Zurakowski D, Micheli LJ: Diagnostic accuracy of magnetic resonance imaging of knee injuries in children and adolescents. Presented at American Orthopaedic Association 32nd Annual Meeting, Chapel Hill, NC, 1999.
185. Konsens RM, Seitz WH Jr: Bilateral fractures through "giant" patellar tendon ossicles: A late sequela of Osgood-Schlatter disease. Orthop Rev 17:797, 1988.
186. Koshino T, Sugimoto K: New measurement of patellar height in the knees of children using the epiphyseal line midpoint. J Pediatr Orthop 9:216, 1989.
187. Krajbich JI: Modified Van Nes rotationplasty in the treatment of malignant neoplasms in the lower extremities of children. Clin Orthop 262:74, 1991.
188. Krajbich JI, Carroll NC: Van Nes rotationplasty with segmental limb resection. Clin Orthop 256:7, 1990.
189. Krause BL, Williams JPR, Cafterall A: Natural history of Osgood-Schlatter disease. J Pediatr Orthop 10:65, 1990.
190. Kujala UM, Kvist M, Heinonen O: Osgood-Schlatter disease and tibial tuberosity development. Clin Orthop 116:180, 1976.
191. Lange R, Vanderby A, Engber W, et al: Biomechanical and histological evaluation of the Herbert screw. J Orthop Trauma 4:275, 1990.
192. Langenskiöld A: Growth disturbance after osteomyelitis of femoral condyles in infants. Acta Orthop Scand 5:1, 1984.
193. Langenskiöld A, Riska EB: Tibia vara (osteochondrosis deformans tibia): A survey of seventy-one cases. J Bone Joint Surg Am 46:1405, 1964.
194. Lanning P, Heikkinen E: Ultrasonic features of the Osgood-Schlatter lesion. J Pediatr Orthop 11:538, 1991.
195. Lazzarone C: Extraarticular reconstruction in the treatment of chronic lesions of the anterior cruciate ligament. Ital J Orthop Trauma 16:459, 1990.
196. Larson RL, Cabaud HE, Slocum DB, et al: The patellar compression syndrome: surgical treatment by lateral retinacular release. Clin Orthop 134:158, 1978.
197. Lavner G: Osteochondritis dissecans: An analysis of forty-two cases and a review of the literature. Am J Roentgen 57:56, 1947.
198. Lee CK, Mercurio C: Operative treatment of osteochondritis dissecans in situ by retrograde drilling and cancellous bone graft: A preliminary report. Clin Orthop 158:129, 1981.
199. Lee CL, Lamont RL, Peterson HE: Fractures of the distal femoral epiphysis. J Bone Joint Surg Am 82:403, 1977.
200. Lephart SM, Kocher MS, Fu F, et al: Proprioception following anterior cruciate ligament reconstruction. J Sport Rehabil 1: 188, 1992.
201. Leveuf J, Pais C: Les dislocations congenitales du genon. Rev Chir Orthop 32:313, 1946.
202. Levine J, Kashyap S: A new conservative treatment of Osgood-Schlatter disease. Clin Orthop 158:126, 1981.
203. Lewis P, Foster B: Herbert screw fixation of osteochondral fractures about the knee. Aust N Z J Surg 60:511, 1990.
204. Linden B: The incidence of osteochondritis dissecans in the condyles of the femur. Acta Orthop Scand 47:664, 1976.
205. Lipscomb AB, Anderson AF: Tears of the anterior cruciate ligament in adolescents. J Bone Joint Surg Am 68:19, 1986.
206. Litchman HM, McCullough RW, Gandsman EJ, et al: Computerized blood flow analysis for decision making in the treatment of osteochondritis dissecans. J Pediatr Orthop 8:208, 1988.
207. Lo IK, Kirkley A, Fowler PJ, Miniaci A: The outcome of operatively treated anterior cruciate ligament disruptions in the skeletally immature child. Arthroscopy 13:627, 1997.
208. Lo IK, Bell DM, Fowler PJ: Anterior cruciate ligament injuries in the skeletally immature patient. Instuct Course Lect 47:351, 1998.
209. Loder AT, Schafter JJ, Bardenstein MB: Late-onset tibia vara. J Pediatr Orthop 11:162, 1991.
210. Lombardo S, Harvey J: Fractures of the distal femoral epiphysis, factors influencing prognosis: A review of thirty-four cases. J Bone Joint Surg Am 59:742, 1977.
211. Lopez Longo FJ, Monteagudo Saez I, Cobeta Garcia JC, et al: Reiter's syndrome: Considerations on the frequency and mid-term course of its juvenile form. Ann Esp Pediatr 29:298, 1988.
212. Lutter LD: Larsen syndrome: clinical features and treatment—A report of two cases. J Pediatr Orthop 10:270, 1990.
213. Maffulli N: Intensive training in young athletes. The orthopaedic surgeon's viewpoint. Sports Med 9:229, 1990.
214. Maffulli N, Chan KM, Bundoc RC, et al: Knee arthroscopy in Chinese and adolescents: An eight-year prospective study. Arthroscopy 13:18, 1997.
215. Mahomed MN, Beaver RJ, Gross AE: The long-term success of fresh, small fragment osteochondral allografts used for intraar-

ticular posttraumatic defects in the knee joint. Orthopedics 15: 1191, 1992.
216. Makela E, Vainiopaa S, Vihtonen K, et al: The effect of trauma to the lower femoral epiphyseal plate. An experimental study in rabbits. J Bone Joint Surg Br 70:187, 1988.
217. Makhdoomi KR, Doyle J, Moloney M: Transverse fracture of the patella in children. Arch Orthop Trauma Surg 112:302, 1993.
218. Manzione M, Pizzutillo PD, Peoples AB, et al: Meniscectomy in children: A long-term follow-up study. Am J Sports Med 11:111, 1983.
219. Marine JM, DiSimone RE, Clancy MJ: Blount's disease: tibia vara. Orthopedics 12:1504, 1989.
220. Matelic TM, Aronsson DD, Boyd DW, et al: Acute hemarthrosis of the knee in children. Am J Sports Med 23:668, 1995.
221. Mayer P, Micheli L: Avulsion of the femoral attachment of the posterior cruciate ligament in an eleven-year old boy. J Bone Joint Surg Am 61:431, 1979.
222. McCarroll JR, Rettig AC, Shelbourne KD: Anterior cruciate ligament injuries in the young athlete with open physes. Am J Sports Med 16:44, 1988.
223. McCarroll JR, Shelbourne KD, Patel DV: Anterior cruciate ligament reconstruction in athletes with an ossicle associated with Osgood-Schlatter's disease. Arthroscopy 12:556, 1996.
224. McCarroll JR, Shelbourne KD, Rettig AC, et al: Patellar tendon graft reconstruction for midsubstance anterior cruciate ligament rupture in junor high school athletes: An algorithm for management. Am J Sports Med 22:478, 1994.
225. McConnell J: The management of chondromalacia patellae: A long term solution. Aust J Physiother 32:215, 1986.
226. Medlar RC, Lyne ED: Sinding-Larsen-Johansson disease. Its etiology and natural history. J Bone Joint Surg Am 60:1113, 1978.
227. Medlar RC, Mandiberg JJ, Lyne ED: Meniscectomies in children: Report of long-term results. Am J Sports Med 8:87, 1980.
228. Mendez AA, Keret D, MacEwen GD: Treatment of patellofemoral instability in Down's syndrome. Clin Orthop 234:148, 1988.
229. Merchant AC: Classification of patellofemoral disorders. Arthroscopy 4:235, 1988.
230. Mesgarzade M, Sapega AA, Bonakdarpour A, et al: Osteochondritis dissecans: Analysis of mechanical stability with radiography, scintigraphy, and MR imaging. Radiology 165:775, 1987.
231. Meyers M, McKeever F: Fractures of the intercondylar eminence of the tibia. J Bone Joint Surg Am 52:1677, 1970.
231b. Micheli LJ: Sports injuries in children and adolescents: Questions and controversies. Clin Sports Med 14:727, 1995.
232. Micheli LJ: Patellofemoral disorders in children. In Fox JM, Del Pizzo W, eds: The Patellofemoral Joint. New York, McGraw-Hill, 1993, pp 105-121.
233. Micheli LJ: Special considerations in children's rehabilitation programs. In Hunter LY, Funk FJ Jr, eds: Rehabilitation of the Injured Knee. St. Louis, Mosby, 1984.
234. Micheli LJ, Foster TE: Acute knee injury in the immature athlete. In Heckman JD, ed: Instructional course lectures, vol. 1 and 2. Park Ridge, IL: American Academy of Orthopaedic Surgeons, pp 1993, 473-481.
235. Micheli LJ, Jupiter J: Osteoid osteoma as a cause of knee pain in the young athlete. A case study. Am J Sports Med 6:199, 1978.
235b. Micheli LJ, Rask B, Gerberg L: Anterior cruciate ligament reconstruction in patients who are prepubescent. Clin Orthop 364:40, 1999.
236. Micheli LJ, Slater JA, Woods E, et al: Patella alta and the adolescent growth spurt. Clin Orthop 213:159, 1986.
237. Micheli LJ, Stanitski CL: Lateral patellar retinacular release. Am J Sports Med 9:330, 1981.
238. Miller GF: Familial recurrent dislocation of the patella. J Bone Joint Surg Br 60:203, 1978.
239. Miller TT, Shapiro MA, Schultz E, et al: Sonography of patellar abnormalities in children. AJR Am J Roengenol 171:739, 1998.
240. Mital MA, Hayden J: Pain in the knee in children: The medial plica shelf syndrome. Orthop Clin North Am 10:713, 979.
241. Mital MA, Matza RA, Cohen J: The so-called unresolved Osgood-Schlatter lesion: A concept based on fifteen surgically treated lesions. J Bone Joint Surg Am 62:732, 1980.
242. Mizuta H, Kubota K, Shiraishi M, et al: The conservative treatment of complete tears of the anterior cruciate ligament in skeletally immature patients. J Bone Joint Surg Br 77:890, 1995.
243. Mok D, Good C: Nonoperative management of acute grade III medial collateral ligament injury of the knee: A prospective study. Injury 20:277, 1989.
244. Molander M, Wallin G, Wikstad I: Fracture of the intercondylar eminence of the tibia. J Bone Joint Surg Br 63:89, 1981.
245. Mori Y, Kuroki Y, Yamamoto R, et al: Clinical and histological study of patellar chondropathy in adolescents. Arthroscopy 7: 182, 1991.
246. Mori Y, Okumo H, Iketani H, et al: Efficacy of lateral retinacular release for painful bipartite patella. Am J Sports Med 23:13, 1995.
247. Morrissy RT, Eubanks RG, Park JP, et al: Arthroscopy of the knee in children. Clin Orthop Rel Res 162:103, 1982.
248. Mubarak SJ, Carroll NC: Familial osteochondritis dissecans of the knee. Clin Orthop 140:131, 1979.
249. Mubarak SJ, Carroll NC: Juvenile osteochondritis dissecans of the knee. Clin Orthop 157:200, 1981.
250. Munk S: Early operation of the dislocated knee in Larsen's syndrome. Acta Orthop Scand 59:582, 1988.
251. Munzinger U, Ruckstuhl J, Scherrer H, et al: Internal derangement of the knee joint due to pathologic synovial folds: The mediopatellar plica syndrome. Clin Orthop 155:59, 1981.
252. Mylle J, Reynders P, Broos P: Transepiphyseal fixation of anterior cruciate avulsion in a child. Report of a complication and review of the literature. Arch Orthop Trauma Surg 112:101, 1993.
253. Nakanishi K, Inoue M, Ishida T, et al: MR evaluation of mediopatellar plica. Acta Radiologica 37:567, 1996.
254. Nakhostine M, Bollen SR, Cross MJ: Reconstruction of midsubstance anterior cruciate rupture in adolescents with open physes. J Pediatr Orthop 15:286, 1995.
255. Nasca RJ: Unicameral bone cyst of the tibia complicated by genu valgum. South Med J 81:1301, 1988.
256. Nietosvaara Y, Aalto K, Kallio PE: Acute patellar dislocation in children: incidence and associated osteochondral fractures. J Pediatr Orthop 14:513, 1994.
257. Noble JW, Heinrich SD, Guanche CA: Midsubstance anterior cruciate ligament rupture in a 7-year old child. Am J Knee Surg 8:32, 1995.
258. Nogi J, MacEwen GD: Congenital dislocation of the knee. J Pediatr Orthop 2:509, 1982.
259. O'Dwyer KJ, Peace PK: The plica syndrome. Injury 19:350, 1988.
260. Ogata K: Painful bipartite patella: A new approach to operative treatment. J Bone Joint Surg Am 76:573, 1994.
261. Ogden JA: Skeletal Injury in the Child. Philadelphia, WB Saunders, 1990.
262. Ogden JA, McCarthy SM, Jokl P: The painful bipartite patella. J Pediatr Orthop 2:263, 982.
263. Ogden JA, Southwick WO: Osgood-Schlatter's disease and tibial tubercle development. Clin Orthop 116:180, 1976.
264. Ogden JA, Tross RB, Murphy MJ: Fractures of the tibial tuberosity in adolescents. J Bone Joint Surg Am 62:205, 1980.
265. O'Neill DB, Micheli U: Overuse injuries in the young athlete. Clin Sports Med 7:591, 1988.
266. Ohl MD, Kean JR, Steensen RN: Arthroscopic treatment of septic arthritic knees in children and adolescents. Orthop Rev 20:894, 1991.
267. Oni OOA, Keswani H: Idiopathic or primary windswept deformity: The etiological significance of the radiological findings. J Pediatr Orthop 4:293, 1984.
268. Oostvogel HJM, Kiasen HJ, Reddingius RE: Fractures of the intercondylar eminence in children and adolescents. Arch Orthop Trauma Surg 107:242, 1988.
269. Opinya GN, Imalingat B: Skeletal and dental fluorosis: Two case reports. East Afr Med J 68:304, 1991.
270. Oyemade GM: The correction of primary knee deformities in children. Int Orthop 5:241, 1981.
271. Paletta GA Jr, Bednarz PA, Stanitski CL, et al: The prognostic value of quantitative bone scan in knee osteochondritis dissecans. A preliminary experience. Am J Sports Med 26:7, 1998.
272. Pappas AM: Osteochondritis dissecans. Clin Orthop 158:59, 1981.
273. Parekh PK: Flexion contractures of the knee following poliomyelitis. Int Orthop 7:165, 1983.
274. Parker AW, Drez D, Cooper JL: Anterior cruciate ligament inju-

ries in patients with open physes. Am J Sports Med 22:44, 1994.
275. Parsch K, Schulz R: Ultrasonography in congenital dislocation of the knee. J Pediatr Orhop Br 3:76, 1994.
276. Patel D: Arthroscopy of the plicasynovial folds and their significance. Am J Sports Med 6:217, 1978.
277. Pavanini G, Turra S, Fama G, et al: Septic arthritis in children. Chir Organi Mov 74:93, 1989.
278. Pellaci F, Montanari G, Prosperi P, et al: Lateral discoid meniscus: Treatment and results. Arthroscopy 8:526, 1992.
279. Pettrone FA, Stay EJ: Chondroma. An unusual presentation of an extraarticular soft tissue mass about the knee. Am J Sports Med 18:536, 1990.
280. Pipkin G: Lesions of the suprapatellar plica. J Bone Joint Surg Am 32:363, 1950.
281. Poulsen TD, Skak SV, Jensen U: Epiphyseal fractures of the proximal tibia. Injury 20:111, 1989.
282. Pressman AE, Letts RM, Jarvis JG: Anterior cruciate ligament tears in children: An analysis of operative versus nonoperative treatment. J Pediatr Orthop 17:505, 1997.
283. Rab GT: Oblique tibial osteotomy for Blount's disease (tibia vara). J Pediatr Orthop 8:715, 1988.
284. Ranawat CS, Bryan WJ, Inglis AE: Total knee arthroplasty in juvenile arthritis. Arthritis Rheum 26:1140, 1983.
285. Ray JM, Hendrix J: Incidence, mechanism of injury, and treatment of fractures of the patella in children. J Trauma 32:464, 1992.
286. Reider B, Marshall J, Warren R: Clinical characteristics of patellar disorders in young athletes. Am J Sports Med 9:270, 1981.
287. Rinaldi E, Mazarella F: Isolated fractures-avulsions of the tibial insertions of the cruciate ligaments of the knee. Ital J Orthop Traumatol 6:77, 1980.
288. Riseborough EJ, Barrett LR, Shapiro F: Growth disturbances following distal femoral physeal fracture separations. J Bone Joint Surg Am 65:885, 1983.
289. Ritchie D: Meniscectomy in children. Aust N Z J Surg 35:239, 1965.
290. Roberts J: Avulsion fractures of the proximal tibial epiphysis. In Kennedy J, ed: The Injured Adolescent Knee. Baltimore, Williams & Wilkins, 1979.
291. Roberts J: Operative treatment of fractures about the knee. Orthop Clin North Am 21:365, 1990.
292. Ronningen H, Bjerkreim I: Larsen's syndrome. Acta Orthop Scand 49:138, 1978.
293. Rorabeck CP, Bobechko WP: Acute dislocation of the patella with osteochondral fracture: a review of eighteen cases. J Bone Joint Surg Br 58:237, 1976.
294. Rosenberg TD, Paulos LE, Parker RD, et al: Discoid lateral meniscus: Case report of arthroscopic attachment of a symptomatic Wrisberg-ligament type. Arthroscopy 3:277, 1987.
295. Ross AC, Chesterman PJ: Isolated avulsion of the tibial attachment of the posterior cruciate ligament in childhood. J Bone Joint Surg Br 68:747, 1986.
296. Rovere GD, Adair DM: Medial synovial shelf plica syndrome. Treatment by intraplical steroid injection. Am J Sports Med 13: 382, 1985.
297. Rovere GD, Nichols AW: Frequency, associated factors, and treatment of breaststroker's knee in competitive swimmers. Am J Sports Med 13:99, 1985.
298. Roy D, Crawford A: Percutaneous quadriceps recession: A technique for management of congenital hyperextension deformities of the knee in the neonate. J Pediatr Orthop 9:717, 1989.
299. Ryu RK, Ting AJ: Arthroscopic treatment of meniscal cysts. Arthroscopy 9:591, 1993.
300. Sanders W, Wilkins K, Neidre A: Acute insufficiency of the posterior cruciate ligament in children. Two case reports. J Bone Joint Surg Am 62:129, 1980.
301. Sandow MJ, Goodfellow JW: The natural history of anterior knee pain in adolescents. J Bone Joint Surg Br 67:36, 1985.
302. Sarkar P, Dasbupta S: Studies in pathogenesis of extra-articular stiffness of knee. J Indian Med Assoc 84:107, 1984.
303. Schaefer RA, Eilert RE, Gillogly SD: Disruption of the anterior cruciate ligament in a 4-year old child. Orthop Review 22:725, 1993.
304. Schmidt DR, Henry JH: Stress injuries of the adolescent extensor mechanism. Clin Sports Med 8:343, 1989.
305. Schneider T, Mene W, Fink B, et al: Recurrent dislocation of the patella and the Goldthwait operation. Arch Orthop Trauma Surg 116:46, 1997.
306. Schoeneker PL, Meade WC, Pierron RL, et al: Blount's disease: A retrospective review and recommendations for treatment. J Pediatr Orthop 5:181, 1985.
307. Schuchmann L, Ftirmaier A, Pernice W: Nuclear spin tomography studies of joints in juvenile chronic arthritis. Kiln Padiatr 202:147, 1990.
308. Scotti DM, Sadhu VK, Heimberg F, et al: Osgood-Schlatter's disease, an emphasis on soft tissue changes in roentgen diagnosis. Skeletal Radiol 4:21, 1979.
309. Sengupta S: Pathogenesis of infantile quadriceps fibrosis and its correction by proximal release. J Pediatr Orthop 5:87, 1985.
310. Seringe R, Reneaud I: Congenital dislocation of the knee in the newborn. J Pediatr Orthop Br 1:182, 1992.
311. Shelton G: Conservative management of patellofemoral dysfunction. Prim Care 19:331, 1992.
312. Shelton WR, Canale ST: Fractures of the tibia through the proximal tibial epiphyseal cartilage. J Bone Joint Surg Am 61: 167, 1979.
313. Sherman M: Physiologic bowing of the legs. South Med J 53: 830, 1960.
314. Sijelmassi R: Chronic pain of the knee in children and adolescents: Diagnosis and therapeutic management. Pediatrics 45:43, 1990.
315. Silverman FN: Larsen's syndrome: Congenital dislocation of knees and other joints, distinctive facies, and frequently, cleft palate. Ann Radiol 15:297, 1972.
316. Silverman J, Mink J, Deutsch A: Discoid menisci of the knee: MR imaging appearance. Radiology 173:351, 1989.
317. Skak S: Valgus deformity following proximal tibial metaphyseal fractures in children. Acta Orthop Scand 53:141, 1982.
318. Skyhar MJ, Mubarak SJ: Arthroscopic treatment of septic knees in children. J Pediatr Orthop 7:647, 1987.
319. Smillie IS: The congenital discoid meniscus. J Bone Joint Surg Am 30:671, 1948.
320. Smillie IS: Treatment of osteochondritis dissecans. J Bone Joint Surg Br 39:24, 1957.
321. Smith JB: Knee problems in children. Pediatr Clin North Am 33:1439, 1986.
322. Soballe K, Hansen AJ: Late results after meniscectomy in children. Injury 18:182, 1987.
323. Sodergard J, Ryoppy S: The knee in arthrogryposis multiplex congenita. J Pediatr Orthop 10:177, 1990.
324. Speer DP: Differential diagnosis of knee pain in children. Ariz Med 34:330, 1977.
325. Sponseller PD, Beaty JH: Fractures and dislocations about the knee. In Rockwood CA Jr, Wilkins KE, Beaty JH, eds: Fractures in Children, 4th ed. Philadelphia, Lippincott-Raven, 1996.
326. Springfield DS: Musculoskeletal tumors. In Canale ST, Beaty JH, eds: Operative Pediatric Orthopaedics. St. Louis, Mosby-Year Book, 1991, pp 1073-1120.
327. Stadelmaier DM, Arnoczky SP, Dodds J, et al: The effect of drilling and soft tissue grafting across open growth plates: A histologic study. Am J Sports Med 23:431, 1995.
328. Stanciu C, Labelle HB, Morin B, et al: The value of computed tomography for the diagnosis of recurrent patellar subluxation in adolescents. Can J Surg 37:319, 1994.
329. Stanisavljevic S, Zemenick G, Miller D: Congenital, irreducible, permanent lateral dislocation of the patella. Clln Orthop 116: 190, 1976.
330. Stanitski CL: Management of sports injuries in children and adolescents. Orthop Clin North Am 19:689, 1988.
331. Stanitski CL: Anterior cruciate ligament injury in the skeletally immature patient: Diagnosis and treatment. J Am Acad Orthop Surg 3:146, 1995.
332. Stanitski CL: Correlation of arthroscopic and clinical examinations with magnetic resonance imaging findings of injured knees in children and adolescents. Am J Sports Med 26:2, 1998.
333. Stanitski CL: Patellar instability in the school age athlete. Instruct Course Lect 47:345, 1998.
334. Stanitski CL, Harvell, Fu F: Observations on acute knee hemarthrosis in chldren and adolescents. J Pediatr Orthop 13:506, 1993.

335. Steere AC: Clinical definitions and differential diagnosis of Lyme arthritis. Scand J Infect Dis Supp 77:51, 1991.
336. Steiner ME: Hypermobility and knee injuries. Phys Sports Med 15:159, 1987.
337. Steiner ME, Grana WA: The young athlete's knee: recent advances. Clin Sports Med 7:527, 1988.
338. Steininger K, Wodick RE, Spate W: Chondropathia patellae: Untersuchung der femoropatellargelenke bei gesunden, sporttribenden kindern. Sportverletzung Sportschaden 4:87, 1990.
339. Stephens D, Louis E, Louis D: Traumatic separation of the distal femoral epiphyseal cartilage plate. J Bone Joint Surg Am 56:1383, 1974.
340. Stilli S, DiGennaro GL, Marchiodi L, et al: Arthroscopic surgery of the discoid meniscus during childhood. Chir Degli Org Mov 82:335, 1997.
341. Strong M, Lejman T, Michno P, et al: Sequelae from septic arthritis of the knee during the first two years of life. J Pediatr Orthop 14:745, 1994.
342. Stulberg SD, Shulman K, Smart S, et al: Breaststroker's knee: Pathology, etiology, and treatment. Am J Sports Med 8:164, 1980.
343. Sullivan JA: Ligamentous injuries of the knee in children. Clin Orthop 255:44, 1990.
344. Suman RK, Stother IG, Illingworth G: Diagnostic arthroscopy of the knee in children. J Bone Joint Surg Br 66:535, 1984.
345. Svendsen RN: High substantial rupture of the anterior cruciate ligament in a 6 year old boy. Injury 26:70, 1995.
346. Takeda Y, Ikata T, Yoshida S, et al: MRI high-signal intensity in the menisci of asymptomatic children. J Bone Joint Surg Br 80:463, 1998.
347. Thabit G, Micheli LJ: Patellofemoral pain in the pediatric patient. Orthop Clin North Am 23:567, 1992.
348. Thiery JA: Arthrosopic drainage in septic arthritides of the knee: A multicenter study. Arthroscopy 5:65, 1989.
349. Thompson GH, Carter JR: Late-onset tibia vara (Blount's disease). Clin Orthop 255:24, 1990.
350. Torg JS, Loughran T, Pavlov H, et al: Osteoid osteoma. Distant, periarticular, and subarticular lesions as a cause of knee pain. Sports Med 2:296, 1985.
351. Torisu T: Avulsion fracture of the tibial attachment of the posterior cruciate ligament: Indications and results of delayed repair. Clin Orthop Rel Res 143:107, 1979.
352. Toupin JM, Lechevallier J: Fractures osteochondrales du condyle femoral externe apres luxation traumatique de la rotule de l'enfant sportif. Rev Chir Orthop 83:540, 1997.
353. Trail IA: Tibia sequestrectomy in the management of Osgood-Schlatter disease. J Pediatr Orthop 8:554, 1988.
354. Tsunoda M: Bilateral Sinding-Larsen-Johansson disease. A case report with histological investigation. Am J Knee Surg 4:127, 1991.
355. Ure BM, Tiling T, Rodecker K: Arthroscopy of the knee in children and adolescents. Eur J Pediatr Surg 2:102, 1992.
356. Vahasarja V, Kinnunen P, Serlo W: Arthroscopy of the acute traumatic knee in children: Prospective study of 138 cases. Acta Orthop Scand 64:580, 1993.
357. Vahasarja V, Kinnunen P, Serlo W: Arthroscopy in the diagnostics and treatment of non-acute knee disorders in children. Eur J Pediatr Surg 6:25, 1996.
358. Vahvanen V, Aalto K: Meniscectomy in children. Acta Orthop Scand 50:791, 1979.
359. Vandermeer RD, Cunningham FK: Arthroscopic treatment of the discoid lateral meniscus: Results of long-term follow-up. Arthroscopy 5:101, 1989.
360. Vaughan-Lane T, Dandy DJ: The synovial shelf syndrome. J Bone Joint Surg Br 64:475, 1982.
361. Victor J, Gielen J, Martens M, et al: Correlation between magnetic resonance imaging and arthroscopy in the diagnosis of anterior cruciate ligament and meniscus lesions. Acta Orthop Belg 57(Suppl):56, 1991.
362. Vizsolyi P, Taunton J, Robertson G, et al: Breaststroker's knee. An analysis of epidemiological and biomechanical factors. Am J Sports Med 15:63, 1987.
363. Vorne M: Septic Haemophilus influenzae polyarthritis demonstrated best with Tc-99m labeled leukocytes. Clin Nucl Med 15:883, 1990.
364. Walker J, Rang M, Daneman A: Ultrasonography of the unossified patella in young children. J Pediatr Orthop 11:100, 1991.
365. Walker P, Harris I, Leicester A: Patellar tendon-to-patella ratio in children. J Pediatr Orthop 18:129, 1998.
366. Watanabe M, Takeda S, Ikeuchi H: Atlas of Arthroscopy, 3rd ed. Berlin, Springer-Verlag, 1979.
367. Warner J, Micheli L: Pediatric and adolescent musculoskeletal injuries. In Grana WA, Kalanek A, eds: Clinical Sports Medicine. Philadelphia, WB Saunders, 1991, pp 490–498.
368. Washington ER III, Root L, Liener UC: Discoid lateral meniscus in children: Long-term follow-up after excision. J Bone Joint Surg Am 77:1357, 1995.
369. Wasilewski S, Frank U: Osteochondral avulsion fracture of femoral insertion of anterior cruciate ligament. Am J Sports Med 20:224, 1992.
370. Weaver JK: Bipartite patellae as a cause of disability in the athlete. Am J Sports Med 5:137, 1977.
371. Webber A: Acute soft-tissue injuries in the young athlete. Clin Sports Med 7:611, 1988.
372. Weiner D, Macnab I, Turner M: The fabella syndrome. Clin Orthop 126:213, 1977.
373. Weiner DS, Macnab I: The fabella syndrome: An update. J Pediatr Orthop 2:405, 1982.
374. Weiss CB, Lundberg M, Hamberg P, et al: Non-operative treatment of meniscal tears. J Bone Joint Surg Am 71:811, 1989.
375. Wenger DR, Mickelson M, Maynard JA: The evolution and histopathology of adolescent tibia vara. J Pediatr Orthop 4:78, 1984.
376. Wester W, Canale ST, Sutkowsky JP, et al: Prediction of angular deformity and leg-length discrepancy after anterior cruciate ligament reconstruction in skeletally immature patients. J Pediatr Orthop 14:516, 1994.
377. White PH: Growth abnormalities in children with juvenile rheumatoid arthritis. Clin Orthop 259:46, 1990.
378. Wijesekera C: Habitual dislocation of the patella. Ceylon Med J 35:57, 1990.
379. Wiley J, Baxter M: Tibial spine fractures in children. Clin Orthop 255:54, 1990.
380. Williams CL: Lyme disease in childhood: Clinical and epidemiologic features of ninety cases. Pediatr Infect Dis J 9:10, 1990.
381. Williams JS, Abate JA, Fadale PD, et al: Meniscal and nonosseous ACL injuries in children and adolescents. Am J Knee Surg 9:22, 1996.
382. Wiss DA, Schilz JL, Zionts L: Type III fractures of the tibial tubercle in adolescents. J Orthop Trauma 5:475, 1991.
383. Woods G, Whelan J: Discoid meniscus. Clin Sports Med 9:695, 1990.
384. Woolfry BF, Chandler EF: Manifestations of Osgood-Schlatter's disease in late teenage and early aduthood. J Bone Joint Surg Am 42:327, 1960.
385. Wright JG, Menelaus MB, Broughton NS, et al: Natural history of knee contractures in myelomeningocele. J Pediatr Orthop 11:725, 1991.
386. Wroble RR, Henderson RC, Campion ER, et al: Meniscectomy in children and adolescents: A long-term follow-up study. Clin Orthop 279:180, 1992.
387. Wu CD, Huang SC, Liu TK: Sleeve fracture of the patella in children. A report of five cases. Am J Sports Med 19:525, 1991.
388. Yashar A, Loder RT, Hensinger RN: Determination of skeletal age in children with Osood-Schlatter disease by using radiographs of the knee. J Pediatr Orthop 15:298, 1995.
389. Yates CK, Grana WA: Patellofemoral pain in children. Clin Orthop 255:36, 1990.
390. Yerys P: Case report. Arthroscopic posterior cruciate ligament repair. J Arthrosc Rel Surg 7:111, 1991.
391. Zaman M, Leonard MA: Meniscectomy in children: results in 59 knees. Injury 12:425, 1981.
392. Zaricznyj B: Avulsion fracture of the tibial eminence: Treatment by open reduction and pinning. J Bone Joint Surg Am 59:1111, 1977.
393. Zionts LE, MacEwen GD: Spontaneous improvement of post-traumatic tibia valga. J Bone Joint Surg Am 68:680, 1986.
394. Ziv I, Carroll NC: The role of arthroscopy in children. J Pediatr Orthop 2:243, 1982.
395. Zobel MS, Borrello JA, Siegel MJ, et al: Pediatric knee MR imaging: Patterns of injuries in the immature skeleton. Radiology 190:397, 1994.

67

Physeal Fractures About the Knee

MARK L. BURMAN • WILLIAM A. GRANA

In the past several years there has been a large increase in participation in organized sports by children due to the growth of club, recreational, and school sports.[13, 62] With this increase comes an increased risk for injury. The knee is the most common site of injury in childhood sports.[16] Sports trauma is considered to be an important cause of physeal injuries about the knee.[62] Although the anatomy of the child's knee is similar to that of the adult, the distal femoral and proximal tibial physes as well as the tibial tubercle apophysis have a unique potential for injury. These structures respond differently to acute and repetitive loads and often provide less resistance to traumatic forces than do surrounding ligament and bone.[13] Treatment of displaced physeal fractures about the knee remains one of the more difficult problems in orthopedics. Even with appropriate conservative or surgical treatment, a successful outcome is not always certain. Accurate recognition of these injuries and prompt treatment are necessary in order to minimize subsequent complications. Several classification systems have been developed, with the Salter-Harris classification being the best known. They provide general guidelines regarding the risk of growth disturbance. There are, however, no good clinical methods for quantifying the true extent of physeal damage in an acute injury. Ultimately, the value of a treatment method must be evaluated on the basis of restoration of articular congruity, physeal anatomy, and physeal function, as evidenced by the continuation of normal growth.

This chapter reviews the epidemiology of physeal fractures about the knee as well as the anatomy, physiology, and biomechanics of the growth plate as it pertains to these unique fractures. The chapter then discusses fractures of the distal femoral physis, tibial tubercle apophysis, and the intercondylar eminence, all in terms of mechanism of injury, presentation, evaluation, treatment, and outcome.

ANATOMY, PHYSIOLOGY, AND BIOMECHANICS OF THE PHYSIS

The distal femoral and proximal tibial physes are the largest and fastest-growing physes[24, 29, 46, 59] They are responsible for approximately 65% of the total growth of the lower extremity. The physis is a cartilaginous layer that lies between the epiphysis at the end of the long bone and metaphyseal region of the bone. The physis is not a uniform structure but an irregular layer. This configuration enhances the stability of the physis and increases its strength to resist sheer forces. The physes can be divided histologically into four distinct layers, or zones (Fig. 67.1). Beginning at the epiphyseal end is the reserve, or germinal, zone, which is followed by the zone of proliferation and the zone of hypertrophy. The zone of hypertrophy can be subdivided into the zone of maturation, the zone of degeneration, and the zone of provisional calcification, which lies directly above the metaphyseal bone. Most physeal fractures generally occur through or near the zone of provisional calcification within the hypertrophic zone.[13] The level and type of fracture, however, vary according to the unique shape of the physeal plate, the amount of axial compression at the time of injury, and the obliquity of the forces causing the fracture.[24] The irregular shape of the physis, which is designed to enhance its stability, also predisposes it to fractures through more than one zone.[46] The frequency of growth disturbance after physeal fracture is explained by several factors. First, the effective growth risk may be exaggerated due to rapid local growth in the injured bone. Second, injury tends to occur during adolescence, when skeletal growth is accelerated. Third, as previously mentioned, the irregularly-shaped physis may predispose to fracture through more than one zone.[13]

The overall prognosis following physeal fracture depends on several factors: the severity of injury, the age of the patient, the anatomic site of injury, and the type of physeal fracture.[39] The severity of injury is the most important prognostic factor; it includes the mechanism of injury (high-energy or low-energy), the amount of comminution, and open or closed fracture. The patient's age is significant in that most physeal fractures around the knee tend to occur during adolescence. This is fortunate: significant leg-length discrepancies and angular deformities are unlikely because the patient is nearing skeletal maturity. Physeal injuries in younger children, however, do have the potential for significant growth arrest and angular deformities. The anatomic site of injury is important because different physes respond to injury depending on their anatomy, location, and vascular supply. Finally, the type of fracture is prognostic because different fracture configurations will lead to varying amounts of damage to the physeal cells. Several classification schemes for physeal fractures have been described, many of which are designed to aid in overall prognosis. These are discussed later in this chapter.

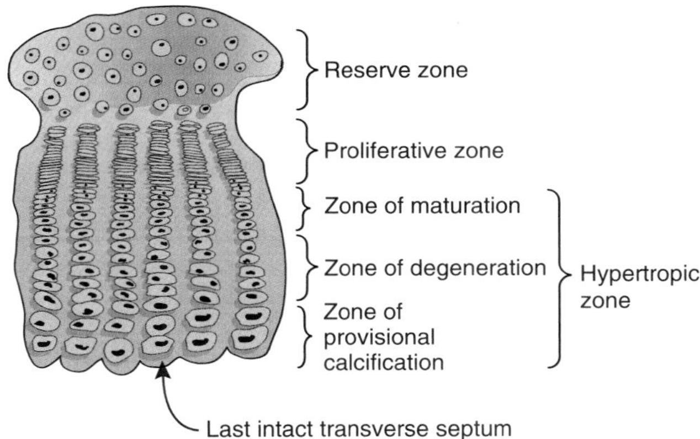

FIGURE 67.1 ➢ Schematic drawing illustrating the layers of the physeal plate. The epiphyseal side of the growth plate is at the top of the drawing. Redrawn from[62].

EPIDEMIOLOGY

Many authors have reported on and tried to quantify the incidence of physeal injuries in children.[4, 12, 26, 31, 44, 62, 66, 70] Values ranging from approximately 15% to 30% of all fractures in children involve the growth plate. An average incidence, calculated at 21.7% of all children's fractures, involved the physis.[66] The upper extremity is involved more often than the lower extremity. Males are injured more frequently than females by a ratio of 2 to 1. The highest rate of physeal fractures occurs in boys aged 14 years and girls aged 11 and 12 years.[40] Although, of all physeal fractures, only 2.2% occur around the knee, they represent a significant amount of all growth arrest, thus requiring surgical correction.

There are many causes of physeal fractures around the knee, high-energy motor vehicle accidents and sports being two common mechanisms. The exact role of sports as a cause for physeal injury is not known; however, some studies have suggested that sports are the major cause of a large proportion of physeal fracture.[24, 60] Two of the most common sports associated with physeal fractures are football and soccer; within these sports, a common mechanism of injury is a clipping-type injury leading to fractures of the distal femoral physis.

CLASSIFICATION OF PHYSEAL FRACTURES

Over the years, many classification systems have been proposed to describe physeal fractures. Foucher,[15] Poland, Johnson and Fahl, Ogden, and Shapiro and Peterson are some of the authors who have proposed classification systems.[20, 23–25, 37, 41, 42, 50] However, the most well-known and widely used classification scheme is that proposed by Salter and Harris in 1963[49] (Fig. 67.2). In this scheme, there are five fracture types, and the classification is based on the anatomic and radiographic appearance of the fracture types. Furthermore, this scheme is useful because treatment can be planned based on fracture type.

In Salter-Harris type I fractures, the fracture line traverses the physes, staying entirely within it. Type II fractures are the most common. The fracture line traverses the growth plate for a variable length and then exits obliquely through the metaphysis. Type III fractures also begin in the physis but exit through the epiphysis toward the joint. Type IV fractures involve a vertical split of the epiphysis, physis, and metaphysis. Type V fractures are crush injuries to the physeal plate and are usually apparent only in retrospect. From a prognostic point of view, types I and II are extra-articular; types III and IV involve an intra-articular fragment and require anatomic reduction. Type V involves crush injuries and often significant damage to the physis, which is only appreciated in retrospect.

The Salter-Harris classification was originally intended to act in a prognostic fashion. Types I, II, and III have an excellent prognosis for avoiding physeal

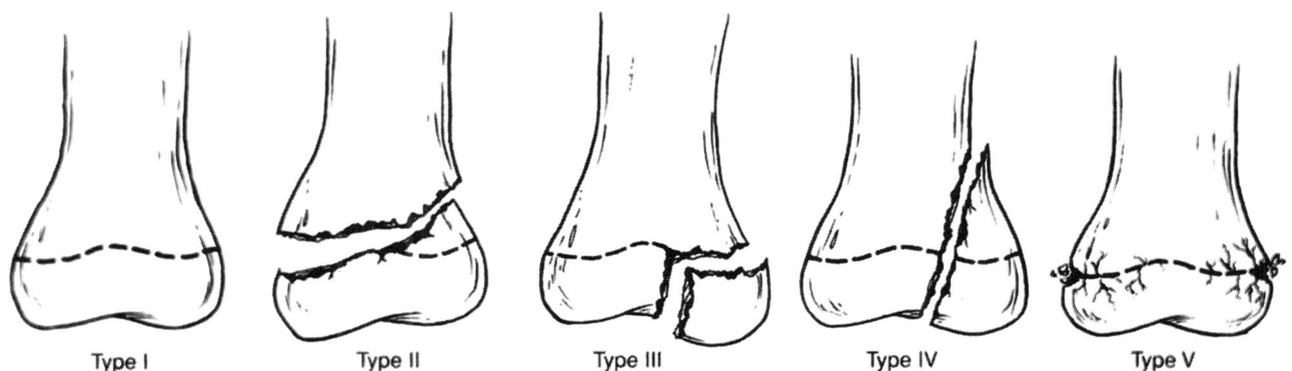

FIGURE 67.2 ➢ The Salter-Harris classification of physeal fractures. In type I fractures, the fracture line traverses the physis, staying entirely within it. In type II injuries, the fracture line traverses the growth plate for a variable length and then exits obliquely through the metaphysis. Type III fractures also begin in the physis but exit throughout the epiphysis toward the joint. Type IV fractures involve a vertical split of the epiphysis, physis, and metaphysis. Type V fractures are crush injuries to the physeal plate.

arrest because the blood supply for the injured physis remains intact. Type III fractures have a poorer prognosis than the first two because there is an intra-articular fragment that requires anatomic reduction. Type IV fractures have a still poorer prognosis if they are not anatomically reduced due to the intra-articular extension and the disruption of the metaphyseal and epiphyseal circulation. Type V injuries have the worst prognosis because of the crushing nature of the injury to the physes. Several subsequent studies have questioned the correlation between the Salter-Harris type and subsequent growth arrests. Overall, however, the Salter-Harris classification is still the most widely accepted classification due to its ease of use and reproducibility.

MANAGEMENT PRINCIPLES

The physician treating a physeal injury as with any other injury should perform a thorough history and physical examination as well as have a high index of suspicion. A careful history must include a detailed mechanism of injury, a history of any underlying bone or metabolic condition that may adversely affect the skeleton, and any history of trauma that may also have had an effect on the bone or physeal area in question. Given that the growth plate is the weak link in structures around the joint, one must have a high index of suspicion and look for physeal injury with any knee injury in a growing child. Certain mechanisms are classically associated with various physeal injuries around the knee, and they must also raise one's suspicions for a physeal injury until proven otherwise. Examples of these mechanisms include football clipping injuries in association with distal femoral physeal injuries[48] and falls from a bicycle associated with fractures of the intercondylar eminence.[27] One must also be ready to consider the possibility of child abuse in any physeal fracture in a young child.

During physical examination, a careful inspection is made of the entire injured extremity, particularly of the joints above and below; in the case of a high-energy trauma, the physician must carefully rule out other systemic and visceral injuries. A careful neurovascular examination of the affected limb is extremely important as significant injuries about the knee may be associated with limb-threatening neurovascular injury. Even though the physis is weaker than the ligamentous structures about the knee, the presence of a physeal injury does not exclude the possibility of a coexisting ligamentous disruption. The incidence of ligamentous instability about the knee in association with physeal injuries has been estimated to be 48%. Of this percentage, 38% is anterior cruciate ligament (ACL) injury, 17% is medial collateral ligament (MCL) injuries, and 7% is combined ACL/MCL instabilities.[3] These findings emphasize the importance of a careful ligamentous examination of the knee, especially once fracture fixation has been carried out.

Diagnosis of a physeal injury is often easily made with simple, plain radiographs. Two orthogonal views are mandatory, and additional oblique views are often quite helpful in picking up more subtle injuries, especially small, metaphyseal fragments in type II injuries (Thurston-Holland sign). As with many other pediatric skeletal injuries, one should not hesitate in requesting a comparison view of the contralateral side in order to better delineate the appearance of the physes in question. Stress views are useful in demonstrating a physeal injury that is not readily apparent on plain views of the knee, especially in a patient with apparent collateral ligament laxity. One must be very cautious with the use of stress views in that any excessive and unnecessary manipulation of a physeal fracture may have a detrimental effect on the already injured growth plate. Tomograms, computed tomography scans, arthrograms, and ultrasonography have all been used to assess physeal fractures; however, they are rarely necessary in physeal fractures about the knee. In recent years, investigators have looked at the usefulness of magnetic resonance imaging (MRI) in the evaluation of acute physeal injuries. MRI may be helpful in cases of complex or radiographically occult physeal injuries.[9, 19, 47, 64]

The treatment of physeal fractures follows several principles based on the unique physiology of the physis. Manipulation of a physeal fracture should be gentle to avoid further damage to the physis. In the tense and apprehensive child, general anesthesia provides the best relaxation and consequently allows the most gentle manipulation. Physeal fractures heal rapidly, with healing time generally half that for nonphyseal fractures in the patient of the same age.[13] Weight-bearing on healing physeal fractures should be discouraged because of risk of further damage to the physeal cartilage.

In cases where internal fixation is deemed necessary, one should make every effort to avoid crossing the growth plate with hardware if at all possible. When the growth plate has to be crossed in order to achieve adequate fixation, small-diameter smooth pins should be placed in as perpendicular an orientation to the physis as possible in order to minimize further damage to the already traumatized growth plate.

FRACTURES OF THE DISTAL FEMORAL PHYSIS

General

The distal femoral physis has a large surface area and a complex undulating contour and shape. These protect the physis and help resist injury. However, this complex design also accounts for the high incidence of growth arrest and angular deformities seen with distal femoral physeal injuries, even with the less severe Salter-Harris type I and II fracture patterns. These injuries may account for a large amount of shear across the physis, which results in greater injury than otherwise expected with these fracture patterns. The distal femoral physis is the largest and most active physis in the body. It is extra-articular and has a rich blood supply. Its orientation is concave in the coronal plane. The distal femoral physis contributes approximately

70% to total femoral growth and approximately 40% to total growth of the entire lower limb. Longitudinal growth occurs at the rate of 0.95 cm per year at the distal femoral physis. This physis fuses between ages 9 and 19 years.[5, 9] Fractures of the distal femoral physis account for 1% to 6% of all physeal injuries.[54, 59] These injuries are most common during adolescence, especially at the time of a growth spurt, with the highest incidence between ages 11 and 15 years. Males predominate over females, but with increased female participation in sports these numbers are changing. Girls' injuries occur most commonly between the ages of 8 and 15 years, and boys' injuries occur between the ages of 12 and 16 years.

Mechanism of Injury

Historically, the distal femoral physis has been recognized as a common and important site of bone injury in children. In the 19th century, "the wagon wheel" or "cart wheel" injury frequently produced neurovascular compromise and severe deformity. A young boy who tried to jump onto a moving cart or wagon would catch his leg or foot in the wheel spokes, causing a forced hyperextension from the rotary force of the wheel. This hyperextension injury caused displacement of the epiphysis anteriorly in the sagittal plane while the distal end of the bone was displaced posteriorly into the popliteal space, resulting in a high incidence of popliteal neurovascular injuries. Over time, the occurrence and complications associated with this fracture have decreased, and vehicular trauma and sports have become the most common causes of injury. According to Tachdjian,[59] motor vehicle accidents account for 50% of all distal femoral epiphyseal fractures, with football accounting for 20%, fall from heights 15%, and miscellaneous causes 15%. Sponseller and Beaty[54] found sports injuries to account for 49% of all distal femoral physeal injuries, with vehicular trauma 30% and falls 12% of injuries.

Excluding birth fractures, there are two types of distal femoral physeal fractures. Juvenile-type injuries (age 2 to 10 years) more commonly follow a high-energy injury, such as a motor vehicle accident.[13] Common associated injuries include other extremity fractures, local vascular injuries, and intra-abdominal and intra-thoracic injuries. Adolescent-type injuries (age 11 years and older) frequently present after a low-energy injury, which is often sports-related. The thinner perichondral ring in the older age group provides less resistance to fracture. Approximately two-thirds of distal femoral physeal injuries have been found to occur in this adolescent group.[54]

The distal femoral physeal fracture is usually a Salter-Harris type II injury with displacement in the coronal plane. This is closely followed by a Salter-Harris type I injury.[24, 29, 46] A valgus force produces medial physeal separation, often with associated sprain of the MCL. The force traverses the physis and exits laterally with an oblique fracture through the metaphysis. A hyperextension mechanism of injury, although rare, can also be responsible, which is important because of the potential for neurovascular injury at the posterior edge of the displaced metaphysis (as in the "wagon wheel" injury).

Presentation and Evaluation

A patient with a distal femoral physeal fracture usually presents with a large hemarthrosis and local swelling of the extremity. The patient is usually unable to bear weight and may describe a "pop" at the time of the injury. There is often circumferential tenderness over the physis and crepitation with motion. The anatomic landmark for the distal femoral physis is at the same level as the superior pole of the patella and the adductor tubercle. One may appreciate abnormal motion above the level of the knee, at the level of the physis, associated with crepitation. The knee is often held in a flexed position due to hamstring spasm, and there is often angular limb malalignment in a varus or valgus direction. The prominence of the metaphyseal edge often causes a deformity that is easily palpable. In the hyperextension injury, there is anterior skin dimpling. Apparent laxity of the knee corresponds to that which would be seen in an adult ligamentous injury. Evaluation should include a thorough examination for associated injuries as well as careful appraisal of the knee itself. A thorough neurovascular examination of the involved extremity is essential. Anterior, posterior, lateral, and oblique radiographs are required to evaluate the fracture. Stress radiographs or MRI may be needed to evaluate laxity of the knee when plain radiographs appear normal, unless the laxity is clearly of ligamentous origin. (However, in the skeletally immature, this is difficult without radiographs.) Care should be exercised with a stress test to prevent additional injury to the growth plate. In displaced hyperextension injuries, a careful neurovascular examination is necessary, and an arteriogram may be required if there is any suspicion of vascular compromise on clinical examination. If arteriography is not performed, careful monitoring with Doppler or another noninvasive modality is recommended.

Treatment

The treatment of distal femoral physeal fractures is dictated by the fracture type and the amount of displacement. Whatever the form of treatment, an anatomic reduction of this fracture is mandatory. When there is displacement of the physis posteriorly, there will often be an associated loss of extension and extensor mechanism dysfunction with possible patellar impingement on the residual anterior deformity.[29]

Nondisplaced fractures are immobilized in a long leg cast or a hip spica, depending on the patient's body type and ability to maintain fracture immobilization.[46, 54, 58] An obese patient typically requires more extensive immobilization. Knee position is dictated by the direction of fracture displacement, given the principle that the forces involved in producing the injury are reversed and that the intact periosteal hinge is tightened.[54] Posteriorly displaced fractures are immobilized in full extension, and anteriorly displaced fractures are immobilized in 30 degrees of flexion. Varus and valgus deformities are corrected for as well.

Displaced Salter-Harris type I or II injuries are gently manipulated with closed techniques and immobilized in a cast.[29, 46, 54, 58] Such injuries are usually stable once reduced. In the adolescent patient, fractures can be manipulated up to 10 days following injury, and repeat reduction is possible 1 week after the primary attempt.[13, 54, 62] As previously mentioned, anatomic reduction is the goal; however, angulation up to 15 degrees in the anteroposterior direction can be well tolerated. Deformity in the varus or valgus plane will usually not remodel with further growth.[54] Riseborough et al[46] reported that up to 80% of Salter-Harris type II injuries can be well managed conservatively. Following closed reduction and casting, radiographs should be repeated after approximately 1 week of immobilization to ensure that displacement has not occurred.[54] The patient is to remain non-weightbearing for 3 to 6 weeks, and isometric exercises may be started once symptoms permit. By 4 to 8 weeks, the patient is removed from the cast and begun on gentle range-of-motion exercises. In the athletic population, return to sports may not be permitted until all symptoms are completely resolved, the knee has regained full range of motion, and the patient has regained full quadriceps strength equivalent to that of the other side.

Displaced Salter-Harris type I or II fractures that are unstable will require fixation. Percutaneous smooth-pin fixation under fluoroscopic imaging is recommended. Preferably, the hardware should not cross the physis. However, displaced, unstable type I injuries and unstable type II injuries with small metaphyseal fragments will require transphyseal pins (Fig. 67.3). In type II injuries, if there is a large metaphyseal fragment (Thurston-Holland fragment), a threaded pin or screw may be directed horizontally across the metaphysis following reduction in order to stabilize the fracture, thereby avoiding crossing the physis (Fig. 67.4). Displaced type I and II fractures that cannot be acceptably reduced closed should be treated with open reduction.[13, 24, 29, 46, 54] The most common reason for irreducibility is trapping of a large periosteal flap in the fracture site.

Aside from failed attempts at closed reduction of Salter-Harris type I and II fractures, other indications for open reduction internal fixation include displaced Salter-Harris type III and IV fractures, open injuries, and injuries with associated neurovascular compromise. Occasionally, displaced type III and IV fractures can be successfully reduced by closed techniques and can be pinned percutaneously parallel to the physis. In the majority of cases, however, open reduction and internal fixation with smooth wires or screws are required to restore articular congruity.[13] These fractures are approached via anteromedial or anterolateral longitudinal incisions. An arthrotomy should be peformed to allow for direct visualization of the articular surface and to properly ascertain an anatomic reduction at the level of the joint. The ideal form of fixation is with pins or screws placed parallel to the physis, above it, below it, or both, depending on the fracture pattern,

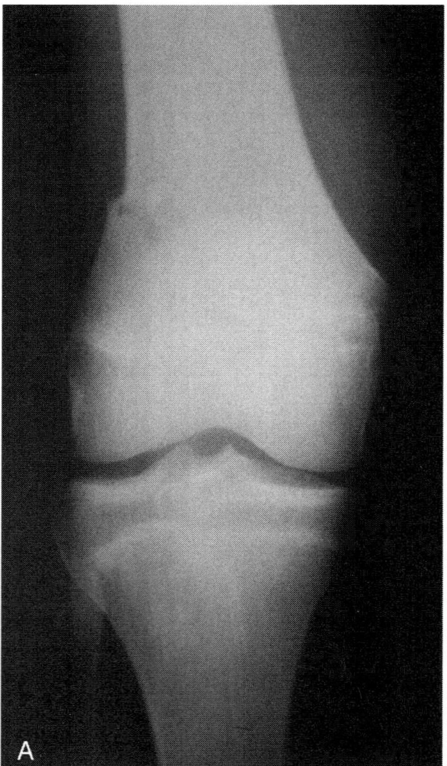

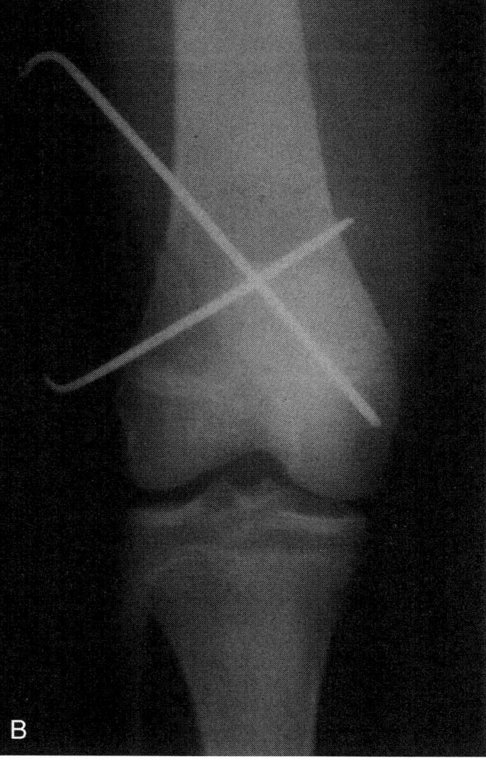

FIGURE 67.3 ➢ *A,* 16-year-old male who suffered a Salter-Harris type II distal femur fracture playing football. *B,* Fixation achieved with crossed smooth Kirschner wires.

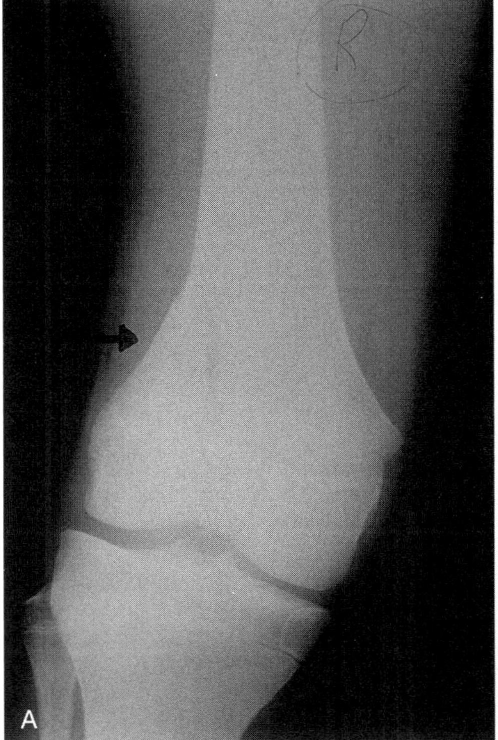

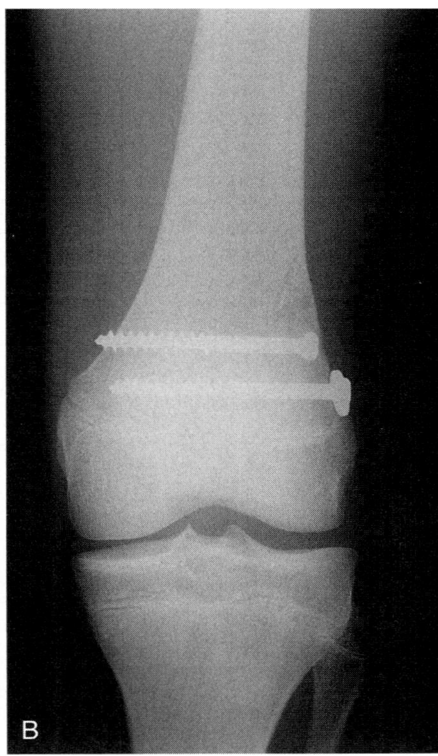

FIGURE 67.4 ➢ *A,* 17-year-old female, injured playing soccer, with Salter-Harris type II distal femoral fracture. Note the large Thurston-Holland fragment *(arrow). B,* Fixation with percutaneous 6.5-mm cancellous screws. Note how the hardware does not cross the growth plate.

in order to stabilize the fracture. Such an approach provides solid fixation and avoids crossing the physis with fixation hardware (Fig. 67.5).

Although damage to the physis at the time of injury is the most common cause of growth arrest, failure to obtain adequate alignment or loss of initial reduction also leads to growth disturbance or angular deformity. Consequently, careful radiographic follow-up is recommended for all fractures. Patients should be monitored until skeletal maturity or until a stable growth patterning is assured to watch for any sequelae such as growth arrest or angular deformity.

Outcome

Distal femoral physeal fractures generally heal predictably with good outcomes. Patients can usually return to normal activities within 4 to 6 months. Complications associated with fractures of the distal femoral physis include popliteal artery injury (1%), peroneal nerve injury (3%), knee stiffness (16%), and angular deformity or leg length discrepancy, which have been the two most common complications seen.[54] Significant shortening is seen in 30% to 50% of adolescent fractures and in more than 50% of juvenile fractures.[13] Lombardo and Harvey[24] found that 36% of patients with distal femoral physeal fractures had shortening greater than 2 cm. Riseborough et al,[46] in their review of 66 distal femoral physeal fractures, found that 37 (56%) had a significant growth arrest. Sponseller and Beaty[54] noted leg length discrepancy in 24% of injuries and angular deformity in 19%. Associated ligamentous injury has also been reported; the incidence varies from 24% to 44% of distal femoral physeal fractures. The ACL is the ligament most often injured.[1, 3, 24, 58]

Loss of reduction is a common occurrence, especially once swelling subsides or if a stable reduction was not achieved initially. For this reason, repeat x-ray films within a week are recommended; if the reduction is lost, then fixation is recommended.

Risk factors for angular deformity and shortening include metaphyseal displacement of greater than half the shaft diameter and relative degrees of skeletal maturity. Although as much as one-third of patients sustain damage to the physis at the time of injury,[54] the adolescent population close to skeletal maturity usually does not have significant shortening or angular deformity. Growth arrest is noted in 6 to 12 months in most cases, but final evaluation 2 years after the injury is recommended to identify atypical growth problems. While yearly follow-up until skeletal maturity will guarantee picking up any growth abnormalities, many authors feel that 2 years is sufficient if there is no evidence of any growth disturbance.[13, 54]

Leg length inequality of less than 2 cm is usually managed conservatively. Larger discrepancies require a contralateral epiphysiodesis or, rarely, an ipsilateral leg lengthening procedure. Other treatment options include physeal stapling, leg shortening procedures, and physeal bar resection. These techniques are beyond the scope of this chapter.

Angular deformity is caused by malunion or asymmetrical growth. An angular deformity greater than 5 degrees may develop in up to one-third of patients

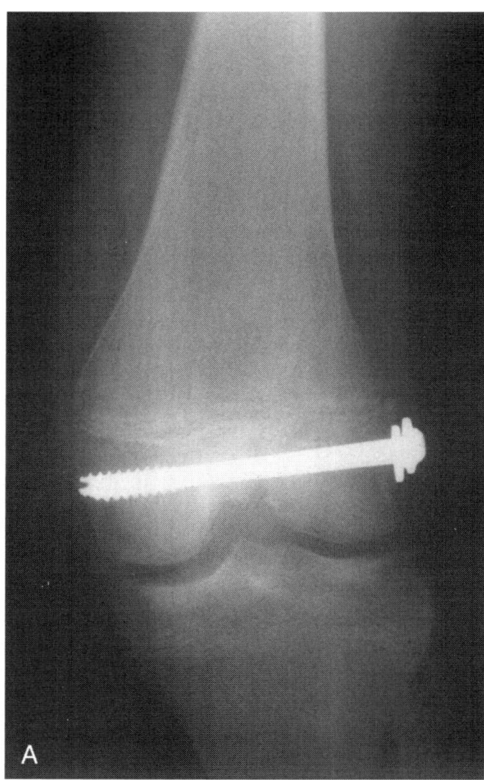

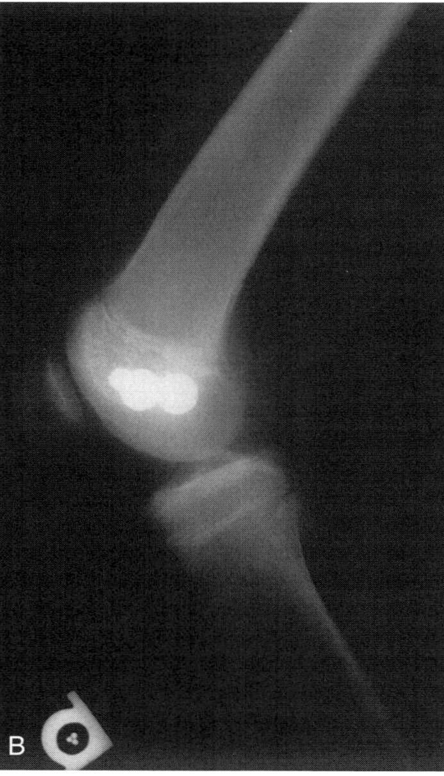

FIGURE 67.5 ➢ 11-year-old female with a Salter-Harris type III distal femur fracture. Note the intra-articular extension. The fracture was fixed with cannulated screw fixation, avoiding the growth plate with the hardware.[13]

with distal femoral physeal fractures,[13] but on average it occurs in 20%.[54] Usually, local growth arrest occurs opposite the metaphyseal (Thurston-Holland) fragment.[49] In the common valgus injury, this causes medial growth arrest with a subsequent varus deformity. Treatment options include excision of the osseous bridge, or osteotomy. In the series of Riseborough et al,[46] 16 of 66 patients required osteotomy because of angular deformity.

In cases of neurovascular injury, the outcome depends on timely initial treatment. Peroneal nerve injury is managed by early closed manipulation of the fracture. Observation with late nerve exploration is indicated if there is no recovery. Popliteal artery injuries that are diagnosed and treated rapidly usually present no long-term problems. The presence of compartment syndrome must be considered, and fasciotomy may be necessary. Circumferential immobilization is to be avoided initially.

FRACTURES OF THE PROXIMAL TIBIAL PHYSIS

General and Mechanism of Injury

Although knee injuries in children are quite common, proximal tibial physeal injuries are not, representing fewer than 1% of all physeal injuries.[16, 26, 59] The majority of these are seen in adolescent boys from the ages of 8 to 15 years. The physis of the proximal tibia is well protected by ligamentous attachments distal to the epiphysis and by the presence of the proximal tibiofibular joint, which buttresses the physis laterally. The tibial tubercle projects down from the epiphysis to overhang the proximal metaphysis anteriorly, and the insertion of the semimembranosus muscle spans the physis on the posteromedial side.

Proximal tibial physeal fractures usually occur as a result of indirect force, with the most common mechanism of injury being a valgus force that produces a Salter-Harris type II fracture and an associated greenstick fracture of the fibula.[7, 29, 51, 59] The physis opens medially, often with concomitant injury to the medial collateral ligament. The fracture line then traverses the physis and exits the lateral metaphysis, creating an oblique fracture. In addition to associated MCL injuries, ACL injuries have also been found in association with these fractures. Bertin and Goble in 1983[3] found this to occur in 62% of their cases. In addition, associated avulsion fractures of the tibial spines resulting in ACL laxity were found in 5 of the 15 patients in Poulsen's series.[43]

As occurs with fractures of the distal femoral physis, hyperextension injuries occasionally involve the potential for serious neurovascular injury, especially with posterior displacement of a metaphyseal fragment into the popliteal fossa. The popliteal artery is tethered to the posterior tibial metaphysis by its articular branches, and the metaphyseal edge can cause local compression or laceration of the artery. The series of 31 patients of Wozasek et al[71] in 1991 had five patients with limb ischemia, four of whom were present before reduction and that resolved once the fracture was reduced.

Due to its soft-tissue protection, fractures of the proximal tibial physis require a significant amount of trauma to cause displacement. Thus, they are not as common as other fractures about the knee, especially in sports.

Presentation and Evaluation

As stated, proximal tibial physeal fractures occur most commonly in adolescent boys.[13, 54] The signs and symptoms include pain, swelling, hemarthrosis, and the inability to bear weight. Typically, the leg is held in flexion due to hamstring spasm, and tenderness is present along the area of the physis just distal to the joint line. The displaced metaphyseal edge may be palpable subcutaneously, and in hyperextension injuries skin dimpling can be seen over the anterior metaphysis. Neurovascular status is carefully evaluated as with fractures of the distal femoral physis. Any suspicion of vascular injury should be thoroughly worked up, including the use of angiogram. In addition to neurovascular injury, other concomitant injuries must be sought out, including ligamentous injury and associated fractures. Injuries to the ipsilateral distal femoral physis may be seen; this is analogous to an adult floating knee. Associated involvement of the tibial tubercle and tibial spines must be ruled out as well.

Anteroposterior, lateral, and oblique radiographs are the standard imaging modalities used in the diagnosis of these injuries. Stress radiographs may be useful when there is a question about the origin of medial laxity (Fig. 67.6). Tomograms and computed tomography scans are also helpful in identifying fractures involving the articular surface (Salter-Harris types III and IV) (Fig. 67.7). MRI is used to identify soft-tissue interposition when closed reduction is found to be difficult. Interposition of the pes anserinus has been reported.[69] Approximately two-thirds of these fractures are Salter Harris type I or II injuries.[13]

Treatment

Salter-Harris type I and II injuries are treated with gentle closed manipulation and application of a long leg cast.[7, 13, 54, 59, 71] The length of immobilization in a cast varies with recommendations varying from 4 to 8 weeks.[54, 59] The position of the knee in the cast will depend on the direction of displacement of the initial fracture. A type II fracture is usually stable after manipulation; when unstable, percutaneous metaphyseal pinning is indicated. Ideally, smooth pins or cannulated screws are placed through the metaphyseal fragment parallel to the physis. If the fragment is too small, however, transphyseal pins are necessary. Once again, as with other physeal fractures, small-diameter smooth pins are used. The pins should cross the physis in as perpendicular a plane as possible and not converge at the physis in order to optimize stability. The use of an intraoperative fluoroscope is helpful to ascertain the position of the pins and to be sure they do not enter the joint. When closed manipulation fails, open reduction is indicated.[7, 13, 51, 54, 59, 71] Soft-tissue interposition such as an interposed periosteal flap in the fracture site is the usual cause of inadequate reduction. Open reduction with pin fixation or the use of cannulated screws followed by a noncircumferential immobilization is then necessary. Radiographs are required to detect early or late displacement of a satisfactorily reduced fracture. Follow-up x-ray films at 1 week are generally obtained.

Salter-Harris type III and IV injuries are usually treated with open reduction and internal fixation[7, 13, 51, 54, 59, 71] (Fig. 67.8). As with any intra-articular fracture, correction of incongruent articular surface is mandatory. Minimally displaced fractures are often quite unstable, and internal fixation should be considered even in these fractures.[51] In performing an open reduction, an anterior incision is often used, and a small arthrotomy is performed to inspect the articular surface. Fixation usually involves pin or screw fixation parallel to the physis, either proximal, distal, or both in order to achieve stable fixation and to avoid disruption of the growth plate. The primary repair of associated ligamentous injuries should also be considered at the time of open reduction. When osseous fixation is achieved, the knee is examined again for ligamentous laxity. Following treatment, the patient is monitored for a minimum of 2 years or until skeletal maturity, looking for signs of angular deformity, growth arrest, or persistent instability.

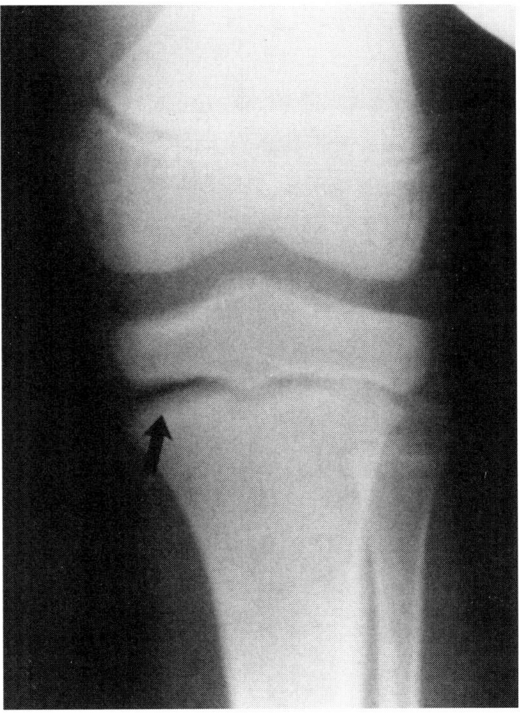

FIGURE 67.6 ➢ Stress radiograph demonstrating physeal separation without joint space widening.[13]

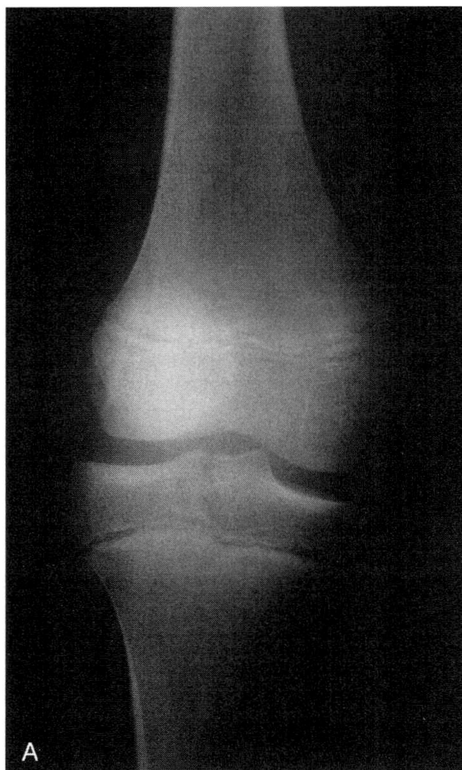

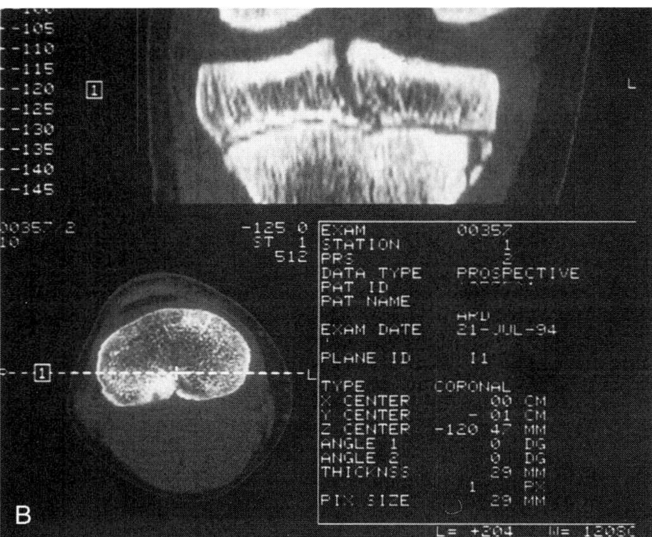

FIGURE 67.7 ➢ *A,* 13-year-old male with a Salter-Harris type IV proximal tibia fracture. *B,* Note the intra-articular extension and that the metaphyseal fragment is only appreciated on the computer tomography image.[13]

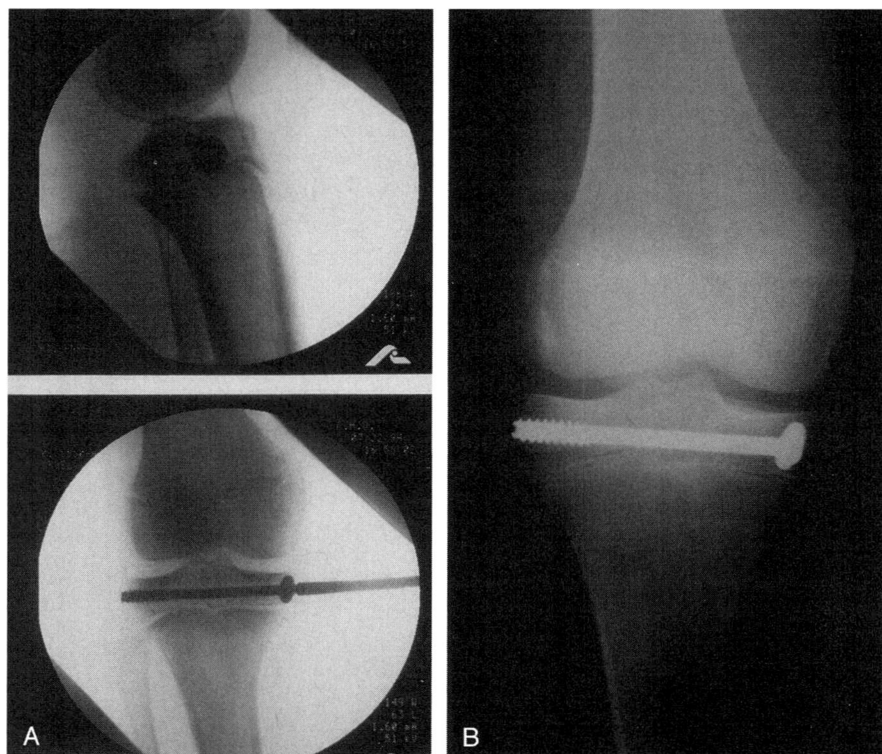

FIGURE 67.8 ➢ *A,* Intraoperative images of cannulated screw fixation of the fracture in Figure 67.7. *B,* Final result with a well-healed fracture and hardware avoiding the physis.

Outcome

Proximal tibial physeal fractures heal predictably, and nonunions are rare. Problems with significant shortening and angulation are less common than with distal femoral injuries because of the smaller contribution of the proximal tibial physis to overall limb growth. The proximal tibial physis contributes approximately one-quarter of an inch of growth per year.[54]

Shelton and Canale[51] reported 86% satisfactory results in their series of 28 patients; however, they also found leg length inequality of more than 1 cm could be expected in 20% of the patients. Burkhart and Peterson[7] found 76% satisfactory results in their subgroup of 21 patients with proximal tibial physeal injuries that were not due to lawnmower injuries. As with the distal femur, growth arrest is more common than elsewhere in the appendicular skeleton, even with Salter-Harris type I and II fractures.[7, 51] Salter-Harris type IV fractures are almost always associated with some amount of growth arrest or angular deformity.[59] Sponseller and Beaty[54] found an overall incidence of growth disturbance of 10%.

Treatment for these growth disturbances is accomplished by contralateral epiphysiodesis or ipsilateral lengthening, depending on the amount of shortening that must be overcome to achieve leg length equality. If the patient is monitored over time with sequential growth measurements on a growth chart, one can fairly accurately predict the amount of leg length discrepancy. In general, leg length discrepancies of less than 2 cm can be treated conservatively. Discrepancies of 2.5 to 5 cm are usually treated with epiphysiodesis of the contralateral side at the appropriate time. Discrepancies of greater than 5 cm often require limb lengthening procedures.[8, 13, 54]

Angular deformity occurs because of asymmetrical growth arrest or malunion. This is treated with physeal bar excision if less than 30% to 50% of the physis is involved. Corrective osteotomy is usually required when a larger physeal bar is present.[21, 54]

Other associated complications with these fractures include vascular impairment (10%), peroneal palsy (3%), and knee instability or degenerative joint disease (20%).[54] The development of degenerative joint changes in the knee are generally related to Salter-Harris type III and IV fractures with intra-articular involvement. Open injuries to the proximal tibia have a much worse prognosis and are frequently the result of lawnmower injuries. Causes of vascular impairment following a tibial physeal fracture include direct popliteal artery injury/disruption or compartment syndrome. Burkhart and Peterson's series[7] included a 12-year-old hurdler, treated with closed reduction and long leg cast, who subsequently developed a compartment syndrome. Nicholson[34] reported on a patient with a completely severed popliteal artery and vein after sustaining a proximal tibial physeal injury while playing football. Vascular injuries are catastrophic, and a high level of suspicion must be maintained for these injuries, especially in hyperextension-type injuries and injuries with posterior metaphyseal displacement. Associated ligamentous instability can involve the MCL or ACL, and one should assess for these injuries immediately following bony stabilization.

FRACTURES OF THE TIBIAL TUBERCLE APOPHYSIS

Acute isolated fracture of the tibial tubercle is quite rare. Stanitski[56] found a total of 106 reported cases. This is in contrast to the high frequency of chronic injury of this anatomic region. As in the juvenile Tillaux fracture, the differential rate of physeal closure of the tubercle apophysis plays an important role. In the period of preclosure of the physis, between the ages of 12 and 16 years, the apophysis matures, and columnar hypertrophic cells become dominant.[30, 37] The columnar cells do not resist traction as well as their fibrocartilaginous precursors. A severe concentric or eccentric contraction of the extensor mechanism produces a fracture through this level of the apophysis.[13, 22, 30, 36, 56, 59] This injury is therefore usually seen in athletic-type activities where the knee is forcibly flexed against a contracted or resisting quadriceps. Common activities include high jump, basketball, and football.[13, 56, 59]

Mechanism of Injury

Certain predisposing risk factors for these fractures include patella infera with tight hamstrings and possibly preexisting Osgood-Schlatter disease.[54] Acute apophyseal fracture must be distinguished from the Osgood-Schlatter condition. Although both conditions involve traction force through the immature physis, the rate of loading and the magnitude of the force are different. Osgood-Schlatter condition is a chronic avulsion of the anterior surface of the tubercle, whereas the tubercle fracture is an acute avulsion through the apophysis.[26, 59] Several reports suggest that Osgood-Schlatter condition may predate apophyseal fracture in 12% to 60% of cases.[56] Ogden et al[36] suggested a biomechanical link between these conditions, but this hypothesis has yet to be documented.

Classification

Acute tibial tubercle avulsion fracture is classified in several ways. Watson-Jones[63] described three fracture types, depending on the amount of tibial epiphyseal involvement. This classification was expanded by Ogden et al[36] (Fig. 67.9). In this system, fractures are divided on the basis of the severity of displacement. Type I is a distal fracture through the physis, with breakout through the secondary ossification center. Type II is a more proximal fracture through the cartilage bridge between the ossification center of the tubercle and the proximal tibial physis. Type III propagates upward through the proximal tibial physis into the knee. This latter type is considered a Salter-Harris type IV fracture (Fig. 67.10). Ogden's classification is subtyped into an A and B category. Subtype A fractures are noncomminuted, and subtype B fractures are

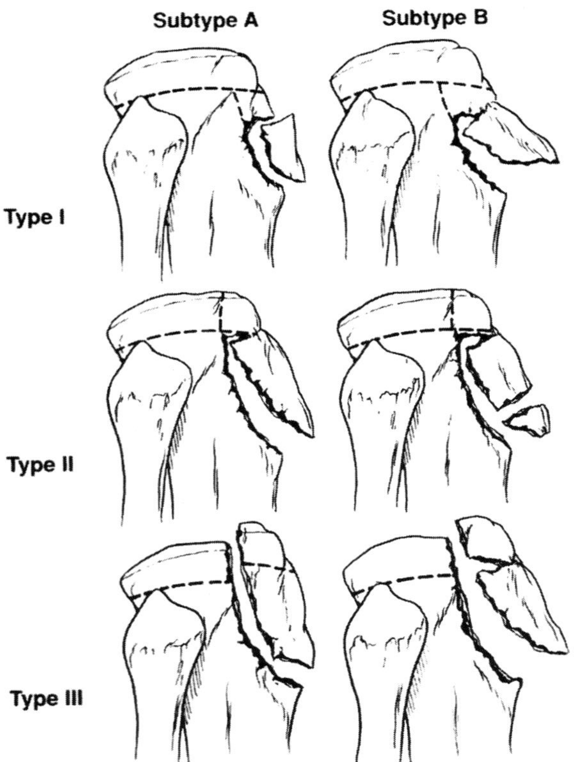

FIGURE 67.9 ➢ Classification of tibial tubercle fractures according to the system developed by Ogden et al. Type I is a distal fracture through the physis with breakout through the secondary ossification center. Type II is a more proximal fracture through the cartilage bridge between the ossification center of the tubercle and the proximal tibial physis. Type III propagates upward through the proximal tibial physis into the knee. Subtype A fractures are noncomminuted; subtype B fractures are comminuted.[13]

comminuted. Type I fractures are the most common, but the exact incidence of this injury is not clear because of the cross-classification with proximal tibial physeal fractures.[36, 46]

Presentation and Evaluation

The typical patient presents with a history of acute injury during participation in a jumping sport: basketball, football, high jump, diving, and competitive running have all been implicated.[13, 54] As previously mentioned, the mechanism is usually a strong contraction of the quadriceps muscle against a fixed tibia or passive flexion of the knee against a contracted quadriceps. This occurs when the athlete takes off or lands during a jump. A sudden acceleration or deceleration of the extensor mechanism is therefore involved.[54, 56] The typical patient is usually male, age 14 to 16 years, and near skeletal maturity.[16, 36, 56] There is often swelling and tenderness over the area of the tibial tubercle. An effusion is seen associated with fractures with an intra-articular involvement or with associated intra-articular injuries, such as meniscal tear, chondral, or cruciate ligament injuries.[5, 14]

Occasionally a mobile, subcutaneous piece of bone is palpated, and crepitus is felt. The knee is held in a flexed position because of the swelling and hamstring spasm. Active knee extension is possible in type I fractures, but not in type II or III injuries as there is often a discontinuity or disruption in the extensor mechanism.[36, 56] Patella alta is observed in fractures with significant displacement.

Evaluation should include standard anteroposterior, lateral, and oblique radiographs of the knee. A lateral view is necessary to classify these fractures adequately. Oblique views may demonstrate unexpected propagation of the fracture into the knee.

Treatment

Nondisplaced type I injuries are treated in a cylinder cast, with the knee in full extension for 4 to 6 weeks.[36, 56] For all displaced fractures (types I, II, and III), most authors advocate open reduction and internal fixation followed by cast immobilization in extension for 4 to 6 weeks.[16, 29, 36, 54, 56] The fracture is usually approached through an anterior vertical incision. Care is taken to clean the fracture bed of all debris. Occasionally, a periosteal flap is found interposed in this fracture site. This flap is removed and repaired with direct suture after fixation of the osseous injury. In the presence of a type III fracture (one that extends into the joint), the menisci are inspected

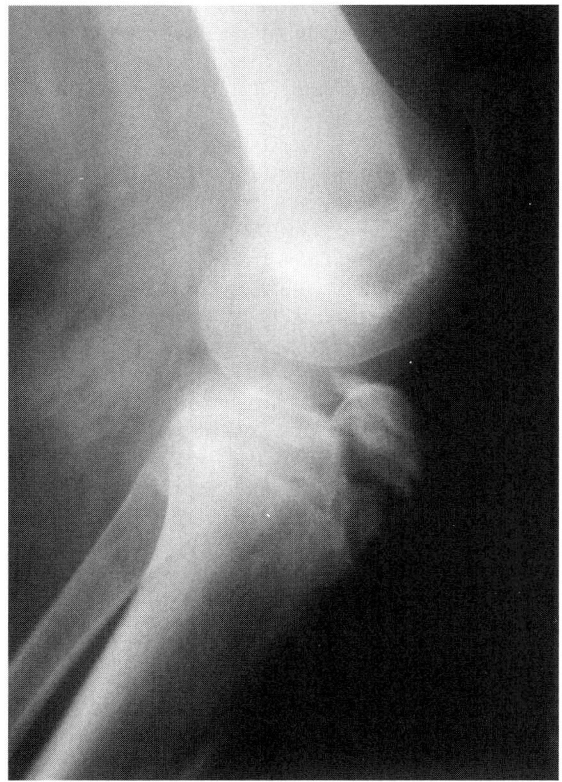

FIGURE 67.10 ➢ 12-year-old male with an Ogden type III tibial tubercle fracture. Note how one may consider this to be a Salter-Harris type IV proximal tibial fracture.

to rule out tears.[54] Closed reduction methods may be used for very minimally displaced fractures when the extensor mechanism is intact and the patient can actively extend the knee fully. When open reduction and internal fixation are necessary, fixation options include direct suturing, pin, screw, or tension band wire fixation.[29, 36, 56] Anatomic reduction is necessary to restore the proper resting length of the extensor mechanism. This decreases the possibility of patella baja or patella alta resulting from inadvertent shortening or lengthening of the extensor mechanism.[2]

Outcome

Complications following tibial apophyseal fracture are quite uncommon. The fracture heals well and essentially by epiphysiodesis, be it naturally or surgically induced. Most, if not all, patients can return to normal function and normal sporting activities.[5, 10, 22, 36] Usually, no leg length discrepancy or genu recurvatum deformity occurs because the injury happens in the age group of patients who are undergoing apophyseal closure.[36, 54, 56] Prominence of the tubercle with local sensitivity[22] and patellofemoral pain due to patella alta or patella baja may occur.[13] Other sequelae can include extension loss[10] and persistent quadriceps atrophy.[17] One devastating but uncommon complication reported with avulsion fractures of the tibial tubercle is anterior compartment syndrome, which results from bleeding into the anterior compartment from vessels around the level of the tubercle.[38, 68] A high level of suspicion for this complication is important, with a careful ongoing evaluation of the neurovascular status of these patients.

FRACTURES OF THE TIBIAL INTERCONDYLAR EMINENCE

General and Mechanism of Injury

Intercondylar eminence fractures are a relatively uncommon injury with a reported occurrence of 3 per 100,000 children per year.[52] Fractures of the intercondylar eminence tend to occur in adolescent patients between the ages of 8 to 15 years.[13, 29] Less commonly, they can also be found in a skeletally mature adult. The usual mechanism of injury is a rotational force combined with hyperextension. The ACL attaches to the tibia in a fossa anterior and lateral to the tibial spines. There are fibrous attachments to the base of the anterior spine and to the anterior horn of the lateral meniscus. In 1980 Rinaldi and Mazzarella[45] stated that the intercondylar eminence offers less resistance to a traction or tensile load than does the ligament itself. Consequently, hyperextension and rotational force that would cause ACL disruption in the adult often results in an intracondylar eminence avulsion fracture in the skeletally immature patient. Although eminence fractures remain more common, isolated ACL disruptions are now being recognized more frequently in skeletally immature athletes. Some have even reported equal incidence of proximal, distal, and midsubstance ACL injuries in children.[57] In eminence fractures, ultimate failure occurs through bone, but interstitial injury and stretching are recognized as significant components of this injury.[2, 53, 72]

Tibial eminence fractures classically have been found to occur as a result of a young child falling from a bicycle, as originally described by Meyers and McKeever in 1959 and 1970. They believed that a young child with a hemarthrosis after a fall from a bicycle should be considered to have an eminence fracture until proven otherwise. Other mechanisms of injury have been described; they include sports and athletic injuries as well as motor vehicle accidents, particularly those involving pedestrian vehicular trauma.[23]

Classification

Fractures of the intracondylar eminence (tibial spine) are typically described according to the classifications of Meyers and McKeever[27] (Fig. 67.11). In their classification scheme, these fractures are divided into four

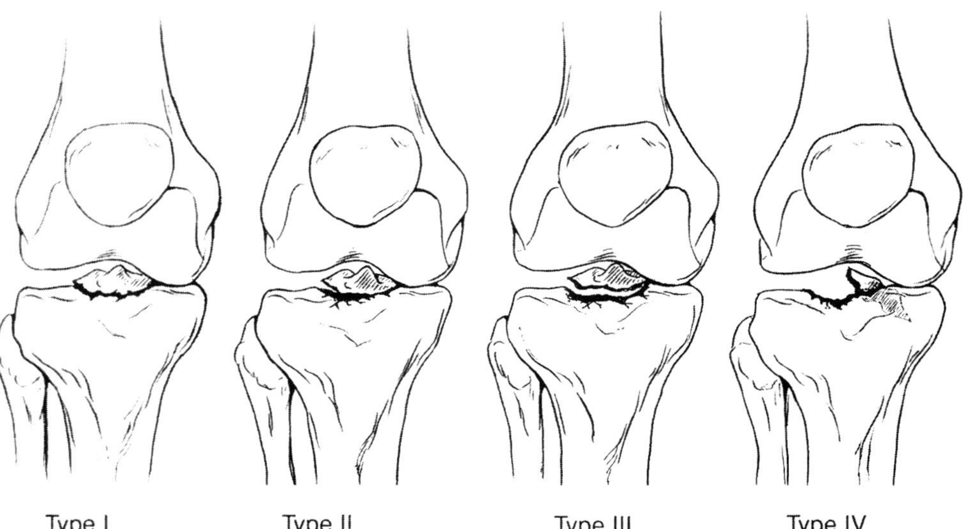

FIGURE 67.11 ➢ Classification of intercondylar eminence fractures according to the system of Meyers and McKeever. Type I fractures are nondisplaced. Type II fractures are partially displaced and are often hinged posteriorly. Type III fractures are displaced completely. Type IV fractures are displaced and rotated.[13]

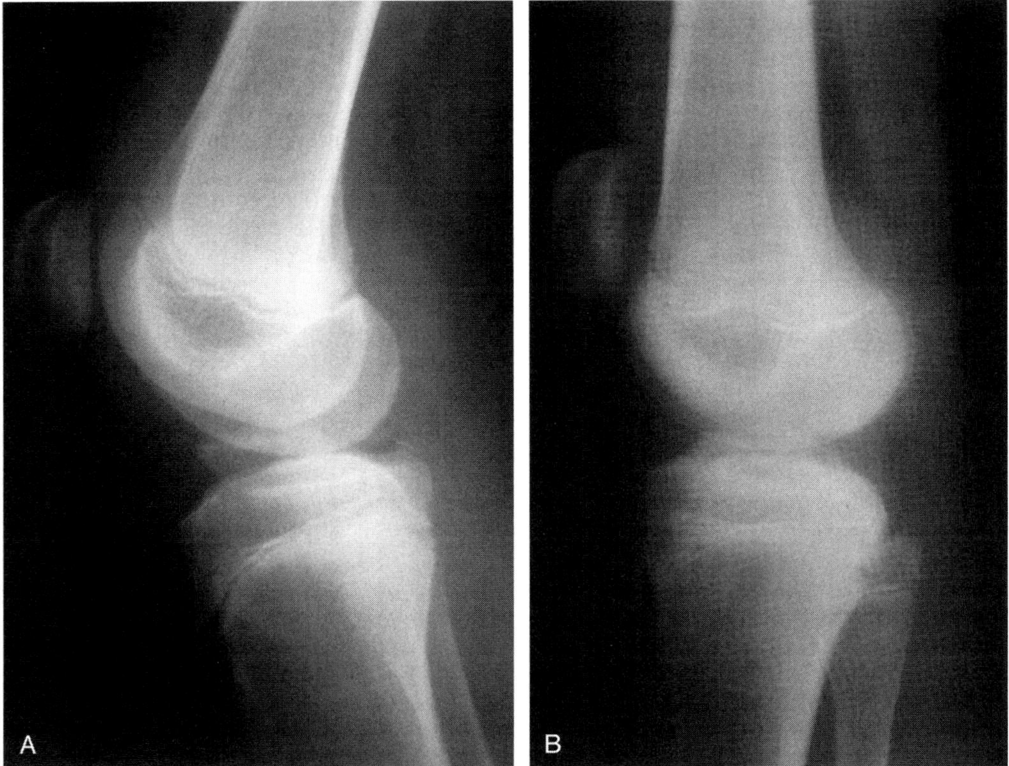

FIGURE 67.12 ➢ *A*, 12-year-old male cut while playing basketball and suffered a type II tibial spine. *B*, Patient underwent a closed reduction casting under anesthesia following aspiration of the hemarthrosis.

types: type I fractures are nondisplaced, type II fractures are partially displaced and are often hinged posteriorly, type III fractures are completely displaced, and type IV fractures are displaced and rotated. Interposition of the transverse meniscal ligament can be noted in type II and III fractures.[29] Others have modified this classification scheme somewhat by labeling the type IV fracture a type III+ and then including a fourth type as described by Zaricznyj,[72] in which the displaced fragment is comminuted.[23]

Presentation and Evaluation

As previously stated, tibial eminence fractures most often occur in patients younger than 15 years. These fractures, however, can also be seen in the adult population. The patient typically presents following either hyperextension or rotational injury to the knee with pain and a hemarthrosis. The knee is often held in a flexed position due to the effusion and hamstring spasm. The patient is either unable to bear weight or has difficulty. These injuries are often not isolated, and several authors have reported the presence of other associated injuries, in particular collateral ligament injuries, meniscal injuries, and ipsilateral extremity fracture.[6, 11, 13, 18, 23, 27–29, 55, 72] This makes it crucial to do a thorough examination of the knee to rule out any of these associated findings.

Routine radiographs (anteroposterior and lateral views) will demonstrate an eminence fracture. Visualization of fracture displacement is best seen on lateral views. Oblique radiographs aid in determining extension of the fracture into the plateau. Radiographs are often deceptive in the young patient, as the eminence may be largely cartilaginous. The visualization of a small flake of bone in the intercondylar notch of a young patient should raise suspicion of an imminence fracture. On occasion, a notch view is useful to better identify a small avulsed fragment. Stress views may be helpful if collateral ligament injury or a physeal fracture, proximal or distal to the joint, is suspected based on clinical examination. This examination should be performed with the patient under adequate sedation or general anesthesia. If one suspects a collateral ligament tear, one may find joint space widening on the stress view; the stress view may also help to show an occult concomitant physeal fracture. Magnetic resonance imaging may also be helpful in evaluation of these associated injuries.[13]

Treatment

Fractures of the tibial spine not only disrupt the ACL but also involve the articular surface of the tibial plateau. The goals of treatment for these injuries, therefore, involve restoration of the appropriate tension to

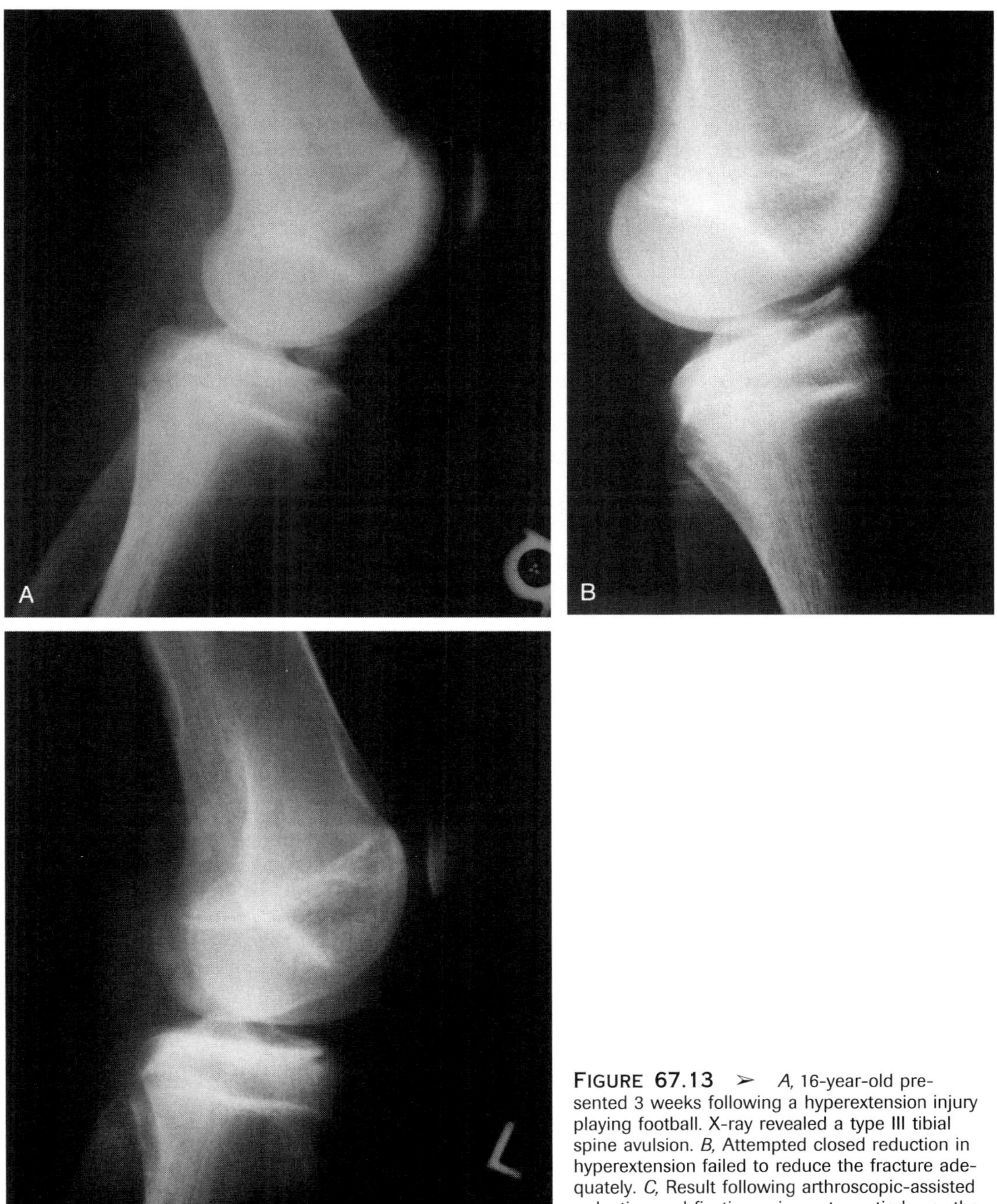

FIGURE 67.13 ➢ *A,* 16-year-old presented 3 weeks following a hyperextension injury playing football. X-ray revealed a type III tibial spine avulsion. *B,* Attempted closed reduction in hyperextension failed to reduce the fracture adequately. *C,* Result following arthroscopic-assisted reduction and fixation using sutures tied over the tibia.

the ACL and anatomic reduction of the articular surface of the joint. Treatment of tibial spine fractures varies according the fracture type. The undisplaced type I injuries are treated by immobilization in a long leg cast, with the knee held in 0 to 20 degrees of flexion.[23, 27, 29, 53, 54] Aspiration of a hemarthrosis is often necessary in order to obtain full extension. Type II and III injuries, even though they are displaced, can also often be treated with closed reduction and immobilization with good results (Fig. 67.12). The position of the knee following closed reduction is somewhat controversial. Many authors recommend immobilization in full extension or hyperextension.[23, 54, 61] This position directly reduces the tibial spine through a direct contact with the femoral condyles.[23] Other authors prefer anywhere from 10 to 15 degrees of flexion.[23, 29, 54] This is because the ACL is thought to be under the least amount of tension at 15 to 20 degrees of flexion.[29] Patients are generally immobilized for a total of 4 to 6 weeks.[23, 54] X-rays films should be taken 1 week after reduction to ensure that the fragment does not redisplace.[54] Open reduction and internal fixation are recommended if closed manipulation does not reduce the fragment[23, 29] (Fig. 67.13). Fixation options include pin fixation, cannulated screw fixation, and direct suture.[13, 23] Suture fixation offers the advantage of avoiding hardware in the knee and allows the surgeon to cross the physis with very small drill holes.[23, 54] Open reduction and internal fixation need not necessitate a formal arthrotomy. The use of arthroscopy or arthroscopic-assisted surgery allows the surgeon to properly reduce the fracture and fix the fracture securely without necessitating a large arthrotomy.[23, 29, 69] If an open reduction and internal fixation are done either via an arthrotomy or an arthroscopically assisted technique, thoroughly débride the fracture bed of any interposed material such as hematoma, interposed meniscus, or cartilage[23] (Fig. 67.14). When using a suture technique, a heavy, absorbable suture is used to weave through the stump of the ACL, and these sutures are then tied on the anterior cortex of the proximal tibia after they are passed through drill holes in the proximal epiphysis of the tibia.[23, 54] A suture in a lasso-type fashion may also be used: loop it posterior to the ACL, pass the free ends through drill holes in the proximal tibial epiphysis, and tie the suture over the anterior cortex of the tibia. One must be sure to have a stable reduction following fixation of the suture. Lo et al[23] recommend 2 weeks of postoperative immobilization and extension followed by gentle range-of-motion exercises, whereas Sponseller and Beaty[54] recommend immobilization in 0 to 20 degrees of flexion for 6 weeks followed by progressive quadriceps- and hamstring-strengthening and range-of-motion exercises. Edwards and Grana[13] recommend 6 to 8 weeks of immobilization in extension postoperatively. It is, therefore, important to realize that despite internal fixation, the fragment or its anterior cartilaginous component can still displace. The key is that all patients require a period of immobilization postoperatively; the length of time will depend somewhat on the security of the fixation.[23]

Outcome

Following satisfactory reduction of tibial spine fractures, results are good to excellent.[23, 54] Meyers and McKeever in 1970[27] reported 86% excellent results; Willis in 1993[67] reported on 56 patients, 84% of whom returned to the same level of sports, and 98% had no subjective complaints of giving way. Complications and sequelae associated with these fractures include persistent ACL laxity and extension loss. Residual collateral ligament laxity can be seen secondary to an associated collateral ligament injury, and an unrecognized physeal fracture can also result in poor long-term results.[13, 54] Late fracture through a fibrous union as well as anterior epiphysiodesis following screw fixation has also been reported.[25, 33] Loss of extension is not an uncommon problem. Wiley and Baxter in 1990[65] reported on 45 patients, all of whom had some loss of extension, 60% of whom had more than 10 degrees' extension loss. This loss of extension may result from a malunion or malreduction, causing the fragment to impinge in the notch.[54, 55] Others maintain that immobilization in flexion may contribute to this problem.[13]

Residual ACL laxity has frequently been cited as a common event following fractures of the intercondylar eminence. This residual laxity may arise from the malunion or malreduction resulting in relative ACL lengthening, from hypertrophy and lengthening of the tibial spine itself, or from associated intrasubstance ACL injury.[2, 13, 16, 23, 29, 53, 54] Studies by Noyes in 1974[35] showed that the normal collagen of the ACL fibers does get disrupted in the presence of a tibial spine injury, even though the site of failure of the ACL is at the tibial spine itself. Grana[16] stated that one-third of patients with malunion or nonunion of tibial spine fractures will present with instability complaints and that two-thirds decrease their activity in order to minimize symptoms. In reviewing the literature, there does appear to be a very high incidence of objective and clinically detectable instability following tibial spine fractures; however, the incidence of functional instability is markedly less. Meyers and McKeever[27] reported only 1 of 35 patients in their series to have residual instability. In 1981 Mollander[32] had no patients with residual instability in his series of 35 patients. Baxter and Wiley[2] in 1988 had 51% of patients with a positive Lachman test; however, no patients subjectively complained of instability. Willis' series of 56 patients in 1993[67] showed that patients with type I fractures had a side-to-side laxity difference of 1 mm. Patients with type II fractures had a difference of 3.5 mm, and patients with type III fractures had a 4.5-mm difference. Overall, 74% of patients had objective signs of laxity, and 64% had clinical signs of instability. However, no patients complained of subjective instability, and 84% were able to return to their same preinjury level of sports. Wiley and Baxter[65] found similar results in objective ligament testing, with type III patients showing a greater side-to-side difference than did type I or type II patients. However, none of their patients complained of objective instability. Of note in this series, many patients did not return to their same level of sports.

SUMMARY

Treatment of displaced physeal fractures about the knee remains one of the more difficult problems in orthopedics. Even with appropriate conservative or surgical treatment, a successful outcome is not always certain. Unfortunately, damage to the physis at the time of the injury is a variable over which the surgeon has no control. The Salter-Harris classification provides a general guideline regarding the risk of growth disturbance, but there are no good clinical methods for quantifying the true extent of physeal damage in an acute injury. Thus, outcomes remain somewhat unpredictable. Fortunately, most physeal fractures above the knee are seen in an adolescent athletic population close to skeletal maturity, which minimizes the chance of significant growth disturbance. Other associated injuries, as well as the occurrence of these fractures in a

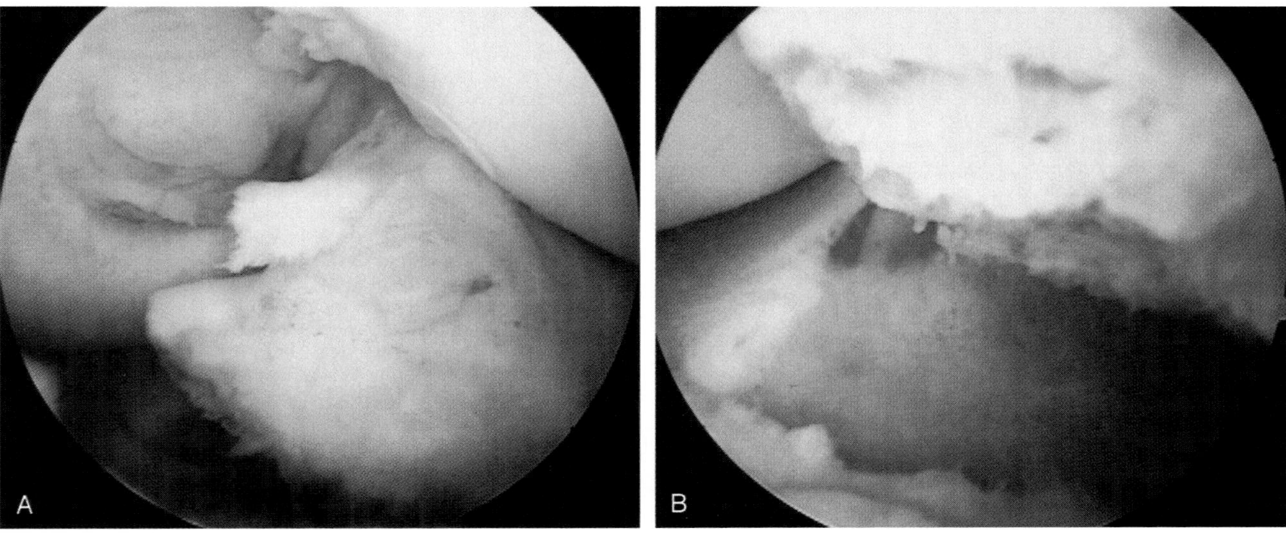

FIGURE 67.14 ➢ Intra-articular arthroscopic views of the loose fragment *(A)* and the fracture bed once it was débrided *(B)*.

younger age population, can lead to disastrous results. Ultimately, the value of a treatment method must be evaluated on the basis of the restoration of articular congruity, physeal anatomy, and physeal function, as evidenced by the continuation of normal growth.

References

1. Aitken AP, Magill HK: Fractures involving the distal femoral epiphyseal cartilage. J Bone Joint Surg Am 34:96, 1952.
2. Baxter MP, Wiley JJ: Fractures of the tibial spine in children: An evaluation of knee stability. J Bone Joint Surg Br 70:228, 1988.
3. Bertin KC, Goble EM: Ligament injuries associated with physeal fractures about the knee. Clin Orthop 177:188, 1983.
4. Bisgard JD, Martenson L: Fractures in children. Surg Gynecol Obstet 65:465, 1937.
5. Bolesta MJ, Fitch RD: Tibial tubercle avulsions, J Pediatr Orthop 6:186, 1986.
6. Bradley GW, Shives TC, Samuelson KM: Ligament injuries in the knees of children. J Bone Joint Surg Am 61:167, 1979.
7. Burkhart SS, Peterson HA: Fractures of the proximal tibial epiphysis. J Bone Joint Surg Am 61:996, 1979.
8. Canale ST, Stanitski DF: Orthopedic Knowledge Update No. 5: Home Study Syllabus—Knee & Leg: Pediatric Aspects, Chapter 38, 1996, pp 437-451.
9. Carey J, Spence L, Blickman H, et al: MRI of pediatric growth plate injury: Correlation with plain film radiographs and clinical outcome. Skeletal Radiol 27:250, 1998.
10. Christie, MJ, Dvonch VM: Tibial tuberosity avulsion fracture in adolescents. J Pediatr Orthop 1:391, 1981.
11. Clanton TO, Delee JC, Sanders B, et al: Knee ligament injuries in children. J Bone Joint Surg Am 61:1195, 1979.
12. Compere EL: Growth arrest in long bones as a result of fracture that include the epiphyseal. JAMA, 105:2140, 1935.
13. Edwards PH, Grana WA: Physeal fractures about the knee. J Am Acad Orthop Surg 3:63, 1995.
14. Falster O, Hasselbalch H: Avulsion fracture of the tibial tuberosity with combined ligament and meniscal tear. Am J Sports Med 20:82, 1992.
15. Foucher JT: De la divulsion des epiphyses. Reprinted in English in Clin Orthop 188:3, 1984.
16. Grana WA: Injuries to the knee. In Sullivan JA, Grana WA, eds: The Pediatric Athlete. Park Ridge, IL: American Academy of Orthopedic Surgeons, 1990.
17. Hand WL, Hand CR, Dunn AW: Avulsion fractures of the tibial tubercle. J Bone Joint Surg Am 53:1579, 1971.
18. Hyndman JC, Brown DC: Major ligamentous injuries of the knee in children. J Bone Joint Surg Br 161:245, 1979.
19. Jaramillo D, Hoffer FA, Shapiro F, et al: MR imaging of fractures of the growth plate. Am J Roentgenol 155:1261, 1990.
20. Johnson EW Jr, Fahl JC: Fractures of the distal epiphysis of the tibia and fibula in children. Am J Surg 93:778, 1957.
21. Kasser JR: Physeal bar resection after growth arrest about the knee. Clin Orthop 255:68, 1990.
22. Levi JH, Coleman CR: Fracture of the tibial tubercle. Am J Sports Med 4:254, 1976.
23. Lo IK, Bell DM, Fowler PJ: Anterior cruciate ligament injuries in the skeletally immature patient. Instr Course Lect 47:351, 1998.
24. Lombardo SJ, Harvey JP Jr: Fractures of the distal femoral epiphyses: Factors influencing prognosis—a review of thirty-four cases. J Bone Joint Surg Am 59:742, 1977.
25. Lombardo SJ: Avulsion of a fibrous union of the intercondylar eminence of the tibia: A case report. J Bone Joint Surg Am 76: 1565, 1994.
26. Mann DC, Rajmaihra S: Distribution of physeal and nonphyseal injuries in 2650 long bone fractures in children aged zero to sixteen. J Pediatr Orthop 10:713, 1990.
27. Meyers MH, Mckeever FM: Fracture of the intercondylar eminence of the tibia. J Bone Joint Surg Am 52:1677, 1970.
28. Meyers MH, McKeever FM: Fracture of the intercondylar eminence of the tibia. J Bone Joint Surg Am 41:209, 1959.
29. Micheli LJ, Foster TE: Acute knee injuries in the immature athlete. Instr Course Lect 42:473, 1993.
30. Mirbey J, Besancenot J, Chambers RT, et al: Avulsion fractures of the tibial tuberosity in the adolescent athlete: Risk factors, mechanism of injury, and treatment. Am J Sports Med 16:336, 1988.
31. Mizuta T, Benson WM, Foster BK, et al: Statistical analysis of the incidence of physeal injuries. J Pediatr Orthop 7:518, 1987.
32. Molander ML, Wallin G, Wikstad I: Fracture of the intercondylar eminence of the tibia: A review of 35 patients. J Bone Joint Surg Br 63:89, 1981.
33. Mylle J, Reynders R, Broos P: Transepiphyseal fixation of anterior cruciate avulsion in a child: Report of a complication and review of the literature. Arch Orthop Trauma Surg 112:101, 1993.
34. Nicholson JT: Epiphyseal fractures about the knee. Instr Course Lect 18:74, 1967.
35. Noyes FR, DeLucas JL, Torvik PJ: Biomechanics of anterior cruciate ligament failure: An analysis of strain-rate sensitivity and

mechanisms of failure in primates. J Bone Joint Surg Am 56:236, 1974.
36. Ogden JA, Tross RB, Murphy MJ: Fractures of the tibial tuberosity in adolescents. J Bone Joint Surg Am 62:205, 1980.
37. Ogden JA: Injury to the growth mechanism of the immature skeleton. Skeletal Radiol 6:237, 1981.
38. Pape JM, Goulet JM, Hensinger RN: Compartment syndrome complicating tibial tubercle avulsion. Clin Orthop 295:201, 1993.
39. Peterson HA: Physeal and Apophyseal Injuries: Fractures in Children. Philadelphia, Lippincott-Raven, 1996.
40. Peterson HA, Madhok R, Benson JT, et al: Physical fractures: I—Epidemiology in Olmsted County, Minnesota, 1979-1988. J Pediatr Orthop 41:423, 1994.
41. Peterson HA: Physeal Fractures: III—Classification. Pediatr Orthop 14:439, 1994.
42. Poland J: Traumatic Separation of the Epiphyses. London, Smith, Elder, & Co., 1898.
43. Poulsen TD, Skak SV, Toftgaard-Jensen T: Epiphyseal fractures of the proximal tibia. Injury 20:111, 1989.
44. Reed MH: Fractures and dislocations of the lower extremities in children, J Trauma 17:351, 1977.
45. Rinaldi E, Mazzarella F: Isolated fracture-avulsions of the tibial insertions of the cruciate ligaments of the knee. Ital J Orthop Traumatol 6:77, 1980.
46. Riseborough EJ, Barrett IR, Shapiro F: Growth disturbances following distal femoral physeal fracture-separations. J Bone Joint Surg Am 65:885, 1983.
47. Rogers LF, Poznanski AK: Imaging of epiphyseal injuries. Radiology 191:297, 1994.
48. Rogers LF, Jones S: "Clipping injury" fracture of the epiphysis in the adolescent football player: An occult lesion of the knee. Am J Radiol 121:69, 1974.
49. Salter RB, Harris WR: Injuries involving the epiphyseal plate. J Bone Joint Surg Am 45:587, 1963.
50. Shapiro F: Epiphyseal growth plate fracture-separation: A pathophysiologic approach. Orthopedics 5:720, 1982.
51. Shelton WR, Canale ST: Fractures of the tibia through the proximal tibial epiphyseal cartilage. J Bone Joint Surg Am 61:167, 1979.
52. Skak SV, Jensen TT, Poulson TD, et al: Epidemiology of knee injuries in children. Acta Orthop Scand, 58:78, 1987.
53. Smith JB: Knee instability after fractures of the intercondylar eminence of the tibia. J Pediatr Orthop 4:462, 1984.
54. Sponseller P, Beaty JH: Fractures and Dislocations About the Knee. Philadelphia, Lippincott-Raven, 1996, p 1233.
55. Stanitski CL: Ligamentous Injury of the Knee. In Stanitski CL, DeLee JC, Drez D Jr, eds: Pediatric and Adolescent Sports Medicine. Philadelphia, WB Saunders, 1994, p 406.
56. Stanitski CL: Acute tibial tubercle avulsion fracture. In Stanitski CL, DeLee JC, Drez D Jr, eds: Pediatric and Adolescent Sports Medicine, vol 3. Philadelphia, WB Saunders, 1994, p 329.
57. Stanitski CL, Harvell JC, Fu F: Observations on acute hemarthrosis in children and adolescents. J Pediatr Orthop 13:506, 1993.
58. Stephens DC, Louis DS: Traumatic separation of the distal femoral epiphyseal cartilage plate. J Bone Joint Surg Am 56:1383, 1974.
59. Tachdjian MO: Fractures involving the distal femoral epiphysis: Fractures and dislocations. Pediatr Orthop 4:3274, 1990.
60. Torg JS, Pavlov H, Morris VB: Salter-Harris type III fracture of the medial femoral condyle occuring in the adolescent athlete. J Bone Joint Surg Am 63:586, 1981.
61. Warner JP, Micheli LJ: Pediatric and adolescent muscoloskeletal injuries. In Grana WA, Kalenak A, eds: Clinical Sports Medicine. Philadelphia, WB Saunders, 1991, p 490.
62. Wascher DC, Finerman GAM: Physeal injuries in young athletes. In Stanitski CL, DeLee JC, Drez D Jr, eds: Pediatric and Adolescent Sports Medicine. Philadelphia, WB Saunders, 1994.
63. Watson-Jones R: Fractures and Joint Injuries, 4th ed. Baltimore, Williams & Wilkins, 1955, p 786.
64. White PG, Mah JY, Friedman L: Magnetic resonance imaging in acute physeal injuries. Skeletal Radiol 23:627, 1994.
65. Wiley JJ, Baxter MP: Tibial spine factures in children. Clin Orthop 255:54, 1990.
66. Wilkins KE: The incidence of fractures in children. In Rockwood CA, Wilkens KE, Beaty JH, eds: Fractures in Children, 4th ed, Philadelphia, Lippincott-Raven, 1996.
67. Willis RB, Blokker C, Stoll TM, et al: Long-term follow-up of anterior tibial eminence fractures. J Pediatr Orthop 13:361, 1993.
68. Wiss DA, Schilz JL: Frontal type III fracture of the tibial tubercle in adolescents. J Orthop Trauma 5:475, 1991.
69. Wood KB, Bradley JP, Ward WT: Pes anserinus interposition in proximal tibial physeal fracture. Clin Orthop 264:239, 1991.
70. Worlock P, Stower M: Fracture patterns in Nottingham children. J. Pediatr 6:656, 1986.
71. Wozasek GE, Moser KD, Haller H, et al: Trauma involving the proximal tibial epiphysis. Arch Orthop Trauma Surg 110:301, 1991.
72. Zaricznyj B: Avulsion fracture of the tibial eminence: Treatment by open reduction and pinning. J Bone Joint Surg Am 59:1111, 1977.

68

Anterior Cruciate Ligament Injuries and Acute Tibial Eminence Fractures in Skeletally Immature Patients

CARL L. STANITSKI

ACUTE INJURY IN SKELETALLY IMMATURE PATIENTS

The anterior cruciate ligament (ACL) is a high-profile ligament thanks to the exposure given by the media reporting ACL injuries in celebrity athletes and their usually successful return to play following reconstructive surgery. The term ACL has entered the lay lexicon, and patients and parents are aware of this structure and the grim athletic portents accompanying its injury. Over the past two decades, major strides have been made in understanding the role of the ACL in normal knee function. As an extension of this information, the natural history of a patient's ACL-deficient knees had been established with the recognition of the consequences of attempting to return to high-demand sports, i.e., progressive intra-articular compromise and onset of premature degenerative joint disease.[4, 23, 26] A subset of patients with ACL injury is now appreciated—the skeletally immature athlete. In the past, ACL injuries in the truly immature patients were considered curiosities, and data on ACL injuries in the more mature adolescent were melded into adult series. The otherwise normal skeletally immature patient was simply considered to not suffer the meniscal and ACL injuries of the adult counterparts. The true prevalence and incidence of ACL injuries in the skeletally immature patient group are unknown, but it is certainly not an uncommon event in the young, school-age athlete, especially with the significant number of children and youth participants in scholastic and community sports. The data suggest that the ACL injury is especially common in female athletes. The precise cause of this gender difference, especially in soccer and basketball participants, is unknown.[3, 4] Theories of notch morphology variability, lower-extremity mechanical alignment abnormalities, underlying conditioning deficits, and hormonal challenges have been proposed and are under scrutiny. Awareness of the ACL tear in this age group has been heightened by a spectrum of circumstances. Improvements in clinical acumen have been made and include the relationship of a "pop" and acute hemarthrosis, return to play limitation, and Lachmann and pivot shift signs with quantitation of sagittal plane translation by arthrometry. Magnetic imaging techniques extend diagnostic capabilities when correlated with clinical findings. Arthroscopic findings are considered the gold standard of diagnosis documentation.

Reports by Angel and Hall,[2] Lo and coworkers,[17] Stanitski and associates,[30] and others[14, 19, 28] have presented significant numbers of cases of arthroscopically documented ACL damage in skeletally immature patients, particularly ones with hemarthrosis and excluding those patients with tibial eminence fractures. Many previous studies of knee injuries in the immature patient suffered from major limitations, including study design, lack of diagnosis specificity and documentation, patient number, length of follow-up, activity modification, outcome quantitation, and imprecision in differentiating physiological from chronological maturity.[8, 10, 22]

The majority of growth in the lower extremity centers around the distal femoral and proximal tibial physes. In immature patients the ACL attaches to the distal femoral and proximal tibial chondroepiphyses through a perichondral cuff that transforms during adolescence to a fibrocartilage-osseous interface at maturity. In the past it was assumed that the ACL was rarely injured in skeletally immature patients because of the relative vulnerability of the chondroepiphysis relative to the ligament resistance. This attitude neglected to appreciate that the junctional tissues involved responded differently to load rate and magnitude. Ligamentous injury is caused by lower magnitude forces at rapid load rates, and physeal damage occurs in response to high-energy forces at lower rates of loading. The nutrition of the ACL in children is via the perisynovial sheath and terminal osseous elements of the femur and tibia. Femoral intercondylar notch configuration and other intra-articular morphology are determined by the effects of use superimposed on a genetically determined template. Although alterations in ACL morphology are often seen in congenital disorders of the lower extremities, e.g., congenital short femur, fibular hemimelia, this chapter will not address those circumstances, and readers are referred to standard texts dealing with those conditions.

NATURAL HISTORY

Few retrospective and no prospective well-done natural history studies exist about isolated ACL tears in truly skeletally immature patients. Angel and Hall[2] used phone and mail questionnaires to retrospectively review the outcome of 27 children (mean age 14.5 years) with arthroscopically documented ACL tears (18 partial) at an average of 51 months postinjury. Twenty-five patients were treated with physical therapy and without immobilization, bracing, or sports limitation. At follow-up, half of the patients reported functional instability and pain, 11 had temporarily returned to full sports activity, and another 7 participated at a reduced level of play; 9 patients were unable to participate. This return to activity distribution is similar to that reported by Noyes and colleagues in their adult patients with ACL tears.[26] Mizuta and coworkers[2] reported the outcome of 18 patients, 10 to 15 years old with an average age of 12.8 years followed up for 36 to 51 months. No comment was made regarding physiological maturity and no patient was placed at diminished athletic activity. One patient was able to return to full activity. Not surprisingly, most patients had poor Lysholm scores. Secondary meniscal tears were arthroscopically documented in six patients, and three others had clinical evidence of a meniscal tear. Pressman and colleagues[28] conducted a 12-year retrospective analysis of 42 patients with arthroscopically documented complete midsubstance ACL tears. Patients were from 5 to 17 years old at the time of injury with an average follow-up evaluation of 5.3 years by either phone survey or clinical exam. Of the 13 patients treated nonoperatively with derotation brace, physiotherapy, and initial casting, outcomes in this group were significantly poorer assessed by functional knee scores than in a similar aged group treated by intra-articular surgical reconstruction.

McCarroll and colleagues[19] followed 38 middle school (13 to 15 years old, average 13.5) with arthroscopically documented midsubstance ACL tears for an average of 4.2 years, with a minimum follow-up of 2 years postinjury. Sixteen of the 38 patients attempted to return to previous levels of athletic participation but all complained of giving way, and 10 of these 16 cases developed documented meniscal tears; 2 of the 16 had chronic knee effusions. In their final analysis, 37 of the 38 patients treated nonoperatively had functional complaints of instability and 27 of the 38 developed symptomatic meniscal tears. In Graf and coworkers'[10] retrospective study of 12 patients with an average age of 14.5 years with arthroscopically proven ACL tears, 8 meniscal tears (4 medial, 4 lateral) were seen in 6 patients. Eight patients underwent rehabilitation and functional bracing, but all developed functional instability and multiple episodes of giving way while attempting to play at an average of 7 months from the injury to the first complaints of instability. This mirrors the 6-month period noted by Noyes and associates.[26] In Graf's small series of 12 patients without documented physiological maturity, 7 patients developed additional meniscal damage at an average of 15 months postprimary ACL injury despite brace use.

The fate of patients with a partial ACL tear is not known in the skeletally immature patient group. The amount of force from either a single episode or as a result of summated submaximal forces needed to convert a partial tear in an attenuated ligament to a complete tear is unknown. The percentage of injury to each of the ACL's bundles to indicate partial tear has not been quantitated and classified.

Clinical Examination

Clinical evaluation in the hands of an experienced surgeon is an extremely accurate diagnostic method for ACL tears, especially in the nonacute setting.[32] Immediately following the injury the patient is usually less than cooperative due to apprehension and pain during the various maneuvers used to determine stability. I characterize the mechanism of injury as contact or noncontact and whether there is a component of deceleration and rotation. It is uncommon to find an ACL tear in someone without elements of rotation and deceleration and knee hyperextension or flexion. The mechanism of injury seems to be similar to the one seen in adults, mainly, a noncontact stress combined with rapid directional change. A sensation of a "pop" in the knee is reported in about a third of the patients with an acute ACL tear. Onset of effusion is rapid, and the patients are usually unable to return to play. In order to get an idea of the acuity of the injury, I group acute tears as ones seen less than 3 weeks; subacute, 3 to 12 weeks; and chronic, more than 12 weeks after the injury.[31] Future sports risks and demands need to be addressed. In addition to the usual characterization of historical points relative to the knee, additional data must be gathered about the patient's level of physiological maturity and projected remaining growth. Knowing parental and sibling heights as well as the growth status of the patient allows an educated guess to be made as to growth remaining when combined with findings of maturity on clinical exam. Onset of menarche should be determined because the growth phase of peak height velocity occurs just before menarche. Determination of secondary sexual development is necessary because physiological and not chronological age is required as a data point in the treatment algorithm. Appearance of curly underarm hair is a clinical sign of maturity in boys, which equates in timing of maturation with menarche in girls.[12, 34] Shoe size stability is a rough guide to impending skeletal maturity.

During the usual clinical tests of knee stability, the opposite uninjured knee should serve as the control for tibial translation with assessment of the magnitude of translation and rotation and the endpoint quality.

Many symptomatic teenage girls have significant knee rotation and translation including positive pivot shifts due to inherent, genetically determined, nonpathological ligamentous laxity. Tenderness to palpation should be sought around the patellar retinaculum (including the patellomeniscal ligament), joint lines, and tibial and femoral physes. Joint line tenderness, particularly mid and posterior, commonly accompanies peripheral meniscal injury. Physeal tenderness may be misinterpreted as the site of collateral ligament injury in the skeletally immature patient. Effusion presence or absence as well as volume of effusion should be noted. An ACL tear of any consequence is always associated with an initial and persisting effusion. Arthrometric examination is usually difficult to perform shortly after injury because of patient guarding due to pain.

Imaging

Initial imaging is via high-quality standard anteroposterior, lateral, notch, and patellar view radiographs. Other than in the case of a tibial eminence fracture, true avulsion of the ACL is a rare event, and the avulsed frgment in this circumstance is usually composed of mostly chondral tissue with only a fleck of bone. Osteochondral femoral and patellar fragments should be sought since the mechanism of injury of an ACL is similar to that causing patellar instability. Unsuspected osteochondritis dissecans lesions may also be seen. In addition to the above-mentioned potential findings, radiographs provide information about notch morphology, physeal injury, and physeal maturity. If an undisplaced physeal injury is suspected, stress views should not be done because they produce further damage to the physis and do not add anything to the treatment plan for this undisplaced fracture. Follow-up radiographs in 10 to 14 days document the periosteal response expected in this type of injury.

Magnetic resonance imaging (MRI) studies should be ordered by the treating surgeon for specific indications, e.g., when the diagnosis cannot be made by clinical exam. MRI studies should not be used as a screening test by nonsurgical physicians. Major errors occur in radiologist interpretations of knee MRI in skeletally immature patients, as evidenced by reports of supposed meniscal tears in normal children. Stanitski[32] noted major discrepancies between clinical examination findings and radiologist reports of knee MRI studies and between these reports and findings at arthroscopy. In this study there was a 75% presence of false-positives and false-negatives of MRI readings and only a 30% coincidence of MRI and arthroscopic findings. Clinical examination proved highly more accurate in this skeletally immature group of patients evaluated in a nonacute setting by a single surgeon. MRI studies provided no significant help in patient management. Acute ACL injury changes on MRI include increases in signal and change in morphology. Late changes are seen in the configuration of the PCL due to the attachment of the fibrotic ACL stump. Transient subchondral changes, especially on the lateral femoral condyle, are commonly seen in the acute phase and reflect marrow edema. Clinical tenderness at these sites should not be confused with meniscal damage.

Treatment

All treatment plans are based on an accurate and complete diagnosis achieved by clinical, imaging and, if necessary, arthroscopic assessments. Treatment goals are a functional knee without progressive intra-articular damage with predisposition to premature osteoarthrosis. There are no well-documented follow-up studies of adequate length of truly skeletally immature patients with complete (or incomplete) ACL tears without initial meniscal injury who have complied with a non–high-demand sport program. In the emerging young athlete, a torn ACL is not a surgical emergency. One must take the time to discuss treatment options and their impact on future sports involvement, vocational and avocational concerns, and the risks, complications, and outcomes of the various management programs. The patient is often under significant pressure from peers, coaches, and often parents to return to play in replication of the professional athlete demands. The orthopedic surgeon should assume the role of a knee counsellor, especially to those patients whom he or she recognizes as "knee abusers" with high-risk activities.

Nonoperative treatment does not mean nontreatment. The goal of the program must be defined from the outset. The plan may be a temporizing measure until the patient is mature enough to undergo an adult-type, complete transphyseal procedure or the nonoperative choice may be the definitive one for a patient willing to accept the athletic functional limitations consigned by not repairing the torn ACL.

The nonoperative program I use for skeletally immature patients is in three phases.[33] Phase I begins shortly after injury, lasts 7 to 10 days, and includes protected partial weightbearing with crutched, out-of-brace daily active knee flexion to comfort with passive knee extension and use of a knee immobilizer for comfort. During this time patient education regarding the consequences of imprudent high-level sports activity is reinforced.

Phase II lasts about 6 weeks. During that time, monitored and documented rehabilitation efforts are done to restore full range of motion and normalize the muscle balance of the lower extremity with focus on the quadriceps/hamstring complex. Active terminal knee extension is avoided but full passive knee extension is emphasized. As the strength ratio is normalized, crutch use is diminished and then abandoned.

Phase III continues the rehabilitation and incorporates functional brace use, and, when quadriceps and hamstring strength and endurance are equal to the oposite normal side by isokinetic testing at functional speeds (>260 degrees/s), return to low to moderated demand sports is allowed. Jogging and swimming are encouraged. The role of functional knee braces in children has not been defined, and issues of brace size, fit, and cost remain. Questions about the timing of brace use are also present relative to the brace's use full time versus only during sports activities. The patient is seen monthly for the first 6 months to assess program compliance and to rule out further knee functional alterations.

The surgical management of an isolated ACL tear in the truly skeletally immature patient is currently controversial.[1, 17, 19, 27, 28, 31, 33] In those with what I term the "ACL plus" knee, i.e., with a combined ACL and meniscal injury, consensus seems to exist for surgical reconstruction in this skeletally immature patient because of the poor prognosis for meniscal repair alone in the face of cruciate compromise. Concerns exist about the consequences of physeal transgression by a variety of surgical methods and also about restoration of ligamentous isometry in the growing skeleton. The percentage of physeal invasion, even when central, that is safe and that will not produce angular and longitudinal deformities in humans is unknown. Experimental laboratory models in various species have been used in an attempt to provide guidance in these aspects.[9, 11, 15, 18, 29] Guzzanti and coworkers[11] used a lapin model with semitendinosus transfer through 2-mm tibial and femoral central transphyseal tunnels. Histological sections of the operative areas up to 6 months postoperatively showed no evidence of premature epiphyseodesis in the tunnels traversed by tendons. Femoral physeal cross-sectional analysis showed an 11% frontal and 3% sagittal plane involvements without alteration in length or axial deviation. Tibial cross-section analysis showed 12% frontal and 4% sagittal plane involvements. Two tibiae developed valgus deformities and one was shortened. Stadelmaier and colleagues[29] studied a small number of canines in whom a tensor fascial autograft was placed through tibial and femoral transphyseal drilled defects. In the control animal in which no fascia was placed through similar-sized defects, a transphyseal bone bridge was histologically apparent within 2 weeks postsurgery. These authors also commented on the potential physeal sparing effect of the biologic material spacer in the tunnel. Janarv and colleagues[15] also studied a lapin model in a pilot model to determine the true area of involvement of the drilled undulant femoral physis as well as the true area of the drill hole compared with a planar model of the physis and found that use of the nonanatomic type of planar system underestimated the areas by 24 and 23%, respectively. In a second phase of the study, they determined that the relative size of a transphyseal drill injury required to cause a true growth disturbance was between 7 and 9%, comparable with data noted by previous investigators. They also found that free tendon grafts as well as grafts in continuity prevented bone bridge formation. However, all grafts were surrounded by a thin cylinder of bone. In a large enough graft, the authors question whether a firm cylinder of bone would cause permanent physeal effects. These authors also pointed out that in their studies as well as in other similar animal model studies, the remaining growth duration was quite brief until maturity in contrast with adolescent humans whose exposure to the effects of transphyseal surgery is more prolonged, especially in boys. It must be pointed out that none of the animal series used transphyseal fixation techniques. Whether the effects of these quadruped models can be translated to the unique anatomy demanded by bipedal gait also remains unanswered. The eventual outcome of any grafted tissue that provides the biological scaffolding for neoligament formation must be assessed in terms of the tissue's orientation, size, strength, growth, and isometric substitution potentials.

There are no data that specifically address the timing of surgery in the acutely injured ACL in the skeletally immature patient. I like to wait 10 to 14 days to allow the initial inflammatory response to abate and restore full passive extension. In the uncommon case of a patient with a blocked knee from a displaced meniscal tear, this delay is not possible. I use this interval to again emphasize the 6-month timeline required for recovery and return to sports, despite the contemporary accelerated rehabilitation programs, and to point out that the reinstitution of high-level sports participation postreconstruction is a function of biology and not arthroscopic technology.

ACL reconstruction requires consideration of the three T's — tissues, tunnels, and techniques. Autograft tissues include patellar or hamstring tendons, usually the semitendinosus with or without gracilis augmentation in the latter case. Although allograft use for ACL reconstruction has been reported in adolescents,[1] concerns of potential viral transmission and sterilization effects on graft strength remain.[25] Synthetic replacement of the ACL either as an isolated structure or in combination as a ligament backup carries concerns about longevity, fixation, and foreign body synovitis from wear particles. The tunnels are technique dependent and may include grooves in the tibial epiphysis, over-the-top capsular placement, or tibial tunnel orientation, which is more vertical, in an attempt to improve isometry or may be via the more traditional tibial and femoral tunnels. In the skeletally immature patient, I consider tunnel choices as physeal sparing, partial transphyseal, or complete transphyseal.[31] Physeal-sparing techniques are used in the quite immature patient, Tanner stage 0–I, usually one with an associated meniscal tear requiring treatment as well. I use partial transphyseal procedures in the slightly more mature individual, i.e., Tanner stage II. Patients who are Tanner stage III (postmenarchal girls, boys with curly axillary and pubic hair) are treated by complete transphyseal techniques because their residual femoral and tibial physeal growth is limited.

Physeal-Sparing Techniques

These procedures attempt to provide a ligament restraint without transgressing either the tibial or femoral physis. The major drawback with these methods is the inability to restore anatomic isometric placement of the neoligament. Either a distally based patellar tendon strip or medial hamstring graft in continuity is used (Fig. 68.1). Brief reported a technique using a hamstring tendon graft passed over the anterior tibia,

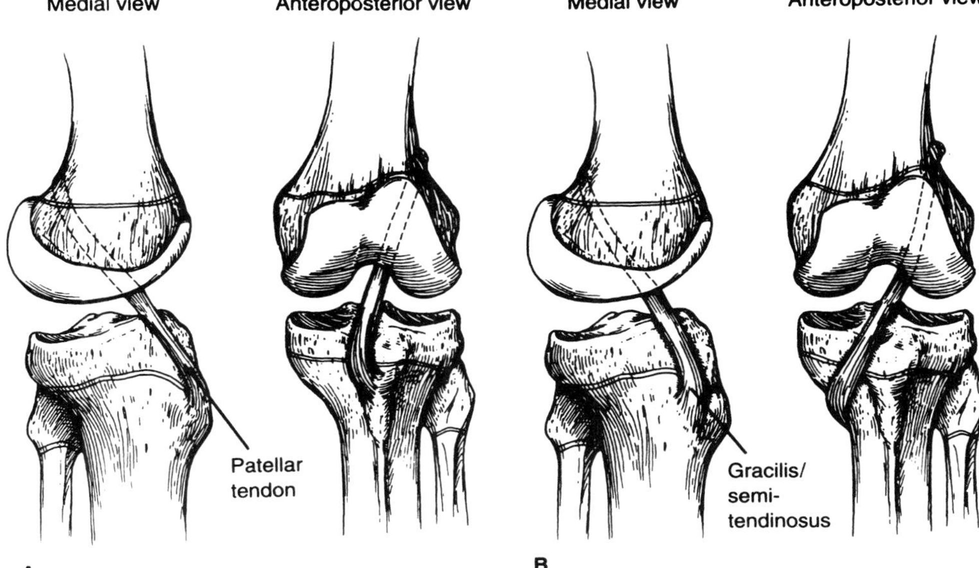

FIGURE 68.1 ➢ Non-transphyseal ACL reconstruction with either *(A)* a patellar tendon segment or *(B)* a gracilis and/or semitendinosus autograft. (From Stanitski CL: ACL injury in the skeletally immature patient. J Am Acad Orthop Surg 3:153, 1995.) Copyright 1995 American Academy of Orthopaedic Surgeons.

under the meniscal coronary ligament, and afixed to the femur in an over-the-top position.[7] In his small series of patients, all of whom were more than 14 years old, they also had an extra-articular iliotibial band tenodesis. During a brief follow-up period, the patients seemed to be doing well, but no functional, objective outcome data were reported. Parker and coworkers[27] described creating a groove in the proximal anterior tibial epiphysis, avoiding the physis, through which is passed a medial hamstring tendon that is attached to the femur in the over-the-top location. The tibial groove's anterior/inferior to superior orientation is designed to place the transfer more centrally and improve its isometry. Each of their six patients had associated meniscal tears and were much younger than those reported by Brief.[7] In the Parker series,[27] outcomes were generally favorable at almost 2-year follow-up.

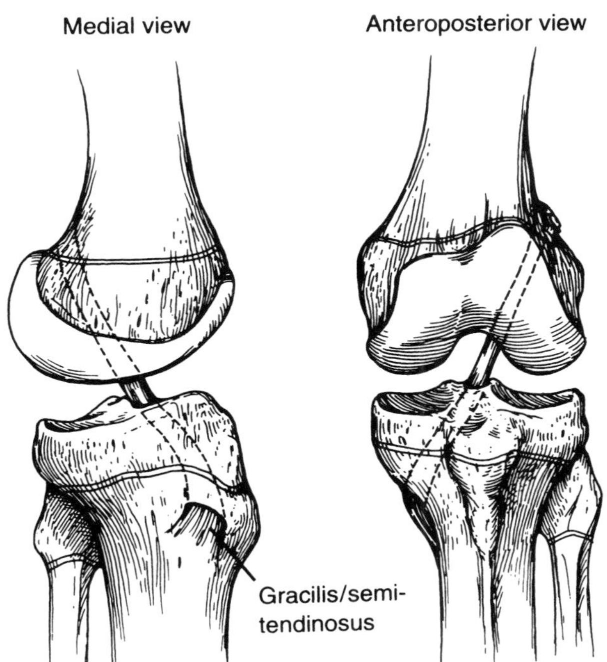

FIGURE 68.2 ➢ Partial transphyseal ACL reception using a hamstring (semitendinosus and/or gracilis) autograft through a transphyseal tibial tunnel with an over-the-top femoral position. A central patellar tendon autograft can be used as an alternative tissue. (From Stanitski CL: ACL injury in the skeletally immature patient. J Am Acad Orthop Surg 3:153, 1995.) Copyright 1995 American Academy of Orthopaedic Surgeons.

Partial Transphyseal Techniques

Patellar or medial hamstring tendon grafts in continuity are usually 6 to 8 mm in diameter and passed intra-articularly through a transphyseal tibial tunnel oriented more vertically than usual in an attempt to improve isometry of the reconstruction. Femoral fixation is at the over-the-top position (Fig. 68.2). As with physeal-sparing techniques, the femoral attachment site must be chosen to not damage the peripheral femoral physis. Lo,[17] reported the largest series using this technique. Their 29 truly skeletally immature patients had excellent functional and objective measurement outcomes at follow-up, which averaged more than 3 years. No clinical or radiographic evidence of limb deformity was seen.

Complete Transphyseal Techniques

ACL reconstruction using complete transphyseal methods is the equivalent of adult-type procedures and is done in patients with advanced skeletal maturity, i.e., Tanner stage III or higher. McCarroll and coworkers[19] reported good results from complete transphyseal reconstructions in mature adolescents. In light of these outstanding results postreconstruction by this highly experienced group of knee surgeons, temporization on reconstruction in the immature patient is advocated

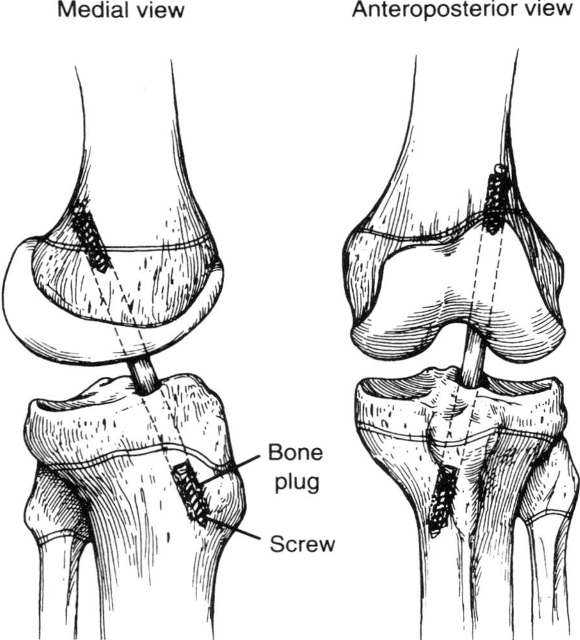

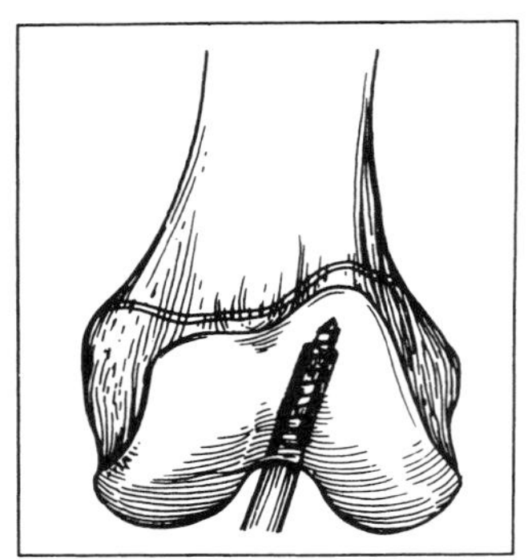

FIGURE 68.3 ➢ Complete transphyseal ACL reconstruction with central patellar tendon autograft with patellar and tibial tubercle bone segments. Fixation is via interference screws. Inset shows an alternative method of femoral fixation. (From Stanitski CL: ACL injury in the skeletally immature patient. J Am Acad Orthop Surg 3: 154, 1995.) Copyright 1995 American Academy of Orthopaedic Surgeons.

until the patient is mature enough to undergo a complete transphyseal procedure.

Graft choice is dependent on the surgeon and may be a patellar bone-patellar tendon-tibial bone construct or a multistrand medial hamstring configuration. Graft fixations are by intra-articular or extra-articular tunnel fixations (Fig. 68.3).

Postoperative Rehabilitation Program

The rehabilitation program is physiologically designed to minimize deleterious effects of immobilization, disuse, and misuse and to encourage maturation of the neoligament and its attachments through physiologically tolerated stresses with progression to the next phase of the program once objective criteria are achieved. The four-phase program I use[33] emphasizes restoration of range of motion and weightbearing; muscle strengthening; increases of speed, agility, power, and endurance; and sports readiness activities. Specific functional objectives must be met prior to return to sports.

Phase I. Immediately postoperative to 6 weeks. A knee immobilizer brace is set from minus 30 to 120 degrees and worn during the day. The patient is encouraged to progressively increase weightbearing with crutch protection with the goal to be crutch free by 6 weeks. Modification of weightbearing and amount of knee flexion is done if concomitant meniscal reconstruction is performed. Active knee flexion is done within the brace's arc of motion. Out-of-brace passive knee extension is done four times daily with emphasis on maintaining full extension. Closed-chain lower extremity-resisted exercises are incorporated for hip flexors and abductors and the gastrocnemius-soleus complex.

Phase II. 6 to 12 weeks postoperatively. This phase focuses on restoring lower extremity muscle strength and endurance using a closed-chain, isokinetic program. At the end of this portion, quadriceps strength should be at least two-thirds of the opposite quadriceps by isokinetic testing at 120 degrees/second from minus 30 to 120 degrees of motion, and knee motion should be full.

Phase IIIA. 12 to 18 weeks postoperatively. Using a functional brace and level ground, straight line running is begun and as quadriceps/hamstring strength ratio is normalized, agility drills begin. Quadriceps strength should be 75% to 80% of normal at the end of this phase.

Phase IIIB. 18 to 24 weeks postoperatively. Advanced agility drills are added as lower extremity strength and endurance are normalized. In the final part of this phase, sports-specific tasks are introduced and are done at progressively higher speeds.

Phase IV. 24 weeks and beyond. Return to full sport participation is permitted when full, painless motion is present and strength, endurance, stability, and agility are equal to the opposite normal side. Functional bracing is continued during sports.

The rehabilitation program is modified according to delays present in each of the phases. No specific complication management results have been presented in large numberrs following ACL reconstruction of skeletally immature patients. Complications similar to ones seen in adults can be expected and include loss of motion, fibroarthrosis, and donor and insertion site problems. With the introduction of current early motion and rehabilitation programs, problems of loss of motion are uncommon. The specter of limb length, rotation, and angular deformity exists if imprudent decision making or technical surgical errors result in physeal compromise. Experimental and limited clinical data suggest that such growth complications are uncommon if appropriate indications and surgical approaches are observed.[1, 17, 27]

In summary, skeletally immature patients do get ACL injuries, and decisions regarding treatment must include the patient's physiological age and amount of growth remaining at the two major lower extremity physes. Nonoperative treatment requires counseling about avoidance of high-demand sports that would lead to further intra-articular injury and premature joint senescence. If meniscal tears requiring surgical management occur concomitant with a complete ACL tear, surgical reconstruction of both structures is recommended, tailoring the ACL technique appropriate for the patient's maturity. Three types of ACL reconstruction are considered: physeal sparing, partial transphyseal, and complete transphyseal. Each case must be assessed independently based on the patient's anatomic and physiological assets and liabilities.

TIBIAL EMINENCE AVULSION FRACTURES

Avulsion fractures of the tibial intercondylar eminence occur because of the modulus mismatch present between the ACL and its insertion to the tibial proximal chondroepiphysis, especially in the 8- 12-year-old age group. This age spread reflects the relative physiological skeletal maturity seen in this chronologic span. The mechanism of injury is almost always knee hyperflexion, particularly associated with falls from a bicycle. Unfortunately, fractures of the tibial eminence have been dismissed as the ACL injury of the immature knee, and true ACL tears are often misdiagnosed as commented on in the previous section. The natural history and outcome of the skeletally immature patient with a tibial eminence fracture are in marked counterdistinction from their counterpart with a complete ACL tear.

Patients with this injury present with acute knee pain, limited knee motion from guarding due to pain, or true mechanical obstruction by the displaced fragment. Tenderness may be diffuse but examination of the joint lines, collateral ligament areas, and femoral and tibial physes helps to identify other sites of associated injury. Because of the acuity of the injury and its attendant diminished patient cooperation with the clinical exam because of pain, muscle spasm, and guarding, the associated sagittal laxity may not be appreciated at the initial assessment.

Standard four-view knee radiographs are the primary imaging studies, taking particular effort to ensure that a true lateral is accomplished so classification of the injury can be done. Because of the often significant chondral segment of the fracture fragment, the injury may be dismissed as being only a small chip and the true extent of the damage underestimated. I find that the anteroposterior and tunnel views usually provide better data about fragment rotation and comminution than does the lateral radiograph. More sophisticated imaging methods, e.g., computed tomography scan and MRI, are usually not required and do not add a significant factor in the treatment decision. The initial radiographic classification of this injury dealt only with the sagittal displacement of the fragment[21] but was later modified to encompass not only the amount of fragment sagittal displacement but also fragment comminution.[38] The fracture types indicate progressive increase in the amount of displacement of the fragment from its bed, with type I being the most benign and type IV representing significant displacement and comminution. Type I has minimal displacement (<3 mm), type II has an anterior flap elevation of one-third to one-half of the fragment, type III has sagittal and usually rotation displacement of the entire fragment, and type IV has comminution of the completely displaced fragment (Fig. 68.4).

The natural history of tibial eminence avulsion fractures is usually quite good, with rapid healing and few functional complaints despite varying amounts of residual sagittal plane laxity and slight limitation of extension demonstrated on follow-up examination.[13, 21, 36, 37, 38] Even though the patients were skeletally mature at follow-up in several series, they were still quite young and had not undergone the vocational and avocational stresses and demands of advancing age. With current enhanced techniques of diagnosis, associated injuries are being recognized with increasing frequency especially in types III and IV fractures. Medial collateral and meniscal (usually medial) damage has been reported in as high as 10% to 20% of tibial eminence fracture cases.[6, 20, 35] No data have been reported that specifically look at the outcome of patients with these associated injuries because these patients' outcomes were incorporated in the ones without associated injuries.

Treatment of tibial eminence avulsion fractures depends on the fracture classification and associated injuries. In undisplaced, uncomplicated type I fractures, if the knee cannot be placed in full extension, local anesthetic is injected intra-articularly after hemarthrosis evacuation to allow full extension. Controversy exists as to the optimal knee casted position, i.e., full extension versus 30 degrees of flexion to diminish ACL tension.[5, 13, 20, 35, 36, 37] I use full extension and avoid hyperextension, which is painful and unnecessary. Placement in 30 degrees of knee flexion in a knee whose ACL is already attenuated does not seem to make physiologic sense to me. The concept of knee extension for fracture reduction was advocated to allow fragment reduction by femoral condylar impingement on the fragment. Although this mechanism may be true for the uncommon case of fragments with large basilar extensions into the lateral and medial tib-

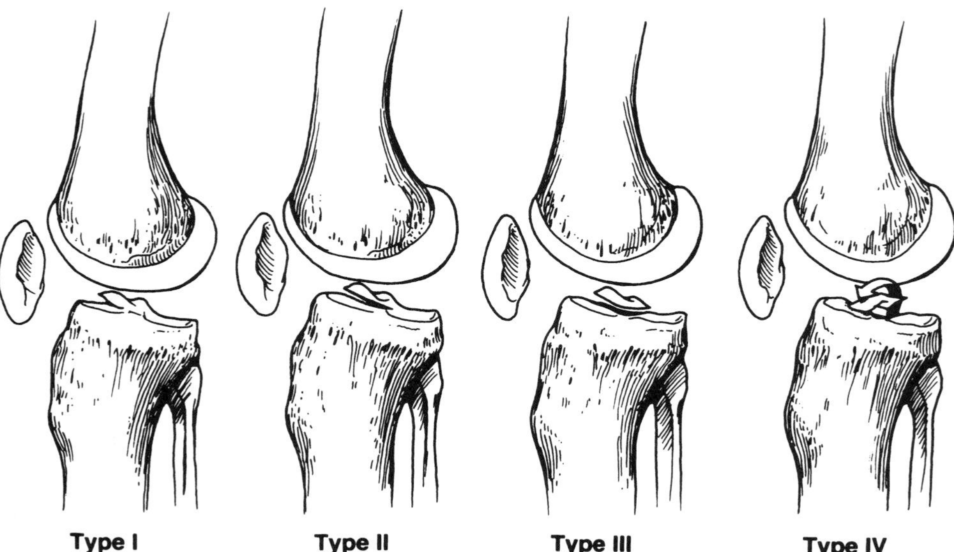

FIGURE 68.4 ➢ Tibial eminence avulsion fracture classification. Type III may be rotated (III+) and type IV represents fragment displacement rotation and comminution. (From Stanitski CL: ACL injury in the skeletally immature patient. J Am Acad Orthop Surg 3: 151, 1995.) Copyright 1995 American Academy of Orthopaedic Surgeons.

ial compartments, in the majority of cases, fragment morphology does not come into contact with the femoral condyles, and reduction and maintenance of the reduction are effected by impingement of the fragment by the femoral intercondylar notch. In type I cases, I immobilize the patient for 4 weeks in a cylinder cast with progressive weightbearing with initial crutch protected gait. Repeat lateral radiographs are done at weekly intervals for the first 2 weeks to ensure that the reduction is maintained. In type II fractures, reduction is done to prevent residual fragment deformity, which will prevent full knee extension. Following knee aspiration and intra-articular injection of local anesthetic, the knee is placed in extension and confirmation of reduction is done by a true lateral knee radiograph. A bolster is used at the ankle to provide knee extension and lateral support at the knee and to prevent the tendency of the limb to externally rotate during the exposure. If anatomic fracture restoration within 2 mm is achieved, cylinder casting treatment is done for 6 weeks with weightbearing with initial crutch protection. Repeat radiographs are done weekly for the first 2 weeks to document fracture reduction. If anatomic reduction is not achieved, I recommend arthroscopic assessment of the fracture to ascertain the reason for fracture malreduction. At surgery, the meniscus (usually medial in my experience) is commonly found trapped in the fracture site. A probe easily removes this obstruction to reduction. Knee extension is then achieved, and if the fragment is well reduced and no other associated injuries are present intra-articularly, the limb is incorporated in a cylinder cast with the knee in extension and the post-cast fracture reduction confirmed by lateral radiograph. If significant comminution of the fragment is present or anatomic restoration of reduction cannot be achieved, arthroscopic reduction and fixation of the fracture are carried out by techniques used for types III and IV fractures.

In type III or IV tibial eminence fractures, fracture reduction and fixation can be done by traditional arthrotomy or by arthroscopic techniques.[5, 16, 20, 35, 38] Meniscal injuries are dealt with by established principles and techniques, taking into account the meniscal injury's site, size, and stability. Fragment reduction is

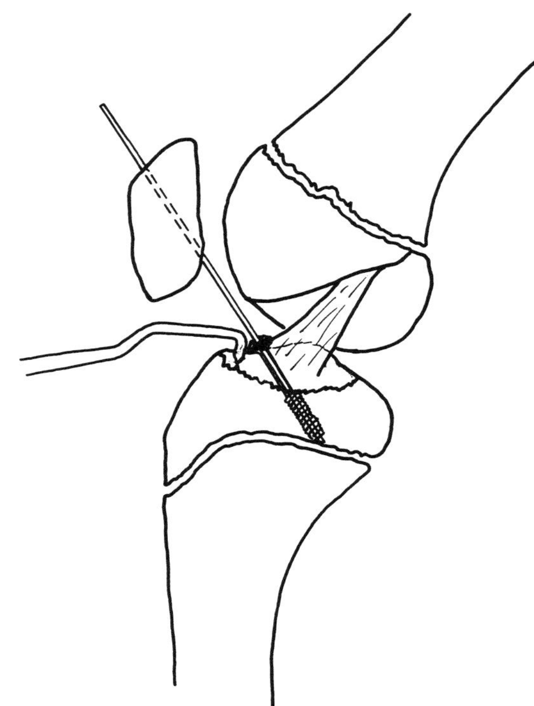

FIGURE 68.5 ➢ Percutaneous fixation of an acute tibial eminence avulsion fracture using a cannulated small fragment screw following arthroscopic fracture reduction. The guided pin is started medially at the upper pole of the patella. Note the prevention of physeal transgression of the fixation system. (From Wall EJ: Tibial eminence fractures in children. Op Tech Sp Med 6:209, 1998.)

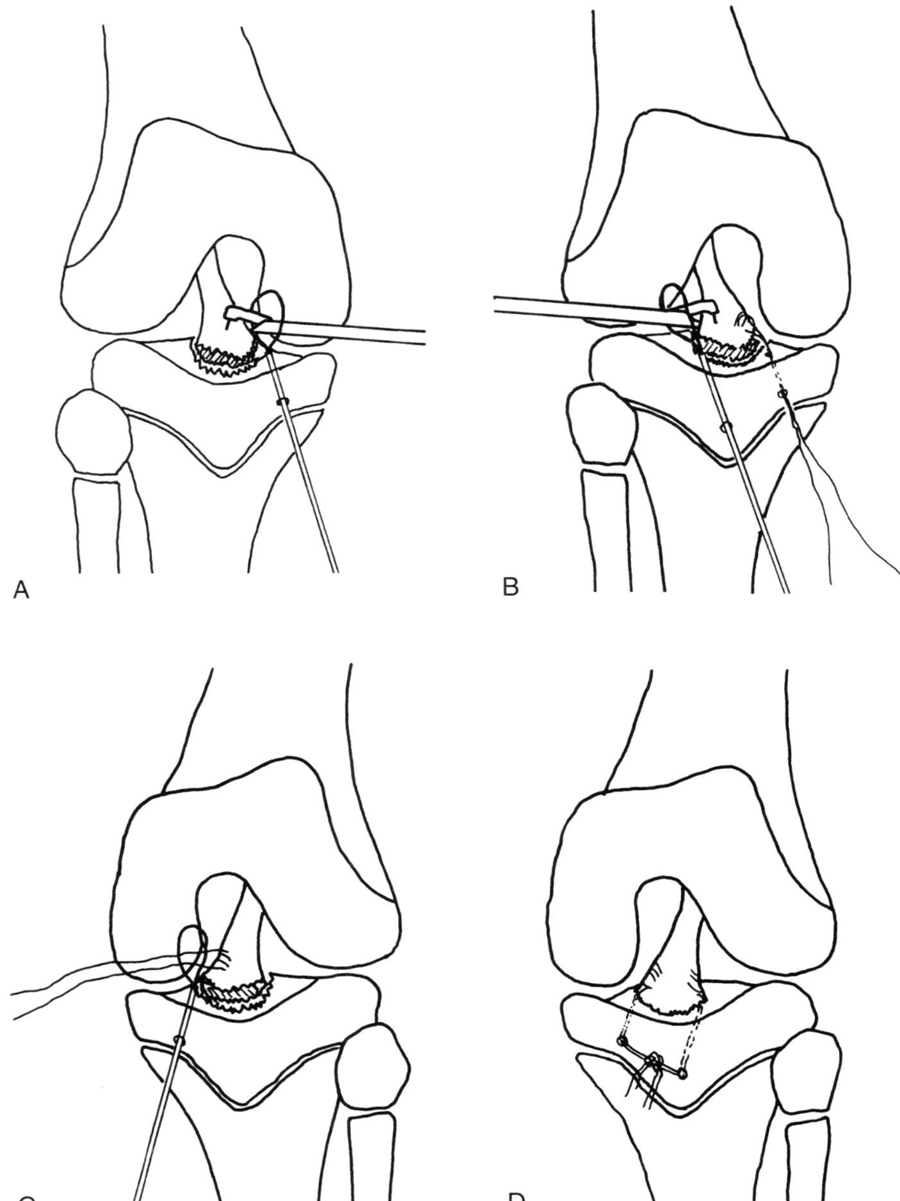

FIGURE 68.6 ➢ Arthroscopic management of a comminuted acute tibial eminence avulsion fracture not amenable to screw fixation. A ligament suture passer is placed through the epiphysis *(A–C);* sparing the physis the sutures provides both reduction and fixation when tied over the anterior tibial epiphysis *(D)*. (From Wall EJ: Tibial eminence fractures in children. Op Tech Sp Med 6:209, 1998.)

done by probe manipulation after any obstructions are removed from the fracture site and the fragment reduction is maintained using an ACL guide. If the fragment is large enough (>1 × 1 cm) and without comminution, fixation can be done using a cannulated screw placed through a percutaneous proximal-medial approach, taking care to not violate the proximal tibial physis.[5, 24, 35] The head of the screw (usually <20 mm) should be seated within the ligament substance to avoid impingement in extension (Fig. 68.5). Countersinking the fragment into the epiphysis in an attempt to restore isometry to the attenuated ligament is not recommended. Type IV comminuted fractures do not lend themselves to screw fixation and are repaired using suture methods about the ACL bone "stump."[6, 16, 35] Once again, care is taken to avoid physeal damage with suture passage through the tibial epiphysis (Fig. 68.6). Postoperatively, patients with types III and IV fractures are immobilized in a cylinder cast with the knee in extension and crutch-protected weight-bearing gait used initially. Lateral knee radiographs are done weekly for the first 2 weeks to document maintenance of fracture reduction. If the fracture fragment was large and uncomminuted and the fixation solid, immobilization is done for only 4 weeks followed by use of controlled motion brace, similar to the ones used following ACL reconstruction. In cases with tenuous screw fixation or in those requiring suture fixation because of fracture comminution, immobilization is continued for 6 weeks.

Complications following tibial eminence fracture are uncommon but include loss of extension, arthrofibrosis, fracture malunion, and nonunion with late reavulsion. The period of immobilization should be as brief as is compatible with fracture healing, and, in noninternally fixed fractures, is usually 6 weeks. Postimmobilization rehabilitation is similar to the type used following ACL reconstruction with emphasis on restoration of full extension. Arthrofibrosis with loss of flexion and extension may occur as a consequence of the inflammatory synovial response to the injury and associated hemarthrosis. If progressive gains in knee range of motion are not seen within the first month postimmobilization with a stable fracture, arthroscopic lysis and débridement of adhesions should be done with postoperative caudal analgesia provided to allow aggressive rehabilitation. Knee manipulation should be avoided in these children because of the potential for femoral and tibial physeal fractures, especially in the postimmobilization period. If symptomatic loss of knee extension occurs due to fracture malunion, notchplasty is done to eliminate the impingement.

In summary, skeletally immature patients with tibial eminence fractures tend to do quite well. This injury should be suspected in 8- to 12-year-old patients with an acute knee injury from a fall from a bicycle. Minor loss of extension and clinical exam sagittal plane laxity are often seen at follow-up but do not cause functional limitations, in general. In the relatively small percentage of patients with associated rotatory instability, the mechanism of injury, i.e., flexion/rotation, caused damage to the secondary restraints with resultant combined instability. This is in contrast to the direct flexion mechanism, which preserves the secondary capsular restraints. Associated meniscal and collateral ligament injuries should be sought, especially in older patients. Treatment is dependent on fracture type, with reduction and fixation needed for the more advanced types. Arthroscopic techniques of fracture reduction and fixation usually produce excellent outcomes. Because the fracture occurs through a chondroepiphysis, awareness of the potential for physeal injury with imprecise fixation methods must be kept in mind.

References

1. Andrews M, Noyes FR, Barber-Westin SD: Anterior cruciate ligament allograft reconstruction in the skeletally immature athlete. Am J Sports Med 22:48, 1994.
2. Angel K, Hall D: Anterior cruciate ligament injury in children and adolescents. Arthroscopy 5:197, 1989.
3. Arendt EA, Dick R: Knee injury patterns among men and women in collegiate basketball and soccer: NCAA data and review of literature. Am J Sports Med 23:694, 1995.
4. Beachy G, et al: High school sports injuries. Am J Sports Med 25:675, 1997.
5. Berg EE: Pediatric tibial eminence fractures: Arthroscopic cannulated screw fixation. Arthroscopy 11:328, 1995.
6. Berg EE: Comminuted tibial eminence anterior cruciate ligament avulsion fractures: Failure of arthroscopic treatment. Arthroscopy 9:446, 1993.
7. Brief LP: Anterior cruciate ligament reconstruction without drilling holes. Arthroscopy 7:350, 1991.
8. DeLee JC, Curtis R: Anterior cruciate ligament insufficiency in children. Clin Orthop 172:112, 1983.
9. Garces GL, Mugica-Garay I, Lopez-Gonzales Coviella N, et al: Growth-plate modifications after drilling. J Pediatr Orthop 14: 225, 1994.
10. Graf BK, Lange RH, Fujisaki K, et al: Anterior cruciate ligament tears in skeletally immature patients: Meniscal pathology at presentation and after attempted conservative treatment. Arthroscopy 8:229, 1992.
11. Guzzanti V, Falciglia F, Gigante A, et al: The effect of intra-articular ACL reconstruction on the growth plates of rabbits. J Bone Joint Surg Br 76:960, 1994.
12. Hensinger RN: Standards in Pediatric Orthopaedics: Tables, Charts, and Graphs Illustrating Growth. New York, Raven Press, 1986.
13. Janarv PM, Wesblad P, Johansson C, et al: Long-term follow-up of anterior tibial spine fractures in children. J Pediatr Orthop 15: 63, 1995.
14. Janarv PM, Nystrom A, Werner S, et al: Anterior cruciate ligament injuries in skeletally immature patients. J Pediatr Orthop 16:673, 1996.
15. Janarv PM, Wikstrom B, Hirsch G: The influence of transphyseal drilling and tendon grafting on bone growth: An experimental study in the rabbit. J Pediatr Orthop 18:149, 1998.
16. Kogan MG, Marks P, Amendola A: Technique for arthroscopic suture fixation of displaced tibial intercondylar eminence fractures. Arthroscopy 10:301, 1997.
17. Lo IKY, Fowler PJ, Miniaci A: The outcome of operative treated anterior cruciate disruptions in the skeletally immature child. Arthroscopy 13:627, 1997.
18. Makela EA, Vainionpaa S, Vihtonen K, et al: The effect of trauma of the lower femoral epiphyseal plate. J Bone Joint Surg Br 70: 187, 1988.
19. McCarroll JR, Shelbourne KB, Rettig AC, et al: Patellar tendon graft reconstruction for midsubstance anterior cruciate ligament rupture in junior high school athletes: An algorithm for management. Am J Sports Med 22:478, 1994.
20. McLennan JG: Lessons learned after second-look arthroscopy in type III fractures of the tibial spine. J Pediatr Orthop 15:59, 1995.
21. Meyers MH, McKeever FM: Fracture of the intercondylar eminence of the tibia. J Bone Joint Surg Am 52: 1677, 1970.
22. Mizuta H, Kubota K, Shiraishi M, et al: The conservative treatment of complete tears of the anterior cruciate ligament in skeletally immature patients. J Bone Joint Surg Br 77: 890, 1995.
23. Moretz JA: Long-term follow-up of knee injuries in high school football players. Am J Sports Med 12:298, 1984.
24. Mylle J, Reynders P, Broos P: Transepiphyseal fixation of anterior cruciate avulsion in a child: Report of a complication and a review of the literature. Arch Orthop Trauma Surg 112:101, 1993.
25. Nemzek JA, Arnoczky S, Swenson CL: Retroviral transmission by the transplantation of connective tissue allografts. J Bone Joint Surg Am 76:1036, 1984.
26. Noyes FR, Mooar PA, et al: The symptomatic anterior cruciate-deficient knee. Part I: The long-term functional disability in athletically active individuals. J Bone Joint Surg Am 65:154, 1983.
27. Parker AW, Drez D Jr, Cooper JL: Anterior cruciate ligament injuries in patients with open physes. Am J Sports Med 22:44, 1994.
28. Pressman AE, Letts RM, Jarvis JG: Anterior cruciate ligament tears in children: An analysis of operative versus nonoperative treatment. J Pediatr Orthop 17:505, 1997.
29. Stadelmailer DM, Arnoczky SP, Dodds J, et al: The effect of drilling and soft tissue grafting across open growth plates: A histologic study. Am J Sports Med 23:431, 1995.
30. Stanitski CL, Harvell JC, Fu F: Observations on acute knee hemarthrosis in children and adolescents. J Pediatr Orthop 3:506, 1993.
31. Stanitski CL: Anterior cruciate ligament injury in the skeletally immature patient: Diagnosis and treatment. J Am Acad Orthop Surg 3:145, 1995.
32. Stanitski CL: Correlation of arthroscopic and clinical examinations with magnetic resonance imaging findings of injured knees in children. Am J Sports Med 26:2, 1998.
33. Stanitski CL: Anterior cruciate ligament injury in the skeletally immature athlete. Op Tech Sports Med 6:228, 1998.

34. Tanner JM, Davies PSW: Clinical longitudinal standards for height and weight velocity for North American children. J Pediatr Orthop 107:317, 1985.
35. Wall EJ: Tibial eminence fractures in children. Op Tech Sports Med 6:206, 1998.
36. Wiley JJ, Baxter MP: Tibial spine fractures in children. Clin Orthop 255:54, 1990.
37. Willis RB, Blokker C, Stoll, TM, et al: Long-term follow-up of anterior tibial eminence fractures. J Pediatr Orthop 13:361, 1993.
38. Zaricznyj B: Avulsion fracture of the tibial eminence: Treatment by open reduction and pinning. J Bone Joint Surg Am 63:1342, 1981.

SECTION X

Joint Replacement and Its Alternatives

69 Surgical Pathology of Arthritis

M.A.R. FREEMAN

The view of the surgical pathology in osteoarthritis and rheumatoid arthritis set out in this chapter is based on my clinical and operative observations. Although this presentation stands mostly on common ground, it is somewhat controversial, to be viewed as a working hypothesis requiring confirmation or refutation. This discussion is limited to my personal view for clarity of exposition, without reference to those generally accepted observations that can be found readily in the literature. I make no claim to originality.

INITIATION OF OSTEOARTHRITIS AND RHEUMATOID ARTHRITIS OF THE KNEE

Osteoarthritis of the knee, as of other joints, is almost certainly attributable fundamentally to mechanical events. For example, a rise in the contact pressures applied to articular cartilage produced by meniscectomy or the malunion of tibial or femoral fractures (Fig. 69.1) may give rise to osteoarthritis in the presumably overloaded compartment, but not initially elsewhere in the knee. The initial changes affect the cartilage, and it is at least probable that fragmentation of the collagen fiber network, caused by fatigue failure in the face of raised contact stresses, is the fundamental event.[4]

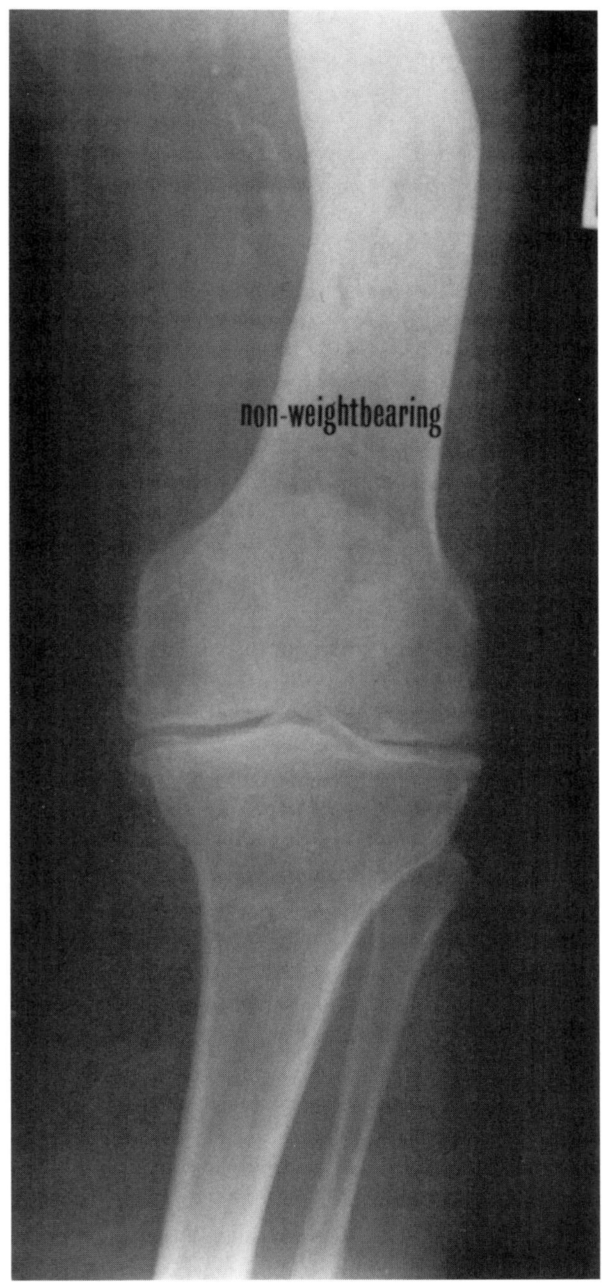

FIGURE 69.1 ➢ Varus malunion of a fracture of the shaft of the femur with medial osteoarthrosis in the ipsilateral knee. It is tempting to suggest that the degenerative changes in this knee were produced by the medial shift in the resultant of the forces acting on the joint after the malunion.

Osteoarthritis

Changes in the bone subjacent to the cartilage are negligible until the cartilage is lost. They then appear to be caused by bone-to-bone contact and by the resultant mechanical disturbances (including abrasive wear and a rise in contact stresses) in the bone; certainly most changes in the bone can be explained on this basis,[3] and pain is not significant until bone is exposed in the articular surface. One bone alteration, osteophyte formation, represents an exception to this generalization, since osteophytes can form at the margin of intact surfaces (in knees displaying degenerative changes in other parts of the joint).

This view of the genesis of osteoarthritis would suggest that abnormalities in the knee might be focal initially, affecting only those areas in which the contact stresses are increased. This expectation is confirmed on the gross scale by the frequent finding of macroscopically unicompartmental degenerative changes (Fig. 69.2); it has now been further shown that the unfibrillated cartilage in knees, such as that

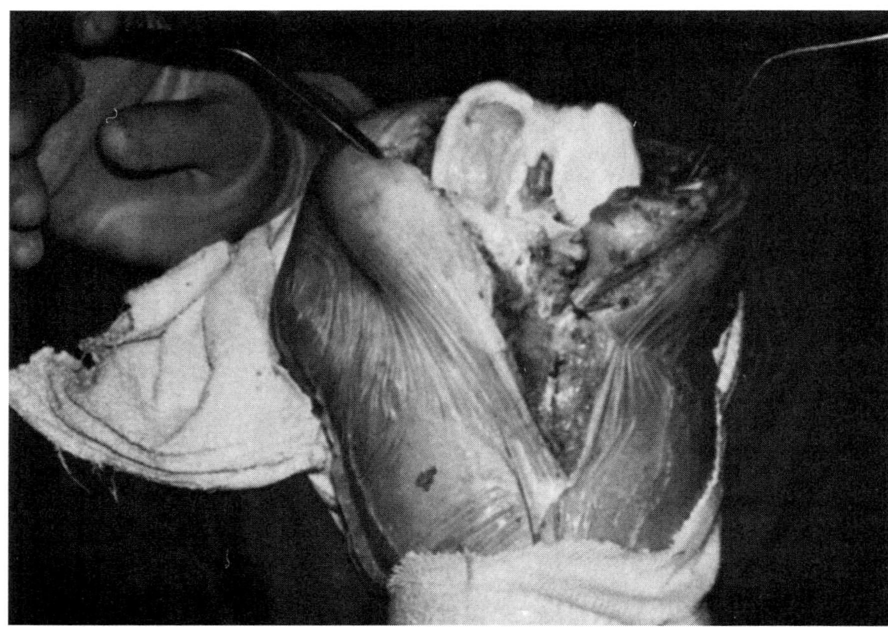

FIGURE 69.2 ➢ Unicompartmental osteoarthrosis of the tibiofemoral joint. Recent work (see text) has demonstrated that if the cartilage in the intact compartment is not fibrillated, it is functionally normal.

shown in Figure 69.2, is, for practical purposes, normal histologically and thus functionally.[1]

Summary

In summary, osteoarthritis may be viewed as a focal mechanical disorder that ends up destroying first the articular cartilage and thereafter the bone. Because the bone starts out in a normal state, its destruction begins slowly and is further retarded by reactive new bone formation.

Adult human articular chondrocytes do not appear to be capable of undergoing mitosis.[15] (Chondrocyte cluster formation has been interpreted as evidence of chondrocyte mitosis, but, in my view, clusters probably arise from the loss of matrix between previously separated cells rather than from cell division.) Thus true healing of an articular cartilage defect cannot occur. Even an effective reactive cellular response to incipient destruction of the matrix seems unlikely, in view of the extreme slowness of collagen turnover in cartilage and the complexity of the organization of the fibers in this tissue.[10, 12] Thus true healing of cartilage ulcers and the regression of fibrillation do not appear to be realistic therapeutic possibilities.

Although true healing cannot (and, in my view, does not) occur, healing by scar formation is a possibility. As a consequence, exposed bone surfaces can be recovered by functionally useful fibrocartilage. This tissue, derived from granulation tissue reaching the exposed bone surface from the marrow spaces, first becomes loosely fibrous and then fibrocartilaginous in response to compression. This sequence implies that gaps in the bone surface are a prerequisite for this process and hence that a dense, sclerotic surface is unlikely to acquire soft-tissue coverage. Equally, soft-tissue coverage cannot be expected if the bone in question is constantly subjected to abrasive wear by the opposing condyle, since this must result in the destruction of any granulation tissue that reaches the surface. These facts imply that in order to achieve healing by fibrocartilage (i.e., by scar formation), two conditions must exist: (1) bone sclerosis must not be far advanced or, if it is, gaps in sclerotic surfaces must be made surgically; and (2) the high contact pressures originally responsible for cartilage destruction must be eliminated to preserve any granulation tissue reaching the surface. The first of these implications provides the rationale for surgical drilling of sclerotic surfaces and the second for osteotomy.

Rheumatoid Arthritis

In contrast to osteoarthritis, rheumatoid arthritis appears to be caused by the generalized destruction of cartilage by lysozymal enzymes, perhaps particularly collagenase derived from leukocytes. Because the cartilage is destroyed as part of a generalized enzymatic attack (much as it is in septic arthritis), its loss is also generalized. Cartilage that has been mechanically weakened by enzymatic attack will of course be more than usually susceptible to mechanical destruction. Thus the cartilage lesions in rheumatoid arthritis may be worse in some places than in others, although the cartilage is nowhere normal, that is, the lesions are both general (enzymatic) and focal (mechanical). This contrasts with the essentially focal nature of the lesions of osteoarthritis.

Two other surgically relevant considerations follow from the generalized inflammatory nature of the cartilage destruction in rheumatoid arthritis: (1) destruction of cartilage, leading to bone exposure, might be expected to occur more rapidly in rheumatoid arthritis; and (2) cartilage healing by scar formation, which might conceivably be induced in osteoarthritis, seems inconceivable in rheumatoid arthritis. Finally, the hyperemia in the joint, disuse, and even medicinal therapy produce osteoporosis; thus bone destruction, like cartilage destruction, is more rapid in rheumatoid arthritis.

The initial cause of the synovitis in rheumatoid arthritis is unknown, but it seems clear that its bad prognosis for the joint can be traced to the resultant enzymatic attack on the cartilage; a synovitis without this enzymatic attack, such as that which occurs in rheumatic fever, leaves the joint unscathed. Thus the prognosis for the joint in rheumatoid arthritis is similar to that in septic arthritis and unlike that in rheumatic fever because in both rheumatoid arthritis and septic arthritis, but not in rheumatic fever, leukocytes reach the joint cavity to produce generalized enzymatic destruction of the cartilage. Enzymatic attack might conceivably be prevented by synovectomy, but clinical experience shows that this procedure is at best unpredictably beneficial. In contrast to the uncertain effect that removal of the synovium has on the cartilage, the removal of the cartilage (by arthrodesis or total knee replacement) predictably aborts, indeed effectively cures, the synovitis. This clinical observation suggests that the synovitis may be in some way attributable to the presence of cartilage in the joint, a speculation now strongly supported by experimental work, as reviewed by Cooke.[2]

Summary

In summary, rheumatoid arthritis appears to be caused by a generalized enzymatic attack on cartilage to which focal mechanical factors may be added. The destruction of both cartilage and bone is not only more generalized than in osteoarthritis, it is also usually more rapid. Because any cartilage that remains in the joint is mechanically very abnormal, osteotomy is unlikely to be useful. Perhaps because residual cartilage is actually responsible for the synovitis in the first place,[2] the only surgical treatments that might, a priori, be expected to be successful are those involving the ablation of cartilage (i.e., arthrodesis and total joint replacement).

If this general view of the surgical pathology in osteoarthritis and rheumatoid arthritis is correct, it should be possible to demonstrate the presence of bone and cartilage loss in the knee and to explain the various misalignments (e.g., varus and valgus) seen in the clinical setting on this basis. This description would constitute a rational anatomic basis for such surgical procedures as osteotomy and knee replacement. Before considering the knee in this way, however, it is helpful to review briefly the presumably similar surgical pathology in osteoarthritis and rheumatoid arthritis of the hip, since this joint has been available for study for many years and the findings are now not a matter of controversy.

RELEVANT CHANGES IN THE HIP

Bone and Cartilage Loss

In osteoarthritis, bone and cartilage loss usually occurs superolaterally at the zenith of the femoral head and acetabulum, but it may occur medially. In the former situation, it accounts for the wandering acetabulum, for lateral subluxation, for a break in Shenton's line, and for true shortening of the leg. Measured by the latter, a loss of 2 cm of bone is not uncommon. Medial bone and cartilage loss leads to protrusio acetabulae, a change that occurs more commonly in rheumatoid arthritis than in osteoarthritis. Just as in the hip, where bone loss may be predominantly lateral or medial, at the knee it will be shown that bone loss may also be predominantly medial or lateral. In this connection there is an interesting but ill-defined similarity between lateral bone loss at the hip (producing lateral subluxation of the femur) and medial bone loss at the knee (producing varus and lateral subluxation of the tibia). Both are common osteoarthrotic patterns in contrast to their opposites (protrusio at the hip and valgus at the knee), which occur mainly in rheumatoid arthritis. If the former is the result of some shared mechanical feature of the hip and knee, it may be speculated that the obliquity of the femoral shaft may have some bearing on the matter. Thus if the lower limb is thought of as a vertical pelvis, an oblique femur, and a vertical tibia, axial compression would tend to "squeeze" the upper end of the femur laterally and the lower end of the femur medially, thereby producing lateral tibial subluxation.

Soft-Tissue Contracture

Soft-tissue contracture affects particularly the muscles on the anterior and medial aspects of the hip, accounting for fixed flexion and fixed adduction. Of these, the most dramatic, well-known example is a contracture of the adductor muscles (especially of adductor longus), accounting for the persistence of an adduction deformity after hip replacement unless corrected by adductor tenotomy. Adhesions around ligaments may also maintain deformities.

Osteophyte Formation

Osteophytes grow by endochondral ossification,[3] (with the possible exception of medial tibial osteophytes in the varus knee, which may be formed in part by "crushing" the bone's articular margin). Thus osteophytosis occurs particularly in osteoarthritis, where peripheral cartilage persists. In rheumatoid arthritis, the generalized loss of cartilage tends to prevent osteophyte formation. Osteophytes grow only in soft-tissue spaces, the best example being the space created in the cavity of the hip inferomedial to the femoral head by bone loss at the zenith and lateral migration of the head. Although osteophytes may limit movement mechanically (and thus help to maintain deformity) it is difficult to conceive that their growth could actually produce deformity by pushing the bones into an abnormal position.

Ligamentous Elongation

Ligamentous elongation appears never to occur to any significant extent in the arthritic hip, even in rheumatoid arthritis. Hypermobility and dislocation, which would be expected if gross elongation did occur, are never seen.

Ligamentous Rupture

Ligamentous rupture affects only the intracapsular ligament in the hip (the ligamentum teres). Whether the ligament is destroyed by enzymatic digestion or by mechanical attrition is unclear. In rheumatoid arthritis both seem possible, whereas in osteoarthritis the latter is more likely.

Summary

At the hip, the processes responsible for the development and maintenance of deformity appear to be the loss of cartilage and bone occurring either laterally or medially and soft-tissue adhesions and contractures (affecting ligaments and muscles, respectively). Ligamentous elongation either does not occur or does so only to a slight extent. Ligament rupture affects only intracapsular ligaments (the ligamentum teres) that can be exposed to mechanical attrition. Osteophytes grow by endochondral ossification into soft-tissue spaces. They thus only appear where cartilage persists.

If bone loss and soft-tissue contracture are the cause of deformity at the hip, and if significant ligamentous elongation does not occur at this joint, it would not be unreasonable to expect that the same would be true of the knee. This view is, however, controversial; valgus and varus instabilities in the arthritic knee have been attributed (presumably by analogy with similar instability after ligamentous injury) to elongated or defective medial and lateral collateral ligaments, respectively. However, although instability in the arthritic knee might theoretically be attributed to elongation, it is equally possible that instability might be caused by bone loss on the concave side of the joint, a view that would be consistent with the morbid anatomy of the arthritic hip. On this view, valgus or varus instability at the arthritic knee could be accounted for by postulating the presence of bone loss, and fixed valgus or varus deformity by postulating a combination of bone loss and soft-tissue contracture.

The existence of these alternative pathologic explanations for valgus and varus deformity is not simply of academic interest, since if these and other misalignments are to be reversed rationally, the nature of the underlying structural abnormalities must first be understood.

NATURE OF MORBID ANATOMIC CHANGES RESPONSIBLE FOR DEFORMITY OF THE KNEE IN OSTEOARTHRITIS AND RHEUMATOID ARTHRITIS

This section considers, first, instability in a varus and valgus direction and, second, the same two malalignments, but with the addition of fixed deformity. Other abnormalities of alignment seen in the arthritic knee are then considered.

Varus Instability

Theoretically, varus instability might be caused by (1) rupture and/or elongation of the lateral soft tissues (as after soft-tissue trauma), or (2) a loss of bone medially, or both. Both pathologic processes would produce the same physical sign on the examination couch, that is, it would be possible to displace the tibia from neutral to varus alignment and back again. In contrast, if the knee were to be compressed axially (as on bearing weight or during muscular contraction), a knee with normal bones would tend to be stabilized in normal alignment, whereas a knee with bone loss would tend to be driven into the position of deformity (Fig. 69.3). It is a commonplace radiologic observation in the arthritic knee (1) that bone loss is present (Fig. 69.4), and (2) that the affected knee falls into a position of deformity on bearing weight (Fig. 69.5). It may be concluded—even without visual inspection of the articular surfaces of the knee—that bony defects are

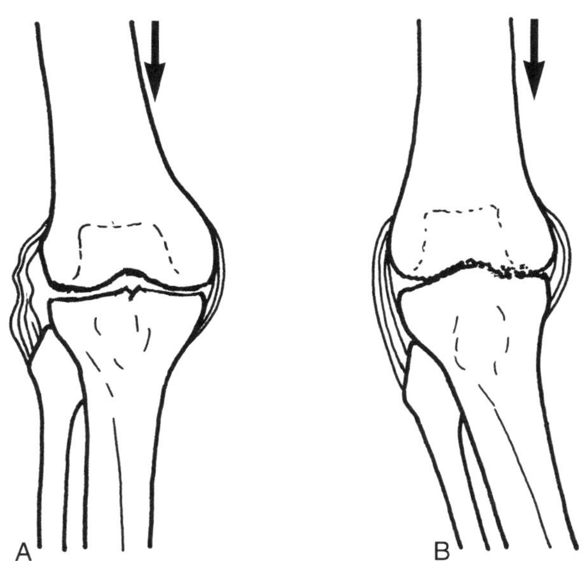

FIGURE 69.3 ➢ *A*, Diagram showing a knee without bone defects but with laxity of the lateral collateral ligament loaded in compression, as during one-leg stance. Because the line of action of the load on the knee passes through the area of contact between the femoral and tibial condyles, there is no tendency for the joint to open laterally; thus normal alignment is maintained. *B*, Diagram showing a knee with a medial bone defect during one-leg stance. The load now acts to close the defect, causing the knee to buckle into varus malalignment. (From Freeman[5].)

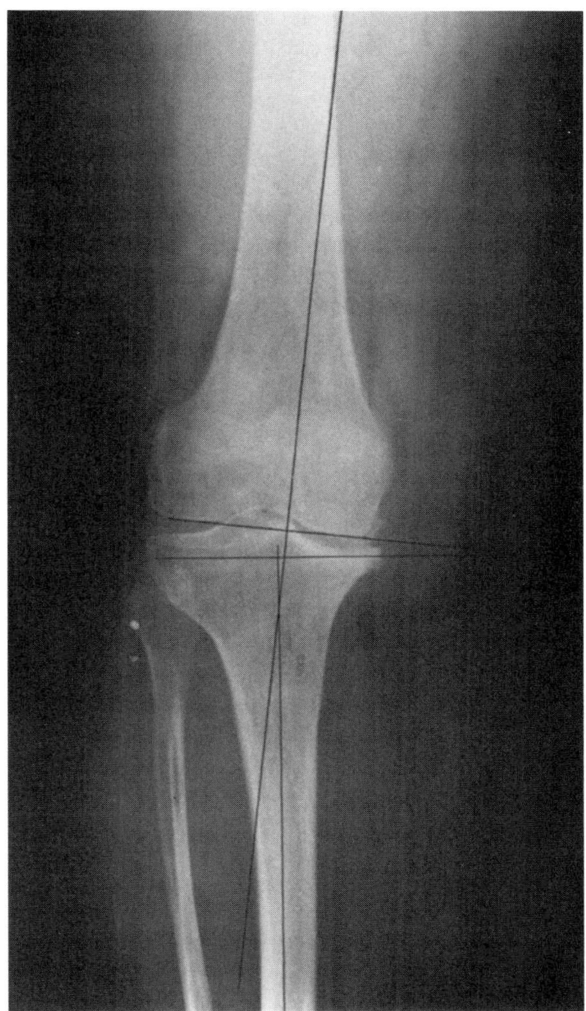

FIGURE 69.4 ➢ Anteroposterior radiograph of the knee, taken with the patient supine. The vertical line over the tibia represents the tibial axis, that is, this line passes from the center of the knee to the center of the ankle. A horizontal line has been drawn perpendicular to this axis. Medially this line passes through the floor of the medial tibial defect. Laterally it passes approximately 1 cm below the lateral tibial condyle. Thus about 1 cm of bone has been lost medially. A second vertical line has been drawn to show the femoral axis. A line drawn perpendicular to this axis passes across the surface of both femoral condyles. Thus no bone has been lost from the femur. Note that the femoral and tibial axes are not parallel, that is, the knee is in varus. Since the knee is unloaded, this implies the presence of a medial soft-tissue contracture.

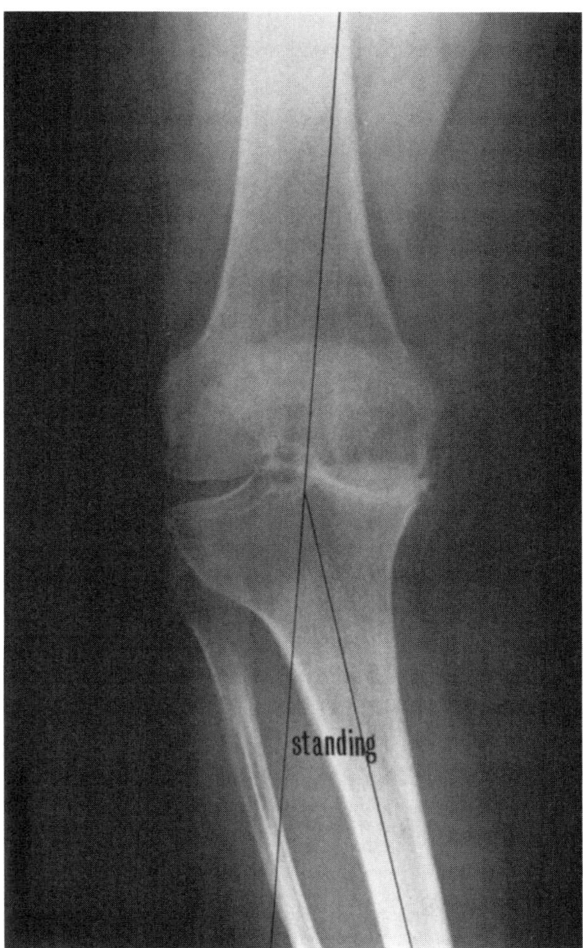

FIGURE 69.5 ➢ Radiograph of the same knee, as shown in Figure 69.4, now taken with the patient standing. Note that the femoral condyle has fallen into the tibial defect to increase the malalignment. Compare this x-ray film with the diagram shown in Figure 69.3B. (From Freeman[5].)

responsible, at least in part if not wholly, for varus instability.

The possibility remains that lateral collateral ligament elongation or rupture may also play a part in the genesis of varus instability. I have never observed a frank rupture of the lateral collateral ligament and capsule at operation in uninjured knees. Although this finding does not exclude the possibility that this lesion occurs, it must mean that if it does occur, it is indeed rare.

Elongation of a collateral ligament (as against rupture) seems to be a more likely possibility; indeed, its existence is strongly suggested by radiographic appearances such as those shown in Figure 69.6. The question has to be asked, however, "What mechanism might be responsible for elongation (especially in osteoarthritis, where damage to the ligament secondary to a prolonged synovitis or by collagenase — both conceivable in rheumatoid arthritis — seem very unlikely)?" A probable answer is that as the deformity on bearing weight increases, a point is reached at which the line of action of the resultant forces acting on the knee passes medial to the most medial point of bony contact in the joint. At or a little before this stage, the knee will tend to hinge open laterally, thus subjecting the lateral and midline soft tissues to persistent tension. Since it seems most unlikely that the collateral and cruciate ligaments are persistently subjected to tensile forces in the normal knee, the result may well be that the collateral ligament is overstressed. According to this analysis, ligamentous elongation might be expected to increase the malalignment in a knee that

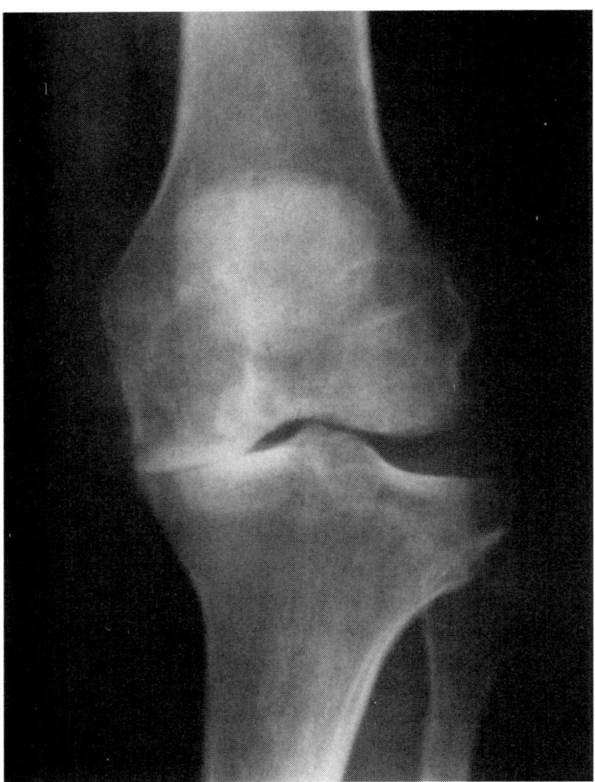

FIGURE 69.6 ➢ Anteroposterior radiograph of a weightbearing varus knee, showing the appearance of opening of the lateral compartment of the joint. This appearance suggests that the lateral collateral ligament has been elongated, perhaps as a consequence of tensile stresses developing in it secondary to the varus malalignment. Although the lateral compartment appears to have opened, the radiologic space between the lateral femoral and tibial condyles is in fact partly occupied by articular cartilage and meniscus. The actual elongation of the lateral collateral ligament is therefore less than it appears on this x-ray film. (From Freeman[5].)

is already significantly malaligned as a consequence of bone loss, but not to initiate the malalignment.

That this is indeed the case may be demonstrated at operation by using a special surgical instrument known as a Tensor. This instrument and its mode of action are illustrated in Figures 69.7 and 69.8. It will be seen that if a Tensor were to be used to tighten the two collateral ligaments in a varus knee that before operation had been unstable (i.e., fully correctable to neutral alignment passively), three possibilities would theoretically arise. First, if the lateral collateral ligament had elongated but not ruptured, the collateral ligaments would tighten to leave the knee in persistent varus (Fig. 69.8A). Second, if only a medial bone defect were present, the medial blade of the Tensor would open more than the lateral, but the two collateral ligaments would then tighten with the knee in anatomic alignment (Fig. 69.8B). Third, if the lateral collateral ligament had ruptured, it would not be possible to tense it, so that the lateral compartment of the knee could be opened indefinitely, turning the knee into ever-increasing varus (Fig. 69.8C). I have never observed the last of these possibilities. The first possible outcome has occurred, suggesting elongation of the ligament on the convex side of the deformity. This happens mainly in osteoarthritis and, less commonly, in rheumatoid arthritis. The usual outcome is the second.

It may be concluded that material elongation of the lateral collateral ligament is a late event and that rupture is rare or nonexistent. Thus varus instability in osteoarthritis (and when it occurs, in rheumatoid arthritis) is initiated by medial bone loss. Simple trigonometry shows that, roughly speaking, 1 cm of medial bone and cartilage loss will result in 10 degrees of varus malalignment. Since 2 cm of tissue loss is commonplace at the hip, 13 degrees of varus (i.e., 20 degrees of deformity relative to an initial 7 degrees valgus) might be a frequent finding at the knee.

The appearances produced by such bone loss in the tibial and femoral condyles of an osteoarthritis varus knee are shown in Figure 69.9. In contrast to the usual femoral defect in a valgus knee, the femoral defect in the varus knee is typically small. This may perhaps be attributed to the fact that the bone of the distal femur is stronger than that of the tibia, and hence less likely to be crushed, and that medial patellar subluxation, leading to damage to the medial femoral condyle by the patella, occurs rarely, if at all.

As bone is lost from the medial side of the joint, the intercondylar eminence of the tibia (1) moves upward relative to the femur and (2) tilts (as the tibia as a whole tilts), so that its apex moves laterally (Fig. 69.10). The combined effect of these two displacements is to produce impingement within the knee between the normally nonarticular central parts of the femur and tibia. By analogy with such abnormal bony contact elsewhere (e.g., between the fibula and os calcis), this process might be expected to be painful and to lead gradually to the formation of a false midline joint in the knee. The latter does indeed occur, so that the knee comes to transmit load medially and centrally, but not laterally (see Fig. 69.10).

The formation of a false midline joint osteoarthritis is encouraged by the formation of osteophytes at the margins of the femoral intercondylar notch, which eventually fuse to bury the cruciate ligaments and produce a continuous, false, central articular surface. Progressive destruction of the weightbearing medial and central areas of the knee may eventually reestablish weightbearing contact between the lateral condyles so that finally the lateral surface also becomes eburnated to produce a "switch-back knee."

Valgus Instability

All the arguments and observations applied above to varus instability apply to valgus instability as well, save that the bony defects are now lateral and the soft-tissue defects are medial. Such bony defects are illustrated in a rheumatoid arthritic knee in Figure 69.11. It should be noted that the tibial defect involves particularly the posterior three-quarters of the condyle, the anterior margin being relatively spared (Fig. 69.11C). This may be attributed to the fact that the femur does

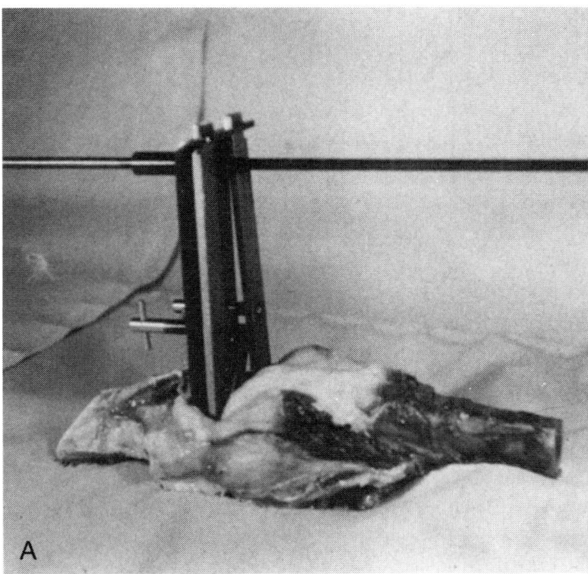

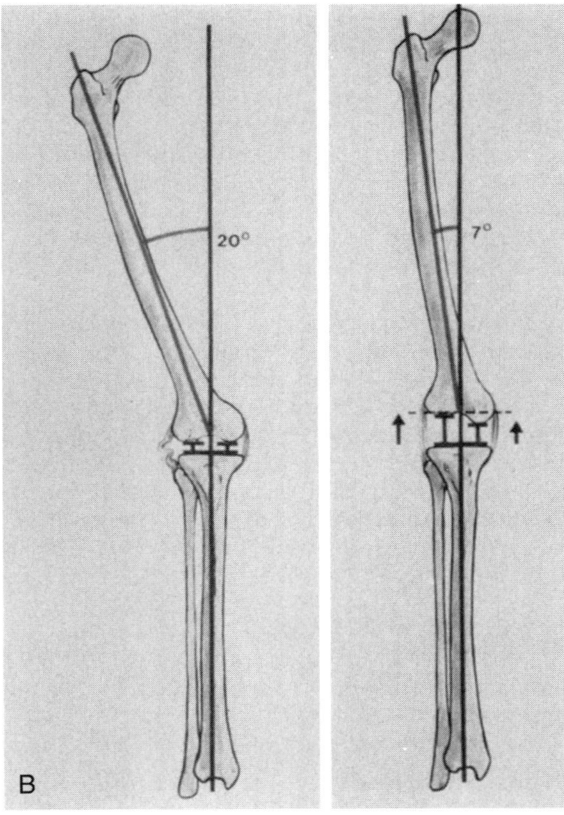

FIGURE 69.7 ➢ The Tensor, an instrument used in arthroplasty of the knee, with which the presence or absence of soft-tissue contractures can be demonstrated at operation. Before insertion of this instrument, the cruciate ligaments are divided, and the tibial plateau is sectioned at right angles to the anatomic axis of the bone. The instrument is used in the *(A)* extended knee to separate first one and then the other femoral condyle from the tibia, thereby tensing the medial and lateral soft tissues in turn. A bar passes through the tibial plate at right angles to the latter. The distal end of this bar must lie over the center of the ankle. The proximal end of the bar will lie over the hip when the soft tissues are tensed only when there is neither contracture nor elongation of these tissues on *(B)* either side of the joint. Thus by tensing the tissues and noting the relationship of the proximal end of the bar to the hip, the surgeon can judge the presence and magnitude of soft tissue contracture or elongation.

not articulate with, and thus will not mechanically damage, the anterior part of the tibial condyle. The lateral femoral condyle is often more grossly destroyed than the lateral tibial plateau (Fig. 69.11B), an observation that may be attributed to the fact that it is exposed to damage, not only from the tibia, but from the laterally subluxated patella as well. Lateral patellar subluxation is often present in such knees; its cause and consequences are discussed in the section on lateral patellar subluxation below.

As with varus instability, it may be concluded that valgus instability is initially caused by bone loss laterally and that this loss can be explained mainly on simple mechanical grounds. Using the Tensor, my experience has been the same as in knees displaying varus instability. This suggests that elongation of the medial collateral ligament is a late secondary event.

Fixed Varus Deformity

Theoretically, a fixed varus deformity could be attributable only to one of two possible events: (1) ligamentous elongation laterally combined with growth of the lateral condyles, or (2) collapse of the bone medially combined with contracture of the medial soft tissues (Fig. 69.12). The former seems inconceivable: growth (as distinct from marginal and intracartilaginous surface osteophytosis) of the condyles is seen neither in rheumatoid arthritis nor in osteoarthritis. In contrast, contractures (e.g., at the hip causing fixed adduction, and at the knee causing fixed flexion), are a common finding. It may be concluded that contracture formation, not growth, is at work, a conclusion that reinforces the view put forward earlier that instability is caused as much by bone loss as by soft-tissue elongation.

It remains to consider the nature of the contractures that may be responsible. Surgeons will be familiar with the concept of a contracture at the hip, as already discussed. Although such lesions are clinically commonplace, the precise nature of the pathologic events responsible for them is unclear; presumably they arise from a mixture of shortening and fibrosis in muscles and adhesion formation around muscles and ligaments.

Whatever their precise pathologic nature, it is now suggested that similar contractures occur in the arthritic knee (and indeed in all arthritic joints) and that they are responsible for the maintenance of fixed tibiofemoral deformities in varus, valgus, flexion, and external rotation, for fixed lateral tibial and patellar subluxation, and in part for an inability to flex the knee fully. In addition, medial osteophytes may tent the medial collateral ligament and hence contribute to the maintenance of deformity by effectively shortening this ligament.

In fixed varus deformity, the presence of such contractures can easily be demonstrated at operation. With the Tensor in place and the condyles fully separated in such a knee, a varus deformity persists and the contracted tissues can be felt and seen to be tight. These tissues include the medial collateral ligament, the medial half of the posterior capsule, and the muscles crossing the medial side of the knee (the cruciate ligaments may also be involved, but they have been resected by the time the Tensor is inserted).

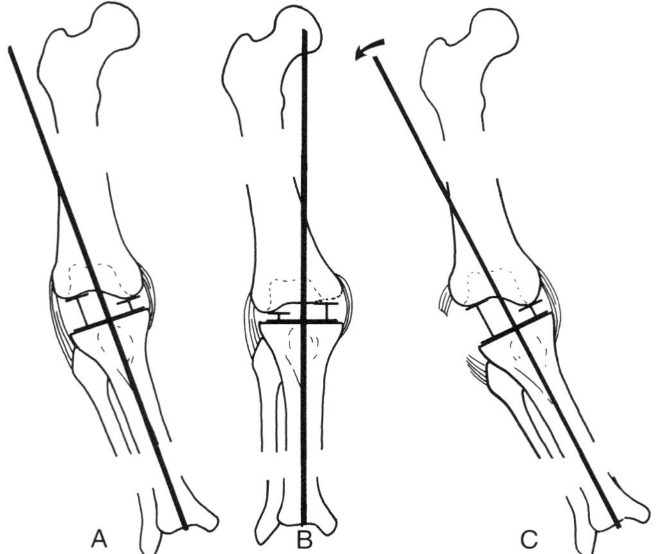

FIGURE 69.8 ➢ Diagrams illustrating the detection of soft-tissue elongation, bone defects, and soft-tissue rupture. *A,* The Tensor in place, with its blades opened, in a knee having no bone defect, but an elongated lateral collateral ligament (such as that shown in Figure 69.3A). The blades of the Tensor could be opened wider in the lateral compartment than in the medial compartment of the knee, turning the joint into varus. *B,* The Tensor in place, with its blades opened, in a joint having preoperatively a medial tibial and femoral defect (such as that shown in Figure 69.3B), but no soft tissue contracture. The blades can now be opened more widely on the medial than on the lateral side of the joint. When the medial and lateral soft tissues are equally tense, this knee will lie in normal alignment. *C,* The Tensor in place, with its blades opened, in a knee having preoperatively a ruptured lateral collateral ligament. In such a knee the lateral blade could theoretically be opened infinitely, turning the knee into progressively increasing varus.

Fixed Valgus Deformity

The fixed valgus deformity is maintained by lateral contractures that affect most obviously the muscles inserted into the iliotibial tract and the biceps. If the tract and the tendinous part of the biceps are divided, their cut ends spring apart (Fig. 69.13) to permit separation of the lateral femoral and tibial condyles with consequent correction of the valgus deformity. In addition to the contractures mentioned above, a fixed valgus deformity may be maintained by adhesions (contractures) between the lateral femoral condyle on the one hand and the posterior capsule and lateral ligament on the other. Contracture of, or adhesions around, the cruciate ligaments may also prevent full correction of the deformity. It should be appreciated that both in valgus and in varus, the extent of the contracture may be less than that of the bone loss: such a knee will display some degree of instability superimposed on an element of fixed deformity. Only the latter is caused by contracture, whereas the bone defect underlies both the instability and the fixed deformity.

Fixed Flexion

The position of comfort in the knee (i.e., the position of maximum intrasynovial volume) is one of about 15 degrees of flexion. If pain prevents the knee from being voluntarily extended beyond this point, contractures (in this case probably caused chiefly by adhesion formation) involving the posterior capsule (becoming adherent both to itself and to the posterior femoral condyles), the hamstring muscles, and, to a lesser extent, the cruciate ligaments may develop and physically prevent full extension. Weightbearing on the flexed knee then loads the distal and posterior femoral condyles, where they articulate with the posterior half of the tibial condyles at loads significantly greater than those borne by the weightbearing extended knee.[14] If, as commonly happens in rheumatoid arthritis, the loaded bone collapses, the femur in effect sinks downward into the posterior part of the tibial condyles until the tibial intercondylar eminence comes to abut against the roof of the femoral intercondylar notch (see Fig. 69.10). Eventually a groove is formed running across the anterodistal aspect of the femoral condyles into which the anterior margin of the tibia locks as the knee is extended (Fig. 69.14). Both bony impingements prevent extension. Midline impingement may cause an attrition rupture of the anterior cruciate ligament—especially in rheumatoid arthritis, when the ligament may be weakened enzymatically and is rarely protected by osteophytes. Such ruptures might be considered analogous to ruptures of the ligamentum teres at the hip.

Loss of Flexion

Loss of flexion is simply the reverse of a flexion deformity, although it is not usually thought of as such. Viewed in this light, however, it may be regarded as being caused by (1) a contracture of the quad-

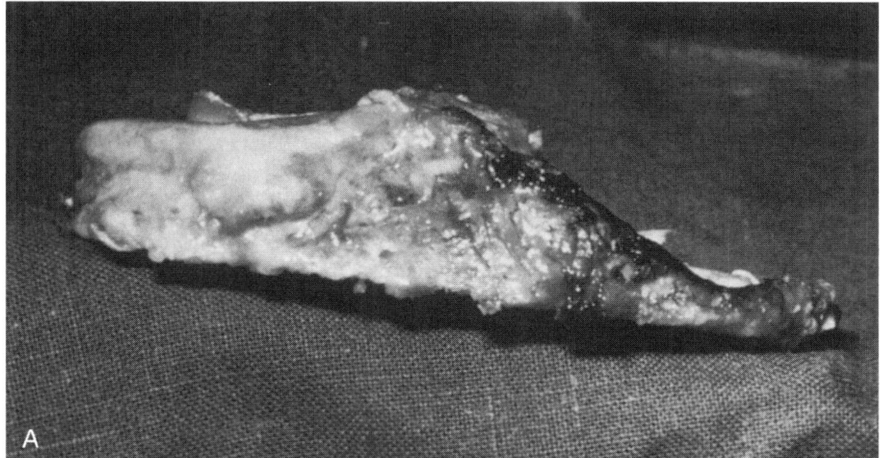

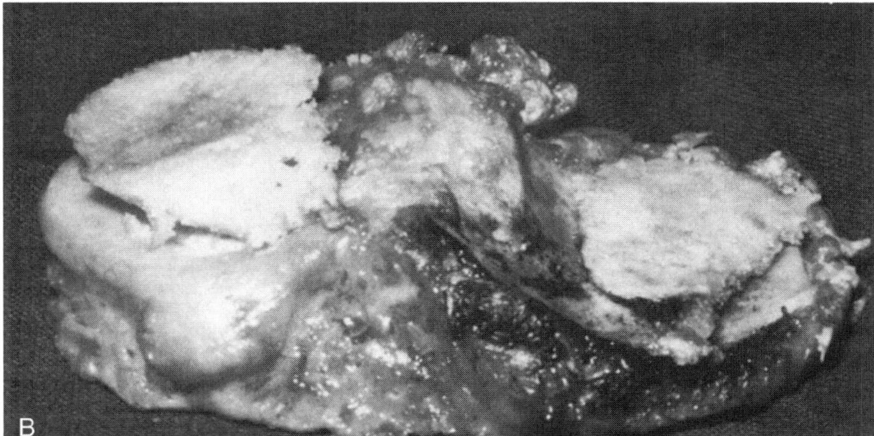

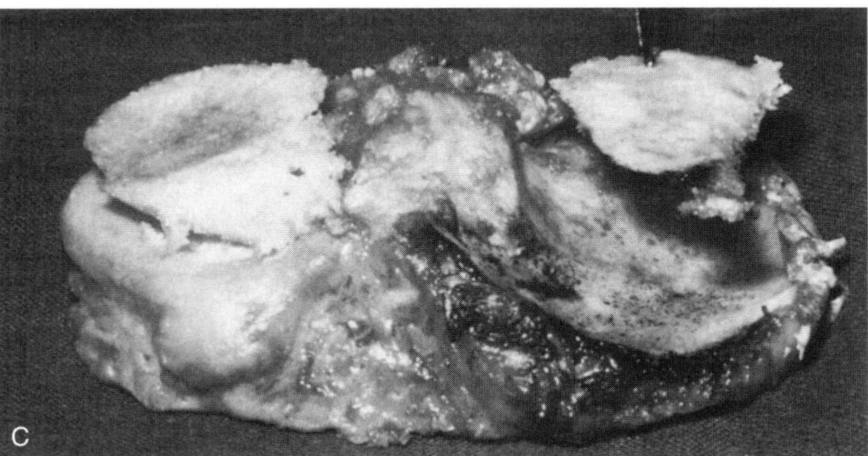

FIGURE 69.9 ➢ Surgical specimens taken from the knee shown in Figure 69.4 and 69.5. *A,* Frontal appearance of the bone removed from the tibia. Note that more bone has been removed laterally than medially, because of the pathologic loss of bone from the medial tibial condyle. The anterior edge of the tibia has been stained with methylene blue. *B,* The fragments of bone resected from the distal aspects of the femoral condyles have now been added to the tibial specimen shown in *A.* The distal femoral condyles have been sectioned at right angles to the mechanical (hip, knee, ankle) axis of the femoral shaft. Here the medial femoral and tibial condyles are in contact, that is, the pathologic specimen is in the position shown in Figure 69.5. *C,* Same specimen shown in *B.* The medial femoral bone fragment has now been lifted to place it on the same horizontal level as the lateral femoral fragment, and the specimen is now in an anatomic position, creating a space on the medial side of the joint due to the loss of about 1 cm of bone and cartilage. Closure of this defect creates the varus malalignment shown in Figure 69.5. (From Freeman[5].)

riceps muscle and cruciate ligaments, (2) adhesions between the collateral ligaments and the sides of the femoral condyles, and perhaps by (3) posterior osteophytosis.

Lateral Subluxation of the Patella

The lateral subluxation of the patella is seen particularly in valgus externally rotated rheumatoid arthritis knees and is presumably caused by the action of the quadriceps muscle, which must have a tendency to pull the patella laterally if the knee is in valgus with external rotation of the tibia (Fig. 69.15). It is permitted by bone loss (as are valgus and varus tibiofemoral deformities), in this case bone being lost from the patella (Fig. 69.16). In my experience, the deformity is usually fixed, as the lateral patellar retinaculum becomes contracted.

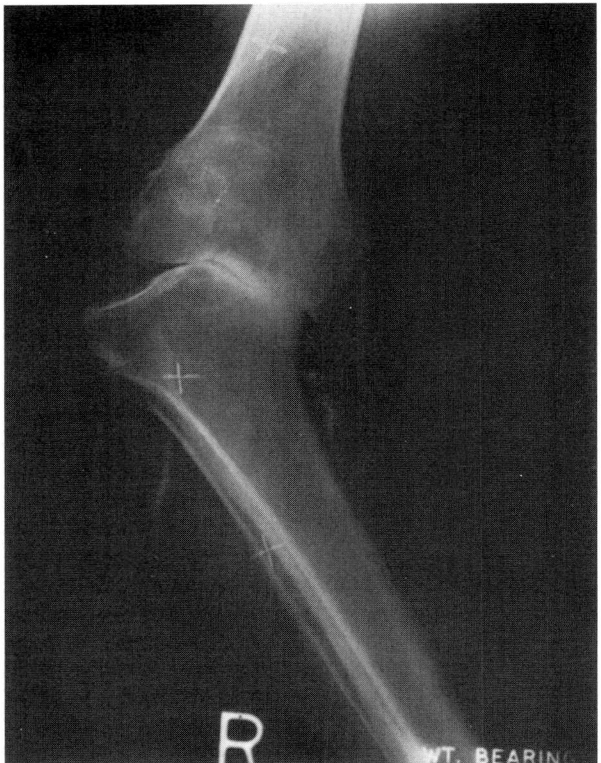

FIGURE 69.10 ➢ Anteroposterior radiograph of a weightbearing knee in varus showing contact between the intercondylar eminence of the tibia and the midline of the femur, resulting in load-carriage medially and centrally but not laterally. Note that the areas of bone-carrying load are relatively sclerotic and that the tibial intercondylar eminence has tilted laterally so as to contact the lateral femoral condyle (see also Figure 69.6). Both this knee and that shown in Figure 69.6 appear to display lateral tibial subluxation, but in the latter the medial side of the medial femoral and tibial condyles are in line, whereas here they are not, partly because the medial flare of the tibial condyle has been destroyed. On the lateral side of the joint, the lateral tibial condyle projects beyond the lateral femoral condyle, and the lateral collateral ligament and capsule are elongated.

External Rotation of the Tibia

External rotation of the tibia is a deformity that is usually seen in rheumatoid arthritis valgus knees in women and is most obvious in the flexed, rather than in the extended, joint. There appear to be three possible sources for a deforming external rotation force: (1) the laterally subluxed extensor mechanism, (2) tensor fasciae lata and gluteus maximus acting via the iliotibial tract, and (3) the biceps muscle. It seems possible that this external rotation thrust is exacerbated by a loss of the internal rotator power of the popliteus muscle, since (in my experience) the intra-articular tendon of this muscle is usually absent from the rheumatoid (but not from the osteoarthrotic) knee. The tendon is presumably damaged enzymatically and ruptured by being ground between the collapsing lateral femoral and tibial condyles. (So-called posterior ruptures of the knee are probably in fact caused by the discharge of synovial contents through the hole in the posterior capsule left by the retraction of this tendon from the joint rather than by a rupture of the capsule. The capsule itself is very strong and is never found to be ruptured at operation. Arthrographically, the synovial leak in posterior ruptures is lateral, that is, it corresponds in position to the point of exit of the popliteus tendon.)

Such unbalanced external rotation forces would themselves be capable of rotating the tibia only to its normal extreme, but not beyond. In my view, the hyperexternal rotation that occurs in these knees is permitted by the lateral tibial and femoral bone loss that occurs in the valgus knee, since this will effectively relax posterior cruciate control over the lateral, but not over the medial compartment of the knee. As a consequence, the equivalent of a posterior drawer sign can occur laterally but not medially; that is, the lateral, but not the medial, tibial condyle is free to sublux posteriorly. Thus the tibia rotates externally. Once rotated, the same contractures that maintain fixed valgus in the extended knee (i.e., contractures of the iliotibial tract and of the biceps) will maintain fixed external rotation in the flexed knee. Finally, the whole circumference of the tibia may become adherent to the capsule in its new position of external rotation.

Hyperextension

Hyperextension is usually seen in knees displaying fixed valgus deformities (i.e., in knees with contractures of the iliotibial tract) (Fig. 69.17). For the first 5 to 10 degrees of flexion, the iliotibial tract passes in front of the axis of rotation of the knee, acting as an extensor. Its contracture in the absence of a fixed flexion deformity may therefore lead to hyperextension. The tendency for this deformity to develop should theoretically be exacerbated by bone loss from both sides of the knee, since this would loosen all those ligaments lying behind the axis of tibiofemoral rotation, normally preventing hyperextension. If, as is frequently the case in the rheumatoid knee, the anterior cruciate ligament has been ruptured, its contribution to the limitation of extension will also be lost.

The Stable Neutral Knee

From what has been said above, it can be seen that a stable arthritic knee in neutral alignment might be attributable either to the absence of both bone loss and soft tissue abnormality or paradoxically to the presence of symmetrical bone loss (medially and laterally) and soft-tissue contracture (medially and laterally).

The Loose Knee

In the loose knee, which is rare, there is both medial and lateral bone loss without soft-tissue contracture. Alternatively, and theoretically, both collateral ligaments might elongate. They are, however, never absent; all knees of this kind that I have treated could be stabilized in neutral alignment with the Tensor.

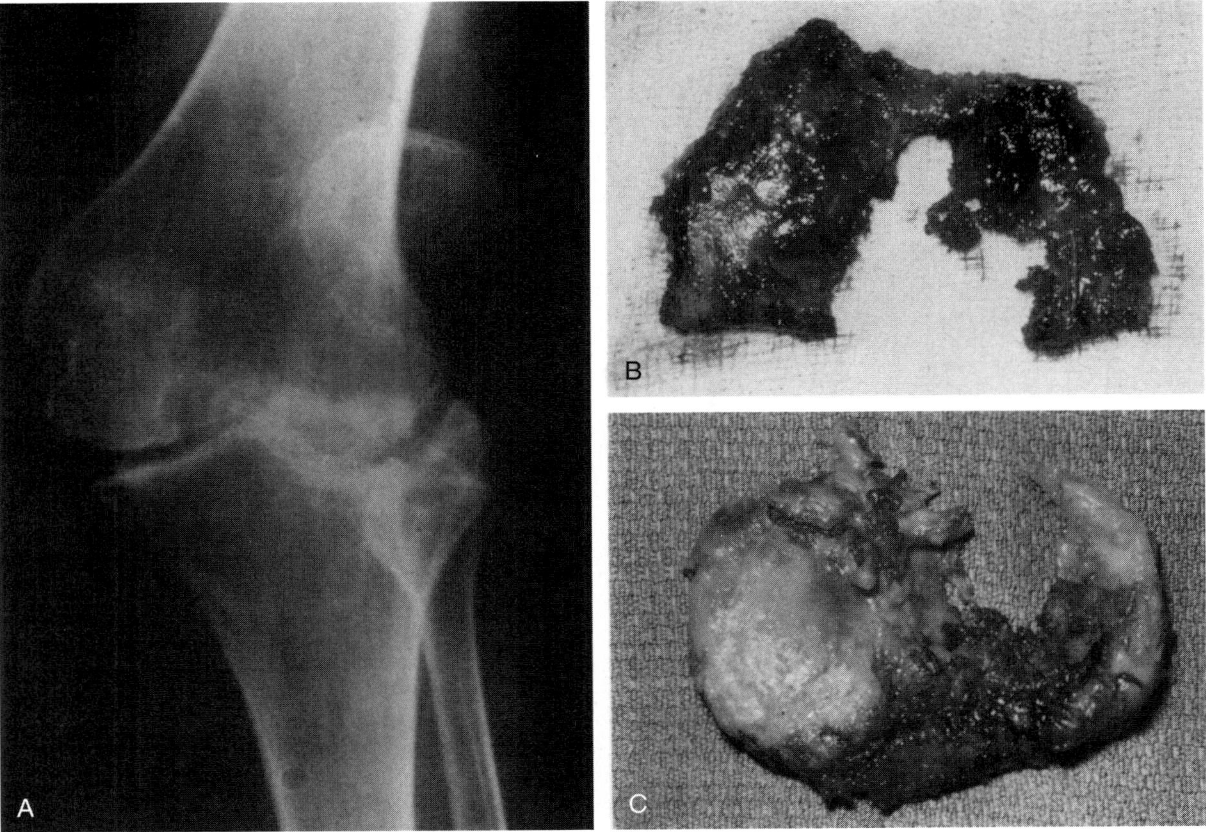

FIGURE 69.11 ➢ A knee in rheumatoid arthritis displaying fixed valgus deformity. *A,* An anteroposterior radiograph of the non-weightbearing knee. The valgus deformity is caused by femoral and tibial defects. It persists in the non-weightbearing knee because it is held, whether the knee is weightbearing or not, by the presence of a lateral soft-tissue contracture. Note the lateral subluxation of the patella. *B,* Surgical specimen removed from the distal femur shown in *(A)* by resection of the bone at 83 degrees to the long axis of the femoral shaft (i.e., at 90 degrees to the mechanical axis of the femur). On the lateral side *(right),* little or no bone has been removed because of the preexisting defect. *C,* Specimen removed from the tibia by transecting it at right angles to the axis of the shaft. Note that once again little or no bone has been removed from the lateral side. Note that the tibial and the femoral defects are mainly posterior. (*B* and *C* from Freeman[5].)

Lateral Subluxation of the Tibia

Although lateral subluxation of the tibia, usually combined with varus, is a well-recognized clinical entity (see Figs. 69.6 and 69.10), it is not clear why in some, but not in all, knees the tibia tends to shift laterally on the femur as the loss of medial cartilage and bone turns the knee into varus. Indeed to some extent the appearance of lateral subluxation may be illusory (see Fig. 69.10). Perhaps in such knees, before the onset of degenerative changes, the long axis of the tibia intersects that of the femur not in the plane of the knee but farther proximally, that is, perhaps the tibia is congenitally somewhat laterally placed in these knees. Whatever the initial cause of lateral tibial subluxation, it is permitted (as are all other abnormalities of alignment) by bone and cartilage loss—in this case from the tibial intercondylar eminence or the medial side of the lateral femoral condyle, or both. A contracture of the popliteus muscle, running from the tibia medially to the femur laterally, then holds the tibia laterally. In support of the view that a popliteus contracture is responsible, division of the popliteus tendon in knees displaying lateral tibial subluxation eliminates the tendency (which otherwise used to be seen after replacement of the knee with the ICLH prosthesis, which lacked medial-lateral constraint) for the tibia to move laterally relative to the femur as the knee nears full extension.

A connection exists between subluxation of the patella and of the tibia. Both occur in a lateral direction, and they might be causally connected, since the extensor mechanism must be carried laterally with the tibia. Thus, at least in theory, a vicious regress may be initiated in the following manner. The tibia subluxes laterally, carrying the patella with it. The resulting increased lateral thrust in the patellofemoral joint promotes the destruction of the anterior aspect of the lateral femoral condyle and of the patella, thereby allowing the patella to sublux even farther laterally.

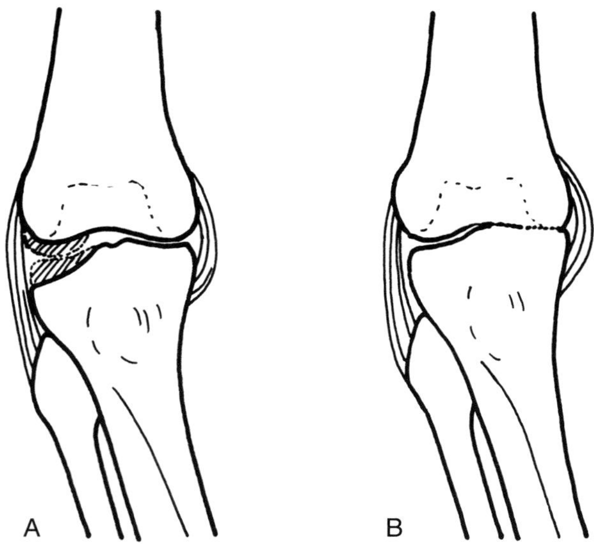

FIGURE 69.12. ➢ Two mechanisms that might theoretically produce a fixed varus deformity. *A,* The varus deformity has been produced by growth of the lateral femoral and tibial condyles combined with elongation of the lateral collateral ligament, which would seem impossible. *B,* The fixed deformity has been produced by a medial tibial defect similar to that shown in Figures 69.3 to 69.5 and 69.9, combined with a medial soft-tissue contracture. This seems likely in reality.

Once the patella has moved laterally, quadriceps activity must tend to pull the tibia laterally. If such a knee already has a medial tibiofemoral defect (as a consequence of which it is in varus), this lateral patellar pull would displace the proximal tibia bodily laterally, rather than turning the bone into valgus, that is, there would be increasing lateral subluxation of the tibia in a varus knee.

It is perhaps significant in this context that the tibia, for practical purposes, always subluxes laterally, not medially, and that both the commonly occurring bone defects (a medial defect in the tibia and a lateral defect in the femur) produce a joint line that slopes upward and laterally, an abnormality that might lead to lateral tibial subluxation.

Conclusions

The fundamental pathologic event, on the gross scale, in the knee in osteoarthritis and rheumatoid arthritis is the destruction first of cartilage and then of bone. If, as is usual, this happens asymmetrically, it manifests itself as malalignment, with lateral tibiofemoral defects causing valgus, medial tibiofemoral defects causing varus, and lateral patellofemoral defects causing lateral patellar subluxation.

When the tibiofemoral or patellofemoral joints become malaligned, the lines of action of the forces acting on both joints are altered—unfortunately, in such a way as to increase the forces acting on the destroyed area of the knee. As a consequence, bone destruction tends to be progressive.

The most important pathologic process in muscle-tendon units is contracture formation; in ligaments it is adhesion formation. Such contractures and adhesions hold the bones in a position of deformity. They also limit movement.

The ligaments of the knee are rarely, if ever, destroyed in arthritis, the only exception to this being the anterior cruciate ligament, which is sometimes destroyed by attrition between the tibia and femur in rheumatoid arthritis. The collateral ligament on the convex side of a valgus or varus deformity may stretch if the deformity is sufficient to generate tensile forces on its convex side. Such elongation is late and secondary to the bone defect.

PROGRESSION OF THE PATHOLOGY

In osteoarthritis the mechanism by which the pathology becomes progressively worse seems clear; that is, the forces that initiated the cartilage and bone damage in the first place continue to act and thus accentuate the defect. Indeed a vicious circle is established because not only does the force accentuate the defect, the defect accentuates the force. Thus, for example, a varus position produced by a medial defect has the effect of moving the resultant of the forces acting on the knee medially, thereby increasing the force acting on the defect. Similarly, a flexion deformity in excess of 10 degrees increases the magnitude of the tibiofemoral compressive forces.[14]

Since this force acts in the flexed knee, the more posterior parts of the tibial condyles are affected (because the femur articulates posteriorly with the tibia in flexion), whereas the anterior tibia is spared. As a result, the femur sinks into the posterior two-thirds of the tibial condyles, leaving the anterior margin of the tibia as an upwardly projecting ridge that strikes the femur as the knee extends. Thus, by a vicious circle similar to that affecting the varus knee, the forces perpetuate and accentuate fixed flexion deformity.

Although precisely similar considerations as those applying to the varus knee might be thought to apply to the valgus knee, gait analysis suggests that contrary to theoretical expectations, the resultant is not always shifted laterally.[7] Possibly, this is because patients can compensate better for a valgus deformity (by altering the placement of their feet as they walk) than they can for a varus deformity.

Misalignment of the patella must of course affect the tibiofemoral joint force. Thus lateral patellar subluxation, which often accompanies tibiofemoral valgus, can be expected to shift the line of action of the quadriceps muscle (and thus the resultant of the tibiofemoral forces) laterally in extension. In flexion, the same lateral patellar subluxation will lead to tibial external rotation to produce the complex deformity often seen in rheumatoid arthritis of valgus, lateral patellar subluxation, external rotation in flexion, and often fixed flexion.

In rheumatoid arthritis, all the same mechanical considerations apply, but in addition it is widely thought that an active synovitis, attributable to some fundamental but unknown causative agent, is at work. In

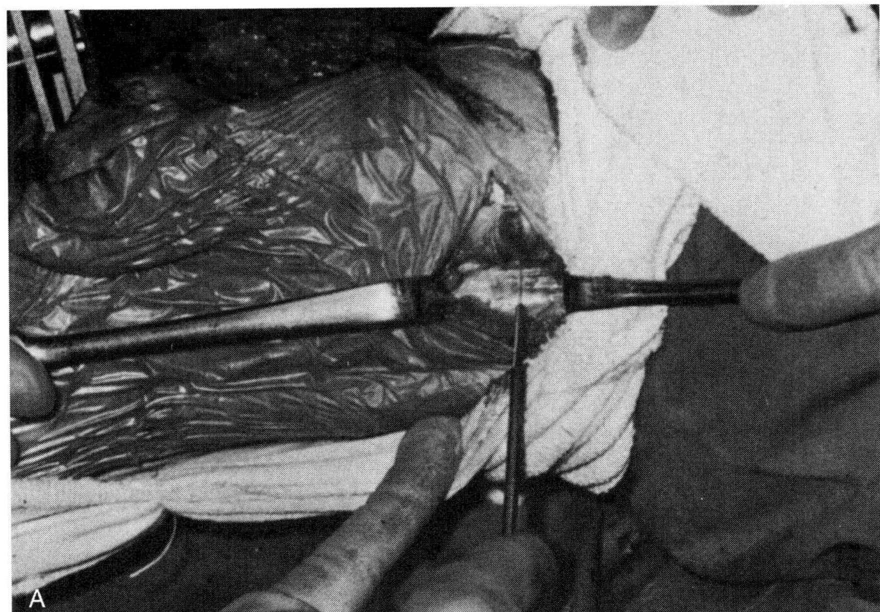

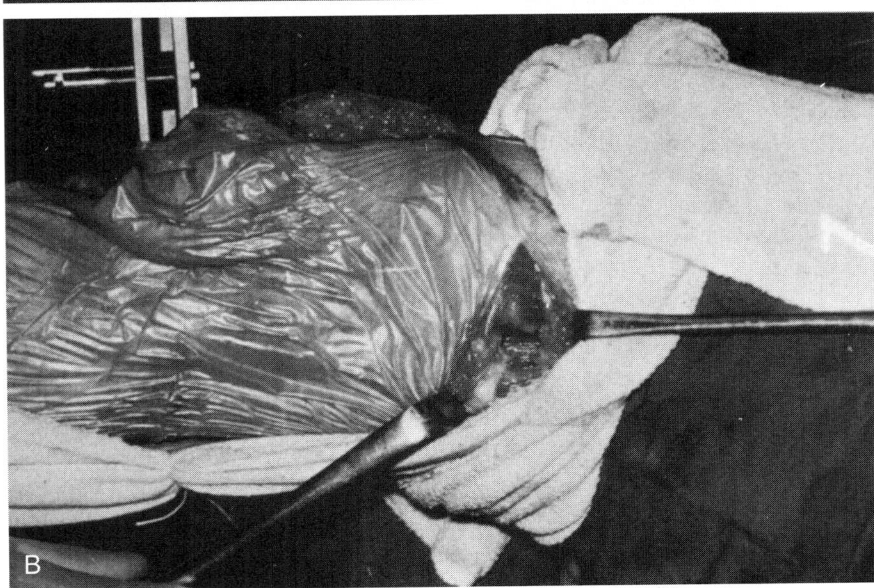

FIGURE 69.13 ➢ *A,* Lateral view of a knee with fixed valgus deformity during operation. The iliotibial tract is about to be divided. At this stage of the operation, the medial and lateral soft tissues had been tensed, but even so the knee lay in valgus. This implies the presence of a lateral soft-tissue contracture. *B,* The iliotibial tract has now been incised, and the lateral blades of the Tensor *(top left)* have been opened farther, separating the lateral tibial and femoral condyles and correcting the valgus deformity. This has caused the cut edges of the iliotibial tract to separate (the proximal edge not seen here). A contracture of the iliotibial tract (perhaps involving particularly the tensor fascia lata muscle) was mainly responsible for the fixed valgus malalignment in this knee. (From Freeman[5].)

my own (admittedly speculative) view, such a primary synovitis continues only as long as cartilage remains in the joint, since it seems to be this tissue that provokes the synovial reaction.[14] This perhaps explains the fact that once the cartilage is entirely lost, the rheumatoid synovitis may burn itself out. It may also explain the clinical observation that a synovitis may recur after a synovectomy (because cartilage persists), but rarely after a total replacement (because cartilage is then absent from the joint). There is, however, another possible cause for an active synovitis in rheumatoid arthritis, and indeed to a lesser extent in osteoarthritis. This is the continuous release of bone and cartilaginous debris into the synovial cavity. According to this argument, the synovitis in rheumatoid arthritis would merely be viewed as a more violent variety of that occurring, for example, in the presence of a torn meniscus and might be thought to be more florid in rheumatoid arthritis than in osteoarthritis because enzymatic attack and osteoporosis (and hence the rate of bone and cartilage destruction) is greater in the former. This synovitis, like the disturbance of joint forces, could be seen as being secondary to the bone defects, not the cause of them.

There is another feature of the arthritic knee that may appropriately be considered here. This feature concerns the magnitude and duration of action of major forces in the joint as contrasted with those in the hip. As regards the magnitude of such forces, gait analysis studies and static analysis suggest (but do not prove, since no direct measurements are available) that peak forces in everyday activities, such as walk-

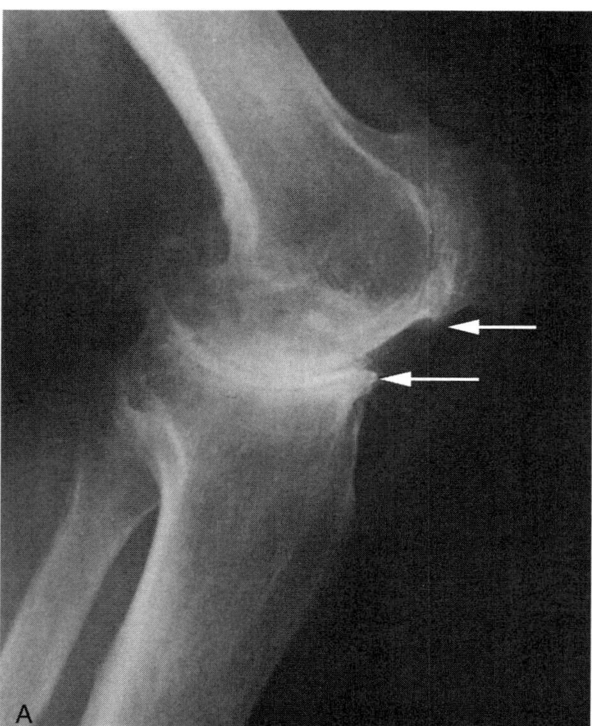

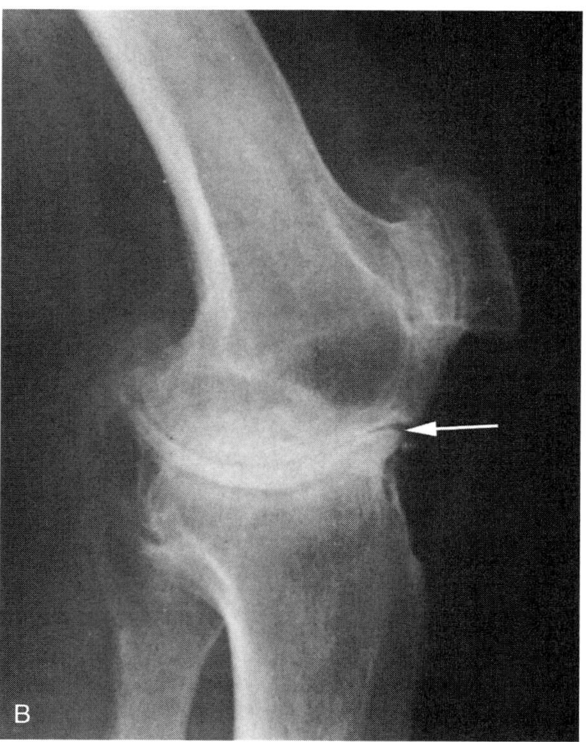

FIGURE 69.14. ➢ Lateral radiographs of an osteoarthritic knee having a fixed flexion deformity. *A,* Note the anterior osteophyte on the tibia *(arrow). B,* A groove is seen on the distal end of the femur *(arrow)* in the slightly flexed knee; the tibial osteophyte and the femoral groove contact each other *(arrow)* to limit extension.

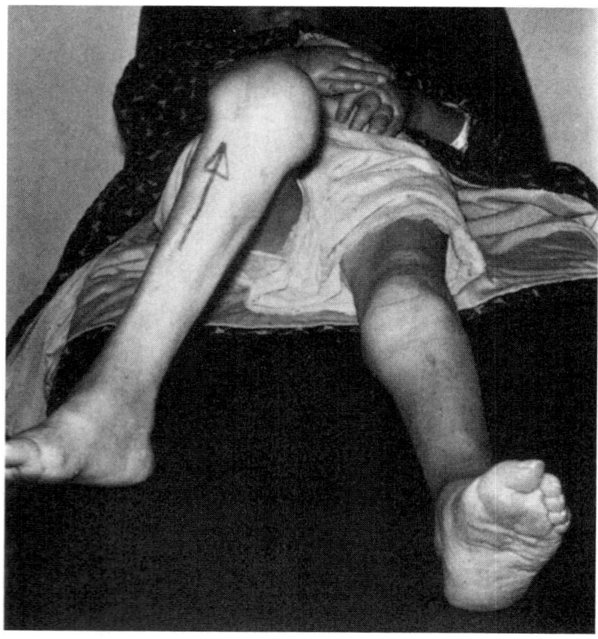

FIGURE 69.15. ➢ Right knee *(arrow)* in rheumatoid arthritis, showing valgus, external rotation, and lateral subluxation of the patella in the flexed knee. (From Freeman[5].)

ing, are greater in the hip than in the tibiofemoral joint. For example, in the hip, Paul[13] finds the maximum force to be about five times the body weight during level walking, and Morrison,[11] in the same laboratory, finds the peak tibiofemoral force to be about three times body weight.

The patellofemoral force may equal or even exceed that in the tibiofemoral joint but only on activities such as unsupported squatting; generally, it is lower.

Not only are the peak forces on activity lower in the knee, there is also evidence that true off-loading is possible in this joint. Thus at the tibiofemoral joint it is well known that the damaged surfaces of the tibia and femur can be seen to separate on an x-ray film when the patient lies down, hence the need to take radiographs of this joint during weightbearing if it is to be fully assessed clinically. At the hip no such separation occurs. This radiologic fact probably accounts for the well-known clinical observation that night pain is an important clinical feature in arthritis of the hip, but not of the knee, since in the latter the structures responsible for the pain (i.e., the exposed bone surfaces) can be off-loaded at night.

That the forces in the knee are probably smaller in magnitude and more intermittent in action than in the hip may account for the generally slower evolution and relatively less severe pain in osteoarthritis of the knee than of the hip. That the tibiofemoral joint can be unloaded when the patient lies down probably ac-

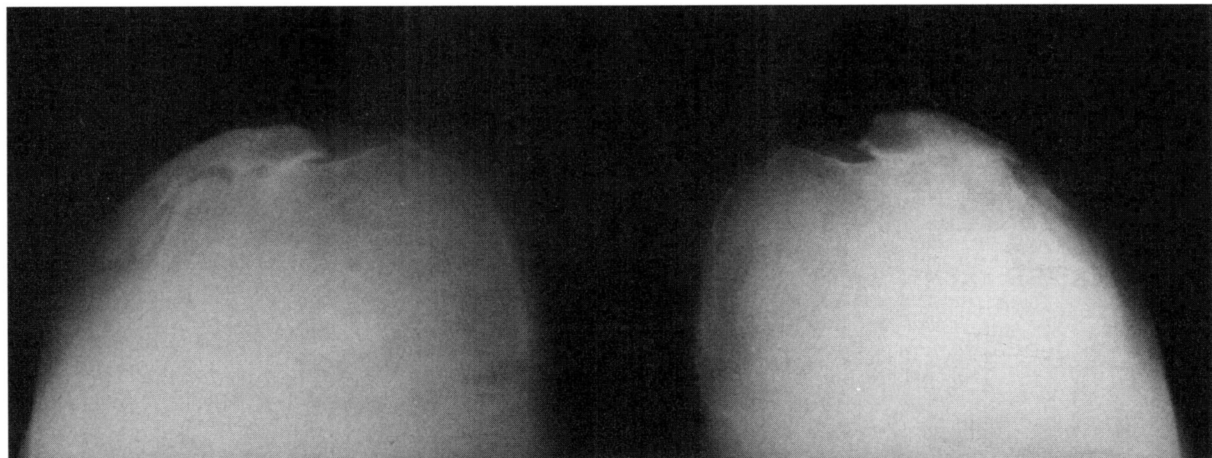

FIGURE 69.16. ➢ Skyline radiograph of the knee shown in Figure 69.15. Note the lateral subluxation of the patella permitted by destruction of the patella itself and of the lateral femoral condyle (see also Fig. 69.11A). It will be recalled that the anterior prominence of the lateral femoral condyle is normally greater than that of the medial femoral condyle, the reverse of the situation seen in this knee. (From Freeman[5].)

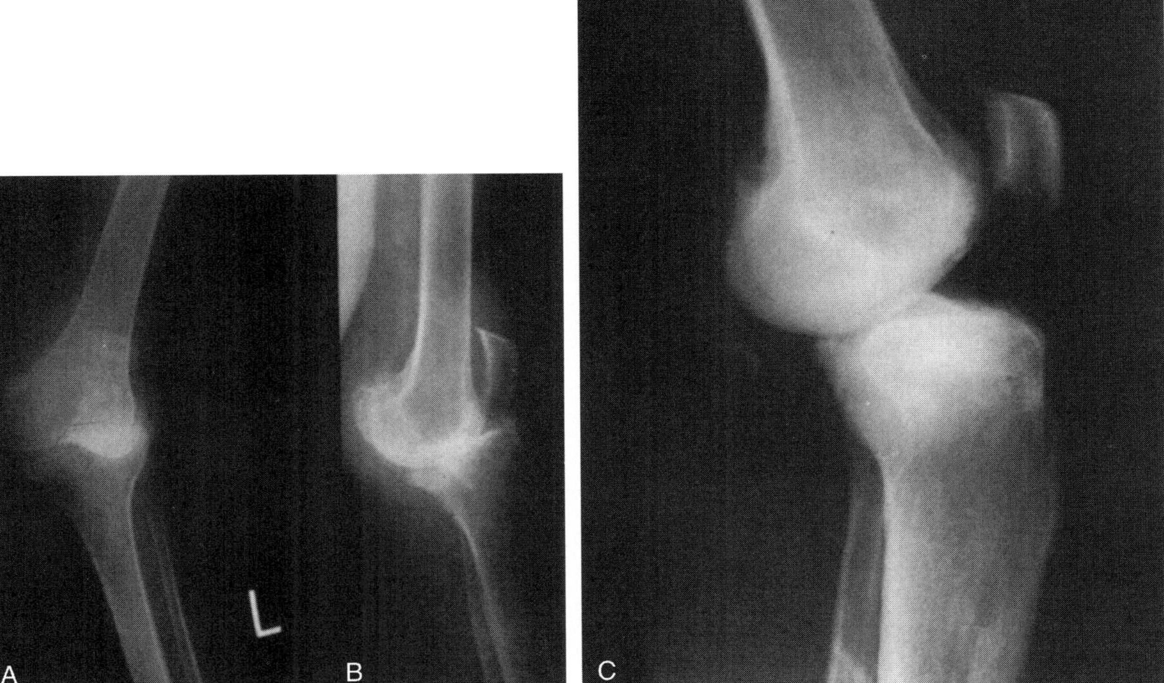

FIGURE 69.17. ➢ *A, B,* Knee in rheumatoid arthritis, showing hyperextension and valgus malalignment, the latter being fixed. *C* Similar anterior subluxation in osteoarthritis. In both knees, the anterior cruciate ligament was found to be ruptured at operation. Hyperextension appears to be caused by a contracture of the iliotibial tract in the absence of fixed flexion (see text). Such a contracture must have been present in the knee illustrated in *(B)* because of (1) the presence of a fixed valgus deformity, and (2) at operation the use of the Tensor demonstrated the contracture (From Freeman[5].)

counts for the rarity of significant night pain in osteoarthritis of the knee as compared with its frequency at the hip. In rheumatoid arthritis, the much greater area of cartilage in the knee and the fact that because the joint is more peripheral its cartilage is more permeable,[9] probably account for the increased incidence of rheumatoid synovitis in the knee as compared with the hip.

IMPLICATIONS FOR TREATMENT

From what has been said above it seems unlikely that a conservative form of treatment for osteoarthritis will ever be found. Other than instructing the patient to reduce body weight, moderate activities, and use a stick, nothing can be done to alter the forces acting on the knee. Once cartilage has been damaged, the inability of the chondrocyte to undergo mitosis makes it as unlikely that new cartilage can be induced pharmacologically as it is that new brain tissue (i.e., new neurons) can be induced after a cerebrovascular accident (CVA). Analgesics can, of course, relieve pain (and I believe there is no convincing evidence that the so-called anti-inflammatory agents have any action whatsoever except insofar as they have analgesic properties). There remains the possibility of surgery.

Osteotomies could be expected to move the line of action of the resultant of the forces acting on the tibiofemoral joint but not to alter its magnitude. From what has been said above, it would seem reasonable to expect that to off-load a defect, say in the medial tibial condyle, in this way might enable fibrocartilage to form on the exposed bone surface (provided that this is not too densely sclerotic, when additional drilling might be helpful). Such an osteotomy might be expected to be more predictably beneficial for a medial defect causing varus than for a valgus knee because recent gait analysis studies[7] (referred to above) show that in the former the resultant force is always displaced medially when the patient walks, whereas in the latter its line of action is not always displaced laterally. This theoretical expectation conforms with clinical experience.

Theoretically, however, and indeed in practice, osteotomy would seem to have limitations. First, it will do nothing for lateral tibial subluxation or for instability unless, in the case of the latter, contractures happen to form postoperatively to stabilize the joint. Second, overcorrection might induce degenerative changes in the opposite compartment, whereas undercorrection will fail to solve the problem in the damaged compartment. A priori it seems impossible to guarantee the achievement of the perfect alignment (whatever that may be), especially when it is borne in mind that some collapse may occur at any loaded fracture site, that is, at the osteotomy as it unites, thereby altering the alignment produced at operation. The symptomatic unpredictability of this procedure may be attributable to the fact that pain relief probably depends on off-loading the damaged compartment enough to permit formation of fibrocartilage, while taking care not to overload the opposite side, a difficult compromise to achieve.

At the patellofemoral joint, the theory behind the Maquet procedure[5] is sound, but in practice the cosmetic and wound-healing problems associated with this operation may represent unacceptable disadvantages.

Thus, in theory, as in practice, osteotomy might be expected to be most useful for the early varus knee, for which it is the tibia that should be angulated, because the defect is tibial. Such an operation might theoretically be expected to produce healing by the formation of functionally useful fibrocartilaginous scars on the surfaces of the exposed bones, provided these are not too sclerotic; indeed, there is arthroscopic evidence that this does happen.[6]

Apart from fibrocartilage formation, the only way in which exposed bone surfaces can be recovered with insensitive material so as to relieve pain is by the use of implants. If such an implant and the subjacent bone on which it rests are not to be destroyed by the same forces as those originally producing the defect, the height of the implants must be adjusted so as to realign the limb perfectly. In a knee with a contracture, the requisite space for the implant cannot be obtained until the contractures have been surgically reversed. Since these objectives can now be achieved technically, there is, theoretically at least, a prospect that properly executed replacement—either total or unicompartmental—can restore the function of an osteoarthrotic knee in the same way that properly executed dentistry can restore the function of a carious tooth.

In rheumatoid arthritis it seems unlikely that anything useful would be gained from transferring load from one compartment to another, because the loss of cartilage is generalized. Thus osteotomy seems unlikely to be helpful in rheumatoid arthritis. In contrast, synovectomy might at first sight have something to offer. But in practice, synovectomy has not proved reliably beneficial. This outcome would be expected on the basis of the views set out above, which imply that the synovitis in rheumatoid arthritis is secondary—either, early in the disease, to an immune mechanism involving cartilage, or later to detritus. Neither of these primary events will be affected by synovectomy. Indeed, according to this analysis, this operation appears to be directed against a consequence of the fundamental pathology, not against the fundamental pathology itself.

Therefore, as in osteoarthritis, replacement seems to offer the only serious prospect of surgical relief and for the same reasons; namely, exposed bone surfaces are covered and the joint realigned. Two points are of special relevance to rheumatoid arthritis, however. First, unicompartmental replacement, which might theoretically be useful in those cases of osteoarthritis in which the cartilage in the apparently uninvolved tibiofemoral compartment is now known to be essentially normal, can have no place in rheumatoid arthritis in which none of the cartilage is normal. Second, if the synovitis in rheumatoid arthritis represented a primary pathologic process, it should continue after the joint surfaces have been replaced so as to eventually loosen the prosthesis and once again destroy the joint. Replacement in these circumstances would be futile. In practice, the synovitis in rheumatoid arthritis remits after resurfacing, and I have not thus far seen a recurrent rheumatoid flare in a satisfactorily replaced joint. This observation is easy to understand, indeed it is predictable, if it is accepted that the two causes of synovitis in rheumatoid arthritis are an autoimmune response to cartilage and the release of detritus, because total resurfacing removes both cartilage and debris from the joint. Thus not only does total replacement control the local symptoms of rheumatoid arthritis, it also "cures" the disease in that joint.

POSTSCRIPT 2000

This chapter was originally written in 1982 for publication in 1984. Since then, nothing has been published to my knowledge to change my view of the pathology of OA and RA at the knee and thus to alter the implications for treatment drawn in this chapter.

However, recent work using MRI to study the shapes of the bones and the way in which they contact each other in the tibiofemoral joint[1] suggests a possible cause for at least one variety of OA (idiopathic anteromedial OA) and a conceivable method for its treatment other than by replacement.

In humans, the medial femoral and tibial condyles are composed of two facets, the anterior pair of which articulate from full extension to $20+/-10°$. At full extension, contact anteriorly is confined to the medial compartment. Dye[2] has reported that in other mammals the knee does not extend beyond 30°, the possible exceptions being the bear and the elephant (author's observation). In conformity with this, the tibial contact area of the femoral condyles of mammals, other than humans, is composed of only one circular surface in sagittal section, not two such surfaces as in humans. Thus, it could be argued that in achieving an erect stance, humans have produced a mode of articulation in or near full extension, which, by reference to other mammals, is "abnormal." This abnormality is located anteromedially in precisely the area where OA commonly begins.[3] Perhaps the price of erect stance is a mode of articulation at the knee that generates contact stresses too high to be tolerated by articular cartilage for a contemporary human lifetime? It has already been suggested that such a possibility may apply to the hip.[4] If this view is correct, the possibility arises that an anteromedial subtraction osteotomy at the tibia, by lowering the tibial extension facet, might improve the prognosis early in anteromedial OA.

Postscript References

1. Iwaki H, Pinskerova V, Freeman MAR: Tibio-femoral movement 1: The shapes and relative movements of the femur and tibia in the unloaded cadaver knee. J Bone Joint Surg 2000 (in press).
2. Dye FS: An evolutionary perspective of the knee. J Bone Joint Surg Am 69:976, 1987.
3. White SH, Ludkowski PF, Goodfellow JW: Anteromedial osteoarthritis of the knee. J Bone Joint Surg Br 738:582, 1991.
4. Freeman MAR: Is collagen fatigue failure a cause of osteoarthrosis and prosthetic component migration? A hypothesis. (The 1998 Steindler Award Lecture). Orthop Res 17:3, 1998.

References

1. Brocklehurst R, Bayliss MT, Maroudas, A, et al: The composition of normal and osteoarthritic articular cartilage from human knee joints. J Bone Joint Surg Am 66:95, 1984.
2. Cooke TDV: How does the mechanism of cartilage destruction influence surgical management of the rheumatoid joint? J Rheumatol 7:119, 1980.
3. Freeman MAR: The pathogenesis of primary osteoarthrosis: An hypothesis. In Apley AG, ed: Modern Trends in Orthopaedics. vol 6. Butterworths, London, 1972, p 40.
4. Freeman MAR, Meachim G: Aging and degeneration. In Freeman MAR, ed: Adult Articular Cartilage. 2nd ed. Pitman Medical, Tunbridge Wells, England, 1979, p 487.
5. Freeman MAR: Arthritis of the Knee. Berlin, Springer-Verlag, 1980.
6. Fujisawa Y, Masuhara K, Matsumoto N, et al: The effect of high tibial osteotomy on osteoarthritis of the knee: An arthroscopic study. Clin Orthop Surg 11:576, 1976.
7. Johnson F, Leitl S, Waugh W: The distribution of load across the knee: a comparison of static and dynamic measurements. J Bone Joint Surg Br 62:346, 1980.
8. Maquet P: Considérations biomécaniques sur l'arthrose du genou: Un traitement biomécanique de l'arthrose femoropatellaire: L'avancement du tendon rotulieu. Rev Rhum 30:779, 1963.
9. Maroudas A: Biophysical chemistry of cartilaginous tissues with special reference to solute and fluid transport. Biorheology 12: 233, 1975.
10. Meachim G, Stockwell RA: The matrix. In Freeman MAR, ed: Adult Articular Cartilage. 2nd ed. Pitman Medical, Tunbridge Wells, England, 1979, p 10.
11. Morrison JB: Biomechanics of the knee joint in relation to normal walking. J Biomech 3:51, 1970.
12. Muir IHM: Biochemistry. In Freeman MAR, ed: Adult Articular Cartilage. 2nd ed. Pitman Medical, Tunbridge Wells, England, 1979, p 187.
13. Paul JP: Bio-engineering studies of the forces transmitted by joints. II. Engineering analysis. In Kenedi RM, ed: Biomechanics and Related Bio-Engineering Topics. Pergamon Press, Oxford, 1964, p 369.
14. Perry J, Antonelli D, Ford W: Analysis of knee-joint forces during flexed-knee stance. J Bone Joint Surg Am 57:961, 1975.
15. Stockwell RA, Meachim G: The chondrocytes. In Freeman MAR, ed: Adult Articular Cartilage. 2nd ed. Pitman Medical, Tunbridge Wells, England, 1979, p 113.

70

Osteotomy About the Knee: American Perspective

ARLEN D. HANSSEN

After initial reports in Europe,[35, 51] the concept of proximal tibial osteotomy for the treatment of arthritis with associated limb malalignment was popularized in North America by Coventry.[22] The basis of realignment osteotomy about the knee is to transfer weightbearing forces from the arthritic portion of the knee to a healthier location of the knee joint. This redistribution of mechanical forces to increase the life span of the knee joint distinguishes osteotomy from other treatment modalities. The prevalence of realignment osteotomy has steadily declined since the introduction and subsequent success of knee arthroplasty, yet osteotomy remains a viable option for some selected patients (Fig. 70.1).

The goals of osteotomy include pain relief, functional improvement, and ability to meet heavy functional demands otherwise precluded by prosthetic replacement. Alternative procedures should be compared with current standards of osteotomy and not historic controls because patients undergoing osteotomy are generally considered worst-case scenarios for a successful long-term outcome with prosthetic replacement. The key to success after osteotomy is careful patient selection combined with skillful surgical technique. Remarkably, the patient selection process and specific indications for osteotomy are more standardized than the various preoperative planning methods and operative techniques currently being used.

PATIENT SELECTION PROCESS

The process of patient selection is possibly the single most important factor determining a successful result after osteotomy. A thorough synthesis of multiple variables is required to formulate the decision to proceed with osteotomy (Table 70.1). The primary indications for realignment osteotomy include pain relief associated with degenerative arthritis or a desired mechanical axis correction in conjunction with ligamentous reconstruction. It is often helpful to start by focusing on the relative and absolute contraindications to corrective osteotomy during the patient selection process (Table 70.2).

Historic Variables

The ideal candidate for osteotomy is a thin active individual in the fifth or sixth decade of life with localized, activity-related unicompartmental knee pain, no patellofemoral symptoms, a stable knee, and full knee extension with flexion of at least 90 degrees.[10] Although many patients do not meet all of these ideal

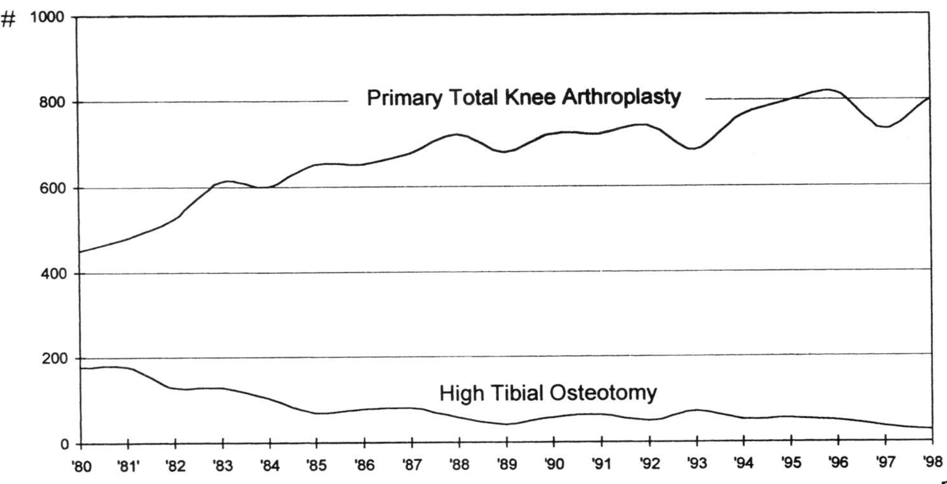

FIGURE 70.1 ➢ Incidence graph depicting the increasing rate of primary total knee arthroplasty and the declining rate of high tibial osteotomy at the Mayo Clinic between 1980 and 1998.

TABLE 70.1 SELECTION FACTORS FOR REALIGNMENT OSTEOTOMY

Historical	Examination	Radiological	Miscellaneous
Age	Malalignment	Anatomic axis	Patient expectations
Chronological	Magnitude	Mechanical axis	Surgeon capabilities
Physiological	Direction	Severity of arthrosis	Dynamic gait factors
Patient's desired activity level	Prior incisions	Magnitude of deformity	Soft tissue tension
Pain	Body habitus	Tibiofemoral subluxation	Upper body shift
Location	Range of motion	Status of other compartments	Potential complications
Character	Total arc	Joint space opening	Postoperative recovery
Patellofemoral?	Flexion contracture	Amount of articular cartilage loss	Immobilization time
Rheumatological status	Ligamentous deficiencies	CPPD	Durability of procedure
Prior meniscectomy	Patellofemoral mechanics	Osseous defects	Ease of revision to TKA
Infection history	Adductor thrust	Deformities away from joint	
		Joint line obliquity	

CPPD = calcium pyrophosphate deposition; TKA = total knee arthroplasty.

guidelines, a careful selection process allows satisfactory results in some of these individuals.

Emphasis on the location and character of pain, desired activity level, and appropriate patient expectations is particularly important when considering osteotomy. Diffuse and nonspecific knee pain reduces the chance of a successful outcome after osteotomy. Symptoms related to knee instability will not be alleviated with osteotomy alone, and moderate or severe laxity is a poor prognostic factor. In young active patients, the combination of degenerative arthritis, malalignment, and knee instability presents a difficult treatment entity beyond the confines of this discussion. Total knee arthroplasty is the treatment of choice for elderly patients with degenerative arthritis and instability.[47]

Patients with osteoarthritis, when compared with those with rheumatoid arthritis, fare better, and realignment osteotomy for inflammatory disorders is not recommended.[21, 39, 54] In the presence of secondary degenerative arthritis from a prior fracture, osteochondritis dissecans, or a prior medial meniscectomy, the results do not seem to be adversely affected, whereas patients with prior medial and lateral meniscectomies have disappointing outcomes.[77, 90]

Degenerative arthritis of the patellofemoral joint may be a cause of failure after corrective osteotomy.[32, 46, 85] Conversely, long-term results have shown a low incidence of unsatisfactory results attributed to the patellofemoral joint, and it is possible that extremity realignment may favorably alter patellofemoral mechanics.[27, 41, 55] Patellofemoral pain can improve after upper tibial osteotomy.[30, 64] Significant retropatellar pain should be a cautionary factor during patient selection, but mild retropatellar pain should not preclude osteotomy if the primary indication for osteotomy is unicompartmental tibiofemoral pain.

TABLE 70.2 CONTRAINDICATIONS TO CORRECTIVE OSTEOTOMY

Absolute	Relative
Diffuse, nonspecific knee pain	Age greater than 60 years
Patellofemoral pain primary complaint	Range of motion arc less than 90 degrees
Moderate or severe ligamentous instability	Obesity (1.32 × ideal body weight)
Meniscectomy in compartment intended for weightbearing	Severe arthrosis
Arthrosis in compartment intended for weightbearing	Tibiofemoral subluxation
Underlying diagnosis of inflammatory disease	
Unrealistic patient expectations	

Age assessment requires consideration of physiological status and lifestyle requirements; many younger and sedentary patients may be better served with arthroplasty, whereas some elderly and active patients may be better suited for osteotomy. Arthroplasty provides more complete pain relief and shorter rehabilitation and is more reliable than osteotomy in most individuals older than 60 years.[47]

Examination

Ipsilateral hip function should be assessed, and hip surgery is preferred before realignment osteotomy to eliminate the possibility of referred pain from the hip region. Limb inspection should confirm the presence of axial malalignment and assess for a lateral thrust. Analysis of preoperative gait adduction moments reveals that patients with high adduction moments, noted by the lateral thrust during gait, have worse outcomes, and overcorrection of extremity alignment is desirable in these individuals.[83] If sufficient correction of alignment is achieved at operation, preoperative peak adduction moments of the knee do not correlate with clinical outcomes of osteotomy.[98]

Particular care should be directed toward any prior skin incisions, which may affect the intended surgical exposure. Knee motion should reveal a flexion arc of at least 90 degrees with less than 10 to 20 degrees of a flexion contracture; however, these criteria have been established only by clinical convention. Patellofemoral symptoms or significant meniscal disease should not be the primary cause of the patient's complaints, and every effort must be pursued to differentiate the potential sources of pain. Moderate or severe knee instability should not be present, but anterior cruciate ligament insufficiency does not adversely affect outcomes if the preoperative symptoms can be specifically attributed to an overloading of the degenerative joint compartment.[43] The preoperative neurovascular status should be documented.

It cannot be overemphasized that osteotomy is technically more difficult in the obese patient, particularly in individuals with peripheral dystrophic weight distribution. Obesity has been associated with lower success rates after high tibial osteotomy because the surgical technique and postoperative immobilization are more difficult in these individuals.[28, 70] The long-term results after high tibial osteotomy are definitely worse in individuals who exceed their ideal body weight by 1.32 times.[28] The activity level of these patients should be carefully assessed because sedentary, overweight individuals of any age may be better served with prosthetic replacement. It should be stressed that significant weight loss may provide enough symptomatic relief to defer any operative intervention.

Counseling

The surgeon needs to discuss all treatment alternatives and convey that neither osteotomy or arthroplasty provide a "normal joint." The long-term results, rehabilitation, pain relief, and durability of realignment osteotomy and arthroplasty should be differentiated for the patient. A longer postoperative recovery period with less pain relief after rehabilitation is expected after osteotomy. These disadvantages need to be balanced against the possible catastrophic complications of infection or prosthetic failure with arthroplasty in the young and active patient.

Specifically, realignment osteotomy is based on the concept that certain high-impact and excessive loading activities are not sanctioned with prosthetic arthroplasty. Functional analysis of young patients after osteotomy reveals that many patients are able to participate in running and jumping activities that would likely lead to damage of a knee prosthesis.[78, 81] Eighty-two percent of patients in this study believed that the osteotomy met their expectations and would choose the operation again given the same situation. Many patients also value the real potential for technological advances in arthroplasty over the expected survival period of an osteotomy and recognize that "buying time" with an osteotomy is a viable concept.

The expected results of total knee arthroplasty after osteotomy also need to be considered. The literature detailing poor results of arthroplasty after osteotomy clearly indicate that technical difficulties or complications associated with osteotomy produce worse results with the subsequent arthroplasty.[11, 100] Surgeons with occasional experience performing corrective osteotomies should consider referral because a suboptimal surgical technique that may compromise subsequent procedures should not be the sole criterion used to abandon osteotomy. The poorer long-term radiographic results of total knee arthroplasty after high tibial osteotomy occur in a specific subset of patients.[53] These patients are younger, heavier, and more active males, which suggests that buying time with an osteotomy to avoid prosthetic replacement as long as possible is a wise choice in these individuals.

Radiographic Evaluation

The location and severity of the arthritis are determined with standing anteroposterior, lateral, intercondylar notch, and skyline patellar views. One should carefully inspect the contralateral tibiofemoral compartment for marginal osteophytes, which indicates the presence of diffuse arthritis. Tibiofemoral subluxation, excessive bony erosion, and diffuse arthritic involvement are associated with poorer outcomes.[21, 32, 48]

A full-length 51 × 14-inch weightbearing radiograph is necessary to determine the mechanical axis. Although there is generally a high correlation between the anatomic and mechanical axes, long films are also helpful to determine whether deformities of the tibia or femur exist and the effect these deformities have on the overall mechanical alignment.[61] Although technetium bone scanning can potentially help assess the location and intensity of bone reaction in the contralateral compartment of the knee joint, some investigators questioned this as a useful means of patient selection.[96]

Preoperative Planning

The principal considerations for osteotomy planning include the location, direction, and magnitude of malalignment (Table 70.3). These variables need to be weighed concurrently during the planning phase to achieve appropriate angular correction. One reason for premature failure after osteotomy is undercorrection or overcorrection of the deformity, which may be due to deficiencies in either the preplanning process or the surgical technique.[28, 33, 41, 55, 70, 85, 98, 102] Clearly, philosophy, training, and experience heavily bias preference for a specific osteotomy technique. The rationale for choosing between these options is delineated in the discussion of these various techniques (Table 70.4). In recent times, varus deformities are corrected by high tibial osteotomy, whereas most valgus deformities are corrected by distal femoral osteotomy. For most surgeons the most pragmatic approach is the closing-wedge osteotomy.

Intra-articular deficiencies require special consideration when calculating the degree of desired angular correction. Slack collateral ligamentous restraint causes angular deformity, and each millimeter of tibiofemoral separation requires subtraction of approximately 1 degree per millimeter to avoid overcorrection.[31] It is important to remember that ligamentous laxity will not be detected on standing radiographs when the laxity exists in the same compartment being overloaded. For example, lateral ligament laxity in a valgus knee or medial collateral ligament laxity in a varus knee, not observed on radiographs, may cause overcorrection of alignment after realignment osteotomy once the load

TABLE 70.3 COMPONENTS OF MALALIGNMENT

Location	Direction	Magnitude
Extra-Articular	***Sagittal***	Mild (<10 degrees)
Femur	Flexion	Moderate (10–20 degrees)
Tibia	Extension	Severe (>20 degrees)
Intra-Articular	***Coronal***	
Joint line obliquity	Varus	
Ligamentous laxity	Valgus	
Articular cartilage deficiency		
Osseous deficiencies	***Rotational***	

has been shifted toward the opposite compartment of the knee.

Some patients with proximal tibial varus deformity have excessive valgus angulation of the distal femoral articular surface.[20, 76] This obliquity of the distal femoral surface affects the magnitude of alignment correction and requires special consideration during preoperative planning because patients with femoral shaft-transcondylar angles of less than 9 degrees have an increased incidence of undercorrection.[85] Extra-articular deformities distant from the knee joint may need to be addressed at the apex of the deformity rather than with periarticular correction.

The magnitude of coronal plane malalignment may dictate the location of the osteotomy or suggest the use of a particular technique. For example, excessive malalignment may contraindicate high tibial osteotomy if the tibial articular surface will be adversely tilted, and for malalignment exceeding 12 to 15 degrees, the supracondylar femoral osteotomy is recommended.[23] Alternatively, the dome or barrel-vault osteotomy allows greater correction with less effect on the resultant joint line obliquity and should be potentially considered for varus deformities exceeding 20 degrees.[4, 68] For severe deformities, a dual (double) osteotomy of both the distal femur and proximal tibia may also be deemed necessary.[9] Sagittal plane deformities can be corrected with proper planning and appropriate adjustment of the osteotomy technique.

Historically, axial limb alignment was determined by measuring the femoral-tibial (anatomic) angle from standing radiographs and then judging the amount of correction required to restore this angle to normal, which typically averages 5 degrees of valgus (Fig. 70.2).[58] The height of a tibial osteotomy wedge was then estimated based on the rule of thumb that each millimeter provided roughly 1 degree of angular correction. This method of calculation is accurate only when the actual width of the tibial flare is 56 mm and is significantly altered by differences in the tibial width or distortion caused by radiographic magnification.[25] Use of this method without considering the actual tibial width invariably leads to undercorrection because the mean tibial width in men is 80 mm and 70 mm in women (Fig. 70.3). The mechanical axis averages 1.2 degrees of varus and is based on a line connecting the centers of the femoral head and tibiotalar joint (see Fig. 70.2). This axis is more accurate than the anatomic axis when defining the load transmission forces across the knee joint; this has been determined to be a more reliable method of measurement when there are femoral or tibial deformities that contribute to the malalignment.[45]

TABLE 70.4 CORRECTIVE OSTEOTOMY TECHNIQUES

Tibial	Femoral
Lateral closing wedge	Medial closing wedge
Medial closing wedge	Medial fixation
Medial opening wedge	Lateral fixation
Graft	Oblique metaphyseal wedge
Staple	Lateral opening wedge
Distraction histogenesis	Lateral closing wedge
Barrel-vault (dome) osteotomy	
Oblique metaphyseal wedge	

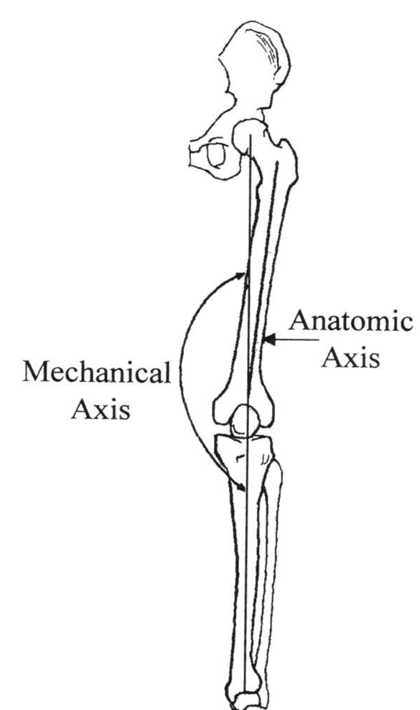

FIGURE 70.2 ➢ The mechanical axis, based on a line connecting the centers of the femoral head and tibiotalar joint, averages 1.2 degrees of varus, whereas the femoral-tibial (anatomic) angle normally averages 5 degrees of valgus.

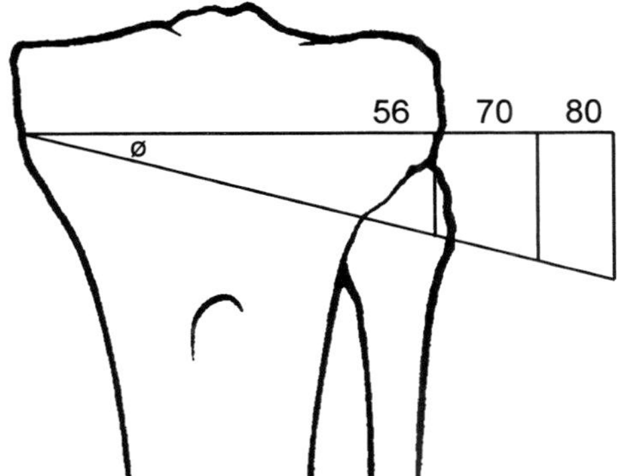

FIGURE 70.3 ➢ Given the same desired angle of correction (ø), the wedge height measurement progressively increases with increasing tibial width. The rule of thumb that 1 mm of wedge height equals 1 degree of angular correction results in undercorrection for tibial widths exceeding 56 mm.

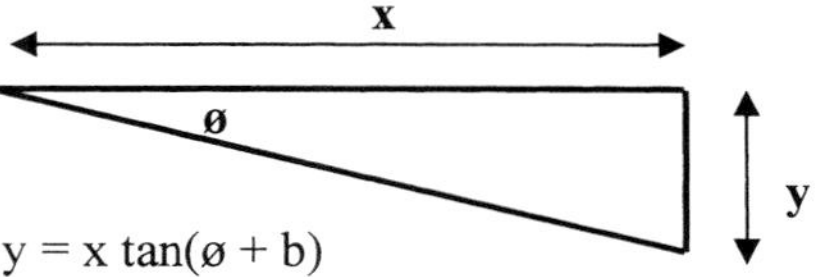

FIGURE 70.4 ➢ The trigonometric method of determining actual wedge height (y) is calculated with a trigonometric formula using known values of desired angle of correction (ø) and actual tibial width (x). A direct measurement of tibial width at a point 2.0 to 2.5 cm distal to the joint line, on radiographs incorporating radiographic markers, is normalized by the amount of magnification present to obtain the actual tibial wedge height (x).

One measurement method for high tibial osteotomy uses the mechanical axis on a full-length standing radiograph with radiographic markers to adjust for magnification. By using trigonometric principles and adjusting for radiographic magnification, the intended wedge height is determined by ascertaining the amount of angular correction required placing the mechanical axis at the desired location within the knee joint. The formula for these calculations is shown in Figure 70.4. A similar method, the weightbearing line method, divides the tibial plateau from 0% to 100% (medial to lateral) to determine the appropriate coordinate for the mechanical axis to intersect the knee joint (Fig. 70.5).[31] Lines to the center of the femoral head and the talar dome connect this coordinate, and the angle formed by these lines is the angle of desired correction. This angle is accordingly adjusted for distraction of the tibiofemoral joint surfaces allowed by ligamentous laxity and articular cartilage deficiency. The height of the wedge is then calculated by tracing the wedge on the radiograph and normalizing the measured height of the wedge by the amount of radiographic magnification. Both of these measurement methods account for the actual width of the tibial plateau.

The use of a full-length radiograph for measurement of the mechanical alignment is a static measurement only. Soft tissue tension, joint line obliquity, and upper body gravity shift also affect tibiofemoral plateau pressure distribution during dynamic gait. A software program, Osteotomy Analysis Simulation Software (OASIS), was developed to provide a comprehensive preoperative assessment of these factors and to assist the surgeon's final determination of the location, magnitude, and type of knee osteotomy most appropriate for the individual patient.[17] The data printout generated by this program details various osteotomy options and seems most useful for several circumstances: (1) the decision whether to perform a periarticular osteotomy or an osteotomy at the apex of the deformity away from the knee joint or (2) to determine whether joint line obliquity may be adversely affected after correction of severe malalignment with a particular technique. Currently, no data suggest the upper limit of acceptance for resultant joint line obliquity, and we often accept up to 10 degrees of resultant joint line obliquity before proceeding with the dual osteotomy (Figs. 70.6 to 70.10).

In contrast with severe or complex deformities, for patients with mild or moderate deformity, the static measurement planning methods seem sufficient and comparable to the OASIS program. Although these preoperative planning schemes provide objective criteria to guide the surgeon, even the most detailed plans

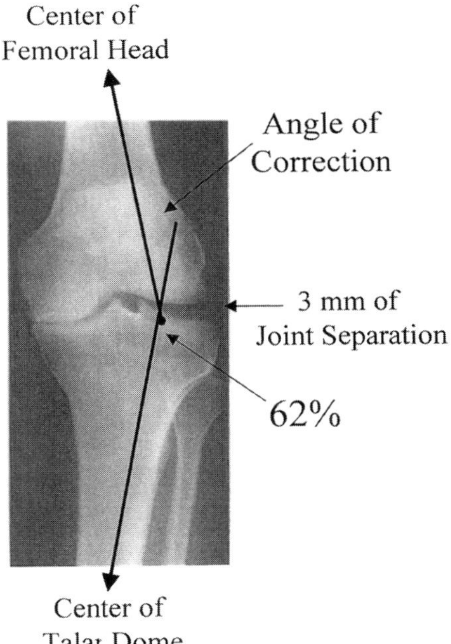

FIGURE 70.5 ➢ The weightbearing line method divides the tibial plateau from 0% to 100% (medial to lateral) to determine the desired intersection coordinate of the mechanical axis through the knee joint. The angle formed by lines drawn from this coordinate to the center of the femoral head and talar dome is corrected for tibiofemoral joint surface distraction allowed by ligamentous laxity to establish the desired angle of correction. The wedge height is calculated by tracing the wedge on the radiograph with the desired angle of correction. The wedge height measurement on the radiograph is then normalized by the radiographic magnification present.

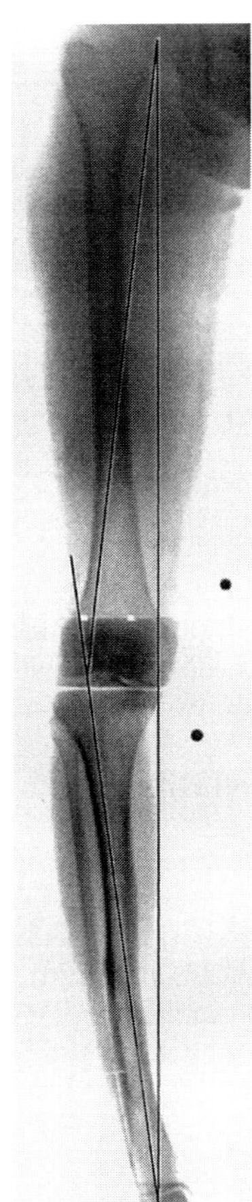

FIGURE 70.6 ➢ Standing full-length radiograph of an active 46-year-old woman with localized medial compartment knee pain. Note the tibial distal malunion.

require accurate performance of the surgical procedure.

SURGICAL TECHNIQUES

Inherent principles of these techniques include appropriate placement of skin incisions, careful handling of soft tissues, respect for neurovascular structures, accurate osteotomy, and adequate skeletal fixation. The options for fixation and a discussion of complications associated with osteotomy are discussed later in this chapter. Preparation for a skin incision should include forethought of an eventual total knee replacement, and longitudinal incisions on the lateral or medial side of the knee should provide large bridges of skin for any future midline or parapatellar approach. Carelessly placed incisions for the osteotomy may provide catastrophic complications of wound healing and infection at a later arthroplasty.

The accuracy of the osteotomy cannot be overemphasized because precise apposition of bone surfaces facilitates prompt healing, whereas proper orientation and resection of bone ultimately determine final mechanical alignment. The use of jig systems to assist the correct placement and orientation of the osteotomy appears particularly useful for many surgeons who have limited experience performing these osteotomies.[42, 60, 63] The use of intra-operative radiographs or fluoroscopy to document that appropriate correction has been achieved seems prudent and is strongly recommended.

Varus Deformity

For varus malalignment of the knee, many surgeons prefer a lateral closing-wedge osteotomy of the proximal tibia.[15, 26, 42, 48, 84, 85] This technique, performed between the knee joint and tibial tubercle, confers the advantages of broad cancellous bone surfaces and correction near the maximal point of deformity and uses the compressive forces of the quadriceps mechanism.[22] Further stabilization is provided by the medial periosteum and cortex, which act as a tether when the osteotomy is closed. Utmost care must be undertaken to avoid medial disruption; if this should occur, insertion of medial staples may be required. The following description, modified from the original report, is currently the preferred technique at our institution and is relatively simple and straightforward compared with other techniques.[22] The primary modification of this technique is the partial resection of the fibular head rather than total fibular head resection combined with advancement of the lateral ligamentous structures.

Lateral Closing Tibial Wedge

The patient is positioned supine with a sandbag positioned beneath the ipsilateral trochanteric region to place the extremity in neutral rotation. The extremity is exsanguinated and, under tourniquet control, the procedure is typically performed with the knee flexed to 90 degrees, although this does not protect the popliteal artery from injury compared with the fully extended position.[103] Although originally described as a long curvilinear incision, a short oblique incision coursing from fibular head toward the tibial tubercle is currently preferred. The iliotibial band is split longitudinally just anterior and parallel to fibular collateral ligament and the peroneal nerve located by palpation only. The anterior tibial musculature is then elevated subperiosteally from the proximal tibia.

Removal of the inner one-third of fibular head and cartilage is then accomplished with an osteotome. The posterior tibia is subperiosteally exposed to allow insertion of a broad malleable retractor to protect the neurovascular structures. An anterior retractor is placed between patellar ligament and tibia just proximal to tibial tubercle. The location of the joint line can be established either with a small arthrotomy or with placement of medial and lateral Kirschner wires. At a point 2.0–2.5 cm below the joint line, a guide wire is inserted from lateral to medial paralleling the tibial articular surface (Fig. 70.11a). The second pin is inserted at a point measured distally from pin 1 based on preoperative calculation of the tibial wedge height. This pin is advanced obliquely to intersect with the

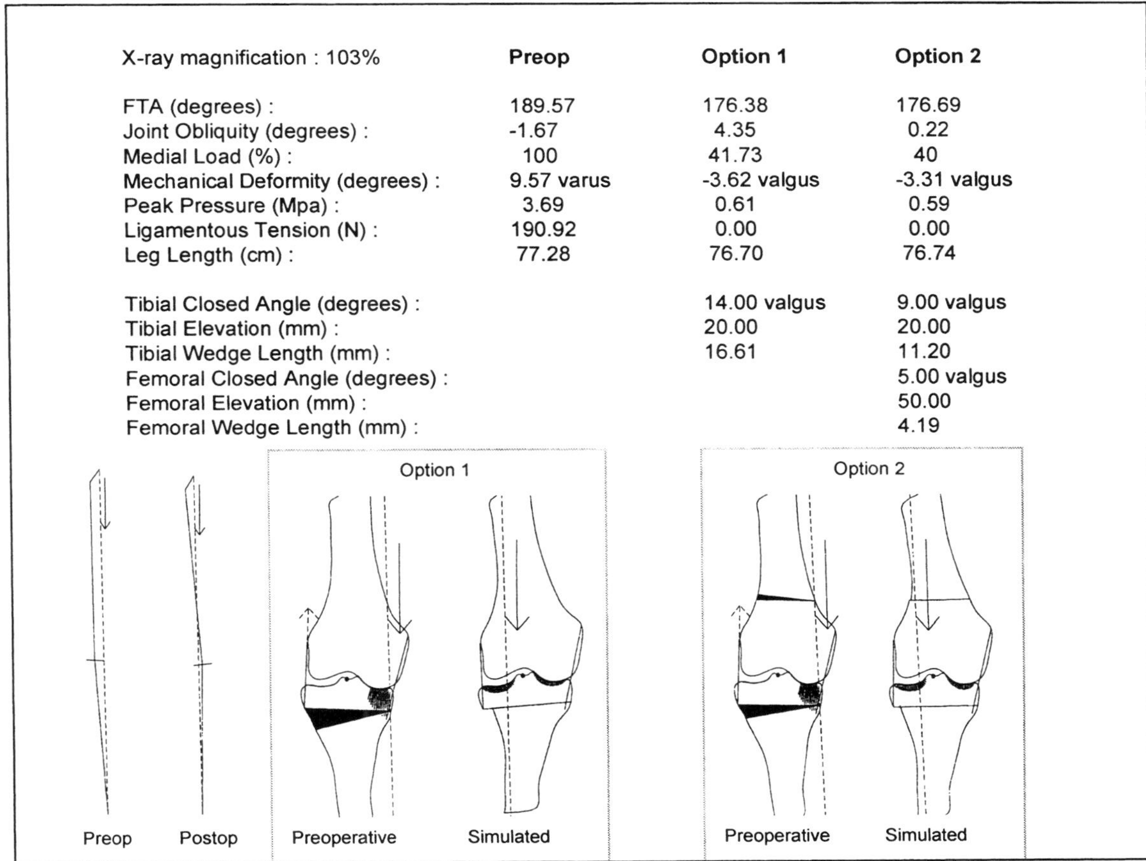

X-ray magnification : 103%	Preop	Option 1	Option 2
FTA (degrees) :	189.57	176.38	176.69
Joint Obliquity (degrees) :	-1.67	4.35	0.22
Medial Load (%) :	100	41.73	40
Mechanical Deformity (degrees) :	9.57 varus	-3.62 valgus	-3.31 valgus
Peak Pressure (Mpa) :	3.69	0.61	0.59
Ligamentous Tension (N) :	190.92	0.00	0.00
Leg Length (cm) :	77.28	76.70	76.74
Tibial Closed Angle (degrees) :		14.00 valgus	9.00 valgus
Tibial Elevation (mm) :		20.00	20.00
Tibial Wedge Length (mm) :		16.61	11.20
Femoral Closed Angle (degrees) :			5.00 valgus
Femoral Elevation (mm) :			50.00
Femoral Wedge Length (mm) :			4.19

FIGURE 70.7 ➢ An Osteotomy Analysis Simulation Software data printout, obtained from the full-length radiograph in Figure 70-6, details the several corrective osteotomy options. Option 1, with a proximal tibial wedge resection of 16.61 mm, is calculated to leave 4.35 degrees of resultant joint line obliquity. Option 2 describes a dual osteotomy designed to minimize resultant joint line obliquity.

first pin at medial tibial cortex. Pin placement should be confirmed radiographically.

Using a broad osteotome or an oscillating saw, the osteotomy is performed parallel to the posterior slope of tibial articular surface in the sagittal plane. The tibia is transected on the undersurface of pin 1 and on the upper surface of pin 2. The width of the wedge can be adjusted to correct for flexion or extension deformity by altering the height of the wedge in the anteroposterior plane. Initially, the osteotomy traverses approximately 50% to 75% of the tibial width so that the outer wedge of bone can be removed to facilitate completion of osteotomy with small osteotomes (Fig. 70.11*B*). It is important that the medial cortex is not transected but rather is perforated four to five times with long drill bit or small osteotome to maintain an intact periosteal hinge. Bone comprising the inner wedge is removed with small curets, taking great care to ensure removal of all cortical bone, especially in posteromedial tibial corner.

Osteoclasis is then achieved by applying a valgus stress to the extremity with the knee in full extension. The fibular head is inspected to verify that it is not preventing complete closure of the osteotomy. Mechanical alignment is verified by fluoroscopy with a rod extending from the femoral head to the talar dome. Fixation is then accomplished with the insertion of two stepped staples, positioning the first staple just anterior to the fibular head and the second staple yet more anteriorly (Fig. 70.11*C*). During staple insertion, it is helpful to start advancing the proximal tine into the tibial plateau until the distal tine rests against the tibial cortex. Using a 3.2 drill bit, a starter hole is made just distally to the tine to facilitate compression at the osteotomy site and avoid propagation of a fracture through the thick tibial cortex.

Counterpressure by a surgical assistant against the medial tibia during final staple insertion helps prevent tibial translation and disruption of the medial periosteum. In overweight individuals, it is often difficult to provide adequate counterpressure against the medial tibia because of the thickness of the subcutaneous tissues. A large provisional pin inserted obliquely across the osteotomy site helps stabilize the tibia during staple insertion in these patients. The accuracy of apposition and integrity of the medial periosteal hinge is then assessed dynamically with fluoroscopy. Bone graft, from the removed wedge of bone, is placed

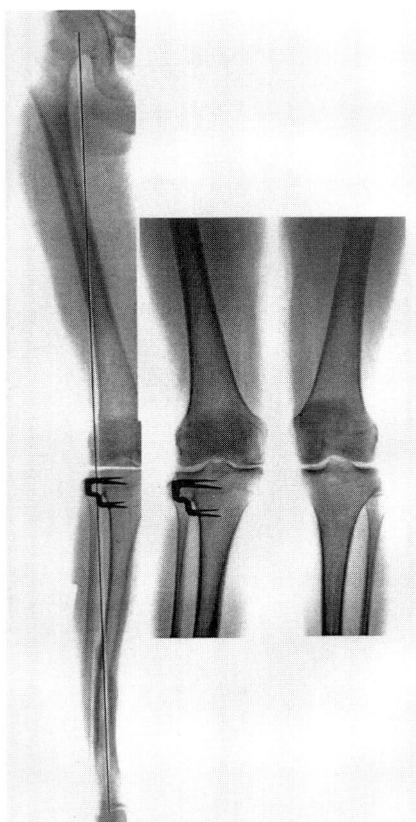

FIGURE 70.8 ➢ Postoperative full-length radiograph of patient after a 16-mm lateral wedge resection osteotomy of the proximal tibia demonstrating that the mechanical axis now intersects the lateral tibial compartment at the 75% coordinate. The inset standing radiograph demonstrates symmetry of the lower extremities.

adjacent to the staples. After tourniquet release, careful hemostasis is obtained, paying particular attention in the region of the anterior tibial musculature. Deep drains are then inserted along the posterior tibia and beneath the anterior compartment musculature. The wound is closed in layers, and the extremity is placed in a compressive dressing.

Medial Opening Tibial Wedge

Correction of malalignment with an opening medial wedge osteotomy has been reported as a successful technique for unicompartmental arthritis of the knee.[41]

The advantages of this technique include the fact that the fibula and tibiofibular joint need not be violated and surgical dissection is away from the peroneal nerve. This method embraces the disadvantages of procuring bone graft or using structural allograft bone, dependence on graft healing, and the risk of graft displacement and subsequent loss of correction. These complications are minimized with the use of rigid internal fixation. An alternative technique uses the insertion of a specialized interpositional stepped plate with or without the use of bone graft (Puddu G, personal communication, February 1998). This opening-wedge technique has been useful for young patients in whom joint line obliquity and malalignment require correction with concomitant ligamentous reconstruction of the knee, but we have not used this technique for isolated correction of malalignment.

An alternative approach includes gradually opening the medial wedge with an external fixation device.[16, 67] The advantages of these distraction histogenesis techniques include accurate correction of the desired mechanical axis at termination of distraction, rapid mobilization of the patient, absence of limb length shortening, and maintenance of soft tissue tension about the knee. The disadvantages include the use of an external fixation device and the attendant problems of pin-site difficulties. We have purposely avoided these external fixation techniques.

Barrel-Vault (Dome) Tibial Osteotomy

The dome osteotomy uses a curved osteotomy, which allows rotation or translation of the distal tibia on the proximal fragment.[4, 44, 68] A fundamental aspect of this procedure requires resection of a portion of the fibula to allow correction of the malalignment. Advantages of this method include avoidance of limb length alteration, potential for anterior displacement of the tibial tubercle to decrease patellofemoral joint reaction forces, and large corrections of malalignment that do not adversely affect the resultant joint line obliquity. This procedure is technically demanding, yet with adequate experience proponents prefer this procedure because of the ability to adjust the mechanical axis exactly. Use of a curved, double-bladed osteotomy guide facilitates an accurate osteotomy.[60] Disadvantages of this technique include a high incidence (33%) of complications, including pin-tract infections, loss of correction after fixator removal, and peroneal palsy.[44] We have limited experience with this osteotomy technique.

Dual (Double) Osteotomy

The dual osteotomy is another alternative for patients with severe deformity in whom osteotomy would potentially and adversely alter the obliquity of the joint line. This procedure is performed by an osteotomy of the femur and tibia to correct malalignment.[9] The use of the OASIS method to determine the correction required in both the femur and tibia to maintain proper joint line obliquity has been particularly useful in these patients.[17] Typically, the femoral wedge is performed as a lateral closing wedge when correcting varus malalignment and a medial closing wedge when correcting valgus malalignment. One of the conspicuous disadvantages of this osteotomy technique is the requirement for simultaneous osteotomy of the femur and tibia. In a comparative study of single and double osteotomy, patients with double osteotomies had fewer successful outcomes, a higher incidence of complications, and more restricted range of knee motion.[49] This additional morbidity must be weighed against the disadvantages of slight joint line obliquity.

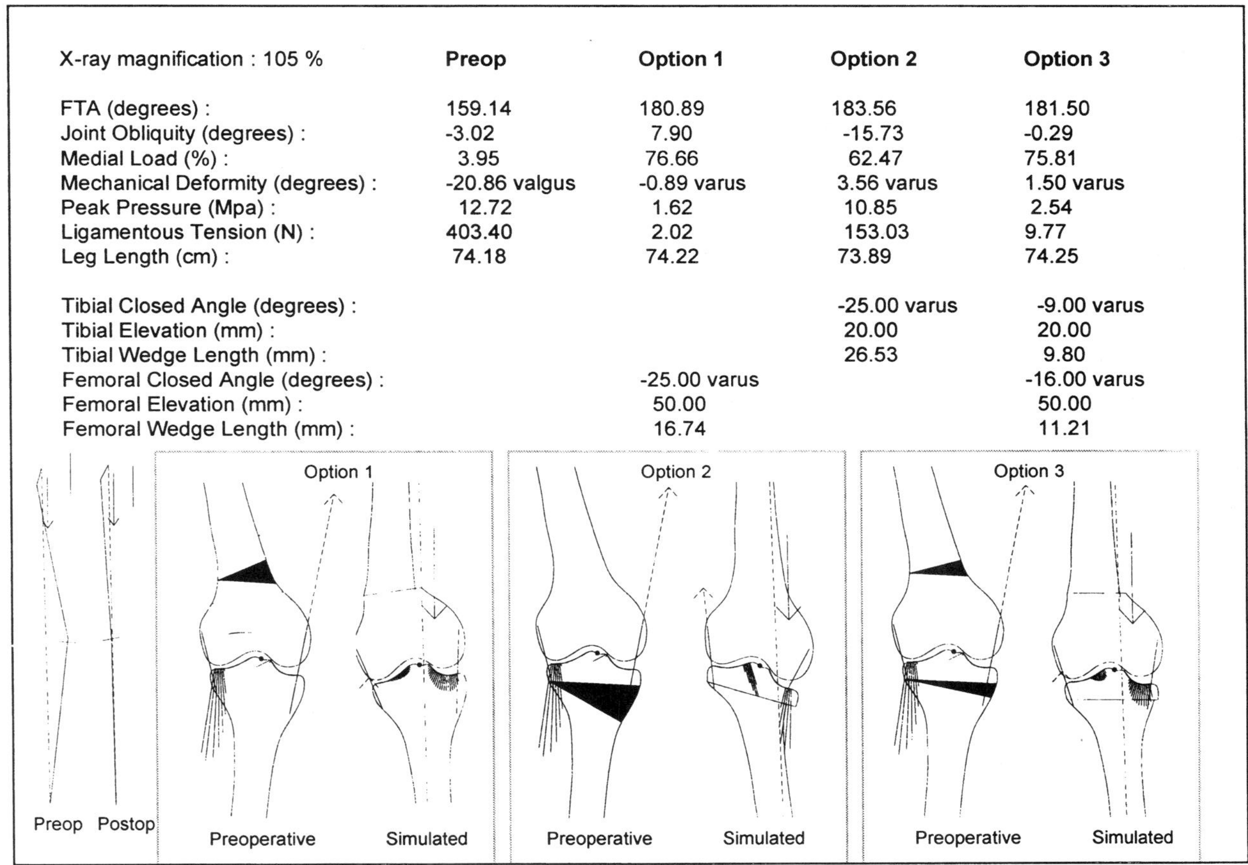

X-ray magnification : 105 %	Preop	Option 1	Option 2	Option 3
FTA (degrees) :	159.14	180.89	183.56	181.50
Joint Obliquity (degrees) :	-3.02	7.90	-15.73	-0.29
Medial Load (%) :	3.95	76.66	62.47	75.81
Mechanical Deformity (degrees) :	-20.86 valgus	-0.89 varus	3.56 varus	1.50 varus
Peak Pressure (Mpa) :	12.72	1.62	10.85	2.54
Ligamentous Tension (N) :	403.40	2.02	153.03	9.77
Leg Length (cm) :	74.18	74.22	73.89	74.25
Tibial Closed Angle (degrees) :			-25.00 varus	-9.00 varus
Tibial Elevation (mm) :			20.00	20.00
Tibial Wedge Length (mm) :			26.53	9.80
Femoral Closed Angle (degrees) :		-25.00 varus		-16.00 varus
Femoral Elevation (mm) :		50.00		50.00
Femoral Wedge Length (mm) :		16.74		11.21

FIGURE 70.9 ➢ An Osteotomy Analysis Simulation Software data printout obtained from a full-length standing radiograph of a 42-year-old active woman with painful genu valgum and osteoarthritis of the lateral compartment of her right knee. Option 2 demonstrates the anticipated resultant joint line obliquity produced by a varus, requiring osteotomy of the proximal tibia.

Valgus Deformity

Genu valgum is a much rarer entity than varus deformity of the knee.[54] The biomechanics of the varus and valgus knee are also different because most valgus knees have inherent superolateral obliquity of the joint line. Classically, distal femoral osteotomy has been recommended for valgus deformities exceeding 12 to 15 degrees or when the joint line obliquity would exceed 10 degrees after correction.[23] Although genu valgum may be corrected by a varus producing proximal tibial osteotomy, the magnitude of the joint line obliquity is increased by the wedge resection and may be a cause of clinical failure.[7, 21, 27, 39, 71, 89] Excessive joint line obliquity produces ineffective weight transfer because some weight is applied as shear forces against the intercondylar eminence when the femur subluxes on the tibia. This problem is aggravated in the presence of the medial collateral laxity produced by the proximal tibial wedge removal, leading to the "teeter effect" of the femur toggling on the intercondylar eminence during gait.[57] The reader is referred to Coventry's description of a closing-wedge varus producing proximal tibial osteotomy.[23]

Although dome osteotomy of the proximal tibia does not increase joint line obliquity, the superolateral obliquity associated with a valgus deformity is not corrected, and the persistent femoral valgus angulation continues to exert valgus forces on the knee joint. Osteotomy in the supracondylar region is the most effective method of addressing this deformity because the transcondylar line becomes perpendicular with the mechanical axis and minimizes medial collateral ligament laxity. For most surgeons today, valgus malalignment about the knee of any magnitude is best managed with femoral osteotomy, and a medial closing-wedge osteotomy, with either lateral or medial fixation, seems to be the preferred technique.[13, 32, 39, 69, 71, 74] Valgus deformity can also be corrected by an opening-wedge osteotomy of the distal femur with insertion of tricortical autograft wedges supplemented by lateral plate fixation.[95]

It has been noted that the supracondylar femoral osteotomy is an "unforgiving" procedure for three specific reasons: (1) difficulty cutting the wedge effectively, (2) effective stabilization of the closed osteotomy, and (3) prediction of the wedge size necessary to ensure proper correction of the limb.[54] In many respects, it is clear that the biomechanics, preopera-

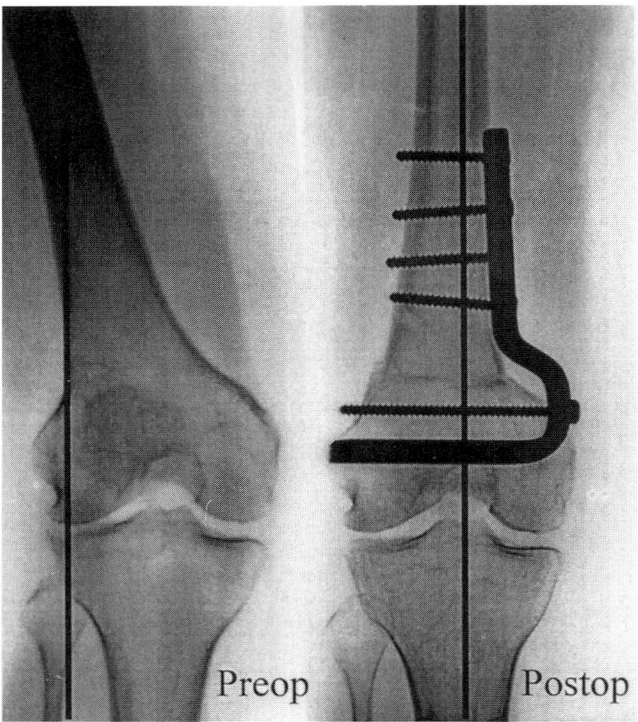

FIGURE 70.10 ➢ Spot views of full-length radiographs described in Figure 70-9. Note the correction of the mechanical axis from the 95% coordinate in the preoperative radiograph to the 50% coordinate (neutral position) in the postoperative radiograph.

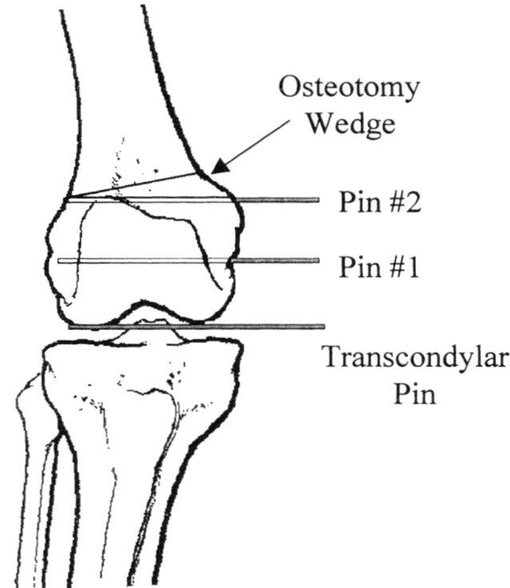

FIGURE 70.12 ➢ Diagram depicting placement of the transcondylar pin, location of pin 1 for entry of the blade plate, and location of pin 2 for the inferior portion of the osteotomy wedge. A truly parallel position of the transcondylar pin and blade plate entry is essential to obtain a neutral mechanical axis.

tive planning, and operative technique of a supracondylar femoral osteotomy is quite different from that of a proximal tibial osteotomy. These three concerns are adequately addressed by the following surgical technique, which is characterized by a simple preoperative planning process, a straightforward surgical technique that minimizes wedge removal difficulties and reproducibly allows accurate extremity realignment.

Medial Closing Femoral Wedge

This technique, which can be performed with either medial or lateral fixation, has been modified from the original description.[8, 71] Essentially, this method uses the transcondylar line and a 90-degree AO blade plate to correct the mechanical axis to neutral. The patient is placed in the supine position; tourniquet control is optional. A 12- to 15-cm longitudinal incision extending from the joint line proximally can be placed anywhere from the midline to the medial side of the thigh. The vastus medialis obliquus is elevated from the medial septum and retracted anteriorly to expose the medial femoral condyle and femoral cortex. The joint line is located with a small arthrotomy or the use of a large needle.

With the knee flexed to 90 degrees, a guide wire is

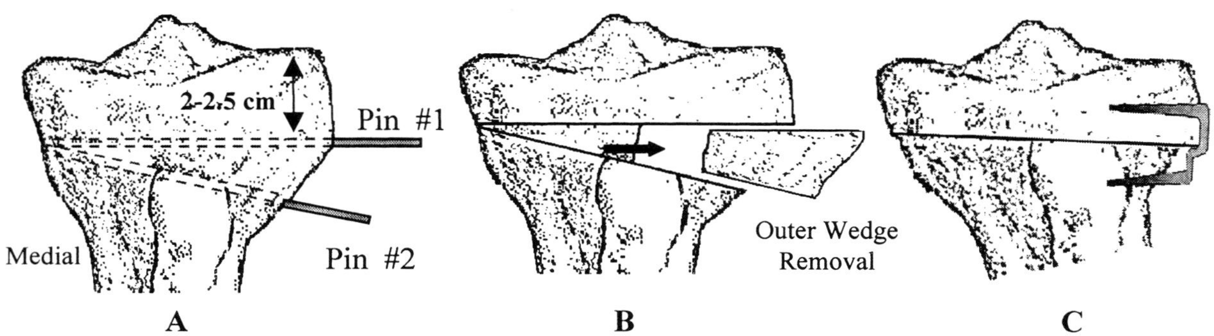

FIGURE 70.11 ➢ *A,* The first guide wire is inserted parallel to the tibial articular surface approximately 2.0 to 2.5 cm below the joint line. The second guide wire, inserted at a point distally based on the preoperative calculation of actual tibial wedge height, is advanced obliquely to intersect at the medial tibial cortex with the first guide wire. *B,* The outer 50% to 75% of the wedge is initially removed to allow completion of the inner portion of the wedge. *C,* The tibia is stabilized with insertion of two stepped staples bridging the osteotomy site.

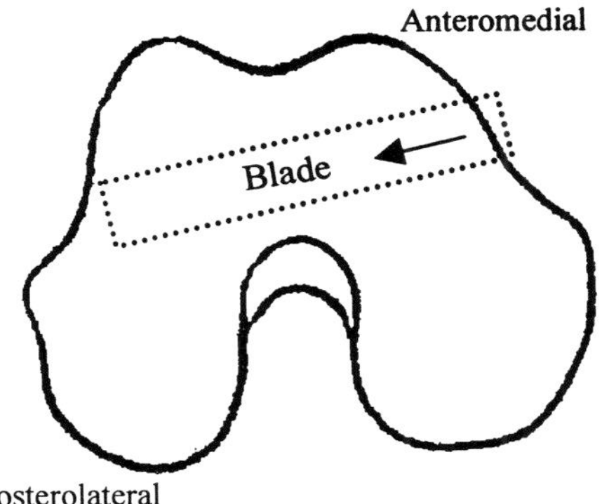

FIGURE 70.13 ➢ The blade plate should be inserted obliquely from anteromedial to posterolateral to avoid penetration of the intercondylar notch or the anterior femoral articular surface.

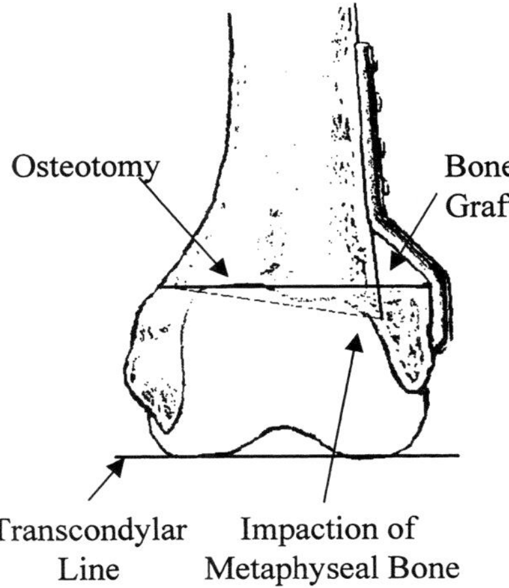

FIGURE 70.14 ➢ After osteotomy closure and impaction of the proximal fragment, the 90-degree AO osteotomy blade plate is secured to the proximal femur, which is now perpendicular with the transcondylar line.

placed across the joint parallel with the articular surface of the distal femur (Fig. 70.12). A second guide wire, inserted approximately 2.0 cm proximal and parallel to the first pin, is directed from anteromedial to posterolateral to aid insertion of the blade plate chisel at the correct angle (Fig. 70.13). The position of the guide wires is verified with radiographs because a truly parallel position of these pins with the transcondylar line is imperative. The guide wire is inserted up to the lateral cortex of the femur to allow measurement of the proper blade plate length, which is usually 50 to 70 mm.

Three 4.5-mm drill holes are then placed just above the second pin in the medial femoral condyle to prevent cortical comminution during chisel penetration. The chisel is impacted along the upper surface of pin 2 to the desired depth. The plate holder attached to the box chisel facilitates proper chisel entry and ensures correct apposition of the blade plate against the proximal femur. Radiographs taken at this point document proper chisel angle and ascertain that the chisel has not penetrated the intercondylar notch or the anterior femoral surface. Large malleable retractors are placed medially and posteriorly to protect the neurovascular structures.

Guide wires, placed form medial to lateral and converging at the lateral cortex, are used to perform the osteotomy. The inferior guide wire is placed parallel with the transcondylar pin in the supracondylar region just proximal to the adductor tubercle (see Fig. 70.12). A longitudinal line extending above and below the site of the osteotomy is placed on the femur with a marking pencil to ensure proper rotation of the limb at the time of osteotomy closure. The medial portion of the osteotomy is performed with an oscillating saw so that the outer 50% to 75% of the wedge can be removed before perforating the lateral cortex with several drill holes. Great care is taken to avoid transection of the lateral cortex and overlying periosteum with the saw. The height of the wedge can be a predetermined measurement, but preferably removal of only a 5- to 10-mm wedge allows impaction of the proximal fragment into the metaphysis of the distal fragment (Fig. 70.14). This impaction promotes maximal bone apposition and improves stability of the osteotomy site.

Use of preoperative templates to determine the proper plate size is prudent. The proper 90-degree AO blade plate, selected by length of the blade and one of three sizes of offset, is then inserted into the femur. Osteoclasis is performed with a varus force to the extremity to close the osteotomy site, impact the proximal fragment, and apply the plate along the medial femoral cortex proximally. The plate is secured to the femur with multiple cortical screws using the dynamic compression technique; however, the AO outrigger compression device should be avoided because of the proximity of the vascular structures in the adductor canal. The medial femoral cortex and distal femoral articular surface should now be perpendicularly aligned, and the resultant mechanical axis is approximately neutral (see Fig. 70.10). The removed bone wedge is then morseled and placed medially and posteriorly along the osteotomy site (see Fig. 70.14). The vastus medialis obliquus is reattached to the medial septum with several interrupted sutures over a drain placed at the osteotomy site. The wound is closed in layers and the limb placed in a compressive dressing.

Because of concerns raised with delayed union, nonunion, and hardware failure after supracondylar osteotomy with medially based fixation, a method of closing-wedge osteotomy with lateral fixation has been proposed.[74] This technique is based on the rationale that the lateral femur becomes the tensile side of the knee after osteotomy, and under these circumstances laterally based fixation is superior to fixation inserted medially. Indeed, these authors reported a higher incidence of implant failure or nonunion with medial fixation compared with lateral fixation. It is important to note that the technique described by these authors incorporates more than just fixation location because the osteotomy is performed obliquely and is stabilized by an interfragmentary screw. Undoubtedly, these technical aspects also contribute to the differences observed between the two techniques.

A major criticism of this report is that medial fixation was definitely adequate with younger patients who had better bone quality, and the technique of lateral fixation was not tried in older patients with osteopenic bone. In their hands, the final postoperative alignment was also more accurate with the lateral fixation technique. Although the authors were unable to explain this latter finding, the learning curve of performing supracondylar osteotomy may be a factor because the lateral fixation technique is actually more difficult, and many of the medial fixation osteotomies were performed years before these lateral fixation osteotomies.

ARTHROSCOPY

Although controversial, it has been reported that arthrotomy and joint débridement done simultaneously with osteotomy enhances the final result.[66, 71] Extrapolation of this experience leads one to believe that some patients might benefit from arthroscopic débridement in conjunction with corrective osteotomy. In one study, osteotomy patients with simultaneous arthroscopic abrasion arthroplasty (Group A) were compared with patients who had osteotomy alone (Group B).[3] At 12-month follow-up, arthroscopic evaluation of Group A knees revealed a significantly higher incidence of grade II cartilage repair; however, there was no difference in the clinical outcome between the two groups at 2- to 9-year follow-up. It has been our experience with high tibial osteotomy that arthroscopy has not been particularly beneficial, and our experience with arthroscopy and distal femoral osteotomy has been too limited to provide any data or recommendations.

Another reason for considering arthroscopy is to evaluate the stage of arthritis in the knee to predict the potential efficacy of osteotomy. Prognostic value has not been demonstrated when using arthroscopy to evaluate the joint before corrective osteotomy.[55, 56] Interestingly, observation of moderate or severe degenerative patellofemoral joint changes has not adversely affected the eventual clinical results. Proliferation of fibrocartilage and regeneration of articular cartilage has been documented by second-look arthroscopy compared with arthroscopic findings visualized preoperatively.[44, 80] Importantly, only overcorrected knees demonstrated cartilage regeneration, supporting the concept of mechanical realignment to facilitate reparative capacity of the knee joint once unloaded.[80]

FIXATION

Skeletal fixation should be sufficiently rigid to allow early knee motion if desired and yet promote bone healing. Many options are available for fixation, and most are in conjunction with the description of a specific osteotomy technique. In general, it is accepted that fixation of the distal femoral osteotomy requires more rigid fixation than osteotomy of the proximal tibia. Difficulties with fixation are more frequently reported with supracondylar osteotomy, and most authors agree that rigid internal fixation is required. In our hands, although staple fixation has been inadequate for the distal femoral osteotomy, they have remained the preferred method of fixation for high tibial osteotomy.[24, 28, 32, 54] The literature suggests a trend toward more rigid fixation techniques in preference to staple fixation when performing high tibial osteotomy. The blade plate appears to be the primary choice of fixation for most surgeons when performing distal femoral osteotomy.

Different methods of fixation described include (1) cast immobilization without internal fixation,[1, 2, 48] (2) external fixation devices,[4, 44, 67, 68, 82] (3) staple fixation,[6, 24, 54, 65, 94] (4) screw fixation,[59] (5) buttress plates,[40, 42] (6) tension band plates,[73, 92] (7) L-plates,[42] and (8) blade plate fixation.[13, 32, 34, 39, 61, 71] Because of the difficulties of loss of correction associated with cast immobilization without internal fixation, the use of internal fixation or an external fixation is preferable.[41]

Disadvantages of specialized buttress or blade plates for fixation of the proximal tibia after osteotomy include additional dissection of the anterior compartment to allow plate positioning, difficulties with precise plate contouring to accommodate the tibial step-off created by the wedge removal. In the presence of a poorly contoured plate, the plate may create undesirable mechanical forces that may predispose toward delayed healing or frank nonunion. Finally, many of these internal fixation devices require removal of the hardware, associated with additional soft tissue dissection, when performing a subsequent total knee arthroplasty. In contrast, staples usually do not require removal during the arthroplasty.

One of the stated advantages of external fixation devices includes the absence of internal hardware. Although undoubtedly true, the premature removal of external fixation is often dictated by pin-site difficulties, and loss of correction may occur in these patients. Pin-site difficulties are definitely more common when using external fixation in the distal femur, and their use in this location for realignment osteotomy cannot be recommended.[32] We have treated patients with septic arthritis of the knee joint related to pin-site difficulties and infected total knee arthroplasty most likely caused by pin-site infections associated with a prior external fixation device. Although the incidence of this phenomenon is unknown, concern about the prognosis of these patients is warranted. As such, we have avoided external fixation techniques for corrective osteotomy. Although no controlled studies compared external fixation devices with internal fixation, it appears that there are higher prevalence of infection, peroneal palsy, delayed healing, and loss of correction associated with the use of external fixation devices. External fixation devices have been useful in the management of osteotomy nonunion or delayed union associated with internal fixation and deep infection.[88]

Under most circumstances, when using internal fixation or an external fixation device, the patient is allowed early knee motion and progressive weightbearing over the ensuing 8 weeks. In particular, staple fixation requires an accurate assessment of stability at surgery to determine postoperative management. Use of a cast brace to supplement rigid staple fixation has provided satisfactory results.[62] If there is any question about the rigidity of staple fixation during the operative procedure, alternative methods of internal fixation or use of a long-leg cast for 4 to 6 weeks postoperatively is advisable.

COMPLICATIONS

The technical difficulties and potential severity of complications associated with realignment osteotomy have undoubtedly contributed to the decline in popularity of this operative procedure. In general, complications can be categorized as major and minor (Table 70.5). Clearly, many complications arise from the quality of the patient selection process, preoperative planning, surgical technique, and postoperative regimen. These have been previously separated into evaluation pitfalls and technical pitfalls.[57] Patient selection considerations and poor postoperative alignment, probably the most common factors in complications of corrective osteotomy, are discussed in the Results section. Some of the other complications such as pin-site infection, fixation, and adverse joint line obliquity have already been discussed.

Neurological injury after osteotomy ranks as one of the most adverse consequences of this procedure. Causative factors include intraoperative injury (resulting from traction, compression, laceration, or penetration by an external fixation pin), tight postoperative dressings or casts, and progressive development of postoperative edema or hematoma. Avoiding dissection of the peroneal nerve, carefully placing retractors, and keeping the knee flexed during the operative procedure are useful. Postoperative dressings should be well padded with the knee in a slightly flexed position.

Postoperative peroneal palsy appears to be associated with the use of an external fixation device.[44, 52, 68]

TABLE 70.5 Complications Associated with Realignment Osteotomy

Major	Minor
Neurologic injury	Superficial wound healing
Vascular injury	Pin site infections
Compartment syndrome	Skin numbness
Deep infection	Neuroma formation
Thromboembolic disease	Arthrofibrosis
Intra-articular fracture	Knee instability
Hardware failure	Adverse joint line obliquity
Nonunion	Patella infera
Malunion	Delayed union
Loss of correction	Inadequate pain relief
Undercorrection	Painful hardware
Overcorrection	Flare-up chondrocalcinosis
	Osteonecrosis of tibial plateau

Many external fixation techniques use a proximal fibular osteotomy, which is another etiological factor.[29, 68] The occurrence of neurological deficit is clearly related to the level of fibular osteotomy.[101] A safe area for proximal fibular osteotomy is located up to 20.5 mm distal to the tip of the fibular head.[91] Distal fibular osteotomy should be performed at the junction of the middle and distal thirds of the fibula.[5] Injury to the posterior tibial nerve has been uniquely associated with the dome osteotomy.[72]

Vascular injury associated with high tibial osteotomy is fortunately quite rare, and most reported cases involve the popliteal artery.[21, 37, 87, 103] As shown in 20 cadaveric dissections, flexion of the knee joint as compared with full knee extension does not protect the surgeon from popliteal artery injury.[103] Injury to the anterior tibial and peroneal arteries has also been reported.[1, 7] The more extensive dissection required for plate and screw fixation predisposes toward anterior tibial artery compromise.[26] We are unaware of any reported cases of vascular injury associated with distal femoral osteotomy. Compartment syndrome is also a rare yet devastating complication after osteotomy. It has been demonstrated that suction drainage of the anterior compartment is helpful; 8 of 10 patients with drains had postoperative compartment pressures of <30 mm Hg compared with pressure elevation >50 mm Hg in 7 of 10 patients without drains.[36] The importance of rapid diagnosis and the potential to avert an impending compartment syndrome before onset of an established compartment syndrome must be emphasized to all members of the health care team when participating in patients' care.

Deep infection is quite rare after corrective osteotomy, but the risk is higher when using external fixation devices.[44, 52] Thromboembolic disease occurs with lower frequency after osteotomy than with total knee arthroplasty, and the proper method of prophylaxis is controversial. We use the same anticoagulation protocol for osteotomy and arthroplasty and currently prefer the use of low-dose warfarin.

Intra-articular fracture of either tibial plateau, occurring during closure of the osteotomy, can be minimized by maintaining at least 2 cm of thickness in the entire proximal fragment, removing the entire bone wedge, and carefully perforating the apical portion of the osteotomy.[22, 57] These fractures are often caused by an inadvertent superomedial osteotomy angle and can be minimized by careful documentation of guide wire or jig placement. If guide wires are used, one should cut on the undersurface of the wire. Evaluation of the osteotomy site with fluoroscopy before osteotomy closure helps ensure complete bone removal of the medial portion of the wedge and allows observation of an osteotomy too close to the joint surface. The lateral tibial plateau can also split during insertion of internal fixation, and predrilling the cortex before staple insertion is recommended. After fixation is complete, radiographs should be taken to ensure that the hardware has not penetrated the joint. Excessive medial bone loss can cause an errant direction of the osteotome or saw and lead to direct osteotomy of the joint surface.[7, 48] Postoperative fracture of the proximal fragment can occur as a result of an excessively thin fragment[7, 48] or secondary to acute trauma.[50] Fracture of the tibial plateau should be accurately reduced and fixed to maintain the proper position of the plateaus for weight distribution. Osteonecrosis of tibial plateau can also occur with a thin proximal tibial fragment.[26]

Joint stiffness has been rarely reported after high tibial osteotomy, whereas this phenomenon has been frequently reported after supracondylar osteotomy.[8, 15, 32, 54, 69] Rigid fixation and early range of motion minimize the prevalence of stiffness, but rapid healing of the osteotomy and maintenance of postoperative alignment should take priority. The stiffness associated with supracondylar osteotomy did make surgical exposure more difficult for a subsequent knee arthroplasty in some patients.[11]

Early range of motion also helps avoid quadriceps atrophy and may aid in the prevention of patellar ligament shortening after osteotomy.[99] It has been questioned whether patellar position is actually lowered after high tibial osteotomy.[75] These authors suggested that traditional tibial reference marker methods to determine patellar height after an osteotomy of the proximal tibia may generate spurious values. Therefore, they recommended a femoral reference point for measurement. Despite this interesting perspective, the scarring and shortening of the patellar ligament often prevents eversion of the patella, and surgical exposure may require specialized exposure techniques during a subsequent total knee arthroplasty.[100]

An acute postoperative flare-up of joint pain may be due to calcium pyrophosphate deposition (CPPD) and has been reported to occur in 4.6% of cases.[21] These flare-ups are generally documented by analysis of synovial fluid and radiographic evidence of crystalline deposition. Management with anti-inflammatory medications or intra-articular injection of corticosteroids is usually sufficient. Coventry[25] believed preoperative evidence of CPPD, with the attendant generalized joint inflammation, to be a contraindication to corrective osteotomy. Recurrence of preoperative deformity over time has been correlated with clinical deterioration.[25, 26, 41, 48, 93] Recurrent deformity should not be confused with loss of postoperative correction, but this phenomenon has been correlated with undercorrection of alignment at surgery.[41, 44] A majority of patients had some recurrence of varus at a minimum of 5 years follow-up, but only 18% had more than 5 degrees of recurrence.[93] In contrast, 83% had significant progression of lateral compartment arthritis.

Difficulties with successful union are mentioned in essentially all reports of corrective osteotomy. Potential causes include the location of osteotomy, the fixation method, bone necrosis caused by use of a power saw, fibular impingement against the proximal tibial fragment, and poorly performed osteotomy cuts. Tibial osteotomy below the tibial tubercle is associated with a four-fold increase of delayed union when compared with tibial osteotomy performed above the tibial tubercle.[97] Nonunion after high tibial osteotomy performed above the tubercle ranges from 2% to 4% in the literature, which is distinctly less than the rates reported for supracondylar osteotomy. Nonunion of the supracondylar osteotomy has been reported to be between 4.2% and 19%.[8, 32, 39, 54, 69, 71, 74] Although previously discussed, the reported 29% rate of nonunion associated with medial fixation is most unfavorable.[74]

For supracondylar delayed unions or nonunions associated with medial fixation, bone grafting with application of a lateral T-plate has provided satisfactory healing.[12] For patients with broken medial hardware, the process of plate removal and bone grafting with application of a lateral plate has been successful.[74] Application of new and rigid internal fixation or the use of an external fixator has been useful in the management of proximal tibial nonunion.[14, 88]

RESULTS

High Tibial Osteotomy

It is clear that reported outcomes of high tibial osteotomy are quite variable. Factors that affect outcome, such as patient selection and surgical technique, have been clarified over the past four decades. The literature suggests that high tibial osteotomy provides durable and satisfactory long-term clinical results if the procedure is accurately performed in carefully selected patients who are typically younger than 60 years and who have an angular deformity less than 12 degrees, pure unicompartmental disease, ligamentous stability, and a preoperative range of motion arc of at least 90 degrees.[10] The importance of patient selection is underscored by the results obtained in 39 osteotomies, many of which were performed without precise indications.[10] Among the 10 poor results, the preoperative diagnoses included four cases of diffuse degenerative arthritis, two cases of inflammatory disease, one case of prior septic arthritis, and one case of post-traumatic arthritis with severe deformity. Clearly, today these patients are considered poor candidates for realignment osteotomy. If these 10 patients were excluded from analysis, the overall satisfactory results at 12-year follow-up would be an impressive 79%.

An equally important consideration for a successful clinical outcome is the quality of the surgical technique. In a series of 30 tibial osteotomies, at 51-month follow-up, 43% were judged satisfactory and 57% were deemed poor.[18] Importantly, in this series, patient selection criteria were quite rigid. In patients with good results, there were no technical errors, and all had good correction of malalignment. Among the 17 poor results, there were 10 technical errors, including five cases of undercorrection, three cases of overcorrection, and two cases involving joint penetration with the osteotomy; there were 11 total complications. These results emphasize the adversity of suboptimal surgical technique on the outcome of corrective osteotomy even in the face of good patient selection.

Many series of high tibial osteotomy reveal satisfactory results at 5 to 7 years of follow-up; the percentage of satisfactory clinical results then diminishes significantly (Table 70.6). Ritter and Fechtman[84] concluded

TABLE 70.6 SURVIVAL SUCCESS OF SELECTED SERIES OF HIGH TIBIAL OSTEOTOMY

Study	No. Patients	Survival (%) 2 Years	5 Years	7 Years	10 Years	15 Years
Berman et al (1991)[10]	39	87	—	—	—	57*
Cass and Bryan (1988)[15]	86	94	87	—	69	—
Coventry et al (1993)[23]	87	—	87	—	66	—
			(96)†		(91)†	
			(94)‡		(94)‡	
Healy and Riley (1986)[38]	31	92	88	91	80§	—
Hernigou et al (1987)[41]	93	—	90	—	45	—
			(100)‖		(100)‖	
Matthews et al (1988)[70]	40	86¶	50	—	28§	—
Ritter and Fechtman (1988)[84]	78	95	80	58	58	58*
Rudan and Simurda (1991)[86]	128	—	—	—	80	70
Yasuda et al (1992)[102]	86	—	88	—	63	—

* Twelve to 13 years.
† Body weight <1.17 × normal.
‡ Postoperative alignment 8 degrees or more of valgus.
§ Nine years.
‖ Twenty patients with appropriate postoperative alignment.
¶ One year.

that the "reliable longevity of the proximal tibial osteotomy is approximately six years." It is often difficult to ascertain the effects of patient selection and technical errors on the long-term outcome when evaluating many of these clinical series. Several of these studies carefully analyzed subgroups of patients to refine further the prognostic factors associated with long-term success. The following quote requires careful consideration: "the passage of time seemed to influence the result only in knees that were undercorrected or overcorrected."[41] In this series of 93 osteotomies, the overall 5-year survival of 90%, which then diminished to 45% at 10 years, hides the results obtained in patients with good postoperative alignment. In these 20 patients, there were no failures at 11.5 years follow-up, which sharply contrasts with the observed deterioration in 51 (75%) of 68 knees with postoperative undercorrection.

Excluding patient selection, accuracy of postoperative alignment does appear to be a primary determining factor of success with the passage of time.[15, 28, 38, 41, 44, 70, 86, 102] The difficulty lies with determining the "appropriate postoperative alignment" because recommendations vary between these reports. In contrast with the recommendation of Hernigou et al[41] for 3 to 6 degrees of valgus, Cass and Bryan[15] suggested 10 to 12 degrees, whereas Rudan and Simurda[85] advocated 6 to 14 degrees. Coventry et al[23] reported that for knees with 8 degrees or more of postoperative valgus the survival rate was 94% at 5- and 10-year follow-up compared with 63% at 5 and 10 years for knees corrected to 5 degrees or less of valgus angulation.

Finally, among 314 patients monitored for 10 to 19 years, of the 170 patients who had undercorrection, 54 subsequently required additional revision surgery for clinical deterioration, whereas in 144 patients with a normalized or overcorrected alignment, only eight patients required surgical revision.[79] Based on this long-term experience, these surgeons suggested that a properly performed high tibial osteotomy rivals the longevity of current prosthetic replacements.

TABLE 70.7 RESULTS OF DISTAL FEMORAL OSTEOTOMY

Study	No. Patients	Success (%)	Follow-up (years)
Beaver et al (1991)[8]	42	83	3.6 (2-11.5)
Cameron et al (1997)[13]	49	87	7*
Conrad et al (1985)[19]	16	62	6.5
Edgerton et al (1993)[32]	24	71	8.3 (5-11)
		(86)†	
Finkelstein et al (1996)[34]	21	64	11 (8-20)
Healy et al (1988)[39]	23	83	4 (2-9)
		(93)‡	
Johnson and Godell (1981)[54]	53	70	3.6 (1-9.3)
Matthews et al (1998)[69]	21	57	3 (1-8)
McDermott et all (1988)[71]	24	92	4 (2-11.5)
Miniaci et al (1990)[74]	35	86	5.4 (2-16.7)
		(100)§	
Terry and Cimino (1992)[95]	35	60	5.4 (2-19)

* End point of survival analysis.
† Isolated compartment disease.
‡ Excluding rheumatoid arthritis patients.
§ Valgus deformity without arthrosis.

Distal Femoral Osteotomy

As with high tibial osteotomy, the reported success with distal femoral osteotomy has been variable (Table 70.7).[8, 13, 19, 32, 34, 39, 54, 69, 71, 74, 95] Patient selection factors, good surgical technique, appropriate postoperative alignment, and passage of time all affect the final clinical outcome. Many reports comment on the fact that some patients were poor candidates for distal femoral osteotomy and reported better success in patients meeting strict selection criteria.[32, 34, 39, 74] In general, patients should be younger than 65 years, have good bone stock and isolated osteoarthritis of the lateral compartment, minimal ligamentous laxity, a range of motion arc of more than 90 degrees, and a flexion contracture of less than 20 degrees.

Proper postoperative alignment appears to be an essential factor for a good long-term result, and again the absolute range for the optimum range of alignment has not been determined. In one study the success rate was 77% if the alignment was corrected to neutral or varus compared with 60% in patients left in some degree of valgus.[32] Another report noted disappointing results when considering pain relief, but only 33% of the patients were corrected to <2 degrees of valgus angulation.[69] It was recommended that a prospective trial is required to determine the optimum postoperative alignment angle. Because of the rarity of supracondylar osteotomy, such a trial is quite unlikely. We agree with others that a tibiofemoral angle of approximately 0 degrees (neutral alignment) is the desired correction for the supracondylar osteotomy.[71]

SUMMARY

Realignment osteotomy about the knee continues to meet many of the original expectations. Although the current indications are relatively narrow, the surgeon should be confident in corrective osteotomy when appropriate criteria are met. The long-term results linked with careful patient selection, accurate surgical technique, and appropriate postoperative alignment portray a favorable outlook for these procedures, particularly because the population at large is more active and is expected to have increasing longevity.

References

1. Aglietti P, Rinonapoli E, Stringa G, et al: Tibial osteotomy for the varus osteoarthritic knee. Clin Orthop 176:239, 1983.
2. Aglietti P, Stringa G, Buzzi R, et al: Correction of valgus knee deformity with a supracondylar V osteotomy. Clin Orthop 217: 214, 1987.
3. Akizuki S, Yasukawa Y, Takizawa T: Does arthroscopic abrasion arthroplasty promote cartilage regeneration in osteoarthritic knees with eburnation? A prospective study of high tibial osteotomy with abrasion arthroplasty versus high tibial osteotomy alone. Arthroscopy 13(1):9, 1997.
4. Aydogdu S, Sur H: High tibial osteotomy for varus deformity of more than 20 degrees. Rev Chir Orthop 84(5):439, 1997.
5. Aydogdu S, Yercan H, Saylam C, et al: Peroneal nerve dysfunction after high tibial osteotomy. An anatomical cadaver study. Acta Orthop Belg 62(3):156, 1996.
6. Bae DK, Mun MS, Kwon OS: A newly designed miniplate staple for high tibial osteotomy. Bull Hosp Jt Dis 56(3):167, 1997.
7. Bauer GC, Insall J, Koshino T: Tibial osteotomy in gonarthrosis (osteo-arthritis of the knee). J Bone Joint Surg Am 51:1545, 1969.
8. Beaver RJ, Jinxiang YU, Sekyi-Otu A, et al: Distal femoral varus osteotomy for genu valgum: A prospective review. Am J Knee Surg 4:9, 1991.
9. Benjamin A: Double osteotomy for the painful knee in rheumatoid arthritis and osteoarthritis. J Bone Joint Surg Br 51:694, 1969.
10. Berman AT, Bosacco SJ, Kirshner S, et al: Factors influencing long-term results in high tibial osteotomy. Clin Orthop 272:192, 1991.
11. Beyer CA, Lewallen DG, Hanssen AD: Total knee arthroplasty following distal femoral osteotomy. Am J Knee Surg 4:25, 1994.
12. Cameron HU: Repair of nonunion of supracondylar femoral osteotomy. Orthop Rev 21(3):349, 1992.
13. Cameron HU, Botsford DJ, Park YS: Prognostic factors in the outcome of supracondylar femoral osteotomy for lateral compartment osteoarthritis of the knee. Can J Surg 40(2):114, 1997.
14. Cameron HU, Welsh RP, Jung YB, et al: Repair of nonunion of tibial osteotomy. Clin Orthop 287:167, 1993.
15. Cass JR, Bryan RS: High tibial osteotomy. Clin Orthop 230:196, 1988.
16. Catagni MA, Guerreschi F, Ahmad TS, et al: Treatment of genu varum in medial compartment osteoarthritis of the knee using the Ilizarov method. Orthop Clin North Am 25(3):509, 1994.
17. Chao EY, Sim FH: Computer-aided preoperative planning in knee osteotomy. Iowa Orthop J 15:4, 1995.
18. Chillag KJ, Nicholls PJ: High tibial osteotomy. A retrospective analysis of 30 cases. Orthopedics 7:1821, 1984.
19. Conrad EU, Soudry M, Insall JN: Supracondylar femoral osteotomy for valgus deformities. Orthop Trans 9:25, 1985.
20. Cooke TD, Pichora D, Siu D, et al: Surgical implications of varus deformity of the knee with obliquity of joint surfaces. J Bone Joint Surg Br 71:560, 1989.
21. Coventry MB: Osteotomy about the knee for degenerative and rheumatoid arthritis. J Bone Joint Surg Am 55:23, 1973.
22. Coventry M: Osteotomy of the upper portion of the tibia for degenerative arthritis of the knee: A preliminary report. J Bone Joint Surg Am 47:984, 1965.
23. Coventry MB: Proximal tibial varus osteotomy for osteoarthritis of the lateral compartment of the knee. J Bone Joint Surg 69: 32, 1987.
24. Coventry M: Stepped staple for upper tibial osteotomy. J Bone Joint Surg Am 51:1011, 1969.
25. Coventry MB: Upper tibial osteotomy for gonarthrosis: The evolution of the operation in the last 18 years and long-term results. Orthop Clin North Am 10:191, 1979.
26. Coventry MB: Upper tibial osteotomy for osteoarthritis. J Bone Joint Surg Am 67:1136, 1985.
27. Coventry MB, Bowman PW: Long-term results of upper tibial osteotomy for degenerative arthritis of the knee. Acta Orthop Belg 48:139, 1982.
28. Coventry MB, Ilstrup D, Wallrichs S: Proximal tibial osteotomy. A critical long-term study of eighty-seven cases. J Bone Joint Surg Am 75:196, 1993.
29. Curley P, Eyres K, Brezinova V, et al: Common peroneal nerve dysfunction after high tibial osteotomy. J Bone Joint Surg Br 72:405, 1990.
30. Dohin B, Migaud H, Gougeon F, et al: Effect of a valgization osteotomy with external wedge removal on patellar height and femoro-patellar arthritis. Acta Orthop Belg 59(1):69, 1993.
31. Dugdale TW, Noyes FR, Styer D: Preoperative planning for high tibial osteotomy: The effect of lateral tibiofemoral separation and tibiofemoral length. Clin Orthop 274:248, 1992.
32. Edgerton BC, Mariani EM, Morrey BF: Distal femoral varus osteotomy for painful genu valgum: A five- to- 11-year follow-up study. Clin Orthop 288:263, 1993.
33. Engel GM, Lippert FG III: Valgus tibial osteotomy: Avoiding the pitfalls. Clin Orthop 160:137, 1981.
34. Finkelstein JA, Gross AE, Davis A: Varus osteotomy of the distal part of the femur: A survivorship analysis. J Bone Joint Surg Am 78:1348, 1996.
35. Gariepy R: Correction du genou flechi dans l'arthrite. Int Soc Orthop Surg Traumatol 8:884, 1960.
36. Gibson MJ, Barnes MR, Allen MJ, et al: Weakness of dorsiflexion and changes in compartment pressures after tibial osteotomy. J Bone Joint Surg Br 68:471, 1986.
37. Griffith JF, Cheng JC, Lung TK, et al: Pseudoaneurysm after high tibial osteotomy and limb lengthening. Clin Orthop 354: 175, 1998.
38. Healy W, Riley LJ: High tibial valgus osteotomy. A clinical review. Clin Orthop 209:227, 1986.
39. Healy WL, Anglen JO, Wasilewski SA, et al: Distal femoral varus osteotomy. J Bone Joint Surg Am 70:102, 1988.
40. Hee HT, Low CK, Seow KH, et al: Comparing staple fixation to buttress plate fixation in high tibial osteotomy. Ann Acad Med Singapore 25(2):233, 1996.

41. Hernigou P, Medevielle D, Debeyre J, et al: Proximal tibial osteotomy for osteoarthritis with varus deformity. A 10 to 13 year follow-up study. J Bone Joint Surg Am 66:332, 1987.
42. Hofmann AA, Wyatt RWB, Beck SW: High tibial osteotomy: Use of an osteotomy jig, rigid fixation, and early motion versus conventional surgical technique and cast immobilization. Clin Orthop 271:212, 1991
43. Holden DL, James SL, Larson RL, et al: Proximal tibial osteotomy in patients who are fifty years old or less. A long-term follow-up study. J Bone Joint Surg Am 70:977, 1988.
44. Hsu R: The study of Maquet dome high tibial osteotomy. Arthroscopic-assisted analysis. Clin Orthop 243:280, 1989.
45. Hsu RWW, Himeno S, Coventry MB, et al: Normal axial alignment of the lower extremity and load-bearing distribution at the knee. Clin Orthop 255:215, 1990.
46. Insall JN: High tibial osteotomy in the treatment of osteoarthritis of the knee. South Surg Ann 7:347, 1975.
47. Insall JN, Joseph DM, Msika C: High tibial osteotomy for varus gonarthrosis: A long-term follow-up study. J Bone Joint Surg Am 66:1040, 1984.
48. Insall JN, Shoji H, Mayer V: High tibial osteotomy. J Bone Joint Surg Am 56:1397, 1974.
49. Iveson JM, Longton EB, Wright V: Comparative study of tibial (single) and tibiofemoral (double) osteotomy for osteoarthrosis and rheumatoid arthritis. Ann Rheum Dis 36(4):319, 1977.
50. Ivey M, Cantrell JS: Lateral tibial plateau fracture as a postoperative complication of high tibial osteotomy. Orthopedics 8(8): 1009, 1985.
51. Jackson JP: Osteotomy for osteoarthritis of the knee. J Bone Joint Surg Br 40:826, 1958.
52. Jackson JP, Waugh W: The technique and complications of upper tibial osteotomy. J Bone Joint Surg Br 56:236, 1974.
53. Johnson BC, Hanssen AD, Morrey BF: Long-term radiographic analysis of cemented condylar total knee arthroplasty in patients who have had a prior high tibial osteotomy. Presented at the meeting of the American Academy of Orthopaedic Surgeons, Orlando, February 1995.
54. Johnson EW Jr, Godell LS: Corrective supracondylar osteotomy for painful genu valgus. Mayo Clin Proc 56:87, 1981.
55. Keene J, Monson D, Roberts J, et al: Evaluation of patients for high tibial osteotomy. Clin Orthop 243:157, 1989.
56. Keene JS, Dyreby JRJ: High tibial osteotomy in the treatment of osteoarthritis of the knee. The role of preoperative arthroscopy. J Bone Joint Surg Am 65:36, 1983.
57. Kettelkamp DB, Leach RE, Nasca R: Pitfalls of proximal tibial osteotomy. Clin Orthop 106:232, 1975.
58. Kettelkamp DB, Wenger DR, Chao EYS, et al: Results of proximal tibial osteotomy: The effects of tibiofemoral angle, stance-phase flexion-extension, and medial-plateau force. J Bone Joint Surg Am 58:952, 1976.
59. Khalfayan EE, Sharkey PF, Alexander AH: High tibial osteotomy: fixation with cannulated screws. Orthop Rev 22(2):259, 1993.
60. Korn MW: A new approach to dome high tibial osteotomy. Am J Knee Surg 9(1):12, 1996.
61. Koshino T, Morii T, Wada J, et al: High tibial osteotomy with fixation by a blade-plate for medial compartment osteoarthritis of the knee. Orthop Clin North Am 20(2):227, 1989.
62. Kreigshauser LA, Bryan RS: Early motion with cast-brace after modified Coventry high tibial osteotomy. Clin Orthop 195:168, 1985.
63. Learmonth ID: A simple technique for varus supracondylar osteotomy in genu valgum. J Bone Joint Surg Br 72:235, 1990.
64. Lootvoet L, Massinon A, Rossillon R, et al: Upper tibial osteotomy for gonarthrosis in genu varum. Apropos of a series of 193 cases. Rev Chir Orthop Reparatrice Appar Mot 79(5):375, 1993.
65. Mabrey JD, McCollum DE: High tibial osteotomy: A retrospective review of 72 cases. South Med J 80(8):975, 1987.
66. MacIntosh DL, Welsh RP: Joint debridement—A complement to high tibial osteotomy in the treatment of degenerative arthritis of the knee. J Bone Joint Surg Am 59:1094, 1977.
67. Magyar G, Toksvig-Larsen S, Lindstrand A: Open wedge tibial osteotomy by callus distraction in gonarthrosis. Operative technique and early results in 36 patients. Acta Orthop Scand 69(2):147, 1998.
68. Maquet P: Valgus osteotomy for osteoarthritis of the knee. Clin Orthop 120:143, 1976.
69. Mathews J, Cobb AG, Richardson S, et al: Distal femoral osteotomy for lateral compartment osteoarthritis of the knee. Orthopedics 21(4):437, 1998.
70. Matthews LS, Goldstein SA, Malvitz TA, et al: Proximal tibial osteotomy: Factors that influence the duration of satisfactory function. Clin Orthop 229:193, 1988.
71. McDermott AG, Finklestein JA, Farine I, et al: Distal femoral varus osteotomy for valgus deformity of the knee. J Bone Joint Surg Am 70:110, 1988.
72. McLaren CAN, Wootton JR, Heath PD, et al: Pes planus after tibial osteotomy. Foot Ankle 9:300, 1989.
73. Miniaci A, Ballmer FT, Ballmer PM, et al: Proximal tibial osteotomy. A new fixation device. Clin Orthop 246:250, 1989.
74. Miniaci A, Grossman SP, Jakob RP: Supracondylar femoral varus osteotomy in the treatment of valgus knee deformity. Am J Knee Surg 2:65, 1990.
75. Miura H, Kawamura H, Nagamine R, et al: Is patellar height really lower after high tibial osteotomy? Fukuoka Igaku Zasshi 88(6):261, 1997.
76. Moreland JR, Bassett LW, Hanker GJ: Surgical implications of varus deformity of the knee with obliquity of joint surfaces. Radiographic analysis of the axial alignment of the lower extremity. J Bone Joint Surg Br 71:560, 1989.
77. Morrey BF: Upper tibial osteotomy for secondary osteoarthritis of the knee. J Bone Joint Surg Br 71:554, 1989.
78. Nagel A, Insall JN, Scuderi GR: Proximal tibial osteotomy. A subjective outcome study. J Bone Joint Surg Am 78:1353, 1996.
79. Odenbring S, Egund N, Knutson K, et al: Revision after osteotomy for gonarthrosis: A 10–19 year follow-up of 314 cases. Acta Orthop Scand 61:128, 1990.
80. Odenbring S, Egund N, Lindstrand A, et al: Cartilage regeneration after proximal tibial osteotomy for medial gonarthrosis. An arthroscopic, roentgenographic, and histologic study. Clin Orthop 277:210, 1992.
81. Odenbring S, Tjornstrand B, Egund N, et al: Function after tibial osteotomy for medial gonarthrosis below aged 50 years. Acta Orthop Scand 60(5):527, 1989.
82. Paley D, Maar DC, Herzenberg JE: New concepts in high tibial osteotomy for medial compartment osteoarthritis. Ortho Clin North Am 25(3):483, 1994.
83. Prodromos CC, Andriacchi TP, Galante JO: A relationship between gait and clinical changes following high tibial osteotomy. J Bone Joint Surg Am 67:1188, 1985.
84. Ritter MA, Fechtman RA: Proximal tibial osteotomy: A survivorship analysis. J Arthroplasty 3:309, 1988.
85. Rudan JF, Simurda MA: High tibial osteotomy. A prospective clinical and roentgenographic review. Clin Orthop 255:251, 1990.
86. Rudan JF, Simurda MA: Valgus high tibial osteotomy: A long-term follow-up study. Clin Orthop 268:157, 1991.
87. Ruebens F, Wellington JL, Bouchard AG: Popliteal artery injury after tibial osteotomy: Report of two cases. Can J Surg 33:294, 1990.
88. Schatzker J, Burgess RC, Glynn MK: The management of nonunions following high tibial osteotomies. Clin Orthop 193:230, 1985.
89. Shoji H, Insall J: High tibial osteotomy for osteoarthritis of the knee with valgus deformity. J Bone Joint Surg Am 55:963, 1973.
90. Slawski DP: High tibial osteotomy in the treatment of adult osteochondritis dissecans. Clin Orthop 341:155, 1997.
91. Soejima O, Ogata K, Ishinishi T, et al: Anatomic considerations of the peroneal nerve for division of the fibula during high tibial osteotomy. Orthop Rev 23(3):244, 1994.
92. Sprenger TR, Weber BG, Howard FM: Compression osteotomy of the tibia. Clin Orthop 140:103, 1979.
93. Stuart MJ, Grace JN, Ilstrup DM, et al: Late recurrence of varus deformity after proximal tibial osteotomy. Clin Orthop 260:61, 1990.
94. Sundaram NA, Hallett JP, Sullivan MF: Dome osteotomy of the tibia for osteoarthritis of the knee. J Bone Joint Surg Br 68:782, 1986.

95. Terry GC, Cimino PM: Distal femoral osteotomy for valgus deformity of the knee. Orthopedics 15(11):1283, 1992.
96. Uematsu A, Kim EE: Role of radionuclide joint imaging in high tibial osteotomy. Clin Orthop 144:220, 1979.
97. Vainionpaa S, Laike E, Kirves P, et al: Tibial osteotomy for osteoarthritis of the knee. A five to ten-year follow-up study. J Bone Joint Surg Am 63:938, 1981.
98. Wada M, Imura S, Nagatani K, et al: Relationship between gait and clinical results after high tibial osteotomy. Clin Orthop 354:180, 1998.
99. Westrich GH, Peters LE, Haas SB, et al: Patella height after high tibial osteotomy with internal fixation and early motion. Clin Orthop 354:169, 1998.
100. Windsor RE, Insall JN, Vince KG: Technical considerations of total knee arthroplasty after proximal tibial osteotomy. J Bone Joint Surg Am 70:547, 1988.
101. Wootton JR, Ashworth MJ, MacLaren CA: Neurological complications of high tibial osteotomy—The fibular osteotomy as a causative factor: A clinical and anatomical study. Ann Royal Coll Surg 77(1):31, 1995.
102. Yasuda K, Majima T, Tsuchida T, et al: A ten to 15-year follow-up observation of high tibial osteotomy in medial compartment osteoarthritis. Clin Orthop 282:186, 1992.
103. Zaidi SH, Cobb AG, Bentley G: Danger to the popliteal artery in high tibial osteotomy. J Bone Joint Surg Br 77:384, 1995.

71

Osteotomy for the Arthritic Knee: A European Perspective

PASCAL POILVACHE

INTRODUCTION

Do high tibial or low femoral osteotomies for the treatment of gonarthrosis belong to the past?

Considering the improvement of the outcome of total[72, 80, 233] and unicompartmental[38, 150, 198, 257] knee arthroplasties reported in the past few years, the question arises whether osteotomies are still necessary.

They seem likely to become an exception, just like hip osteotomies in the case of coxarthritis. This trend clearly emerges—at least in the United States—when the number of osteotomies is compared with that of the number of prostheses.[285]

Rather than become the exception, should not the indication for osteotomy be redefined? From the review of the literature, which follows, it emerges that osteotomies should be aimed at young—at least physiologically—active subjects who present a moderate deformation as well as arthrosis in its early stages.

By maintaining these criteria, are we at risk of making osteotomies—which are not without complications—only prophylactic operations and, perhaps, superfluous? The orthopedic literature is particularly lacking in longitudinal studies, assessing in the long term the outcome of an early gonarthrosis arising from axial deviation. Two Swedish studies, however, provide information on this subject. Hernborg and Nilsson[107] reviewed, in a 10- to 17-year follow-up, 71 patients (94 knees) who had suffered from gonarthrosis in the 1950s. More than half of the knees had deteriorated, particularly in the case of young patients and when axial deviation was present. Preexisting instability also made the prognosis worse. The femorotibial compartment that was intact at the time of the first radiography remained so more often than not at the last control.

Between 1972 and 1988, Odenbring et al[211] monitored 189 knees presenting a medial arthrosis. After 14 years, tibial osteotomy had been performed in 85 knees and arthroplasty in another 33 knees. No major surgery had been undertaken in 71 knees. Of these 71 knees, 31 patients (40 knees) died, and in the majority of the remaining 23 patients (31 knees), the results were unsatisfactory; they managed only on a low-activity level. The authors concluded that the natural course of medial gonarthrosis had a poor prognosis as the majority of patients suffering from this condition would eventually have to undergo major knee surgery.

Given this bad prognosis, the good long-term results of osteotomy when strict selection criteria are implemented, and compliance with a rigorous technique, it appears that these procedures do have their place in the treatment of the early stages of gonarthrosis arising from axial deviation. This is all the more true now that multiple techniques for the early treatment of knee arthrosis have been developed: administration of chondroprotective substances, reimplantation of cultured chondrocytes, meniscal grafts, cartilage transplantation, ligament reconstruction in the presence of mild arthritis, and so on. These techniques aim at preventing the ulterior radical surgery of articular replacement. They cannot, however, be crowned with success unless the charges imposed on the damaged compartment are below the bearable threshold, and thus they often require an axial correction. Osteotomy of the knee has a long past,[28, 50, 64, 85, 132, 186] dating back to the 19th century[271]; now that it has crossed the threshold of a new millennium, a description of its merits is worthwhile.

HIGH TIBIAL OSTEOTOMY

Biomechanical Principles

Osteoarthrosis can be considered the consequence of the loss of balance between the biological resistance of the joint and its mechanical stressing. The direct deleterious effect of excessive pressure on articular cartilage has been repeatedly documented in animal models.[213, 228, 235, 287]

McKellop et al,[183, 184] using pressure-sensitive films in cadaver limbs, demonstrated a relationship between the level and magnitude of the deformity and the contact pressure across the knee.

Treatment must reduce the articular stresses sufficiently to make them tolerable.

Maquet[169–171, 173, 174, 176, 177] proposed a biomechanical theory stating that the joint stability in a normal knee is the result of the equilibrium between two forces (Fig. 71.1). The force P, eccentrically exerted by the part of the body supported by the knee, must be balanced by active muscular forces L and by passive ligamentous forces. Force R is the resultant or the vectorial sum of all these forces. It creates compressive stresses and must act perpendicular to the weight-

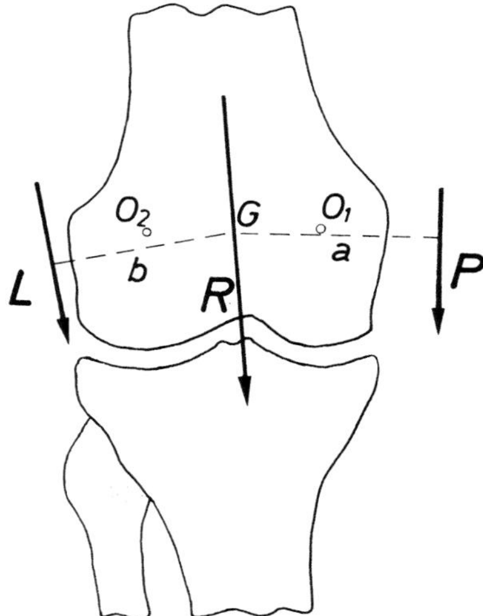

FIGURE 71.1 ➢ Loaded knee projected on the coronal plane. P, force exerted by the part of the body supported by the knee; L, lateral muscle stay; a, lever arm of P; b, lever arm of L; R, resultant of P and L; O1, center of curvature of the medial condyle; O2, center of curvature of the lateral condyle; G, central point on the axis of flexion of the knee. (From Maquet P: Osteotomy. In Freeman MAR, ed: Arthritis of the Knee: Clinical Features and Surgical Management. Berlin, Springer-Verlag, 1980, p 148.)

bearing surfaces through their center of gravity[172, 174] (Fig. 71.2).

Indeed, according to Pauwels' law,[217] the quantity and the structure of osseous tissue depends on the magnitude of the stresses applied to it. The symmetrical subchondral dense bone, of even thickness throughout, that underlies the tibial plateaus of a normal knee shows an even distribution of the articular compressive stresses. Akamatsu et al,[8] in a series of 144 knees, in which 23 were treated with high tibial osteotomy (HTO), measured by dual x-ray absorptiometry that the bone mineral density of the medial femoral and tibial condyles was greater than that of the lateral femoral and tibial condyles in all knees with medial compartmental osteoarthritis. The ratios of bone mineral density of the medial condyles to that of the lateral condyles were found to increase significantly with the progression of osteoarthritis and the increase of varus deformity. These ratios decreased sharply within 1 year after HTO. This agrees with the results of Koshino and Ranawat,[149] who studied remodeling of the femoral condyles before and after HTO using bone scintimetry. They demonstrated that the raised uptake of strontium-85 in the medial condyle before osteotomy decreased markedly at more than 1 year after osteotomy in knees with adequate correction of the varus deformity.

Force R can be displaced medially by a weakening of the muscles L, by an increase of the force P, by a varus deformity, or by a medial displacement of the center of gravity of the body (Fig. 71.3). This will alter the distribution and magnitude of the stresses in the joint and soon decrease its effective weightbearing surfaces.

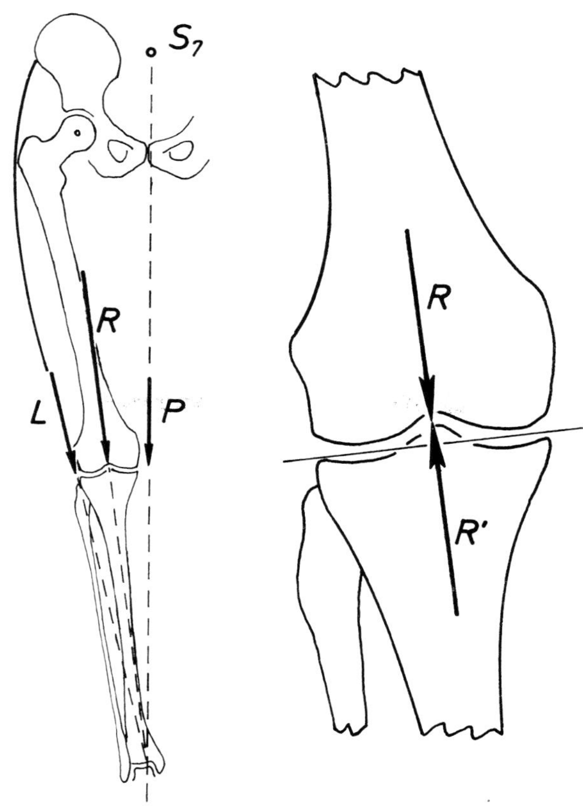

FIGURE 71.2 ➢ Normal knee. Force R acts perpendicular to the plane tangential to the tibial plateau. (From Maquet P: Osteotomy. In Freeman MAR, ed: Arthritis of the Knee: Clinical Features and Surgical Management. Berlin, Springer-Verlag, 1980, p 148.)

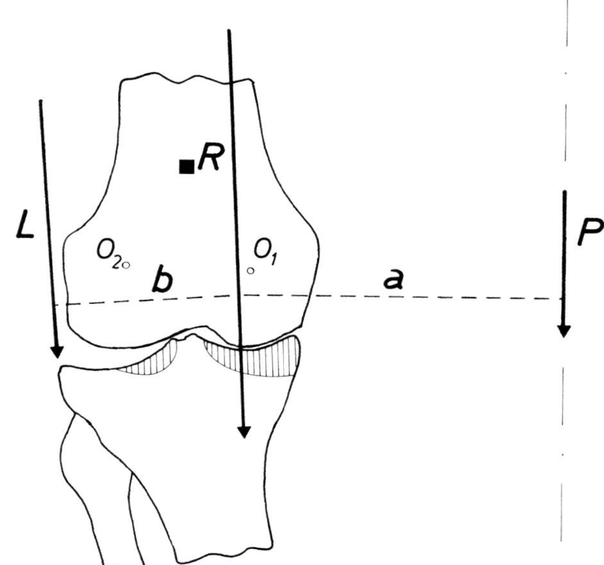

FIGURE 71.3 ➢ Increased stresses in the medial compartment of the knee resulting from a medial displacement of resultant R. P, force exerted by the mass of the body supported by the knee; L, lateral muscle stay; R, resultant of P and L; O1, center of curvature of the medial condyle; O2, center of curvature of the lateral condyle; a, lever arm of P; b, lever arm of L. (From Maquet P: Osteotomy. In Freeman MAR, ed: Arthritis of the Knee: Clinical Features and Surgical Management. Berlin, Springer-Verlag, 1980, p 148.)

Blaimont[23, 24] demonstrated the role of the muscles in balancing the medially-exerted gravity forces. Through radioscopic and electrophysiological studies, he stated that the tensor fascia latae and the biceps femoris were the main stabilizers of the knee in the frontal plane. They act as a lateral shroud. Their moment of force is the product of their forces by their lever arm (Fig. 71.4). Blaimont determined the maximum moment of force by measuring, under fluoroscopic control, the maximal load against which subjects were able to actively close the lateral opening of their knee joints. The force of the biceps and the tensor was always diminished in medial arthritic knees. According to Blaimont, the aim of a valgus osteotomy should be to reduce the lever arm of the gravity force P in order to allow the weakened lateral muscles to adequately stabilize the joint and distribute the compressive stresses among the medial and lateral compartments of the knee.

If the role of the muscles is not taken into account, and accepting that the center of gravity of the body lies in S2,[81, 232] one should admit that, even in a perfectly aligned knee, in the midstance phase of gait, the medial compartment would be compressed whereas the lateral compartment would be distracted and that the knee would gap laterally at every step. Moreover, in this case, the valgus deformity that should be created to effectively unload the medial compartment during gait would be unacceptable, as stated by Shaw and Moulton,[246] who used a cadaver osteotomy model.

The action of the lateral muscles can explain why a normally aligned knee can develop medial osteoarthrosis, provided that the muscles are insufficient, and why some varus knees never wear, provided a good muscular activity.

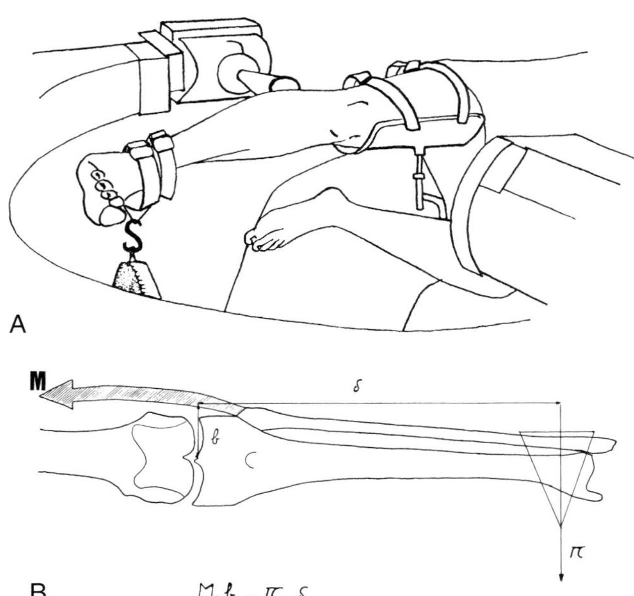

FIGURE 71.4 ➢ Under fluoroscopic control, the maximal load against which the subject is able to actively close the lateral opening of the knee joint is measured. M, lateral muscular force; b, lever arm of M; P, varus force applied on the ankle; d, lever arm of P. (From Blaimont P, Burnotte J, Baillon JM, et al: Contribution biomécanique à l'étude des conditions d'équilibre dans le genou normal et pathologique: Application au traitement de l'arthrose varisante. Acta Orthop Belg 1971; 37:573.)

Blaimont et al[24] also reported that a varus thrust, secondary to an insufficiency of the biceps and the tensor, was often observed in incipient medial gonarthrosis. They showed that, at this early stage of the disease, provided that the varus is minimal and that the subject is not overweight, reinforcing the lateral muscles can bring the knee back to equilibrium. Yasunaga[290] demonstrated that the lateral thrust was significantly greater in medial compartmental osteoarthritic knees than in normal knees and that a properly performed HTO was effective in restraining the lateral thrust.

Thomine et al[261] further refined the concept of the adduction moment about the knee during gait. They divided the lever arm a of the gravity force P into two parts: an extrinsic one, which is independent of the axial alignment of the leg, and an intrinsic one, which reflects the axial alignment of the knee. Figure 71.5 schematizes this theory of the varus moment.

In a neutral knee (mechanical axis at 180 degrees), the distance between the line of force of gravity and the center of the knee is the extrinsic varus distance. In a varus knee, an intrinsic varus distance, consisting of the distance between a theoretical neutral mechanical axis and the center of the knee, is added to the extrinsic varus distance, thus forming the global varus distance. This concept clarifies the effect of the morphology of the patient on the adduction moment, independently of the axial alignment of the knee (Fig. 71.6): a broad pelvis, a coxa vara, a short femur, and a hip adduction will increase the extrinsic varus distance. Conversely, a narrow pelvis, a coxa valga, a long femur, and a hip abduction will decrease the extrinsic varus distance. The extrinsic varus distance plays a major role in the development of medial gonarthrosis. It explains why, in a varus arthritic knee, in which the lateral muscles are weakened,[23, 24] some overcorrection is necessary to reestablish the balance between the varus gravity stresses and the valgus muscular stresses applied on the joint. The amount of overcorrection necessary is a function of the body weight, of the extrinsic varus distance, and of the force of the lateral muscles.

However, this static way of considering the adduction moment about the knee does not account for the dynamic variations that occur during gait. Studies of gait have shown that the distribution of joint loads within the knee during gait is highly dependent on the static angular deformity and on dynamic factors.[100, 138, 223, 272, 278]

Prodomos et al[223] and Wang et al[278] have demonstrated that the importance of the adduction moment, measured through gait analysis, plays a major role in the results of proximal tibial osteotomy. A patient who has a low adduction moment preoperatively has a higher probability of a good result for a longer time than one who has a high adduction moment.

Some patients with a varus knee seem to develop

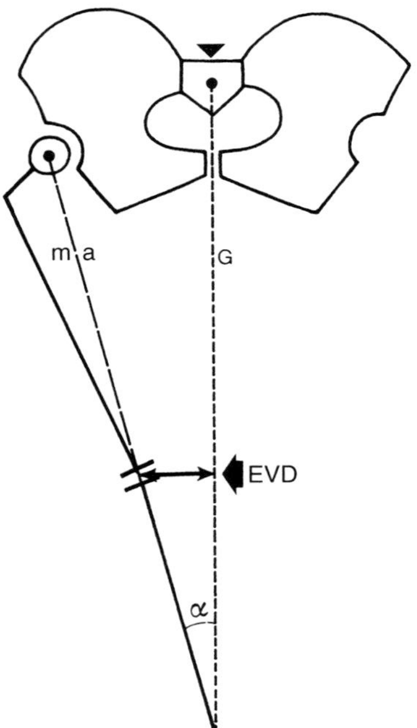

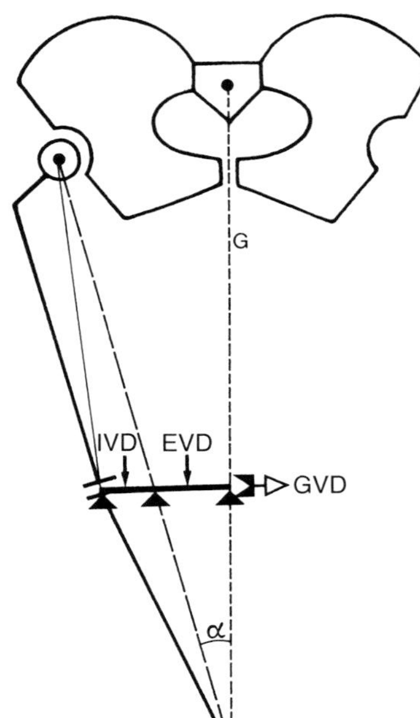

FIGURE 71.5 ➢ In a neutral knee, the mechanical axis passes through the center of the knee. The distance between the line of force of gravity and the center of the knee is the extrinsic varus distance (EVD). In a varus knee, an intrinsic varus distance, consisting of the distance between a theoretical neutral mechanical axis and the center of the knee, is added to the EVD, thus forming the global varus distance. (From Thomine JM, Boudjemaa A, Gibon Y, et al: Les écarts varisants dans la gonarthrose: Fondement théorique et essai d'évaluation pratique. Rev Chir Orthop 1981; 67:319. © Masson Editeur.)

compensatory mechanisms that reduce the adduction moment. These mechanisms, which may continue postoperatively, include shortening of the stride and toeing-out (Fig. 71.7).

Wada et al[272] demonstrated that, provided sufficient valgus alignment is achieved at surgery, the preoperative peak adduction moment does not correlate with the clinical or radiographic outcome of HTO, whereas only alignment is associated significantly with long-term clinical results. This supports the importance of overcorrection at surgery and the need for an accurate osteotomy technique.

Preoperative gait analysis should become a part of patient assessment when an osteotomy is considered. It could help to customize the amount of overcorrection needed for every individual knee in a way similar to that of Blaimont 20 years ago by measuring the force of the lateral muscles. Knees with a high adduction moment should be overcorrected to a greater extent than knees with a low adduction moment. A

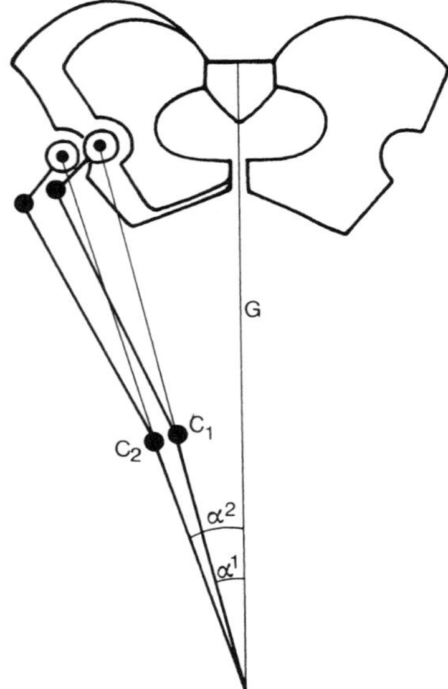

FIGURE 71.6 ➢ A broad pelvis increases the distance between the center of the knee (C) and the line of force of gravity (G), even if the mechanical axis is through the center of the knee. This increases the extrinsic varus distance. (From Thomine JM, Boudjemaa A, Gibon Y, et al: Les écarts varisants dans la gonarthrose: Fondement théorique et essai d'évaluation pratique. Rev Chir Orthop 1981; 67:319. © Masson Editeur.)

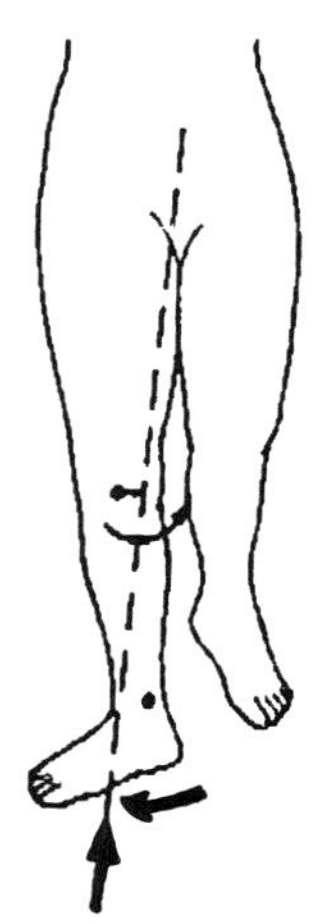

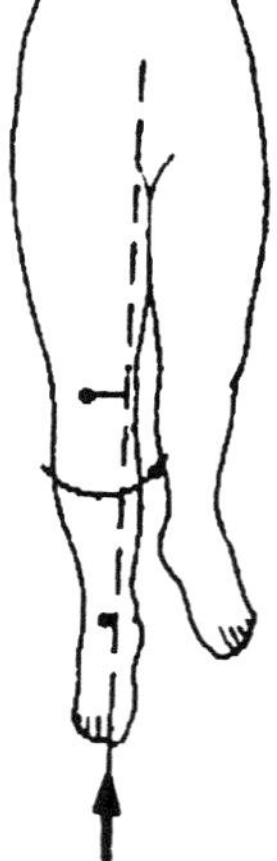

FIGURE 71.7 ➢ The toe-out of the foot is an adaptive mechanism that is used to lower the adduction moment during gait. (From Wang JW, Kuo KN, Andriacchi TP, et al: The influence of walking mechanics and time on the results of proximal tibial osteotomy. J Bone Joint Surg Am 1990; 72:905.)

future perspective could be the development of rehabilitation techniques for reducing the adduction moment. This gait training could be coupled with reinforcement of the lateral muscles: the biceps femoris and the tensor fascia latae.

Another important factor in the pathogenesis of gonarthrosis is the rotational alignment of the lower limbs. Eckoff et al[75, 76] and Goutallier et al[94] have shown that rotational malalignment should be considered as a mechanical cause of arthrosis. Rotational malalignment can alter the pressure distribution in an otherwise normal joint. There is a positive correlation between decreased rotation in the femur and increased arthrosis of the medial femorotibial articulation[75, 196] as well as between increased femoral anteversion and patellar arthrosis.[75, 76, 102, 120] There is more version in the arthritic knee than in the normal knee.[75] The observation of a relationship between malrotation of the lower limbs and gonarthrosis is not new: in 1977 Blaimont[25] reported two cases of medial compartmental arthrosis secondary to an abnormal internal tibial torsion and treated by a corrective osteotomy. The correlation of internal tibial torsion or decreased femoral external torsion with medial arthritic changes in the knee could aid in understanding why toeing-out is one of the compensatory mechanisms adopted by some patients to decrease the adduction moment during gait.

Patient Selection and Preoperative Evaluation

Patient selection is the most critical factor in planning and achieving a successful HTO. Selection criteria have become more restrictive in the last 15 years, given the excellent alternatives offered by the advent of total[72, 233, 251] or unicompartmental[38, 198, 224, 257, 279, 280] knee arthroplasties. Despite the increasing success of knee arthroplasty, tibial osteotomy may still be the more appropriate procedure for younger, active patients with unicompartmental arthritis, as an arthroplasty implies limitations on postoperative physical activities and has a limited life expectancy.

Clearly, there is no general agreement among surgeons concerning the choice between osteotomy and knee arthroplasty. This has been illustrated by the study by Wright et al,[286] comparing the rates of tibial osteotomies in Canada and the United States. Although there are national or even continental tendencies, this choice still remains in the hands of each individual surgeon and patient.

Some broad outlines can nevertheless be drawn. They concern not only the status of the knee but also the general status of the patient.

Age

Notwithstanding that the physiological rather than the chronological age should be considered, HTO is nowadays an operation reserved for the reasonably young and active patient. There is no agreement about the meaning of "reasonably young." Langlais[245] showed that, even after 70 years, the failure rate of an HTO is not higher, given a preoperative Ahlbäck's grade I or II osteoarthritis. On the other hand, Matthews et al,[181] Lootvoet et al,[163] and Odenbring et al,[212] analyzing the factors that influence the duration of satisfactory function following proximal tibial osteotomy, concluded that relative youth is a strong predictor of long function for the osteotomy-treated knee. This disagreement about the influence of age is secondary to the difficulty of separate age from other negative factors. Like other surgeons,[104] I reserve osteotomy for patients younger than 55 to 60 years of age, but exceptions are made to this rule.

Level of Activity

The preoperative activity level is probably more determinant than the age in guiding the choice between osteotomy and arthroplasty, especially when the patient is between 50 and 60 years of age. Indeed, the preoperative level of activity is the best predictor for the postoperative level of activity.[201] As a total or even a unicompartmental knee replacement can be a reasonable option in this age group, it is important to spot the patients whose activity level precludes an arthroplasty. However, a very high level of activity has potential adverse effects on the durability of the polyethylene articular surface of a knee arthroplasty[1] and on the fixation of the implant. Nagel et al,[201] in a retrospective study of the results of proximal tibial osteotomy in 34 men age 28 to 60 years, found that 17 engaged in manual labor to an extent that would have been of concern if they had had a total knee arthroplasty (TKA). Nineteen continued to take part in sports involving running and jumping. Odenbring et al[212] examined, after 7 to 18 years, 27 patients (28 knees), with a median age of 42 years, treated with an HTO for early medial gonarthrosis (Ahlbäck's stage I). At follow-up, 22 knees were satisfactory; 9 patients managed high-activity sports or heavy work (Tegner[258] score: 9-10); and 3 patients performed industrial work and walked in forested terrain (Tegner score: 8).

Personality

As much as possible, the patient should take an active part in the decision process. The patient should, therefore, be clearly informed about the pros and cons of the possible options. The advantages and the disadvantages of these options might be perceived differently by each patient. If an osteotomy is planned, the patient should be aware that the pain relief could be incomplete and that it will not be everlasting. The patient should also realize that the alignment of the limb will be modified. The patient's acceptance of these limitations is mandatory.

Other Joints

As a rule, the prerequisite to major knee surgery is a well-working ipsilateral hip. Weakness of the hip abductors, restricted hip mobility, and hip ankylosis have a detrimental effect on the knee[82, 169, 232, 261] and should, when possible, be corrected first.

An osteotomy requires a prolonged period of protected weightbearing. For this reason, the status of the contralateral lower limb and of the superior limbs should be assessed.

Weight

Matthews,[181] analyzing the factors that influence the duration of satisfactory function after proximal tibial osteotomy, stated that obesity has a negative impact on the outcome of this procedure. Coventry,[51] Brueckmann and Kettelkamp,[29] and Levigne and Bonnin[162] share the same opinion. Obese patients are also not ideal candidates for a knee arthroplasty[130, 150]; it is, therefore, difficult to make a decision based on this criterion. A multidisciplinary approach is advisable for these patients, and the problem of obesity should be considered at the same time as the gonarthrosis. An overweight female patient older than 65 years is certainly not a valid candidate for an osteotomy.[245] I recommend a total knee replacement if the patient is older than 60 years and is not willing to lose weight.

Inflammatory Diseases

Rheumatoid arthritis is a definite contraindication for osteotomy.[7, 42, 51, 53] The efficacy of HTO has not been specifically studied in the other inflammatory diseases of the joints, but one should expect similarly bad results.

Job et al[137] compared the 5-year results of HTO in 146 osteoarthritic knees without chondrocalcinosis and in 94 osteoarthritic knees with chondrocalcinosis. There were 73% good clinical results in the first group and only 34% good results in the second.

Examination of the Knee

Clinical examination of the knee is decisive in the selection of the appropriate patient.

During gait, the angular deformity, the torsional pattern of the limb, the position of the foot, a possible limp, a flexion deformity, and the presence or absence of a varus thrust[123] should all be assessed.

In this chapter, the alignment is expressed as the hip-knee-ankle angle, the neutral alignment being arbitrarily numbered zero for practical purposes.

There are limits of deformity that can be reliably corrected by a proximal tibial osteotomy. The results of proximal tibial osteotomy are best when the varus deformity is 10 degrees or less,[4, 123, 163] the reason being that the greater the deformity, the more severe the arthritic changes. HTO is best suited for knees with moderate arthritic changes, in which the deformity is secondary to proximal tibial bowing rather than to medial bone loss.[65, 161–163, 245] Varus deformity greater than 15 degrees is generally associated with increased medial bone loss,[163] bicompartmental deterioration, and lateral subluxation at the tibiofemoral joint.[104, 163]

The torsional pattern of the limb and the position of the foot during gait influence the varizing distances and the adduction moment, and they should be taken into account for planning the correction.

A major limp, a flexion deformity, and a frank varus thrust generally reflect a more advanced stage of arthritis,[65, 123] and the indication for an HTO should, therefore, be considered cautiously. As stated by Andriacchi,[10] the varus thrust places all of the reaction force on the medial compartment and greatly increases the rate of degenerative changes associated with higher-than-normal medial compartment loads.

In the standing position, in addition to the static deformities one should look for the presence of a popliteal cyst, varicose veins, and marked muscular atrophy.

The clinical examination should continue with the patient in the sitting position. Inflammatory signs should be ruled out. Pain should be located predominantly on the medial side of the knee, and signs of patellofemoral arthritis should be sought. Possible arterial insufficiency should be detected.

Knee stability should also be tested. Medial laxity is seldom important in medial arthritic knees and is often secondary to bone loss.[22, 52] Because even after correction of the mechanical axis into valgus there remains an adduction moment about the knee during gait,[10, 90, 100, 223, 246, 272, 278] mild-to-moderate medial laxity should not contraindicate a valgus tibial osteotomy. However, in this situation, failure to take the laxity into account during surgery could lead to undercorrection, if the amount of correction is visually estimated by the intraoperative alignment of the limb.[24] Indeed, a valgus stress manually applied to the knee could open the joint medially, which would not occur during gait because of the persistence of the adduction moment. For marked medial laxity associated with a varus knee, Cameron and Saha[37] recommend performing a combined opening and closing wedge osteotomy. Vielpeau[245] considers that medial laxity does not specifically indicate an opening wedge osteotomy as it would not retension the deep medial collateral ligament (MCL) and because attempts to tighten the superficial MCL could lead to undercorrection.

The lateral collateral ligament (LCL) may be stretched as the varus deformity develops. Active muscular contraction, primarily of the biceps[10, 23, 24] and of the tensor fasciae latae,[23, 24, 170, 174] and secondarily of the quadriceps,[10] will produce dynamic stabilization against lateral joint opening but at the expense of a greater joint contact force. Correction of the axis will not suppress the lateral laxity, but it will restrain the lateral thrust of the knee,[290] reducing the high medial forces secondary not only to malalignment but also to lateral joint opening. LCL laxity can not, therefore, be considered as a contraindication for valgus tibial osteotomy, even if it usually reflects a more advanced stage of arthritis. Paley et al[215] proposed a technique for tightening the LCL. Although I have no experience with this technique, I believe that tightening the LCL is usually unnecessary provided sufficient overcorrection has been achieved. The effect of lateral tibiofemoral separation should be taken into account for calculating the desired amount of correction.[74, 154]

The association of an old anterior cruciate ligament (ACL) rupture with medial gonarthrosis may justify a valgus tibial osteotomy, especially when there is an added lateral laxity. The ACL is a secondary restraint against lateral joint opening, and the conjunction of lateral and anterior laxity considerably increases the stresses on the medial compartment.[10] The relative indication of isolated osteotomy, isolated ligament reconstruction, and simultaneous or staged procedures is beyond the scope of this chapter.[67, 155, 160, 204, 205]

Radiographic Examination

Preoperative radiographs are necessary at one and the same time to select the appropriate patient and to plan the surgery.

The radiological evaluation should include the following:

- Anteroposterior and lateral radiographs on long films (18 x 43 cm), with the patient in the supine position, knees extended.
- Skyline views.
- "Shuss" anteroposterior radiographs (standing anteroposterior x-ray films, knees flexed to 30 degrees).[229]
- Valgus and varus and stress anteroposterior radiographs made with the patient supine and the knee flexed to 20 degrees.
- Hip-knee-ankle radiographs, with the patient standing on both legs.

The first goal of the radiographic assessment is to confirm the indication for an osteotomy.

The aim of knee osteotomy is to modify the axis of the limb in order to shift compressive forces from a diseased compartment to a more normal compartmental joint space. The radiographs should therefore demonstrate unicompartmental joint space deterioration, associated with an abnormal lower extremity alignment and abnormal force transmission through the knee.

An increase of contact stresses in one compartment will induce joint space narrowing, subchondral bone densification, and osteophyte formation. In the absence of these signs of overload, even in the case of axial malalignment, the origin of the knee pain should be further investigated. A bone scan, a magnetic resonance image, or an arthrogram should help to determine the cause of the symptoms and to plan the appropriate treatment.

If the opposite compartment is not intact, the indication for an osteotomy should be questioned. A metabolic or inflammatory disease should be suspected. As already mentioned, rheumatoid arthritis is a clear contraindication for knee osteotomy.[7, 42, 53, 104] Chondrocalcinosis[137] also significantly affects the longevity of the osteotomy.

The patellofemoral joint should also be investigated. Although mild-to-moderate patellofemoral osteoarthrosis does not contraindicate an osteotomy,[73, 108, 111, 123, 125, 128] the patellar height and the patellar alignment could influence the technique of the osteotomy.[73, 197, 244]

Varus and valgus stress x-ray films are essential. They provide useful information about the condition of both compartments and of the ligaments. Joint space narrowing when stressing the presumably healthy compartment precludes the osteotomy. A preoperative reliable recording of the knee alignment is also necessary to plan the osteotomy.

The full-length radiographs should determine the global alignment of the knee and evaluate the varizing distances[261] in order to calculate the adductor moment.

There are many ways to perform full-length radiographs.[97] Originally, full-length radiographs were made with the patient in the supine position. But this position did not provide any information concerning the ligamentous laxity, and therefore the amount of deformity could be underestimated in the case of bony defects or ligament overstretching. On the other hand, unipodal standing full-length radiographs also have some disadvantages. Although walking is a succession of unipodal stances, a static unipodal station does not reproduce the dynamic aspect of the loading of the knee during the normal gait. When standing on one leg, the patient tilts the pelvis to bring the center of gravity of the body nearer to the hip of the weight-bearing limb. This attitude decreases the extrinsic varizing distance and the adductor moment.[261] Another drawback of unipodal standing x-ray films is the difficulty of positioning elderly or disabled patients for them. Finally, ligament integrity is better evaluated with stress radiographs, obtained with a constant and predetermined force instead of unipodal standing radiographs.[11, 261]

An acceptable compromise is the bipodal standing radiograph, which gives a correct estimation of the axial alignment of the lower limb and can be realized in almost every candidate for an osteotomy.

Errors in rotational positioning of the limb will alter the reliability of the standing radiographs.[11, 96, 136, 154, 206, 231, 261, 270] Several landmarks have been advocated to correctly position the patient. The most usual technique is to position the patient with the patella forward in order to obtain a true anteroposterior view of the knee. This technique is not valid in the case of marked femoropatellar dysplasia. The most reproducible technique[11, 154, 206, 231] is to define the frontal projection as perpendicular to a lateral view of the knee, which is monitored by superimposing the posterior aspects of the femoral condyles under fluoroscopic control (Fig. 71.8). Using a similar technique, Odenbring et al[206] demonstrated that the assessment of the hip-knee-ankle angle had a variability of 2 degrees at the most. A drawback of this technique is that the position imposed on the limb is not necessarily the same as when the patient is walking.

On a bipodal standing radiograph several landmarks are drawn:

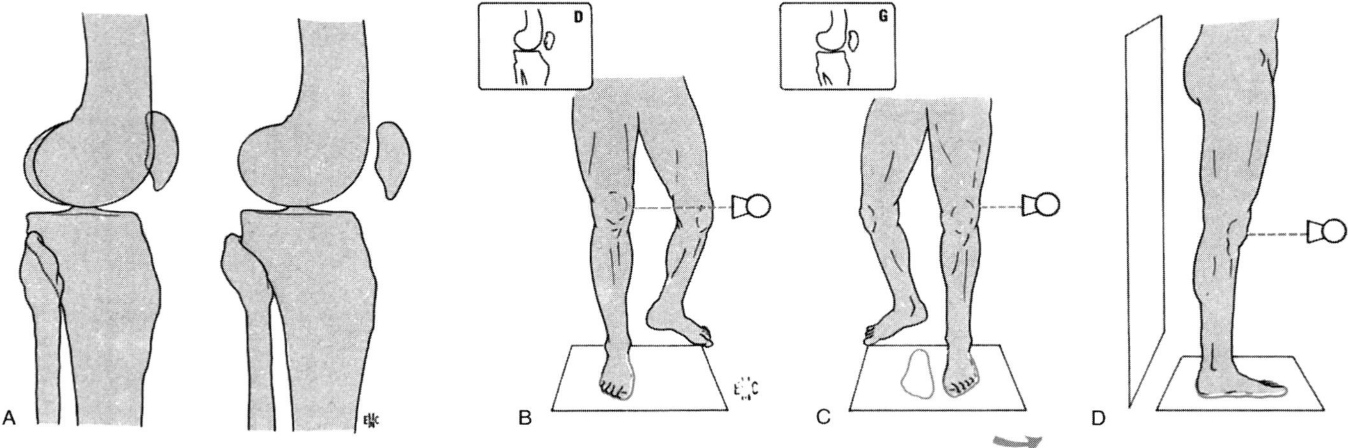

FIGURE 71.8 ➢ *A,* The superimposition of the posterior aspect of the condyles defines the reference profile. *B,* The patient stands on a cardboard sheet, his weight on one leg. The leg is turned under fluoroscopic control until a true profile is obtained. The outline of the foot is traced on the carton. *C,* The procedure is repeated for the other limb. If the patient stands on the two traced outlines, both knees are perfectly in profile. *D,* The carton is turned 90 degrees, and the camera is replaced by a large-size x-ray plate. The knees are thus x-rayed strictly full-face. (From Langlais F, Thomazeau H: Ostéotomies du genou. In Encyclopédie médico-chirurgicale. Paris, Editions scientifiques et médicales Elsevier, 1989, p 1.)

- The center of the second sacral vertebra, which is a rough approximation of the center of gravity of the supported part of the body.[23, 81, 232]
- The center of the hip.
- The center of the ankle.
- The mechanical axis of the femur, joining the center of the hip to the center of the intracondylar notch.[81]
- The mechanical axis of the tibia, joining the center of the proximal epiphysis to the center of the ankle.[81]
- The mechanical axis of the lower extremity, joining the center of the hip to the center of the ankle.[230]

This allows the measurement of the following (Fig. 71.9):

- The hip-knee-ankle angle, defined as the angle between the mechanical axis of the femur and the mechanical axis of the tibia.[47, 194] The normal value is close to 0 degrees.[47, 194, 231]
- The transcondylar angle, defined as the angle between the tangent line of the condyles and the mechanical axis of the femur.[43, 48, 220, 291]
- The tibial plateau - tibial shaft angle, defined as the angle between the tangent line of the tibial plateau and the mechanical axis of the tibia[43, 47, 220, 291]
- The tibiofemoral separation, defined as the angle between a line tangent to the distal aspect of the femoral condyles and a line tangent to the tibial plateau.[47, 74]
- The varizing distances[261] (extrinsic, intrinsic, and global).

On the full-length radiographs or on long anteroposterior x-ray films, the constitutional tibial varus can also be measured (Fig. 71.10). The constitutional tibial varus was described by Dejour and Levigne.[161] It represents the epiphyseal bony component of the tibial varus. Its value is that of the angle formed by the mechanical axis of the tibia and the axis of the upper tibial epiphysis. In the absence of bone loss, the axis of the upper tibial epiphysis can be described as a line perpendicular to the tangent of the tibial plateaus. In the presence of bone wear, this epiphyseal axis can be estimated by drawing a line from the center of the tibial spines to the middle of the old physeal line. From the study of a group of 110 nonosteoarthritic patients, Levigne[161] demonstrated that this way of determining the epiphyseal axis is reliable.

The angle between the epiphyseal axis and the mechanical axis of the tibia allows one to distinguish the part of the deformity attributable to the tibial bone loss from that secondary to the bowing of the proximal tibia. This distinction is important for correctly selecting the candidates for an HTO, as the result of an HTO is better when the varus deformity is mainly due to bowing than when the deformity is essentially due to wear.[65, 162, 163]

Another goal of the radiologic assessment is to select the site of the osteotomy. The normal upper tibia has a 3-degree varus slope.[48, 104, 141, 193, 194] In most varus knees, this varus slope is increased,[161, 220] whereas it is decreased or even inverted in valgus knees.[161, 220] In varus or neutral knees, the line tangent to the distal extent of the femoral condyles is perpendicular to the mechanical axis of the femur, but it is inclined medially and distally in valgus knees.[48, 51, 154, 220, 247] Cooke et al[49] described a subgroup of patients with varus arthritic knees showing excessive valgus angulation of the femoral joint surface together with proximal tibia vara. This pattern of deformity warrants special consideration because it could, in some ex-

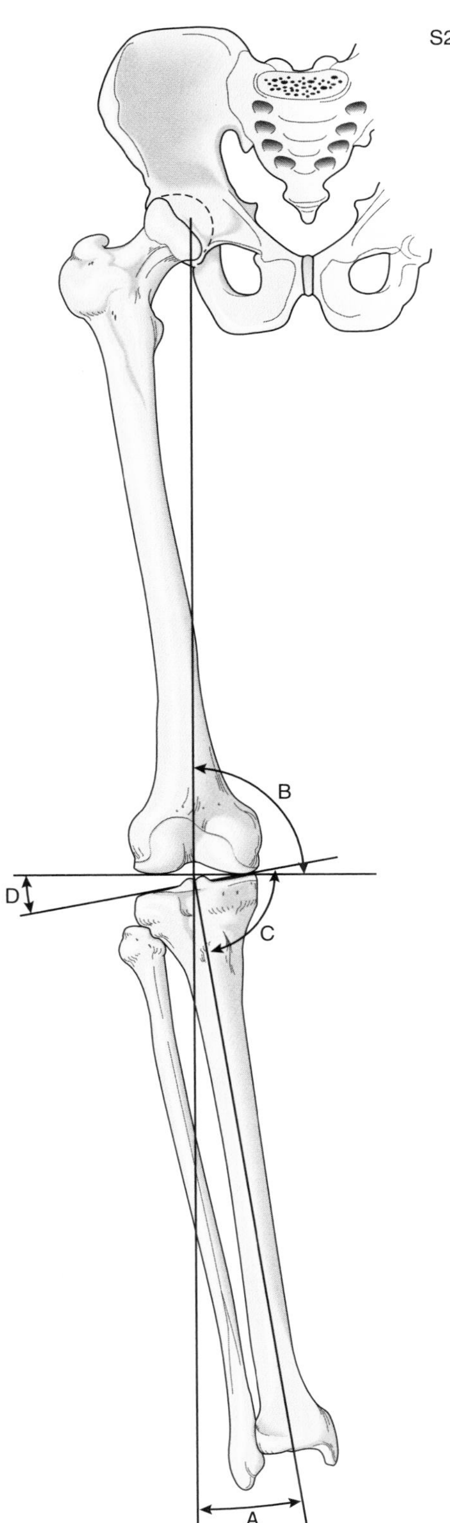

FIGURE 71.9 ➢ Schematic drawing of a bipodal standing radiograph. S2, center of the second sacral vertebra; *A,* Hip-knee-ankle angle. *B,* Transcondylar angle. *C,* Tibial plateau-tibial shaft angle. *D,* Tibiofemoral separation.

treme cases, require combined femoral and tibial osteotomies to restore the horizontality of the joint surfaces.

The hip-knee-ankle angle is the sum of the angles between the mechanical axes of each bone and the corresponding articular surfaces and of the lateral or medial tibiofemoral separation, which is the angle between the articular surfaces of the femur and the tibia.

In theory, the correction should be performed at the site of the maximal deformity in order to keep the joint line as perpendicular to the ground as possible. With a few exceptions, the osteotomy should be tibial in varus knees and femoral in valgus knees. Several authors[14, 55, 66] have reported good results when a tibial osteotomy is performed to correct a moderate valgus deformity. It seems, therefore, reasonable to correct mixed tibial and femoral deformities on the tibial side, insofar as the resultant obliquity of the joint line will not exceed 10 degrees.

Gait Analysis

Peak adduction moments at the knee are indicative of the resultant loading in the medial compartment of the knee joint.

Gait analysis can measure the distribution of load during walking.[10, 90, 138, 223, 272, 278] Johnson et al[138, 139]

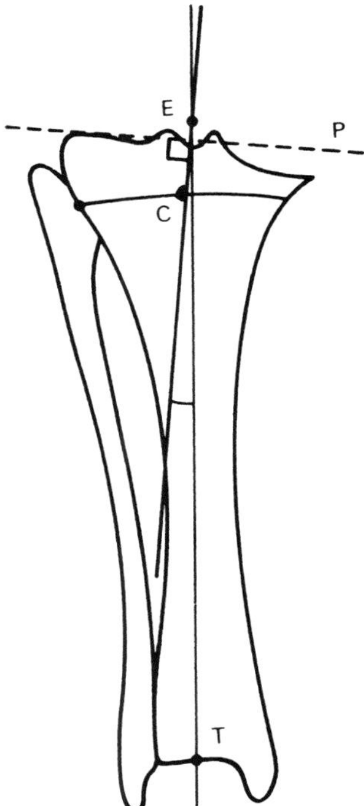

FIGURE 71.10 ➢ Constitutional tibial varus (CTV), after Levigne.[161] E, center of spines; C, center of vestige of the epiphyseal growth plate; P, line tangential to the tibial plateaus before medial wear; T, center of the ankle; EC, epiphyseal axis; ET, mechanical axis; EC-ET, constitutional tibial varus in degrees. (From Lootvoet L, Massinon A, Rossillon R, et al: [Upper tibial osteotomy for gonarthrosis in genu varum: Apropos of a series of 193 cases reviewed 6 to 10 years later]. Rev Chir Orthop Reparatrice Appar Mot 1993; 79:375. © Masson Editeur.)

have shown that there is a lack of correlation between static analysis based on the mechanical axis and weightbearing in the knee calculated from gait analysis. Results from this study also showed a poor correlation between the mechanical axis and the peak adduction moment about the knee. Several authors[10, 90, 100, 138, 223, 278] postulated that an individual can adapt gait and compensate dynamically for joint deformity. These compensatory mechanisms include slowing walking speed, shortening stride length, displacing the trunk toward the affected limb, and toeing out.

Prodomos et al[223] and Wang et al[278] showed that the compensatory gait pattern that reduces the joint load may continue postoperatively and that this reduction of the adduction moment is a key factor for the long-term clinical outcome. Wada et al[272] suggested, on the basis of a prospective study of 32 patients with primary osteoarthritis of the medial compartment of the knee who underwent an HTO, that, on the contrary, provided sufficient valgus alignment is obtained at surgery, the preoperative peak adduction moment of the knee does not correlate with clinical or radiographic outcomes of HTO. In this group, the average postoperative femorotibial angle was 167 to 169 degrees, which roughly corresponds to a 5- to 7-degree mechanical axis, whereas in the study groups of Prodromos and Wang the average mechanical axis was 2 degrees valgus immediately after surgery and 1.2 degrees varus at follow-up. From those studies, one can infer that some overcorrection is necessary to provide good long-term results of HTO and that the amount of overcorrection should be larger in knees with a high preoperative adduction moment.

Therefore, a gait analysis should probably become a part of the preoperative assessment for all patients undergoing HTO in order to adapt the amount of overcorrection according to the importance of the adduction moment. Another field of investigation is the development of gait training techniques for reducing the adduction.

Arthroscopy and Joint Débridement

The usefulness of arthroscopy as a diagnostic tool before planning an osteotomy is very limited. When the integrity of the supposed unaffected joint space is questionable, stress radiographs, arthrograms possibly combined with computed tomography scans, or magnetic resonance imaging should provide adequate information, eliminating the need for more invasive investigations.

The role of routine preosteotomy arthroscopy has been studied by Keene et al.[143] They concluded that there was no correlation between preosteotomy arthroscopic findings and the clinical result of osteotomy.

Hsu[119] also stated that preoperative arthroscopic grading, according to the criteria of Fujisawa et al,[83] did not adequately predict the knee's functional outcome but that postoperative arthroscopic grading was of some prognostic value.

Odenbring et al[209] performed diagnostic arthroscopy at the time of HTO and 2 years after surgery in 16 patients. They found cartilage regeneration in eight medial tibial condyles and in nine medial femoral condyles. The main repair feature was proliferation of fibrocartilage that covered bone, areas of fibrillated cartilage, and filled clefts in hyaline cartilage. Cartilage regeneration was correlated to the degree of knee alignment achieved after proximal tibial osteotomy but not with the clinical outcome.

Débridement has been advocated as a complement to osteotomy.[166]

In keeping with Johnson,[139] who reported that the combination of degeneration with varus deformity could be relieved by abrasion arthroplasty, Tippet[262] combined arthroscopic arthroplasty and dome osteotomy and reported satisfactory results in 90% of his cases. Korn[147] also combined the two procedures, with an interval of 4 to 6 weeks between the arthroscopy and the dome osteotomy, and claimed that prior arthroscopic abrasion arthroplasty provides early medial compartment resurfacing with fibrocartilage and that correction of varus deformity protects the developing fibrocartilage.

On the contrary, based on a large review of the literature, Goldman et al[91] concluded that in degenerative knee arthritis abrasion arthroplasty does not appear to offer any additional benefit to arthroscopic débridement alone.

Rand and Ritts,[234] based on a series of eight patients with persistent pain after upper tibial osteotomy subsequently treated with abrasion arthroplasty, concluded that this procedure was not a satisfactory salvage for a failed upper tibial osteotomy.

Finally, whether arthroscopic débridement in conjunction with upper tibial osteotomy is more beneficial when compared with osteotomy alone has not been clearly determined. Arthroscopy in conjunction with osteotomy should be reserved for patients with mechanical symptoms suggestive of meniscal abnormalities or loose bodies, in addition to unicompartmental osteoarthritis associated with deformity.[104]

Surgical Techniques

Closing Wedge Proximal Tibial Valgus Osteotomy With Internal Fixation by Blade Plate

My preferred technique for closing wedge proximal tibial valgus osteotomy remains internal fixation by a "swan-neck" blade plate, as described by Postel and Langlais,[221] Merle d'Aubigné,[185] and Langlais and Thomazeau,[154] and in use at the Hospital Cochin in Paris since 1967. Large series[71, 163, 221, 245] have demonstrated the precision and the reliability of the procedure. Lootvoet et al[163] analyzed the results of a series of 193 osteotomies performed with the same technique. In this series the hip-knee-ankle angle was 7.7 degrees ± 3.8 degrees of varus preoperatively, 2.7 degrees ± 3.1 degrees of valgus at union, and 0.1 degree ± 5.1 degrees of valgus at review 6 to 10 years postoperatively.

This method not only provides a rigid internal fixation to allow early motion but also offers an "automatic" correction as opposed to other methods of fixation, like the buttress plate.[116] The complication rate—which was feared to increase secondary to the larger surgical exposure required for plate fixation[54]—remains quite low. Lemaire[158] reported a series of 207 osteotomies fixed with an angled blade plate in which the complication rate was 7%. The most frequent complication was a transient partial peroneal nerve palsy (nine cases), with a full recovery seven times and a residual weakness of the great-toe extensor twice. In this series, the fibula was osteotomized at the junction of its middle and upper thirds.

The principle of the swan-neck blade plate is to use a special jig and a guide wire, over which the blade plate is driven once the osteotomy is completed. The orientation of the guide wire sets the amount of correction. The correction is thus dependent on two angles: the angle of the jig and the angle of the blade plate (Fig. 71.11).

A vertical incision is usually made beginning midway between the patella and the fibular head and extending distally for about 12 cm to the crest of the tibia. Make the incision closer to the midline in order to facilitate a possible revision. The upper tibia is exposed by making a fascial incision 5 mm away from the crest of the tibia, extending proximally into the iliotibial band, in line with its fibers. This creates a posteriorly hinged fasciomuscular flap in order to protect the peroneal nerve. This flap then covers the blade plate at the end of the procedure. The flap consists of the posterior part of the iliotibial band and of the tibialis anterior muscle.

The fascial incision may be continued proximally through the patellar retinaculum as far as the vastus lateralis, if a lateral patellar release is needed.

The tethering effect of the fibula is removed either by fibular shaft osteotomy or by separation of the superior tibiofibular joint.

The lateral joint line is identified with a needle. The guide wire is inserted in the upper tibia 10 to 15 mm distal to the joint line, using the special jig. The jig, which has the same profile as the blade plate and which perfectly fits the lateral proximal tibia, is set for a predetermined amount of correction. This jig is normally set for use with a 90-degree blade plate, but when greater correction is required, an alternative 100-degree blade plate can be used.

The insertion point of the guide wire should be located midway between the posterior and the anterior aspect of the tibia in the sagittal plane. The guide wire should be inserted strictly in the plane of flexion of the knee. It should be parallel to the joint line or slightly ascendant from medial to lateral in the frontal plane. The track for the blade plate is started in the proximal fragment with a cannulated cutting tool, which is passed over the guide wire and aligned with the jig. Two guiding pins should be used to figure the wedge resection. The proximal limb of the osteotomy should be parallel with the guide wire and situated 15 to 20 mm distal to it. With the help of a template, a distal diaphyseal pin should be placed at an angle relative to the guide wire equal to the desired amount of resection. At the end of the procedure, these two pins should become parallel.

After wedge removal and completion of the osteotomy, the angular correction is performed by manually exerting a valgus force on the leg, with the knee in extension. The selected blade plate is driven over the guide wire and fixed to the tibial cortex with three screws.

It is mandatory to obtain the correction without applying any constraint on the blade plate, as this would lead to a loss of correction either by sweeping the blade into the cancellous bone or by bending the plate.

When calculating the correction, one should take into account that the level of the osteotomy is distal relative to the joint line. The effect of the osteotomy on the hip-knee-ankle angle is therefore smaller than if the same angular correction was performed at the level of the joint line. One should therefore add approximately two degrees to the correction calculated on the basis of the hip-knee-ankle angle.[27, 71]

Radiographic checks are made at two stages, the first after insertion of the guide wire and the second after insertion of the plate.

The fascia is closed nonhermetically over a suction drain. Continuous passive motion can be started in the recovery room. Active exercises begin on the first postoperative day. Walking is permitted with crutches, and weightbearing should be restricted to 15 kg until union of the osteotomy. This technique of osteotomy permits more complex corrections, such as an extension or an internal rotation coupled to a valgization.

Closing Wedge Proximal Tibial Valgus Osteotomy With Internal Fixation by Plate

Hofmann et al[116] developed special instruments to resect the bone wedge with an improved precision. They recommend a standard lateral approach with division of the proximal tibiofibular capsule. Keith needles are used to identify the joint line, and a transverse osteotomy jig is fixed with 3.2-mm drill points. The transverse limb portion of the osteotomy is performed keeping the medial cortex intact (Fig. 71.12).

The desired correction is achieved using a slotted osteotomy jig with 2-degree increments to perform the oblique portion of the osteotomy (Fig. 71.13). An L buttress plate is applied to the proximal tibia with fully threaded cancellous screws, and an external compressor device is used to draw the osteotomy close before screws are placed in the plate distally. Postoperatively, the patients are started on immediate continuous passive motion and allowed 50% weightbearing.

This technique is very similar to the blade plate technique. I maintain that, if the inner cortex of the tibia is disrupted, the risk of overcorrection is higher with a plate and a compressor than with a rigid blade plate and that the stability of the fixation is lower (Fig. 71.14).

Surer[255, 256] developed a device to improve the stabil-

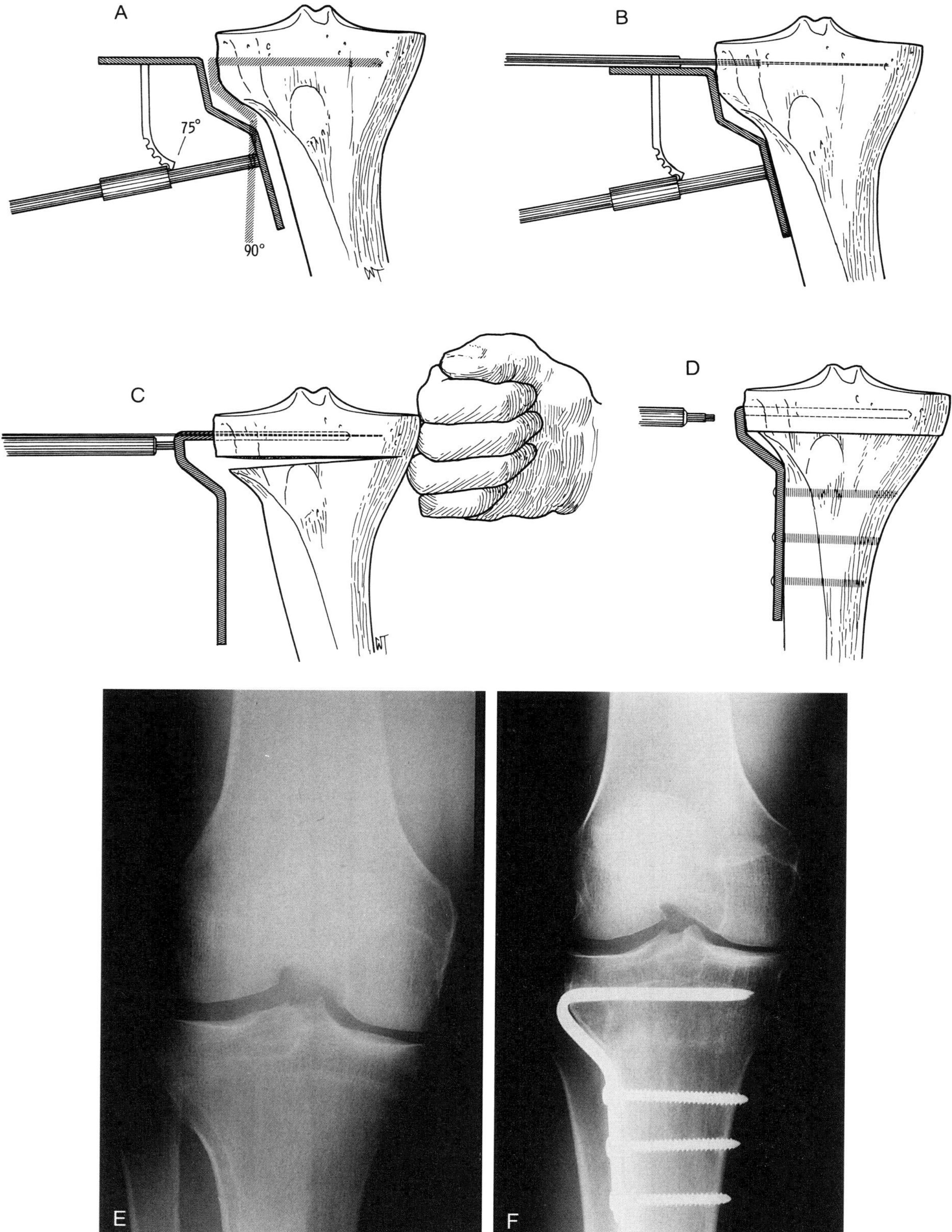

FIGURE 71.11 ➢ Blade-plate fixation. *A,* The guide instrument is set for the correction angle desired. *B,* A guide wire is drilled into the proximal tibia. *C,* After completion of the osteotomy, the blade plate is driven into the proximal tibia over the guide wire. *D,* The blade is screwed to the tibia. (From Merle d' Aubigné R: Joint realignment in the management of osteoarthritis. In Straub LR, Wilson PD Jr, eds: Clinical trends in orthopaedics. New York, Thieme-Stratton, 1982, p 246.) *E–F,* 10-year follow-up of a closing wedge osteotomy with blade-plate fixation.

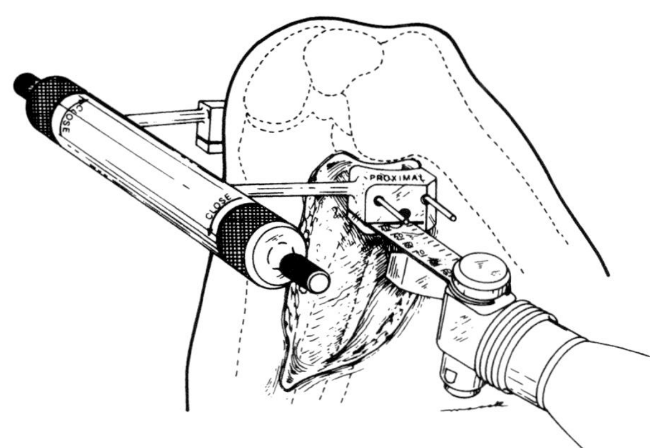

FIGURE 71.12 ➢ Transverse tibial osteotomy jig. (From Hofmann AA, Wyatt RW, Beck SW: High tibial osteotomy: Use of an osteotomy jig, rigid fixation, and early motion versus conventional surgical technique and cast immobilization. Clin Orthop 1991; 271: 212.)

ity of screw fixation. It uses a set screw to fix the screw to the plate (Fig. 71.15). Fixing the screw to the plate modifies the action of the screw, which then becomes directly involved in anchoring the implant. The stability of the fixation no longer depends on the simple application of the plate to the surface of the bone but benefits from the hold of the screw in the bone. A series of plates using this principle has been designed and can be used for distal femoral osteotomies and for tibial opening or closing wedge osteotomies.

Several other fixation devices and guiding jigs are available,[140, 143, 148, 187, 197, 199, 214] but most of them do not combine the advantages of a rigid fixation and a precise and reliable correction.

The other blade plates available[148, 197] are not guided by a wire as in the Postel-d'Aubigné technique. The precision of the correction relies, therefore, only on the exact measurement of the wedge and on the integrity of the medial tibial cortex.

Staple fixation, although advocated by several authors,[13, 54, 106, 283, 293] is not reliable enough to authorize early rehabilitation and often necessitates complementary cast immobilization. There is no advantage in using staples as a mean of fixation because the plates and blade plates now available are more stable and do not carry additional risks of complication.

Opening Wedge Osteotomy

TECHNIQUE

Debeyre et al have employed a medial opening wedge osteotomy proximal to the tibial tubercule since 1951.[61, 62, 64] Hernigou et al[113] published the long-term results of this technique in 1987. The technique of the opening wedge osteotomy is straightforward. A longitudinal skin incision of approximately 8 cm is made over the anteromedial aspect of the tibia, along the anterior edge of the MCL. The hamstring tendons are dissected, and the superficial MCL is exposed and is separated from bone proximally as far as the level of the osteotomy, which should be started at least 3.5 cm distal to the medial joint line and directed laterally and proximally toward the tip of the fibula. A Steinmann pin can be inserted under fluoroscopic control to figure the osteotomy line. The fibula and tibiofibular joint do not need to be disturbed. The medial tibial cortex is cut with osteotomes, or the osteotomy can be initiated with an oscillating saw. The lateral tibial cortex should remain intact. The bone at the site of the osteotomy is forced open, and three bicortical wedges of appropriate size, obtained from the iliac crest, are inserted. Hernigou et al recommend fixation of the osteotomy with a T-plate and screws, as the lateral part of the cortex may crack during the osteotomy or postoperatively. The wound is closed by repairing the divided tendons and superficial MCL and then approximating the subcutaneous tissue and skin.

Goutallier et al[95] reported their experience in substituting cement for full-thickness iliac crest wedges, combined with the use of buttress-plate fixation (Fig. 71.16). By reviewing 107 osteotomies performed with this technique, they stated that using a cement wedge instead of an iliac bone graft does not expose to any special complication and improves the accuracy of axial correction.

Puddu[225] designed a special plate, which combines the roles of the buttress plate and of cement wedge (Fig. 71.17). This plate has two holes for one stainless steel 6.5-mm cancellous screw proximally and one 4.5-mm cortical screw distally. A plate with four holes can be used if the bone is soft. A set of five presized plates has been designed. The plates have metal blocks 4 mm deep and are of varying height (5, 7.5, 10, 12.5, 15 mm). The aim of these plates is to fix and stabilize the osteotomy. Once the block is inserted into the osteotomy site, it prevents loss of correction. The opening osteotomy is facilitated by the use of a specially designed wedge-shaped instrument (Fig. 71.18).

Once the plate is fixed and the osteotomy stabilized, a bone graft is obtained and inserted into the defect. Puddu advises taking the bone graft from the tibia itself if the osteotomy is 7.5 mm or less and from the iliac crest if the opening wedge is 1 cm or more. The distal part of the MCL is left open, and the wound is closed.

The knee is protected in a brace that permits a full range of motion. A suction drain is left in place for 24 hours postoperatively. Partial weightbearing is permitted after 40 days, and full weightbearing is allowed after 60 days if the x-ray films show good healing at the operative site.

CALCULATION OF WEDGE SIZE

Hernigou et al[114] mathematically analyzed the orientation of the superior tibial epiphysis in the frontal and sagittal planes. They determined the opening wedges and established tables expressing the height of the

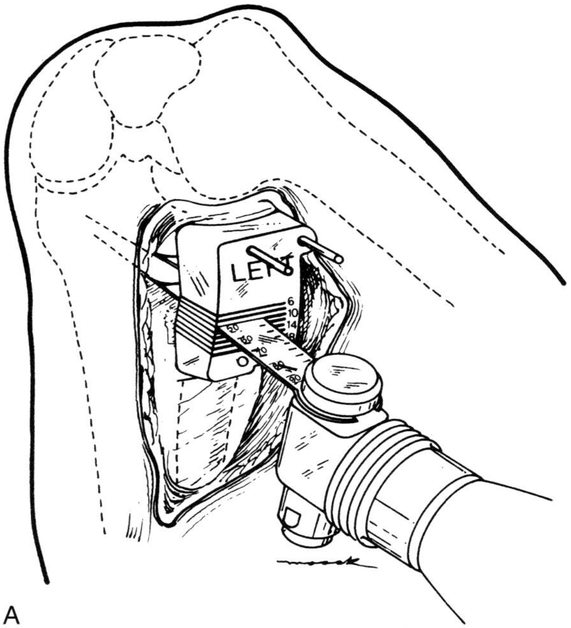

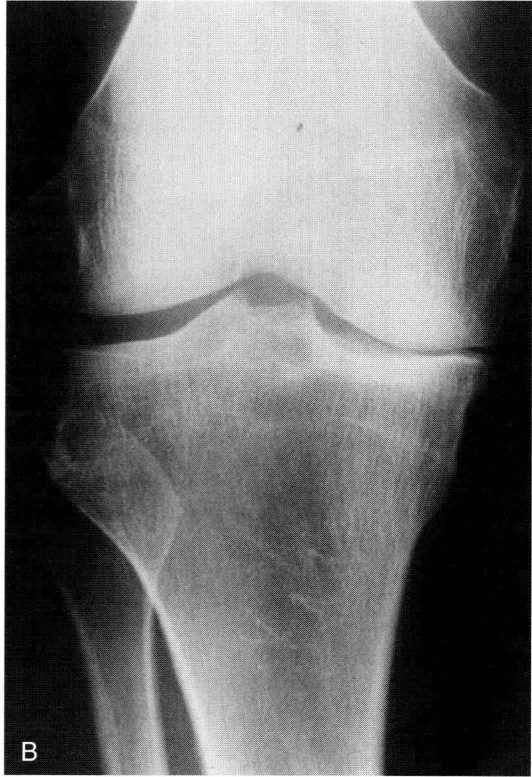

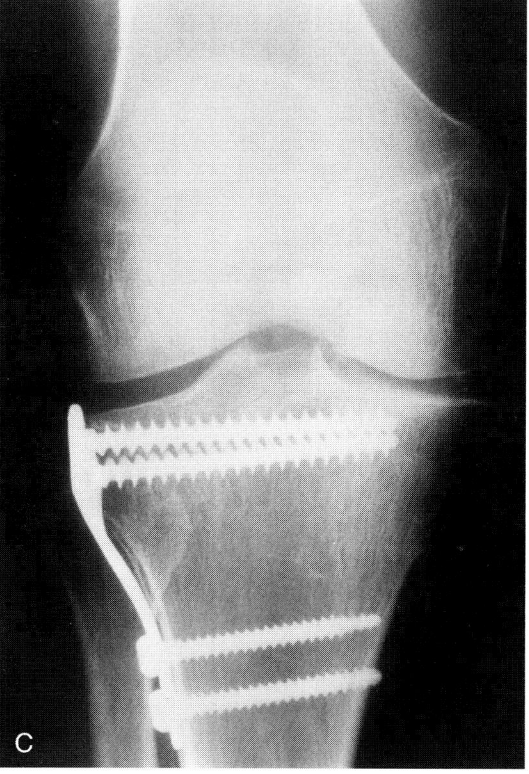

FIGURE 71.13 ➢ *A,* Oblique tibial osteotomy jig with 2-degree increments. (From Hofmann AA, Wyatt RW, Beck SW: High tibial osteotomy: Use of an osteotomy jig, rigid fixation, and early motion versus conventional surgical technique and cast immobilization. Clin Orthop 1991; 271:212.) *B,* Severe medial joint space narrowing in a 45-year-old female, secondary to a previous medial meniscectomy and a 5-degree varus deformity. *C,* Weightbearing anteroposterior radiograph of the same knee 5 years after closing wedge osteotomy with internal fixation by plate.

wedge's base as a function of the tibial width and the desired angular correction. The height of the wedge's base can also be determined graphically.[61] For a tibia 55 to 60 mm wide at the level of the osteotomy, 1 mm of opening produces roughly 1 degree of correction. As the proximal tibia has a triangular cross-section, the base of the wedge should be higher posteriorly than anteriorly to avoid a posterior tilt of the tibial plateaus.

ADVANTAGES AND DISADVANTAGES

The main advantage is leaving the fibula untouched. Another advantage is that this osteotomy can be combined with an ACL reconstruction through the same incision.[225]

The disadvantages are a longer uniting time and the necessity for bone grafting.

I have used freeze-dried cancellous bone grafts[68, 69] several times in opening wedge osteotomies stabilized

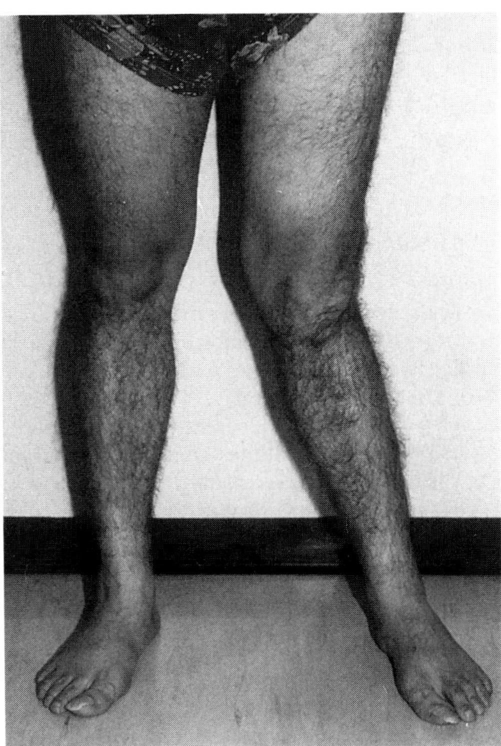

FIGURE 71.14 ➢ Severe overcorrection resulting in an unacceptable valgus malalignment. The closing wedge osteotomy had been performed with the help of a compression clamp that excessively crushed the lateral metaphyseal bone.

by Puddu's plate. This seems a reasonable option, provided that the wedge's size is small. If the wedge height is greater than 7.5 mm, a bone graft should be taken from the iliac crest. In this situation, the other osteotomy techniques should be considered.

Dome-Shaped Proximal HTO

TECHNIQUE

The dome or curviplane HTO was introduced by Blaimont[21, 22] and popularized by Maquet.[173, 177] This osteotomy is proximal to the tibial tubercule. It is semicylindrical, and its concavity is downward, circumscribing the tibial tuberosity (Fig. 71.19).

After oblique division of the fibula in its middle third, two Steinmann pins are inserted in the tibia, one proximal and the other distal to the osteotomy curve. The angle between the two pins should correspond to the planned correction. This can be facilitated by the use of a special guide.[135, 173, 174, 276] The barrel-vault tibial osteotomy is performed through a 5-cm longitudinal incision centered on the tibial tuberosity.

Special curved osteotomes (Fig. 71.20) that can easily glide behind the patellar tendon can be used to initiate the osteotomy.[276] An alternative technique is to mark a curved line on the proximal tibia and to make holes along this line, with either Kirschner wires[173] or 3-mm drills.[254] Korn[147] designed a curved double-bladed osteotomy guide, which directs the wires in the frontal plane and in the sagittal plane.

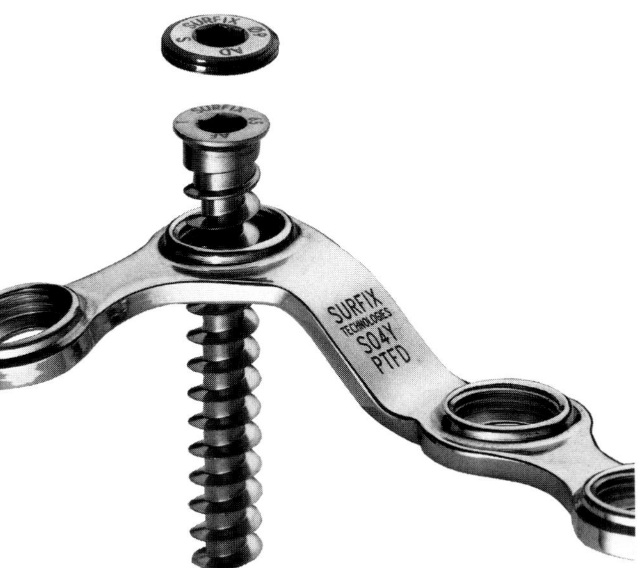

FIGURE 71.15 ➢ The fixation of the screw to the plate is achieved by the set screw, which is screwed into the plate. To be effective, the blockage requires two conditions: respecting coaxial alignment and cleaning all debris interposed between the plate, the screw, and the set screw. (From Surer P: Reliability of fixation with the Surfix plate: Analysis of the first 100 osteotomies. Eur J Orthop Surg Traumatol 1997; 7:47.)

The osteotomy is completed with a thin osteotome, along the curved line formed by the Kirschner wire holes or the curved osteotome. The tibial fragments are rotated until both Steinmann pins are parallel. Two Charnley clamps[173] or a Müller external fixator[276] linking the two pins fix the fragments under compression. Unilateral external fixators placed on the lateral side of the tibia have also been used.[45, 222]

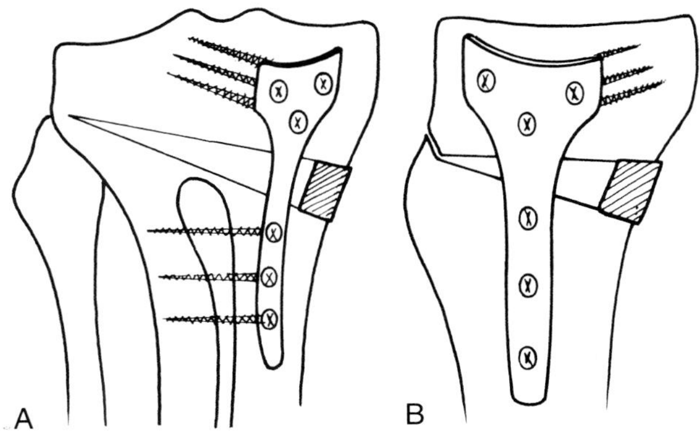

FIGURE 71.16 ➢ Opening wedge osteotomy with a cement wedge and a T-plate. The cement wedge should be posterior because the base of the opening wedge should be higher posteriorly than anteriorly to avoid a posterior tilt of the tibial plateaus. (From Goutallier D, Julieron A, Hernigou P: Cement wedge replacing iliac graft for medial opening wedge tibial osteotomy. Rev Chir Orthop 1992; 78:138. © Masson Editeur.)

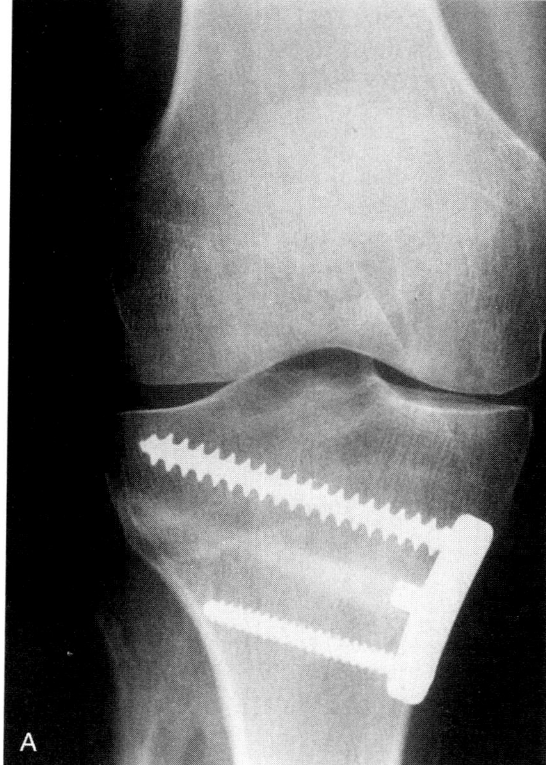

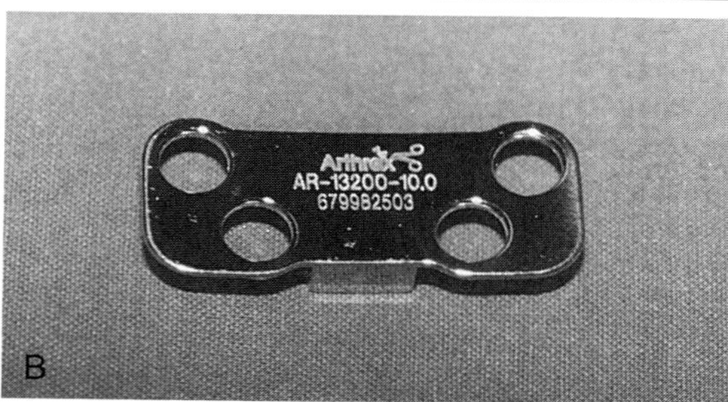

FIGURE 71.17 ➢ *A,* Medial opening wedge osteotomy combined with an ACL reconstruction, using freeze-dried cancellous bone allograft and fixed with a two-hole Puddu plate. *B,* Alternatively, a four-hole plate can be used.

Another method to assess intraoperatively that the appropriate correction has been obtained was described by Blaimont.[22] A long and straight metallic rod is aligned, under fluoroscopy, on the mechanical axis of the tibia. The position of the proximal end of the rod is then checked: it should be medial to the femoral head and should project radiologically over the obturator hole. This ensures that enough overcorrection has been obtained, provided that, during this fluoroscopic control, the possible medial collateral laxity has been annulled by maintaining the contact between the medial femoral condyle and the medial tibial plateau (Fig. 71.21). A suction drainage is left in place for 24 hours to reduce the risk of an anterior compartment syndrome,[177, 276] and the tibial and fibular wounds are closed.

Postoperatively, the knee is passively and actively flexed from the day after surgery. On the second day the patient stands and walks with two crutches, putting some weight on the operated knee. After 8 weeks and x-ray film evidence of healing, the Steinmann pins are removed. The crutches are discarded as soon as the patient feels stable on the operated leg.

ADVANTAGES AND DISADVANTAGES

Maquet,[173, 177] Blaimont,[21, 22] and Lemaire[158] claimed that the dome osteotomy was more accurate than the other techniques. Maquet recommended combining an anterior displacement of the patellar tendon with correction of the varus deformity. This can be easily performed with a barrel vault osteotomy. Whether this association has any advantage is subject to debate.

The application of an external fixator allows postoperative correction of axial alignment, if necessary, as well as compression.

The amount of correction using a dome osteotomy is theoretically unrestricted,[12, 21, 22, 174, 177] whereas it is limited by the amount of bone available when a closing wedge osteotomy is performed. The dome osteotomy tightens the MCL, without affecting the position of the tibial tubercle relative to the joint line, as opposed to the opening wedge osteotomy.[22]

The main disadvantages are related to the use of the external fixator. The external fixator is cumbersome and is not easily accepted by some patients. The percutaneous Steinmann pins can damage the peroneal nerve or its branches,[59, 146, 175] and can give rise to an

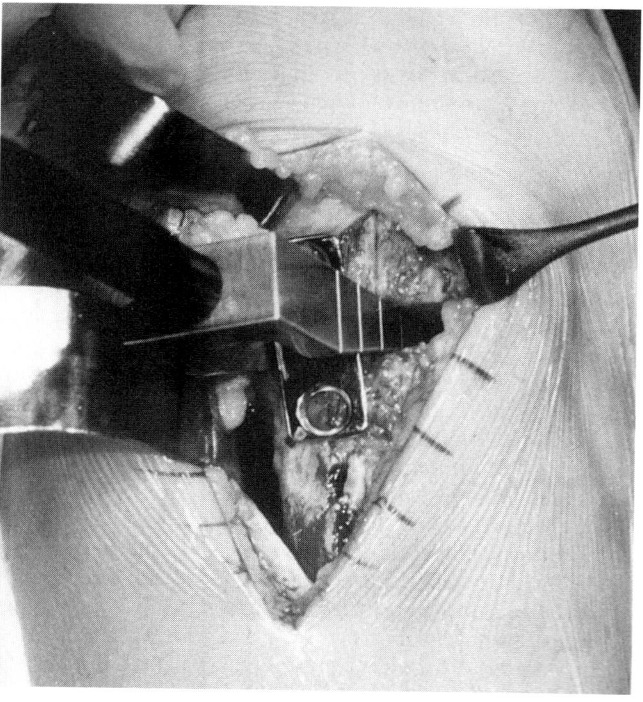

FIGURE 71.18 ➢ Graduated wedge-shaped instrument used to open the osteotomy. The plate is inserted between the two limbs of the instrument.

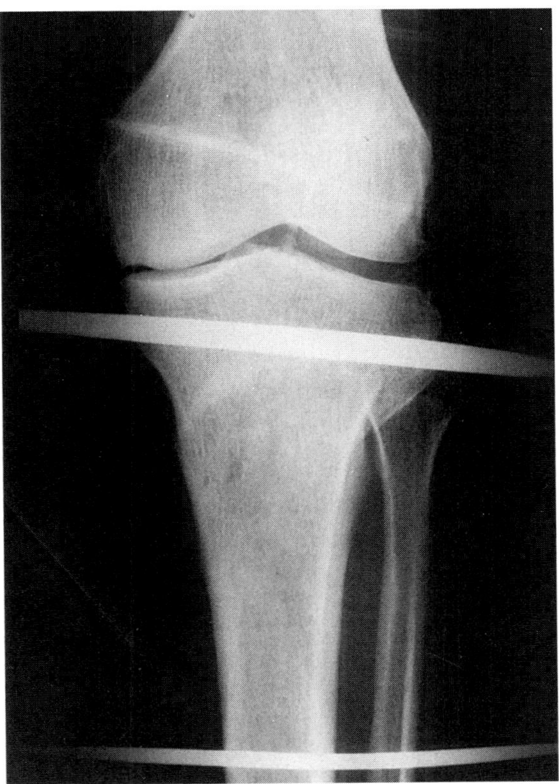

FIGURE 71.19 ➢ Dome high tibial osteotomy. The use of one proximal and one distal Steinmann's pin is generally recommended, but two proximal and two distal pins can be used if extra stability is deemed necessary. Insertion of four Steinmann's pins increases the risk of neurological complications.

infection[125, 178] with a risk of late recurrence if the osteotomy has to be converted to a total knee replacement.

Open Wedge Tibial Osteotomy by Callus Distraction

TECHNIQUE

During the last few years, the technique of progressive opening wedge osteotomy by hemicallotasis has raised considerable interest.[31, 60, 167, 189, 190, 218, 222, 243, 248]

The external fixator used in this technique can be either a ventral T-shaped fixator or a medial fixator (Fig. 71.22). These fixators have a lockable ball joint and a distraction device in order to make a progressive medial opening possible, keeping the lateral tibial cortex as a hinge. The use of an Ilizarov circular external fixator for progressive correction has also been described.[243]

The osteotomy can be performed above the tibial tubercle[189, 218, 248] or at the distal part of it.[31, 167, 243] Some authors[218] advise performing a fibular osteotomy, but most[167, 189, 248] claim that fibular osteotomy is not required.

Partial weightbearing is allowed immediately. The distraction process starts 7 to 10 days after surgery. The gradual distraction is performed by the patient, usually at the speed of 1 mm per day (a quarter turn four times a day). The distraction phase lasts about 2 weeks, and a weekly radiological control is necessary during that period.

When the desired correction is achieved, the fixator is locked and left in place until union is obtained. The fixator is usually removed about 3 months after surgery. The pins are removed at the outpatient clinic.

ADVANTAGES AND DISADVANTAGES

The supporters of this technique claim that it is relatively simple to perform; that it allows precise correction, early mobilization, and weightbearing; and that it is a benign procedure performed through a very short incision, not requiring a fibular osteotomy in most cases.

The main drawback of hemicallotasis is the risk of pin-tract infection. Perusi et al,[218] in a series of 58 osteotomies, reported ten pin-tract infections treated by local antibiotics and two cases of septic arthritis.

A second disadvantage, shared with the opening

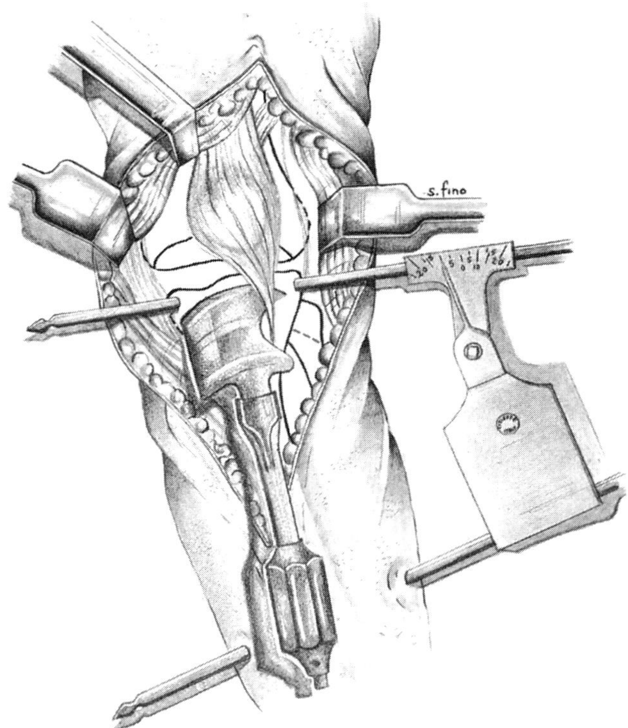

FIGURE 71.20 ➢ Tibial osteotomy using curved osteotomes and an angular guide. Under fluoroscopy, a Steinmann pin is inserted through the upper part of the tibial epiphysis, proximal to the osteotomy. The desired angle of correction is fixed on the guide. The guide, being slid on the first upper pin, gives the direction for the second Steinmann pin. After completion of the osteotomy, the exact correction is obtained by setting the Steinmann pins in parallel. (From Wagner J: Curvilinear osteotomy of the tibia. In Aichroth PM, Cannon WD Jr, eds: Knee Surgery: Current Practice. London, Martin Dunitz, 1992, p 608.)

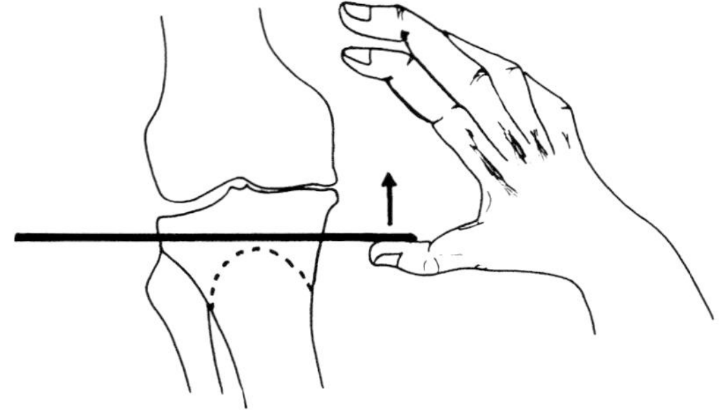

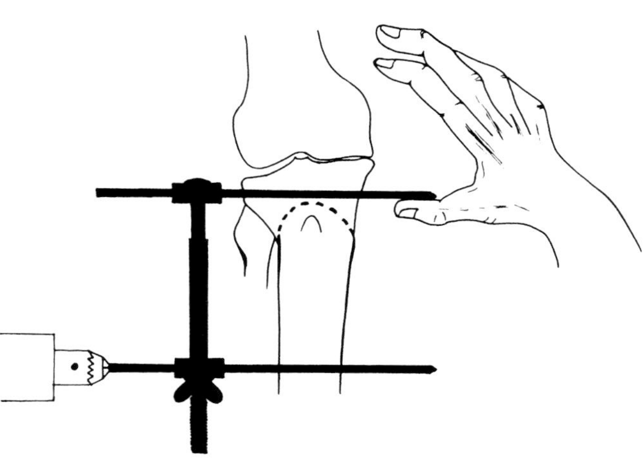

FIGURE 71.21 ➢ If the amount of correction is visually estimated by the intraoperative alignment of the limb, one should manually maintain the contact between the medial femoral condyle and the medial tibial plateau. In the presence of medial laxity, a valgus stress applied to the knee could open the joint medially, which would not occur during gait because of the persistence of the adduction moment. Failure to take the laxity into account during surgery could lead to undercorrection. (From Blaimont P: [Curviplane osteotomy in the treatment of gonarthrosis]. Acta Orthop Belg 1982; 48:97.)

wedge osteotomy, is the lowering of the tibial tubercle relative to the joint line.

Another risk is the potential loss of correction, as the mechanical properties of the newly formed bone are unknown at the time of the removal of the fixator.

Finally, the published follow-ups cover a very short time (average follow-up of 18 months,[218] 14 months,[167] 5 to 36 months,[189] 2 years[248]). One of the teams[248] that performed this technique stopped using it because of unsatisfactory results. I recommend waiting for more clinical data and longer follow-ups before extensive use of the hemicallotasis.

Other Techniques

Wagner et al[273–275] described an oblique metaphyseal proximal tibial osteotomy just below the tibial tubercle. This technique is still popular in Germany[219]; it does not modify the patellar height. The main drawback of this technique is a longer healing time and a higher risk of nonunion.

Catagni et al[40] developed a technique using the Ilizarov apparatus for correction and stabilization. The osteotomy is distal to the tubercle and combines a valgus angulation and a small amount of translation. The time before removing the fixator averaged 85 days. The series described is small (55 patients). The drawbacks of this technique are the risk of pin-tract infection (10%), the bulkiness of the frame, and the required familiarity with the Ilizarov technique in order to avoid neurovascular complications.

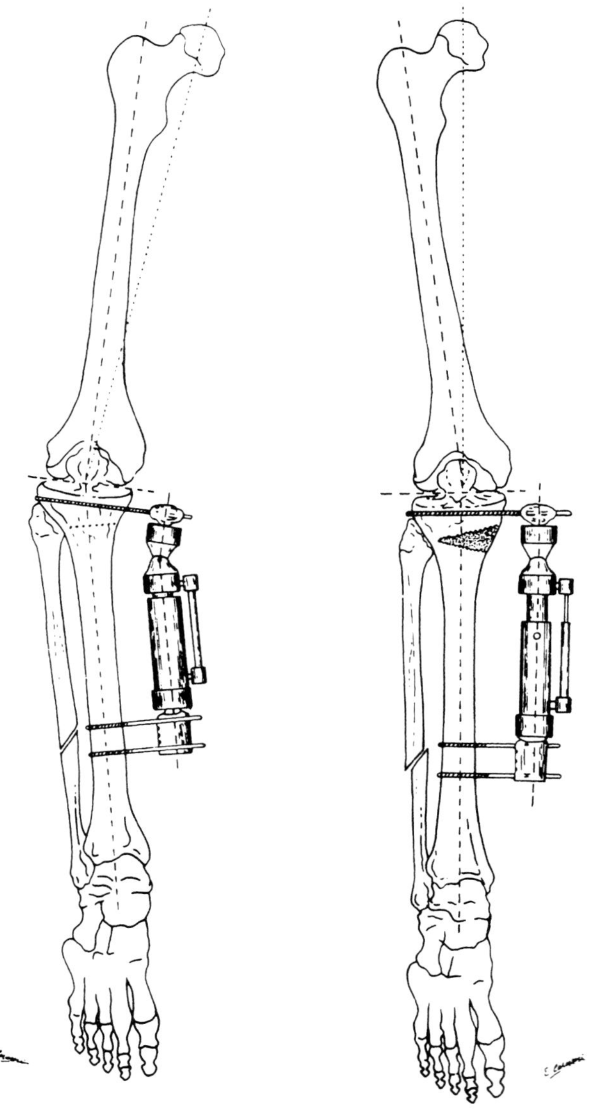

FIGURE 71.22 ➢ Medial external fixator used for progressive opening wedge osteotomy by hemicallotasis. (From Perusi M, Baietta D, Pizzoli A: [Surgical correction of osteoarthritic genu varum by the hemicallotasis technique]. Rev Chir Orthop Reparatrice Appar Mot 1994; 80:739. © Masson Editeur.)

Fibular Osteotomy Versus Division of the Superior Tibiofibular Joint or Excision of the Fibular Head

Opening wedge osteotomies, with immediate or gradual correction, usually leave the fibula untouched. Closing wedge osteotomies and the dome osteotomies require relieving the tethering effect of the fibula, for which three methods can be used: fibular head excision, division of the superior tibiofibular joint, or osteotomy of the fibular shaft (Fig. 71.23).

In agreement with Maquet,[169, 172, 174] Blaimont et al,[23, 24] Andriacchi[10] and others, I maintain that the lateral muscles — tensor fascia lata, biceps cruris — play a major role in counterbalancing the body mass acting eccentrically on the knee during the stance phase of gait.

In principle, division of the superior tibiofibular joint or excision of the fibular head are susceptible to further weakening those dynamic stabilizers, already insufficient in the varus arthritic knee,[24] and to affecting the LCL.[197] This could partly contribute to some unpredictable results of HTO.

Moreover, Wagner et al[277] demonstrated the role of the fibula as a weightbearing bone, together with the tibia. This role is even more important in the case of valgus or varus knee deformity.

The fibular head excision[51, 85] necessitates detaching the lateral ligament, the fabellofibular ligament, the arcuate ligament, to which the popliteus tendon is attached, and the biceps tendon.

Although a repair of the lateral soft tissues is possible after the osteotomy, it seems doubtful that this repair could be able to reproduce the complex anatomy and function of the posterolateral corner of the knee. Another disadvantage of fibular head excision is the risk of peroneal nerve injury. Coventry[51] did not have any peroneal palsy in his series, but Harris and Kostuik,[101] using a similar technique, reported 2 in 44 osteotomies.

Division of the superior tibiofibular joint implies proximal migration of the fibular head relative to the proximal tibial fragment after the osteotomy. This aggravates preexisting lateral collateral laxity or creates new laxity that did not exist previously. This also destabilizes and proximalizes the point of action of the biceps. The increased lateral collateral laxity, together with the weakening of the biceps, impairs the improved load distribution achieved with the tibial osteotomy.[10, 216] This is especially true if the secondary restraints to lateral laxity, i.e., the ACL, the posterior capsule, and the fascia lata, are damaged[10] (Fig. 71.24).

The amount of proximal migration of the fibular head that is detrimental to the knee stability and to the action of the biceps has to be determined, but I believe that division of the tibiofibular joint should be restricted to the correction of small varus deformities, i.e., when the wedge height is less than or equal to 5 mm.

Fibular osteotomy avoids destruction of a normal joint, avoids proximal migration of the fibular head and loosening of the point of action of the biceps, and avoids increasing the laxity of the LCL.[197] The level of the osteotomy of the fibula influences the rate of peroneal nerve injuries.[59, 146] High-risk regions can be located relative to the fibular head[146] (Fig. 71.25).

Curley et al,[59] in a study of 16 patients assessed by electrophysiological recordings and intracompartmental pressure recording before and after HTO, observed that patients who had a proximal fibular osteotomy had greater electrical abnormalities postoperatively. Two of them developed common peroneal palsies.

More commonly, an iatrogenic, isolated weakness or paralysis of the extensor hallucis longus muscle can occur in patients who have had a proximal tibial and fibular osteotomy. To investigate why this complication occurs, Kirgis and Albrecht[146] dissected the deep peroneal nerve and neighboring structures in 29 specimens from cadavers, paying special attention to the

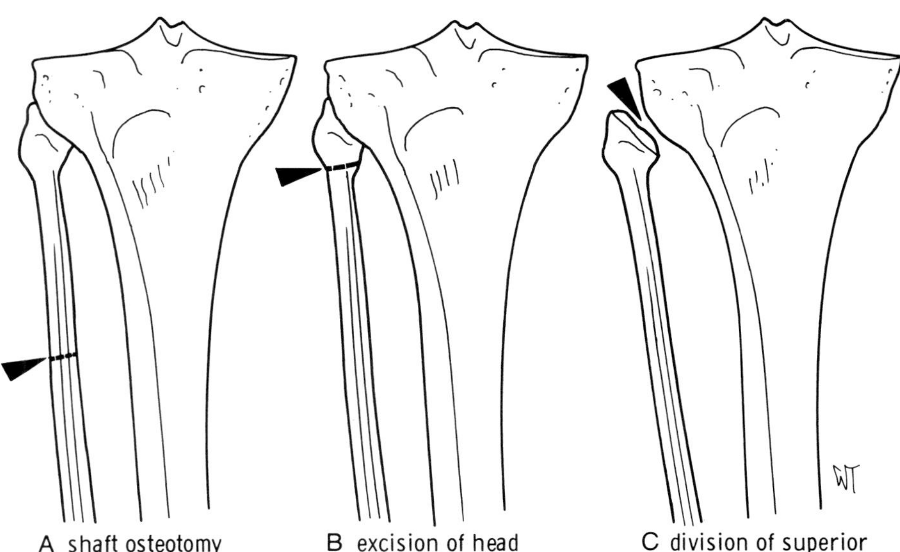

FIGURE 71.23 ➢ Methods of relieving the tethering effect of the fibula. *A*, Osteotomy of the fibular shaft. *B*, Excision of the fibular head. *C*, Division of the superior tibiofibular ligaments. (From Bauer GC, Insall J, Koshino T: Tibial osteotomy in gonarthrosis (osteoarthritis of the knee). J Bone Joint Surg Am 1969; 51:1545.)

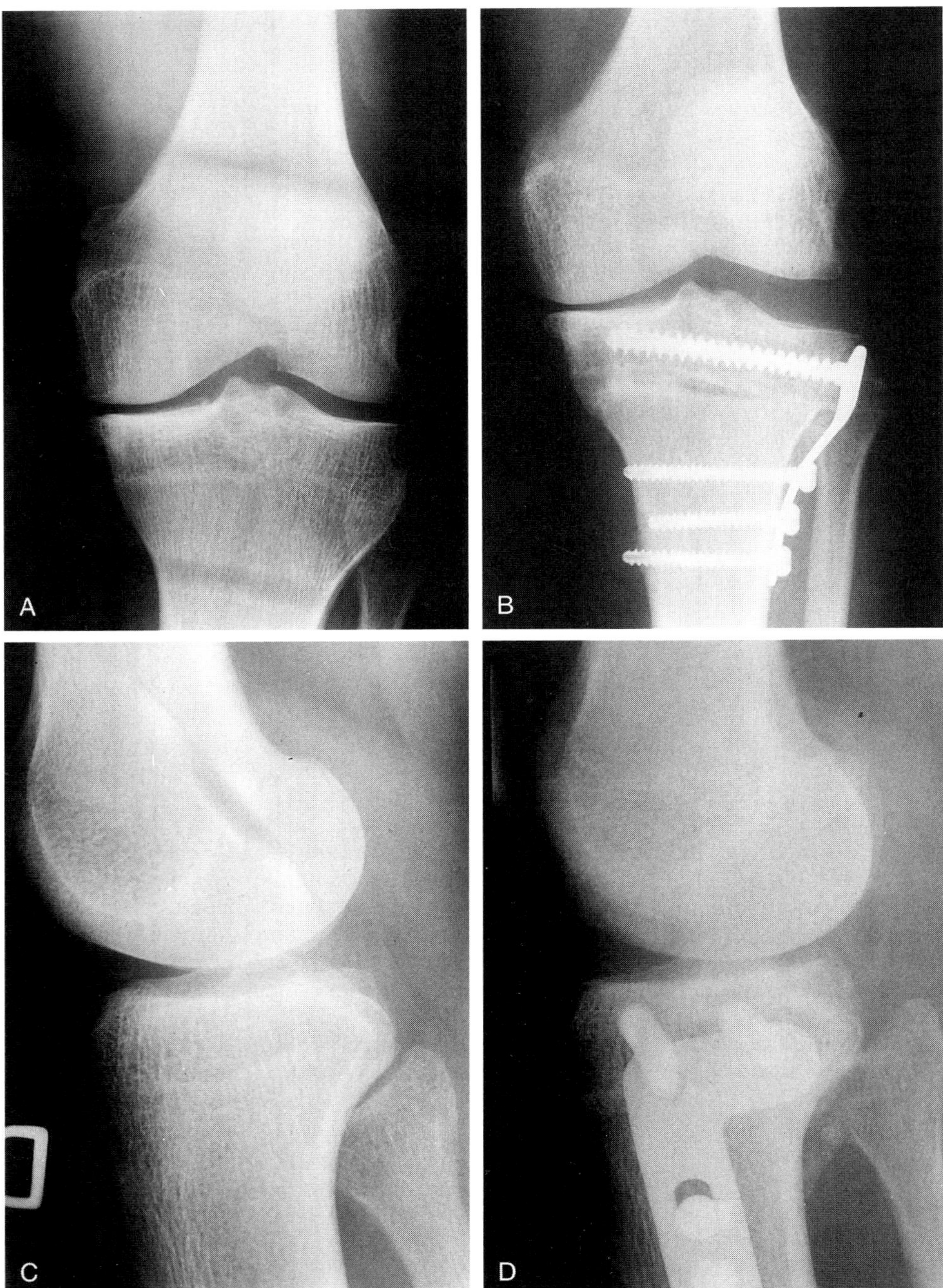

FIGURE 71.24 ➢ *A,* Medial gonarthrosis in a 33-year-old man, with an ACL-deficient knee but without significant lateral laxity. *B,* Severe LCL laxity after lateral closing wedge osteotomy with division of the superior tibiofibular joint. *C,* Preoperative lateral x-ray of the same knee, showing the tibiofibular joint. *D,* Postoperative lateral x-ray demonstrating the posterior and superior dislocation of the tibiofibular joint.

motor branches supplying the extensor hallucis longus. Of 46 motor nerves that were identified, 8 entered the muscle from the lateral side in an area 70 to 150 mm distal to the fibular head; all of them ran close to the fibular periosteum. They suggested that, in some patients, the nerve supply to the extensor hallucis longus is at high risk of injury during a fibular osteotomy because of the proximity of the bone to the motor branches. Fibular osteotomy can be performed safely in the region between the middle and distal thirds of the fibula, about 160 mm distal to the fibular head.

Influence of Osteotomy on the Tibial Slope in the Sagittal Plane

The normal upper tibia has a posterior slope.[129] As the proximal tibia is triangular in section at the level of the osteotomy site, a wedge having the same height ventrally and dorsally will affect not only the alignment in the frontal plane but also the tibial slope. In this case, an opening wedge would increase the posterior slope, whereas a closing wedge would reduce the posterior slope.[245]

An excessive posterior slope is detrimental for the long-term result of the osteotomy.[112, 245] It can provoke

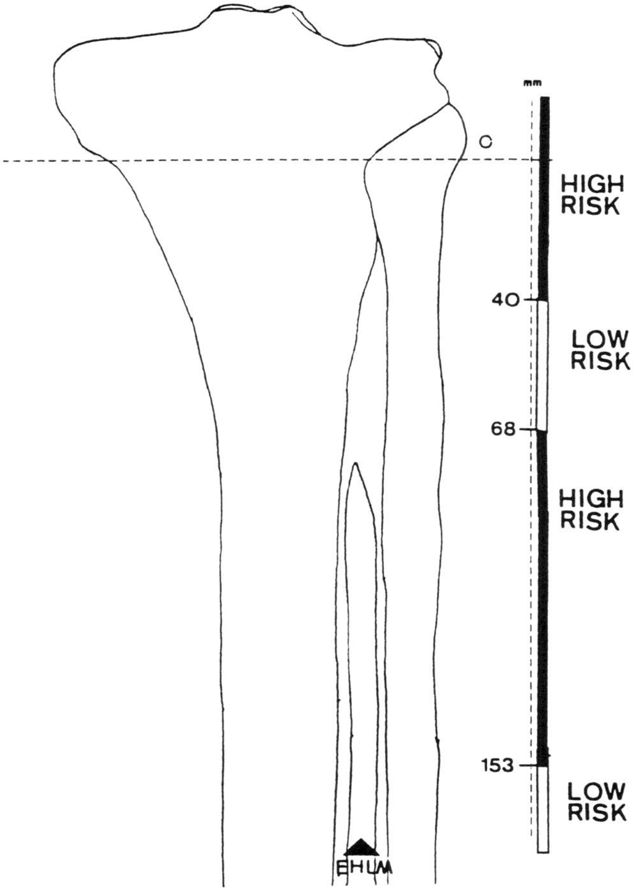

FIGURE 71.25 ➢ Frontal view showing a leg with a longitudinal scale. The scale illustrates regions that are at high and low risk for intraoperative injury relative to the presence of the motor branches from the truncus of the deep peroneal nerve. EHLM, extensor hallucis longus muscle. (From Kirgis A, Albrecht S: Palsy of the deep peroneal nerve after proximal tibial osteotomy: An anatomical study. J Bone Joint Surg Am 1992; 74:1180.)

an anterior subluxation of the tibia, particularly when the ACL is deficient. For this reason, Hernigou et al[113] advise that, when performing an opening wedge osteotomy, the posterior wedge should have a base that is exactly the height that is needed, whereas the base of the middle wedge should measure about 2 mm less and the most anterior one about 6 mm less.

On the other hand, a closing wedge osteotomy will tend to decrease the posterior tibial slope if the base of the wedge has the same height posteriorly and anteriorly. This does not induce an anterior subluxation of the tibia, except if the posterior cruciate ligament (PCL) is damaged.

These changes in the normal tibial slope will complicate the conversion of the osteotomy to a total knee replacement.

HTO and the Patellofemoral Joint

Most authors agree that mild patellofemoral arthritis does not contraindicate an HTO and is of little prognostic significance.[57, 61, 104, 125, 128, 145, 174]

On the other hand, moderate-to-severe patellofemoral arthritis has a negative influence on prognosis.[111, 226, 239, 245, 264] As stated by Insall,[125] an osteotomy should be avoided in patients with marked patellofemoral arthritis, given the excellent alternative of TKA.

An HTO acts on the patella in different ways: it changes the patellar height, the Q-angle, and the medial lateral position of the tibial tubercle.

The change in the Q-angle and in the medial lateral position of the tibial tubercle is minimal,[92, 111, 245] whatever the osteotomy technique, except for major angular corrections.

The patellar height is, in principle, affected differently by the various osteotomy techniques. A dome osteotomy or an osteotomy below the tibial tuberosity should not modify the proximal distal position of the tubercle, whereas an opening wedge should render it more distal and a closing wedge more proximal. The length of the patellar tendon can also be altered after an HTO, as a consequence of scarring or immobilization.

Scuderi et al[244] observed, in a study group of 66 patients who had had a proximal closing wedge tibial osteotomy, that 89% of the patellae as measured by the Insall-Salvati[122] index, and 76.3%, as measured by the Blackburne-Peel[20] index, were lowered on the postoperative lateral radiograph. All knees were immobilized in a cylinder cast during healing of the osteotomy.

More recently, Westrich et al[282] demonstrated that, in a study group of 65 patients having undergone an HTO with a closing wedge osteotomy above the tibial tubercle, 33 patients who underwent some type of internal fixation and received early range of motion postoperatively had less postoperative shortening of the patellar tendon, according to the Insall-Salvati index, than the patients who were postoperatively immobilized with a cast.

Dohin et al,[73] in a group of 59 closing wedge osteotomies fixed by a blade plate and immediately mobilized, showed that the patellar height was not modified, as measured by the index of Caton et al.[41]

This is a strong argument for using rigid internal fixation and early range of motion, as this should result in a better knee and facilitate any subsequent TKA. It also suggests that a closing wedge osteotomy should be preferred to an opening wedge osteotomy in case of preoperative patella baja or patellofemoral arthritis. Nevertheless, Hernigou and Goutallier,[111] studying the radiological changes in the patellofemoral joint 10 to 13 years after upper tibial valgus opening wedge osteotomy, found only minimal deteriorations that were not correlated with the functional results.

Whether advancement or medial transfer of the tibial tubercle in addition to HTO has any value in the presence of patellofemoral arthritis is doubtful.

Although Maquet[177] recommended this combination, Nguyen et al,[203] in a prospective study of similarly matched patients with medial and patellofemoral osteoarthritis, were unable to demonstrate any benefit from the addition of tubercle elevation to the osteotomy. Jackson and Waugh,[133] Hofmann et al,[117] Goutallier et al,[93] Hernigou et al,[111] and the members of the symposium of the Société Française de Chirurgie Orthopédique et Traumatologique, concerning the failures of HTOs,[245] reached the same conclusion.

Postoperative Complications

The complication rates of HTO vary considerably according to different series.

They include undercorrection, overcorrection, loss of correction, patella baja, restricted range of motion, intra-articular fractures, nonunion, infection, peroneal nerve dysfunction, compartment syndrome, vascular injury, and thromboembolic disease.

Insall[125] analyzed the complications in 10 clinical series totaling 804 osteotomies. Of the 60 infections reported, 55 were superficial, and 5 were deep; 37 of the infections occurred in association with transfixion pins and an external frame. Eight intra-articular fractures occurred, most of which were caused by a proximal tibial fragment that was too thin. Fifty-six peroneal-nerve palsies were reported, 37 associated with transfixion pins.

Hofmann et al,[116] comparing 19 patients (group A) who underwent osteotomies with staple fixation or cast immobilization, and 21 patients (group B) whose osteotomies were rigidly fixed by a buttress plate and not immobilized, found that 8 patients in group A had associated complications, as opposed to 1 in group B. The only complication in group B was a nondisplaced intra-articular fracture from overcompression of the buttress plate; in group A, there were two transient peroneal nerve palsies, one compartment syndrome, one nonunion, three delayed unions, one superficial infection, two nondisplaced intra-articular fractures, and two losses of correction.

The complication rate is technique-dependent: cast immobilization, proximal fibular osteotomy or fibular head excision, and transfixion pins appear to increase the operative risk.

Undercorrection, Overcorrection, Loss of Correction

Under- and overcorrection are secondary to incorrect preoperative planning or technical errors. Late recurrence of varus deformity was studied by Stuart et al[252] in a series of 113 knees monitored for a minimum of 5 years. Varus recurred in 18%, lateral compartment arthritis progressed in 60%, and medial compartment arthritis occurred in 83% by 9 years after surgery. They concluded that the probability of arthritic progression is much higher than the probability of significant varus recurrence. In this report, the relationship between the postoperative hip-knee-ankle angle and the risk of recurrence of the deformity was not analyzed.

Hernigou,[108] reviewing a series of 35 opening wedge osteotomies with a 20-year follow-up, stated that osteotomy rarely avoids the problem of recurrent deformity, which appears before 10 years when the initial correction is less than 3 degrees of valgus. Even correction between 3 and 6 degrees of valgus is not immune to recurrent varus deformity at long term (20 years): among knees 3 to 6 degrees of valgus at the 1-year postoperative follow-up, most of them remained in this range of correction at 10 years, but half of them had lost some correction at 20 years. Hernigou also reported that a second valgus tibial osteotomy can be successful: 13 repeated tibial osteotomies produced a good result 20 years after the principle osteotomy.

In a large multicentric study,[245] it appeared that the deformity recurred in 14% of cases when the preoperative hip-knee-ankle angle ranged between 3 and 6 degrees valgus, and in 38% of cases when this angle was between 0 and 2 degrees valgus. Overcorrection superior to 6 degrees valgus did not improve the result, was not well accepted by the patients, and should, therefore, be avoided. Overcorrection superior to 10 degrees is not compatible with a normal gait and necessitates a revision of the osteotomy.[245]

Patella Baja and Reduced Range of Motion

As already discussed, lowering of the patella can be minimized by early range of motion allowed by rigid internal or external fixation. In the case of preoperative patella infera, an opening wedge osteotomy should be avoided.

Odenbring et al,[210] in a prospective study, randomized 32 knees in 32 patients to either a cylinder plaster cast or a hinged cast-brace after HTO for medial gonarthrosis. At 6 weeks, 3 months, and 1 year after surgery, the range of motion was better in the cast-brace group. Hofmann et al,[116] comparing a group of 19 osteotomies with cast immobilization and a group of 21 osteotomies with rigid internal fixation and early motion, noted that 3 patients had less than 90 degrees flexion at 6 months in the first group, and all patients had gained 90 degrees flexion at 6 weeks in the second group.

There are clear advantages in favor of early motion after HTO, and this should guide the choice for a strong fixation.

Intra-Articular Fractures

Fracture of the tibial plateau can usually be avoided or corrected if recognized during surgery. The risk of fracture can be decreased if the proximal fragment is appropriately 2 cm or more thick,[56, 144] if the osteotomy is continued to the opposite periosteum,[144] or if the opposite cortex is sufficiently weakened. The reported incidence rate is 2%.[104]

This complication seems to be more frequently encountered in opening wedge osteotomies. Hernigou et al[113] reported 10 undisplaced lateral plateau fractures in a series of 93 opening wedge osteotomies. There was no evidence that these undisplaced fractures had had any effect on the final results.

When using a blade plate for fixation, care should be taken that the entry point of the blade is at least 10 to 15 mm distal to the joint line[154] and that its course is not too ascendant toward the sclerotic medial tibial plateau.[221] In this condition, Descamps et al[70] did not observe any tibial plateau fracture in a series of 544 osteotomies with blade-plate fixation.

Nonunion

Delayed union or nonunion of the osteotomy is rare (Fig. 71.26). The reported rate of nonunion ranges from 0% to 3%.[39, 124, 200, 263, 264] Most authors report a 0.5% to 1% nonunion rate.[36, 57, 70, 128, 158, 163] Jackson and Waugh[133] reported a threefold increase in the nonunion rate when the osteotomy was performed below the tuberosity rather than above it.

Insall[125] believes that a thin proximal fragment is a risk factor for nonunion, perhaps because of avascular necrosis.

Mammi et al[168] investigated the effect of electromagnetic field stimulation in a group of 40 consecutive patients treated with valgus tibial osteotomy, randomly receiving an active or a dummy stimulator postoperatively. They concluded that electromagnetic field stimulation had positive effects on the healing of tibial osteotomies. Coventry[54] reported that electrical stimulation has been effective in treating nonunion if the position is acceptable.

However, treatment of nonunion following osteotomy usually consists of bone grafting alone if rigid fixation is maintained or bone grafting and compression fixation in cases where rigid fixation was not used initially.[104] This fixation may be internal, or an external fixator may be used.[54]

Cameron et al[36] recommends a double T-plate technique when the proximal bone fragment is small, soft, or relatively avascular.

Infection

Deep infection is rare after HTO. Compiling the complications of 10 clinical series, for a total of 804 osteotomies, Insall[125] took a census of 5 deep and 55 superficial infections; 37 occurred when an external fixator was used.

Maquet et al,[178] in a series of 700 osteotomies, the majority of which were dome osteotomies, noted a 2.8% rate of skin necrosis and a 7.7% infection rate. The respective incidence rates of deep and superficial infections were not mentioned.

Lortat-Jacob et al[164] reported six cases of early reintervention for infection after HTO. In four cases the internal fixation was left in place, with a good end result. One patient with gas gangrene required amputation, and another died from septic shock.

The hemicallotasis technique necessitates the use of an external fixator for a prolonged period of time. As already mentioned, Perusi,[218] in a series of 58 osteotomies, reported 10 pin-tract infections treated by local antibiotics and 2 cases of septic arthritis.

However, septic complications related to the use of an external fixator should not be overestimated. Lemaire,[158] in a series of 201 dome osteotomies fixed by a compression frame, reported 3 infections: 1 was successfully treated by general antibiotics, and 2 were treated by curettage and antibiotic-impregnated polymethylmethacrylate beads left temporarily in the wound.

The infection rate after HTO justifies routine antibiotic prophylaxis.[104]

Peroneal Nerve Dysfunction

Fibular osteotomy or resection of the fibular head can induce a common peroneal nerve palsy[59] or an isolated weakness of the extensor hallucis longus muscle.[146]

From the studies of Curley et al[59] and Kirgis and Albrecht,[146] the fibular osteotomy should be performed distally at the junction of the middle and distal thirds of the leg. Kirgis and Albrecht defined two high-risk regions for an isolated injury of the motor branches to the extensor hallucis longus, the first one about 30 mm and the second one 68 to 153 mm distal to the fibular head. Kirgis and Albrecht stressed the danger consecutive to the application of an external fixation device after a proximal tibial osteotomy. The nerve can be damaged directly by the pin or by the stab incision created for it. The distal Steinmann pin should always be placed in the safe region, 40 to 60 mm distal to the fibular tubercle, and it should always be inserted from the medial side.

In a large series of osteotomies, Maquet[175] recorded a 3.1% rate of motor deficits and a 4.1% rate of sensory deficits, of which 1.2% and 1.5%, respectively, were definitive.

Idusuyi and Morrey[121] documented 32 postoperative peroneal nerve palsies in a retrospective review of 10,361 consecutive TKAs performed at the Mayo Clinic. They demonstrated that epidural anesthesia for postoperative control of pain was significantly associated with peroneal nerve palsy. They postulated that the decrease in proprioception and sensation postoperatively allows the limb to rest in an unprotected state, thereby making it susceptible to neurological ischemia from local compression. Although this association has not been documented in HTO, the neurological status of the patient should be carefully monitored if epidural anesthesia is used postoperatively. External rotation of the limb should be avoided to decrease the pressure on the nerve where it courses around the head of the fibula. The anesthesia should not produce prolonged sensory and motor blockade.

The peroneus superficialis nerve could also be damaged when the fibular osteotomy is performed distally. The nerve should be carefully avoided at the time of the fascial incision.[154]

The technique of the tibial osteotomy itself also influences the rate of neurological complications. Fierl et al[79] and Sabo et al[242] retrospectively investigated 132 cases of closing wedge HTOs using an external fixation device. When the osteotomy was performed through consecutive drill holes of increasing diameter

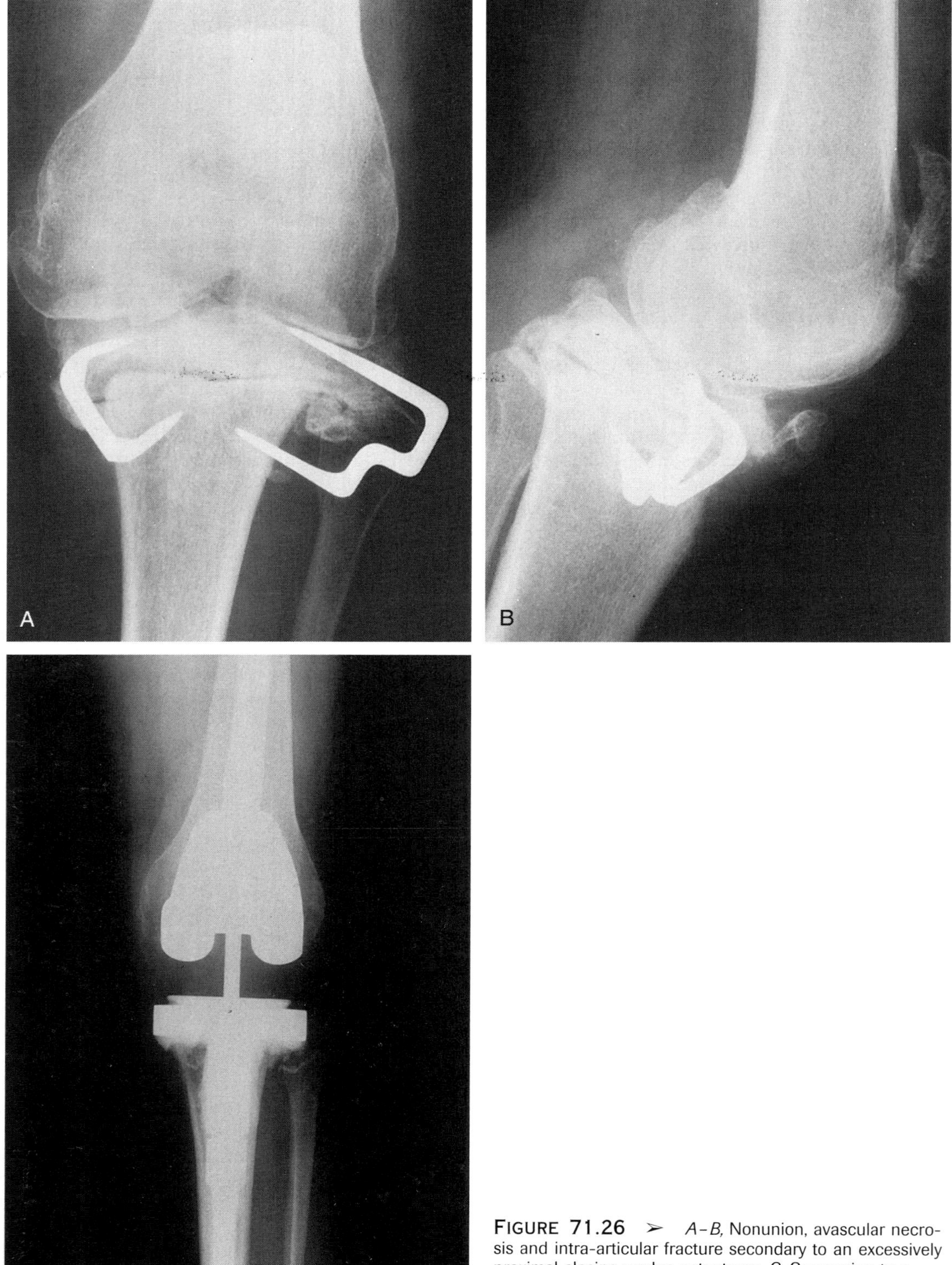

FIGURE 71.26 ➢ *A–B,* Nonunion, avascular necrosis and intra-articular fracture secondary to an excessively proximal closing wedge osteotomy. *C,* Conversion to a total knee arthroplasty, requiring the use of a custom-constrained condylar implant.

followed by osteoclasis, persistent neurological deficits were encountered in 4.7% of cases, as opposed to 12.4% of cases when the osteotomy was performed with an oscillating saw. They concluded that the reduction of neurological complications was related to the less extensive approach of the drilling technique. I prefer using bone chisels instead of an oscillating saw for closing wedge osteotomies, as the trajectory of the chisels is more easily controlled than that of a saw. Another advantage of chisels is that they do not cause any thermal damage to bone.

Compartment Syndrome

The exact incidence rate of compartment syndrome after HTO is not known.[87]

Several technical precautions can help to decrease this risk. The tibialis anterior muscle should not be damaged during the approach and should not be crushed by the retractors. The proximal tibia should be accessed subperiosteally. The tourniquet should be released before closure, and careful hemostasis should be performed. The fascial incision should not be tightly closed.[154] A suction drain should be left in place[87, 154, 177, 276] and, if a separate incision is made for the fibular osteotomy, the incision should also be drained. Tight dressings should be avoided. Epidural anesthesia can mask the signs of an impending ischemia. For that reason, I prefer to use patient-controlled analgesia rather than an epidural in the postoperative phase of HTO. If epidural anesthesia is used, the amount of local anesthetic that is given should be sufficient to make the patient comfortable without producing prolonged sensory and motor blockade, and the status of the leg should be even more closely observed.

If in doubt, the tissue pressure should be monitored. Impending tissue ischemia must be considered when the tissue pressure reaches between 30 and 10 mm Hg below the diastolic pressure. A higher pressure is a strong indication that fasciotomy should be undertaken.

Vascular Injury

Vascular injuries following osteotomy of the proximal tibia are rare. Two cases of false aneurysm of the popliteal artery after upper tibial osteotomy have been reported.[238] Lang et al[153] described a case of iatrogenic popliteal arteriovenous fistula after dome HTO. This complication was diagnosed following an angiography 8 weeks postoperatively and was surgically treated.

Zaidi et al[292] reported a case in which the popliteal artery was divided, although the osteotomy was performed with the knee at 90 degrees flexion. Using Doppler ultrasonography in ten healthy volunteers to define the relationship of popliteal artery to the back of the tibia and to assess the protection afforded by flexing the knee, they demonstrated that the distance between the popliteal artery and the posterior tibial cortex varied from 3.9 mm to 10.8 mm in normal knees in full extension. This distance became smaller with 90 degrees flexion in 12 knees and minimally larger in the other 8. They also stressed that, although in most cases the artery is protected by the bulk of the popliteus muscle, in a minority of cases high branching implies that the anterior tibial artery is closely applied to the tibia anterior to this muscle.

Haddad et al[98] treated an arteriovenous fistula of the peroneal artery acquired after a dome osteotomy with midshaft fibular osteotomy. This was undetected at first and presented as a recurrent hemarthrosis after a total knee replacement. It was treated by percutaneous embolization. To avoid this complication, Haddad et al recommended that fibular osteotomy should be carried out as distally and in the least traumatic manner as possible.

Thromboembolic Disease

In a review of the English-language literature, Heatley et al[105] found 19 cases of pulmonary embolism, 5 of them fatal, among 1647 upper tibial osteotomies: an incidence rate of emboli of 1.2% and a mortality rate of 0.3%. The reported incidence rate of deep-vein thrombosis was 2.8%, which is very low in relation to the number of emboli. This low incidence rate can be explained by the sparse recourse to ultrasonography or venography in the reviewed series. Matthews et al[181] reported an incidence rate of clinical thrombosis of 6%.

Turner et al[267] performed postoperative venography on 84 consecutive patients who had undergone upper tibial osteotomy and demonstrated deep-vein thrombosis in 41%. Only 15% of the cases were diagnosed clinically, all in the calf veins, whereas 3 proximal thromboses and 12 mixed-vein thromboses were only revealed by venography. One nonfatal pulmonary embolism also occurred in this series, in which prophylaxis with heparin 5000 IU, given subcutaneously, was delayed until the second postoperative day.

Leclerc et al[157] randomly assigned a consecutive cohort of 129 patients undergoing knee arthroplasty or tibial osteotomy into two groups. In the first group, 30 mg enoxaparin was administered subcutaneously every 12 hours, generally starting on the morning of the first postoperative day; the patients in the second group received an identical-looking placebo. Deep vein thrombosis was detected by either venography or noninvasive tests in 58% of patients in the placebo group and in 17% of patients in the enoxaparin group. Proximal vein thrombosis was found in 19% of the placebo patients and in none of the enoxaparin patients. There were no differences in bleeding complications or in the amount of blood loss. One patient in the placebo group developed nonfatal pulmonary embolism.

Routine prophylaxis with low-molecular-weight heparin, starting 12 hours before surgery, has been my standard postoperative regimen for the last 10 years, in the aftercare of patients undergoing major surgery of the lower limbs, and I have not detected increased bleeding secondary to this protocol. I strongly recommend the use of some form of thromboembolic prophylaxis following osteotomy.

Revision Surgery for Late Failure of HTO

Numerous reports deal with revision of failed HTO. Most describe the results and the technical pitfalls of revision using a TKA,[9, 16, 26, 88, 109, 115, 142, 151, 159, 179, 191, 192, 202, 245, 250, 265, 268, 284] but some of them also consider the possibility of repeated osteotomy[108, 245] and of revision with a unicompartmental knee arthroplasty.[245]

Based on the existing literature, I suggest some answers to the following questions: What are the indications for the different revision procedures available? What technical mistakes at the time of osteotomy will make the revision difficult? What tips at the time of repeated surgery can ease the revision? What results can be expected from the revision of a valgus tibial osteotomy?

The largest series of repeated surgeries after failed HTO, including 225 knees, was reported at the 1991 annual meeting of the Société Française de Chirurgie Orthopédique et Traumatologique.[245] This report is, with the exception of the iterative osteotomies reported by Hernigou,[108] the only one specifically dealing with techniques other than TKA to revise a failed HTO. This series includes 48 repeated osteotomies, 25 unicompartmental knee arthroplasties, 11 bicompartmental arthroplasties, and 141 TKAs. The authors confirm the good results of repeated HTO also reported by Hernigou. The condition for a successful repeated proximal tibia valgus osteotomy is that the failure of the initial osteotomy was exclusively secondary to undercorrection or loss of correction. Other causes of failure, like inflammatory joint disease, chondrocalcinosis, painful femoropatellar arthritis, and lateral compartment degradation, should be ruled out. Reiterated osteotomy is also indicated in cases of severe hypercorrection (Fig. 71.27). In this situation, the second osteotomy should be performed early to prevent the advent of degenerative changes in the lateral compartment. This is less difficult if the first osteotomy was an opening wedge. In this case, a medial closing wedge is the right solution. When the hypercorrection was secondary to a closing wedge osteotomy, correction with a lateral opening wedge exposes to the risk of peroneal nerve palsy, whereas a medial closing wedge increases the proximal tibial bone loss. A dome osteotomy could be an appropriate compromise for solving this difficult problem.

Revision with a unicompartmental knee arthroplasty gave good or excellent results in 24 of the 25 cases reported in this series. The prerequisites are roughly the same as for repeated valgus osteotomy, with the added condition of a normal ACL. The other factors being identical, a more advanced age could push the indication toward a unicompartmental or a TKA, whereas this series and the one reported by Hernigou[108] demonstrate that, provided a strict selection is made, repeated osteotomy may be the appropriate solution in the young, active patient.

From the group of total or bicompartmental arthroplasties in this series, no clear conclusions can be drawn concerning the choice of the implant except that hinge prosthesis should definitely be abandoned. From the other series of condylar TKAs after failed HTO available, it is not possible to affirm the superiority of cruciate-retaining or cruciate-substituting designs for revision of HTO.

Several factors can make revision of a tibial osteotomy a difficult procedure. Most of them can be avoided by a proper realization of the osteotomy. They include previous incisions, flexion contracture, decreased range of motion, patella infera, epiphyseal malrotation or translation, hypercorrection, severe alteration of the normal posterior tibial slope, nonunion, avascular necrosis, sepsis, peroneal nerve palsy, collateral ligament laxity, and hardware removal.

The incision for a tibial osteotomy should be performed in such a manner that it will not complicate a future TKA. A midline or close-to-midline longitudinal incision should be chosen in order to allow the same incision to be used at the time of revision.

The fixation of the osteotomy should be stable in order to authorize immediate motion and to avoid secondary displacement. Indications for combined valgus and rotation osteotomies are exceptional in arthritic knees; when severe patellofemoral pain in a medial arthritic knee is involved, a TKA should be performed directly.

The shape of the wedge should be calculated in order to keep the posterior tibial slope within the normal range. One should not attempt to correct a flexion deformity through an extension osteotomy. A flexion deformity exceeding 15 degrees contraindicates a tibial osteotomy. A minor flexion contracture can usually be solved by resecting the anterior and intercondylar osteophytes.[245]

Nonunion and avascular necrosis are often due to a too-thin proximal tibial fragment,[125] and care should be taken to osteotomize the tibia at least 2 cm distal to the joint line.

If the anatomy of the peroneal nerve and of its branches is taken into account, the rate of neurological complications can be significantly lowered, provided there is adequate surgical technique and postoperative care.

Hypercorrection is the main cause of collateral ligament instability at reoperation. This stresses the imperative necessity of accurate preoperative planning and a reliable operation.

Large fixation devices such as blade plates generally need to be removed at the time of revision. If the skin incision was adequate at the time of the osteotomy, hardware removal and knee arthroplasty can be performed in one session; otherwise the removal and the arthroplasty should be staged.

The infection rate is increased when using transfixion pins, and if this technique is used, a strict aftercare protocol is mandatory. When in doubt at the time of revision, torpid bone infection can be diagnosed by resorting to C-reactive protein determination, magnetic resonance imaging,[266] or leucocyte scintigraphy.[152, 236, 241]

Now consider the solutions to the technical difficul-

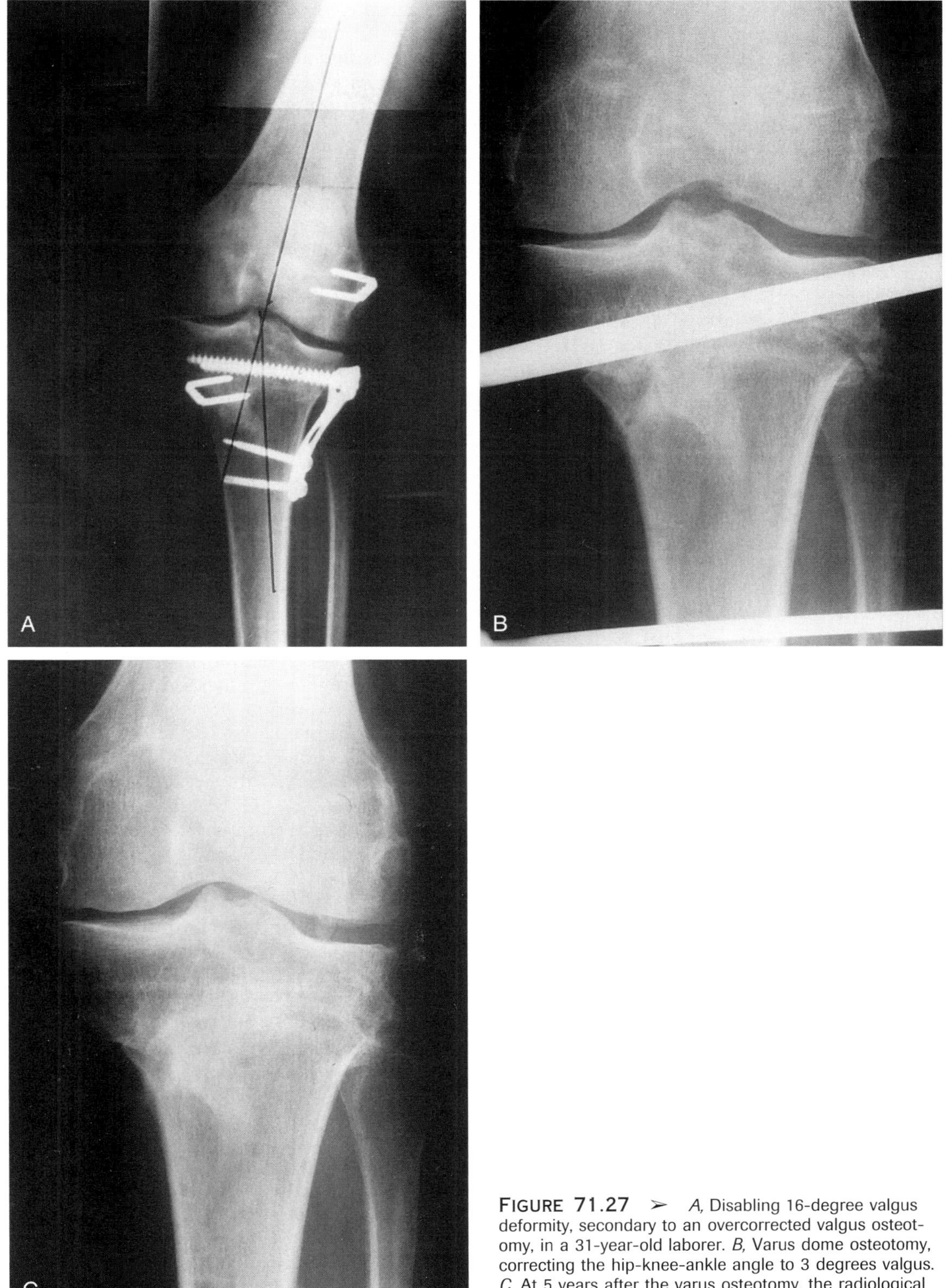

FIGURE 71.27 ➢ *A,* Disabling 16-degree valgus deformity, secondary to an overcorrected valgus osteotomy, in a 31-year-old laborer. *B,* Varus dome osteotomy, correcting the hip-knee-ankle angle to 3 degrees valgus. *C,* At 5 years after the varus osteotomy, the radiological and clinical outcome remains good.

ties that can be faced when performing a TKA in a knee in which a previous suboptimal proximal tibial osteotomy has been done.

A midline longitudinal incision should be used, regardless of whether the previous osteotomy was through a lateral, longitudinal, or short horizontal incision.[284] When the osteotomy scar is lateral longitudinal, close to the midline, it can be reopened to enter the joint medially, raising a short skin flap, or laterally through the approach described by Buechel.[30] Segal et al[245] advise the use of this lateral approach, particularly when the reason for failure of the tibial osteotomy is hypercorrection, as it allows the removal of the hardware through the same incision, to correct the valgus deformity without creating excessive instability, to medially displace the patella if needed, and to close the joint with the fat pad if the lateral retinaculum is left open. Because of soft-tissue scarring, subperiosteal exposure of the proximal tibia is more difficult in the postosteotomy knee, and the dissection should be performed with a scalpel rather than with a periosteal elevator or an osteotome.[142, 192, 284] If a medial approach is used, care should be taken to extend the incision to the tibial periosteum 1 cm medial to the tibial tubercle in order to leave a cuff of tissue that helps prevent inadvertent avulsion of the patellar ligament.[284]

Eversion of the patella can be difficult in a knee that has had a previous osteotomy because of scarring, patella infera, or, after a closing wedge osteotomy, the decreased distance from the tubercle to the joint line.[191, 244] A lateral retinacular release early in the operation may facilitate eversion.[191, 202, 284] In some instances, this will not be sufficient, and a decision should be taken among three options: a quadriceps snip,[86, 126, 127] a quadriceps turndown,[88, 191, 192, 284] or a tubercle osteotomy.[142, 159, 202, 245] This choice seems to be mainly a matter of personal preference, although in the specific situation of a failed tibial osteotomy, tibial tubercle elevation seems more logical, as it allows to correct the iatrogenic patella baja.

After a closing wedge osteotomy, the bone stock available from the proximal part of the tibia is reduced, and extra care should be taken to resect the least amount of bone from the tibial plateau that is necessary to obtain a satisfactory surface for fixation of the tibial component. Severe defects in the lateral plateau may require bone grafting[191, 284] or metal wedges.[126] Angulation of the tibial plateau in the sagittal plane may have been significantly altered. In case of tibial recurvatum, even if care is taken not to overresect the proximal tibia, the tibial insertion of PCL may be divided. This situation is best treated with a cruciate-substituting implant.[126, 245]

In case of epiphyseal translation[159, 202] or truncated metaphysis,[142, 191] the use of prostheses that have a tibial component with a central peg may result in impingement of the tip of the peg on the lateral part of the tibial cortex. A custom-made tibial component[284] or an offset stem may be needed to accommodate the altered anatomy of the tibia.

In severe cases, a second osteotomy to reverse the extra-articular deformity produced by the first osteotomy may be required.[35, 191, 245] This is the case when facing a hypercorrection of more than 10 degrees. Cameron and Welsh[35] advise performing a dome osteotomy to prevent further shortening of the extremity and an osteotomy of the fibula to permit adequate correction. A stemmed component should be used to bridge the osteotomy site,[35, 268] if the reosteotomy and the arthroplasty are carried out at the same time, although some authors[89] have advised, in the same operative session, to implant the prosthesis first, regardless of the deformity, and to correct the axis afterward by a second osteotomy.

Ligament imbalance is especially prevalent in knees with overcorrected valgus. Krackow and Holtgrewe[151] have developed a complex ligament reconstruction for this subset of patients to allow simultaneous implantation of a minimally constrained total knee prosthesis. This reconstruction associates advancement of the MCL and of the PCL and posteromedial capsule. In the described series of five patients, although the preoperative femorotibial alignment averaged 25 degrees valgus, the postoperative alignment and function were comparable to that with a standard primary TKA. The series available are too small to give clear guidelines about when a lateral approach, a ligament reconstruction, or a second osteotomy should be performed.

Diverging conclusions have been presented concerning the outcome of TKA after HTO. Several authors[9, 16, 179, 202, 250] have reported that the results of TKA after HTO are comparable to the results of primary TKA. In contrast other groups[109, 142, 192, 284] have cited inferior results, with an increased incidence rate of complications and technical pitfalls.

As HTO and unicompartmental arthroplasty are often in competition, Jackson et al[134] and Gill et al[88] compared the results of revision arthroplasty following these two procedures. The results of these two studies were conflicting. Jackson et al reported a higher complication rate in the post-tibial osteotomy group, mainly because of wound healing problems. This stresses again the importance of planning the osteotomy, including the skin incision, with a future total knee in mind. On the contrary, Gill et al estimated that difficulty with exposure was not significantly greater in the osteotomy group and concluded that the functional level, complication rate, and technical results of revision TKA following unicompartmental knee arthroplasty for the initial treatment of unicompartmental arthritis approached, but did not equal, those obtained after HTO.

Although this is not formally established, I agree with the conclusions reached by Segal et al,[245] who inferred from a review of 225 revisions for failed HTOs that the results of revision are affected mainly when the initial osteotomy was incorrectly performed and, more specifically, when hypercorrection exceeded 10 degrees of mechanical valgus. Like Staheli et al,[250] my opinion is that an HTO, properly performed, does not "burn any bridges" insofar as a future arthroplasty is concerned (Fig. 71.28). The long-term fixation of the tibial component after failure of a tibial osteotomy should not be a concern, as Toksvig et al,[265] using roentgen stereophotogrammetric analysis, demonstrated that there was no difference in the prosthetic fixation for implants after primary TKA and for implants after TKA secondary to failed closing wedge osteotomy.

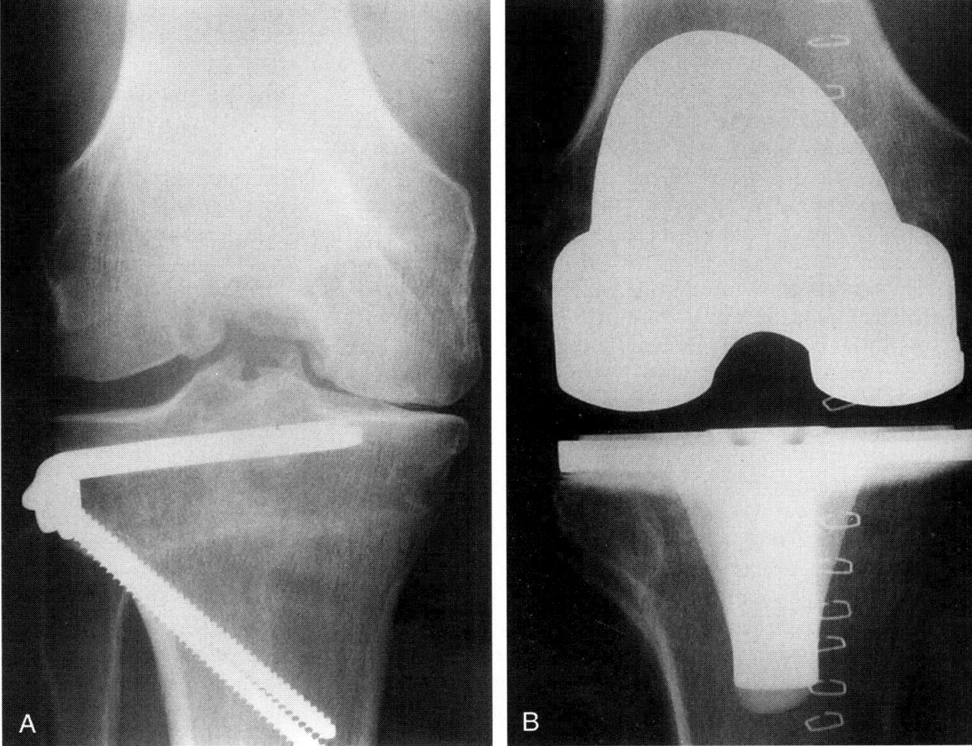

FIGURE 71.28 ➢ *A,* Late failure of a closing wedge high tibial osteotomy, internally fixed with a Giebel blade plate. *B,* Uneventful one-step conversion to a TKA.

Results and Conclusions

The results of HTO have been extensively studied and reported over the past 40 years. Insall[125] and Healy and Wilk[104] reviewed the experience of those first 3 decades.

The main conclusions that Insall drew from his review were the following:

1. Following an HTO, pain recurs in most knees, and most will eventually require TKA.[181]
2. Younger patients with moderate varus deformities give the best results; obesity, undercorrection, and overcorrection[51, 181] are adverse factors.
3. The ideal correction is a femorotibial angle between 170 degrees and 165 degrees.
4. The overall preoperative state of the knee is the most important determinant of an eventual good result.[118]
5. Preoperative arthroscopic assessment of the knee is not useful.[143]
6. Previous medial meniscectomy[212] and anterior cruciate deficiency are not contraindications, but previous lateral meniscectomy may be.
7. The addition of tibial tubercle elevation to the osteotomy in the case of associated patellofemoral arthritis is not necessary, and it increases the complication rate.[119, 203]

Taking into account the reports of the last decade, my opinion remains very similar to that of Insall, although some complementary information has been added, most of which has been developed in the previous paragraphs.

The negative influence of the passage of time on the results of high tibial osteotomy has been repeatedly confirmed.[18, 27, 58, 108, 131, 163, 208, 237, 252, 288, 289]

However, it does not appear clearly from the long-term follow-up studies available that a TKA will be the end point for the majority of the osteotomized knees, but rather that a conversion to TKA will be necessary in 5% to 15% of the osteotomized knees (although some authors report a relatively higher revision rate of about 20% to 25% at 10 years[17, 58]). Holden et al,[118] in a group of 51 proximal tibial valgus osteotomies reviewed with an average follow-up of 10 years, reported that 3 knees needed revision to a total arthroplasty. In a retrospective study of 128 osteoarthritic knees treated by valgus HTO, Rudan and Simurda[240] reported a relatively low revision rate of 10.9% over 15 years. Bouharras et al[27] reported 4 conversions to TKAs in a group of 118 HTOs with an average follow-up of 8 years. Hernigou[108] reported 15 TKAs following 93 osteotomies with a minimal follow-up of 20 years. Ivarsson et al[131] reported 8 reoperations in a group of 65 knees reviewed at a mean of 11.9 years. Levigne and Bonnin,[162] in a study group of 217 osteotomies with an average follow-up of 9 years, reported 17 reoperations, including 5 repeated osteotomies, 1 unicompartmental knee arthroplasty, and 11 TKAs. Lootvoet et al[163] analyzed the results of a series of 193 upper tibial valgus osteotomies reviewed with an average follow-up of 8 years. Fourteen knees were operated on again because of a failure of their osteotomy: 3 had a repeated osteotomy, 1 had a unicompartmental arthroplasty, and 10 had a TKA. Yasuda et al[288, 289] observed a group of 56 osteotomies at a 10- to 15-year follow-up and reported 4 conversions to TKA. Odenbring et al[208] reported the revision by reosteotomy or arthroplasty after tibial osteotomy in a consecutive series of 314 osteotomies at follow-up after 10 to 19 years: 52 knees had been revised by arthroplasty and 10 knees by reosteotomy.

The importance of precise postoperative alignment has been stressed in many reports.[3, 17, 58, 108, 119, 131, 143, 162, 163, 207, 208, 239, 240, 249, 269, 288, 289] However, there is no general agreement about the optimal postoperative femorotibial alignment. If one tries to define a consensus ideal postoperative hip-knee-ankle angle, the obtained value approximates 3 to 6 degrees valgus, although Yasuda et al[288, 289] recommend a larger overcorrection of up to 10 degrees valgus.

The influence of the preoperative grade of osteoarthritis on the long-term result of HTO has also been confirmed.[17, 27, 108, 131, 162, 163, 208, 239, 240] A preoperative Ahlbäck grade I or II is predictive of a good long-term result. Lootvoet et al[163] reported an 84% rate of good long-term results when the height of the preoperative medial joint space equaled or exceeded 50% of the normal height, whereas a narrowing greater than 50% reduced this rate to 60%. This is confirmed by the excellent long-term results of HTO in young patients with Ahlbäck grade I medial gonarthrosis reported by Odenbring et al.[212] By measuring the constitutional tibial varus, Lootvoet et al[163] and Levigne and Bonnin[161, 162] also demonstrated that when the cartilage lesion is secondary to bony deviation of the epiphysis in varus, a correction, even if incomplete, will immediately bring mechanical relief. On the other hand, when there is a primary degeneration of cartilage, this "sick" cartilage will not tolerate any undercorrection.

The negative influence of age, obesity, hip disease, inflammatory diseases, preoperative deformity exceeding 10 degrees varus, femorotibial subluxation, and postoperative immobilization was discussed earlier. The mutual relationships between patellofemoral joint disorders and HTO have also been analyzed as well as the advantages and disadvantages of the various osteotomy techniques and ways to deal with the fibula.

From the numerous reported series of HTOs, it is extremely difficult to draw a precise estimate of the quality of the long-term results of this procedure: the selection criteria, the surgical techniques, the postoperative evaluation and rating scales are extraordinarily disparate. Moreover, as most of the series are retrospective, very few have reported the results of this procedure in a selected cohort of "ideal" candidates by currently accepted standards. As rigorous comparison between the series is impossible, I want to conclude by quoting the results and conclusions of two long-term follow-up studies carried out by Odenbring et al. The first study[212] describes the function after HTO for medial gonarthrosis in a group of 27 patients (28 knees) between 27 and 50 years of age. Of the 27 patients, 25, with an average follow-up of 11 years, had experienced improvement or even great improvement, and 12 could participate in at least recreational exercise. Three-fifths gained a Lysholm[165] score of 84 points or more, and no revision to knee arthroplasty had been performed; sagittal instability or previous medial meniscectomy did not alter the results. This study demonstrates that HTO is a beneficial procedure for young patients with gonarthrosis, including the increasing group of patients with gonarthrosis secondary to meniscal and ligamentous lesions, even if these patients maintain their active lifestyle.

The second study[208] underlines the importance of the surgical accuracy and appropriate correction of the angular deformity, as the revision rate, in a group of 314 osteotomies at follow-up after 10 to 19 years, was 54/170 in undercorrected knees and 8/144 in normo- or overcorrected knees. These knees were affected by early stages of gonarthrosis (Ahlbäck stages I–III).

In summary, HTO for medial gonarthrosis is a successful procedure in active, relatively young patients, with a good preoperative function and a low stage of arthritis. The results are better if the preoperative deformity is secondary to varus deviation of the epiphysis rather than to medial wear of the joint. The axial correction should be accurate, and stable internal fixation with an early range of motion is advisable. The accuracy of the osteotomy and of its planning can be improved by a strict radiographic protocol, by the use of gait analysis and, in future, by computer-aided analysis[44] or by computer-assisted surgery.[227] The posterior tibial slope should not be altered by the osteotomy. Small corrections are easily performed with an opening wedge osteotomy. Closing wedge osteotomies are suitable for corrections of 10 to 15 degrees. In this case, a fibular shaft osteotomy seems biomechanically more logical than excision of the fibular head or division of the superior tibiofibular joint. The osteotomy of the fibula should be carefully performed at the junction of its middle and lower thirds. Given the risks related to transfixion pins, dome osteotomies should be set apart for the rare instances where a very large correction is necessary. Despite the remarkable results of knee arthroplasty, a place should remain for a surgical procedure aimed at maintaining the natural knee, as this effort goes in the direction of the development of conservative treatment of arthritis, which is clearly the way of the future.

TREATMENT FOR VALGUS DEFORMITY

Principles

Valgus deformity of the knee is usually secondary to a valgus orientation of the distal part of the femur with regard to its long axis.[47, 220, 291] In this case, the line tangent to the distal extent of the femoral condyles is tilted medially and distally. In order to bring the joint line parallel to the floor through osteotomy, the deformity has to be corrected where it lies, i.e., in the distal femur.[47, 104, 125, 247]

In some knees, the valgus deformity has a dual origin: the distal condyles are sloped medially, whereas the tibial plateau is sloped laterally.[161, 220] In these knees, if the deformity is mild and the correction less than 10 degrees, a tibial osteotomy can be successful.[14, 55, 66]

However, a tibial osteotomy should not be used for larger corrections, as the resultant tilt of the joint line would, in time, cause medial subluxation of the femur on the tibia,[99, 125, 247] whereas a tibial closing wedge osteotomy proximal to the tibial tubercle would create or increase laxity of the superficial medial ligament.[125]

Valgus deformities are better tolerated than varus deformities and develop arthritic changes later on.[154, 170] This is explained by the adduction moment that places the gravity forces predominantly on the medial compartment during gait.[10, 23, 90, 100, 138, 170, 172, 223, 261, 272] A severe valgus deformity is necessary to shift the gravity stresses toward the lateral compartment.[246] Moreover, in the varus knee, the adduction moment is counteracted by the contraction of the lateral muscles.[10, 23, 172, 174] This results in higher loading of the knee joint.[10] On the contrary, in the valgus knee, the activity of the lateral muscles may decrease,[154, 170] resulting in lower compressive forces across the joint.

A pathological ipsilateral hip joint can increase the stresses on the lateral compartment of the knee by two main mechanisms.[82, 125, 154, 232, 261] The gluteus major, the tensor fasciae latae, and the biceps act on the hip and the knee. If their activity is augmented in order to stabilize an abnormal hip, it will increase the compressive forces on the lateral compartment of the knee at the same time.[170] On the other hand, if the hip is abducted during the stance phase of gait, i.e., if the pelvis tilts upward on the unaffected side, the center of gravity of the body will be displaced laterally, also enhancing the stresses on the lateral compartment of the knee.[261] Therefore, whenever possible, a hip disorder should be treated before undertaking an osteotomy of the underlying knee.[125]

In varus knees, overcorrection is necessary because of the presence of an adduction moment during gait. On the contrary, in valgus knees, there is no need for hypercorrection, as it has been demonstrated that in a neutrally aligned knee most of the gravity forces are transmitted through the medial compartment.[10, 172, 174, 246] The goal of a varus osteotomy should be to bring the hip-knee-ankle angle close to 0 degrees.

Patient Selection

The criteria of age and activity level should be even more restrictive for femoral supracondylar varus osteotomy than for proximal tibial valgus osteotomy, because the time the bone takes to heal and the period of partial weight-bearing on crutches are longer.

Because lateral compartmental arthrosis usually develops later in life than medial compartmental arthrosis, it is often better tolerated and has a lower incidence rate,[6, 107] the indications for varus osteotomy of the knee are less frequent, and a TKA will often be preferred. The procedure should be performed relatively early in the disease process before severe compromise of function has occurred,[77, 180] and the arthrosis should be limited to the lateral compartment.[77, 78, 180]

Severe instability is a contraindication to osteotomy,[125] as there are no dynamic restraints to medial laxity, which will persist even if the alignment is correct. Extension loss of more than 15 degrees and flexion less than 90 degrees are also contraindications.[182, 195]

Hernigou et al,[110] in a retrospective study of 96 valgus arthritic knees, noticed that femoral osteotomy or lateral unicompartmental arthroplasty led to poor results if undertaken in the presence of a preoperative recurvatum. Recurvatum seldom occurs as a consequence of valgus gonarthrosis and appears at a late stage of arthritic evolution. At this stage, a TKA is the appropriate option.

Stubbs[253] described a specific pattern of valgus knees in which the degenerative changes are confined to the posterolateral portion of the knee. The symptoms often begin at a young age, the pain is posterolateral, and a history of trauma and a previous lateral meniscectomy are frequently noted. Bone-on-bone contact in the posterolateral corner of the knee can be seen with a posteroanterior flexion weightbearing view but is not detected with standing radiographs in extension. Based on three failures in three osteotomized knees, Stubbs considers that posterolateral arthritis of the knee may be a contraindication to valgus osteotomy, as this offers an angular solution for a rotatory problem.

Surgical Techniques

There are several techniques available for the correction of a valgus deformity at the femur. The surgical procedure may be performed from a lateral approach employing an opening wedge osteotomy, or a medial wedge can be resected from a medial approach. Supracondylar dome osteotomies,[281] V osteotomies,[5] and intercondylar osteotomies[63] have also been described. A medial closing wedge osteotomy is the most commonly used procedure (Fig. 71.29).

Medial Closing Wedge Supracondylar Osteotomy

The patient is placed in the supine position. A tourniquet is generally applied. A longitudinal medial or straight midline incision is made along the femur, beginning from just distal to the joint line and extending proximally for 15 cm. The fascia over the vastus medialis is incised, and the muscle is deflected forward and laterally. Dissection is carried distally to the joint capsule, but the joint is not entered. If the blade plate that is to be used is cannulated and guided by a wire,[84, 154, 221] the technique is very similar to that described for the closing wedge proximal tibial valgus osteotomy with internal fixation by blade plate (Fig. 71.30). The guide wire is inserted using a special jig, set for a predetermined amount of correction. The track for the blade is initiated, the desired wedge of

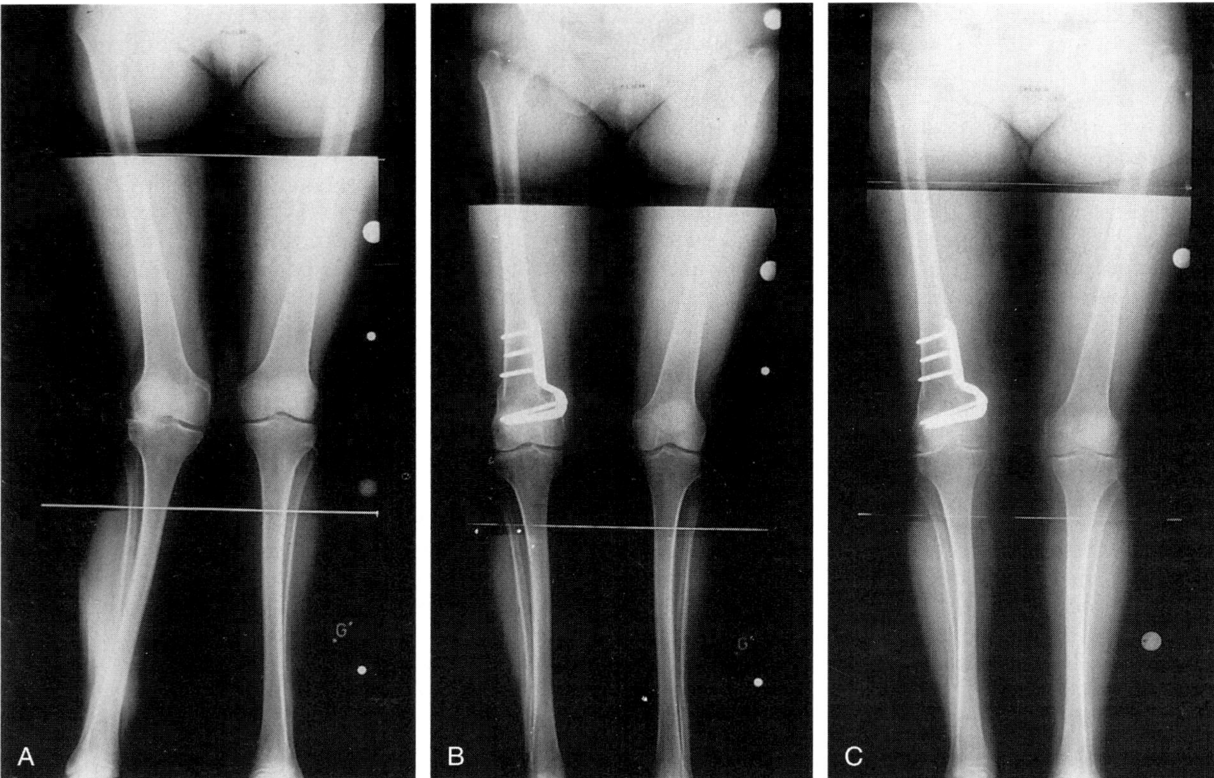

FIGURE 71.29 ➢ *A*, A 17-degree valgus deformity in a 55-year-old female. *B*, Bipodal standing radiograph at 9 months after medial closing wedge supracondylar osteotomy. *C*, Satisfactory radiological and functional result at 10 years.

bone is removed, the osteotomy is closed, and the blade plate is driven over the guide wire and fixed to the femoral cortex with screws. The obtained angular correction is the complementary angle between the angle set on the guide and the 90-degree angle of the blade plate. More often than not, the blade plate used is not cannulated and is a AO-type 90-degree offset dynamic-compression blade plate.[182] The correction relies in this case on the accurate positioning of pins under fluoroscopic control, but special jigs have also been designed in order to guide a 90-degree AO blade plate.[156] The first pin guides the osteotomy blade plate. It is inserted across the distal femoral metaphysis, approximately 2.5 cm proximal to the femoral articular surfaces, using fluoroscopy. McDermott et al[182] advises placing the blade parallel to the articular surfaces. This results in approximately 6 degrees of mechanical varus, which seems excessive, as already discussed. I believe the guiding pin should not be strictly parallel to the joint line, but slightly oblique distally and laterally, which is facilitated by using a guide. A second pin is then placed proximally across the diaphysis, perpendicular to the long axis of the femur. These first two pins should become parallel at the end of the procedure. Then two pins are inserted, with the help of a goniometer or templates, to figure the wedge which will be removed. The proximal side of the wedge is perpendicular to the shaft of the femur. Care should be taken to keep a medial cortical bridge of at least 2 cm between the osteotomy line and the blade. An oscillating saw is used to perform the osteotomy. The lateral cortex is weakened with a thin osteotome but is not interrupted with the saw. As mentioned by Insall,[125] there is a tendency to overestimate the necessary wedge, which leads to overcorrection. It is wiser to start with a slightly thinner osteotomy than might ultimately be required.[195] If a greater correction is necessary, this can usually be obtained by crutching the distal femur in the softer metaphyseal bone rather than by taking additional bone from the distal segment. The blade plate is driven across the distal metaphysis along the line of the initially placed pin, and the wedge is closed by manually exerting a varus force on the knee. Before an AO angled blade plate can be inserted into bone, a channel must be drilled and precut with the U-profile chisel. This is performed more easily before completion of the osteotomy. Three to four screws secure the plate to the femur. The removed bone can serve as a graft. The tourniquet is released, careful hemostasis is performed, a suction drain is placed, and the wound is closed.

Continuous passive motion is started immediately, and weightbearing is restricted until bony union is confirmed on radiographs.

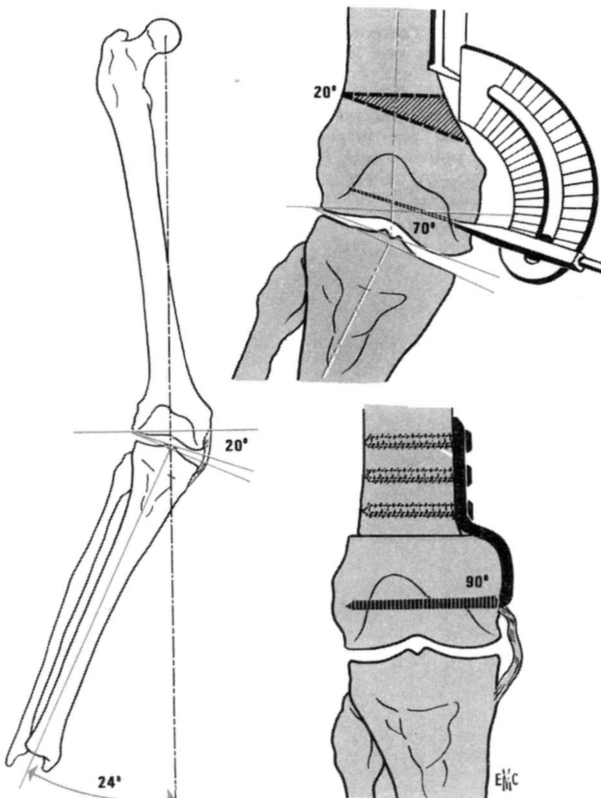

FIGURE 71.30 ➢ Medial closing wedge supracondylar osteotomy with the use of a cannulated blade plate, guided by a wire. In this case, the 24-degree valgus deformity is secondary to a 20-degree distal femoral valgus deviation and to a 4-degree medial laxity. If the goal is to bring the hip-knee-ankle angle to 0 degrees, the correction and the resected wedge should be 20 degrees. The jig used to insert the guide wire should be set at 70 degrees because the blade-plate has a 90-degree angle. (From Langlais F, Thomazeau H: Ostéotomies du genou. In Encyclopédie médico-chirurgicale. Paris, Editions scientifiques et médicales Elsevier, 1989, p 1.)

Lateral Opening Wedge Supracondylar Osteotomy

This technique has been described by Postel and Langlais[221] and by Langlais and Thomazeau.[154] It requires a lateral approach and the use of a guided blade plate angled at 95 degrees (Fig. 71.31). The patient is in the lateral position. The lateral side of the distal femur is exposed by a straight lateral approach, reflecting the vastus lateralis anteriorly. Using a jig, the guide wire is inserted in the epiphysis, 20 to 30 mm proximal to the joint line. As the blade plate has a 95-degree angle, the angle between the guide wire and the lateral femoral cortex should equal the sum of the desired correction and 95 degrees. This wire should be parallel to the axis of flexion of the knee. Another wire figures the osteotomy line, which should leave a lateral cortical bridge of 25 mm proximal to the blade. The position of these two wires is checked under fluoroscopy. The osteotomy is performed with an oscillating saw, keeping the medial cortex intact temporarily. The blade plate is inserted on the guide wire and partly driven into the epiphyseal bone, and the osteotomy is completed using thin chisels. The insertion of the blade plate is achieved, opening the wedge laterally. Impaction can be realized manually by striking the flexed knee. The plate is fixed to the femur by three screws in the proximal fragment and one additional screw in the distal fragment. An AO 95-degree condylar blade plate can also be used, losing the advantage offered by the "automatic" correction. This opening wedge osteotomy does not require autologous bone grafting, as medial impaction is created. It should not be used for corrections greater than 15 to 20 degrees, given the risk of stretching the peroneal nerve. Postoperative care is similar to that of closing wedge osteotomy.

Complications

Supracondylar femoral osteotomy is technically demanding and is not frequently performed. It has, therefore, a rather high rate of complications.

Teinturier et al,[259] in a series of 131 lateral supracondylar osteotomies, reported four infections treated by removal of the blade plate, one nonunion successfully treated by iterative plating, and five deep-vein thromboses. Weill and Jacquemin,[281] in a series of 39 dome supracondylar varus osteotomies internally fixed by a lateral blade plate, reported one nonunion, one fracture secondary to a subsequent trauma, one hypocorrection with early reintervention, and one severe loss of motion. Aglietti et al,[5] in a preliminary report of 14 V-shaped supracondylar osteotomies followed by an immobilization period of 8 weeks, did not report any complication. Edgerton et al,[77, 195] in a group of 24 knees treated by supracondylar osteotomies usually fixed by staples, reported complications in 15 patients (63%). These included a pin-tract infection in one patient treated with an external fixator, loss of correction and failure of fixation in nine patients, and delayed or nonunion in seven patients. McDermott et al,[182] out of 24 medial closing wedge supracondylar osteotomies, reported one failure of fixation that required reoperation, one manipulation for stiffness at 6 months postoperatively, one superficial wound infection, and one nonfatal pulmonary embolism.

Learmonth[156] had no complications in 12 consecutive valgus knees corrected by a femoral closing wedge osteotomy performed with the help of a special jig.

Cameron et al,[33] reporting on 49 consecutive patients treated by supracondylar varus closing wedge osteotomy stabilized with a blade plate, had six cases of delayed union, one loss of fixation, and one rotatory deformity. All delayed unions were successfully treated with lateral compression plating and occasionally with autogenous bone grafting from the iliac crest.[32] Healy et al[103] evaluated the results of 23 distal femoral varus osteotomies and reported two nonunions, one fracture, and one stiffness that necessitated a manipulation under anesthesia. Mathews et al,[180] in a group of 21 supracondylar osteotomies, had a complication rate of 57%, including severe knee stiff-

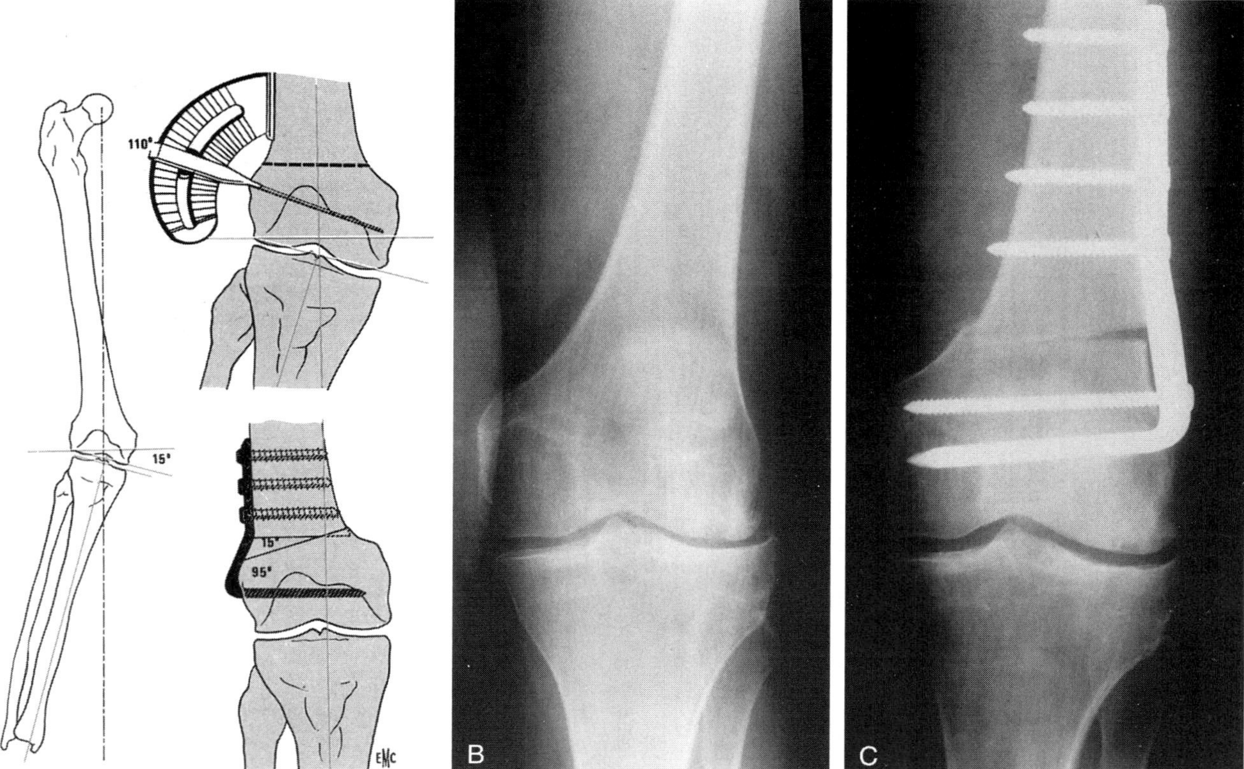

FIGURE 71.31 ➢ *A,* Lateral opening wedge osteotomy with the use of a cannulated blade plate guided by a wire. In the absence of medial laxity, the correction should equal the preoperative valgus deformity. Because the blade plate has a 95-degree angle, the jig should be set at 110 degrees to correct a 15-degree valgus deformity. (From Langlais F, Thomazeau H: Ostéotomies du genou. In Encyclopédie médico-chirurgicale. Paris, Editions scientifiques et médicales Elsevier, 1989, p 1.) *B,* 9-degree valgus deformity in a 44-year-old female. *C,* Immediate postoperative x-ray film demonstrates the medial impaction and the lateral opening created by the osteotomy.

ness requiring manipulation under anesthesia (48%), nonunion/delayed union (19%), infection (10%), and fixation failure (5%). Five knees (19%) required total knee replacement within 5 years of surgery.

Mironneau[188] analyzed the results of 28 supracondylar osteotomies, including 5 closing wedges, 4 opening wedges, and 19 domes, all fixed by a blade plate. The morbidity rate was high, with three losses of fixation, one fracture, one nonunion, and one arthrofibrosis.

The reported complication rate is variable and is certainly technique-dependent. As stated by Aglietti et al,[5] avoiding entering the knee joint should reduce the incidence rate of stiffness. A rigid internal fixation is mandatory, given the high rate of loss of fixation and nonunion when staples are used. It is not certain whether the fixation provided by a medial blade plate is sufficient, and one could look for better implants. The use of an oscillating saw could increase the risk of nonunion, because of its thermal effect, and osteotomes or special saw blades with irrigation should be used. The lateral cortex should not be interrupted when performing a closing wedge osteotomy, and this could be eased by the use of a device for progressive closure of the osteotomy. McDermott et al[182] feared that the use of the outrigger AO compression could endanger the femoral vessels in the Hunter canal, but a compression clamp similar to the ones designed for closing wedge HTO could be efficient to close the resection site in a slow, controlled manner while under compression. The use of the resected bone as a graft is recommended.

Results of Supracondylar Osteotomy

There are few reports that allow a clear estimation of the anticipated results of supracondylar osteotomy—the series are small, and the average of follow-ups is short. The average follow-up in the series of McDermott et al[182] was 4 years. It was 2 years in Aglietti and Buzzi's series,[2] 4 years for Healy and Wilk,[103] 3.5 years for Cameron et al,[33] 41 months for Learmonth,[156] and 3 years for Teinturier et al[259] and Mathews et al.[180]

Despite a high complication rate, the reported long-term results are generally good. Mironneau[188] reported 8 excellent, 13 good, 4 fair, and 3 poor results in 28 patients, with an average 7-year follow-up. He stated that the key factor was a precise axial correction and recommended bringing the mechanical axis to neutral,

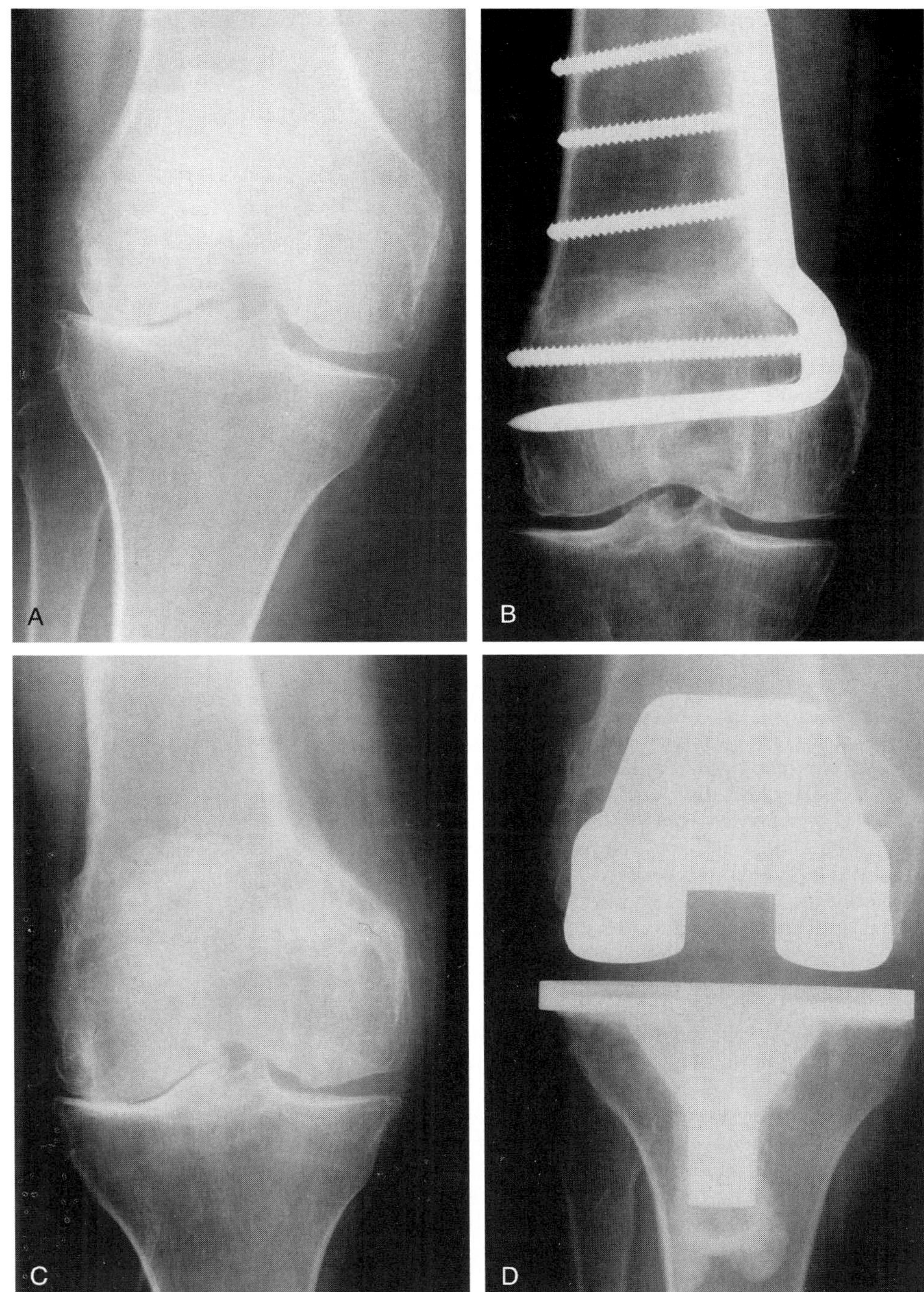

FIGURE 71.32 ➢ *A,* Severe lateral gonarthrosis in a 57-year-old female. *B,* Result of a medial closing wedge osteotomy at 1 year. *C,* Deterioration at 11 years. *D,* Successful conversion to a TKA.

except in the case of medial laxity. In this situation, some hypercorrection is necessary. In the presence of medial laxity and severe wear of the lateral tibial plateau, an arthroplasty rather than an osteotomy should be performed.

Cognet et al[46] reported the results of 75 closing wedge supracondylar osteotomies fixed by a guided blade plate, with an average follow-up of 8.7 years (range 5 to 14 years). The mechanical axis at follow-up was 0.1 degrees varus. Of all the patients, 77% were satisfied or very satisfied. The ideal candidate is active, has less than 15 degrees of flexion contracture, and has an isolated lateral arthritis at an Ahlback[6] stage inferior or equal to stage II.

Terry and Cimino[260] monitored a series of 36 knees for an average of 5.4 years, on which a medial closing wedge (14 knees) or a lateral opening wedge osteotomy with bone grafting (22 knees) had been performed. Postoperative correction of the anatomic axis averaged 3.8 degrees valgus, with a wide dispersion (range from 8 degrees varus to 20 degrees valgus). Pain decreased or resolved in 21 of 35 knees (60%), and activity level improved in 24 of 35 knees (69%). One patient was unavailable for follow-up evaluation.

Using the Hospital for Special Surgery knee score in a group of 24 knees with an average follow-up of 8.3 years (range 5 to 11 years), Edgerton et al[77] reported 71% good or excellent results. The severity of the disease was a statistically significant prognostic factor, as reflected by the pre- and postoperative knee scores. The results were better when the disease was limited to the lateral compartment. This study did not document a tendency for a good result, once attained, to deteriorate with time, in contrast to the experience with proximal tibial osteotomy for varus deformity.

Finkelstein et al[78] monitored 21 knees long-term or until failure. At an average follow-up of 11 years, 13 osteotomies were still successful, 7 had failed, and 1 patient had died. The probability of survival at 10 years was 64%. All of the patients who had a failure subsequently underwent a TKA. The three early failures were attributed to poor selection of patients or failure of the fixation. The remaining four patients who had a failure were able to function for 72 to 98 months before they needed a conversion to a TKA. The authors did not find that a previous varus osteotomy of the distal part of the femur made a subsequent TKA more technically demanding, in contrast with Beyer et al,[19] who reported increased technical difficulty when total joint arthroplasty was performed after supracondylar varus osteotomy. Cameron and Park[34] reviewed eight cases of total knee replacement following supracondylar varus femoral osteotomy and stated that, although in each case the distal femur was offset medially on the femoral diaphysis, it did not prove difficult to achieve correct mechanical alignment. Cameron and Park advised hardware removal 6 months before total knee replacement. They stressed the importance of carefully templating the position of the femoral guidance system and of carrying out an intraoperative radiograph of the femoral guidance rod if there is any doubt about its accurate positioning. In these three series of conversion of supracondylar osteotomies to TKA, the ultimate result of arthroplasty was not compromised (Fig. 71.32).

From these reports, it appears that, with proper selection of patients, exact correction of the femorotibial alignment, and stable fixation, varus osteotomy of the distal part of the femur is a reliable and effective procedure for the treatment of gonarthrosis of the lateral compartment in valgus knees. The ideal candidate is physiologically young and active, has an isolated grade I or II lateral compartmental arthrosis, and has good preoperative function and range of motion. The candidate should not have recurvatum, posterolateral arthritis, marked medial laxity, or severe wear of the lateral tibial plateau. These criteria are very stringent and will be attained by a limited number of patients, most valgus arthritic knees being more suitable for a total knee replacement.

References

1. Wright TM, Goodman SB, eds: Implant Wear: The Future of Total Joint Replacement. Chicago, American Academy of Orthopaedic Surgeons, 1996.
2. Aglietti P, Buzzi R: Idiopathic osteonecrosis of the knee. Ital J Orthop Traumatol 1984; 10:217.
3. Aglietti P, Buzzi R, Gaudenzi A, et al: [Accuracy in high tibial osteotomy in varus gonarthrosis]. Arch Putti Chir Organi Mov 1989; 37:271.
4. Aglietti P, Rinonapoli E, Stringa G, et al: Tibial osteotomy for the varus osteoarthritic knee. Clin Orthop 1983; 176:239.
5. Aglietti P, Stringa G, Buzzi R, et al: Correction of valgus knee deformity with a supracondylar V osteotomy. Clin Orthop 1987; 217:214.
6. Ahlback S: Osteoarthrosis of the knee: A radiographic investigation. Acta Radiol (Stockh) 1968; 227(S):1.
7. Ahlberg A, Scham S, Unander SL: Osteotomy in degenerative and rheumatoid arthritis of the knee joint. Acta Orthop Scand 1968; 39:379.
8. Akamatsu Y, Koshino T, Saito T, et al: Changes in osteosclerosis of the osteoarthritic knee after high tibial osteotomy. Clin Orthop 1997; 334:207.
9. Amendola A, Rorabeck CH, Bourne RB, et al: Total knee arthroplasty following high tibial osteotomy for osteoarthritis. J Arthroplasty 1989; 4(S):11.
10. Andriacchi TP: Dynamics of knee malalignment. Orthop Clin North Am 1994; 25:395.
11. Augereau B: [Radiological assessment before femoral and tibial osteotomies]. Ann Radiol Paris 1993; 36:252.
12. Aydogdu S, Sur H: [High tibial osteotomy for varus deformity of more than 20 degrees]. Rev Chir Orthop Reparatrice Appar Mot 1997; 84:439.
13. Bae DK, Mun MS, Kwon OS: A newly designed miniplate staple for high tibial osteotomy. Bull Hosp Jt Dis 1997; 56:167.
14. Bauer GC, Insall J, Koshino T: Tibial osteotomy in gonarthrosis (osteoarthritis of the knee). J Bone Joint Surg Am 1969; 51: 1545.
15. Beachy AM, Stuart MJ, Grabowski JJ, et al: Evaluation of a new device for proximal tibial osteotomy. Personal communication, 1998.
16. Bergenudd H, Sahlstrom A, Sanzen L: Total knee arthroplasty after failed proximal tibial valgus osteotomy. J Arthroplasty 1997; 12:635.
17. Berman AT, Bosacco SJ, Kirshner S, et al: Factors influencing long-term results in high tibial osteotomy. Clin Orthop 1991; 272:192.
18. Bettin D, Karbowski A, Schwering L, et al: Time-dependent clinical and roentgenographical results of Coventry high tibial valgisation osteotomy. Arch Orthop Trauma Surg 1998; 117:53.
19. Beyer CA, Lewallen DG, Hanssen AD: Total knee arthroplasty following prior osteotomy of the distal femur. Am J Knee Surg 1994; 7:25.
20. Blackburne JS, Peel TE: A new method of measuring patellar height. J Bone Joint Surg Br 1977; 59:241.
21. Blaimont P: The curviplane osteotomy in the treatment of the knee arthrosis. SICOT, 11th meeting, Mexico, 1969.
22. Blaimont P: [Curviplane osteotomy in the treatment of gonarthrosis]. Acta Orthop Belg 1982; 48:97.
23. Blaimont P, Burnotte J, Baillon JM, et al: Contribution biomécanique à l'étude des conditions d'équilibre dans le genou normal et pathologique: Application au traitement de l'arthrose varisante. Acta Orthop Belg 1971; 37:573.
24. Blaimont P, Burnotte J, Halleux P: La préarthrose du genou: Pathogénie biomécanique et traitement prophylactique. Acta Orthop Belg 1975; 41:177.
25. Blaimont P, Schoon R: A propos de 2 cas de gonarthrose associée à un vice de torsion interne du tibia. Acta Orthop Belg 1977; 43:476.
26. Booth REJ: TKA revision after osteotomy. Orthopedics 1994; 17:859.
27. Bouharras M, Hoet F, Watillon M, et al: [Results of tibial valgus osteotomy for internal femorotibial arthritis with an average 8-year follow-up]. Acta Orthop Belg 1994; 60:163.
28. Bouillet R, Van Gaver PH: L'arthrose du genou: Étude pathogénique et traitement. Acta Orthop Belg 1961; 27:1.

29. Brueckmann FR, Kettelkamp DB: Proximal tibial osteotomy. Orthop Clin North Am 1982; 13:3.
30. Buechel FF: A sequential three-step lateral release for correcting fixed valgus knee deformities during total knee arthroplasty. Clin Orthop 1990; 260:170.
31. Calista F, Pegreffi P: High tibial osteotomy: Osteotomy in minus or hemicallotasis with EAF? Chir Organi Mov 1996; 81:155.
32. Cameron HU: Repair of nonunion of supracondylar femoral osteotomy. Orthop Rev 1992; 21:349.
33. Cameron HU, Botsford DJ, Park YS: Prognostic factors in the outcome of supracondylar femoral osteotomy for lateral compartment osteoarthritis of the knee. Can J Surg 1997; 40:114.
34. Cameron HU, Park YS: Total knee replacement after supracondylar femoral osteotomy. Am J Knee Surg 1997; 10:70.
35. Cameron HU, Welsh RP: Potential complications of total knee replacement following tibial osteotomy. Orthop Rev 1988; 17: 39.
36. Cameron HU, Welsh RP, Jung YB, et al: Repair of nonunion of tibial osteotomy. Clin Orthop 1993; 287:167.
37. Cameron JC, Saha S: Management of medial collateral ligament laxity. Orthop Clin North Am 1994; 25:527.
38. Carr A, Keyes G, Miller R, et al: Medial unicompartmental arthroplasty: A survival study of the Oxford meniscal knee. Clin Orthop 1993; 295:205.
39. Cass JR, Bryan RS: High tibial osteotomy. Clin Orthop 1988; 230:196.
40. Catagni MA, Guerreschi F, Ahmad TS, et al: Treatment of genu varum in medial compartment osteoarthritis of the knee using the Ilizarov method. Orthop Clin North Am 1994; 25:509.
41. Caton J, Deschamps G, Chambat P, et al: Les rotules basses: A propos de 128 observations. Rev Chir Orthop 1982; 68:317.
42. Chan RN, Pollard JP: High tibial osteotomy for rheumatoid arthritis of the knee: A one- to six year follow-up study. Acta Orthop Scand 1978; 49:78.
43. Chao EY, Neluheni EVD, Hsu RW, et al: Biomechanics of malalignment. Orthop Clin North Am 1994; 25:379.
44. Chao EY, Sim FH: Computer-aided preoperative planning in knee osteotomy. Iowa Orthop J 1995; 15:4.
45. Christodoulou N, Moussas T, Karaindros C, et al: [Osteosynthesis of tibial valgus osteotomies by goniometric CH-N external fixator]. Rev Chir Orthop Reparatrice Appar Mot 1996; 82: 331.
46. Cognet JM, Rouvillain JL, Mousselard HP, et al: Résultat des ostéotomies fémorales de varisation pour genu valgum: A propos de 75 cas revus à plus de cinq ans de recul. Rev Chir Orthop Reparatrice Appar Mot 1998; 84:46.
47. Cooke TD, Bryant JT, Scudamore RA: Biomechanical factors in alignment and arthritic disorders of the knee. In Fu FH, Harner CD, Vince KG, eds: Knee Surgery. Baltimore, Williams and Wilkins, 1994, p 1061.
48. Cooke TD, Li J, Scudamore RA: Radiographic assessment of bony contributions to knee deformity. Orthop Clin North Am 1994; 25:387.
49. Cooke TD, Pichora D, Siu D, et al: Surgical implications of varus deformity of the knee with obliquity of joint surfaces. J Bone Joint Surg Br 1989; 71:560.
50. Coventry MB: Osteotomy of the upper portion of the tibia for degenerative arthritis of the knee: A preliminary report. J Bone Joint Surg Am 1965; 47:984.
51. Coventry MB: Osteotomy about the knee for degenerative and rheumatoid arthritis. J Bone Joint Surg Am 1973; 55:23.
52. Coventry MB: Upper tibial osteotomy for gonarthrosis: The evolution of the operation in the last 18 years and long-term results. Orthop Clin North Am 1979; 10:191.
53. Coventry MB: Upper tibial osteotomy. Clin Orthop 1984; 182: 46.
54. Coventry MB: Upper tibial osteotomy for osteoarthritis. J Bone Joint Surg Am 1985; 67:1136.
55. Coventry MB: Proximal tibial varus osteotomy for osteoarthritis of the lateral compartment of the knee. J Bone Joint Surg Am 1987; 69:32.
56. Coventry MB: Osteotomy of the upper portion of the tibia for degenerative arthritis of the knee: A preliminary report. Clin Orthop 1989; 248:4.
57. Coventry MB, Bowman PW: Long-term results of upper tibial osteotomy for degenerative arthritis of the knee. Acta Orthop Belg 1982; 48:139.
58. Coventry MB, Ilstrup DM, Wallrichs SL: Proximal tibial osteotomy: A critical long-term study of eighty-seven cases. J Bone Joint Surg Am 1993; 75:196.
59. Curley P, Eyres K, Brezinova V, et al: Common peroneal nerve dysfunction after high tibial osteotomy. J Bone Joint Surg Br 1990; 72:405.
60. de Pablos J, Gonzalez-Herranz P, Barrios C: Progressive opening-wedge osteotomy for severe tibia vara in adults. Orthopedics 1998; 21:1253.
61. Debeyre J, Artigou JM: [Long-term results of 260 tibial osteotomies for frontal deviations of the knee]. Rev Chir Orthop Reparatrice Appar Mot 1972; 58:335.
62. Debeyre J, Artigou JM: [Indications and results of tibial osteotomy: Influence of laxity]. Rev Chir Orthop Reparatrice Appar Mot 1973; 59:641.
63. Debeyre J, Frain P: [An intercondylar femoral osteotomy technique in the management of knee deviations due to arthrosis]. Ann Chir 1967; 21:548.
64. Debeyre J, Patte D: Place des osteotomies de correction dans le traitement de la gonarthrose. Acta Orthop Belg 1961; 27:374.
65. Dejour, H: Indications thérapeutiques dans l'arthrose fémoro-tibiale. 7th Journées lyonnaises de chirurgie du genou 1991; 404.
66. Dejour, H: L'ostéotomie tibiale de varisation—Résultats: à propos de 118 cas. 7th Journées lyonnaises de chirurgie du genou 1991; 169.
67. Dejour H, Neyret P, Boileau P, et al: Anterior cruciate reconstruction combined with valgus tibial osteotomy. Clin Orthop 1994; 299:220.
68. Delloye Ch: Les implants osseux lyophilisés. Rev Chir Orthop 1988; 74:149.
69. Delloye Ch, Allington N, Munting E, et al: L'os de banque lyophilisé: Technique et résultats après trois années d'utilisation. Acta Orthop Belg 1987; 53:2.
70. Descamps L, Jarsaillon B, Schuster P, et al: [Angular synthesis in upper tibial valgus osteotomy in osteoarthritis: Apropos of a series of 544 cases]. Rev Chir Orthop 1987; 73:231.
71. Descamps L, Jarsaillon B, Schuster P, et al: [Angular synthesis in upper tibial valgus osteotomy in osteoarthritis: Apropos of a series of 544 cases]. Rev Chir Orthop 1987; 73:231.
72. Diduch D, Insall JN, Scott WN, et al: Total knee replacement in young, active patients: Long-term follow-up and functional outcome. J Bone Joint Surg Am 1997; 79:575.
73. Dohin B, Migaud H, Gougeon F, et al: [Effect of a valgization osteotomy with external wedge removal on patellar height and femoro-patellar arthritis]. Acta Orthop Belg 1993; 59:69.
74. Dugdale TW, Noyes FR, Styer D: Preoperative planning for high tibial osteotomy: The effect of lateral tibiofemoral separation and tibiofemoral length. Clin Orthop 1992; 274:248.
75. Eckhoff DG: Effect of limb malrotation on malalignment and osteoarthritis. Orthop Clin North Am 1994; 25:405.
76. Eckhoff DG, Montgomery WK, Kilcoyne RF, et al: Femoral morphometry and anterior knee pain. Clin Orthop 1994; 302: 64.
77. Edgerton BC, Mariani EM, Morrey BF: Distal femoral varus osteotomy for painful genu valgum: A 5- to 11-year follow-up study. Clin Orthop 1993; 288:263.
78. Finkelstein JA, Gross AE, Davis A: Varus osteotomy of the distal part of the femur: A survivorship analysis. J Bone Joint Surg Am 1996; 78:1348.
79. Flierl S, Sabo D, Hornig K, et al: Open wedge high tibial osteotomy using fractioned drill osteotomy: A surgical modification that lowers the complication rate. Knee Surg Sports Traumatol Arthrosc 1996; 4:149.
80. Font-Rodriguez DE, Scuderi GR, Insall JN: Survivorship of cemented total knee arthroplasty. Clin Orthop 1997; 345:79.
81. Frain PH: Retentissement sur le genou des atteintes de la hanche: Bases théoriques. Rev Chir Orthop 1967; 53:713.
82. Frain PH, Mazas F, Kerboul M, et al: Retentissement sur le genou des atteintes de la hanche. Rev Chir Orthop 1967; 53: 713.
83. Fujisawa Y, Masuhara K, Shiomi S: The effect of high tibial osteotomy on osteoarthritis of the knee: An arthroscopic study of 54 knee joints. Orthop Clin North Am 1979; 10:585.

84. Gardes JC: [Distal femoral osteotomy with internal closure for the correction of gonarthroses with genu valgum]. Rev Chir Orthop Reparatrice Appar Mot 1983; 69(S2):110.
85. Gariépy R: Genu varum treated by high tibial osteotomy. J Bone Joint Surg Br 1964; 46:783.
86. Garvin KL, Scuderi GR, Insall JN: Evolution of the quadriceps snip. Clin Orthop 1995; 321:131.
87. Gibson MJ, Barnes MR, Allen MJ, et al: Weakness of foot dorsiflexion and changes in compartment pressures after tibial osteotomy. J Bone Joint Surg Br 1986; 68:471.
88. Gill T, Schemitsch EH, Brick GW, et al: Revision total knee arthroplasty after failed unicompartmental knee arthroplasty or high tibial osteotomy. Clin Orthop 1995; 321:10.
89. Godeneche A, Besse JL, Moyen B, et al: Prothèse totale du genou et ostéotomie dans le même temps opératoire pour déviation axiale majeure (à propos de 11 cas). Rev Chir Orthop 1998; 84:42.
90. Goh JC, Bose K, Khoo BC: Gait analysis study on patients with varus osteoarthrosis of the knee. Clin Orthop 1993; 294:223.
91. Goldman RT, Scuderi GR, Kelly MA: Arthroscopic treatment of the degenerative knee in older athletes. Clin Sports Med 1997; 16:51.
92. Goutallier D, Delepine G, Debeyre J: [The patello-femoral joint in osteoarthritis of the knee with genu varum (author's transl)]. Rev Chir Orthop Reparatrice Appar Mot 1979; 65:25.
93. Goutallier D, Delepine G, Debeyre J: [The patello-femoral joint in osteoarthritis of the knee with genu varum (author's transl)]. Rev Chir Orthop Reparatrice Appar Mot 1979; 65:25.
94. Goutallier D, Garabedian JM, Allain J, et al: Influence of lower limb torsional deformities on the development of femoro-tibial degenerative arthritis. Rev Chir Orthop 1997; 83:613.
95. Goutallier D, Julieron A, Hernigou P: Cement wedge replacing iliac graft for medial opening wedge tibial osteotomy. Rev Chir Orthop 1992; 78:138.
96. Green SA, Green HD: The influence of radiographic projection on the appearance of deformities. Orthop Clin North Am 1994; 25:467.
97. Grelsamer RP: Unicompartmental osteoarthrosis of the knee. J Bone Joint Surg Am 1995; 77:278.
98. Haddad FS, Prendergast CM, Dorrell JH, et al: Arteriovenous fistula after fibular osteotomy leading to recurrent haemarthroses in a total knee replacement. J Bone Joint Surg Br 1996; 78:458.
99. Harding ML: A fresh appraisal of tibial osteotomy for osteoarthritis of the knee. Clin Orthop 1976; 114:223.
100. Harrington IJ: Static and dynamic loading patterns in knee joints with deformities. J Bone Joint Surg Am 1983; 65:247.
101. Harris WR, Kostuik JP: High tibial osteotomy for osteoarthritis of the knee. J Bone Joint Surg Am 1970; 52:330.
102. Harrison MM, Cooke TD, Fisher SB, et al: Patterns of knee arthrosis and patella subluxation. Clin Orthop 1994; 309:56.
103. Healy WL, Anglen JO, Wasilewski SA, et al: Distal femoral varus osteotomy. J Bone Joint Surg Am 1988; 70:102.
104. Healy WL, Wilk RM: Osteotomy in treatment of the arthritic knee. In Scott WN, ed: The Knee. St. Louis, Mosby, 1994, p 1019.
105. Heatley FW, Lea Thomas ML, Giddins GEB, et al: Deep vein thrombosis in barrel vault tibial osteotomy: A pilot study. J Bone Joint Surg Br 1989; 71:729
106. Hee HT, Low CK, Seow KH, et al: Comparing staple fixation to buttress plate fixation in high tibial osteotomy. Ann Acad Med Singapore 1996; 25:233.
107. Hernborg JS, Nilsson BE: The natural course of untreated osteoartritis of the knee. Clin Orthop 1977; 123:130.
108. Hernigou P: [A 20-year follow-up study of internal gonarthrosis after tibial valgus osteotomy: Single versus repeated osteotomy]. Rev Chir Orthop Reparatrice Appar Mot 1996; 82:241.
109. Hernigou P, Bassaine M: Prothèse totale de genou après ostéotomie tibiale d'addition et de soustraction. Rev Chir Orthop 1998; 84:43.
110. Hernigou P, Duparc F, de-Ladoucette A, et al: [Recurvatum in arthritic genu valgum: Contraindication for osteotomy and unicompartmental prosthesis]. Rev Chir Orthop Reparatrice Appar Mot 1992; 78:292.
111. Hernigou P, Goutallier D: [Outcome of the femoropatellar joint in osteoarthritic genu varum after tibial wedge osteotomy for angulation: 10- to 13-year regression]. Rev Chir Orthop 1987; 73:43.
112. Hernigou P, Goutallier D: Usure osseuse sous chondrale des plateaux tibiaux dans les gonarthroses fémoro-tibiales: Aspect radiologique sur l'incidence de profil—corrélations anatomiques et conséquences. Rev Mal Osteoartic 1990; 57:67.
113. Hernigou P, Medevielle D, Debeyre J, et al: Proximal tibial osteotomy for osteoarthritis with varus deformity: A 10- to 13-year follow-up study. J Bone Joint Surg Am 1987; 69:332.
114. Hernigou P, Ovadia H, Goutallier D: Modelisation mathématique de l'ostéotomie tibiale d'ouverture et tables de correction. Rev Chir Orthop 1992; 78:258.
115. Hofmann AA, Kane KR: Total knee arthroplasty after high tibial osteotomy. Orthopedics 1994; 17:887.
116. Hofmann AA, Wyatt RW, Beck SW: High tibial osteotomy: Use of an osteotomy jig, rigid fixation, and early motion versus conventional surgical technique and cast immobilization. Clin Orthop 1991; 271:212.
117. Hofmann AA, Wyatt RW, Jones RE: Combined Coventry-Maquet procedure for two-compartment degenerative arthritis. Clin Orthop 1984; 190:186.
118. Holden DL, James SL, Larson RL, et al: Proximal tibial osteotomy in patients who are fifty years old or less: A long-term follow-up study. J Bone Joint Surg Am 1988; 70:977.
119. Hsu RW: The study of Maquet dome high tibial osteotomy: Arthroscopic-assisted analysis. Clin Orthop 1989; 243:280.
120. Huberti HH, Hayes WC: Patellofemoral contact pressures: The influence of Q-angle and tendofemoral contact. J Bone Joint Surg Am 1984; 66:715.
121. Idusuyi OB, Morrey BF: Peroneal nerve palsy after total knee arthroplasty: Assessment of predisposing and prognostic factors. J Bone Joint Surg Am 1996; 78:177.
122. Insall J, Salvati E: Patella position in the normal knee joint. Radiology 1971; 101:101.
123. Insall J, Shoji H, Mayer V: High tibial osteotomy: A five-year evaluation. J Bone Joint Surg Am 1974; 56:1397.
124. Insall JN: High tibial osteotomy in the treatment of osteoarthritis of the knee. Surg Annu 1975; 7:347.
125. Insall JN: Osteotomy. In Insall JN, Windsor RE, Scott WN, et al, eds: Surgery of the Knee. New York, Churchill Livingstone, 1993, p 635.
126. Insall JN: Surgical techniques and instrumentation in total knee arthroplasty. In Insall JN, Windsor RE, Scott WN, et al, eds: Surgery of the Knee. New York, Churchill Livingstone, 1993, p 739.
127. Insall JN: Knee arthroplasty: Limits and other problems—extensor mechanism complications. Orthopedics 1996; 19:809.
128. Insall JN, Joseph DM, Msika C: High tibial osteotomy for varus gonarthrosis: A long-term follow-up study. J Bone Joint Surg Am 1984; 66:1040.
129. Insall JN, Kelly MA: Anatomy. In Insall JN, Windsor RE, Scott WN, et al, eds: Surgery of the Knee. New York, Churchill Livingstone, 1993, p 1.
130. Insall JN, Stern SH: Total knee arthroplasty in obese patients. J Bone Joint Surg Am 1990; 72:1400.
131. Ivarsson I, Myrnerts R, Gillquist J: High tibial osteotomy for medial osteoarthritis of the knee. A 5- to 7- and 11-year follow-up. J Bone Joint Surg Br 1990; 72:238.
132. Jackson JP: Osteotomy for osteoarthritis of the knee. J Bone Joint Surg Br 1958; 40:826.
133. Jackson JP, Waugh W: The technique and complications of upper tibial osteotomy: A review of 226 operations. J Bone Joint Surg Br 1974; 56:236.
134. Jackson M, Sarangi PP, Newman JH: Revision total knee arthroplasty: Comparison of outcome following primary proximal tibial osteotomy or unicompartmental arthroplasty. J Arthroplasty 1994; 9:539.
135. Jiang CC, Hang YS, Liu TK: A new jig for proximal tibial osteotomy. Clin Orthop 1986; 226:118.
136. Jiang CC, Insall JN: Effect of rotation on the axial alignment of the femur: Pitfalls in the use of femoral intramedullary guides in total knee arthroplasty. Clin Orthop 1989; 248:50.
137. Job DC, Languepin A, Benvenuto M, et al: [Tibial valgization osteotomy in gonarthrosis with or without chondrocalcinosis: Results after 5 years]. Rev Rhum Mal Osteoartic 1991; 58:491.

138. Johnson F, Leitl S, Waugh W: The distribution of load across the knee: A comparison of static and dynamic measurements. J Bone Joint Surg Br 1980; 62:346.
139. Johnson LL: Arthroscopic arthroplasty historical and pathological perspectives: Present status. Arthroscopy 1986; 2:54.
140. Jokio PJ, Lindholm TS: The angle-measuring device: A practical resource in high tibial osteotomy. Ann Chir Gynaecol 1991; 80: 54.
141. Kapandji IA: The Physiology of the Joints. New York, Churchill Livingstone, 1970.
142. Katz MM, Hungerford DS, Krackow KA, et al: Results of total knee arthroplasty after failed proximal tibial osteotomy for osteoarthritis. J Bone Joint Surg Am 1987; 69:225.
143. Keene JS, Monson DK, Roberts JM, et al: Evaluation of patients for high tibial osteotomy. Clin Orthop 1989; 243:157.
144. Kettelkamp DB, Leach RE, Nasca R: Pitfalls of proximal tibial osteotomy. Clin Orthop 1975; 232.
145. Kettelkamp DB, Wenger DR, Chao EY, et al: Results of proximal tibial osteotomy: The effects of tibiofemoral angle, stance-phase, flexion-extension, and medial-plateau force. J Bone Joint Surg Am 1976; 58:952.
146. Kirgis A, Albrecht S: Palsy of the deep peroneal nerve after proximal tibial osteotomy: An anatomical study. J Bone Joint Surg Am 1992; 74:1180.
147. Korn MW: A new approach to dome high tibial osteotomy. Am J Knee Surg 1996; 9:12.
148. Koshino T, Morii T, Wada J, et al: High tibial osteotomy with fixation by a blade plate for medial compartment osteoarthritis of the knee. Orthop Clin North Am 1989; 20:227.
149. Koshino T, Ranawat NS: Healing process of osteoarthritis in the knee after high tibial osteotomy through observation of strontium-85 scintimetry. Clin Orthop 1972; 82:149.
150. Kozinn SC, Scott RD: Current concepts review: Unicondylar knee arthroplasty. J Bone Joint Surg Am 1989; 71:145.
151. Krackow KA, Holtgrewe JL: Experience with a new technique for managing severely overcorrected valgus high tibial osteotomy at total knee arthroplasty. Clin Orthop 1990; 258:213.
152. Krznaric E, Roo MD, Verbruggen A, et al: Chronic osteomyelitis: Diagnosis with technetium-99m-d, l-hexamethylpropylene amine oxime labelled leucocytes. Eur J Nucl Med 1996; 23:792.
153. Lang W, Ott R, Haas P, et al: Popliteal arteriovenous fistula after corrective upper tibial osteotomy. Arch Orthop Trauma Surg 1993; 112:99.
154. Langlais F, Thomazeau H: Ostéotomies du genou. In Encyclopédie médico-chirurgicale. Paris, Editions scientifiques et médicales Elsevier, 1989, p 1.
155. Lattermann C, Jakob RP: High tibial osteotomy alone or combined with ligament reconstruction in anterior cruciate ligament-deficient knees. Knee Surg Sports Traumatol Arthroscopy 1996; 4:32.
156. Learmonth ID: A simple technique for varus supracondylar osteotomy in genu valgum. J Bone Joint Surg Br 1990; 72:235.
157. Leclerc JR, Geerts WH, Desjardins L, et al: Prevention of deep vein thrombosis after major knee surgery: A randomized, double-blind trial comparing a low-molecular-weight heparin fragment (enoxaparin) to placebo. Thromb Haemost 1992; 67:417.
158. Lemaire R: [Comparative study of 2 series of tibial osteotomies with blade-plate fixation or with compression frame]. Acta Orthop Belg 1982; 48:157.
159. Lemaire R, Gillet P, Rondia J: [Semi-constrained prosthetic arthroplasty of the knee following tibial osteotomy]. Acta Orthop Belg 1991; 57:130.
160. Lerat JL, Moyen B, Garin C, et al: [Anterior laxity and internal arthritis of the knee: Results of the reconstruction of the anterior cruciate ligament associated with tibial osteotomy]. Rev Chir Orthop Reparatrice Appar Mot 1993; 79:365.
161. Levigne CH: Interêt de l'axe épiphysaire dans l'arthrose. 7th Journées lyonnaises de chirurgie du genou 1991; 127.
162. Levigne, CH, Bonnin M: Ostétomie tibiale de valgisation pour arthrose fémoro-tibiale interne: Résultats d'un échantillon de 217 ostéotomies revues avec un recul de 1 à 21 ans. Journées lyonnaises de chirurgie du genou 1991; 7:142.
163. Lootvoet L, Massinon A, Rossillon R, et al: [Upper tibial osteotomy for gonarthrosis in genu varum: Apropos of a series of 193 cases reviewed 6 to 10 years later]. Rev Chir Orthop Reparatrice Appar Mot 1993; 79:375.
164. Lortat JA, Hardy P, Benoit J: [Early reoperation for infection in orthopedic surgery of the leg (arthroplasties and hip surgical procedures excluded)]. Rev Chir Orthop Reparatrice Appar Mot 1990; 76:321.
165. Lysholm J, Gillquist J: Evaluation of knee ligament surgery results with special emphasis on use of a scoring scale. Am J Sports Med 1982; 10:150.
166. MacIntosh DL, Welsh RP: Joint debridement: A complement to high tibial osteotomy in the treatment of degenerative arthritis of the knee. J Bone Joint Surg Am 1977; 59:1094.
167. Magyar G, Toksvig LS, Lindstrand A: Open wedge tibial osteotomy by callus distraction in gonarthrosis: Operative technique and early results in 36 patients. Acta Orthop Scand 1998; 69: 147.
168. Mammi GI, Rocchi R, Cadossi R, et al: The electrical stimulation of tibial osteotomies: Double-blind study. Clin Orthop 1993; 288:246.
169. Maquet P: Biomécanique des membres inférieurs. Acta Orthop Belg 1966; 32:705.
170. Maquet P: Biomécanique du genou et gonarthrose. Rev Chir Orthop 1967; 53:111.
171. Maquet P: La solicitation mécanique du genou durant la marche. Acta Orthop Belg 1975; 41:119.
172. Maquet P: Biomechanics of the Knee. New York, Springer Verlag, 1976.
173. Maquet P: Valgus osteotomy for osteoarthritis of the knee. Clin Orthop 1976; 120:143.
174. Maquet P: Osteotomy. In Freeman MAR, ed: Arthritis of the Knee: Clinical Features and Surgical Management. Berlin, Springer Verlag, 1980, p 148.
175. Maquet P: [Surgical treatment of femoro-tibial arthrosis]. Acta Orthop Belg 1982; 48:172.
176. Maquet P: Pathogénie de la gonarthrose. Acta Orthop Belg 1982; 48:45.
177. Maquet P: The treatment of choice in osteoarthritis of the knee. Clin Orthop 1985; 192:108.
178. Maquet P, Watillon M, Burny F, et al: [Conservative surgical treatment of arthrosis of the knee]. Acta Orthop Belg 1982; 48: 204.
179. Marcacci M, Iacono F, Zaffagnini S, et al: Total knee arthroplasty after proximal tibial osteotomy. Chir Organi Mov 1995; 80:353.
180. Mathews J, Cobb AG, Richardson S, et al: Distal femoral osteotomy for lateral compartment osteoarthritis of the knee. Orthopedics 1998; 21:437.
181. Matthews LS, Goldstein SA, Malvitz TA, et al: Proximal tibial osteotomy: Factors that influence the duration of satisfactory function. Clin Orthop 1988; 229:193.
182. McDermott AG, Finklestein JA, Farine I, et al: Distal femoral varus osteotomy for valgus deformity of the knee. J Bone Joint Surg Am 1988; 70:110.
183. McKellop HA, Llinas A, Sarmiento A: Effects of tibial malalignment on the knee and ankle. Orthop Clin North Am 1994; 25: 415.
184. McKellop HA, Sim FH, Redfern FC, et al: The effect of simulated fracture-angulations of the tibia on cartilage pressures in the knee joint. J Bone Joint Surg Am 1991; 73:1382.
185. Merle d' Aubigné R: Joint realignment in the management of osteoarthritis. In Straub LR, Wilson PD Jr, eds: Clinical Trends in Orthopaedics. New York, Thieme-Stratton, 1982, p 246.
186. Merle d'Aubigné R, Ramadier JO, Van Houtte H: Arthroses du genou et surcharge articulaire. Acta Orthop Belg 1961; 27:365.
187. Miniaci A, Ballmer FT, Ballmer PM, et al: Proximal tibial osteotomy: A new fixation device. Clin Orthop 1989; 246:250.
188. Mironneau A: L'ostéotomie fémorale de varisation dans l'arthrose fémoro-tibiale externe essentielle. 7th Journées lyonnaises de chirurgie du genou 1991; 181.
189. Mollica Q, Leonardi W, Longo G, et al: Surgical treatment of arthritic varus knee by tibial corticotomy and angular distraction with an external fixator. Ital J Orthop Traumatol 1992; 18: 17.
190. Mollica Q, Leonardi W, Travaglianti G: Correction of lower limb deformity using external fixation. Ital J Orthop Traumatol 1992; 18:297.
191. Mont MA, Alexander N, Krackow KA, et al: Total knee arthro-

plasty after failed high tibial osteotomy. Orthop Clin North Am 1994; 25:515.
192. Mont MA, Antonaides S, Krackow KA, et al: Total knee arthroplasty after failed high tibial osteotomy: A comparison with a matched group. Clin Orthop 1994; 299:125.
193. Moreland JR: Mechanisms of failure in total knee arthroplasty. Clin Orthop 1988; 226:49.
194. Moreland JR, Basset LW, Hanker GJ: Radiographic analysis of the axial alignment of the lower extremity. J Bone Joint Surg Am 1987; 69:745.
195. Morrey BF, Edgerton BC: Distal femoral osteotomy for lateral gonarthrosis. Instr Course Lect 1992; 41:77.
196. Moussa M: Rotational malalignment and femoral torsion in osteoarthritic knees with patellofemoral joint involvment. Clin Orthop 1994; 304:176.
197. Murphy SB: Tibial osteotomy for genu varum: Indications, preoperative planning, and technique. Orthop Clin North Am 1994; 25:477.
198. Murray DW, Goodfellow J, O'Connor J: The Oxford medial unicompartmental arthroplasty. J Bone Joint Surg Br 1998; 80:983.
199. Myrnerts R: The SAAB jig: An aid in high tibial osteotomy. Acta Orthop Scand 1978; 49:85.
200. Myrnerts R: High tibial osteotomy with overcorrection of varus malalignment in medial gonarthrosis. Acta Orthop Scand 1980; 51:557.
201. Nagel A, Insall JN, Scuderi GR: Proximal tibial osteotomy: A subjective outcome study. J Bone Joint Surg Am 1996; 78:1353.
202. Neyret P, Deroche P, Deschamps G, et al: [Total knee replacement after valgus tibial osteotomy: Technical problems]. Rev Chir Orthop Reparatrice Appar Mot 1992; 78:438.
203. Nguyen C, Rudan J, Simurda MA, et al: High tibial osteotomy compared with high tibial and Maquet procedures in medial and patellofemoral compartment osteoarthritis. Clin Orthop 1989; 245:179.
204. Noyes FR, Barber SD, Simon R: High tibial osteotomy and ligament reconstruction in varus angulated, anterior cruciate ligament-deficient knees: A two- to seven-year follow-up study. Am J Sports Med 1993; 21:2.
205. O'Neill DF, James SL: Valgus osteotomy with anterior cruciate ligament laxity. Clin Orthop 1992; 278:153.
206. Odenbring S, Berggren AM, Peil L: Roentgenographic assessment of the hip-knee-ankle axis in medial gonarthrosis: A study of reproducibility. Clin Orthop 1993; 289:195.
207. Odenbring S, Egund N, Hagstedt B, et al: Ten-year results of tibial osteotomy for medial gonarthrosis: The influence of overcorrection. Arch Orthop Trauma Surg 1991; 110:103.
208. Odenbring S, Egund N, Knutson K, et al: Revision after osteotomy for gonarthrosis: A 10- to 19-year follow-up of 314 cases. Acta Orthop Scand 1990; 61:128.
209. Odenbring S, Egund N, Lindstrand A, et al: Cartilage regeneration after proximal tibial osteotomy for medial gonarthrosis: An arthroscopic, roentgenographic, and histologic study. Clin Orthop 1992; 277:210.
210. Odenbring S, Lindstrand A, Egund N: Early knee mobilization after osteotomy for gonarthrosis. Acta Orthop Scand 1989; 60:699.
211. Odenbring S, Lindstrand A, Egund N, et al: Prognosis for patients with medial gonarthrosis: A 16-year follow-up study of 189 knees. Clin Orthop 1991; 266:152.
212. Odenbring S, Tjornstrand B, Egund N, et al: Function after tibial osteotomy for medial gonarthrosis below aged 50 years. Acta Orthop Scand 1989; 60:527.
213. Ogata K, Whiteside LA, Lester PA, et al: The effect of varus stress on the moving rabbit knee joint. Clin Orthop 1977; 129:313.
214. Ortlepp K, Siegling CW: [Results of follow-up studies following proximal corrective osteotomy of the tibia]. Beitr Orthop Traumatol 1989; 36:563.
215. Paley D, Bhatnagar J, Herzenberg JE, et al: New procedures for tightening knee collateral ligaments in conjunction with knee realignment osteotomy. Orthop Clin North Am 1994; 25:533.
216. Paley D, Maar DC, Herzenberg JE: New concepts in high tibial osteotomy for medial compartment osteoarthritis. Orthop Clin North Am 1994; 25:483.
217. Pauwels F: Biomécanique de l'appareil locomoteur: Contribution à l'étude de l'anatomie fonctionnelle. Berlin, Springer Verlag, 1979.
218. Perusi M, Baietta D, Pizzoli A: [Surgical correction of osteoarthritic genu varum by the hemicallotasis technique]. Rev Chir Orthop Reparatrice Appar Mot 1994; 80:739.
219. Pfeiffer M, Griss P: The valgisation osteotomy of the tibia: Results of a comparative follow-up study of the Coventry versus the Wagner technique. Zeitschrift Orthop 1990; 128:51.
220. Poilvache PL, Insall J, Scuderi GR, et al: Rotational landmarks and sizing of the distal femur in total knee arthroplasty. Clin Orthop 1996; 331:35.
221. Postel M, Langlais F: Osteotomies du genou pour gonarthrose. in Encyclopédie médico-chirurgicale. Paris, Editions Techniques, 1977, p 1.
222. Price CT: Unilateral fixators and mechanical axis realignment. Orthop Clin North Am 1994; 25:499.
223. Prodromos CC, Andriacchi TP, Galante JO: A relationship between gait and clinical changes following high tibial osteotomy. J Bone Joint Surg Am 1985; 67:1188.
224. Psychoyios V, Crawford RW, O'Connor J, et al: Wear of congruent meniscal bearings in unicompartmental knee arthropasty: A retrieval study of 16 specimens. J Bone Joint Surg Br 1998; 80:976.
225. Puddu G, Cerullo G, Cipolla M, et al: A plate for open wedge tibial osteotomy. Personal communication, 1997.
226. Putnam MD, Mears DC, Fu FH: Combined Maquet and proximal tibial valgus osteotomy. Clin Orthop 1985; 197:217.
227. Radermacher K, Portheine F, Anton M, et al: Computer-assisted orthopaedic surgery with image-based individual templates. Clin Orthop 1998; 354:28.
228. Radin EL, Paul IL, Rose RM: Role of mechanical factors in pathogenesis of primary osteoarthrits. Lancet 1972; 1:519
229. Railhac JJ, Fournie A, Gay A, et al: Exploration radiologique du genou de face en légère flexion et en charge: Son intérêt dans le diagnostic de l'arthrose fémoro-tibiale. J Radiol 1981; 62:157.
230. Ramadier JO: Etude radiologique des déviations dans la gonarthrose. Rev Chir Orthop 1967; 53:139.
231. Ramadier JO, Buard JE, Lortat-Jacob A, et al: Mesure radiologique des déformations frontales du genou: Procédé du profil vrai radiologique. Rev Chir Orthop 1982; 68:75.
232. Ramadier JO, Merle d'Audigne R: Genou: Gonarthroses avec déviations transversales du genou. In Merle DR, Postel M, eds: Chirurgie du Rhumatisme, tome 2. Paris, Masson, 1978, p 232.
233. Rand JA, Ilstrup DM: Survivorship analysis of total knee arthroplasty: Cumulative rates of survival of 9200 total knee arthroplasties. J Bone Joint Surg Am 1991; 73:397.
234. Rand JA, Ritts GD: Abrasion arthroplasty as a salvage for failed upper tibial osteotomy. J Arthroplasty 1989; 4(S):45.
235. Reimann I: Experimental osteoarthritis of the knee in rabbits induced by alteration of the load-bearing. Acta Orthop Scand 1973; 44:496.
236. Reynolds JH, Graham D, Smith FW: Imaging inflammation with 99Tcm HMPAO-labelled leucocytes. Clin Radiol 1990; 42:195.
237. Rinonapoli E, Mancini GB, Corvaglia A, et al: Tibial osteotomy for varus gonarthrosis. A 10- to 21-year follow-up study. Clin Orthop 1998; 353:185.
238. Rubens F, Wellington JL, Bouchard AG: Popliteal artery injury after tibial osteotomy: Report of two cases. Can J Surg 1990; 33:294.
239. Rudan JF, Simurda MA: High tibial osteotomy: A prospective clinical and roentgenographic review. Clin Orthop 1990; 255:251.
240. Rudan JF, Simurda MA: Valgus high tibial osteotomy: A long-term follow-up study. Clin Orthop 1991; 268:157.
241. Ruther W, Hotze A, Moller F, et al: Diagnosis of bone and joint infection by leucocyte scintigraphy: A comparative study with 99Tcm-HMPAO-labelled leucocytes, 99Tcm-labelled antigranulocyte antibodies, and 99Tcm-labelled nanocolloid. Arch Orthop Trauma Surg 1990; 110:26.
242. Sabo D, Flierl S, Thomsen M, et al: Fractioned drilling: A technique for wedge osteotomy of the knee. Int Orthop 1995; 19:352.
243. Schwartsman V: Circular external fixation in high tibial osteotomy. Instr Course Lect 1995; 44:469.
244. Scuderi GR, Windsor RE, Insall JN: Observations on patellar

height after proximal tibial osteotomy. J Bone Joint Surg Am 1989; 71:245.
245. Segal P, Burdin PH, Cartier PH, Vielpeau CL: Les échecs des ostéotomies tibiales de valgisation pour gonarthrose et leurs reprises: Symposium. Rev Chir Orthop 1992; 78(S):85.
246. Shaw JA, Moulton MJ: High tibial osteotomy: An operation based on a spurious mechanical concept. Am J Orthop 1996; 25:429.
247. Shoji H, Insall J: High tibial osteotomy for osteoarthritis of the knee with valgus deformity. J Bone Joint Surg Am 1973; 55: 963.
248. Siegrist O, Fritschy D, Manueddu C, et al: Osteotomie de valgisation progressive du tibia proximal. 56th Congrès annuel de la Société suisse d'orthopédie, 3-14 June 1996.
249. Specchiulli F, Laforgia R, Solarino GB: Tibial osteotomy in the treatment of varus osteoarthritic knee. Ital J Orthop Traumatol 1990; 16:507.
250. Staeheli JW, Cass JR, Morrey BF: Condylar total knee arthroplasty after failed proximal tibial osteotomy. J Bone Joint Surg Am 1987; 69:28.
251. Stern SH, Insall JN: Posterior stabilized prosthesis: Results after follow-up of nine to twelve years. J Bone Joint Surg Am 1992; 74:980.
252. Stuart MJ, Grace JN, Ilstrup DM, et al: Late recurrence of varus deformity after proximal tibial osteotomy. Clin Orthop 1990; 260:61.
253. Stubbs BT: Posterolateral arthritis of the knee. J Arthroplasty 1995; 10:427.
254. Sundaram NA, Hallett JP, Sullivan MF: Dome osteotomy of the tibia for osteoarthritis of the knee. J Bone Joint Surg Br 1986; 68:782.
255. Surer P: Un nouveau matériel d'ostéosynthèse—la plaque à ancrage "surfix": Son utilisation dans les ostéosynthèses métaphyso-épiphysaires du genou. Ann Orthop Ouest 1995; 27:127
256. Surer P: Reliability of fixation with the Surfix plate: Analysis of the first 100 osteotomies. Eur J Orthop Surg Traumatol 1997; 7: 47.
257. Tabor OB Jr, Tabor OB: Unicompartmental arthroplasty: A long-term follow-up study. J Arthroplasty 1998; 13:373.
258. Tegner Y, Lysholm J: Rating systems in the evaluation of knee ligament injuries. Clin Orthop 1985; 198:43.
259. Teinturier P, Boulleret J, Terver S, et al: [Supracondylar osteotomy]. Rev Chir Orthop Reparatrice Appar Mot 1975; 61(S2): 291.
260. Terry GC, Cimino PM: Distal femoral osteotomy for valgus deformity of the knee. Orthopedics 1992; 15:1283.
261. Thomine JM, Boudjemaa A, Gibon Y, et al: Les écarts varisants dans la gonarthrose: Fondement théorique et essai d'évaluation pratique. Rev Chir Orthop 1981; 67:319.
262. Tippett JW: Articular cartilage drilling and osteotomy in osteoarthritis of the knee. In McGinty JB, Caspari RB, Jackson RW, et al, eds: Operative Arthroscopy. Philadelphia, Lippincott-Raven, 1996, p 411.
263. Tjornstrand B, Hagstedt B, Persson BM: Results of surgical treatment for non-union after high tibial osteotomy in osteoarthritis of the knee. J Bone Joint Surg Am 1978; 60:973.
264. Tjornstrand BA, Egund N, Hagstedt BV: High tibial osteotomy: A seven-year clinical and radiographic follow-up. Clin Orthop 1981; 124.
265. Toksvig LS, Magyar G, Onsten I, et al: Fixation of the tibial component of total knee arthroplasty after high tibial osteotomy: A matched radiostereometric study. J Bone Joint Surg Br 1998; 80:295.
266. Totty WG: Radiographic evaluation of osteomyelitis using magnetic resonance imaging. Orthop Rev 1989; 18:587.
267. Turner RS, Griffiths H, Heatley FW: The incidence of deep-vein thrombosis after upper tibial osteotomy: A venographic study. J Bone Joint Surg Br 1993; 75:942.
268. Uchinou S, Yano H, Shimizu K, et al: A severely overcorrected high tibial osteotomy: Revision by osteotomy and a long-stem component. Acta Orthop Scand 1996; 67:193.
269. Valenti JR, Calvo R, Lopez R, et al: Long-term evaluation of high tibial valgus osteotomy. Int Orthop 1990; 14:347.
270. Van De Berg AJ, Collard PH, Quiriny M: Gonarthrose et déviation angulaire du genou dans le plan frontal. Acta Orthop Belg 1982; 48:8.
271. Volkmann R: Osteotomy for knee joint deformity. Edinburgh Med J.
272. Wada M, Imura S, Nagatani K, et al: Relationship between gait and clinical results after high tibial osteotomy. Clin Orthop 1998; 354:180.
273. Wagner H: Principles of corrective osteotomies in osteoarthrosis of the knee. Orthopade 1977; 6:145.
274. Wagner H: Principles of corrective osteotomy in osteoarthritis of the knee. Prog Orthop Surg 1980; 4:75.
275. Wagner H, Zeiler G, Baur W: [Indication, technique and results of supra- and infracondylar osteotomy in osteoarthrosis of the knee joint]. Orthopade 1985; 14:172.
276. Wagner J: Curvilinear osteotomy of the tibia. In Aichroth PM, Cannon WD Jr, eds: Knee Surgery: Current Practice. London, Martin Dunitz, 1992, p 608.
277. Wagner J, Bourgois R, Hermanne A: Comportement mécanique du cadre tibio-péronier dans les genoux varum et valgum. Acta Orthop Belg 1982; 48:57.
278. Wang JW, Kuo KN, Andriacchi TP, et al: The influence of walking mechanics and time on the results of proximal tibial osteotomy. J Bone Joint Surg Am 1990; 72:905.
279. Weale AE, Newman JH: Unicompartmental arthroplasty and high tibial osteotomy for osteoarthrosis of the knee: A comparative study with a 12- to 17-year follow-up period. Clin Orthop 1994; 302:134.
280. Weidenhielm L, Olsson E, Brostrom LA, et al: Improvement in gait one year after surgery for knee osteoarthrosis: A comparison between high tibial osteotomy and prosthetic replacement in a prospective randomized study. Scand J Rehabil Med 1993; 25:25.
281. Weill D, Jacquemin MC: [Cylindrical femoral supracondylar varisation osteotomy in the surgical treatment of gonarthrosis]. Acta Orthop Belg 1982; 48:110.
282. Westrich GH, Peters LE, Haas SB, et al: Patella height after high tibial osteotomy with internal fixation and early motion. Clin Orthop 1998; 354:169.
283. Wildner M, Peters A, Hellich J, et al: Complications of high tibial osteotomy and internal fixation with staples. Arch Orthop Trauma Surg 1992; 111:210.
284. Windsor RE, Insall JN, Vince KG: Technical considerations of total knee arthroplasty after proximal tibial osteotomy. J Bone Joint Surg Am 1988; 70:547.
285. Wright J, Heck D, Hawker G, et al: Rates of tibial osteotomies in Canada and the United States. Clin Orthop 1995; 319:266.
286. Wright JG, Coyte P, Hawker G, et al: Variation in orthopedic surgeons' perceptions of the indications for and outcomes of knee replacement. Can Med Assoc J 1995; 152:687.
287. Wu DD, Burr DB, Boyd RD, et al: Bone and cartilage changes following experimental varus or valgus tibial angulation. J Orthop Res 1990; 8:572.
288. Yasuda K, Majima T, Tanabe Y, et al: Long-term evaluation of high tibial osteotomy for medial osteoarthritis of the knee. Bull Hosp Jt Dis Orthop Inst 1991; 51:236.
289. Yasuda K, Majima T, Tsuchida T, et al: A ten- to 15-year follow-up observation of high tibial osteotomy in medial compartment osteoarthrosis. Clin Orthop 1992; 282:186.
290. Yasunaga M: [The study of lateral thrust of the knee in normal and osteoarthritic knees: Evaluation with an accelerometric technique]. Fukuoka Igaku Zasshi 1996; 87:242.
291. Yoshioka Y, Siu D, Cooke TD: The anatomy and functional axes of the femur. J Bone Joint Surg Am 1987; 69:873.
292. Zaidi SH, Cobb AG, Bentley G: Danger to the popliteal artery in high tibial osteotomy. J Bone Joint Surg Br 1995; 77:384.
293. Zuegel NP, Braun WG, Kundel KP, et al: Stabilization of high tibial osteotomy with staples. Arch Orthop Trauma Surg 1996; 115:290.

72 Scoring Systems and Their Validation for the Arthritic Knee

JOSE ALICEA

HISTORICAL PERSPECTIVE

Development of the modern total knee arthroplasty (TKA) began in the 1960s. The polycentric knee designed by Frank H. Gunston was the first to use two cemented polyethylene tibial components articulating on two cemented femoral components. The design was revolutionary for its time and introduced specialized instrumentation to insert the prosthesis. The combination of a reliable fixation agent and a metal-on-polyethylene articulation led to a proliferation of designs in knee arthroplasties.

Different prostheses were designed that incorporated varying degrees of tibiofemoral conformity and that emphasized the designer's belief in the merits of sacrifice or retention of the anterior and posterior cruciate ligaments. Investigators developed various methods of evaluating TKA performance. Over time, investigators standardized reporting methods by selecting those they found most useful. The Hospital for Special Surgery Knee Score[7, 9–11] and the Knee Society[8] Score are the scales most commonly used in the medical literature to report TKA results.

The substantial changes in health care and funding have stimulated development of additional methods for measuring the results of medical therapeutics. It has become increasingly important to quantify the results of a procedure from the patient's perspective; these evaluations are called outcome studies. Outcome studies in total joint arthroplasty are composed of two basic measurements, a health status questionnaire and a pain and function questionnaire. Standard Form (SF) 36, Health Care, attempts to measure the patient's quality of life. The pain and function questionnaire most often used is the Western Ontario and MacMaster Osteoarthritis Index or WOMAC[2–5] score. The WOMAC score was used by the Patient Outcome Research team at the University of Indiana in their evaluation of TKA.

Each score, the Hospital for Special Surgery Knee Score, the Knee Society Score, and the Western Ontario and MacMaster Osteoarthritis Index, will now be considered in detail.

TOTAL KNEE REPLACEMENT SCORES

The two most commonly used scores for reporting the results of knee arthroplasty in the medical literature are the Hospital for Special Surgery (HSS) Knee Score (HSS Knee Score) and the Knee Society Score (KSS). The KSS can be thought of as a derivation of the HSS Knee Score because it incorporates most aspects of the HSS Knee Score and it was created at a later date. The HSS Knee Score and the KSS are evaluations performed by an observer (usually a health care professional) through an interview and physical examination.

The HSS Knee Score

The HSS Knee Score (Fig. 72.1) was introduced in the late 1970s. Physicians and investigators at the HSS evaluated surgical results of different prostheses. The differences in prostheses were reflected in the measurement parameters for each device. The measurement schemes were modified and the most valuable information standardized into the data collected by the HSS Knee Score.

The HSS Knee Score is based on a total of 100 points. The score is divided into seven categories: pain, function, range of motion, muscle strength, flexion deformity, instability, and subtractions. The knee is initially given a score of 0; points are awarded or subtracted according to specific criteria. A high score indicates a better outcome. Half the score is based on information received by interviewing the patient and half on the results of a physical examination. The categories and point scores were those found to be most useful from previous measurement schema. Analysis of HSS Knee Score data has been the cornerstone of much medical research evaluating various designs, techniques, and instrumentation.

Researchers have found the HSS Knee Score valuable in evaluating the merits of different prostheses and instrumentation. Individual physicians may benefit from a standardized evaluation of surgical outcomes. To assess the patient's improvement over time, the evaluation is typically conducted at several different times: preoperatively, 6 months and 1 year after surgery, and each year thereafter. There may be several factors that can affect outcome data such as a patient's well-being, interobserver bias, evolving techniques, and different prostheses. As a result, the measurements are most useful when used to evaluate a specific technique or prosthesis or to quantify a patient's progress over time. There are several software programs that allow physicians to input their data and the SF-36

THE HOSPITAL FOR SPECIAL SURGERY
KNEE SERVICE
Knee Rating Sheet

Name ______________________ HSS# __________ Preoperative date ______________

		LEFT						RIGHT					
	Score	pre	6 mo	1 yr	2 yr	3 yr	4 yr	pre	6 mo	1 yr	2 yr	3 yr	4 yr
PAIN (30 points)													
Walking: None	15												
Mild	10												
Moderate	5												
Severe	0												
At rest: None	15												
Mild	10												
Moderate	5												
Severe	0												
FUNCTION (22 points)													
Walk: Walking and standing unlimited	12												
5–10 blocks, standing >30 min	10												
1–5 blocks, standing 15–30 min	8												
Walk <1 block	4												
Cannot walk	0												
Stairs: Normal	5												
With support	2												
Transfer: Normal	5												
With support	2												
ROM (18 points)													
Each 8° = 1 point													
MUSCLE STRENGTH (10 points)													
Cannot break quadriceps	10												
Can break quadriceps	8												
Can move through arc of motion	4												
Cannot move through arc of motion	0												
FLEXION DEFORMITY (10 points)													
None	10												
5–10°	8												
10–20°	5												
>20°	0												
INSTABILITY (10 points)													
None	10												
0–5°	8												
6–15°	5												
>15°	0												
TOTAL													
SUBTRACTIONS:													
One cane	1												
One crutch	2												
Two crutches	3												
Extension lag of 5°	2												
10°	3												
15°	5												
Deformity (5° = 1 point)													
Varus													
Valgus													
TOTAL SUBTRACTIONS													
KNEE SCORE													

FIGURE 72.1 ➢ The Hospital for Special Surgery Knee Score. (Courtesy Hospital for Special Surgery, New York City.)

score to a national data base and compare results with a national norm.

Whether an individual practitioner or a researcher uses the score, care should be given to ensure consistency. Health care professionals who administer the outcome data collection should be familiar with its significance and implementation. This will minimize differences in evaluation and scoring between observers.

It takes approximately 15 to 30 minutes to complete the evaluation. To conduct the examination requires only a copy of the score sheets and a goniometer. An explanation of the individual categories follows.

Pain

Thirty points are used to describe the amount of pain while ambulating and resting. The patient is asked to describe level of pain as "none," "mild," "moderate," or "severe" when walking and resting. A response of "no pain" is given 15 points, "mild pain" 10 points, "moderate" pain 5 points, and "severe" pain no points.

Function

Twenty-two points are used to quantify the knee's function. The examiner asks the patient how far she or he can walk before having to stop. The distance is measured in Manhattan city blocks, where a city block is 1/20 mile long. If the patient is able to walk and ambulate indefinitely, 12 points are awarded. If the patient is able to walk 5 to 10 blocks (distances from 1/4 to 1/2 mile), or stand for 30 minutes, 10 points are awarded. A decreasing schedule of points is awarded for shorter distances. Eight points are given if the patient can walk 1 to 5 blocks and stand 15 to 30 minutes, 4 points are given for walking less than 1 block, and no points are awarded if the patient is unable to walk.

The remaining ten points in the function category are used to determine the patient's ability to walk up and down stairs and to transfer. If the patient is able to go up and down stairs without assistance and without holding the railing, the knee is given five points; if the patient holds on to the railing or needs minimal assistance, the knee is given two points. The patient's ability to transfer is evaluated next. If the patient is able to rise from a chair without assistance or pushing off the arms of the chair, the knee is awarded five points. If the patient needs minimal assistance in rising from a chair, the knee is awarded two points.

Range of Motion

Eighteen points are used to quantify the patient's range of motion. To determine the value for this category, the health care professional measures the range of motion of the knee. Range of motion is measured against a maximum are of 144 degrees. One point is awarded for each 8 degrees of motion. The observer measures the patient's range of motion and divides that value by 8 to obtain the final score. A patient must gain 8 degrees of motion before a point is awarded. For example, if a patient's range of motion is from 0 to 95 degrees, the total range of motion is 95 degrees. Divide the value of 95 by 8 for a final score of 11 points; the remainder of 7 is discarded.

Muscle Strength

Ten points are used to measure the strength of the quadriceps muscles. It is easier to evaluate quadriceps strength if the patient is sitting. The examiner asks the patient to extend the leg to the maximum point. The observer then tries to break the quadriceps muscle contracture by pushing down on the leg. If the examiner cannot break the quadriceps contracture, ten points are awarded. If the quadriceps contracture can be broken, eight points are awarded. If the patient cannot extend the knee against gravity, but can lie on the side and move the knee through its arc of motion, four points are awarded. If the patient cannot move the knee through the arc of motion, no points are awarded.

Flexion Contractures

Ten points are used to assess flexion contractures. If there are no flexion contractures, 10 points are given; a 5- to 10-degree flexion contracture carries a value of 8 points; 11 to 20 degrees of flexion contracture receives a value of 5 points, and a 20-degree or greater contracture carries a value of zero.

Instability

Ten points are used to categorize knee instability in the varus/valgus plane. The examiner applies varus and valgus stresses to the knee in two different positions, at maximum extension and at 90 degrees of flexion. The examiner may place a goniometer in front of the knee to estimate the degree of instability. A finding of no instability carries a value of 10 points. A zero- to 5-degree instability to varus/valgus stress carries a value of eight points. A 6- to 15-degree instability carries a value of 5 points. More than 15 degrees of instability carries a value of 0.

Subtractions

Add the point values for the first six categories to obtain the subtotal score. This score is now subject to subtractions. Subtractions are divided into three parts: the need of the patient to use ambulatory aids; the degree of extensor lag associated with the knee; and the amount of deformity from the normal anatomic axis of 7 degrees of valgus. If the patient ambulates with a cane, one point is deducted. If the patient ambulates with a crutch, two points are deducted. If two crutches are used, three points are deducted. An extension lag of 5 degrees incurs a 2-point deduction, of 10 degrees carries a 3-point deduction, and of 15 degrees carries a 5-point deduction.

For every 5 degrees of deviation from the normal

anatomic axis of 7 degrees in either the valgus or varus directions, one point is subtracted. The amount of deviation is determined by using a goniometer to measure the alignment of the knee when the knee is at maximum extension. Values in varus are considered negative numbers. The obtained angle is then subtracted from 7 and then divided by 5. The absolute value of the calculation is used. For example, if a patient has a varus alignment of 3, the calculation of (7 − 3)/5 is performed to arrive at a value of 2. Two points would be the applied deduction in this example.

To obtain the final HSS Knee Score, make all necessary subtractions from the subtotal score. The final HSS Knee Score offers a high-level evaluation of the surgical outcome. Scores between 100 and 85 points are considered excellent results; scores between 84 and 70 points are good results; scores between 69 and 60 points are fair, and scores less than 60 are considered poor results. However, these scores are considered against an ideal of 100 points. Given the patient's medical history and physical findings, for example, under specific conditions of arthritis, physical limitations may constrain the maximum score. In addition, scores improve with time, with the maximum gains typically made in the first year postoperatively.

THE KNEE SOCIETY SCORE

Founded in 1983, the Knee Society is a private society of renowned physicians and scientists with special interest in total knee replacements. In 1989, the Knee Society introduced a new rating score for TKA. It attempted to address some of the shortcomings of the HSS Knee Score. The KSS (Fig. 72.2) added an instability evaluation in the anteroposterior plane and a classification system for patients with associated medical conditions. The KSS also applies different point values to the criteria. The KSS is divided into three sections. It consists of the Knee Score (100 points), the Knee Function Score (100 points), and a patient classification system. The classification system assigns patients to three categories depending on their associated medical conditions. Both point scores are initially valued at 0, and points are awarded or deducted according to specific criteria.

The Knee Score

The Knee Score of the KSS evaluates pain, range of motion, and stability in the anteroposterior plane and mediolateral plane. It also offers deductions for flexion contractures, extension lag, and malalignment. Like its predecessor, the Knee Score is based on the interview and physical examination of the patient as conducted by a health care professional.

Pain

Fifty points are used to evaluate pain. The interviewer asks the patient to categorize level of pain as "none," "mild," "moderate," or "severe." There are subclassifications for responses of mild or moderate pain. Based on the patient's answer, the interviewer selects the most appropriate score. If the patient has no pain, the knee is given 50 points. If the patient has occasional pain that is not associated with specific physical activity, the knee is given 45 points. If the patient has pain while climbing or descending stairs, the knee is given 40 points, or while walking and using stairs, 30 points. Should the patient have moderate pain, the examiner follows up by asking if the pain is either occasional, which is awarded 20 points, or continuous, which is awarded 10 points.

Range of Motion

Twenty-five points are awarded for range of motion. One point is given for every 5 degrees of motion. For example, if a patient has an 84-degree range of motion, 16 points are recorded. In those rare instances when the range of motion exceeds 125 degrees, the maximum score of 25 points is awarded.

Stability

Stability is measured in the anteroposterior plane and mediolateral plane. The stability on the anteroposterior plane is measured by the maximum degree of translation of the tibia on the femur. The purpose of this measurement is to determine the stability of the posterior cruciate ligament or its mechanical substitute. To conduct this measurement, ask the patient to sit on an examining table; the examiner then places posterior forces on the proximal tibia. A perceived motion of less than 5 mm receives 10 points. If the knee moves between 5 and 10 mm, the knee is awarded 5 points. If the knee translates more than 1 cm, it receives no points.

Stability in the mediolateral plane is also evaluated in degrees. The stability on the mediolateral plane is measured by the maximum degree of alignment change to varus/valgus stress. The examiner may place a goniometer in front of the knee to estimate the degree of instability. If the knee opens less than 5 degrees, it is given 15 points. If it opens between 6 and 9 degrees, it gets 10 points. Mediolateral instability between 10 and 14 degrees is given 5 points. A mediolateral instability of more than 15 degrees is given no points.

Deductions

Deductions are taken in three major areas: flexion contractures, extension lag, and malalignment. If the knee has a flexion contracture of less than 5 degrees, no deductions are taken. Contractures between 5 and 10 degrees receive a 2-point deduction. Contractures between 11 and 15 degrees receive a 5-point deduction. Flexion contractures between 16 and 20 degrees receive a 10-point deduction. Contractures more than 20 degrees receive a 15-point deduction.

Name ______________________ Operative date ________

	Score	LEFT						RIGHT					
		pre	1 yr	2 yr	3 yr	4 yr	5 yr	pre	1 yr	2 yr	3 yr	4 yr	5 yr
PAIN None	50												
Mild or Occ	45												
Stairs only	40												
Walking and stairs	30												
Moderate Occ	20												
Cont	10												
Severe	0												
ROM: (5° = 1 point)	25												
STABILITY (max mov any pos)													
A/P <5	10												
5–10mm	5												
10mm	0												
M/L <5°	15												
6–9°	10												
10–14°	5												
15°	0												
TOTAL													
Deductions (minus)													
FLEXION CONTRACTURE													
None	0												
5–10°	2												
10–15°	5												
16—20°	10												
>20°	15												
EXTENSION LAG													
None	0												
<10°	5												
10–20°	10												
>20°	15												
ALIGNMENT													
5–10° (None)	0												
0–4° (3 pt each deg)													
11–15° (3 pt each deg)													
Other	20												
Total Deductions													
KNEE SCORE													
(If total is a minus, score is zero)													
FUNCTION													
WALKING: Unlimited	50												
>10 blocks	40												
5 to 10 blocks	30												
<5 blocks	20												
Housebound	10												
Unable	0												
STAIRS: Norm up and down	50												
Norm up: down rail	40												
Up and down rail	30												
Up rail: unable down	15												
Unable	0												
TOTAL													
Deductions (minus)													
Cane	5												
Two canes	10												
Crutches/Walker	20												
Total Deductions													
FUNCTION SCORE													

Patient category: A. Unilateral or bilateral (opposite knee successfully replaced)
B. Unilateral - other knee symptomatic
C. Multiple arthritis or medical infirmity

FIGURE 72.2 ➢ The Knee Society Score. (From Insall JN et al: Rationale of the Knee Society clinical rating system. Clin Orthop 248: 13, 1989.)

The next category of deductions concerns the extension lag of the knee. If the knee does not exhibit an extension lag, zero points are deducted. If the extension lag is less than 10 degrees, 5 degrees are deducted. If the lag is between 10 and 20 degrees, 10 points are deducted. Extension lags over 20 degrees receive a 15-point deduction.

Alignment of the knee between 5 and 10 degrees of valgus receives no deduction. If the knee is malaligned between 0 and 4 degrees of valgus, the alignment value is subtracted from 5 and then multiplied by 3 to calculate the correct deduction. For example, if a knee has a valgus alignment of 3 degrees, 3 is subtracted from 5 and the result, 2, is multiplied by 3, giving a final deduction of 6 points. An analogous procedure is used for larger values of valgus alignment. If the knee has a valgus alignment between 11 and 15 degrees, 10 is subtracted from the alignment value and the result is multiplied by 3 to calculate the correct point deduction. Knees that are placed in varus, or in more than 16 degrees of valgus, receive a deduction of 20 points.

The points for the pain, range of motion, stability, flexion contracture and lag, and alignment categories are summed to obtain the Knee Score. This is a subtotal of the KSS.

Knee Function Score

The Knee Function Score of the KSS is based on an interview between the health care professional and the patient. The score measures the patient's ability to function as defined by walking and by going up and down stairs. Walking and stair climbing are considered in two separate categories. The ability to walk is measured in city blocks. Again, Manhattan city blocks are used as the standard, with one city block equaling 1/20 mile.

Walking

If the patient is able to walk an unlimited number of blocks, 50 points are given. For distances more than 10 blocks, but not unlimited, 40 points are given. The ability to walk between 5 and 10 blocks receives 30 points, less than 5 blocks, 20 points; household ambulators receive 10 points, and patients unable to ambulate receive zero points.

Stair Climbing

If the patient is able to go up and down stairs without assistance, the knee is given 50 points. If the patient holds on to the rail going downstairs but can climb normally, the knee is given 40 points. If the patient is able to climb stairs but cannot descend, the knee is given 15 points. If the patient cannot go up and down stairs, zero points are given.

Deductions

Deductions are made if the patient needs ambulatory aids to walk. Five points are deducted if the patient uses a cane, ten if two canes are used. If the patient uses crutches or a walker, 20 points are deducted.

Patient Category

Recognizing that the outcome of a knee replacement is dependent on many variables, the Knee Society devised a categorical score to try to distinguish medical conditions that can affect the patient's surgical outcome. The patient is assigned to three different categories, depending on her or his functional impairment with relation to medical infirmity or diseases of other joints in the body.

CATEGORY A

Patients are assigned to this category if they have a unilateral total knee replacement or a bilateral replacement in which the knee not being measured has been successfully replaced. This category would also apply to asymptomatic total hip arthroplasties.

CATEGORY B

Patients are assigned to this category if they have a unilateral total knee replacement and their contralateral knee is symptomatic.

CATEGORY C

Patients are assigned to this category if they have multiple arthritic sites or have a significant medical infirmity compromising their function.

Total Scores

The Knee Score and Knee Function Score are considered separately. Scores between 100 and 85 points are considered excellent results; between 84 and 70 points are good results; between 69 and 60 points are considered fair; and scores less than 60 are poor results. These scoring guidelines apply to patients who are otherwise in good health. If a patient has compromising illness that would affect the surgical outcome, it is most useful to compare that patient's preoperative score to the postoperative score. The patient category is used as an explanatory variable to address how other physical conditions can affect the Knee Score and Knee Function Score.

THE WESTERN ONTARIO AND MACMASTER (WOMAC) OSTEOARTHRITIS INDEX SCORE

The WOMAC Score was designed to study the effectiveness of nonsteroidal anti-inflammatory agents in the treatment of osteoarthritis. However, the Patient Outcome Research Team at the University of Indiana found it to be a useful tool to study TKA. The WOMAC Score is based on a questionnaire completed by the patient without the help or intervention of the health care provider. It has proven to be an effective and reproducible vehicle in medical research.

The WOMAC score is based on a maximum of 96 points and is composed of 3 sections. There are 24 questions: 5 questions evaluate pain, 2 evaluate stiffness, and 17 evaluate function. The patient answers each question with a response of "none," "mild," "moderate," "severe," or "extreme." The patient is asked to read each question and mark the response that best describes his or her condition. Once the patient has completed the questionnaire, an examiner totals the score. The answer "none" carries a value of 0, "mild" carries a value of 1 point, "moderate" carries a value of 2 points, "severe" carries a value of 3 points, and "extreme" carries a value of 4 points. It typically takes a patient 20 minutes to complete the questionnaire. The questions are as follows:

Section A (Pain)

How much pain do you have?

1. *Walking on a flat surface.*
2. *Going up or down stairs.*
3. *At night while in bed.*
4. *Sitting or lying.*
5. *Standing upright.*

Section B (Stiffness)

6. *How severe is your stiffness after first wakening in the morning?*
7. *How severe is your stiffness after sitting, lying, or resting later in the day?*

Section C (Function)

What degree of difficulty do you have with:

8. *Descending stairs?*
9. *Ascending stairs?*
10. *Rising from sitting?*
11. *Standing?*
12. *Bending to floor?*
13. *Walking on flat?*
14. *Getting in/out of car?*
15. *Going shopping?*
16. *Putting on socks/stockings?*
17. *Rising from bed?*
18. *Taking off socks/stockings?*
19. *Lying in bed?*
20. *Getting in/out of bath?*
21. *Sitting?*
22. *Getting on/off toilet?*
23. *Heavy domestic duties?*
24. *Light domestic duties?*

Total Score and Interpretation

Unlike the HSS Knee Score and the KSS, a high total score from the WOMAC questionnaire represents a poor result. Scores higher than 38 points represent poor results; scores from 29 to 38 are considered fair results; scores between 15 and 28 can be considered good results; and scores between 14 and 0 are excellent results.

COMPARISON BETWEEN OUTCOME MEASURES

The three scores discussed in this chapter are the outcome measures most often used to evaluate TKA. The HSS Knee Score and the KSS are interview-based and dependent on a physical examination. When using these scores, the physician should be cognizant that the scores are subject to examiner bias; the values obtained from the physical examination may vary considerably between examiners.[6] However, the HSS Knee Score and the KSS provide detailed information about the physical dynamics of the prosthesis, an area not addressed by the WOMAC Score. As a result, the KSS and the HSS Score are powerful tools for comparing specific dynamics of a knee replacement and are useful for evaluating the performance dynamics of TKA. The WOMAC Score is a valuable tool in evaluating the patient's level of function and pain postsurgery.

Although the HSS Knee Score and the KSS are different in organization and technique from the WOMAC Score, the three scales have proven to correlate well with each other in their measurement of total knee replacement outcomes.[1] The WOMAC Score does not provide data on the performance parameters of a prosthesis; it quantifies a patient's functioning following TKA.

USES OF TOTAL KNEE REPLACEMENT SCORES

Historically, these scores were most often used by researchers to report the results of TKA. These researchers evaluated the preoperative function of their patients prior to TKA and compared their preoperative score with the postoperative score. This permitted the researcher to evaluate patient variables (comorbidities) as well as different types of prostheses.

Because of changes in medical care and most notably medical coverage plans, there has been increased pressure to decrease the cost of medical treatments. As a result, it has become increasingly important to evaluate the outcomes of different medical treatments. The evaluation often takes the form of outcome studies that attempt to measure the patient's quality of life and the therapeutic result. In 1989, the Agency for Health Policy and Research funded several Patient Outcome Research teams to study different medical therapeutics. This type of research has two objectives: to document the value of a specific therapy relative to its cost and to determine its impact on the patient's quality of life. If this type of research is successful, the government and eventually third-party billers may use the results to ration or direct medical care into more "effective" therapeutic means. Many health care providers are concerned that these data may eventually be used to judge the ability to deliver health care.

This has convinced many physicians to begin measuring the results of their TKAs. Unfortunately, there is no one score used to gather or one method used to analyze outcome data. There are different commercial products that collect a multitude of information, including the scores discussed in this chapter, financial data on the cost of the prosthesis, length of stay, and several other parameters. Most of these products are computer database software that provides a variety of reports. Practitioners can use these reports to study their own data and analyze the results. Some programs allow the practitioners to join a national data bank and compare their data with others in the country.

Physicians in conjunction with orthopedic companies have designed most of these programs. These companies want to ensure that physicians who use their products stay competitive. Some companies collect and analyze the data free of charge for physicians using that company's products. Other companies sell the software, permitting physicians to use the data and reports as they wish. Unfortunately, this adds cost to the business operations because data collection and analysis may require a separate dedicated computer system. If outcome data are eventually required of all practitioners, business software packages will most likely incorporate outcome data subroutines into their products.

APPENDIX

The following is a list of some of the suppliers of outcome software and their affiliated companies.

American Academy of Orthopedic Surgeons—*MODEMS*—Musculoskeletal Outcomes Data Evaluation and Management System: The program enables physicians to collect data on patients' demographics, general health status, musculoskeletal function, and resource utilization. Physicians can store and use the data and make them part of the national data bank, which will allow participants to compare their practice to national norms.

Biomet: Provides forms for data collection for physicians. Analyzes data and provides feedback to the physician through reports. Able to compare user to other physicians and normative data. Only available to Biomet product users.

DePuy—*Capture Ware:* Data collection database for total joint arthroplasty to be used by physicians in their offices. Incorporates several outcome measures and delivers predesigned reports. Comparison with other physicians available through DePuy. The software targets DePuy products.

Howmedica—*Orthopedic Resource Patient Advisory Software:* Software designed to expand patient education by delivering documents written in clear and detailed manner that are designed for take-home use.

Intermedics—*Velocity Healthcare Infomatics:* Software database program that allows comparisons against other orthopedic surgeons and normative data. The data input is done in the physician's office, and the analysis and reporting is done by Intermedics and sent back to the physician.

Osteonics—*Outcomes Performance Users System (OPUS):* Data collection database for total joint arthroplasty to be used by physicians in their offices. Incorporates several outcome measures and delivers predesigned reports. The software targets Osteonics products.

Smith & Nephew—*The Summit Solution:* Data collection database for total joint arthroplasty to be used by physicians in their offices. Incorporates several outcome measures and delivers predesigned reports. Outcome data organized in three categories: clinical/functional; cost; patient satisfaction. This product is not vendor dependent.

Wright Medical—*Quick Trak:* Computer database software designed to keep information on operative cases in the form of index cards. No reports or data comparisons are available.

References

1. Alicea JA, Insall JN, Scuderi GR: Comparative Analysis of Outcome Scores in Total Knee Arthroplasty. Presented at AAOS, Orlando, FL, 1995.
2. Bellamy N: Pain assessment in osteoarthritis: Experience with the WOMAC osteoarthritis index. Semin Arthritis Rheum 18:14, 1989.
3. Bellamy N, Buchanan WW, Goldsmith CH, et al: Validation study of WOMAC: A health status instrument for measuring clinically important patient relevant outcomes to antirheumatic drug therapy in patients with osteoarthritis of the hip or knee. J Rheumatol 15:1833, 1988.
4. Bellamy N, Goldsmith CH, Buchanan WW, et al: Prior score availability: Observations using the WOMAC osteoarthritis index (letter). Br J Rheumatol 30:150, 1991.
5. Bellamy N, Kean WF, Buchanan WW, et al: Double blind randomized controlled trial of sodium meclofenamate (Meclomen) and diclofenac sodium (Voltaren): Post validation reapplication of the WOMAC Osteoarthritis Index. J Rheumatol 19:153, 1992.
6. Cartwright J, Oronoz J, Stevens W, et al: Reproducibility and reliability of the Knee Society Score. Presented at Society of Military Orthopaedic Surgeons, Vail, CO, 1996.
7. Insall J, Scott WN, Ranawat CS: The total condylar knee prosthe-

sis. A report of two hundred and twenty cases. J Bone Joint Surg Am 61:173, 1779.

8. Insall JN, Dorr LD, Scott RD, et al: Rationale of the Knee Society clinical rating system. Clin Orthop 248:13, 1989.
9. Insall JN, Hood RW, Flawn LB, et al: The total condylar knee prosthesis in gonarthrosis. A five- to nine-year follow-up of the first one hundred consecutive replacements. J Bone Joint Surg Am 65:619, 1983.
10. Insall JN, Lachiewicz PF, Burstein AH: The posterior stabilized condylar prosthesis: A modification of the total condylar design. Two- to four-year clinical experience. J Bone Joint Surg Am 64: 1317, 1982.
11. Insall JN, Ranawat CS, Aglietti P, et al: A comparison of four models of total knee replacement prostheses. J Bone Joint Surg Am 58:754, 1976.

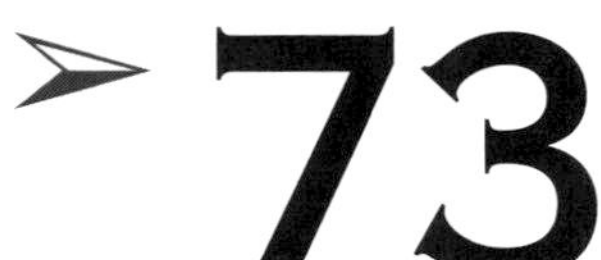

73 Historic Development, Classification, and Characteristics of Knee Prostheses

JOHN N. INSALL • HENRY D. CLARKE

The evolution of total knee replacement—in its modern form about 30 years old—is not merely of historic interest. Those surgeons with some years of experience will have noticed that fashion tends to repeat itself. For example, in the early years (1970 to 1974) a range of prostheses (unicondylar, bicondylar, and hinged) were used according to the preoperative condition and deformity. These prostheses fell into disrepute, and for a while tricondylar prostheses were in vogue for virtually all procedures. In recent years, successful results have been obtained with unicondylar prostheses in selected patients, and the use of both constrained and hinged prostheses have found a place in the surgical armamentarium for revision and complex primary surgery. In addition, interest in mobile-bearing prostheses has been rekindled as the limits of current fixed-bearing prostheses, both cruciate retaining and cruciate substituting, are defined. In order to help advances in the field of total knee arthroplasty (TKA), we believe it is useful to look at what has worked and what has not worked.

EARLY PROSTHETIC MODELS

Interposition and Resurfacing Prostheses

The concept of improving knee joint function by modifying the articular surfaces has received attention since the 19th century. In 1860, Verneuil[220] suggested the interposition of soft tissues to reconstruct the articular surface of a joint. Subsequently, pig bladder, nylon, fascia lata, prepatellar bursa, and cellophane were some of the materials used for this purpose. The results were disappointing. In 1860, Ferguson[61] resected the entire knee joint, which resulted in mobility of the newly created subchondral surfaces (Fig. 73.1). When more bone was removed, the patients enjoyed good motion but lacked the necessary stability, whereas with less bone resection, spontaneous fusions often resulted. These early attempts were usually performed on knees damaged by tuberculosis or other infectious processes, with concomitant ankylosis and deformity. The results of this procedure were sufficiently poor to discourage anything more than occasional attempts in severe cases.

Encouraged by the relative success of hip cup arthroplasty, Campbell[36] reported the successful use of the metallic interposition femoral mold in 1940. A similar type of arthroplasty was developed and used at the Massachusetts General Hospital. The results, published by Speed and Trout[209] in 1949 and by Miller and Friedman[156] in 1952, were not very good, and this type of knee arthroplasty never achieved wide recognition.

In 1958, MacIntosh[143] described a different type of hemiarthroplasty he had used in treating painful varus or valgus deformities of the knee. An acrylic tibial plateau prosthesis was inserted into the affected side

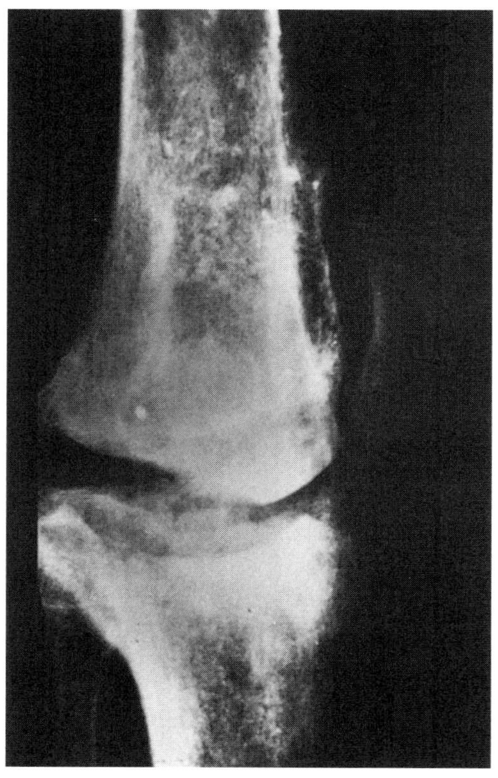

FIGURE 73.1 ➢ Resection arthroplasty creates a mobile but usually unstable joint.

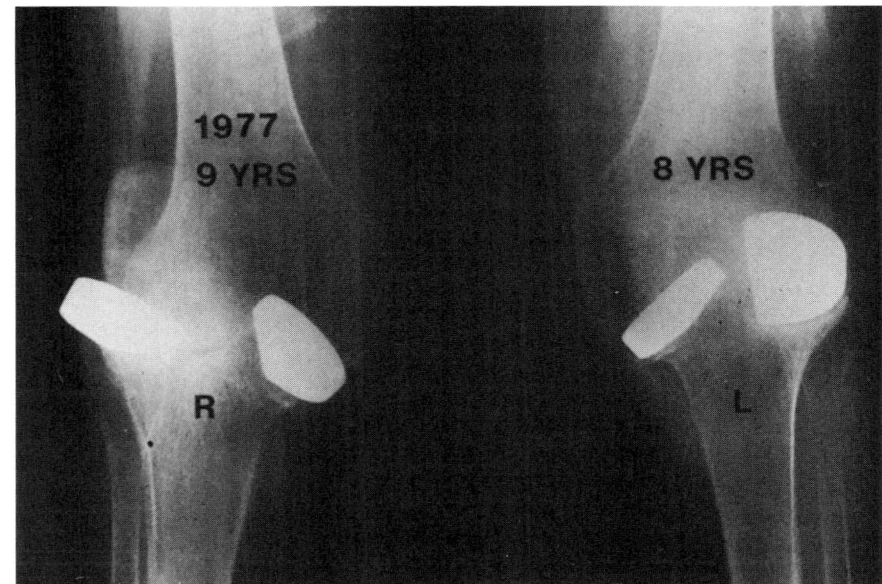

FIGURE 73.2 ➢ MacIntosh hemiarthroplasty used in rheumatoid arthritis often restores alignment and stability for a few years. However, as in this bilateral case, late dislocation and sinkage are common.

to correct deformity, restore stability, and relieve pain. Later versions of this prosthesis[144] were made of metal (Fig. 73.2), and the somewhat similar McKeever prosthesis[54, 154, 188] showed considerably more success and was extensively used, particularly in rheumatoid arthritis. Gunston[85] carried MacIntosh's ideas a step further and, instead of using a simple metal disk interposed within the joint, substituted metallic runners embedded in the femoral condyles, articulating against polyethylene troughs attached to the tibial plateau. To make a four-part system of this kind feasible, it was necessary to find a means of fixing the components rigidly to the bone. The solution was provided by acrylic cement.

Although the Gunston polycentric prosthesis[85] was the first cemented surface arthroplasty of the knee joint, the work of Freeman and colleagues[66] has had an even greater influence on the direction of both prosthetic design and surgical technique. The design objectives for a prosthesis (Fig. 73.3A,B) were outlined in 1973 by Freeman and colleagues.[66] The most important of these objectives are the following:

1. A salvage procedure should be readily available. The implantation of the prosthesis should require the removal of no more bone than for primary arthrodesis and should leave large, flat surfaces of cancellous bone.

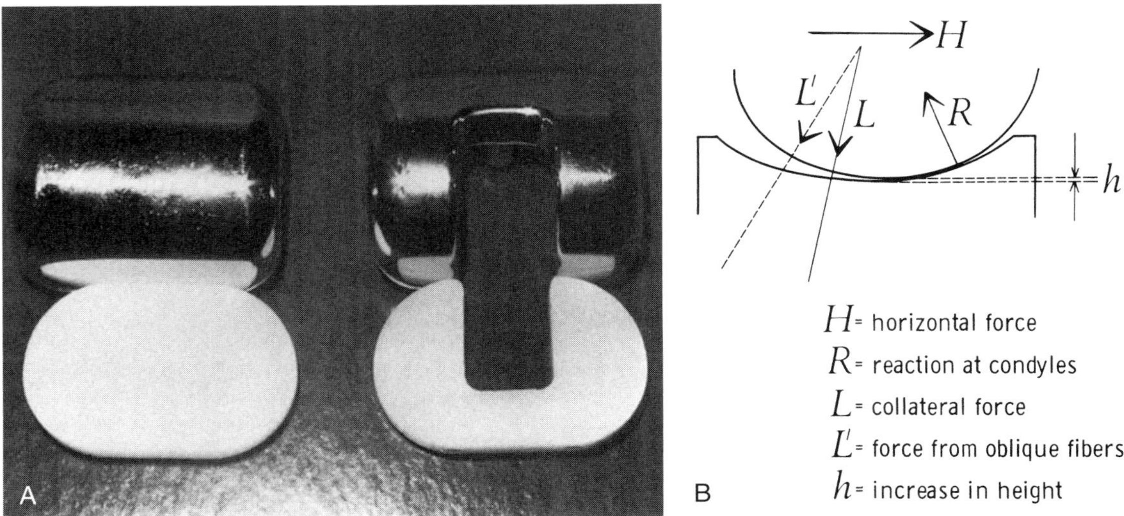

FIGURE 73.3 ➢ *A,* The original Freeman-Swanson prosthesis used two one-piece components. *B,* Stability is obtained by the roller-in-trough concept; dislocation can occur only if one component runs uphill on the other. Distraction is resisted by capsular and collateral ligament tension.

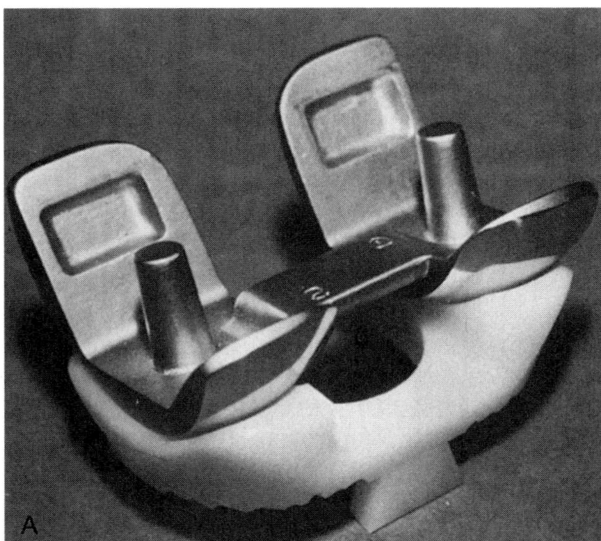

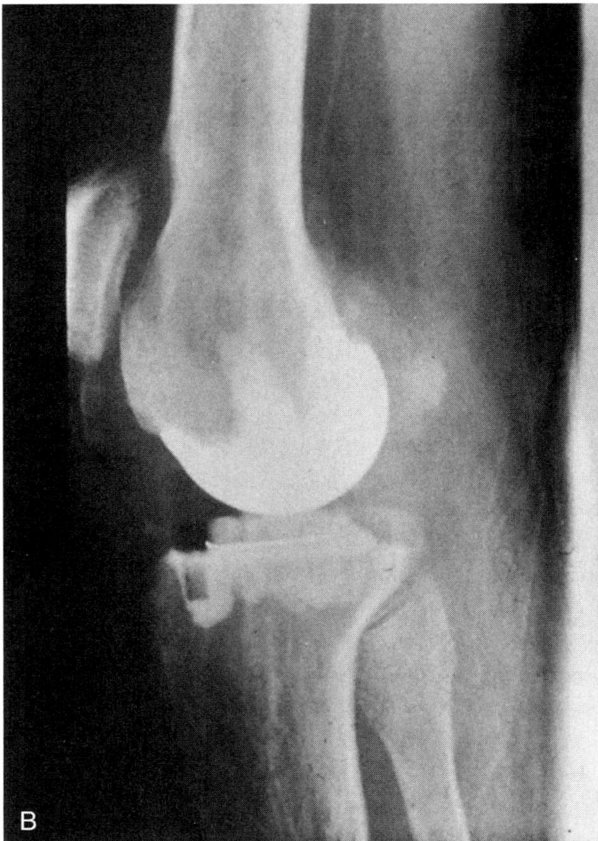

FIGURE 73.4 ➢ *A* and *B*, An early and widely used surface replacement was the geometric prosthesis.

2. The chances of loosening should be minimized.
   a. The femoral and tibial components should be incompletely constrained relative to each other so that twisting, varus, or valgus moments cannot be transmitted to the bonds between prosthesis and skeleton.
   b. The friction between the components should be minimized.
   c. Any hyperextension-limiting arrangement should be progressive and not sudden in action.
   d. The prosthetic component should be fitted to the bone by means that spread the loads over the largest possible areas of the bone prosthesis interface.
3. The rate of production of wear debris should be minimized, and the debris produced should be as innocuous as possible. This leads to a preference for metal-on-plastic-bearing surfaces, which should be as large as possible to keep the surface stresses low.
4. The probability of infection should be minimized by having compact prosthetic components with few dead spaces.
5. The consequences of infection should be minimized by avoiding long intramedullary stems and intramedullary cement.
6. A standard insertion procedure should be available.
7. The prosthesis should give motion from 5 degrees of hyperextension to at least 90 degrees of flexion.
8. Some freedom of rotation should be resisted.
9. Excessive movements in any direction should be resisted by the soft tissues, particularly the collateral ligaments.

Most of these objectives remain valid today, although two additional points cited in the Freeman report remain issues for debate. These are (1) the place of the cruciate ligaments in TKA and (2) the need to replace the patellofemoral joint and the desirability of patellar resurfacing.

Other early examples of resurfacing prostheses (Figs. 73.4 and 73.5) were the Geometric,[45, 46, 218] Duocondylar,[170, 202] UCI (University of California at Irvine),[229] and Marmor.[147-149, 151]

Constrained Prostheses

A second line of development in knee arthroplasty occurred parallel to the concepts of interposition and, later, surface replacement. In 1951, Walldius[227] devel-

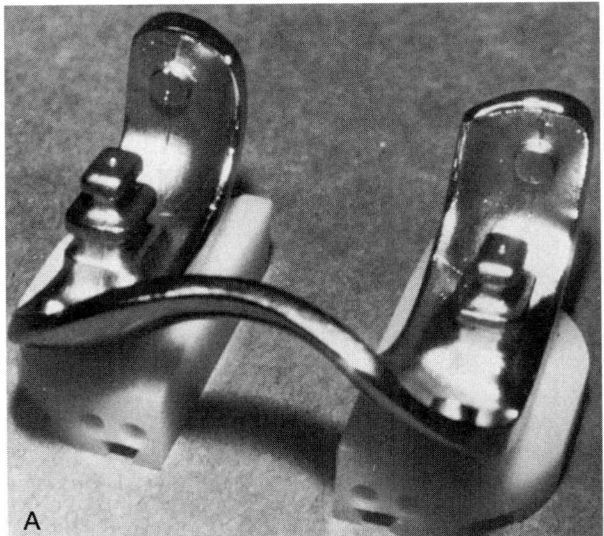

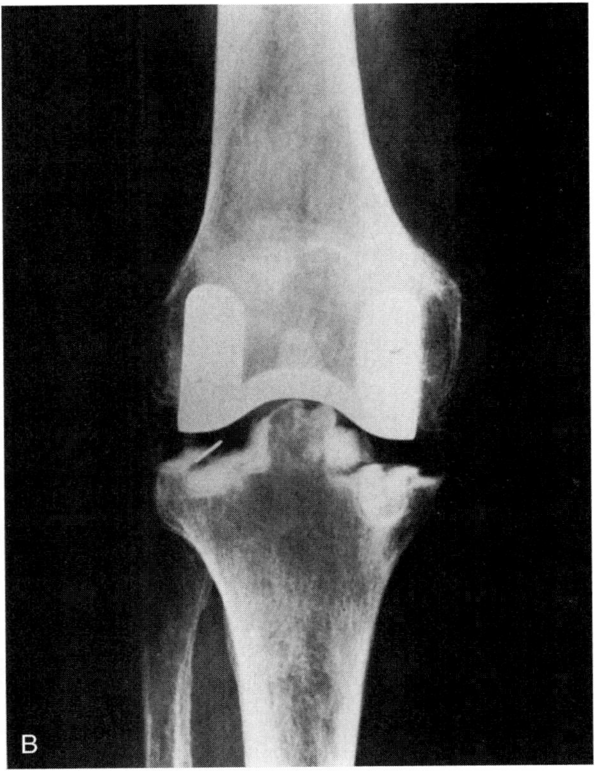

FIGURE 73.5 ➢ *A,* The Duocondylar prosthesis was anatomic in concept, retained both cruciate ligaments when these were present, but did not resurface the patellofemoral joint. Sinkage and loosening of the tibial components were an eventual problem with this design. *B,* An anteroposterior radiograph with the duocondylar prosthesis inserted. Radiolucent lines around both tibial components are visible.

oped the hinged prosthesis that bears his name. The device was initially made of acrylic and later of metal.

Shortly thereafter, Shiers[196] described a similar device with even simpler mechanical characteristics (Fig. 73.6). A hinged prosthesis has considerable appeal. Technically it is easy to use as the intramedullary stems make the prosthesis largely self-aligning, and all the ligaments and other soft-tissue constraints can be sacrificed because the prosthesis is self-stabilizing. The extent of damage of the knee is therefore of no consequence, and even the most extreme deformities can be corrected by dividing the soft tissues and resecting sufficient bone. Of course, the early hinged designs were uncemented, although later developments such as the GUEPAR (Fig. 73.7) were designed from the outset to be used with methyl methacrylate cement. The current models that have evolved from this lineage are the kinematic rotating hinge, the spherocentric (Fig. 73.8), and a model that is a crossbreed, the TCP III (total condylar prosthesis)[50] (Fig. 73.9), now known as the constrained condylar knee (CCK). There has been a return to *uncemented stems,* particularly for revision surgery.

EVOLUTION OF PROSTHETIC DESIGN

The prostheses discussed up to this point are now more or less obsolete. Although the early results were quite encouraging, further follow-up demonstrated various problems that have to this day given total knee arthroplasty a bad reputation.

The literature relevant to total knee arthroplasty includes many articles that report the clinical results of designs no longer in common use.[5, 10-14, 16, 30, 32, 35, 38, 39, 42, 47, 48, 50, 52, 58-60, 64, 68-70, 72, 73, 76, 77, 83, 86, 92, 97, 98, 100, 103-106, 109-113, 116, 130, 132, 138-140, 145, 152, 153, 161, 162, 165, 166, 173, 175, 176, 179, 184, 194, 195, 197, 198, 200, 201, 203, 205, 213, 217, 219, 230, 231, 236, 237, 242] These published reports on results using early models are somewhat difficult to compare because different rating methods were used. A review conducted at the Hospital for Special Surgery (HSS) between 1971 and 1973 is probably representative. This review[98] compared four different models (Fig. 73.10): the unicondylar (Fig. 73.11), Duocondylar, Geometric, and GUEPAR (see Fig. 73.7). The results were expressed using the HSS 100-point knee-rating scale.

The postoperative knees were classified into four groups, according to their scores on the HSS scale:

Excellent: 85+. These knees approached the normal, and were obviously much improved in the opinion of both the patient and the examiner.

Good: 70 to 84. These knees showed obvious improvement after arthroplasty, but the result was not as good as in the Excellent group.

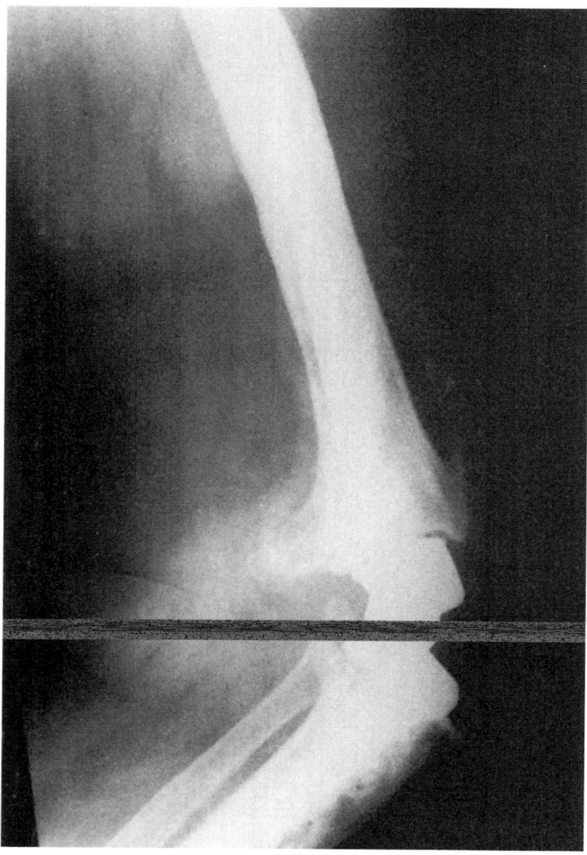

FIGURE 73.6 ➢ The Shiers prosthesis was a simple uniaxial metallic hinge.

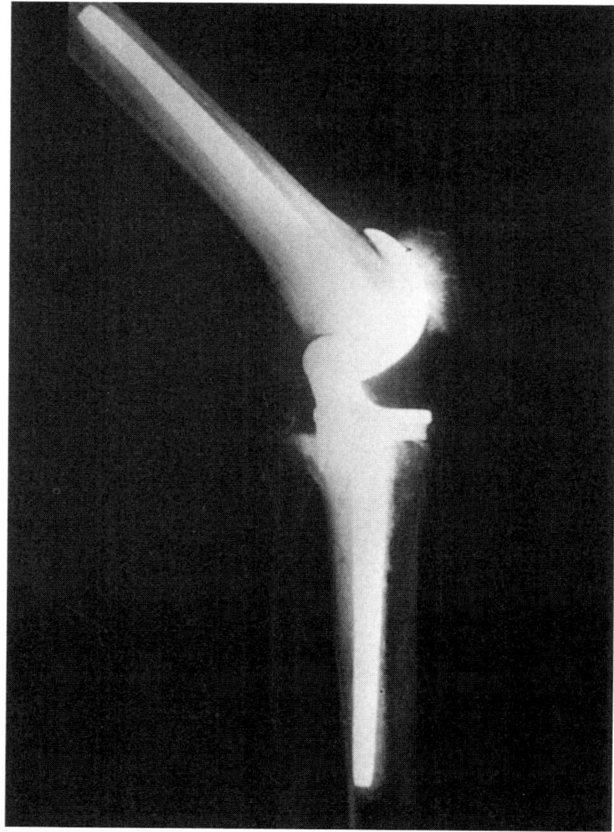

FIGURE 73.7 ➢ The GUEPAR hinge was like the Shiers uniaxial metallic hinge, but with the axis placed more posteriorly and femoral resurfacing for the patellar articulation.

Fair: 60 to 69. This group mostly comprised knees in which the result of the arthroplasty was deficient in some way (persistent pain, moderate instability, or unsatisfactory range of motion), but also included some in which the rating of the arthroplasty was downgraded by the patient's general condition (e.g., multiple joint involvement in rheumatoid arthritis or systemic disease).

Failure: Less than 60. These knees were evidently unsatisfactory and below the rating achieved by knee fusion (which scores a 60 on the HSS knee-rating scale). This classification included knees in which the prosthesis had been removed or replaced and knees in which the improvement, if any, did not seem to justify the risk of arthroplasty.

Considering the entire group of 178 arthroplasties studied in the four different models (23 unicondylar, 60 Duocondylar, 50 geometric, and 45 GUEPAR), the results were considered excellent in 47 (26%), good in 66 (37%), fair in 37 (21%), and poor in 28 (16%) (Fig. 73.12). There was no statistically significant difference between the results obtained with each of the four prostheses studied. However, because it is easier to improve a bad knee than a relatively good one, the percentage of improvement was much greater with the GUEPAR than with the unicondylar (120% versus 45%).

Three specific problems were identified from this study: patellar pain, component loosening, and surgical technique. However, because the GUEPAR hinge was inserted into the worst knees originally, it gave the greatest percentage of improvement in the HSS knee-rating scale. At the time of the study, the conclusion reached was that the GUEPAR prosthesis appeared superior in a number of ways. It had been selected for use in the most severely involved knees and yet equaled any of the other prostheses in the quality of results both in rheumatoid arthritis and in osteoarthritis. It also gave the lowest proportion of failures and was the only model to improve range of motion postoperatively. However, the potential problems of loosening and mechanical failure with the GUEPAR prosthesis were noted. More than 100 GUEPAR prostheses were used at the Hospital for Special Surgery 15 to 20 years ago, and these expected problems have now to a large extent materialized. Approximately 80% of the prostheses are loose both clinically and radiographically, although they are not necessarily symptomatic (Fig. 73.13A). There have also been seven cases of stem breakage (four femoral and three tibial) (Fig. 73.13B) and, as noted later, infection became a major

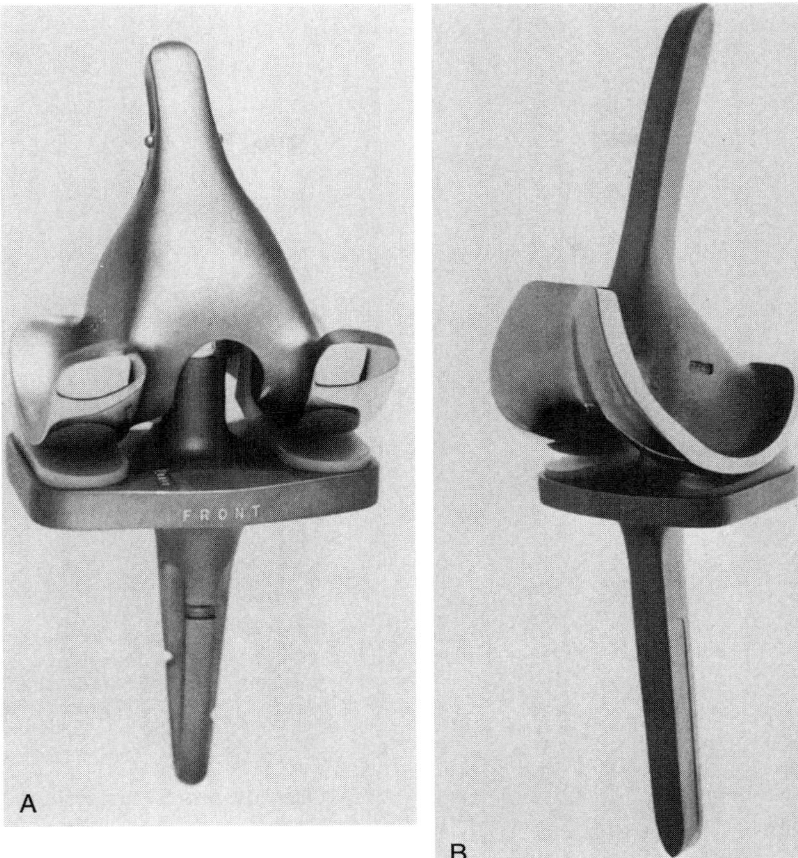

FIGURE 73.8 ➢ Spherocentric prosthesis. *A*, Standard version. *B*, Long-stemmed variant with patellar flange. (Courtesy of Drs. Kauffer and Matthews.)

problem. This study therefore reached some erroneous conclusions because of a short follow-up—a point of great relevance today when many new prostheses are being used in patients with scanty clinical follow-up to support their merits.

Patellar Pain

None of the four early prosthetic models studied made any provision for patellofemoral function. Patellectomy did not seem to offer a solution to the problem of patellofemoral arthritis (Fig. 73.14). In our study, 38 patellectomies were performed in the group as a whole, 3 of which were done at a later date than the arthroplasty because of persistent patellar pain. A complaint of pain after patellectomy was as frequent as in patients in whom patellectomy had not been performed. In addition, patients with a patellectomy suffered from inadequacy of the extensor mechanism. In the GUEPAR group of 45 knees, pain on patellar compression was found in 22 on follow-up, and patellar erosion was observed in 5 patients. Patellar subluxation frequently occurred with the GUEPAR prosthesis in spite of a wide lateral release of the patellar retinaculum at the time of arthroplasty (Fig. 73.15). However, this was often not apparent to the patient and may be considered an incidental finding. Subluxation of the patella did not necessarily correlate with complaints of postoperative pain. However, with the geometric prosthesis, 29 of 50 knees had pain on patellofemoral compression. Patellar subluxation was found in nine knees, and all were painful.

Loosening

A radiolucent line surrounding the prosthetic components was seen with great frequency. With the condylar replacements, the radiolucency was usually observed around the tibial component. It was present in 70% of knees with the unicondylar, 50% with the Duocondylar, and 80% with the geometric prosthesis. A radiolucent line was observed around the femoral component in 45% of the patients with a GUEPAR prosthesis. The radiolucent line was slightly more frequent in osteoarthritis than in rheumatoid arthritis patients; it was observed in all knees with osteoarthritis in which the geometric prosthesis was used. Radiolucent lines are by no means always symptomatic, but when complete, progressive, and associated with pain on weightbearing, they generally indicate failure of fix-

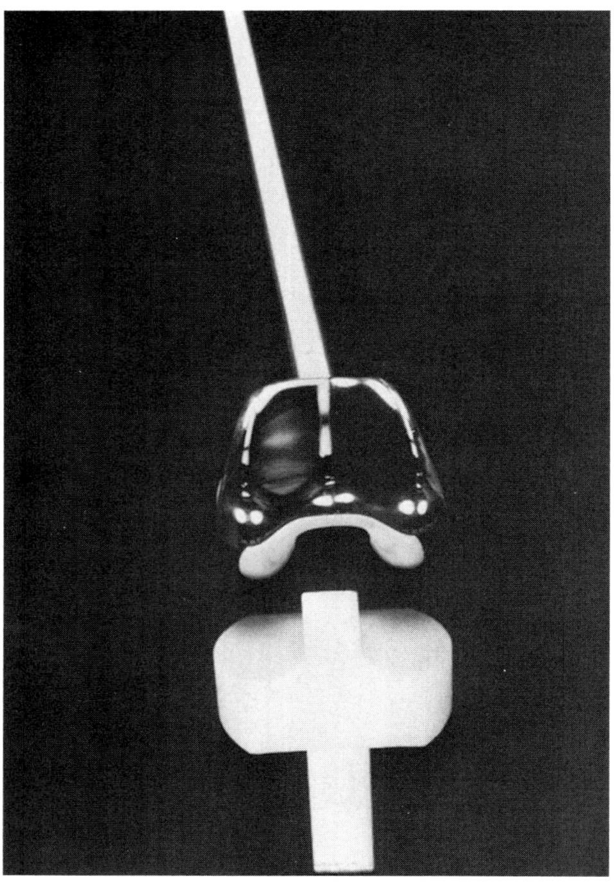

FIGURE 73.9 ➢ The constrained but unlinked TCP III. Varus and valgus constraint is provided by the rectangular central peg on the tibial component.

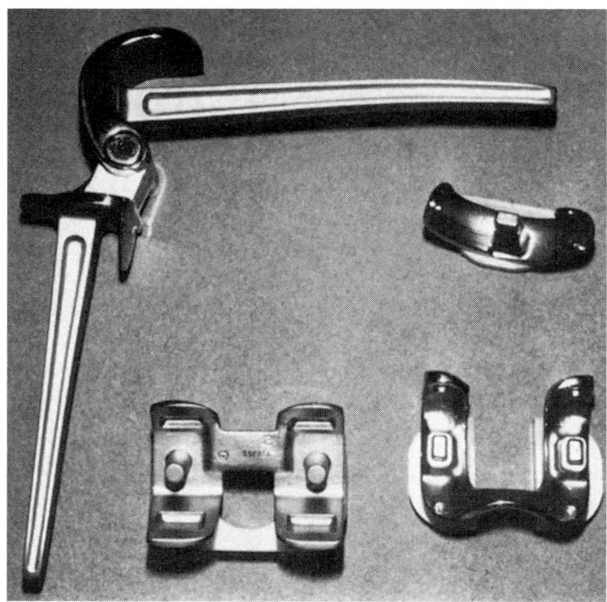

FIGURE 73.10 ➢ The graduated system concept selected the prosthesis according to the degree and extent of damage. The prostheses shown here in a clockwise direction are the unicondylar, Duocondylar, geometric, and GUEPAR prostheses.

ation. Our subsequent experience has shown that the incidence of partial radiolucencies for a particular prosthesis does not correlate with the eventual amount of component loosening. On the basis of a 10- to 12-year follow-up on one particular cemented prosthesis (the total condylar), we recently concluded that a detailed study of partial radiolucent lines is worthless

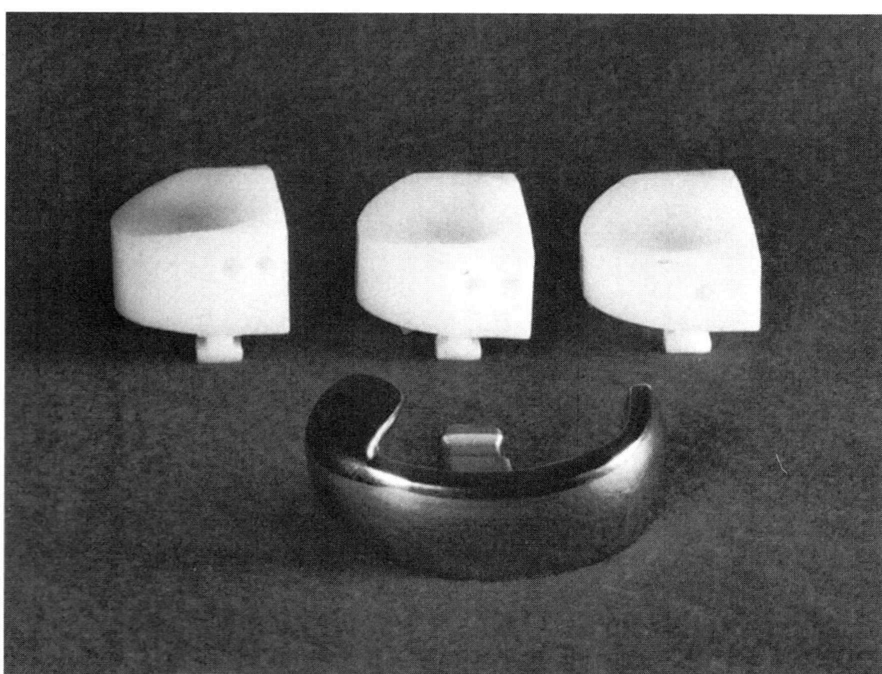

FIGURE 73.11 ➢ The unicondylar prosthesis was designed to resurface only the affected femorotibial compartment. The shape and curvature of the component were similar to the duocondylar design.

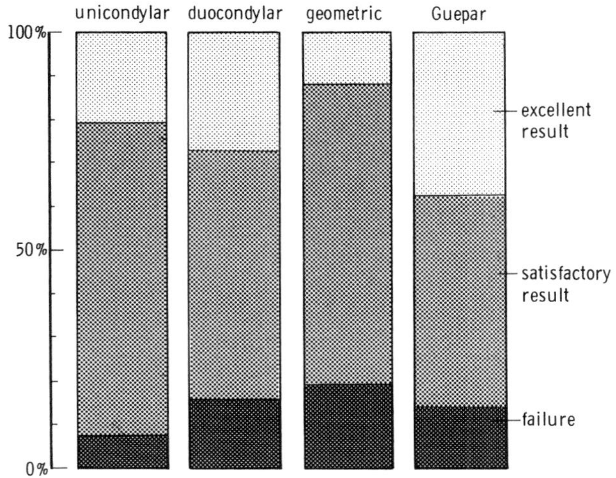

FIGURE 73.12 ➢ Graph showing comparative results of four early prosthetic models.

and a poor predictor of future failure (Fig. 73.16). Whether the same observation holds true for uncemented prostheses remains to be seen.

On the basis of early analysis of these data, it was clear that tibial loosening represented a failure in prosthetic design. The flat, cancellous surface of the upper tibia is not a suitable bed for a flat prosthetic component because of poor resistance to shear stress. Moreover, this bone is not of sufficient strength to resist subsidence of the tibial component, even if excavations are made to accommodate fixation fins or lugs on the bottom of the tibial prosthesis (Figs. 73.17 and 73.18). It was concluded that some form of cortical fixation would be essential for a successful series of TKAs.

Prosthesis Selection and Surgical Technique

Like many others, we initially believed in the concept of a graduated system in which selection of a prosthesis depended upon the severity of damage found in the arthritic knee (see Fig. 73.10). For example, knees with cartilage erosion restricted to one femorotibial compartment were replaced with a unicondylar pros-

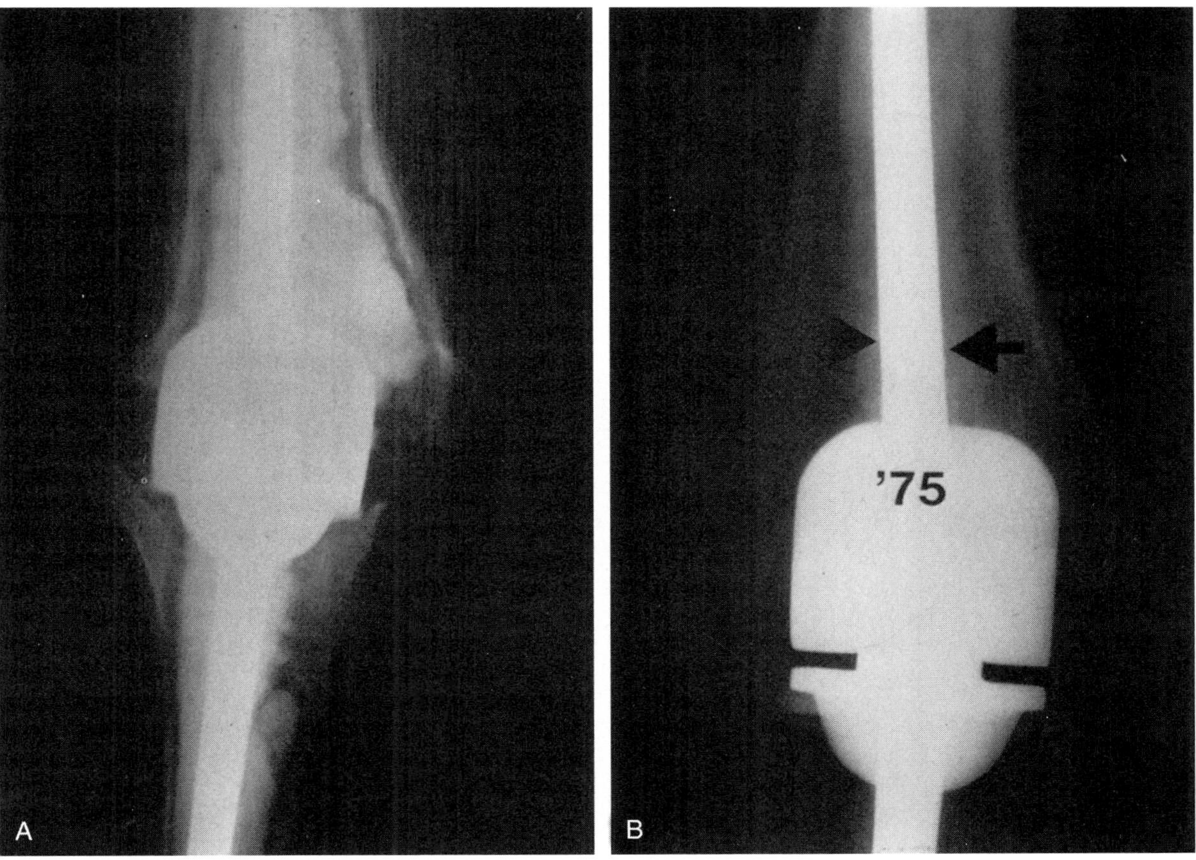

FIGURE 73.13 ➢ *A,* Radiograph of a grossly loose GUEPAR prosthesis 5 years after the initial insertion. *B,* Stem breakage occurred with the GUEPAR prosthesis, usually at the site shown here in the radiograph 5 cm proximal to the joint.

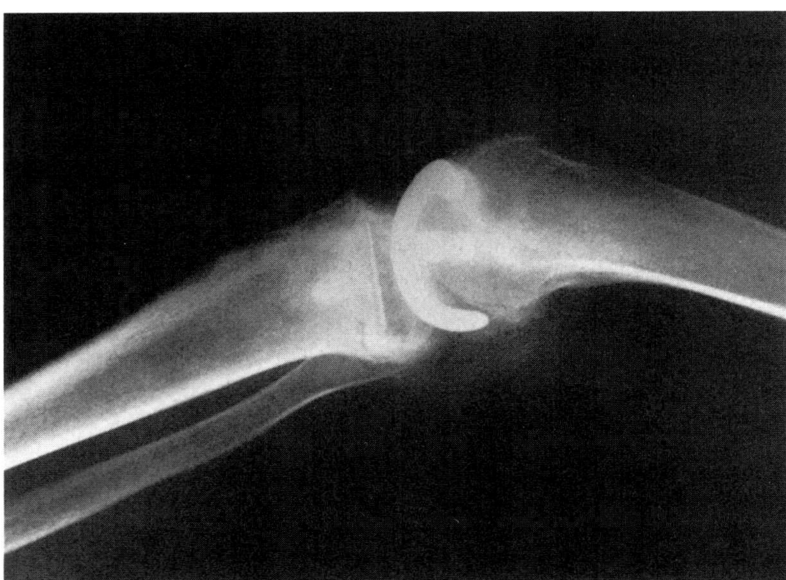

FIGURE 73.14 ➢ Patellectomy is not a satisfactory solution to patellofemoral pain. Patellectomy was done in conjunction with a unicondylar prosthesis.

thesis, whereas in the most severely damaged and deformed knees, a hinged prosthesis was used. The bicondylar prosthesis occupied an intermediate position with respect to the severity of arthritis. While the use of a hinged prosthesis is not technically demanding, the early condylar designs were difficult to insert and align and there was very little margin for error. Obviously the advantage of even the most sophisticated prosthetic design is lost if the surgical placement is incorrect. Furthermore, an inherent drawback in a graduated system of prostheses is that a model may be used for degrees of deformity exceeding the limits for which the prosthesis was intended. This error can itself be a cause for failure (e.g., dislocation) (Fig. 73.19). Clearly, there is no purpose in selecting one prosthetic design over another unless some advantage can be shown. For example, in our comparative study we did not find that the unicondylar prosthesis offered any advantage over bicondylar models. The merits of graduated knee systems remain a source of debate today.

Infection

Although deep periprosthetic infection was not a frequent cause of failure for the condylar designs, it has subsequently proved a major problem with the GUEPAR prosthesis. With further follow-up, 15 of 108 prostheses became infected (4 early and 8 late). This incidence of 16% is likely to rise as late infection oc-

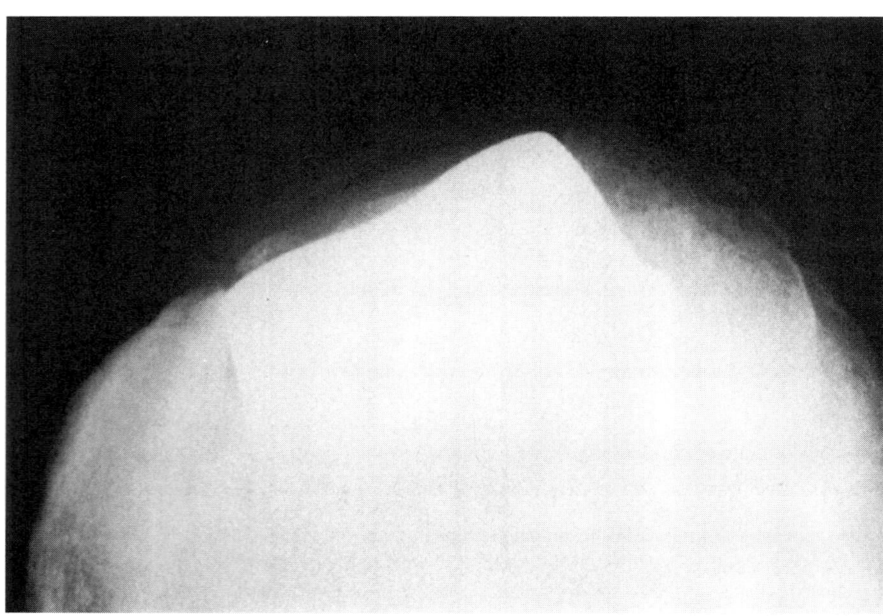

FIGURE 73.15 ➢ Patellar subluxation and dislocation often occurred with the GUEPAR prosthesis. It was not always symptomatic.

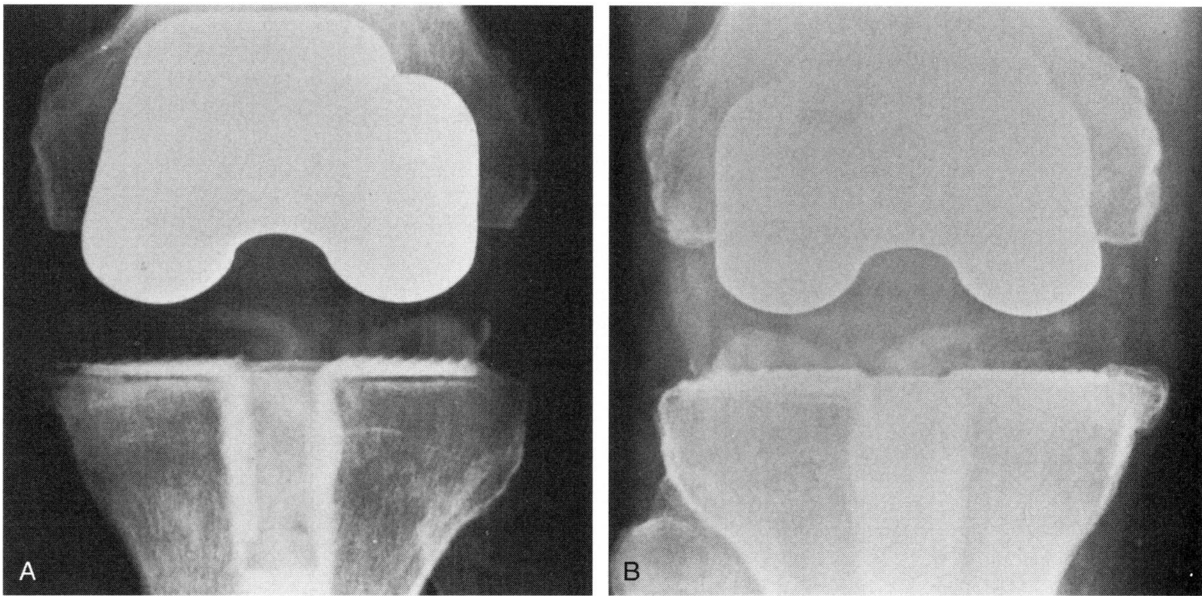

FIGURE 73.16 ➢ *A*, Radiograph taken 1 year after implantation shows a pronounced radiolucent line beneath medial and lateral tibial plateaus. *B*, Radiograph of the same knee taken at 5 years shows a barely visible radiolucency.

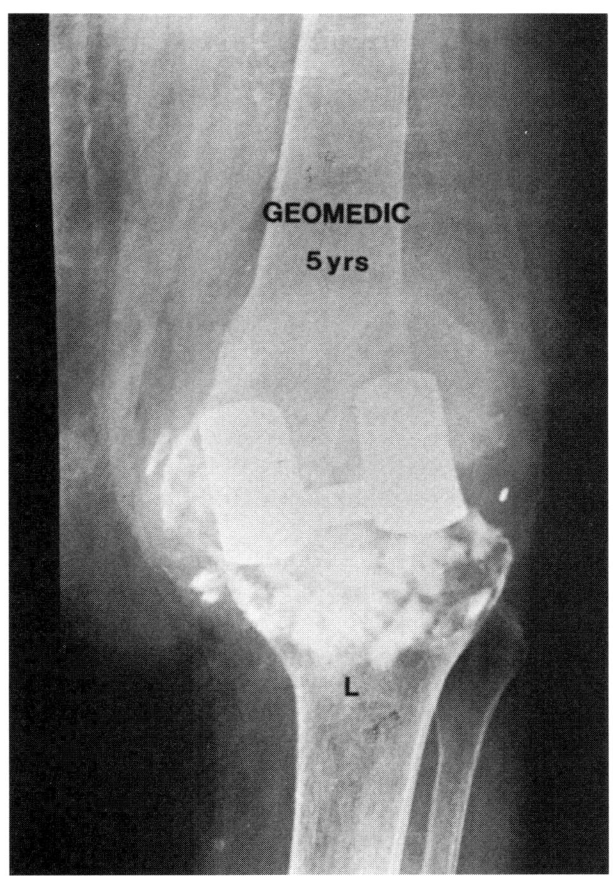

FIGURE 73.17 ➢ Failure of tibial fixation was a frequent problem with many early prosthetic designs. The problem was primarily attributable to collapse of the cancellous bone of the upper tibia, with sinkage of the component.

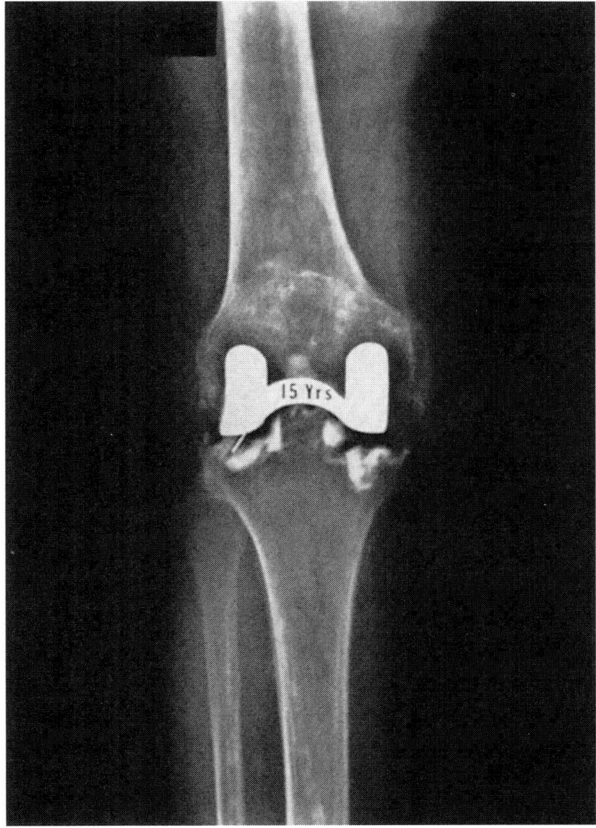

FIGURE 73.18 ➢ Radiograph of a 15-year follow-up of a duocondylar prosthesis, which had two separate tibial components. There is the appearance of osteopenia around the femoral component runners. The knee continued to function well.

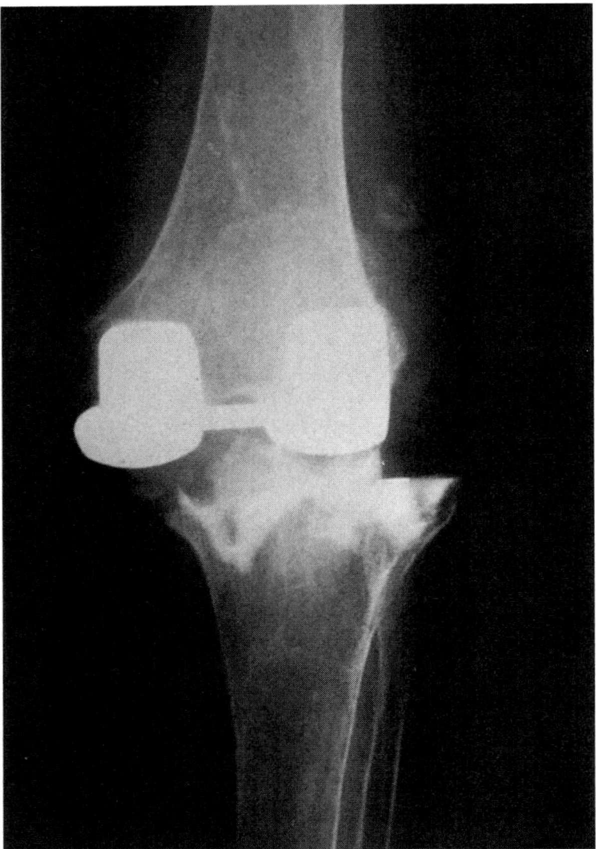

FIGURE 73.19 ➢ This geometric prosthesis translocated and dislocated. This was the condition of the knee before the prosthesis was inserted and represents an error of selection of prosthesis.

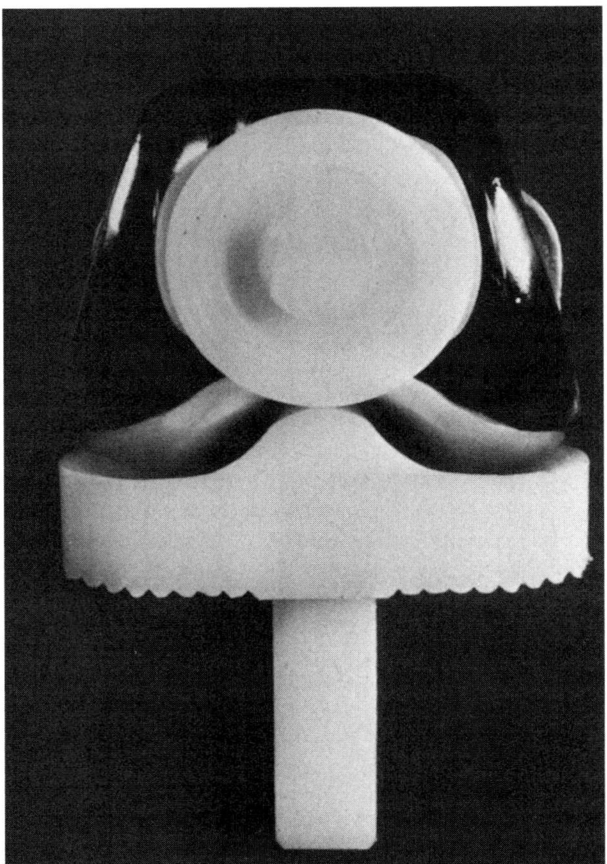

FIGURE 73.20 ➢ The total condylar prosthesis.

curs even many years after the arthroplasty. An example was an 85-year-old woman who had a GUEPAR prosthesis inserted in 1972. She did very well for 8 years until onset of acute deep sepsis. There was no obvious focus elsewhere to suggest a metastatic infection. Because of her age and the extreme toxicity caused by virulent infection, a midthigh amputation had to be performed. More recently a second amputation was performed for late-onset sepsis: the extreme devitalization of the tissues caused by metallic debris made any thought of salvage impossible. There have been reports of similar occurrences in the literature.[11]

This experience has led to a convergence of prosthetic designs, particularly in the United States.

At the Hospital for Special Surgery, dissatisfaction with the early prostheses led to the design of the total condylar and duopatellar prostheses.

TYPES OF PROSTHESES

Most simply, a prosthesis can be a surface replacement or a constrained design. These two categories may be further subdivided. Surface replacements comprise unicondylar and bicondylar designs. Unicondylar prostheses are discussed elsewhere in this text.[15, 37, 88, 124, 125, 129, 131, 146, 150, 158, 159, 186, 187] Bicondylar prostheses can be cruciate retaining, cruciate excising, or cruciate substituting. Constrained prostheses can be loose or rigid. Loose designs allow some degree of rotation and varus-valgus rock, and they have a bearing surface usually made of metal on polyethylene. Rigid designs have a fixed-axis metal hinge.

Early Surface Replacement Designs

In the following sections we discuss early surface replacement designs[224] and the role of the cruciates.

Total Condylar Prosthesis

Although coined as the name of a specific prosthesis, the term total condylar prosthesis has more recently been used generically to describe a whole range of surface prostheses that share general characteristics with the original (Fig. 73.20).[2, 9, 56, 62, 78, 91, 95, 96, 99, 101, 102, 105, 108, 115, 118, 122, 135, 171, 185, 191, 221, 222] Some of these later models differ in design details that may prove important in the long run.

The total condylar prosthesis, designed in 1973, was a true total replacement of the knee in that the patellofemoral joint was replaced as well as the femorotibial compartment. The salient features of the design are discussed in the following sections.

Femoral Component. Made of cobalt chromium alloy, the femoral component contains a symmetrically grooved anterior flange separating posteriorly into two symmetric condyles, each of decreasing radius posteriorly and having a symmetric convex curvature in the coronal plane.

Tibial Component. The tibial component is made of high-density polyethylene in one piece with two separate biconcave tibial plateaus that mate (articulate) precisely with the femoral condyles in extension, thus permitting no rotation in this position. In flexion the fit ceases to be exact and rotation and gliding motions are possible. The symmetric tibial plateaus are separated by an intercondylar eminence designed to prevent translocation or sideways sliding movements. The peripheral margin of the articular concavities is of an even height both anteriorly and posteriorly. The deep or bony surface of the component has a central fixation peg 35 mm in length and 12.5 mm in width. The anterior margin of the peg is vertical, but the posterior margin is oblique, conforming with the posterior cortex of the tibia.

Patellar Component. Made of high-density polyethylene, the patellar component is dome-shaped on its articular surface, conforming closely to the curvature of the femoral flange. A dome was selected because this shape does not require rotary alignment as would an anatomic prosthesis. The bony surface of the prosthesis has a central, rectangular fixation peg.

Duopatellar Prosthesis

The total condylar prosthesis was designed for cruciate excision. In contrast, the duopatellar prosthesis,[59] a sibling prosthesis designed at the Hospital for Special Surgery as a replacement for the duocondylar model, was intended to preserve existing cruciate ligaments, particularly the posterior cruciate. The general shape of the tibial runners was anatomic in the sagittal plane. Coronally, the condyles were flat with a median curvature.

The anterior connecting bar of the duocondylar prosthesis was extended into a femoral flange. The initial version of the Duopatellar model had two separate tibial plateaus identical to the Duocondylar design: flat in the sagittal plane, but with a median curvature coronally to prevent translocation. The deep surface was dovetailed for cement fixation. Later the two components were joined, and a central fixation peg similar to that of the total condylar prosthesis was added. A posterior cruciate cutout was provided. The patellar component of the duopatellar prosthesis was identical to that of the total condylar prosthesis.

Cruciate Excision, Retention, and Substitution

The total condylar and duopatellar prostheses were designed for cruciate excision and retention, respectively.[8, 9, 51, 68, 74] Subsequent modifications to the total condylar prosthesis incorporated a cam on the femoral component and a central post on the tibial polyethylene (Fig. 73.21). This cam-and-post mechanism was designed to act as a functional substitute for the posterior cruciate ligament (PCL), producing femoral rollback during flexion. With the development of this so-called posterior stabilized prosthesis, it was apparent that cruciate excision alone was not optimal. However, the relative merits of PCL retention versus PCL substitution have been debated vigorously by opposing groups within the orthopedic community for many years. Development of total knee prostheses has occurred along two distinct evolutionary paths based

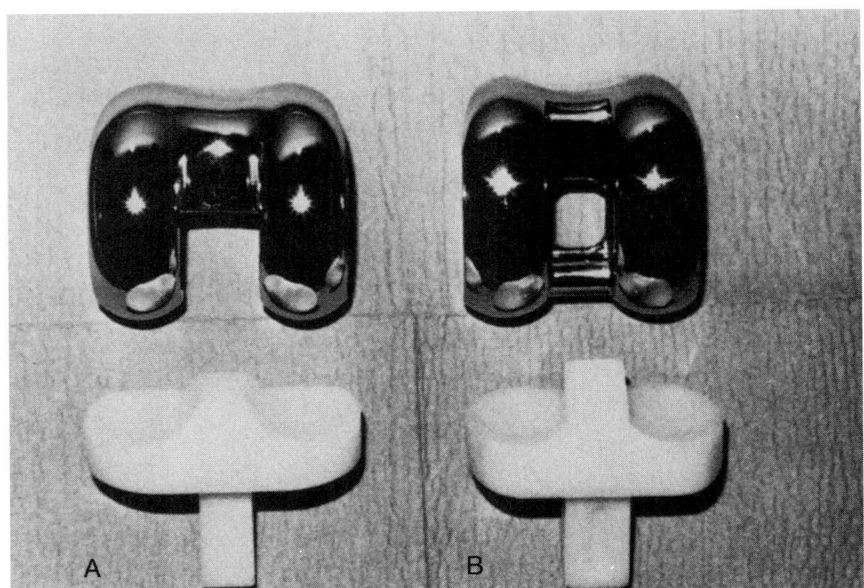

FIGURE 73.21 ➢ *A,* Total condylar prosthesis. *B,* Posterior stabilized condylar knee, a newer derivative providing posterior cruciate substitution by means of a central cam mechanism. (From Insall et al.[107])

upon these quite different principles. In the following section, the anatomic function of the cruciate ligaments, the relative advantages and disadvantages of cruciate excision, and the subject of PCL retention versus PCL substitution will be reviewed.

ANATOMIC FUNCTIONS OF THE CRUCIATE LIGAMENTS

One function of the cruciate ligaments, in addition to providing static anterior and posterior stability, is to impose certain movements on the joint surfaces relative to one another. The anterior cruciate ligament (ACL) is often absent in arthritic knees and has not been thought to be of much consequence in TKA. The importance of the ACL may have been underestimated as unconstrained prostheses have increased sagittal plane laxity and fail more often when the ACL is absent.[232] Although the PCL is often attenuated in arthritic knees, it is usually present. It has been considered as the collateral ligament for the medial compartment of the knee.[53] The PCL causes the femoral condyles to glide and roll back on the tibial plateau as the knee is flexed.[114] In the normal knee the shape of the plateau does not restrain this motion, and the laxity of the meniscal attachments allows the menisci to move posteriorly with the femur. This femoral rollback is crucial in prosthetic design. If the cruciates are excised, a more conforming tibial polyethylene component can be used, which provides some degree of anterior and posterior stability. However, without the function of the PCL, femoral rollback will not occur, which theoretically limits the ultimate flexion that can be obtained. If the PCL is retained the tibial surface must be flat or even posteriorly sloped[232] (Fig. 73.22). If a more conforming component is used in these circumstances, then posterior impingement will occur (Fig. 73.23). Substitution of the PCL with a cam-and-post mechanism not only re-creates femoral rollback but also allows a conforming articulation to be used without risk of posterior impingement. These considerations were reflected in the design of the total condylar, Duopatellar posterior stabilized, and various PCL-retaining prostheses.

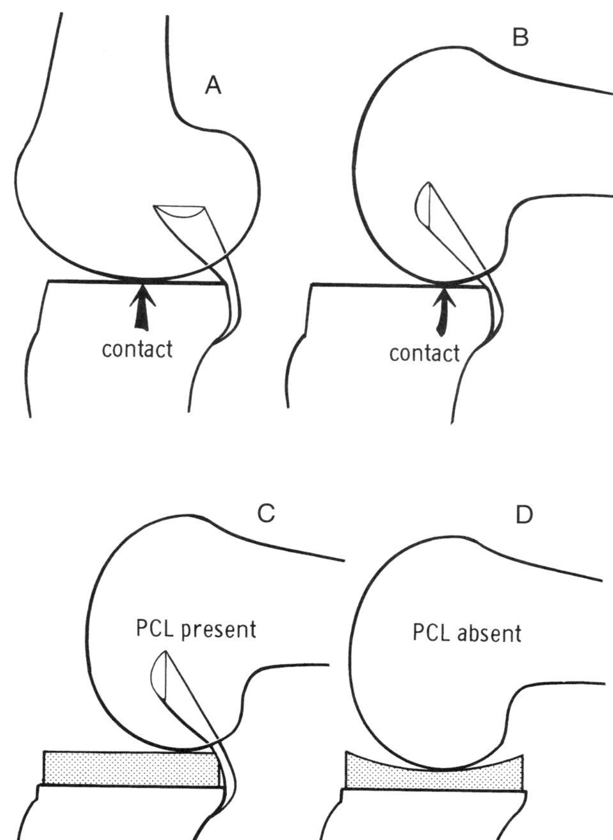

FIGURE 73.22 ➢ The effect of posterior cruciate retention on prosthetic design. *A & B*, Because of the rollback enforced by the posterior cruciate ligament, the prosthetic tibial surface must be flat to allow this movement. *C & D*, When the posterior cruciate ligament is absent, a dished tibial plateau is used.

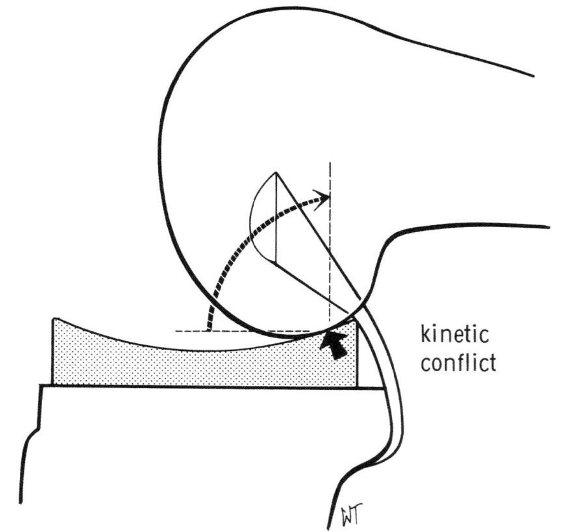

FIGURE 73.23 ➢ Kinematic conflict occurs if concepts are mismatched. In this case the posterior cruciate ligament is preserved, using a dished tibial component. Impingement occurs posteriorly with flexion.

ARGUMENTS FOR CRUCIATE EXCISION

Correction of Deformity

Removal of the cruciate ligaments is an important element in the soft-tissue release of fixed varus or valgus deformities. Correction of these deformities is therefore facilitated by cruciate excision. Also, clearance of the intercondylar notch provides clear visualization of the posterior capsule, which facilitates release and osteophyte removal during correction of flexion deformities.

Simpler Technique

Release of the cruciate ligaments facilitates surgical exposure, especially in tight knees, which makes the procedure less demanding. It is also technically easier to cut straight across the tibia than around the cruciate insertions. These factors make it easier to make the correct bone cuts and obtain accurate placement of the prosthesis.

Wear

Cruciate excision allows use of a more conforming articulation, which increases contact area and reduces contact stresses.

ARGUMENTS AGAINST CRUCIATE EXCISION

Range of Motion

Without a functional PCL or PCL-substituting mechanism, rollback of the femoral component does not occur. This theoretically limits the ultimate flexion obtainable with prostheses such as the total condylar prosthesis.

Instability

Failure to obtain flexion and extension balance can result in anterior-posterior laxity that may exceed the stability imparted by the moderately conforming articular surfaces. This may lead to symptomatic instability.

Loosening

The increased conformity of the articular surfaces used in the total condylar prosthesis theoretically results in increased stress at the bone-cement-prosthesis interface, which provoked concern that it would ultimately cause loosening. However, as discussed later in the section on PCL substitution, these concerns have not become clinically significant.

PCL RETENTION VERSUS SUBSTITUTION

Kinematics

Retention of the PCL was initially believed to allow preservation of normal knee kinematics following total knee replacement (TKR). In particular, preservation of the normal femoral rollback caused by tightening of the PCL, which acts to move the tibiofemoral contact point posteriorly during flexion, thereby increasing quadriceps efficiency and range of motion, was felt to be critical in activities such as stair climbing. The natural PCL was initially perceived to be superior in performing this kinematic function than the cam-and-post mechanism used in posterior stabilized knee prostheses. However, recent fluoroscopic studies by Stiehl and coauthors[209a] and Dennis and colleagues,[48a] have demonstrated that PCL-retaining prostheses do not replicate the kinematics of the normal knee. Instead, in many cases a paradoxical roll forward of the femur with anterior translation of the tibiofemoral contact area occurs. This motion, which is directly opposite normal knee kinematics, may result from improper tension of the PCL (Fig. 73.24). Adverse consequences may include decreased flexion, reduced quadriceps efficiency, and posterior tibial polyethylene wear. In addition, Dennis and coauthors demonstrated that although posterior stabilized prostheses did not completely reproduce normal knee kinematics, reliable rollback did occur. Surgeons who advocate the use of PCL-retaining prostheses have emphasized the importance of balancing the PCL with techniques such as PCL release and recession.[178, 185a] However, the success of utilizing these techniques to restore normal knee kinematics has not yet been proven. Based upon current knowledge it seems that PCL substitution more reliably results in desirable kinematics after TKR.

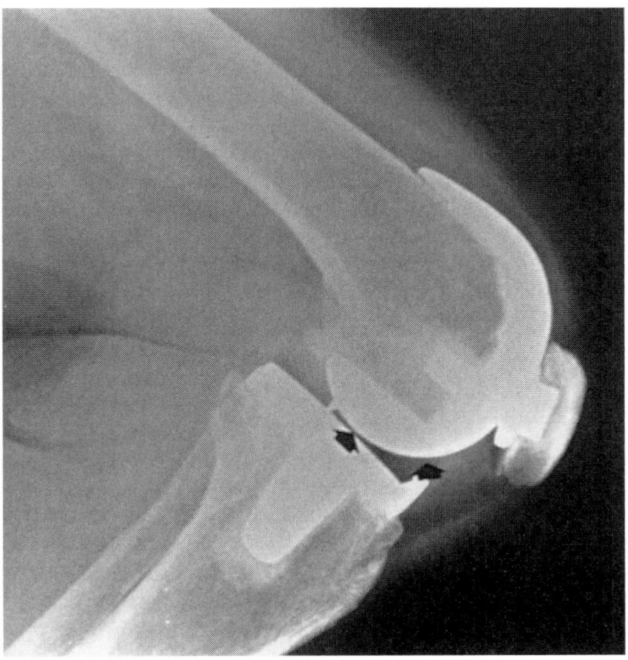

FIGURE 73.24 ➢ Sagittal radiograph of a "nonfunctional" posterior cruciate ligament. There has been "roll forward" rather than "roll back" with knee flexion. The anterior margin of the femoral component abuts the anterior margin of the tibial component as it does in a total condylar-type design.

Range of Motion

Early experience with the use of the cruciate-sacrificing total condylar prosthesis produced flexion of about 90 to 95 degrees, which is near the theoretical limit for this type of prosthesis. Improved flexion with both posterior stabilized and PCL-retaining prostheses has been reported. Pooled data from numerous studies demonstrate mean flexion of approximately 100 to 115 degrees with both types of prosthesis.[19a, 164a] Again, the importance of PCL recession and balancing in helping to allow optimal results with PCL-retaining prostheses has been advocated.[178, 185a] With careful surgical technique, reliable flexion of 110 to 115 degrees should be obtainable with either type of prosthesis. However, due to the experience and attention that seem to be required to correctly tension the PCL, we believe the posterior stabilized prosthesis is less technically challenging and produces more consistent results. The consequences of inadequately tensioning the PCL have been reported. Arthroscopic release of tight PCLs seems to be successful in improving flexion in select patients with PCL-retaining prostheses.[236a]

Modifications to the latest generation of posterior stabilized prostheses, which included redesign of the trochlea to accommodate the natural patella, necessitated posterior translation of the cam-and-post mechanism. As a result of this change the cam engages the post at approximately 70 degrees and then rides down the post, prior to eventually moving up the post with extreme flexion. This has effectively increased the "jump distance," thereby allowing greater flexion prior to dislocation. In conjunction with increased intraoperative attention to removing posterior osteophytes, in order to reduce posterior impingement, and slight changes to the sagittal radii of the posterior femoral condyles, this modification has increased attainable flexion. These concepts, in addition to further modifications to the radii of curvature of the posterior femoral condyles, are being incorporated into a new generation of "high flexion" posterior stabilized prostheses designed to attain greater motion.

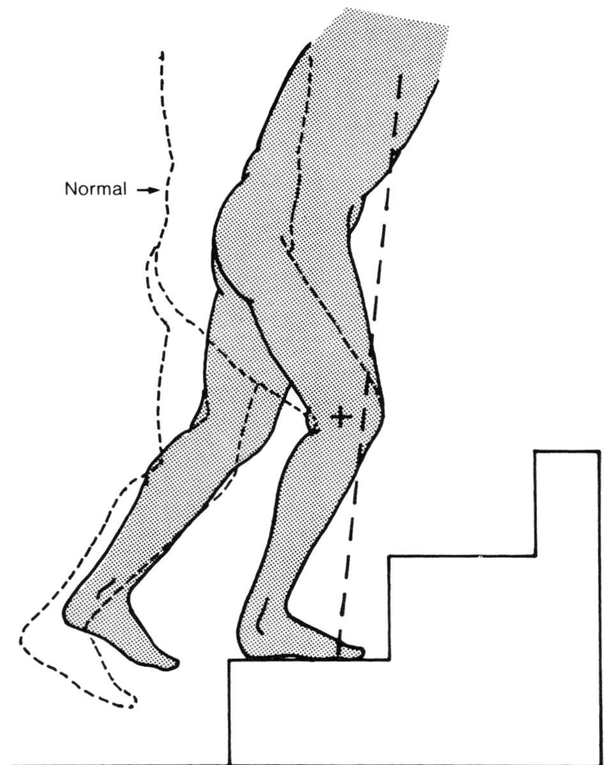

FIGURE 73.25 ➢ According to some gait analysis studies, there is a difference in stair climbing between cruciate-retaining and cruciate-sacrificing knee prostheses. It is reported that the latter climb stairs using less knee flexion and a compensatory forward lean of the trunk. (From Andriacchi et al.[7])

Proprioception

Both cruciate ligaments contain mechanoreceptors, and therefore advocates of PCL retention have proposed that preserving the natural ligament would lead to superior proprioception after TKR. However, the current literature has not demonstrated a clear advantage. Simmons and coauthors were unable to identify any advantage in proprioception in patients who had a PCL-retaining prosthesis versus those with a PCL-substituting prosthesis.[200a] Warren and coauthors found slightly different results.[228a] Following TKR all patients experienced improved proprioception regardless of whether a PCL-retaining or PCL-substituting prosthesis had been used. However, the improvement was greater in patients with a PCL-retaining prosthesis. The improved proprioception in both groups was speculated to be due to elimination of pain, restoration of articular congruity, and retensioning of the collateral ligaments and soft tissues. These inconclusive results may be due to the inherent qualities of the PCL in patients with arthritic knees. Kleinbart and coauthors have observed significant degenerative changes in the PCLs of patients with arthritic knees that exceed those in age-matched controls.[122b] Therefore, the PCL that is preserved in a patient with a PCL-retaining prosthesis is likely to be abnormal and should not be expected to function normally either biomechanically or proprioceptively. The effects of PCL recession on the proprioceptive function of the ligament are not known.

Gait Analysis

Initial studies suggested that the mechanics of walking and stair climbing, in particular, are different in patients with PCL-retaining and PCL-substituting prostheses.[6, 118] Andriacchi and Galante have described a characteristic forward lean of the trunk with less knee flexion in patients with PCL-substituting prostheses during stair climbing when compared with patients with PCL-retaining prostheses (Fig. 73.25).[6] This was suggested to represent a compensatory mechanism for the absence of the PCL. However, recent gait analysis by Wilson and coauthors and by Bolanos and coworkers dispute these findings. Bolanos and coauthors were unable to identify any significant differences in spatiotemporal gait parameters or knee range of motion during level walking or stair climbing in patients with PCL-retaining or PCL-substituting prostheses.[26b] Wilson and coauthors also did not identify any differences in these parameters during stair climbing between patients with PCL-substituting prostheses and normal age-matched controls.[237a] However, differences between the patients after TKR and the controls were identified during level walking and descending stairs. This evidence suggests that although after TKR patients do exhibit differences in gait pattern compared with normal controls, there is no clear effect of prosthesis type.

Correction of Deformity

Patients with significant preoperative fixed varus, valgus, or flexion deformities can be successfully managed with the use of PCL-retaining prostheses. However, as the PCL is one deforming factor in these cases, careful balancing with PCL release or recession may be required in order to achieve flexion and extension space symmetry.[84a, 178, 185a] Balancing of the PCL may be difficult and is experience dependent. Laskin has reported inferior results in patients with fixed varus deformities exceeding 15 degrees in whom PCL-retaining rather than PCL-substituting designs were used.[135a] In most circumstances, we believe that use of a posterior stabilized prosthesis is technically less challenging and allows more reliable correction of the preoperative deformity. Failure to appropriately tension the PCL may lead to either reduced flexion or flexion instability.[164b, 228b, 236a]

Stability

The more conforming tibial insert and cam-and-post mechanism of posterior stabilized prostheses do not provide any constraint in the medial/lateral directions (Fig. 73.26). Neither the PCL-retaining nor the PCL-substituting designs are designed to compensate for instability in this plane and therefore require intact collateral ligaments. In the anterior and posterior directions, the inherent characteristics of the designs are different and different problems are encountered if flexion-extension balance is not achieved. As previously discussed, a less conforming tibial polyethylene insert should be used in PCL-retaining prostheses due to the kinematic conflict that results during femoral rollback in flexion if a more conforming insert is used. If the PCL is functionally incompetent or stretches, posterior instability may occur because the minimally conforming or flat insert does little to prevent posterior translation of the femur. The phenomenon of symptomatic flexion instability in patients with PCL-retaining prostheses, due to an incompetent PCL, has recently gained more widespread recognition.[164b, 228b] The consequences of overtensioning of the PCL have been previously discussed. Recent biomechanical studies have suggested that it is difficult to obtain the appropriate tension in the PCL.[97a, 144a] However, the results of techniques used to balance the PCL have not been directly evaluated.

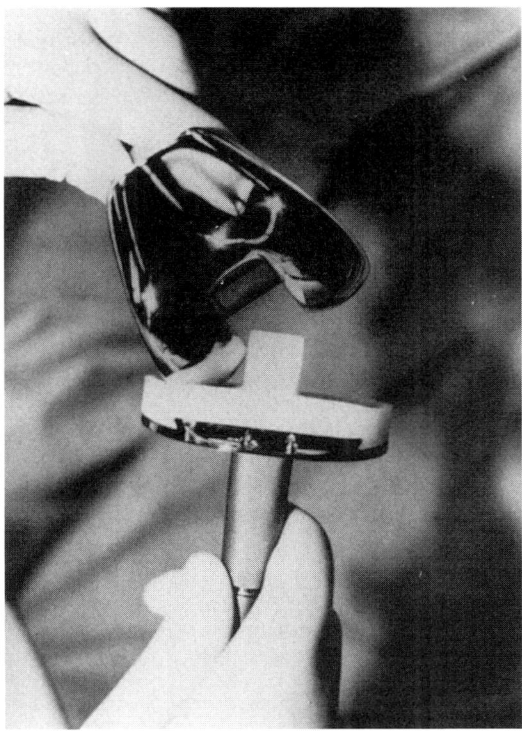

FIGURE 73.26 ➢ Posterior stabilized prosthesis showing that the post-and-cam mechanism offers no restraint to varus or valgus stability.

While posterior stabilized prostheses eliminate the PCL as a factor in preventing adequate flexion-extension balancing, anterior and posterior instability can still occur. In some cases with significant flexion instability, the jump distance of the cam-and-post mechanism may be exceeded during extreme flexion, resulting in acute dislocation (Fig. 73.27). In prior series, a dislocation rate of 2% to 3% has been reported.[48b, 171a] In one series, changes in the design of the cam-and-post mechanism eliminated subsequent dislocations over a 2-year period.[171a] Due to the uncertainties in achieving optimal tension in the PCL, we believe PCL-substituting prostheses produce more reliable long-term anterior-posterior stability.

Polyethylene Wear

Polyethylene wear in current posterior stabilized designs that have moderately conforming articular surfaces has not been a major clinical problem in older, less-active patients.[42a, 171a] In contrast, the higher contact stresses encountered in the unconstrained flat-on-flat articulations, in conjunction with heat pressed, thin polyethylene inserts used in PCL-retaining prostheses during the 1980s, have led to documented rapid wear.[26, 55, 120, 217a] Failure to balance the PCL may also result in severe posteromedial polyethylene wear. Based upon these results, the more conforming surfaces of the posterior stabilized implants seem better suited to optimizing long-term wear Fig. 73.28).

Loosening

The increased constraint imposed by the moderately conforming articular surfaces of posterior stabilized prostheses was initially considered to be detrimental to long-term fixation at the cement-bone-prosthesis interface, due to increased stress transmission versus the relatively less conforming PCL-retaining prostheses. However, by proper design this shear stress can be altered to forces that are compressive (73.29).

A theoretical seesaw motion may occur in PCL-retaining prostheses (Fig. 73.30). The rolling motion of the femur changes the metal-plastic contact point from anterior in extension to posterior in flexion. Thus, in extension the anterior portion of the tibia is compressed and in flexion the situation is reversed. This

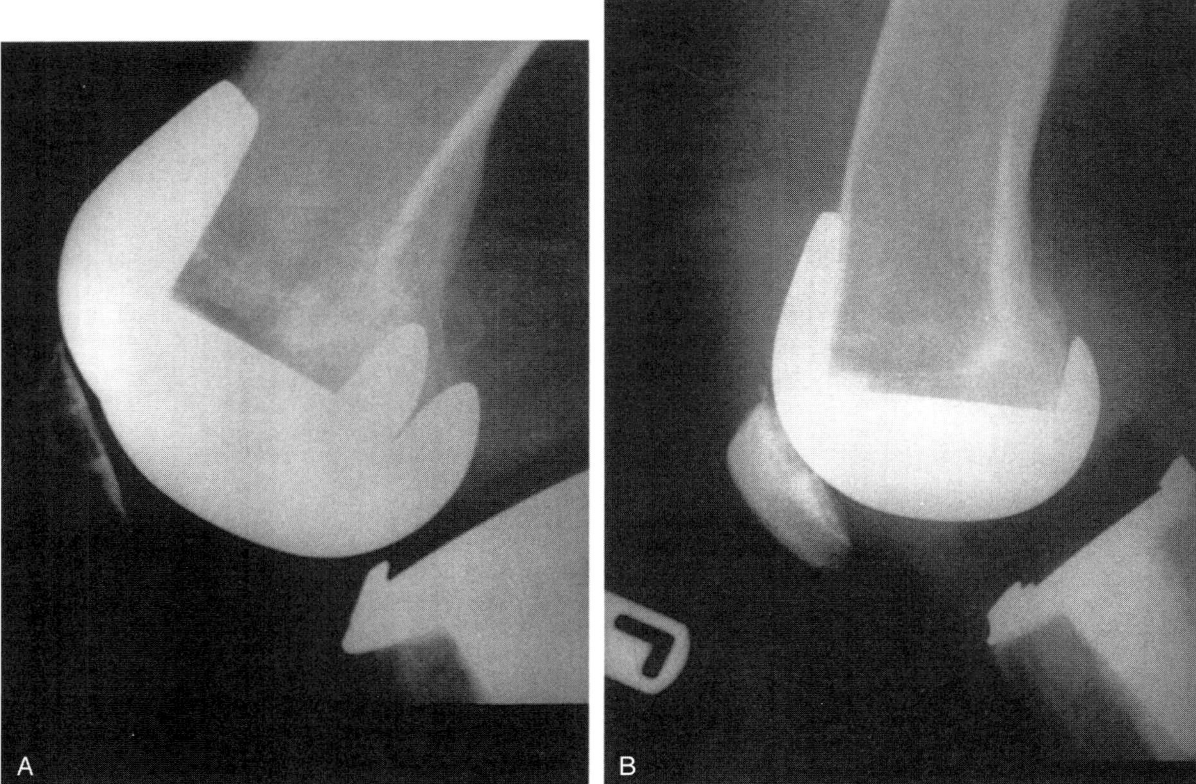

FIGURE 73.27 ➢ *A,* Radiograph of a dislocated posterior stabilized prosthesis. The post of the tibial component has displaced posteriorly behind the cam of the femoral component. *B,* Radiograph after reduction.

alternating compression-distraction may theoretically affect long-term fixation.

Long-term follow-up studies have failed to identify a significant clinical problem caused by these theoretical concerns, with only rare cases of aseptic loosening with both types of prosthesis. In the senior author's experience, with posterior stabilized prostheses, no cases of aseptic loosening of the tibial component and only two cases of femoral component loosening occurred among 165 primary TKRs at a mean of 10 years' follow-up.[42a] These are similar to the results obtained using PCL-retaining designs. Malkani and coauthors, from the Mayo Clinic, have reported a 96% survival rate at 10 years' follow-up.[144b] In summary, at 10- to 15-year follow-up there is little evidence to suggest that posterior stabilized prostheses are at increased risk of aseptic loosening.

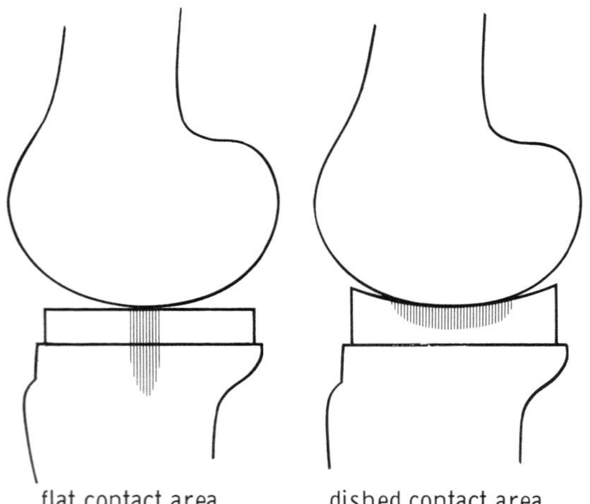

FIGURE 73.28 ➢ A dished component permits greater conformity, hence a larger contact area. The smaller contact area with a flat tibial component increases the stresses on the polyethylene.

Current Surface Replacement Designs

The prostheses described in the preceding section have given rise to derivatives. The total condylar prosthesis led to a series of posterior stabilized designs (see Figs. 73.24 to 73.26 and 73.31).[3, 4, 63, 84, 87, 107, 192, 193, 210–212, 234] The duopatellar prosthesis evolved into the Kinematic I and II and the Press-Fit condylar (Fig. 73.32).

Cementless Designs

In addition, a new series of prostheses appeared that were designed for cementless use. The first was the porous coated anatomic (Fig. 73.33),[20, 40, 44, 49, 65, 93, 94,

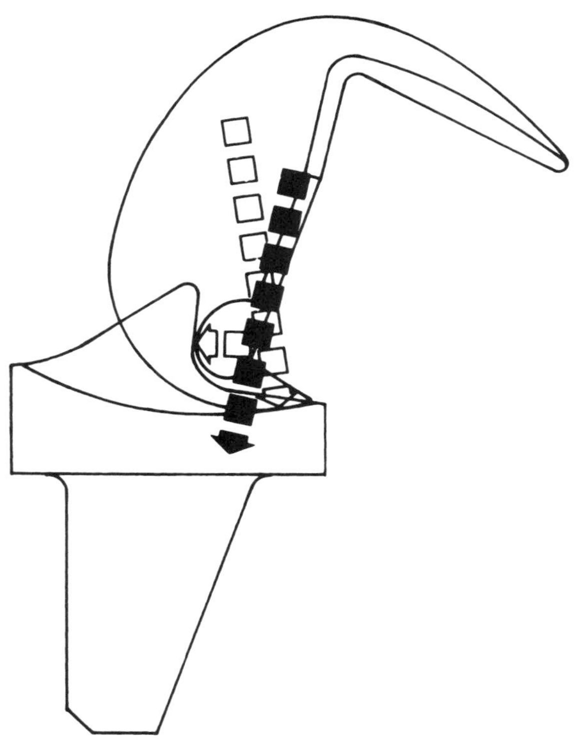

FIGURE 73.29 ➢ The cam mechanism of the posterior stabilized knee simulates the function of the posterior cruciate ligament and causes a rollback of the femur on the tibia with flexion. The resulting vector of forces passes distally through the fixation peg. (From Insall et al.[107])

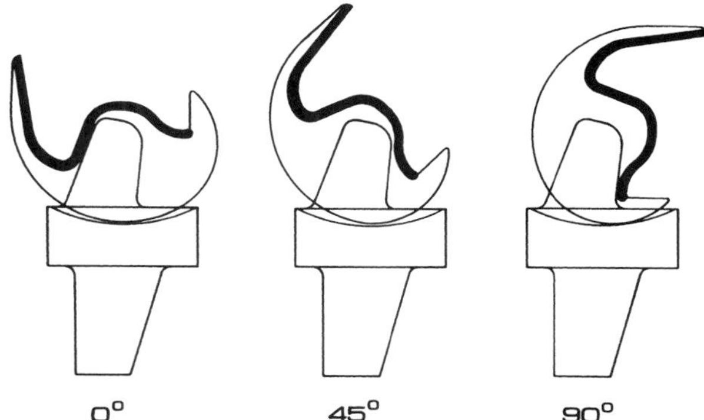

FIGURE 73.31 ➢ The TCP II was a precursor of the posterior stabilized knee that provided a passive stop against posterior displacement in flexion, as well as a hyperextension stop in extension. (From Insall et al.[101])

[123, 160, 180, 182, 208] and other examples of this type are the porous coated anatomic II, the Miller-Galante (Fig. 73.34),[126, 127, 181] the Miller-Galante II, Tricon M,[133, 163] Genesis (Fig. 73.35), and Ortholoc. Cementless prostheses have all been PCL-retaining designs with very unconstrained surfaces (either curved-on-flat or flat-on-flat to minimize fixation stresses that might interfere with bone ingrowth).

The Freeman-Swanson prosthesis[73, 75] has been modified into the Freeman-Samuelson prosthesis[71, 183] (Fig. 73.36), still using serrated polyethylene pegs for cementless fixation but now offering a metal base plate with intramedullary rods for the tibia and an intramedullary rod on the femoral component.

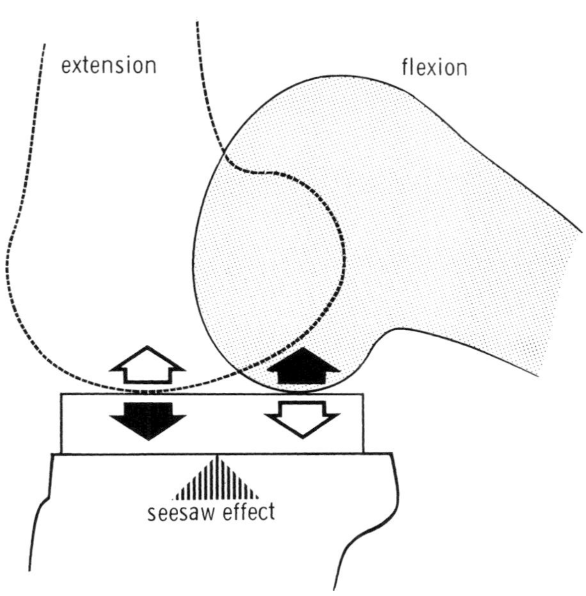

FIGURE 73.30 ➢ The seesaw effect. The back-and-forth movement on the tibial component caused by posterior cruciate ligament retention creates a rocking motion that may cause loosening.

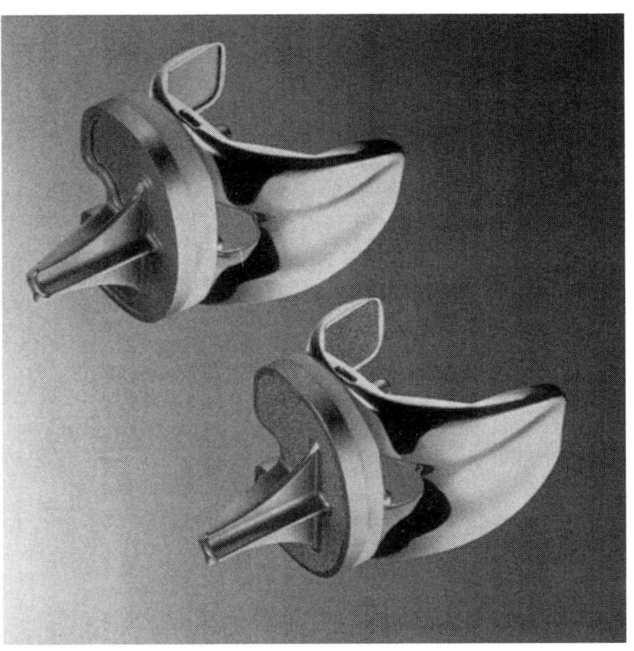

FIGURE 73.32 ➢ Press-Fit condylar prosthesis. (Courtesy of Johnson & Johnson.)

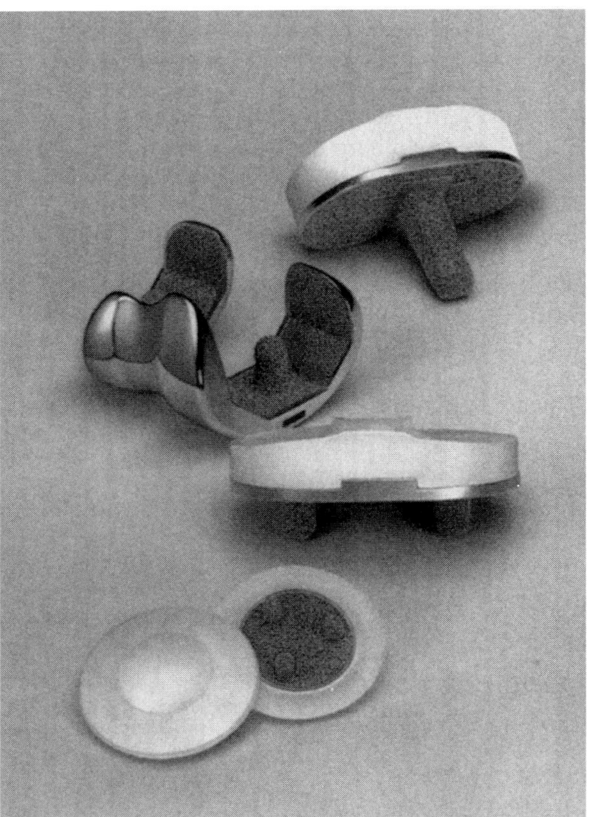

FIGURE 73.33 ➢ Porous-coated anatomic prosthesis. (Courtesy of Howmedica.)

Meniscal-Bearing Prostheses

Conventional fixed-bearing knee prostheses have proved clinically successful with very favorable results at 10 to 15 years.[42a] However, with only a few exceptions, these results have been obtained in older, less active patient populations.[48b, 52a] Concerns exist regarding the long-term durability of current prostheses in younger, more demanding patients, especially regarding problems related to polyethylene wear and osteolysis. Polyethylene wear may be reduced by radical improvements in the inherent qualities of the material itself, which have not yet been realized, or by decreasing the contact stresses at the articular surfaces. Reduction in contract stresses could be accomplished by increasing the conformity of the femoral component and polyethylene insert. However, due to the inherent trade-off that exists in fixed-bearing prostheses between conformity and freedom of motion, significant improvements in contact stresses are not feasible. Therefore, at the present time a mobile-bearing prosthesis seems to represent the only plausible solution to this problem. A mobile-bearing prosthesis eliminates the relationship between articular conformity and freedom of rotation that exists in fixed-bearing prostheses, as rotation occurs at the interface between the superior surface of the tibial baseplate and the inferior surface of the polyethylene insert, whereas articular conformity is a property of the shape of the femoral component and superior surface of the polyethylene insert. In a mobile-bearing prosthesis articular conformity can be maximized, thereby reducing contact stresses and wear on the superior surface of the polyethylene, while freedom of rotation is maintained.

The many nuances of mobile-bearing prosthesis design and our interest in the development of these prostheses will be reviewed more thoroughly in a subsequent chapter. Briefly, the concepts behind these

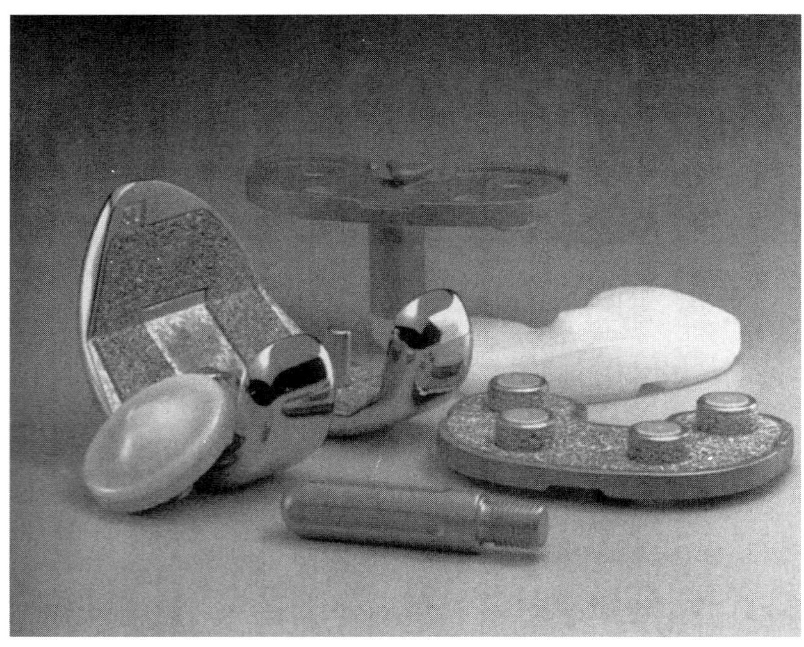

FIGURE 73.34 ➢ The Miller-Galante prosthesis. (Courtesy of Zimmer.)

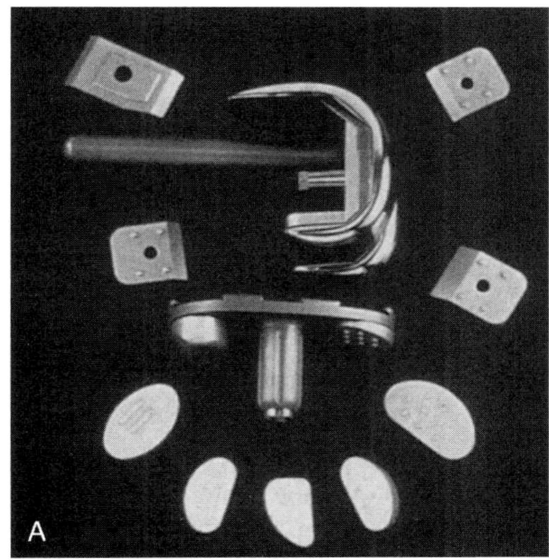

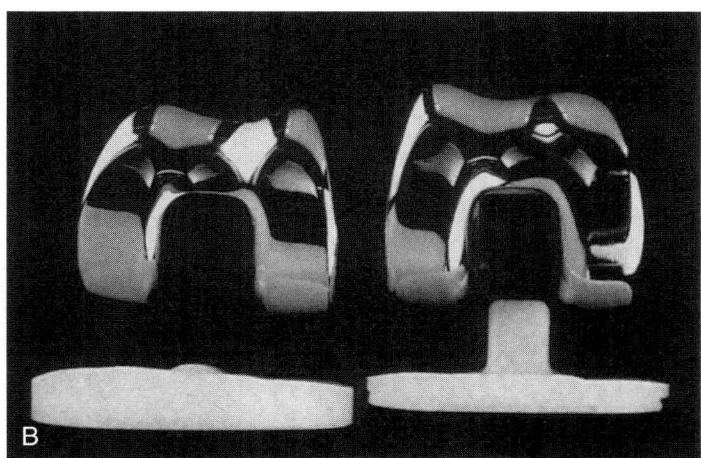

FIGURE 73.35 ➢ *A&B,* The Genesis prosthesis. (Courtesy of Richards.)

prostheses are not new, as borne out by the Oxford prostheses.[17, 27, 28, 79–82, 216, 235]

In 1976 Goodfellow and O'Connor introduced a bicondylar knee that attempted to solve the potential problem of polyethylene wear by providing a meniscal bearing, that is, a polyethylene tibial component that is fully congruent with the femoral component but free to move on a metallic tibial base tray. This concept hopes to provide the best possible wear characteristics with complete lack of constraint.

The designers of the Oxford knee now recommend that this prosthesis be used only as a unicompartmental prosthesis when both anterior and posterior cruciate ligaments are present and can be preserved: An absent anterior cruciate ligament is now considered a contraindication to the Oxford knee. Buechel and associates have developed the meniscal-bearing concept into a series of prostheses known as the low-contact stress (LCS)[21, 33, 34] knee prostheses (Fig. 73.37). These devices possess a femoral component similar to the total condylar prosthesis, which is mated to meniscal-bearing tibial components resembling those of the Oxford knee or, alternatively, a rotating platform for use when cruciate excision is indicated. There is also a metal-backed patellar component with a swiveling polyethylene surface of anatomic design.

Unlike the Oxford knee, the low-contact stress model has a femoral component of decreasing radius posteriorly; congruency is less when the knee is flexed so the contact area decreases in flexion, thereby losing a major advantage of the original design.

A puzzle created by meniscal designs, particularly the Oxford model, is in deciding the position of the actual joint axis. Flexion takes place between the femur and the superior surface of the polyethylene bearing, wheareas anteroposterior sliding and rotation occur at the inferior surface (a position 8 to 10 mm distal to the true joint line). Whether this curious anomaly has clinical significance has not been much studied. (The low-contact stress design, because of its lack of flexion congruence, may behave more like the total condylar prosthesis than a true meniscal-bearing type).

Meniscal-bearing designs have the disadvantage of increased complexity, with movement occurring both proximal and distal to the polyethylene bearing and the potential of wear at both surfaces. Dislocation of the bearings has been reported.[21]

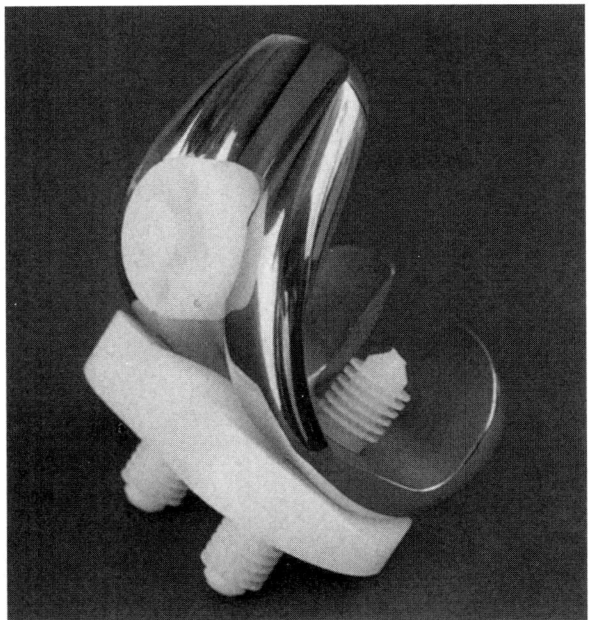

FIGURE 73.36 ➢ The current version of the Freeman-Samuelson prosthesis. (Courtesy of MAR Freeman.)

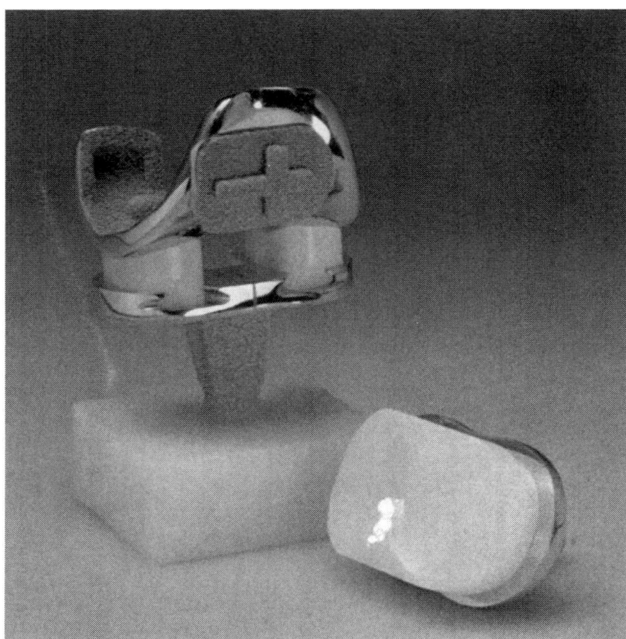

FIGURE 73.37 ➢ Low-contact stress prosthesis. (Courtesy of Depuy).

Constrained Prostheses

Constrained Condylar Knee

A derivative of the total condylar prosthesis (TCP) III[23, 41, 50, 90, 117, 121] design, the constrained condylar knee (CCK) provides both posterior stability and medial-lateral stability by means of an enlarged post articulating closely with a femoral recess (Fig. 73.38). This prosthesis can be used for most situations in which a hinge would be otherwise indicated, except for recurvatum deformity. In its TCP III form, Donaldson and coworkers[50] found no loosening in 15 primary cases followed for more than 2 years; all stems were cemented. The TCP III has evolved into the constrained condylar knee for use with modular, Press-Fit stems. More than 100 of these prostheses have been used at the time of writing without loosening: 70% followed for more than 1 year show evidence of stem tip reaction. The constrained condylar knee was initially used primarily for revision cases, but, based on the good experience with the TCP III in primary knees, the CCK has proved very successful in managing difficult valgus knees in elderly low-demand patients. The avoidance of extensive release procedures and possible peroneal-nerve complications has hastened recovery and lessened morbidity. Although the follow-up period is still relatively short, the lack of adverse fixation effects has led us to continue use of the prosthesis for this type of primary knee deformity.

The constrained condylar knee metal components can be used with both its own polyethylene tibial insert and the posterior stabilized insert. Thus, in a difficult knee arthroplasty, a final intraoperative decision can be made concerning the degree of constraint needed; for example, in severe valgus knees, we use the constrained condylar knee metal components, but where possible we use a posterior stabilized tibial insert. Constrained condylar knee metal components can also be used in cases of poor bone quality and arguably in patients who are younger than the usual age for arthroplasty.

Kinematic Rotating Hinge

Rand and colleagues[172] give results on 50 Kinematic rotating hinge TKAs done at the Mayo Clinic. The

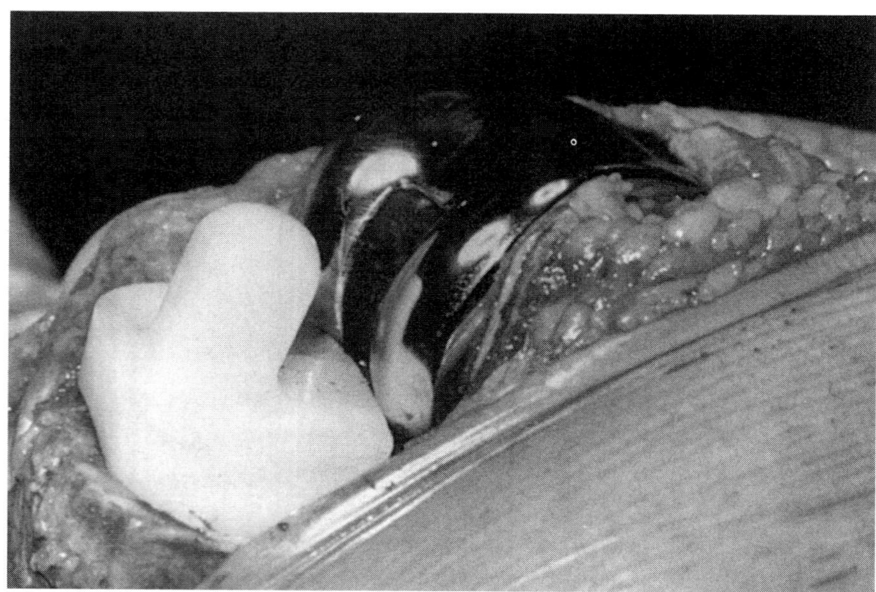

FIGURE 73.38 ➢ Articulation of the TCP III, a constrained condylar knee. A rectangular tibial post fits within a central femoral box or cavity, providing varus-valgus stability as well as posterior restraint.

indications were either ligamentous instability, loss of bone, or both. The follow-up was 50 months (range 29 to 79 months). There were 14 excellent, 12 good, 5 fair, and 5 poor results. Progression of radiolucent lines was observed in 13 knees, and 5 knees probably had radiographic loosening. The rate of sepsis was 16%, patellar instability, 22%, and breakage of the implant, 6%. In these patients, 64% of the operations were revisions: a first revision in 17, a second revision in 16, a third revision in 3, and a fourth revision in 1. The results were similar to previous experience with the GUEPAR prosthesis at the Mayo Clinic, although in this series the high percentage of revisions probably contributed to the poor results, especially the high rate of sepsis. Rand and coworkers combined the incidence of complications reported for several series, comprising 2099 hinged implants. In these combined series, loosening was reported in 27% of knees, sepsis in 7% and wound healing problems in 5.5%. The authors concluded that the Kinematic rotating hinge prosthesis, although possessing theoretical advantages, gave no better results than the older nonrotating hinges. Mechanical failures have also been reported.[119]

GENERAL PROSTHETIC FEATURES

Interchangeability of Sizes

The natural variation that occurs between individual knee joints means that prosthetic components based on average dimensions do not always fit the femur and tibia of a particular joint equally well. Interchangeability of sizes, so that the femoral, tibial, and patellar components can be selected independently of each other according to the fit on their respective bones, becomes an attractive feature. Although it has long been possible to match patellar components with various femoral sizes, similar adaptability between the femoral and tibial components is a relatively new feature. As with other aspects of knee arthroplasty, some compromises are involved. Matching a smaller femur with a larger tibia (the usual combination) requires that the intercondylar distance, or, more correctly, the bearing spacing between the femoral runners, be constant for all sizes and that the tibial surface be almost flat. As we have seen, articulating a curved femur against a flat tibia produces a small contact patch with the attendant disadvantage of high localized stresses on the polyethylene. The contact patch can be enlarged by also flattening the femoral surfaces (Fig. 73.39). However, malalignment or any situation that leads to asymmetric loading, even those occurring during the normal gait cycle, shifts the loading area to the periphery. This type of "edge" loading has been shown experimentally[18, 223, 225] to produce the greatest stresses at the prosthesis-bone interface, perhaps offsetting any benefits obtained from more complete tibial coverage.

Articular Geometry

Conforming joint surfaces should have the best wear resistance, particularly when the polyethylene is relatively thick.[19] However, conforming articulations are not fully interchangeable, may conflict with the PCL kinematics, and theoretically cause greater fixation stresses.

Thatcher and colleagues,[214] discussing inherent laxity in knee prostheses, state that laxity is a function of joint conformity. They believe the implanted prosthesis should compensate for soft-tissue structures that are deficient or removed. They believe that the optimal laxity profile has not yet been determined but suggest that the articular geometry should possess partial conformity and comment upon the classic inherent design compromise. The greater the conformity the larger the contact area and the less the intrinsic stresses and wear. However, conforming prostheses will create greater fixation stresses, which may lead to loosening.

Wear is an increasing problem in TKA. Several fac-

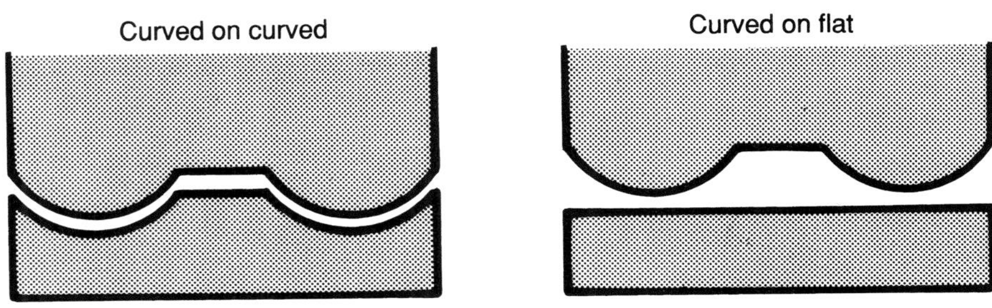

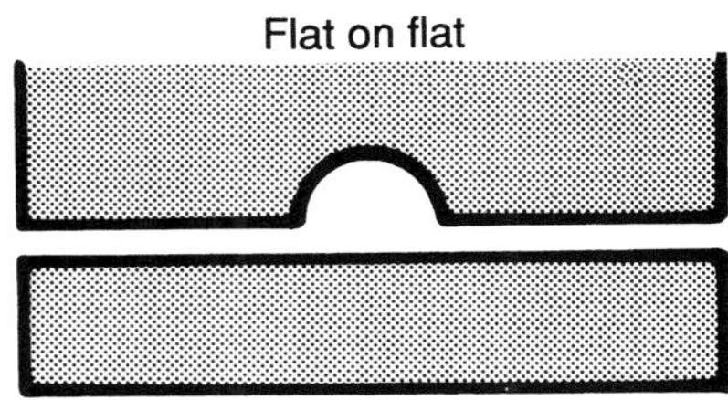

FIGURE 73.39 ➢ The more conforming the articulation the larger the contact area and the less stress on the polyethylene. In the frontal plane, curved-on-curved geometries are the best. Curved-on-flat geometry is the worst. Flat-on-flat surfaces can give a good area of contact but are sensitive to edge loading whenever the prosthesis is loaded unevenly, such as in leaning or pivoting movements.

tors have been implicated, including the quality of the polyethylene, the manufacturing process, the thickness of the tibial components as well as the articular geometry.[206] It is also true that in the best of circumstances polyethylene is not an ideal bearing material,[239] but attempts to improve its performance have not been successful.[240]

Many cases of severe wear and delamination of tibial components have been reported,[55, 120] mainly involving thinner polyethylene components. The manufacturing process (which involved heat pressing[26] the polyethylene to give a smoother surface) has been implicated, particularly in causing the most severe phenomenon of delamination, although design factors giving high-contact stresses are probably equally important, as other models from the same manufacturer using similar polyethylene treatment have not shown the same degree of damage.

Design and Fixation of the Tibial Component

An important difference between prostheses is the method of tibial fixation.[141] The total condylar, posterior stabilized condylar, and Kinematic prostheses employ a central peg. The Press-Fit condylar has a central tri-fin post. These prostheses are primarily designed for cement fixation. Others that can be inserted with or without cement have two to four short studs, augmented in most cases by screws. Long-term studies using central peg fixation and cement show tibial component loosening to be rare (Fig. 73.40).

There is good evidence from early experience with knee arthroplasty that separate tibial components are susceptible to fixation failure. Neither an anterior bar nor the use of fixation studs is helpful. Walker and coworkers[225] tested a variety of tibial components by applying compressive load with anteroposterior force, rotational torque, or varus-valgus moment (Fig. 73.41). The relative deflections, both compressive and distractive, were measured between the component and the bone. The fewest deflections occurred with one-piece metal components. Whether a central peg or two lateral studs were used did not seem to make much difference. Thick plastic components behaved much like metal-backed ones, except when a cruciate cutout was made. Metal backing seems particularly desirable for cruciate-retaining implants.

Railton and coworkers[168] found that metal backing of the polyethylene without a central stem to be of little value in enhancing fixation. They did not address the question of optimal stem length or the use of cement. Yamamoto and coworkers,[241] discussing the results of the Kodama-Yamamoto Mark II prosthesis, which has an all-polyethylene tibial component with four small studs and is inserted without cement, express the opinion that a stem is unnecessary. They report a 4.4% incidence of femoral loosening accompanied by tibial sinkage in some. Cases with only tibial sinkage were not observed.

Lewis and colleagues[141] tested the fixation of six tibial component configurations, using finite element analysis, and concluded that metal-backed single post designs provided the lowest system stresses overall when cement was used.

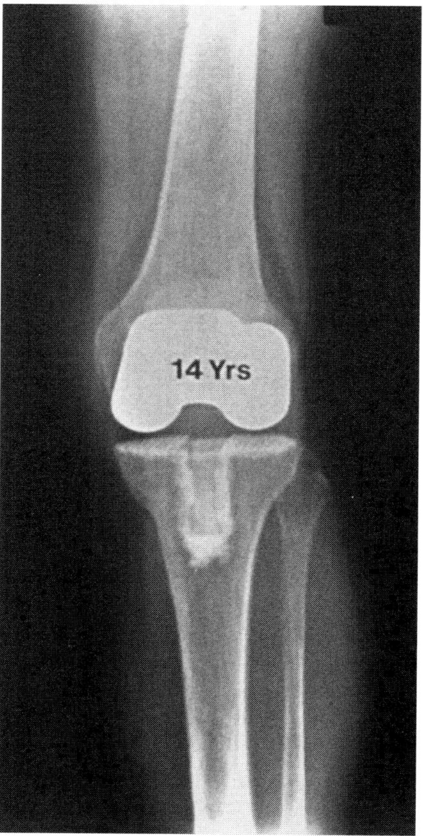

FIGURE 73.40 ➢ A radiograph of a total condylar prosthesis 14 years postoperatively. Note the thin cement mantle clearly showing ridges in the cement caused by the design of the tibial polyethylene. There is no evidence of cracking or fragmentation of the cement. This type of appearance was seen frequently in the more than 10-year follow-up of this prosthesis and indicates that a thick cement mantle is unnecessary.

Clinical data on more recent implants using metal tray and small stud fixation are mostly short-term and applicable to cementless fixation. Computer simulations of bone remodeling around porous coated implants[164] stress concentrations around small tibial pegs; this resulted in denser bone, with a decrease in density in more peripheral locations. This agrees with the clinical observation that bone ingrowth occurs most predictably around fixation pegs.

Walker and colleagues,[226] in a comparative study of uncemented tibial component designs found that central stemmed and bladed designs performed better than short pegs placed near the periphery.

Support of the plastic by means of a metal tray or endoskeleton is certainly desirable when the bone of the upper tibia is deficient (severe erosive arthritis or revision operations), but when the bone is of good quality, metal backing may not offer an advantage. One-piece plastic components with a central peg have a low rate of loosening, but in 30% to 40% of cases a partial radiolucency develops. For the most part, these

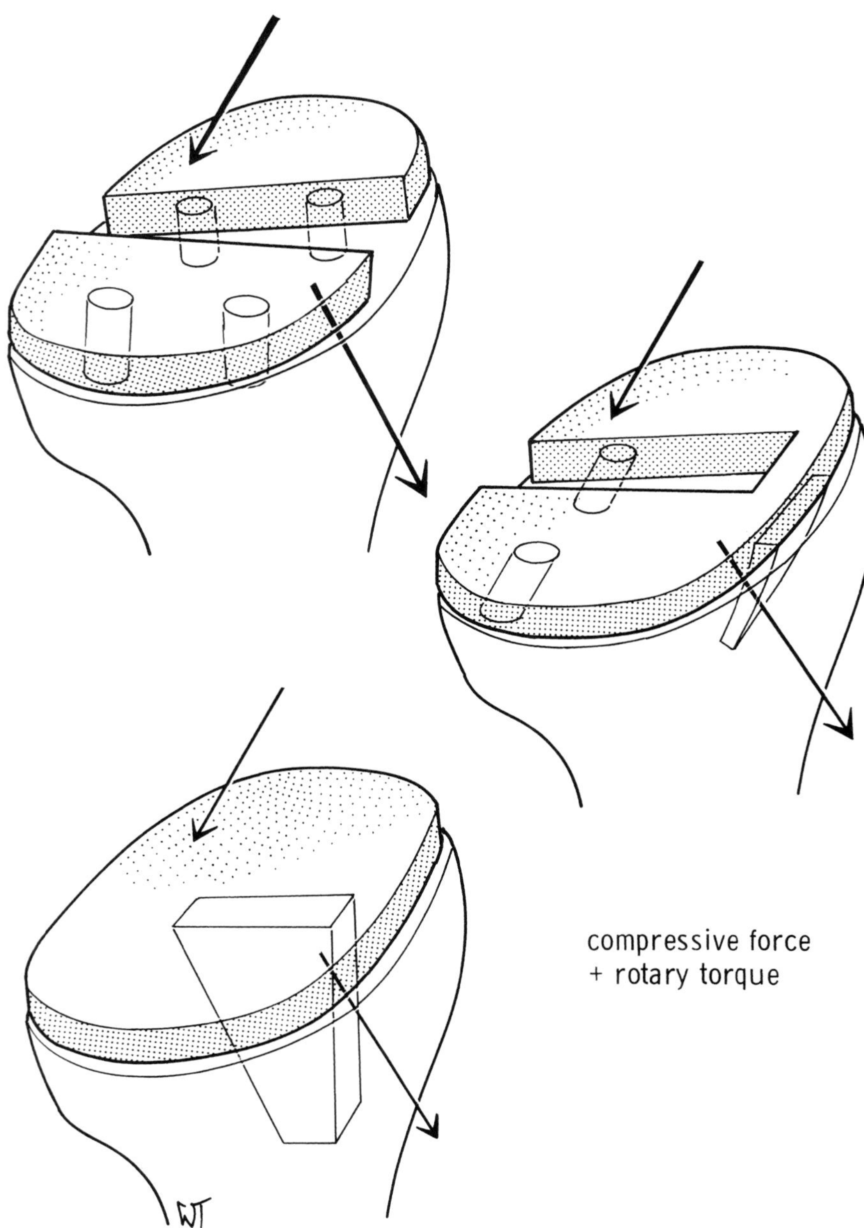

FIGURE 73.41 ➢ Deflections at the bone-cement interface showing different configurations of tibial component. (Courtesy of Dr. Peter Walker.)

radiolucencies appear within the first year, are nonprogressive, and are of dubious clinical significance. The addition of a metal tray reduces the incidence of radiolucency and it seems may also reduce the incidence of late tibial loosening. However, metal backing of the component has not been in use as long as the all-polyethylene designs, and the application of metal-backed tibial components for all cases cannot yet be unequivocally recommended (Fig. 73.42).

Modularity

Modularity, in the sense under discussion, refers to the ability to add stems, augments, and wedges to standard components so that, to a degree, the surgeon is able to make a custom prosthesis intraoperatively. At least one model (Genesis) allows conversion from cruciate retention to cruciate substitution, although conversion adds 4 mm to the distal femur thickness. Other designs (I-B II, Press-Fit condylar[238]) permit the addition of stems, wedges, and augments (Fig. 73.43) to both tibial and femoral components as well as intraoperative conversion from posterior stabilizing to constrained condylar by alterations of the tibial polyethylene shape.

Modularity is particularly useful for revision surgery when the bone deficiencies cannot be completely anticipated. It is also of value for primary knee replacement, for dealing with bone defects, and when prosthetic stability cannot be obtained. Modularity does not necessarily imply interchangeability, although both features may be present in a particular design.

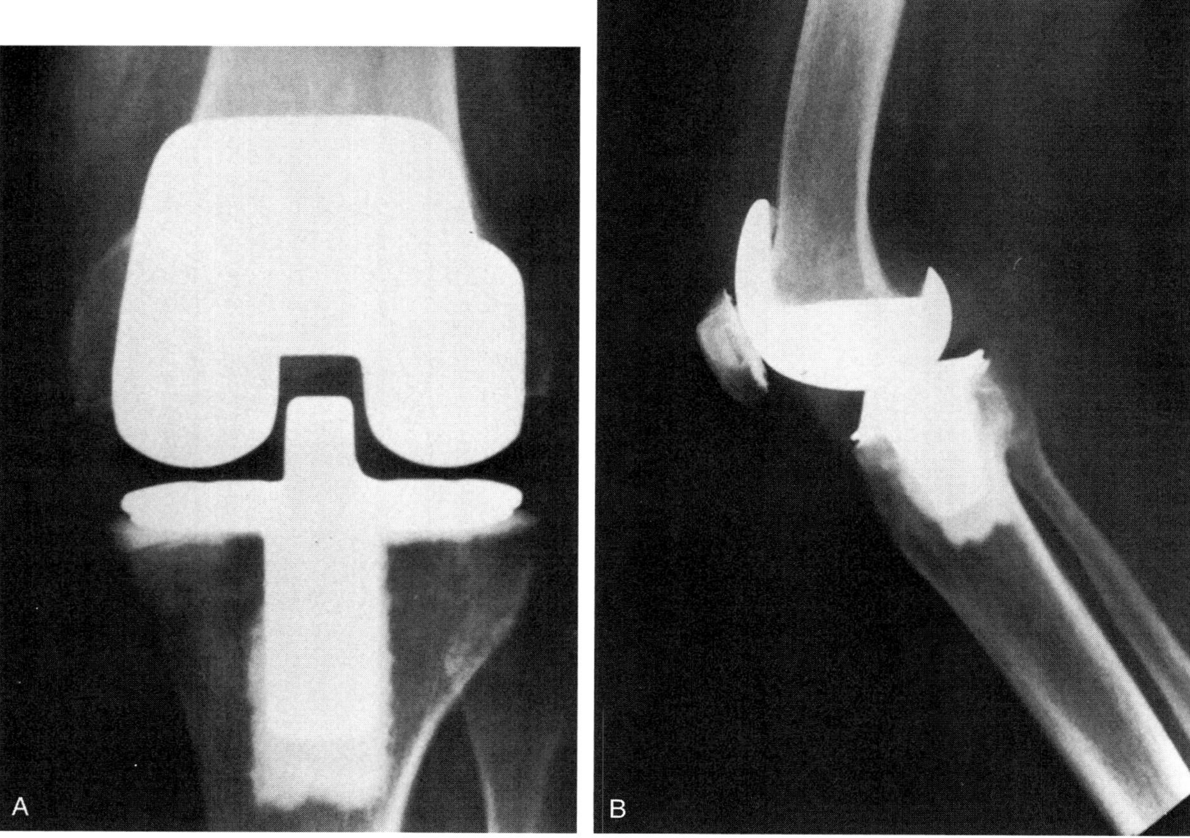

FIGURE 73.42 ➢ *A&B,* Anteroposterior and lateral radiographs of a tibial component with an endoskeleton. Metal backing of this type may in the long run enhance fixation.

Component Augmentation for Bone Defects

Cement,[142] cement and screws,[177] or bone grafts can be used to compensate for small bone defects.[31]

The senior author's experience indicates that onlay bone grafts should not be used on the femoral condyles or for revision defects. Cancellous grafting for contained defects is of course applicable in these circumstances. The advantage of bone grafting lies in the potential improvement of bone stock.

Another method is to use metal wedges (Fig. 73.44) and augments that can be adapted to fit existing defects without the need to remove sclerotic areas to expose bleeding cancellous surfaces. In this sense one can view them as more conservative. If they fail, bone deficiency is not made worse. The metal pieces are either screwed or cemented to their components. Screw fixation, although mechanically satisfying, creates the possibility of metallic debris formation by micromotion (fretting). Cement also may not be the ideal bonding material between metal surfaces. At present, one or the other method must be used.

Prosthetic

Prosthetic stems about the knee have a stigma that is related to their use with hinges and other constrained models, especially when the stems are cemented. However, Blauth and Hassenpflug and Bohm and Holy report continuing good results with the hinge knee prosthesis that bears Blauth's name.[25, 26a] Reporting on the Stanmore hinge replacement, Lettin and colleagues[139, 140] found 83% survivorship at 6 years (survivorship defined as prosthesis in situ) and Kaufer and Matthews[116] found an infection rate of 5% and revision rate of 15% of the spherocentric prosthesis followed for an average of 8 years. Nonetheless, these reports appeared to be exceptions. In our experience, 15 of 108 GUEPAR prostheses became infected. All but 4 of them were late infections, and uncontrollable sepsis led to 2 above-the-knee amputations. Young[242] found that in a series of hinge prostheses all had failed by the end of 10 years. Hui and Fitzgerald[92] reported an 11.7% infection rate in 77 GUEPAR arthroplasties followed for 2 or more years. They comment on the difficulty of obtaining arthrodesis if the prosthesis has to be removed. Deburge[48] had a failure rate of 34% with the GUEPAR prosthesis attributable to major complications. Grimer and colleagues[83] recommend against the routine use of the Stanmore prosthesis as a primary arthroplasty. Of 103 Stanmore knee replacements, they had 7 cases of infection and 4 of fracture around the prosthesis, contributing to major complications. Eight knees were revised for aseptic loosening

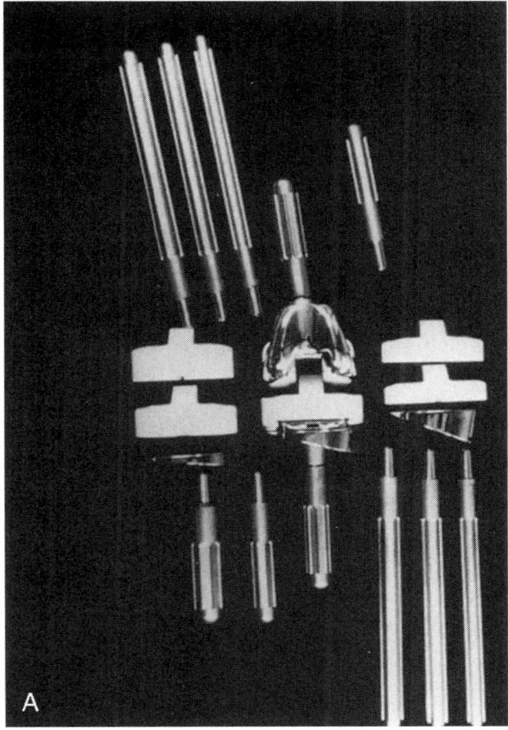

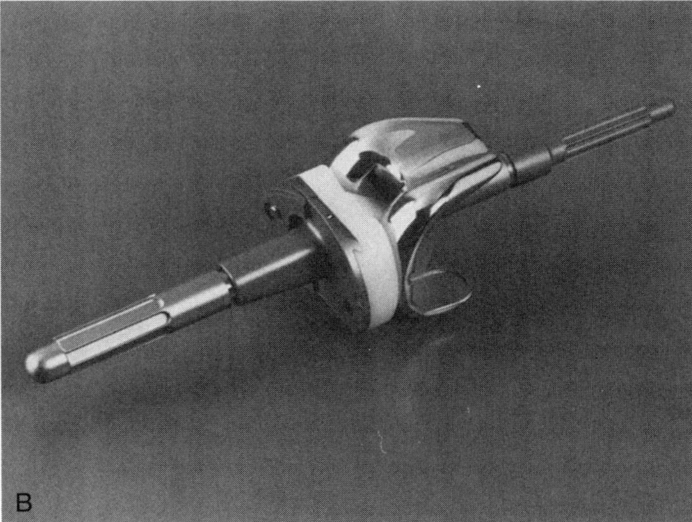

FIGURE 73.43 ➢ *A,* A modular prosthesis (I-B II). The components offer stems, augments, and wedges, which are fixed with screws. There is also a choice of polyethylene components for posterior stabilization or for varus and valgus constraint. *B,* A revision-type, constrained condylar modular prosthesis, assembled in the operating room. (Courtesy of Zimmer.)

and a further 14 were found to have radiologic signs of loosening. There were two cases of amputation for fracture and sepsis. Only Wilson and colleagues[237] have reported favorable results over a long period using an uncemented Walldius prosthesis. The overall infection rate was 3.2%, and clinical evidence of loosening occurred infrequently. The 20 knees followed for an average of 10 years showed little evidence of progressive deterioration. They attribute this to the absence of cement. Walldius[228] himself has written on 27 years' experience with his prosthesis and states that good results are obtained in 80% of patients with a high degree of preoperative disability. No details are given.

In assessing these results, it must be pointed out that all relate to constrained prostheses with cemented stems (excepting the Walldius), and the worst results were obtained with metal-on-metal-bearing surfaces, which generate large volumes of metallic debris.[167] Complete constraint of the degree provided by a hinge is rarely needed in knee arthroplasty, and lesser degrees of constraint such as provided by the total condylar prosthesis III or constrained condylar knee do not seem to have particular disadvantages.[50] Murray and coauthors, from the Mayo Clinic, have reported 5-year results with the use of cemented stems in conjunction with the Kinematic Stabilizer prosthesis, in 40 revision TKRs.[162a] The incidence of radiolucent lines was 13% about the femoral stems and 32% about the tibial stems. However, the majority were incomplete, nonprogressive and less than 1 mm. Only one femoral and 1 tibial component were radiographically loose. Theoretical concerns regarding stress shielding were not noted in these cases. Therefore, it appears that in this time frame cemented stems function adequately without significant complications. However, concerns regarding bone loss and increased surgical difficulties at revision still remain. If the intention is merely to provide additional component support, in the case of deficient bone, stems need not be associated with constraint and do not need to be cemented.[157] The senior author has used uncemented stems since 1977 with both custom and modular components, and Bertin and colleagues have reported on Freeman's experience with uncemented stems in revision surgery.[22, 86a] In neither report was there any increase in the infection rate. Freeman used a stem of fixed diameter and did not attempt to obtain a press-fit (the so-called dangle stem) (Fig. 73.45). Bertin and colleagues noted the development of radiopaque lines adjacent to the stem in 88% of cases. In our study similar lines were observed about 67% of femoral rods and 69% of tibial rods. A sclerotic halo about the tip of the prosthesis has also been noted in some cases (Fig. 73.46).[22] The importance of these findings is not fully understood but may be interpreted as evidence of the stem's func-

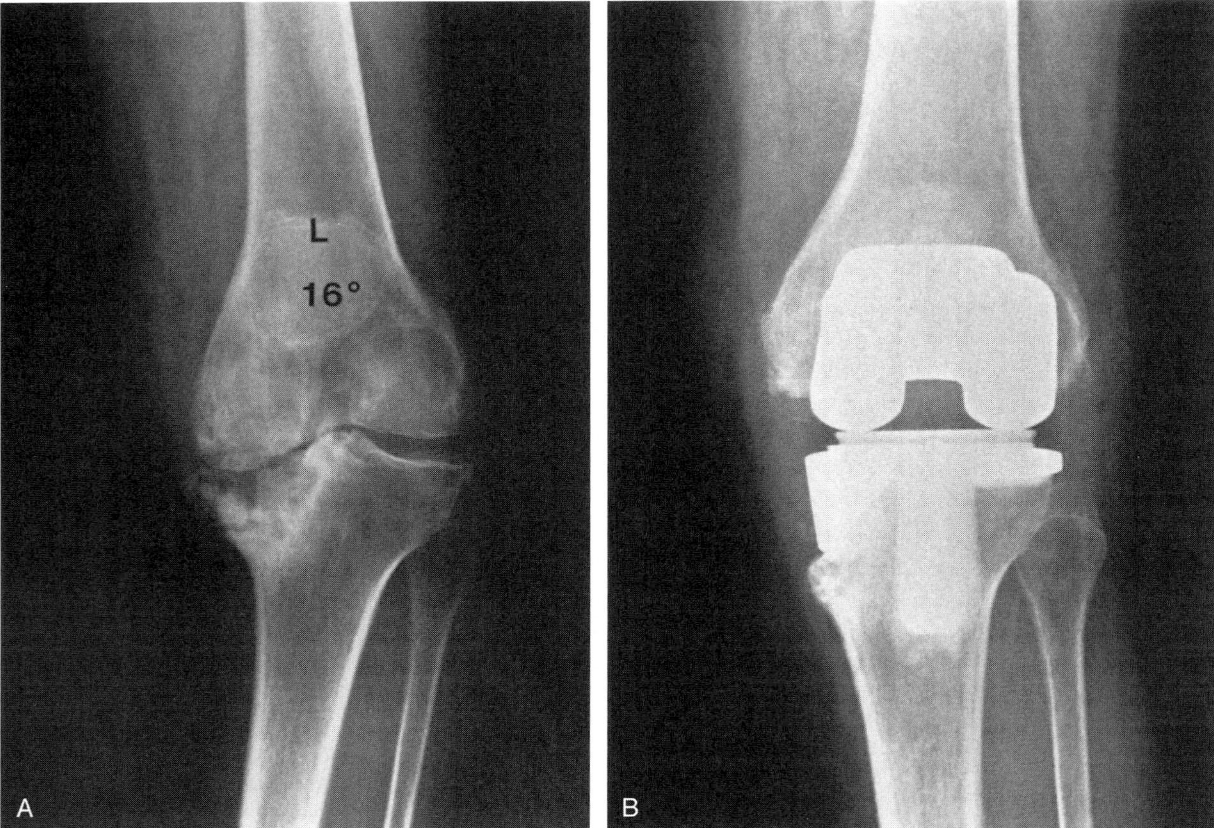

FIGURE 73.44 ➢ *A,* Radiograph of a knee with osteonecrosis of the medial tibia and a massive tibial defect. *B,* Replacement of the knee with a custom prosthesis with medial wedge.

tion in resisting moments and load sharing. While the stems need not have rigid fixation in the shaft, medial tilting and slight displacement noticed in one case suggests that press-fitting the stems is desirable, especially in cases with more extensive bone loss (Fig. 73.47). In revision and reimplant surgery we now routinely use hand reamers to select a stem that makes contact with the cortices but do not attempt to expand the canal. With the flexibility of the current modular systems, and the development of offset stems, this can routinely be accomplished without major difficulty.

Custom Prostheses

Modular components have greatly reduced the need for custom prostheses for primary and revision surgery. However, custom devices are occasionally needed, most frequently in our experience, for cases in which a previous high tibial osteotomy has been done. The problem in these knees is when the osteotomy has produced an offset in the diaphysis and a tibial stem is desired (Fig. 73.48). The development of offset stems as part of current modular prosthesis systems has significantly reduced the number of custom components required in our experience.

Patellar Prostheses

Resurfacing

In rheumatoid arthritis the patella should always be replaced to remove all articular cartilage from the joint. Some surgeons recommend selective resurfacing of the patella in osteoarthritis.[189, 199, 204] Others think the result more predictable with routine patellar resurfacing (Fig. 73.49).[57, 174, 190, 207] Undoubtedly patellar resurfacing has its share of iatrogenic complications such as fracture[215] and soft-tissue overgrowth with impingement.[89] Fixation holes into the patella weaken its structure, central holes probably more so than peripheral (Fig. 73.50).

Configuration

Until recently most patellar components were dome-shaped. This configuration is not ideal because the convex contour might be expected to wear poorly on the basis of engineering experience (in an articulation the softer material should be concave). A component that is anatomic (e.g., porous coated anatomic and low-contact stress) has a more desirable configuration in this respect but requires careful rotary alignment to prevent binding against the femur (Fig. 73.51). In addi-

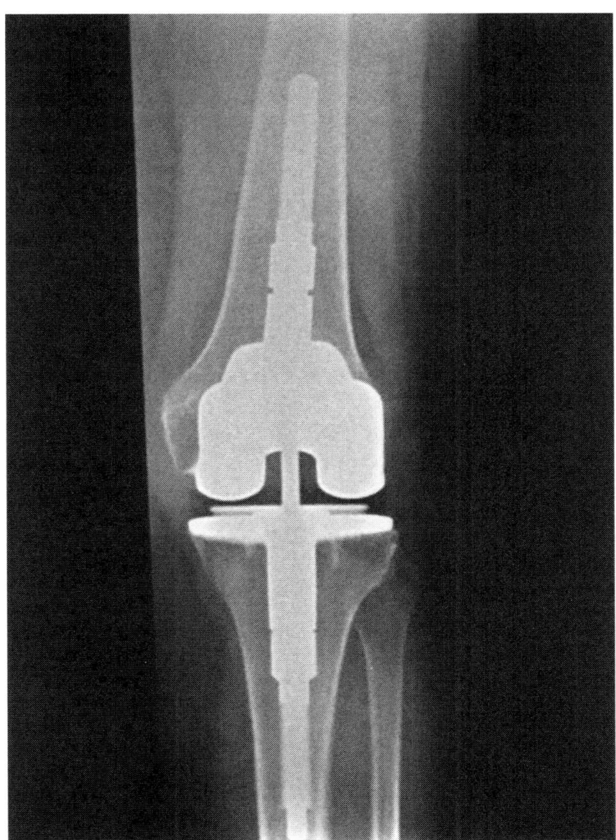

FIGURE 73.45 ➢ Radiograph of a knee prosthesis showing so-called dangle stems. These are uncemented stems that rest in the intramedullary canal and do not make contact with the cortices. Even so, roentgen stereophotogrammatic analysis data have shown on the tibial side that uncemented stems of this type have the lowest rates of migration and inducible displacement.

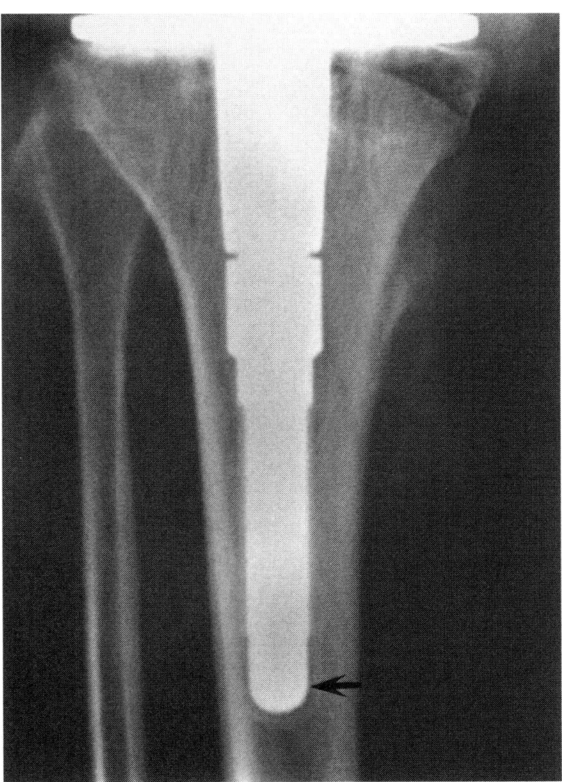

FIGURE 73.46 ➢ Radiograph showing sclerosis at the tip of an uncemented stem (*arrow*). The interpretation of this finding, which is fairly constant, is arguable. In part, it is probably due to bending of the more flexible bone, but it may also be indicative of the stem's role in resisting tilting movements.

tion, correct static alignment, even if achieved at operation, may not predict the functional pull of the quadriceps in active use, and the more desirable wear characteristics can be offset by increased torque on the component caused by malalignment. The low-contact stress patellar design attempts to solve this problem by having an anatomic polyethylene articulation swivel upon a metal baseplate. This design has been in use for 10 years and is apparently very successful. The tendency of the universal patellar dome to deform has led to the use of oval and sombrero shapes.[29] An oval patella provides greater coverage of the patellar bone, and a sombrero shape has theoretically more attractive wear characteristics. Other workers advocate inlaying the prosthesis into the central portion of the patellar bone[136] (Fig. 73.52), stating that the peripheral bony rim in contact with the femoral condyles does not cause symptoms. If this is so, the inlay patella is attractive, but the concept does not appear to be entirely rational. In any event, wear with a dome-shaped patellar component has not been seen as a problem in long-term clinical studies, but retrieval analysis raises some cause for concern (Fig. 73.53).

Metal-Backed Patellar Component

Metal backing of the polyethylene (polyethylene dissociation and wear-through) (Fig. 73.54) has become a serious clinical problem whose full dimension has not yet been realized. It is apparent that many patellae were designed with inadequate polyethylene thickness.

Metal backing of the patellar component was inspired in part by the good experience with tibial component design and in part by the wish to obtain bone ingrowth.[65] This feature of design introduced very serious complications in the form of polyethylene wear-through or dissociation from the metal baseplate. It is impossible to design an onset patellar component with the necessary thickness of polyethylene to avoid wear-through without producing an unacceptably bulky component. This design difficulty has caused a widespread return to all-polyethylene patellar components generally used with cement, although press-fit inlaid components are used without cement.[24] The optimal patellar design remains uncertain.[43] However, Laskin and Bucknell[136] and others believe metal-backed failures are due to a design problem that can be solved by increasing the thickness on the polyethylene and countersinking the base within the patellar bone. The

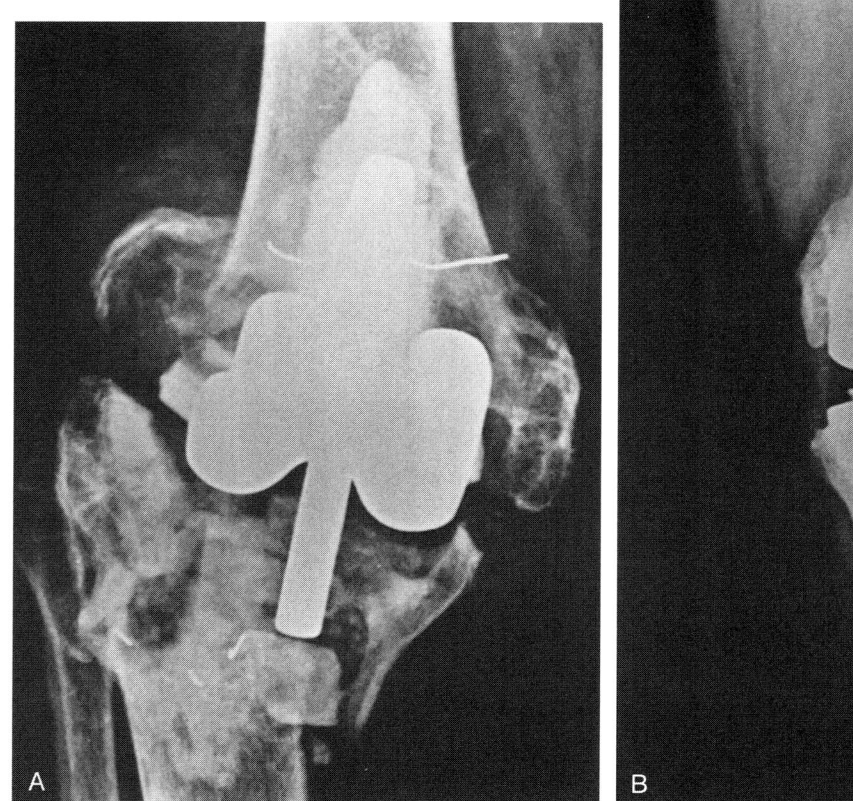

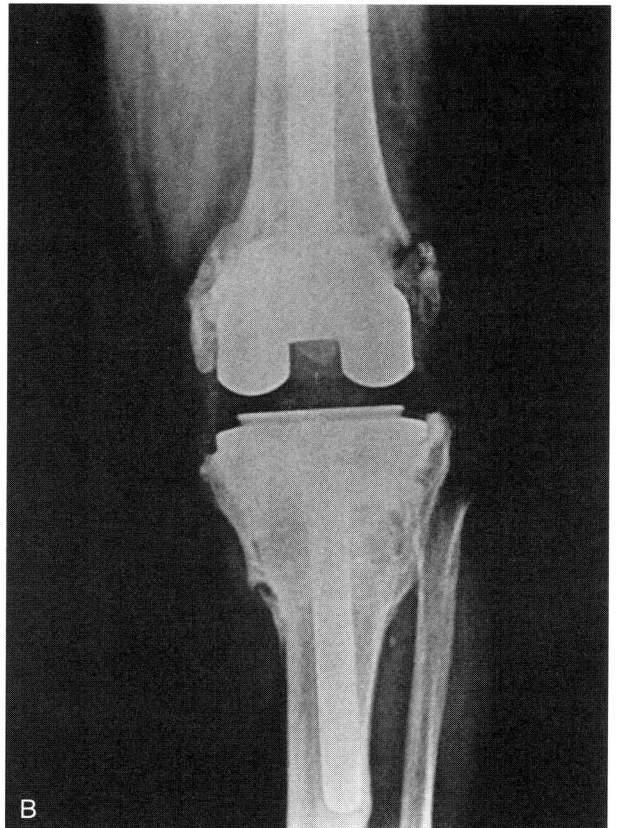

FIGURE 73.47 ➢ *A,* Failed Attenborough prosthesis with great loss of bone and fragmentation of the upper tibia. *B,* Reconstruction with a custom prosthesis, using a femoral head allograft in the tibia. The intramedullary rod was passed through a hole in the femoral head. Morselized cancellous graft was used to fill in remaining defects. The custom rod was undersized and has migrated into slight varus and stabilized in this position. Some cortical reaction is seen. This indicates the need for precise sizing of the intramedullary rods for this type of revision case, an advantage of modular systems. However, this knee functioned well until the patient's death 8 years postoperatively.

low-contact stress design continues to use a rotating platform with a metal base.

Prosthetic Patellar Problems

However the patella is treated, patellofemoral symptoms on stair climbing and other flexed knee activities remain a troublesome problem not yet fully resolved. Avoidance of a "high shoulder" profile of the femoral component in the junctional area between flange and condylar runners in favor of a smooth, uniformly curved patellar sulcus reduces patellofemoral strain.[155] Technical factors, such as the orientation of the patellar osteotomy and the thickness of the patellar prosthesis composite, are important, as is avoidance of patellar infera due to proximal alteration of the prosthetic joint line.

Should the Patella Be Resurfaced?

Some of the patellar problems can be avoided if the patellar prosthesis is omitted altogether (Fig. 73.55). Abraham and coworkers studied 100 knees, of which 47 had patellar resurfacing.[1] The prosthesis used was the variable axis. The two groups were similar in diagnosis, age, and sex. They were unable to find significant differences between the two groups with regard to walking distance, ability to climb stairs, ability to rise from a chair, motion, extensor lag, and quadriceps strength. One patient in the resurfacing group required reoperation for subluxation, and two in the unresurfaced group required subsequent resurfacing. A number of more recent studies have noted similar findings. Keblish and colleagues reported on patients who had undergone bilateral TKR with patellar resurfacing on one side and retention of the natural patella on the other.[122a] The patients expressed no preference between the two sides, and there were no differences in stair climbing or the incidence of anterior knee pain. Barrack and coauthors have also reported results of a prospective, randomized study on patellar resurfacing involving 87 patients.[16a] They were unable to detect a difference in the overall Knee Society Score, function score, or patient satisfaction. Thirty-two patients had

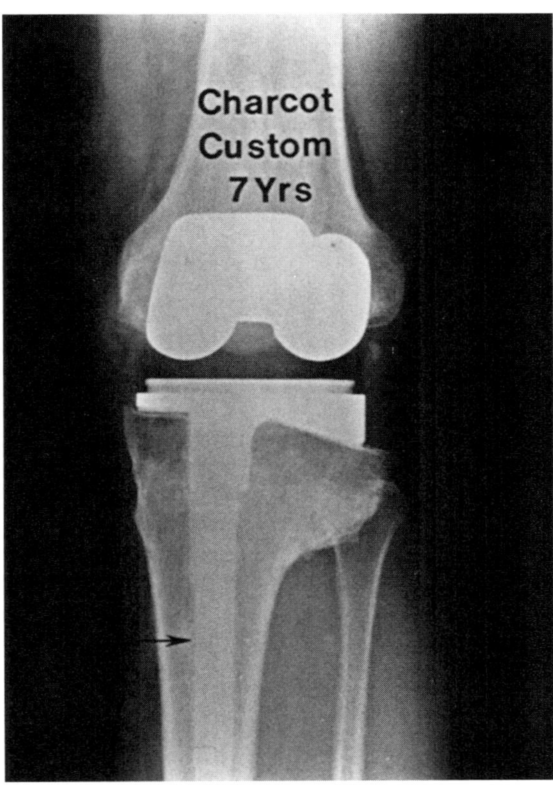

FIGURE 73.48 ➢ Radiograph of a custom prosthesis with a lateral wedge and offset stem. The prosthesis was designed for a patient with a neuropathic joint who had previously undergone high tibial osteotomy. The knee migrated into excessive valgus, leaving a lateral defect and an offset to the tibial diaphysis. A standard modular prosthesis would not have fit in this case.

OVERALL GROUP

PERCENT

100
80
60
40
20
0

EXCELLENT
GOOD
FAIR
POOR

NO PATELLA
(37 KNEES)

PATELLA
(188 KNEES)

FIGURE 73.49 ➢ The clinical results are slightly better when a patellar component is used.

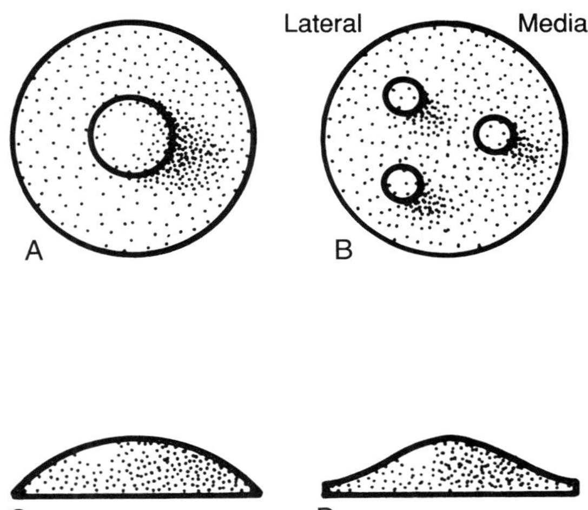

FIGURE 73.50 ➢ Patella shapes and methods of fixation. *A & C,* A dome patella with a central fixation lug. *B & D,* A sombrero patella with three fixation pegs.

undergone bilateral TKR with resurfacing of the patella on one side and retention of the natural patella on the other side. This subgroup of patients expressed no clear preference. Whereas the results were not significantly different between the two groups, a clear difference in complications was noted. A significantly higher rate of anterior knee pain was detected in the group with retention of the natural patella (13% versus 7%) that resulted in a 10% prevalence of subsequent patellar resurfacing. Boyd and coworkers also reported that in early to midterm follow-up, increased complications occur in patients with a retained natural patella.[27a] At a mean of 3 years, the overall complication rate in the group with patellar resurfacing was 4% versus 12% in the unresurfaced group. Among patients with rheumatoid arthritis who had undergone patellar resurfacing, loosening of the patellar prosthesis was 1%, whereas a 13% reoperation rate for subsequent resurfacing occurred in the group who initially had been left with the natural patella. Recently, Kajino and colleagues have reported superior pain relief in pa-

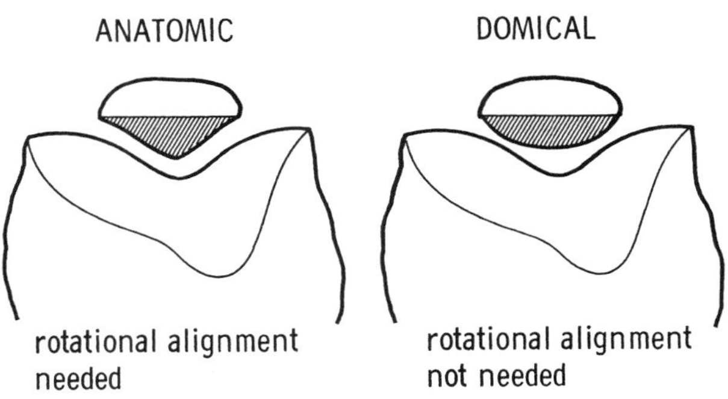

FIGURE 73.51 ➢ Rotational alignment is needed with a patellar replacement of anatomic shape.

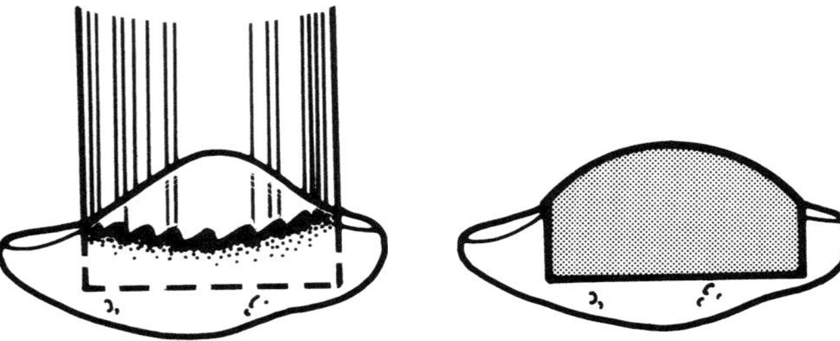

FIGURE 73.52 ➢ Insetting the patella allows greater thickness of polyethylene and the use of metal backing. There is a rim of peripheral exposed bone, which can impinge against the femur.

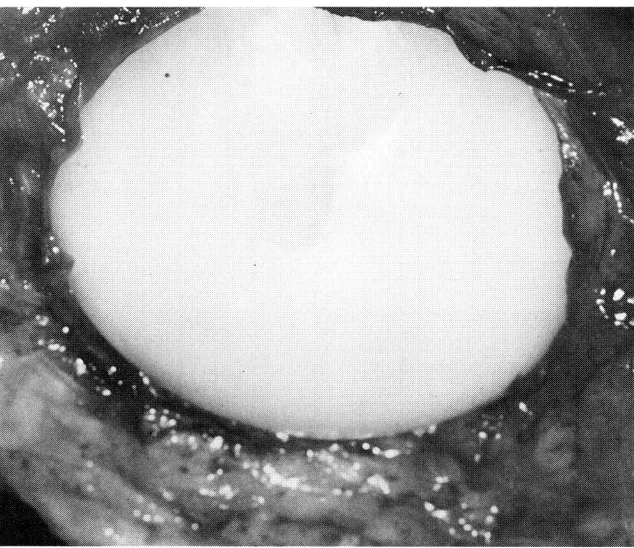

FIGURE 73.53 ➢ A patella showing considerable lateral polyethylene wear. This amount of polyethylene damage is unusual and was caused by lateral subluxation of the patella. Normally, only slighter flattening and deformation of dome-type patellae are noted.

tients with rheumatoid arthritis after patellar resurfacing.[113a] In this prospective, randomized study of patients who underwent bilateral TKR, only one knee was selected for patellar resurfacing. Although knee scores were not significantly different, patients only experienced pain on standing or during stair climbing on the side with a retained natural patella.

Enis and coauthors[57] have also reported a slight preference among 25 patients with bilateral arthroplasties in whom the patella was resurfaced, with the Townley prosthesis, on one side but not the other. The majority of patients expressed a preference for the resurfaced side, which they found to be relatively pain-free and stronger during flexed knee activities, such as stair climbing. However, the difference was not very great. Our experience agrees with these results, which suggest slightly better results following patellar resurfacing, particularly in patients with inflammatory arthritis. However, in certain circumstances it may be preferable to leave the natural patella intact. It may be advisable to omit patellar resurfacing when:

1. The patellar articular surface is near normal.
2. The patient is obese. Stern and Insall have shown that with resurfacing, pain and complications are higher in obese patients.[212]
3. The patella is too small or eroded to accept a prosthesis.
4. The patient is young and active, which theoretically increases the risk of loosening and wear.

In order to allow the option to omit patellar resurfacing, it seems wise to design the femoral component

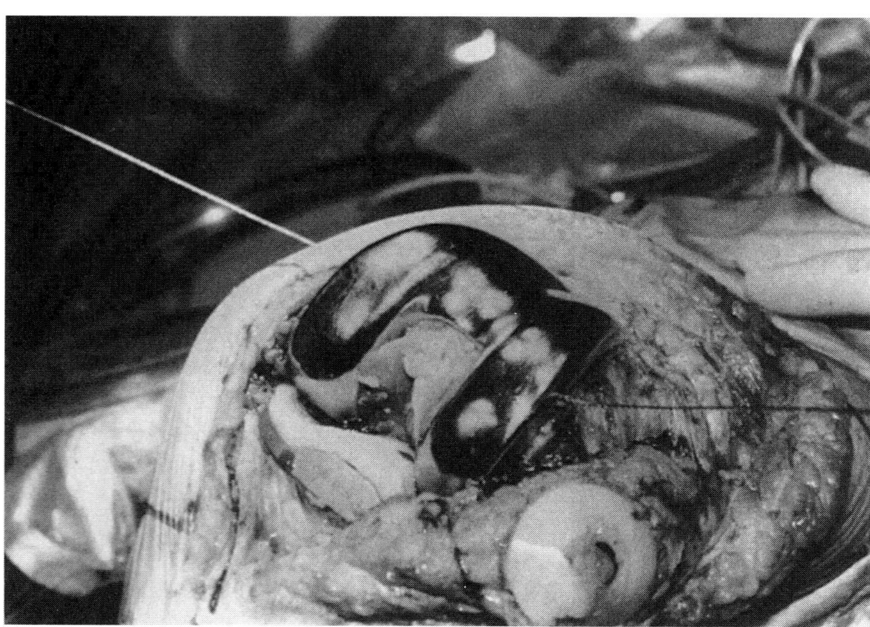

FIGURE 73.54 ➢ A Kinematic prosthesis showing central wear-through of a metal-backed patellar component.

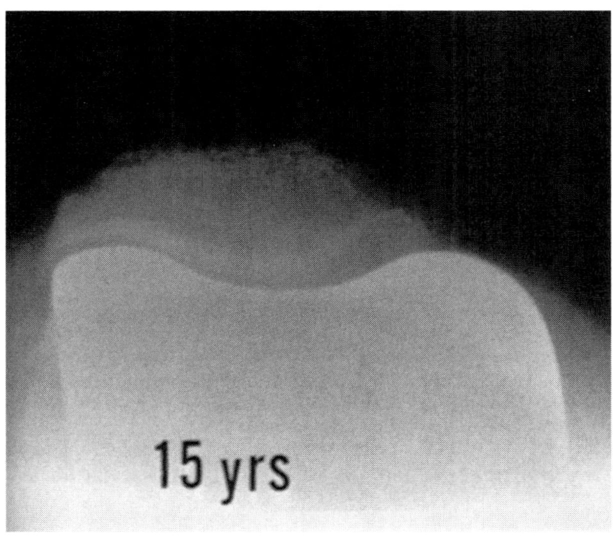

FIGURE 73.55 ➢ Skyline radiograph showing an unresurfaced patella, 15 years postoperatively. In this case the patella has remodeled to fit the femoral groove. The knee is functioning satisfactorily, has good function on stairs, and is pain-free. Unfortunately, this is not always the result in patellae that are left unresurfaced.

to be compatible with the natural patella. The latest generation of posterior stabilized prosthesis that we use is side specific with an extended trochlea that has a more gradual transition with the distal condyles in order to accommodate the natural patella. In order to facilitate these changes it was necessary to move the cam posteriorly.

Effect of Patellectomy on Total Knee Arthroplasty

Lennox and colleagues[137] described 11 patients who underwent TKA after a previous patellectomy. Good to excellent results were obtained in 5 of the 11 knees, compared with 11 of 11 in a control group with intact patellae. They did not find that presence or absence of the PCL was of importance. Two patients later had an arthrodesis for continued complaints of pain. They found that a patient who preoperatively had more than three previous operations with minimal or moderate tibiofemoral arthritic changes and with severely compromised quadriceps function was unlikely to achieve an acceptable result from TKA.

Other investigators have reported their studies of knee arthroplasty following patellectomy with similar results.[128, 169]

The senior author's experience has been that when extensor mechanism function was good before knee arthroplasty, the result was also functionally satisfactory. However, postoperative pain from the patellar tendon area could not be accurately predicted.

References

1. Abraham W, Buchanan JR, Daubert H, et al: Should the patella be resurfaced in total knee arthroplasty? Efficacy of patellar resurfacing. Clin Orthop 236:128, 1988.
2. Aglietti P, Rinonapoli E: Total condylar knee arthroplasty: A five-year follow-up study of 33 knees. Clin Orthop 186:104, 1984.
3. Aglietti P, Buzzi R, Gaudenzi A: Patellofemoral functional results and complications with the posterior stabilized total condylar knee prosthesis. J Arthroplasty 3:17, 1988.
4. Aglietti P, Buzzi R: Posteriorly stabilised total-condylar knee replacement: Three to eight years' follow-up of 85 knees. J Bone Joint Surg Br 70:211, 1988.
5. Andersen JL: Knee arthroplasty in rheumatoid arthritis: An analysis of 240 cases of hemi-, hinge and resurfacing arthroplasties. Acta Orthop Scand, Suppl 180:1, 1979.
6. Andriacchi TP, Galante JO: Influence of total knee replacement design on walking and stair climbing. J Bone Joint Surg Am 64: 1328, 1982.
7. Andriacchi TP, Galante JO, Draganich LF: Relationship between knee extensor mechanics and function following total knee replacement. In Dorr LD, ed: The Knee: Papers of the First Scientific Meeting of the Knee Society. University Park Press, Baltimore, 1985, p 83.
8. Andriacchi TP, Stanwyck TS, Galante JO: Knee biomechanics and total knee replacement. J Arthroplasty 1:211, 1986.
9. Andriacchi TP, Galante JO: Retention of the posterior cruciate in total knee arthroplasty. J Arthroplasty, suppl S13, 1988.
10. Arciero RA, Toomey HE: Patellofemoral arthroplasty: A three- to nine-year follow-up study. Clin Orthop 236:60, 1988.
11. Arden GP: Total replacement of the knee. J Bone Joint Surg Br 57:119, 1975.
12. Attenborough CG: Total knee replacement using the stabilized gliding prosthesis. Ann R Coll Surg Engl 58:4, 1976.
13. Attenborough CG: The Attenborough total knee replacement. J Bone Joint Surg Br 60:320, 1978.
14. Bain AM: Replacement of the knee joint with the Walldius prosthesis using cement fixation. Clin Orthop 94:65, 1973.
15. Barck AL: 10-year evaluation of compartmental knee arthroplasty. J Arthroplasty, suppl S49, 1989.
16. Bargar WL, Cracchiolo A III, Amstutz HC: Results with the constrained total knee prosthesis in treating severely disabled patients and patients with failed total knee replacements. J Bone Joint Surg Am 62:504, 1980.

16a. Barrack RL, Wolfe MW, Waldman DA, et al: Resurfacing of the patella in total knee arthroplasty: A prospective, randomized, double-blind study. J Bone Joint Surg Am 79:1121, 1997.

17. Barrett DS, Biswas SP, MacKenney RP: The Oxford knee replacement: A review from an independent centre. J Bone Joint Surg Br 72:775, 1990.
18. Bartel DL, Burstein AH, Santavicca EA, et al: Performance of the tibial component in total knee replacement: Conventional and revision designs. J Bone Joint Surg Am 64:1026, 1982
19. Bartel DL, Bicknell VL, Wright TM: The effect of conformity, thickness, and material on stresses in ultra-high molecular weight components for total joint replacement. J Bone Joint Surg Am 68:1041, 1986.

19a. Becker MW, Insall JN, Farris PM: Bilateral total knee arthroplasty: One cruciate retaining and one cruciate substituting. Clin Orthop 271:122, 1991.

20. Bernasek TL, Rand JA, Bryan RS: Unicompartmental porous-coated anatomic total knee arthroplasty. Clin Orthop 236:52, 1988.
21. Bert JM: Dislocation/subluxation of meniscal bearing elements after New Jersey low-contact stress total knee arthroplasty. Clin Orthop 254:211, 1990.
22. Bertin KC, Freeman MAR, Samuelson KM, et al: Stemmed revision arthroplasty for aseptic loosening of total knee replacement. J Bone Joint Surg Br 67:242, 1985.
23. Bisla RS, Inglis AE, Lewis RJ: Fat embolism following bilateral total knee replacement with the GUEPAR prosthesis: A case report. Clin Orthop 115:195, 1976.
24. Blaha JD, Insler HP, Freeman MAR, et al: The fixation of a proximal tibial polyethylene prosthesis without cement. J Bone Joint Surg Br 64:326, 1982.

25. Blauth W, Hassenpflug J: Are unconstrained components essential in total knee arthroplasty? Long-term results of the Blauth knee prosthesis. Clin Orthop 258:86, 1990.
26. Bloebaum RD, Nelson K, Dorr LD, et al: Investigation of early surface delamination observed in retrieved heat-pressed tibial inserts. Clin Orthop 269:120, 1991.
26a. Bohm P, Holy T: Is there a future for hinged prostheses in primary total knee arthroplasty? A 20 year survivorship analysis of the Blauth prosthesis. J Bone Joint Surg Br 80:302, 1998.
26b. Bolanos AA, Colizza WA, McCann PD, et al: A comparison of isokinetic strength testing and gait analysis in patients with posterior cruciate-retaining and substituting knee arthroplasties. J Arthroplasty 13:906, 1998.
27. Bourne RB, Rorabeck CH, Finlay JB, et al: Kinematic I and Oxford knee arthroplasty: A 5-8-year follow-up study. J Arthroplasty 2(4):285, 1987.
27a. Boyd AD, Ewald FC, Thomas WH, et al: Long term complications after total knee arthroplasty with or without resurfacing of the patella. J Bone Joint Surg Am 75:674, 1993.
28. Bradley J, Goodfellow JW, O'Connor JJ: A radiographic study of bearing movement in unicompartmental Oxford knee replacements. J Bone Joint Surg Br 69:598, 1987.
29. Brick GW, Scott RD: The patellofemoral component of total knee arthroplasty. Clin Orthop 231:163, 1988.
30. Brodersen MP, Fitzgerald RH, Jr, Peterson LFA et al: Arthrodesis of the knee following failed total knee arthroplasty. J Bone Joint Surg Am 61:181, 1979.
31. Brooks PJ, Walker PS, Scott RD: Tibial component fixation in deficient tibial bone stock. Clin Orthop 184:302, 1984.
32. Bryan RS, Peterson LFA: Polycentric total knee arthroplasty: A prognostic assessment. Clin Orthop 145:23, 1979.
33. Buechel FF, Pappas MJ: Long-term survivorship analysis of cruciate-sparing versus cruciate-sacrificing knee prostheses using meniscal bearings. Clin Orthop 260:162, 1990.
34. Buechel FF, Pappas MJ, Makris G: Evaluation of contact stress in metal-backed patellar replacements: a predictor of survivorship. Clin Orthop 273:190, 1991.
35. Callihan SM, Halley DK: Prospective analysis of Sheehan total knee arthroplasty. Clin Orthop 192:124, 1985.
36. Campbell WC: Interposition of vitallium plates in arthroplasties of the knee: preliminary report. Am J Surg 47:639, 1940.
37. Cartier P, Cheaib S: Unicondylar knee arthroplasty: 2-10 years of follow-up evaluation. J Arthroplasty 2:157, 1987.
38. Cartier P, Sanouiller J-L, Grelsamer R: Patellofemoral arthroplasty: 2-12-year follow-up study. J Arthroplasty 5(1):49, 1990.
39. Cavendish ME, Wright JTM: The Liverpool Mark II knee prosthesis: a preliminary report. J Bone Joint Surg Br 60:315, 1978.
40. Cheng CL, Gross AE: Loosening of the porous coating in total knee replacement. J Bone Joint Surg Br 70:377, 1988.
41. Chotivichit AL, Cracchiolo A III, Chow GH et al: Total knee arthroplasty using the total condylar III knee prosthesis. J Arthroplasty 6:341, 1991.
42. Cloutier JM, Gauthier F, Rizkallah R: Arthroplasty of the knee using the Marmor prosthesis. J Bone Joint Surg Br 58:142, 1976.
42a. Colizza WA, Insall JN, Scuderi GR: The posterior stabilized total knee prosthesis: Assessment of polyethylene damage and osteolysis after a ten-year-minimum follow-up. J Bone Joint Surg Am 77:1713, 1995.
43. Collier JP, McNamara JL, Surprenant VA, et al: All-polyethylene patellar components are not the answer. Clin Orthop 273:198, 1991.
44. Cooke TDV, Collins A, Wevers HW: Failure of a knee prosthesis accelerated by shedding of beads from the porous metal surface. Clin Orthop 258:204, 1990.
45. Coventry MB, Finerman GAM, Riley LH, et al: A new geometric knee for total knee arthroplasty. Clin Orthop 83:157, 1972.
46. Coventry MB, Upshaw JE, Riley LH, et at: Geometric total knee arthroplasty. II. Patient data and complications. Clin Orthop 94:177, 1973.
47. Deane G: The evolution and clinical use of the Deane intercondylar knee. J Bone Joint Surg Br 63:476, 1981.
48. Deburge A, GUEPAR: GUEPAR hinge prosthesis: Complications and results with two years follow-up. Clin Orthop 120:47, 1976.
48a. Dennis DA, Komistek RD, Hoff WA, et al: In vivo knee kinematics derived using an inverse perspective technique. Clin Orthop 331:107, 1996.
48b. Diduch DR, Insall JN, Scott WN, et al: Total knee replacement in young active patients: Long-term follow-up and functional outcome. J Bone Joint Surg Am 79:575, 1997.
49. Dodd CAF, Hungerford DS, Krackow KA: Total knee arthroplasty fixation: Comparison of the early results of paired cemented versus uncemented porous coated anatomic knee prostheses. Clin Orthop 260:66, 1990.
50. Donaldson WF III, Sculco TP, Insall JN, et al: Total condylar III knee prosthesis: Long-term follow-up study. Clin Orthop 226:21, 1988.
51. Dorr LD, Ochsner JL, Gronley J, et al: Functional comparison of posterior cruciate-retained versus cruciate-sacrificed total knee arthroplasty. Clin Orthop 236:36, 1988.
52. Ducheyne P, Kagan A II, Lacey JA: Failure of total knee arthroplasty due to loosening and deformation of the tibial component. J Bone Joint Surg Am 60:384, 1978.
52a. Duffy GP, Trousdale RT, Stuart MJ: Total knee arthroplasty in patients 55 years old or younger: 10 to 17 year results. Clin Orthop 356:22, 1998.
53. Elias SG, Freeman MAR, Gokcay EI: A correlative study of the geometry and anatomy of the distal femur. Clin Orthop 260:98, 1990.
54. Emerson RH, Jr, Potter T: The use of the McKeever metallic hemiarthroplasty for unicompartmental arthritis. J Bone Joint Surg Am 67:208, 1985.
55. Engh GA: Failure of the polyethylene bearing surface of a total knee replacement within four years: A case report. J Bone Joint Surg Am 70:1093, 1988.
56. England SP, Stern SH, Insall JN, et al: Total knee arthroplasty in diabetes mellitus. Clin Orthop 260:130, 1990.
57. Enis JE, Gardner R, Robledo MA, et al: Comparison of patellar resurfacing versus nonresurfacing in bilateral total knee arthroplasty. Clin Orthop 260:38, 1990.
58. Evanski PM, Waugh TR, Orofino CF, et al: UCI knee replacement. Clin Orthop 120:33, 1976.
59. Ewald FC, Thomas WH, Poss R, et al: Duo-patella total knee arthroplasty in rheumatoid arthritis. Orthop Trans 2:202, 1978.
60. Ewald FC, Jacobs MA, Miegel RE, at al: Kinematic total knee replacement. J Bone Joint Surg Am 66:1032, 1984.
61. Ferguson W: Excision of the knee joint: Recovery with a false joint and a useful limb. Med Times Gaz 1:601, 1861.
62. Figgie HE III, Davy DT, Heiple KG, et al: Load-bearing capacity of the tibial component of the total condylar knee prosthesis: An in vitro study. Orthop Clin 183:288, 1984.
63. Figgie HE III, Goldberg VM, Heiple KG, et al: The influence of tibial-patellofemoral location on function of the knee in patients with the posterior stabilized condylar knee prosthesis. J Bone Joint Surg Am 68:1035, 1986.
64. Finerman GAM, Coventry MB, Riley LH, et al: Anametric total knee arthroplasty. Clin Orthop 145:85, 1979.
65. Firestone TP, Teeny SM, Krackow KA, et al: The clinical and roentgenographic results of cementless porous-coated patellar fixation. Clin Orthop 273:184, 1991.
66. Freeman MAR, Swanson SAV, Todd RC: Total replacement of the knee using the Freeman-Swanson knee prosthesis. Clin Orthop 94:153, 1973.
67. Freeman MAR, Insall JN, Besser W, et al: Excision of the cruciate ligaments in total knee replacement. Clin Orthop 126:209, 1977.
68. Freeman MAR, Sculco T, Todd RC: Replacement of the severely damaged arthritic knee by the ICLH (Freeman-Swanson) arthroplasty. J Bone Joint Surg Br 59:64, 1977.
69. Freeman MAR, Todd RC, Bamert P, et al: ICLH arthroplasty of the knee: 1968-1977. J Bone Joint Surg Br 60:339, 1978.
70. Freeman MAR, Insall JN: Tibio-femoral replacement using two unlinked components and cruciate resection (the ICLH and total condylar prostheses). In Freeman, MAR, ed: Arthritis of the Knee: Clinical Features and Surgical Management. Springer-Verlag, New York, 1980, p 254.
71. Freeman MAR, Samuelson KM, Bertin KC: Freeman-Samuelson total arthroplasty of the knee. Clin Orthop 192:46, 1985.
72. Freeman MAR, Levack B: British contribution to knee arthroplasty. Clin Orthop 210:69, 1986.

73. Freeman MAR, Samuelson KM, Levack B, et al: Knee arthroplasty at the London Hospital: 1975–1984. Clin Orthop 205:12, 1986.
74. Freeman MAR, Railton GT: Should the posterior cruciate ligament be retained or resected in condylar nonmeniscal knee arthroplasty? The case for resection. J Arthroplasty, suppl S3, 1988.
75. Freeman MAR, Samuelson KM, Elias SG, et al: The patellofemoral joint in total knee prostheses: Design considerations. J Arthroplasty, suppl S69, 1989.
76. Gibbs AN, Green GA, Taylor JG: A comparison of the Freeman-Swanson (ICLH) and Walldius prostheses in total knee replacement. J Bone Joint Surg Br 61:358, 1979.
77. Goldberg VM, Henderson BT: The Freeman-Swanson ICLH total knee arthroplasty: Complications and problems. J Bone Joint Surg Am 62:1338, 1980.
78. Goldberg VM, Figgie MP, Figgie HE III, et al: Use of a total condylar knee prosthesis for treatment of osteoarthritis and rheumatoid arthritis: Long-term results. J Bone Joint Surg Am 70:802, 1988.
79. Goodfellow J, O'Connor J: Kinematics of the knee and the prosthetic design. J Bone Joint Surg Br 59:119, 1977.
80. Goodfellow JW, O'Connor J: Clinical results of the Oxford knee: Surface arthroplasty of the tibiofemoral joint with a meniscal bearing prosthesis. Clin Orthop 205:21, 1986.
81. Goodfellow JW, Tibrewal SB, Sherman KP, et al: Unicompartmental Oxford meniscal knee arthroplasty. J Arthroplasty 2:1, 1987.
82. Goodfellow JW, Kershaw CJ, D'A Benson MK, et al: The Oxford knee for unicompartmental osteoarthritis: The first 103 cases. J Bone Joint Surg Br 70:692, 1988.
83. Grimer RJ, Karpinski MRK, Edwards AN: The long-term results of Stanmore total knee replacements. J Bone Joint Surg Br 66: 55, 1984.
84. Groh GI, Parker J, Elliott J, et al: Results of total knee arthroplasty using the posterior stabilized condylar prosthesis: A report of 137 consecutive cases. Clin Orthop 269:58, 1991.
84a. Firestone TP, Krackow KA, Davis JD IV, et al: The management of fixed flexion contractures during total knee arthroplasty. Clin Orthop 284:221, 1992.
85. Gunston FH: Polycentric knee arthroplasty: Prosthetic simulation of normal knee movement. J Bone Joint Surg Br 53:272, 1971.
86. Gunston FH, MacKenzie RI: Complications of polycentric knee arthroplasty. Clin Orthop 120:11, 1976.
86a. Haas SB, Insall JN, Montgomery W III, et al: Revision total knee arthoplasty with use of modular components with stems inserted without cement. J Bone Joint Surg Am 77:1700, 1995.
87. Hanssen AD, Rand JA: A comparison of primary and revision total knee arthroplasty using the kinematic stabilizer prosthesis. J Bone Joint Surg Am 70:491, 1988.
88. Hernigou PH, Goutallier D: GUEPAR unicompartmental lotus prosthesis for single-compartment femorotibial arthrosis: A five- to nine-year follow-up study. Clin Orthop 230:186, 1988.
89. Hirsh DM, Sallis JG: Pain after total knee arthroplasty caused by soft tissue impingement. J Bone Joint Surg Am 71:591, 1989.
90. Hohl WM, Crawfurd E, Zelicof SB, et al: The total condylar III prosthesis in complex knee reconstruction. Clin Orthop 273: 91, 1991.
91. Hood RW, Vanni M, Insall JN: The correction of knee alignment in 225 consecutive total condylar knee replacements. Clin Orthop 160:94, 1981.
92. Hui FC, Fitzgerald RH, Jr: Hinged total knee arthroplasty. J Bone Joint Surg Am 62:513, 1980.
93. Hungerford DS, Kenna RV, Krackow KA: The porous-coated anatomic total knee. Orthop Clin North Am 13:103, 1982.
94. Hungerford DS, Krackow KA: Total joint arthroplasty of the knee. Clin Orthop 192:23, 1985.
95. Hvid I, Nielsen S: Total condylar knee arthroplasty: Prosthetic component positioning and radiolucent lines. Acta Orthop Scand 55:160, 1984.
96. Hvid I, Kjaersgaard-Andersen P, Wethelund J-O, et al: Knee arthroplasty in rheumatoid arthritis: Four- to six-year follow-up study. J Arthroplasty 2:233, 1987.
97. Ilstrup DM, Coventry MB, Skolnick MD: A statistical evaluation of geometric total knee arthroplasties. Clin Orthop 120:27, 1976.
97a. Incavo SJ, Johnson CC, Beynnon BD, et al: Posterior cruciate ligament strain biomechanics in total knee arthroplasty. Clin Orthop 309:88, 1994.
97b. Insall JN: Adventures in mobile-bearing knee design: A mid life crisis. Orthopaedics 21:1021, 1998.
98. Insall JN, Ranawat CS, Aglietti P, et al: A comparison of four models of total knee replacement prostheses. J Bone Joint Surg Am 58:754, 1976.
99. Insall JN, Ranawat CS, Scott WN, et al: Total condylar knee replacement: Preliminary report. Clin Orthop 120:149, 1976.
100. Insall JN, Walker P: Unicondylar knee replacement. Clin Orthop 120:83, 1976.
101. Insall JN, Tria AJ, Scott WN: The total condylar knee prosthesis: The first five years. Clin Orthop 145:68, 1979.
102. Insall JN, Scott WN, Ranawat CS: The total condylar knee prosthesis: A report of two hundred and twenty cases. J Bone Joint Surg Am 61:173, 1979.
103. Insall JN, Tria AJ: The total condylar prosthesis type II. Orthop Trans 3:300, 1979.
104. Insall JN, Aglietti P: A five- to seven-year follow-up of unicondylar arthroplasty. J Bone Joint Surg Am 62:1329, 1980.
105. Insall JN, Freeman MAR, Matthews LS, et al: Present status of total knee replacement. [Symposium]. Contemp Orthop 2:592, 1980.
106. Insall JN: Reconstructive surgery and rehabilitation of the knee. In Kelley WN, Harris ED, Jr, Ruddy S, et al, eds: Textbook of Rheumatology. WB Saunders, Philadelphia, 1980, p 1980.
107. Insall JN, Lachiewicz PF, Burstein AH: The posterior stabilized condylar prosthesis: A modification of the total condylar design: Two to four year clinical experience. J Bone Joint Surg Am 64:1317, 1982.
108. Insall JN, Kelly M: The total condylar prosthesis. Clin Orthop 205:43, 1986.
109. Jones EC, Insall JN, Inglis AE, et al: GUEPAR knee arthroplasty results and late complications. Clin Orthop 140:145, 1979.
110. Jones GB: Arthroplasty of the knee by the Walldius prosthesis. J Bone Joint Surg Br 50:505, 1968.
111. Jones GB: Walldius arthroplasty of the knee. J Bone Joint Surg Br 52:390, 1970.
112. Jones WT, Bryan RS, Peterson LFA, et al: Unicompartmental knee arthroplasty using polycentric and geometric hemicomponents. J Bone Joint Surg Am 63:946, 1981.
113. Jonsson B, Astrom J: Alignment and long-term clinical results of a semiconstrained knee prosthesis. Clin Orthop 226:124, 1988.
113a. Kajino A, Yoshino S, Kameyama S, et al: Comparison of the results of bilateral total knee arthroplasty with and without patellar replacement for rheumatoid arthritis: A follow-up note. J Bone Joint Surg Am 79:570, 1997.
114. Kapandji IA: The Physiology of the Joints. vol. 2: The Lower Limb. Churchill Livingstone, London, 1970, p 120.
115. Katz MM, Hungerford DS, Krackow KA, et al: Results of total knee arthroplasty after failed proximal tibial osteotomy for osteoarthritis. J Bone Joint Surg Am 69:225, 1987.
116. Kaufer H, Matthews LS: Spherocentric arthroplasty of the knee. J Bone Joint Surg Am 63:545, 1981.
117. Kavolus CH, Faris PM, Ritter MA, et al: The total condylar III knee prosthesis in elderly patients. J Arthroplasty 6:39, 1991.
118. Kelman GJ, Biden EN, Wyatt MP, et al: Gait laboratory analysis of a posterior cruciate-sparing total knee arthroplasty in stair ascent and descent. Clin Orthop 248:21, 1989.
119. Kester MA, Cook SD, Harding AF, et al: An evaluation of the mechanical failure modalities of a rotating hinge knee prosthesis. Clin Orthop 228:156, 1988.
120. Kilgus DJ, Moreland JR, Finerman GAM, et al: Catastrophic wear of tibial polyethylene inserts. Clin Orthop 273:223, 1991.
121. Kim Y-H: Salvage of failed hinge knee arthroplasty with a total condylar III type prosthesis. Clin Orthop 221:272, 1987.
122. Kjaersgaard-Andersen P, Hvid I, Wethelund J-O, et al: Total condylar knee arthroplasty in osteoarthritis: A four- to six-year follow-up evaluation of 103 cases. Clin Orthop 238:167, 1989.
122a. Keblish PA, Varma AK, Greenwald AS: Patellar resurfacing or retention in total knee arthroplasty. J Bone Joint Surg Br 76: 930, 1994.
122b. Kleinbart FA, Bryk E, Evangelista J, et al: Histologic compari-

son of posterior cruciate ligaments from arthritic and age-matched knee specimens. J Arthroplasty 11:726, 1996.
123. Knahr K, Salzer M, Schmidt W: A radiological analysis of uncemented PCA tibial implants with a follow-up period of 4–7 years. J Arthroplasty 5:131, 1990.
124. Kozinn SC, Marx C, Scott RD: Unicompartmental knee arthroplasty: A 4.5–6-year follow-up study with a metal-backed tibial component. J Arthroplasty, suppl S1, 1989.
125. Kozinn SC, Scott R: Unicondylar knee arthroplasty. J Bone Joint Surg Am 71:145, 1989.
126. Kraay MJ, Meyers SA, Goldberg VM, et al: "Hybrid" total knee arthroplasty with the Miller-Galante prosthesis: A prospective clinical and roentgenographic evaluation. Clin Orthop 273:32, 1991.
127. Landon GC, Galante JO, Maley MM: Noncemented total knee arthroplasty. Clin Orthop 205:49, 1986.
128. Larson KR, Cracchiolo A III, Dorey FJ, et al: Total knee arthroplasty in patients after patellectomy. Clin Orthop 264:243, 1991.
129. Larsson S-E, Larsson S, Lundkvist S: Unicompartmental knee arthroplasty: A prospective consecutive series followed for six to 11 years. Clin Orthop 232:174, 1988.
130. Laskin RS: Modular total knee replacement arthroplasty: A review of eighty-nine patients. J Bone Joint Surg Am 58:766, 1976.
131. Laskin RS: Unicompartmental tibiofemoral resurfacing arthroplasty. J Bone Joint Surg Am 60:182, 1978.
132. Laskin RS: RMC total knee replacement: A review of 166 cases. J Arthroplasty, 1:11, 1986.
133. Laskin RS: Tricon-M uncemented total knee arthroplasty: A review of 96 knees followed for longer than 2 years. J Arthroplasty 3:27, 1988.
134. Laskin RS: Total knee arthroplasty in the presence of large bony defects of the tibia and marked knee instability. Clin Orthop 248:66, 1989.
135. Laskin RS: Total condylar knee replacement in patients who have rheumatoid arthritis: A ten-year follow-up study. J Bone Joint Surg Am 72:529, 1990.
135a. Laskin RS: Total knee replacement with posterior cruciate ligament retention in patients with a fixed varus deformity, Clin Orthop 331:29, 1996.
136. Laskin RS, Bucknell A: The use of metal-backed patellar prostheses in total knee arthroplasty. Clin Orthop 260:52, 1990.
137. Lennox DW, Hungerford DS, Krackow KA: Total knee arthroplasty following patellectomy. Clin Orthop 223: 220, 1987.
138. Lettin AWF, Deliss LJ, Blackburne JS, et al: The Stanmore hinged knee arthroplasty. J Bone Joint Surg Br 60:327, 1978.
139. Lettin AWF, Kavanagh TG, Craig D, et al: Assessment of the survival and the clinical results of Stanmore total knee replacements. J Bone Joint Surg Br 66:355, 1984.
140. Lettin AWF, Kavanagh TG, Scales JT: The long-term results of Stanmore total knee replacements. J Bone Joint Surg Br 66:349, 1984.
141. Lewis JL, Askew MJ, Jaycox DP: A comparative evaluation of tibial component designs of total knee prostheses. J Bone Joint Surg Am 64:129, 1982.
142. Lotke PA, Wong RY, Ecker ML: The use of methyl-methacrylate in primary total knee replacements with large tibial defects. Clin Orthop 270:288, 1991.
143. MacIntosh DL: Hemiarthroplasty of the knee using a space occupying prosthesis for painful varus and valgus deformities. J Bone Joint Surg Am 40:1431, 1958.
144. MacIntosh DL: Arthroplasty of the knee in rheumatoid arthritis. J Bone Joint Surg Br 48:179, 1966.
144a. Mahoney OM, Noble PC, Rhoads DD, et al: Posterior cruciate function following total knee arthroplasty: A biomechanical study. J. Arthroplasty 9:569, 1994.
144b. Malkani AL, Rand JA, Bryan RS, et al: Total knee arthroplasty with the Kinematic condylar prosthesis: A ten year follow-up study. J Bone Joint Surg Am 77:423, 1995.
145. Manchester Knee Arthroplasty [Editorial]. J Bone Joint Surg Br 61:225, 1979.
146. Marks KE, Nelson CL, Lautenschlager EP: Antibiotic-impregnated acrylic bone cement. J Bone Joint Surg Am 58:358, 1976.
147. Marmor L: The modular (Marmor) knee: Case report with a minimum follow-up of two years. Clin Orthop 120:86, 1976.
148. Marmor L: Results of single compartment arthroplasty with acrylic cement fixation: a minimum follow-up of two years. Clin Orthop 122:181, 1977.
149. Marmor L: Marmor modular knee in unicompartmental disease: minimum four-year follow-up. J Bone Joint Surg Am 61:347, 1979.
150. Marmor L: Total knee arthroplasty in a patient with congenital dislocation of the patella: Case report. Clin Orthop 226:129, 1988.
151. Marmor L: Unicompartmental knee arthroplasty: Ten- to 13-year follow-up study. Clin Orthop 226:14, 1988.
152. Matthews LS, Goldstein SA, Kolowich PA, et al: Spherocentric arthroplasty of the knee: A long-term and final follow-up evaluation. Clin Orthop 205:58, 1986.
153. Mazas FB, GUEPAR: GUEPAR total knee prosthesis. Clin Orthop 94:211, 1973.
154. McKeever DC: Tibial plateau prosthesis. Clin Orthop 18:86, 1960.
155. McLain RF, Bargar WF: The effect of total knee design on patellar strain. J Arthroplasty 1:91, 1986.
156. Miller A, Friedman B: Fascial arthroplasty of the knee. J Bone Joint Surg Am 34:55, 1952.
157. Miura H, Whiteside LA, Easley JC, et al: Effects of screws and a sleeve on initial fixation in uncemented total knee tibial components. Clin Orthop 259:160, 1990.
158. Moller JT, Weeth RE, Keller JO, et al: Unicompartmental arthroplasty of the knee: Cadaver study of the importance of the anterior cruciate ligament. Acta Orthop Scand 56:120, 1985.
159. Moller JT, Weeth RE, Keller JO: Unicompartmental arthroplasty of the knee: Cadaver study of tibial component placement. Acta Orthop Scand 56:115, 1985.
160. Moran CG, Pinder IM, Lees TA, et al: Survivorship analysis of the uncemented porous-coated anatomic knee replacement. J Bone Joint Surg Am 73:848, 1991.
161. Moreland JR, Thomas RJ, Freeman MAR: ICLH replacement of the knee: 1977 and 1978. Clin Orthop 145:47, 1979.
162. Murray DG, Webster DA: The variable-axis knee prosthesis: Two-year follow-up study. J Bone Joint Surg Am 63:687, 1981.
162a. Murray RB, Rand JA, Hanssen AD: Cemented long-stem revision total knee arthroplasty. Clin Orthop 309:116, 1994.
163. Nilsson KG, Karrholm J, Ekelund L: Knee motion in total knee arthroplasty: A roentgen stereophotogrammetric analysis of the kinematics of the Tricon-M knee prosthesis. Clin Orthop 256: 147, 1990.
164. Orr TE, Beaupré GS, Carter DR, et al: Computer predictions of bone remodeling around porous-coated implants. J Arthroplasty 5:191, 1990.
164a. Pagnano MW, Cushner FD, Scott WN: Role of the posterior cruciate ligament in total knee arthroplasty. J Am Acad Orthop Surg 6:176, 1998.
164b. Pagnano MW, Hanssen AD, Lewallen DG, et al: Flexion instability after primary posterior cruciate retaining total knee arthroplasty. Clin Orthop 356:39, 1998.
165. Phillips H, Taylor JG: The Walldius hinge arthroplasty. J Bone Joint Surg Br 57:59, 1975.
166. Rackemann S, Mintzer CM, Walker PS, et al: Uncemented Press-Fit total knee arthroplasty. J Arthroplasty 5(4):307, 1990.
167. Rae T: A study on the effects of particulate metals of orthopaedic interest on murine macrophages in vitro. J Bone Joint Surg Br 57:444, 1975.
168. Railton GT, Waterfield A, Nunn D, et al: The effect of a metal-back without a stem upon the fixation of a tibial prosthesis. J Arthroplasty, suppl 5:S67, 1990.
169. Railton GT, Levack B, Freeman MAR: Unconstrained knee arthroplasty after patellectomy. J Arthroplasty 5:255, 1990.
170. Ranawat CS, Insall J, Shine J: Duo-condylar knee arthroplasty: Hospital for Special Surgery design. Clin Orthop 120:76, 1976.
171. Ranawat CS, Boachie-Adjei O: Survivorship analysis and results of total condylar knee arthroplasty. Eight- to 11-year follow-up period. Clin Orthop 226:6, 1988.
171a. Ranawat CS, Luessenhop CP, Rodriguez JS: The Press-Fit condylar modular total knee system: Four to six year results with a posterior-cruciate-substituting design. J Bone Joint Surg Am 79: 342, 1997.
172. Rand JA, Chao EYS, Stauffer RN: Kinematic rotating-hinge total knee arthroplasty. J Bone Joint Surg Am 69:489, 1987.

173. Rand JA, Coventry MB: Ten-year evaluation of geometric total knee arthroplasty. Clin Orthop 232:168, 1988.
174. Rand JA: Patellar resurfacing in total knee arthroplasty. Clin Orthop 260:110, 1990.
175. Riley LH, Hungerford DS: Geometric total knee replacement for treatment of the rheumatoid knee. J Bone Joint Surg Am 60: 523, 1978.
176. Riley D, Woodyard JE: Long-term results of geomedic total knee replacement. J Bone Joint Surg Br 67:548, 1985.
177. Ritter MA: Screw and cement fixation of large defects in total knee arthroplasty. J Arthroplasty 1:125, 1986.
178. Ritter MA, Faris PM, Keating EM: Posterior cruciate ligament balancing during total knee arthroplasty. J Arthroplasty 3:323, 1988.
179. Ritter MA, Campbell E, Faris PM, et al: Long-term survival analysis of the posterior cruciate condylar total knee arthroplasty: A 10-year evaluation. J Arthroplasty 4(4):293, 1989.
180. Rorabeck CH, Bourne RB, Nott L: The cemented kinematic-II and the non-cemented porous-coated anatomic prostheses for total knee replacement: A prospective evaluation. J Bone Joint Surg Am 70:483, 1988.
181. Rosenberg AG, Barden RM, Galante JO: Cemented and ingrowth fixation of the Miller-Galante prosthesis: Clinical and roentgenographic comparison after three- to six-year follow-up studies. Clin Orthop 260:71, 1990.
182. Rosenqvist R, Bylander B, Knutson K, et al: Loosening of the porous coating of bicompartmental prostheses in patients with rheumatoid arthritis. J Bone Joint Surg Am 68:538, 1986.
183. Samuelson KM: Bone grafting and noncemented revision arthroplasty of the knee. Clin Orthop 226:93, 1988.
184. Samuelson K, Nelson L: An all-polyethylene cementless tibial component: A five- to nine-year follow-up study. Clin Orthop 260:93, 1990.
185. Schurman DJ, Parker JN, Ornstein D: Total condylar knee replacement: A study of factors influencing range of motion as late as two years after arthroplasty. J Bone Joint Surg Am 67: 1006, 1985.
185a. Scott RD, Thornhill TS: Posterior cruciate supplementing total knee replacements using conforming inserts and cruciate recession: Effect on range of motion and radiolucent lines. Clin Orthop 309:146, 1994.
186. Scott RD, Welsh RP, Thomas WH: Unicompartment unicondylar total knee replacement in osteoarthritis of the knee. Orthop Trans 2:203, 1978.
187. Scott RD, Santore RF: Unicondylar unicompartmental replacement for osteoarthritis of the knee. J Bone Joint Surg Am 63: 536, 1981.
188. Scott RD, Joyce MJ, Ewald FC, et al: McKeever metallic hemiarthroplasty of the knee in unicompartmental degenerative arthritis: Long-term clinical follow-up and current indications. J Bone Joint Surg Am 67:203, 1985.
189. Scott RD, Volatile TB: Twelve years' experience with posterior cruciate-retaining total knee arthroplasty. Clin Orthop 205: 100, 1986.
190. Scott WN, Rozbruch JD, Otis JC, et al: Clinical and biomechanical evaluation of patella replacement in total knee arthroplasty. Orthop Trans 2:203, 1978.
191. Scott WN, Tria A, Insall JN: Total knee arthroplasty: Past present, future. Orthop Surv 3:135, 1979.
192. Scott WN, Rubinstein M: Posterior stabilized knee arthroplasty. Six years' experience. Clin Orthop 205:138, 1986.
193. Scott WN, Rubinstein M, Scuderi G: Results after knee replacement with a posterior cruciate-substituting prosthesis. J Bone Joint Surg Am 70:1163, 1988.
194. Shaw NE, Chatterjee RK: Manchester knee arthroplasty. J Bone Joint Surg Br 60:310, 1978.
195. Sheehan JM: Arthroplasty of the knee. J Bone Joint Surg Br 60: 333, 1978.
196. Shiers LGP: Arthroplasty of the knee: Preliminary report of a new method. J Bone Joint Surg Br 36:553, 1954.
197. Shindell R, Neumann R, Connolly JF, et al: Evaluation of the Noiles hinged knee prosthesis: A five-year study of seventeen knees. J Bone Joint Surg Am 68:579, 1986.
198. Shoji H, D'Ambrosia RD, Lipscomb PR: Failed polycentric total knee prostheses. J Bone Joint Surg Am 58:773, 1976.
199. Shoji H, Yoshino S, Kajino A: Patellar replacement in bilateral total knee arthroplasty: A study of patients who had rheumatoid arthritis and no gross deformity of the patella. J Bone Joint Surg Am 71:853, 1989.
200. Simison AJM, Noble J, Hardinge K: Complications of the Attenborough knee replacement. J Bone Joint Surg Br 68:100, 1986.
200a. Simmon S, Lephart S, Rubash H, et al: Proprioception after unicondylar knee arthroplasty versus total knee arthroplasty. Clin Orthop 331:179, 1996.
201. Skolnick MD, Bryan RS, Peterson LFA: Unicompartmental polycentric knee arthroplasty. Description and preliminary results. Clin Orthop 112:208, 1975.
202. Sledge CB, Stern P, Thomas WH, et al: Two-year follow-up of the duo-condylar total knee replacement. Orthop Trans 2:193, 1978.
203. Sledge CB, Ewald FC: Total knee arthroplasty experience at the Robert Breck Brigham Hospital. Clin Orthop 145:78, 1979.
204. Smith SR, Stuart P, Pinder IM: Nonresurfaced patella in total knee arthroplasty. J Arthroplasty, suppl S81, 1989.
205. Sonstegard DA, Kaufer H, Matthews LS: The spherocentric knee: Biomechanical testing and clinical trial. J Bone Joint Surg Am 59:602, 1977.
206. Soudry M, Walker PS, Reilly DT, et al: Effects of total knee replacement design on femoral-tibial contact conditions. J Arthroplasty 1:35, 1986.
207. Soudry M, Mestriner LA, Binazzi R, et al: Total knee arthroplasty without patellar resurfacing. Clin Orthop 205:166, 1986.
208. Spector M: Historical review of porous-coated implants. J Arthroplasty 2:163, 1987.
209. Speed JS, Trout PC: Arthroplasty of the knee: A follow-up study. J Bone Joint Surg Br 31:53, 1949.
209a. Stiehl JB, Komistek RD, Dennis DA, et al: Fluoroscopic analysis of kinematics after posterior-cruciate-retaining knee arthroplasty. J Bone Joint Surg Br 77:884, 1995.
210. Stern SH, Insall JN, Windsor RE, et al: Total knee arthroplasty in patients with psoriasis. Clin Orthop 248:108, 1989.
211. Stern SH, Bowen MK, Insall JN, et al: Cemented total knee arthroplasty for gonarthrosis in patients 55 years old or younger. Clin Orthop 260:124, 1990.
212. Stern SH, Insall JN: Total knee arthroplasty in obese patients. J Bone Joint Surg Am 72:1400, 1990.
213. Tew M, Waugh W, Forster IW: Comparing the results of different types of knee replacement: A method proposed and applied. J Bone Joint Surg Br 67:775, 1985.
214. Thatcher JC, Zhou X-M, Walker PS: Inherent laxity in total knee prostheses. J Arthroplasty 2:199, 1987.
215. Thompson FM, Hood RW, Insall JN: Patellar fractures in total knee arthroplasty. Orthop Trans 5:490, 1981.
216. Tibrewal SB, Grant KA, Goodfellow JW: The radiolucent line beneath the tibial components of the Oxford meniscal knee. J Bone Joint Surg Br 66:523, 1984.
217. Townley CO: The anatomic total knee resurfacing arthroplasty. Clin Orthop 192:82, 1985.
217a. Tsao A, Mintz L, McRae CR, et al: Failure of the porous-coated anatomic prosthesis in total knee arthroplasty due to severe polyethylene wear. J Bone Joint Surg Am 75:19, 1993.
218. Turner RH, Matza R, Hamati YI: Geometric and anametric total knee replacements. In Savastano AA, ed: Total Knee Replacement. Appleton-Century-Crofts, New York, 1980, p 171.
219. Vanhegan JAD, Dabrowski W, Arden GP: A review of 100 Attenborough stabilised gliding knee prostheses. J Bone Joint Surg Br 61:445, 1979.
220. Verneuil A: De la création d'une fausse articulation par section ou résection partielle de l'os maxillaire inférieur, comme moyen de rémedier a l'ankylose vraie ou fausse de la machoire inférieure. Arch Gen Med 15(ser. 5):174, 1860.
221. Vince KG, Insall JN, Kelly MA: The total condylar prosthesis: 10- to 12-year results of a cemented knee replacement. J Bone Joint Surg Br 71:793, 1989.
222. Vince KG, Insall JN, Bannerman CE: Total knee arthroplasty in the patient with Parkinson's disease. J Bone Joint Surg Br 71: 51, 1989.
223. Walker PS, Ranawat C, Insall JN: Fixation of the tibial components of condylar replacement knee prostheses. J Biomech 9: 269, 1976.

224. Walker PS: Human joints and their artificial replacements. Charles C Thomas, Springfield, IL, 1977.
225. Walker PS, Greene D, Reilly D, et al: Fixation of tibial components of knee prostheses. J Bone Joint Surg Am 63:258, 1981.
226. Walker PS, Hsu H-P, Zimmerman RA: A comparative study of uncemented tibial components. J Arthroplasty 5:245, 1990.
227. Walldius B: Arthroplasty of the knee joint using endoprosthesis. Acta Orthop Scand [Suppl]24:19, 1957.
228. Walldius B: Arthroplasty of the knee—twenty-seven years' experience. In Savastano AA, ed: Total Knee Replacement. Appleton-Century-Crofts, New York, 1980, p 195.
228a. Warren PJ, Olanlokun TK, Cobb AG, et al: Proprioception after total knee arthroplasty: The influence of prosthetic design. Clin Orthop 297:182, 1993.
228b. Waslewski GL, Marson BM, Benjamin JB: Early, incapacitating instability of posterior cruciate ligament-retaining total knee arthroplasty. J Arthroplasty 13:763, 1998.
229. Waugh TR, Evanski PM: University of California, Irvine (UCI) knee replacement—Design, operative technique, and results. In Savastano AA, ed: Total Knee Replacement. Appleton-Century-Crofts, New York, 1980, p 217.
230. Waugh W, Tew M: Total replacement of the knee. [Letter to the Editor]. J Bone Joint Surg Br 61:225, 1979.
231. Webster DA, Murray DG: Complications of variable axis total knee arthroplasty. Clin Orthop 193:160, 1985.
232. White SH, O'Connor JJ, Goodfellow JW: Sagittal plane laxity following knee arthroplasty. J Bone Joint Surg Br 73:268, 1991.
233. Whiteside LA, Amador DD: The effect of posterior tibial slope on knee stability after Ortholoc total knee arthroplasty. J Arthroplasty, suppl S51, 1988.
234. Whiteside LA, Amador DD: Rotational stability of a posterior stabilized total knee arthroplasty. Clin Orthop 242:241, 1989.
235. Whittle MW, Jefferson RJ: Functional biomechanical assessment of the Oxford meniscal knee. J Arthroplasty 4:231, 1989.
236. Williams EA, Hargadon EJ, Davies DRA: Late failure of the Manchester prosthesis: Its relationship to the disease process. J Bone Joint Surg Br 61:451, 1979.
236a. Williams RJ III, Westrich GH, Siegel J, et al: Arthroscopic release of the posterior cruciate ligament for stiff total knee arthroplasty. Clin Orthop 331:185, 1996.
237. Wilson FC, Fajgenbaum DM, Venters GC: Results of knee replacement with the Walldius and geometric prostheses: A comparative study. J Bone Joint Surg Am 62:497, 1980.
237a. Wilson SA, McCann PD, Gotlin RS, et al: Comprehensive gait analysis in posterior-stabilized knee arthroplasty. J Arthroplasty 11:359, 1996.
238. Wright RJ, Lima J, Scott RD, et al: Two- to four-year results of posterior cruciate-sparing condylar total knee arthroplasty with an uncemented femoral component. Clin Orthop 260:80, 1990.
239. Wright TM, Bartel DL: The problem of surface damage in polyethylene total knee components. Clin Orthop 205:67, 1986.
240. Wright TM, Astion DJ, Bansal M, et al: Failure of carbon fiber-reinforced polyethylene total knee-replacement components. J Bone Joint Surg Am 70:926, 1988.
241. Yamamoto S, Nakata S, Kondoh Y: A follow-up study of an uncemented knee replacement: The results of 312 knees using the Kodama-Yamamoto prosthesis. J Bone Joint Surg Br 71:505, 1989.
242. Young HH: Use of a hinged vitallium prosthesis (Young type) for arthroplasty of the knee. J Bone Joint Surg Am 53:1658, 1971.

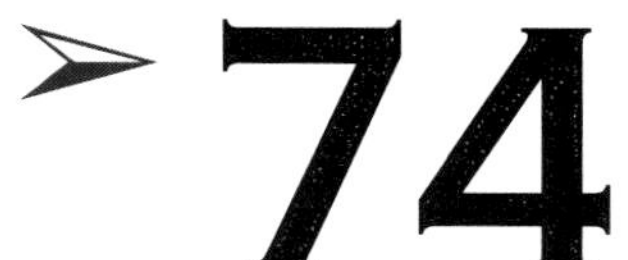

74 Surgical Techniques and Instrumentation in Total Knee Arthroplasty

JOHN N. INSALL • MARK E. EASLEY

RELEVANT KNEE ANATOMY AND ALIGNMENT

There is considerable variation in body habitus, and one must be cautious in describing what is "normal." However, the following description represents consensus.[71, 98]

Static Alignment

The mechanical axis of the leg (Fig. 74.1) is formed by a line that passes from the center of the hip through the center of the knee into the center of the ankle joint. Because of the offset caused by the femoral neck, there is a valgus angle of 7 degrees between the femoral and tibial shafts. The proximal-to-distal mechanical axis forms an angle of 3 degrees with the midline vertical axis of the body. The transverse axis of the knee joint is perpendicular to the midline vertical axis of the body and thus forms a 3-degree angle with the axis of the tibial shaft and a 10-degree angle with the axis of the femoral shaft. Hungerford and Krackow[67] and Townley[159] have pointed out that the "normal" angle of varus is variable due to anatomic factors such as pelvic width, femoral neck varus, femoral and tibial bowing, and femoral length. Because of this arrangement, the distribution of body weight when standing is more medial than lateral in each knee.[65, 70, 108, 159]

Dynamic Alignment

During normal walking, the center of gravity of the body moves toward the supporting leg during each gait cycle. However, the distribution of contact forces across the knee joint is not symmetric; it is estimated that between 60% and 75% of these forces are carried by the medial compartment of the knee.[61, 76, 108]

Johnson et al[76] noted that during normal walking, a greater medial load than would be predicted is observed because of the laterally directed ground reaction force. The forces do not rest on a perpendicular tibial plateau; the anatomic tibial plateau is sloped 2 to 10 degrees posteriorly and distally. However, when the menisci are taken into account, tibial plateaus are not posteriorly sloped; only the bony surfaces give the appearance of posterior slope. Furthermore, the medial tibial subchondral bone is concave ("dished") relative to the more convex lateral tibial subchondral surface. Combined with the 3-degree angle of the tibial anatomic axis relative to the transverse knee axis, a varus moment is imparted during normal gait. This lateral "thrust" is resisted by the lateral stabilizing force arising from the lateral collateral ligament (LCL), the cruciate ligaments, the ligamentum patellae, and the iliotibial band (ITB).[98]

OBJECTIVES OF PROSTHETIC REPLACEMENT

The above description applies to the normal condition, but it must be appreciated that many patients developing osteoarthritis of the knee have contributing anatomic variations such as habitual varus or valgus alignment. One must ask how closely prosthetic components should duplicate normal anatomy; for example, should the forces across a knee arthroplasty be borne predominantly by the medial compartment?

It is our opinion that the objective of prosthetic replacement is to distribute contact stresses across the artificial joint as symmetrically as possible, even if this implies deviation from normal anatomy in general and from individual anatomy in particular. For example, it is likely that many patients who develop medial compartment arthritis of the knee have been bowlegged since childhood; to restore prearthritic alignment, although "normal" for these people, would result in a position of more varus than is generally considered acceptable after knee arthroplasty.

There are also practical considerations. Given the factor of human error, reproducibility is important. For most of us, it is easier to make a right-angle bone cut than an oblique one, and it is easier (and thus more reproducible) to make a cut across the upper tibia at right angles to the tibial shaft rather than to make a cut that is inclined 3 degrees medially and 10 degrees posteriorly (Fig. 74.2). Additionally, if angle cuts are not appropriately adjusted from a rotational perspective, further inaccuracies result; for example, an intended 10-degree posterior slope may result in a combination of posterior and valgus slope if the cutting guide is internally rotated (Fig. 74.3).

The same considerations apply to the precise anatomy of the knee-joint surfaces. Duplication of the original intact joint surfaces is a worthy goal, but, in real-

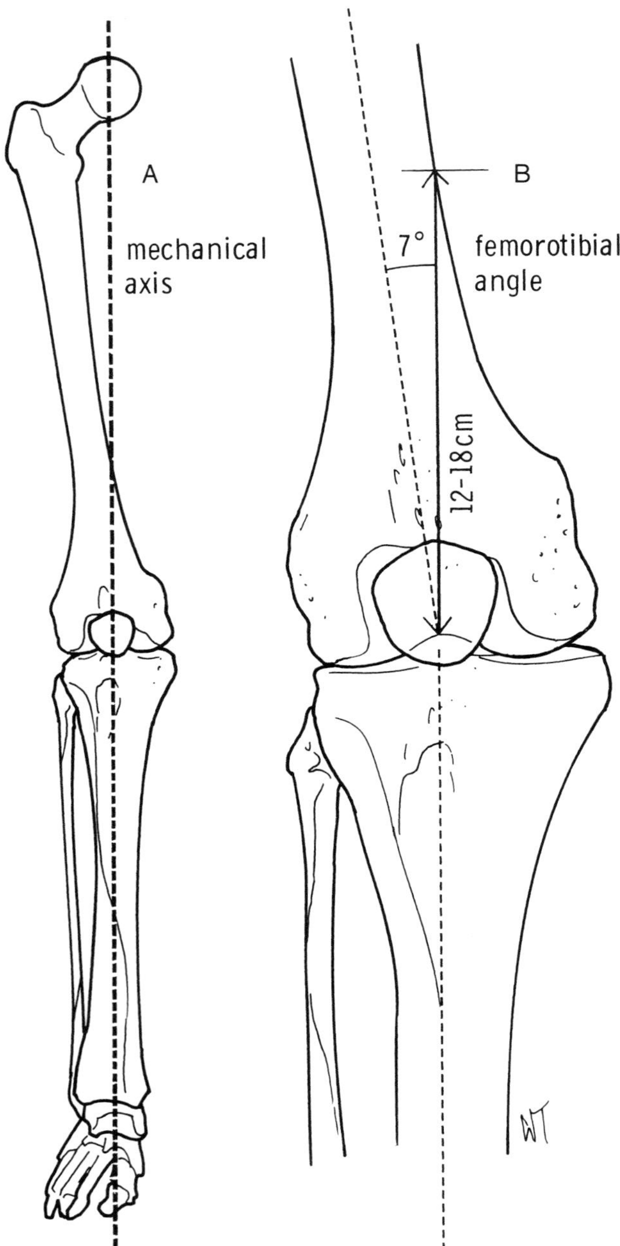

FIGURE 74.1 ➢ The mechanical axis usually corresponds to a femorotibial angle of about 7 degrees, and the mechanical axis intersects the medial femoral cortex 12 to 18 cm proximal to the knee.

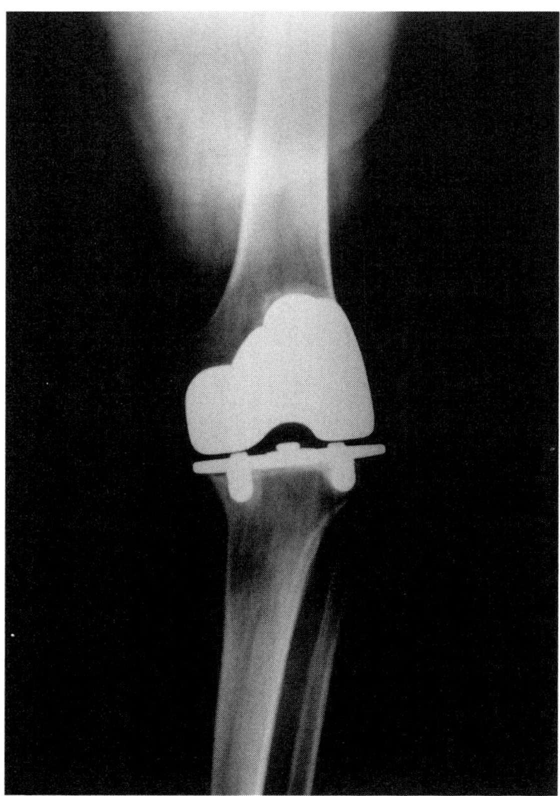

FIGURE 74.2 ➢ Radiograph of a prosthesis with a varus tibial cut. The instrument system designed for this prosthesis recommended a 3-degree tibial cut because this slope more closely duplicates normal anatomy. In practice, it often led to a greater and undesirable sloping cut to the tibia.

ity, is it possible? Human knee joints are formed in such a variety of sizes and shapes that, even given an infinite number of prosthetic components, it is unlikely that an individual joint could be exactly recreated. In pathological states, which in themselves create secondary changes in the ligaments, this difficulty is obviously compounded. Practical and economic considerations dictate that inventory should be limited to five to seven sizes.

It is nonsense to believe that restoration of normal anatomy is always or even often achieved. Does this matter? On present evidence, probably not. Early models of knee prostheses were crude, often grossly mismatched in size, incompatible with ligamentous structures, and often inexpertly inserted. Many of these devices failed, but a surprising number not only worked well but continued to do so for many years, proving the human body's remarkable resilience (Fig. 74.4). As clinical experience increased, surgical expertise improved, and prosthetic design became more sophisticated, more durable, and more "natural." Today,

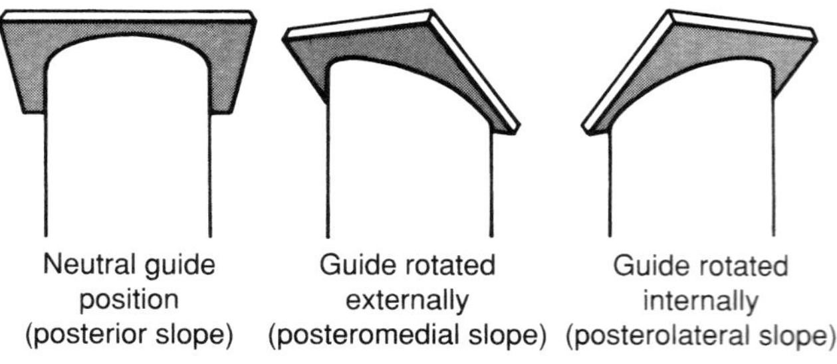

FIGURE 74.3 ➢ Care must be taken when making a 10-degree posterior slope on the tibial cut. The guide must be placed in the neutral position. When it is externally rotated, a posteromedial slope (varus) will be produced. When the guide is internally rotated, a posterolateral slope (valgus) will result.

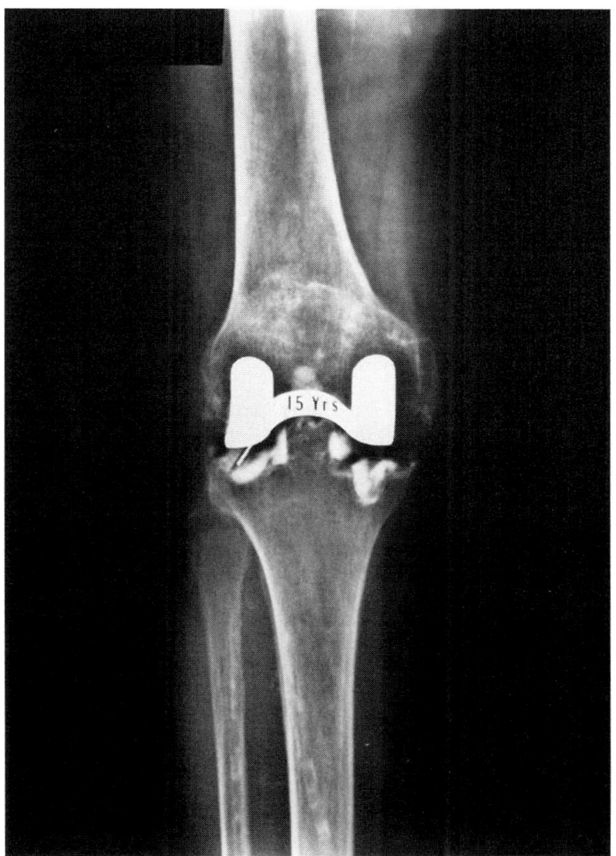

FIGURE 74.4 ➢ Radiograph of a 15-year follow-up of a duocondylar prosthesis with two separate tibial components. There is the appearance of osteopenia around the femoral component runners. The knee continued to function well.

in addition to painlessness, normality of feel and function are expected. Furthermore, some individuals require a more naturally functioning knee, such as Middle Eastern and Asian patients who need significant knee flexion during prayer; currently, we are involved in developing a more natural "high flexion" knee prosthesis to accommodate these demands. High flexion can be combined with mobile bearing designs that may provide even greater approximation of the natural knee.

Materials remain a problem: Polyethylene wear is emerging as a major clinical issue, and ideal "anatomic" joint surfaces may conflict with the bioengineering requirements needed to reduce wear. At least partial conformity between the components is considered necessary to reduce high polyethylene stresses and to provide acceptable durability. In addition, modularity has introduced the potential for wear secondary to micromotion between the polyethylene insert and the tibial tray.[51, 116, 162]

In life, the mobile menisci allow conformity of the joint in different positions, and, apart from meniscal-bearing prostheses (which have their own potential problems), all current designs are compromises between conformity and mobility.

THEORIES OF SURGICAL TECHNIQUE

In part because of differing concepts in prosthetic design, there are currently two distinct and sometimes conflicting schools of surgical technique.[34] The first, which developed in conjunction with the design of cruciate substituting prostheses, is based on the "gap" technique. The second, developed by surgeons and designers who favor cruciate retention, emphasizes measured femoral and tibial resection as the primary consideration.

Gap Technique

The gap technique[50, 69, 71] is used in conjunction with cruciate substituting prostheses and some cruciate retaining devices (often accompanied by posterior cruciate release from the posterior tibia). Ligament releases (see below) are performed to correct fixed deformity, bringing the limb into approximate alignment before the bone cuts are made (Fig. 74.5).

The gap technique was developed at a time when a limited number of anteroposterior femoral sizes were available, frequently dictating that a relatively small femoral component be fitted onto a larger distal femur. This typically necessitated over-resection of the posterior femoral condyles. To appropriately balance the flexion gap, less proximal tibia was resected. In fact, the largest available tibial polyethylene insert was approximately 15 mm. Leaving a substantial amount of proximal tibial bone was in accordance with the belief that the proximal tibial bone weakened significantly with resection greater than 5 mm. The gap technique is still used, but because most systems have a full complement of component sizes, posterior femoral over-resection is less likely, and the flexion gap may be balanced even with proximal tibial resection greater than 10 mm.

A particular sequence of steps in balancing the flexion gap is not essential; the femur or tibia may be osteotomized first; the goal is to create a balanced flexion gap (Fig. 74.6). Although we traditionally perform the tibial cut first, we often begin with contouring the femur when referencing instruments can be adequately placed on the posterior femoral condyles.

The proximal tibial osteotomy is performed 10 mm below the least compromised articular cartilage (Fig. 74.7). A perpendicular tibial cut will establish proper limb alignment with reference to a properly performed distal femoral cut. Harada et al[60] suggested that the proximal tibia weakens below a depth of 5 mm, prompting many surgeons to resect as little bone as possible. Because this requires use of thinner polyethylene inserts, the potential risk of stress-related wear is introduced.[173] However, we have little reservation resecting an average of 10 mm of proximal tibia. As early as 1983, Goldstein et al[54] demonstrated that significantly weaker tibial bone is observed only beyond a depth of 20 mm. When the gap theory is applied to cruciate retaining designs, the posterior cruciate ligament (PCL) may be retained if it is appropriately recessed, permitting the proper joint line position to be reestablished with modular tibial inserts.

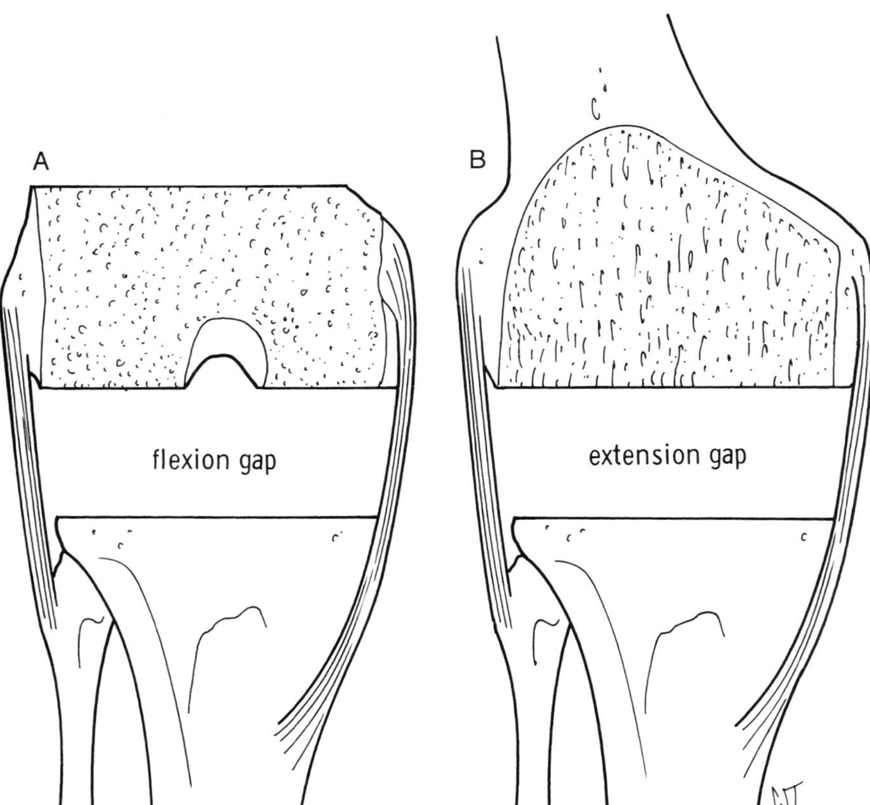

FIGURE 74.5 ➢ The extension gap must exactly equal the flexion gap.

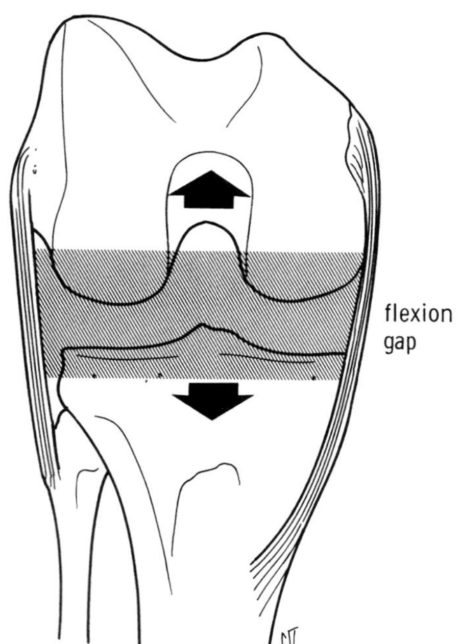

FIGURE 74.6 ➢ The flexion gap is created first, removing bone from the tibial plateaus and posterior femoral condyles.

Rotational Alignment of the Femur

The rotational alignment of the femoral component is decided by the anatomy of the distal femur but is influenced to some degree by the condition of the medial soft tissues. When a medial release is not required for axial alignment, some external rotation of the femoral template is needed to compensate for the normal medial inclination of the tibial plateau and the flexion laxity of the lateral ligamentous structures (Fig. 74.8). Only by this external rotation can a rectangular "flexion gap" be produced (Figs. 74.9 and 74.10). However, when a medial soft-tissue release is done, a rectangular flexion gap is created by the ligament release itself, and the femoral template can be positioned anatomically with regard to the distal femoral anatomy.

Proper femoral rotation is essential because inappropriate femoral component rotation may result in flexion imbalance and patellofemoral problems.[6, 10, 122] Although an arbitrary predetermined external rotation of 3 degrees is often satisfactory,[47, 123] several methods have been developed in an effort to accurately determine appropriate femoral rotation (Fig. 74.11):

1. Medial and lateral epicondyles.[11, 118]
2. Posterior femoral condyles.[58]
3. Anteroposterior femoral axis ("Whiteside's line").[7, 168]

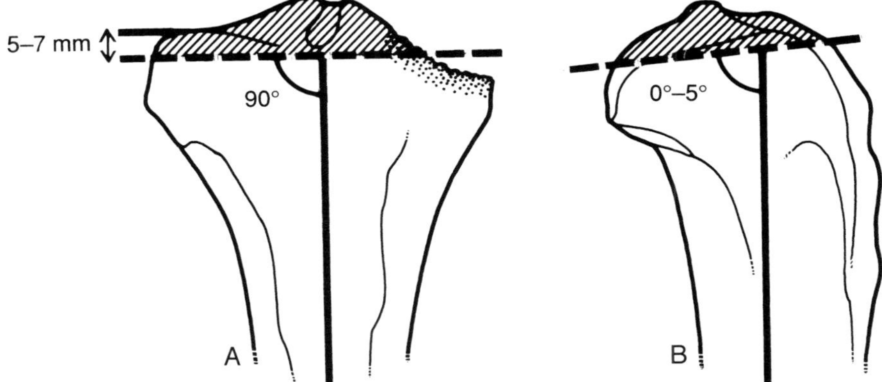

FIGURE 74.7 ➢ The correct cut on the tibia ignores defects and removes 10 mm from the normal side, cut at right angles to the long axis in the coronal plane *(A)* and sloped posteriorly no more than 5 degrees in the sagittal plane *(B)*.

4. Tibial shaft axis.[151]
5. Ligament tension.

Femoral rotation is difficult to instrument precisely because of landmark inconsistencies and obscurities; the surgeon must form her or his own judgment, making sure to err on the side of external rotation, *never* internal rotation.[6, 10, 122]

The posterior condylar axis is frequently used as the reference for femoral rotation; however, posterior condylar erosion as part of the arthritic process often distorts this reference angle, and so it should probably not be relied on as the sole method of determining femoral rotation.[58, 151] The anteroposterior axis of the femoral sulcus, described by Whiteside,[7, 168] has also been shown to be an accurate reference point for determining femoral rotation; however, it has been shown to be less reliable in cases of trochlear dysplasia and some valgus knees.[118] The tibial shaft axis has also been described as an effective reference axis for defining femoral rotation.[151] Using the anatomic axis of the tibia is particularly useful because it should facilitate balancing the flexion space when perpendicular proximal tibial cuts are used for total knee arthroplasty (TKA).

We use the epicondylar axis to most closely recreate the patient's natural femoral rotation.[11, 118] Identifying the epicondylar axis requires some additional soft-tissue dissection to define the anatomic postitions of the medial and lateral epicondyles. The center of the me-

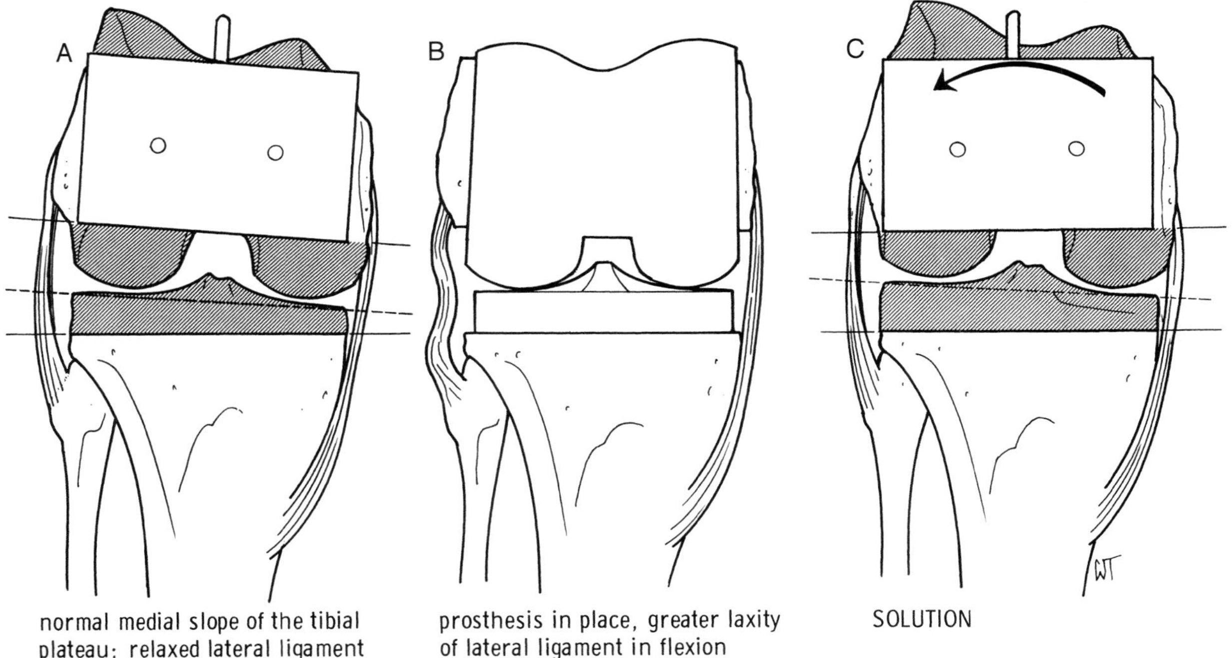

FIGURE 74.8 ➢ Imitating the normal anatomy results in lateral laxity in flexion.

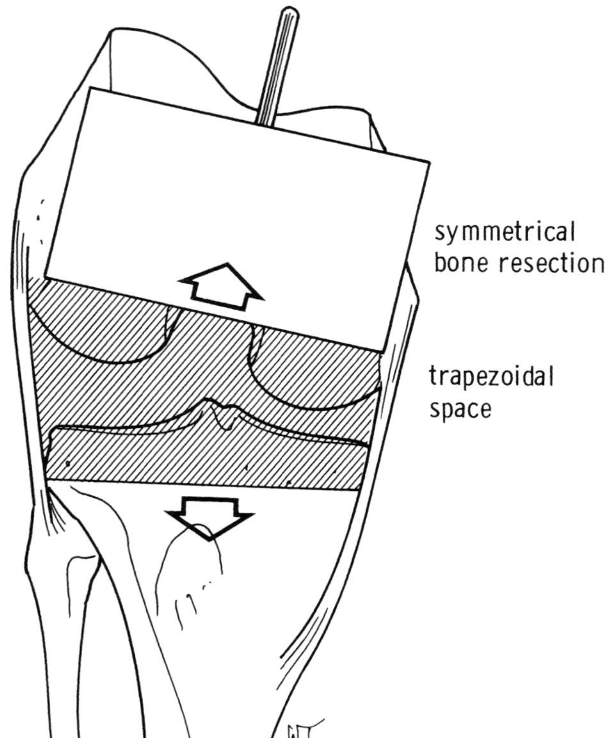

FIGURE 74.9 ➢ In the osteoarthritic knee, lateral laxity is accentuated; when symmetric bone is excised from the posterior femoral condyles, the resulting space on distraction is trapezoidal.

dial epicondyle is located in the sulcus, which lies between the proximal origin of the superficial deep medial collateral ligament (MCL) and the distal origin of the deep MCL. The medial epicondylar ridge at the origin of the superficial MCL can be identified by isolating the condylar vessels that lie proximal and anterior to the medial epicondylar ridge. From these vessels the epicondylar ridge can readily be outlined; the center of this outline is the sulcus, which can typically be palpated (Fig. 74.12). The lateral epicondyle is the most prominent point on the lateral aspect of the distal femur. Here, too, following the leash of condylar vessels confirms the exact location of the lateral epicondyle that lies immediately distal to the vessels (Fig. 74.13).

The benefit of having several different methods of assessing femoral rotation is that one or more can be used to confirm the surgeon's preferred method (Fig. 74.14). Several investigators have compared these various methods. Poilvache et al[118] correlated the transepicondylar, anteroposterior, and posterior condylar axes. Berger et al[11] and Griffin et al[57] described the relationship of the epicondylar axis to the posterior condylar axis. Whiteside[7, 168] defined the relationship of the anteroposterior and posterior condylar axes. Finally, Stiehl et al[151] demonstrated that referencing from the tibial shaft axis is more accurate than referencing from the posterior condylar axis.

Reference Point: Anterior Cortex or Posterior Femoral Condyles?

CLASSIC GAP TECHNIQUE

Given that there will seldom be an exact match between the sagittal dimension of the femoral component and the actual size of the bone, some compromise may be necessary. With anterior referencing, adjustments are made in the amount of the posterior femoral condyles that is removed, and thus the flexion gap is somewhat variable. Conversely, with posterior referencing (Fig. 74.15), the flexion gap is constant, but there is danger of "notching" the anterior femoral cortex or of having the femoral flange sit proud of the bone. Anterior referencing implies a willingness to make small adjustment cuts from the distal femur in extension. However, the virtue of a constant flexion gap cannot be denied, particularly when the PCL is preserved.

Unless sizing exactly matches component availability, adjustments made purely with posterior condylar

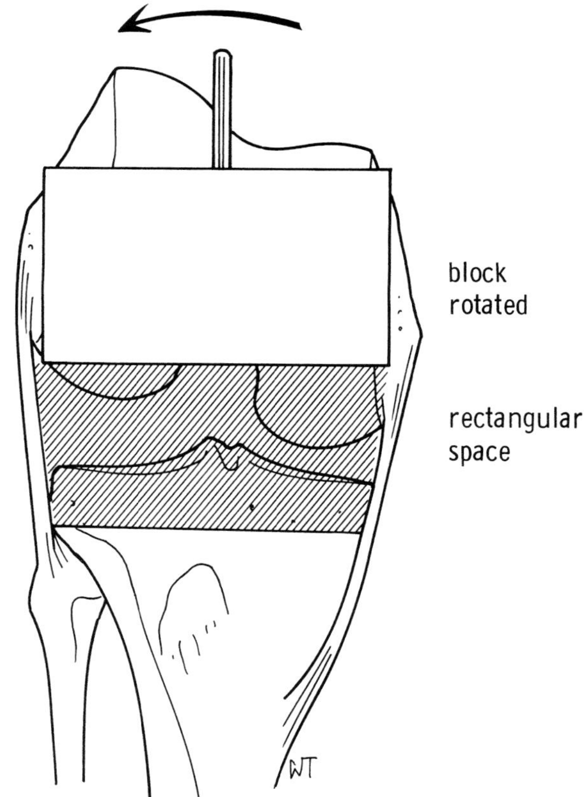

FIGURE 74.10 ➢ By externally rotating the femoral component and removing an asymmetric amount of bone from the posterior femoral condyles, soft-tissue length is equalized and the resulting space is rectangular.

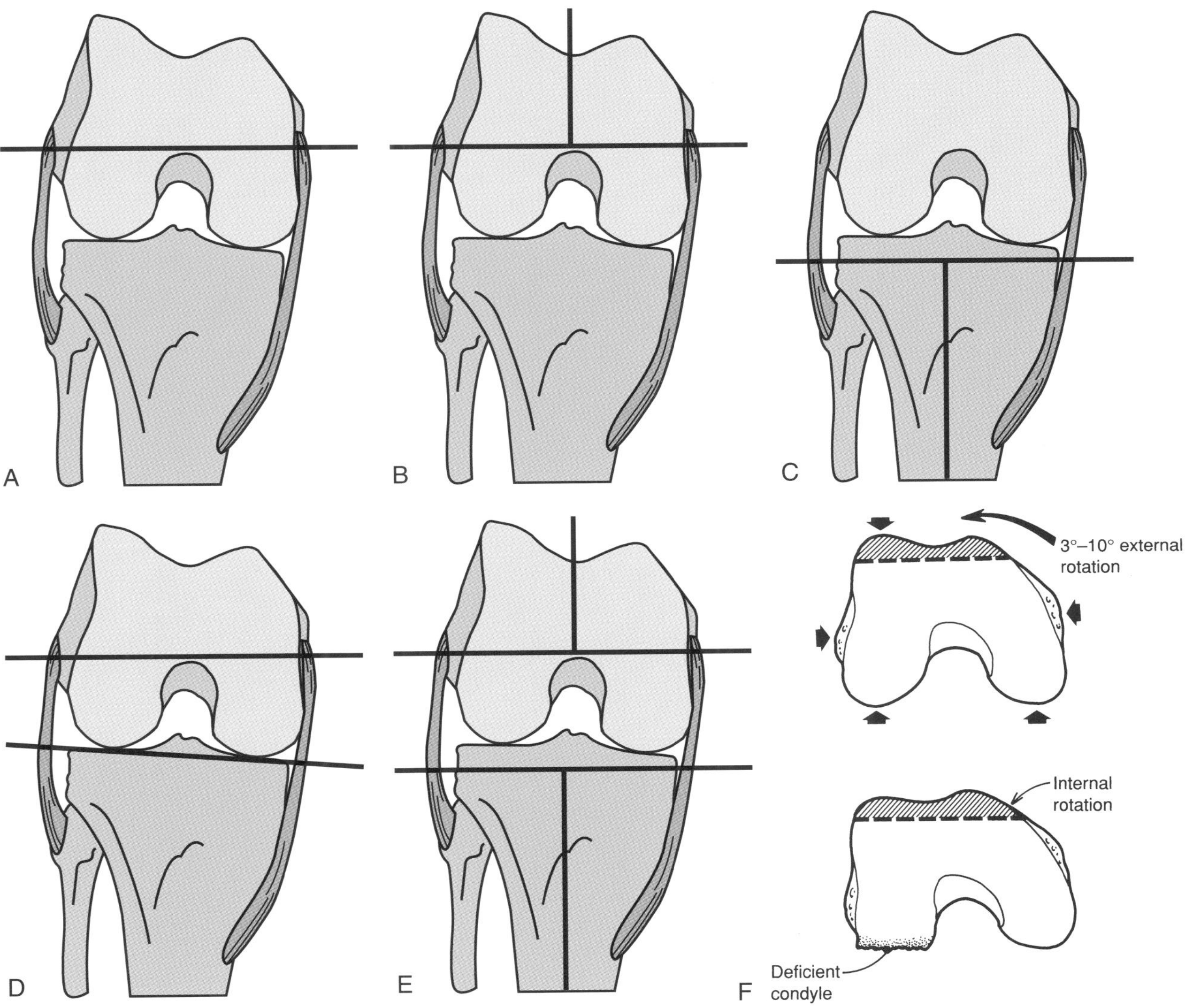

FIGURE 74.11 ➢ Reference points for rotational positioning of the femoral component are the epicondyles, the trochlear surface, the tibial shaft, and the posterior condyles. *A,* The transepicondylar axis. *B,* The anteroposterior trochlear sulcus ("Whiteside's line"). *C,* The tibial shaft axis. *D,* The posterior condylar angle. *E,* The transepicondylar axis is perpendicular to the anteroposterior sulcus line and the tibial shaft axis. *F,* When the posterior condyles are used for rotational reference, one must beware of erosion of the condyles. For example, in valgus knees, posterior erosion of the lateral femoral condyle is often present, which may result in internal rotation of the femoral component.

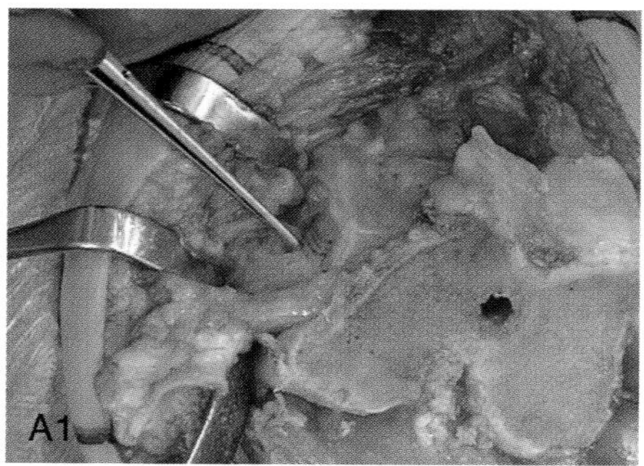

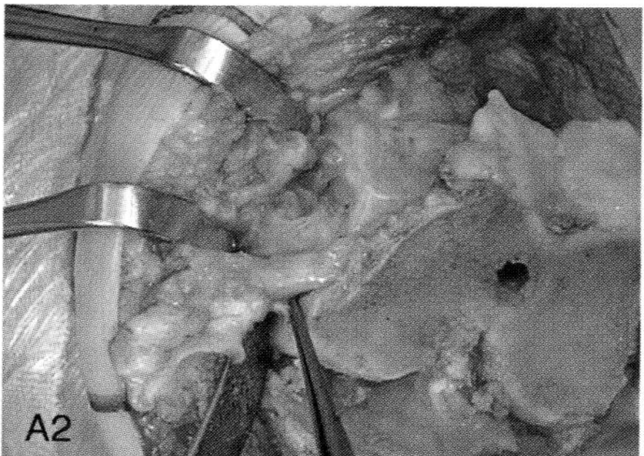

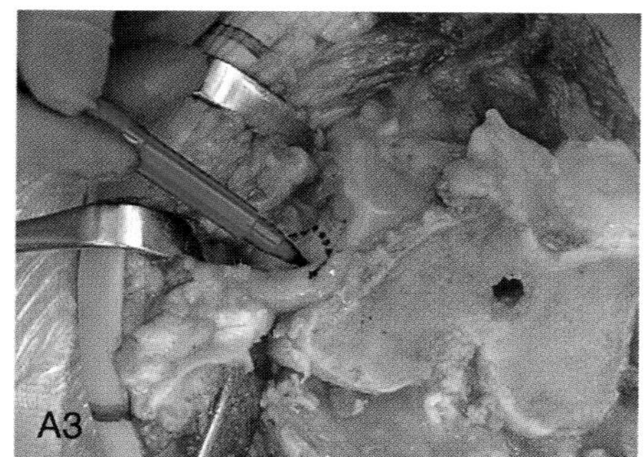

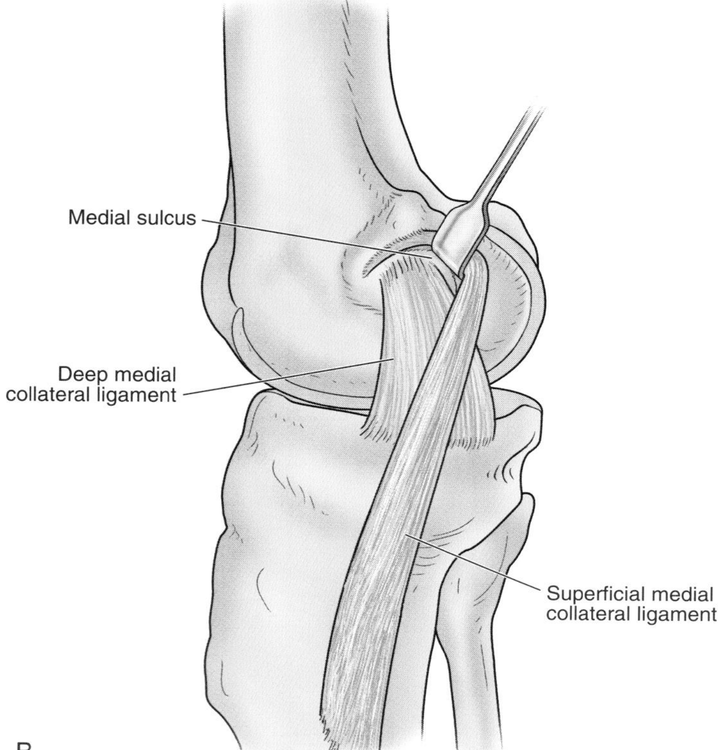

FIGURE 74.12 ➢ *A,* Intraoperative photos of the medial epicondyle. *A1,* leash of vessels over the insertion of the superficial medial collateral ligament (MCL). *A2,* Instrument placed to define the insertion of the deep MCL. *A3,* Between the two MCL insertions, at the medial sulcus, the medial epicondyle is marked in a "bull's eye" fashion. *B,* Deep to the superficial MCL, the deep MCL overlies the medial sulcus, the palpable focus of the medial epicondyle.

resection risk tightness in flexion when too little bone is removed and flexion instability when too much posterior bone is resected. To compensate for in-between sizing, we downsize components and favor instrument systems that allow for slight flexion of the femoral component (typically 3 degrees), to lessen the risk of anterior notching (Fig 74.16).

The gap between the cut surfaces of the posterior femoral condyles and proximal tibia is measured. We use spacer blocks to determine the gap size (Fig. 74.17), but some knee specialists still use tensor devices in primary and revision TKA (Figs. 74.18 and 74.19). Using tensors, the proximal tibial cut is made first to properly tension the flexion space (Fig. 74.20). The size of this space corresponds to the combined thickness of tibial and femoral components and determines the thickness of the tibial component required to stabilize the knee in flexion.

If the flexion gap is asymmetric, then further ligament release procedures, described later, may be necessary to establish flexion space balance. Alternatively, flexion space incongruity may be the result of improper femoral rotation. Although some accuracy of the cut surfaces is forfeited, small adjustment cuts of the distal femur to allow for a change in rotation may be necessary to balance the flexion gap.

EXTENSION GAP

As with the flexion gap, sizing of the extension gap is performed using either spacers or a tensioning device. The distal femoral osteotomy is performed early in the procedure at a predetermined level corresponding to the thickness of the femoral component (Fig. 74.21). The extension space so formed is then assessed with a spacer, and the distal femur is recut when necessary to match the flexion gap. The amount of additional resection is decided by using a series of

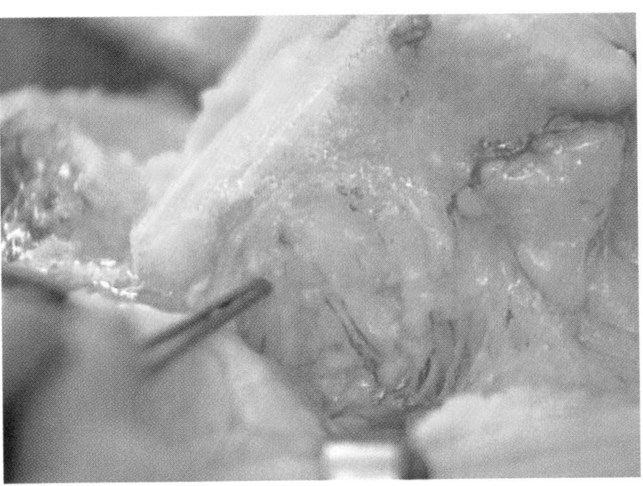

FIGURE 74.13 ➢ Intraoperative photo of the lateral epicondyle, the most prominent point on the distal lateral femur.

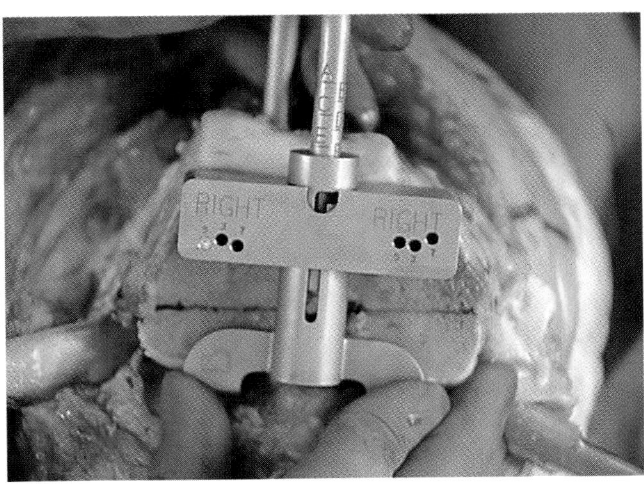

FIGURE 74.15 ➢ An instrument used for sagittal sizing of the femur.

thinner spacers (and, when necessary, the so-called minus spacers) (see Fig. 74.18). In this way, the amount of additional resection can be calculated from the difference between the flexion spacer and the thinner spacer that is used to assess the preformed extension gap. (For example, if an 8-mm spacer is needed in flexion and a minus 3 spacer is needed to stabilize the bone in extension, the additional resection will be 3 mm.) Rarely do we recut the distal femur after the initial osteotomy at the predetermined level; the flexion and extension gaps can usually be balanced with appropriate soft-tissue balancing and posterior release when a preoperative flexion contracture is present.

Alternatively, the knee is extended and axial traction is applied on the limb by using a mechanical device inserted in the knee, such as a tensor (see Figs. 74.18 to 74.20). The level of distal femoral osteotomy is determined by the selected thickness of spacers used for the flexion gap. A distal femoral osteotomy is performed at this level perpendicular to the mechanical axis (Figs. 74.22, 74.23, and 74.24) (approximately 7 degrees of valgus measured from the femoral axis).

The essential point of the gap technique is that it builds on the state of the soft tissues. This technique can be readily applied to standard primary TKA, primary TKA with severe deformity, and revision TKA. In contrast to the measured resection method described later, the amount of bone osteotomized from the femur may or may not be greater than the thickness of the femoral component.

Disadvantages of the gap technique include the following:

1. The joint line (referenced from the femur) may be moved proximally. This is most likely to happen when there is a preoperative flexion contracture or when the chosen femoral component is smaller than the anteroposterior dimension of the femur. Joint line alteration can be minimized by correct femoral measurement, a full range of femoral component sizes, and posterior capsulotomy to correct flexion contractures.
2. The method ensures soft-tissue balance and correct tensioning in full extension and at 90 degrees of flexion, but midrange laxity may occur at other positions. The clinical significance of

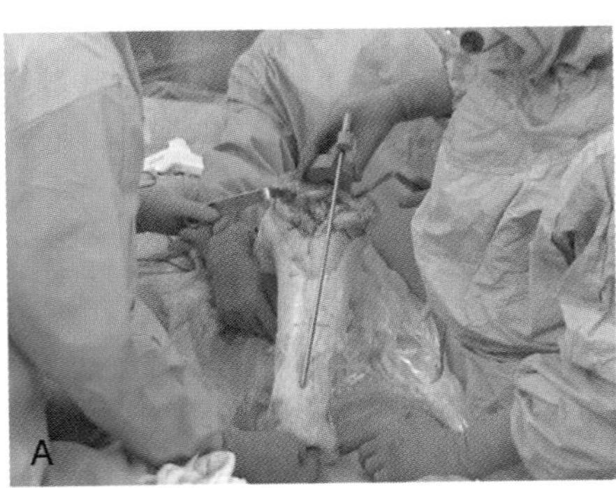

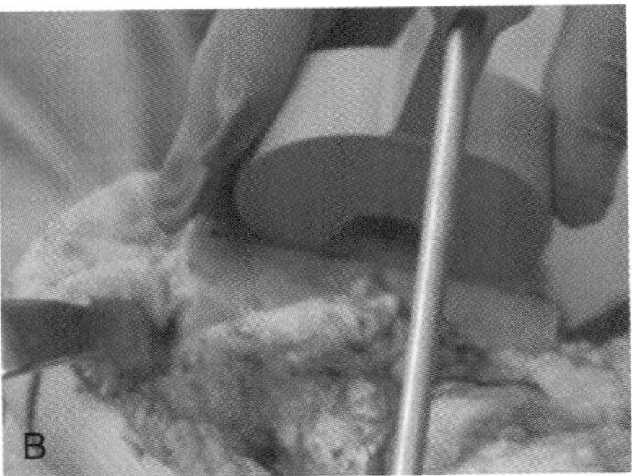

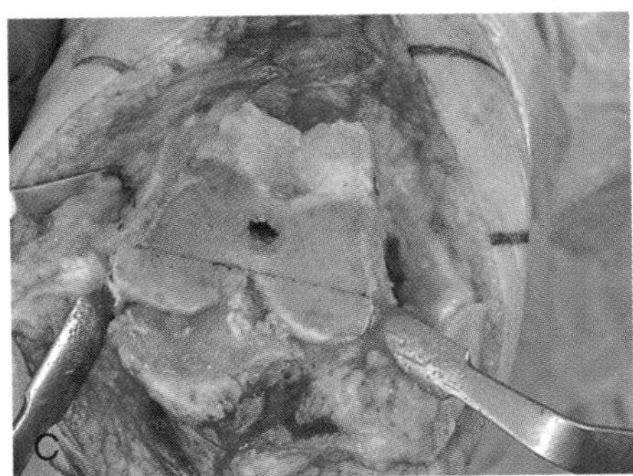

FIGURE 74.14 ➢ Confirming proper femoral rotation. *A*, Tibial shaft axis. *B*, Comparing transepicondylar and tibial shaft axes. *C*, Transepicondylar axis.

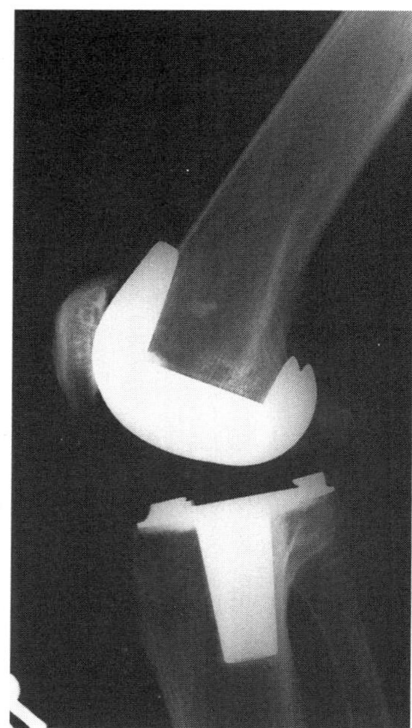

FIGURE 74.16 ➢ Lateral radiograph demonstrating the femoral component cemented in 3 degrees of flexion to avoid anterior notching of the femur.

this (if any) is not known, although it is certain that long-term clinical results have not been affected.

Classic Measured Resection Technique

The second theory of surgical technique, the measured resection theory, argues strongly for cruciate retention — especially the PCL.[100] Hungerford developed the method of measured resection, and in its original form it was used in conjunction with principles of anatomic alignment (see next section).[67]

Posterior Cruciate Ligament

A proportion of arthritic knees are without significant ligament abnormalities, and it is argued that preservation of the PCL offers many advantages because this ligament

1. is an important stabilizer of the knee,
2. is a strong structure that can absorb stresses that might otherwise be transmitted to the prosthesis-bone interface,
3. controls the rollback of the femur on the tibia that occurs with flexion of the knee and can maximize flexion,

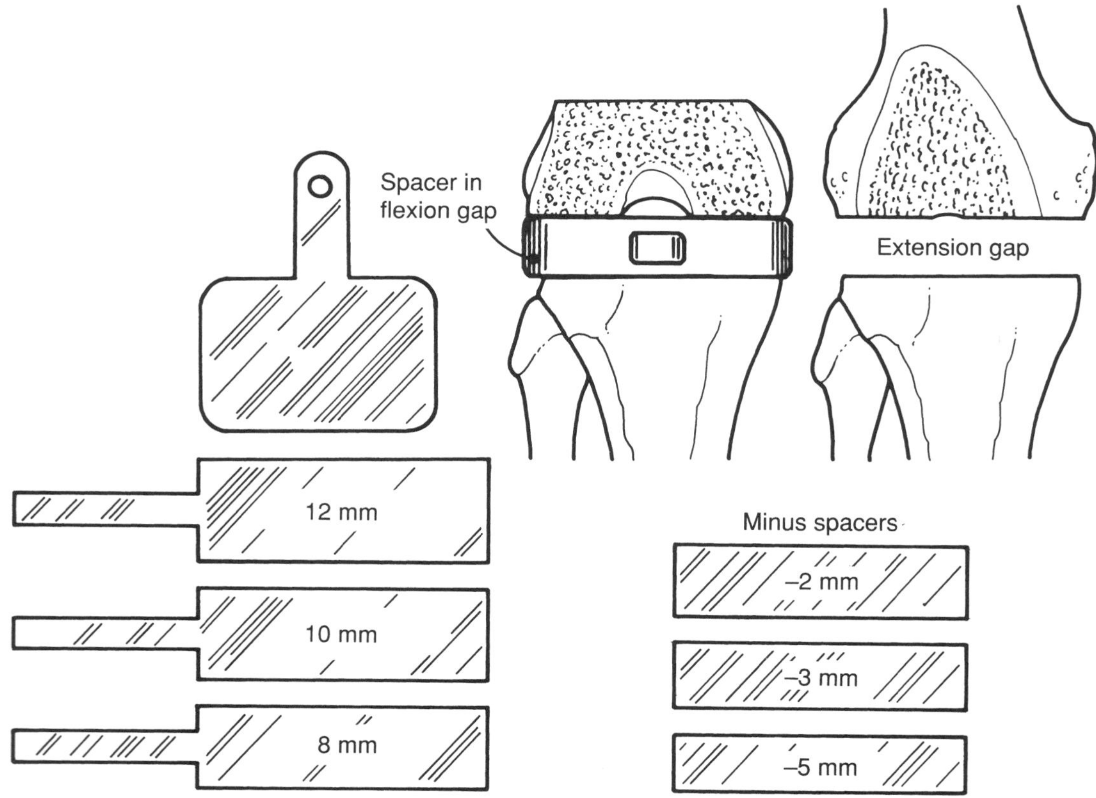

FIGURE 74.17 ➢ The flexion and extension gaps are assessed by a series of spacers. When the extension gap is smaller than the flexion gap, it must be equalized by the resection of extra distal femoral bone. The amount needed is assessed using the spacer system. Minus spacers are available when the flexion gap requires the thinnest (8 mm) spacer.

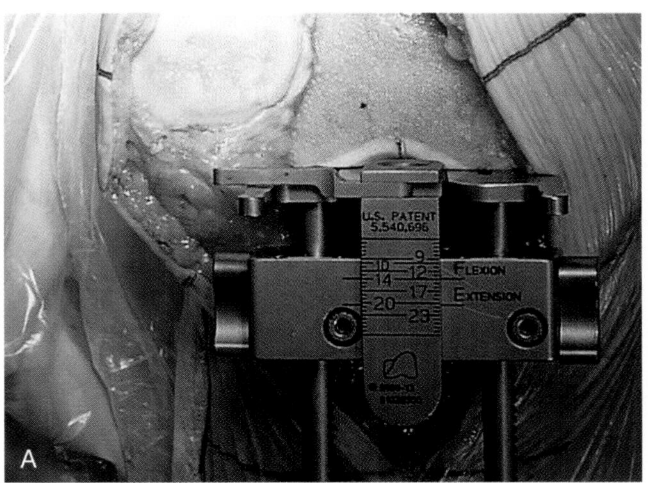

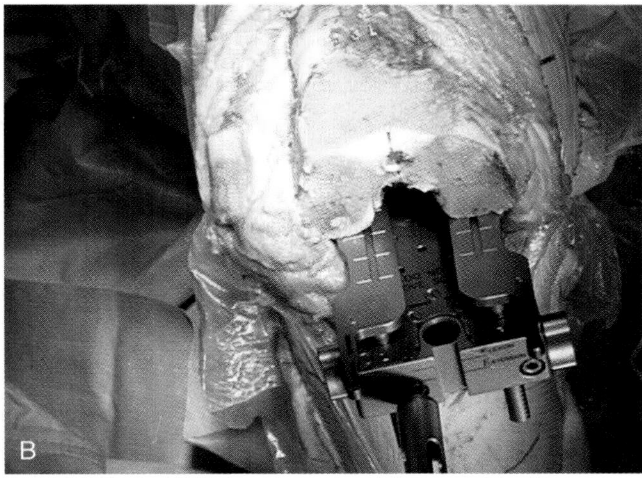

FIGURE 74.18 ➢ Close-up intraoperative view of a tensor. *A,* In extension. *B,* In flexion.

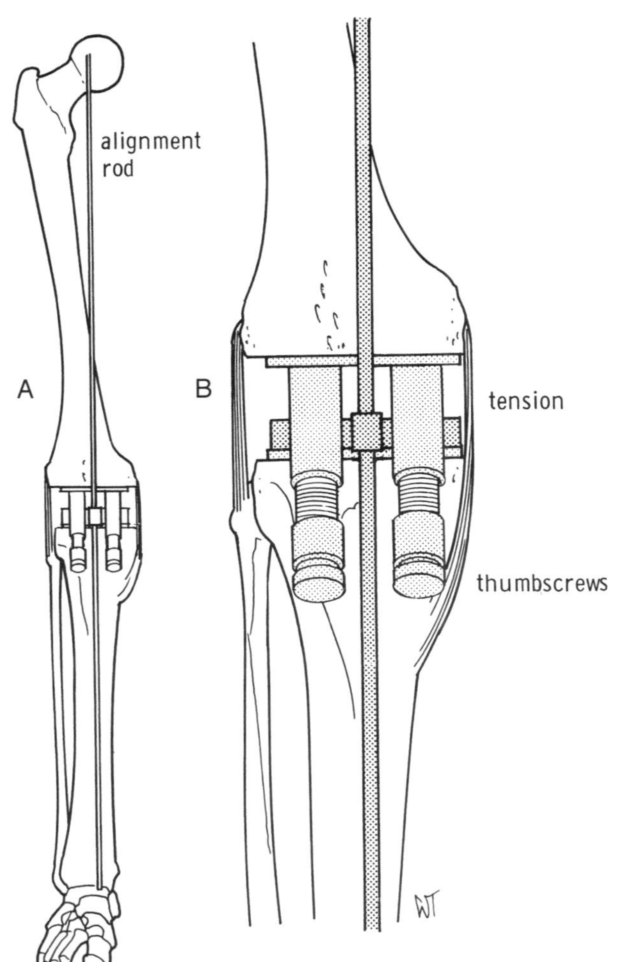

FIGURE 74.19 ➢ By adjusting the medial and lateral thumbscrews of the tensor, the alignment rod is brought into the mechanical axis.

4. may be important for stair-climbing activities, and
5. may have a proprioceptive function.

However, to possess these attributes, the PCL must be accurately tensioned during knee replacement, because if it is too tight it will impede flexion, and, conversely, if it is too loose the PCL loses its functional significance (Fig. 74.25).

For the PCL to fulfill its anatomic purposes, the joint surfaces must be kept at or very close to their original anatomic position, and this implies the following:

1. The joint line or axis must be restored to its prearthritic condition.
2. The shape and size of the femoral condyles must likewise be restored.
3. The tibial plateau surface must be at the correct level, sloped approximately 10 degrees posteriorly and approximately 3 degrees medially.
4. The tibial surface must be flat or nearly so, offering no impedance to rotation and gliding movements.

In practice, techniques that are aimed at preserving the PCL meet these requirements to varying degrees. A few systems mimic the medial slope of the normal tibia, and some cut the tibia at right angles to its shaft. However, all share the objective of closely preserving or restoring the anatomic joint line with reference to the femur. If this is achieved and the PCL is retained, the arc of motion should also be close to normal with correct ligament tensioning throughout the range of motion, bringing the attendant benefits of better "feel" and useful function.

The position of the femorotibial joint axis also has a bearing on the function of the patellar mechanism. Patellofemoral dysfunction remains the cause of most unsatisfactory knee arthroplasties, and it is in stair-climbing and flexed-knee activities that the prosthetic joint deviates the most from normal. Maintenance of

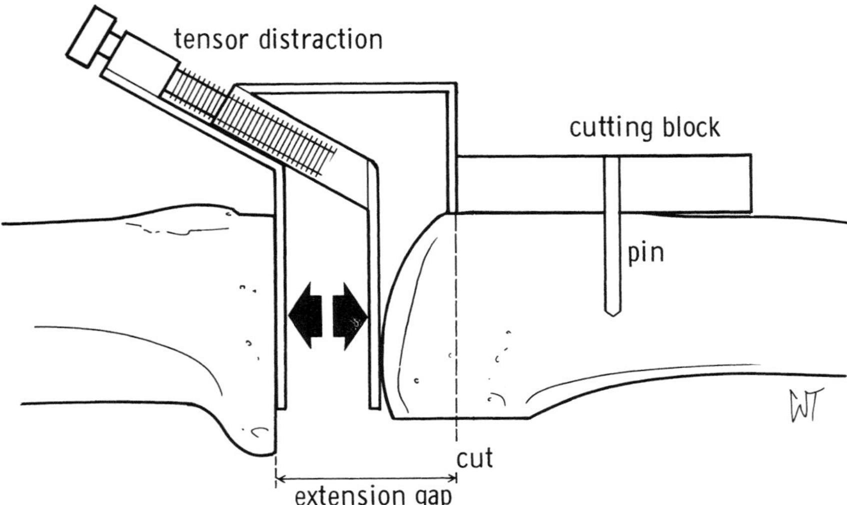

FIGURE 74.20 ➢ The distal femoral cutting guide is controlled by the tensor and positioned to create an extension gap of the correct dimensions.

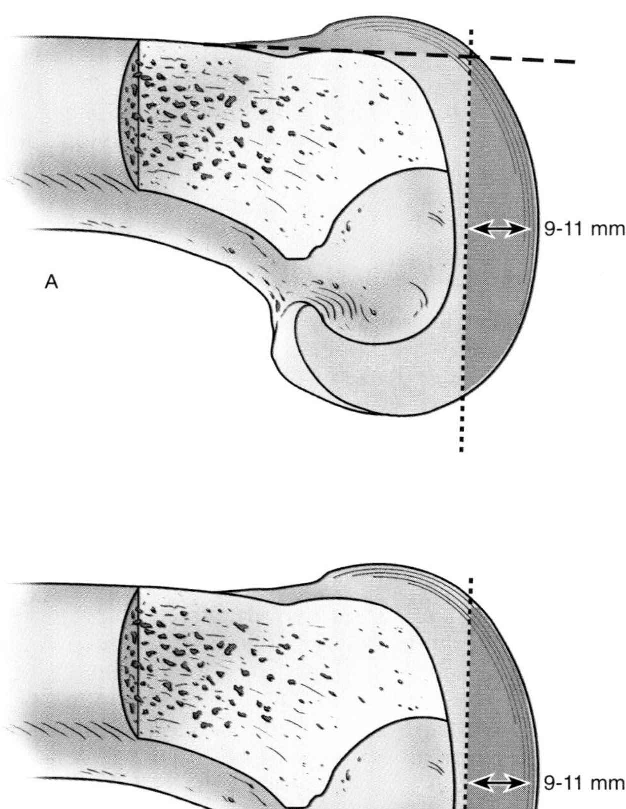

FIGURE 74.21 ➢ The thickness of the prosthesis, normally somewhere between 9 and 11 mm, is removed from the distal femur.

the anatomic joint line avoids patella infera (Fig. 74.26); Figgie et al[47] demonstrated that if the patella is not within a defined sagittal "neutral zone" (10 to 30 mm above the joint line), a greater number of patellar problems is observed (Fig. 74.27).

PCL retention in TKA has limitations. Although some investigators have demonstrated that the PCL is typically intact in most arthritic knees,[141, 143] others demonstrated that the PCL degenerates and contracts as part of the arthritic process,[4, 82] often rendering the ligament nonfunctional. Even proponents of PCL retention acknowledge that it is not applicable to all arthritic knee deformities.[87, 143] Corces and Lotke[26] demonstrated that, even for a skilled surgeon, it may be difficult to achieve the aims of successful PCL retention. In their small series of knees evaluated intraoperatively, the PCL was often too tight or too loose following prosthetic implantation. A PCL that is too tight limits flexion and may cause increased posterior stresses, risking posterior polyethylene compromise and anterior femoral component displacement. A tight PCL may also result in "booking" as the femur subluxes posteriorly, causing the knee to "open like a book" (Fig. 74.28). Recognition of this phenomenon is possible by observing anterior tibial component "lift-off" with trial components that are free to move with applied stresses (Fig. 74.29). To avoid excessive tightness in flexion, ligament balancing techniques have been developed that permit PCL retention when the ligament is contracted but remains competent.[128, 137, 142] The technique is similar to the medial release performed for balancing varus deformity; a graduated PCL release (Fig. 74.30A) is performed from the posterior aspect of the tibia using a periosteal elevator until the PCL tension is deemed appropriate (Fig. 74.30B). The PCL may also become too loose and lose its functional significance. Provided this problem is observed intra-

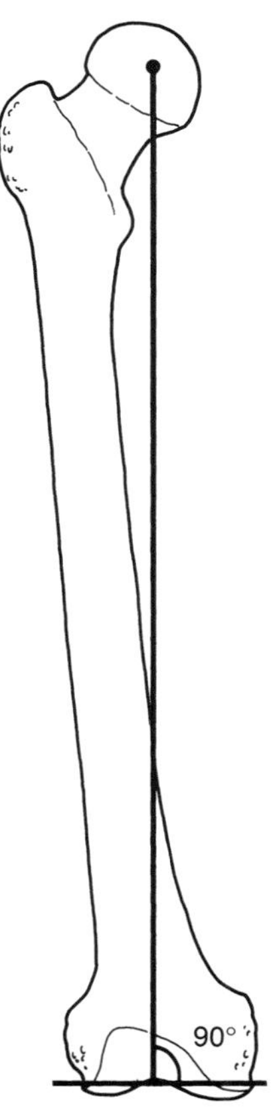

FIGURE 74.22 ➢ The distal femoral cut should be templated by measuring from the center of the femoral head to the center of the knee on a full-length radiograph of the femur. A second line passing into the intramedullary canal of the femur will indicate the angulation of the distal femoral cut.

operatively, a transition to a PCL substituting design can be made; however, after a partial PCL release, the PCL occasionally becomes incompetent postoperatively, rendering the prosthesis unstable.[114, 163]

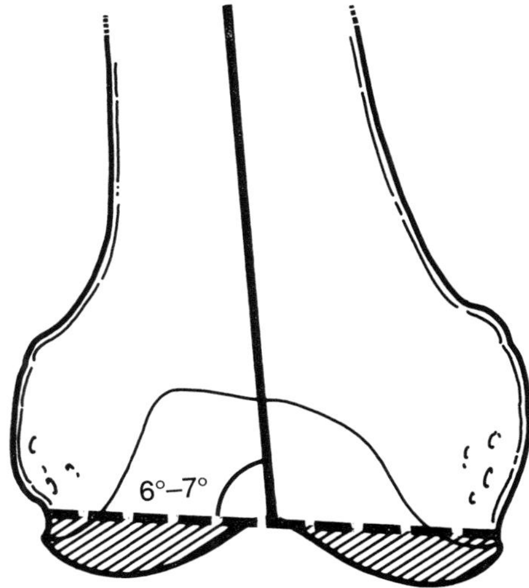

FIGURE 74.23 ➢ The distal femoral cut is normally aligned 6 to 7 degrees of valgus from the intramedullary alignment rod.

Anterior Cruciate Ligament

The anterior cruciate ligament (ACL) is an important functional element in the normal knee, and its absence causes not only instability but an abnormal pattern of motion, including rotational and sliding movements (e.g., pivot shift). Together with the PCL, the ACL forms a "four-bar linkage" at the center of the knee, and the absence of either component destroys this mechanism. Only a few knee prostheses are designed to preserve both cruciate ligaments, and the use of one, the meniscal-bearing Oxford knee, is not recommended unless both ligaments are present.[56]

In many arthritic knees, the ACL is damaged or absent, and most cruciate preserving systems advocate removal of the ACL when it is there. Thus "cruciate retention" refers only to the PCL and is not a truly accurate term. It is probable that knee prostheses preserving only the PCL will not move normally even

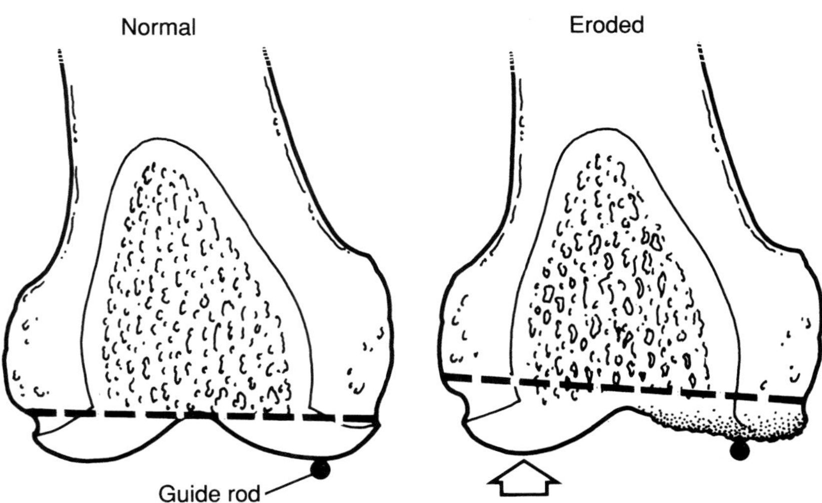

FIGURE 74.24 ➢ Ideally, the amount of distal femoral resection should be judged from the normal side. When measurement is made from the medial femoral condyle, regardless of the pathology, extra distal femoral resection will occur.

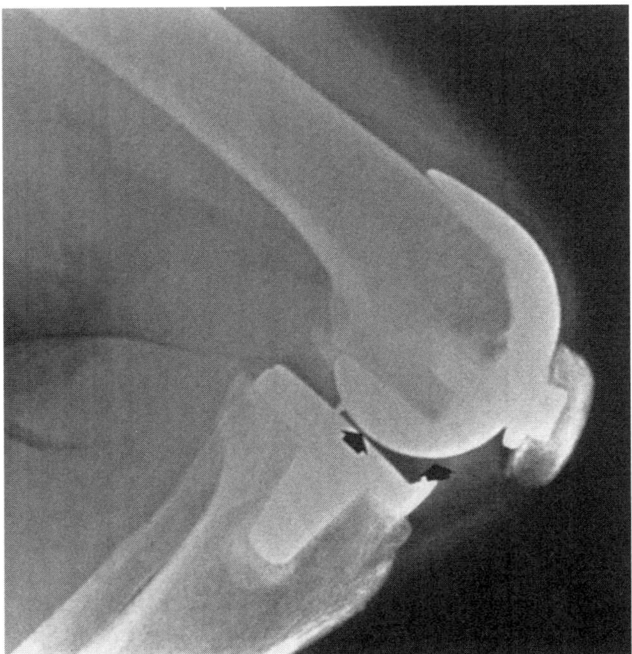

FIGURE 74.25 ➢ Sagittal radiograph of a "nonfunctional" posterior cruciate ligament. There has been "roll-forward" rather than "rollback" with knee flexion. The anterior margin of the femoral component abuts the anterior margin of the tibial component as it does in a total condylar-type design.

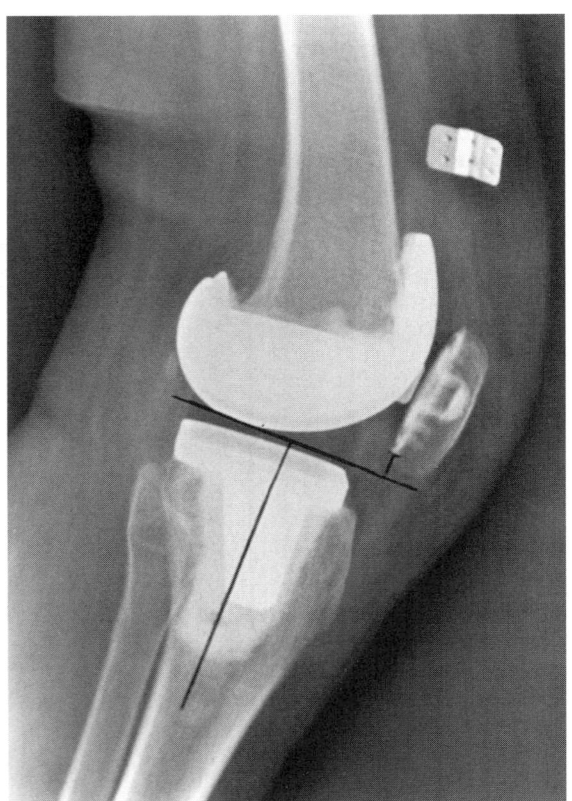

FIGURE 74.26 ➢ Lateral radiograph of a posterior stabilized prosthesis showing a patella infera. The distal pole of the patella lies just proximal to a projection of the joint line. Patella infera may be associated with an increased frequency of patellar symptoms.

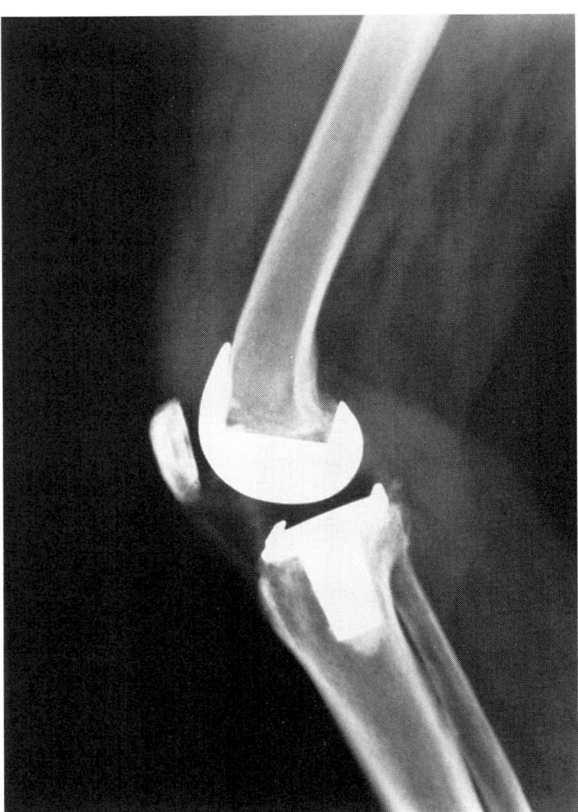

FIGURE 74.27 ➢ Lateral radiograph showing a satisfactory patellar position postoperatively. The patella lies in its normal position in relation to the joint line. The patellar prosthesis composite is of the correct thickness. Note the sclerosis that has developed in the remaining patellar bone. This is a common finding that develops several years postoperatively and is an example of Wolff's law.

when the geometry and surgery are precise. Abnormal sliding movements, in particular, can be expected.[29, 30, 80, 152]

INFLUENCE OF SURGICAL PHILOSOPHY ON SURGICAL TECHNIQUE AND INSTRUMENTATION

From the previous discussion, it is apparent that a philosophical gulf exists between the gap school of thought and the measured resection school of thought. The classic gap method emphasizes preservation of tibial bone and conforming joint surfaces and accepts, when it occurs, proximal migration of the joint surface. The classic measured resection school emphasizes, above all, preservation of the joint axis and accepts lower congruence of the articulation. The PCL, in effect, "drives" the knee.

The differing philosophies are also reflected in technique and instrument systems. Although the instruments used for making bone cuts are generally similar, gap systems depend on a tensor or a series of spacers, and *adjustment* cuts for extension balance are made on the distal femur. Ligament releases are generally performed before the bone cuts or perhaps after the

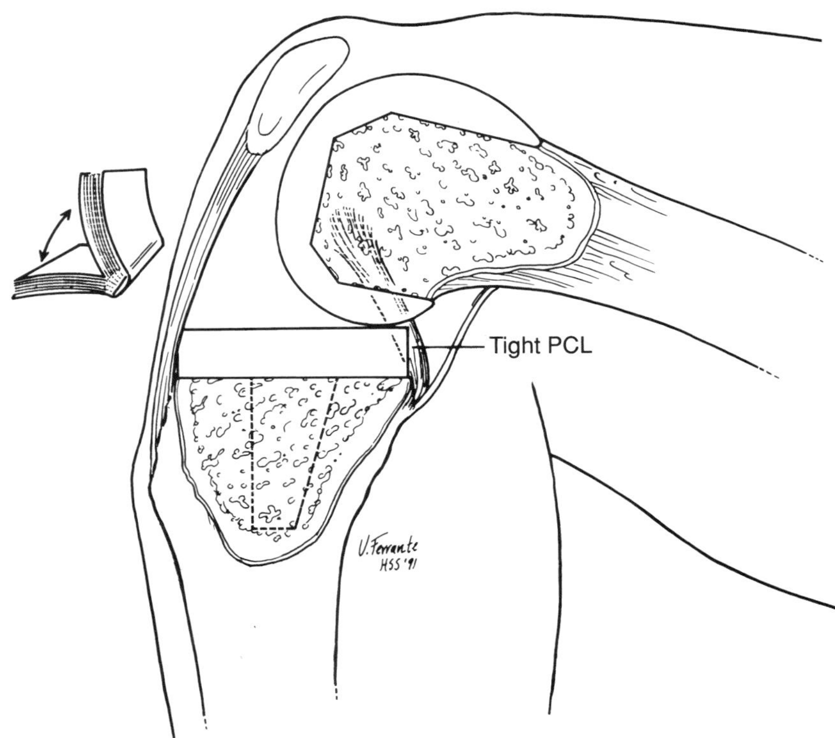

FIGURE 74.28 ➢ An overtight posterior cruciate ligament causes "booking." There is excessive rollback of the femur, and the knee hinges open.

upper tibia has been osteotomized (technique using tensors or laminar spreaders). In contrast, measured resection systems osteotomize the tibia and femur independently, aiming to remove only enough bone to accommodate the components. The tensor or spacing function is performed by the components themselves, and ligament releases are done after the trial components have been inserted. Flexion contractures, when present, are corrected either by posterior capsulotomy or by "working out" the contracture with postoperative physiotherapy. Preservation of the PCL and constant bone resection may necessitate that some degree of flexion contracture be accepted in the measured resection technique. In contrast, the varying amount of femoral bone resection in combination with posterior capsulotomy and PCL resection of the gap technique permits intraoperative correction of flexion contractures. Tanzer and Miller[154] have argued that postoperative flexion deformities tend to decrease with time and claim that a small residual contracture is not a problem to the patient. We have not found this to be true, and we believe that intraoperative correction of all deformities is very important.

INTEGRATING MEASURED RESECTION AND GAP TECHNIQUES

The distinctions between the gap and the measured resection techniques have blurred. Methods of PCL recession or release have made the two techniques more similar. Because PCL release opens both the flexion and the extension gaps approximately 1 to 4 mm (Griffin F, unpublished data), measured resection used with PCL release creates larger gaps. In our view, the importance of femoral rollback attributed to the PCL has been overemphasized. In fact, there should be very little rollback medially and less than 10 mm later-

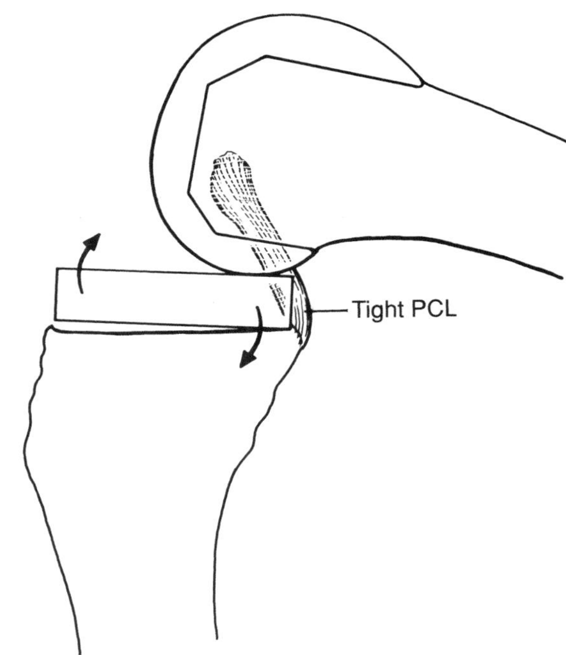

FIGURE 74.29 ➢ A method of demonstrating a tight posterior cruciate ligament intraoperatively. The tibial trial component does not have undersurface fixation, and the component lifts anteriorly.

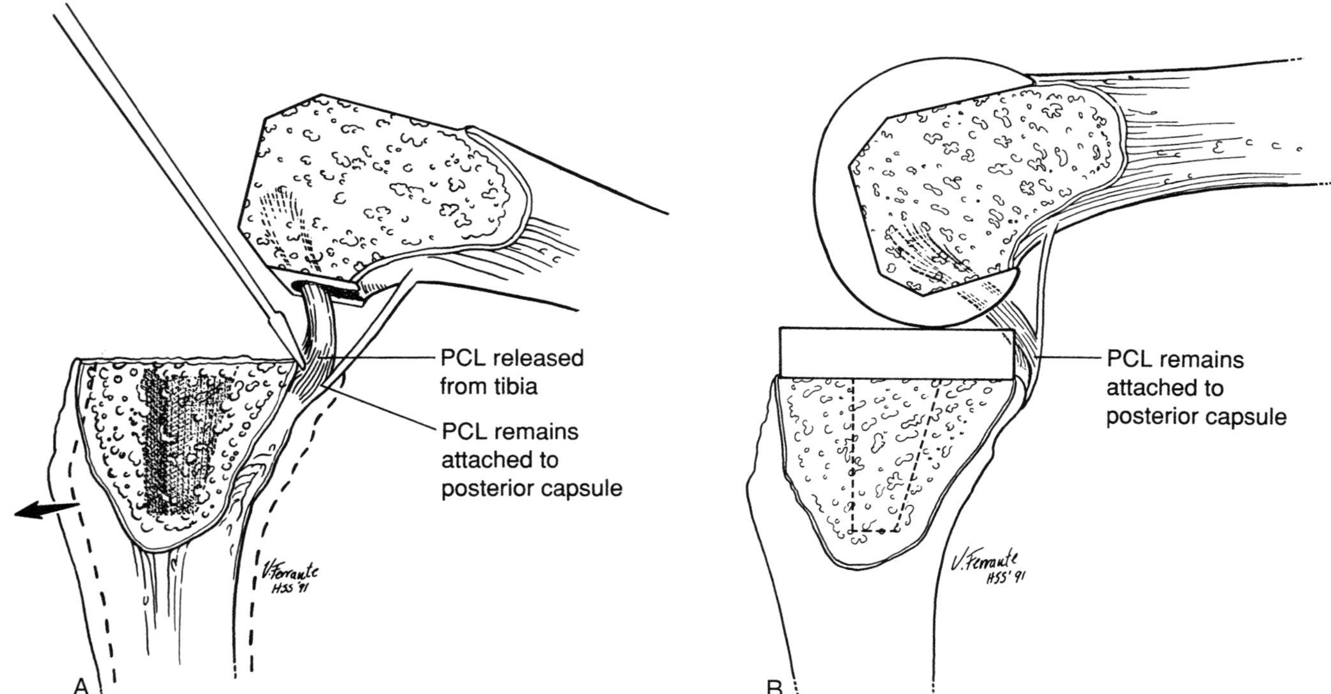

FIGURE 74.30 ➢ Posterior cruciate ligament (PCL) release from the posterior tibia lengthens a tight PCL. *A,* The release can be done progressively until correct tension is obtained. *B,* The PCL remains attached to the posterior capsule.

ally; that is, the so-called femoral rollback is actually axial rotation of the tibia. Using fluoroscopic analysis, several investigators have demonstrated that femoral rollback does not occur with flexion in cruciate retaining prostheses[80, 152]; in fact, some authors report better femoral rollback using posterior stabilized prosthetic designs (depending on the cam-post mechanism).[29, 30] Furthermore, flat tibial surfaces are not a prerequisite for PCL retention.[142] In long-term follow-up evaluations of cruciate retaining knees with conforming articular surfaces, satisfactory results have been reported.[131, 143, 164] Therefore, completely flat tibial surfaces for PCL retaining designs are not necessary, and cupping of some degree is acceptable (provided the PCL is "balanced"). If this degree of articular conformity is permissible and compatible with PCL retention, then a major objection (polyethylene wear) to retaining the PCL is negated.

For this melding of theories to occur, it is necessary for surgeons and prosthetic designers to become less rigid in their attitude toward the so-called PCL controversy. It must also be accepted that not all arthritic knees are suitable for PCL retaining designs, and there must be more objective methods for deciding when the PCL is too tight or so loose as to be rendered nonfunctional. Some PCL retaining systems have "markers" on the trial components to indicate proper kinematics. When the PCL is not fulfilling its purpose within acceptable and defined limits, a PCL release may be performed or, alternatively, a posterior stabilized design may be adopted. Most newer knee systems afford flexibility in functioning as either cruciate retaining or cruciate substituting systems, permitting an intraoperative switch to posterior stabilization when the PCL is deemed nonfunctional or detrimental.

Current Preference

Our current preference is a modified gap technique that has elements of both the gap and the measured resection methods. We perform measured resections of both the distal femur and the proximal tibia. We avoid the need for a variable distal femoral cut with PCL resection and an extensive posterior capsular release when appropriate. Through posterior referencing, we are able to perform a measured resection of the flexion gap as well. To avoid notching of the anterior cortex, the femoral component is either placed in 3 degrees of flexion or permitted to be proud anteriorly to a minor degree (see Fig. 74.16).

Because PCL release opens the flexion and extension gaps, modifications of the measured resection technique are possible. If the PCL is appropriately adjusted, strict adherence to anatomic alignment is no longer required, and the classic alignment traditionally assigned to the gap technique can be applied. As noted previously, some degree of articular congruency is permissible, rendering nonconforming polyethylene inserts obsolete.

Summary of Modified Gap Technique

Femoral preparation is done initally as follows:

1. Balance ligaments.
2. Establish proper femoral rotation (using the transepicondylar axis).
3. Cut anterior and posterior femur.
   a. Posterior referencing (1) 3-degree flexion cut and (2) correct preoperative flexion contractures by posterior release.
   b. Anterior referencing recut femur if downsizing leads to over-resection of femur.
4. Choose femoral component (downsize for in-between sizing).
5. Make proximal tibial cut.
6. Reassess ligament balance.
7. Adjust distal femoral cut to match the flexion and extension gaps. (Note that *under*-resection of the distal femur is seldom needed.)

Tibial preparation is performed initially as follows:

1. Balance ligaments.
2. Cut 10 mm from proximal tibia.
3. Balance with tensioner.
4. Cut distal femur 10 mm.
5. Rotate femur.
6. Cut anterior and posterior femur.

CEMENTED VERSUS UNCEMENTED FIXATION

Another conceptual divergence in TKA has been cemented and uncemented designs. Cemented designs afford the benefit that slight incongruities of the bone-prosthesis interface can be eliminated with the cement, whereas cementless prostheses require almost perfect bone cut congruency to optimize bony ingrowth.

We continue to favor cemented TKA. Long-term follow-up studies of cemented TKA have consistently demonstrated successful clinical results and survivorship, particularly when used in combination with a posterior stabilized design (Fig. 74.31A).[23, 31, 144, 149] Although failure of initial cemented TKA was most likely a result of excessive prosthetic tibiofemoral constraint, concerns over polymethylmethacrylate degradation, bone-cement interface deterioration, and resultant third-body wear led to the development of minimally constrained, PCL retaining TKA designs that featured cementless fixation.[66] Although the initial results of cementless and cemented TKA were comparable, a decline in satisfactory results was observed with cementless fixation.[3, 106, 110]

Cement fixation appears to provide an advantage over press-fit techniques. In a prospective comparison of cemented and cementless fixation using the same implant, Duffy et al[37] demonstrated better durability of femoral and tibial fixation with cemented techniques. At an average follow-up of 10 years, survival rates of the cemented prostheses were 94% versus 72% for the uncemented group. Although these results suggest that nonuse of cement fixation alone is responsible for a higher failure rate, failure of cementless TKA is probably multifactorial. PCL retention and thin, flat polyethylene inserts frequently used in combination with cementless designs created high-contact stresses, resulting in polyethylene wear and osteolysis.[15, 46, 77, 138, 153] However, all failures of cementless TKA cannot be attributed to PCL retention and nonconforming polyethylene inserts alone. Retrieval studies of cemented components revealed minimal bone ingrowth, resulting in component loosening and migration. To enhance fixation, pegs were added to the femoral component and screws to the tibial component. Although femoral component fixation improved, screw osteolysis was observed under the tibial component, resulting in proximal tibial bone resorption.[41, 92] Other studies have shown that tracks on the tibial baseplate undersurface serve as conduits that permit polyethylene debris to reach the cancellous tibial surface.[166] Renewed efforts have resulted in the development of methods to improve bony ingrowth, including uniform porous coating of the tibial baseplate[166] and fixation enhanced by hydroxyapatite.[113, 114] The results of Ritter et al's series[131] of cemented cruciate retaining total condylar knees and Scott et al's[141] series of cemented cruciate retaining TKA approach those of cemented posterior stabilized designs. Improvements in design have enhanced results in cementless TKA as well; Whiteside's[164] series of cementless, cruciate retaining prostheses with conforming articular surfaces and intramedullary alignment techniques common to posterior stabilized cemented designs demonstrated outcome matching that of cemented cruciate substituting prostheses. Longer follow-up is required to determine if cementless designs maintain satisfactory results. Until this longer follow-up of cementless designs is available, cemented TKA remains the gold standard against which other methods of fixation are measured.

Theoretically, the cement mantle at the edge of the bone-prosthesis interface serves as a protective "skirt" preventing the particles responsible for osteolysis from accessing the cancellous bone surfaces. Although this concept is appealing, use of cement in TKA does not eliminate the risk of osteolysis. Cases of osteolysis have been observed in cemented TKA.[21, 57, 122, 133] As noted previously, we attribute our two cases of osteolysis to modularity as polyethylene insert micromotion occurs within the tibial tray, a phenomenon originally described in cementless, cruciate retaining designs.[117] Regardless of how polyethylene debris is generated, it may have access to the cancellous surfaces, and the cement mantle is not necessarily a barrier.

Cement Technique

Cement fixation is achieved as polymethylmethacrylate penetrates the porous cancellous bony surfaces. Pulsatile lavage is used to remove blood, fat, and debris,

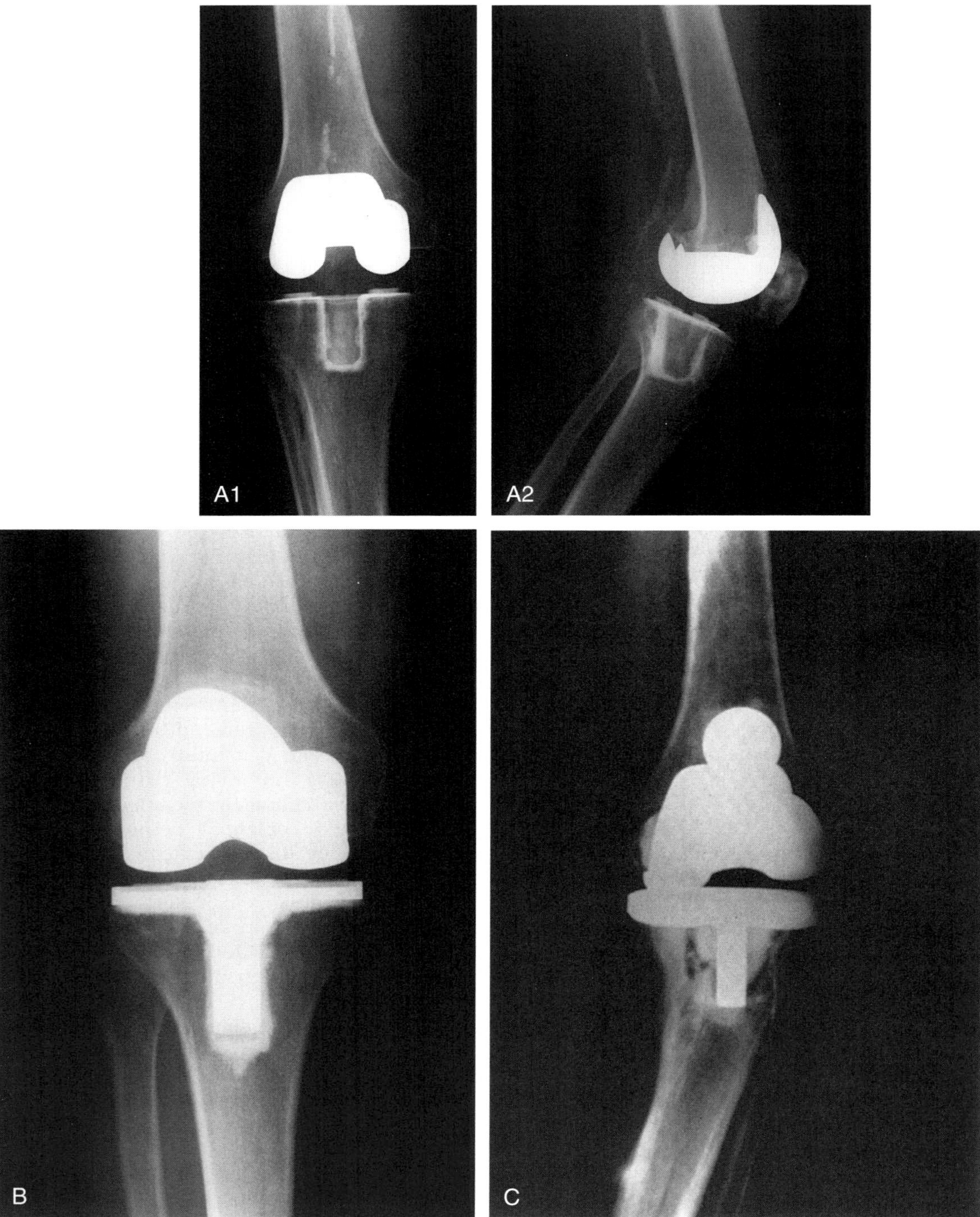

FIGURE 74.31 ➢ *A,* Anteroposterior and lateral radiographs of an Insall-Burstein I prosthesis at 19-year follow-up. *B,* Radiograph of a knee prosthesis that has been correctly cemented. The amount of cement is minimal. This type of cement fixation is obtained by using cement in the doughy stage. *C,* Radiograph of a knee prosthesis showing undesirable cement technique. In addition to the varus positioning, there is excessive cement in the proximal tibia and around the stem.

and proper cleaning of the cancellous bone permits uninhibited penetration of cement.[130] Based on our experience, the cement should be used in the doughy tactile state, which allows for easy handling and manual pressurization (Fig. 74.31B, C). Centrifugation is unnecessary in TKA because the cement layer is thin and air bubbles escape readily. Ideal cement penetration into bone is 1 to 2 mm; caution should be exercised in softer rheumatoid bone where deeper penetration may occur. Sclerotic surfaces may be drilled,

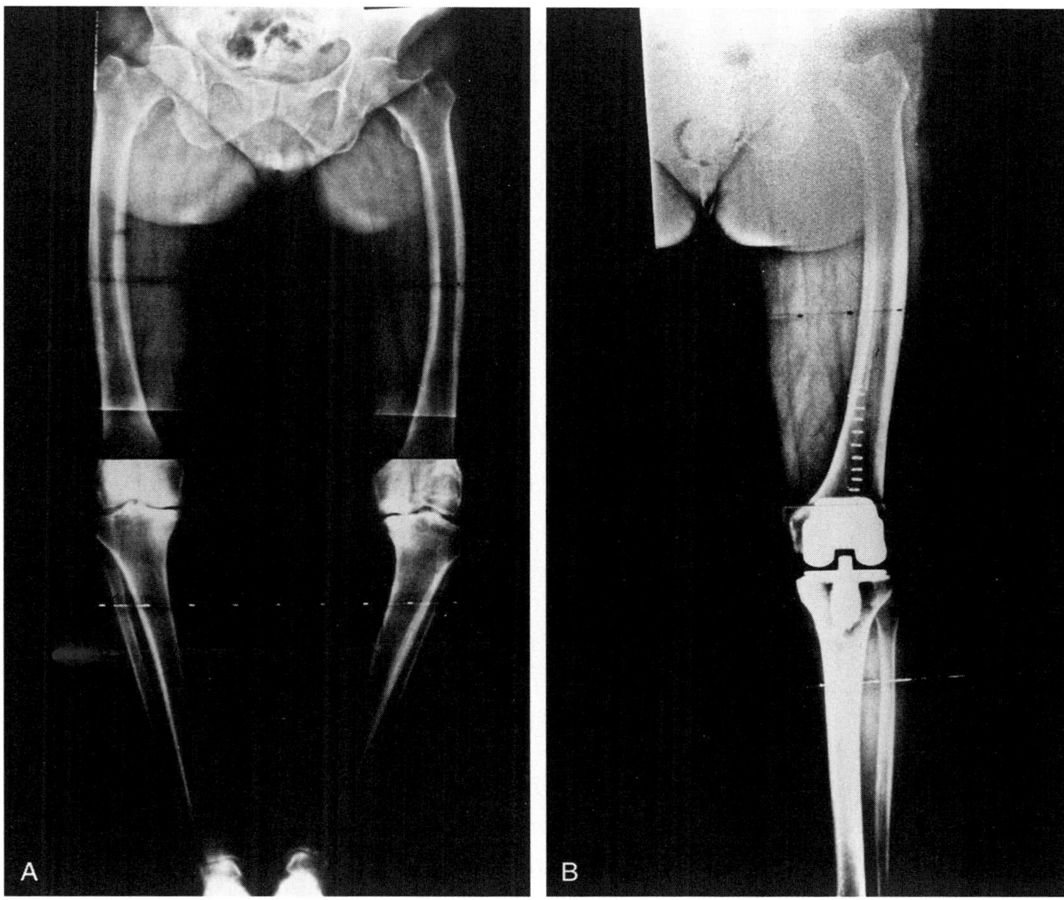

FIGURE 74.32 ➢ *A,* Long, 52-in radiograph of a preoperative patient with varus osteoarthritis. From preoperative planning, a 14-degree valgus cut on the femur was predicted. *B,* Postoperative radiograph of the same patient. Extramedullary alignment check showed that the 14-degree prediction was grossly incorrect; in fact, the femur was resected at 7 degrees of valgus. The apparent lateral bowing was, in fact, excessive anterior bowing of the femur seen in a position of some external rotation.

but drilling should be limited to no more than 1 to 2 mm because deeper cement penetration transfers the bone-cement interface away from the tibial surface into the cancellous bone where cancellous strength tends to be less. Furthermore, in the event that revision is required, cement removal may result in excessive bone loss, especially when the prosthesis and cement must be removed for infection.

Summary of the Authors' Preferred Surgical Principles

1. Cemented, posterior stabilized design.
2. Measured resection for the osteotomies.
3. Epicondylar axis to determine femoral component rotation.
4. Posterior referencing for AP sizing.
5. Appropriate balance of flexion and extension gaps (spacer block technique).
6. When a problem occurs while equal flexion and extension gaps are being established, making the femoral chamfer cuts should be delayed until the gaps are properly balanced (to simplify recutting the distal femur).

PREOPERATIVE PLANNING

Full-length radiographs that show hip, knee, and ankle joints are desirable for preoperative planning but require special equipment. Alternatively, full-length radiographs of the femur (and of the tibia if an intramedullary guide is used) may be taken. Radiographs are position sensitive, and care must be taken to obtain the films in neutral rotation (Figs. 74.32 and 74.33).[75] Information concerning the angle of femoral and tibial cuts and the desired entry hole position (which may not be in the bone center) is obtained. Unusual shaft bowing is noted (Fig. 74.34).

Templates made from the lateral radiograph provide information about the approximate size of the prosthesis (when a full inventory is not kept in the hospital). Unusual anatomic variations that could cause intraop-

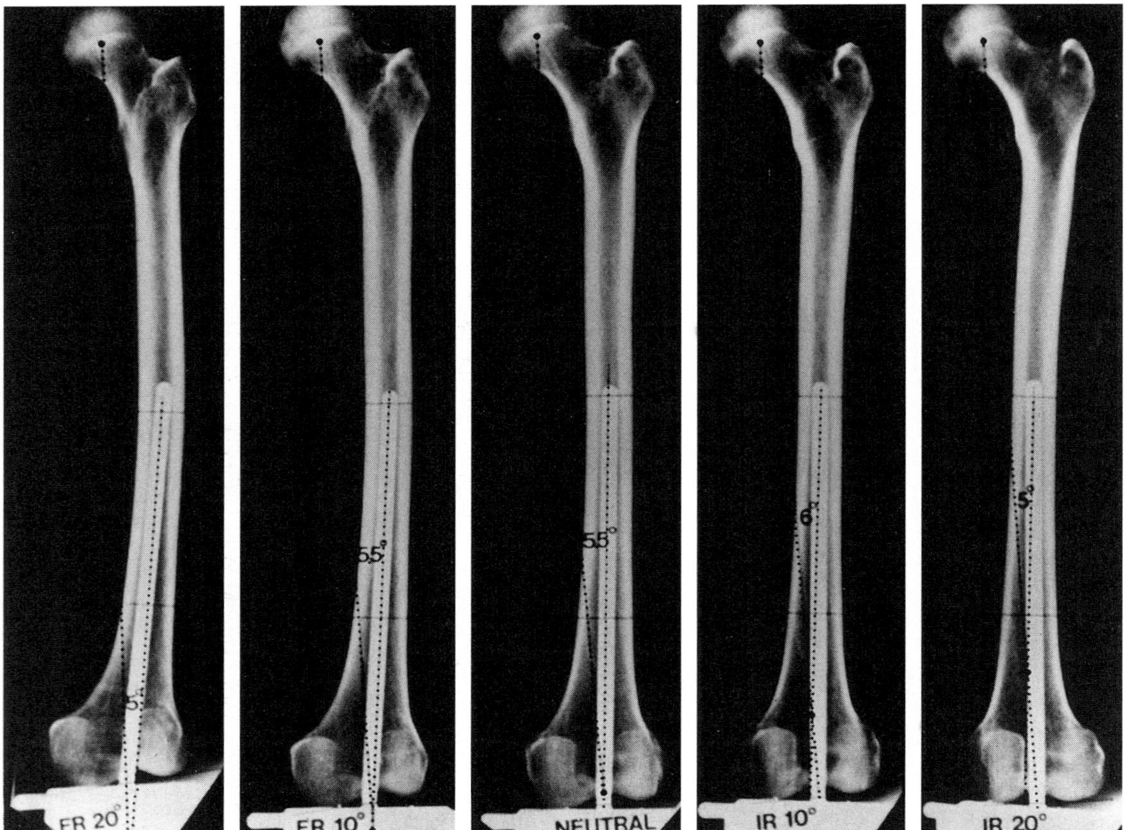

FIGURE 74.33 ➢ Radiographs of femur in internal and external rotation. It can be seen that internal rotation is perceived as medial bowing and external rotation as lateral bowing. This is a normal femur, and the effect would be accentuated if the femur had excessive anterior bowing.

erative difficulty are sought (e.g., very small or large intramedullary canal) (Fig. 74.35).

EXPOSURE

Routine Exposure

Medial Parapatellar Approach

A midline skin incision centered over the patella is typically 20 to 25 cm in length to avoid retraction of the skin edges during the procedure. Distally, the incision is approximately 1 cm medial to the tibial tubercle. We perform the medial parapatellar arthrotomy as straight as possible, usually crossing the medial border of the patella to avoid transecting longitudinal fibers of the extensor mechanism. Proximally, the capsular incision is positioned along the medial margin of the vastus medialis; distally, the arthrotomy parallels the patellar tendon approximately 5 to 10 mm medial to the tibial tubercle. A medial periosteal sleeve that includes the deep MCL is elevated from the tibia to allow the proximal tibia to be translated anteriorly, and when the ACL is present, it is divided to improve this translation.

TECHNIQUES TO ENHANCE EXPOSURE IN STANDARD MEDIAL PARAPATELLAR APPROACH

We routinely use several techniques to improve exposure with the standard medial parapatellar approach:

1. Elevation of a small cuff of periosteum immediately adjacent to the patellar tendon insertion at the tibial tubercle. This diminishes the risk of transverse patellar tendon avulsion during exposure.
2. Division of the lateral patellofemoral ligament, which permits slightly greater patellar eversion.
3. Longitudinal split of the fat pad. Although some surgeons excise the fat pad, we routinely remove only the amount needed to visualize the tibial plateau; during exposure; longitudinally splitting the fat pad on the lateral side allows the patella to be everted more easily.
4. Posterior extension of the medial periosteal elevation of the tibia. We strip the medial soft-tissue sleeve to the posterior aspect of the proximal

medial tibia, reflecting the medial capsule, the deep MCL, and the semimembranosus. Although some surgeons consider this medial soft-tissue elevation a medial release, it is not. A medial release would also involve elevation of the medial soft-tissue sleeve toward the distal attachment of the superficial MCL. Instead, this medial reflection of tissues allows for significantly greater external rotation and anterior translation of the tibial tubercle, thereby improving exposure and patellar eversion (Fig. 74.36).

Other accepted methods of exposing the knee for TKA, such as the subvastus (Hoffman), vastus splitting (Engh), trivector (Fisher), and lateral parapatellar (Keblish) methods are discussed elsewhere in this text.

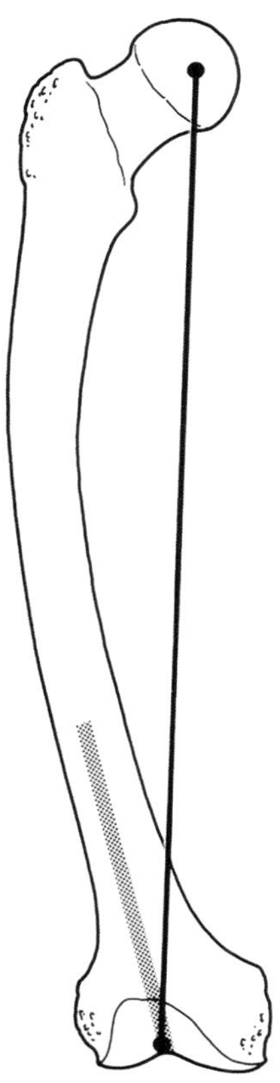

FIGURE 74.34 ➢ When the femur is bowed, the angle of the distal femoral cut will be increased. When templating the femur, beware excessive valgus cuts because the bowing may represent external rotation of the femoral bone on the radiograph. An external alignment check is advisable.

Difficult Exposures

When exposing a stiff or ankylosed knee, the standard exposure will often result in damage to the patellar ligament attachment to the tibial tubercle; before this complication can occur, preventive measures should be taken. Difficult surgical exposures are briefly reviewed here and are discussed in detail elsewhere in this text.

Quadriceps Turndown

Coonse and Adams originally described the quadriceps turndown as a narrow inverted V incision based distally with the apex in the quadriceps tendon. This incision has been variously modified so that it can be used intraoperatively by *conversion* of the standard midline or medial parapatellar capsular incision. We feel that this approach is obsolete and that there are essentially no indications to use it.

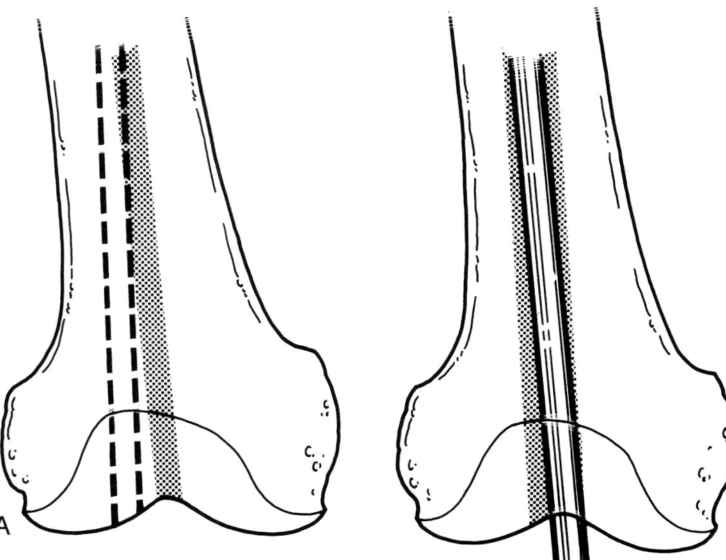

FIGURE 74.35 ➢ Malposition of the entry hole into the femur introduces an error into the valgus cut. *A*, Lateral entry hole increases the valgus of the cut. *B*, Oversized canal allows the intramedullary rod to toggle, and a 1- to 2-degree error in both varus and valgus can be produced.

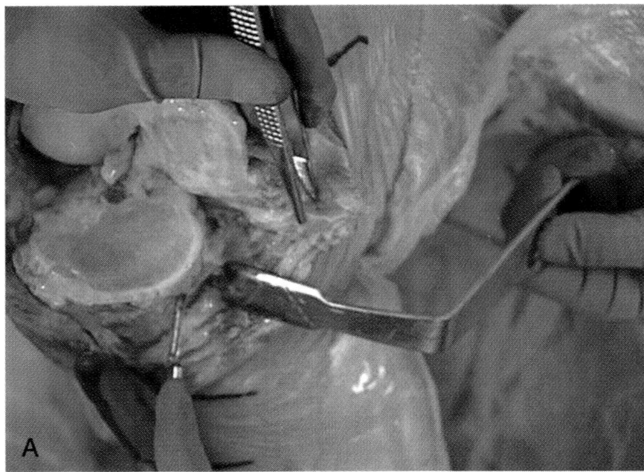

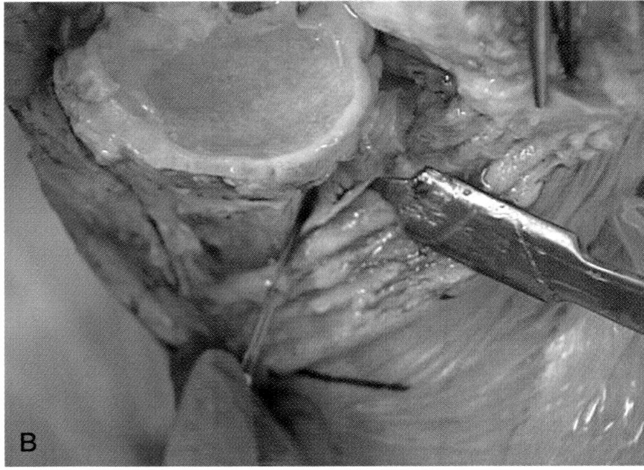

FIGURE 74.36 ➢ Routine exposure includes release of all soft tissues from the medial tibia at the joint line. A medial release involves distal stripping of the superficial medial collateral ligament, which was not performed in this case. *A,* Exposure to the posteromedial proximal tibia. *B,* Close-up view.

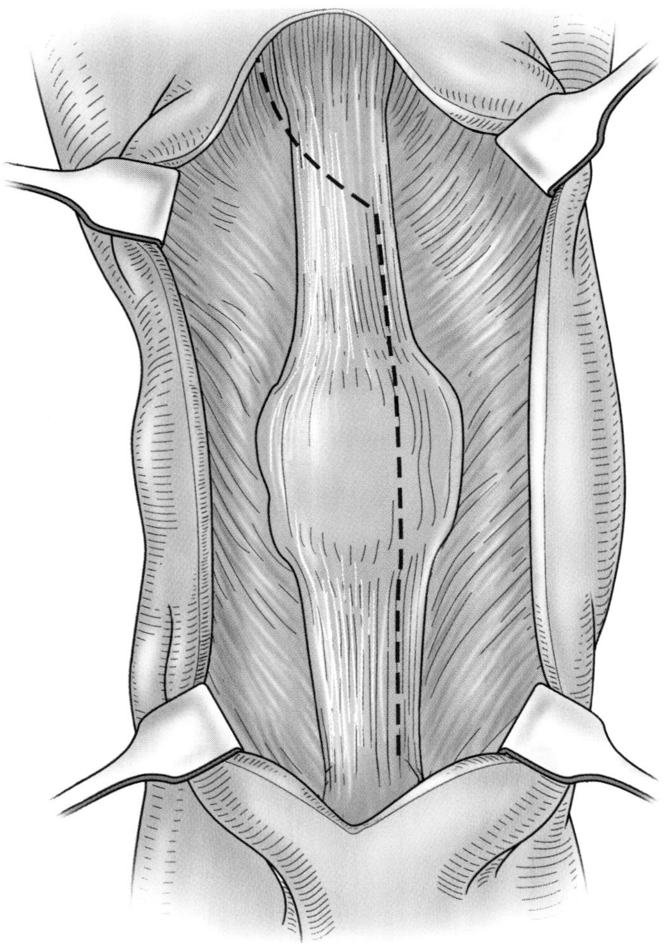

FIGURE 74.37 ➢ The rectus "snip." The medial parapatellar incision is continued proximally across the apex of the rectus femoris tendon into the fibers of the vastus lateralis. Division of the rectus tendon in and of itself allows elasticity and takes stress off the patellar ligament insertion into the tibial tubercle. When combined with a lateral patellar release, but retaining a bridge of tissue consisting of the vastus lateralis insertion into the quadriceps tendon, the result is equivalent to a quadriceps turndown.

Rectus "Snip"

The rectus snip is the extensile proximal exposure for the medial parapatellar approach[52] and is readily adopted intraoperatively (Fig. 74.37). The medial incision is the same as that described for the standard midline approach. At the apex of the quadriceps tendon, the arthrotomy is continued laterally across the thin proximal portion of the tendon into the vastus lateralis, dividing the rectus tendon and deep to it contributions made to the trilaminar tendon by the vasti. More distally, a lateral retinacular patellar release may also be done at this stage. The superior lateral genicular vessels are isolated as they run at the lower border of the vastus lateralis and are preserved. Thus the remaining proximal attachment is from the more distal fibers of the vastus lateralis.

This approach is suitable for most purposes—even ankylosed knees have been exposed. The advantage lies in the proximal continuity now provided by both the vastus medialis and the vastus lateralis when the incision is repaired. Thus, postoperatively, continuous passive motion can begin in the usual manner, and problems with extension lag are minimal.

Tibial Tubercle Osteotomy

Whiteside and Ohl[169] recommended a tibial tubercle osteotomy, emphasizing that to obtain reliable healing a large portion, measuring 3 to 6 cm in length, must be detached from the anterior tibia (Fig. 74.38). A tibial fragment of this size may be securely reattached by wires or screws at the conclusion of the operation, whereas small fragments in osteoporotic bone afford insufficient substance for successful reattachment. Whiteside[167] reported on use of this technique in 136 knees—both primary and revision TKAs. Complications were few, and no further release of the quadriceps mechanism was necessary in any procedure. However, Wolff and colleagues[172] reported a 23% com-

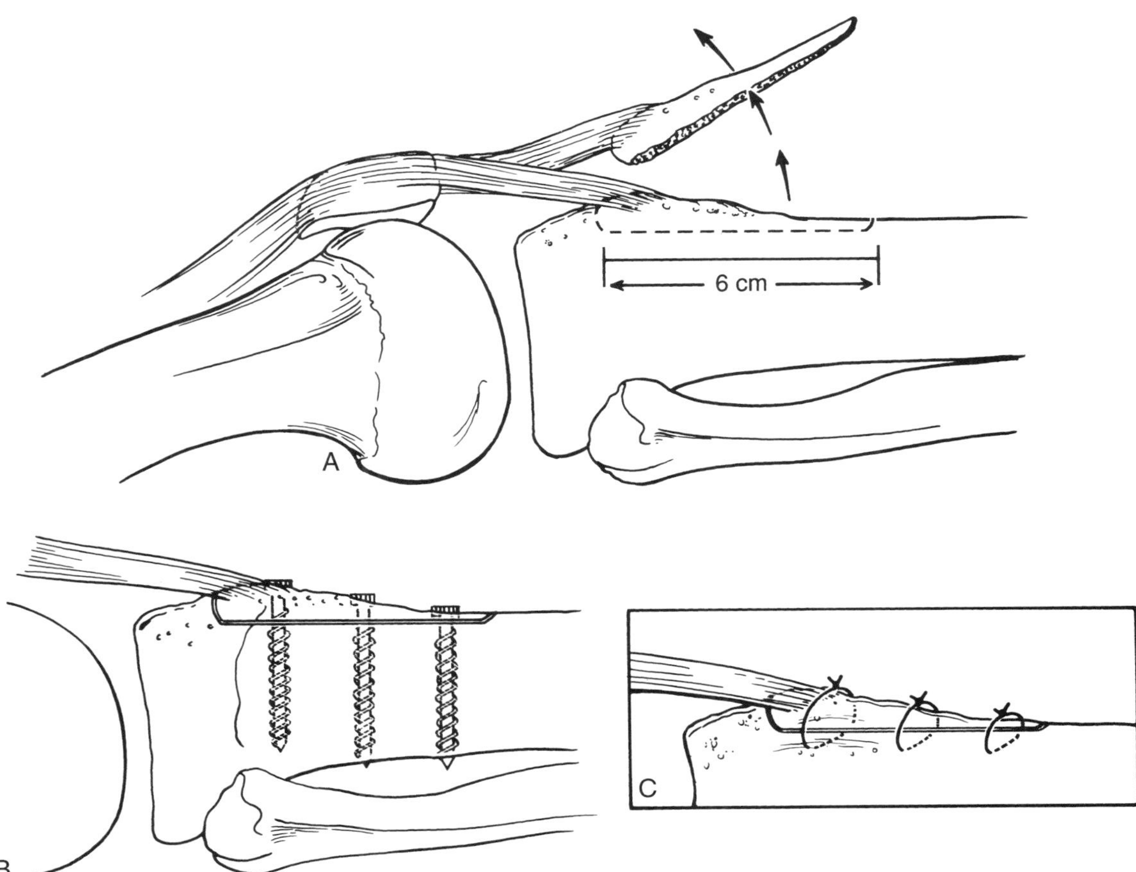

FIGURE 74.38 ➢ A method of exposure for difficult or ankylosed knees. *A,* Tibial tubercle is osteotomized by taking a large fragment of bone, at least 6 cm long. *B,* This allows firm reattachment with either screws or wire sutures.

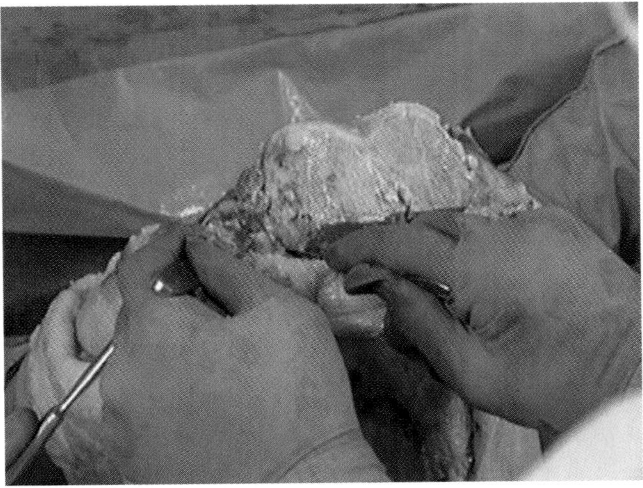

FIGURE 74.39 ➢ A skeletonized femur. The collateral ligaments, together with the adjacent periosteum of the distal femur, have been stripped posteriorly, allowing the distal femur to be buttonholed anteriorly. The soft tissues remain in continuity, and, after the operation has been completed, the soft-tissue sleeve remains intact, providing stability. This type of exposure, combined with subperiosteal stripping of the proximal tibia and quadriceps turndown or modification thereof, is very useful in dealing with ankylosed knees and for reimplantation after infection.

plication rate when using a similar technique. These authors also emphasized the need to osteotomize a sufficiently large fragment.

Subperiosteal Peel

In ankylosed knees, it may be necessary to perform a subperiosteal exposure of the femur or tibia. It is advisable to begin with a subperiosteal exposure of the medial tibia while attempting to flex the knee, being careful not to avulse the femoral attachment of the MCL. If this is not successful, the periosteum of the supramedial and supralateral lower femur is incised, and the lower femur is "skeletonized" by subperiosteal dissection (Fig. 74.39). The entire soft-tissue envelope is peeled from the bone and retracted posteriorly, allowing the distal femur to be buttonholed forward. This, combined with the medial subperiosteal dissection of the upper tibia, allows the knee to be flexed without danger of damaging or tearing important soft-tissue structures. When the incision is eventually closed, the soft-tissue envelope falls back around the bones. The soft-tissue sleeve usually provides sufficient medial-lateral stability, and only occasionally is a constrained condylar prosthesis needed. The technique is

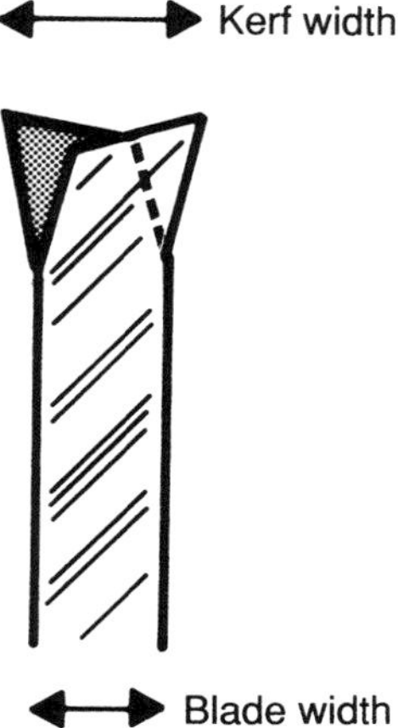

FIGURE 74.40 ➢ Saws used with cutting slots must use appropriately designed blades with a reduced offset to the cutting tips so that the kerf width and the slot width are nearly the same reducing "slot."

useful for long-standing ankylosis of the knee and for reimplantation after infection.[105]

Closure

The wound is closed over a suction or reinfusion drain in standard fashion. During closure, the vastus medialis obliquus (VMO) should never be allowed to translate proximally relative to the lateral extensor mechanism tissues. To optimize extensor mechanism function, we routinely perform a modified VMO advancement, in which the medial soft-tissue envelope is advanced several millimeters distally relative to the lateral soft tissues. Because the VMO is important in terminal extension, this advancement should theoretically reduce the risk of a postoperative extension lag.

There has been some debate about closing the extensor mechanism in flexion rather than in extension. Some authors feel that closing the knee in flexion promotes a more rapid recovery of knee function.[39] However, others suggest that the degree of knee flexion during closure of the arthrotomy has no influence on early rehabilitation after TKA.[101] We routinely close the knee in extension (with the precaution noted above), believing that accurate reapposition is the key to capsular closure.

TECHNIQUES AND INSTRUMENTATION

It is not the purpose here to describe in detail any one particular instrument system. Instruments change and evolve, but all have generic resemblances that differ only according to the two philosophies described previously, and many of the instruments used for making the actual osteotomies are similar.

Cutting Blocks

Bone cuts may be made from the free edge of the cutting block or through slotted capture guides that reduce human error. We have used both methods and believe that bone cuts made through cutting slots are more accurate. The slots may afford some degree of safety by limiting the excursion of saw blades; however, in practice they obscure the saw blade tip, potentially increasing the risk of compromising important structures such as the MCL. Although saw blades designed for the capture guides function well in the cutting slots, their cutting "teeth" are less efficient when used freehand because they have less offset to allow the blade to pass within the cutting slot (Fig. 74.40).

Milling frames probably create the smoothest bone surface through the improved precision provided by their rotary blades. In addition, the rotary blades have been shown to generate less heat than standard saw blades, thereby creating less damage to the cut bony surface (Fig. 74.41). As noted previously, these advancements are less important in cemented prostheses;

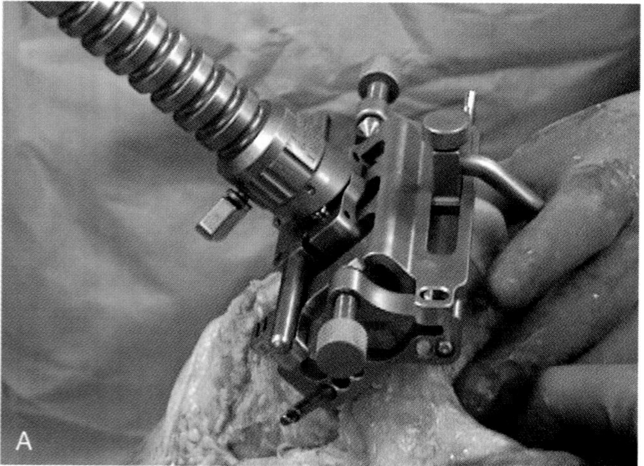

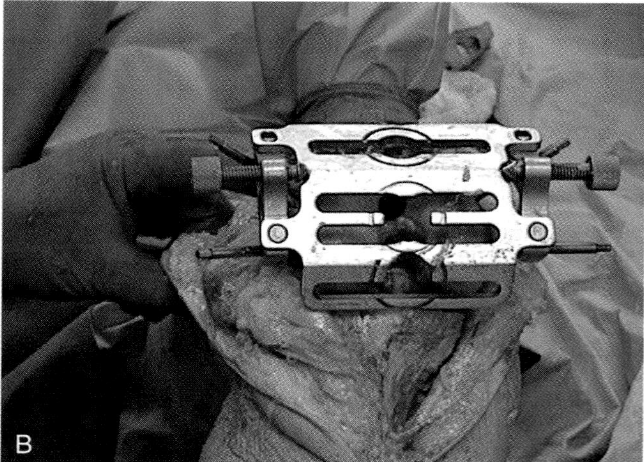

FIGURE 74.41 ➢ Milling frame. *A,* Frame secured. *B,* After milling with rotary blade.

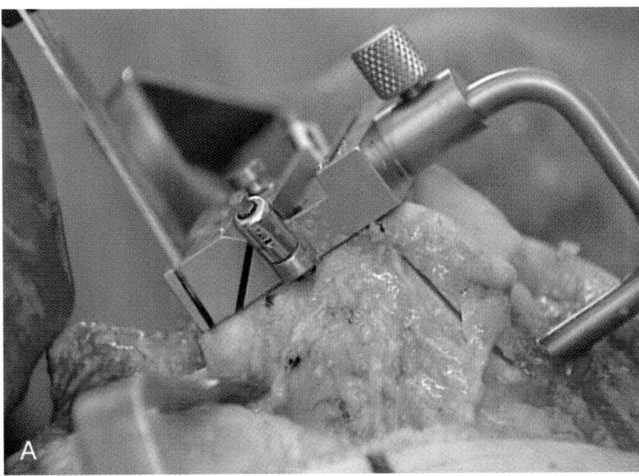

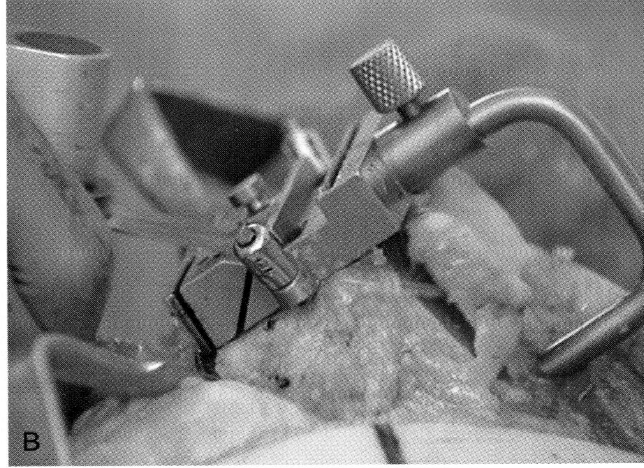

FIGURE 74.42 ➢ Universal femoral cutting block. *A,* Anteroposterior cuts. *B,* Chamfer cuts.

however, they may improve the amount of bone ingrowth in cementless designs.

Efficiency in femoral and tibial preparation has been advanced through improved instrumentation. Traditionally, the multiple femoral cuts were made with individual cutting blocks. Newer universal cutting blocks allow for multiple steps of bone surface preparation to be performed using a single block (Fig. 74.42). Most newer femoral cutting blocks provide slots for the anteroposterior and chamfer cuts and guides for creation of the lug holes; typically, the notch cut for posterior stabilized designs is still created from a separate block. Milling frames also permit efficient femoral preparation, with the slots for AP and chamfer cutting located on the same frame.

Although performing multiple femoral cuts from the same cutting block is convenient, chamfer cuts should be performed only at the same time as AP cuts when difficulty balancing the extension and flexion gaps is not anticipated. If all femoral contouring is done before establishing proper gap balance, the surgeon may be tempted to accept a tighter extension gap and use a thinner polyethylene spacer rather than recontour the distal femur. If, however, making the chamfer cuts is delayed until proper balance is established, appropriate distal femoral resection can be easily performed without recontouring the distal femur.

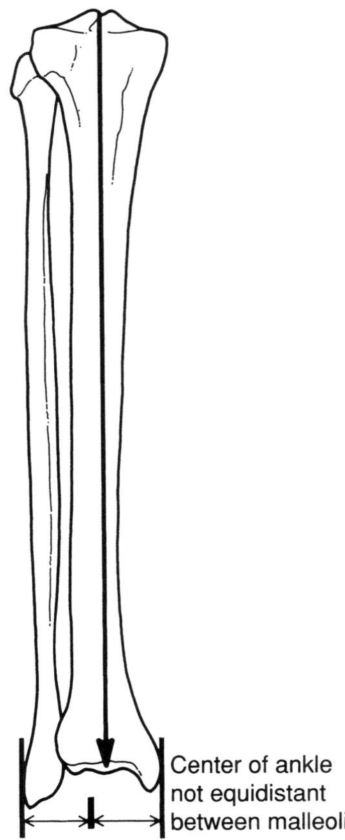

FIGURE 74.43 ➢ Center of the knee. Center of the talus axis lies a few millimeters medial to the center point between the malleoli.

Alignment Guides

It is generally agreed that restoration of the mechanical axis of the limb should be achieved. (As previously discussed, "restoration" may be an incorrect description for some individuals with habitual deviation from normal alignment.) Alignment is obtained by making appropriate cuts on the femur and tibia plus soft-tissue adjustments to provide the necessary stability (ligament balancing).

Alignment guides may be placed according to external landmarks such as the anterosuperior iliac spine or the center of the hip joint[125] proximally and the ankle mortise distally (Fig. 74.43). Because the above landmarks can sometimes be hard to identify, intramedullary guides have become more popular than extramedullary guides for making the distal femoral osteotomy.

Method of Alignment

Classic Method (Authors' Preferred Method)

It is more convenient and thus our preference (Fig. 74.44) to initially create appropriate distal femoral valgus, but either the tibial or the femoral osteotomy may be performed first. We tend to vary the distal femoral valgus depending on the patient's body habitus. Varus knees are routinely cut in 7 degrees of valgus, whereas valgus knees are cut in 4 to 5 degrees of valgus. Nondeformed knees are cut at 6 to 7 degrees of valgus. In obese patients, we limit the amount of valgus to 5 degrees even when the patient presents with a varus deformity to avoid contact between the medial knee soft tissues. The tibial cut is made neutral to the tibial anatomic axis. Our desired alignment has essentially remained unchanged since Lotke and Ecker reported that distal femoral valgus of 4 to 6 degrees and a perpendicular proximal tibial cut resulted in the most favorable outcome.[94] Hsu et al[64] confirmed that 7 degrees of femoral valgus matched with 0 degrees of proximal tibial alignment resulted in the most even load distribution across a total condylar knee prosthesis.

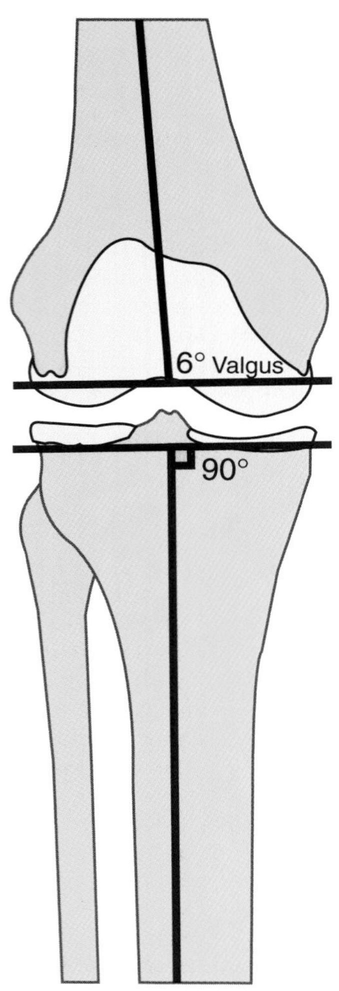

FIGURE 74.44 ➢ Classic alignment.

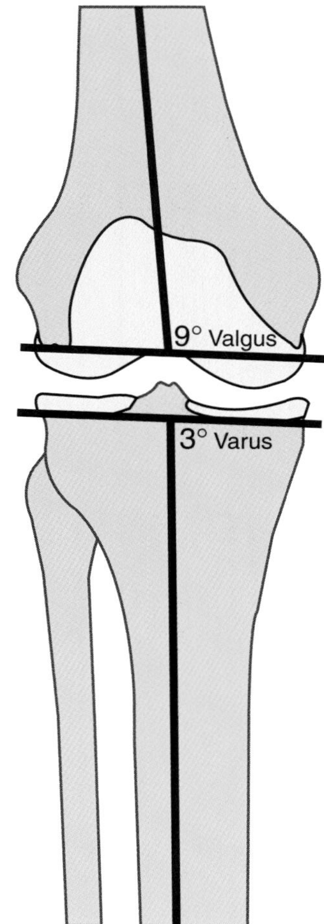

FIGURE 74.45 ➢ Anatomic alignment.

Anatomic Method

In an attempt to recreate natural knee kinematics with a PCL retaining prosthesis, Hungerford used an anatomic method (Fig. 74.45) of lower limb alignment for TKA.[66] Femoral valgus is set at an anatomic 9 to 10 degrees, and the tibial cut is made in 2 to 3 degrees of varus, thereby creating an anatomic 6 to 7 degrees of lower extremity valgus. Hsu et al[64] demonstrated that these angles produce even load distribution across the knee joint in a cruciate retaining design. As noted above, if the surgeon is not experienced in this technique, intentional varus tibial cuts can easily result in accidental excessive tibial varus, creating uneven load distribution and ligament imbalance.

Tibial Guides

Background

Most systems continue to use an extramedullary guide for the upper tibial osteotomy. Advocates of intramed-

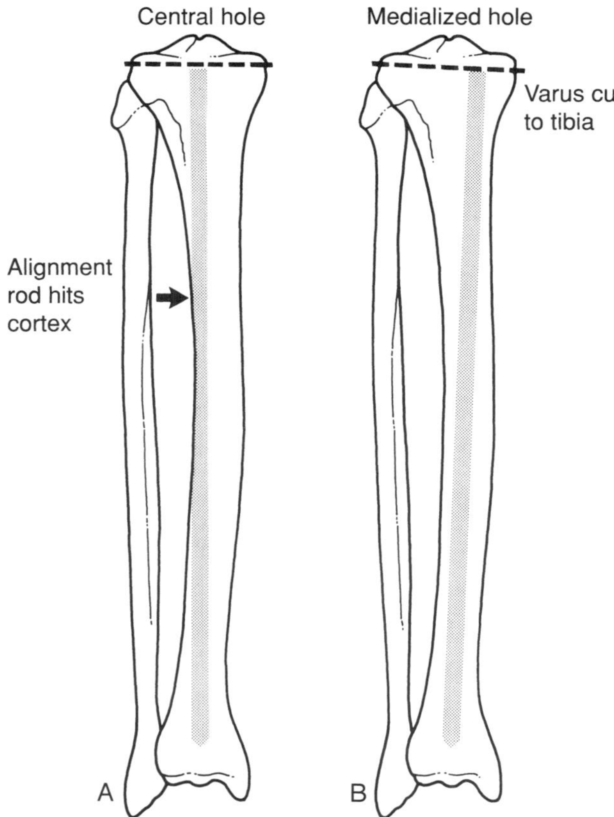

FIGURE 74.46 ➢ Intramedullary guides are not satisfactory when the tibia is bowed. *A,* The guide passed through a central hole abuts the lateral cortex. *B,* To pass the guide down the shaft to the ankle, the entry hole has to be medialized. This produces a varus cut to the tibia.

ullary tibial guides maintain that a rod of sufficient length reaching well into the tibial diaphysis will reliably align the tibial-cutting guide. This may be so when there is no bow or offset to the tibial shaft, but we have found that the shape of the tibia is inconsistent. A central entry hole will often cause the intramedullary rod to impact against the tibial cortex (usually lateral), and placing the entry hole so that this does not happen alters the angle of the proximal guide (Fig. 74.46). For the extramedullary tibial guide, the distal end attaches above the ankle, while the proximal end is pinned to the center of the proximal tibia. Some guides allow adjustment at the ankle in both mediolateral and anteroposterior directions. The center of the ankle does not exactly correspond to the midpoint between the malleoli but instead is slightly medial to this point (5 to 10 mm) (see Fig. 74.43). In obese patients, anteroposterior guide adjustment at the ankle may be necessary to make the guide parallel to the tibial shaft. Locating the proper proximal position of the extramedullary guide may be difficult; the natural tendency is to place the guide medially, producing a varus cut. However, referencing off the tibial plateau center, the tibial shaft axis, and the center of the ankle, proper alignment for the proximal tibial osteotomy is usually possible. Proper exposure of the proximal tibia is essential. In our experience, a tendency toward valgus is desirable, because empirically it is very difficult to cut the tibia in valgus using extramedullary methods.

A third alternative is to use "bogus" intramedullary alignment (Fig. 74.47)—that is, to place an intramedullary rod into the upper tibia and use it to anchor an upright alignment rod proximally and then make adjustments at the ankle. We have problems with this technique but concede that it works best for many surgeons. Intramedullary guides are 8 to 10 mm in diameter and 15 to 20 cm in length. Shorter rods are available for special circumstances.

Several investigators have demonstrated that extra- and intramedullary systems are equally accurate in establishing tibial alignment.[28, 89] However, intramedul-

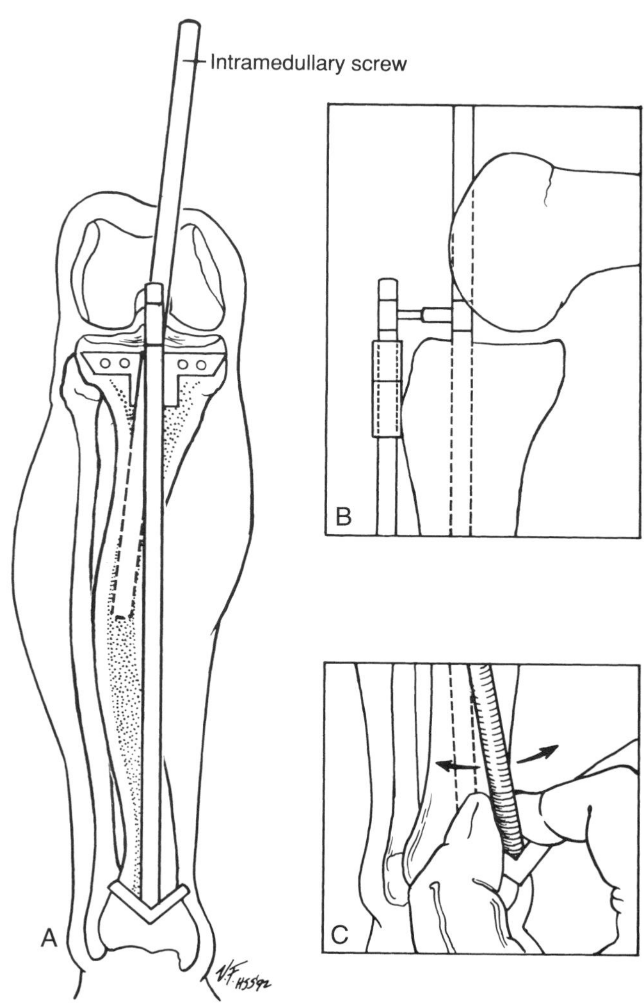

FIGURE 74.47 ➢ *A,* Diagram showing a combination internal-external tibial alignment guide. The intramedullary alignment guide is passed as far as possible through a central entry hole. *B and C,* Sometimes the intramedullary and extramedullary guides will coincide, but often they will not, in which case the extramedullary guide is adjusted to the center of the ankle, using the proximal attachment as an anchor or pivot point.

lary instrumentation forfeits some of its accuracy in the face of tibial bowing or offset of the tibial shaft, especially when used for valgus knees. Simmons et al[147] noted that accuracy for intramedullary tibial alignment systems was 83% for varus knees versus 37% for valgus knees; they attributed the poor accuracy to tibial bowing observed in two thirds of valgus knees.

Posterior slope of the proximal tibia may also be incorporated into the tibial osteotomy. As noted previously, we favor an essentially perpendicular cut relative to the tibial shaft. However, some systems, especially cruciate retaining designs, function more effectively with posterior slope. The 7 degrees of posterior slope is anatomic when considering the subchondral bone, but, taking the posterior menisci into consideration, the proximal tibial surface is actually perpendicular to the shaft (Fig. 74.48).

Authors' Preferred Technique of Tibial Preparation

The upper tibial osteotomy is made at right angles to the tibial shaft both in the coronal plane and sloped posteriorly about 3 to 5 degrees in the sagittal plane. The extramedullary guide is provisionally secured to the tibia in alignment with the tibial shaft, the center of the tibial plateau, and the middle of the ankle. Adjustments to the tibial cutting block are then performed at the ankle. The depth of proximal tibial resection depends on the type of system that is used. Obviously, enough bone must be removed to accommodate the tibial component. Because of the risk of polyethylene wear, we do not stock modular polyethylene inserts thinner than 10 mm (including the metal tray). Given the few additional millimeters of laxity produced following PCL excision, we typically resect 1 cm of proximal tibia to accommodate at least a 10-mm tibial component. The 10 mm of resection are typically measured using a stylus placed on the articular surface with the most residual cartilage; alternatively, the stylus can measure 2 mm of resection from the most eroded articular surface (Fig. 74.49). The cutting block is then fixed, and the proximal tibial osteotomy is performed. Although studies have shown that resection of up to 20 mm is acceptable,[54] care must be taken to avoid detaching the ITB at the level of Gerdy's tubercle. Rarely, alignment may still not be ideal despite careful assessment using the extramedullary technique. In this case, we adjust the proximal tibial osteotomy using a freehand method to compensate for any malalignment (typically slight varus). Tibial recutting instruments are also available.

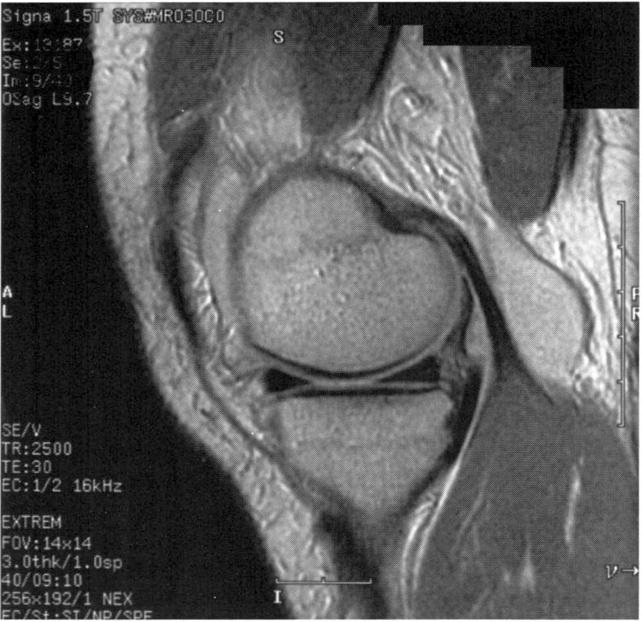

FIGURE 74.48 ➢ Lateral magnetic resonance image of the knee demonstrating that the posterior slope is present when considering the subchondral surface; however, with the menisci intact, the 5 to 7 degrees of "physiological posterior slope" is reduced to essentially neutral.

Femoral Guides

Background

Intramedullary femoral alignment to determine the angle of the distal femoral cut is generally favored because reliable external landmarks are not readily palpable. The thigh musculature and commonly associated thigh obesity make defining femoral shaft orientation difficult. The femoral head is not palpable, and the anterior superior iliac spine is frequently obscured by surgical drapes and soft-tissue redundancy. Multiple investigations have demonstrated that both intra- and extramedullary alignment systems are accurate; however, most studies suggest that intramedullary femoral alignment systems are more commonly used because of limitations of extramedullary alignment noted previously.[97] Although Engh and colleagues initially suggested that no significant difference existed in a comparative study of intra- and extramedullary alignment systems,[157] they subsequently recanted their original findings following a second, similar investigation.[42] Both investigations compared a standard intramedullary technique with an extramedullary method verifying femoral head location radiographically with an intraoperative radioopaque marker. Longer x-ray cassettes were used in the second study, and intramedullary and extramedullary alignment techniques proved 88% and 69% accurate, respectively. Femoral alignment should probably be determined using intramedullary methods and confirmed with extramedullary methods if any uncertainty exists (e.g., unusual femoral bowing, wide intramedullary canal).

Preoperative radiographic evaluation with a three-joint view allows for identification of extra-articular deformity, such as abnormal femoral bowing. With extra-articular deformity, the starting hole position for femoral canal access can be altered slightly to properly position the intramedullary guide. If the extra-articular deformity is too great to allow for standard femoral guide placement, then a modified (shorter) intramedul-

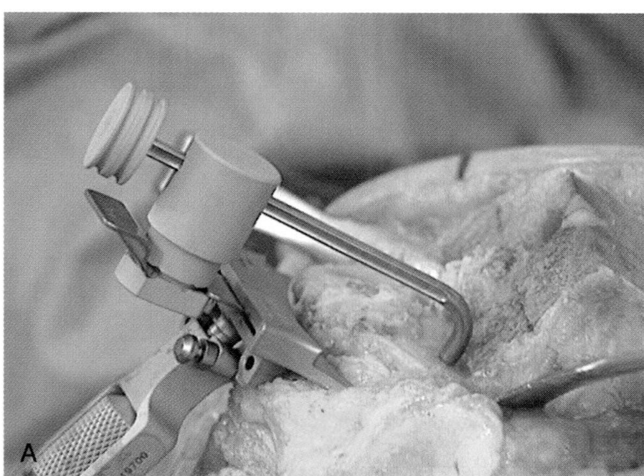

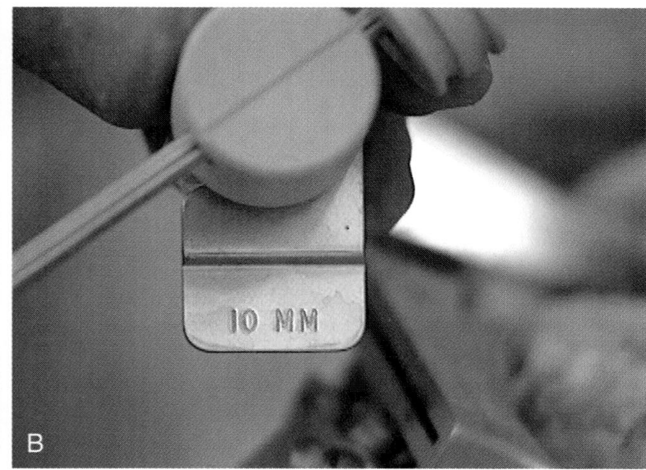

FIGURE 74.49 ➢ *A,* Intraoperative photo of the stylus used to determine the amount of proximal tibial bone resection. *B,* In this case, a 10-mm resection is measured off the least affected articular surface.

lary alignment rod may be used, although it may not be as accurate because referencing is not performed off the length of the femoral canal. If any concern about position exists, femoral intramedullary guide position can be confirmed with extra-articular alignment or intraoperative radiographic techniques using opaque markers.

FIGURE 74.50 ➢ A 52-in radiograph showing the position of entry holes from preoperative templating. Note that the femoral entry hole is slightly medial and that the tibial entry hole is slightly lateral.

Another advantage of using intramedullary methods over extramedullary techniques to determine femoral alignment is that referencing from the femoral canal typically avoids placing the femoral component in either flexion or extension. Control of flexion and extension is more difficult using extramedullary referencing points.

A disadvantage of intramedullary guides is that if the angle of entry into the canal is incorrect, the intramedullary rod may contact the femoral cortices rather than pass directly into the canal's center (see Fig. 74.35). If the rod contacts the lateral cortex, the valgus angle may be reduced, and if the medial cortex is contacted, the valgus angle may be increased. This problem may be encountered using systems with a fixed intramedullary rod length; some instrument systems have variable rod lengths to avoid these problems.

Depending on the particular instrument system and

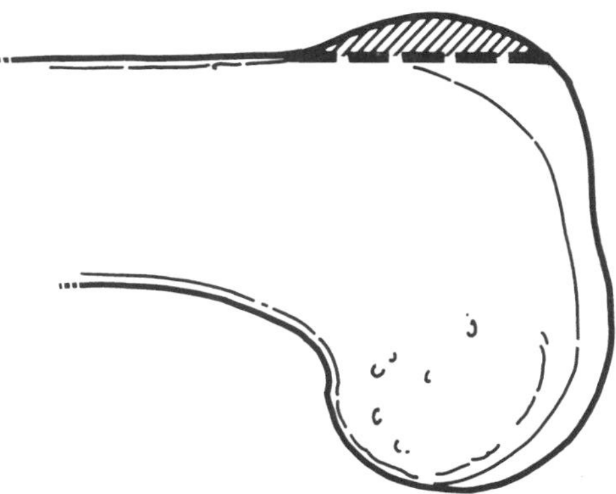

FIGURE 74.51 ➢ An anterior rough cut is often made on the distal femur before the distal cut is made, enabling firmer fixation to the anterior femur of the femoral cutting guide.

arthritic pattern, an intramedullary rod may cause the distal femoral cutting block (or its attachment) to contact either the medial or the lateral condyle first. If attempts are made to fully seat the instrumentation on both condyles, errors in the distal femoral cut may occur. For example, in valgus knees (associated with lateral femoral condylar erosion), the distal femoral cutting block attachment typically contacts the medial femoral condyle first. If the surgeon allows the instrumentation to contact both condyles in this situation, the valgus angle of the distal femoral cut will be exaggerated. To avoid such errors, the surgeon must be aware of the arthritic pattern and use the intramedullary guide to establish proper position of the distal femoral cutting block, even if the instrumentation contacts only a single condyle (see Fig. 74.24).

Authors' Preferred Technique of Femoral Preparation

The entering hole for a femoral intramedullary guide is made about 1 cm anterior to the origin of the PCL, although this position can be adjusted to accommodate any abnormalities noted on preoperative radiographs; usually the entry hole is directed slightly medially (Fig. 74.50). Overdrilling the entry to 12 mm is recommended because of increased intramedullary pressure during intramedullary rod insertion; use of a fluted rather than a round intramedullary rod has also been shown to diminish intramedullary pressure during rod insertion.[124] Some systems remove the trochlear surface of the femur (Fig. 74.51). If such an anterior "rough cut" is used for rotational alignment, then the guide must be positioned using the landmarks described. The distal femoral osteotomy guide is attached to the intramedullary guide at an angle derived from the preoperative radiograph; normally, this is 6 to 7 degrees. When intramedullary assessment appears unreliable, an extramedullary rod should be used to confirm that the proposed osteotomy is appropriate. When this step provides conflicting information, the preoperative radiographs should be reevaluated; rarely, intraoperative radiographic determination of the proper femoral valgus angle is necessary.

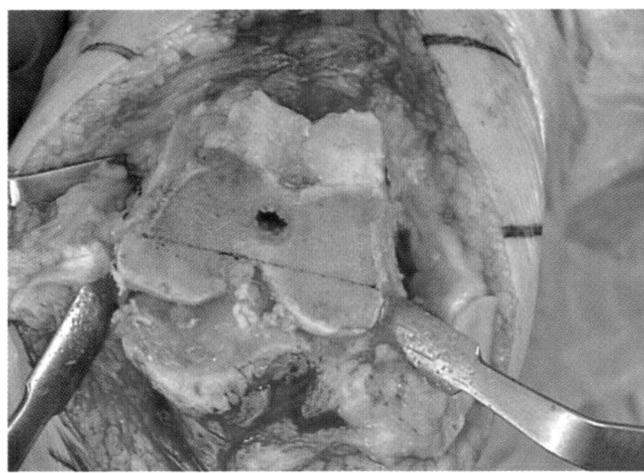

FIGURE 74.53 ➢ Intraoperative photograph demonstrating the epicondylar axis drawn across the cut distal femoral surface.

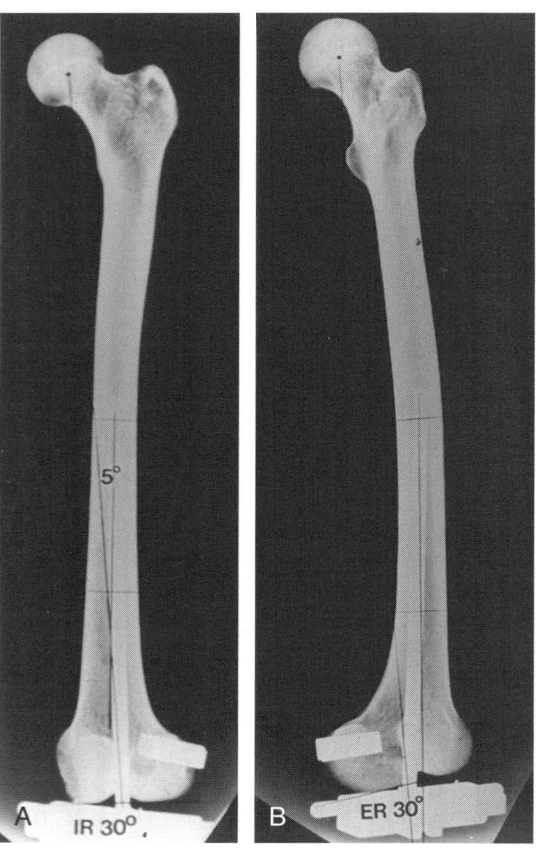

FIGURE 74.52 ➢ Radiographs of femur in *(A)* internal and *(B)* external rotation. It can be seen that internal rotation is perceived as medial bowing and external rotation as lateral bowing. This is a normal femur, and the effect would be accentuated if the femur had excessive anterior bowing.

Rotation of the femur in the preoperative full-length radiograph can create a false impression of varus or valgus bowing (Fig. 74.52). In this sense, the planning of alignment for full-length radiographs may be no more accurate than using shorter films or relying on external landmarks, such as the hip or the external iliac spine. To enhance our ability to accurately determine femoral component rotation, we currently mark the epicondylar axis on the distal femoral surface (Fig. 74.53).

The distal femoral osteotomy is made by removing precisely the amount of bone that will be replaced by the femoral prosthesis. Some systems measure this amount from the uninvolved condyle, whereas others key off the medial femoral condyle regardless of the knee pathology (see Fig. 74.24).

The distal femur is then sized, and anterior and posterior femoral resections are made, using appropriate templates (Fig. 74.54). Rotational alignment, if not already done at an earlier stage, is adjusted when posi-

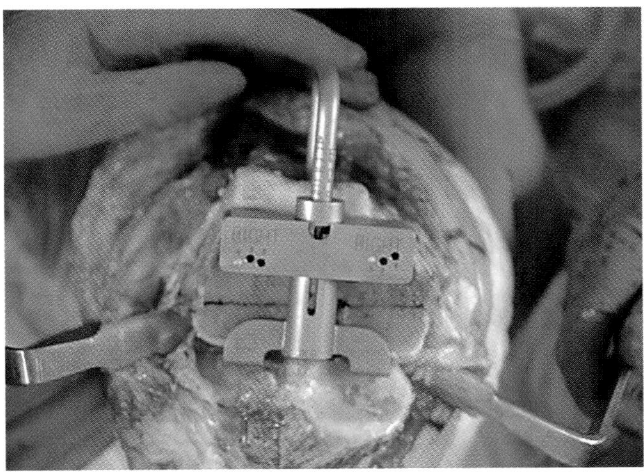

FIGURE 74.54 ➢ Sizing the femoral condyle.

FIGURE 74.55 ➢ The instrumentation is aligned with the epicondylar axis (pins are parallel to epicondylar axis, as indicated by ruler placed across them).

tioning the femoral template. We align the femoral AP cutting block with the epicondylar axis (Fig. 74.55).

For cruciate substituting prostheses, flexion and extension gaps are now measured with spacers, and additional distal femoral bone is removed when indicated, using a recutting instrument (Fig. 74.56A, B). More recently, we have performed a predetermined measured resection of the distal femur that rarely warrants readjustment (typically only with severe flexion contractures). Adjustment cuts should be made before the bone-sculpting or chamfer stage to save tedious reshaping of the entire distal femur (Fig. 74.56B, C, D). As noted previously, this is especially true when using universal cutting blocks with which AP and chamfer cuts are made early in the procedure. Apart from creating extra work, more important is the temptation to accept the fit as it is (flexion contracture because of tight components) or to use a thinner tibial insert (flexion instability) (Fig. 74.57).

Tensor systems perform this "recutting" function at an earlier stage of the operation by indicating the level of distal femoral resection. Thus, when a tensor is incorporated into the system, the spacers confirm the accuracy of the bone cuts, and additional bone resection should not be necessary (see Fig. 74.20). Although the distal femoral cut determined using a tensor system typically addresses flexion contractures,

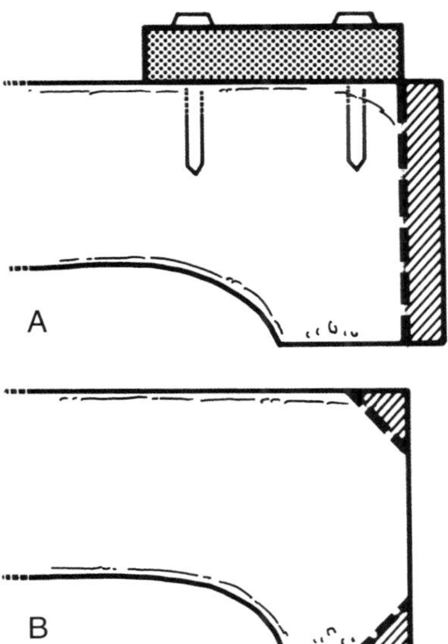

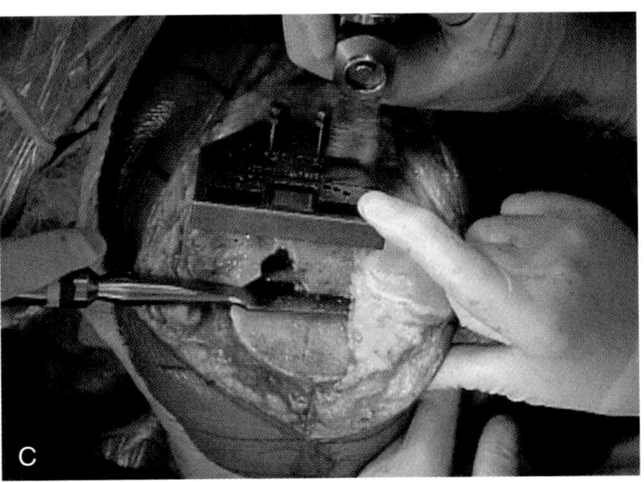

FIGURE 74.56 ➢ *A,* Femoral recutting should be done before the chamfer cuts are made, an important reason for incorporating spacers into the system. It is simple to remove 2 to 3 mm from the end of the distal femur. *B,* When the femur has been sculpted to receive the prosthesis, recutting is much more complex. *C,* The distal femoral recutter allowing 2, 3, and 5 mm of additional resection. (The cut tibial surface should be protected.)

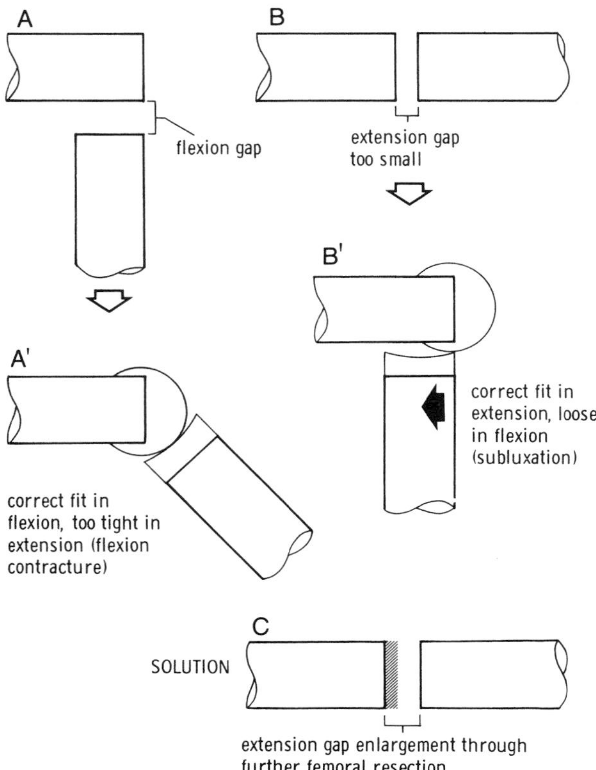

FIGURE 74.57 ➢ Unequal gap size is a frequent technical error. When the extension gap is too small, the knee will not fully extend; if a thinner tibial component is used, the prosthesis will be too loose in flexion. The solution is to excise more bone from the distal femur.

adequate posterior capsular release usually obviates the need for excessive distal femoral resection.

Both types of instrument systems then proceed to the bone-sculpting stage. Chamfer, notch, and fixation holes are made on the distal femur (Fig. 74.58) and proximal tibia (Fig. 74.59). The lower femur is shaped to fit the prosthesis, using appropriate instruments.

Rotational Positioning of Prosthetic Components

Rotational alignment of the femoral component has already been decided, as previously discussed. Rotational positioning of the tibial component remains to be determined. The landmarks that can be used are the posterior surface of the cut tibia, the anterior surface of the tibia, the tibial tubercle, and the ankle mortise. Assessment can be done with the knee in flexion, in extension, or in both.

We prefer to determine proper tibial component rotation with the knee flexed. This way, tibial component rotation can be related to the anterior surface of the tibia and to the position of the tibial tubercle, which should lie slightly lateral to the midposition of the component (Fig. 74.60). Reference is then made to the ankle and to the position of the malleoli, which should lie approximately 30 degrees externally rotated to the tibial component position. An alignment rod can be suspended from the tibial guide. When a symmetric tibial component is used, there is often some overhang posterolaterally (Fig. 74.61) because the medial tibial plateau is larger than the lateral (by approximately 10% in our studies); for this reason, we do not favor using the posterior margins of the tibial plateau as alignment landmarks.

Rotational alignment can also be assessed in extension, allowing the tibial component position to be related to the patellar groove of the femoral component, the tibial tubercle, and the ankle mortise. With the femoral trial prosthesis in position, a range of motion is performed and patellar tracking is observed before the final fixation holes for the tibial component are made. A tibial trial component without fixation pegs allows the component to "find" its correct position. We do not use this technique and prefer to use the anatomy of the proximal tibia.

Consequences of tibial tray malrotation are detrimental to patellar tracking, especially with excessive internal rotation of the tibial component. Excessive internal rotation of the tibial component increases the risk of patellar subluxation.[10] Conversely, excessive external tibial component rotation may also result in abnormal tracking of the patella[111] as well as a kinematic conflict in the femorotibial articulation.

Mediolateral Positioning of Prosthetic Components

The medial-lateral positioning of both femoral and tibial components is important. Generally, they should be positioned anatomically on their respective bones and when correctly sized there is little leeway. On the femoral side, the component should ideally coincide with the resected margin of the lateral femoral condyle. For prostheses systems that allow separate sizing of the femur and tibia (interchangeable components), the tibial component selected will normally and quite precisely coincide with the resected tibial plateau. However, for some cruciate substituting designs, the option exists for some medial or lateral translation of the tibial component. This option is useful when marginal bony defects exist, to reduce the size of the bony defect (Fig. 74.62).

Patellar Cuts and Cutting Guides

The patellar osteotomy is perhaps the most difficult to instrument and still is often done by the "eyeball" technique (Fig. 74.63).[93] Patellar cutting guides have been developed but are mostly unsatisfactory or not widely available (Fig. 74.64). In our hands, reaming devices[55] (Fig. 74.65), traditionally used for inset patellar components, are also effective in establishing the proper resection level for onset patellar components. The objective of the patellar osteotomy is to produce an even resection of a thickness that will leave sufficient bone to anchor the patellar prosthesis without being too bulky (Fig. 74.66). Caliper measurements of the patellar size before and after resection are essen-

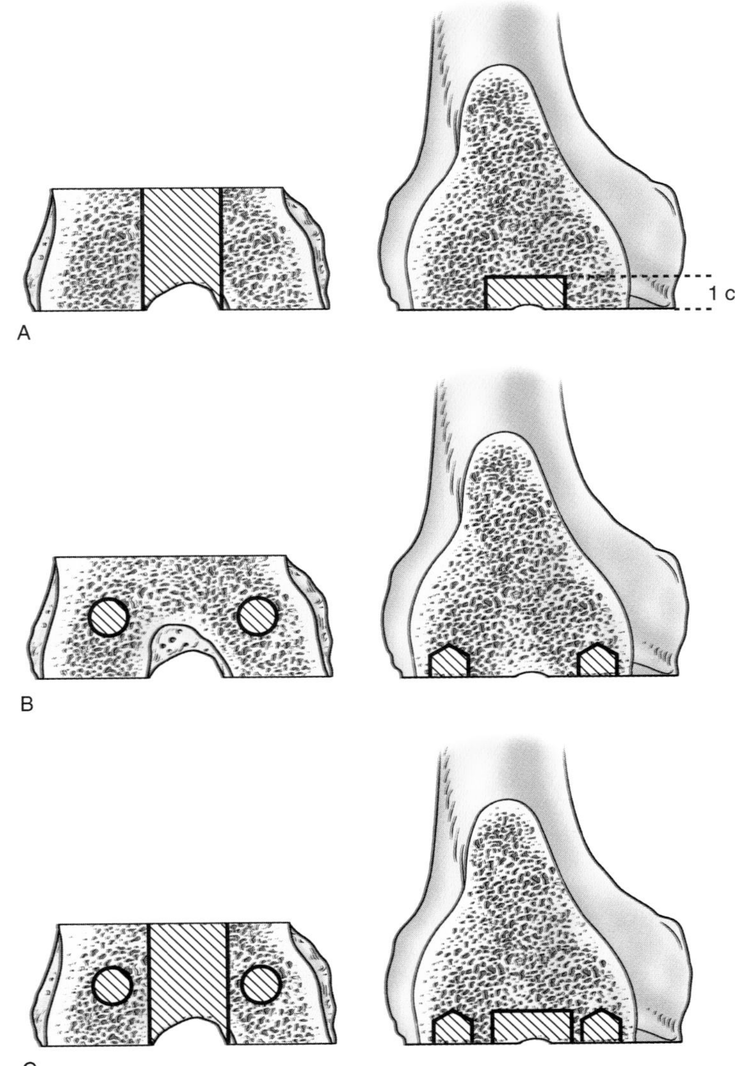

FIGURE 74.58 ➢ Femoral fixation can be enhanced by a central box usually found with *(A)* posterior stabilized designs, *(B)* medial and lateral fixation lugs, or *(C)* both.

tial, and with the prosthesis inserted, the patellar measurements should be equal to or slightly less than the original thickness of the patellar bone (Fig. 74.67).

The patella does not have to be resurfaced. Investigators have reported acceptable results without patella resurfacing,[8, 12, 13, 99] especially when the patellar articular cartilage has limited articular wear. Patella resurfacing is recommended in patients with osteoarthrosis involving the patellofemoral joint, crystalline disease, or inflammatory arthropathy.[121] On the other hand,

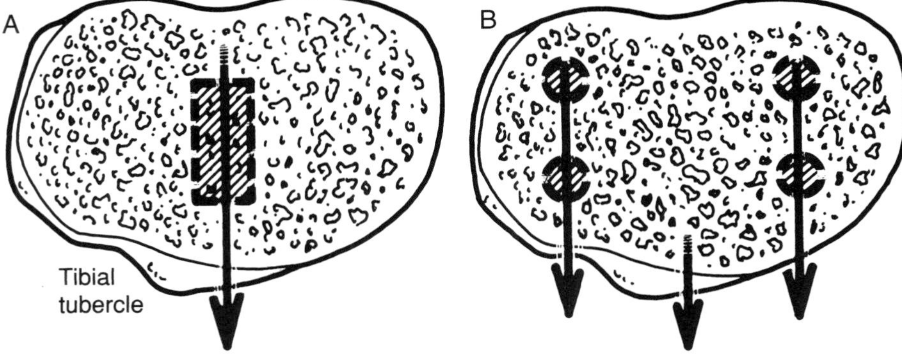

FIGURE 74.59 ➢ *A,* Alignment of the tibial component is projected at a point slightly medial to the tibial tubercle. *B,* Alignment of a symmetric component with the posterior margin of the tibial plateau will usually result in some internal rotation of the tibial component. One should err on the side of external rotation.

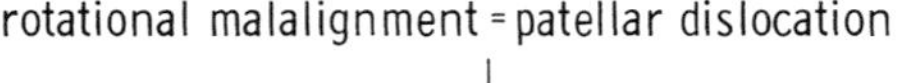

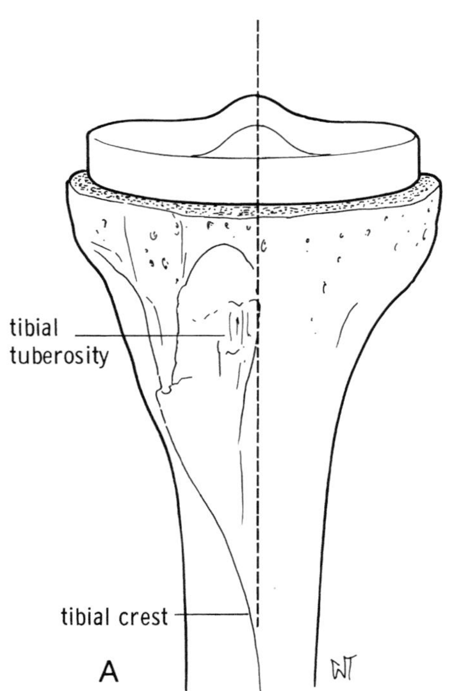

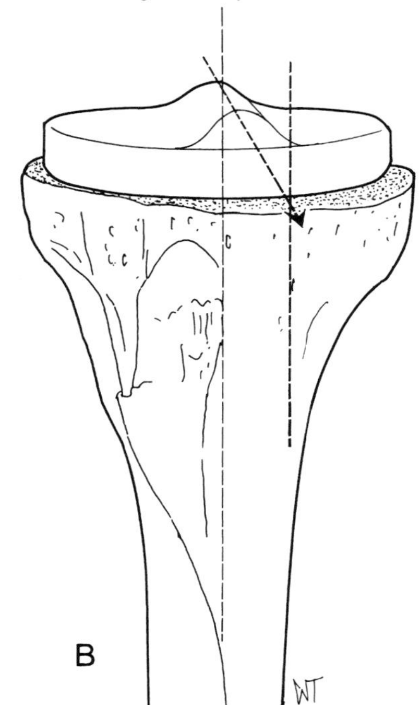

FIGURE 74.60 ➢ The tibial component should be aligned with the tibial tubercle. *A*, Correct position. *B*, Tibial component internally rotated on the tibia.

extreme patellar articular erosion makes use of a patellar component difficult or impossible. In these cases, contouring of the residual patellar bone ("patelloplasty") is performed. We typically resurface the patella, except in significantly obese patients and in young, active patients without eburnation of the patellar articular surface. We are not sure if this practice is justified, but TKA without patella resurfacing in these patients has been reported with satisfactory results in short-term follow-up.[99, 121] Longer-term follow-up will determine if the natural patellar articular surface is compatible with the metal femur; an anatomic trochlea is obviously necessary.

Lug or fixation holes are made into the patella. Most designers currently favor three 3- to 4-mm holes placed in a triangular fashion rather than a larger, centrally placed fixation point (Fig. 74.68). A round dome patellar prosthesis should be positioned to the medial side of the oblong patellar osteotomy and is sized by the superior-inferior dimension of the bone (Fig. 74.69).

Insetting designs of 28 or 32 mm in diameter have been tried with some success (Fig. 74.70). These designs require central reaming of the patella, leaving the periphery intact. This technique is not quite as easy as reaming for onset patellae. We have found that reamers work well when the bone is relatively soft but cause difficulty with sclerotic bone when a preliminary osteotomy with an oscillating saw is needed. The reamers have sharp teeth and can cause inadvertent damage to peripheral bone if not carefully controlled.

FITTING OF TRIAL COMPONENTS

Fitting of the trial components is now done. Stability and alignment are checked in both flexion and exten-

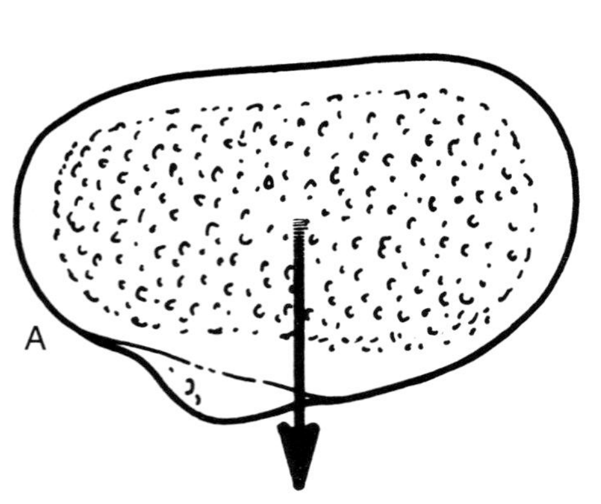

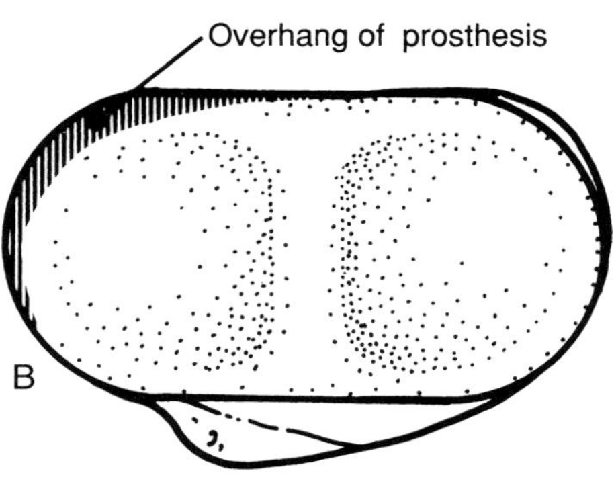

FIGURE 74.61 ➢ *A* and *B*, With a symmetric component, some degree of posterolateral overhang of the prosthesis is expected.

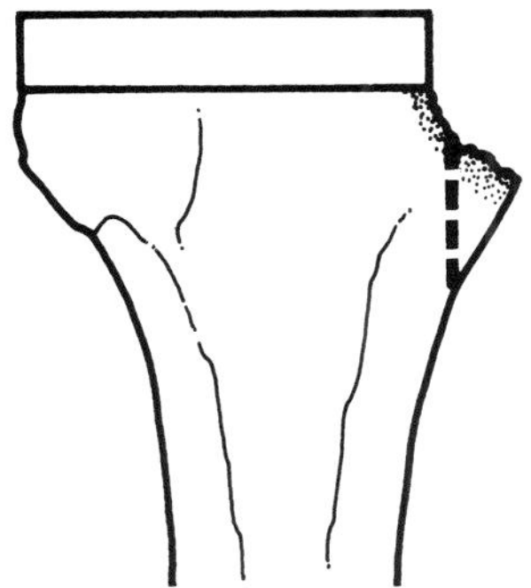

FIGURE 74.62 ➢ Lateralization of the tibial component can be done with cruciate substituting designs. The tibia is deliberately undersized and placed at the lateral margin of the tibia. The medial defect is reduced, and overhanging bone can be excised vertically.

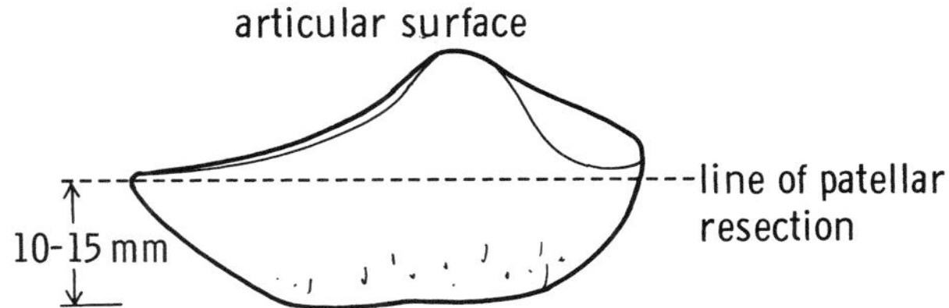

FIGURE 74.63 ➢ The line of patellar resection.

sion. For cruciate substituting designs, little further adjustment should be required. For cruciate retaining prostheses, ligament balancing is done at this stage, using different thicknesses of tibial trial components until satisfactory stability is obtained.

Particular attention must be paid to the PCL, and a posterior release from the tibia is performed when tightness in flexion is observed. At this stage, if optimal balance cannot be obtained, it is wise to make an intraoperative change to a PCL substituting design. An inadequate PCL will not prevent flexion instability when the tibial design is flat.

PATELLAR TRACKING

When the correct tibial component thickness has been selected, patellar tracking is observed with the patellar component in place. The "no thumb" test is applied: the patella should track with its medial border in contact with the femoral component throughout the range of motion without the surgeon maintaining it in this position manually (Fig. 74.71). It is permissible to take the slack out of the quadriceps tendon by applying longitudinal tension (Fig. 74.72) or by using a single stitch to reapproximate the vastus medialis to the proximal patellar margin. If this suture ruptures, or if there is any doubt about patellar tracking, a lateral retinacular release is performed. After isolating the lateral superior genicular vessels (Fig. 74.73), which can be found distal to the lower border of the vastus lateralis, and protecting these vessels, a lateral retinacular release is done approximately 1 to 2 cm from the lateral patellar margin from inside out (Fig. 74.74). In our opinion, the tendinous part of the vastus lateralis should be included in the release.

The patellar position in the sagittal plane is also important, but it is for the most part determined by the bone cuts of the femur and tibia. There is a tendency toward producing patella infera with whatever technique is used (even when the femoral geometry is restored, the tibia may be "over-replaced" by the need to use a thicker tibial component to achieve stability). The observation of a postoperative patella infera may not always be related to surgical technique. Koshino et al[83] have observed a gradual lowering of patellar position similar to that seen after high tibial osteot-

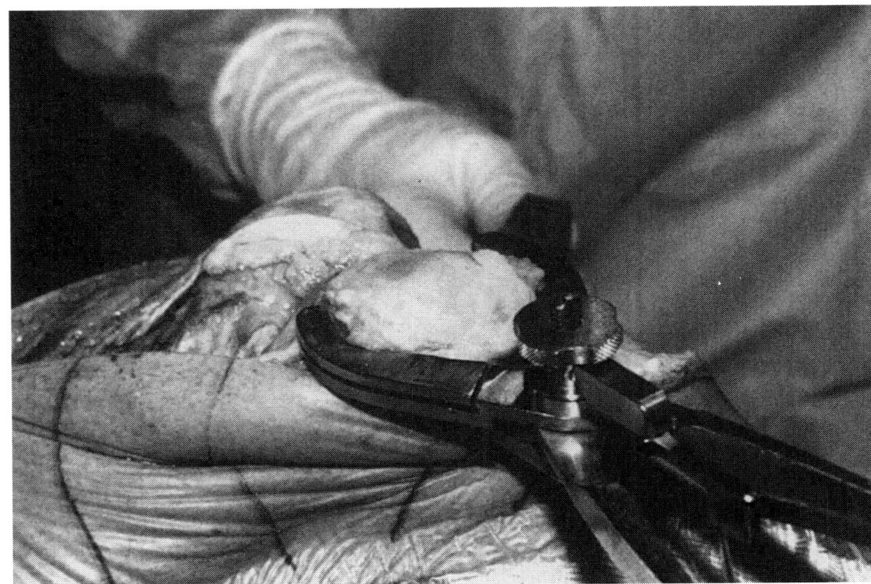

FIGURE 74.64 ➢ A slotted patellar cutting guide. The depth of the resection is selected by the knurl knob. The jaws grasp the patella, and the slots direct the cutting blade.

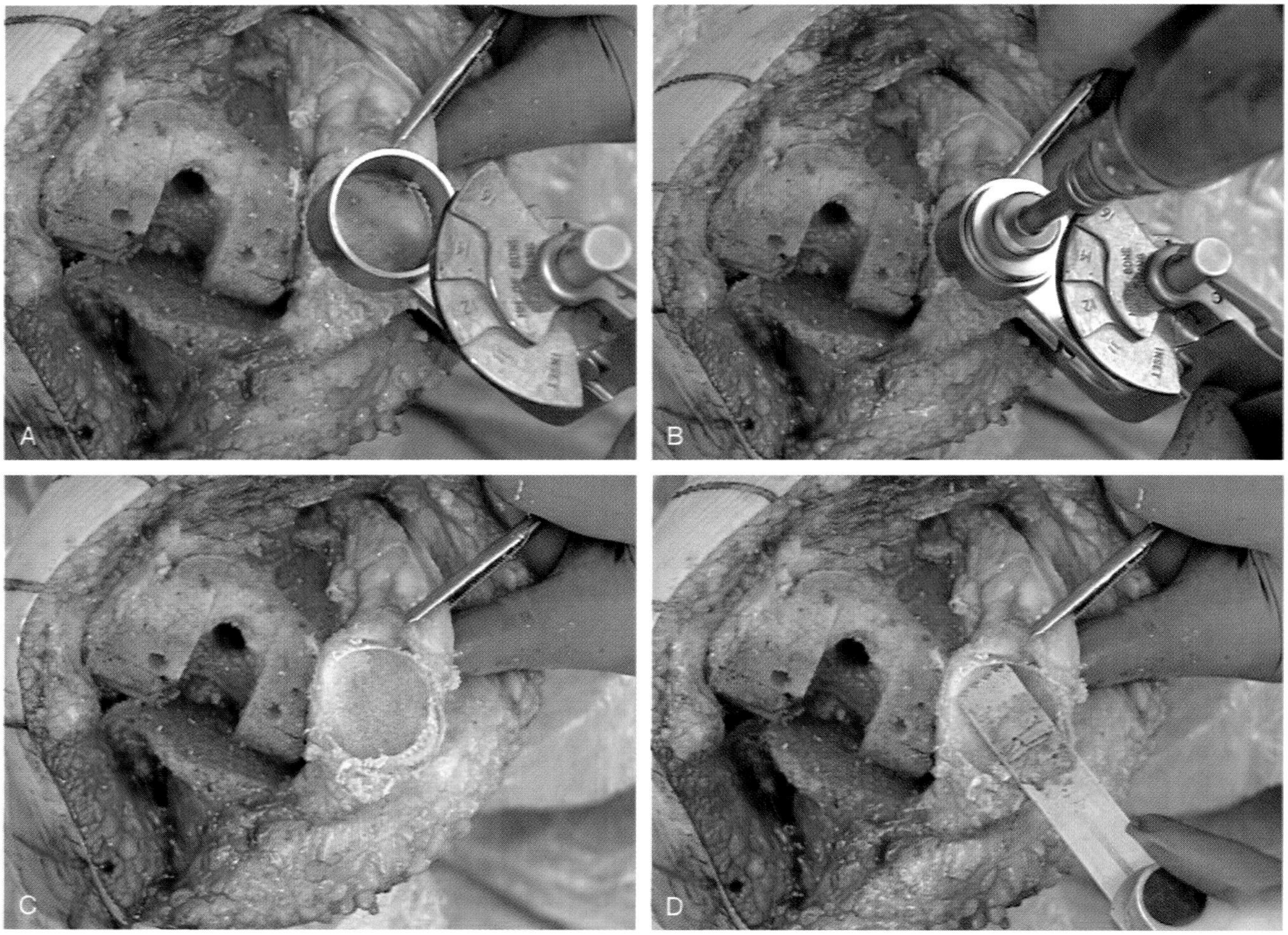

FIGURE 74.65 ➢ Although the reamer is traditionally used for insetting patellar components, it may also be used in creating an accurate flat cut for an onset component. *A,* Patellar clamp balanced on the patella. *B,* Reamer positioned within the clamp. *C,* Patella reamed to desired resection level. *D,* Resection completed with the saw blade.

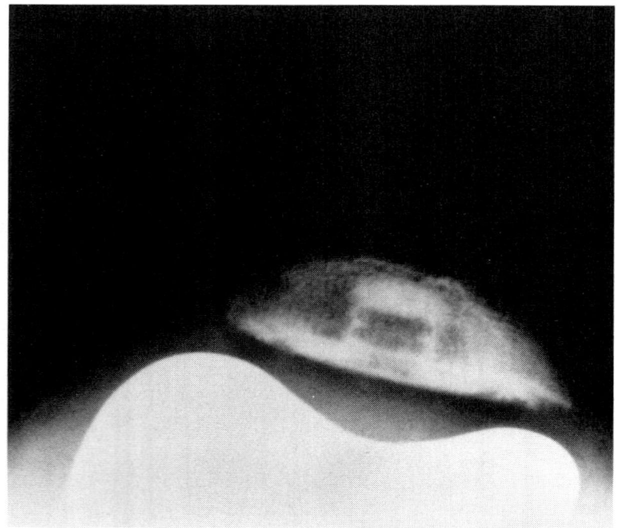

FIGURE 74.66 ➢ Radiograph showing a patellar component with "ideal" patellar tracking, orientation, and thickness.

omy; they attribute the low position to fibrosis around the patellar ligament.

Before final fixation of the components, we recommend an overall check of limb alignment using external, proximal, and distal landmarks.

MANAGEMENT OF INSTABILITY OR DEFORMITY

Principles

In most arthritic knees, some degree of instability, deformity, contracture, or a combination of these elements will be found.[22, 74] Moreover, even in knees without initial deformity, some change in alignment may be required (for example, in the patient who is habitually bowlegged). Although some minor degree of postoperative ligament asymmetry or laxity may be tolerated, it is better to obtain near-perfect stability through surgical technique.

Although several investigators have suggested that residual malalignment is not detrimental to the out-

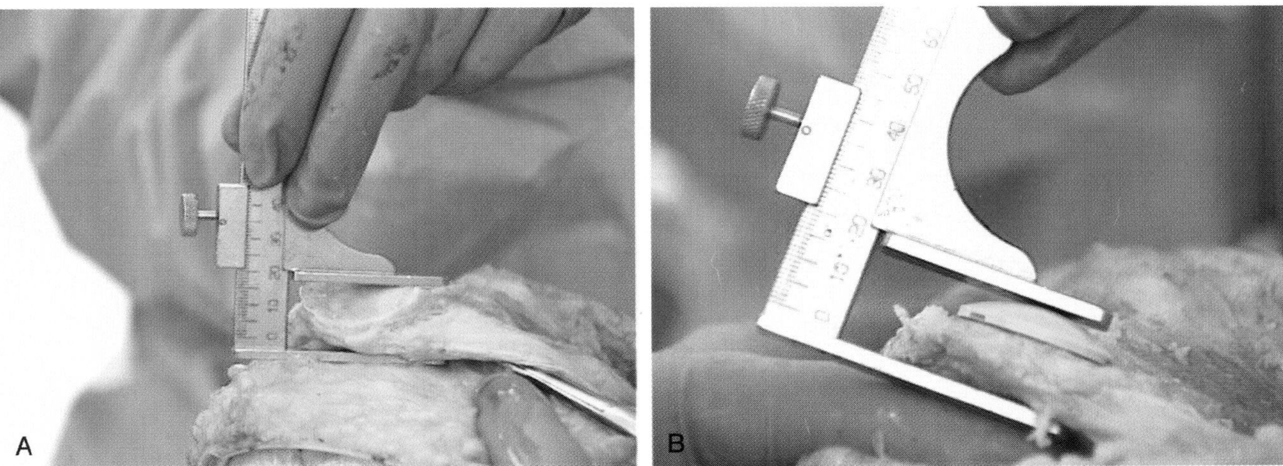

FIGURE 74.67 ➢ *A and B,* Caliber measurements of patella thickness should be made before and after patellar osteotomy. The thickness of the patella composite should not be increased; rather, a thickness of 2 to 3 mm less is preferred. Between 10 and 15 mm of patellar bone should remain.

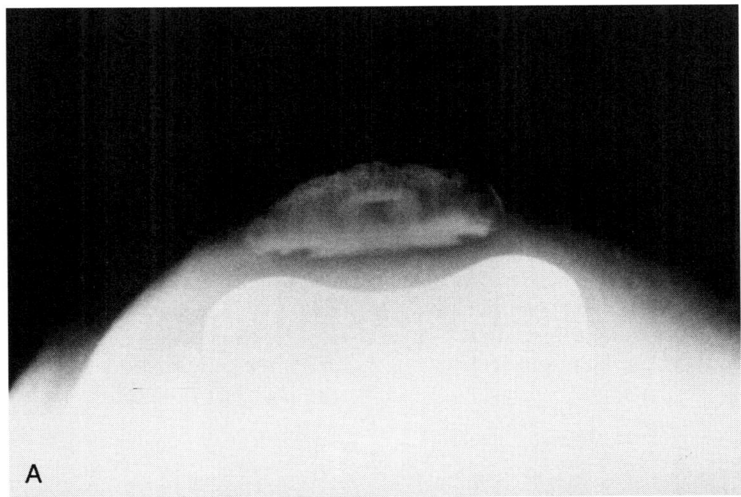

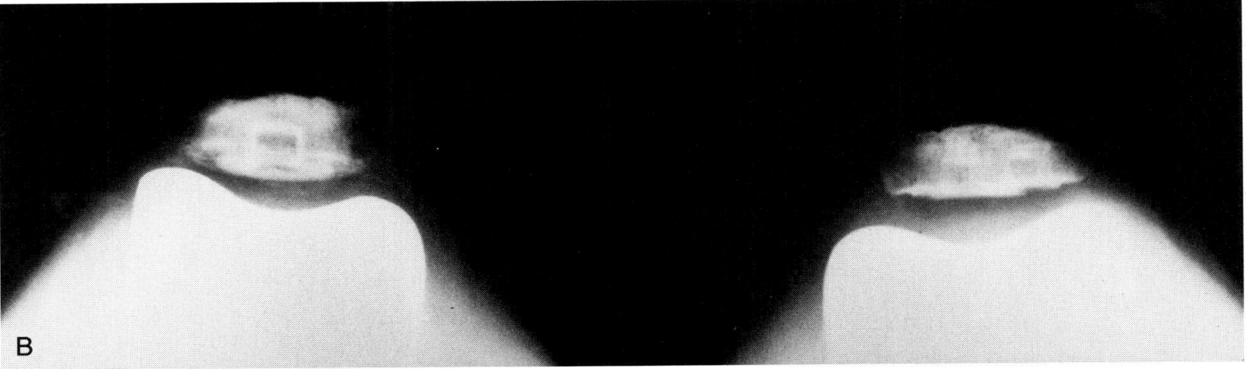

FIGURE 74.68 ➢ *A,* Merchant's view radiograph of a well-aligned and well-positioned polyethylene patellar implant. The thickness of the bone polyethylene composite restores the original thickness of the patellar bone. *B,* Patellar implants done some years apart. On the left, the patellar cut was made by eye and a single-peg patellar implant was used. The patella is too thick and the patellar osteotomy is not quite symmetric. On the right, the arthroplasty was done more recently, a slotted patellar cutting guide was used, and a three-peg patellar implant was inserted. Although there is a slight tilt, the patellar cut is symmetric and the patellar thickness is correct.

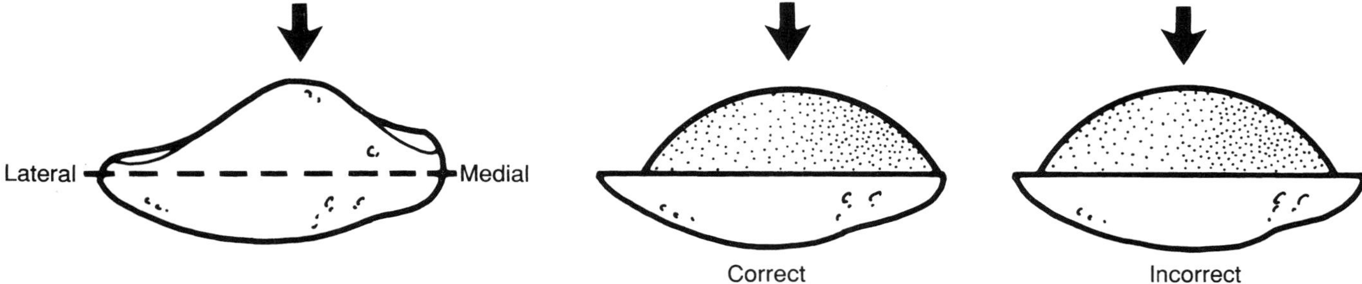

FIGURE 74.69 ➢ With a conventional patellar dome onset on the patella, the component should be medialized. This has the advantage of placing the apex of the dome in the correct position for patellar tracking but has the disadvantage of leaving peripheral lateral bone exposed.

come of TKA,[27, 43, 132, 148] other authors have demonstrated that malalignment has a negative influence on long-term results of TKA.[17, 63, 64, 73, 91, 107, 159, 171] These investigations suggest that the most important factor for maintaining satisfactory long-term outcome in TKA is anatomic alignment, which depends significantly on ligamentous balance. As early as 1977, Lotke et al[95] observed that the most favorable results are observed with femorotibial alignment in 3 to 7 degrees of valgus, the tibial component in neutral, and the femoral component in 4 to 6 degrees of valgus. Although the bone cuts can be made to establish anatomic alignment, proper ligamentous balance is required to maintain alignment in the dynamic state. In a polyethylene retrieval study, Wasielewski et al[161] noted that increased wear occurred when preoperative varus or valgus was present. Polyethylene wear and cold flow tended to be greater in the tightest prearthroplasty compartment. These observations were made despite correction of the lower extremity to the normal anatomic axis. However, the authors recognized that the majority of failures occurred when ligament releases were inadequate.

Instability of the arthritic knee may be viewed as being symmetric or asymmetric. Symmetric instability is a result of erosion of cartilage or bone without associated adaptive ligamentous changes. This type of deformity is common in early arthritis of the knee and is typically how the arthritic process begins. Standard surgical techniques and prosthesis spacing of TKA are typically adequate to restore ligamentous balance (Fig. 74.75). Asymmetric instability, common to advanced knee arthritis, occurs when bone and cartilage compromise are associated with adaptive ligamentous changes (Figs. 74.76 and 74.78). Standard surgical technique and prosthesis spacing prove inadequate in balancing asymmetric instability because of fixed ligamentous contractures.

Operative management of asymmetric instability and contracture cannot be accomplished by bone cuts alone. Although postoperative bracing has been described for the management of instability following TKA, it is seldom optimal. Two surgical methods, which can be used in isolation or in combination, have been described for correction of asymmetric instability: (1) controlled ligament release from the con-

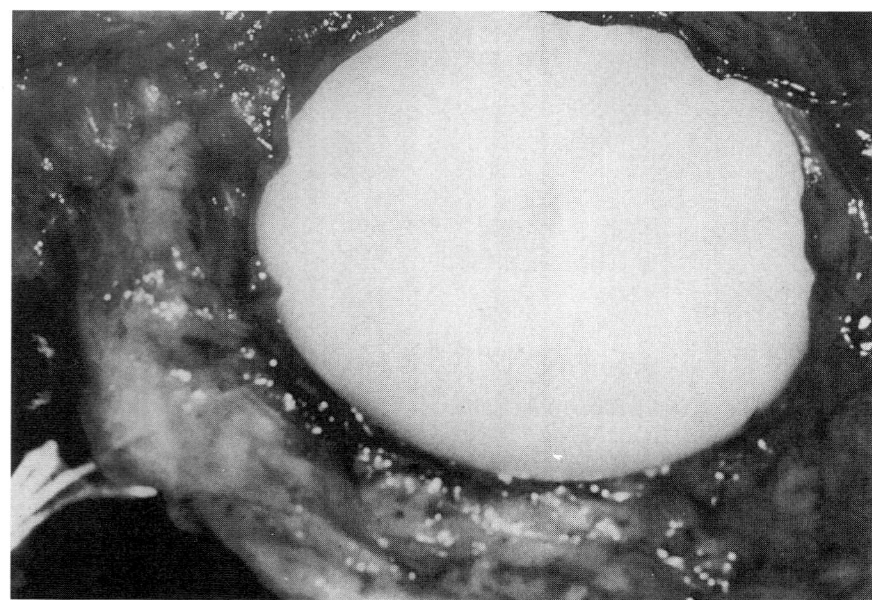

FIGURE 74.70 ➢ Insetting the patella allows greater thickness of polyethylene and use of metal backing. There is a rim of peripheral exposed bone that can impinge against the femur.

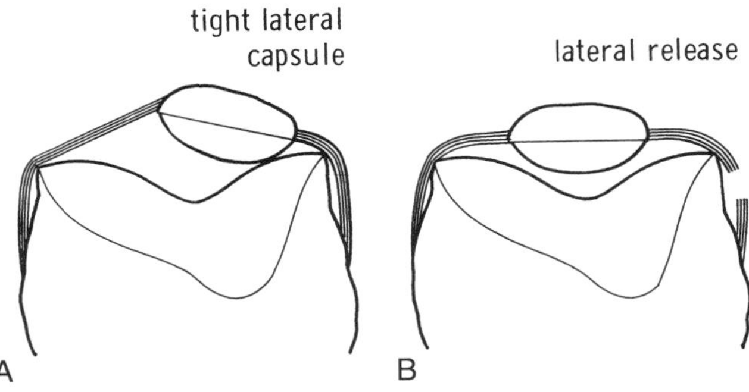

FIGURE 74.71 ➢ If the patella does not track smoothly without a tendency to displace, a lateral release is done.

tracted concave side of the deformity and (2) ligament advancement on the attenuated convex side. Ligament release of the contracted structures is adequate in correction of most deformities, although there are limits to the amount of correction that can be gained with ligament release. This is particularly true for valgus deformities where the amount of correction is restricted by the fear of stretching the peroneal nerve.

Every attempt should be made to balance the knee before increasing the constraint in TKA, especially in younger, active patients. When extreme deformity cannot be balanced with controlled ligament release, the options are as follows:

1. Correct and balance to the maximum degree, and then brace the knee for about 6 weeks postoperatively. This option applies only to fixed varus knees.
2. Reconstruct the elongated ligament. Krackow has described techniques for both medial and lateral reconstruction (discussed later).
3. Use a prosthetic device (such as a constrained condylar knee [CCK]) that provides for collateral ligament substitution (Figs. 74.79, 74.80, and 74.81).

Asymmetric Varus Instability

Pathophysiology

Development of asymmetric varus instability typically follows a common sequence. Loss of medial compartment bone and cartilage imparts a varus moment to the joint that ultimately results in pathological shortening of the MCL. The bony deficits typically occur on the medial tibial plateau, although both the medial tibia and the femur may be involved in advanced disease. The MCL contracture is worsened by medial osteoarthritic overgrowth that impinges on the ligament, thereby causing relative shortening. Eventually, the effect of contracture of the MCL is a fixed varus deformity (Fig. 74.77; see also Fig. 74.76). Simultaneously, adaptive changes occur in the LCL and capsule, resulting in attenuation of these lateral soft-tissue structures. This combination of elements results in a "lateral thrust" of the knee. Varus contracture may be associated with a flexion contracture (described later).

Varus deformity is defined by any preoperative femorotibial angle less than naturally occurring anatomic valgus. The definition is not absolute because of the variability of human limb alignment; in patients with habitual genu varum, this malalignment is typically exaggerated. Generally, TKA in patients with arthritis and habitual genu varum involves realignment to physiological valgus. Moderate to severe varus has been arbitrarily defined as greater than 15 to 20 degrees of varus deviation from the mechanical axis.[87, 155]

Management

PRINCIPLES

MCL release is essential to achieve soft balance in TKA with fixed varus deformity. Several authors have

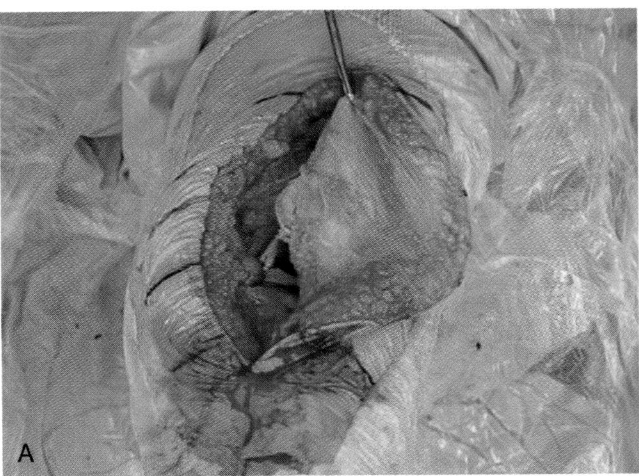

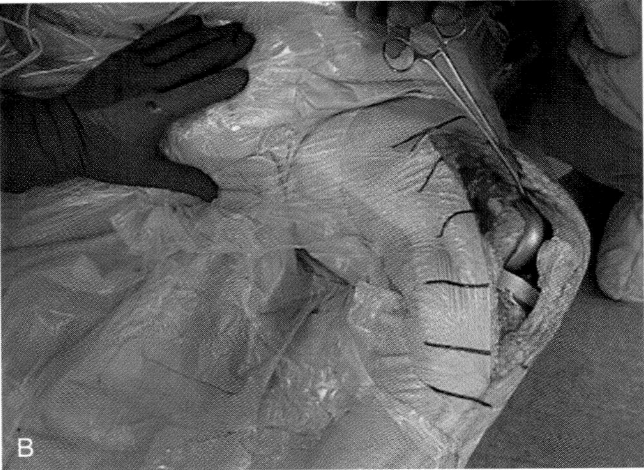

FIGURE 74.72 ➢ *A and B,* When assessing patellar traction, the "rule of no thumb" must be observed, but it is advisable to take longitudinal slack out of the extensor mechanism because, on bringing the knee from flexion into extension, the patellar ligament tends to buckle and can cause a misleading lateral tilt to the patella.

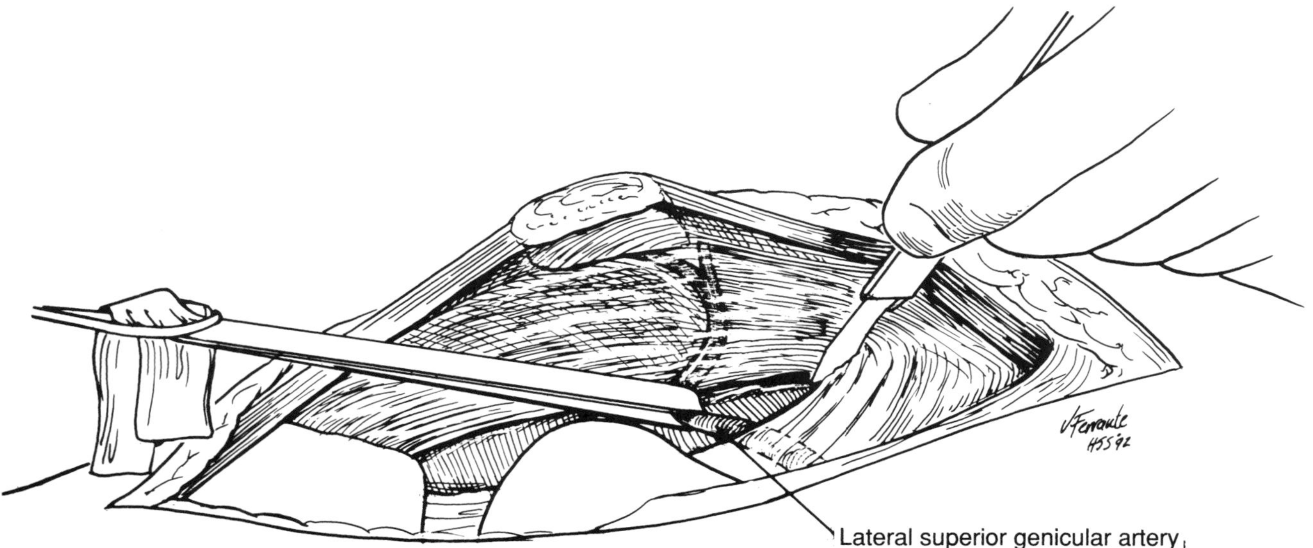

FIGURE 74.73 ➢ The patellar release is performed vertically about 1 in from the lateral border of the patella from inside out while retracting and preserving the lateral genicular vessels. The release may include the lower fibers of the vastus lateralis.

shown that residual varus deformity in TKA increases the failure rate.[17, 63, 64, 73, 91, 107, 159, 171] Wasielewski et al[161] observed increased posteromedial polyethylene wear in knees with preoperative varus deformity, especially if the medial release was inadequate. Sambatakakis et al[136] described a radiographic "wedge sign" characteristic of incompletely corrected varus deformity; this finding has been confirmed by Laskin[87] and correlates with our observations that the majority of failures occur because of medial tibial collapse.

Although some investigators have reported success with PCL balancing procedures in TKA with a fixed varus deformity,[155] other studies have demonstrated that moderate to severe varus deformity warrants PCL resection because of its contribution to varus malalignment. In fact, Alexiades et al[4] demonstrated that without the balance of the ACL, the PCL tends to contract. Laskin[87, 88] (Fig. 74.82) demonstrated that for fixed varus deformities exceeding 15 degrees, the best results in terms of pain relief, correction, and range of motion are obtained by excision of the PCL and use of a cruciate substituting prosthesis. Teeney et al[155] noted that 40% of knees with preoperative varus tended to remain in varus; their series included more than 50% of knees with cruciate retaining prostheses. Both Laskin[87] and Teeney et al[155] observed that functional outcome of varus knees approached but did not equal the results of nondeformed knees.

FIGURE 74.74 ➢ The lateral release is done obliquely to preserve the distal genicular arteries.

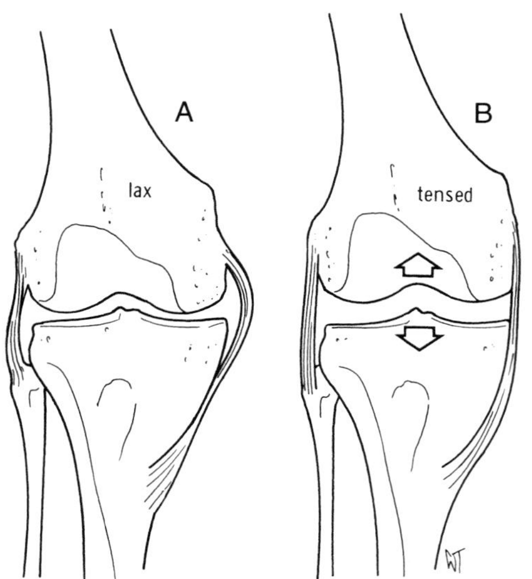

FIGURE 74.75 ➢ Symmetric instability. The ligaments, although lax, are of equal length. Both alignment and stability are restored by tensioning the ligaments.

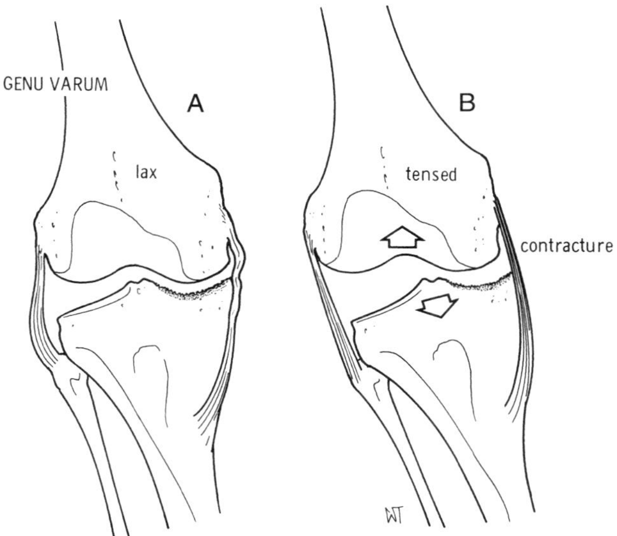

FIGURE 74.76 ➢ Asymmetric instability in varus. The medial ligament is shorter than the lateral ligament.

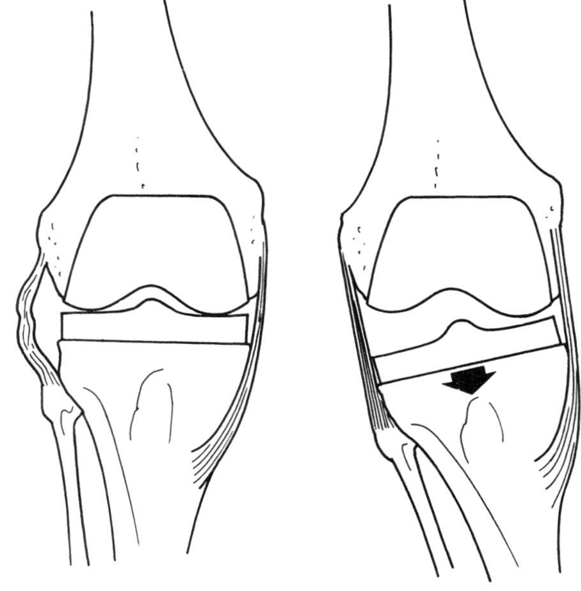

FIGURE 74.77 ➢ The medial ligament was not released; hence, an asymmetric instability remains.

TECHNIQUE

Ligament balance is achieved by progressively releasing the medial soft tissues until they reach the length of the lateral ligamentous structures. The extent of the release can be monitored by periodically inserting laminar spreaders (Fig. 74.83) and judging alignment with the aligning rod or plumb line. The endpoint of the release is a stable position in which a plumb line will extend from the hip through the center of the knee to the ankle joint. The cruciate ligaments, being in the center of the knee, usually retain approximately normal length regardless of alterations in the collateral ligaments and thus will not permit the stretching that is the objective of the release procedure. If the PCL is tethering the release, it should be excised or lengthened by a posterior release from the tibia. For techniques that use the prosthetic components themselves to test the balancing process, the ligament release will be done after the bone cuts and after insertion of the trial components; for cruciate substituting designs, the ligament releases will be done before the bone cuts or after the tibial cut has been made. The latter technique is preferable for very large deformities because the laxity in the knee joint after release may occasionally suggest the need for under-resection of the distal femur (Fig. 74.84). A full MCL release will not only correct fixed varus but also open the medial space in flexion (whereas the normal knee in flexion has more lateral than medial laxity). Although the flexion gap symmetry is influenced by the medial release, the femoral component rotational alignment is determined relative to the femoral anatomy and *not* by the ligament release.

The medial release (Fig. 74.85) is done by removing medial osteophytes from the femur and tibia, including the protruding flare of the tibial plateau, and raising a sleeve of soft tissue from the upper medial tibia that is allowed to slide proximally. The sleeve consists of periosteum, deep medial ligament, superficial medial ligament, and insertion of the pes anserinus tendons. More posteriorly, at the joint surface, the sleeve is continuous with the semimembranosus insertion and posterior capsule.

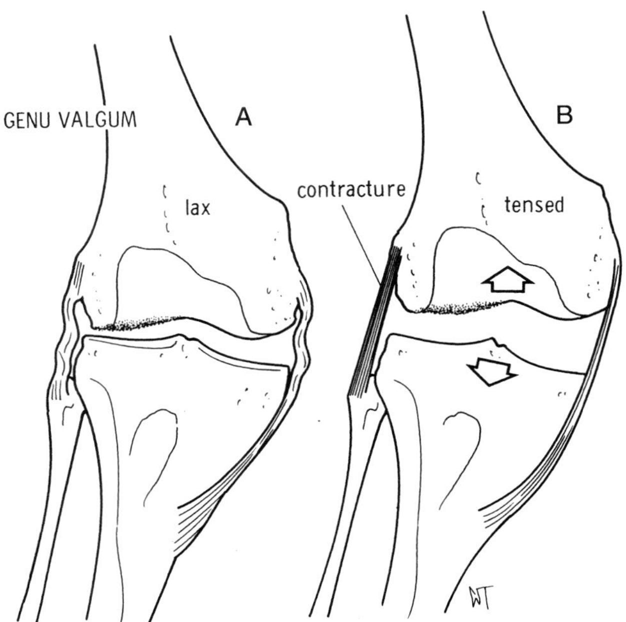

FIGURE 74.78 ➢ Asymmetric instability in valgus.

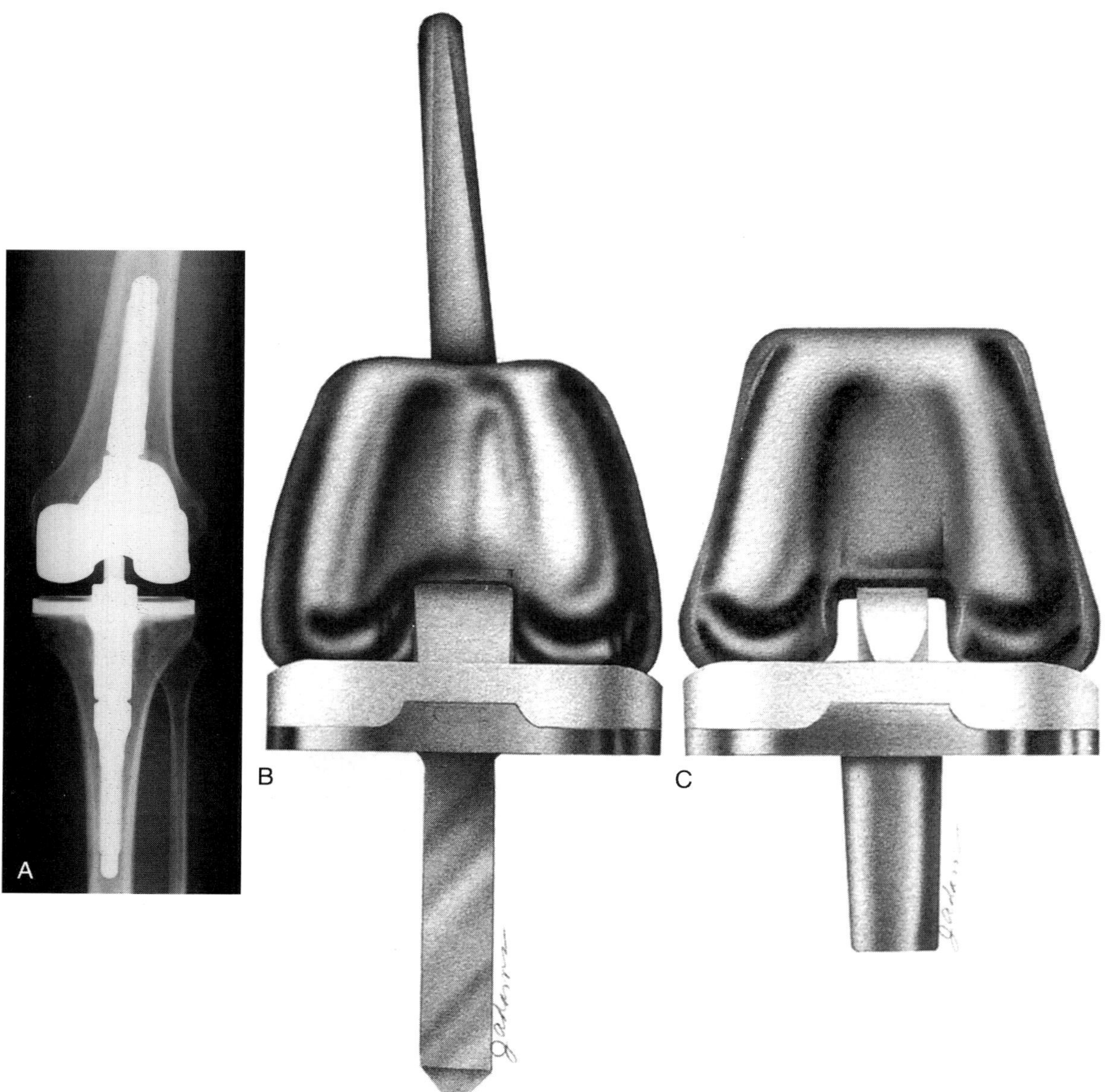

FIGURE 74.79 ➢ Constrained condylar knee prosthesis. *A*, Radiograph. *B*, The constrained condylar device is an unlinked constrained design that places limitations on varus-valgus deflection, anteroposterior displacement, and rotation within the flexion-extension axis of the knee. Restriction of varus-valgus deflection and rotation is provided by a large tibial spine within an intracondylar femoral box, while posterior subluxation is prevented by engagement of the spine on the femoral cam. *C*, Posterior stabilized device. Nonlinked, semiconstrained posterior stabilized devices prevent posterior subluxation via a tibial spine that engages a femoral cam. Slight rotational constraint is afforded by the degree of conformity of the femorotibial articulation. (*B* and *C*, from Scott WN: The Knee, vol 2. St. Louis, Mosby–Year Book, 1994, p 1308.)

Distally, the release may include the deep fascia investing soleus and popliteus muscles. The sleeve is made by stripping the periosteum medially from the tibia 10 to 15 cm distal to the standard arthrotomy. The knee is flexed, and the tibia is progressively externally rotated to gain posterior access. The distal attachment of the superficial medial ligament can be left intact initially; in moderate deformities this will be the extent of the release needed. When this is not enough, the release is continued posteriorly and distally by further subperiosteal stripping. Correction of deformity occurs in a graduated manner and is aided by the intermittent stretching action of a medial laminar spreader. With a progressive release, there is no discontinuity between the medial soft-tissue structures, but rather a progressive shredding of the periosteal layer at a point some way distal to the MCL attachment to the tibia (Fig. 74.86). The result is balancing, with some overall lengthening of the limb (the amount of lengthening depends on the degree of preoperative

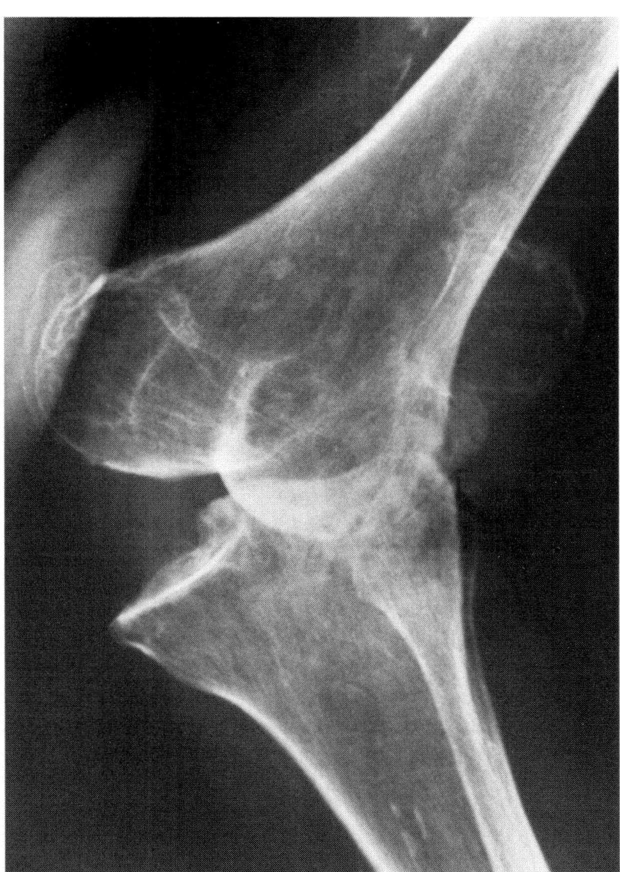

FIGURE 74.80 ➢ Radiograph of a very unstable valgus knee. This degree of ligamentous instability cannot be managed by any type of ligament release. Reconstruction will involve either a medial ligament tightening procedure or a constrained prosthesis.

stretching of the lateral structures). The released medial soft tissues ideally should give way imperceptibly rather than with an obvious "pop" (which indicates that the distal insertion of the ligament has been forcibly separated from its tibial attachment). To gain access with the laminar spreader, the proximal tibial osteotomy may be done first. When varus is combined with flexion contracture, it is helpful to divide transversely the medial portion of the posterior capsule; laterally the posterior capsule is often sufficiently stretched to prevent tethering. Posterior osteophytes should be removed, and it may be necessary to make posterior femoral cuts to gain access to do this. The occasional need for under-resection of the femur should be carefully judged, because it is wise to be conservative about the amount of bone resection; the distal femur can always be recut.

As stated earlier, the ideal postoperative alignment with regard to prosthetic placement and function is independent of the original anatomy. In a patient who has always been bowlegged and has later developed unilateral osteoarthritis, it is not sufficient to match the alignment of the replaced knee with that of the opposite "normal" (which in this case means varus) knee. Whatever the original appearance may have been, the relationship of hip, knee, and ankle must be correct after prosthetic replacement (femorotibial alignment of 6 to 7 degrees). Otherwise, the prosthetic components will be unequally loaded and subjected to excessive stress.

At the completion of a varus release, the limb is already aligned in the proper position. No further correction is needed, and the bone cuts can be made in a standard manner to place the components in position. After insertion of components of the correct size, the knee should be fully stable and not require immobilization because of the release. Motion can be started immmediately, and walking with full weightbearing is permitted as tolerated.

Ligament advancement procedures have also been described to correct varus deformity.[155] We have found that essentially all deformity can be corrected with ligament releases in posterior stabilized TKA without resorting to ligament reconstruction procedures. However, we acknowledge that limits to ligament release procedures exist. When varus knees cannot be fully corrected with medial release and are associated with lateral laxity, consideration may be

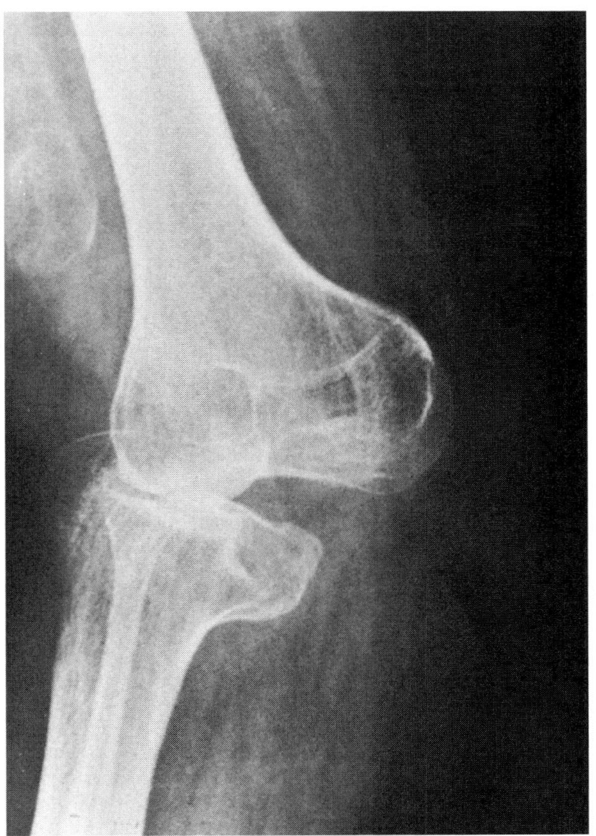

FIGURE 74.81 ➢ In this valgus knee, although the medial ligament is not absent, it is so elongated that soft-tissue balancing by lateral release is impractical. This is an indication for a constrained prosthesis.

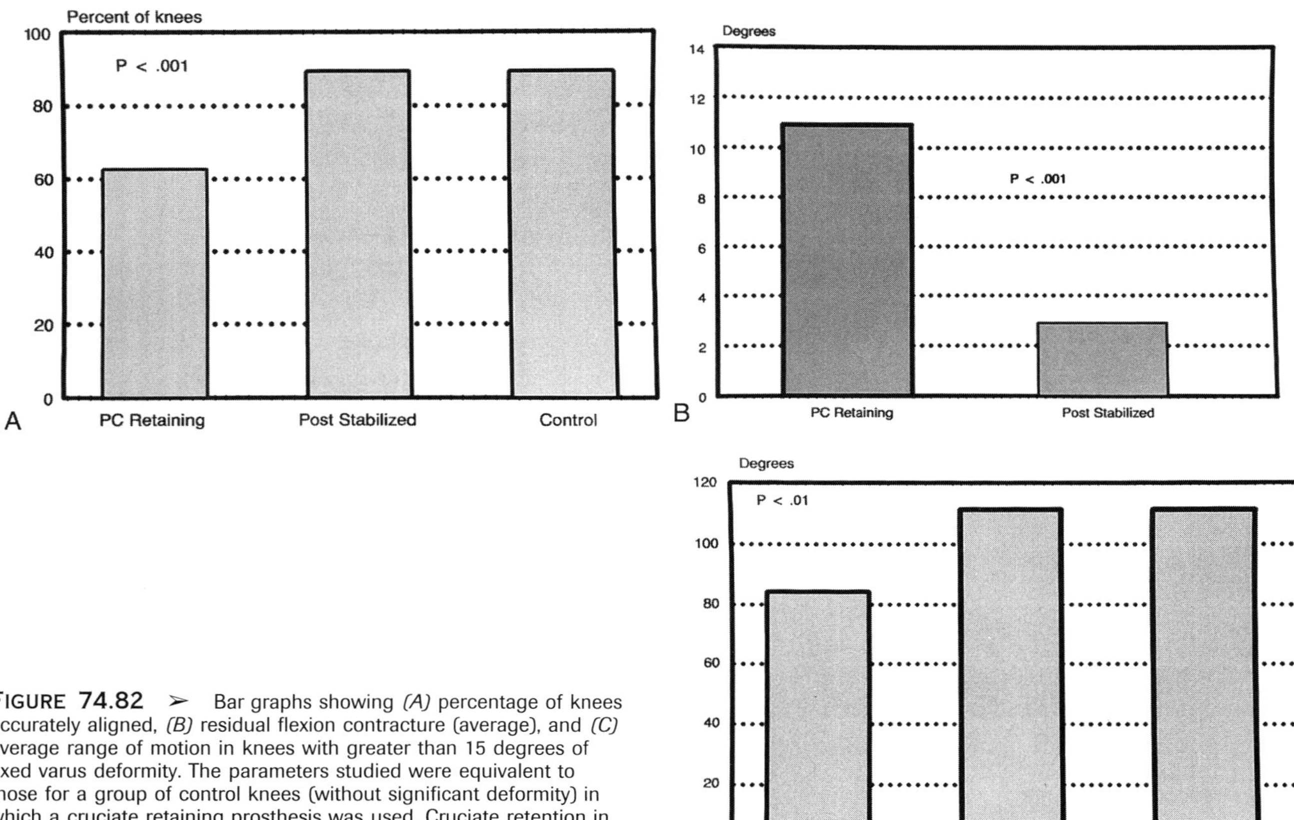

FIGURE 74.82 ➢ Bar graphs showing *(A)* percentage of knees accurately aligned, *(B)* residual flexion contracture (average), and *(C)* average range of motion in knees with greater than 15 degrees of fixed varus deformity. The parameters studied were equivalent to those for a group of control knees (without significant deformity) in which a cruciate retaining prosthesis was used. Cruciate retention in deformed knees led to a less satisfactory correction of alignment and flexion contracture and an inferior range of motion.

given to lateral ligament reconstruction (as discussed later).

Asymmetric Valgus Instability

Pathophysiology

In the valgus knee, the lateral soft-tissue structures, including the LCL, ITB, and lateral capsule, contract while the medial soft tissues become stretched. The lateral femoral condyle has been shown to be dysplastic in the valgus deformity, and therefore most of the bony deficit occurs on the femoral side.[150] However, in advanced disease, cartilage and bone erosion may be observed on the tibial side as well. In long-standing deformity, the lateral contracture and medial lengthening become permanent (see Fig. 74.78). This combination of elements may result in a "medial thrust." As for varus deformities, valgus contractures may be associated with a flexion contracture; however, presumably because of the contracture of the ITB, a fixed external rotation deformity often accompanies asymmetric valgus instability, particularly in patients with inflammatory arthritis.

Valgus deformity is defined as malalignment exceeding natural femorotibial valgus orientation, typically greater than 7 to 10 degrees.[104, 150, 165] Krackow classified valgus deformity into three distinct types.[85] Type I involves lateral femoral bone loss, lateral soft-tissue contracture, and intact medial soft tissues. Type II is type I with lengthened medial soft tissues. Type III is a severe valgus deformity with malpositioning of the proximal tibial joint line (e.g., secondary to high tibial osteotomy).

Management

PRINCIPLES

Valgus release has traditionally been performed by elevating the lateral capsule, LCL, arcuate ligament, popliteus tendon, lateral femoral periosteum, distal ITB, and adjacent lateral intermuscular septum from their bony attachments. Except for the ITB, the release is performed from the lateral femoral condyle; the ITB is released from Gerdy's tubercle. Because desired postoperative alignment is physiological valgus, some degree of lateral laxity after an extensive lateral release is typically well tolerated. The sequence of lateral release has been the focus of some controversy.[1, 15, 79, 90, 104, 150, 165] We have traditionally managed lesser deformities with simple release of the ITB from its insertion on Gerdy's tubercle (Fig. 74.87). For moderate to severe fixed deformities, we formerly stripped the lateral femoral condyle of its soft-tissue attachments proximally for about 9 cm and at this level divided the

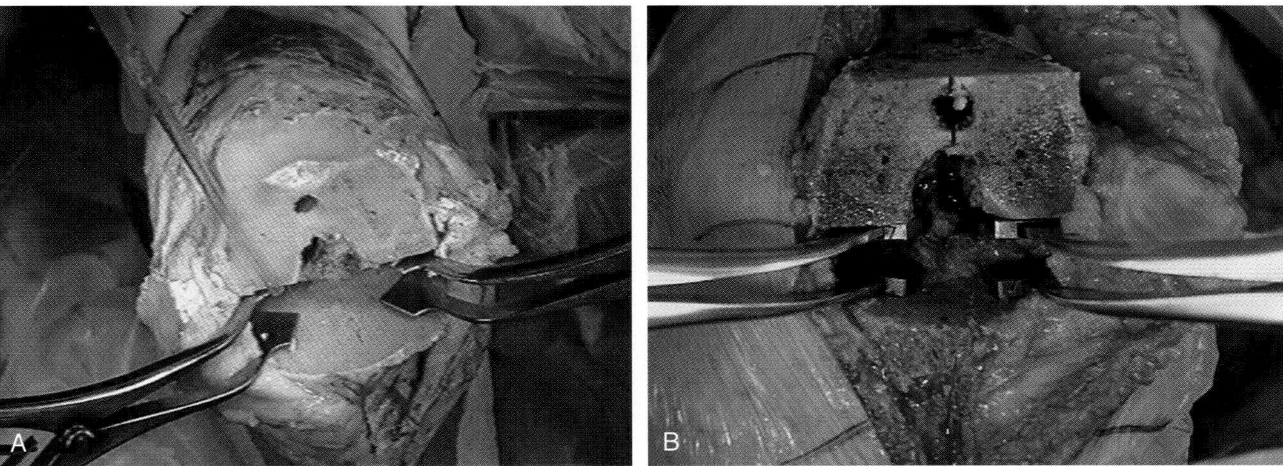

FIGURE 74.83 ➢ *A and B,* Laminar spreaders are useful in monitoring soft-tissue balance and the performance of ligament releases.

periosteum, the iliotibial tract, and the lateral intramuscular septum transversely from inside out (Figs. 74.88 and 74.89). Any part of the lateral intramuscular septum that remained attached to the distal femur was divided longitudinally until the entire "flap" was free to slide. Although such an extensive release generally corrects any severity of deformity, posterolateral flexion instability may occur postoperatively.[70, 104] Furthermore, case reports exist in which extensive soft-tissue stripping has devascularized the lateral femoral condyle, resulting in osteonecrosis.

Because of the risk of posterolateral instability (and osteonecrosis) following extensive soft-tissue stripping from the lateral femoral condyle, "stab-incision"[104] and "pie-crusting" (our preference) techniques have been developed. These techniques permit a graduated intra-articular release of the posterolateral capsule and ITB. Although both techniques involve transverse punctures (pie-crusting) of the ITB well above the joint line and some degree of transverse release of the posterolateral capsule, the stab-incision technique includes a more extensive transverse release of the arcuate complex immediately above the joint line and posterior to the ITB (Fig. 74.90). Releasing at the joint line leaves only the LCL for lateral restraint; perforations of the lateral capsule and ITB above the joint line in combination with a limited transverse posterolateral capsular release maintain greater soft-tissue continuity. Both techniques typically allow for preservation of the popliteus tendon, affording greater stability to the posterolateral corner. Whereas Miyasaka et al[104] observed a 24% incidence of posterolateral instability with extensive lateral femoral condylar release for valgus deformity, by using the stab-incision technique they limited the incidence to 6%. In our experience with the pie-crusting technique, we have had a similar reduction in the incidence of posterolateral instability.

Correction of valgus deformity in TKA has been associated with patellofemoral instability and peroneal palsy. The incidence of patellofemoral instability has been reported to be as high as 4%[90]; however, the incidence using the stab-incision technique and preserving the popliteus has been reported as 0%.[104] Although the overall incidence of peroneal nerve palsy after TKA has been estimated as less than 1%, the incidence in valgus knees has been reported at 3% to 4%.[85, 150] In the most recent investigation using the stab-incision technique, no cases of peroneal nerve compromise were observed.[104]

In elderly patients or those with low physical demands, the use of a CCK may avoid postoperative morbidity. In our small series of primary CCK implants (with up to 10 years of follow-up), there has been uniform success without prosthetic loosening (Insall,

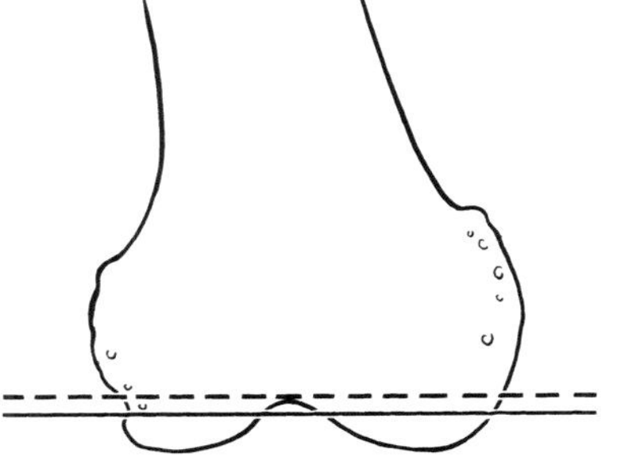

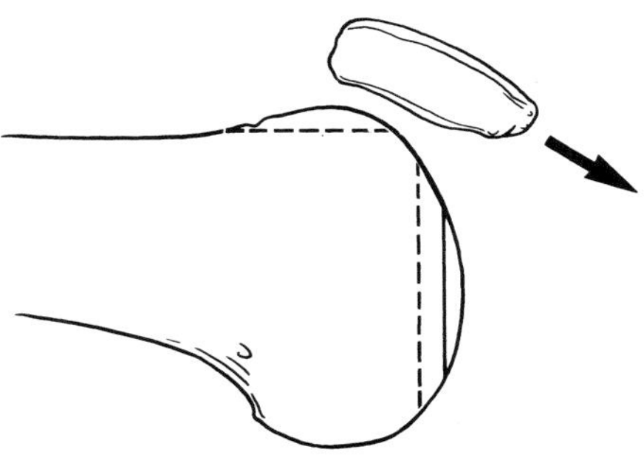

FIGURE 74.84 ➢ In cases with considerable ligamentous laxity, an under-resection of the distal femur may be preferable. The standard femoral resection will necessitate a thicker tibial component to take up the slack in the soft tissues and may cause distal migration of the patella. By under-resecting the femur, desirable patellar position is maintained.

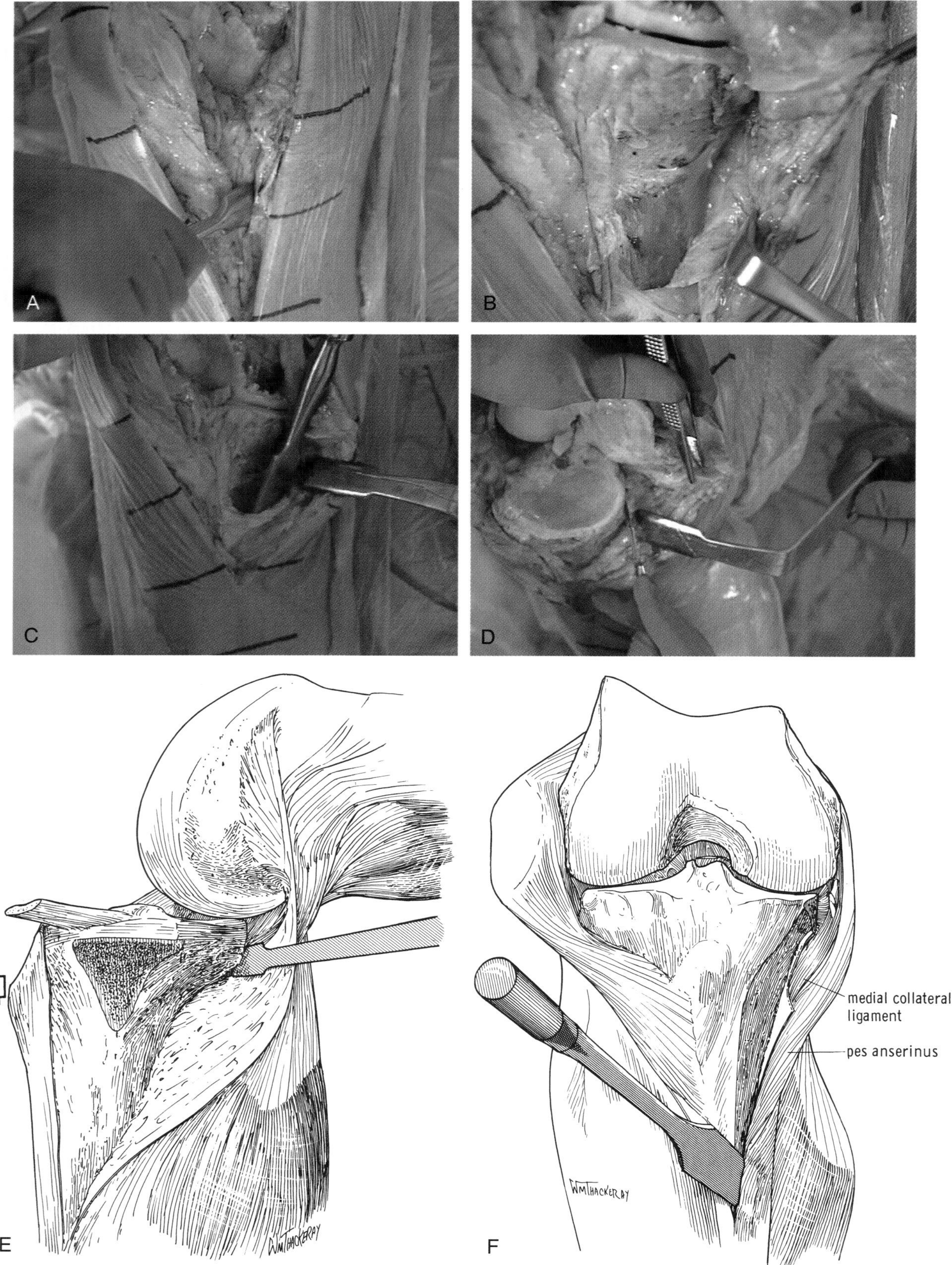

FIGURE 74.85 ➢ Varus release. *A and B,* The exposure is begun by subperiosteal stripping beneath the superficial medial collateral ligament. *C,* Completed release. Only the superficial medial collateral ligament remains intact, but this too can be detached if necessary. *D,* The tibia is externally rotated with a complete posteromedial release.

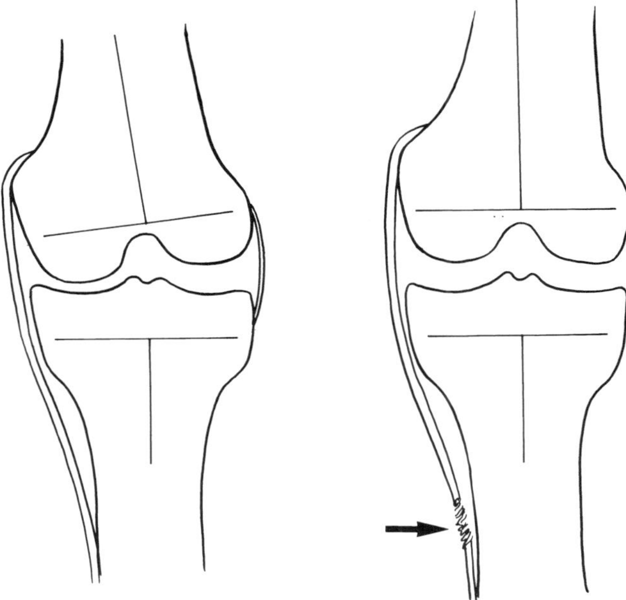

FIGURE 74.86 ➢ The ideal medial collateral ligament (MCL) release occurs distal to the insertion of the ligament into the tibia through the periosteum and in continuity with the MCL. At this level, a controlled release is obtained.

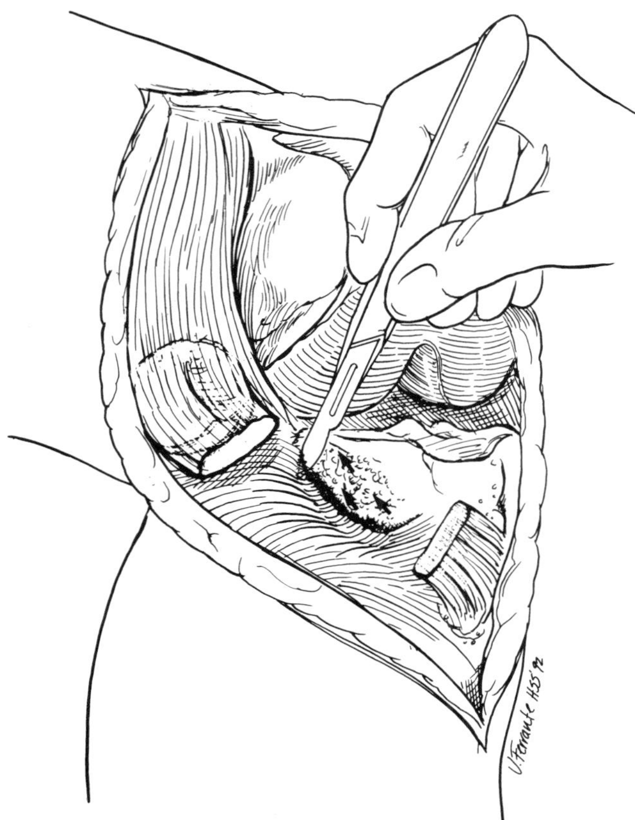

FIGURE 74.87 ➢ First stage of a lateral release. The iliotibial band is separated from its attachment to Gerdy's tubercle and the capsular attachments from the lateral margin of the tibia.

unpublished data). Although we do not recommend indiscriminate use of the CCK, our experience suggests that this implant may be a reasonable option in selected cases.

TECHNIQUE

Pie-Crusting Method (Insall)

First, bone cuts are made to gain access and to create congruent surfaces to assess gap symmetry. Because erosion occurs on the lateral femoral condyle in long-standing valgus malalignment, relatively more bone should be resected from the medial femoral condyle. Appropriate femoral rotation is imperative to ensure proper balancing in flexion. Although the PCL can be preserved, we favor posterior stabilized designs that avoid the need for PCL balancing techniques. Furthermore, the PCL often contributes to the deformity and requires resection to appropriately balance the knee.[70, 104] The posterolateral capsule and arcuate complex lateral to the popliteus are cut transversely at the level of the tibial cut, and titrated intra-articular and extra-articular releases of the lateral capsule and the ITB are performed using a knife blade. The technique is performed with a moderate amount of stress in the lateral compartment using a laminar spreader or the help of an assistant. Multiple stab incisions are made in the contracted lateral soft tissues (particularly the ITB) within and above the joint until the deformity is corrected (see Fig. 74.90A, B). Spacer blocks are used to frequently check the balance to avoid overcorrection. As noted above, the popliteus and the LCL are preserved if possible to limit posterolateral instability. The technique of ligament advancement will be described later.

Correction Through a Lateral Parapatellar Approach (Keblish)

In our experience, valgus deformity can be adequately corrected using a medial parapatellar approach; however, Keblish[79] and Buechel[17] have described a three-step lateral release through a lateral parapatellar approach. The tibial tubercle is osteotomized and reflected medially, retaining a medial periosteal hinge. The infrapatellar fat pad is maintained on the patellar tendon to facilitate closing of the lateral retinacular defect. The three steps of lateral release are as follows:

1. The anterior compartment musculature and the iliotibial tract are elevated from Gerdy's tubercle to the level of the fibular head. The amount of correction is tested at this point.
2. With the knee flexed to 90 degrees, the LCL and the popliteus are elevated as a subperiosteal flap based proximately on the lateral femoral shaft. If needed, the entire periosteum is elevated. If the peroneal nerve is observed to sublux, then the fibular head is resected.
3. With the knee maintained at 90 degrees of flexion, the entire periosteum of the fibular head is

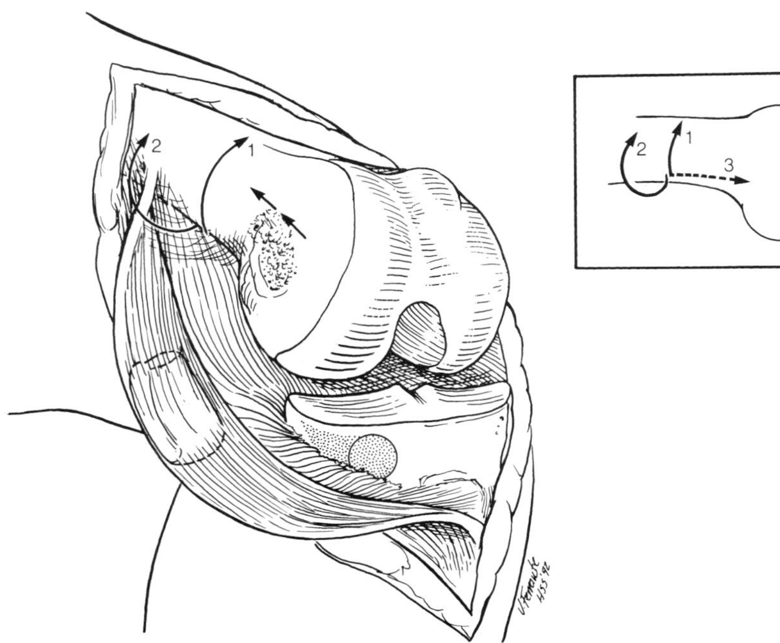

FIGURE 74.88 ➢ *A*, Further stages of lateral release include raising a flap from the lateral femoral condyle to a point 3 in proximal to the joint. *B*, The periosteum is incised transversely *(1)*; the lateral intramuscular septum and proximal iliotibial tract are divided transversely at the same level *(2)*; and the remaining distal attachment of the lateral intramuscular septum is divided vertically and separated from the femur *(3)*.

elevated while the peroneal nerve at the fibular neck is protected, and the fibular head is resected. The extension position of the peroneal nerve is checked to ensure that the nerve is situated in the space created by femoral head resection.

As emphasized by Buechel,[16] lateral instability that occurs with extensive lateral release is corrected with compensatory femoral component external rotation. Although this may create patellofemoral malalignment in extension, the associated lateral retinacular release typically eliminates this problem.

Flexion Contracture

Pathophysiology

Flexion contractures involve the posterior capsule, the PCL, and the musculotendinous units crossing the posterior aspect of the knee joint. In osteoarthritis, the deformity is typically limited to soft-tissue contracture with minimal posterior bone involvement (Fig. 74.91), whereas in inflammatory arthritis, it may result in significant posterior femoral condylar erosion. In fact, the erosion may be so much more extensive posteriorly than distally that the distal femur resembles a "chicken drumstick" when viewed on lateral radiographs (Fig. 74.92). Extreme posterior femoral condylar erosion generally occurs in patients who have been unable to walk for years and have spent most of their time in wheelchairs, resulting in fixed flexion deformities that may exceed 90 degrees. Because of posterior condylar erosion, in addition to posterior capsular contracture, flexion contracture may be paradoxically associated with flexion instability. This situation represents a considerable technical challenge and typically warrants application of revision TKA principles.

Flexion contractures may be classified according to severity; however, the system is somewhat arbitrary. Mild-to-moderate deformity is typically reported to be less than 20 degrees, whereas severe deformity exceeds 30 degrees; the purpose of establishing a distinction is to decide when greater distal femoral resection is required to correct the deformity, which is generally classified as a severe deformity.

Several authors have suggested that full intraoperative correction of flexion contractures in TKA is not essential because postoperative correction is possible[49, 102, 154] and clinical outcome is not affected by residual flexion contractures of up to 30 degrees.[102, 156] However, we have not found this to be the case and support current consensus among knee surgeons that flexion contractures should be completely corrected at the time of TKA. We agree with Firestone et al[49] that if a flexion contracture remains at the completion of TKA, then the residual deformity will persist and worsen with time, especially if the PCL is preserved.

TECHNIQUE

Small flexion contractures can be reduced by removal of posterior osteophytes and elevation of the posterior capsule (Fig. 74.93).[154, 156] Correction by bone resection alone unbalances the collateral ligaments so that stability in extension is provided by the tight posterior capsule. This clearly results in kinematic abnormalities. Posterior capsulotomy is the preferred method for moderate-to-severe contractures and should be performed with the knee flexed. The shortened posterior capsule is first elevated from the central posterior aspect of the femoral calcar. Next, the medial and lateral capsule is cut transversely with a curved-on-flat osteotome or with a knife if the capsule is too thick. In severe cases, the capsule must be separated from the collateral structures by making ver-

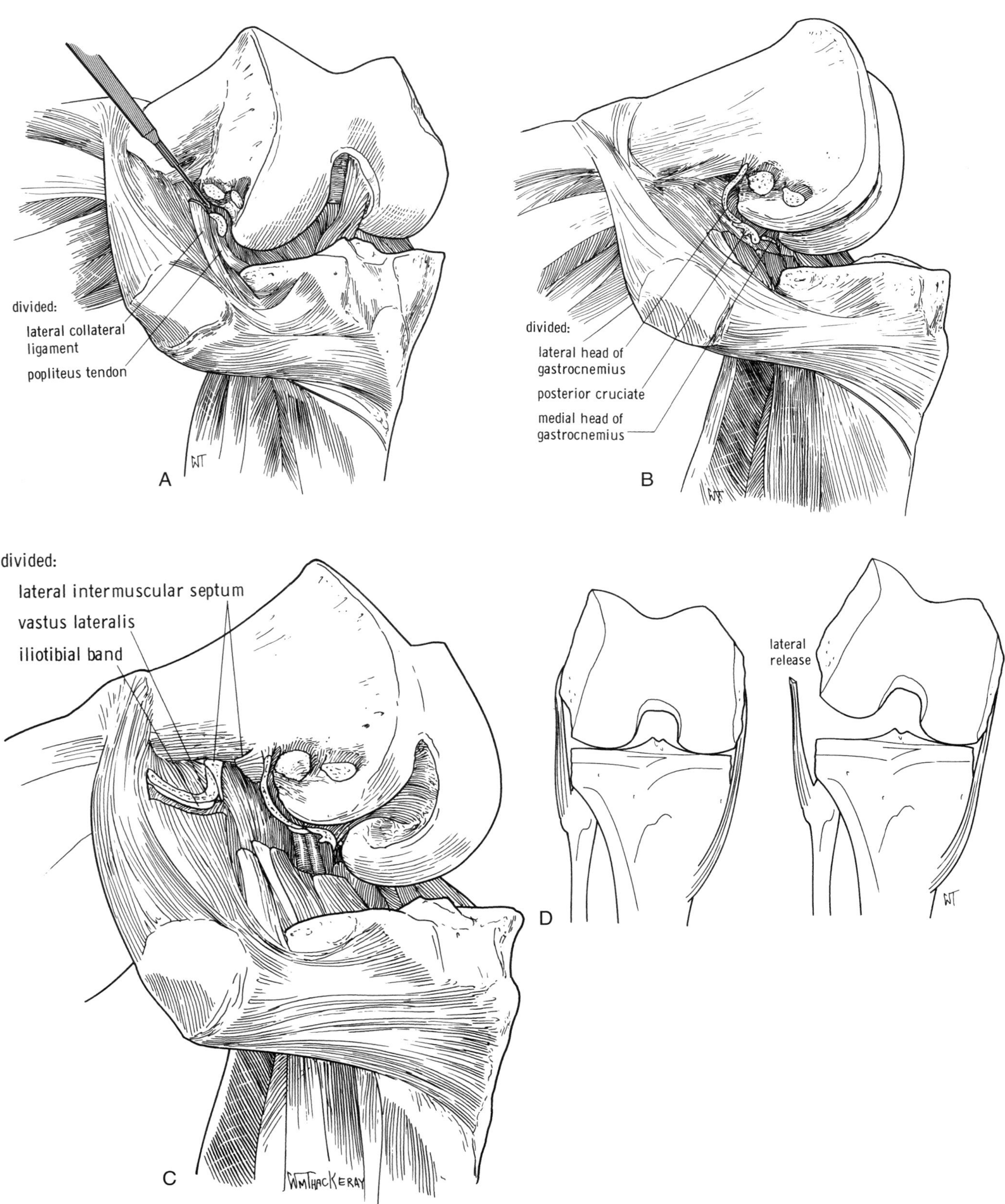

FIGURE 74.89 ➢ *A–C,* Valgus release is done on the femur, completely releasing the soft tissues from the lateral femoral condyle and, if necessary, transversely dividing the iliotibial band. *D,* After lateral release for the correction of valgus, the knee is always inherently unstable in flexion. A lateral rotary instability may develop that will be exacerbated if there is any malrotation of the tibial component.

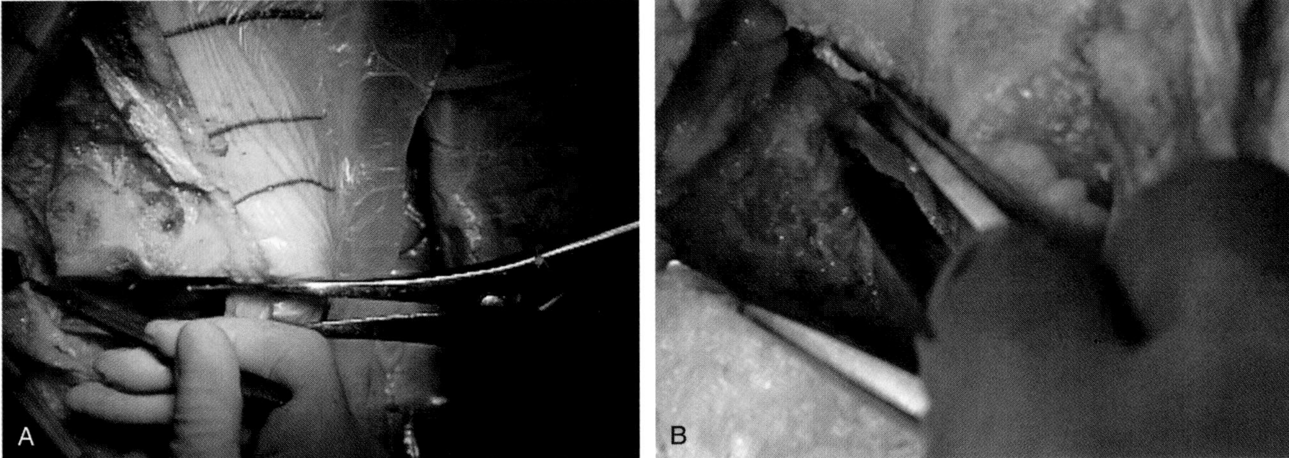

FIGURE 74.90 ➢ Intraoperative photo of lateral release using the "pie-crusting" technique. *A,* Joint distracted using a laminar spreader placed medially. *B,* Close-up view of multiple intra-articular punctures in the contracted lateral soft tissues proximal to the joint line.

tical incisions at the medial and lateral corners. Resection of the PCL is most likely necessary and aids in the division of the midline fibers. Posterior capsular release should be done after the bone cuts because until they are made, posterior visualization is poor and impeded by the posterior femoral condyles. Initially, distal femoral and proximal tibial bone cuts should be conservative. After the capsulotomy, the components are inserted and the knee brought into as much extension as possible. If extension is still not complete, further bone can be removed from the distal femur. This procedure may require use of a constrained prosthesis when the collateral ligaments are removed from their origins because extreme cases may require resection of so much bone that the knee becomes completely unbalanced. We no longer recommend postoperative splinting and now favor aggressive range of motion with an emphasis on extension in the immediate postoperative period.

Extension Contracture ("Stiff Knee")

Overview

Primary TKA in stiff and ankylosed knees, although technically demanding, has been shown to provide excellent pain relief and significantly improved range of motion.[2, 105, 109] Stiff knees are typically defined as having less than 50 degrees of motion, while ankylosed knees have essentially no motion (Fig. 74.94). In the largest reported series, Montgomery et al[105] studied 82 stiff or ankylosed knees in 71 patients at an average follow-up of 5.3 years. The investigators noted an average Hospital for Special Surgery (HSS) knee score improvement of from 38 to 80 points and an average arc of motion improvement of from 36 degrees to 93 degrees. All prostheses were posterior stabilized, with the majority being nonconstrained. Only one quadricepsplasty was necessary. Two patients with flexion-

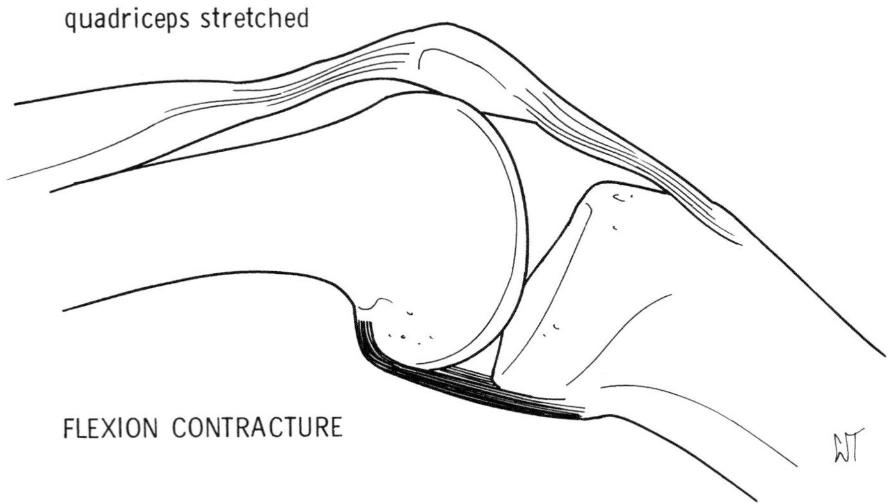

FIGURE 74.91 ➢ In a flexion contracture, the posterior capsule is shortened and adherent.

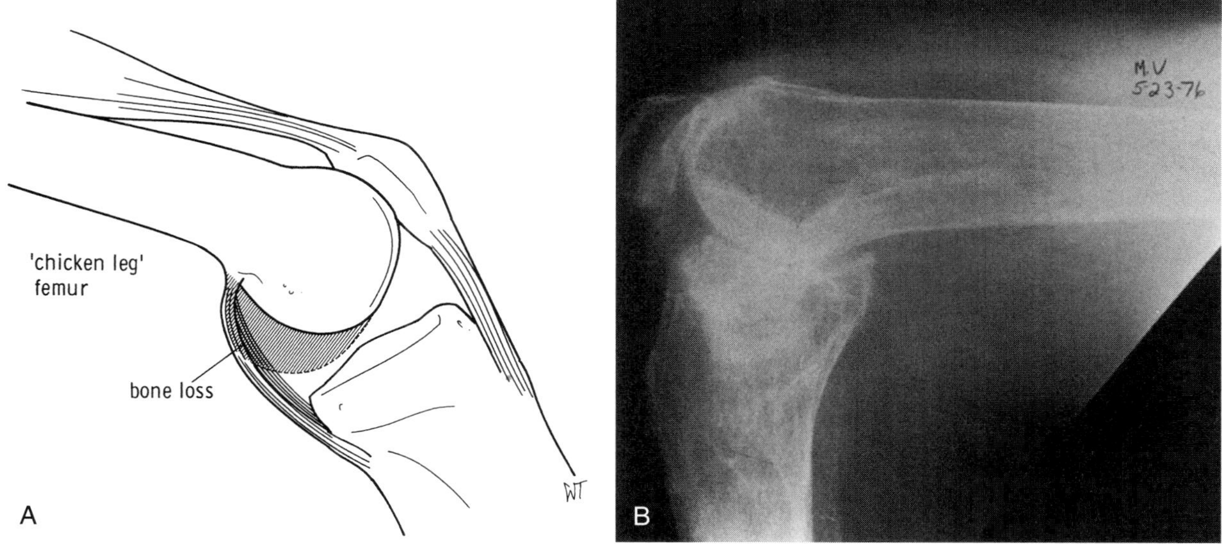

FIGURE 74.92 ➢ *A,* In rheumatoid arthritis, there is excessive loss of bone on the posterior aspect of the femoral condyles. *B,* Lateral radiograph showing this condition. Unless the technique recognizes and adjusts for it, flexion instability will result.

valgus deformities developed peroneal nerve palsies that resolved spontaneously, and one patient had an inferior pole of the patella fracture managed conservatively. This investigation is reflective of previous, smaller series,[2, 109] although one series reported that quadricepsplasty was required in 42% of cases.

TECHNIQUE

Our technique is described in a series by Montgomery et al.[105] The approach is made using a midline longitudinal incision and medial parapatellar arthrotomy. Typically, the techniques described in "Difficult Exposures" are necessary. Eversion of the patella is generally challenging. Early release of the lateral retinaculum and lateral patellofemoral ligaments is commonly performed. Soft-tissue releases are performed in the same fashion as they are for the varus, valgus, and flexion deformities described above; however, extensive soft-tissue releases are routinely required. In varus knees, an extensile proximal medial tibial release is performed, whereas valgus knees are managed with lateral release, including that of the LCL. Flexion contractures require posterior capsule release; because of its contribution to contractures, we favor routine excision of the PCL. Occasionally, complete subperiosteal reflection of the soft tissues from the distal femur (femoral peel) is necessary (see Fig. 74.39). Adequate bone cuts are then performed to create balanced flexion and extension gaps. Despite extensive releases, constrained prostheses are not typically required unless ligament stability is forfeited.

Ligament Advancement or Tightening

It should now be obvious that there are limits to ligament release procedures. For example, in the correction of a valgus knee, a lateral ligament release may

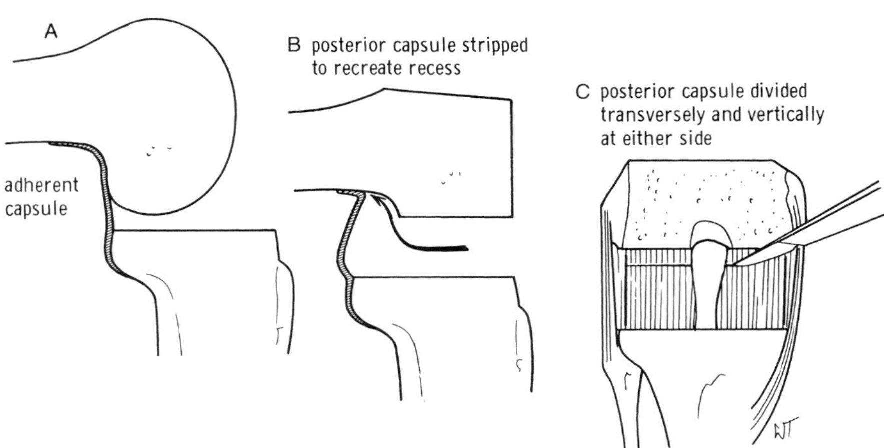

FIGURE 74.93 ➢ Posterior capsulotomy for flexion contracture. *A,* The posterior capsule is adherent. *B,* The original recess is reestablished. *C,* The cruciate ligaments have already been excised; only the medial and lateral parts of the posterior capsule need division. Often the underlying gastrocnemii are adherent and must be divided as well. At the margin of the collateral ligaments, vertical incisions in the capsule must be made.

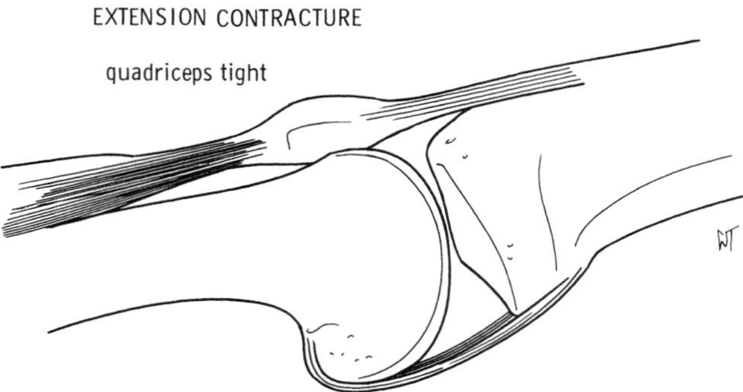

FIGURE 74.94 ➢ In an extension contracture, not only are there intra-articular adhesions, but the quadriceps muscle itself is shortened and tight.

allow overlengthening of perhaps 5 mm to compensate for 5 mm of stretching of the MCL (Fig. 74.95). However, when MCL elongation is 10 mm or more, it is simply not possible to achieve this much stretching by a lateral release alone. The same argument can be applied to varus deformities, although there are differences (notably that there is no counterpart to the peroneal nerve). It is possible to overlengthen the medial side a greater amount and, provided axial alignment is correct, some degree of lateral laxity is tolerable. As a rule of thumb, balance is acceptable provided the knee alignment cannot be passively brought into varus.

Krackow[84] has described techniques for ligament tightening for both the medial and the lateral soft tissues and estimates that he has performed them in 1% to 2% of knee arthroplasties.

Medial Tightening

The MCL can be tightened either by detaching its distal insertion into the tibia with a bone block and advancing this to a more distal position on the tibia or by proximally advancing the femoral attachment. Although we have had no experience with the techniques Krackow describes, we believe the proximal procedures, in particular, have merit and are preferred over constrained prostheses in younger patients. In support of Krackow's methods, Healy et al[62] reported success with lateral soft-tissue release and proximal MCL advancement with bone plug recession into the medial femoral condyle to correct valgus deformity in a small group of patients.

Medial and Lateral Proximal Advancement

Krackow's Method

The proximal attachment of the MCL to the medial femoral epicondyle is detached from the bone over a fairly wide area (Fig. 74.96).[84] Removing a flake of bone with the attachment is not recommended. The flap of tissue is advanced to a more proximal and slightly anterior position. It is secured by passing a special interlocking stitch through the flap and tying

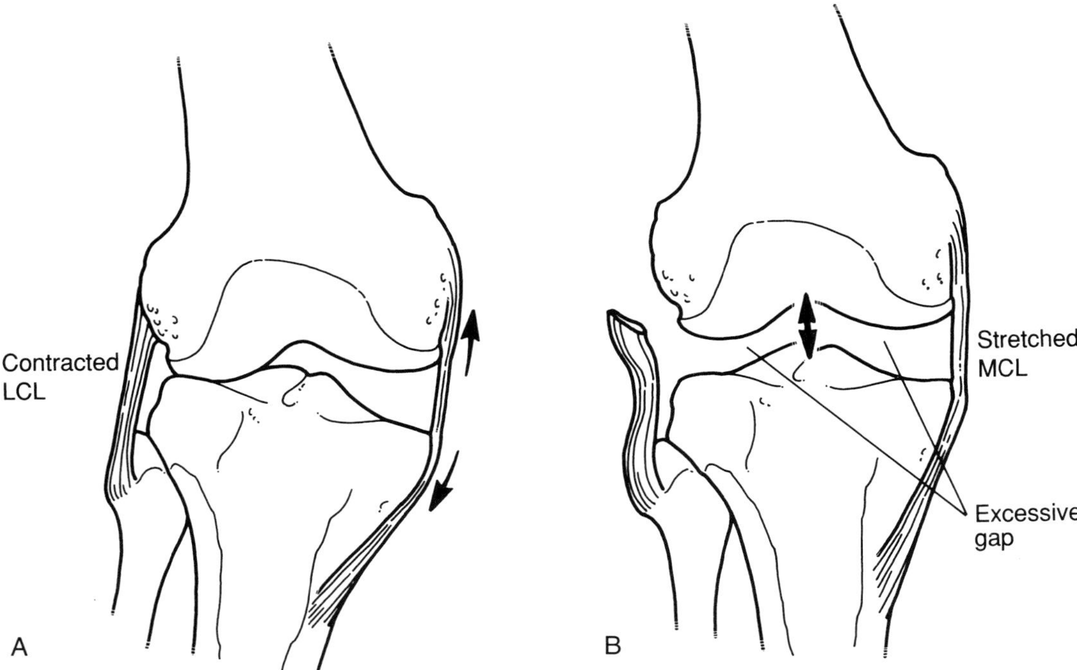

FIGURE 74.95 ➢ *A and B,* There are limits to ligament balancing. In this case, the medial collateral ligament is stretched beyond its normal length and, after lateral release, the knee will be distracted abnormally. Stabilizing this knee with thicker components involves actual lengthening of the limb, and there are clearly limits to how much lengthening can be tolerated without damage to the neurovascular structures.

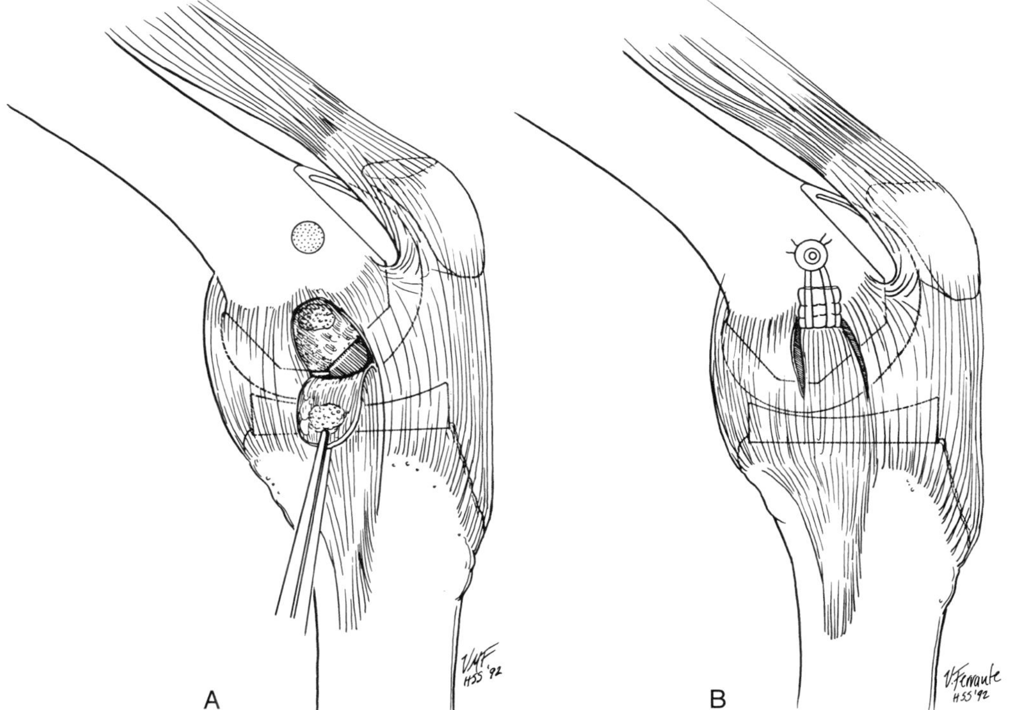

FIGURE 74.96 ➢ Krackow's technique of proximal medial collateral ligament (MCL) advancement. *A,* The proximal attachment of the MCL is removed en bloc without bone. A screw and washer are placed proximal and slightly anterior. *B,* Using the locking loop ligament fixation suture, the MCL is tightened proximally by tying the sutures around the screw and washer, which is then tightened. A second screw may be placed through the MCL's new attachment.

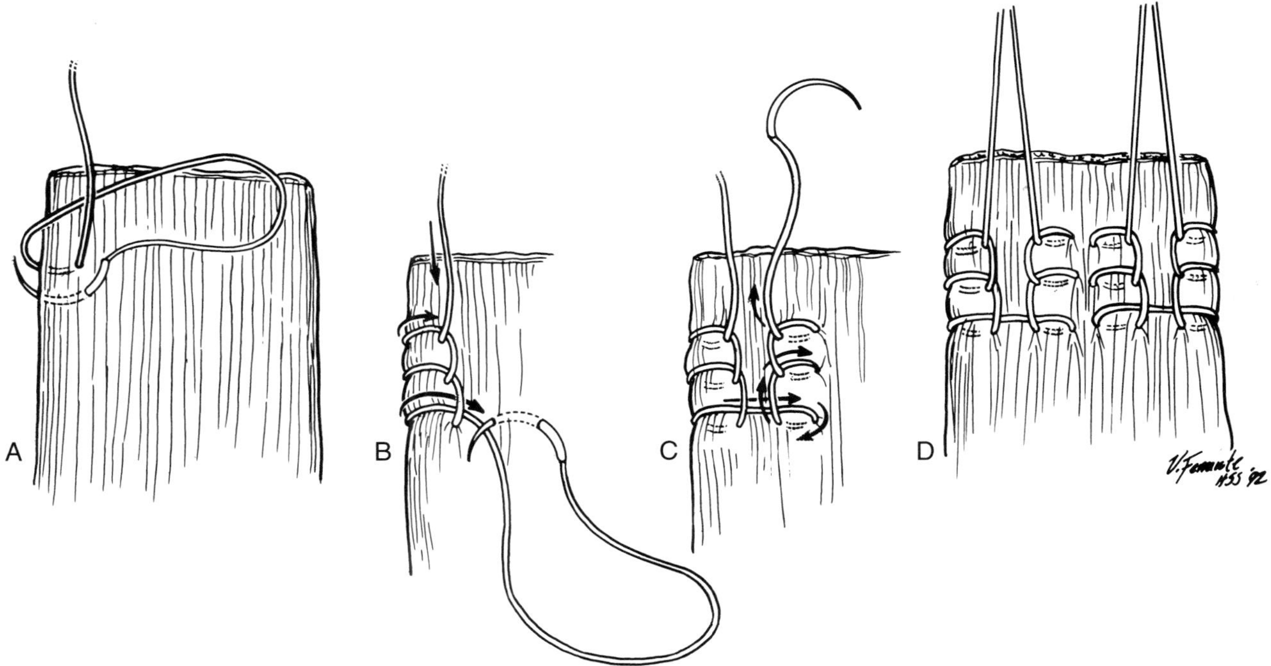

FIGURE 74.97 ➢ *A–D,* Krackow's locking loop ligament fixation suture.

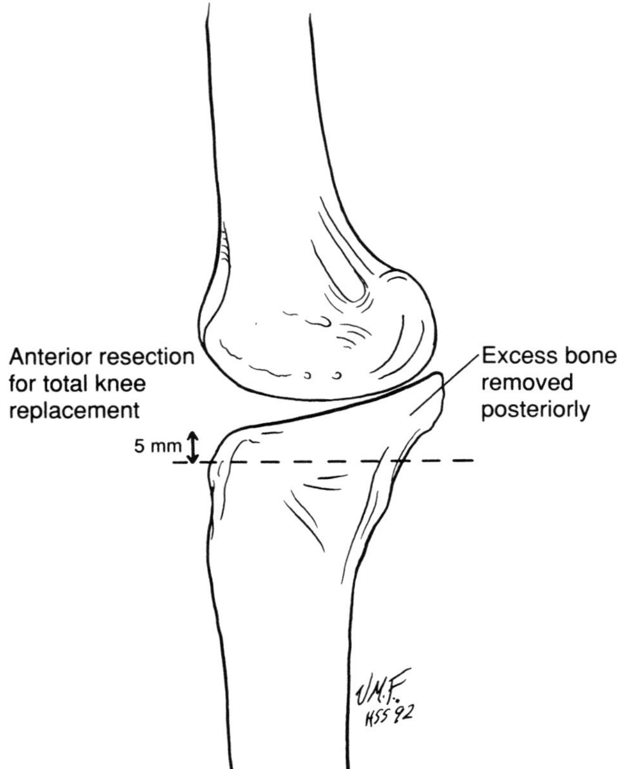

FIGURE 74.98 ➢ "Tibial recurvatum" after high tibial osteotomy. The osteotomy has healed with the distal fragment extended on the proximal, resulting in an anterior tilt to the anterior surface. Unless care is taken performing the tibial resection for total knee replacement, excessive bone may be removed.

this tightly over a proximally placed screw and washer (Fig. 74.97). A staple is then placed into the flap in the area of the original femoral epicondyle.

Healy's Method

This technique involves recession of the MCL attachment in its anatomic position at the medial femoral condyle rather than translocation of the proximal ligament.[67] The recessed proximal bone plug is secured over a bony bridge or button on the lateral side. For lax lateral structures, Krackow's method has been described for the varus knee; reports are not available describing Healy's method of proximal recession of the LCL.

Krackow also described a technique for reconstructing deformed knees using a minimally constrained prosthesis. The essence of this technique is as follows:

1. Resect the tibia to level the lateral defect; that is, the bone removed will be much thicker medially than laterally.
2. Preserve the PCL and posterior capsule with a small fragment of attached bone, which is reattached to the back of the tibia at a lower level through anteroposterior sutures passed through drill holes in the tibia.
3. Remove the MCL from its insertion with a predrilled bone block. The insertion will be advanced distally and slightly anteriorly. The MCL is pulled taut, and a bone trough is made in the new area of attachment and fixed with an A-O 4.5-mm malleolus screw. Krackow commented that this reconstruction can be technically demanding.

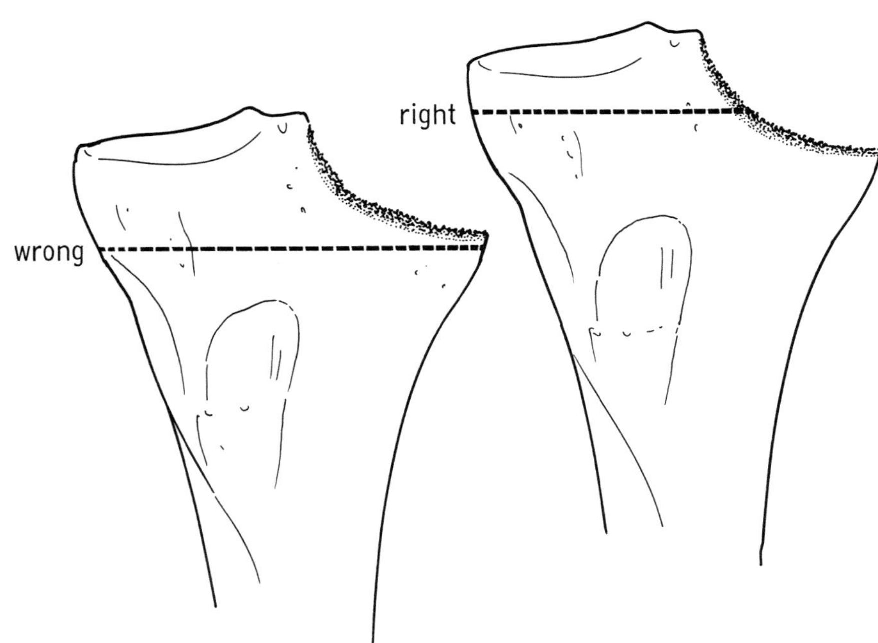

FIGURE 74.99 ➢ When there is asymmetric bone loss from the upper tibia, the tibial resection must not be too distal but rather at the usual level.

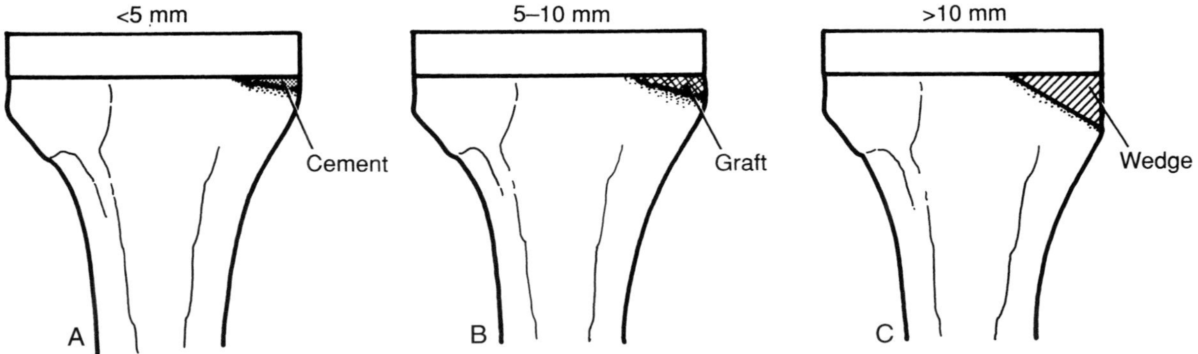

FIGURE 74.100 ➢ Bone defects are frequently seen in the medial tibia. It is incorrect to make the tibial cut at the base of the defect. It is correct to resect a normal amount from the upper tibia and fill the remaining defect. *A*, Small defects of less than 5 mm can be filled with cement. *B*, Defects between 5 and 10 mm are suitable for bone grafting. *C*, Defects larger than 10 mm are best treated with a metal wedge or augment.

Correction of Genu Recurvatum

Genu recurvatum is an uncommon deformity and is seldom severe except in poliomyelitis. Operative correction is easily obtained by under-resection of the bone ends and use of thicker components. However, paralytic types tend to recur and may require the use of a hinge or a similarly constrained prosthesis (this being one of the few indications for such a device). Krackow[84] has described a technique whereby the proximal ligament insertions are transferred proximally and posteriorly; this repositioning causes the collateral ligaments to tighten in extension. We have no experience with this technique.

Occasionally after a previous tibial osteotomy, recurvatum will be found because of deformity of the tibia itself (tibial recurvatum) (Fig. 74.98). The anterior cortices have impacted, and the result is an anterior slope to the tibia. This should be evident from a study of the radiographs, and the level of the tibial cut should be adjusted accordingly.

MANAGEMENT OF BONE DEFECTS

Principles

Although bone defects are more common in revision TKA, they do occur in primary TKA. The etiology of bone defects in primary TKA includes erosion secondary to angular arthritic change, inflammatory arthritis, osteonecrosis, and fracture. Bone defects in primary TKA are typically asymmetric and peripheral, although contained deficiencies caused by cyst formation may occur. The base of contained and peripheral defects in primary TKA typically comprises condensed sclerotic bone, in contrast to revision surgery, in which removal of components often leaves osteopenic surfaces. In our experience, most bone defects in primary TKA occur on the tibia. A major concern with tibial defects is that subchondral bone strength diminishes substantially distal to the subchondral plate.[9, 60, 68] Several authors have advised that the level of lateral tibial resection should not exceed 1 cm to avoid compromising implant durability,[35, 119] yet others have demonstrated that proximal tibial bone strength is adequate to 20 mm.[54]

Management

Various techniques are available to compensate for bone defects in primary TKA, including (1) translation of the component away from a defect, (2) lower tibial resection, (3) cement filling, (4) autologous bone graft, (5) allograft, (6) wedges or augments, and (7) custom implants. Use of stems in primary TKA is necessary when the bone defect renders the resurfacing component unstable without the added support of intramedullary fixation.

Lower Tibial Resection

A lower tibial resection is often effective in elimination of bony defects (Fig. 74.99). Based on Goldstein et al's investigation, resection of up to 20 mm of proximal tibia does not significantly compromise the strength of the residual tibial metaphysis.[54] When more than 10 mm of bone is removed, however, the resection must

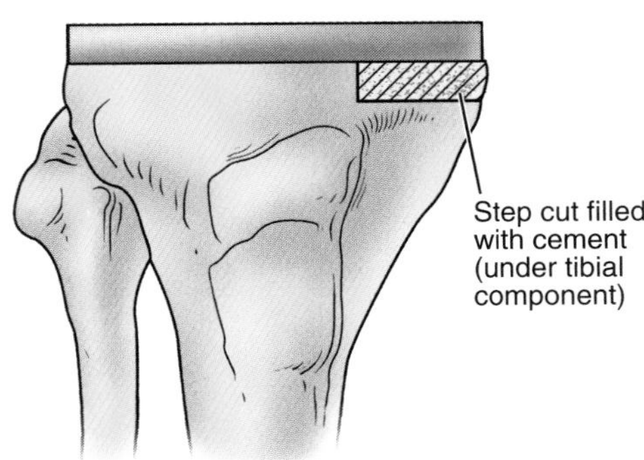

FIGURE 74.101 ➢ Step-cut technique for cement filling of a peripheral proximal tibial defect.

be proximal to Gerdy's tubercle, or else ITB function may be compromised.

Lateral Translation

Lateralizing a smaller tibial component size may effectively eliminate a bony defect (see Fig. 74.62).[72, 94] However, the largest tibial tray size and polyethylene insert should always be favored to create the largest reasonable contact surface to distribute load.

Cement Filling

Lotke et al[96] demonstrated satisfactory long-term results with cement fill (Fig. 74.100), provided tibial bone defects are no deeper than 20 mm and involve less than 50% of either plateau. Although Ritter[126] reported good results filling defects with cement supported by a screw, the results of Lotke et al[96] suggest that a screw within the cement fill is not necessary. The obvious advantages of cement are its availability and capacity to contour perfectly to any given defect. The disadvantage is that it is feasible only in defects not exceeding the size criteria established by Lotke et al.[96] Despite the satisfactory results of Lotke and Ritter, other authors recommend that use of cement be limited to smaller peripheral defects that do not compromise tibial component support, because biomechanical testing suggests that cement fill with or without screw reinforcement is an inferior method of defect management.[15] Clinical results have demonstrated that radiolucent lines are commonly observed under defects filled with cement.[33, 74] Furthermore, larger volumes of cement introduce the risk of thermal necrosis of the cement-bone interface, and net cement shrinkage during polymerization may diminish the cement-prosthesis and cement-bone interface contact areas.[15] To increase the surface area contact and reduce the potential shear stresses on the cement, our preferred method of cement fill is the step-cut method described by Krackow (Fig. 74.101).

Bone Grafting

Both autologous bone and allograft (Figs. 74.102, 74.103, and 74.104) are readily available in primary TKA. Both have demonstrated high rates of incorporation that are particularly important in reestablishing proximal tibial bone strength and restoring bone stock, should revision surgery be required. Autografting is generally favored because of its osteoinductive properties and lack of potential disease transmission.

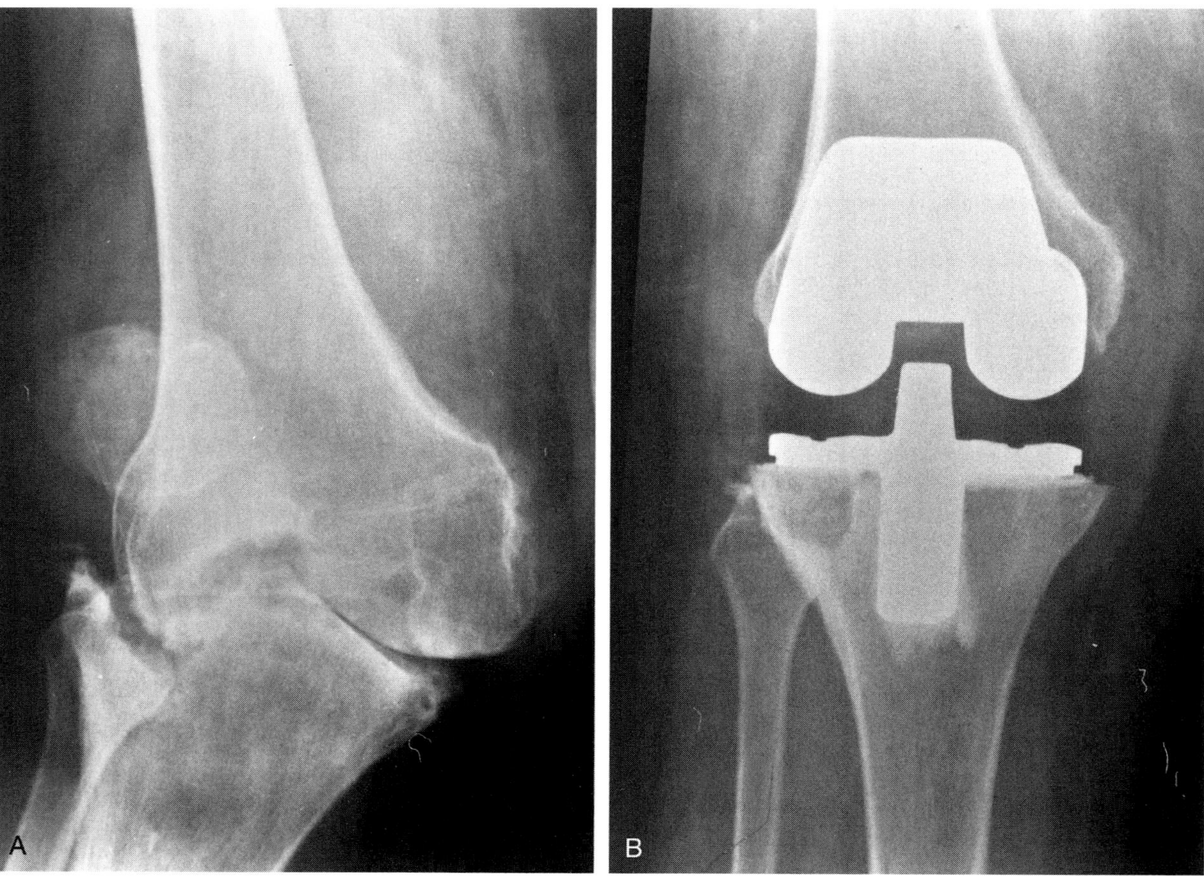

FIGURE 74.102 ➢ *A*, Radiograph showing large defect in lateral tibial plateau. *B*, Radiograph showing appearance after packing defect with cancellous bone graft. The graft can be either autologous or homologous.

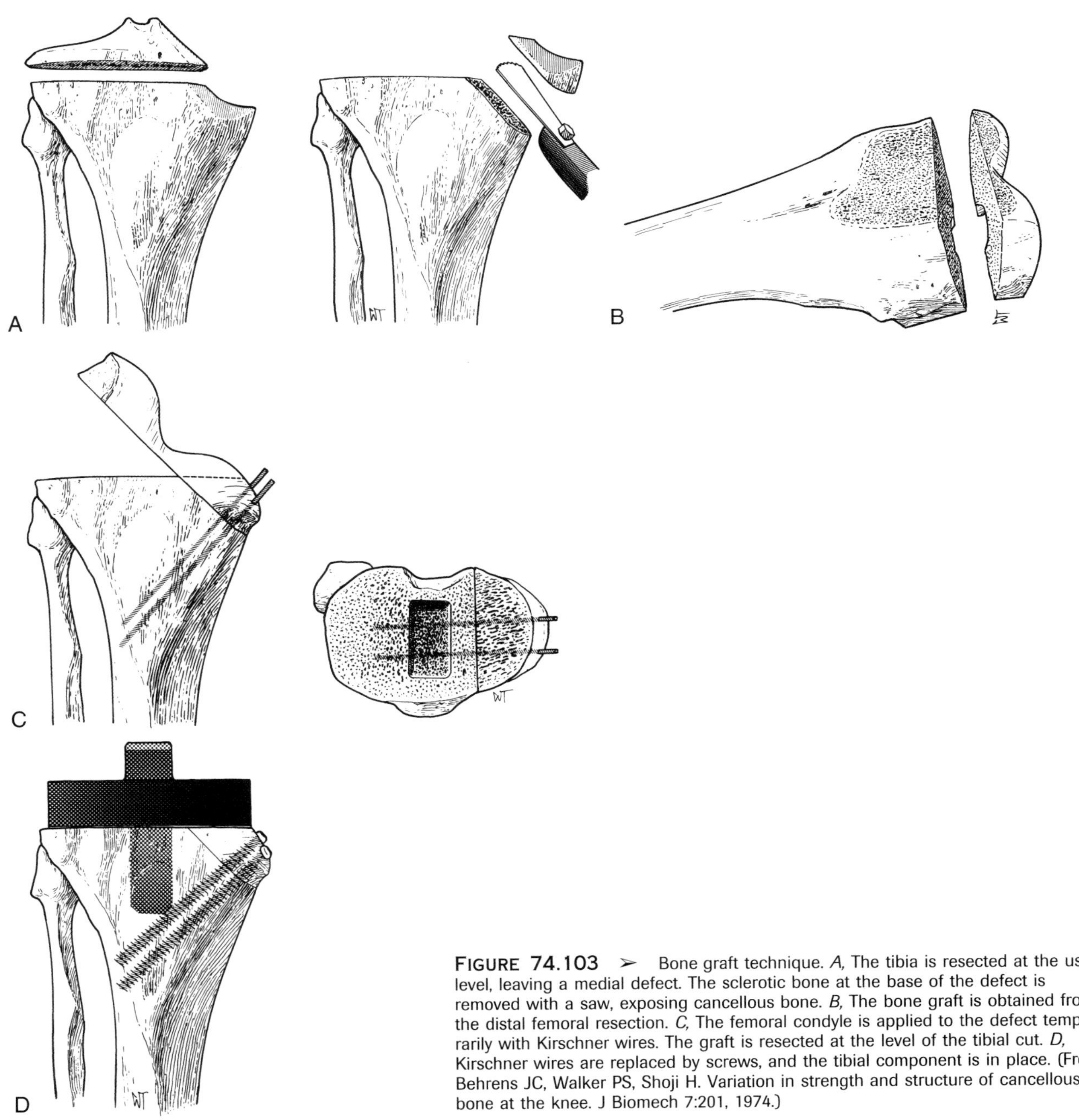

FIGURE 74.103 ➢ Bone graft technique. *A,* The tibia is resected at the usual level, leaving a medial defect. The sclerotic bone at the base of the defect is removed with a saw, exposing cancellous bone. *B,* The bone graft is obtained from the distal femoral resection. *C,* The femoral condyle is applied to the defect temporarily with Kirschner wires. The graft is resected at the level of the tibial cut. *D,* Kirschner wires are replaced by screws, and the tibial component is in place. (From Behrens JC, Walker PS, Shoji H. Variation in strength and structure of cancellous bone at the knee. J Biomech 7:201, 1974.)

Bone graft is typically used when the size criteria for cement fill are exceeded. Dorr et al[36] identified criteria that promote improved outcome, as follows: (1) creation of a viable/bleeding bed of host bone, (2) proper fit and finish of graft in host bed, (3) complete coverage of graft by the component to avoid graft resorption secondary to stress shielding, (4) optimal alignment of components for even load distribution, (5) limited weightbearing when larger grafts are used to allow for graft union, and (6) grafts protected with stems when required. Advantages of bone graft are its availability, its adaptability to size or shape of defect, and its biological compatibility.[145]

Although contained defects are easily filled with bone graft, peripheral defects are more challenging. Several techniques have been developed to address peripheral defects using bone graft. Dorr et al[36] described a technique in which the peripheral defect is converted into a single oblique cut at the base of the deficiency and is filled using bone from the larger distal femoral condylar resection. The graft is secured to the oblique surface using screw fixation (see Fig. 74.103). Their series of 24 cases using this technique included 10 primary knees, all of which had evidence of graft incorporation. Eight varus knees had peripheral defects of the medial tibial plateau, while two valgus knees had central tibial defects. Altcheck et al[5] reported good to excellent results at an average fol-

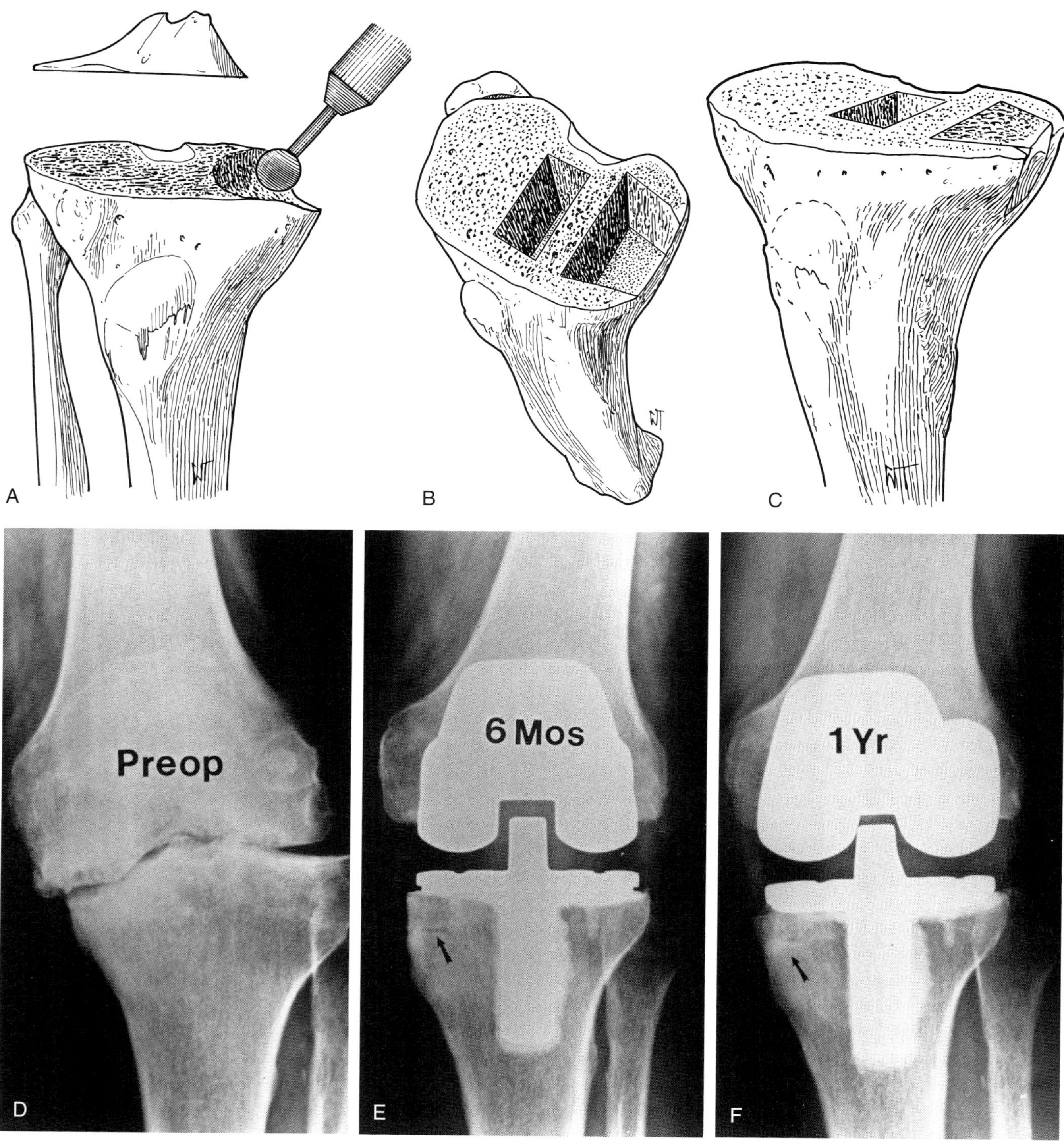

FIGURE 74.104 ➢ Autogenous tibial bone graft technique. *A,* The tibial defect is resected at the standard level. The remaining medial defect is reshaped with a burr. *B,* A trapezoidal defect is formed medially; usually, there is intact bone anteriorly and posteriorly to make this possible. *C,* A self-locking bone graft is fashioned to fit in the trapezoidal defect. The bone graft can be obtained from local resection in the knee; in the case of the posterior stabilized prosthesis, bone removed from the intercondylar notch makes an ideal source. *D,* Preoperative radiograph of a medial defect. *E,* Radiograph taken 6 months after medial bone grafting using the interlocking technique. *F,* Bone graft after 1 year; arthroplasty appears to be fully incorporated.

low-up of 4 years in 14 patients with severe angular deformity managed with this technique. All grafts consolidated without evidence of collapse, resorption, or prosthetic subsidence.

Laskin[86] used the resected posterior femoral condyles as bone graft to fill tibial defects in a similar manner. The success rate of the 24 knees studied was 67% at 5-year follow-up, with eight grafts demonstrating no evidence of incorporation. Laskin concluded that the long-term prognosis for this method of bone grafting was not satisfactory.

Insall originally described the inlay autogeneic bone-grafting technique. An interference fit for a contoured bone graft is created by converting the dish-shaped peripheral defect into a trapezoidal shape (see Fig. 74.104). Because of the interlocking fit, this method of bone grafting does not require fixation. After preliminary results were reported by Windsor et al,[170] Scuderi et al[145] reviewed 26 primary TKAs treated using this technique, reporting 96% good to excellent results at an average follow-up of 3 years. Graft position either medially or laterally did not influence the results. With restoration of anatomic knee alignment, no tibial component loosened. One medial bone graft collapsed with an obvious radiolucency, but the tibial component had not changed position at 4.5 years of follow-up.

Although bulk allografts and morselized cancellous allograft techniques can be applied to primary TKA, they are largely described as methods to manage bone loss in revision TKA. These techniques are reviewed elsewhere in this text.

Custom Prostheses and Metal Wedge Augmentation

Custom prostheses (Figs. 74.105, 74.106, 74.107, and 74.108) provide the most effective fit and force transmission of the various methods of managing bone deficiencies, especially larger defects[15]; however, custom prostheses have limitations of practicality and cost. Metal wedge augmentation permits an intraoperative construction of a custom implant to address a bone defect, affording load transfer from the implant to the bone.[115] Brooks et al[16] demonstrated that metal wedge augmentation of tibial trays provided similar support to custom prostheses. Advantages of metal wedges are that they need not incorporate into host bone and do not carry a risk of nonunion or collapse. Augments are available in triangular and rectangular shapes. Although the mechanical support afforded by triangular and rectangular wedges has been shown to be similar,[158] load transfer across a larger defect is probably best managed with a rectangular block.[45] Because of the risk of shear stresses at the cement interface, triangular wedge angles are typically restricted to 15 degrees[19]; stem augmentation improves biomechanical support.[158] Although rectangular wedges avoid shear stresses, they

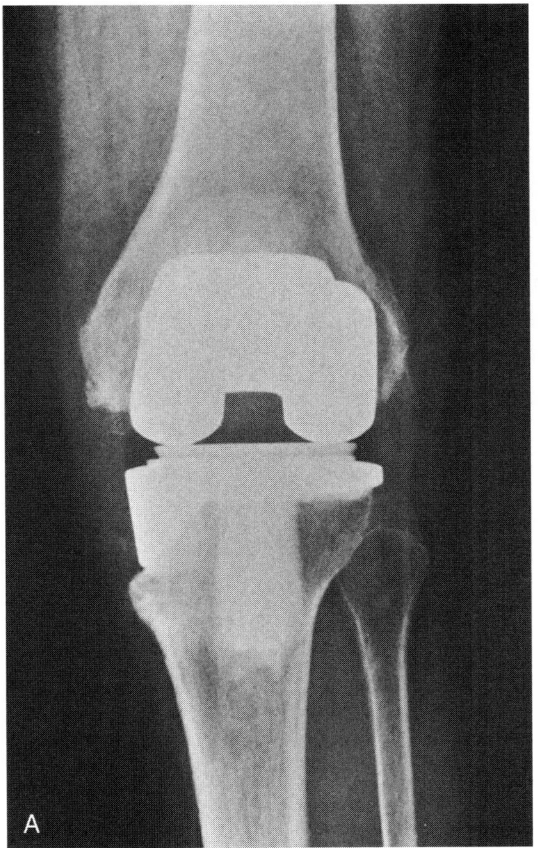

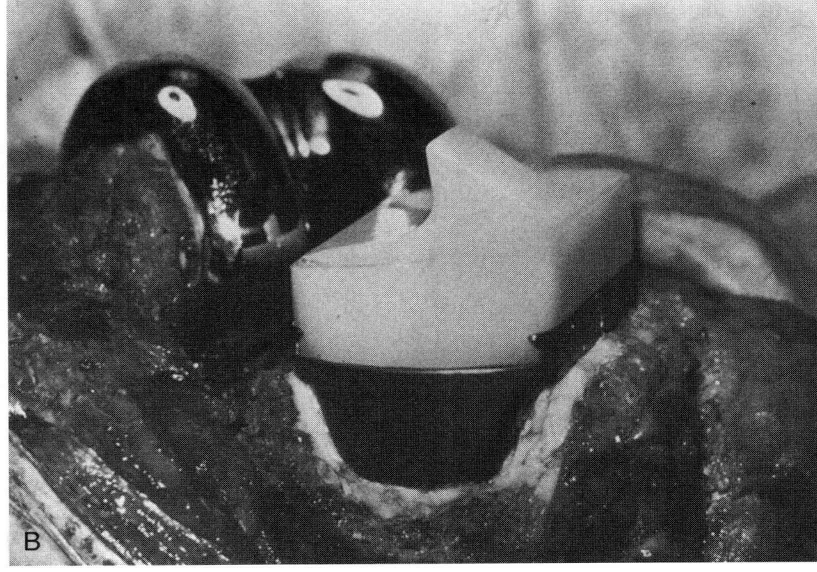

FIGURE 74.105 ➢ *A and B,* Asymmetric bone loss should be compensated for by an asymmetric tibial component.

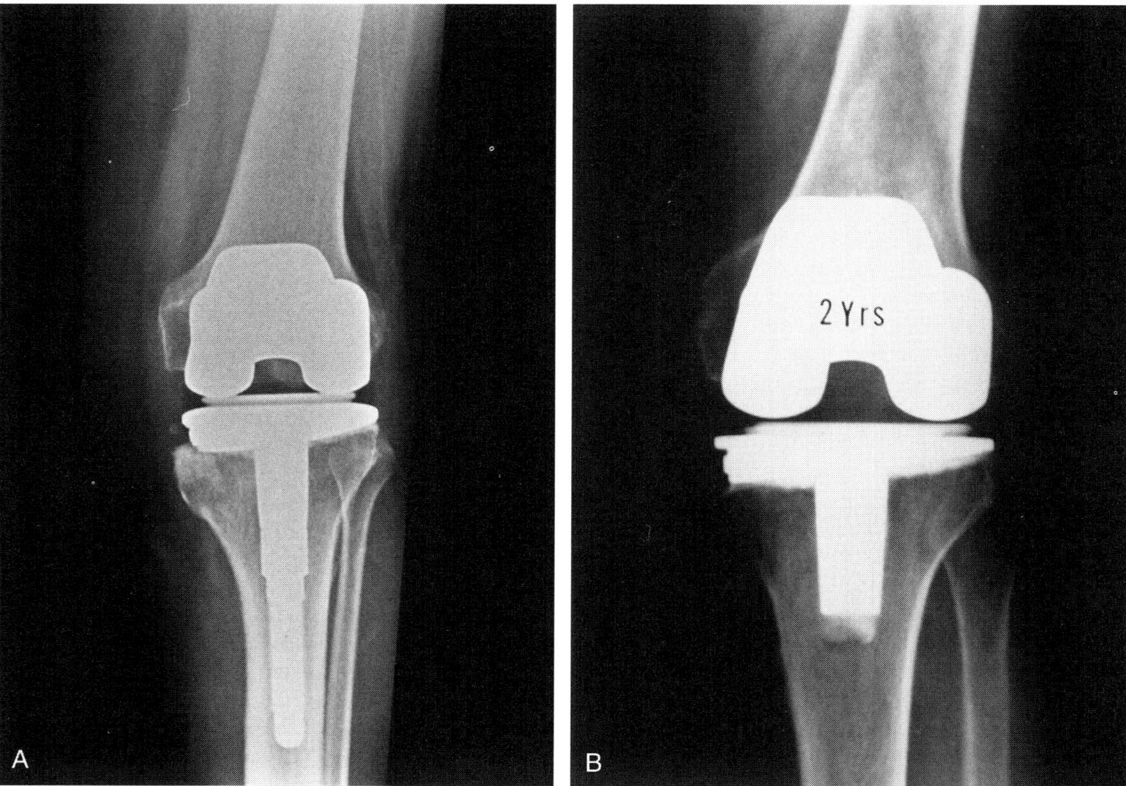

FIGURE 74.106 ➢ *A,* Full wedge applied to a tibial component for a medial tibial defect. In this case, an uncemented stem has been added. *B,* Full wedge applied to a tibial component. No stem extension has been added. It is not known at present whether a stem extension is necessary to resist possible shearing effects.

generally necessitate removal of some intact host bone. Attachment of wedges using cement has been recommended because of the potential for fretting when screws are used. We have not observed any problems with screw fixation of modular wedges and support the good results using wedges attached with screw fixation reported by Schemitsch et al.[139] In Pagnano et al's series of 24 primary cemented TKAs performed using metal wedge augmentation for tibial bone deficiency, clinical results were 96% good to excellent at an average follow-up of approximately 5 years.[115] Although radiolucent lines at the cement-bone interface beneath the metal wedge were noted in 13 knees, no deterioration of the prosthesis-wedge or wedge-cement-bone interface was observed. Defects of less than 25 mm can be managed effectively with metal wedge augmentation,[14] especially with stem augmentation. Custom prostheses may be required for larger defects.

Stem extensions should be used when the bony support beneath the resurfacing prosthesis is weakened (see Fig. 74.106). Most commonly, stem extensions are applied when bone graft or augments do not provide adequate support to the resurfacing prosthesis. As noted above, intramedullary stems serve to diminish potential shear forces that are observed when using a full wedge.[158] In our experience, squared half-wedges do not require stem support. Brooks et al[16] demonstrated that tibial component stem extensions greater than 70 mm support approximately 30% of the weight-bearing load.

Management of bone defects is reviewed in greater detail elsewhere in this text.

Authors' Preferred Method in the Management of Bone Defects

Tibial Defects

CONTAINED DEFECTS

When the bony defect, cavity, or cyst is enclosed within the bone, it is known as a contained defect. The treatment of choice is bone grafting, using local bone graft from the osteotomies. In the rare event that local autograft is insufficient, supplementary allograft may be added. In our anecdotal experience, this is the most satisfactory application for bone grafting.

PERIPHERAL DEFECTS

Peripheral defects are typically located in the posteromedial aspect of the tibial plateau. Although small and intermediate-size defects are relatively shallow and elliptical and are bound anteriorly, medially, and poste-

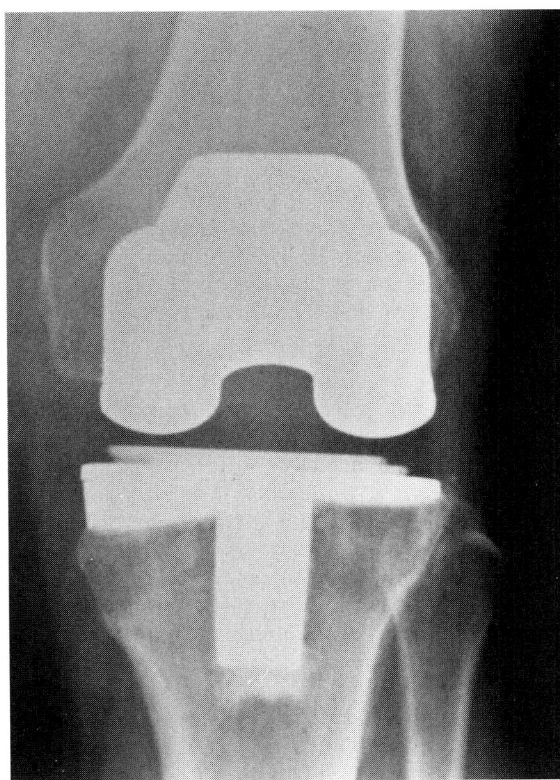

FIGURE 74.107 ➢ A modular medial wedge is attached to the prosthesis to fill a medial defect in the tibia.

riorly by a solid rim of cortical bone, severe defects have a steeper pitch and may involve the entire medial plateau. Several management options exist, as follows:

1. If possible, we translate the tibial tray away from the location of the peripheral defect. Although simple and attractive, this method results in use of a smaller polyethylene tray that may not distribute load as effectively as a larger tibial tray (see Fig. 74.62).[72, 94]
2. Occasionally, the defect can be eliminated by resecting the tibia at a lower level. As noted above, we routinely remove 10 mm of bone with proximal tibial osteotomy. In most knees with deformity, this adequately eliminates the defect such that the residual defect may be filled with cement. However, when a larger defect is present, we increase the resection to 12 to 14 mm (see Fig. 74.99).
3. Although the literature suggests that defects of up to 20 mm can be managed with cement fill technique, we typically limit the use of cement to fill residual defects of 5 mm. We often convert the dished defect into a rectangular shape with a horizontal base and three vertical borders. Theoretically, this defect configuration creates an interference fit for the cement, provided it does not extrude from the free peripheral edge. The defect base should be cleaned to permit cement interdigitation (see Fig. 74.100).
4. We generally perform bone grafting for defects between 6 and 10 mm, measured after the proximal tibial osteotomy. In our experience, such massive residual defects are rare because patients generally undergo TKA before developing severe deformity and because research has shown that a greater proximal tibial resection is permissible without compromising tibial metaphyseal support. All methods of bone grafting tend to perform best when the principles outlined by Dorr et al[36] are followed. Although we have applied all the bone-grafting techniques described, we have traditionally favored the inlay bone-grafting method reviewed by Scuderi et al,[145] because it allows for an interference fit of the graft and does not require fixation that may interfere with tibial stem placement. For inlay autogeneic bone grafting, the saucer-shaped peripheral defect is converted to a trapezoidal defect (see Fig. 74.104). The trapezoidal shape affords the advantage of allowing a stable fit so that uniform compressive forces may be exerted over the entire graft recipient site. The widest base of the trapezoidal defect is directed toward the center of the tibia to create the interlocking fit. Traditionally, the bone that is routinely removed from the intercondylar notch during posterior stabilized TKA is suitable for grafting; however, with newer prosthetic instrumentation, this bone is compromised because of the entry hole that is created for intramedullary guide placement. Furthermore, because our method of TKA now also includes a predetermined measured resection of the distal femur, only a limited amount of autologous bone is available from the distal femoral osteotomy. In these situations with massive defects, we are

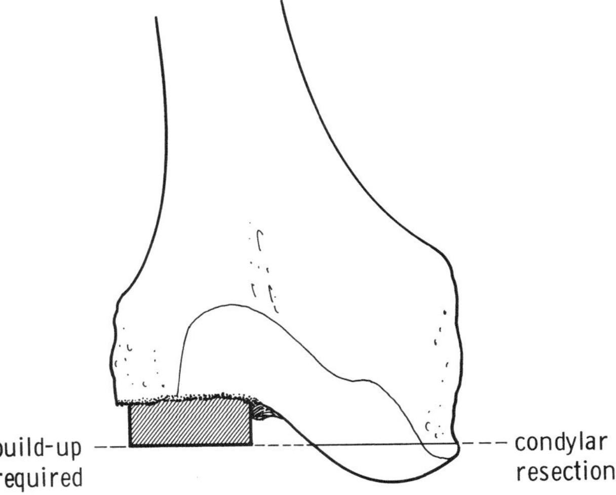

FIGURE 74.108 ➢ In some valgus knees, the level of femoral resection may pass distal to the lateral femoral condyle. Lateral augmentation of the femoral component is required.

forced to use alternative sources of bone graft (allograft) or metal augmentation. When bone can be used, the bone block is tapped into place and should fit snugly into the defect to prevent cement from entering the graft-tibia interface. Proper fit is assessed with a trial prosthesis. In Dorr et al's technique, the anterior and posterior margins of the defect are excised to create a single oblique cut to the base of the tibial deficiency.[36] The base of the cut should comprise a bleeding cancellous surface. To fill this defect, local autograft is obtained from the larger condyle of the distal femoral resection that is rotated so that its cancellous surface is matched to the cancellous surface of the tibial defect. The graft is provisionally fixed, and then a fully cancellous tibial surface is reconstituted by cutting the excess graft flush with the intact surface. The provisional fixation is then replaced with screws, which are positioned without interfering with the stem of the tibial baseplate. The junction of intact tibia and graft is "caulked" to prevent cement entering the space between the graft and the tibia.

5. When inlay bone grafting is not feasible, we use modular wedges attached to resurfacing prostheses. Despite the concern for fretting, we favor screw fixation of the wedges to the prosthesis because of its convenience. To diminish shear forces, we may add an intramedullary stem to the tibial component when a full or half oblique wedge is used. Our experience with oblique wedges has been satisfactory (Gold, unpublished data), and we typically do not use block-shaped half wedges that necessitate removal of a greater amount of intact proximal tibia.

Distal Femoral Defects

CONTAINED DEFECTS

Contained femoral defects are managed in the same manner as contained tibial defects.

PERIPHERAL DEFECTS

Surface or peripheral defects of the femur are categorized as (1) affecting the chamfer cuts, (2) distal surface, or (3) major bone loss. Loss of femoral condylar bone is most frequently observed in valgus deformities when the lateral femoral condyle is dysplastic. As with the tibia, defects can be managed with cement, bone graft, and metal augments.

Femoral deficiencies can be viewed in increasing stages of bone loss.

Stage 1

Stage 1 is observed when the femoral osteotomy includes a portion of the lateral distal femur but contouring to accommodate the femoral component results in chamfer "air cuts" anteriorly and posteriorly. In our experience, cement fill is acceptable for filling anterior and posterior spaces between bone and prosthesis.

Stage 2

Stage 2 occurs when the level of the femoral osteotomy passes distal to the lateral femoral condyle even without chamfer cuts. In this situation, cement fill is typically unsatisfactory unless combined with a femoral stem extension. Even in this instance, a metal augment to the distal femur is preferred.

Stage 3

Stage 3 refers to massive bone loss of one femoral condyle. Substantial bone loss can be managed with allograft, which has been shown to incorporate well but requires a period of non-weightbearing postoperatively. The advantage of allograft is that if a revision is required, bone stock has been restored. Another option is combining block augmentation and stem extension with a cemented prosthesis that allows for immediate weightbearing in the postoperative period. The cement typically fills the small residual defect between the bone and the implant.

Rarely is posterior augmentation required without distal augmentation. This unique situation is typically encountered only in the rheumatoid patient with longstanding flexion contracture that results in posterior condylar erosion. Most cases requiring posterior augmentation are also deficient distally. As noted above, we have not observed problems with fretting and thus attach these augments using screws. Anterior augmentation is rarely required. However, some prostheses do allow for anterior wedge placement. The advantage of these modular augments is that the natural anatomy can be restored despite bone loss. Although thicker polyethylene spacers can compensate for deficits in both flexion and extension gaps, we prefer to restore the natural anatomy, optimizing collateral ligament stability to avoid resorting to using constrained prostheses.

INTRAOPERATIVE PROBLEMS AND THEIR SOLUTIONS

Many of the basic elements of technique, bone cutting, soft-tissue balancing, and overall alignment have already been addressed. There remain a few intraoperative situations to be discussed (Fig. 74.109):

1. Templating of the femoral cut suggests an unusual angle outside the 4- to 7-degree range. Sometimes such an angle is necessary because of internal or external bowing of the femoral shaft (see Fig. 74.34), but more often the radiograph has been taken with the femur in a rotated position and an accentuated anterior bow is perceived as either a medial or a lateral bow. When the angle appears unusual, it should be checked

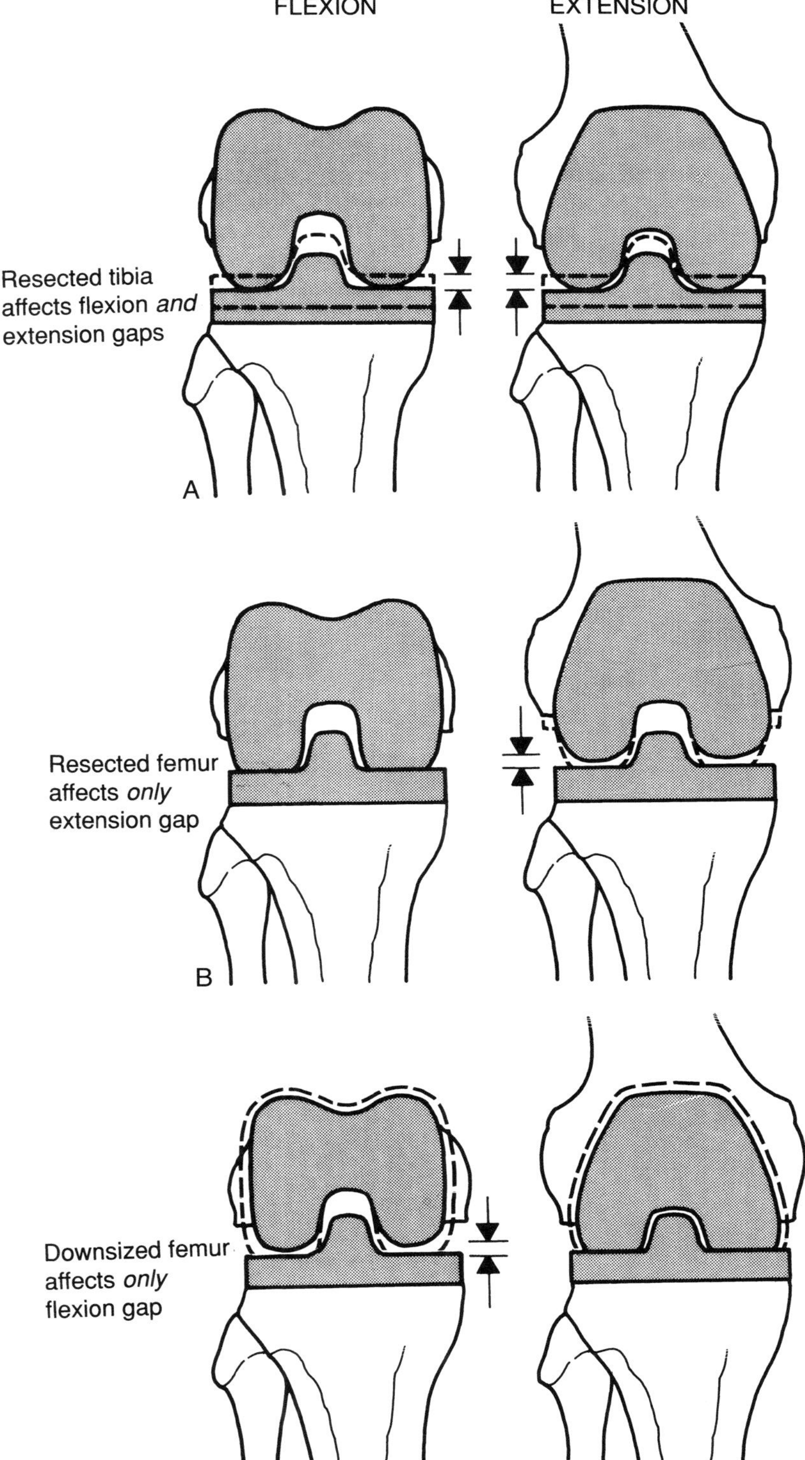

FIGURE 74.109 ➢ The effect of the bone cuts on prosthetic fit. *A,* The level of tibial resection affects both flexion and extension gaps equally. Under-resection of the tibia will make the joint tight in both positions. Over-resection of the tibia can be compensated for by using a thicker tibial component. *B,* Distal resection of the femur affects only the extension gap, which may cause instability in extension. If the knee is too tight in flexion to admit a thicker tibial component, distal femoral buildup is the solution. *C,* Over-resection of the femur in the sagittal plane affects only the flexion gap, causing laxity in flexion. This cannot be overcome by a thicker tibial component because the knee will be too tight in extension. The solutions are *(1)* to restore the proper sagittal dimension of the femur by using a larger femoral component with a posterior buildup or *(2)* to resect additional distal femur. The former is preferred.

with an external guide before making the cut. Although it is desirable to routinely use a marker for the femoral head, there are often logistic difficulties in doing this, so we depend on finding the anterior superior iliac spine and then place the tip of the external guide 1 in medial to it. At least we are assured that the overall alignment will be within an acceptable range.

2. The flexion gap is too small to admit the thinnest tibial component. If spacers are used, as we think they should be, this error will be identified early on. It is caused by either under-resection of

the proximal tibia or oversizing of the femoral component. Therefore, the size of the tibial fragment should be measured, and if 7 to 8 mm have already been removed from the normal side, then the problem lies in oversizing of the femur, and it will be necessary to recut the posterior femoral condyles so that one size smaller can be used.

3. The flexion gap is unequal—that is, tighter either medially or laterally. The cause is an error in the tibial cut into either varus or valgus, a malrotation of the femoral component, or an excessive ligament release. If the cause is either of the first two, it should be corrected. However, sometimes the necessary medial or lateral release will cause an asymmetric flexion gap that must be accepted. A larger-than-normal medial gap is not of clinical consequence, but an excessive lateral gap can lead to a posterolateral subluxation. The soft tissues must be given time to readhere, which means pursuing postoperative flexion rehabilitation less vigorously than normal.
4. The extension gap is larger than the flexion gap (Fig. 74.110). This is an unusual situation and is created by standard bone resection in a knee with excessive ligamentous laxity. A tensor obviates this occurrence because the need for femoral under-resection will be indicated; if one has committed to a standard femoral cut, the solution is to augment the distal femur (a thicker tibial component cannot be used because the flexion gap will not admit it). Augments on the distal femur usually require the use of a stemmed femoral component to get proper fixation. The "tightness" of the fit in extension is arguable. Edwards et al[38] found that with a PCL retaining prosthesis, some collateral ligament laxity improved the clinical result. We agree up to a point. The laxity must be symmetric and limited to a few millimeters of passive motion. No "thrust" on weight-bearing is permissible. Conversely, the components should not be so tight as to produce a flexion contracture.

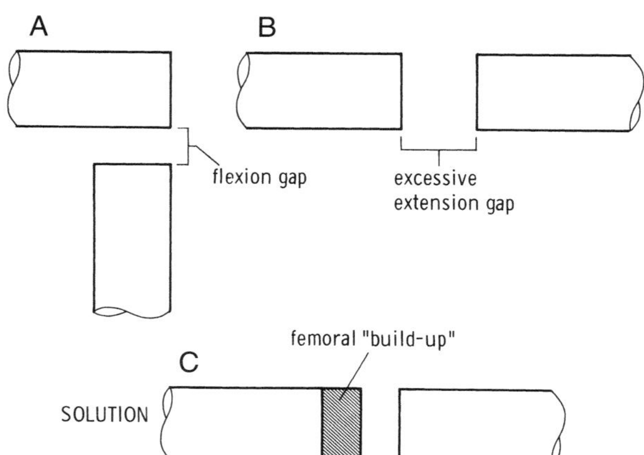

FIGURE 74.110 ➢ When the extension gap is too large, equalization cannot be obtained by further bone resection. The prosthesis must be built up on the femoral side.

5. The patella cannot be made to track in spite of an extensive lateral retinacular release. The causes are (1) femoral malrotation, (2) tibial malrotation, and (3) overly thick patella. The latter two causes are readily correctable, but the first is more difficult and will result in a malfit of the femoral component. A stemmed component and cement are needed to give adequate fixation.
6. The alignment fit and motion with the trial components are satisfactory, but this is not so when the final components are inserted. There are several reasons for this:
   a. The knee does not reach full extension. The probable explanation is that the femoral component has been put on flexed so that it is sitting proud of the bone. This problem has been virtually eliminated with the use of pegs that engage the femur, ensuring proper sagittal position of the femoral component.
   b. The knee is too loose in extension after satisfactory trial reduction. This can happen even with a proper fit because the finished components are polished and become slightly less bulky than the trials; adjustment to the thickness of the tibial component will remedy the situation. A more serious occurrence is when the femoral component has been driven into soft rheumatoid or osteoporotic bone. A thicker tibial component may upset the flexion-extension balance and a stemmed femoral component, possibly with augments, may be needed to restore the proper femoral position.
   c. The varus-valgus alignment and balance are incorrect. This is also due to compacting one or the other of the components (usually the femoral component) asymmetrically into soft bone. The correction is the same as previously described.
   d. Patellar tracking is unsatisfactory. The cause is insertion of the final components in a different position to the trials. This usually happens when the bone is soft, and it is most likely to happen when a central stem tibial design is used and the tibial component is allowed to spin into internal rotation. It is, of course, correctable but can be prevented if the position of the tibial trial on the tibia is marked with methylene blue, so that the surgeon can be certain that both the trial and the final components are correctly inserted.
   e. Excessive bleeding occurs. Opinions differ about the timing of tourniquet release or even on whether to release it at all. There have been studies that show blood loss to be similar with and without tourniquet release. However, we believe tourniquet release serves two purposes: (1) Occasional profuse bleeding, usually from the lateral genicular artery, can be secured (see Fig. 74.50) (we know of cases that have been returned to the operating the-

ater for this cause) and (2) very occasionally, blood flow may not return through an arteriosclerotic femoral artery when the tourniquet is let down. This is usually due to clotting in the femoral artery, and if treated early has an uneventful outcome. Release of the tourniquet alerts the surgeon to this possibility, whereas identification of this potentially catastrophic event may be delayed in the recovery room.

AFTERCARE OF TOTAL KNEE ARTHROPLASTY

At the conclusion of the operation, a light dressing is applied and radiographs of the knee are obtained either in the operating room itself or in the recovery room. We use a postoperative drain for approximately 24 hours. Continuous passive motion is initiated in the recovery room; simultaneous continuous passive motion machines are used in bilateral cases. The patient is encouraged to flex the knee as much as is tolerated; recent investigations suggest that high flexion in the immediate postoperative period accelerates postoperative rehabilitation and is not associated with wound complications.[78] The objective is to reach active flexion of 90 degrees in 5 to 7 days.

With a cemented knee, full weightbearing under the supervision of a therapist is allowed on the first or second postoperative day. The protocol for a cementless prosthesis, however, calls for weightbearing to be restricted for 6 weeks. Some surgeons recommend protected weightbearing even when cement is used. Generally, we allow the patient to stand on the first occasion, and if this is well accepted, a few steps with a walker are encouraged. Progression of walking is variable and age dependent and is initially done with a walker until the patient is steady enough to use canes (usually between the fourth and seventh days). The use of night splints is unnecessary except for knees with troublesome flexion contractures.

General muscle exercises are for the feet and ankles, and isometric exercises are for the thigh and buttock muscles. Because of the possibility of disrupting the surgical repair and causing a dislocation of the patella, our policy is to avoid deliberate exercising of the quadriceps muscle for the first 2 weeks. Quadriceps exercises and straight-leg raising, using light weights, can be commenced after this as tolerated. Hamstring exercises should be avoided in the seated position and when using a posterior stabilized prosthesis because dislocation can occur. Bicycle exercises are most useful as soon as the patient has sufficient flexion.

The patient is discharged from the hospital when walking unaided, when flexing to approximately 90 degrees, and when able to climb stairs using a handrail. Physical therapy with emphasis on bicycling, range of motion, and quadriceps strength is continued at home for approximately 1 month.

Our protocol for thromboembolic conditions is described elsewhere in this text.

References

1. Aglietti P, Buzzi R, Giron F, et al: The Insall-Burstein posterior stabilized total knee replacement in the valgus knee. Am J Knee Surg 9:8, 1996.
2. Aglietti P, Windsor RE, Buzzi R, et al: Arthroplasty for the stiff or ankylosed knee. Clin Orthop 143:115, 1979.
3. Albredtsson BEJ, Carlsson LV, Freeman MAR, et al: Proximally cemented versus uncemented Freeman Samuelson knee arthroplasty. A prospective randomized study. J Bone Joint Surg Br 74:233, 1992.
4. Alexiades M, Scuderi G, Vincent V, et al: A histologic study of the posterior cruciate ligament in the arthritic knee. Am J Knee Surg 2(4):153, 1989.
5. Altcheck D, Sculco TP, Rawlins B: Autogenous bone grafting for severe angular deformity in total knee arthroplasty. J Arthroplasty 4(2):151, 1989.
6. Anouchi YS, Whiteside LA, Kaiser AD, et al: The effects of axial rotational alignment of the femoral component on instability and patellar tracking in total knee arthroplasty demonstrated on autopsy specimens. Clin Orthop 287:170, 1993.
7. Arima J, Whiteside LA, McCarthy DS, et al: Femoral rotational alignment, based on the anteroposterior axis in total knee arthroplasty in a valgus knee. J Bone Joint Surg Am 77: 1331, 1995.
8. Barrack RL, Wolfe MW, Waldman DA, et al: Resurfacing of the patella in total knee arthroplasty. A prospective, randomized, double-blind study. J Bone Joint Surg Am 79:1121, 1997.
9. Behrens JC, Walker PS, Shoji H: Variation in strength and structure of cancellous bone at the knee. J Biomech 7:201, 1974.
10. Berger RA, Crossett LS, Jacobs JJ, et al: Malrotation causing patellofemoral complications after total knee arthroplasty. Clin Orthop 356:144, 1998.
11. Berger RA, Rubash HE, Seel MJ, et al: Determining the rotational alignment of the femoral component in total knee arthroplasty using the epicondylar axis. Clin Orthop 286:40, 1993.
12. Bourne RB, Rorabeck CH, Vaz M, et al: Resurfacing versus not resurfacing the patella during total knee replacement. Clin Orthop 321:156, 1995.
13. Boyd AD, Ewald FC, Thomas WH, et al: Longterm complications after total knee arthroplasty with or without resurfacing of the patella. J Bone Joint Surg Am 75(5):674, 1993.
14. Brand MG, Daley RJ, Ewald FC, et al: Tibial tray augmentation with modular metal wedges for tibial bone stock deficiency. Clin Orthop 248:71, 1989.
15. Brooks PJ, Walker PS, Scott RD: Tibial component fixation in deficient tibial bone stock. Clin Orthop 184:302, 1984.
16. Buechel FF: A sequential three-step lateral release for correcting fixed valgus knee deformities during total knee arthroplasty. Clin Orthop 260:170, 1990.
17. Cameron HU: Tibial component wear in total knee replacement. Clin Orthop 309: 29, 1994.
18. Cameron HU, Hunter GA: Failure in total knee arthroplasty. Mechanisms, revisions, and results. Clin Orthop 170:141, 1982.
19. Cates HE, Ritter MA, Keating EM, et al: Intramedullary versus extramedullary femoral alignment systems in total knee replacement. Clin Orthop 286:32, 1993.
20. Chen F, Krackow KA: Management of tibial defects in total knee arthroplasty. A biomechanical study. Clin Orthop 305:249, 1994.
21. Chiba J, Schwendeman LJ, Booth RE Jr, et al: A biomechanical, histologic, and immunohistologic analysis of membranes obtained from failed cemented and cementless total knee arthroplasty. Clin Orthop 299: 114, 1994.
22. Clayton ML, Thompson TR, Mack RP: Correction of alignment deformities during total knee arthroplasties: Staged soft-tissue releases. Clin Orthop 202:117, 1986.
23. Colizza WA, Insall JN, Scuderi GR: The posterior stabilized total knee prosthesis. Assessment of polyethylene damage and osteolysis after a ten year minimum followup. J Bone Joint Surg Am 77:1713, 1995.
24. Cook SD, Thomas KA, Kay JF, et al: Hydroxyapatite-coated titanium for orthopedic implant applications. Clin Orthop 232: 225, 1988.
25. Coonse K, Adams JD: A new operative approach to the knee joint. Surg Gynecol Obstet 77:344, 1943.

26. Corces A, Lotke PA, Williams JL: Strain characteristics of the posterior cruciate ligament in total knee replacement. Orthop Trans 13(3):527, 1989.
27. Coventry MD: Two-part total knee arthroplasty: Evolution and present status. Clin Orthop 145:29, 1979.
28. Dennis DA, Channer M, Susman MH, et al: Intramedullary versus extramedullary tibial alignment systems in total knee arthroplasty. J Arthroplasty 8(1):43, 1993.
29. Dennis DA, Komistek RD, Colwell CE, et al: In vivo anterior-posterior femorotibial translation of total knee arthroplasty: A multicenter analysis. Clin Orthop 356:47, 1998.
30. Dennis DA, Komistek RD, Hoff WA, et al: In vivo knee kinematics derived using an inverse perspective technique. Clin Orthop 331:107, 1996.
31. Diduch DR, Insall JN, Scott WN, et al: Total knee replacement in young, active patients. Long-term followup and functional outcome. J Bone Joint Surg Am 79: 575, 1997.
32. Donaldson WF III, Sculco TP, Insall JN, et al: Total condylar III knee prosthesis: Long-term follow-up study. Clin Orthop 226: 21, 1988.
33. Dorr LD: Bone grafts for bone loss with total knee replacement. Orthop Clin North Am 20:179, 1989.
34. Dorr LD, Boiardo RA: Technical considerations in total knee arthroplasty. Clin Orthop 205:5, 1986.
35. Dorr LD, Conaty JP, Schreiber R, et al: Technical factors that influence mechanical loosening of total knee arthroplasty. In Dorr LD, ed: The Knee. Baltimore, University Park Press, 1985, pp 121-135.
36. Dorr LD, Ranawat CS, Sculco TA, et al: Bone graft for tibial defects in total knee arthroplasty. Clin Orthop 205:153, 1986.
37. Duffy GP, Berry DJ, Rand JA: Cement versus cementless fixation in total knee arthroplasty. Clin Orthop 356: 66, 1998.
38. Edwards E, Miller J, Chan KH: The effect of postoperative collateral ligament laxity in total knee arthroplasty. Clin Orthop 236:44, 1988.
39. Emerson RH, Ayers C, Head WC, et al: Surgical closure in primary total knee arthroplasty. Flexion versus extension. Clin Orthop 331:74, 1996.
40. Engh GA, Dwyer KA, Hanes CK: Polyethylene wear of metal backed tibial components in total and unicompartmental knee prostheses. J Bone Joint Surg Br 74:9, 1998.
41. Engh GA, Parks NL, Ammeen DJ: Tibial osteolysis in cementless total knee arthroplasty. A review of 25 cases treated with and without tibial component revision. Clin Orthop 309:33, 1994.
42. Engh GA, Petersen TL: Comparative experience with intramedullary and extramedullary alignment in total knee arthroplasty. J Arthroplasty 5:1, 1990.
43. Faris PM, Herbst SA, Ritter MA, et al: The effect of preoperative knee deformity on the initial results of cruciate-retaining total knee arthroplasty. J Arthroplasty 7(4):527, 1992.
44. Faris PM, Ritter MA, Keating EM: Sagittal plane positioning of the femoral component in total knee arthroplasty. J Arthroplasty 3(4):355, 1988.
45. Fehring TK, Peindl RD, Humble RS, et al: Modular tibial augmentations in total knee arthroplasty. Clin Orthop 327:207, 1996.
46. Feng EL, Stulberg DS, Wixon RS: Progressive subluxation and polyethylene wear in total knee arthroplasty with flat articular surfaces. Clin Orthop 299:60, 1993.
47. Figgie HE III, Goldberg VM, Heiple KG, et al: The influence of tibial-patellofemoral location on function of the knee in patients with the posterior stabilized condylar knee prosthesis. J Bone Joint Surg Am 68:1035, 1986.
48. Finerman GAM, Coventry MB, Riley LH, et al: Anametric total knee arthroplasty. Clin Orthop 145:85, 1979.
49. Firestone TP, Krackow KA, Davis JD, et al: The management of fixed flexion contractures during total knee arthroplasty. Clin Orthop 284:221, 1991.
50. Freeman MAR: Arthritis of the Knee: Clinical Features and Surgical Management. New York, Springer-Verlag, 1980.
51. Gabriel SM, Dennis DA, Honey MJ, Scott RD: Polyethylene wear on the distal tibial insert surface in total knee arthroplasty. The Knee 5:221-228, 1998.
52. Garvin KL, Scuderi GR, Insall JN: Evolution of the quadriceps snip. Clin Orthop 321:131, 1995.
53. Geesink RGT, de Groot K, Klein CPAT: Bonding of bone to apatite-coated implants. J Bone Joint Surg Br 70:17, 1988.
54. Goldstein SA, Wilson DL, Sostengard DA, et al: The mechanical properties of human tibial trabecular bone as a function of metaphyseal location. J Biomech 16(12):965, 1983.
55. Gomes LSM, Bechtold JE, Gustilo RB: Patellar prosthesis positioning in total knee arthroplasty: A roentgenographic study. Clin Orthop 236:72, 1988.
56. Goodfellow JW, O'Connor JJ: The anterior cruciate ligament in knee arthroplasty: A risk factor with unconstrained meniscal prostheses. Clin Orthop 276:245, 1992.
57. Griffin FM, Insall JN, Scuderi GR: The posterior condylar angle in osteoarthritic knees. J Arthroplasty 13(7):812, 1998.
58. Griffin FM, Scuderi GR, Gillis AM, et al: Osteolysis associated with cemented total knee arthroplasty. J Arthroplasty 13(5): 592, 1998.
59. Haddad RJ, Jr, Cook SD, Thomas KA: Biological fixation of porous-coated implants. J Bone Joint Surg Am 69:1459, 1987.
60. Harada Y, Wevers HW, Cooke TDV: Distribution of bone strength in the proximal tibia. J Arthroplasty 3(2):167, 1988.
61. Harrington IJ: A bioengineering analysis of force actions at the knee in normal and pathologic gait. Biomed Engin 11(5):167, 1976.
62. Healy WL, Iorio R, Lemos DW: Medial reconstruction during total knee arthroplasty for severe valgus deformity. Clin Orthop 356:161, 1998.
63. Hood RW, Vanni M, Insall JN: The correction of knee alignment in 225 consecutive total condylar knee replacements. Clin Orthop 160:94, 1981.
64. Hsu HP, Garg A, Walker PS, et al: Effect of knee component alignment on tibial load distribution with clinical correlation. Clin Orthop 248:135, 1989.
65. Hsu WW, Himeco S, Coventry MB, et al: Normal axial alignment of the lower extremity and load bearing distribution of the knee. Clin Orthop 255:215, 1990.
66. Hungerford DA, Kenna RV: Preliminary experience with a total knee prosthesis with porous coating used without cement. Clin Orthop 176:96, 1983.
67. Hungerford DS, Krackow KA: Total joint arthroplasty of the knee. Clin Orthop 192:23, 1985.
68. Hvid I: Trabecular bone strength at the knee. Clin Orthop 227: 210, 1988.
69. Insall JN: Choices and compromises in total knee arthroplasty [presidential address to The Knee Society]. Clin Orthop 226:43, 1988.
70. Insall JN: Surgical techniques and instrumentation in total knee arthroplasty. In Insall JN, ed: Surgery of the Knee. New York, Churchill Livingstone, 1993.
71. Insall JN: Technique of total knee replacement. American Academy of Orthopaedic Surgeons. Instr Course Lect 30:324, 1981.
72. Insall JN: Total knee replacement. In Insall JN, ed: Surgery of the Knee. New York, Churchill Livingstone, 1984, pp 587-695.
73. Insall JN, Lachiewicz PF, Burstein AH: The posterior stabilized condylar prosthesis: A modification of the total condylar design: Two to four year clinical experience. J Bone Joint Surg Am 64:1317, 1982.
74. Insall JN, Hood RW, Flawn LB: The total condylar knee prosthesis is gonarthrosis. A five to nine-year followup of the first one hundred consecutive replacements. J Bone Joint Surg Am 65:619, 1983
75. Jiang CC, Insall JN: Effect of rotation on the axial alignment of the femur: Pitfalls in the use of femoral intramedullary guides in total knee arthroplasty. Clin Orthop 248:50, 1989.
76. Johnson F, Leitl S, Waugh W: The distribution of load across the knee. J Bone Joint Surg Br 62: 346, 1980.
77. Jones SMG, Inder IM, Moran CG, et al: Polyethylene wear in uncemented knee replacements. J Bone Joint Surg Br 74:18, 1992.
78. Jordan LR, Siegel JL, Olivio JL: Early flexion routine. An alternative method of continuous passive motion. Clin Orthop 315: 231, 1995.
79. Keblish PA: The lateral approach to the valgus knee. Surgical technique and analysis of 53 cases with over two-year followup evaluation. Clin Orthop 271:52, 1991.
80. Kim H, Pelker RR, Gibson DH, et al: Rollback in posterior

cruciate ligament-retaining total knee arthroplasty. A radiographic analysis. J Arthroplasty 12(5):553, 1997.
81. King TV, Scott RD: Femoral component loosening in total knee arthroplasty. Clin Orthop 194:285, 1985.
82. Kleinbart FA, Bryk E, Evangelista J, et al: Histologic composition of posterior cruciate ligaments from arthritic and age-matched specimens. J Arthroplasty 11(6):726, 1996.
83. Koshino T, Ejima M, Okamoto R, et al: Gradual low riding of the patella during postoperative course after total knee arthroplasty in osteoarthritis and rheumatoid arthritis. J Arthroplasty 5(4):323, 1990.
84. Krackow KA: The Technique of Total Knee Arthroplasty. St. Louis, CV Mosby, 1990.
85. Krackow, KA, Jones MM, Teeny SM, et al: Primary total knee arthroplasty in patients with fixed valgus deformity. Clin Orthop 273:9, 1991.
86. Laskin RS: Total knee arthroplasty in the presence of large bony defects of the tibia and marked knee instability. Clin Orthop 248:66, 1989.
87. Laskin RS: Total knee replacement with posterior cruciate ligament retention in patients with a fixed varus deformity. Clin Orthop 331:29, 1996.
88. Laskin RS, Rieger M, Schob C, et al: The posterior-stabilized total knee prosthesis in the knee with a severe fixed deformity. Am J Knee Surg 1(4):199, 1988.
89. Laskin RS, Turtel A: The use of an intramedullary tibial alignment guide in total knee replacement. Am J Knee Surg 2(3): 123, 1989.
90. Laurencin CT, Scott RD, Volatile TB, et al: Total knee replacement in severe valgus deformity. Am J Knee Surg 5:135, 1992.
91. Lewallen DG, Bryan RS, Peterson LFA: Polycentric total knee arthroplasty. J Bone Joint Surg Am 66:1211, 1984.
92. Lewis PL, Rorabeck CH, Bourne RB: Screw osteolysis after cementless total knee replacement. Clin Orthop 321:173, 1995.
93. Lombardi AV Jr, Mallory TH, Maitino PD, et al: Freehand resection of the patella in total knee arthroplasty referencing the attachments of the quadriceps tendon and patellar tendon. J Arthroplasty 13(7):788, 1998.
94. Lotke PA: Tibial component translation for bone defects. Orthop Trans 9:425, 1985.
95. Lotke PA, Ecker ML: Influence of positioning of prosthesis in total knee replacement, J Bone Joint Surg Am 59(1):77, 1977.
96. Lotke PA, Wong RY, Ecker ML: The use of methylmethacrylate in primary total knee replacements with large tibial defects. Clin Orthop 270:288, 1991.
97. Manning M, Elloy M, Johnson R: The accuracy of intramedullary alignment in total knee replacement. J Bone Joint Surg Br 70: 852, 1988.
98. Maquet PGJ: Biomechanics of the Knee. New York, Springer-Verlag, 1976.
99. Marcacci M, Iacono F, Zaffagnini S, et al: Total knee arthroplasty without patellar resurfacing in active and overweight patients. Knee Surg Sports Trauma Arthroscopy 5(4):258, 1997.
100. Martin JW, Whiteside LA: The influence of joint line position on knee stability after condylar knee arthroplasty. Clin Orthop 259:146, 1990.
101. Masri BA, Laskin RS, Windsor RE, et al: Knee closure in total knee replacement. A randomized prospective trial. Clin Orthop 321:81, 1996.
102. McPherson EJ, Cushner FD, Schiff CF, et al: Natural history of uncorrected flexion contractures following total knee arthroplasty. J Arthroplasty 9(5):499, 1994.
103. Mintzer CM, Robertson DD, Rackemann S, et al: Bone loss in the distal anterior femur after total knee arthroplasty. Clin Orthop 260:135, 1990.
104. Miyasaka KC, Ranawat CS, Mullaji A: 10- to 20-year followup of total knee arthroplasty for valgus deformities. Clin Orthop 345: 29, 1997.
105. Montgomery WH, Insall JN, Haas SB, et al: Primary TKA in stiff and ankylosed knees. Am J Knee Surg 11(1):20, 1998.
106. Moran CG, Pinder IM, Lees TA, et al: 121 cases in survivorship analysis of the uncemented porous coated anatomic knee replacement. J Bone Joint Surg Am 73:848, 1991.
107. Moreland JR: Mechanisms of failure in total knee arthroplasty. Clin Orthop 226:49-64, 1988.
108. Morrison JB: Bioengineering analysis of force actions transmitted by the knee joint. Biomed Engin 3:164, 1968.
109. Muller JO: Range of motion following total knee arthroplasty in ankylosed joints. Clin Orthop 179:200, 1983.
110. Nafei A, Neilsen S, Kristensen O, et al: The press fit Kinemax knee arthroplasty. High failure rate of noncemented implants. J Bone Joint Surg Br 74:243, 1992.
111. Nagamine R, Whiteside LA, White SE, et al: Patellar tracking after total knee arthroplasty. The effect of tibial tray malrotation and articular surface configuration. Clin Orthop 304:262, 1994.
112. Nelissen RG, Valstar ER, Rozing PM: The effect of hydroxyapatite on the micromotion of total knee prostheses. A prospective, randomized, double-blind study. J Bone Joint Surg Am 80: 1665, 1998.
113. Onsten I, Norqvist A, Carlsson AS, et al: Hydroxyapatite augmentation of the porous coating improves fixation of tibial components. A randomized RSA study in 116 patients. J Bone Joint Surg Br 80:417, 1998.
114. Pagnano MW, Hanssen AD, Lewallen DG, et al: Flexion instability after primary posterior cruciate retaining total knee arthroplasty. Clin Orthop 356:39, 1998.
115. Pagnano MW, Trousdale RT, Rand JA: Tibial wedge augmentation for bone deficiency in total knee arthroplasty. Clin Orthop 321:151, 1995.
116. Parks NL, Engh GA, Topoleski LDT, et al: Modular tibial insert micromotion: A concern with contemporary knee implants. Clin Orthop 356:10, 1998.
117. Peters PC, Engh GA, Dwyer KA, et al: Osteolysis after total knee arthroplasty without cement. J Bone Joint Surg Am 74: 864, 1992.
118. Poilvache PL, Insall HN, Scuderi GR, et al: Rotational landmarks and sizing of the distal femur in total arthroplasty. Clin Orthop 331:35, 1996.
119. Rand JA: Bone deficiency in total knee arthroplasty. Use of metal wedge augmentation. Clin Orthop 271:63, 1991.
120. Rand JA: Cement or cementless fixation in total knee arthroplasty? Clin Orthop 273:52, 1991.
121. Rand JA: The patellofemoral joint in total knee arthroplasty. J Bone Joint Surg Am 74(4):612, 1994.
122. Rhoads DD, Noble PC, Reuben JD, et al: The effect of femoral component position on patellar tracking after total knee arthroplasty. Clin Orthop 260:43, 1990.
123. Rhoads DD, Noble PC, Reuben JD, et al: The effect of femoral component position on the kinematics of total knee arthroplasty. Clin Orthop 286:122, 1993.
124. Ries MD, Guiney W, Lynch F: Osteolysis associated with cemented total knee arthroplasty. J Arthroplasty 9:555, 1994.
125. Ries MD, Rauscher LA, Hoskins S, et al: Intramedullary pressure and pulmonary function during total knee arthroplasty. Clin Orthop 356:154, 1998.
126. Ritter MA: Screw and cement fixation of large defects in TKA. J Arthroplasty 1:125, 1986.
127. Ritter MA, Campbell ED: A model for easy location of the center of the femoral head during total knee arthroplasty. J Arthroplasty (Suppl):59, 1988.
128. Ritter MA, Faris PM, Keating EM: Posterior cruciate ligament balancing during total knee arthroplasty. J Arthroplasty 3(4): 323, 1988.
129. Ritter MA, Gandolf VS, Holston KS: Continuous passive motion versus physical therapy in total knee arthroplasty. Clin Orthop 244:239, 1989.
130. Ritter MA, Herbst SA, Keating EM, et al: Radiolucency at the bone cement interface in total knee replacement. The effects of bone surface preparation and cement technique. J Bone Joint Surg Am 76:60, 1994.
131. Ritter MA, Herbst SA, Keating EM, et al: Long-term survival of a posterior cruciate-retaining total condylar total knee arthroplasty. Clin Orthop 309:136, 1994.
132. Ritter MA, Stringer EA: Predictive range of motion after total knee replacement. Clin Orthop 143:115, 1979.
133. Robinson EJ, Muluken BD, Bourne RB, et al: Catastrophic osteolysis in total knee replacement. A report of 17 cases. Clin Orthop 321:98, 1995.
134. Romness DW, Rand JA: The role of continuous passive motion following total knee arthroplasty. Clin Orthop 226:34, 1988.

135. Salter RB: The biologic concept of continuous passive motion of synovial joints: The first 18 years of basic research and its clinical application. Clin Orthop 242:12, 1989.
136. Sambatakakis A, Wilton TJ, Newton G: Radiographic sign of persistent soft-tissue imbalance after knee replacement. J Bone Joint Surg Br 73:751, 1991.
137. Sany MR, Scott RD: Posterior polyethylene wear in posterior cruciate ligament-retaining total knee arthroplasty. A case study. J Arthroplasty 8(4):439, 1993.
138. Schai PA, Thornhill TS, Scott RD: Total knee arthroplasty with the PFC system. Results at a minimum of ten years and survivorship analysis. J Bone Joint Surg Br 80:850, 1998.
139. Schemitsch EH, Scott RD, Ewald FC, et al: Tibial tray augmentation with modular wedges for tibial bone stock deficiency. J Bone Joint Surg Br 77(Suppl):79, 1995.
140. Scott RD: Duopatellar total knee replacement: The Brigham experience. Orthop Clin North Am 13:17, 1982.
141. Scott RD: Posterior cruciate ligament retaining designs and results. In Insall JN, Scott WN, Scuderi GR, eds: Current Concepts in Primary and Revision Total Knee Arthoplasty. Philadelphia, Lippincott-Raven, 1996, pp 37–40.
142. Scott RD, Thornhill TS: Posterior cruciate supplementing total knee replacement using conforming inserts and cruciate recession: Effect on range of motion and radiolucent lines. Clin Orthop 309:146, 1994.
143. Scott RD, Volative TB: Twelve years' experience with posterior cruciate-retaining total knee arthroplasty. Clin Orthop 205:100, 1986.
144. Scott WN, Rubinstein M, Scuderi GR: Results after knee replacement with a posterior cruciate substituting prosthesis. J Bone Joint Surg Am 70:1163, 1988.
145. Scuderi GR, Insall JN, Haas SB, et al: Inlay autogeneic bone grafting of tibial defects in primary total knee arthroplasty. Clin Orthop 248:93, 1989.
146. Siegel JL, Shall LM: Femoral instrumentation using the anterosuperior iliac spine as a landmark in total knee arthroplasty. An anatomic study. J Arthroplasty 6(4):317, 1991.
147. Simmons ED Jr, Sullivan JA, Rackemann S, et al: The accuracy of tibial intramedullary alignment devices in total knee arthroplasty. J Arthroplasty 6(1):45, 1991.
148. Smith JL, Tullos HS, Davidson JP: Alignment of total knee arthroplasty. J Arthroplasty (Suppl):55, 1989.
149. Stern SH, Insall JN: Posterior stabilized prosthesis. Results after followup of nine to twelve years. J Bone Joint Surg Am 72: 1400, 1992.
150. Stern SH, Moeckel BH, Insall JN: Total knee arthroplasty in valgus knees. Clin Orthop 273:5, 1991.
151. Stiehl JB, Cherveny PM: Femoral rotational alignment using the tibial shaft axis in total knee arthroplasty. Clin Orthop 331:47, 1996.
152. Stiehl JB, Komistek RD, Dennis DA, et al: Fluoroscopic analysis of kinematics after posterior-cruciate retaining total knee arthroplasty using fluoroscopy. J Bone Joint Surg Br 77:884, 1995.
153. Swany MR, Scott RD: Posterior polyethylene wear in posterior cruciate ligament retaining total knee arthroplasty. J Arthoplasty 8:439, 1993.
154. Tanzer M, Miller J: The natural history of flexion contracture in total knee arthroplasty: a prospective study. Clin Orthop 248: 129, 1989.
155. Teeny SM, Krackow KA, Hungerford DS, et al: Primary total knee arthroplasty in patients with severe varus deformity. Clin Orthop 273:19, 1991.
156. Tew M, Forster IW: Effect of knee replacement on flexion deformity. J Bone Joint Surg Br 69:395, 1987.
157. Tillett ED, Engh GA, Petersen T: A comparative study of extramedullary and intramedullary alignment systems in total knee arthroplasty. Clin Orthop 230:176, 1988.
158. Touchi H, Lock DA, Genuino VS, et al: The effect of metal wedges on the strain distribution in the proximal tibia following total knee arthroplasty. Trans Orthop Res Soc 42:731, 1996.
159. Townley CO: The anatomic total knee resurfacing arthroplasty. Clin Orthop 192: 82, 1985.
160. Trent PS, Besser W, Dueland R, et al: Total knee prosthesis combining porous ingrowth and initial stabilization. Trans Orthop Res Soc 3:164, 1978.
161. Wasielewski RC, Galante JO, Leighty RM, et al: Wear patterns on retrieved polyethylene tibial inserts and their relationship to technical considerations during total knee arthroplasty. Clin Orthop 299:31, 1994.
162. Wasielewski RC, Parks NL, Williams I, et al: The tibial insert undersurface as a contributing source of polyethylene wear debris. Clin Orthop 345:53, 1997.
163. Waslewski GL, Marson BM, Benjamin JB: Early, incapacitating instability of posterior cruciate ligament-retaining total knee arthroplasty. J Arthroplasty 13(7):763, 1998.
164. Whiteside LA: Cementless total knee replacement. Nine- to 11-year results and 10-year survivorship analysis. Clin Orthop 309: 185, 1994.
165. Whiteside LA: Correction of ligament and bone defects in total arthroplasty of the severely valgus knee. Clin Orthop 288:234, 1993.
166. Whiteside LA: Effect of porous-coating configuration on tibial osteolysis after total knee arthroplasty. Clin Orthop 321:92, 1995.
167. Whiteside LA: Exposure in difficult total knee arthroplasty using tibial tubercle osteotomy. Clin Orthop 321:32, 1995.
168. Whiteside LA, Arima J: The anteroposterior axis for femoral rotational alignment in valgus total knee arthroplasty. Clin Orthop 321:168, 1995.
169. Whiteside LA, Ohl MD: Tibial tubercle osteotomy for exposure of the difficult total knee arthroplasty. Clin Orthop 260:6, 1990.
170. Windsor RE, Insall JN, Sculco TP: Bone grafting of tibial defects in primary and revision total knee arthroplasty. Clin Orthop 205:132, 1986.
171. Windsor RE, Scuderi GR, Moran MC, et al: Mechanisms of failure of the femoral and tibial components in total knee arthroplasty. Clin Orthop 248:15, 1989.
172. Wolff AM, Hungerford DS, Krackow KA, et al: Osteotomy of the tibial tubercle during total knee replacement: A report of twenty-six cases. J Bone Joint Surg Am 71:848, 1989.
173. Wright TM, Bartel DL: The problem of surface damage in polyethylene total knee components. Clin Orthop 205:67, 1986.
174. Wright RJ, Lima J, Scott RD, et al: Two- to four-year results of posterior cruciate-sparing condylar total knee arthroplasty with an uncemented femoral component. Clin Orthop 260:80, 1990.
175. Yashar AA, Venn-Watson E, Welsh T, et al: Continuous passive motion with accelerated flexion after total knee arthroplasty. Clin Orthop 345:38, 1997.

75 Unicompartmental Total Knee Arthroplasty

RICHARD D. SCOTT

Despite more than two decades of controversy, the status of unicompartmental knee replacement remains uncertain. In the early 1970s several authors reported early discouraging results with unicondylar arthroplasty and questioned its role except perhaps in lateral compartmental disease.[15, 22] During the next 10 years, more favorable results began appearing.[1, 25, 37] These were largely the result of refined surgical technique and the narrowing of patient selection to those candidates better suited for the procedure.

The concept of unicompartmental total knee replacement is attractive as an alternative to tibial osteotomy or tricompartmental replacement in the osteoarthritic patient with unicompartmental disease confirmed at arthrotomy.[12, 19, 42] Compared with osteotomy, unicompartmental arthroplasty has a higher initial success rate and fewer early complications.[16, 37] Any internal derangement can be relieved at the time of arthrotomy. Intra-articular débridement can lead to an improvement in range of motion. Patients with bilateral disease can have both knees operated on during the same anesthetic with full recovery within 3 months of surgery. Osteotomies in the same patient are often spaced 3 to 6 months apart, and as much as a year may be required to achieve full recovery from the time of the initial procedure.

Compared with tricompartmental arthroplasty, unicompartmental replacement has the advantage of preserving both cruciate ligaments, yielding a knee with nearly normal kinematics.[19, 31, 42] A study of 42 patients with a bi- or tricompartmental arthroplasty on one side and a unicompartmental replacement on the other showed that more patients preferred the unicompartmental side because it felt more like a normal knee and had better function.[8, 27]

Another potential advantage over tricompartmental replacement is the preservation of bone stock in the patellofemoral joint and opposite compartment. Theoretically, this should make revision easier to perform should it become necessary. This advantage, however, has not been supported by several studies of revision of unicompartmental replacements.[2, 21, 28] Results of revision were not superior to those seen after revision of bi- or tricompartmental replacement, and bone stock deficiency in the femoral condyle or tibial plateau often had to be augmented with bone graft or special components. These deficiencies are frequently the result of poor surgical techniques or prostheses that invade the bone stock unnecessarily. More modern techniques using surface replacements on the femoral and tibial sides have made the procedure as conservative in practice as it is in theory.

In a study by Levine and associates the results of revision of failed unicompartmental replacements performed with bone-sparing components were similar to those published for primary knee arthroplasty.[23]

Survivorship analyses have been reported for tricompartmental replacement, indicating that survivorship with or without cruciate retention can be above 90% after 10 years of follow-up.[29, 30, 33, 38] Survivorship studies generated from early unicompartmental series show that survivorship is not as good at 10 years, dropping into the 85% range.[5, 13, 25, 35, 40, 41] These series were generated, however, at a time when patient selection was still evolving and surgical techniques were not yet perfected. Later reports may show better survivorship into the second decade.[7]

PATIENT SELECTION

Osteotomy remains the procedure of choice in the young, heavy, active male patient with unicompartmental osteoarthritis. Rest pain and poor range of motion are relative contraindications to osteotomy. Internal derangement is not a contraindication to osteotomy but should be relieved by an arthroscopic procedure before or after the osteotomy. Subluxation and extreme angular deformity are contraindications to both osteotomy and unicompartmental replacement. Metallic interpositional arthroplasty may occasionally be advisable when osteotomy is contraindicated and the patient is considered too young or too heavy to be a candidate for total knee arthroplasty (Fig. 75.1).[9, 36] Until recently the ideal candidate for unicompartmental replacement was the osteoarthritic patient with a physiologic age greater than 60 and a sedentary lifestyle.[19, 39] With survivorship studies of tricompartmental arthroplasty superior to unicompartmental arthroplasty after the first decade, the selection process must be reconsidered. Patients in their 60s and 70s would seem to have a greater chance of living out their life without a revision if they undergo a tricompartmental procedure. Unicompartmental replacement now might assume its role in two groups of patients. One is the middle-aged osteoarthritic patient (especially female undergoing a "first arthroplasty"). Advantages include a reliable initial result, anatomic realignment (versus osteotomy with clinical valgus that can be cosmetically objectionable), retention of both cruciates for higher performance, and easy salvage. A published report of

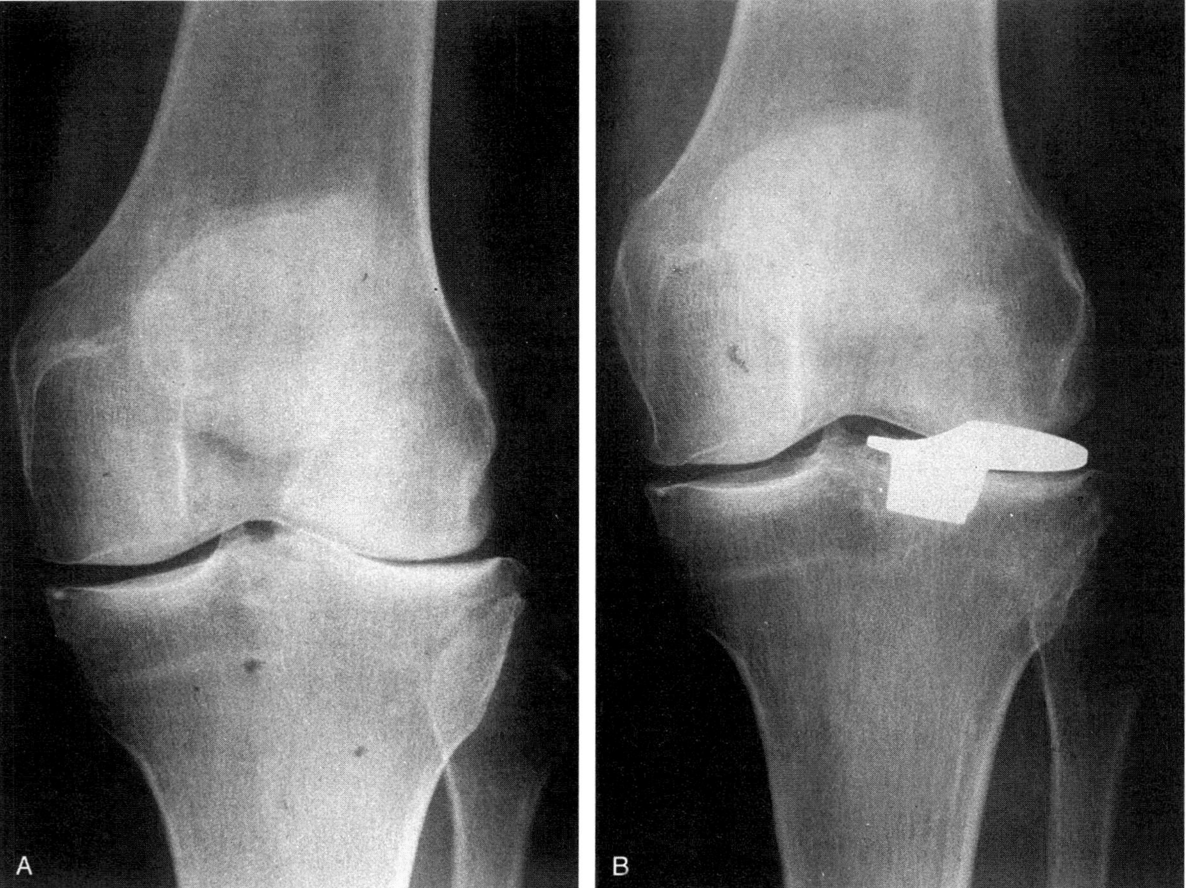

FIGURE 75.1 ➢ *A,* Preoperative anteroposterior (AP) radiograph of a 50-year-old ski instructor with advanced lateral compartmental osteoarthritis and early medical changes. *B,* AP radiograph 8 years after McKeever hemiarthroplasty. The patient returned to downhill skiing.

early results in middle-aged patients supported this concept but recommended caution in the heavy, active middle-aged male.[32]

The second group of potential candidates comprises osteoarthritic octagenarians having their "first and last" arthroplasty. Advantages include faster surgery, faster recovery, less blood loss, less energy consumption, and a less expensive prosthesis. An unpublished series of 42 octagenarians from my clinic shows that at 5 to 10 years after surgery, the prostheses survived the patient in all but 1 case.

Once an arthroplasty has been chosen over osteotomy, the final decision between unicompartmental replacement versus bi- or tricompartmental replacement is made at arthrotomy.[19, 37, 42] Although the patient may be an ideal candidate for unicompartmental arthroplasty, as indicated by clinical examination and radiography, several contraindications to the procedure may be discovered at the time of arthrotomy. I consider an absent anterior cruciate ligament to be a significant (although not absolute) contraindication to unicompartmental replacement because this is usually accompanied by ligamentous laxity that can promote eventual lateral subluxation of the tibia on the femur and secondary opposite compartment disease. Inspection of the opposite compartment and patellofemoral joint may show significant degenerative changes that make unicompartmental arthroplasty inadvisable.

Mild chondromalacia in the opposite compartment can be accepted, but areas of eburnated bone are definite contraindications. In a varus osteoarthritic knee with medial compartment arthritis, a secondary lesion appears on the medial aspect of the lateral femoral condyle with early lateral subluxation. This is usually accompanied by intercondylar osteophyte formation (Fig. 75.2). If the subluxation is slight and the lesion is small, it can be débrided and corrected by unicompartmental arthroplasty. If the subluxation is great and the lesion large, bi- or tricompartmental arthroplasty is advisable.

Eburnated bone in the patellofemoral compartment is also a contraindication to unicompartmental arthroplasty. There are some surgeons, however, who will accept patellofemoral degeneration, including areas of eburnated bone, and still proceed with unicompartmental arthroplasty. I will accept significant chondromalacia but usually not eburnated bone.

A third contraindication discovered at arthrotomy

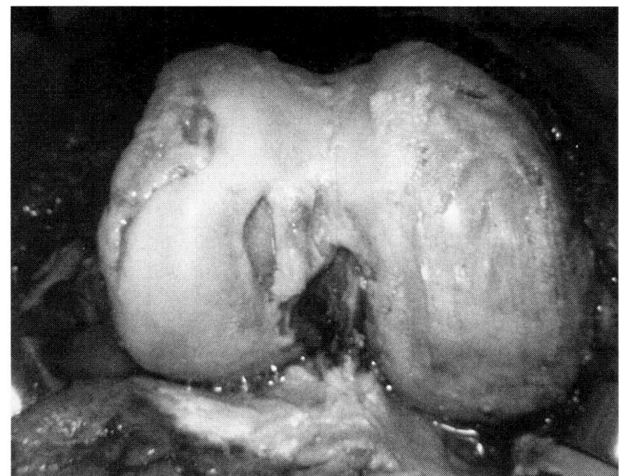

FIGURE 75.2 ➢ Erosion of the medial aspect of the lateral femoral condyle secondary to tibial spine impingement.

consists of a significant inflammatory component to the patient's disease. This may be in the form of a very strong synovial reaction or the discovery of diffuse crystal deposits from either gout or pseudogout. Inflammatory disease in any form substantially increases the risk of secondary degeneration of the opposite compartment in subsequent years.

IMPLANT DESIGN

Over the past two decades many lessons have been learned concerning the ideal design features of a unicompartmental arthroplasty. Many early femoral components were narrow in their mediolateral dimension and suffered a high incidence of subsidence of the component into the condylar bone.[35, 37] The ideal component should be wide enough to maximally cap the resurfaced condyle, widely distributing the weightbearing forces and decreasing the chance of subsidence and loosening. For this reason, multiple sizes should be available to accommodate both small and large patients. Revision studies have shown the inadvisability of deeply invading the condyle with fixation methods.[2, 21, 28] Relatively small fixation lugs appear to be sufficient as long as there are two lugs to gain rotational fixation to the bone or some sort of fin provided for this purpose. The posterior metallic condyle should fully cap the posterior condyle of the patient to allow physiological range of motion without impingement. The amount of bone resection required for insertion should be minimal. Preferably, the femoral component can be supported on top of the distal subchondral bone without any resection, but this requires sacrifice of more bone from the tibial side. The ideal compromise is perhaps to resect 4 to 6 mm of distal condyle, still preserving adequate distal femoral bone to allow easy conversion to a bicompartmental prosthesis. At the same time, this distal femoral resection preserves an equivalent amount of proximal tibial bone.

The coronal articulating topography of the prosthetic components must also consist of a compromise. A flat surface on the femoral component articulating with flat surface on the tibial component may potentially improve metal-to-plastic contact, but is difficult to technically line up precisely enough to avoid edge contact throughout the range of motion. An articulating surface with a small radius of curvature articulating on the tibial side with a flat surface creates too much point contact. A femoral surface with a small radius of curvature matched to a similarly small radius on the tibial side can create too much constraint. The ideal surfaces of both components therefore are probably those with a relatively large radius of curvature that

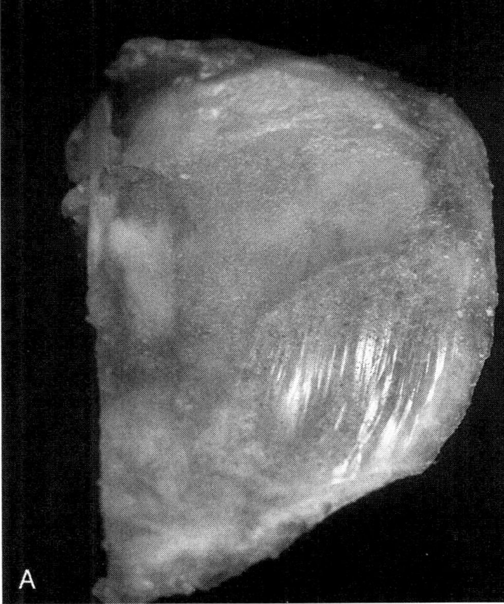

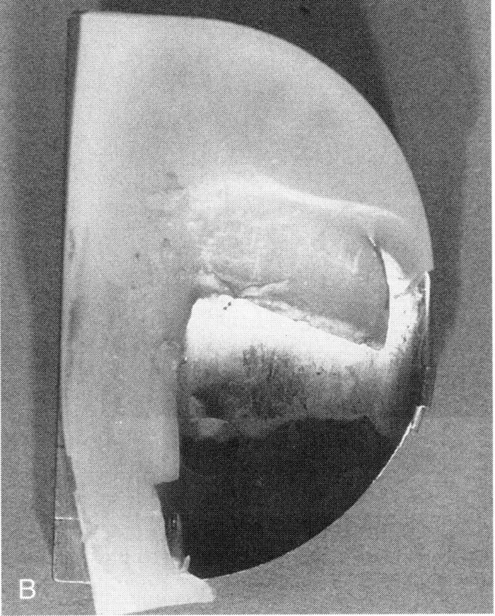

FIGURE 75.3 ➢ *A,* A typical anterior and peripheral wear pattern in medial osteoarthritis. *B,* A worn medial metal-backed tibial component showing an anterior and peripheral wear pattern.

allows adequate metal-to-plastic contact without excessive constraint.

In the sagittal plane, conformity might at first seem attractive to increase contact area and lower stresses that cause polyethylene wear. Retrievals of worn unicompartmental tibial components have yielded important information regarding wear patterns and their implications on prosthetic design (Fig. 75.3). It appears that the polyethylene wear pattern tends to reproduce the preoperative wear pattern of the osteoarthritic knee.[26] As noted by White and associates,[43] this tends to be anterior and peripheral on the medial tibial plateau in a varus knee. If a fixed-bearing unicompartmental knee is too conforming, a higher incidence of component loosening is reported.[14, 32]

The mobile- or meniscal-bearing articulation is an attractive way to maximize contact area and decrease contact stresses while avoiding excessive constraint.[10, 11] This technique, however, usually requires slightly more tibial resection to accommodate the thinnest bearing and runs the slight additional risk of bearing subluxation.

The shape of the tibial component as it sits on the tibial plateau should probably be anatomic. This will maximize contact between the prosthesis and the bone and widely distribute the weightbearing forces to resist subsidence and loosening. It will also provide maximum plastic for an anterior and peripheral wear pattern. This will necessitate an asymmetrical shape with right and left components (Fig. 75.4). As is necessary on the femoral side, multiple sizes will be required on the tibial side to accommodate both small and large patients.

Metal backing of the tibial component is controversial. This was initiated in the early 1980s in order to distribute the weightbearing forces more uniformly on the cut surface of the plateau. Early results with metal-backed components were superior to those with all polyethylene components, but possibly because of improved patient selection and operative technique rather than the use of the metal backing.[20] When metal-backed components were followed for more than 5 years, failures were seen in 6-mm components because of wear-through of the polyethylene to the metal backing. This resulted when therere were areas of polyethylene thickness of less than 4 mm and design flaws in the method of fixation of the polyethylene to metal. These problems were similar to those seen with metal-backed patellar components.[3, 24] Depending on the type of metal used (titanium versus chrome cobalt), the minimal composite thickness of a metal-backed tibial component must be 8 to 10 mm. This necessity makes metal backing less attractive than previously thought, and there appears to be a trend back to all polyethylene tibial components.

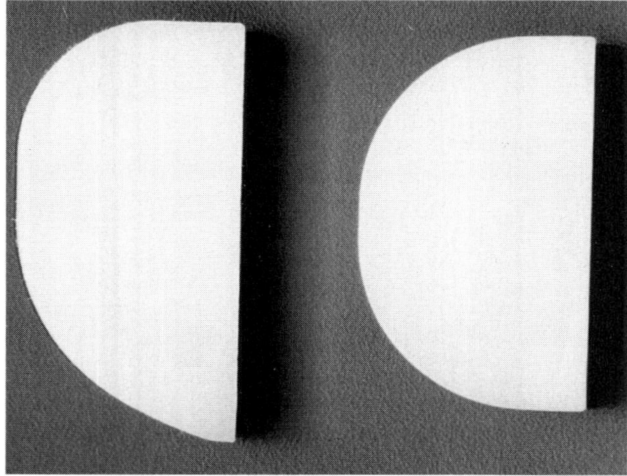

FIGURE 75.4 ➢ A comparison of anatomic symmetric and asymmetric tibial components.

SURGICAL TECHNIQUE

The surgical technique is critical to the success of the procedure.[34, 37, 42] A vertical incision centered over the medial one-third of the patella is recommended. It is usually about 12 cm long and begins proximally over the midshaft of the femur and ends distally just medial to the tibial tubercle. A medial parapatellar capsulotomy is performed to allow eversion of the patella and adequate exposure.

For medial compartmental arthroplasty, the coronary ligament is incised at the anterior horn of the medial meniscus, and a periosteal sleeve is elevated from the anteromedial aspect of the tibia. To allow eversion of the patella, the lateral dissection is performed within the fat pad anterior to the coronary ligament, avoiding derangement of the anterior horn of lateral meniscus. For lateral compartmental replacement, the coronary ligament is left intact medially, avoiding derangement of the anterior horn of the medial meniscus. The ligament is incised lateral to the midline and a periosteal sleeve is elevated from the anterolateral aspect of the tibia as far as Gerdy's tubercle.

Alternatively, some surgeons recommend a lateral parapatellar incision for a valgus deformity and lateral compartment arthroplasty.[17] This will provide excellent exposure of the lateral compartment but may make bicondylar replacement more difficult if this is deemed necessary and the surgeon is not familiar with the lateral approach.

After adequate exposure has been achieved, the three compartments of the knee are carefully inspected and a decision is made concerning the number of compartments that need replacement. Unicompartmental arthroplasty is contraindicated if there is an inflammatory synovitis or there are crystalline deposits of uric acid or calcium pyrophosphate. The anterior cruciate should be intact. The cartilage in the opposite compartment should appear to be healthy. Chondromalacia in the patellofemoral compartment is not a contraindication to unicompartmental arthroplasty, but eburnated bone on the patella or trochlea probably mandates tricompartmental replacement.

INTERCONDYLAR OSTEOPHYTES

As osteoarthritis of the medial compartment progresses, there is usually a tendency for lateral subluxation of the tibia on the femur during weightbearing. As a result, the lateral tibial spine impinges on the medial aspect of the lateral femoral condyle, and "kissing" osteophytes develop, accompanied by erosion of the medial aspect of the lateral femoral condyle (see Fig. 75.2). If these osteophytes are not removed, intercondylar impingement can persist after unicompartmental arthoplasty with pain on weightbearing. If the kissing lesion is large, bicompartmental or tricompartmental arthroplasty may be necessary.

As lateral compartment osteoarthritis progresses, lateral subluxation of the tibia on the femur usually does not occur until the deformity is so severe that unicompartmental arthroplasty is not appropriate. The medial collateral ligament and medial capsule gradually elongate as the valgus deformity progresses (Fig. 75.5). With significant medial laxity, the knee can no longer be stabilized by unicompartmental arthroplasty, and bicompartmental arthroplasty accompanied by lateral release is necessary.

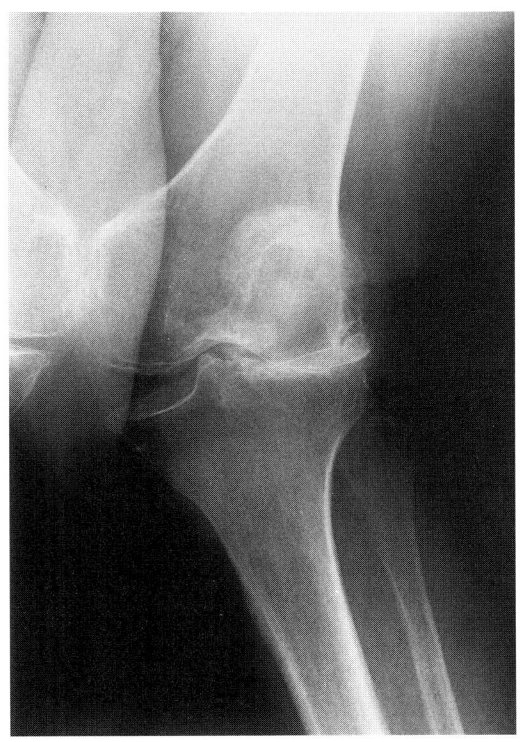

FIGURE 75.5 ➢ Lateral unicompartmental osteoarthritis with significant laxity of the medial collateral ligament.

PERIPHERAL OSTEOPHYTES

In an osteoarthritic knee with a varus deformity, peripheral osteophytes build up on the periphery of the medial femoral condyle and medial plateau of the tibia. The medial collateral ligament and capsule may be tented over these osteophytes, resulting in relative shortening of these structures, preventing passive correction of a varus deformity. When the osteophytes are removed, there is relative lengthening of the medial collateral ligament and capsule allowing passive correction of the varus deformity (Fig. 75.6). A formal medial ligament release is rarely necessary, because this need would imply that there is a varus deformity too great for unicompartmental arthroplasty.

FEMORAL COMPONENT

Placement

The femoral component should be placed in the center of the mediolateral dimension of the femoral condyle, measured after removal of peripheral and intercondylar osteophytes. If the femoral component is placed laterally in a medial compartmental arthroplasty (too close to the intercondylar notch), the procedure may fail for the following reasons. If the tibial component used provides no mediolateral constraint, the femoral component can impinge on the medial tibial spine. If, however, the laterally placed femoral component is mated to a medial tibial component with intercondylar constraint, the tibia will move laterally on the femur when the components are seated and the lateral tibial spine will impinge on the lateral femoral condyle.

The femoral component should extend far enough anteriorly to cover the weightbearing surface that comes in contact with the tibia in full extension. The anterior extent of the weightbearing surface is usually well defined by the junction between the eburnated bone of the femoral condyle and the intact cartilage remaining in the trochlear groove. The leading edge of

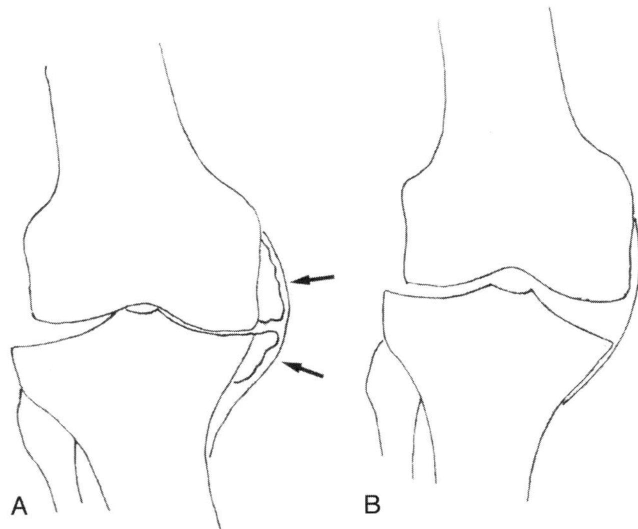

FIGURE 75.6 ➢ *A,* A diagram showing how medial osteophytes on the femur and tibia tent up the medial collateral ligament and capsule. *B,* After removal of osteophytes, the varus deformity can be corrected.

the femoral component must be countersunk into this junction to prevent patellar impingement during flexion of the knee. The same principles apply to placement of a femoral component onto the lateral femoral condyle.

Size

The femoral component used should be of a size that reproduces most accurately the anteroposterior dimension of the femoral condyle. In borderline cases, the larger size should always be inserted first to conserve bone. The posterior condylar bone should be resected to at least the thickness of the metallic implant. It is better to resect slightly too much of the posterior condyle than too little to avoid making the components too tight in flexion.

TIBIAL COMPONENT

Placement

The tibial component should be positioned on the tibia so that with the knee correctly aligned this component is directly under the femoral component in the mediolateral dimension and the articulating surfaces of the two components are rotationally congruent during weightbearing (Fig. 75.7). The congruency of components should be determined with the knee in full extension. It should not be judged while the knee is flexed and the patella is everted, because in that position the displaced quadriceps mechanism artificially externally rotates and laterally subluxes the tibia on the femur. If there is a preoperative quadriceps contracture, the force of the displaced quadriceps is even greater. After placement of the tibial component, proper congruency in the frontal plane should be judged by observing the tracking of the components as the knee is flexed and extended with the patella located in the trochlear groove. Viewed from the front, the line of resection of the tibial plateau should be within 5 degrees of right angle to the longitudinal axis of the tibia. Viewed from the side, the line of resection varies from 0 to 10 degrees of posterior slope, depending on the individual case; 3 to 5 degrees of posterior slope is usually appropriate.

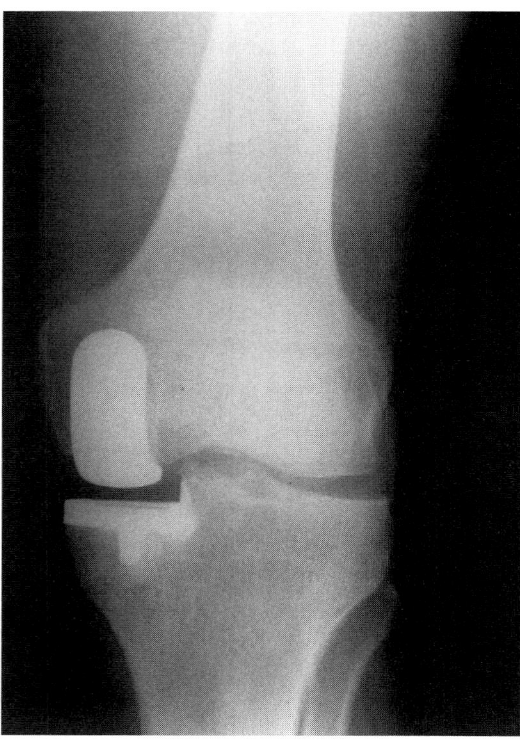

FIGURE 75.7 ➢ AP radiograph showing well-positioned components after medial unicompartmental arthroplasty.

Size

Ideally, the proper thickness of the tibial component is that which is necessary to restore the worn tibial plateau to its normal height after resection. In a varus knee, if the medial collateral ligament and capsule have been properly released by removal of medial osteophytes, correction of the deformity should be possible without resorting to thicker tibial components. If the articulated components are too tight, the tibia will subluxate toward the opposite compartment and produce excessive pressure there. After the medial compartment replacement, the medial joint space should open up 1 or 2 mm when valgus stress is applied with the knee in full extension. The same principles apply to replacement of the lateral compartment.

The alignment goals for unicompartmental arthroplasty are different from those for osteotomy or tricompartmental replacement. The deformity should not be overcorrected as advocated for osteotomy.[18]

POSTOPERATIVE REHABILITATION

A postoperative regimen following unicompartmental arthroplasty will be similar to that following bi- or tricompartmental arthroplasty. It is often noted, however, that rehabilitation goals are met faster and the patients suffer from less postoperative pain, swelling, and blood loss.[8] Following closure of the capsule, a note is made of the patient's potential flexion against gravity, since it is unreasonable to expect improvement on this during the initial postoperative period. My current postoperative protocol includes the use of low-dose Coumadin (started the night before surgery) combined with pulsatile compression stockings to minimize the chance for postoperative venous thrombosis.

Continuous passive motion is begun immediately in the recovery room, starting at 30 to 40 degrees of flexion if a general anesthetic has been used or 70 to 90 degrees if a long-acting spinal or continuous epidural anesthetic has been administered. The motion machine is used during the day and a knee immobilizer is applied at night to minimize the chance for the development of a significant flexion contracture. The continuous passive motion machine is advanced 10 to 20 degrees per day as tolerated until 90 degrees is achieved and maintained. Quadriceps-setting exercises and attempts at straight-leg raising are initiated on the second postoperative day when the patient also begins bed-chair transfers. By the third day the patient ambulates with a walker or crutches and 50% weightbearing.

A knee immobilizer is used during ambulation until the patient has a secure ability to straight-leg raise. Most patients remain on protected weightbearing with full-time support until 4 to 6 weeks following surgery when they graduate to a cane outdoors and no support for short distances. The cane is discontinued completely at 3 months postsurgery.

CEMENTLESS UNICOMPARTMENTAL ARTHROPLASTY

The role of cementless unicompartmental arthroplasty is uncertain. In theory, it is appealing if it could be shown to be conservative compared with cemented unicompartmental arthroplasty. In practice, a cementless unicompartmental arthroplasty is actually more radical than a cemented procedure. For most cementless components, more bone resection is required on the femoral side. Failure rates are reported to be higher in terms of loosening on both the femoral and tibial sides.[4] Metal-backed components are most likely required on the tibial side. Cementless unicompartmental arthroplasty must remain experimental until better methods and results are reported.

SUMMARY

Despite almost three decades of experience, the role of unicompartmental arthroplasty remains controversial. It appears to offer an attractive alternative to osteotomy or tricompartmental arthroplasty in selected osteoarthritic patients. The procedure can be conservative with preservation of cruciate ligaments along with bone stock in the opposite compartment and patellofemoral joint.

With appropriate patient selection, prosthetic design, and operative technique, unicompartmental replacement can function as the initial conservative replacement in middle-aged osteoarthritics, especially females. It may also be appropriate in the very elderly patient with a life expectancy of less than 10 years. Osteotomy should still be considered in the young, heavy-active individual, especially males.

References

1. Bae KK, Guhl JF, Keane SP: Unicompartmental knee arthroplasty for single compartment disease. Clin Orthop 176:235, 1983.
2. Barrett WH, Scott RD: Revision of failed unicondylar arthroplasty. J Bone Joint Surg Am 69:1328, 1987.
3. Bayley JC, Scott RD, Ewald FC, et al: Failure of the metal-backed patellar component after total knee replacement. J Bone Joint Surg Am 70:668, 1988.
4. Bernasek TL, Rand JA, Bryan RS: Unicompartmental porous coated anatomic total knee arthroplasty. Clin Orthop 236:52, 1988.
5. Bert JM: Ten year survivorship of metal-backed unicompartmental arthroplasty. J Arthroplasty 13:901, 1998.
6. Broughton NS, Newman JH, Bailey RA: Unicompartmental replacement osteoarthritis of the knee. J Bone Joint Surg Br 68: 447, 1986.
7. Cartier P, Sanouiller JL, Grelsamer RP: Unicompartmental knee arthroplasty surgery. J Arthroplasty 11:782, 1996.
8. Cobb AG, Kozinn SC, Scott RD: Unicondylar or total knee replacement: The patient's preference. J Bone Joint Surg Br 72: 166, 1990.
9. Emerson RH, Potter T: The use of the metallic McKeever hemiarthroplasty for unicompartmental arthritis. J Bone Joint Surg Am 67:208, 1985.
10. Goodfellow JW, O'Connor JJ: Clinical results of the Oxford knee: Surface arthroplasty of the tibiofemoral joint with a meniscal-bearing prosthesis. Clin Orthop 205:21, 1986.
11. Goodfellow JW, Tribewal MB, Sherman KP, et al: Unicompartmental Oxford meniscal knee arthroplasty. J Arthroplasty 2:1, 1987.
12. Grelsamer RP: Unicompartmental osteoarthritis of the knee. J Bone Joint Surg Am 77:278, 1995.
13. Heck DA, Marmos L, Gibson A, et al: Unicompartmental knee evaluation. Clin Orthop 28:6:154, 1993.
14. Hodge WA, Chandler HP: Unicompartmental knee replacement: A comparison of constrained and unconstrained designs. J Bone Joint Surg Am 74:877, 1992.
15. Insall JN, Walker PS: Unicondylar knee replacement. Clin Orthop 120:83, 1976.
16. Jackson M, Sarongi PP, Newman JH: Revision total knee arthroplasty: Comparison of outcome following primary proximal tibial osteotomy or unicompartmental arthroplasty. J Arthroplasty 9: 539, 1994.
17. Keblish PA: Valgus deformity in total knee replacement: The lateral retinacular approach. Orthop Trans 9:28, 1985.
18. Kennedy W, White R: Unicompartmental total knee arthroplasty of the knee: Postoperative alignment and its influence on overall results. Clin Orthop 221:278, 1997.
19. Kozinn SC, Scott RD: Current concepts review: Unicompartmental total arthroplasty. J Bone Joint Surg Am 71:145, 1989.
20. Kozinn SC, Marx C, Scott RD: Unicompartmental knee arthroplasty. J Arthroplasty 4:1, 1989.
21. Lai, Rand JA: Revision of failed unicompartmental total knee arthroplasty. Clin Orthop 287:193, 1993.
22. Laskin RS: Unicompartmental tibiofemoral resurfacing arthroplasty. J Bone Joint Surg Am 60:182, 1978.
23. Levine WN, Ozuna RM, Scott RD, et al: Conversion of failed modern unicompartmental arthroplasty to total knee arthroplasty. J Arthroplasty 11:797, 1996.
24. Lombardi AV Jr, Engh Ga, Volz RG, et al: Fracture/dissociation of the polyethylene in metal-backed patellar components in total knee arthroplasty. J Bone Joint Surg Am 70:675, 1988.
25. Marmor L: Unicompartmental knee arthroplasty: Ten to thirteen year follow-up study. Clin Orthop 226:24, 1987.
26. McCallum JD, Scott RD: Duplication of medial erosion in unicompartmental knee arthroplasties. J Bone Joint Surg Br 77:726, 1995.
27. Newman JH, Ackroyd CE, Shah NA: Unicompartmental or total knee replacement? Five-year results of a prospective randomized trial of 102 osteoarthritic knees with unicompartmental arthritis. J Bone Joint Surg Br 80:862, 1998.
28. Padgett DE, Stern SH, Insall JN: Revision total knee arthroplasty for failed unicompartmental replacement. J Bone Joint Surg Am 73:186, 1991.
29. Ranawat CS, Oheneba BA: Survivorship analysis and results of total condylar knee arthroplasty. Clin Orthop 226:6, 1988.
30. Rand JA, Illstrup DM: Survivorship analysis of total knee arthroplasty: Cumulative rates of survival of 9200 total knee arthroplasties. J Bone Joint Surg Am 73:397, 1991.
31. Rougraff BT, Heck DA, Gibson AE: A comparison of tricompartmental and unicompartmental arthroplasty for the treatment of gonarthrosis. Clin Orthop 273:157, 1991.
32. Schai PA, Suh JT, Thornhill TS, et al: Unicompartmental knee arthroplasty in middle-aged patients. J Arthroplasty 13:365, 1998.
33. Schai PA, Thornhill TS, Scott RD: Total knee arthroplasty with the PFC system. J Bone Joint Surg Br 80:850, 1998.
34. Scott RD: Robert Brigham unicondylar knee surgical techniques. Tech Orthop 5:15, 1990.

35. Scott RD, Cobb AG, McQueary FG, et al: Unicompartmental knee arthroplasty: Eight- to twelve-year follow-up with survivorship analysis. Clin Orthop 271:96, 1991.
36. Scott RD, Joyce MJ, Ewald PC, et al: McKeever metallic hemiarthroplasty of the knee in unicompartmental degenerative arthritis. J Bone Joint Surg Am 67:203, 1985.
37. Scott RD, Santore R: Unicondylar unicompartmental replacement for osteoarthritis of the knee. J Bone Joint Surg Am 63:536, 1981.
38. Scuderi GR, Insall JN, Windsor RE, et al. Survivorship of cemented knee replacement. J Bone Joint Surg Br 71:798, 1989.
39. Stern SH, Becker MW, Insall JN: Unicondylar knee arthroplasty: An evaluation of selection criteria. Clin Orthop 286:143, 1993.
40. Swant M, Stulberg SD, Jiganti J, et al. The natural history of unicompartmental arthropalsty: An eight-year follow-up study with survivorship analysis. Clin Orthop 286:130, 1993.
41. Tabor OB Jr, Tabor OB: Unicompartmental arthroplasty: A long-term follow-up study. J Arthroplasty 13:373, 1998.
42. Thornhill TS, Scott RD: Unicompartmental total knee arthroplasty. Orthop Clin 20:25, 1989.
43. White SH, Ludkowski PF, Goodfellow JW: Anteriomedial osteoarthritis of the knee. J Bone Joint Surg Br 73:582, 1991.

76 Results of Posterior Cruciate-Preserving Total Knee Arthroplasty*

JAMES A. RAND • KAYVON S. RIGGI

There are many implant designs that preserve the posterior cruciate ligament (PCL). Early designs that saved the PCL include the Polycentric, Geometric, Duocondylar, Duopatellar, cruciate-sparing total condylar, Kinematic, Townley, Miller-Galante, PCA (porous-coated anatomic), and Cloutier total knee arthroplasties (TKAs). Recent examples of PCL-preserving designs include the Genesis, Press-Fit condylar, AMK (anatomic), AGC, and Kinemax prostheses. The role of the cruciate ligaments is an important feature in the design of TKA. Most authors now favor resection of the anterior cruciate ligament (ACL). The status of the PCL, however, remains controversial.[2, 22]

Proponents of PCL retention argue that preservation improves function, range of motion, strength, and stability, and reduces interface stresses. Many authors have found that PCL preservation results in a more normal and efficient gait pattern, especially with stair climbing.[3, 18, 40] The PCL may induce femoral rollback with knee flexion resulting in posterior translation of the tibiofemoral contact point. In an in vitro study, greater rollback was identified in posterior cruciate retaining than posterior cruciate sacrificing or posterior stabilized total knees.[81] Rollback improves potential range of motion by preventing impingement of the posterior tibial plateau on the femur. Rollback increases the dynamic quadriceps lever arm for improved strength. The PCL is the strongest ligament in the knee joint and stabilizes the knee against a predominantly posteriorly directed shear force during activities of daily living. When the PCL is not present, this shear force must be transmitted to the fixation interfaces where shear stress is not well tolerated. In addition, retention of the PCL helps maintain the joint line and may provide some proprioceptive function. The joint line is more likely to be maintained with PCL-preserving than PCL-sacrificing designs.

Proponents of PCL resection argue that removal greatly simplifies correction of deformity, allows for less tibial bone resection for a given thickness of prosthesis, and permits placement of a prosthesis with greater articular conformity and thus improved polyethylene wear characteristics.[22] The PCL is not histologically normal in the arthritic knee.[1] In one series, 23 of 27 PCLs removed at surgery were abnormal and correlated with patient age greater than 70 years and the extent of deformity.[1] In another study, 24 PCLs obtained at the time of TKA were compared with a control group of 36 PCLs from age-matched controls.[42] Marked degenerative changes were identified in 63% of the PCLs from the TKA group compared with none of the controls. Late rupture of the PCL may occur, leading to symptomatic instability.[57] Late PCL rupture has been reported with a prevalence of 2% in a series of 150 total knee replacements.[57] Comparative studies of PCL-retaining, PCL-sacrificing, and unicompartmental TKAs have shown no difference in proprioception.[8, 47, 77] However, one study found better proprioception in PCL-retaining than posterior stabilized knees.[88] In vitro, normal PCL strain was achieved in only 37% of knees undergoing PCL-retaining TKA.[52] In another study, PCL strain was increased in three, decreased in two, and was normal in two knees.[35] In vitro, extensor efficiency was best and rollback greatest with a posterior stabilized compared with PCL-preserving or PCL-sacrificing TKA design.[52] A PCL-sacrificing design is applicable to a wide variety of potential clinical problems and has more versatility than a PCL-retaining design. In vivo fluoroscopic studies of TKA have shown inconsistent motion patterns in PCL-retaining or PCL-sacrificing designs with the most consistent patterns in posterior stabilized designs.[16, 83] Ultimately the dilemma is between a PCL-retaining, low-conformity prosthesis with reduced interface stresses and a PCL-substituting semiconstrained prosthesis with reduced polyethylene stresses. Continued long-term study is necessary to determine where the proper balance lies. This chapter describes the evolution and results of cruciate-retaining TKAs. The results of PCL-retaining designs provide an important baseline for comparison and establish a minimum standard that future designs must meet.

POLYCENTRIC KNEE ARTHROPLASTY

The Polycentric (Howmedica, Rutherford, NJ) knee arthroplasty was the first cruciate-sparing, resurfacing TKA[25, 34] (Fig. 76.1). Gunston recognized that movement in the normal knee consists of rocking, gliding, and axial rotation and follows a multiple center, or

*Modified from Riggi KS, Rand JA: Posterior cruciate ligament-retaining total knee arthroplasty. In Scott WN: The Knee, vol 2, St. Louis, Mosby-Year Book, 1994, pp 1117-1141.

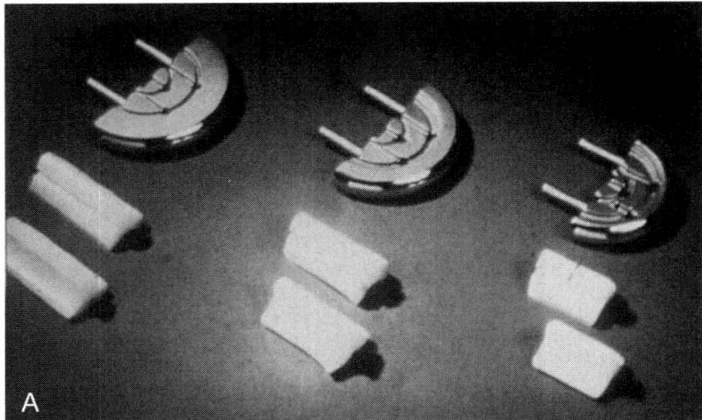

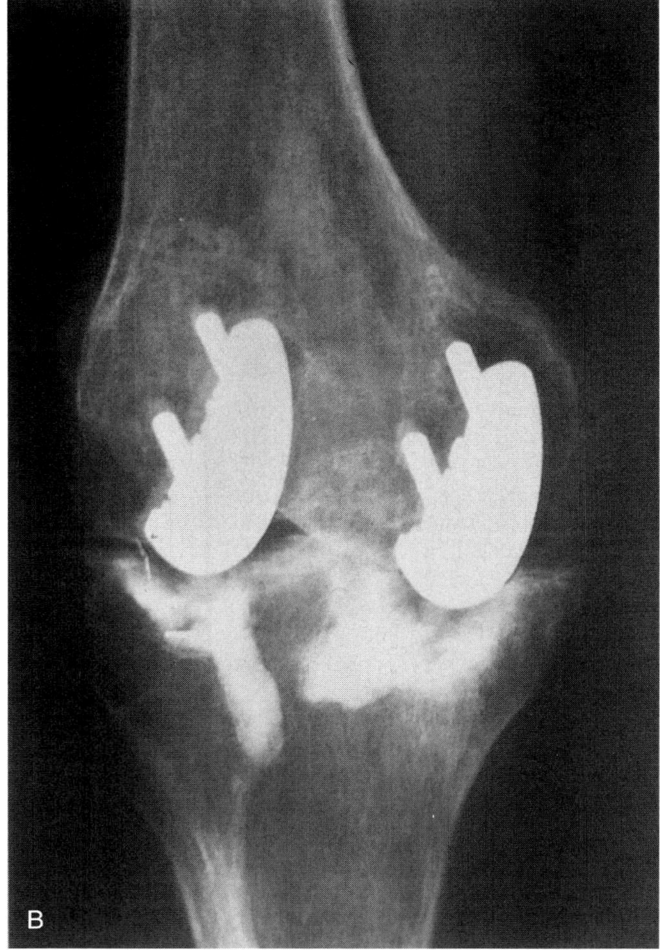

FIGURE 76.1 ➢ *A*, Photograph and *B*, anteroposterior (AP) radiograph of the Polycentric prosthesis. (From Scott WN: The Knee, vol 2, St. Louis, Mosby-Year Book, 1994, p 1118.)

polycentric pathway. The instant center for each increment of flexion moves posteriorly in a spiral pattern. Thus the concept of the Polycentric knee was to simulate normal knee motion by separate prosthetic replacement of each joint surface. The circular configuration of the femoral runners was a compromise between ease of manufacturing and the spiral curve of the femoral condyle in the normal knee. The length of the tibial track allowed both rocking and gliding movements and the articular groove allowed 20 degrees of axial rotation in an effort to reduce rotational stresses on the cemented-bone interface. Gunston in 1971 reported on 22 Polycentric TKAs in 20 patients, all with rheumatoid arthritis except for 2 patients with osteoarthritis and a previous contralateral knee arthrodesis.[25] With 1 to 2.5 years follow-up, all patients had excellent pain relief. One knee, however, in a patient with a previous patellectomy required reoperation to an arthrodesis for residual lateral instability. Thirteen knees recovered a motion arc of greater than 90 degrees and 19 of 20 patients benefited from an increased overall mobility. Operative complications included delayed wound healing in four knees and peroneal nerve palsy in one.

In 1976 Skolnick reported on 500 Polycentric TKAs performed at the Mayo Clinic between July 1970 and October 1971 and followed for 2 years.[79] Patients' ages ranged from 20 to 83 years, with a mean of 60 years; 68% were women, and 32% were men. The diagnosis was rheumatoid arthritis in 60%, osteoarthritis in 34%, and miscellaneous diagnoses in the remaining 6%. Of the 500 knees, 432 (86%) obtained excellent pain relief, with similar improvement in function for those with rheumatoid arthritis and those with osteoarthritis. The number of patients able to ambulate without aids improved from 23% to 64% and the number of patients unable to walk at all decreased from 8% to 2%. The average postoperative arc of motion was 95 degrees, an average increase of 5 degrees of motion. Overall, 96% of patients expressed satisfaction with their surgical results. Complications included malalignment or imprecise apposition of the components in 19 knees (3.8%), deep infections in 14 (2.8%), 12 instances of loosening (2.4%), and instability in 7 knees (1.4%). A total of 59 reoperations were performed on 51 knees for an overall failure rate of 10.2%.

Gunston[26] in 1980 reported the results of 204 Polycentric knee arthroplasties in 172 patients 2 to 10 years after operation. Patients' ages ranged from 29 to

79 years with a mean of 60 years with the diagnosis of rheumatoid arthritis in 80% and osteoarthritis in 20%. Pain relief was obtained in only 59%; 39% of patients had residual pain from the patellofemoral joint. Loosening occurred in 10% and infection in 6.4% of patients. Overall, 24 patients required reoperation (12%), including 7 revisions and 13 arthrodeses.

Lewallen and colleagues[50] in 1984 reported the 10-year results of 209 Polycentric TKAs performed in 159 patients at the Mayo Clinic between July 1970 and November 1971. Fifty-two men and 107 women ranged in age from 20 to 82 years, with a mean of 56 years. Sixty-seven percent had rheumatoid arthritis, 26% osteoarthritis, and 4% post-traumatic arthritis. Based on the Kaplan-Meier survival curve, the probability of still having a successful Polycentric TKA declined to 66% at 10 years. Important determinants of success or failure were the existence of a previous operation and axial alignment. Knees with previous surgery had only a 48% probability of success at 10 years compared with a 75% probability of success in the knee without prior surgery. If components were implanted in any varus angulation or valgus angulation greater than 8 degrees, the failure rate was approximately doubled. Malalignment often led to ligamentous laxity and instability, which were the most common causes of failure in 27 knees (13%). Loosening, usually of the tibial component, was the cause of failure in 15 knees (7%). Deep infection developed in 7 knees (3%). Overall, 71 knees had a failed result (34%), 58 requiring reoperation, with most undergoing a revision arthroplasty.

Although the early reports were encouraging, once longer follow-up was obtained it became apparent that instability and loosening would claim many of these prostheses and that only slightly more than half of the patients would retain a successfully functioning arthroplasty at 10 years (Table 76.1).

GEOMETRIC TKA

In the early 1970s, Coventry and colleagues designed the Geometric (Howmedica) TKA[13, 14, 33] (Fig. 76.2). The goals of this resurfacing, cruciate-sparing design were to avoid the early recognized deficiencies of the hinge prostheses while at the same time providing improved stability compared with the Polycentric prosthesis. Unfortunately, it was not recognized in that era that a geometrically partially constrained implant with a single axis of rotation that preserves the cruciate ligaments represents a kinematic mismatch and is predisposed to loosening. Skolnick and colleagues[78] reported the 2-year follow-up of 119 knees in 85 patients with geometric TKAs implanted at the Mayo

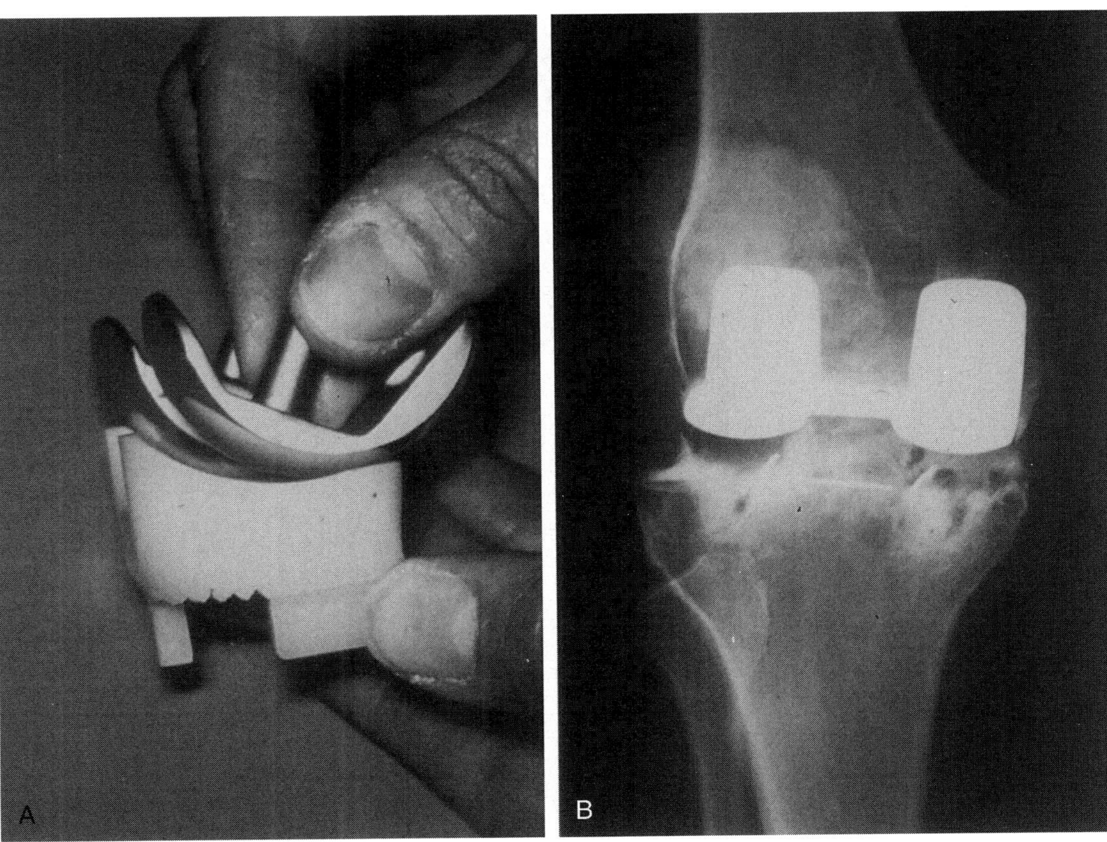

FIGURE 76.2 ➢ *A,* Photograph and *B,* AP radiograph of the Geometric prosthesis. (From Scott WN: The Knee, vol 2, St. Louis, Mosby-Year Book, 1994, p 1120.)

TABLE 76.1 Polycentric Total Knee Arthroplasty

Authors	No. of Knees/Patients	Mean Age (yr; range)	Rheumatoid Arthritis (%)	Osteoarthritis (%)	Follow-up (yr)	Successful Results (%)	Instability (%)	Loosening (%)	Infection (%)	Reoperations/ Failures (%)
Gunston (1971)[25]	22/20	—	91	9	1–2.5	95	27	—	—	4.5
Skolnick et al (1976)[79]	500 knees	$\overline{X}$ = 60 (20–83)	60	34	2	86	1.4	2.4	2.8	10.2
Gunston (1980)[26]	204/172	$\overline{X}$ = 60 (29–79)	80	20	2–10	59	—	10	6.4	39
Lewallen et al (1984)[50]	209/159	$\overline{X}$ = 56 (20–82)	67	26	10.5	66 (actuarial analysis)	13	7	3	34

Clinic between April 1971 and June 1972; 38% were men and 62% were women with an age range from 25 to 84 years, and a mean of 61 years. Fifty-three percent of patients had rheumatoid arthritis, and 41% had osteoarthritis. Satisfactory relief of pain was obtained in 84% of knees with comparable rsults in those with rheumatoid arthritis and with osteoarthritis; 93% of the patients expressed overall satisfaction with their results. Complications included tibial component loosening in 13 knees (11.8%), 8 of which had persistent varus deformity. Deep infection occurred in only 2 knees (1.8%). In contrast to the Polycentric knee, instability was not a significant problem, with only one case of dislocation occurring in a patient with rheumatoid arthritis and absence of both cruciate ligaments. Overall, 17 of 110 knees (15.5%) required a total of 22 reoperations.

In 1981, Lowe and McNeur[51] reported on 150 knee arthroplasties in 106 patients implanted at the Alfred Hospital in Melbourne, Australia, between 1973 and 1977. Forty-eight percent of the arthroplasties were performed for rheumatoid arthritis in patients with an average age of 55 years; 52% of the arthroplasties were performed for osteoarthritis in patients, with an average age of 74 years. Follow-up ranged from 2 to 6 years postoperatively. In the osteoarthritis group 89% of the arthroplasties were considered satisfactory or better and 79% of the knees in the rheumatoid group were satisfactory or better. Complications included loosening in 5 knees (3.3%), deep infection in 7 (4.7%), and patellofemoral pain in 1 knee. Overall, 17 knees (11%) were considered unsatisfactory leading to seven revisions arthroplasties (5%).

Riley and Woodyard[66] in 1985 published the results of 71 Geometric knees implanted in 48 patients at the Stafford District Hospital (England) with follow-up of 2 months to 8 years. There were 37 women and 11 men in the study, 68% with rheumatoid arthritis and 32% with osteoarthritis. Ages ranged from 25 to 79 years with a mean of 61 years. Pain relief was considered to be 72% of the maximum possible. Complications included 11 knees (15.5%) with mechanical loosening and 2 knees (2.8%) with deep infection. Overall, 18.3% of knees either had severe pain or underwent revision arthroplasty and were considered failures. By an actuarial technique, a 21% probability of success was predicted at 8 to 9 years.

Rand and Coventry[63] reported the results of 193 Geometric prostheses implanted in 129 patients between February 1972 and March 1975. The study comprised 63 men and 66 women, all with osteoarthritis, with a mean age at operation of 69 years. Final follow-up evaluation occurred at an average of 10.8 years, with a minimum of 8 years. The actuarial survival of a retained implant was 78% at 10 years. Using implant removal or pain as an endpoint, the success rate dropped to 69% at 10 years. Loosening occurred in 24 knees (12.5%), necessitating revision. These authors evaluated the development of lucent lines, which almost always occurred at the bone-cement interface of the tibial component. Radiolucent lines wider than 1 mm were present in 38% and progressed in 34%. The initial postoperative axial alignment significantly influenced the development of lucent lines: 9 of 15 knees with greater than 3 degrees of varus alignment compared with 17 of 53 knees with a greater valgus alignment had progressive radiolucent lines. In addition, varus tibial component positioning was associated with the development of lucent lines: 21 of 45 knees with greater than 4 degrees of varus alignment compared with 5 of 23 with a more valgus component orientation. Other complications included infection in 8 (4.1%), and instability in 3 (1.5%). Overall, revision procedures were performed in 38 (20%) of the 193 knees.[63]

Compared with modern standards, the Geometric prosthesis was lacking in design, with an inherent kinematic mismatch, as well as in instrumentation to provide for consistent implant positioning. Even so, the geometric knee provided approximately 70% successful results at 10 years. These results are important because they serve as a baseline with which the results of more contemporary designs can be compared (Table 76.2).

DUOCONDYLAR AND DUOPATELLAR TKAs

In the early 1970s Walker, Insall, and Ranawat at the Hospital for Special Surgery in New York City developed the Duocondylar (Johnson & Johnson Orthopaedics, Braintree, MA) total knee[36, 60] (Fig. 76.3). The metal femoral condylar surfaces closely matched the shape of the normal femoral condyles in an effort to reproduce a normal polycentric motion pattern. The condylar surfaces were connected by an anterior bar providing increased stability and making insertion easier. Two separate polyethylene tibial components each had upward-sloping curves toward the intercondylar area in an effort to provide mediolateral stability, but were flat in the sagittal plane to provide no constraint in the anteroposterior direction. The tibial intercondylar eminence and PCL were preserved and there was no replacement of the patellofemoral joint.

In 1976 Ranawat and colleagues[59] reported the results of 94 Duocondylar knees in 88 patients with an average 3-year follow-up. Seventy-five percent of patients had rheumatoid arthritis and 25% had osteoarthritis. Ages ranged from 25 to 72 years, with an average of 65 years. As judged by the Hospital for Special Surgery knee rating system, good or excellent results were obtained in 75% of the knees. Complications included significant instability in 9.3% and loosening in 5.3%. There were no cases of deep infection. Lucent lines occurred under the tibial component in 76% and were progressive in 26% of knees. Overall, 5.5% required revision arthroplasty. The main causes of failure were under- or overcorrection of deformity leading to instability, loosening of the tibial components, and patellofemoral pain.

Sledge and coworkers[81] in 1978 reported the results of 135 Duocondylar prostheses with an average of 2.7 years' follow-up. The patients ranged in age from 39 to 80 years, with a mean of 62 years. Seventy-nine

TABLE 76.2 GEOMETRIC TOTAL KNEE ARTHROPLASTY

Authors	No. of Knees/Patients	Mean Age (yr; range)	Rheumatoid Arthritis (%)	Osteoarthritis (%)	Follow-up (yr)	Successful Results (%)	Instability (%)	Loosening (%)	Infection (%)	Reoperations/ Failures (%)
Skolnick et al (1976)[78]	119 knees	$\bar{X}$ = 61 (25–84)	53	41	2	84	.8	11.8	1.8	15.5
Lowe and McNeur (1981)[51]	150/106	OA 74; RA 55	48	52	2–6	OA 89; RA 79	—	3.3	4.7	11
Riley and Woodyard (1985)[66]	71/48	$\bar{X}$ = 61 (25–79)	68	32	0–8	72	—	2.8	2.8	18.3
Rand and Coventry (1988)[63]	193/129	$\bar{X}$ = 69	—	100	10.8	69 (acturial analysis)	1.5	12.5	4.1	20

OA = osteoarthritis, RA = rheumatoid arthritis.

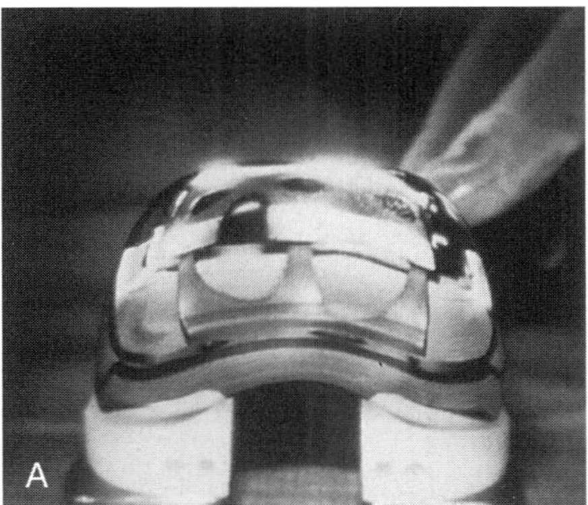

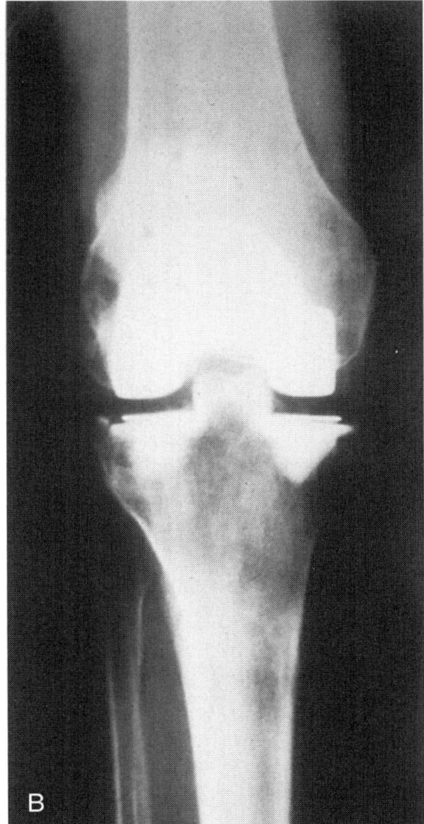

FIGURE 76.3 ➢ *A*, Photograph and *B*, AP radiograph of the Duocondylar prosthesis. (From Scott WN: The Knee, vol 2, St. Louis, Mosby-Year Book, 1994, p 1122.)

percent of patients had rheumatoid arthritis and 21% had osteoarthritis. Overall, 67% of patients were considered to have good or excellent results. Complications included two knees with component loosening (one tibial and one femoral), instability in one, and residual patellofemoral pain in 20%. Lucent lines occurred at the tibial bone-cement interface in 22%, but in all were less than 1 mm thick, incomplete, and not associated with clinical loosening. Revision operations were required in five knees (3.7%), and patellofemoral pain was noted to be the most common cause of poor results (Table 76.3).

Based on these observations from Harvard Medical School and the Hospital for Special Surgery, the Duocondylar evolved into the Duopatellar total knee with incorporation of an anterior patellar flange on the femur. The tibial component initially remained as two separate components, and the surface contour was changed from a flat to a curved surface in the sagittal plane conferring added inherent articular constraint.[20, 76, 80] In 1978, initial 2-year results were reported from both institutions.

Ewald and associates[20] in Boston reviewed 167 knees (70% with rheumatoid arthritis and 30% with osteoarthritis) and found 85% of patients with good or excellent results. The incidence of patellofemoral pain was reduced from 20% with the Duocondylar to only 5% with the Duopatellar prosthesis. Loosening occurred in only 0.9%; however, incomplete lucent lines less than 1 mm in thickness were discovered in 45%. This was a twofold increase in lucent lines at 2 years compared with the Duocondylar knees reviewed at the same institution (45% versus 22%). As the patellar flange and the dished tibial articular surface were the only two design changes, the most likely explanation for the increased incidence of lucent lines was that the higher degree of constraint transferred greater stress to the bone-cement interface.[20, 79] Inglis and Lane[36] in New York made similar observations in 53 Duopatellar knees at 2 years with 90% overall good and excellent results, but also with incomplete lucent lines less than 2 mm in thickness in 45%.

In 1980 Thomas and colleagues[84] evaluated 493 knees with Duopatellar prostheses out of 747 performed with an average 2.7-year follow-up. Overall, 93% of patients experienced marked pain relief. Average preoperative and postoperative scores according to the Hospital for Special Surgery system improved from 39 to 87 in the rheumatoid population and from 39 to 90 in the osteoarthritis population. Clinical loosening occurred in only 7 of 747 knees (0.9%). However, in 344 radiographs studied, incomplete lucent lines were present in 50%, and lines greater than 1 mm wide or involving greater than 90% of the surface were present in 3% of tibial components. The overall revision rate for the 747 knees was 2.8%.

Extensive biomechanical laboratory testing performed in 1979 demonstrated that a one-piece tibial component with a central stem enhanced tibial component fixation through increased surface area contact

TABLE 76.3 Duocondylar Total Knee Arthroplasty

Authors	No. of Knees/Patients	Mean Age (yr; range)	Rheumatoid Arthritis (%)	Osteoarthritis (%)	Follow-up (yr)	Good or Excellent Results (%)	Instability (%)	Loosening (%)	Lucent Lines (%)	Infection (%)	Reoperations/ Failures (%)
Ranawat et al (1976)[59]	94/88	$\overline{X}$ = 65 (25–72)	75	25	2–4	75	9.3	5.2	76* 26† 22	—	5.5
Sledge and Ewald (1979)[80]	135 knees	$\overline{X}$ = 62 (30–80)	79	21	2.7	67	.75	1.5		—	3.7

* Incomplete lucent lines <1 mm.

† Lucent lines >1 mm and complete, or progressive.

and better distribution of the weightbearing force. As a result, the two-piece Duopatellar tibial components were abandoned in favor of the one-piece design.[80] At the same time the tibial component was made flat in the sagittal plane, imparting less constraint and allowing femoral rollback in flexion.[76]

Scott[76] in 1982 reported the results of the first 100 Duopatellar replacements using the flat one-piece all polyethylene tibial components, with a minimum 2-year follow-up. Fifty percent were implanted in patients with rheumatoid arthritis and 45% in patients with osteoarthritis. Ninety-five percent of patients had excellent pain relief with an average of 106 degrees of motion. The incidence of incomplete lucent lines less than 1 mm thick decreased to 24%, and only 3% had lucent lines greater than 1 mm in thickness. Two reoperations were necessary for patellar resurfacing, but no revisions were required for tibial loosening (Table 76.4).

Duocondylar and Duopatellar arthroplasties marked a significant era in the evolution of TKA. Important concepts and design considerations that were introduced and confirmed were (1) the use of an anterior femoral flange to resurface the femoral trochlea; (2) flat tibial surface geometry in the sagittal plane in concert with a retained PCL to preseve motion and reduce interface stresses; and (3) use of a one-piece tibial component with a central stem for improved component stability and fixation.

CRUCIATE-SPARING TOTAL CONDYLAR KNEE REPLACEMENT

The posterior cruciate condylar knee (Howmedica) was introduced in 1975. The design was essentially identical to the total condylar knee with the exception of a central posterior cruciate cutout section that allowed preservation of the PCL (Fig. 76.4). The aim of the design change was to improve posterior stability for improved function (e.g., stair climbing) while retaining the wear and motion characteristics of the total condylar knee.[68] Potential disadvantages expressed by Insall and colleagues[38] included the possibility of impingement of the femur on the posterior aspect of the upper tibial plateau during flexion, which could limit flexion, deform the plastic, and increase interface stresses. In addition, correction of the deformity may be rendered more difficult with retention of the PCL.[38]

Ritter and associates[68] in 1984 reoprted the 5-year follow-up results of 94 cruciate condylar knee replacements. Sixty-three percent of patients had osteoarthritis and 27% had rheumatoid arthritis. The average age was 67 years (range, 21 to 85 years). Overall, 96.8% of patients had excellent or good results, which compares well with the 90% rate reported by Insall and colleagues for the totally condylar design and 96% for the posterior-stabilized design.[37, 38] The average preoperative flexion was 104 degrees and average postoperative flexion was 101 degrees. Postoperatively, only one knee showed varus deformity and only one knee had a valgus deformity greater than 10 degrees. Incomplete, nonprogressive tibial radiolucencies less than 1 mm wide occurred in 22%, and only one knee demonstrated tibial loosening with a complete radiolucency around the prosthesis. Six percent of knees had a 2+ anterior drawer and 5% had a 2+ posterior drawer; there were no cases of 3+ instability. One knee developed a deep infection requiring revision.

Bourne and coworkers[5] reported the results of 164 cruciate condylar arthroplasties with an average 5.3-year follow-up. Sixty-one percent of patients had osteoarthritis and 32% had rheumatoid arthritis. The average age was 65 years (range, 26 to 88 years). Seventy percent of tibial components were solid polyethylene and 30% were metal backed. Overall, good or excellent results were obtained in 95%, and 97% of knees had no posterior instability. The percentage of patients who could climb stairs without support increased from 37% to 69%. Maximum flexion averaged 107 degrees preoperatively and 101 degrees postoperatively. Ninety-nine knees demonstrated a preoperative deformity of more than 3 degrees of varus or 10 degrees of valgus alignment. Postoperatively, only eight knees had such a deformity. Lucent lines greater than 1 mm in length or width occurred in only 6% and progressed in only 3%. Lucent lines occurred in 5.6% of all-polyethylene tibiae, and in 2.7% of tibiae with metal backing. Of note, no fluoroscopic radiographs were used. Nevertheless, this rate of radiolucency compares well with the 22% incidence of lucent lines seen with the total condylar prosthesis.[38] No knees developed clinical loosening, deep infection occurred in one, and revision was required in three knees (one supracondylar fracture, one tibial component malrotation, and one residual varus malalignment).

A survivorship study of 190 cruciate-sparing total condylar knee prostheses was performed.[61] Sixty-one knees with an all-polyethylene tibial component were compared with 129 knees with a metal-backed tibal component at a mean of 10 years. Using an endpoint of revision, survivorship was 96% for the all-polyethylene compared with 93% for the metal-backed tibial component, which was not statistically significant. Using an endpoint of moderate or severe pain or revision, survivorship was 83% at 10 years overall (86% in all-polyethylene versus 79% in metal-backed tibial components). Of 134 knees in 108 patients available for follow-up at 10 years, the Hospital for Special Surgery knee scores were good or excellent in 88%. Radiolucent lines were present adjacent to 59% of the all-polyethylene and 52% of the metal-backed tibial components, which was not statistically significant.

Another study of 144 knees at a mean of 9 years found 94.5% good or excellent results.[48] The mean range of motion was 106 degrees. Radiolucent lines were identified in 41%, of which 12% were progressive. There were eight failures leading to three revisions. Elevation of the joint line by greater than 8 mm correlated with aseptic loosening. The same surgeons at a mean follow-up of 4.8 years[68] reported an evaluation of 394 knees derived from an original group of 440 total knee arthroplasties. The average patient age was 70 years. The diagnosis was osteoarthritis in 76% and rheumatoid arthritis in 21%. Using an endpoint of

TABLE 76.4 DUOPATELLAR TOTAL KNEE ARTHROPLASTY

Authors	No. of Knees/Patients	Mean Age (yr)	Rheumatoid Arthritis (%)	Osteoarthritis (%)	Follow-up (yr)	Good or Excellent Results (%)	Instability (%)	Loosening (%)	Lucent Lines (%)	Infection (%)	Reoperations/ Failures (%)
Ewald et al (1978)[20]	167 knees	63	70	30	2	85	—	.9	45*	—	2.7
Inglis and Lane (1978)[36]	53/42	54	85	12	2	90	—	—	45*	—	3.8
Thomas et al (1980)[84]	493 knees	—	70	30	2.7	93 pain relief	—	.9	50* 3†	.4	2.8
Scott (1982)[76]	100 knees (one-piece tibial component)	—	50	45	2	95	—	—	24* 3†	—	2

* Incomplete lucent lines <1 mm.
† Lucent lines >1 mm and complete, or progressive.

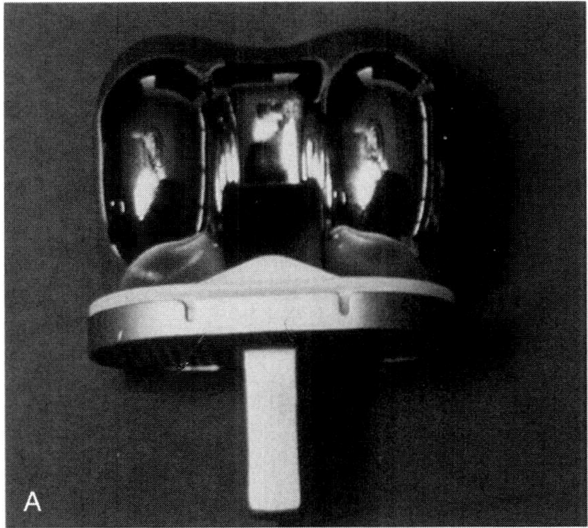

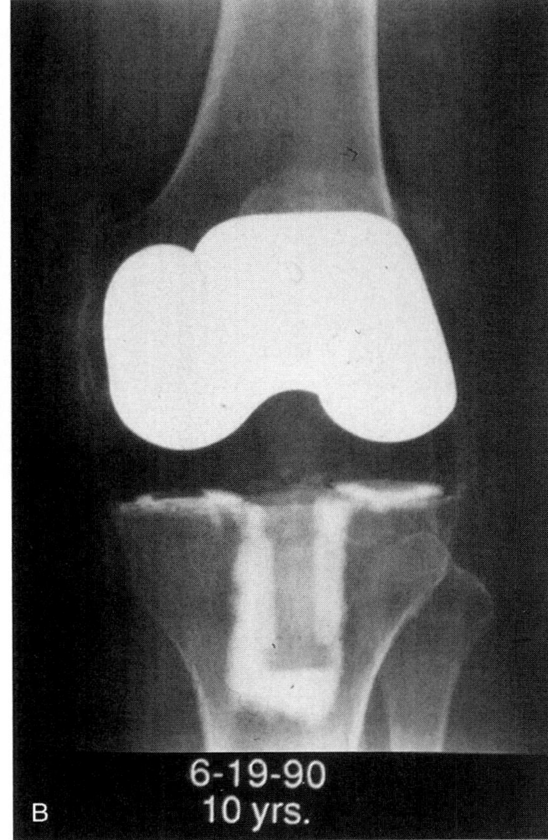

FIGURE 76.4 ➢ *A*, Photograph and *B*, AP radiograph of a cruciate condylar prosthesis. (From Scott WN: The Knee, vol 2, St. Louis, Mosby-Year Book, 1994, p 1125.)

revision, survivorship was estimated at 95% at 10 years. Using an endpoint of revision, pain, or radiographic loosening, survivorship was estimated at 81% at 10 years.

Another study of 42 total knees followed for a mean of 11 years was reported.[15] The mean patient age was 63 years. The diagnoses were equally divided between osteoarthritis and rheumatoid arthritis. Good or excellent knee scores were achieved in 93%. The range of motion was 104 degrees. Incomplete, nonprogressive radiolucent lines were identified adjacent to 75% of the tibial components. Complications occurred in six patients and consisted of patellar fracture in two, patellar dislocation in two, and one each of patellar implant loosening, extensor mechanism dislocation with posterior instability, and supracondylar fracture. Two revisions were performed, one for patellar instability and one for posterior instability in a patient with a prior patellectomy.

The posterior cruciate condylar prosthesis provided good or excellent results in 90% to 95% of knees at 5 or more years' follow-up. Thus the evolution of knee arthroplasty continues to demonstrate benefits. Concerns that cruciate retention would lead to diminished motion, tibial loosening, and persistent deformity were not substantiated by these studies. Despite the excellent results, a subtle kinematic mismatch exists with this prosthesis and a change to a flat tibial plateau in the sagittal plane was reommended[67] (Table 76.5).

KINEMATIC TOTAL KNEE

The Kinematic (Howmedica) total knee is a PCL-sparing prosthesis designed in an attempt to further refine the advancements made in the cruciate-sparing condylar knee (Fig. 76.5). The tibial component was flattened in the sagittal plane, allowing unconstrained femoral rollback, which clears the posterior structures and avoids femoral impingement.[80] A metal-backed, short-stemmed tibial component was designed to improve tibial component fixation and load transmission.[87] Finally, the patellar groove in the anterior flange was placed in slight valgus alignment to improve patellar tracking.

In 1984, Ewald and associates[21] from Harvard Medical School reported the results of 124 Kinematic knee replacements with an average of 2.25 years' follow-up. Fifty-four percent of patients had rheumatoid arthritis, 5% had juvenile rheumatoid arthritis, and 41% had osteoarthritis. The average age of the patients was 76 years (range, 25 to 86 years). The patella was resurfaced in all patients with rheumatoid arthritis and in 68% of patients with osteoarthritis. Overall, 90% (111 knees) had excellent or good results. The average

TABLE 76.5 Cruciate Condylar Total Knee Arthroplasty

Authors	No. of Knees/Patients	Mean Age (yr)	Rheumatoid Arthritis (%)	Osteoarthritis (%)	Follow-up (yr)	Good or Excellent Results (%)	Instability (%)	Loosening (%)	Lucent Lines (%)	Infection (%)	Reoperations/ Failures (%)
Ritter et al (1984)[67]	94/63	67	27	63	5	96.8	—	1	22	1	1
Bourne et al (1989)[5]	164/131	65	32	61	5.3	95	4.2	—	6 3	.6	3.7
Rand (1993)[61]	134/108	63	33	62	10	88	—	1	59	1	1.5
Lee et al (1990)[48]	144/193	67	21	72	9	94	—	12	42	—	2
Dennis (1992)[15]	42/35	63	50	50	11	93	2.3	—	75	—	4.7

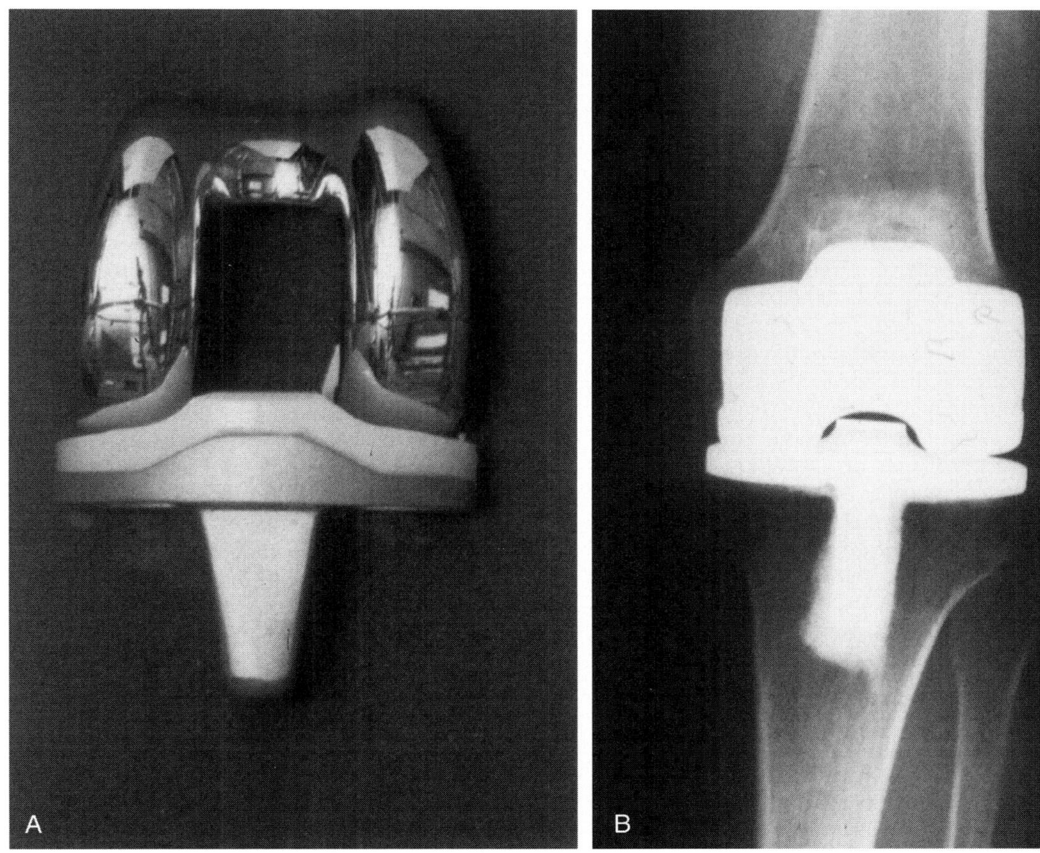

FIGURE 76.5 ➢ *A,* Photograph and *B,* AP radiograph of Kinematic condylar prosthesis. (From Scott WN: The Knee, vol 2, St. Louis, Mosby-Year Book, 1994, p 1127.)

postoperative range of motion was 106 degrees of flexion, and extension to 2 degrees short of full extension. Overall, the average postoperative alignment was 5.3 ± 2.9 degrees of valgus angulation. Radiolucent lines occurred beneath the tibial component in 22 knees (18%), all of which were less than 1 mm wide, incomplete, and nonprogressive. Lucencies occurred in 19 knees with osteoarthritis and in only 3 with rheumatoid arthritis. A statistically significant correlation was found between the development of lucent lines and knees with incompletely corrected varus malalignment in which the tibial component was placed in excessive varus angulation. Two knees required reoperation, for an overall rate of 1.6%. One was for a patellar dislocation and one was a revision for loosening of the tibial component (.8%). This occurred in a knee with a 30-degree preoperative varus angulation in which a large medial tibial plateau defect was filled with unreinforced cement, the tibial component was placed in 10 degrees of varus angulation, and the overall postoperative alignment was zero degrees of valgus angulation. There were no cases of instability or infection.

A subsequent study from the same group reported 192 knees followed for a mean of 6 years.[89] The mean age of the patients with rheumatoid arthritis was 61 years and 70 years in those with osteoarthritis. Knee motion improved from 104 degrees preoperatively to 109 degrees at last follow-up evaluation. Good or excellent results were achieved in 88% of the knees. The joint line was shifted an average of 1 mm. Radiolucent lines were present adjacent to 40% of the tibial, 30% of the femoral, and 60% of the patellar components. Complications consisted of four deep and four superficial infections, four patellar implant loosening, one tibial tray fracture, one patellar fracture, one peroneal nerve palsy, and one patellar subluxation. Reoperations were performed in 10 knees (4 patellar loosenings, 1 tibial tray fracture, 1 patellar fracture, and 4 deep infections).

Another study reported the results of 119 of an original group of 168 knees that were followed for 10 years.[53] The diagnoses were osteoarthritis in 68% and rheumatoid arthritis in 30%. The mean age was 64 years, and range of motion was 105 degrees. Using the Hospital for Special Surgery rating system, the results were good or excellent in 75%. Radiolucent lines were present adjacent to the tibial component in 60%, and femoral component in 39%. Complications consisted of loosening of the patellar component in four, loosening of the femoral and tibial components in two, supracondylar fracture in one, and deep infection in one knee. Using an endpoint of revision, survivorship was 96% at 10 years. Using an endpoint of revision, poor knee score, or a complete radiolucent line, survivorship was 76% at 10 years.

The Kinematic condylar prosthesis was modified to the Kinemax prosthesis by creation of a symmetric femoral component and a modular tibial component. A study of 356 knees was performed at 5 years following arthroplasty.[27] The diagnoses were osteoarthritis in 68% and rheumatoid arthritis in 31%. The mean patient age was 65 years, and range of motion was 113 degrees. Using the Hospital for Special Surgery rating system, the results were good or excellent in 95%. Reoperations were performed for wound necrosis in three, deep infection in three, patellar fracture in 1, and patellar subluxation in 1 knee. Using an endpoint of revision, survivorship was 97.5% at 10 years.

This experience with the Kinematic total knee replacement not only confirms the excellent results obtained with design changes as total knee prostheses evolve, but also continues to elucidate the imporant principles of surgical technique, namely component position and axial alignment. Patellar implant fixation remained a problem (Table 76.6).

TOWNLEY AND CLOUTIER RESURFACING DESIGNS

The original Townley (DePuy, Warsaw, IN) (Fig. 76.6) and Cloutier (Fig. 76.7) prostheses had similar design concepts and hence are discussed together here. The stated goal of both systems was to reproduce as accurately as possible the normal joint anatomy, mechanics, and kinematics of the human knee.[9, 86] Both systems were designed to preserve both cruciate ligaments. Both employed a U-shaped tibial component without a stem that was flat in the sagittal plane so as to provide constrained motion to minimize stress transfer to the cement-bone interface. Finally, both designers emphasized the importance of implant position and axial alignment. Each employed unique instrumentation using an extramedullary alignment system based on intraoperative localization of the femoral head to obtain accurate and reproducible component implantation.

In 1985, Townley[86] reviewed 532 total knees with 1.5 to 11 years' follow-up out of more than 700 implants that had been performed since 1972: 73% were performed for osteoarthritis, 18% for rheumatoid arthritis, and 9% were revision operations for a previously failed arthroplasty. The tibial component was nonmetal-backed and was ideally placed in 2 degrees of varus angulation so that the joint line would remain horizontal during the single-leg stance phase of ambulation to minimize shear stresses.

Overall, excellent or good results were obtained in 89% of knees (i.e., motion beyond 90 degrees, mild or no pain, and no walking aid). Tibial loosening occurred in 10 knees (1.9%) requiring revision; 6 knees (1.1%) had patellofemoral complications necessitating a reoperation. Clinical instability occurred in 3 knees, and deep infection occurred in 9 knees (1.2%). Townley noted that the majority of loosening complications were associated with some degree of technical malalignment of the joint. Overall, 19 knees (3.6%) required reoperation.

A study of 88 Townley knee arthroplasties in 72 patients followed a mean of 2.5 years.[54] The mean relative age of the patients was 68 years. Pain relief was achieved in 94% with "acceptable" results in 86%. Reoperation was performed for tibial loosening in 3, deep infection in 1, and patellar loosening in 1. Incomplete radiolucent lines were identified in 18% (Table 76.7).

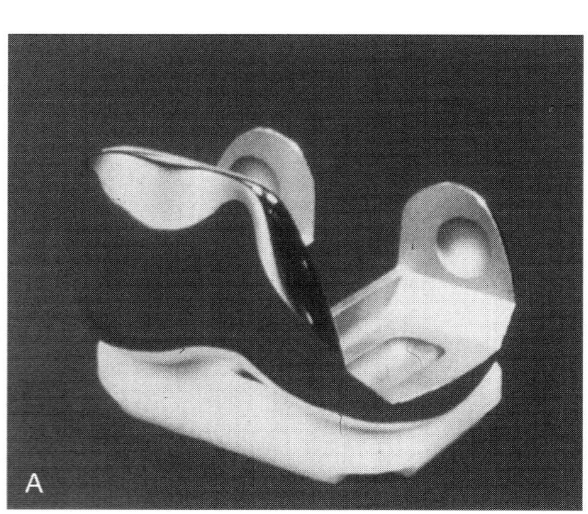

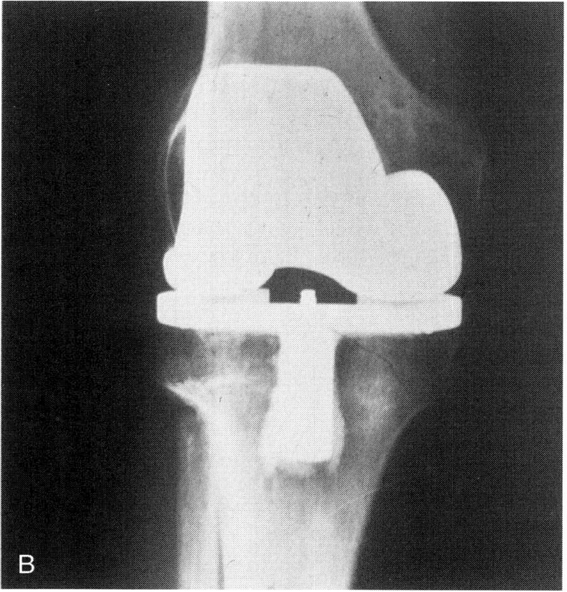

FIGURE 76.6 ➢ *A,* Photograph and *B,* AP radiograph of Townley prosthesis. (From Scott WN: The Knee, vol 2, St. Louis, Mosby-Year Book, 1994, p 1129.)

TABLE 76.6 KINEMATIC CONDYLAR TOTAL KNEE ARTHROPLASTY

Authors	No. of Knees/Patients	Mean Age (yr)	Rheumatoid Arthritis (%)	Osteoarthritis (%)	Follow-up (yr)	Successful Results (%)	Lucent Lines (%)	Infection (%)	Reoperations/ Failures (%)
Ewald et al (1984)[21]	121/91	76	59	41	2.2	90	18	—	1.6
Wright et al (1990)[89]	192/147	70	54	44	6	88	30-40	2	5.7
Malkani et al (1995)[53]	119/84	64	30	68	10	75	60	1	4.8
Harwin (1998)[27]	356	65	31	68	5	95	—	.8	2.8

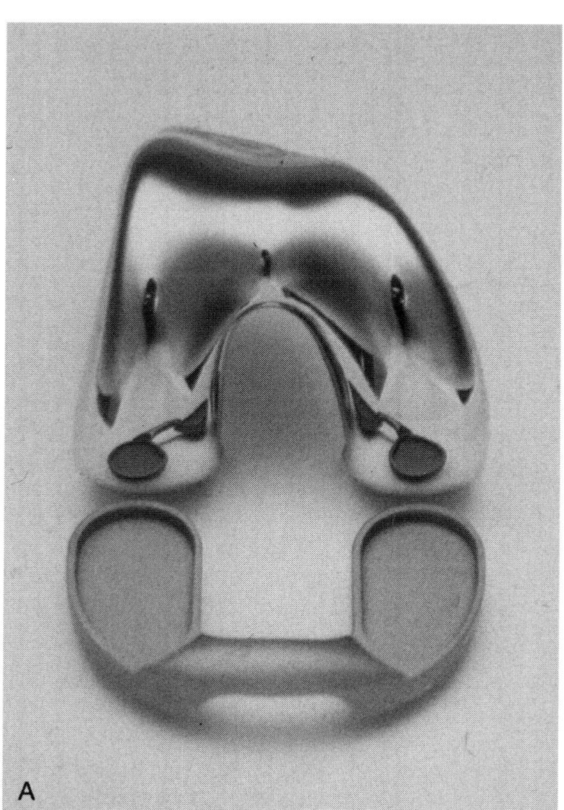

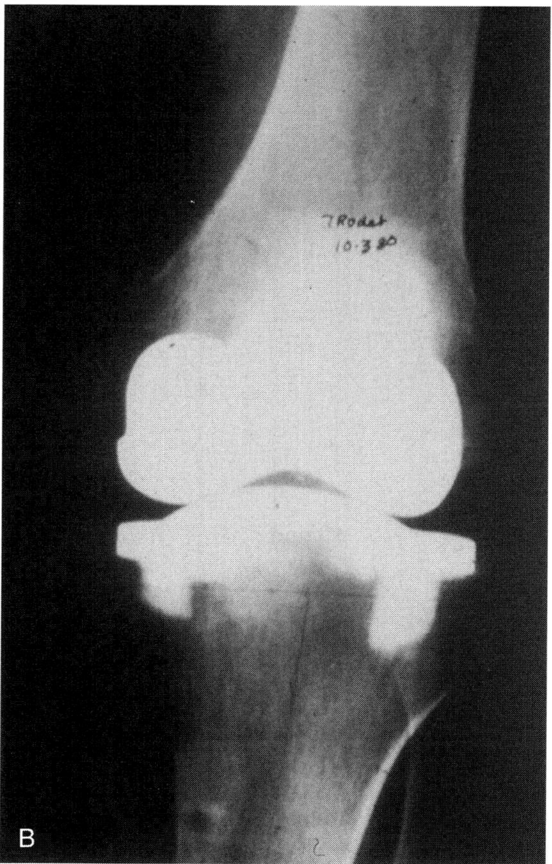

FIGURE 76.7 ➢ *A,* Photograph and *B,* AP radiograph of Cloutier prosthesis. (From Scott WN: The Knee, vol 2, St. Louis, Mosby-Year Book, 1994, p 1130.)

The Townley prosthesis was modified to include metal backing for the tibial component as well as a design that sacrificed both cruciate ligaments. A study of 360 total knees consisted of 153 bicruciate-retaining with an all-polyethylene tibial component; 50 bicruciate with a metal-backed tibial component; 60 with cruciate sacrifice with an all-polyethylene tibial component; and 97 with cruciate sacrifice and a metal-backed tibial component.[58] The diagnoses were osteoarthritis in 167 and rheumatoid arthritis in 193 knees. The mean follow-up was 8 years. Revision was performed for loosening in 18, instability in 6, and infection in 5 knees. Using an endpoint of revision, a survivorship of 89% at 10 years was predicted.

The Cloutier prosthesis was developed at the St. Luc Hospital in Montreal in 1975.[9] Unique features include metal-backed U-shaped tibial plateau into which two separate polyethylene inserts are press-fitted. In addition, the technique for component implantation relies on a knee joint distractor, which maintains axial alignment and ligament tension while the osteotomies are performed.

In 1983, Cloutier published the results of 107 total knee replacements, with follow-up of 2 to 4.5 years.[9] Sixty-four percent were performed for rheumatoid arthritis and 33% for osteoarthritis in patients with an average age of 58 years (range, 35 to 81 years). The ACL was found to be attenuated or destroyed in 57% of knees. The PCL was always preserved, and was not found to prevent adequate component positioning or correction of even severe deformities. Using the Hospital for Special Surgery rating system, 91% of knees had good or excellent results at final follow-up. Complications included instability in three knees and deep infection in 3 knees. Twenty-four percent of knees were found to have lucent lines beneath the tibial component, which were less than 1 mm in width and nonprogressive. Only one progressive tibial lucency occurred, which led to the one case of tibial component loosening and required revision. Overall, reoperations were required in 8 knees (7.5%). A subsequent study of 85 knees in 61 patients followed for 10 to 12 years was performed.[10] The mean patient age was 59 years; good or excellent results were achieved in 79%. The results wre good or excellent in 93% of the ACL-intact knees and in 62.5% of the ACL-deficient knees. Aseptic loosening occurred in 1.2%. Revision was performed in 7 knees (13%): for infection in 2, instability in 3, aseptic loosening in 1, and pain of indeterminate cause in 1. Radiolucent lines were identified in 25% of the knees. The most recent evaluation was of 107 knees in 89 patients derived from an initial group of 163 knees

TABLE 76.7 TOWNLEY TOTAL KNEE ARTHROPLASTY

Authors	No. of Knees/Patients	Mean Age (yr)	Rheumatoid Arthritis (%)	Osteoarthritis (%)	Follow-up (yr)	Good or Excellent Results (%)	Instability (%)	Loosening (%)	Lucent Lines (%)	Infection (%)	Reoperations/ Failures (%)
Mallory et al (1982)[54]	88/72	68	12	81	2.5	86	—	4.1	18	1.3	6.9
Townley (1985)[86]	532/426	—	18	73	1.5–1.1	89	0.6	1.9	—	1.2	3.6
Partio et al (1994)[58]	360/—	—	54	46	8.0	—	—	—	—	2.2	6.9

in 130 patients.[11] At a mean follow-up of 10 years, the results were good or excellent in 97% of the surviving knees. The mean range of motion was 107 degrees. Using an endpoint of revision, the survivorship was 95% at 10 years. Revision was required for 7 knees, 3 for infection, 2 for polyethylene wear, 1 for instability, and 1 for loosening of the femoral component. Additional complications included a medial collateral ligament rupture, a fracture of the medial tibial plateau, and two patellar fractures. Radiolucent lines were seen adjacent to 10% of the femoral and 18% of the tibial components (Table 76.8).

Gait studies were performed on 17 patients with Cloutier prostheses that had excellent results and a minimum of 1 year follow-up.[3] Gait was compared with gait of a matched set of 17 patients with a cruciate-sacrificing total condylar knee prosthesis, excellent results, and at least 1 year follow-up. The results demonstrated that both groups walked on level ground with a shorter than normal stride length and used a smaller than normal flexion during stance phase. However, while ascending and descending stairs, knee flexion was significantly greater in patients with the Cloutier prosthesis and did not differ significantly from normal controls. This suggests that preservation of the PCL may lead to improved function in stair climbing and possibly in other activities of daily living.

The Townley and Cloutier resurfacing prostheses have been carefully studied by their designers and have demonstrated excellent and good results in approximately 90% of patients at midrange follow-up. Lew and Lewis[49] demonstrated in the laboratory the importance of low-conformity, low-constraint articular surfaces when the cruciate ligaments are preserved. These clinical studies not only document the behavior of a particular prosthesis but also add in vivo confirmation of these important concepts.

MILLER-GALANTE PROSTHESIS

The Miller-Galante total knee (Zimmer, Warsaw, IN) (Fig. 76.8), one of the first knee replacements designed for use with cement or cementless fixation, was first implanted in 1986.[46] A titanium fiber composite was chosen for the bony ingrowth surface because of its well-recognized biocompatibility in primates, as well as its previous use in limb-salvage tumor surgery. To replicate normal knee kinematics as closely as possible, the deisgners believed that the slope of the replaced femoral condyles must match that of the native condyles in addition to preservation of the PCL. Seven different femoral component sizes (right and left) were made available. In order to place the tibial component on the cortical rim to avoid subsidence, five sizes of tibial components were designed.[71] Modularity of polyethylene inserts was incorporated in order to allow fine-tuning of ligamentous tension, the degree of articular constraint, and the possibility of future isolated polyethylene replacement. Landon and coworkers in 1986 reported early 1- to 4-year follow-up on the first 37 cementless knees implanted in 35 patients, 54% of whom had osteoarthritis and 26% rheumatoid arthritis.[46] Using the modified rating of the Hospital for Special Surgery, 32 patients (86%) obtained good or excellent results. Five patients were considered failures: 3 for proven infections and 1 for tibial component loosening. No progressive lucencies were observed in the patients with satisfactory results.

In 1989 Rosenberg and colleagues reported the results of 133 cemented and 134 cementless total knee arthroplasties.[71] The series was prospective but not randomized. Patients of older age, with poorer bone stock, and with questionable ability to comply with a touch weightbearing-only rehabilitation were selected for a cemented arthroplasty. The average age in the cemented group was 70 years (range, 31 to 97 years); the average age in the cementless group was 58 years (range, 19 to 75 years). In both groups, osteoarthritis accounted for 80% and rheumatoid arthritis for 15% of patients. The patients were evaluated at a mean of 22 months for the cemented and 23 months for the cementless arthroplasty group.

Using the modified rating of the Hospital for Special Surgery, 93% of cemented and 95% of cementless knees showed good or excellent results. Postoperative range of motion was similar for groups, 104 and 107 degrees, respectively. More patients in the cementless group complained of slight pain at final follow-up (34% versus 19%). Failures requiring revision occurred in 5% (7 knees) of cemented arthroplasties and 3% (4 knees) of cementless arthroplasties. Four additional cemented knees required reoperation for extensor mechanism complications (two patellar realignments, one patellar revision, and one quadriceps repair). Eleven cementless knees required reoperation for failure of the cementless patellar component. In all instances there was ingrowth of the patellar pegs and failure of ingrowth of the patellar plate, with subsequent shear failure of the peg-plate junction. There were two cases of infection in each group, one tibial loosening in the cementless group, and two cases of instability in the cemented group.

Of the 125 cementless knees evaluated for interface radiolucencies, almost no complete or partial lucencies occurred about the femoral component. Evaluation of the patellar components demonstrated only two complete lucencies: 13% showed partial lucencies, 55% showed no lucencies, and in 30% the radiographs could not be evaluated. Partial tibial radiolucencies were seen in 36%, complete lucencies in 8%, no lucencies in 47%, and 10% had inadequate radiographs. In 10 cementless tibial components removed for reasons other than mechanical loosening, the mean extent of plate bone ingrowth was 25%. In all ten, bony ingrowth was present on at least three of the four pegs. A subsequent report by Rosenberg and associates compared 116 cemented with 123 cementless knees at 44 months following arthroplasty.[72] Good or excellent results were achieved in 92% of the cementless compared with 88% of the cemented knees. The range of motion was 105 degrees in the cemented and 109 degrees in the cementless knees. Incomplete radiolucent lines were identified in 26% of cementless and in 16% of cemented knees. Three cementless knees had

TABLE 76.8 CLOUTIER TOTAL KNEE ARTHROPLASTY

Authors	No. of Knees/Patients	Mean Age (yr)	Rheumatoid Arthritis (%)	Osteoarthritis (%)	Follow-up (yr)	Good or Excellent Results (%)	Instability (%)	Loosening (%)	Lucent Lines (%)	Infection (%)	Reoperations/ Failures (%)
Cloutier (1983)[9]	107/83	58	64	33	2–4.5	91	2.8	1	24* 1†	2.8	7.5
Cloutier (1991)[10]	85/61	59	55	39	10–13	79	3.5	1.2	25	2.3	13
Cloutier (1998)[11]	107/89	67	25	75	10	97	.6	.6	18	1.7	4.3

* Incomplete lucent lines <1 mm.

† Lucent lines >1 mm and complete, or progressive.

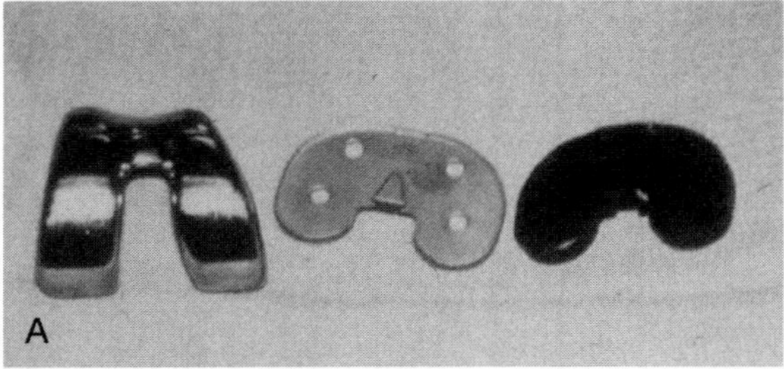

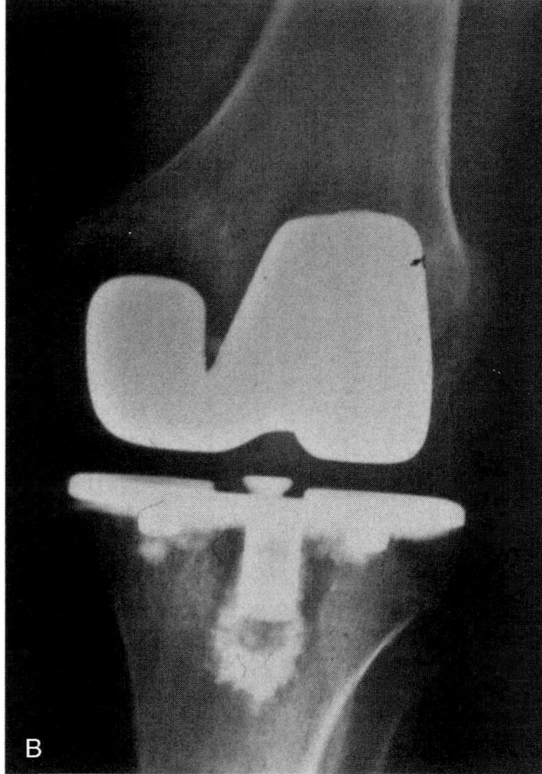

FIGURE 76.8 ➢ *A*, Photograph and *B*, AP radiograph of Miller-Galante prosthesis. (From Scott WN: The Knee, vol 2, St. Louis, Mosby-Year Book, 1994, p 1132.)

complete radiolucent lines. Reoperation was performed in 11% of cementless and in 9% of cemented knees. Revision occurred in 5% of cementless and in 6% of the cemented knees.

Kraay and coworkers reported on 29 knees in 22 patients with hybrid fixation, which were followed for a mean of 28 months.[45] The mean age of the patients was 71 years. The diagnoses were osteoarthritis in 19, traumatic arthritis in 2, and rheumatoid arthritis in 1 patient. The range of motion was 110 degrees. The Knee Society pain score averaged 47 and the function score 79. Radiolucent lines were seen in 39% of knees.

In another study, Kobs and Lachiewicz reported the results of 41 TKA with a cementless femur and cemented tibial component (hybrid fixation) at 46 months' follow-up evaluation.[44] The diagnoses were rheumatoid arthritis in 49% and osteoarthritis in 46%. The mean age was 52 years. The results were good or excellent in 88%, and range of motion was 107 degrees. Radiolucent lines were identified adjacent to the tibial component in 20%, femoral component in 15%, and patellar component in 27%. Complications consisted of failure of six metal-backed patellar components, deep infection in one, and wound necrosis in two knees.

A series of 392 TKA in 344 patients were reported at a follow-up of 3 years.[70] Fixation was with cement in 183 knees and hybrid fixation in 181 knees. The diagnosis was osteoarthritis in all patients. The Hospital for Special Surgery knee rating score was 87 in the hybrid knees and 85 in the cementless knees. Range of motion was 109 in the hybrid and 110 in the cemented knees. Radiolucent lines were seen adjacent to 22% of the hybrid and 34% of the cemented knees. Reoperations were performed in 8% of the hybrid and 9% of the cemented knees. Complications consisted of patellar instability in 13, wear of the patellar component in 12, patellar fractures in 8, patellar tendon rupture in 2, and unexplained pain in 2 knees.

These studies demonstrate equally good short-term results with both the cemented and cementless PCL-sparing Miller-Galante knee with the exception of the cementless metal-backed patellar component. The results closely match those of the previously discussed unconstrained resurfacing designs with at least 90% good and excellent results (Table 76.9).

POROUS-COATED ANATOMIC TOTAL KNEE ARTHROPLASTY

The PCA total knee (Howmedica) was designed with the objective of reconstituting normal kinematic function of the knee through minimal articular surface replacement (Fig. 76.9).[29] Each of the components simulated the normal anatomy of the surface it replaced. Each of the fixation interfaces was porous-coated with a double layer of sintered cobalt-chromium beads and could be implanted with or without cement. The femoral condyles were flattened in the mediolateral dimension to improve loading characteristics. There were three separate instant centers of rotation and three different radii of curvature, which were unique for the

TABLE 76.9 Miller-Galante Total Knee Arthroplasty

Authors	No. of Knees/Patients	Mean Age (yr)	Rheumatoid Arthritis (%)	Osteoarthritis (%)	Follow-up (yr)	Good or Excellent Results (%)	Instability (%)	Loosening (%)	Lucent Lines (%)	Infection (%)	Reoperations/ Failures (%)
Landon et al (1986)[46]	37/35	57	26	54	1-4	86		2.7		8.1	14
Rosenberg et al (1989)[71]	Cemented: 133/113	70	15	80	1-4	93	1.5	—	—	1.5	9
	Uncemented: 134/126	58				95	—	.75	36* 6†	1.5	12
Kobs and Lachiewicz (1993)[44]	Hybrid 41/27	52	49	46	3.5	88	—	—	20	2.4	10
Rorabeck et al (1993)[70]	392/344	—	—	100	3	—	—	—	34	—	9

*Incomplete lucent lines <1 mm.
† Lucent lines >1 mm and complete, or progressive.

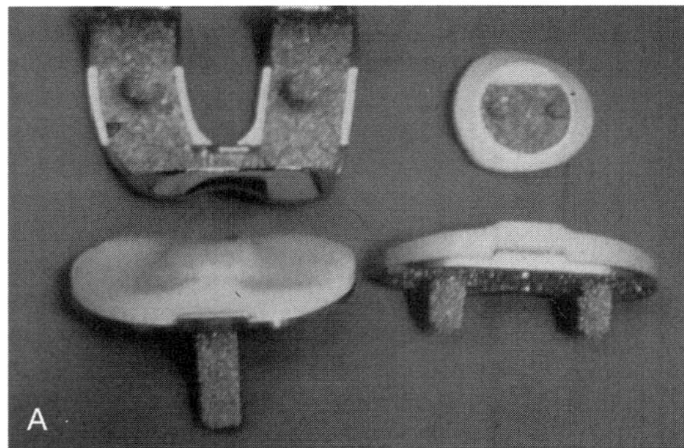

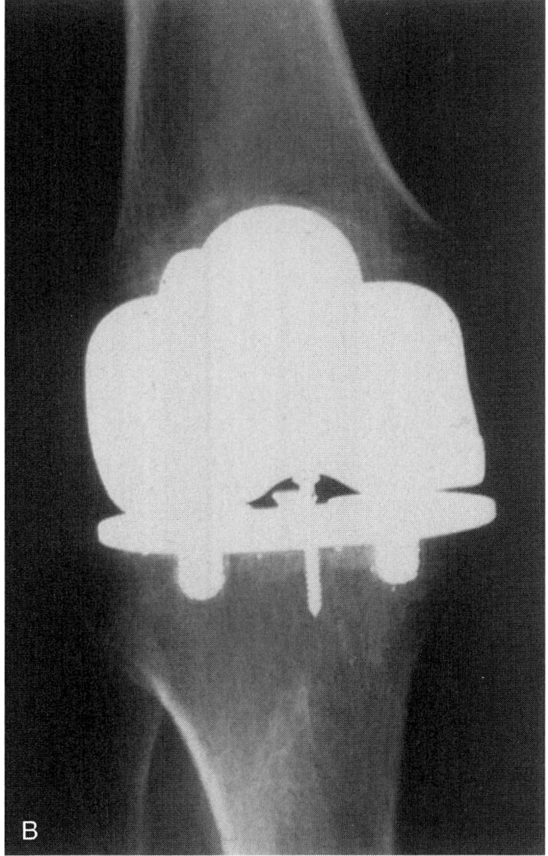

FIGURE 76.9 ➢ *A,* Photograph and *B,* AP radiograph of porous coated anatomic prostheses at 10 years. (From Scott WN: The Knee, vol 2, St. Louis, Mosby-Year Book, 1994, p 1134.)

medial and lateral condyles, thereby mimicking the normal knee. The intercondylar notch was curved to simulate normal anatomy, which contributed to the screw-home mechanism. The tibial component was asymmetric, flat, and sloped posteriorly. The curved posterior slope, which was more anterior on the medial side, also contributed to the automatic rotational or screw-home mechanism. The trochlea was in 3 degrees of valgus angulation, and the lateral facet of both the trochlea and patella was more prominent than the medial facet, again simulating the normal knee.

In 1987, Hungerford and colleagues[30] reported 2- to 5-year follow-up results of 93 cementless PCA knees in 82 patients. Sixty-three percent had osteoarthritis, with a mean age of 68 years; 30% had rheumatoid arthritis, with a mean age of 56 years. Patients were selected for ingrowth arthroplasties if there were less than 25 degrees of axial malalignment, good bone stock, and satisfactory implant stability intraoperatively. These cementless knees represented less then 50% of all knees performed by the authors, the remainder being cemented knees. However, the authors note that this proportion gradually increased until approximately 90% of femoral components and 80% of tibial and patellar components were being implanted without cement.

Overall, 94.5% of patients obtained excellent or good results, using a 100-point evaluation scale that assigns a total of 50 points for pain, 20 points for range of motion, and 10 points each for alignment, stability, and strength. There were no cases of aseptic loosening of femoral or tibial components and no cases of instability. Aseptic loosening of the patellar component requiring revision occurred in six knees and infection occurred in one knee. Using fluoroscopic imaging of the tibial interface, 83% of components showed no radiolucent zones, 17% demonstrated incomplete lucent lines, and no components showed a complete radiolucent line. In addition, the authors noted that interfaces that appeared radiographically stable at 6 months postoperatively remained stable throughout the follow-up period.

In another study, Hungerford and associates compared the results of cemented and cementless PCA knees at 2- to 5-year follow-up.[31] In 186 knees implanted for osteoarthritis (54% cementless), 96% showed good or excellent results. In 92 knees implanted for rheumatoid arthritis (59% cementless), 92% of the cementless knees were rated good or excellent, whereas only 81% of the cemented knees demonstrated good or excellent results. The difference, however, was attributed to the selection criteria, with the more severe bone loss and deformity in the cemented group.

Rand and associates[65] in 1987 also compared the results of cemented versus cementless PCA total knee arthroplasties. Fifty cemented knees wih greater than 2 years' follow-up showed 97% good or excellent results, whereas only 83% of 41 cementless knees showed good or excellent results. There were no differences in function or range of motion between the two groups. Reoperation was required in four cementless knees, including three revision arthroplasties; one each for tibial component breakage, tibial component loosening, and infection. There were no reoperations in the cemented arthroplasty group. Progressive lucent lines occurred in 3% of cemented components and in 18% of cementless components. It is noteworthy, however, that fluoroscopic views were used in the cementless group and not in the cemented group; thus the validity of this comparison is questionable. In the cemented group there were no significant changes in component position. However, in the cementless group, three knees sustained significant shifts in the position of the tibial component. This study demonstrates satisfactory results in both cemented and cementless PCA knees, but raises questions about cementless tibial component fixation.

A study of 48 knees in 39 patients with cementless fixation and an age of less than 50 years was performed.[32] Good or excellent results were achieved in 39 knees (81%), at 4 years after arthroplasty. The mean range of motion was 105 degrees, and radiolucent lines were observed in 35%. Complications consisted of instability in four, patellar loosening in three, subsidence in two, patellar subluxation in two, arthrofibrosis in one, and fat pad impingement in one knee.

A comparative prospective study of 26 cementless and 25 cemented knees was performed.[12] At 3 years following arthroplasty, good or excellent results were achieved in 18 (69%) of the cementless and in 17 (68%) of the cemented knees. Lucent lines of 2 mm in width were seen adjacent to 44% of the cementless and 12% of the cemented knees (p = .02). Tibial component subsidence occurred in 50% of the cementless and 8% of the cemented knees. Reoperation was performed for one knee in each group.

A study of 18 patients with a cemented knee on one side and a cementless knee on the other was performed.[17] At 5 years following arthroplasty there were no differences in knee scores or radiolucent lines. There was one reoperation for cemented tibial component loosening and one for cementless patellar component loosening.

Another study reported the results of 106 knees in patients with osteoarthritis at 6.3 years after arthroplasty.[85] The mean patient age was 73 years. At last evaluation, 79 of 91 knees had good or excellent knee scores using the Hospital for Special Surgery rating system. There were a total of 25 reoperations in the original group of 141 knees. Complications affected the extensor mechanism in 10 knees; 7 knees required revision of the tibial component alone, 6 for wear, and 1 for loosening. There was one revision of the tibial and patellar components for loosening. Wear was calculated at 1 mm. Survivorship to revision was 84% at 10 years; survivorship to reoperation was 76% at 10 years.

In yet another study of 105 knees in 94 patients, fixation was cementless in 73%, cemented in 11%, and hybrid in 16%.[28] The diagnoses were osteoarthritis in 91% and rheumatoid arthritis in 10%. The mean patient age was 59 years. Using the Hospital for Special Surgery scoring system, the results were good or excellent in 92%. Complications occurred in 22% consisting of loosening in 8, patellar instability in 4, delayed wound healing in 4, infection in 4 (1 deep), arthrofibrosis in 1, and patellar fracture in 1.

A review of 158 of an original group of 304 knees at a mean of 84 months was performed.[73] The diagnoses were osteoarthritis in 70% and rheumatoid arthritis in 30%. The mean patient age was 68 years. Using the Hospital for Special Surgery scoring system, the results were good or excellent in 70%. Mean range of motion was 87 degrees. Using an endpoint of revision, survivorship of 86% was estimated at 8 years. Complications from the original group of 304 knees consisted of wear in 11, loosening in 10, infection in 6, instability in 1, and unexplained pain in 1.

The PCA knee was modified to the PCA modular design by placing a 3-degree posterior slope on the tibia, improving capture mechanism for the polyethylene, and manufacturing five sizes of the femoral component. A report of 78 knees in 71 patients was performed at a mean follow-up of 5 years.[43] The diagnoses were osteoarthritis in 85% and rheumatoid arthritis in 12%. The mean patient age was 72 years. Using the Hospital for Special Surgery scoring system, the results were good or excellent in 89%. Complications consisted of loosening in one, extensor mechanism in five, delayed wound healing in five, infection in one, loosening in one, and instability in one. Radiolucent lines were identified adjacent to the femoral component in 13%, tibial component in 44%, and patellar component in 6%.

The PCA prosthesis demonstrates that with the reproduction of normal knee surface anatomy and kinematics, satisfactory results can be expected with a resurfacing, PCL-preserving, unconstrained design (Table 76.10). However, the combination of a low-conformity prosthesis and heat-pressed polyethylene led to an unacceptable rate of wear.

MENISCAL-BEARING PROSTHESIS

The concept of a meniscal-bearing prosthesis is to provide congruity of the articulating surfaces and unconstrained tibiofemoral movement[23] (Fig. 76.10). The conforming articular surfaces minimize wear, but the bearing motion allows knee motion and ligament function. The original Oxford meniscal-bearing prosthesis had a spherical femoral surface of a single size. No soft tissue balancing was performed. Of 125 knees treated with the Oxford prosthesis and reviewed at a mean of 4 years, pain relief was achieved in 89%. Mean motion was 99 degrees. Complications consisted of four loosenings, one deep infection, five dislocated meniscal bearings, one tibial plateau fracture, and two subluxated meniscal bearings. The revision rate was 7%. Radiolucent lines beneath the tibial component were present in 96%. A survivorship study of 327 TKA with follow-up to 9 years was performed.[24] The diag-

TABLE 76.10 Porous Coated Anatomic Total Knee Arthroplasty

Authors	No. of Knees/Patients	Mean Age (yr)	Rheumatoid Arthritis (%)	Osteoarthritis (%)	Follow-up (yr)	Good or Excellent Results (%)	Instability (%)	Loosening (%)	Lucent Lines (%)	Infection (%)	Reoperations/ Failures (%)
Hungerford et al (1985)[31]	OA 186/162					Cementless 96 Cemented 96					7.2
	RA 92/74	—	—	—	2-5	Cementless 92 Cemented 81	—	—	—	—	7.2
Rand et al (1987)[65]	50/33 (cemented)	65	32	68	2.2	97	—	—	3*	—	—
	41/33 (cementless)	56	34	61	2.4	83	4.8	2.4	18*	2.4	9.7
Hungerford et al (1987)[30]	93/82 (cementless)	56	30	63	2-5	94.5	—	—	17†	1.1	8.6
Toksvig-Larsen et al (1996)[85]	106	73	—	100	6.3	87	.7	3.5	—	—	18
Kim (1990)[41]	60/44 (cementless)	56	28	55	5	—	5	5	68	—	—
Hsu et al (1995)[28]	105/94	59	10	91	5.8	92	—	8	—	1	17
Sanzén et al (1996)[73]	158/142	68	30	70	7	70	.3	3.3	—	2	6
Knight et al (1997)[43]	78/71	72	12	85	5	89	1.2	1.2	44	1.3	8

OA = osteoarthritis, RA = rheumatoid arthritis.
* Incomplete lucent lines <1 mm.
† Lucent lines >1 mm and complete, or progressive.

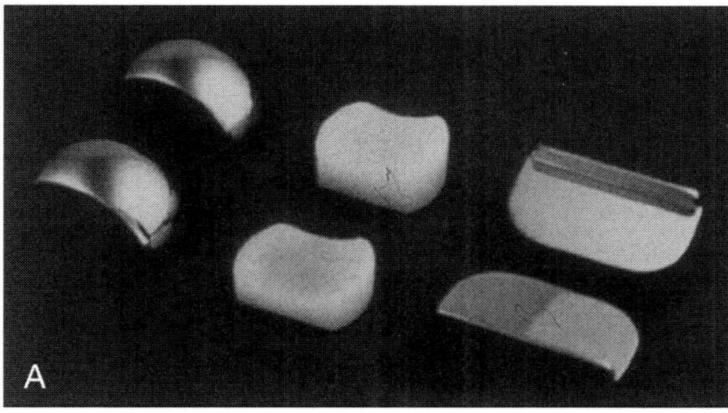

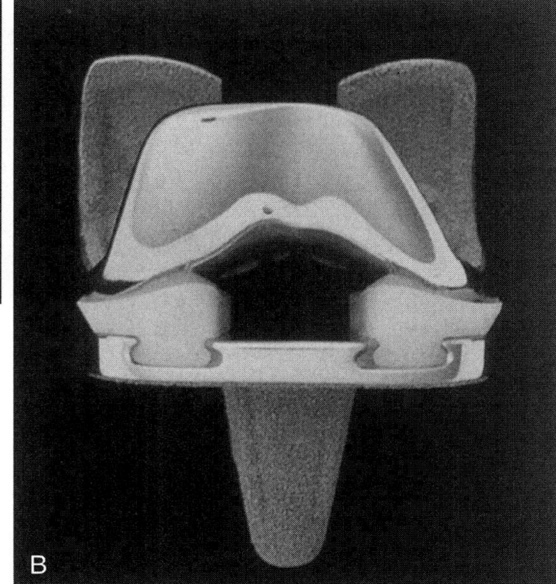

FIGURE 76.10 ➢ *A*, The Oxford meniscal-bearing prosthesis and *B*, low-contact stress (LCS) prosthesis. (From Scott WN: The Knee, vol 2, St. Louis, Mosby-Year Book, 1994, p 1137.)

nosis was osteoarthritis in 66% and rheumatoid arthritis in 32%. Knees with a diagnosis of rheumatoid arthritis had a survivorship of 95% at 6 years compared with 83% for knees with a diagnosis of osteoarthritis. Knees with an intact anterior cruciate ligament (ACL) had a survivorship of 95% at 6 years compared with 81% if the ACL was absent. Failures occurred in 25 (8.3%).

The low-contact stress (LCS) prosthesis differs from the Oxford prosthesis by having a decreased posterior femoral condyle radius, which results in slight incongruence in the tibial articulation.[6] In patients with a mean age of 60 years, 170 knees were treated with cementless fixation[6]: 95% good or excellent results were achieved at 4.5 years; 108 knees were treated with cement fixation in patients with a mean age of 64 years; 89% good or excellent results were obtained at a mean of 7.6 years. Complications were numerous, affecting 32% of the cemented and 27% of the cementless knees. Reoperation was required in 11% of the cemented and 2.9% of the cementless knees. A subsequent study used survivorship analysis with an endpoint of poor knee score or revision.[7] A 91% survivorship of 57 PCL-retaining designs at 6 years was predicted. Another 1-year study of 43 LCS knees found 39 knees (91%) good or excellent.[4] However, there was a 9.3% incidence of dislocation of the meniscal bearings. The mean range of motion was 94 degrees.

A study of 410 of an initial group of 473 TKA with cementless fixation was performed at 2 to 9 years following operation.[39] The diagnosis was osteoarthritis in 90% and rheumatoid arthritis in 10%. The mean patient age was 68 years. The Knee Society pain score was 93 and the function score 92. Using an endpoint of revision, survivorship was estimated at 95% at 8 years. Complications consisted of bearing dislocations in 5 (1%), bearing breakage in 7 (1.5%), subluxation in 5 (1.1%), subsidence of the tibia and femur in 1 each, and infection in 5. Reoperations were performed for infection in 5 and instability in 5 knees.

The concept of meniscal bearings is therefore attractive for managing problems of polyethylene wear. The clinical results of 90% to 95% good or excellent appear to be similar to other designs. Whether the long-term results suggest a lower wear rate and greater durability than other condylar prostheses is unknown (Table 76.11).

PRESS-FIT CONDYLAR PROSTHESIS

The Press-Fit Condylar (PFC) prosthesis (Johnson & Johnson Orthopaedics, Braintree, MA) was designed with a finned keel on the tibial component in an attempt to provide improved resistance to offset loading with minimal removal of tibial bone (Fig. 76.11). The implant was designed for cemented or cementless fixation. The results of 114 PFC knees with hybrid fixation (cementless femur, cemented tibia) followed for 2.8 years were reported.[90] The Knee Society scoring system improved from a preoperative value of 35 to a postoperative value of 92. Ninety-three percent had good or excellent results. The average flexion was 112 degrees. Radiolucent lines were identified adjacent to 30% of the femoral, 30% of the tibial, and 23% of the patellar components. Complications consisted of one wound hematome, two deep infections, three deep venous thromboses, and two pulmonary emboli. The reoperation rate was 3%.

Another study compared 59 knees with cementless fixation with 59 knees with cemented fixation using the PFC prosthesis.[62] At 2.8 years following arthroplasty, good or excellent results were achieved in 98% of the cemented compared with 90% of the cementless knees. Motion was 101 degrees in the cementless and 103 degrees in the cemented knees. Complica-

TABLE 76.11 **MENISCAL-BEARING TOTAL KNEE ARTHROPLASTY**

Authors	No. of Knees/Patients	Mean Age (yr)	Rheumatoid Arthritis (%)	Osteoarthritis (%)	Follow-up (yr)	Successful Results (%)	Lucent Lines (%)	Infection (%)	Reoperations/ Failures (%)
Goodfellow and O'Connor (1986)[23]	125/107	65	40	53	4	89	96	1	7
Buechel and Pappas (1989)[6]	170 (cementless)	60	23	69	4.5	95	—	—	2.9
	106 (cemented)	64	41	58	7.6	89	—	2.5	11
Goodfellow and O'Connor (1992)[24]	301	—	32	66	—	—	—	—	8.3
Jordan et al (1997)[39]	410	68	10	90	4.7	—	—	1.1	2.1

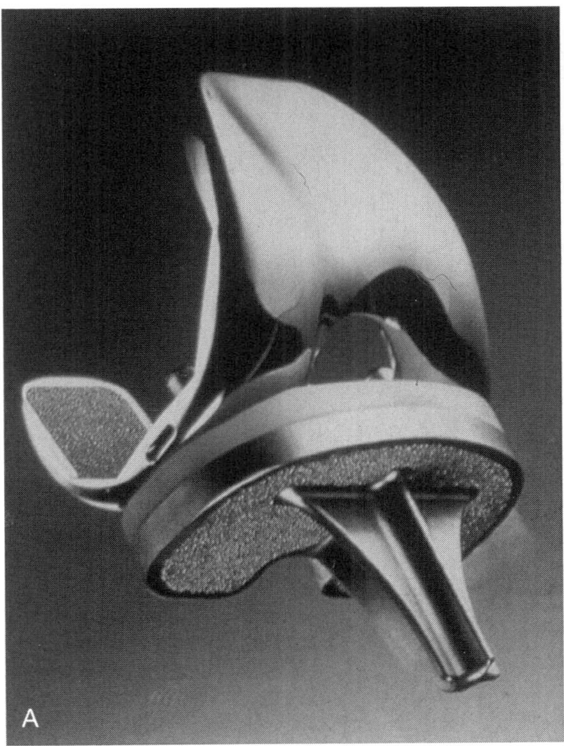

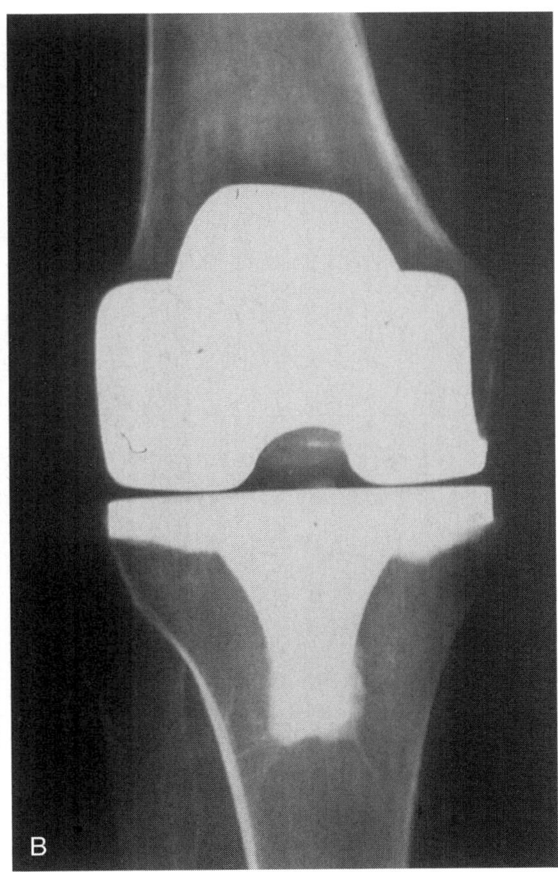

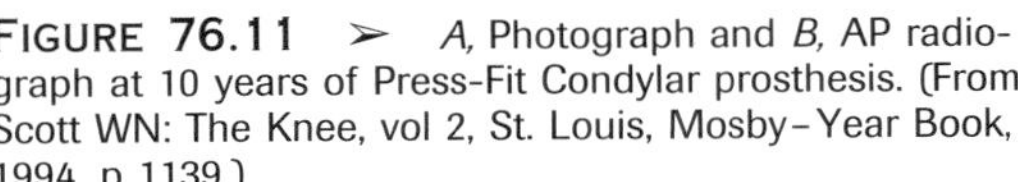
FIGURE 76.11 ➢ *A,* Photograph and *B,* AP radiograph at 10 years of Press-Fit Condylar prosthesis. (From Scott WN: The Knee, vol 2, St. Louis, Mosby-Year Book, 1994, p 1139.)

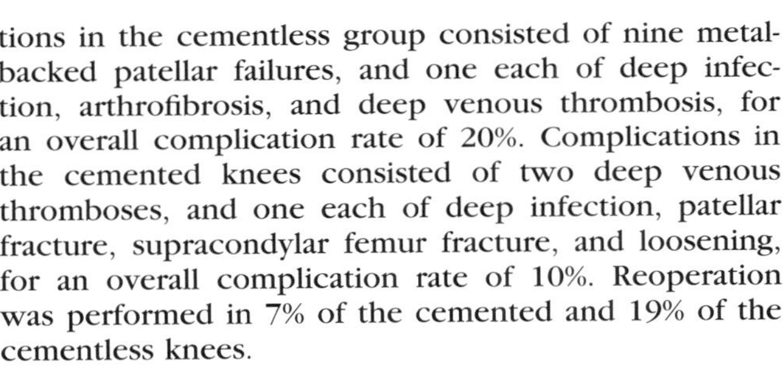

tions in the cementless group consisted of nine metal-backed patellar failures, and one each of deep infection, arthrofibrosis, and deep venous thrombosis, for an overall complication rate of 20%. Complications in the cemented knees consisted of two deep venous thromboses, and one each of deep infection, patellar fracture, supracondylar femur fracture, and loosening, for an overall complication rate of 10%. Reoperation was performed in 7% of the cemented and 19% of the cementless knees.

Another study reviewed 306 knees from an initial group of 378 knees at a mean of 6.5 years following surgery.[55] The mean patient age was 67 years. The diagnoses were osteoarthritis in 66% and rheumatoid arthritis in 30%. Cementless fixation was used for 7% of the tibial components and 70% of the femoral components. The Knee Society scores were 88 for pain and 72 for function. Range of motion was 110 degrees. Radiolucent lines were identified adjacent to the femoral component in 5%, the tibial component in 20%, and patellar component in 8%. Complications occurred in 5.5%, consisting of wear of a metal-backed patellar component in 8, deep infection in 2, patellar pain in an unresurfaced patella in 1, patellar implant loosening in 1, wear of tibial polyethylene in 3, hemarthrosis in 2, and persistent rheumatoid synovitis in 1. A subsequent study by the same surgeons reported the results of 155 of an initial group of 235 knees followed for 10 years.[74] Cementless fixation was used on the femoral component in 54% and on the tibial component in 4%. The Knee Society score was 95 for pain and 84 for function. Radiolucent lines were present adjacent to the tibial component in 16% and the femoral component in 3%. Reoperations were required in 19 knees. Complications consisted of wear of a metal-backed patella in nine, wear of a tibial polyethylene in nine, sepsis in three, hemarthrosis in two, synovectomy for rheumatoid arthritis in one, and patellar resurfacing in one. Using an endpoint of reoperation, survivorship was 92% at 10 years.

A comparison of 51 cemented and 55 cementless knees was performed at a follow-up of 10 years.[19] The Knee Society pain score was 92 for the cemented and 88 for the cementless knees; the Knee Society function score was 72 for the cemented and 66 for the cementless knees. Range of motion was 100 degrees in the cementless and 102 in the cemented knees. Complications consisted of failure of 19 of 53 metal-backed patellar components, loosening in 10 (8 cementless), osteolysis in 2, and infection in 3, patellar fracture in 1, and arthrofibrosis in 1 knee. Using an endpoint of revision of the femoral or tibial component, survivorship at 10 years was estimated at 88% for the cementless and 96% for the cemented knees.

The PFC prosthesis provides satisfactory results in 93% to 94% of knees with or without cement fixation. The complication and reoperation rates are similar to other current condylar prostheses. The use of a metal-

TABLE 76.12 PRESS-FIT CONDYLAR TOTAL KNEE ARTHROPLASTY

Authors	No. of Knees/Patients	Mean Age (yr)	Rheumatoid Arthritis (%)	Osteoarthritis (%)	Follow-up (yr)	Successful Results (%)	Lucent Lines (%)	Infection (%)	Reoperations/ Failures (%)
Wright et al (1990)[89]	112 knees	65	32	68	2.8	93	30	1.8	3
Rand (1991)[62]	118/102	66	13	62	2.8	94	75	1.8	13
Martin et al (1997)[55]	306/231	67	30	66	6.5	95	20	.7	5.5
Schai et al (1998)[74]	155/122	69	33	62	10	—	16	1.2	8
Duffy et al (1998)[19]	106/93	65	14	79	10	—	—	2.8	30

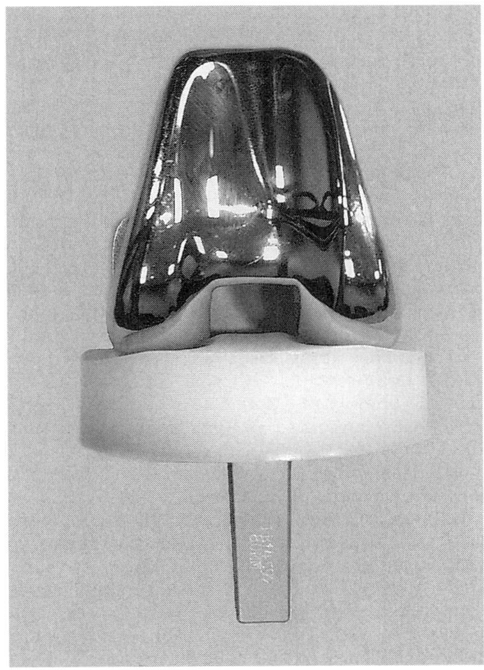

FIGURE 76.12 ➢ Photograph of AGC prosthesis.

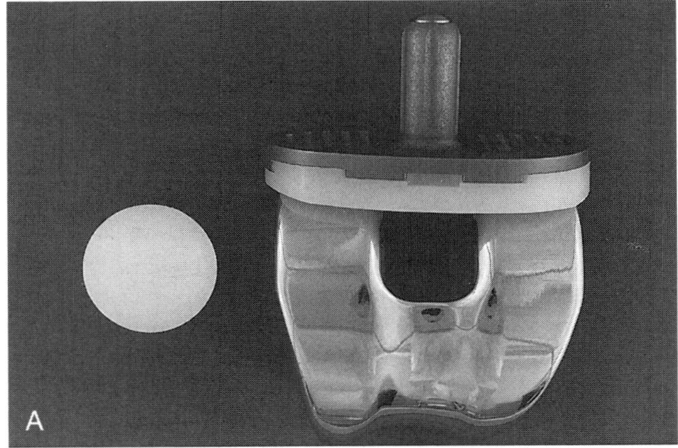

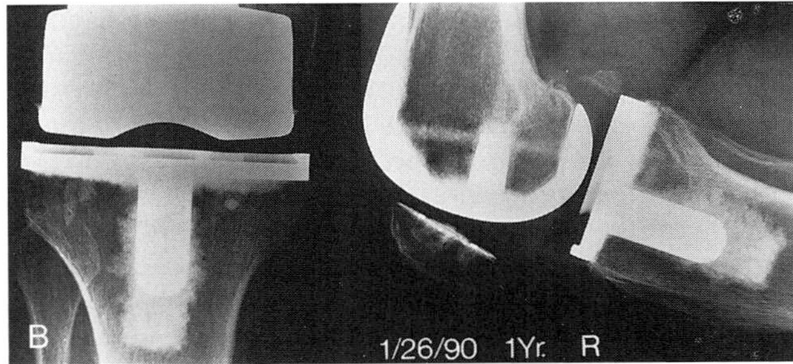

FIGURE 76.13 ➢ *A*, Photograph and *B*, AP radiograph of Genesis prosthesis.

backed patella of this design should be avoided (Table 76.12).

OTHER DESIGNS

The AGC (Biomet Warsaw, IN) is a posterior cruciate-retaining design with a molded one-piece metal-backed tibial component (Fig. 76.12). A study of 41 of an initial group of 51 knees with cementless fixation was performed at a mean of 54 months after operation.[75] The results were good or excellent in all 41 knees. The range of motion was 110 degrees. Radiolucent lines were identified adjacent to the tibial component in 5 knees. Using an endpoint of revision, survivorship was estimated at 100% at 5 years. Complications consisted of loosening in 1, and wound necrosis in 5 knees. In another multicenter study, 2001 TKA were reviewed at 3 to 10 years, with 71 knees having a 10-year evaluation.[69] The diagnoses were osteoarthritis in 91% and rheumatoid arthritis in 6%. The mean age was 69 years. The Knee Society score improved from 38 to 75 and the function score from 49 to 86. The mean flexion was 99 degrees. Complications consisted of failure of 27 metal-backed patellar components of which 2 had concomitant tibial component revision; femoral component loosening in 4; tibial component loosening in 3; instability in 3; patellar loosening in 2; and patellar fracture in 2 knees. Survivorship excluding the metal-backed patellar components and using an endpoint of revision was 98% at 10 years. The Genesis TKA is a cruciate-retaining design with an extended trochlear groove and a modular metal-backed tibial component (Fig. 76.13). A study of 105 knees was performed at a mean of 4.3 years after operation.[56] Fixation was with cement in 52%, hybrid in 47%, and cementless in 1%. The diagnosis was osteoarthritis in 92% and rheumatoid arthritis in 6%. The mean age was 69 years. Good or excellent results were obtained in 99%. The range of motion was 116 degrees. Complications occurred in 12% consisting of deep venous thrombosis in 3, patellar subluxation in 3, infection in 2, patellar fracture in 2, wound necrosis in 1, and cerebrovascular accident in 1.

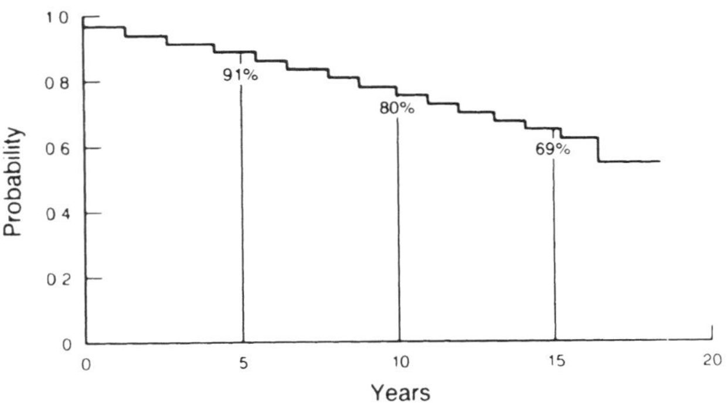

FIGURE 76.14 ➢ Survivorship of 9200 total knee arthroplasties was 69% at 15 years. (From Rand JA, Ilstrup DM: Survivorship analysis of total knee arthroplasty: Cumulative rates of survival of 9200 total knee arthroplasties. J Bone Joint Surg Am 73:397, 1991, with permission.)

SUMMARY

In 1991 Rand and Illstrup[64] reported the results of 9,200 TKAs implanted between 1971 and 1987 using survivorship analysis, with revision of an implant chosen as the endpoint of survival (Fig. 76.14). Of these, 2947 primary TKAs were performed using older resurfacing designs, including the Polycentric and Geometric knees. Cumulative rates of survival were 95% at 2 years, 89% at 5 years, and 78% at 10 years. Primary arthroplasties using condylar-resurfacing PCL-retaining designs with metal-backed tibial components were performed in 3620 knees. These designs included the cruciate condylar (Howmedica), Kinematic condylar, Townley, Cloutier, Miller-Galante, PCA, PFC, and Orthomet (Minneapolis, MN) prostheses. Cumulative rates of survival were 99% at 2 years, 98% at 5 years, and 91% at 10 years. Risk of failure was significantly greater for the early resurfacing designs compared with the metal-backed condylar designs. When metal-backed PCL-retaining arthroplasties were compared with PCL-substituting designs (234 posterior-stabilized knees), the results did not differ significantly for primary or revision arthroplasties. However, when primary and revision knees were combined, the PCL-substituting knees had a statistically significant higher cumulative failure rate: 3.8% versus 1.6% ($p < .03$). Considering all 9200 knees implanted, use of a proportional-hazard general linear model identified four indepent variables associated with a significantly lower risk of failure: (1) primary arthroplasty, (2) diagnosis of rheumatoid arthritis, (3) age of 60 years or more, and (4) use of a condylar PCL-retaining prosthesis with a metal-backed tibial component.

The results of these studies confirm that PCL-retaining TKAs have evolved and improved to become one of the most successful orthopedic operations, with greater than 90% satisfactory results at up to 10 years' follow-up. Continued long-term study is necessary to determine the relative benefits of various design modifications.

References

1. Alexiades M, Scuderi G, Vigorita V, et al: A histologic study of the posterior cruciate ligament in the arthritic knee. Am J Knee Surg 2:153, 1989.
2. Andriacchi TP, Galante JO: Retention of the posterior cruciate in total knee arthroplasty. J Arthroplasty 3:S13, 1998.
3. Andriacchi TP, Galante JO, Fermier RW: The influence of total knee replacement design on walking and stair climbing. J Bone Joint Surg Am 64:1328, 1982.
4. Bert JM: Dislocation/subluxation of meniscal bearing elements after New Jersey low-contact stress total knee arthroplasty. Clin Orthop 254:211, 1990.
5. Bourne MH, Rand JA, Ilstrup DM: Posterior cruciate condylar total knee arthroplasty: Five year results. Clin Orthop 234:147, 1989.
6. Buechel FF, Pappas MJ: New Jersey low-contact stress knee replacement system. Orthop Clin North Am 20:147, 1989.
7. Buechel FF, Pappas MJ: Long-term survivorship analysis of cruciate-sparing versus cruciate-sacrificing knee prostheses using meniscal bearing. Clin Orthop 260:162, 1990.
8. Cash RM, Gonzales MH, Garst J, et al: Proprioception after arthroplasty. Role of the posterior cruciate ligament. Clin Orthop Rel Res 331:172, 1996.
9. Cloutier JM: Results of total knee arthroplasty with a nonconstrained prosthesis. J Bone Joint Surg Am 65:906, 1983.
10. Cloutier JM: Long-term results after nonconstrained total knee arthroplasty. Clin Orthop 273:63, 1991.
11. Cloutier, JM: Long-term results of total knee arthroplasty with retention of both cruciate ligaments. J Bone Joint Surg. In press 1998.
12. Collins DN, Heim SA, Nelson CL, et al: Porous coated anatomic total knee arthroplasty. Clin Orthop 267:128, 1991.
13. Coventry MB, Upshaw JE, et al: Geometric total knee arthroplasty. I. Conception, design, indications and surgical technique. Clin Orthop 94:171, 1973.
14. Coventry MB, et al: Geometric total knee arthroplasty. II. Patient data and complications. Clin Orthop 94:177, 1973.
15. Dennis DA, Clayton ML, O'Connel S, et al: Posterior cruciate condylar total knee arthroplasty. Average 11-year follow-up evaluation. Clin Orthop Rel Res 281:168, 1992.
16. Dennis DA, Komistek RD, Hoff WA, et al: In vivo knee kinematics derived using an inverse perspective technique. Clin Orthop Rel Res 331:107, 1996.
17. Dodd CAF, Hungerford DS, Krackow KA: Total knee arthroplasty fixation. Clin Orthop 260:66, 1990.
18. Dorr LD, et al: Functional comparison of posterior-cruciate-retained versus cruciate-sacrificed total knee arthroplasty. Clin Orthop 236:36, 1988.
19. Duffy GP, Berry DJ, Rand JA: Cemented versus cementless fixation in total knee arthroplasty: Results at 10 years of a matched group. In press 1998.
20. Ewald FC, et al: Duo-patella total knee arthroplasty in rheumatoid arthritis. Orthop Trans 2:202, 1978.
21. Ewald FC, et al: Kinematic total knee replacement. J Bone Joint Surg Am 66:1032, 1984.
22. Freeman MAR, Railton GT: Should the posterior cruciate ligament be retained or resected in condylar nonmeniscal knee arthroplasty: The case for resection. J Arthroplasty 3:83, 1988.
23. Goodfellow JW, O'Connor J: Clinical results of Oxford knee. Clin Orthop 205:21, 1986.
24. Goodfellow JW, O'Connor J: The anterior cruciate ligament in knee arthroplasty. Clin Orthop Rel Res 276:245, 1992.
25. Gunston FH: Polycentric knee arthroplasty. Prosthetic stimulation of normal knee movement. J Bone Joint Surg Br 53:272, 1971.
26. Gunston FH: Ten-year results of polycentric knee arthroplasty. In Proceedings of the Canadian Orthopaedic Association. J Bone Joint Surg Br 62:133, 1980.
27. Harwin SF: Patellofemoral complications in symmetrical total knee arthroplasty. J Arthroplasty 13:753, 1998.
28. Hsu RW, Fan GF, Ho WP: A follow-up study of porous-coated anatomic knee arthroplasty. J Arthroplasty 10:29, 1995.
29. Hungerford DS, Kenna RV, Krackow KA: The porous-coated anatomic total knee. Symposium on Total Knee Arthroplasty. Orthop Clin North Am 13:103, 1982.
30. Hungerford DS, Krackow KA, Kenna RV: Two to five year experience with cementless porous-coated total knee prosthesis. In Rand JA, Dorr LD, ed: Total Arthroplasty of the Knee. Proceedings from the Knee Society, 1985-1986, Aspen, 1987. Rockville, MD, pp 215-235.
31. Hungerford DS, Krackow KA, Kenna RV: Clinical experience with the PCA prosthesis without cement. Orthop Trans 9:424, 1985.
32. Hungerford DS, Krackow KA, Kenna RV: Cementless total knee replacement in patients 50 years old and under. Orthop Clin North Am 20:131, 1989.
33. Ilstrup DM, Coventry MB, Skolnick MD: A statistical evaluation of geometric total knee arthroplasties. Clin Orthop 120:37, 1976.
34. Ilstrup DM, Combs, JG, Bryan RS, et al: A statistical evaluation of polycentric total knee arthroplasties. Clin Orthop 120:18, 1976.
35. Incavo SJ, Johnson CC, Beynnon BD, et al: Posterior cruciate ligament strain biomechanics in total knee arthroplasty. Clin Orthop Rel Res 309:88, 1994.
36. Inglis AE, Lane LB: Total knee replacement using the duo-patella prosthesis. Orthop Trans 2:202, 1978.
37. Insall JN, Lachiewicz PF, Burstein AH: The posterior stabilized condylar prosthesis: A modification of total condylar design. Two to four year clinical experience. J Bone Joint Surg Am 64: 1317, 1982.

38. Insall JN, Scott WN, Ranawat CS: The total condylar knee prosthesis. A report of two hundred twenty cases. J Bone Joint Surg Am 61:173, 1979.
39. Jordan LR, Olivo JL, Voorhost PE: Survivorship analysis of cementless meniscal bearing total knee arthroplasty. Clin Orthop Rel Res 338:119, 1997.
40. Kelman GJ, et al: Gait laboratory analysis of posterior cruciate-sparing total knee arthroplasty in stair ascent and descent. Clin Orthop 248:21, 1989.
41. Kim YH: Knee arthroplasty using a cementless PCA prosthesis with a porous-coated central tibial stem. J Bone Joint Surg Br 72: 412, 1990.
42. Kleinbart FA, Bryk E, Evangelista J, et al: Histologic comparison of posterior cruciate ligaments from arthritic and age-matched knee specimens. J Arthroplasty 11:726, 1996.
43. Knight JL, Atwater RD, Grothaus L: Clinical results of the modular porous-coated anatomic (PCA) total knee arthroplasty with cement: A 5-year prospective study. Orthopedics 20:1025, 1997.
44. Kobs JK, Lachiewicz PF: Hybrid total knee arthroplasty. Clin Orthop Rel Res 226:78, 1993.
45. Kraay MJ, et al: Hybrid total knee arthroplasty with the Miller-Galante prosthesis. Clin Orthop 273:32, 1991.
46. Landon GC, Galante JO, Maley MM: Noncemented total knee arthroplasty. Clin Orthop North Am 205:49, 1986.
47. Lattanzio PJ, Chess DG, MacDermid JC: J Arthroplasty 13:580, 1998.
48. Lee JG, Keating M, Ritter MA, et al: Review of the all polyethylene tibial component in total knee arthroplasty. Clin Orthop 260:87, 1990.
49. Lew WD, Lewis JL: The effect of knee-prosthesis geometry on cruciate ligament mechanics during flexion. J Bone Joint Surg Am 66:1211, 1984.
50. Lewallen DG, Bryan RS, Peterson LFA: Polycentric total knee arthroplasty. A ten year follow-up study. J Bone Joint Surg Am 66:1211, 1984.
51. Lowe GP, McNeur JC: Results of geometric arthroplasty for rheumatoid and osteoarthritis of the knee. Aust NZ J Surg 51:528, 1981.
52. Mahoney OM, Nobel PC, Rhoads DD, et al: Posterior cruciate function following total knee arthroplasty. J Arthroplasty 9:569, 1994.
53. Malkani AL, Rand JA, et al: J Bone Joint Surg Am 77:423, 1995.
54. Mallory TH, Smalley D, Dray J: Townley anatomic total knee arthroplasty using total tibial component with cruciate release. Clin Orthop 169:97, 1982.
55. Martin SD, McManus JL, Scott RD, et al: Press-fit condylar total knee arthroplasty. J Arthroplasty 12:603, 1997.
56. Mokris JG, Smith SW, Anderson SE: Primary total knee arthroplasty using the Genesis total knee arthroplasty system, J Arthroplasty 12:91, 1997.
57. Montgomery RL, Goodman SB, Csongradi J: Late rupture of the posterior cruciate ligament after total knee replacement. Iowa Orthop J 13:167,
58. Partio E, Orava T, Lehto M, et al: Survival of the Townley knee. Acta Orthop Scand 65:319, 1994.
59. Ranawat CS, Insall J, Shine J: Duo-condylar knee arthroplasty. Hospital for Special Surgery design. Clin Orthop 120:76, 1976.
60. Ranawat CS, Shine JJ: Duo-condylar total knee arthroplasty. Clin Orthop 94:185, 1973.
61. Rand JA: A comparison of metal backed and all polyethylene tibial components in cruciate condylar total knee arthroplasty. J Arthroplasty 8:307, 1993.
62. Rand JA: Cement or cementless fixation in total knee arthroplasty? Clin Orthop 273:52, 1991.
63. Rand JA, Coventry MB: Ten-year evaluation of geometric total knee arthroplasty. Clin Orthop 232:168, 1988.
64. Rand JA, Ilstrup DM: Survivorship analysis of total knee arthroplasty: Cumulative rates of survival of 9200 total knee arthroplasties. J Bone Joint Surg Am 73:397, 1991.
65. Rand JA, et al: A comparison of cemented versus cementless porous-coated anatomic total knee arthroplasty. In Rand JA, Dorr LD, eds: Total arthroplasty of the knee. Proceedings of the Knee Society, 1985, 1986, Rockville, MD, Aspen, 1987, p 195.
66. Riley D, Woodyard JE: Long-term results of total knee replacement. J Bone Joint Surg Br 67:548, 1985.
67. Ritter MA, Gioe TJ, Stringer EA, et al: The posterior cruciate condylar total knee prosthesis: A five year follow-up study. Clin Orthop 184:265, 1984.
68. Ritter MA, Campbell E, Faris PM, et al: Long-term survival analysis of the posterior cruciate condylar total knee arthroplasty. A 10-year evaluation. J Arthroplasty 4:293, 1989.
69. Ritter MA, Worland R, Saliski J, et al: Flat-on-flat, nonconstrained compression molded polyethylene total knee replacement. Clin Orthop Rel Res 321:79, 1995.
70. Rorabeck CH, Bourne RB, Lewis PL, et al: The Miller-Galante knee prosthesis for the treatment of osteoarthrosis. J Bone Joint Surg Am 75:402, 1993.
71. Rosenberg AG, Barden R, Galante JO: A comparison of cemented and cementless fixation with the Miller-Galante total knee arthroplasty. Orthop Clin North Am 20:97, 1989.
72. Rosenberg AG, Barden RM, Galante JO: Cemented and ingrowth fixation of the Miller-Galante prosthesis. Clin Orthop 260:71, 1990.
73. Sanzén L, Sahlström A, Gentz CF, et al: Radiographic wear assessment in a total knee prosthesis. J Arthroplasty 11:738, 1996.
74. Schai PA, Thornhill TS, Scott RD: Total knee arthroplasty with the PFC system. Results at a minimum of ten years and survivorship analysis. J Bone Joint Surg Br 80:850, 1998.
75. Schroder HM, Aaen K, Hansen EB, et al: Cementless total knee arthroplasty in rheumatoid arthritis. J Arthroplasty 11:18, 1996.
76. Scott RD: Duopatellar total knee replacement: The Brigham experience. Orthop Clin North Am 13:89, 1982.
77. Simmons S, Lephard S, Rubash H, et al: Proprioception following total knee arthroplasty with and without the posterior cruciate ligament. J Arthroplasty 11:763, 1996.
78. Skolnick MD, Coventry MB, Ilstrup DM: Geometric total knee arthroplasty. A two-year follow-up study. J Bone Joint Surg Am 58:749, 1976.
79. Skolnick MD, et al: Polycentric total knee arthroplasty. A two-year follow-up study. J Bone Joint Surg Am 58:743, 1976.
80. Sledge CB, Ewald FC: Total knee arthroplasty experience at the Robert Breck Brigham Hospital. Clin Orthop 145:78, 1979.
81. Sledge CB, et al: Two-year follow-up of the Duocondylar total knee replacement. Orthop Trans 2:193, 1978.
82. Sorger JI, Federle D, Kirk PG, et al: The posterior cruciate ligament in total knee arthroplasty. J Arthroplasty 12:869, 1997.
83. Stiehl JB, Komistek RD, Dennis DA, et al: Fluoroscopic analysis of kinematics after posterior-cruciate-retaining knee arthroplasty. J Bone Joint Surg Br 77:884, 1995.
84. Thomas WH, et al: Duopatella total knee arthroplasty. Orthop Trans 4:329, 1980.
85. Toksvig-Larsen S, Ryd L, Stenström A, et al: The porous-coated anatomic total knee experience. J Arthroplasty 11:11, 1996.
86. Townley CO: The anatomic total knee resurfacing arthroplasty. Clin Orthop 192:82, 1985.
87. Walker DS, et al: Fixation of tibial components of knee prosthesis. Trans Orthop Res Soc 4:95, 1979.
88. Warren PJ, Olanlokun TK, Cobb AG, et al: Proprioception after knee arthroplasty. The influence of prosthetic design. Clin Orthop Rel Res 297:182, 1993.
89. Wright J, et al: Total knee arthroplasty with the kinematic prosthesis. J Bone Joint Surg Am 72:1003, 1990.
90. Wright RJ, et al: Two to four year results of posterior cruciate sparing condylar total knee arthroplasty with an uncemented femoral component. Clin Orthop 260:80, 1990.

77 Total Knee Arthroplasty With Posterior Cruciate Ligament Substitution Designs

STEVEN H. STERN • JOHN N. INSALL

Posterior cruciate ligament (PCL) substitution remains one of the most enduring innovations in total knee arthroplasty. While the original prosthesis has undergone several modifications, the basic mechanism of cruciate ligament substitution remains essentially unchanged.

At the time of its introduction, some surgeons postulated that the intrinsic stability of the Posterior Stabilized prosthesis might result in an increased incidence of aseptic component loosening.[72] However, clinical results with this implant have been uniformly excellent[1, 2, 8, 21, 22, 28, 33, 40, 53, 62, 73, 74, 75, 82, 84] and offer further testimony to the value of PCL substitution. In contrast, some other prosthetic knee designs have been unable to achieve predictable long-term results.[10, 16, 18, 25, 29, 51, 68, 71]

The concept of PCL substitution is now widely accepted, and most prosthesis manufacturers currently include some version of a Posterior Stabilized implant in their knee arthroplasty line. The contemporary modular NexGen Legacy arthroplasty continues the basic concept of ligament substitution, now into the third decade of clinical use. The original Posterior Stabilized implant persists as one of the few to achieve excellent long-term clinical results and continues to offer a standard of comparison for the multitude of so-called modern component designs available at this time.

Nomenclature Note. One confusing aspect of posterior cruciate substituting knee arthroplasties is the terminology to describe the concept. Specifically, the original posterior substituting design introduced at The Hospital for Special Surgery (HSS) in the late 1970s was called the Posterior Stabilized implant. However, the term posterior stabilized has gained widespread acceptance as a generic description of posterior cruciate substituting arthroplasties. In most cases, the interchangeable use of these words does not cause problems. However, to minimize confusion in this chapter, the terms are used with explicit, distinct definitions. Specifically, the phrases "posterior substituting" or "posterior substitution" refer to a generic type of knee arthroplasty but not to a specific implant. "Posterior Stabilized" is used strictly in reference to the original or subsequent descendant implants (Insall-Burstein Posterior Stabilized or Insall-Burstein II Posterior Stabilized) designed at the HSS.

RATIONALE FOR AND EVOLUTION OF POSTERIOR SUBSTITUTING KNEE ARTHROPLASTY BY THE INSALL GROUP

Total Condylar Prosthesis

The modern age of total knee arthroplasty was ushered in during the early 1970s with the advent of the total condylar prosthesis. The original total condylar prosthesis was a semiconstrained, nonlinked condylar replacement. This design involved sacrifice of both cruciate ligaments. Component fixation was achieved with the use of bone cement. The femoral component's curvature roughly approximated that of the average knee. An anterior flange on the device allowed for articulation with an all-polyethylene patellar dome. The tibial tray had concave surfaces that offered some inherent stability to the device.[36, 37] The tibial tray had a single central intramedullary post to optimize fixation. Cruciate excision was originally undertaken to allow for extensive exposure and to afford easy correction of angular deformities. The total condylar device was one of the first designs to yield predictable and durable results.[37, 41] The long-term clinical results with this prosthesis still offer a standard of comparison for more modern knee designs.[63, 64, 93]

Certain weaknesses, however, became apparent with the total condylar prosthesis as clinicians accumulated experience with its use. Specifically, early reports indicated that "only" 90 degrees of flexion was attained with this particular design.[37, 41] In addition, in cases where the flexion gap was inadequately balanced, the tibial component had a propensity to sublux posteriorly. It was thought that sacrifice of the PCL played an intrinsic role in these problems. An intact ligament would allow the femur to roll back on the tibia during knee flexion and hence promote a greater arc of motion. In addition, an intact ligament would tend to act against posterior tibial subluxation. It was these issues that provided the impetus to design a cruciate substituting device.

The initial attempt at a posterior cruciate substituting knee prosthesis was the Total Condylar 2, introduced in 1976. This construct featured a central post on the tibial component to prevent posterior tibial subluxation. However, it was not designed to substitute for the collateral ligaments or to promote femoral rollback. Early results with the Total Condylar 2 were poor, with a relatively high rate of tibial component loosening.[38] It was believed that this loosening was caused by design problems inherent in this particular device.

Posterior Stabilized Prosthesis

The original Posterior Stabilized prosthesis was introduced at the HSS in 1978 as a further modification of the original total condylar design (Fig. 77.1).[40] The developers of this prosthesis built a PCL substituting mechanism into their device. The designers of the Posterior Stabilized arthroplasty adhered to the basic surgical principles of cruciate ligament excision, which had helped make the total condylar prosthesis successful. Thus, the Posterior Stabilized prosthesis was designed to substitute for the sacrificed cruciate ligament while still retaining the advantage of ligament excision. The prosthesis was intended to improve stair climbing, increase range of motion, and prevent posterior tibial subluxation.

Posterior cruciate substitution was accomplished by interaction of a central tibial polyethylene spine with a transverse femoral cam. The femoral component was composed of chrome-cobalt, and the tibial component was made entirely of ultrahigh-molecular-weight polyethylene. The patellar bone was resurfaced, using an all-polyethylene dome with a central round peg. All components in this arthroplasty were implanted with the use of polymethylmethacrylate.

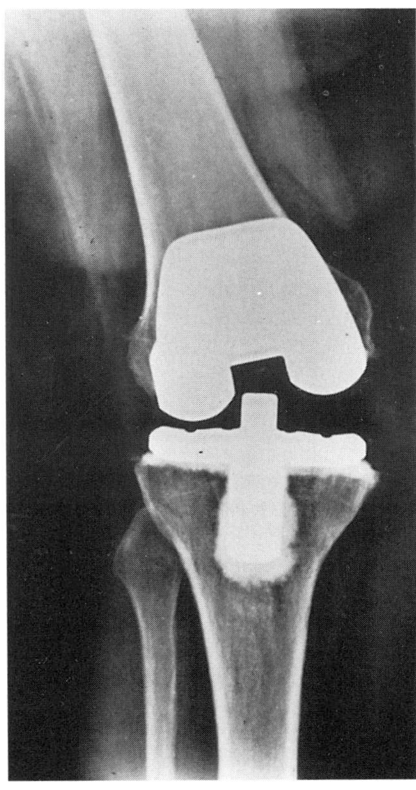

FIGURE 77.2 ➢ A posterior stabilized prosthesis implanted in a patient with medial collateral ligament insufficiency. The posterior substituting mechanism does not prevent medial laxity.

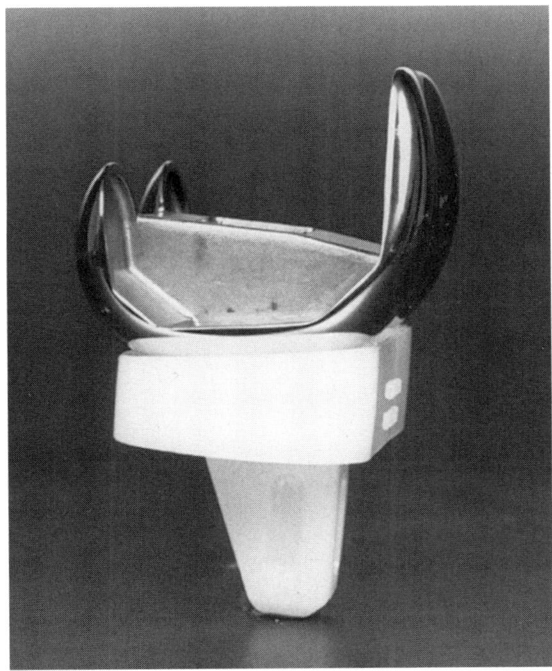

FIGURE 77.1 ➢ The original Insall-Burstein Posterior Stabilized prosthesis composed of a chrome-cobalt femoral component articulating with an all-polyethylene tibial tray.

The tibial component of the Posterior Stabilized arthroplasty employed an articulating surface composed of bicondylar wells that roughly conformed to the condyles on the femoral component. The tibial tray had a posterior slope built directly into the design of the component. This posterior tilt was incorporated so that the component would more closely resemble the proximal portion of the tibia, which also has a posterior angulation. This incline improved knee flexion by helping to clear the posterior tibial condyles at maximum flexion angles. The posterior slope also acted to enhance knee stability, especially in resisting posterior subluxation through the full flexion arc.

The cam mechanism of the Posterior Stabilized prosthesis was designed so that the cam would contact the tibial spine at about 70 degrees of flexion. Therefore, the cam had no effect on knee stability in extension, because it did not articulate at these lesser flexion angles. Knee stability was dependent on both the soft-tissue balance and the inherent conformity of the components. The ligament substitution mechanism did not prevent anterior tibial subluxation, nor did it substitute in any way for the collateral ligaments (Fig. 77.2).

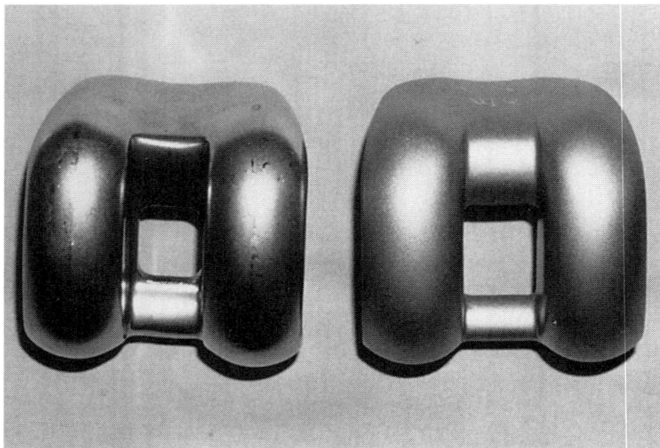

FIGURE 77.3 ➢ Original Insall-Burstein femoral component *(left)* and modified component *(right)*. The femoral groove has been deepened and the anterior aspect more rounded.

Consequently, mediolateral stability of the joint was entirely dependent on intact collateral ligaments. If a knee was unstable to varus or valgus stresses, the Posterior Stabilized prosthesis would not provide sufficient support. These cases would need to be addressed with a more constrained implant.

Several design alterations of the Insall-Burstein Posterior Stabilized prosthesis have been made over the years. One of the first changes involved modification of the composition of the original all-polyethylene tibial tray to include metal backing of the tibial component. This was done in the latter half of 1980 after finite element analysis demonstrated enhanced load transmission to the underlying bone with the addition of metal backing to the tibial component.[4] By 1981, the all-polyethylene tibial component had been totally replaced by its metal-backed counterpart at the HSS.

The early 1980s also marked the advent of carbon-reinforced tibial components. Theoretically, carbon reinforcement would increase the strength of the polyethylene that composed the tibial tray. However, the clinical results with this polyethylene biomaterial proved disappointing and failure of the carbon-reinforced tibia was reported.[74, 75, 76] Thereafter, the plain (nonreinforced) polyethylene tibial tray returned to routine use with the Posterior Stabilized prosthesis.

The next major prosthetic change occurred in 1983 with the introduction of modified Posterior Stabilized components, which was, in part, the practical result of a concern regarding the patellofemoral joint. At that time, the femoral component was altered to allow for a smoother patellofemoral transition (Fig. 77.3). This transition occurs when the patellofemoral contact point moves from the anterior flange to the distal runners as the knee goes through an arc of motion from extension to flexion. Modifications included rounding of the anterior portion of the femoral component, as well as deepening of the femoral groove in an attempt to enhance patellar tracking. Additionally, the implant was produced in various sizes. Because the original version was available in only one intermediate size, mismatches between the component and the host bone occurred; this was corrected with the introduction of multiple sizes.

Insall-Burstein II Posterior Stabilized Prosthesis

The Posterior Stabilized prosthesis continued in use without major change until the late 1980s, when the Insall-Burstein II (IB II) Posterior Stabilized prosthesis was introduced (Fig. 77.4). This prosthesis incorporated several major changes in both component design and instrumentation. Intramedullary instruments were used for prosthetic implantation, and the original

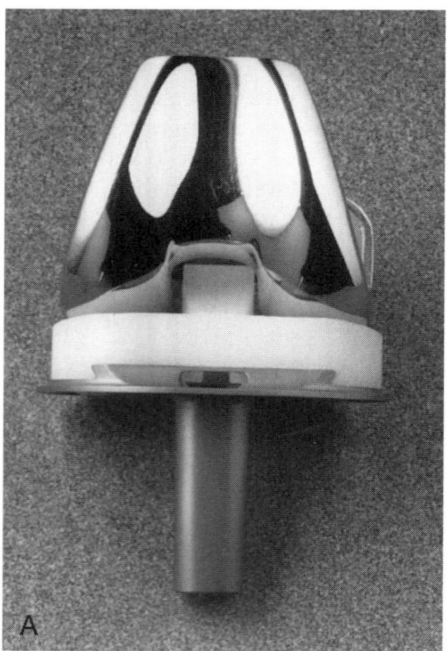

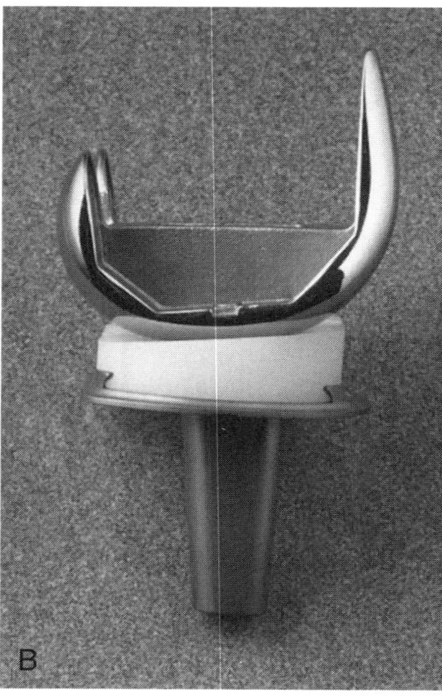

FIGURE 77.4 ➢ The Insall-Burstein II prosthesis. *A,* Front view. *B,* Side view. The tibial component is modular, allowing interchange of the plastic on each metallic tray. The kinematics of the design were altered slightly to improve rollback and knee flexion. Note the posterior incline to the tibial plastic, which acts to enhance knee stability.

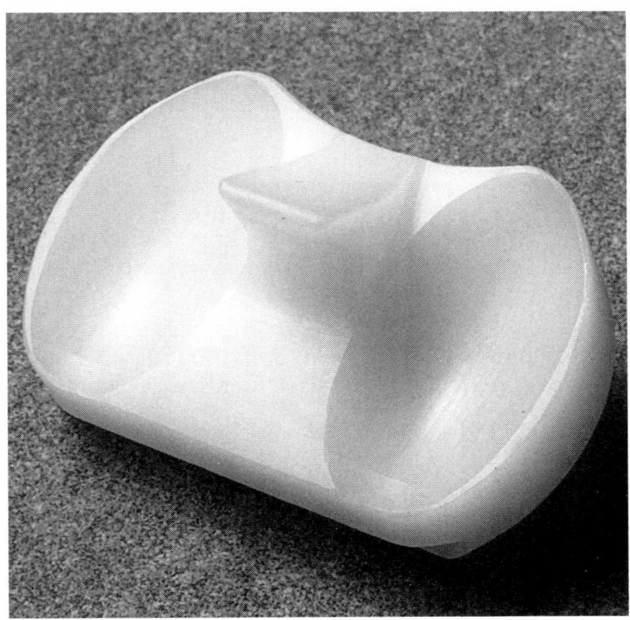

FIGURE 77.5 ➢ The Insall-Burstein II tibial tray has bicondylar wells that conform to the shape of the femoral component.

"tenser," used in the past to ensure balance between the flexion and extension gaps, was abandoned. However, the concept of ligamentous balance was not discarded, and it still remains an essential factor for successful arthroplasty. The IB II prosthesis also introduced modularity to the Posterior Stabilized components. Thus, depending on the clinical needs of an individual case, various metallic trays, polyethylene tibial inserts, intramedullary rods, and wedges could be assembled at the time of surgery.

Additionally, the inauguration of the IB II prosthesis heralded a slight modification in the mechanism of ligament substitution. This was done in an attempt to further enhance femoral rollback and to increase knee flexion. Unfortunately, this new design required further fine-tuning secondary to reports of component dislocation.[6, 54, 55, 59, 96] Although rare, dislocations were especially worrisome in knees with a preoperative valgus deformity or in those that achieved large flexion angles.[23] Because of widespread concern regarding this problem, a modification of the tibial insert was undertaken. Changes, restricted to the tibial insert, included elevation as well as relative anterior translation of the tibial spine. These alterations served to increase the inherent stability of the device.[46, 55]

Thus, the IB II prosthesis offers the advantages of a modular design while maintaining the basic mechanism of ligament substitution (Fig. 77.5). It employs essentially the same arthroplastly philosophy that has been used successfully since the 1980s and is one of the few prosthetic designs to remain fundamentally unchanged after more than a decade in use.

NexGen Legacy

Introduced in the mid-1990s, the NexGen Legacy prosthesis is the most recent evolution of the Posterior Stabilized lineage. The prosthesis incorporates several major design and instrumentation changes. The NexGen Legacy prosthesis includes an anatomic design with both right and left femoral components. This differs from previous Posterior Stabilized designs, which were nonanatomic. In addition, the femoral prosthesis has a raised lateral phalange and a deeper trochlear groove. These design modifications were instituted partly to further optimize patellofemoral kinematics (Fig. 77.6).

Another design modification made with the NexGen Legacy was the addition of lugs to the femoral component's condyles. These were instituted to help stabilize the prosthesis during implantation. Specifically, the femoral component lugs help prevent flexion of the femoral component during flexion. On occasion, this "femoral flex" occurred with the Insall-Burstein design and resulted, if the prosthesis was left flexed, in a gap between the component's femoral flange and the femur's anterior cortex. If correction was attempted by

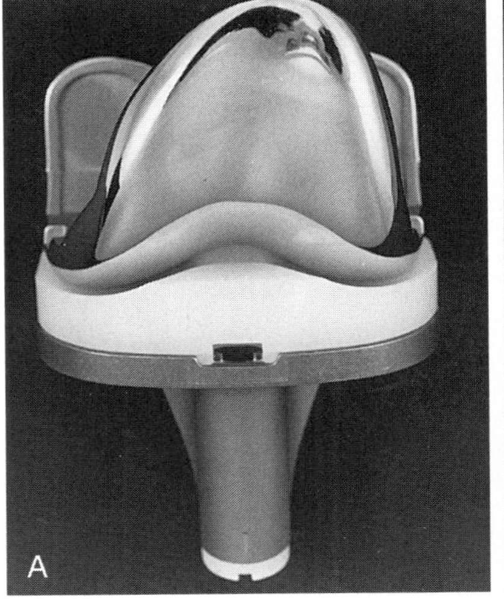

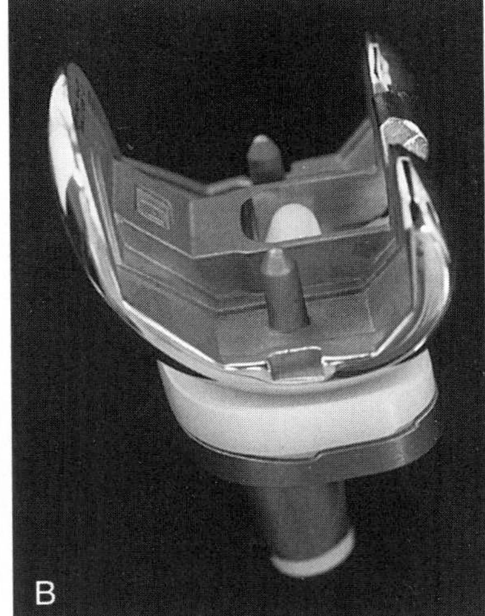

FIGURE 77.6 ➢ NexGen Legacy prosthesis (Zimmer, Warsaw, IN). *A*, Front view. *B*, Oblique view.

twisting the component into extension, the surgeon risked the possibility of creating a gap between the femur's posterior condyle and the component's posterior condyles. The advent of the lugs prevents flexion of the component during insertion, thereby preventing the femoral flex phenomenon.

The NexGen Legacy's tibial baseplates are designed to accept multiple different-sized polyethylene inserts. This contrasts with previous Posterior Stabilized designs, in which each femoral component was paired exclusively with its size-matched tibial component. On occasion, this could lead to intraoperative difficulties if a patient's bone required different femoral and tibial component sizes. The current design of the NexGen Legacy prosthesis allows the surgeon to independently pick both the femoral and the tibial components. Multiple tibial inserts are available for each tibial baseplate. The inserts are designed so that the plastic undersurface mates with the tibial baseplate while the articulating surface corresponds to the particular femoral component. This allows designers to maintain conformity at the femoral-tibial articulation while maintaining flexibility in tibial component sizing.

Finally, the spine cam interaction was modified slightly in the NexGen Legacy prosthesis. The designers attempted to maintain the well-established benefits of posterior cruciate substitution while building increased stability into the substituting mechanism to minimize the dislocation risks associated with the previous prostheses at high flexion angles.[6, 46, 54, 55, 59, 96] Thus, the NexGen Legacy's spine-cam interaction has a similar pathway and angle of contact as the successful previous Posterior Stabilized designs. However, the femoral cam is positioned farther posterior and proximal in the NexGen Legacy's femoral component. This increases knee stability by allowing the femoral cam to ride down the tibial spine as the knee flexes. This differentiates this implant from the previous Posterior Stabilized designs (and most other designs), in which the femoral cam rides up along the tibial spine as the knee bends into deep flexion.[11, 46]

The instrumentation options available for implantation were also modified and increased with the NexGen Legacy prosthesis. The modifications allow for increased flexibility and surgical preference in choosing the manner to implant the prosthesis. Traditional intramedullary instrumentation, which incorporates the classic IB II surgical techniques, is available. In addition, epicondylar instruments that reference the femur's epicondylar axis to optimize femoral component rotation can be used. These instruments also permit both anterior and posterior femoral referencing to aid in positioning the femoral component. Finally, for surgeons desiring an alternative to the traditional sawblade technique, instrumentation is available that allows for preparation of the femur and tibia using a milling technique.

CONTEMPORARY POSTERIOR CRUCIATE LIGAMENT SUBSTITUTION DEVICES

(Table 77.1)

Duracon PS

The Duracon PS (Howmedica, Rutherford, NJ) is an anatomic posterior cruciate substituting design that is part of the Duracon total knee system (Fig. 77.7) The Duracon system uses a versatile tibial baseplate that accepts polyethylene inserts for either cruciate substitution or cruciate retention. As with other modern prostheses, one of the goals of the implant developers was optimizing articular conformity and thereby minimizing contact stresses and polyethylene wear.

The femoral component has a closed-box design, which the designers felt would prevent cement extrusion and reduce polyethylene wear particle migration. The femoral component's closed box is posteriorly located, which corresponds to the posteriorly positioned tibial post. Theoretically, this posterior placement helps preserve anterior femoral bone stock. In addition, the femoral component has a deep trochlear groove with an anatomic lateral flare. The designers felt that this would enable the patella to track naturally during knee motion.

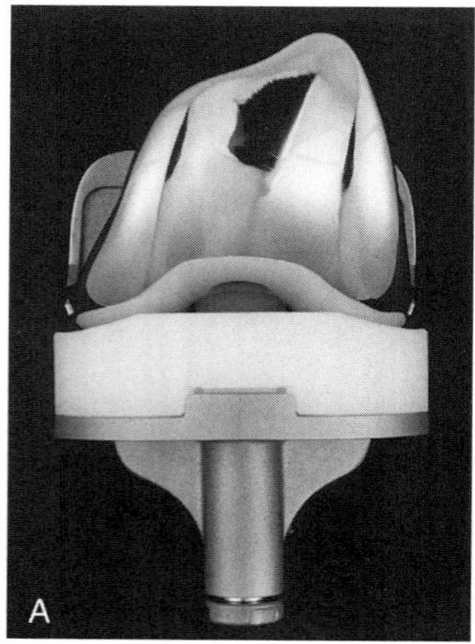

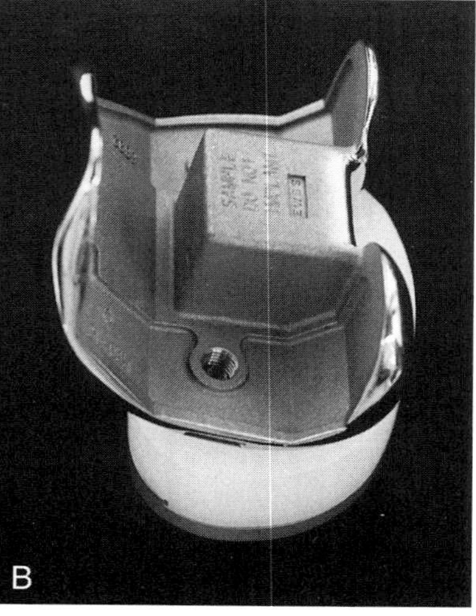

FIGURE 77.7 ➢ Duracon PS (Howmedica, Rutherford, NJ). *A*, Front view. *B*, Oblique view.

TABLE 77.1 COMPARISON OF POSTERIOR CRUCIATE SUBSTITUTING PROSTHESES

Prosthesis Name	NexGen Legacy	Duracon PS	PFC Sigma	Genesis II	Maxim	ADVANCE	OPTETRAK
Manufacturer	Zimmer	Howmedica	Johnson & Johnson	Richards	Biomet	Wright Medical	Exactech
Femoral component	Anatomic	Anatomic	Anatomic	Anatomic	Anatomic	Symmetric	Symmetric
Femoral box design	Open	Closed	Closed	Open	Closed	Open	Open
Tibia	Nonanatomic	Nonanatomic	Nonanatomic	Anatomic	Nonanatomic	Symmetric	Symmetric
Medial-lateral stability with primary implant	No	Yes	No	No	No	No	No
Modularity (primary implant)							
Femur (wedges/blocks)	Yes	Yes	Yes	Yes	Yes	No	No
Femur (IM rods)	Requires different component	Requires different component	Yes	Yes	Requires different component	No	No
Tibia (wedges/blocks)	Yes*	Yes	Requires different component	Yes	Requires different component	Yes	Yes***
Tibia (IM rods)	Yes	Yes	Yes	Yes	Depends**	Yes	Yes***
Ability to up- or downsize	1 to 2 sizes	1 to 2 sizes	1 to 2 sizes	1 to 2 sizes	All sizes	1 size	1 size
Tibial component	Up or down	Up or down	Up or down	Up or down	Up or down	Up	Up or down
Comon sizes							
Femur	5	6	6	8	4	6	6
Tibia	6	8	6	8	6	6	6
Spine-cam kinematics	Femoral cam rolls *down* spine at high knee flexion angles	Early spine-cam contact (~10 degrees flexion), similar to Kinematic Stabilizer	Similar to traditional Insall-Burstein spine-cam mechanism	Spine-cam contact at ~60 to 70 degrees, more stable than original Insall-Burstein		Similar to traditional Insall-Burstein spine-cam mechanism	Similar to traditional Insall-Burstein spine-cam mechanism
Miscellaneous				Femoral component has asymmetric posterior condyles			

* Not all NexGen primary baseplates allow for wedge-block use.
** Maxim one-piece baseplate does not allow IM rods. Other Maxim baseplates do.
*** Trapezoidal tray allows use of wedges and IM rods.

The Duracon PS spine-cam interaction is distinctly different from other modern posterior cruciate substituting designs. Most posterior substituting components are designed to have the femoral cam contact the tibial spine at a knee flexion angle of approximately 60 to 70 degrees. This results in posterior substituting mechanisms that resemble the original Posterior Stabilized spine-cam interaction. At lesser knee flexion angles, the spine does not contact the cam. Thus, at these lower angles, stability depends on implant conformity and soft-tissue tension. In contrast, the Duracon PS is designed for spine-cam interaction to commence at 10 degrees of flexion. The spine and cam then remain in contact throughout the entire range of knee motion. This spine-cam mechanism appears similar to the previous design (Kinematic Stabilizer) from the same company. The developers of these prostheses felt that spine-cam interaction throughout the knee's arc of motion would increase component stability at low flexion angles. Theoretically, this could also increase stress to the tibial spine because of the increased contact. In fact, the tibial component of the Duracon PS is reinforced with a Vitallium endoskeleton specifically to increase its strength and stability. A locking screw is used to secure the reinforced tibial post to the baseplate, thereby augmenting the basic polyethylene snap-lock mechanism.

PFC Sigma

The PFC Sigma knee system (Johnson & Johnson, Raynham, MA) was one of the first comprehensive knee arthroplasty systems widely available. The implants are designed to take advantage of the benefits of modularity and to allow for simple intraoperative interchange between components. Specifically, the tibial tray accepts either cruciate retaining, cruciate supplementing, or cruciate substituting polyethylene tibial inserts. The tray is modular and can be augmented with tibial wedges, blocks, or various-size tibial stems (Fig. 77.8).

The femoral component differs depending on whether it is designed for cruciate retaining or cruciate substituting knee arthroplasty. However, both the cruciate retaining and the cruciate substituting femoral components share the same coronal geometry. The implant developers used this geometry to increase contact area and protect against edge loading, thereby minimizing peak stresses. The similar coronal geometry theoretically aids in easy intraoperative switching between cruciate retaining and posterior substituting implants.

Similar to many other modern cruciate substituting designs, the P.F.C. Sigma femoral components are anatomic, coming in both rights and lefts. The femoral spine interaction is similar to the original Insall-Burstein Posterior Stabilized design. In addition, the femoral components mate either with the identical-sized tibial baseplate or with tibial trays one size larger or smaller. This permits the surgeon to up- or downsize the tibial component by one size, allowing for a three-size spread. Conceptually, this optimizes contact at the femoral-tibial articulation, as well as between tibial baseplate and host bone.

Genesis II

The Genesis II total knee was designed as a comprehensive knee system with a modern posterior cruciate substituting option. The components are anatomic and are designed to promote versatility in matching femoral and tibial component sizes. In general, the system allows the femoral prosthesis to mate with four different-sized tibial components. Additionally, the implant design incorporates several innovative features in an attempt to optimize knee kinematics. One goal was for the femoral component's trochlear groove to gently encourage lateral patellar motion as the knee comes into extension. Thus, the femoral component's trochlear groove was elongated to maximize contact with the patella throughout the arc of motion (full contact through 85 degrees of flexion). In addition, in a fur-

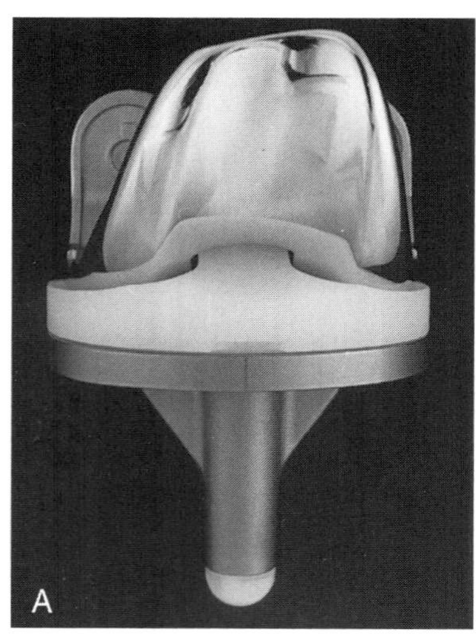

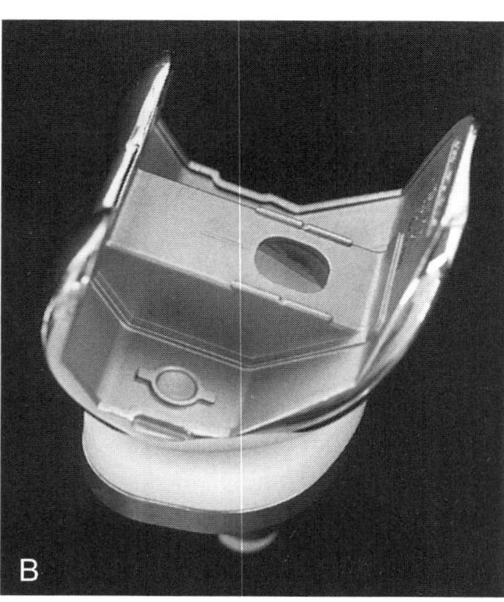

FIGURE 77.8 ➢ Press-Fit Condylar (Johnson & Johnson, Raynham, MA). *A*, Front view. *B*, Oblique view.

ther attempt to facilitate patellar tracking, the trochlear groove of the Genesis II femoral component was lateralized (Fig. 77.9).

An innovative design concept employed in the Genesis II is the design of the femoral component's posterior condyles. Most conventional knee system designs require external rotation of the femoral component to achieve a trapezoidal-shaped flexion gap. External rotation of the femoral cut results in more bone resected from the posterior medial femur than from the posterior lateral femur. The asymmetric femoral bone resections help compensate for the traditional asymmetric tibial resection that occurs with a perpendicular tibial cut. This traditional cut results in more bone resected from the lateral than from the medial tibial plateau. Thus, in the traditional method of component implantation, the bone cuts counterbalance each other and result in a rectangular flexion space. Traditional components are designed for this and have symmetric posterior femoral condyles.

As opposed to traditional symmetric medial and lateral posterior condyles, the Genesis II posteromedial femoral condyle is thinner than the posterolateral condyle. This is because the femoral component is designed to be implanted with a symmetric posterior femoral cut (no external rotation of the femoral component). The Genesis II designers hoped to minimize some of the theoretical limitations associated with traditional external femoral rotation. Limitations include unnecessary anterolateral femoral bone removal, rotational malalignment of the femoral and tibial components, and excessive medial patella tracking at high flexion angles. The Genesis II asymmetric posterior femoral condyles allow for a neutral cut. Conceptually, the flexion space remains balanced because the smaller medial posterior condyle on the Genesis II femoral component compensates for the smaller posterior medial flexion space. In addition, the femoral component's built-in lateralized trochlear groove compensates for the neutral cut in extension and theoretically aids patella tracking.

Stability of the Genesis II posterior cruciate substituting knee depends on both the component's articular geometry and the spine-cam interaction. The implants are designed to articulate freely through the first 60 degrees of flexion, with stability dependent on the surface geometry and soft-tissue balance. Spine-cam engagement occurs at approximately 60 to 70 degrees of knee flexion. Theoretically, the Genesis II spine-cam interaction is designed to minimize dislocations because at high flexion angles it has greater inherent stability, as defined by the dislocation safety factor,[11, 46] than does the Insall-Burstein design.

Maxim Knee

The Maxim Knee (Biomet, Warsaw, IN) is a PCL substituting prosthesis that was introduced in the 1990s. The developers of the Maxim Knee attempted to design components that minimized point loading and maximized component interchangeability (Fig. 77.10). In addition, the prosthesis was designed to maximize congruity at the femoral-tibial articulation but theoretically still allow 30 degrees of rotation.

The femoral component has a "unique condylar radius design" that comprises a 1.5-in radius and a 2-in center that is constant throughout all implant sizes. This design concept is patented with matching femoral and tibial radius in the medial-lateral plane. This allows for complete interchangeability among all tibial and femoral components. The Maxim prosthesis is anatomically designed with both right and left components.

The tibial tray has a built-in 3-degree posterior slope permitting a flat tibial bone cut. The tibial component's post is moved progressively posteriorly as the baseplate size increases. Conceptually, this modification of the spine-cam mechanism allows for a potential maximum flexion angle of approximately 130 degrees. Finally, the implant's instrumentation is posterior referencing to optimize the flexion space.

ADVANCE PS

Of the modern posterior cruciate substituting knee designs, the ADVANCE PS knee (Wright Medical, Arlington, TN) is one of the most similar to the Posterior Stabilized and IB II Posterior Stabilized implants. The ADVANCE knee is a nonanatomic, symmetric knee and thus does not come in rights and lefts (Fig. 77.11). It maintains conformity of the articular surfaces by exclusively mating the femoral component with only one polyethylene tibial insert. However, each polyethylene insert can seat into two tibial baseplates (regular and "plus" size). Functionally, this allows the femoral component to be paired with either the corresponding size tibial baseplate or one a size larger.

The spine-cam mechanism resembles the one used in the Posterior Stabilized and IB II Posterior Stabilized designs, with some modifications. The tibial spine was moved posteriorly and is designed to engage the cam at 70 degrees. The spine-cam interaction allows for theoretic maximum flexion of more than 120 degrees for all sizes, with only a 5-degree variation across all sizes. Cam-spine congruency was designed to more uniformly distribute forces to the polyethylene as compared to the IB II prosthesis. The spine-cam mechanism was adjusted to increase resistance to dislocation at high flexion angles compared with the IB II design.

The developers attempted to optimize patellar tracking by producing a femoral implant with a deepened and posteriorly extended trochlear groove. This modification was undertaken to maximize patellar contact at high flexion angles. The femoral component's anterior phalange was designed with a low profile to decrease retinacular soft-tissue tension, improve patella tracking, and decrease the need for lateral release.

OPTETRAK

Of the modern posterior cruciate substituting designs, the OPTETRAK (Exactech, Gainesville, FL) knee is the other design with the most similarity to the Posterior Stabilized and IB II Posterior Stabilized implants. The similarity between these designs is not unexpected be-

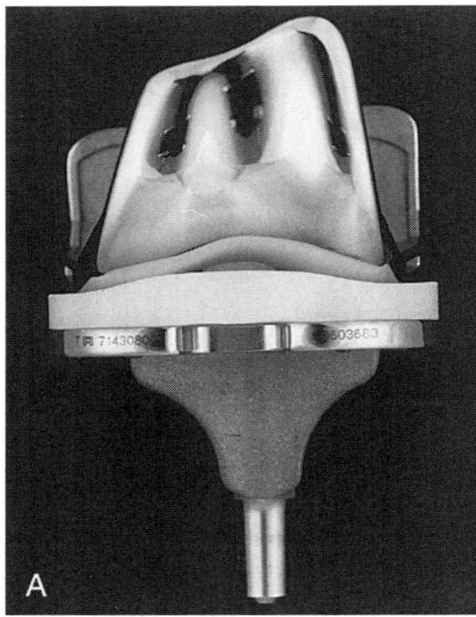

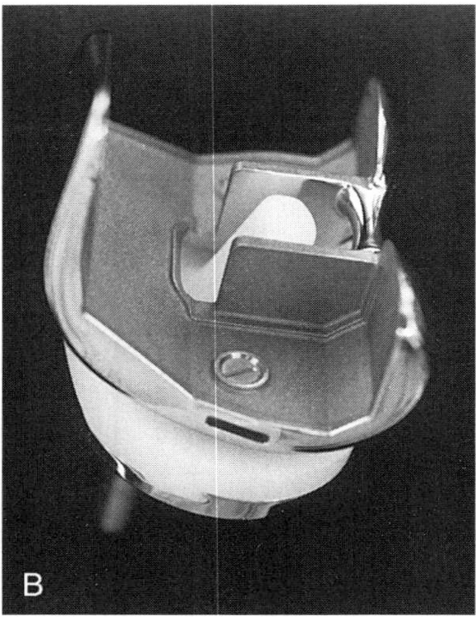

FIGURE 77.9 ➢ Genesis II (Smith & Nephew, Richards, Memphis, TN). *A,* Front view. *B,* Oblique view.

cause some of the same engineers were involved in the development of all these prostheses. Like the ADVANCE PS, the OPTETRAK is a nonanatomic, symmetric knee and does not come in rights and lefts (Fig. 77.12). Conformity of the articular surface is maintained by exclusively mating the femoral component with only one polyethylene tibial insert. However, each polyethylene insert can seat into multiple tibial baseplates. Effectively, this allows most femoral components to be paired with three different-size tibial baseplates.

The spine-cam mechanism resembles the one used in the Posterior Stabilized and IB II Posterior Stabilized designs, with some modifications. The cam box width was reduced to minimize bone resection, and the spine-cam articulation was curved to reduce contact stress on the tibial spine. Finally, the tibial spine height was designed to improve stability and minimize the risk of dislocation.

As with the ADVANCE PS knee, the designers attempted to optimize patellar tracking. This was accomplished by creating a femoral implant with a less prominent femoral flange and a deeper trochlear groove. Softening of the femoral component edges was undertaken to decrease retinacular soft-tissue tension, improve patella tracking, and decrease the need for lateral release.

ADVANTAGES OF POSTERIOR CRUCIATE LIGAMENT SUBSTITUTION

There are several advantages in implanting a PCL substituting prosthesis.

The surgical technique is easier to perform. Sacrifice of the cruciate ligament is a straightforward and reproducible surgical technique. The cruciate ligament can be sharply excised from its femoral attachment. Thus, ligamentous balancing is not complicated by the possible tethering effect of this posterior structure.

Minimal tibial resection is possible. Because there

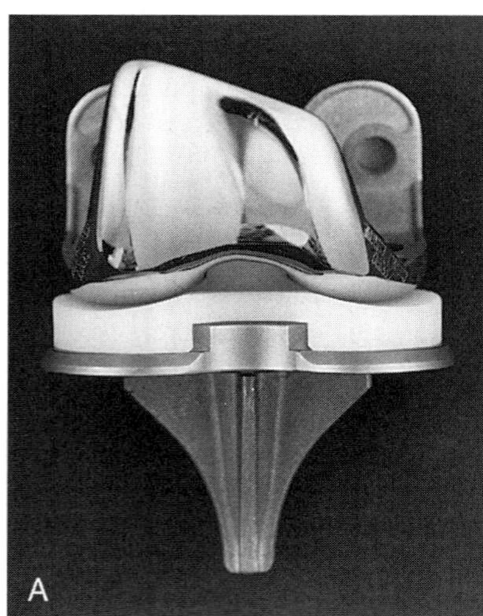

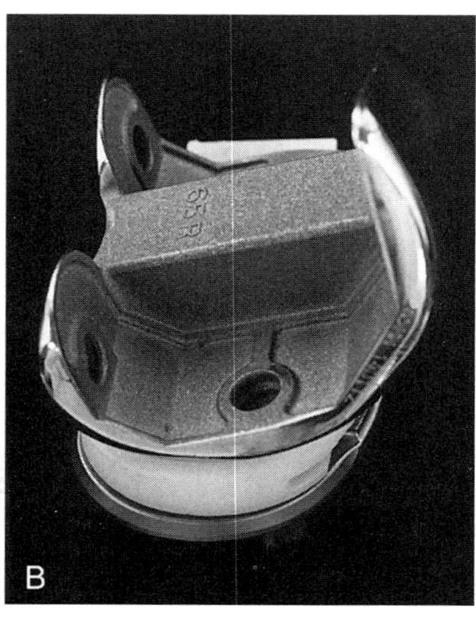

FIGURE 77.10 ➢ Maxim (Biomet, Warsaw, IN). *A,* Front view. *B,* Oblique view.

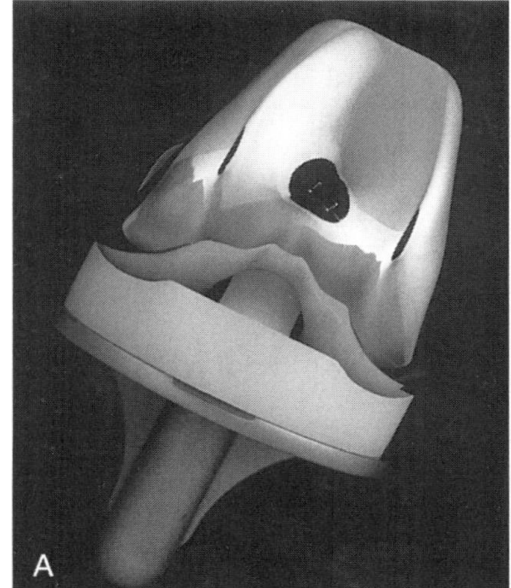

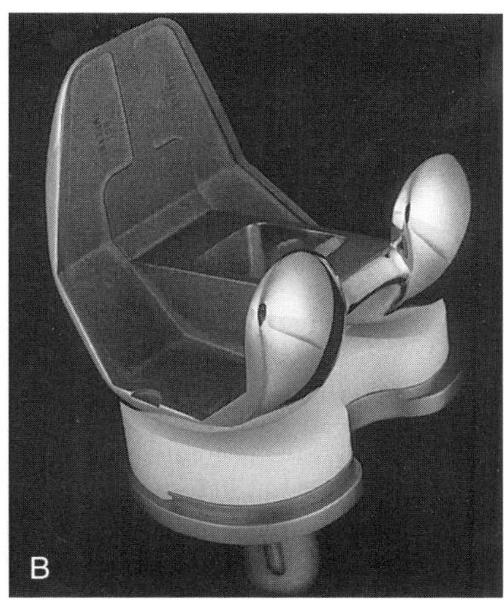

FIGURE 77.11 ➢ ADVANCE PS (Wright Medical, Arlington, TN). *A,* Front view. *B,* Oblique view.

is no need to balance the PCL, the surgeon is not restricted to a particular depth of tibial bone resection. It is thus possible to effect a minimal tibial resection. This allows placement of the tibial component in stronger host bone, as opposed to the weaker metaphyseal cancellous bone encountered with larger tibial resections.

Knees have more normal kinematics. Posterior cruciate substitution results in total knee arthroplasty with more normal knee kinematics. Fluoroscopic studies have shown that cruciate substituting knees have femoral rollback patterns that most closely resemble those of normal knees.[13, 85] Conversely, fluoroscopic analysis has shown cruciate retaining designs demonstrating erratic rollback patterns, with some cruciate retaining knee arthroplasties paradoxically rolling forward in flexion.

Polyethylene wear is decreased when a conforming articular surface is implanted. Because the long-term survival of total knee prostheses is now theoretically possible, the limiting effects of polyethylene wear have become an increasing concern.[34, 47, 67, 95, 98] PCL substitution allows the implantation of a conforming articular polyethylene surface. The increased contact area provided by the conforming surface acts to decrease the stress to which the plastic is subjected. Evidence of significant polyethylene failures in PCL retaining devices with less conforming tibial articular surfaces has already been reported.[9, 45, 60, 90]

The deformity can be corrected more easily. Cruciate ligament excision allows easier deformity correction in severely deformed knees.[48]

SURGICAL TECHNIQUE FOR NEXGEN LEGACY PROSTHESIS

The basic surgical technique for implanting posterior cruciate substituting prostheses has been well documented.[39, 43, 95] The basic objective is to produce a knee that has equal soft-tissue tension on the medial

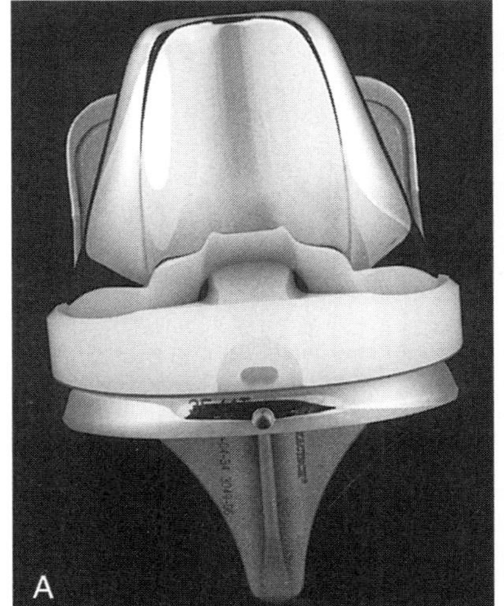

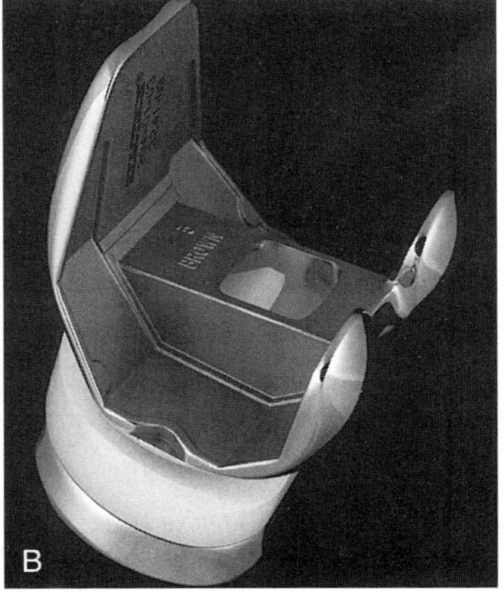

FIGURE 77.12 ➢ OPTETRAK (Exactech, Gainesville, FL). *A,* Front view. *B,* Oblique view.

and lateral sides in both flexion and extension. The axis of flexion is designed to be in the central portion of the knee and shared equally by both the medial and the lateral compartments.

The basic concepts behind knee arthroplasty with cruciate substitution remain virtually unchanged. However, the original Posterior Stabilized prosthesis was inserted with the use of a tenser (Fig. 77.13). This instrument applied tension to the collateral ligaments and helped align the knee. The tenser has been replaced with intramedullary instrumentation. However, it still remains imperative to pay strict attention to soft-tissue tension of the collateral ligaments.

The modern surgical technique begins with an anteroposterior radiograph of the involved extremity obtained on a long film (Fig. 77.14). This radiograph is used to ensure that there are no "surprises" that would preclude the use of intramedullary instruments, as well as to help determine the angle between the anatomic and mechanical axes of the knee (Fig. 77.15). The goal of surgery is to reproduce this angle intraoperatively. This is achieved by executing tibial and femoral bone cuts, which are parallel to each other while remaining perpendicular to the mechanical axis.

The knee is exposed with a straight anterior skin incision. A straight medial parapatellar capsular incision is used for the arthrotomy. The periosteum of the proximal medial tibia is raised in a continuous layer off the tibial bone. Laterally, a small cuff of periosteum is raised in continuity with the patellar ligament to provide some protection against tibial tubercle avulsion. The patellar is everted and the knee flexed.

With the knee in the flexed position, any remnants of the anterior cruciate ligament are carefully excised. The tibia is now subluxed anteriorly. It is sometimes necessary, especially on varus knees, to continue the release of the structures of the proximal medial aspect of the tibia, including a portion of the semimembranosus, to allow adequate tibial subluxation.

After adequate exposure has been achieved, attention is turned to the bone cuts. Depending on surgeon's preference, the bone cuts can commence with either the tibia or the femur. The order of the cuts is

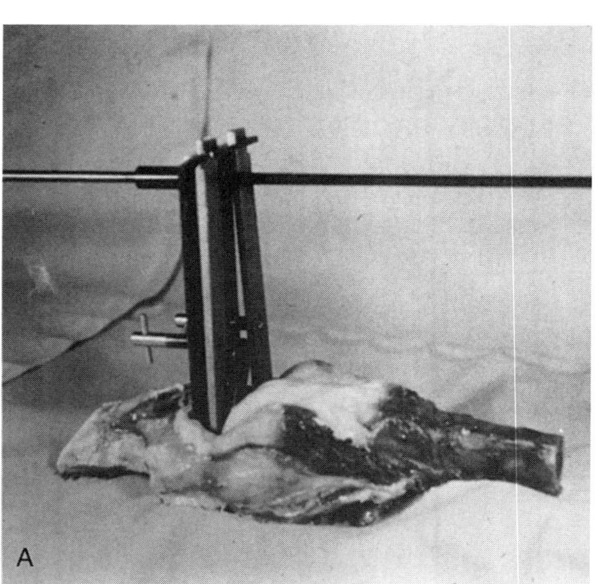

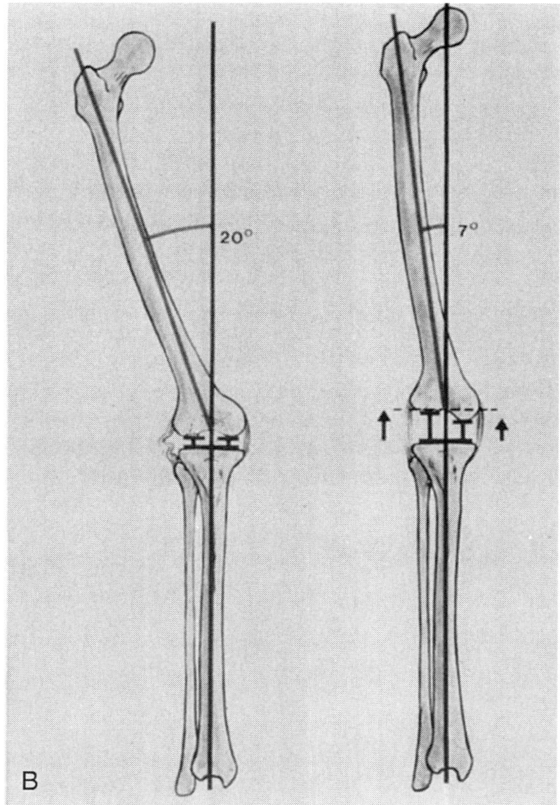

FIGURE 77.13 ➢ The tenser is an instrument used in ICLH arthroplasty of the knee, with which the presence or absence of soft-tissue contractures can be demonstrated at operation. Before insertion of this instrument, the cruciate ligaments are divided, and the tibial plateau is sectioned at right angles to the anatomic axis of the bone. *A,* The instrument is used in the extended knee to separate first one and then the other femoral condyle from the tibia, thereby tensing the medial and lateral soft tissues in turn. A bar passes through the tibial plate at right angles to the latter. The distal end of this bar must lie over the center of the ankle. *B,* The proximal end of the bar will lie over the hip when the soft tissues are tensed only when there is neither contracture nor elongation of these tissues on either side of the joint. Thus, by tensing the tissues and noting the relationship of the proximal end of the bar to the hip, the surgeon can judge the presence and magnitude of soft-tissue contracture or elongation.

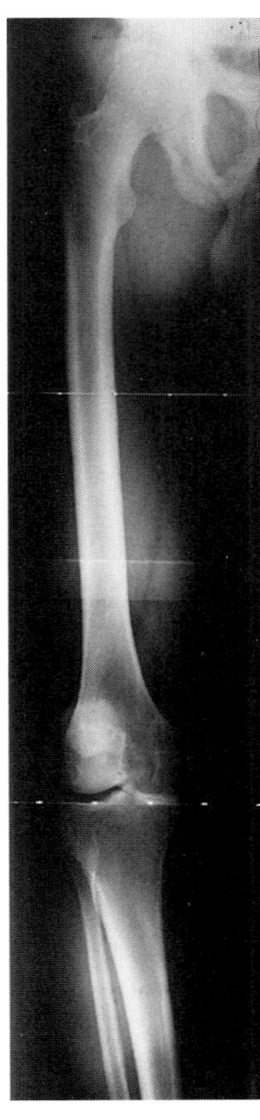

FIGURE 77.14 ➢ Standing anteroposterior long film of knee.

not as important as is adherence to the basic principles of knee arthroplasty in attempting to optimize alignment, balance, and stability.

The first step in cutting the distal femur is to make a small intramedullary hole. This hole should be slightly (3 to 5 mm) medial to the center of the femoral groove to allow easy drilling of the intramedullary portion of the femur. Because of concern regarding physiological changes associated with intramedullary instrumentation,[19] the hole is routinely vented. This is accomplished by overdrilling the hole (Fig. 77.16) with a step drill and using a fluted intramedullary rod. This helps reduce intramedullary pressure during the placement of subsequent intramedullary guides. The femoral alignment guide is then inserted into this intramedullary channel. It should be set at the proper valgus angle as determined by preoperative radiographs. The vast majority of knees fall between 6 and 8 degrees of anatomic valgus. On knees with a preoperative valgus alignment, the tendency is to set the guide at 5 degrees.

For most knees, the standard cutting block is attached to the intramedullary femoral alignment guide before its insertion in the femoral canal. However, for knees with a significant preoperative flexion deformity, it may be beneficial to resect an additional 3 mm of distal femoral bone. This can be accomplished by removal of the standard cutting block, which will allow for this additional distal bone resection. At this point, the femoral alignment guide is inserted into the intramedullary channel. Although this step does not set the final rotation of the femoral component, it is useful to place the guide carefully to achieve reasonable rotation of the distal femoral cut. The epicondylar axis can be used to aid in optimizing this rotation. Desired rotation is neutral to slight external rotation to ensure that the posterior femoral condylar cut will parallel the cut surface of the proximal tibia. In addition, slight external rotation will also enhance patella tracking (Fig. 77.17).

After the intramedullary alignment guide is placed within the femoral canal, the femoral cutting block is attached to the 0-degree distal placement guide. Optionally, a 3-degree distal placement guide can be employed to cut the distal femur in slight flexion and protect the anterior cortex from notching (Fig. 77.18). They are then both inserted into the intramedullary

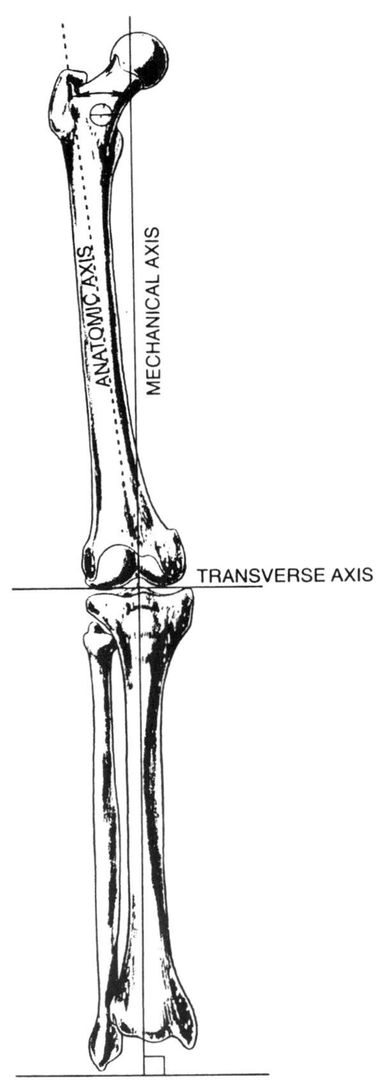

FIGURE 77.15 ➢ Calculation of angle between anatomic and mechanical axis.

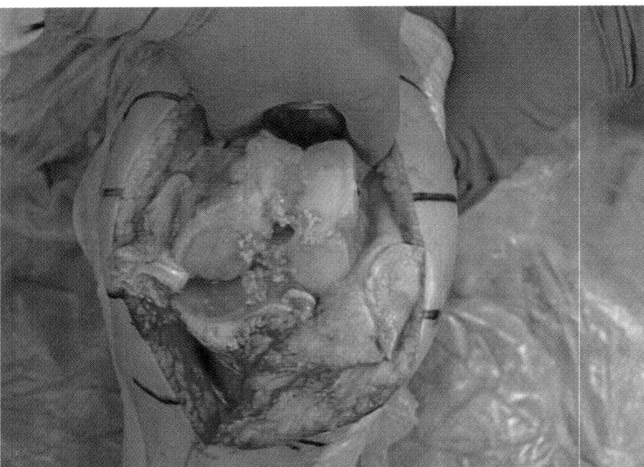

FIGURE 77.16 ➢ An entry hole for the intramedullary femoral rod is made with a step drill. The exact site of the entry hole is a few millimeters anterior to the insertion of the posterior cruciate ligament and situated centrally, medially, or laterally, depending on the preoperative templating on the long film radiograph.

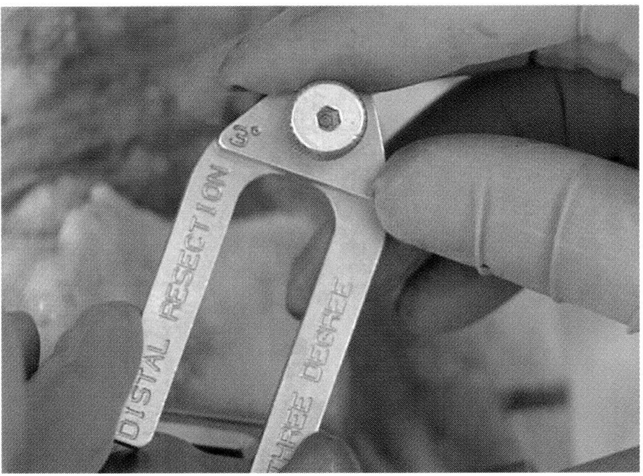

FIGURE 77.18 ➢ The 3-degree distal placement guide can be employed to cut the distal femur in slight flexion and to protect the anterior cortex from notching.

alignment guide until the cutting block rests on the anterior femoral cortex (Fig. 77.19). To further stabilize the guide, the anterior thumbscrew is hand tightened until it contacts the anterior femoral cortex. Two pins are placed in the femoral cutting block for the 0-mm resection. Finally, the distal placement guide is loosened, and a slap hammer is used to remove both the distal placement guide and the intramedullary femoral alignment guide. The distal femur is then cut through the cutting slot in the femoral cutting block.

The next step is sizing and establishing rotation of the femoral component. The anteroposterior (AP) sizing guide is used to determine which of the component sizes will give the best reconstructive result. Ideally, the body of the guide will contact the resected distal femur. Both of the guide's "feet" should rest on the posterior femoral condyles. The guide's anterior boom should contact the anterior cortex of the femur. The boom should be positioned so it does not contact abnormal bony anatomy, such as an osteophyte or a depression. The femoral size should then be read directly from the guide (Fig. 77.20). If the guide falls between sizes, the boom can be adjusted (normally by moving it medially) until the guide directly aligns with a size. This maneuver essentially allows the AP sizing guide to be used in a posterior referencing manner. By adjusting the boom, the surgeon can optimize the AP position of the implant using either strict anterior or posterior referencing or a combination of both techniques. Two headless holding pins are placed in the AP sizing guide's holes. These pins are used to estab-

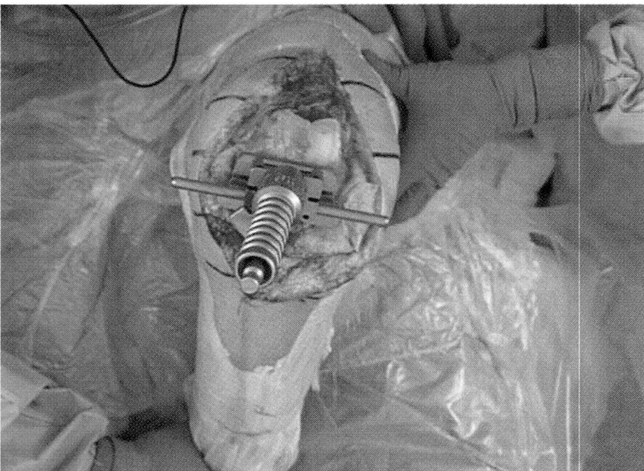

FIGURE 77.17 ➢ The femoral alignment guide is slightly externally rotated. Desired rotation is neutral to slight external rotation to ensure that the posterior femoral condylar cut parallels the cut surface of the proximal tibia. The epicondylar axis can be used to help optimize rotation.

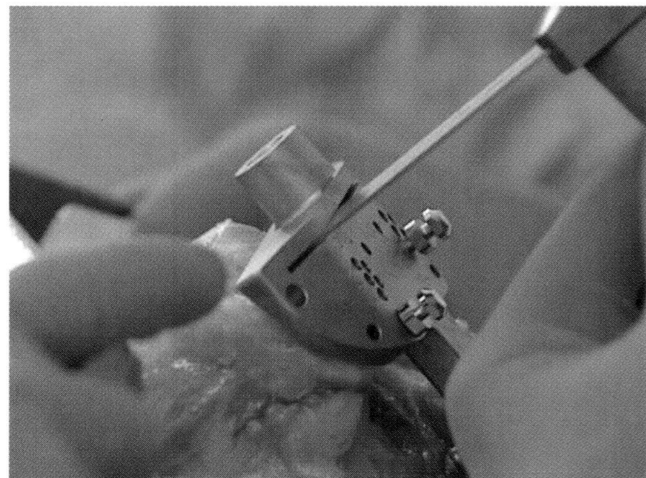

FIGURE 77.19 ➢ The cutting block rests on the anterior femoral cortex. Two pins are placed in the femoral cutting block to further stabilize the guide for the zero-millimeter resection.

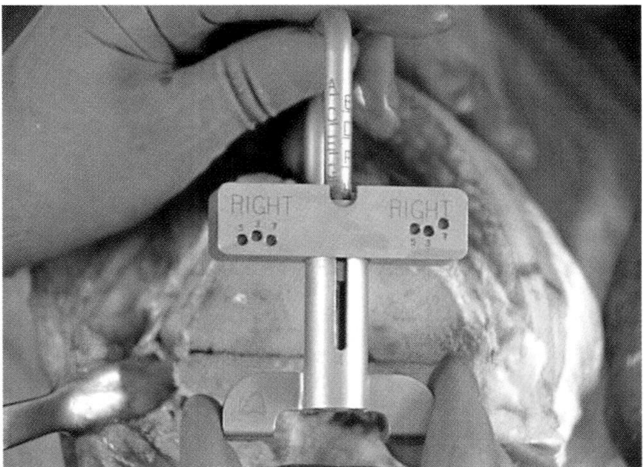

FIGURE 77.20 ➢ The anteroposterior sizing guide guide determines the size of the femoral component. The guide's "feet" should rest on the posterior femoral condyles, and the anterior boom should contact the anterior cortex of the femur. In general, the closer size is chosen, although if there is any question, the smaller size should be selected.

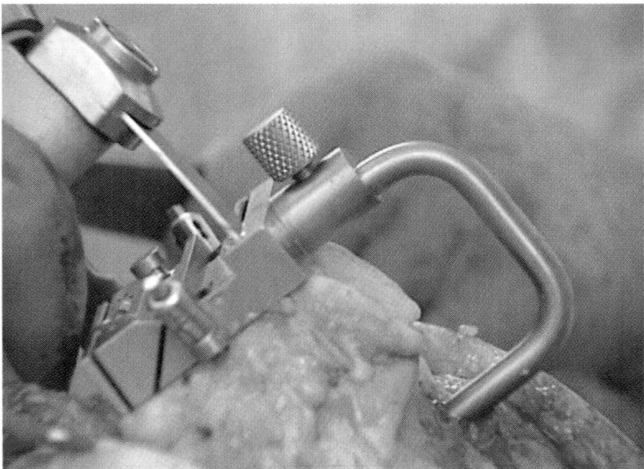

FIGURE 77.22 ➢ The slots are used to cut the posterior condyles, posterior chamfers, anterior condyles, and anterior chamfers. The femoral lug holes are drilled through the appropriate holes in the guide.

lish the AP position of the femoral component as well as to place it in 3 degrees of external rotation (referenced from the posterior condyles). The pins should be checked to ensure that they are parallel to the epicondylar axis. If the headless pins do not align with the epicondylar axis, the pins should be fine-tuned (commonly the lateral one is adjusted) so the pins and axis correspond.

At this point, the correct size 4-in-1 femoral finishing guide (as determined by the previous AP sizing guide) is placed onto the distal femur over the already-positioned headless pins (Fig. 77.21). The 4-in-1 femoral finishing guide is then pinned to the distal femur. The distal femur is then cut in a sequential order (Fig. 77.22). The most common cutting sequence is posterior condyles, posterior chamfers, anterior condyles, and anterior chamfers. Finally, the femoral lug holes are drilled through the appropriate holes in the guide.

The next step is to cut the proximal tibia. This is done with either an extramedullary or an intramedullary guide system, depending on the surgeon's preference and the knee anatomy (Fig. 77.23). The ideal cut is 90 degrees to the long axis of the tibia in the mediolateral plane, with a slight posterior slope in the AP plane. Resection of the PCL allows for a minimal tibial resection. Therefore, in the posterior cruciate substituting knee arthroplasty, the proximal tibial bone cut should ideally be only 5 to 9 mm below the articular surface of the normal side (Fig. 77.24). Excess tibial resection should be avoided because this will place the tibial component in a weaker cancellous bone bed.

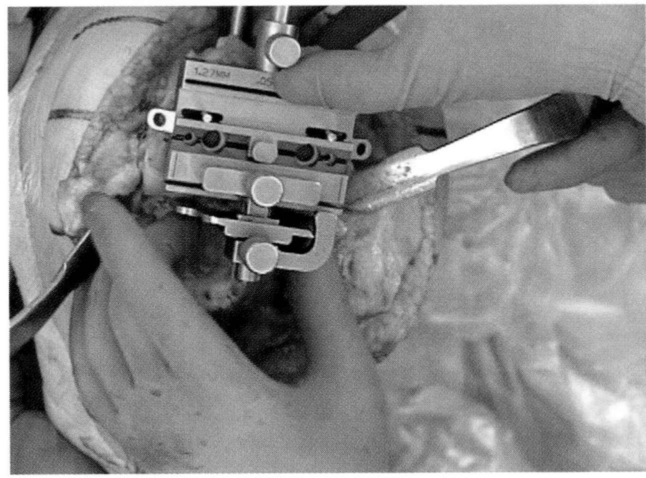

FIGURE 77.21 ➢ The 4-in-1 femoral finishing guide is pinned to the distal femur.

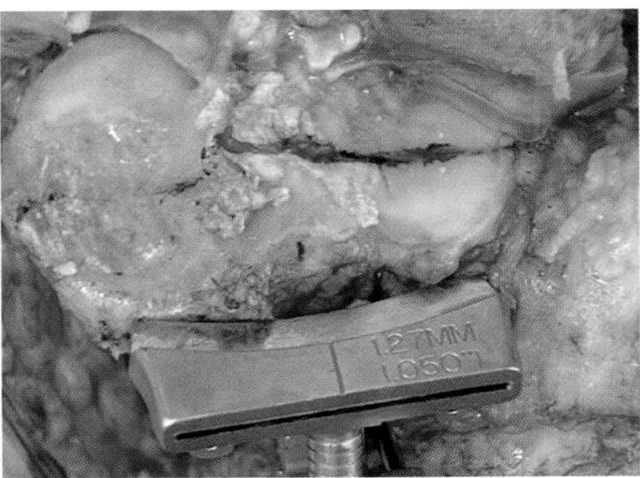

FIGURE 77.23 ➢ The tibial cutter is positioned to make a right-angle cut across the top of the tibia.

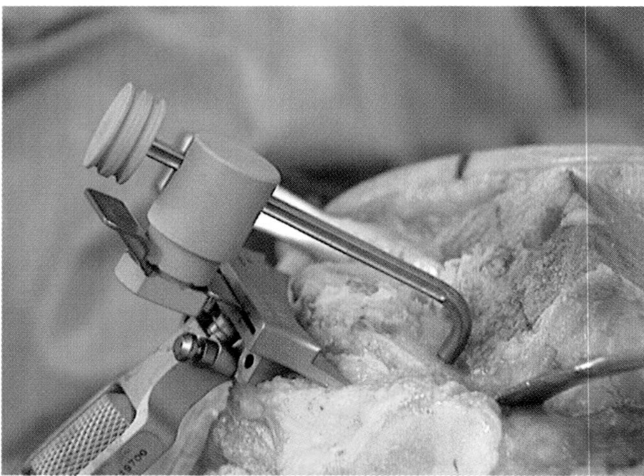

FIGURE 77.24 ➢ The depth of tibial resection should be between 5 and 9 mm, depending on the size of the patient and the desired thickness of the tibial component.

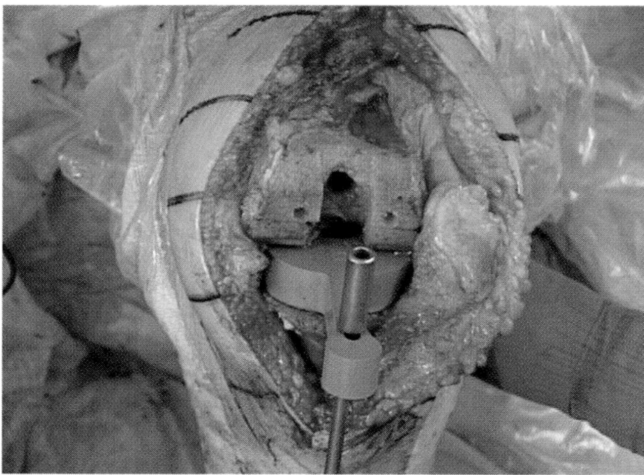

FIGURE 77.26 ➢ The flexion space is judged by selecting the thickest spacer that will fit comfortably between the posterior femur and the proximal tibia. The inclination of the tibial cut can be judged by passing an alignment rod through the spacer.

Laminar spreaders are then inserted, and the intercondylar notch is examined. The remainder of the anterior and posterior cruciate ligaments is excised directly off their femoral attachments (Fig. 77.25). Remnants of the medial and lateral meniscus are also removed. Great care is used with meniscal excision in the region of the deep medial collateral ligament because it is vulnerable to injury at this step in the procedure.

Next, the flexion and extension gaps are carefully measured and balanced. Various spacer blocks are used in the flexed knee until proper soft-tissue balance is achieved. An alignment rod is placed through the end of a block and checked to ensure that its distal end aligns with the center of the ankle (Fig. 77.26). Malalignment of the rod is corrected by adjusting the proximal tibial bone cut. With the correct size block inserted to adequately balance soft-tissue tension in flexion, the knee is brought into extension (Fig. 77.27). If it does not fully extend, the optional distal femoral resector is used to remove additional bone until full extension is achieved (Figs. 77.28). Bone from the distal femur can be resected back to the insertion of the collateral ligaments. It is imperative that additional femoral resection be undertaken if required to achieve full knee extension. The alternative choice of using a thinner tibial tray is unacceptable because it will promote laxity in flexion and increase the chance of knee dislocation.

At this point in the operative procedure, the collateral ligaments should be assessed to ensure correct knee balance. Two laminar spreaders are useful in this

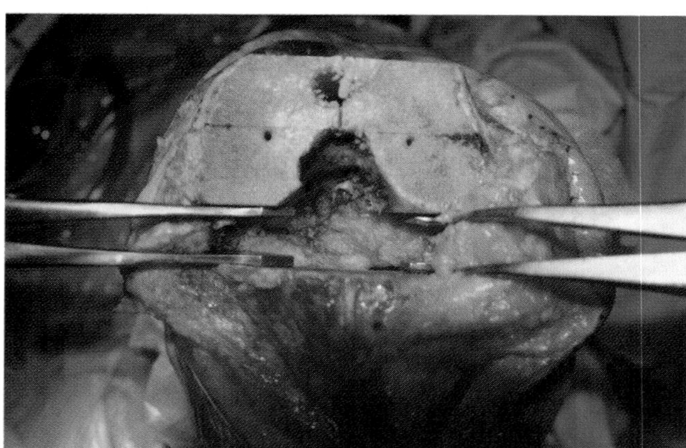

FIGURE 77.25 ➢ Laminar spreaders are inserted, and the intercondylar notch is examined. The cruciate ligaments and meniscal remnants are removed.

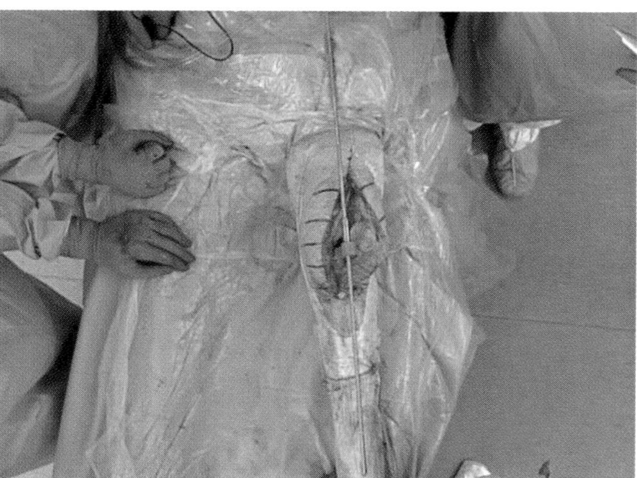

FIGURE 77.27 ➢ The knee is extended, using the same spacer that was used to estimate the flexion space. If the fit is excessively tight or if the knee will not come into full extension, a thinner spacer is selected to judge the amount of extra distal femoral resection required. (If necessary, minus spacers should be used.) Extremity alignment is also assessed.

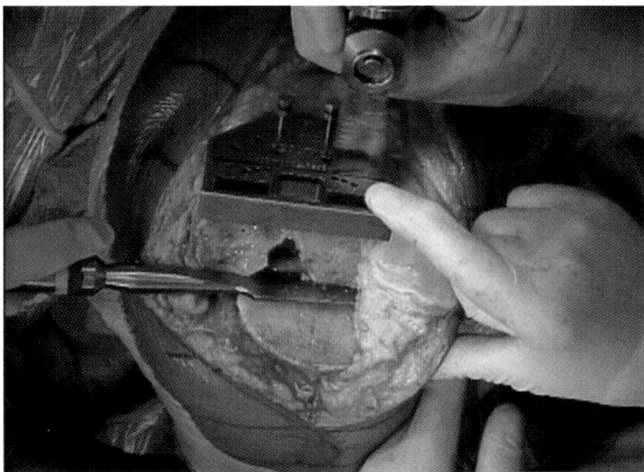

FIGURE 77.28 ➢ The distal femoral recutter is positioned by placing pins through appropriate holes (2, 3, or 5 mm of extra resection). The pins are placed flush against the previous distal femoral cut.

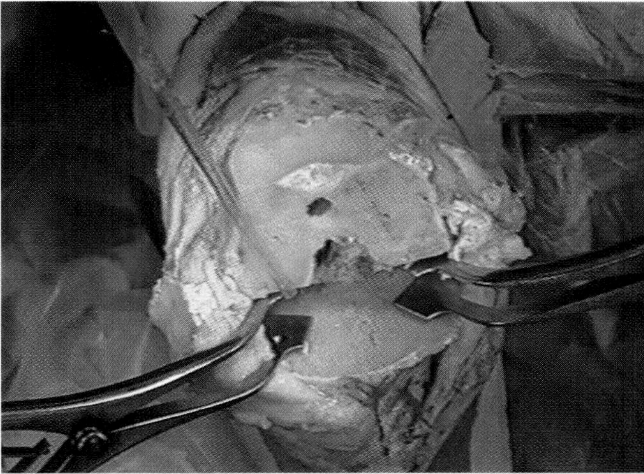

FIGURE 77.29 ➢ Medial and lateral laminar spreaders are useful in judging ligament balance.

assessment (Fig. 77.29). In general, there are three situations that the surgeon will face:

1. *Neutral knee:* Knees with a preoperative alignment between 0 and 10 degrees are usually relatively easy to balance. In most cases, no further releases are required other than those done initially to achieve adequate exposure.
2. *Varus knee:* In general, knees with a severe varus deformity require a more extensive medial release. An osteotome is used to subperiosteally strip the distal insertion of the superficial medial collateral ligament. If necessary, the deep portion of the medial collateral ligament and a portion of the semimembranosus insertion on the tibia are often released.
3. *Valgus knee:* Knees with greater than 10 degrees of anatomic valgus often require a release of the lateral structures. There are multiple methods for performing the ligamentous releases necessary for balancing valgus knees. Currently, a laminar spreader is used to tension the tight lateral structures. These are then sequentially released using multiple stab wounds in a "pie-crusting" manner. In addition, it is usually necessary to perform a lateral retinacular release in knees with a severe valgus deformity. This can also enhance ligamentous balance.

After the soft tissues are adequately balanced, the remaining bone cuts are completed. An intercondylar notch cutting guide is now used (Fig. 77.30). This guide should be lined up with the already-drilled femoral lug holes. This serves to correctly position the guide mediolaterally. In general, the guide should be centered or placed slightly lateral to the midpoint in the mediolateral plane. The intercondylar guide should not be placed medially. Lateral placement of the notch guide decreases the chances of intraoperative fracture of the medial femoral condyle and enhances patellar tracking. Bone from the intercondylar notch can be removed with a mill, oscillating saw, reciprocating saw, or osteotome. Optionally, if the chamfer cuts have not already been performed, the anterior and posterior chamfer cuts can also be made through slots in the intercondylar notch guide.

Attention is then returned to the tibia. The largest tibial template that fits on the resected proximal tibia without excessive overhang is chosen. The template is carefully placed to ensure correct tibial component rotation (Fig. 77.31). The template should align with the anterior aspect of the tibia, with the handle pointing slightly medial to the tubercle. Care is taken to place the template as posteriorly as possible. Correct rotation of the template, coupled with a posterior placement, often causes slight overhang in the poste-

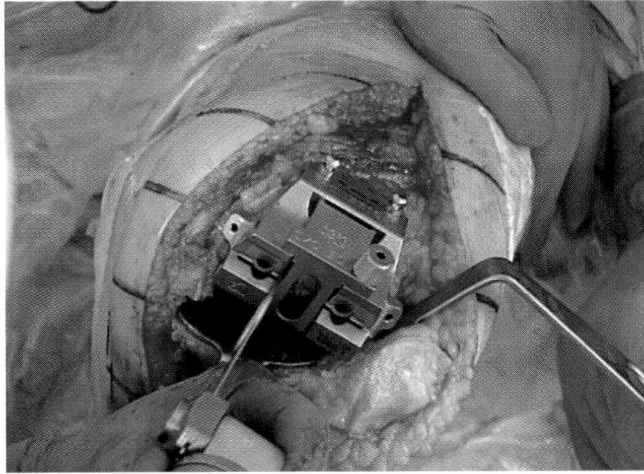

FIGURE 77.30 ➢ The intercondylar cutting guide applied on the distal femur. The guide should be lined up with the already-drilled femoral lug holes. In general, the guide should be centered or placed slightly lateral to the midpoint in the mediolateral plane.

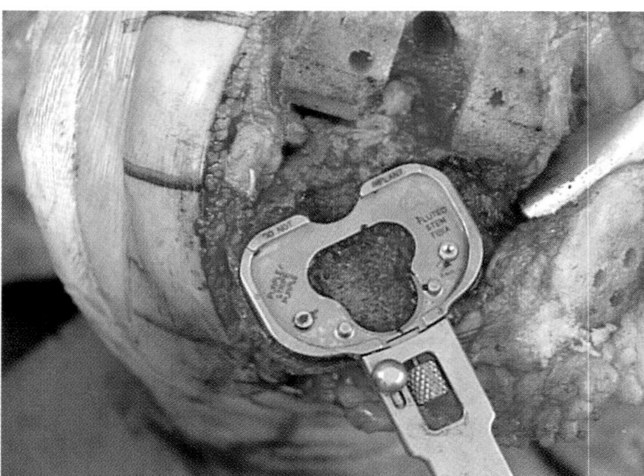

FIGURE 77.31 ➢ Tibial template in place. Note that correct position often results in slight overhang of the template in the posterior lateral corner.

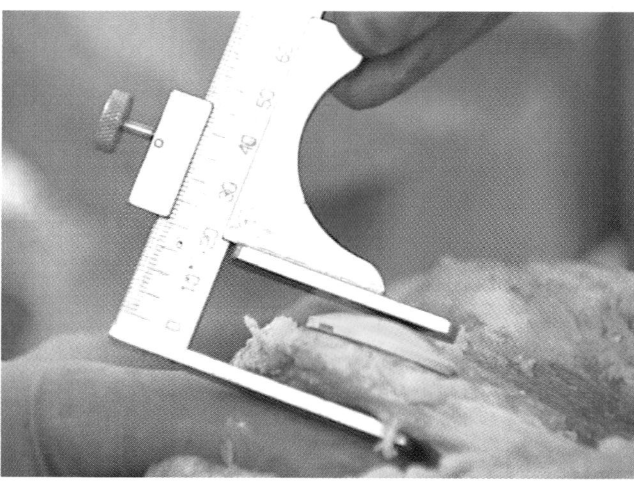

FIGURE 77.33 ➢ The patellar thickness with the patellar component inserted is measured with a caliper. The thickness of the patellar bone prosthesis composite should not exceed the preoperative measurement of patellar thickness.

rior lateral corner. After the template is positioned and pinned in place, the tibial stem hole is prepared. This is done by first drilling through the tibial drill guide and then completing tibial preparation with impaction of the appropriate-sized tibial broach.

Attention is finally turned to the patella. Synovium around the patella is carefully débrided to minimize the patella "clunk" syndrome.[35, 39] This is especially important in the region of the quadriceps tendon. The width of the patella is assessed with calipers (Fig. 77.32), and the aim is to restore the prosthesis-bone composite to the same width as the preresection patellar bone (Fig. 77.33). Traditionally, the bone is prepared with the use of an oscillating saw aligned with a patellar clamp or with a patellar reaming system (Fig. 77.34).

After preparation of the host patellar bone, the appropriate-size patellar implant is chosen. Fixation holes are then fashioned compatible with the prosthetic patellar design employed. A trial component is put in place and thickness once again assessed. This new thickness should be within 1 to 2 mm of the original width. If it is too thick, additional bone is removed.

At this point, trial components are put in place and a trial reduction is carried out. The knee is checked to ensure adequate balance of the collateral ligaments. The knee is inspected to ensure a full range of motion without excessive tightness or laxity.

Patella tracking is also examined (Fig. 77.35), making sure not to use towel clips or thumb pressure, to assess patellar stability and lateral retinacular tightness. If the patella is noted to sublux laterally, a retinacular release is performed. After the release is performed, the tracking of the patella is rechecked.

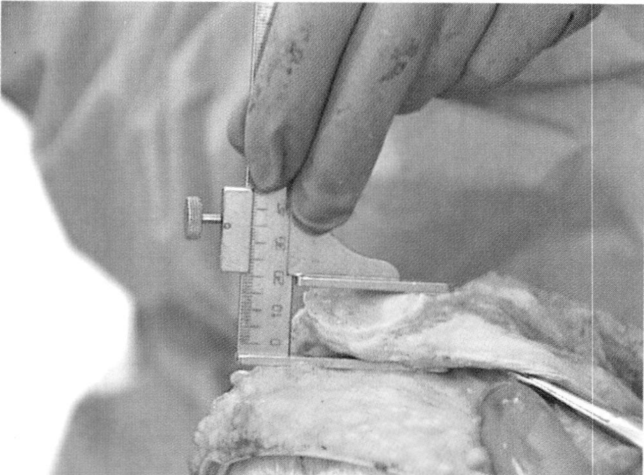

FIGURE 77.32 ➢ The thickness of the original patella is measured with a caliper. Note that the soft tissues surrounding the patella have been removed.

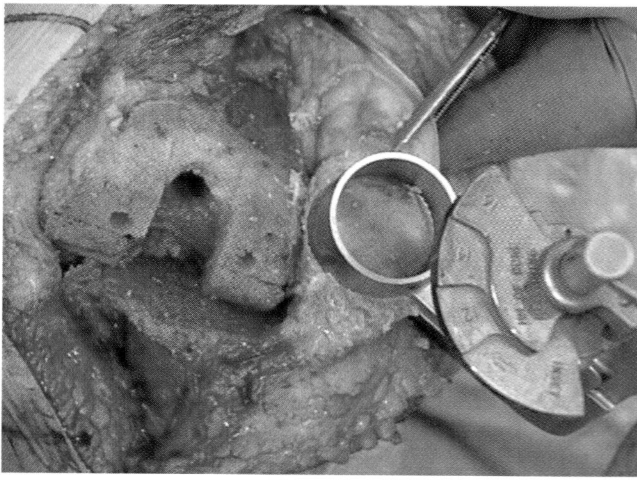

FIGURE 77.34 ➢ A patella reaming system for preparation of the patella.

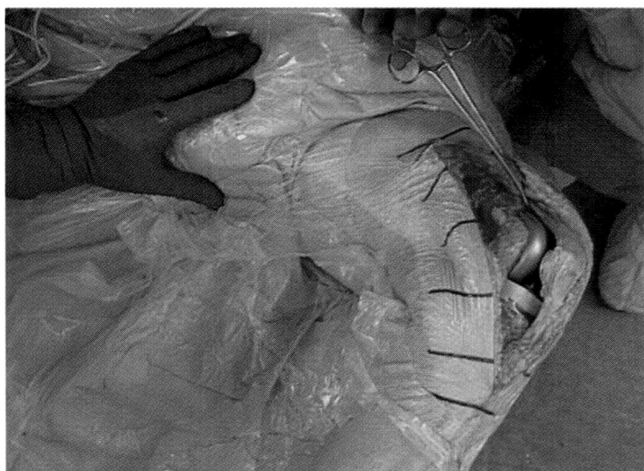

FIGURE 77.35 ➢ At the time of insertion of trial components, the patellar tracking should be observed. The medial edge of the patellar component should not lift away from the medial femoral runner.

The trial components are removed. If desired, the tourniquet can be taken down and bleeding vessels identified and coagulated before tourniquet reinflation. Conversely, if significant soft-tissue dissection has not been required, the tourniquet can be left inflated. The components are cemented in place in either one or two stages. The patellar and femoral components are cemented first. The tibial component is implanted last, using either the same batch or a second batch of cement. Pressure is maintained on the components as the cement polymerizes, and excess cement is trimmed away. The knee is then copiously irrigated and the arthrotomy carefully closed. After the skin is closed, a bulky dressing is applied, and the patient is transferred to the recovery room.

CLINICAL RESULTS OF POSTERIOR SUBSTITUTING DESIGNS

Insall-Burstein Posterior Stabilized Prosthesis

The "Insall Group" Experience

INITIAL REPORTS

There have been multiple reports on the clinical results achieved by the Insall Group at the HSS with the Posterior Stabilized prosthesis (Tables 77.2 and 77.3). Because this design has been in continuous use since the late 1970s, data are now available on numerous cases in which the prosthesis has been implanted for more than 10 years. Interestingly, the earliest report on this arthroplasty appeared in 1981. The title of this paper, "The Correction of Knee Alignment in 225 Consecutive Total Condylar Knee Replacements," was misleading because it actually dealt with the Posterior Stabilized arthroplasty.[33] At that time, the Posterior Stabilized prosthesis was being referred to as a generic type of "total condylar" replacement. This confusion was not repeated in later reports, where the term Posterior Stabilized was clearly used. The initial article, a report on 225 knees, emphasized the importance of soft-tissue releases in knee arthroplasty. Its main point was the excellent correction of clinical malalignment that could be achieved with this prosthesis even in cases of severe malalignment. The report did not otherwise mention clinical or functional results, beyond alluding to three clinical failures: One failure was due to sepsis, and the other two were secondary to tibial component loosening in obese patients undergoing revision procedures.

INTERMEDIATE FOLLOW-UP INSALL-BURSTEIN POSTERIOR STABILIZED KNEE (ALL-POLYETHYLENE TIBIAL COMPONENT)

In 1982, the first widely reviewed report on the Posterior Stabilized knee appeared.[40] It evaluated 118 arthroplasties that had been followed 2 to 4 years from their surgical procedure. The HSS knee-scoring system was used to evaluate these knees. At that period of follow-up, 88% achieved an excellent result; 9%, good or fair results; and 3%, poor results. The range of motion was noted to have significantly increased from 95 degrees preoperatively to 115 degrees postoperatively. The knees with the Posterior Stabilized prostheses rated higher than those from previous reports with the total condylar prosthesis: 76% of patients with a Posterior Stabilized arthroplasty achieved what the authors called "normal function," as compared with 22% who reached this level after a total condylar arthroplasty.

There was, however, a surprisingly high incidence of patellar complications (11%) seen with the original arthroplasty design. Stress fractures of 10 (8.4%) patellas were noted. The vast majority of these (8 of 10) were, nevertheless, asymptomatic and not associated with any quadriceps weakness or extensor lag. The fracture incidence was noted to be 13% in patellas replaced with a 38-mm prosthesis and 7.7% in knees with a 35-mm prosthesis, whereas no fractures were seen in knees with a 32-mm component. As has been pointed out by others,[74] it is not clear whether this distinction is related to the size of the prosthesis or to the size and weight of the patient. Two knees (1.7%) had symptomatic patellar subluxation requiring reoperation. One knee had a peripatellar nodule that required surgical excision because it impinged against the anterior margin of the intercondylar box of the femoral component. The authors mentioned two other instances of presumed patellar impingement, which were asymptomatic at the time of the initial report.

INTERMEDIATE FOLLOW-UP INSALL-BURSTEIN POSTERIOR STABILIZED KNEE (METAL-BACKED COMPONENT)

In part because of concern over the patellofemoral articulation, the Posterior Stabilized prosthesis was modified in the early 1980s. These changes included deepening the femoral component's patellar groove, as

TABLE 77.2 Comparison of HSS Knee Score

Institution	Ref.	Prosthesis	Tibial Composition	F/U (years)	No. of Knees	Excellent (%)	Good (%)	Fair (%)	Poor (%)
Insall Group									
1982	40	Original PS	All-polyethylene	2-4	118	88	8	1	3
1991	84	Original PS	All-polyethylene	9-12	194	61	26	6	7
1990	82	Modified PS	Metal-backed	2-6	257	87.5	11	1	0.5
1995	8	Modified PS	Metal-backed	10-11	101	73	23	0	4
Lenox Hill									
1986	74	Original PS	All-polyethylene	3-6	56	87	7	2	4
1988	75	Mixed group	All-polyethylene[a]	2-8	119	83	15	0	2
Florence, Italy, 1988	2	Mixed group[b]	Mixed group[c]	3-8	85	57	33	5	5
Case Western	21	Original PS	All-polyethylene	2.5-5	116	65	23	3	9
VA Columbia, MO	28	Mixed group	Metal-backed[d]	1-6	137	91	7	0.5	1.5
Mayo Clinic	30	Kinematic Stabilizer	Metal-backed	2-6	26	54	38	4	4
Lenox Hill	65	PFC	Modular metal-backed	4-6	125	82	10	2	5

[a] 17 of these knees were carbon reinforced polyethylene.
[b] (Original PS: 41 knees/modified PS: 44 knees.)
[c] (All-polyethylene: 52 knees/metal-backed: 33 knees.)
[d] (As best determined from paper.)
F/U = follow-up; HSS = The Hospital for Special Surgery; PS = posterior stabilized; VA = Veterans Administration.

TABLE 77.3 **PATELLOFEMORAL PROBLEMS**

Institution	Ref.	Prosthesis	Tibial Composition	F/U (years)	Fracture (%)	Impingement (%)		Miscellaneous (%)
						Mild	*Severe*	
Insall Group								
1982	40	Original PS	All-polyethylene	2-4	8		1	1.7[a]
1991	84	Original PS	All-polyethylene	9-12	4	11	1	
1990	82	Modified PS	Metal-backed	2-6	2	16	1	0.5[b]
1995	8	Modified PS	Metal-backed	10-11	6	10	5	
Lenox Hill								
1986	74	Original PS	All-polyethylene	3-6	5			
1988	75	Mixed group	All-polyethylene	2-8	5			
Florence, Italy 1988	1	Entire group		3-8	2.7			1.4[c]
		Original PS				10	15	
		Modified PS				12	3	
Case Western	21	Original PS	All-polyethylene	2.5-5	116	5	7	
VA Columbia, MO	28	Mixed group		1-6	0.7	21[d]	0	0.7[e]
Lenox Hill	65	PFC	Modular metal-backed	4-6	1	8		

[a] Two knees with subluxation.
[b] One knee with a loose patellar component.
[c] One knee with subluxation.
[d] This includes all knees with mild postoperative pain (26 knees) because the authors stated that most patients with mild pain had anterior knee pain.
[e] One knee with patellar dislocation.
F/U = follow-up; The HSS = Hospital for Special Surgery; PS = posterior stabilized; VA = Veterans Administration.

well as altering the shape of the patellar flange (see Fig. 77.3). The alterations gave the component a more rounded shape in the anterior region. The prosthesis was also made available in multiple sizes to achieve a more congruent match between prosthesis and knee. Finally, metal backing was added to the tibial baseplate to enhance load transfer.

We[82] reported on the results of this modified Posterior Stabilized prosthesis. We followed up 257 knees for 2 to 6 years: 225 knees (87.5%) were rated as excellent, 28 were good (11%), 3 were fair (1%), and 1 was poor (0.5%). The knee for which the result was poor had required a revision because of a delayed infection attributed to a urinary tract infection, but the result was rated excellent at 5 years' follow-up.

The function of the patellofemoral joint was analyzed separately for each knee in this report on the modified Posterior Stabilized arthroplasty. Clinical scores were recorded for flexed knee symptoms that were believed referable to the patellofemoral joint.[82] A grade of 0 meant no symptoms; grade 1, a mild ache anteriorly, perceived only with stair climbing; and grade 2, moderate or severe pain with rising from a chair or pain that limits stair climbing to a nonreciprocal gait. Knees with patellar fractures were graded with the same criteria, but the fracture was also noted: 213 knees (83%) were rated grade 0 and thus had no anterior knee complaints attributable to the patellofemoral joint, 41 knees (16%) were grade 1, and 3 knees (1%) were grade 2. There were four patellar fractures in the group, and one loose patellar component without evidence of fracture. In this study, patellofemoral symptoms were found to be statistically higher in moderately and severely obese patients as compared with their counterparts of more average weight. These results were quite encouraging, in that the overall excellent function of the arthroplasty was confirmed, whereas the incidence of severe patellofemoral problems was clearly reduced. The reduction in frequency of these problems serves as confirmation that the prosthesis after modifications functioned as theorized.

LONG-TERM FOLLOW-UP INSALL-BURSTEIN POSTERIOR STABILIZED KNEE (ALL-POLYETHYLENE TIBIAL COMPONENT)

In addition to the intermediate-term results discussed above for both the original and the modified Posterior Stabilized arthroplasty, long-term results are also available. The long-term report on the original prosthesis reviewed 289 Posterior Stabilized knees (218 patients) implanted with an all-polyethylene tibial tray at the HSS.[84] The diagnosis, as in other studies from the HSS, was predominantly osteoarthritis (73%) and female (73%).

Follow-up assessment was made between 9 and 12 years postarthroplasty for each patient. There were 180 intact knee prostheses in 139 patients available for analysis: 14 patients (14 knees) had undergone knee revision procedures (5 patients with bilateral arthroplasties had 1 knee that required revision and an intact implant on the contralateral side); 48 patients (66 knees) had died before their 9-year follow-up; and 22 patients (29 knees) were lost to follow-up before a 9-year evaluation.

Of the 194 knees studied, the average age at arthroplasty was 63 years. The results were rated excellent for 117 knees (61%), good for 51 knees (26%), fair for 12 knees (6%), and poor for 14 knees (7%). The average range of motion that the knees achieved postoperatively was 110 degrees (range, 40 to 135 degrees).

Because of failure of their index arthroplasty, 14 Posterior Stabilized knees were revised. Five of these arthroplasties were treated by removal of all components because of septic failure. In four of these, knee revisions were successfully performed after removal of the prosthesis, intravenous antibiotics, and reimplantation of the femoral and tibial components. One knee became reinfected 26 months after reimplantation and was treated by removal of the prosthesis and successful arthrodesis of the knee. It should be noted that two of these patients with septic loosening had acquired immunodeficiency syndrome (AIDS). Of the rest of the 14 revised knees, 3 had aseptic loosening of their femoral components, and the remaining 6 had aseptic loosening of the tibial component (Fig. 77.36). All of these were successfully revised in one-stage procedures to prostheses with stemmed components (see Fig. 77.36).

In this long-term study, there were fewer excellent results (61%) than the 88% seen in the original study of the Posterior Stabilized arthroplasty. The original report[40] dealt with a smaller group of patients with shorter (2 to 4 years) follow-up. One possible explanation for this difference is the increasing age of patients at their last follow-up (average age, 73 years) in long-term studies. Knee scores would be expected to decrease with advancing age and increasing frailty, and this phenomenon has indeed been reported by other authors.[7, 26]

The 180 intact prostheses were also rated with the new Knee Society scoring system (Table 77.4).[44] In this system, patients are stratified into one of three categories, depending on their overall musculoskeletal status. Separate scores are then obtained for each of the three groups, providing better assessment of the prosthetic knee function and of the overall functional status of individual patients. The average postoperative knee score was 92 points (range, 35 to 100 points), whereas the average function score was 66 points (range, 0 to 100 points). Figure 77.37 stratifies both the knee and the function scores by patient musculoskeletal status. Analysis of this newer rating system revealed that the knee scores were essentially the same in the three different patient categories. However, as might be expected, the function scores in each subgroup declined as medical infirmity increased. Therefore, the Posterior Stabilized implants yielded relatively uniform results with respect to motion and pain relief, but their functional results varied depending on overall musculoskeletal condition.

The function of the patellofemoral articulation was analyzed separately for each knee. As in the study on the modified Posterior Stabilized prosthesis, a specific clinical score was recorded for flexed knee symptoms

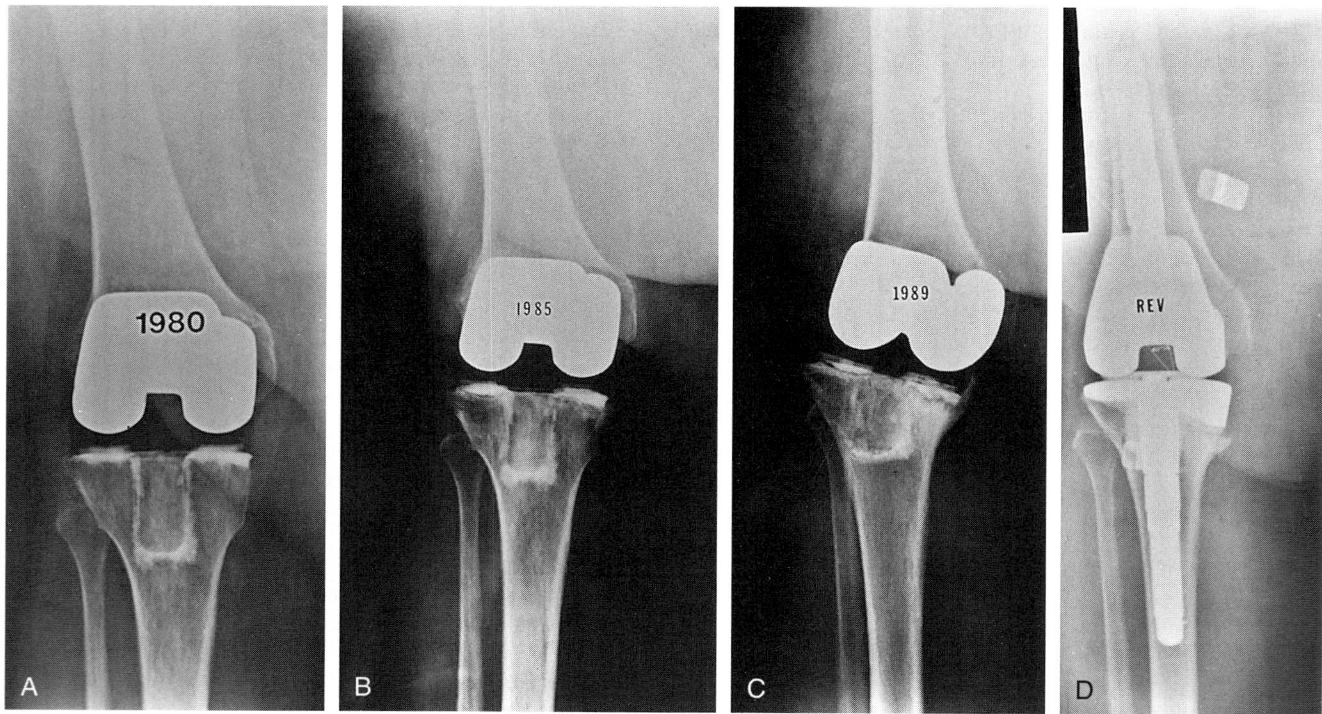

FIGURE 77.36 ➢ *A,* All-polyethylene posterior stabilized component implanted in an obese female in 1980. Note technically good results with satisfactory radiography. *B,* At 5 years, the tibial component is beginning to show signs of migration. *C,* At 9 years, the component has shown a shift in location and evidence of loosening. *D,* Revision to a constrained condylar implant with wedges and stems.

TABLE 77.4 **KNEE SOCIETY CLINICAL RATING SYSTEM**

Patient Category			
A. Unilateral or bilateral with opposite knee successfully replaced			
B. Unilateral with other knee symptomatic			
C. Multiple joints with arthritis or medical infirmity			
Knee Score	***Assigned Points***	***Function Score***	***Assigned Points***
Pain	0–50	Walking	0–50
Motion	0–25	Stairs	0–50
Stability	0–25		
Subtotal	0–100	*Subtotal*	0–100
Deductions	***Points Subtracted***	***Deductions***	***Points Subtracted***
Flexion contracture	0–15	Cane(s)/walker	0–20
Extension lag	0–15		
Malaignment	0–20		
Maximum knee score	100	*Maximum function score*	100

that were believed referable to the patellofemoral joint.[82] The clinical function of the patellofemoral articulation was grade 0 in 88%, grade 1 in 11%, and grade 2 in 1%. Thus, there was an overall incidence of anterior knee complaints believed referable to the patellofemoral joint in 12% of the knees. In these 180 knees, 7 patellar fractures (4%) were noted. All these knees were asymptomatic at long-term follow-up and received a patellar score of 0.

LONG-TERM FOLLOW-UP INSALL-BURSTEIN POSTERIOR STABILIZED KNEE (METAL-BACKED COMPONENT)

The most recent long-term study from the Insall Group reviewed the long-term results with the modified Posterior Stabilized prosthesis.[8] This is one of the first long-term reports in which a nonmodular, metal-backed tibial tray was implanted. The authors reported on 165 primary cemented Posterior Stabilized total knee arthroplasties (120 patients) that were implanted between 1981 and 1983. From the original cohort, 37 patients (53 knees) subsequently died, 5 patients (6 knees) were lost to follow-up, and 3 patients (3 knees) refused evaluation. One patient (two knees) was excluded from analysis because of severe debilitation. This left 101 knees (74 patients) available for analysis at a mean follow-up duration of 10 years and 8 months (range, 10 years to 11 years and 10 months). The mean age of the patients at the time of their initial arthroplasty was 64 years (range, 22 to 81 years). The demographics of this cohort, as in other studies from the Insall Group, were predominantly osteoarthritis (67%) and female (80%).

Of the 101 knees studied, the results were rated excellent for 74 knees (73%), good for 23 knees (23%), fair for 0 knees (0%), and poor for 4 knees (4%) (all of which were revised). The average range of motion that the knees achieved postoperatively was 110 degrees (range, 90 to 145 degrees). Four of the knees (all of which were rated a poor result) underwent revision procedures. None of the revisions were for early or late infections. In addition, no tibial component appeared radiographically or clinically loose. Two knees were revised because of aseptic loosening of the femoral component. One revision was undertaken because of recurrent hemarthrosis from an unknown cause. The final revision was secondary to a technical error that was corrected by implantation of a thicker tibial component.

This was also one of the first long-term studies in which radiographs were specifically scrutinized for evidence of polyethylene wear. This was done in response to the alarming reports of osteolysis seen with

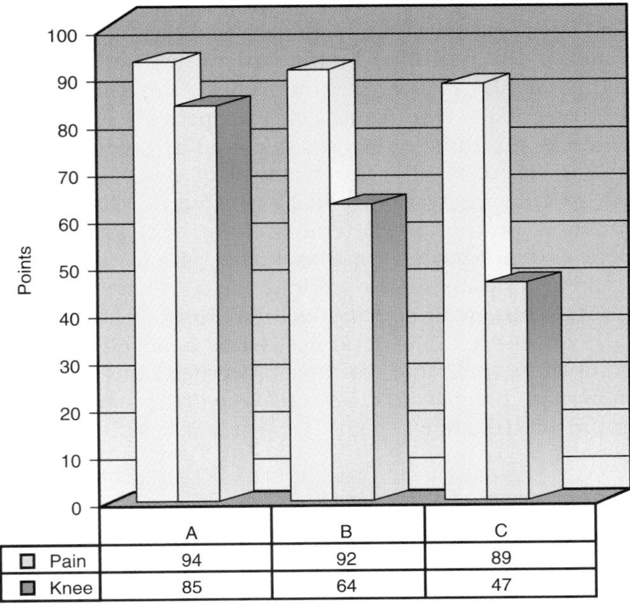

FIGURE 77.37 ➢ Knee Society scoring system. Results at 9- to 12-year follow-up for the original group of knees implanted with an all-polyethylene tibial component. Note that knee scores remain constant despite musculoskeletal categories. As expected, function scores decline with advancing medical and musculoskeletal morbidity.

some other designs at shorter follow-up intervals.[60, 71, 90] Analysis of the follow-up radiographs with the Insall-Burstein Posterior Stabilized prosthesis revealed no evidence of massive osteolysis, which the authors defined as lesions greater than 1 cm. However, they did note three knees that had focal, minimally progressive (a few millimeters) lesions at the latest follow-up. All three of these knees achieved excellent knee scores. Slight asymmetry (less than 1 mm) was noted in eight knees on the AP weightbearing films. No asymmetry was seen in the remaining 93 arthroplasties. Radiolucent lines were present in 11% of these knees (implanted with the nonmodular, metal-backed tibial component). This contrasts with the previous long-term study on the Insall-Burstein Posterior Stabilized prosthesis with an all-polyethylene tibial component, in which minor radiolucencies were seen in 49% of the knees.[84]

Analogous to the reports on the Insall-Burstein all-polyethylene tibial prosthesis,[84] this long-term study of the Insall-Burstein prosthesis[8] with a metal-backed tibial tray found fewer excellent results (73%) than the 87.5% seen in the previous report with intermediate follow-up (2 to 6 years).[82] As discussed earlier, one possible explanation for this difference is increasing patient age with longer follow-up (average age, 74 years). As already stated, knee scores would be expected to decline with increasing age.[7, 26]

As in the previous long-term report on the Insall-Burstein prosthesis,[84] these knees were also analyzed with the Knee Society scoring system (see Table 77.2).[44] When the four knees that underwent revision are excluded, the average knee score was 92 (range, 67 to 100 points) and the average function score was 71 points (range, 0 to 100 points) at latest follow-up. The knee and function scores are graphically shown in Figure 77.38, stratified by the patient's musculoskeletal status. Similar to the previous report, the knee scores are essentially the same in the patient categories, whereas the function scores declined as medical debility increased. Finally, the function of the patellofemoral articulation was specifically analyzed. The clinical function of the patellofemoral joint was grade 0 in 85% (asymptomatic) of the knees, grade 1 in 10% (mild symptoms), and grade 2 in 5% (severe symptoms). Thus, with specific examination of patellofemoral symptoms, 15% of knees were believed to have complaints referable to the patellofemoral joint. Finally, six patellar fractures (6%) were noted in this group of 101 knees.

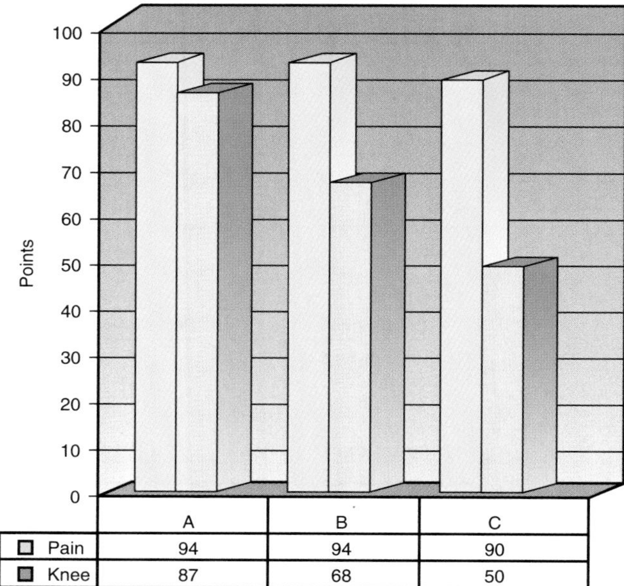

FIGURE 77.38 ➢ Knee Society scoring system. Results at 10- to 11-year follow-up for the group of knees implanted with a metal-backed tibial component. These results are similar to those with the all-polyethylene tibial component. Once again, the knee scores remain constant and the function scores decline with advancing medical and musculoskeletal morbidity.

Experiences of Other Institutions

An extensive experience with the Posterior Stabilized prosthesis has been reported from Lenox Hill Hospital in New York, NY. Early reports from Norman Scott and associates[73, 74] appeared in 1982 and 1986. Although the 1982 report was clearly preliminary, the paper from 1986 detailed results on 56 of the original Posterior Stabilized knees followed for 3 to 6 years. The average age (68 years) and predominance of osteoarthritis (79%) were consistent with the patient population seen in other reports. There was, however, a smaller percentage of women (53%) in this study. The HSS knee score yielded 87% excellent, 7% good, 2% fair, and 4% poor results. Patellar problems remained a major concern with fractures in three cases (5%). As in the HSS study, these were associated with larger patellar prosthetic sizes, because all fractures were in knees implanted with a 41-mm patellar dome.

In a further report in 1988, Scott and colleagues[75] reported their results with a series of knees, including both the original and the modified versions of the Insall-Burstein Posterior Stabilized prosthesis. They reported on 119 knees with a follow-up ranging from 2 to 8 years (average follow-up, 5 years). Patients averaged 67 years of age, and the diagnosis was osteoarthritis in 74%. The average postoperative range of motion achieved was 107 degrees. With the use of the HSS knee score, 83% of the knees were rated excellent, 15% good, none fair, and 2% poor. The authors stratified their results by preoperative diagnosis and found that the patients with osteoarthritis had statistically better results than did patients who had rheumatoid arthritis. In addition, they also showed statistically better outcomes with preoperative varus alignment than did those knees that had preoperative valgus alignment. Survivorship analysis showed 93% intact satisfactory prostheses at 8 years. The authors also analyzed their results over time. They had 98% good or excellent results at 2-year follow-up in 119 knees. Another group had 96% good or excellent results for 41 knees followed up to 6 years.

Aglietti and colleagues[1, 2] reviewed their results with the Posterior Stabilized prosthesis implanted at the University of Florence in two similar studies published in 1988. The larger series[2] reviewed 85 knees that had been replaced with either the original or the modified Posterior Stabilized knee. The average age of patients in their series was 66.5 years. The patient population, as in the studies from the HSS, was predominantly osteoarthritic (72%). Follow-up averaged 5 years (range, 3 to 8 years): 49 knees (57%) had excellent, 28 knees (33%) had good, 4 knees (5%) had fair, and 4 knees (5%) had poor results.

Aglietti's[1] second study on 73 knees paid specific attention to complaints originating from the patellofemoral articulation. Joints were examined for catching and locking ("impingement"), arising at 30 to 40 degrees of flexion as the knee was extended; 15 (21%) of the joints showed evidence of impingement. In only one knee were the symptoms severe enough to require surgical intervention; this knee had a peripatellar synovial frond that was catching on the anterior edge of the femoral component's intercondylar box. Interestingly, the incidence of overall impingement symptoms decreased from 25% with the original design to 15% in knees implanted with the modified prosthesis. The authors felt that locking, which they classified as the most severe problem, decreased from 15% to 3% after the alterations. Only two patellar fractures were noted (one after a motor vehicle accident), and both were asymptomatic at the time of last follow-up.

Figgie and coworkers[21] studied the results of tibiopatellofemoral location on knee function with the original Posterior Stabilized prosthesis. This report dealt with 116 implants followed for 2.5 to 5 years. Average age at arthroplasty was 65 years. Their patient population was fairly typical, with females (70%) and osteoarthritis (70%) predominant. The knees were assessed with a modified Mayo Clinic knee score, as opposed to the more traditional HSS scoring system. Evaluation with this rating system yielded 65% excellent, 23% good, 3% fair, and 9% poor results. The arc of motion averaged 101 degrees. Patellofemoral symptoms were present in 12% of knees, with 7% manifesting severe, persistent symptoms requiring revision procedures. The authors critically analyzed the tibiopatellofemoral mechanical axis and identified a "neutral range" for surgical variables that would maximize functional results of the prosthesis. These included a posterior position of the prosthesis in the AP plane, a joint line change of less than 8 mm, and a patellar height of 10 to 30 mm. Of the 41 knees that fell within this "neutral range," 95% were rated excellent, and 5% were good. No knee within this so-called neutral range had symptoms attributed to the patellofemoral articulation. Although these results are compelling, the concept of a neutral range has not been confirmed in other reports.[20]

Lombardi and colleagues[53] reported on the Columbus, OH experience of Thomas Mallory with the Posterior Stabilized arthroplasty. This study reported on 47 knees with 85% survival at 6 years. As in multiple other studies, their patient population averaged 67 years of age and was predominantly female (71%) and osteoarthritic (83%). The HSS knee score averaged 85, but results were not stratified into the four categories. The average arc of flexion was 97 degrees. There were four failures in their study: one deep infection, two aseptic component loosenings, and one stiff, chronically painful knee. No mention was made of patellar fractures.

Groh and colleagues[28] reported on their results of 137 Insall-Burstein Posterior Stabilized knee arthroplasties performed in a Veterans Hospital. The average age at time of arthroplasty was 61 years. Follow-up was from 1 to 6 years, with an average of 29 months. The authors reported 124 excellent results (91%), 11 good results (7%), 1 fair result, and 3 poor results. A revision procedure was required in three knees: one was for a deep infection, and there were two aseptic tibial loosenings, both of which occurred in obese patients. The authors carefully analyzed pain complaints in these arthroplasties, and found 19% of knees had mild pain, most often patellar in origin; 2% had moderate pain; and no knees had severe pain. They observed one patellar fracture (1%) and one asymptomatic (1%) lateral patellar dislocation. Of particular interest from this study is that the overall excellent results were achieved in a Veterans Hospital setting.

Patel et al[62] reported on 157 total knee arthroplasties (118 patients) performed at the Westminister Hospital in England with the Insall-Burstein Posterior Stabilized prostheses. The average follow-up was 3.5 years (range, 2 to 7 years). The mean age at arthroplasty was 69 years (range, 47 to 85 years). The "BASK" knee function assessment was used to evaluate the knees. There were 86% with excellent or good results, 10% with fair results, and 4% with poor results using this system for evaluation. The authors felt that 90% of the patients were pleased or satisfied with their functional result. They concluded that this was a safe, reliable, and versatile prosthesis.

The results of these institutional experiences are summarized in Tables 77.2 and 77.3.

Specific Conditions

There have been several articles demonstrating the application of the Posterior Stabilized prosthesis to various knee conditions. In a small series of patients with Charcot's arthropathy and Charcot-like joints, the Posterior Stabilized prosthesis yielded all excellent and good results at an average follow-up of 3 years.[78] In these knees, severe bone loss was corrected by either bone grafting or custom augmentation of the prosthesis along with ligamentous balancing. In another small series of patients, the Posterior Stabilized prosthesis was used in a majority of patients with Parkinson's disease.[94] These knees also produced excellent and good results at an average follow-up of 4 years. In knees with post-traumatic arthritis,[102] the Posterior Stabilized prosthesis had 90% good and excellent results at an average follow-up of 4 years. The prosthesis also yielded highly satisfactory results when implanted in patients with diabetes,[17] psoriasis,[80] obesity,[82] and osteonecrosis.[79]

PATIENTS YOUNGER THAN 55 YEARS

Of particular interest are the knee arthroplasties implanted in a younger group of patients. The Posterior Stabilized components were used in a majority of knees with gonarthrosis in patients younger than 55 years at the time of their index arthroplasty.[81] In this study, 68 cemented knee arthroplasties were followed up for an average of 6 years postoperatively: 81% of the knees were rated excellent and 19% were rated fair at the time of follow-up. The results in this study were comparable to those in published reports on older age groups. In addition, no deterioration in results was noted over time, which contrasts sharply with the functional decline seen after high tibial osteotomy in multiple studies.[31, 32, 42]

A second follow-up study was performed on a larger cohort of young patients who underwent total knee arthroplasties.[14] This study represented the combined experiences of Drs. Scott and Insall. Only patients with diagnosis of osteoarthritis or post-traumatic osteoarthritis were included in this report. At the time of surgery, the average age of patients in this group was 51 years (range, 22 to 55 years). There were 108 knees (84 patients) analyzed with a mean follow-up of 8 years (range, 3 to 18 years). All but one of the prostheses were posterior substituting designs. Fifteen components had an all-polyethylene tibial component, with the remainder having metal backing of the tibial tray.

At latest follow-up, there were 103 unrevised knees. All these knees were rated as good or excellent according to the HSS score. All but two patients had improvement in the activity score of Tegner and Lysholm[86] postoperatively. Prosthetic survival was 94% at 18 years, with endpoint-defined femoral or tibial component revision. When the endpoint definition was expanded to include patellar revision and spacer exchange, the survival rate was 87% at 18 years.

The authors concluded that insertion of a cemented posterior cruciate substituting knee replacement was an acceptable option for younger patients with osteoarthritis who have not responded to nonoperative treatment. However, they cautioned that longer follow-up could alter their conclusion. In addition, they stressed that total knee arthroplasty in young patients should be done with discretion and that impacting activity should be avoided.

PATIENTS OLDER THAN 80 YEARS

Knee arthroplasty results in elderly patients were reviewed in a separate study in which the majority of implants (71%) were Posterior Stabilized.[52] For an average of 4.5 years, 98 patients who were 80 years or older at the time of surgery (average age, 82 years) were followed up. Additionally, the patients were divided into two groups based on their tibial component design: 38 all-polyethylene tibial components and 60 metal-backed tibial components. The results were 62% excellent, 31% good, 2% fair, and 5% poor. Stratifying the results by component composition revealed 97% survival for both types of tibial trays. These results were obtained at 12 years for the all-polyethylene components and at 8 years for the metal-backed prosthesis.

In this report, total knee arthroplasty proved to be a reliable and durable procedure in the treatment of knee arthritis in the elderly. Because elderly patients are generally less active, it was generally thought that they may represent a special subset of people that place less stress on their prosthesis. Thus, they may be at less risk for mechanical failure, making an all-polyethylene tibial component a viable option in the thin, sedentary, elderly patient.

VALGUS KNEES

One study evaluated the results of arthroplasty in knees with a preoperative valgus alignment in which the predominant prosthesis implanted was Posterior Stabilized.[83] Because varus knees predominate in the population, most studies have tended to focus on this type of alignment.[8, 26, 37, 40, 41, 44, 92, 93, 97]

In reality, the technique for implanting a knee arthroplasty in a valgus leg differs significantly from that used with a varus orientation. Specifically, the ligamentous releases involved are different, as are the bone defects that are present.[37] Valgus knees tend to have a significant erosion of the lateral femoral condyle, in contrast to varus knees, in which deformity is more likely found in the tibia. These different bone deformities may make achievement of correct external rotation of the femoral component more difficult. Although difficult to quantify, it was felt that valgus knees represented a greater challenge to the surgeon in terms of the intraoperative balancing required. This was believed to be a function of the greater difficulty in achieving ligamentous equilibrium, as well as the relative rarity of valgus knees.

The overall results achieved in this subgroup of valgus knees were satisfactory; 91% achieved an excellent or good result at 4.5 years follow-up. However, the number of excellent results represented only 71% of the overall total, which sharply contrasts with the better outcomes achieved in other studies of patients implanted with the Posterior Stabilized prosthesis.

A second study by Aglietti reported on his experience with the Insall-Burstein prosthesis in knees with a preoperative valgus deformity greater than 10 degrees.[3] Fifty-one knees were available for review at an average follow-up of 6 years. The results, according to the Knee Society rating system, were excellent in 53%, good in 39%, fair in 6%, and poor in 2%. A lateral retinacular release was required in 49% of the knees. The mechanical axis was within 5 degrees of neutral in 88% of knees. The authors reported their cumulative success as 95% at 10 years. However, as in the report from the Insall Group,[83] the clinical function results achieved by Aglietti in these patients was not as good as the outcomes reported in other studies with this prosthesis.[1, 2]

One option to consider in knees with severe valgus deformity is implantation of either a constrained knee arthroplasty or modular components that allow for an "easy" conversion to a constrained knee arthroplasty. Constrained components have inherent stability in both the anteroposterior and the mediolateral planes. Thus, they can be especially useful in severe valgus knees because of the increased incidence of collateral ligament insufficiency and the difficulty in achieving acceptable ligamentous balance in these situations. Therefore, in severe valgus knees, one protocol to consider is implantation of a constrained femoral component. These components interface either with a constrained tibial insert or, if balance is believed to be satisfactory, with a standard tibial component. With this construct, if instability becomes a problem at a later date, it is possible to exchange the tibial inserts without proceeding with a full knee revision.

Peroneal-nerve palsy remains a significant worry in a valgus knee and was seen postoperatively in 3% of patients in one series.[83] Patients are now placed in a continuous passive motion machine in the recovery room. This acts to place the knee in a flexed position, which tends to decrease stress on the nerve and may lower the incidence of this complication.

Kinematic Stabilizer Prosthesis

There have been few reports on the results of posterior substituting designs other than the Insall-Burstein Posterior Stabilized prothesis. In 1988, Hanssen and Rand[30] reported on the Mayo Clinic experience with the Kinematic Stabilizer prosthesis. Both the Insall-Burstein and Kinematic Stabilizer (Howmedica) prostheses are designs that allow for a substitution of the cruciate ligament with the addition of a central tibial post articulating with a femoral housing mechanism. However, the two prostheses differ in several characteristics. In the Insall-Burstein prosthesis, the component substitution mechanism engages only in a knee flexion. The articulation of the cam on the spine causes femoral rollback with flexion. This allows for an increased range of motion, an improved lever arm for the quadriceps, and prevention of the posterior tibial subluxation. The Kinematic Stabilizer has a central tibial post in the femoral housing restraining anterior as well as posterior motion of the tibia between 0 and 30 degrees of flexion. Past 30 degrees of flexion, as in the Insall-Burstein prosthesis, the substituting mechanism replaces only the function of the PCL in enhancing femoral rollback. Neither design substitutes for the collateral ligament.

The Hanssen and Rand[30] report involved 79 arthroplasties (66 patients) with an average follow-up of 37 months. There were 53 revisions and 26 primary arthroplasties in their series. Postoperatively of the entire group, 34 knees (43%) rated excellent; 33 (42%), good; 7 (9%), fair, and 5 (6%), poor. However, in this group of arthroplasties, a majority were undergoing revision procedures. Separate analysis of the results of the 26 knees undergoing index procedures revealed 54% with excellent results, 38% good, 4% fair, and 4% poor. Postoperative motion averaged 101 degrees.

Despite the good results reported by these authors, their patient population differs in several important characteristics from the population implanted with Insall-Burstein Posterior Stabilized knees at the HSS. The Mayo Clinic surgeons are advocates of PCL retention whenever possible. Therefore, the knees reported in their study were either revisions or index arthroplasties performed in knees with preoperative instability or alignment problems. Preoperatively, moderate or severe instability was present in 42% of their knees, while 12 of the 26 primary knees had preoperative flexion contractures greater than 10 degrees. In addition, the diagnoses were osteoarthritis in 37 knees, rheumatoid arthritis in 36 knees, and post-traumatic arthritis in 6 knees. Therefore, they had a relatively high percentage of rheumatoid and traumatic arthritic cases in their series, reserving the use of this prosthesis for their most difficult cases. Accordingly, their results must be viewed in light of the fact that knees with inflammatory arthropathy,[37, 49, 80] post-traumatic arthritis,[102] or preoperative valgus alignment[14, 83] tend to have slightly poorer results. Therefore, while the 92% excellent and good results seen with the Kinematic Stabilizer and primary knee arthroplasties is quite encouraging, one would expect even better results if this prosthesis had been used routinely, as is done in other institutions.

Press-Fit Condylar

The Press-Fit condylar modular knee prosthesis (Johnson and Johnson) is another posterior cruciate substituting prosthesis for which clinical results are now available. In 1997, Ranawat et al reported on their experience with the posterior cruciate substituting version of the PFC.[65] The similarities between the PFC and the IB II prostheses are much more profound than are their relatively minor design differences. The shape of the tibial spine, as well as that of the femoral component, in the PFC is comparable to the corresponding parts in the IB II prosthesis. Finally, the spine-cam interaction is similar in the IB II and PFC designs.

The main differences between the two prostheses involve the patellofemoral articulation. Designers of the IB II specifically fashioned a noncongruent patellofemoral joint (Fig. 77.39). The space in the IB II system between the patellar and femoral components is intended to minimize soft-tissue impingement. Conversely, the PFC patellofemoral articulation is congruent, with symmetric contact between patella and femur. This design characteristic produces a more constrained patellofemoral joint and theoretically accommodates oblique placement of the patellar component.

The report by Ranawat et al[65] reviewed the results of 150 consecutive primary total knee replacements (118 patients) performed between 1988 and 1990.

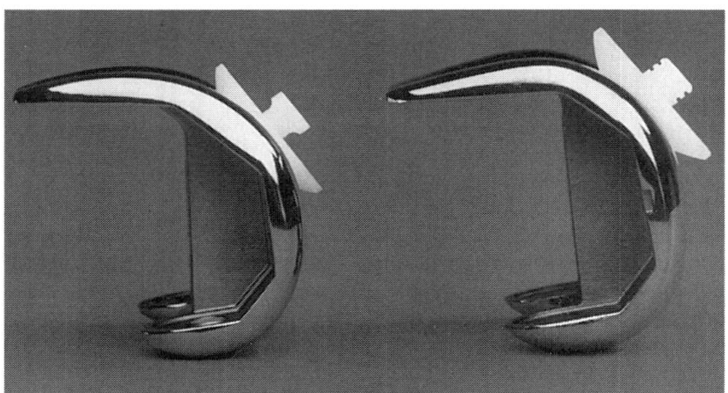

FIGURE 77.39 ➢ Press-Fit Condyle (PFC) *(left)*. Insall-Burstein II (IB II) Posterior Stabilized prosthesis *(right)*. Note the similarities between the PFC and the IB II prostheses. The shape of the femoral component and the cam mechanism are similar in the two prostheses. The PFC design incorporates more constraint into the patellofemoral joint, theoretically accommodating an oblique patellar placement. The IB II design allows for a space between femur and patella to minimize soft-tissue catching in this region.

There were 16 bilateral procedures. All the knees in this study were posterior cruciate substituting PFC modular knees implanted with the use of cement. As in most studies on total knee arthroplasty, the predominant diagnosis was osteoarthritis in 98 patients (83%). Mean age at the time of the index procedure was 70 years (range, 29 to 85 years). Of the knees implanted, the authors felt that 125 knees were followed up for an adequate time interval (mean, 4.8 years; range, 3.8 to 6.2 years) for meaningful analysis. The clinical result was felt to be excellent for 103 knees (82%), good for 13 (10%), fair for 3 (2%), and poor for 6 (5%). At the most recent follow-up, the Knee Society's[44] average functional score was 78 points (range, 0 to 100 points), and the average knee score was 93 points (range, 57 to 100 points). The mean preoperative range of motion increased from 107 degrees to 111 degrees after arthroplasty.

Survivorship analysis was performed with revision operation or a recommendation for revision as an endpoint. The rate of survival was 97% in 6 years. The standard error of the mean for this calculation was 1.6%. Three revision operations were necessary; two of these were for infection, and one was for femoral-tibial instability. Patellofemoral symptoms were noted in 8% (10 knees). The authors concluded that the posterior cruciate substituting PFC modular knee system resulted in excellent relief of pain, excellent range of motion, and restoration of function with a low prevalence of patellofemoral problems.

These intermediate-term results for the posterior cruciate substituting PFC implants[65] are similar to those achieved with the Insall-Burstein prosthesis at comparable follow-up intervals.[8, 40, 74, 75, 82, 84] This is not surprising considering the similarity in both the prosthetic designs and the surgical indications. Specifically, the senior author in the PFC report does not routinely preserve the PCL in any of his index arthroplasties. The regular use of a cruciate substituting PFC prosthesis was akin to what was done by the Insall Group.[8, 40, 82, 84] The routine use of cruciate substitution in both instances would tend to result in similar patient cohorts, as well as minimize any selection bias that may have been present in reports from other institutions on cruciate substituting knee replacements.[30] Finally, the Insall-Burstein and PFC component designs are alike except for minor differences in the patellofemoral articulation (undertaken to minimize anterior knee symptoms). In fact, the reported incidence of patellofemoral symptoms with the PFC design[65] was slightly less than with other cruciate substituting designs.[8, 82, 84] However, the differences were minor and not strictly comparable because patellofemoral symptoms were assessed differently in the various reports.[8, 65, 82, 84]

CLINICAL FUNCTION COMPARISON ANALYSIS OF POSTERIOR SUBSTITUTING DESIGNS

Because long-term results are available for Posterior Stabilized arthroplasty, it is possible to analyze them in the context of earlier reports of other designs. However, it is always difficult to directly compare results with different prostheses because of the large number of confounding variables. These variations include possible differences in preoperative populations (diagnosis, age, extent of preoperative disease, etc.), institutional protocols, surgical skill or experience, and knee evaluation methods employed. Nevertheless, comparisons are useful in critically examining implant function over time.

Comparison With Total Condylar Prosthesis

Long-term reports for both the Total Condylar[93] and the Posterior Stabilized prostheses (all-polyethylene tibial component[84] and metal-backed tibial component[8]) from the Insall Group are now available. Because all these surgeries were done under the direction of the same senior author at the same institution, had similar patient populations, and had similar evaluation methods, confounding variables among the reports are minimized. Of course, they represent results from arthroplasties performed over different time periods. The two Posterior Stabilized groups represent patients implanted several years after the Total Condylar cohort. Over this interval, advancement in surgical techniques and instrumentation occurred, in addition to improvement in prosthetic design. On the other hand, as the senior surgeon gained confidence and experience with successful knee arthroplasty, the number of severely deformed knees believed to be candidates for reconstruction increased.[95]

The Total Condylar report details the 10- to 12-year follow-up of 130 prostheses implanted from 1974 to 1975.[93] The first Posterior Stabilized study examines 289 knee arthroplasties performed from 1978 to 1981 with the Posterior Stabilized prosthesis with an all-polyethylene tibial component.[84] The second paper on the Posterior Stabilized prosthesis with a metal-backed tibial component reviewed 165 knees operated on between 1981 and 1983.[8] The patient populations in the three reports are comparable, with similar ages, weights, diagnosis distribution, and predominance of female patients (Table 77.5).

At 10 to 12 years post arthroplasty, 74 of the original 130 Total Condylar prostheses were evaluated.[93] Of these, 51% (38 knees) were rated excellent, 37% (27 knees) were good, 4% (3 knees) were fair, and 8% (6 knees) were poor. The average flexion arc achieved was 91 degrees. Of the six knees with poor results, five required revisions; four of these were secondary to tibial loosening related to technical errors. One femoral component insidiously loosened over time in a knee with a preoperative valgus deformity. One knee was categorized as poor after a stroke dropped the rating, though the knee had scored as excellent before the infirmity.

Results for 194 of the original 289 Insall-Burstein Posterior Stabilized prostheses available for analysis at 9 to 12 years post arthroplasty have already been described.[84] The results were rated excellent in 61%, good in 26%, fair in 6%, and poor in 7%. The average range of motion that the knees achieved postoperatively was 110 degrees.

Finally, the results for 101 of the 165 Insall-Burstein Posterior Stabilized prostheses with metal-backed tibial trays with 10 to 12 years' follow-up have also already been described.[8] The results were rated excellent in 73%, good in 23%, and poor in 4%. The average range of motion that the knees achieved postoperatively was 110 degrees.

Thus, the functional results in the two Posterior Stabilized series showed either 87% or 96% good and excellent results after long-term follow-up. This is comparable to the rate of excellent and good results (88%) seen in the long-term Total Condylar study (Table 77.6 and Fig. 77.40). However, the percent of knees in the excellent category increased from 51% with the Total Condylar prosthesis to 61% with the original all-polyethylene Posterior Stabilized prosthesis to 73% with the Posterior Stabilized prosthesis with a metal-backed tibial component. Additionally, the average flexion of the knees with the Total Condylar implant was 91 degrees compared with 110 degrees of average flexion in the knees with either Posterior Stabilized design. Consequently, although each prosthesis achieved excellent results at extended follow-up, there was a clear trend to better motion and functional outcomes in patients implanted with a Posterior Stabilized device.

Comparison With Posterior Cruciate Retention Arthroplasty

Kinematic-I Condylar

Surprisingly, there are relatively few long-term results of cruciate retaining knees to compare with the Insall-Burstein Posterior Stabilized arthroplasty. Wright and colleagues[97] reviewed the Brigham and Women's Hospital experience with the Kinematic-I Condylar prosthesis (Howmedica, Rutherford, NJ). They reported on 192 knees with 5- to 9-year follow-up. However, the average follow-up was only 6 years. Of note, their patient population had a high percentage of rheumatoid arthritis (54%). The Brigham knee scoring system was used to evaluate these arthroplasties. There were 59% excellent, 29% good, 6% fair, and 6% poor results. A more appropriate comparison may be in examining only the subset of 85 patients with osteoarthritis. In this group, as might be expected, the results were significantly better: 71% excellent, 24% good, 4% fair, and 1% poor results.

Malkani et al[57] reported on the Mayo Clinic's experi-

TABLE 77.5 COMPARISON OF TOTAL CONDYLAR AND POSTERIOR STABILIZED PROSTHESIS

Features	Total Condylar	Posterior Stabilized All-Polyethylene	Posterior Stabilized Metal-Backed
Interval	1974-1975	1978-1981	1981-1983
Knees	130	289	165
No. of patients	104	218	120
Females (%)	82 (79)	160 (73)	59 (80)*
Males (%)	22 (21)	58 (27)	15 (20)*
Age (range)	67 (39-87)	66 (17-87)	64 (22-81)*
Weight (range)	76 kg (43-113 kg)	77 kg (43-139 kg)	
Diagnosis			
Osteoarthritis/osteonecrosis (%)	100 (77)	223 (77)	73 (72)*
Rheumatoid arthritis (%)	30 (23)	41 (14)	22 (22)*
Traumatic (%)	—	15 (5)	2 (2)*
Miscellaneous (%)	—	10 (4)	4 (4)*

* Demographics of the 74 patients (101 knees) available for analysis at long-term follow-up.

TABLE 77.6 LONG-TERM FOLLOW-UP OF TOTAL CONDYLAR AND POSTERIOR STABILIZED PROSTHESIS

Features	Total Condylar	Posterior Stabilized All-Polyethylene	Posterior Stabilized Metal-Backed
Follow-up	10–12 years	9–12 years	10–11 years
Original no. of knees	130	289	165
Dead (%)	45 (34)	66 (23)	53 (32)
Lost to follow-up (%)	2 (2)	29 (10)	6 (4)
Refused evaluation (%)	—	—	3 (2)
Debilitated (%)	9 (7)	—	2 (1)
Knees available (%)	74 (57)	194 (67)	101 (61)
Range of motion	90 degrees	110 degrees	110 degrees
HSS knee score			
Excellent (%)	51	61	73
Good (%)	37	26	23
Fair (%)	4	6	0
Poor (%)	8	7	4

HSS = The Hospital for Special Surgery.

ence with the Kinematic-I condylar prosthesis. At the time of their review, there were 119 knees (84 patients) available with a mean long-term follow-up of 10 ±0.7 years. They found a significant increase in the HSS knee score from a preoperative average 55 ±12 points to a postoperative average of 81 ±9 points at 10-year follow-up ($p < .0001$). The authors reported

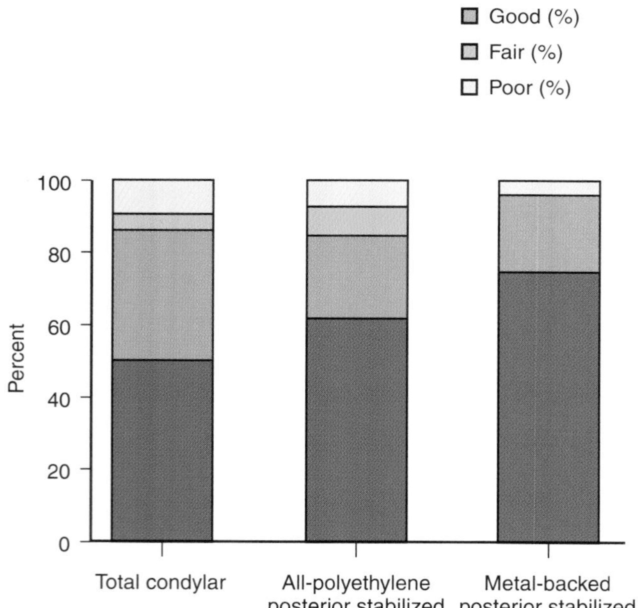

FIGURE 77.40 ➢ Comparison of long-term total condylar and posterior stabilized results by The Hospital for Special Surgery score.

that there were 41 excellent (40%), 48 good (47%), 13 fair (13%), and no poor results. Seventeen knees had inadequate data for score calculation. Six revisions were performed. It is unclear why knees undergoing revision for septic or aseptic loosening were not classified as poor results, as is the convention in reports on the Insall-Burstein Posterior Stabilized prosthesis.[8, 40, 82, 84] Four revisions were for loose patellar components, while two were for loose femoral and tibial components. There was one deep infection. The Knee Society scoring system was also used. At 10-year follow-up, the knee score was 79 ±13 and the function score was 64 ±26. When survival analysis was performed with revision as the endpoint, the rate of prosthesis survival was estimated to be 96% (confidence interval, 93% to 99%) at 10 years.

The clinical results with the Kinematic-I condylar prosthesis (HSS scores and Knee Society scores) in these two studies[57, 97] were slightly lower than those reported in studies on cruciate substituting arthroplasties.[8, 40, 65, 82, 84] Although this may point to an advantage with cruciate substituting arthroplasties, care must be taken in trying to compare subjective scores of clinical evaluations done by different authors at different institutions. In contrast, prosthesis survival in the Mayo Clinic report on the Kinematic-I condylar prosthesis was comparable to previously reported survival rates for posterior cruciate sacrificing[93] or posterior cruciate substituting prosthesis.[8, 22, 76, 84]

Cruciate Condylar

The other cruciate retaining design for which long-term results are available is the cruciate condylar prosthesis (Howmedica, Rutherford, NJ). In many respects, this design has more in common with the original posterior sacrificing Total Condylar prosthesis than with most modern cruciate retaining designs. It has similar geometry to the Total Condylar prosthesis with a posterior cutout on the tibial tray to allow for ligament retention. However, the tibial component retains the relatively high degree of conformity found in the Total Condylar design and subsequently employed with the Posterior Stabilized implants.

Ritter and associates[69] reported on survival results with a posterior cruciate condylar knee arthroplasty. They found 94.6% survival at 10 years with this posterior cruciate retaining device. Although this report is quite encouraging, it must still be viewed as preliminary data. Even though the paper is subtitled "A 10-Year Evaluation," the average follow-up period for the 394 knees was only 4.75 years. Ten-year data were available for 31 knees, representing only 8% of the knees studied. In addition, the authors mentioned that there were four infections noticed less than 1 year after surgery, and these were deleted from the study. Ritter et al[70] did a follow-up report on 418 posterior cruciate condylar knee arthroplasties. Twenty-four patients were excluded, 15 for lack of follow-up data, 6 for infection during follow-up, and 3 for revision surgery. The remaining 394 knees were followed up for an average 8.08 years (range, 1 to 18 years). The Kaplan-Meier survival curves estimated survival at 12 years as 96.8% (95% confidence interval, 90.77 to 99.37). In both these reports, the authors excluded failures secondary to infections because they were attempting "to measure the success of the design and the surgical placement of the prosthesis."[70] Inclusion of these knees would decrease the survival rates reported for the posterior cruciate condylar arthroplasty at all follow-up intervals. Septic knees are routinely counted as failures in survival studies on the Insall-Burstein Posterior Stabilized knees[76, 84] and are not excluded from analysis.

Long-term results with the cemented cruciate condylar prosthesis are also available from the Mayo Clinic.[66] Rand reported on a group of 78 knees (63 patients) with clinical and radiographic follow-up at a mean of 10 ± 7 years (range, 8 to 11.5 years). The mean patient age at the time of surgery was 62 years (range, 26 to 83 years). As in other studies,[8, 84, 93] the majority of patients were female patients (60%), and the most common preoperative diagnosis was osteoarthritis (64%). The knees were implanted with either an all-polyethylene tibial component (22 knees) or a metal-backed tibial component (56 knees). At the latest follow-up evaluation, there were 58% excellent, 35% good, 2% fair, and 5% poor results. There was no significant difference in the scores between the two types of tibial components. Using the Knee Society's scoring system,[44] at last follow-up the pain score was 77 ± 16 points and the function score was 69 ± 27 points. Once again, there was no significant difference in these scores between the two types of tibial components. Survivorship analysis using an endpoint of revision revealed 96% survival at 10 years for knees implanted with either an all-polyethylene tibial tray or a metal-backed component.

Finally, Dennis et al[12] reported long-term results on a small cohort of patients (42 knees) who underwent arthroplasty with posterior cruciate condylar prosthesis between 1975 and 1978. The average follow-up was 11 years. The preoperative diagnosis was equally split between patients with osteoarthritis and those with rheumatoid arthritis. The average postoperative knee score was 85 points; 55% of knees were rated excellent, 38% good; 2% fair; and 5% poor. Range of motion averaged 104 degrees. There was one case that required revision because of posterior instability from an insufficient PCL 10 months after the index procedure. This study represented a relatively small number of patients although the follow-up period was long.

In general, the prosthetic survival rate for the cruciate condylar prosthesis was comparable to the rates seen with the Kinematic-I condylar[57, 97] prosthesis and those with posterior substituting designs.[8, 22, 76, 84] Conversely, the clinical function and pain scores (HSS and Knee Society scores) were slightly lower with the cruciate condylar prosthesis than with posterior substituting designs.[8, 65, 84] However, there was a relatively high percentage of rheumatoid patients in the cruciate condylar reports,[12, 66] which may have helped contribute to this finding. In addition, it is worth pointing out again the difficulty in trying to accurately compare subjective clinical scores performed by different observers at different institutions.

Survivorship Analysis Comparison

Survivorship analysis has been advocated by many as a way to evaluate the results of joint arthroplasties.[15, 27, 50, 51, 76, 87, 88] Long-term survival curves have been generated for the Posterior Stabilized prosthesis in the standard fashion of Armitage. Success was defined as a prosthesis still in place at the end of follow-up. Failure was defined as a prosthesis revised for any cause, or one in which a revision had been recommended.

The survival curve for the original Posterior Stabilized prosthesis with an all-polyethylene tibial component was generated in the comprehensive long-term study (Fig. 77.41).[84] The prosthesis had 14 failures with an average annual failure rate of 0.4% and a 12-year overall success rate of 94%.

Survival analysis for the Posterior Stabilized prosthesis with a metal-backed tibial component was performed in the Insall Group's long-term study.[8] The authors reported both a best-case and a worst-case scenario. The statistical method employed to generate the survival curves in the best-case scenario was similar to the traditional methods used in previous studies on survivorship analysis.[76, 84, 93] In the best-case scenario, the six knees lost to follow-up were considered withdrawals, and overall cumulative prosthesis survival was 96.4% (95% confidence interval, 91.9% to 100%) at 11 years. With the six knees lost to follow-up considered failures (worst case), the overall cumulative prosthesis survival was 92.6% (95% confidence interval, 86.4% to 98.8%) at 11 years.

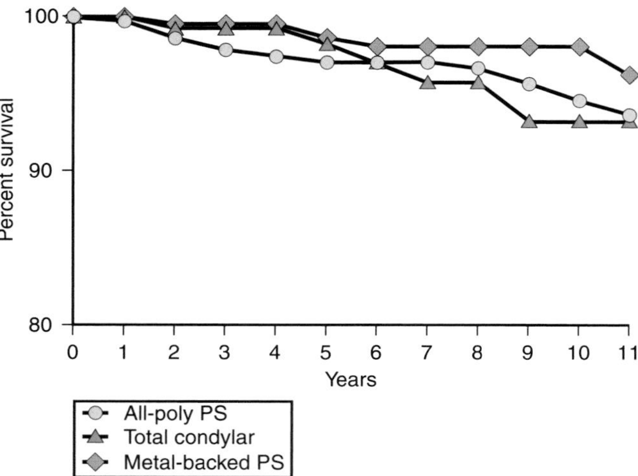

FIGURE 77.41 ➢ Comparison of survival curves for total condylar, all-polyethylene posterior stabilized, and metal-backed posterior stabilized prostheses.

Finally, survivorship analysis was also performed for the PFC posterior cruciate substituting implant.[65] In this report, the failure endpoint was defined as either revision operation or recommendation for revision. This statistical method was similar to the best-case scenario defined above. The survival curves generated with this technique resulted in a calculated prosthetic survival of 97% at 6 years' follow-up. The standard error of the mean for this calculation with the posterior cruciate substituting PFC was 1.6%.

The survival curve for the Total Condylar prosthesis yielded a survival rate of 93% at 11 years, with an average annual failure rate of 0.6% in the long-term study of 130 prostheses (see Fig. 77.41).[95]

Survivorship results for posterior cruciate substituting prostheses with either an all-polyethylene or a metal-backed tibial component are virtually identical to those seen with the Total Condylar design, while producing an improved functional outcome as discussed above. Despite the concern expressed by some regarding the inherent constraint with these designs,[72] there is no evidence from these survival data that long-term substitution for the PCL causes failure at the bone-cement interface.

COMPLICATIONS OF POSTERIOR CRUCIATE LIGAMENT SUBSTITUTION

All patients who undergo knee arthroplasty are at risk for general, as well as local, knee complications. However, there are certain complications that are believed to be more common in patients who undergo posterior cruciate substituting knee arthroplasty. These include component dislocation, intercondylar fractures, and the "patellar clunk" syndrome.

Dislocations

Although knees implanted with a posterior cruciate retaining implant are susceptible to subluxation, this problem is unlikely with a posterior cruciate substituting device. This is because of the inherent stability of the design provided by the interaction between the femoral cam and the tibial spine. However, although the problem of component subluxation is essentially eliminated with cruciate substitution, it is possible for the femoral cam to dislocate anteriorly over the tibial spine (Fig. 77.42).

Reports of dislocations have included knees implanted with the Insall-Burstein Posterior Stabilized prosthesis,[23, 54, 55] the IB II prosthesis,[6, 55, 59, 96] the Kinemax posterior substituting prosthesis,[61] the Kinematic II Stabilizer prosthesis,[24] and other designs (Fig. 77.43).[96] It is not surprising that this problem has been seen most commonly with the Insall-Burstein and Kinematic II Stabilizer designs because they have the longest track record with the posterior cruciate substituting concept.

Dislocations have been described in knees with a preoperative valgus alignment[6, 23, 24, 55, 61] and in those after patellectomy.[24] Although preoperative valgus appears to increase the incidence of this problem, it can also occur in varus knees.[55, 61] There is some controversy over whether the actual component dislocation occurs with the knee in mild flexion with a straight

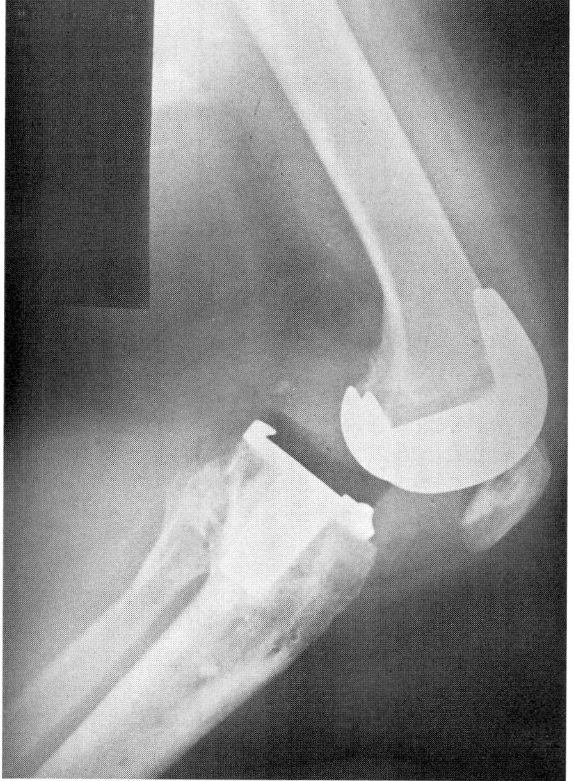

FIGURE 77.42 ➢ Dislocated Insall-Burstein II component.

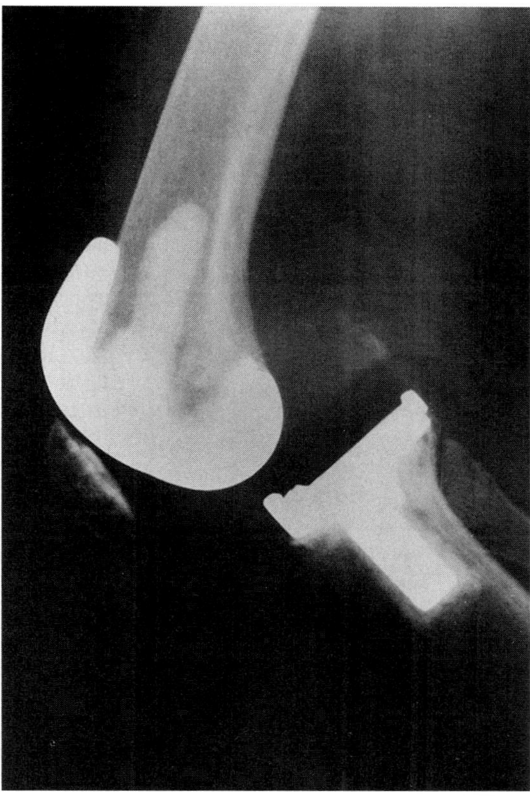

FIGURE 77.43 ➢ Dislocated Kinematic Stabilizer prosthesis.

posterior mechanism or occurs at high flexion angles with a combination of posterior and rotatory stress.[54, 55]

A knee with a dislocated implant normally presents acutely with inability to extend. In many cases, the patients are unable to explain the exact mechanism, nor the position of the knee, when the actual dislocation occurred. In fact, this problem can occur during sleep, causing the patient to awaken with an acute inability to extend the knee. On physical examination, an obvious knee deformity is commonly found. Radiographs reveal the femoral cam translated anterior to the polyethylene tibial spine.

Lombardi et al[55] analyzed the incidence of dislocations in 3032 primary knees implanted with the Insall-Burstein prosthesis series. The incidence of this problem was very rare with the original Insall-Burstein Posterior Stabilized prosthesis (0.2%, or 1 in 494). However, with the advent of the IB II prosthesis, the problem became more apparent (2.5%, or 1 in 40). Knees that dislocated were found to have achieved statistically significant higher average flexion (118 degrees) compared with control knees (105 degrees) ($p < .001$). In addition, they tended to reach high flexion angles rapidly in the postoperative period. In response to this problem, the tibial plastic was modified by raising the tibial spine and moving it anteriorly (Fig. 77.44). This increased the inherent stability of the component and decreased the incidence of dislocation (0.2%, or 1 in 656).

A computer analysis of this phenomenon analyzed the propensity of cruciate substituting knee components to dislocate in the sagittal plane.[11, 46] Kocmond et al defined a dislocation safety factor (DSF) as the jump distance between the bottom of the femoral cam and the top of the tibial spine. The DSF was found to vary with the knee flexion angle. For knees with the Insall-Burstein cruciate substitution mechanism, the DSF increases as knee flexion increases and peaks at about 70 degrees. Knee flexion beyond this angle causes the DSF to decrease and theoretically increases the risk of dislocation. Figure 77.45 lists the DSF curves for the original Insall-Burstein Posterior Stabilized prosthesis, the original IB II prosthesis, and the IB II prosthesis with the modified tibial insert. Many contemporary designs have attempted to minimize the risk of dislocation by ensuring a DSF equal to or greater than that of the original Insall-Burstein Posterior Stabilized prosthesis at high flexion angles.

In general, to prevent knee dislocations, it is imperative that the surgeon balance the knee in both flexion and extension, with a special emphasis on knees with a preoperative valgus alignment. In addition, it may be undesirable to achieve large flexion angles (greater than 100 degrees) in the first postoperative week.

Intercondylar Fractures

Femoral fractures, although a relatively rare occurrence, can occur at the time of knee arthroplasty. Because posterior cruciate substituting components require removal of extra bone from the intercondylar region, the possibility of distal femoral fracture with this technique is increased. Risk factors for fractures include inadequate, as well as excessive, intercondylar bone notch resection. Although it is self-evident that

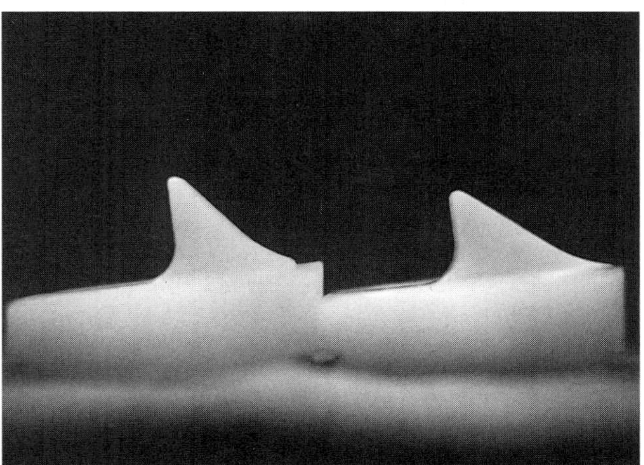

FIGURE 77.44 ➢ Modification of Insall-Burstein II tibial spine by anterior translation and increased height. Original Insall-Burstein plastic *(right)* and modified plastic *(left)*.

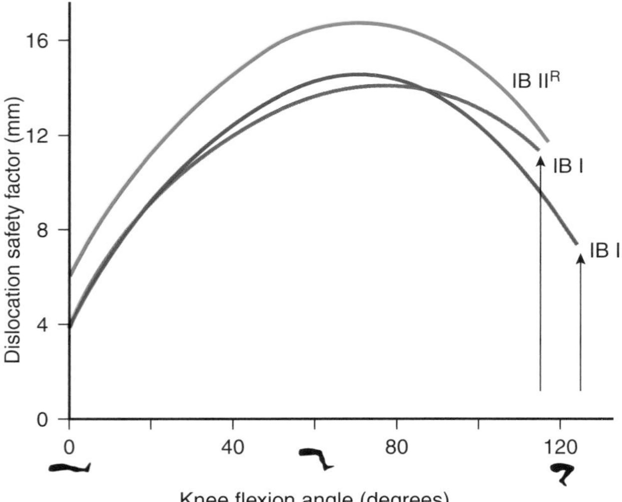

FIGURE 77.45 ➢ Dislocation safety factor curves for the original Insall-Burstein Posterior Stabilized prosthesis, the original Insall-Burstein II prosthesis, and the Insall-Burstein II prosthesis with the modified tibial insert. (Redrawn from Kocmond JH et al: Stability and range of motion of Insall-Burstein condylar prostheses: A computer simulation study. J Arthroplasty 10:386, 1995.)

excessive bone removal results directly in stress risers and deficient bone, the risks associated with incomplete bone resection are not as clear-cut. Nonetheless, if insufficient notch bone is removed, the intercondylar region of the femoral component (or trial) can act like a wedge during insertion and induce a distal femoral fracture. Although this complication has been reported,[56] the exact incidence of this phenomenon has not been well defined.

Lombardi et al[56] reported on this complication in comparing two large series of posterior cruciate substituting knees. In this report, 898 nonconsecutive primary knee arthroplasties performed with a posterior cruciate substituting prosthesis were compared to a second nonconsecutive series of 532 posterior cruciate substituting knee arthroplasties. In the second series, an intercondylar sizing guide was used to confirm the intercondylar resection size. Forty distal femoral fractures were noted in the initial series (approximate rate, 1:22; nondisplaced, 35; displaced, 5). This was in contrast to the second series, in which only one displaced fracture was noted (rate, 1:532). The rate difference between the two series was statistically significant. The authors advocate careful resection technique and intercondylar notch size verification to minimize this complication. Of note, no change in postoperative rehabilitation was required either for patients identified with a nondisplaced intercondylar fracture or for those with an intercondylar fracture treated with intraoperative stabilization.

Patellar Clunk Syndrome

The patellar clunk syndrome is a well-known entity in total knee arthroplasty.[5, 35, 40, 58, 77, 91] Commonly, it is felt to be associated with posterior cruciate substituting arthroplasty,[5, 35, 40, 58, 91] but it has also been reported in association with cruciate retaining components.[77] Historically, a case of patellar catching was mentioned by Insall in his original report on the posterior stabilized knee. However, Hozack et al[35] appear to be the first authors to define the term "patellar clunk syndrome." They described a prominent fibrous nodule at the junction of the proximal patellar pole and the quadriceps tendon. They felt that during flexion this fibrous nodule would enter the femoral component's intercondylar notch but not restrict flexion. However, as the knee extended, the nodule would remain within the notch while the rest of the extensor mechanism slid proximally. They felt that at 30 to 45 degrees of flexion, the tension on the fibrous nodule would be sufficient to cause the nodule to jerk out of the notch as it returned to its normal position. This sudden displacement would cause the audible and palpable clunk found with this entity. Treatment recommendations for patellar clunk syndrome have included physical therapy,[5] surgical removal of the nodule,[35] patellar prosthesis revision,[5, 35] open resection through a limited lateral incision,[58] and arthroscopic débridement.[5, 91]

The largest series on treatment of patellar clunk syndrome appears to be by Beight et al.[5] They reported on 14 operative procedures (11 arthroscopic débridements and 3 patellar component revisions) performed in 12 patients. As in other reports,[35] they found a suprapatellar fibrous nodule that wedged into the intercondylar notch during flexion and dislodged as the knee extended, causing the clunk. The authors related that the symptoms resolved after nodule excision. However, four of the knees that were treated with arthroscopic débridement had recurrence of symptoms. None of the knees that underwent arthrotomy and patella button revisions had recurrence. The authors recommended a treatment protocol that commenced with a short course of nonoperative physical therapy, although they acknowledged that their results were disappointing with this. Arthroscopic débridement was suggested for knees without radiographic component abnormalities. Arthrotomy was suggested for recurrent clunks or malpositioned or loose components.

CONCLUSION

The concept of substitution for the PCL has proven to be versatile and durable, with excellent long-term clinical and survival results. Concern at the time of the concept's introduction that the inherent increased constraint of the components would lead to increased loosening has proved unfounded. PCL substitution has allowed for an increased range of knee motion while preventing posterior tibial subluxation. Modern knee systems make it easier to switch between cruciate retaining and cruciate substituting implants at the time of surgery. Modular components allow for easy intraoperative customization of posterior cruciate substituting components. This allows the surgeon to easily achieve the benefits of posterior cruciate substitution and customization while meeting the individual needs of any particular case.

References

1. Aglietti P, Buzzi R, Gaudeni A: Patellofemoral functional results and complications with the posterior stabilized total condylar knee prosthesis. J Arthroplasty 3(1):17, 1988.
2. Aglietti P, Buzzi R: Posterior stabilized total condylar knee replacement: Three to eight years' follow-up of 85 knees. J Bone Joint Surg Br 70:211, 1988.
3. Aglietti P, Buzzi R, Giron F, et al: The Insall-Burstein posterior stabilized total knee replacement in the valgus knee. Am J Knee Surg 9(1):8, Winter 1996.
4. Bartel DL, Burstein AH, Santavicca EA, et al: Performance of the tibial component in total knee replacement: Conventional and revision designs. J Bone Joint Surg Am 64:1026, 1982.
5. Beight JL, Yao B, Hozack WJ, et al: The patellar "clunk" syndrome after posterior stabilized knee arthroplasty. Clin Orthop 299:139, 1994.
6. Cohen B, Constant CR: Subluxation of the posterior stabilized total knee arthroplasty. A report of two cases. J Arthroplasty 7(2):161, 1992.
7. Cohn BT, Krackow KA, Hungerford DS, et al: Results of total knee arthroplasty in patients 80 years and older. Orthop Rev 19(5):451, 1990.
8. Colizza WA, Insall JN, Scuderi GR: The posterior stabilized total knee prosthesis. Assessment of polyethylene damage and osteolysis after a ten-year-minimum follow-up. J Bone Joint Surg Am 77:1713, 1995.
9. Collier JP, Mayor MB, McNamara JL, et al: Analysis of the failure of 122 polyethylene inserts from uncemented tibial knee components. Clin Orthop 273:232, 1991.
10. Coventry MB: Two-part total knee arthroplasty: Evolution and present status. Clin Orthop 145:29, 1979.
11. Delp SL, Kocmond JH, Stern SH: Tradeoffs between motion and stability in posterior substituting knee arthroplasty design. J Biomech 28:1155, 1995.
12. Dennis DA, Clayton ML, O'Donnell S, et al: Posterior cruciate condylar total knee arthroplasty. Average 11-year follow-up evaluation. Clin Orthop 281:168, 1992.
13. Dennis DA, Komistek RD, Hoff WA, et al: In vivo knee kinematics derived using an inverse perspective technique. Clin Orthop 331:107, 1996.
14. Diduch DR, Insall JN, Scott WN, et al: Total knee replacement in young, active patients. Long-term follow-up and functional outcome. J Bone Joint Surg Am 79:575, 1997.
15. Dobbs HS: Survivorship of total hip replacements. J Bone Joint Surg Br 62:168, 1980.
16. Ducheyne P, Kagan A, Lacey JA: Failure of total knee arthroplasty due to loosening and deformation of the tibial component. J Bone Joint Surg Am 60:384, 1978.
17. England SP, Stern SH, Insall JN, et al: Total knee arthroplasty in diabetes mellitus. Clin Orthop 260:130, 1990.
18. Evanski PM, Waugh TR, Orofino CF, et al: UCI knee replacement. Clin Orthop 120:33, 1976.
19. Fahmy NR, Chandler HP, Danylchuk K, et al: Blood-gas and circulatory changes during total knee replacement. J Bone Joint Surg Am 72:19, 1990.
20. Faris PM, Insall JN, Stern SH: Patellar symptoms in the posterior stabilized knee: A critical analysis. Presented at the 57th Annual Academy of Orthopaedic Surgeons, New Orleans, 1990.
21. Figgie HE, Goldberg VM, Heiple KG, et al: The influence of tibialpatellofemoral location on function of the knee in patients with the posterior stabilized condylar knee prosthesis. J Bone Joint Surg Am 68:1035, 1986.
22. Font-Rodriguez DE, Scuderi GR, Insall JN: Survivorship of cemented total knee arthroplasty. Clin Orthop 345:79, 1997.
23. Galinat BJ, Vernace JV, Booth RE Jr, et al: Dislocation of the posterior stabilized total knee arthroplasty: A report of two cases. J Arthroplasty 3(4):363, 1988.
24. Gebhard JS, Kilgus DJ: Dislocation of a posterior stabilized total knee prosthesis: A report of two cases. Clin Orthop 254:225, 1990.
25. Goldberg VM, Henderson BT: The Freeman-Swanson ICLH total knee arthroplasty: Complications and problems. J Bone Joint Surg Am 62:1138, 1980.
26. Goldberg VM, Figgie MP, Figgie HE III, et al: Use of a total condylar knee prosthesis for treatment of osteoarthritis and rheumatoid arthritis: Long-term results. J Bone Joint Surg Am 70:802, 1988.
27. Grimer RJ, Karpinski MRK, Edwards AN: The long-term results of Stanmore total knee replacements. J Bone Joint Surg Br 66: 55, 1984.
28. Groh GI, Parker J, Elliott J, et al: Results of total knee arthroplasty using the posterior stabilized condylar prosthesis: A report of 137 consecutive cases. Clin Orthop 269:58, 1991.
29. Hamilton LR: UCI total knee replacement: A follow-up study. J Bone Joint Surg Am 64:740, 1982.
30. Hanssen AD, Rand JA: A comparison of primary and revision total knee arthroplasty using the Kinematic stabilizer prosthesis. J Bone Joint Surg Am 70:491, 1988.
31. Hernigou PH, Medevielle D, Debeyre J, et al: Proximal tibial osteotomy for osteoarthritis with varus deformity: A ten to thirteen-year follow-up study. J Bone Joint Surg Am 69:332, 1987.
32. Holden DL, James SL, Larson RL, et al: Proximal tibial osteotomy in patients who are fifty years old or less. J Bone Joint Surg Am 70:977, 1988.
33. Hood RW, Vanni M, Insall JN: The correction of knee alignment in 225 consecutive total condylar knee replacements. Clin Orthop 160:94, 1981.
34. Howie DW, Vernon-Roberts B, Oakeshott R, et al: A rat model of resorption of bone at the cement-bone interface in the presence of polyethylene wear particles. J Bone Joint Surg Am 70: 257, 1988.
35. Hozack WJ, Rothman RH, Booth RE, et al: The patellar clunk syndrome. Clin Orthop 241:203, 1989.
36. Insall JN, Ranawat CS, Scott WN, et al: Total condylar knee replacement: Preliminary report. Clin Orthop 120:149, 1976.
37. Insall JN, Scott WN, Ranawat CS: The total condylar knee prosthesis: A report of two hundred and twenty cases. J Bone Joint Surg Am 61:173, 1979.
38. Insall JN, Tria AJ: The total condylar knee prosthesis type II. Presented at the Annual Meeting of the American Academy of Orthopaedic Surgeons, San Francisco, CA, 1979.
39. Insall JN: Technique of total knee replacement. Instr Course Lect 30:324, 1981.
40. Insall JN, Lachiewicz PF, Burstein AH: The posterior stabilized condylar prosthesis: A modification of the total condylar design. J Bone Joint Surg Am 64:1317, 1982.
41. Insall JN, Hood RW, Flawn LB, et al: The total condylar knee prosthesis in gonarthrosis: A five to nine-year follow-up of the first one hundred consecutive replacements. J Bone Joint Surg Am 65:619, 1983.
42. Insall JN, Joseph DM, Msika C: High tibial osteotomy for varus gonarthrosis. J Bone Joint Surg Am 6:1040, 1984.
43. Insall JN: Total knee replacement. In Insall JN, ed: Surgery of the Knee. New York, Churchill Livingstone, 1984, p 587.
44. Insall JN, Dorr LD, Scott RD, et al: Rationale of the Knee Society clinical rating system. Clin Orthop 248:13, 1989.
45. Kilgus DJ, Moreland JR, Finerman GA, et al: Catastrophic wear of tibial polyethylene inserts. Clin Orthop 273:223, 1991.
46. Kocmond JH, Delp SL, Stern SH: Stability and range of motion of Insall-Burstein condylar prostheses. A computer simulation study. J. Arthroplasty 10:383, 1995.
47. Landy MD, Walker PS: Wear of ultra-high molecular weight polyethylene components of ninety retrieved knee prostheses. J Arthroplasty 3(Suppl 1):573, 1988.
48. Laskin RS, Rieger M, Achob C, et al: The posterior stabilized total knee prosthesis in the knee with a severe fixed deformity. Am J Knee Surg 1:199, 1988.
49. Laskin RS: Total condylar knee replacement in patients who have rheumatoid arthritis: A ten-year follow-up study. J Bone Joint Surg Am 72:529, 1990.
50. Lettin AWF, Kavanagh TG, Craig D, et al: Assessment of the survival and the clinical results of Stanmore total knee replacements. J Bone Joint Surg Br 66:355, 1984.

51. Lewallen DG, Bryan RS, Peterson LFA: Polycentric total knee arthroplasty: A ten-year follow-up study. J Bone Joint Surg Am 66:1211, 1984.
52. L'Insallata JC, Stern SH, Insall JN: Total knee arthroplasty in elderly patients: Comparison of tibial component designs. J Arthroplasty 7(3):261, 1992.
53. Lombardi AV, Sydney SV, Mallory TH, et al: Six year survivorship analysis of the Insall-Burstein posterior stabilized knee: A clinical and radiographic evaluation. Orthop Trans 12:711, 1988.
54. Lombardi AV, Krugel R, Honkala TK, et al: Dislocation following primary posterior stabilized total knee arthroplasty. Presented at the 58th Annual Meeting of the American Academy of Orthopaedic Surgeons, Anaheim, CA, 1991,
55. Lombardi AV Jr, Mallory TH, Vaughn BK, et al: Dislocation following primary posterior-stabilized total knee arthroplasty. J Arthroplasty 8:633, 1993.
56. Lombardi AV Jr, Mallory TH, Waterman RA, et al: Intercondylar distal femoral fracture. An unreported complication of posterior-stabilized total knee arthroplasty. J Arthroplasty 10(5):643, 1995.
57. Malkani AL, Rand JA, Bryan RS, et al: Total knee arthroplasty with the kinematic condylar prosthesis. A ten-year follow-up study. J Bone Joint Surg Am 77:423, 1995.
58. Messieh M: Management of patellar clunk under local anesthesia. J Arthroplasty 11:202, 1996.
59. Mills HJ, McKee MD, Horne G, et al: Dislocation of posteriorly stabilized total knee arthroplasties. Can J Surg 37:225, 1994.
60. Mintz L, Tsao AK, McCrae CR, et al: The arthroscopic evaluation and characteristics of severe polyethylene wear in total knee arthroplasty. Clin Orthop 273:215, 1991.
61. Ochsner JL Jr, Kostman WC, Dodson M: Posterior dislocation of a posterior-stabilized total knee arthroplasty. A report of two cases. Am J Orthop 25:310, 1996.
62. Patel DV, Aichroth PM, Wand JS: Posteriorly stabilized (Insall-Burstein) total condylar knee arthroplasty. A follow-up study of 157 knees. Int Orthop 15:211, 1991.
63. Ranawat CS, Boachie-Adjei O: Survivorship analysis and results of total condylar knee arthroplasty: Eight- to eleven-year follow-up period. Clin Orthop 226:6, 1988.
64. Ranawat CS, Hansraj KK: Effect of posterior cruciate sacrifice on durability of the cement-bone interface. Orthop Clin North Am 20:63, 1989.
65. Ranawat CS, Luessenhop CP, Rodriguez JA: The press-fit condylar modular total knee system. Four-to-six-year results with a posterior-cruciate-substituting design. J Bone Joint Surg Am 79: 342, 1997.
66. Rand JA: Comparison of metal-backed and all-polyethylene tibial components in cruciate condylar total knee arthroplasty. J Arthroplasty 8(3):307, 1993.
67. Revell PA, Weightman B, Freeman MAR, et al: The production and biology of polyethylene wear debris. Arch Orthop Trauma Surg 91:167, 1978.
68. Riley D, Woodyard JL: Long-term results of geomedic total knee replacement. J Bone Joint Surg Br 67:548, 1985.
69. Ritter MA, Campbell MS, Faris PM, et al: Long-term survival analysis of the posterior cruciate condylar total knee arthroplasty. J Arthroplasty 4(4):293, 1989.
70. Ritter MA, Herbst SA, Keating EM, et al: Long-term survival analysis of a posterior cruciate-retaining total condylar total knee arthroplasty. Clin Orthop 309:136, 1994.
71. Robinson EJ, Mulliken BD, Bourne RB, et al: Catastrophic osteolysis in total knee replacement. A report of 17 cases. Clin Orthop 321:98, 1995.
72. Scott RD, Volatile TB: Twelve years' experience with posterior cruciate retaining total knee arthroplasty. Clin Orthop 205:100, 1986.
73. Scott WN, Schosheim P: Posterior stabilized knee arthroplasty. Orthop Clin North Am 20:71, 1982.
74. Scott WN, Rubinstein M: Posterior stabilized knee arthroplasty: Six year experience. Clin Orthop 205:138, 1986.
75. Scott WN, Rubinstein M, Scuderi G: Results after knee replacement with a posterior cruciate-substituting prosthesis. J Bone Joint Surg Am 70: 1163, 1988.
76. Scuderi GR, Insall JN, Windsor RE, et al: Survivorship of cemented knee replacement. J Bone Joint Surg Br 71:798, 1989.
77. Shoji H, Shimozaki E: Patellar clunk syndrome in total knee arthroplasty without patellar resurfacing. J Arthroplasty 11:198, 1996.
78. Soudry M, Binazzi R, Johanson NA, et al: Total knee arthroplasty in Charcot and Charcot-like joints. Clin Orthop 208:199, 1986.
79. Stern SH, Insall JN, Windsor RE: Total knee arthroplasty in osteonecrotic knees. Orthop Trans 12:722, 1988.
80. Stern SH, Insall JN, Windsor RE, et al: Total knee arthroplasty in patients with psoriasis. Clin Orthop 248:108, 1989.
81. Stern SH, Bowen MK, Insall JN, et al: Cemented total knee arthroplasty for gonarthrosis in patients 55 years old or younger. Clin Orthop 260:124, 1990.
82. Stern SH, Insall JN: Total knee arthroplasty in obese patients. J Bone Joint Surg Am 72:1400, 1990.
83. Stern SH, Moeckel BH, Insall JN: Total knee arthroplasty in valgus knees. Clin Orthop 273:5, 1991.
84. Stern SH, Insall JN: Posterior stabilized prosthesis: Results after 9-12 years follow-up of nine to twelve years. J Bone Joint Surg Am 74:980, 1992.
85. Stiehl JB, Komistek RD, Dennis DA, et al: Fluoroscopic analysis of kinematics after posterior-cruciate-retaining knee arthroplasty. J Bone Joint Surg Br 77:884, 1995.
86. Tegner Y, Lysholm J: Rating systems in the evaluation of knee ligament injuries. Clin Orthop 198:43, 1985.
87. Tew M, Waugh W: Estimating the survival time of knee replacements. J Bone Joint Surg Br 64:579, 1982.
88. Tew M, Waugh W, Forster IW: Comparing the results of different types of knee replacement: A method proposed and applied. J Bone Joint Surg Br 67:775, 1985.
89. Thorpe CD, Bocell JR, Tullos HS: Intra-articular fibrous bands: Patellar complications after total knee replacement. J Bone Joint Surg Am 72:811, 1990.
90. Tsao AK, Mintz L, McCrae CR, et al: Severe polyethylene wear in PCA total knee arthroplasties. Presented at Knee Society Meeting, Anaheim, CA, 1991.
91. Vernace JV, Rothman RH, Booth RE Jr, et al: Arthroscopic management of the patellar clunk syndrome following posterior stabilized total knee arthroplasty. J Arthroplasty 4:179, 1989.
92. Vince KG, Kelly MA, Insall JN: Posterior stabilized knee prosthesis: Follow-up at five to eight years. Orthop Trans 12:157, 1988.
93. Vince KG, Insall JN, Kelly MA: The total condylar prosthesis: 10 to 12 year results of a cemented knee replacement. J Bone Joint Surg Br 71:793, 1989.
94. Vince KG, Insall JM, Bannerman CE: Total knee arthroplasty in the patient with Parkinson's disease. J Bone Joint Surg Br 71: 51, 1989.
95. Vince KG: The posterior stabilized knee prosthesis. In Laskin RS, ed: Total Knee Replacement. New York, Springer-Verlag, 1991, p 113.
96. Wang CJ, Wang HE: Dislocation of total knee arthroplasty. A report of 6 cases with 2 patterns of instability. Acta Orthop Scand 68:282, 1997.
97. Wright J, Ewald FC, Walker PS, et al: Total knee arthroplasty with the Kinematic prosthesis. J Bone Joint Surg Am 72:1003, 1990.
98. Wright TM, Bartel DL: The problem of surface damage in polyethylene total knee components. Clin Orthop 205:67, 1986.
99. Wright TM, Rimnac CM, Faris PM, et al: Analysis of surface damage in retrieved carbon fiber-reinforced and plain polyethylene tibial components from posterior stabilized total knee replacements. J Bone Joint Surg Am 70(9):1312, 1988.
100. Wright TM, Astion DJ, Bansal M, et al: Failure of carbon fiber-reinforced polyethylene total knee replacement components: A report of two cases. J Bone Joint Surg Am 70(6):926, 1988.
101. Wright TM, Rimnac CM, Stulberg SD, et al: Wear of polyethylene in total joint replacements: Observations from retrieved PCA knee implants. Clin Orthop 276:126, 1992.
102. Zelicof SB, Scuderi GR, Vince KG, et al: Total knee arthroplasty in post-traumatic arthritis. Orthop Trans 12:547, 1988

78 Fluoroscopic Analysis of Total Knee Replacement

RICHARD D. KOMISTEK • DOUGLAS A. DENNIS

PRINCIPLES OF FLUOROSCOPY

Most previous kinematic studies involving total knee arthroplasty (TKA) have been conducted under in vitro conditions using cadavers or under noninvasive conditions using gait laboratory systems.[1, 15, 16, 18, 20, 28, 44, 45] Unfortunately, cadaveric studies do not allow for in vivo simulations because the actuators applying the muscle loads are unable to produce in vivo motions. Gait laboratory systems are effective in determining in-plane rotations but induce significant out-of-plane rotational and translational error.[29, 33] Therefore, it became imperative that a new procedure be developed if implanted joints were to be accurately analyzed.

Video fluoroscopy allows for visualization of human joints in two dimensions under dynamic, weightbearing conditions. Through the use of model-fitting techniques, it has become possible to accurately recover the three-dimensional (3-D) motions of implanted joints from the two-dimensional (2-D) video fluoroscopic images.[2, 9, 11, 19, 38, 40, 41] The objective of our research was to develop an automated 3-D model-fitting process that would be accurate, precise, nonbiased, and expedient and could be used on any implanted joint in the human body.

A feature of "full perspective" projection (x-ray) images is that objects closer to the radiation source appear larger than those that are placed farther away. This property allows measurement of out-of-plane translation (depth) as well as determination of correct poses for symmetric implant components. Because one side of the implant is positioned farther from the radiation source than the other, the portion of the implant silhouette corresponding to the nearer side will appear larger than that of the distant side.

X-Ray Image Prediction

The use of fluoroscopy has evolved from 2-D attempts[25, 26, 40] at predicting in-plane motions into 3-D techniques that recover accurate 3-D kinematics. Initial attempts at 3-D kinematics relied on library matching techniques,[2, 9, 19, 41] but, more recently a 3-D, computer-automated, iterative model-fitting technique has been developed.[38]

To determine implanted TKA component poses from an x-ray image, the actual fluoroscope is modeled within the computer by representing its components with their computer counterparts. The radiation source is replaced by a virtual camera, the image intensifier is represented by the x-ray image itself, and the patients' implants are replaced with 3-D, solid, computer-assisted-design (CAD) models. Finally, the field of view (FOV) of the virtual camera is set equal to the FOV of the actual fluoroscope (Fig. 78.1).

Once the fluoroscope has been modeled, viewing the CAD models through the virtual camera is equiva-

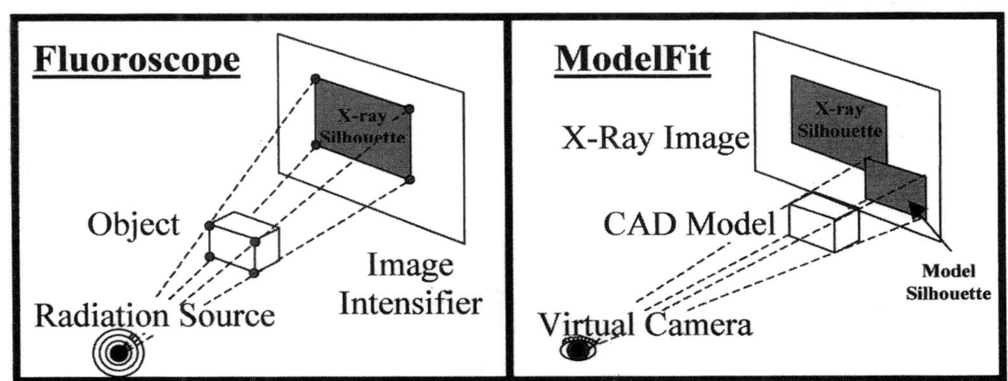

FIGURE 78.1 ➢ Using fluoroscopy, a perspective projection image of an object was created, whereby silhouette size of the object depends on the proximity of the object to the radiation source (*left*). A computer algorithm was used to duplicate the fluoroscopic process to create a predicted x-ray image (*right*). The model is then manipulated by the computer algorithm to align the predicted x-ray image with the actual object silhouette. Once this process is completed, a three-dimensional overlay of a two-dimensional fluoroscopic image can be analyzed.

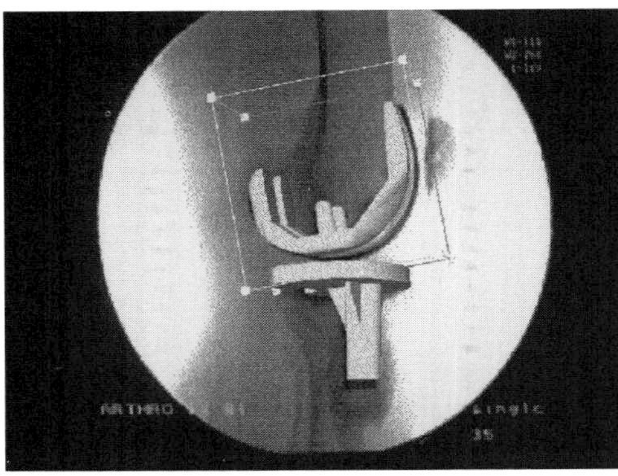

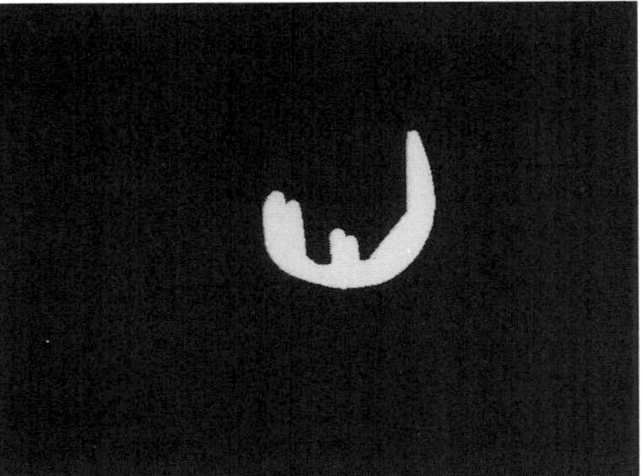

FIGURE 78.2 ➢ Two images produced by the virtual camera are used in the model-fitting process. The first image displays the three-dimensional, solid, computer-assisted–design (CAD) models of the femoral and tibial components overlayed onto the two-dimensional fluoroscopic image, which is viewed by the operator for supervisory purposes (*left*). The second view is used by the computer algorithm to manipulate the pose of the CAD model (*right*). While the computer algorithm is numerically calculating various overlay positions, the operator can watch as the computer chooses the best fit.

lent to viewing the patient's anatomy through the fluoroscope. Viewing the CAD models from this perspective provides two important images that are used in the pose estimation process. The first image is a view of the CAD models superimposed (overlaids) on top of the x-ray image. This image is displayed in the graphical user interface and allows for human supervision of the pose estimation process. The second image is a synthetic x-ray image of the CAD models, consisting of only their silhouettes (Fig. 78.2). This image represents a prediction of the x-ray image corresponding to the selected implant component's current 3-D position and is used in the matching process by rendering the CAD. This rendering is stored by the computer in the frame buffer as numerical values. These values are then copied into a 2-D array and stored as the synthetic x-ray image.

Modeling Methods

In our early analyses of 3-D kinematics of TKA using video fluoroscopy, we used template matching to determine the poses of implants within x-ray images. In template matching, 3-D models of the implant components are used to create silhouette libraries (templates), which contain multiple representations of the implants at various known poses.[2, 9, 19, 41] This method uses computer models of the implants, oriented at varying incremental degrees of out-of-plane rotations, to generate images of the implant at varying poses.[19] Using canonization, these images are then scaled, translated, and rotated so that all silhouettes are 15,000 pixels in size and centered in the image, and the principal axis of the silhouette is aligned with the horizontal axis of the image.

The actual fluoroscopic image is then processed. The image is filtered to reduce noise, and then the contour of the implant silhouette is traced manually by a human operator. An image is then created from the traced contour of the actual implant silhouette. At this point, the x-ray contour is compared with the appropriate template and the closest match is selected from the previously developed silhouette library (it can interpolate between one-degree images). From this match, the 6 degrees of freedom (DOF) position of the implant components can be obtained. The x-axis and y-axis rotations are obtained directly from the template image. The remaining 4 DOFs are then determined from the scaling, rotation, and translation values that were required to canonize the image.

We chose to develop a model-fitting methodology because of significant limitations of using the template-matching technique. Because the created library images are of the full femoral and tibial components, template matching fails if one component obstructs the other component or if portions of either component are out of the FOV. The model-fitting approach requires only one femoral and one tibial component, whereas template matching requires more than 1000 femoral and tibial images in the library. These libraries are generally created at 1-degree increments; thus, actual in vivo orientations between the library orientations are determined using interpolation schemes. Most importantly, the model-fitting approach allows a human to supervise the overlay process, in contrast to the template-matching technique, which provides only numerical determination without direct visualization.[38]

To overcome the limitations of the template-matching methods, a more accurate and reliable 3-D automated interactive kinematic analysis system (ModelFit) was developed (Fig. 78.3).[38] The automated method is faster than the manual technique and removes human error by using a computer algorithm to align the models with implant silhouettes. Using an energy minimization routine to maximize the correlation value, the computer very quickly and accurately determines the correct positions and orientations of the TKA implants.

An unbiased error analysis comparison was initially conducted with the same operator using the three methods (template matching, manual model fitting, and automated model fitting) and then with multiple operators using the three methods. The results from the error analysis determined that the automated model-fitting process is more accurate than the manual model-fitting or template-matching methods (Table 78.1). The automated method also had a higher repro-

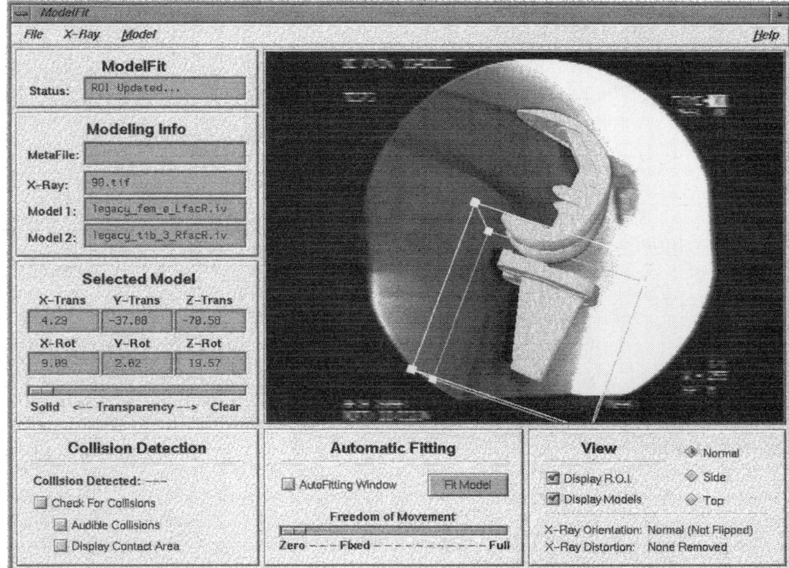

FIGURE 78.3 ➢ An example of the automated model-fitting process showing the three-dimensional femoral and tibial component models being fit by the computer onto the two-dimensional fluoroscopic image. Once the models are fit, the three-dimensional orientation of the femur relative to the tibia is determined.

ducibility that the manual method had: manual (1.1 mm in translation, 0.7 degrees in rotation), automated (0.2 mm in translation, 0.2 degrees in rotation). The automated approach was also statistically faster in total times (p = .2) and user times (p = .005) compared with the manual method.[38]

The developed model-fitting techniques have been used to accurately determine femoral component rotations and translations relative to the tibial component in three dimensions. After implantation with TKA, patients are analyzed while performing weightbearing, dynamic activities under fluoroscopic surveillance. The video images, recorded at frame rates of either 30 or 60 Hz, are downloaded digitally onto a computer network. Initially, the 3-D femoral component is placed over the fluoroscopic image of the 2-D femoral component, and the model-fitting software package determines the best 3-D fit. Next, the 3-D tibial component is precisely positioned over the 2-D fluoroscopic image of the tibia and is fitted. Then the femoral and tibial components are grouped together and oriented with the tibia in the pure sagittal view, and the medial and lateral femorotibial condylar contact positions are determined relative to the midline of the tibia in the sagittal plane. Analysis of multiple video fluoroscopic images then allows determination of 3-D knee kinematics throughout an entire range of flexion.

CLINICAL APPLICATIONS OF FLUOROSCOPY

Using our automated model-fitting approach, we have analyzed the kinematics for posterior cruciate retaining (PCR), posterior cruciate substituting (PS), and mobile bearing (MB) TKA during deep knee bend activity and gait. We have routinely analyzed each implant for anteroposterior femorotibial translation, axial rotation, incidence of femoral condylar lift-off, and maximum range of motion. We have also determined the anteroposterior motions of normal and anterior cruciate ligament-deficient (ACLD) knees in 2-D using digitization so that a control group could be established.[9]

Anteroposterior Translation

Because CAD models for normal and ACLD knees are unavailable, patients with normal and ACLD knees were analyzed in 2-D using digitization. We initially analyzed the motion of the lateral condyle of normal knees during a deep knee bend to maximum flexion.[9]

TABLE 78.1 **ERROR ANALYSIS OF THE TEMPLATE-MATCHING, MANUAL MODEL-FITTING, AND AUTOMATED MODEL-FITTING TECHNIQUES USING A SYNTHETIC IMAGE**

Technique	In-Plane Translation (mm)	σ	Out-of-Plane Translation (mm)	σ	Rotation (Degrees)	σ
Template matching	0.5	0.3	3.5	4.0	0.5	0.3
Manual model fitting	0.5	0.3	3.5	4.0	0.5	0.3
Automated model fitting	0.005	0.02	0.02	0.03	0.002	0.01

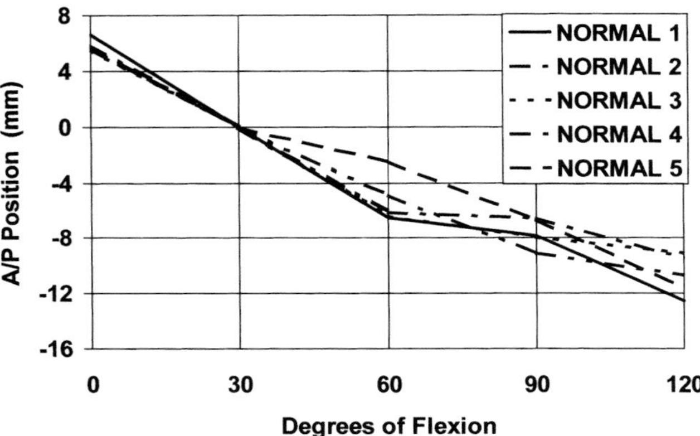

FIGURE 78.4 ➢ Sagittal femorotibial contact positions of five randomly selected normal knees.

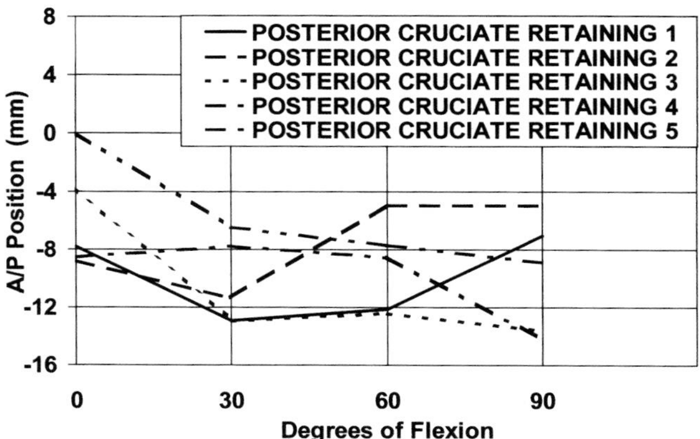

FIGURE 78.6 ➢ Sagittal femorotibial contact positions of five randomly selected posterior cruciate retaining total knee replacements.

At full extension, the femorotibial contact position was anterior to the midline in the sagittal plane. With knee flexion, the lateral femorotibial contact point translated posteriorly (posterior femoral rollback) approximately 14 mm. Analysis of multiple subjects demonstrated very similar femorotibial contact pathways (Fig. 78.4).

The same methodology was used to analyze patients having an ACLD knee. At full extension, the lateral condyle in ACLD knees typically contacted the tibia posterior to the midline in the sagittal plane and, throughout flexion, did not move in a distinct direction. In some, femorotibial contact would remain relatively stationary throughout flexion, whereas others would move in the posterior direction, and, in a third group, femorotibial contact would translate anteriorly with progressive flexion, opposite of the normal knee (Fig. 78.5).

Using the 3-D model-fitting process, lateral femorotibial contact patterns with deep knee bends were studied in patients implanted with both PCR and PS TKA.[9] The PCR knees demonstrated kinematic patterns similar to those ACLD knees (Fig. 78.6). In all subjects, the femorotibial contact position was posterior at full extension. Many subjects experienced a paradoxical anterior translation of femorotibial contact at either 30 to 60 or 60 to 90 degrees of knee flexion. This anterior motion was the opposite of the posterior femoral rollback observed in normal knees. A high degree of variability in femorotibial contact pathways was observed among subjects. Similar to the normal knee, the PS knees routinely experienced posterior femoral rollback averaging 7.7 mm, with increasing knee flexion (Fig. 78.7), although less in normal knees because of a midsagittal position in full extension (Fig. 78.8). In contrast to subjects implanted with PCR TKA, those implanted with PS TKA demonstrated similar and reproducible femorotibial contact patterns.

The described video fluoroscopic evaluation demonstrated that traditional posterior femoral rollback does not occur routinely after PCR TKA; femorotibial contact is posterior at full extension and shifting anteriorly in flexion ranges beyond 30 to 60 degrees in a majority of patients implanted with PCR TKA. Although patients implanted with PS TKA more closely duplicated

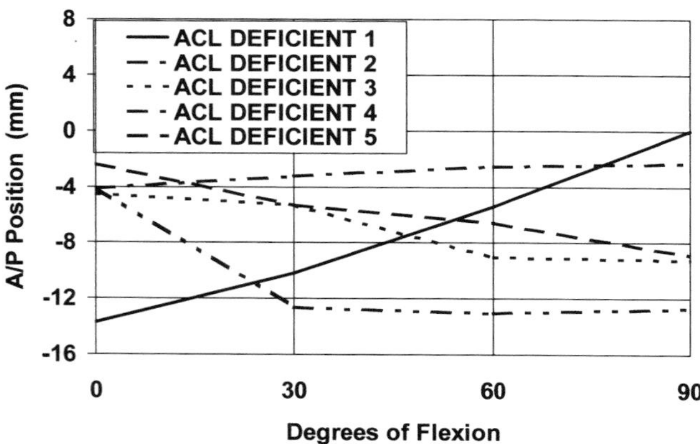

FIGURE 78.5 ➢ Sagittal femorotibial contact positions of five randomly selected anterior cruciate ligament-deficient knees.

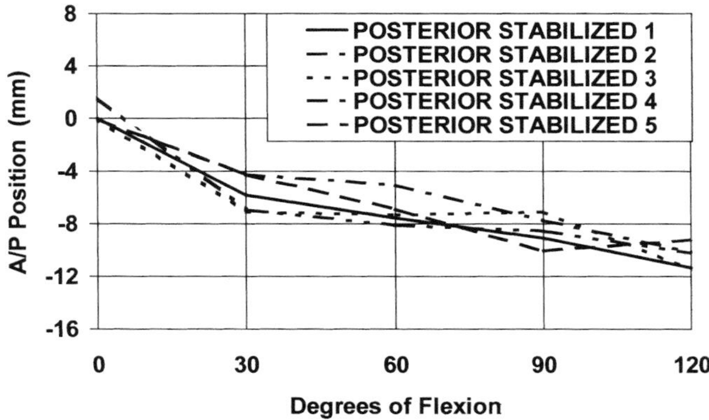

FIGURE 78.7 ➢ Sagittal femorotibial contact positions of five randomly selected posterior stabilized total knee replacements.

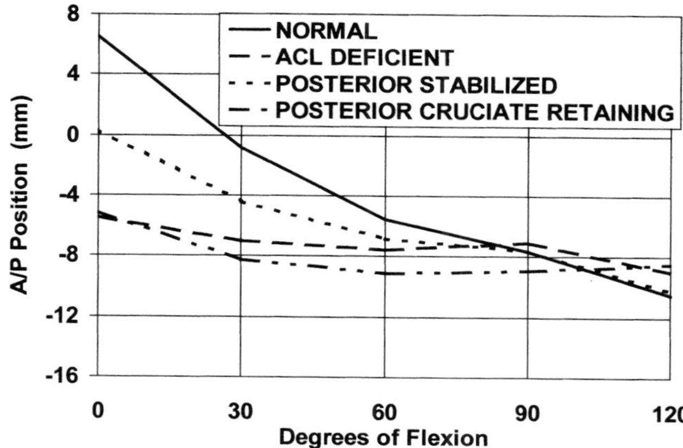

FIGURE 78.8 ➢ Average sagittal femorotibial contact positions of normal, anterior cruciate ligament-deficient, posterior cruciate retaining, and posterior stabilized total knee arthroplasties during a deep knee bend activity.

normal knee kinematics, neither TKA design duplicated the posterior femoral rollback of the normal knee.

A similar analysis of 15 subjects having a PCR TKA and 15 subjects having a PS TKA was performed during gait. The kinematic patterns for both groups were similar. On average, PCR and PS TKA remained posterior during the gait cycle, and neither group demonstrated posterior femoral rollback. Subjects having PCR and PS TKA demonstrated significant anteroposterior translation throughout the stance phase of gait (maximum, PCR = 16.8 mm; PS = 16.3 mm). Because knee flexion is limited during gait, the cam and post mechanism typically does not engage in PS designs. Therefore, similar abnormal anteroposterior translation patterns were observed in both PCR and PS TKA when analyzed during gait.

We also analyzed two MB TKA designs that had polyethylene bearings that were free to rotate or translate relative to the tibial tray (LCS, DePuy Inc., Warsaw, IN).[41] Initially, 20 subjects were analyzed while performing a deep knee bend. Ten subjects were implanted with a PCR (meniscal-bearing) TKA, and 10 subjects were implanted with a posterior cruciate sacrificing (PCS) (rotating-platform) TKA. The subjects having a PCR TKA experienced motions similar to those of the fixed-bearing PCR TKA. As the knee flexed, the medial and lateral condyles would often translate in the anterior direction. The subjects having a PCS TKA experienced a posterior femoral rollback from 0 to 30 degrees of knee flexion but translated in an anterior direction with increased flexion from 30 to 90 degrees. We then performed a second study where 20 subjects having a PCS (rotating-platform) TKA were analyzed during normal gait. The kinematics for each implant were assessed at heel-strike, at 33% and 66% of stance phase, and also at toe-off. On average, both the medial and the lateral condyles remained near the midline of the tibia throughout the weightbearing portion of the gait cycle (Fig. 78.9), which was attributed to the increased sagittal conformity of this MB TKA design.

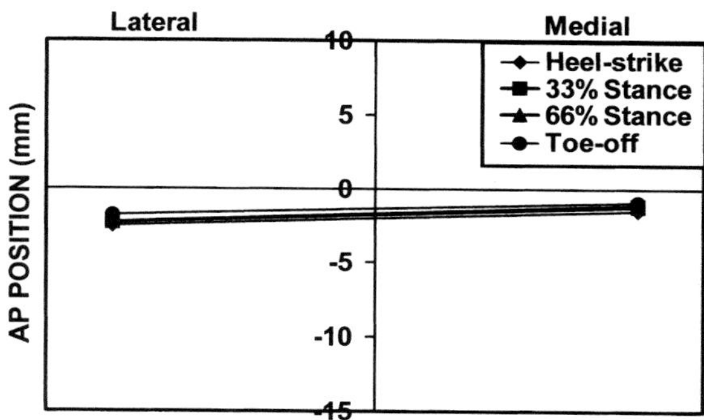

FIGURE 78.9 ➢ Average medial and lateral femorotibial contact patterns of subjects having a rotating platform total knee arthroplasty during gait.

Axial Femorotibial Rotation

We later analyzed subjects implanted with fixed-bearing PS and PCR TKA from an axial perspective, allowing determination of both the medial and the lateral condylar contact patterns. Using this method, axial femorotibial rotation could also be assessed by determining the relative angle between the medial and lateral condyle contact points.[24] On average, the PS-implanted knees experienced rollback of both the medial and the lateral condyles and demonstrated a normal axial femorotibial rotational pattern (Fig. 78.10). The medial condyles translated posteriorly from 0 to 30 degrees of knee flexion but then translated in an anterior direction from 30 to 60 and from 60 to 90 degrees of knee flexion. The lateral condyle translated posteriorly throughout flexion. We speculate that the anterior slide of the medial femoral condyle is a result of axial rotation of the femoral component as it pivots around the tibial post, rather than a paradoxical anterior slide, because it appeared that the cam and post

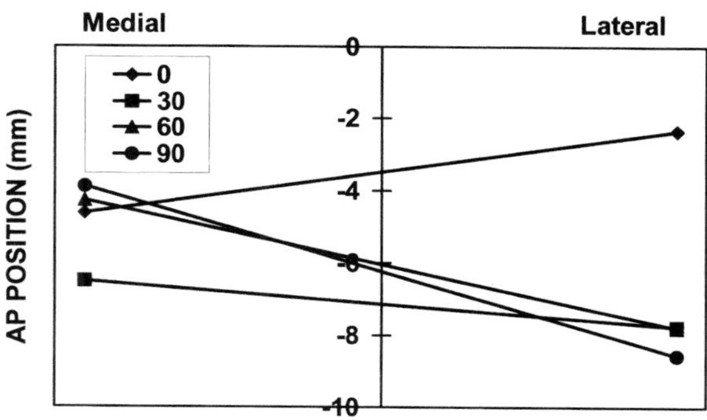

FIGURE 78.10 ➢ Average medial and lateral femorotibial contact patterns of subjects having a posterior stabilized total knee arthroplasty during a deep knee bend.

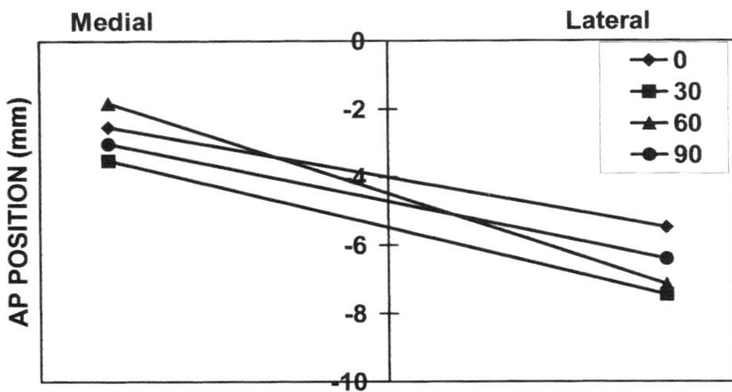

FIGURE 78.11 ➢ Average medial and lateral femorotibial contact patterns of subjects having a posterior cruciate retaining total knee arthroplasty during a deep knee bend.

were engaged and the lateral condyle continued roll in the posterior direction.

On average, the PCR-implanted group did not display a normal axial tibiofemoral rotational pattern.[24] The medial condyle translated posteriorly from 0 to 30 degrees of knee flexion, slid in an anterior direction from 30 to 60 degrees of knee flexion, and translated posteriorly again from 60 to 90 degrees of knee flexion (Fig. 78.11). The lateral condyle experienced a posterior motion from 0 to 30 degrees of knee flexion but translated anteriorly from 30 to 60 and from 60 to 90 degrees of knee flexion, therefore demonstrating a reverse screw home rotational pattern (tibia rotating externally relative to the femur during progressive flexion).

The average amount of axial rotation from full extension to 90 degrees of flexion for subjects in this

TABLE 78.2 AXIAL ROTATION VALUES FOR PCR- AND PS-IMPLANTED KNEES AT VARIOUS FLEXION RANGES

Implant	0 to 30 Degrees	30 to 60 Degrees	60 to 90 Degrees
PCR	1.3	1.8	−2.6*
PS	4.9	3.1	1.8

* Negative numbers denote a reverse screw home rotational pattern at that flexion range.
PCR = posterior cruciate retaining; PS = posterior stabilized.

study was 9.74 and 0.55 degrees for PS- and PCR-implanted knees, respectively (Table 78.2). All 19 subjects having a PS-implanted knee (100%) and 9 of 13 subjects having a PCR-implanted knee (69.2%) exhibited a normal screw home rotational pattern from 0 to 90 degrees of knee flexion. Rotational patterns in both TKA groups were erratic, however, with 10 of 16 subjects with a PS TKA (62.5%) and 10 of 13 subjects with a PCR TKA (76.9%) demonstrating a reverse screw home pattern at one of the three evaluated flexion ranges, most commonly at 60 to 90 degrees of flexion.

Femoral Condylar Lift-Off

Forty subjects were analyzed under fluoroscopic surveillance to assess the incidence of femoral condylar lift-off.[8, 10] Twenty subjects were implanted with a fixed-bearing PCR TKA, and 20 subjects received a PS TKA. Thirty of the 40 subjects (75%) experienced fem-

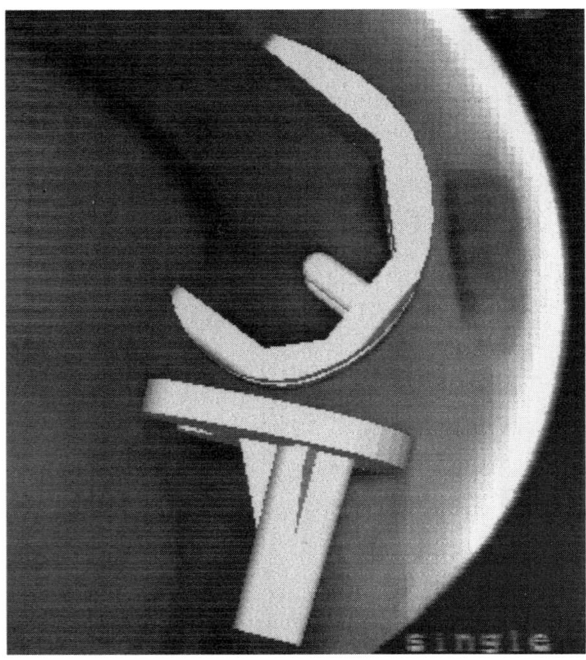

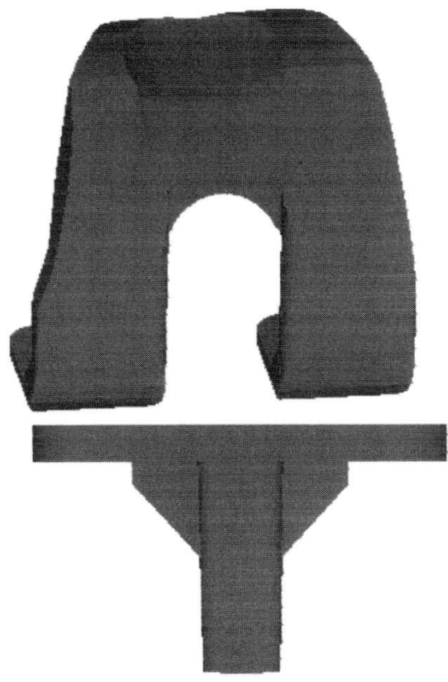

FIGURE 78.12 ➢ Sagittal (*left*) and frontal (*right*) images of a posterior cruciate retaining-implanted knee demonstrating femoral condylar lift-off.

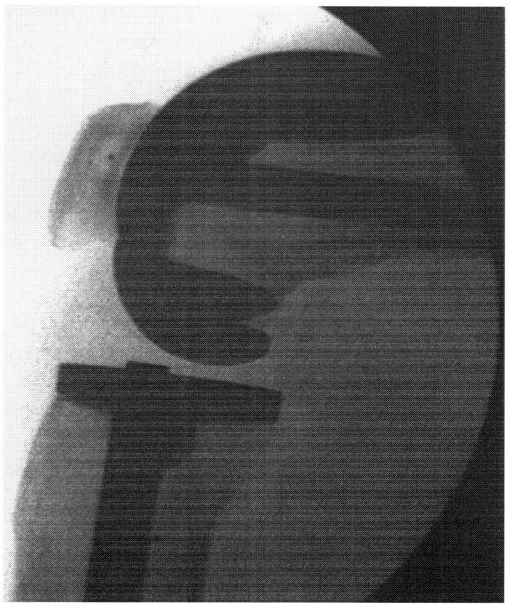

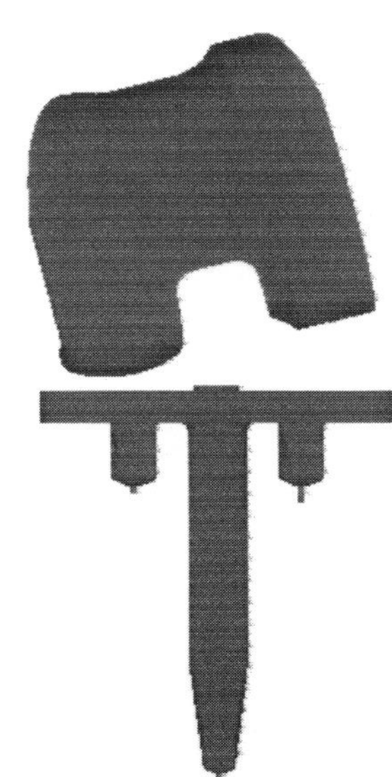

FIGURE 78.13 ➢ Sagittal (*left*) and frontal (*right*) images of a posterior cruciate retaining-implanted knee demonstrating severe femoral condylar lift-off.

oral condylar lift-off during a deep knee bend (Fig. 78.12). Fourteen of the 20 subjects (70%) having a PCR-implanted knee and 16 of the 20 subjects (80%) having a PS-implanted knee experienced femoral condylar lift-off at some increment of knee flexion. Thirteen subjects having a PCR-implanted knee experienced femoral condylar lift-off on their lateral side, and two subjects exhibited medial condylar lift-off. Twelve subjects having a PS-implanted knee experienced femoral condylar lift-off on their lateral side, and nine subjects had medial condylar lift-off. Two subjects having a PCR-implanted knee and five subjects having a PS-implanted knee experienced both medial and lateral femoral condylar lift-off at differing increments of knee flexion. These subjects would lift off from one condyle and then, at a different flexion angle, would reestablish femoral condylar contact on the side that had previously lifted off, but would have condylar lift-off of the opposite femoral condyle. Therefore, during a deep knee bend, these subjects would experience a rocking motion of the knee in the frontal plane.

For both PCR and PS TKA designs, femoral condylar lift-off occurred most commonly at 60 degrees of flexion. The maximum amount of femoral condylar lift-off measured was 1.8 mm for subjects having a PCR-implanted knee and 2.7 mm for subjects implanted with a PS TKA. The mean values for those demonstrating femoral condylar lift-off were 1.2 mm for subjects implanted with PCR TKA and 1.4 mm for those implanted with PS TKA.

Femoral condylar lift-off was also evaluated in subjects having a PCS TKA (MB, rotating platform). Similar to fixed-bearing TKA, 85% of the subjects evaluated having an MB PCS TKA experienced femoral condylar lift-off. The maximum amount of condylar lift-off was 3.5 mm, which occurred during normal gait. Similar to subjects having a fixed-bearing PS TKA, lift-off was determined to occur both medially and laterally.

Although all patients evaluated in the above study were considered clinically excellent, we have also examined other TKAs of various designs with suboptimal function and have observed femoral condylar lift-off as high as 10 mm (Figs. 78.13 and 78.14).

Range of Motion

We have analyzed the in vivo, passive (non-weightbearing), and active (weightbearing) range of motion for patients with normal, PCR-implanted, and PS-implanted knees.[12] All three knee subgroups demonstrated a statistically significant decline in range of motion when measured during weightbearing as compared with non-weightbearing conditions (normal, $p < .045$; PS, $p < .001$; PCR, $p < .001$). This reduction in motion was greatest in the PCR TKA subgroup (20 degree reduction). The normal knee subgroup exhibited superior flexion over both TKA subgroups whether measured under passive, non-weightbearing ($p < .001$) or active, weightbearing conditions ($p < .001$).

The maximum mean postoperative flexion for PCR (123 degrees) and PS (127 degrees) TKA subgroups was similar when evaluated under passive, non-weightbearing conditions ($p > .176$). When measured under weightbearing conditions, patients implanted with PS TKA exhibited significantly greater mean flexion than did those with PCR TKA (113 degrees versus 103 degrees, $p < .024$). This finding occurred despite the fact that the PCR subgroup demonstrated greater knee flexion (118 degrees versus 108 degrees) and had

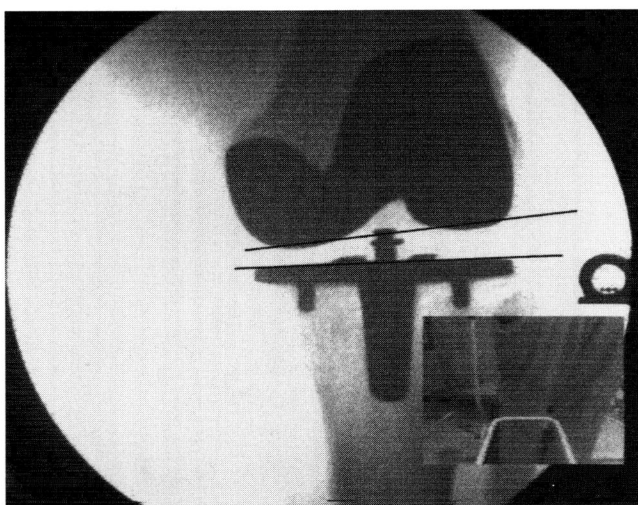

FIGURE 78.14 ➢ Frontal fluoroscopic image of a posterior cruciate retaining-implanted knee demonstrating substantial femoral condylar lift-off.

higher Hospital for Special Surgery (HSS) scores (65.2 points versus 58.7 points) than did the PS subgroup preoperatively and also were of younger age (53.7 years versus 65.5 years), although these differences were not statistically significant.

CLINICAL SIGNIFICANCE

Anteroposterior Translation

The anterior translation of the femur on the tibia observed in the present investigation has numerous, potentially detrimental consequences. First, anterior femoral translation results in a more anterior axis of flexion, lessening maximum knee flexion.[12] Second, the quadriceps moment arm is decreased, resulting in reduced quadriceps efficiency. Last, anterior sliding of the femoral component on the tibial polyethylene surface risks accelerated polyethylene wear. Blunn et al,[4] in a sophisticated laboratory evaluation of polyethylene wear, found dramatically increased polyethylene wear with cyclic sliding as compared with compression or rolling because of increased subsurface shear stresses.

Numerous authors[1, 7, 42] have shown that anteroposterior femorotibial translation is related to the integrity of the cruciate ligaments and the mechanics of the extensor mechanism, particularly in the direction of pull of the patellar ligament and the degree of knee flexion. At lesser degrees of flexion, the direction of the patellar ligament pull is anterior, creating an anterior pull on the tibia. This anteriorly directed shear force on the tibia is normally resisted by the anterior cruciate ligament. At greater degrees of flexion (>45 to 60 degrees), however, the direction of patellar ligament pull on the tibia changes to posterior. This creates a posterior shear force on the tibia, which is normally resisted by tension in the posterior cruciate ligament. This may explain the abnormal posterior contact observed at full extension. At this flexion range, shear stresses on the tibia are directed anteriorly, allowing posterior femorotibial contact to occur because of the absence of the anterior cruciate ligament. Beyond midflexion, the shear forces on the tibia are directed posteriorly, allowing anterior translation of femorotibial contact to occur, possibly because of inadequate function and tension in the posterior cruciate ligament.

Draganich et al[14] found a similar relationship between femorotibial contact position and cruciate ligament integrity. In a cadaveric analysis, they also observed a posterior shift in femorotibial contact after sectioning of the anterior cruciate ligament. After the addition of posterior cruciate ligament sectioning, an anterior shift in femorotibial contact occurred as knee flexion progressed, as was observed in the PCR TKA groups in our analyses.

Axial Femorotibial Rotation

Using our model-fitting process, we determined that normal axial-tibiofemoral rotational patterns are not always present following TKA. Although a mean positive screw home rotational pattern was observed in both TKA groups when analyzed at full extension versus 90 degrees of flexion, average axial rotation was less than that reported for normal knees,[23, 28, 37] particularly in the PCR TKA group (0.55 degrees positive screw home rotation). Additionally, a negative (reverse) screw home pattern was observed in 30.8% (4 of 13) of the PCR TKA group.

Erratic rotational patterns were observed in both TKA design groups, with 62.5% (10 of 16) of subjects with a PS TKA and 76.9% (10 of 13) of those with a PCR TKA demonstrating a negative (reverse) screw home pattern at one of the three evaluated flexion ranges, most commonly at 60 to 90 degrees of flexion (see Table 78.1). The negative screw home pattern found in this analysis may be related, in part, to the abnormal anterior femoral translation laterally during knee flexion observed in our previous kinematic studies of anteroposterior femorotibial translation.[9, 11, 40] The negative (reverse) screw home rotation observed is potentially detrimental, enhancing the risk of patellofemoral instability because of a relative lateralization of the tibial tubercle.

Femoral Condylar Lift-Off

Numerous knee kinematic analyses support the potential occurrence of femoral condylar lift-off in roentgenstereophotogrammetric, cadaveric, or ligament laxity studies,[5, 6, 13, 17, 21, 22, 27, 31, 32, 34-36, 39, 43] Our research has documented that femoral condylar lift-off commonly occurs following both PCR and PS TKA, most commonly at flexion ranges greater than 60 degrees. Lift-off occurred both medially and laterally in subjects with PS TKA but was observed predominantly on the lateral side in those implanted with PCR TKA. This may be related to the presence or absence of the cruciate ligaments. In the knee with intact cruciate ligaments, the anterior cruciate ligament originates at the lateral femoral condyle, whereas the femoral attachment of the posterior cruciate ligament is medial. We theorize, therefore, that the anterior cruciate ligament acts as a "checkrein," limiting the presence of later femoral lift-off, with the posterior cruciate ligament similarly resisting femoral lift-off medially. In PS TKA with both cruciate ligaments resected, the incidence of femoral condylar lift-off was similar both medially and laterally. In PCR TKA, femoral condylar lift-off predominantly occurred laterally, resisting lift-off medially, possibly because of the preservation of the posterior cruciate ligament.

These findings support the importance of coronal femorotibial curvature and conformity in TKA design. Miller et al,[32] in a laboratory analysis, evaluated peak tibial polyethylene stresses under eccentric loading conditions in both flat-on-flat and more coronally curved femorotibial implant geometries. They observed substantially higher polyethylene stresses in flat-on-flat designs, often exceeding the yield strength of polyethylene, whereas designs with increased coronal curvature and conformity proved less sensitive to eccentric loading conditions, with lower peak polyethylene stresses.

Additionally, the results of this study support the use of metal-backed tibial components to reduce peak subchondral cancellous bone loads should femoral condylar lift-off occur. Bartel et al[3] conducted a finite element analysis to determine the effect of metal backing on peak subchondral cancellous stresses. They reported reductions in peak cancellous stresses of 16% to 39% with metal-backed versus all-polyethylene tibial components when evaluated under eccentric loading conditions, as would be present if femoral condylar lift-off occurred.

Range of Motion

Weightbearing range of motion was significantly diminished in all our subjects, presumably resulting from the complex interaction of dynamic muscle forces, soft-tissue constraints, posterior soft-tissue impingement, and articular congruity. Under passive, nonweightbearing conditions, on the other hand, the knee seeks the course of least resistance and may not reflect normal weightbearing articulated motion. The importance of weightbearing in kinematic evaluation of the knee is supported by the work of Hsieh and Walker, who discovered that in the unloaded knee joint, joint laxity is primarily determined by soft-tissue constraints, whereas in the loaded knee joint, the geometric conformity of the joint surfaces is the primary determinant in controlling knee joint laxity.[20]

When tested under weightbearing conditions, patients with PCR TKA exhibited significantly lower postoperative motion than did those with PS TKA. The inferior flexion observed with PCR TKA can be explained by the paradoxical anterior femoral translation occurring with progressive flexion, as previously discussed. This anterior translation of femorotibial contact with progressive flexion may limit maximum flexion because of anteriorization of the axis of flexion, earlier impingement of the posterior soft-tissue structures, and tightening of the extensor mechanism (from anterior femoral displacement). Alternatively, patients implanted with PS TKA demonstrate posterior femoral rollback, dictated by interaction of the femoral cam and tibial post mechanism of the PS design, regardless of weightbearing status.[9]

Because a substantial portion of activities of daily living is performed by subjects under weightbearing conditions, measurement of knee motion in a weightbearing fashion may be a superior method of assessment of functional capabilities.

SUMMARY

The previously described kinematic analyses have demonstrated that numerous kinematic abnormalities are present following TKA. An advantage of the experimental model used is its allowance of analysis under in vivo, weightbearing conditions. The 3-D kinematic method reduces potential error caused by motion between external skin markers and the underlying bone.[29, 33] Methods that allow assessment during dynamic muscle contraction provide a superior estimation of true knee kinematics.[30] Critical evaluation of in vivo, weightbearing kinematic analyses is necessary to develop improvements in implant design and surgical techniques to ultimately increase the durability and longevity of TKA.

References

1. Andriacchi T, Stanwyck T, Galante J: Knee biomechanics and total knee replacement. J Arthroplasty 1:211, 1986.
2. Banks SA, Hodge WA: Accurate measurement of three-dimensional knee replacement kinematics using single plane fluoroscopy. IEEE Trans Biomed Eng 43, 1996.
3. Bartel D, Burstein A, Santavicca E, et al: Performance of the tibial component in total knee replacement. J Bone Joint Surg Am 64:1026, 1982.
4. Blunn G, Walker P, Joshi A, et al: The dominance of cyclic sliding in producing wear in total knee replacements. Clin Orthop 273:253, 1991.
5. Bourne R, et al: In vivo strain distribution in the proximal tibia. Clin Orthop 188:285, 1984.
6. Burgioni D, Andriacchi T, Galante J: A functional and radiographic analysis of the total condylar knee arthroplasty. J Arthroplasty 5:173, 1990.
7. Daniel D, Stone M, Barnett P, et al: Use of the quadriceps active test to diagnose posterior cruciate-ligament disruption and measure posterior laxity of the knee. J Bone Joint Surg Am 70:386, 1988.
8. Dennis D, Komistek R, Cheal C, et al: In vivo determination of femoral condylar lift-off using dynamic fluoroscopic images and an inverse perspective technique, Knee Society-Closed Meeting, Cleveland, OH, 1996.
9. Dennis D, Komistek R, Hoff W, et al: In vivo knee kinematics derived using an inverse perspective technique. Clin Orthop 331:107, 1996.
10. Dennis D, Komistek R, Hoff W, et al: A determination of lateral

condyle lift-off from the tibia plateau using fluoroscopy. European Society of Biomechanics, Belgium, 1996.
11. Dennis D, Komistek R, Colwell C, et al: In vivo anteroposterior femorotibial translation of total knee arthroplasty: A multicenter analysis. Clin Orthop 356:47, 1998.
12. Dennis D, Komistek R, Stiehl J, et al: Range of motion following total knee arthroplasty: The effect of implant design and weight-bearing conditions. J Arthroplasty 13:748, 1998.
13. Dorr L, Ochsner J, Gronley J, et al: Functional comparison of posterior cruciate-retainer versus cruciate sacrificed total knee arthroplasty. Clin Orthop 236:36, 1988.
14. Draganich L, Andriacchi T, Andersson G: Interaction between intrinsic knee mechanics and the knee extensor mechanism. J Orthop Res 5:539, 1987.
15. Fukubayashi T, Torzilli P, Sherman M, et al: An in vitro biomechanical evaluation of anterior-posterior motion of the knee. Tibial displacement, rotation, and torque. J Bone Joint Surg Am 64:258, 1982.
16. Garg A, Walker P: Prediction of total knee motion using a three-dimensional computer-graphics model. J Biomech 23:45, 1990.
17. Goh J, Bose K, Khoo B: Gait analysis study on patients with varus osteoarthritis of the knee. Clin Orthop 294:23, 1993.
18. Grood E, Suntry W: A joint coordinate system for the clinical description of three-dimensional motions: Application to the knee. J Biomech Eng 105:136, 1983.
19. Hoff W, Komistek R, Dennis D, et al: Three-dimensional determination of femoral-tibial contact positions under in vivo conditions using fluoroscopy. Clin Biomech 13:455, 1998.
20. Hsieh H, Walker P: Stabilizing mechanisms of the loaded and unloaded knee joint. J Bone Joint Surg Am 58:87, 1976.
21. Insall J, ed: Surgery of the Knee: Biomechanics of the Knee. New York, Churchill Livingstone, 1984, pp 21–30.
22. Johnson F, Leitl S, Waugh W: The distribution of loads across the knee. A comparison of static and dynamic measurements. J Bone Joint Surg Br 62:346, 1980.
23. Karrholm J, Jonsson H, Nilsson K, et al: Kinematics of successful knee prostheses during weight-bearing: Three-dimensional movements and positions of screw axes in the Tricon-M and Miller-Galante designs. Knee Surg Sports Traumatol Arthrosc 2:50, 1994.
24. Komistek R, Dennis D, Walker S, et al: In vivo analysis of tibiofemoral rotation: Does screwhome rotation occur after TKA? Annual Meeting of the AAOS, New Orleans, LA, 1998.
25. Komistek R, Stiehl J, Dennis D, et al: Mathematical model of the lower extremity joint reaction forces using Kane's method of dynamics. J Biomechanics 31:185, 1998.
26. Komistek R, Dennis D, Mabe J, et al: An in vivo determination of patellofemoral contact positions. Clin Biomech 15:29, 2000.
27. Kostuik J, Harris W, Woodridge C: A study of weight transmission through the knee joint with applied varus and valgus loads. Clin Orthop 108:95, 1975.
28. Kurosawa H, Walker P, Abe S, et al: Geometry and motion of the knee for implant and orthotic design. J Biomech 18:487, 1985.
29. Lafortune M, Cavanagh P, Sommer I III, et al: A three-dimensional kinematics of the human knee during walking. J Biomech 25:347, 1992.
30. Markolf K, Graff-Radford A, Amstutz H: In vivo knee stability. A quantitative assessment using an instrumented clinical testing apparatus. J Bone Joint Surg Am 60:664, 1978.
31. Markolf K, Kochan A, Amstutz H: Measurement of knee stiffness and laxity in patients with documented absence of the anterior cruciate ligament. J Bone Joint Surg Am 66:242, 1984.
32. Miller G, Perry W, Goll C: Congruency and varus/valgus loading effect on prosthetic knee contact stress. San Diego, CA, Combined Orthopedic Research Society, 1995.
33. Murphy M: Geometry and the Kinematics of the Normal Human Knee [Ph D thesis]. Cambridge, MA, Department of Mechanical Engineering, Massachussetts Institute of Technology, 1990.
34. Nilsson K, Kaarholm J: Increased varus-valgus tilting of screw-fixated knee prosthesis. J Arthroplasty 8:529, 1993.
35. Noyes F, Schipplein O, Andriacchi T, et al: The anterior cruciate ligament deficient knee with varus alignment. Amer J Sports Med 20:707, 1992.
36. Prodromos C, Andriacchi T, Galante J: A relationship between gait and clinical changes following high tibial osteotomy. J Bone Joint Surg Am 76:1188, 1985.
37. Reuben H, Rovick J, Schrager R, et al: Three-dimensional dynamic motion analysis of the anterior cruciate ligament deficient knee joint. Am J Sports Med 17:463, 1989.
38. Sarojak M, Hoff W, Komistek R, et al: Utilization of an automated model fitting process to determine kinematics of TKA. ORS Anaheim, CA, 1999.
39. Soudry M, Walker P, Reilly D, et al: Effects of total knee replacement design on femoral-tibial contact conditions. J Arthroplasty 1:35, 1986.
40. Stiehl J, Komistek R, Dennis D, et al: Fluoroscopic analysis of kinematics after posterior cruciate retaining knee arthroplasty. J Bone Joint Surg Br 77:884, 1995.
41. Stiehl J, Dennis D, Komistek R, et al: In vivo kinematic analysis of a mobile bearing total knee prosthesis. Clin Orthop 345:60, 1997.
42. Van Eijden T, DeBoer W, Weijs W: The orientation of the distal part of the quadriceps femoris angle. J Biomech 18:803, 1985.
43. Wang C, Walker P: The effects of flexion and rotation on the length patterns of the ligaments of the knee. J Biomech 6:587, 1973.
44. Whiteside L, Kasselt M, Haynes D: Varus-valgus and rotational instability in rotationally unconstrained total knee arthroplasty. Clin Orthop 219:147, 1987.
45. Whiteside L, Amador D: Rotational stability of a posterior stabilized total knee arthroplasty. Clin Orthop 242:241, 1989.

79

Cementless Total Knee Designs

LEO A. WHITESIDE

Cement use in total knee arthroplasty remains a controversial issue. Many cemented total knee replacement designs introduced through the years have failed and have been removed from the market. Those that remain are the few select designs that have performed reasonably well because of specific design characteristics that include a well-fixed tibial component with an effective stem, multiple sizes of femoral components, a generous curvature on each femoral condyle, and a conforming polyethylene surface with a large articular contact surface area.[17] With the advent of new instruments, these cemented implants, even when placed by inexperienced arthroplastic surgeons, have had a high rate of success. Cement fixation, however, remains a source of consternation for implant designers. Attempts to produce a cemented all-polyethylene tibial component resulted in a loosening rate in excess of 20% at 5 years.[10]

The primary goal of noncemented fixation of total joint arthroplasty is to improve longevity of the implant. Many cementless designs were unsuccessful even at early follow-up periods, but others have been highly successful. In fact, the femoral component in almost all of the cementless designs reliably achieves fixation to bone and is commonly used in hybrid total knee arthroplasty.[20] The tibial component in cementless total knee arthroplasty, as in cemented arthroplasty, has been the greatest source of problems related to fixation because most designs begin with inadequate fixation.

Quality of fixation and load transfer characteristics of the implant-bone interface are two of the most important factors in determining implant longevity. The implants must be designed to apply load in compression to ensure bone hypertrophy and to avoid shear or tensile failure of the interface between the porous surface and base metal. The fixation system must achieve the best immediate fixation possible to allow early weightbearing.

The tibial component has traditionally been considered to present the major load transfer and fixation problems. Adherence of the stem and pegs to the supporting cancellous bone may cause proximal stress shielding as well as high shear stresses at the bone-prosthesis interfaces and high bending stresses in the stem.[30] According to Murase et al[30] in a study of cemented designs, the best configuration to achieve stability and yet avoid proximal stress shielding included a short central stem for toggle control. Tibial component fixation systems without a central stem do not achieve adequate toggle control to prevent liftoff and sinking of the tibial component in response to an eccentrically applied load.[1, 22, 23, 35, 45] Eccentric and tangential loading also cause shear stresses at the interface between the bone and the undersurface of the tray.[13, 19, 20, 27, 29, 46]

Although fixation of the femoral component has generally not been as difficult as that of the tibial component, femoral component design is far from simple. Weightbearing with the knee in extension can generate high shear stresses at the anterior and posterior flange surfaces if the surfaces are adherent to the bone.[44] Weightbearing in flexion can generate high shear stresses at the distal surfaces if the bone is not seated posteriorly and the component is not fixed rigidly against shear loading.[44]

Strain gauge data and clinical radiographic data of the tibial component were in close agreement in a study by Whiteside and Pafford.[55] Low-strain readings around the peripheral rim corresponded to peripheral atrophy seen in the radiographic study, and the area of high-strain readings on the metaphyseal flare corresponded to the area where the hypertrophic cancellous bone joined the metaphyseal cortex. These findings suggested that tibial load-bearing occurs primarily during compression and that the load is transferred through the cancellous bone of the proximal tibia to the cortical bone of the tibial metaphysis, to a certain extent bypassing the proximal peripheral rim of the tibia. The high strain in the anterolateral area of the tibia suggests that the surface fibers of the bone in this area deform to a greater extent than do other areas after total knee arthroplasty. This may be explained by the relatively soft central bone in the anterolateral tibial metaphysis. This softer bone should transfer relatively less of the load, allowing the peripheral surface bone to deform more than other areas.

In the medial condylar area, the bone is denser than in the central condylar area and is therefore more capable of transferring axial load. The radiographic study confirmed this to be a significant clinical pattern.[55] The most likely cause of sinking is inadequate stem fixation that results in compressive failure of the soft cancellous bone in the anterolateral cut surface of the tibia. The sleeve around the tibial stem appeared to control anterolateral sinking of the tibial tray. The relatively soft cancellous bone in the upper surface of the tibia[18] makes this area especially vulnerable to compressive failure, and the need for a stem on the tibial tray to protect this area is abundantly documented in the biomechanical literature. Bartel et al[1] demonstrated in a finite element analysis that prostheses without a stem are likely to sink into the soft areas of the tibial surface when the component is loaded eccentrically. Walker et al[44] and Lewis et al[23] found in separate studies that fixation of the tibial component was best achieved by a rigid tray and central metal stem. Results of the study by Bartel et al[1] also suggest that peripheral contact between the tray and the cortex of the upper tibia would alleviate this problem of sinking. However, the peripheral rim of the proximal tibia does not have a true cortex,[43] and the hardest bone is not arranged around the periphery but instead is usually found on both medial and lateral posterior surfaces and medially just beneath the articular cartilage. Therefore, a finite element model that includes a substantial cortex likely would predict inappropriate benefits from rim contact with the upper tibial surface. All the tibiae in the study that developed sinking of the tibial component had good rim contact.

The load transfer characteristics of the femoral component observed in a clinical radiographic study[55] are predictable from the study by Walker et al[44] on fixation of the femoral component. If the anterior and posterior flange surfaces of the femoral component are bonded to the bone, the femoral shaft transfers weightbearing loads in the form of shear stresses through the flange surfaces during weightbearing in extension, but the load can be transferred to the distal surfaces in the form of compressive stresses if the anterior and posterior flange surfaces are not bonded to bone. Compressive loading is desirable because it encourages ossification at the porous metal-bone interface and promotes hypertrophy of the adjacent cancellous bone. Whiteside and Pafford found it interesting that gaps at the distal surface failed to close and developed a surrounding halo of cancellous bone atrophy, but this is not surprising because the hypertrophy produced by compressive loading on either side of the gap leads to stiffening of the bone and thus increases its ability to transfer load. As the load is transferred in increasing proportion through the hypertrophic bone, the atrophic bone overlying the gap becomes less capable of bearing load, thus transferring more load to the areas that contact the metal surface. It is difficult to see how load sharing and equalization of stresses could be expected to occur, and it is not surprising that gaps, when carefully scrutinized, were seldom seen to close.

Walker et al[44] further predicted that unbonding of the posterior flange surfaces would cause stress relief of these surfaces during weightbearing in flexion. In the study by Whiteside and Pafford,[55] all the specimens showed evidence of greater hypertrophy at the posterior bevel and posterior flange surfaces than at any other surface. The observed pattern of cancellous hypertrophy suggested that the weightbearing loads were transmitted primarily in compression through the cancellous bone and through the interfaces of both components. The smooth posterior femoral flange surface did not appear to prevent posterior femoral condylar hypertrophy. The smooth flange surfaces and the smooth stem and pegs on the femoral component did not appear to bear significant axial load.

The loading pattern of the tibia during normal gait is complex. Although eccentric anterior and posterior loading occurred during weightbearing in flexion and extension in Whiteside and Pafford's[55] study, no attempt was made to quantify this effect. In general, it appeared possible to achieve reliable fixation of the femoral and tibial components without clinically significant stress shielding in either the distal femur or proximal tibia.

Applying a rigid metal tray to a flat surface of cancellous bone does not provide adequate resistance to compressive failure of cancellous bone, liftoff of the opposite side, and toggling micromotion of the component. When early results showed problems with fixation, stems and peripheral screws began to appear on these implant designs. Biomechanical studies clearly indicated that peripheral screws and stems on the tibial component were highly effective and that micromotion of the tray was unacceptably large without these fixation-enhancing features.[28, 42] An aspect of tibial component fixation that is commonly overlooked, but is probably the most important, is the preparation of the upper tibial surface. Small surface irregularities and incongruities can have a devastating effect on fixation, but this aspect of fixation has received little attention in most cementless tibial component designs.

Biomechanical studies have shown that when tibial components are fixed to the bone surface with only short pegs, they sink on the loaded side and lift off on the opposite side.[42] Both stem and screws were effective in controlling sinking and liftoff in the study by Volz et al.[42] Radiographic and histological studies have shown that bone ingrowth into a tibial tray is infrequent,[12] which suggests that micromotion may be unacceptably large. Achieving rigid initial fixation is the most important factor in promoting bone ingrowth. Miura et al[28] evaluated the effect of screws through the tibial tray and a sleeve on the stem to improve tibial component fixation. Bone strength appeared to affect tibial component fixation. It was a major factor in preventing both subsidence and micromotion. Without mechanical fixation, low bone quality was associated with unacceptably large micromovement. The anterolateral portion showed the lowest bone strength in the proximal tibial surface. Hvid and Hansen also reported that bone strength at the anterolateral and intercondylar regions was very low.[16]

In the study by Miura et al,[28] screws were effective in controlling micromovement under axial and sheer loading. When components with screws were compared with those without screws, liftoff was found to be reduced more than 90%. Screws shifted the tilting center lines posteriorly. This finding suggested that the main effect of the screws was to prevent liftoff. Screws also ensured initial bone-implant contact. Miura et al reported that they frequently observed the component to settle on the tibial surface when the screws were tightened. Screws did not eliminate micromotion under axial loads, but they did change the pattern of micromotion. Without screws, micromotion was associated with liftoff and sinking, whereas with screws, sinking and liftoff were minimized, but downward bending of the tray was significantly greater. Although it is uncertain how much micromotion is acceptable while bone ingrowth occurs, it should be minimized as much as possible. A material with elastic modulus similar to that of cancellous bone may be optimal for stress distribution beneath the tibial tray but also may increase the micromotion caused by bending. The results of the study by Miura et al[28] suggest that techniques to lessen bending of the tibial tray minimize micromotion. Mechanisms to prevent bending of the tibial tray might include a material with higher elastic modulus and the addition of an arch to support the tibial tray.

The mechanical effect of a tight stem appeared in the study by Miura et al[28] to improve the keel effect by packing the surrounding soft cancellous bone and thus improving the press-fit effect, increasing the surface area and placing the stem closer to the inner surface of the posterior cortex. Use of a tight stem alone was effective in preventing liftoff and sinking under axial loads, but the use of screws had an overriding effect on sinking and subsidence. Addition of the stem to a screwed-down tibial component had a small (but statistically significant) effect only during liftoff. Location of the tilting axis varied with each specimen and with each group. The effect of screws was to shift the tilting axis posteriorly compared to groups without screws. This is an important mechanical effect and probably is a result of the resistance to liftoff afforded by the screws. It is also the cause of low subsidence found in components fixed with screws. If liftoff was unchecked, the tilting axis shifted toward the point of load application, thus decreasing the area through which the load was transferred. This increased the pressure and aggravated sinking.

Micromotion, as strictly defined in Miura et al's[28] study, was not markedly affected by the use of screws or a tight stem. However, had micromotion been defined as the sum of subsidence (downward or upward) and recoverable motion, the effect of both screws and a stem would have been remarkable. Use of screws or a tight stem alone affected movement of the tray, but a significant additive effect of screws and a stem was also seen in minimizing liftoff.

DESIGN-RELATED FAILURE

Implant material and design features that have occurred coincidentally with cementless total knee replacement designs that are responsible for implant failure are flat polyethylene,[4] heat-pressed polyethylene,[3] and patch porous-coated surfaces.[53] The combination of these features, along with poor quality assurance of polyethylene and gamma irradiation of this material, has caused remarkable wear problems that have led to clinically significant osteolysis.[8, 40, 48, 53] This type of wear and osteolysis is not a function of fixation method; instead, it is caused by design features that incidentally have been associated with cementless fixation.

Tibial Component Design

Inflammatory response to particulate debris has been identified as the primary cause of osteolysis in total knee arthroplasty.[33] Debris contained within the joint minimally affects the surrounding bone, but once it gains access, the osteolytic attack is aggressive. Design features of implants contribute to this phenomenon by the amount of particulate debris released in wear conditions, including the configuration of the porous coating and other modes of joint fluid access to periprosthetic bone, the stability of the locking mechanism that secures the polyethylene articulating surface to the tibial tray, and the amount of intra-articular pressure within the joint.

Smooth metal surfaces that separate pads of porous coating have been shown in experimental and clinical studies to produce metaphyseal and diaphyseal osteolytic lesions by conducting debris into areas of bone that are not protected by the mechanisms that capture wear debris and transfer it to the local lymphatic system.[5, 8, 24, 47, 57] Although these osteolytic lesions have been ascribed to cementless fixation and to the use of screws,[8] they are rare unless the tibial component design includes patch porous coating on the undersurface of the tray, inadequate fixation of the tibial component, and mechanisms that produce large amounts of particulate debris in the knee. As has been seen in cementless total hip arthroplasty, osteolysis occurs when patches of porous coating on the implant are separated by smooth metal surfaces. These smooth metal surfaces form fibrous tissue bridges that conduct polyethylene debris and joint fluid to the diaphyseal endosteal area, where no mechanism exists to diminish the inflammatory response. Porous-coated patches on the Harris-Galante cementless total hip femoral prosthesis appeared to be the cause of a high rate of femoral diaphyseal osteolysis, regardless of method of fixation to bone.[24, 57]

This phenomenon can be explained by a study by Ward et al[47] in which porous coating around the extraosseous portion of proximal tibial prostheses was observed to seal the bone-cement interface from invasion by polyethylene debris, whereas prostheses with smooth surfaces connecting the joint to the bone-cement interface had a high rate of osteolysis and loosening.

This observation also was supported in a laboratory study by Bobyn et al,[5] who reported the effect of porous coating and smooth metal surfaces on migration of particulate debris from the joint cavity in rabbits. Partially porous-coated rods readily conducted polyethylene debris from the knee joint into the medullary canal of the femur, but circumferentially porous-coated rods had bone and tissue penetration into the porous coating that acted as a barrier to migration of the polyethylene debris.

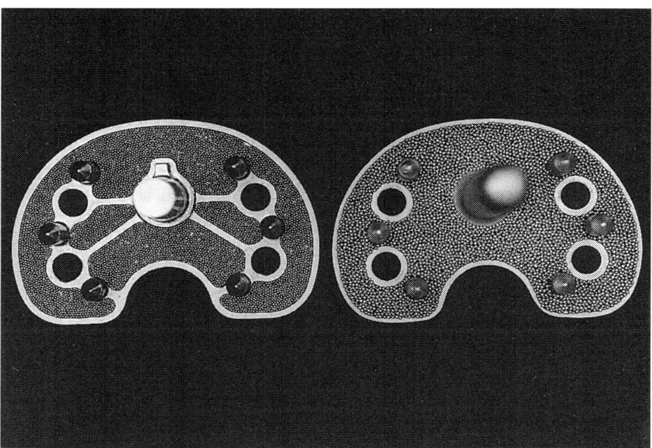

FIGURE 79.1 ➢ Undersurfaces of the Ortholoc Modular (left) and Ortholoc II (right) tibial components. The Ortholoc Modular has smooth metal bridges around the pegs and screw holes that converge on the central stem. Porous coating covers the entire undersurface of the Ortholoc II component. No bridges of smooth metal connect the joint cavity or screw holes to the smooth stem. (From Whiteside LA: Effect of porous-coating configuration on tibial osteolysis after total knee arthroplasty. Clin Orthop 321:93, 1995.)

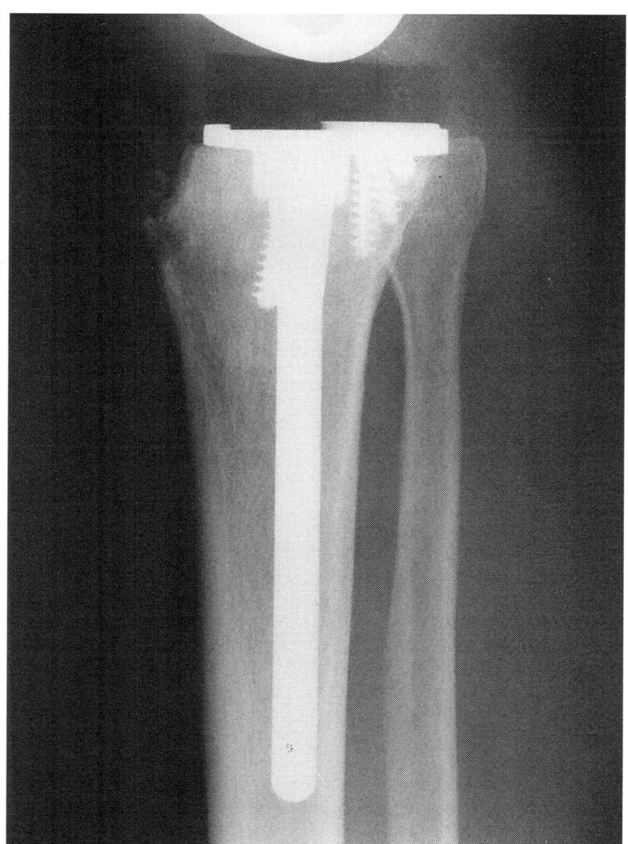

FIGURE 79.2 ➢ Lateral radiograph of an Ortholoc Modular tibial component 1 month after surgery. No sign of osteolysis is evident around the stem, screws, or pegs. (From Whiteside LA: Effect of porous-coating configuration on tibial osteolysis after total knee arthroplasty. Clin Orthop 321:95, 1995.)

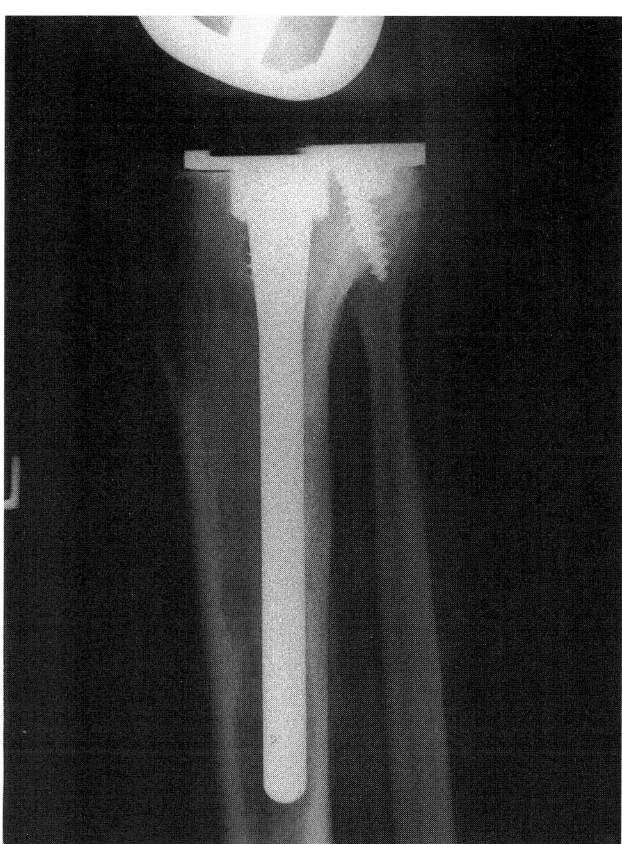

FIGURE 79.3 ➢ Lateral radiograph of an Ortholoc Modular tibial component with osteolysis surrounding the 150-cm stem 2 years after surgery. No evidence of osteolysis is present around the screws or pegs. (From Whiteside LA: Effect of porous-coating configuration on tibial osteolysis after total knee arthroplasty. Clin Orthop 321:95, 1995.)

The Ortholoc Modular tibial component (Wright Medical Technology, Arlington, TN), which has patches of porous coating separated by smooth metal bridges on its undersurface, was clinically compared with the Ortholoc II tibial component (Wright Medical Technology), which has continuous porous coating on the undersurface. The rate of osteolysis was found to be statistically significantly greater in the knees with the patch porous coating design[53] (Fig. 79.1). Osteolysis did not occur around the tibial stem or pegs in 675 patients whose knees were replaced with the Ortholoc II design, but three nonprogressive osteolytic lesions were found around screws on postoperative radiographs. Partial radiolucency was seen beneath the tibial surface in 27 knees. None have been revised for osteolysis.

In contrast, radiographically detectable osteolysis was seen around the tibial stem in 28 (23%) of 124 Ortholoc Modular total knee prostheses with long (150-mm) stems (Figs. 79.2 and 79.3). Of those 28, none had radiographically identifiable osteolysis around the screws or pegs, but 15 (54%) had partial radiolucent lines that extended beneath at least half of the tray on either the anteroposterior or lateral view, and 4 (14%) had radiolucency beneath the entire tibial surface on either radiographic view. An additional 15 (12%) of the 124 knees had radiographically identifiable radiolucency around the stem. Radiographically detectable osteolysis was seen around the tibial stem in 19 (17%) of 112 Ortholoc Modular total knee prostheses with short (75-mm) stems. Thirty (27%) knees had radiolucent lines that extended halfway across the undersurface of the tray, and nine (8%) knees had complete radiolucent lines under the tray on the anteroposterior or lateral radiographic view.

Two Ortholoc Modular knees (one with a short-stem prosthesis, one with a long-stem prosthesis) underwent revision for progressive osteolytic defects around the stem. The knee with a short stem had severe, persistent pain, whereas the knee with a long stem had no pain. Both knees had hypertrophic synovial tissue that filled the cyst around the stem and connected freely with the undersurface of the tibial tray and with the joint cavity, following along the smooth metal surfaces between the porous-coated patches. Histological analysis of the biopsy tissue revealed abundant polyethylene-laden macrophages and free polyethylene particles throughout the tissue, but no metallic debris (Fig. 79.4).

It was postulated that the gasket effect of the continuous porous coating on the Ortholoc II tibial tray prevented access of uncontained polyethylene debris and joint fluid to the surrounding bone. However, in the knees with an Ortholoc Modular component, the smooth metal bridges connecting the screw holes and joint cavity with the stem provided access to migration of fluid and debris to the diaphyseal medullary canal. In the biopsy specimens taken from the two knees that underwent revision, polyethylene debris was present around the stems and in all the osteolytic cysts.

Another group also reviewed the effect of osteolytic attack in cementless total knee arthroplasty and found that smooth metal surfaces provided little resistance to progressive invasion of osteolytic tissue, whereas porous-coated metal interfaces with bone were highly resistant to osteolytic attack.[8]

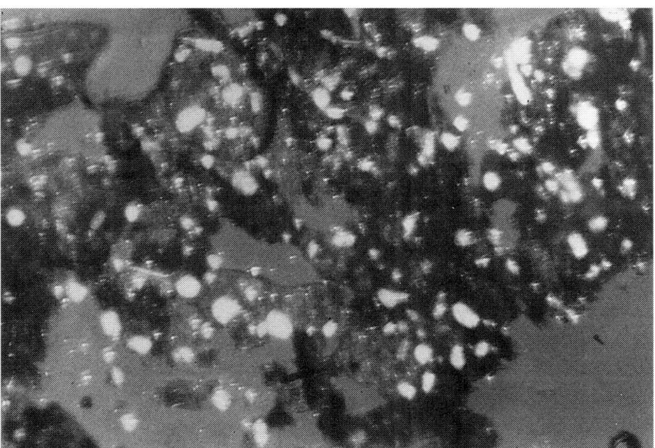

FIGURE 79.4 ➢ Photomicrograph of histological section under polarized light. Abundant polyethylene-laden macrophages and free polyethylene particles are present throughout the tissue. No metal debris could be found. (Original magnification ×100.) (From Whiteside LA: Effect of porous-coating configuration on tibial osteolysis after total knee arthroplasty. Clin Orthop 321:96, 1995.)

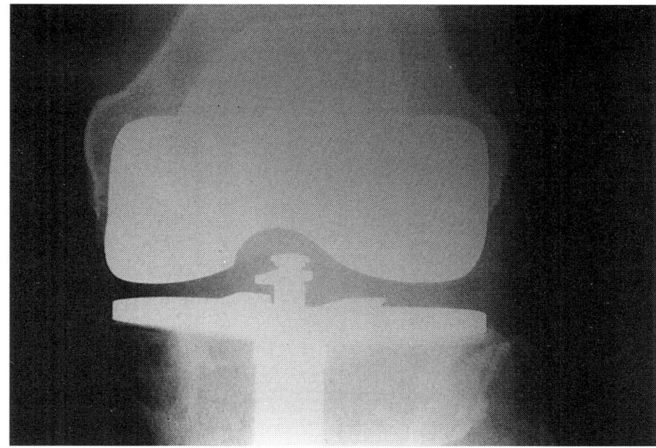

FIGURE 79.5 ➢ Radiograph of a knee with evidence of osteolysis in the femur and tibia. At the time of revision surgery, the locking mechanism of the polyethylene to the tibial component was found to allow at least 1 mm of micromotion between the components, thus creating a pumping action that forced joint fluid into surrounding tissue.

Polyethylene Locking Mechanism

Design of the locking mechanism that secures the polyethylene articulating surface to the tibial component appears to be another factor in migration of debris from the joint to surrounding bone stock. In a study of four failed knee implants (one Synatomic, three AMK; DePuy, Warsaw, IN) retrieved at the time of revision surgery for osteolysis, gross motion of more than 1 mm between the polyethylene piece and metal component was observed. Osteolysis had appeared on radiograph between 18 and 36 months after the original implantation and progressed rapidly (Fig. 79.5). At the time of revision surgery, connection between the joint cavity and the intraosseous cyst was always found at the synovial attachment to the bone in implants fixed with or without screws. The bone-cement interface was eroded severely in the two cemented tibial components. In the two cases in which the prostheses were fixed with cementless technique, the bone-metal interface remained intact, but the synovial fluid and inflamed synovial tissue attacked the bone at the synovial attachment. Severe wear was found in three tibial components, and the cysts were filled with a thick, friable, synovial pannus. The other knee had no visible sign of wear. Pumping of the loose polyethylene appeared to create a wave of synovial fluid that was conducted directly to the capsular attachment to bone.[25]

A laboratory study was undertaken in retrieved knees whose implants were intact to simulate the piston-like motion of a loose locking mechanism and to determine the amount of hydrostatic pressure generated at the interface. Polyethylene articulating components with locking tabs removed were tested first to simulate a loose locking mechanism; then they were exchanged for components with locking tabs intact to simulate a secure locking mechanism. Pressures measured beneath the anteromedial screw hole were nearly the same or higher than intra-articular pressure in the knees with a mobile polyethylene component, whereas pressure beneath the screw hole was a fraction of the intra-articular pressure in knees with a fixed polyethylene component.

Intra-Articular Pressure

In relation to the effect of hydraulic pressures created by a poorly fixed locking mechanism, bone cysts and tissue necrosis are thought to occur as a result of joint fluid forced under high pressure through cartilage defects into the subchondral bone. Intra-articular pressures were measured in the laboratory in 10 normal knees and 10 knees retrieved at autopsy with total knee implants intact. The testing conditions were set to determine whether pressures were high enough during range of motion and with effusion to force reactive joint fluid and particulate debris into surrounding tissues and bone and cause osteolysis. Although the normal and retrieved knees had similar trends in intra-articular pressure throughout range of motion, the retrieved knees had statistically significantly higher intra-articular pressure at every flexion angle except 30 degrees without effusion. Joint pressures were especially high in the suprapatellar and posterior regions of the retrieved knees and required significantly more time to diminish than did the pressures in the normal knees.

Pressures in the retrieved knees occasionally were high enough to cause tissue necrosis and bone cysts, which may suggest a mechanism for osteolytic cyst formation around components even when wear is minimal. These findings suggest that intra-articular pressures can be transmitted to the bone-implant interface and that a poorly fixed polyethylene component can trap synovial fluid and act as a pump to generate high pressures.[7]

Amount or size of particulate debris in the progression of osteolysis therefore does not appear to matter as much as does free access to the joint. In the Ortholoc Modular knees revised for osteolysis, neither had severe polyethylene wear, and the knees with radiographically detectable osteolysis did not appear to have radiographic evidence of severe wear.[53] In the knees retrieved for gross motion between the polyethylene articulating surface and tibial tray, destruction of bone was present even without severe component wear.[25]

Patellar Design

Attempts to produce a metal-backed cementless patellar component led to further problems that were unrelated to a specific method of fixation but were nonetheless attributed to cementless technology. Wear through the polyethylene to the metal backing and subsequent contamination of the articular surface with metal and polyethylene debris led to further damage of already compromised tibial polyethylene components and also to massive osteolysis and loss of bone stock. This cascade of events often is attributed to cementless fixation of the femoral and tibial components, whereas it really indicates that the design concepts and performance of the patellar component were poor. It is clear that the patellar surface is difficult to replace with either a cemented or a cementless component, and use of a metal backing on a thin polyethylene patellar component is a treacherous undertaking.

Femoral Component Design

Fracture of the metal femoral component has rarely been a problem in development of total knee designs, but those that fractured usually were cementless designs that generated excessive stresses through an attempt to conserve bone. Stresses in noncemented knees are different from those generated in knees fixed with cement,[44, 55] and these differences in point and direction of load application may focus high stresses on critical cross-sectional dimensions. Porous coating decreases the strength of metal implants because it thins the cross-sectional dimension, especially at corners and junction areas, where the metal already may be at critical dimensions.

When the Ortholoc II knee femoral component was designed in the mid-1980s, a double porous bead layer was applied to the inner surface for cementless fixation.[54] The design was changed soon after to a single layer of beads to improve strength characteristics. However, within a year of implantation, the manufacturer received reports that fracture of the femoral component had occurred in the design with a double layer of beads, especially those of smaller size (Figs. 79.6 to 79.8). In the author's series of 613 Ortholoc II prostheses with a double bead layer on the femoral component, four fractures occurred. All four implants fractured at the junction between the posterior bevel and the distal surface of the medial femoral condyle.[54]

When a geometric design is shaped with a saw to fit into a curved surface that follows the normal contours of the knee surface, thin sections are formed at the corners. Thin metal at this critical area predisposes the piece to fracture, and porous coating of the inner surface requires that these critical sections be thinned even further. The sintering process can degrade the quality of the base metal itself and thus weaken the implant, and the notch effect caused by the porous coating also can be important in weakening the implant if the porous surface is loaded in tension.

Loads applied to the outer surface of the implant by body weight and muscle force cause bending moments that tend to close the implant and apply tensile stresses to the outer surface. However, loads applied to the inner surface are likely to have the opposite effect. If the anterior and posterior surfaces are not

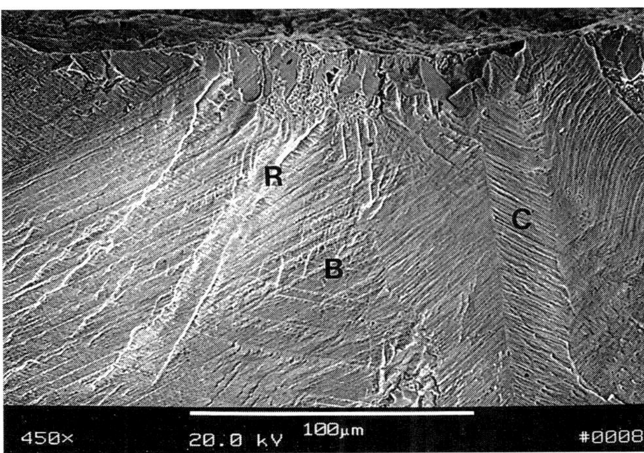

FIGURE 79.6 ➢ Beach marks (B) on the fractured surface of an Ortholoc II femoral component. The concentric beach mark lines converge at a point on the inner surface of the implant where the crack initiated. Radial lines (R) were found on all fractured surfaces. They are oriented in a radial pattern from the point of crack initiation on the inner beaded surface of the component. Chevron zones (C) were found consistently on the fractured surface. These markings are typical of bending fatigue failure. (From Whiteside LA, Fosco DR, Brooks JG Jr: Fracture of the femoral component in cementless total knee arthroplasty. Clin Orthop 286:74, 1993.)

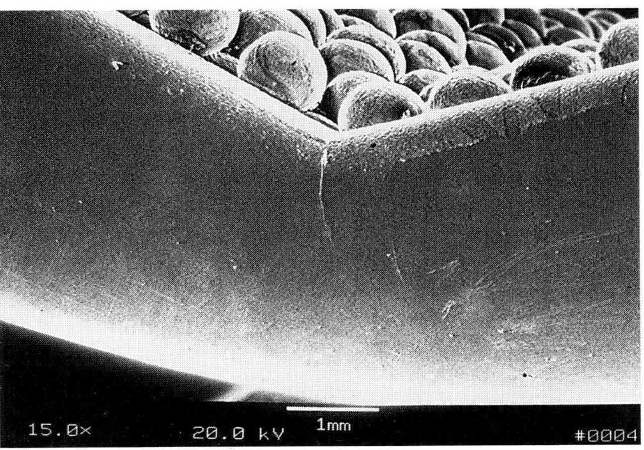

FIGURE 79.7 ➢ A crack originates from the inner beaded surface at the junction between the posterior bevel and distal surface of the nonfractured lateral side in a femoral condyle. (From Whiteside LA, Fosco DR, Brooks JG Jr: Fracture of the femoral component in cementless total knee arthroplasty. Clin Orthop 286:75, 1993.)

allowed to adhere to the bone, load is borne on the distal surfaces preferentially.[44, 55] Because the Ortholoc II femoral component was designed to avoid axial load-bearing by its anterior and posterior flange surfaces, surgical technique that over-resected the distal surface in relation to the bevel surfaces could have resulted in load-bearing exclusively through the inner bevel surfaces. If the implant contacted only the anterior and posterior bevel surfaces and also was not adherent to the surfaces, a wedge would be created, and the femoral component would straighten slightly with weightbearing loads. Application of these cyclic bending loads in the distal portion of the implant probably produced a bending moment that generated tensile load to the inner surfaces.

Surgical bone preparation of the femoral surface for the Ortholoc II implant apparently created a mechanical environment that exposed the porous inner surface to tensile loads. Although the inner surface of the femoral component is generally not considered to be the site of significant tensile stresses, the combination of cementless technique and smaller size of implant predisposed the implants with a double layer of beads to fracture.

INSTRUMENTATION

The instrumentation that has made cemented arthroplasty successful for most surgeons was developed primarily to ensure correct alignment for cementless knee replacement.[15, 49] Aside from instrumentation, many of the principles that resulted in successful cemented knee arthroplasty were not applied to the newer cementless components. Early in the process, developers often stated that implants designed for cemented installation could not simply be porous coated and then used for cementless fixation to bone. In fact, that was exactly what should have been done. Ignoring established criteria of successful total knee arthroplasty design led to experimentation in design that culminated in poor short-term results and in catastrophic long-term results of many of the early cementless knee components. The early failure of cemented tibial components led to extensive research on fixation of the tibial component, and finally the published literature arrived at a consensus that the cancellous bone of the upper tibia was incapable of supporting the tibial component unless an effective stem was incorporated in the design. Nevertheless, the majority of the early cementless designs did not have a stem and also

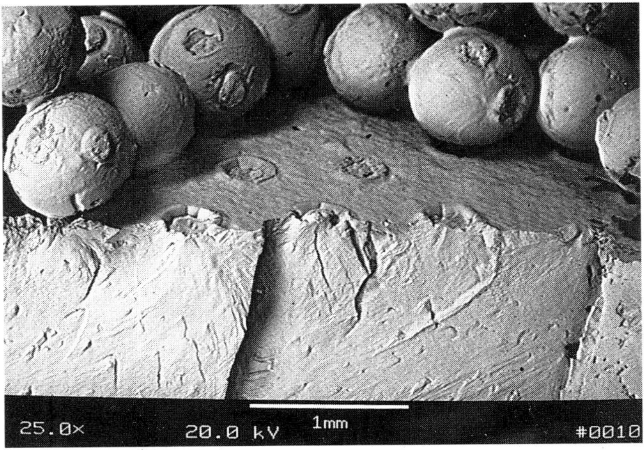

FIGURE 79.8 ➢ Scanning electron micrograph of the inner beaded surface. The fracture joint remnants of several bead craters can be seen. (From Whiteside LA, Fosco DR, Brooks JG Jr: Fracture of the femoral component in cementless total knee arthroplasty. Clin Orthop 286:76, 1993.)

failed to achieve adequate peripheral fixation of the tibial component to the cancellous-cortical structure of the upper tibia. It is not surprising that large numbers of these tibial components loosened and necessitated revision arthroplasty.

RESULTS

Results of cementless total knee replacement since the mid-1980s have proved to be highly dependent on design. Prostheses with excellent fixation of the tibial component, minimal constraint at the articular surface, or both have had very low rates of loosening and have been reliable in all age groups and in cases of inflammatory as well as degenerative arthritic conditions. The rates of 15-year survival of the Ortholoc total knee replacement[52] and the LCS (DePuy)[6] are similar in terms of loosening and wear. The Natural Knee (Intermedics Orthopaedics, Austin, TX) also has continued to deliver excellent clinical results with cementless fixation techniques.[14] The Performance total knee design (Biomet, Warsaw, IN) and the PFC total knee design (Johnson and Johnson Orthopaedics, Raynham, MA) have been reported to perform similarly when fixed with cemented or osteointegrated techniques. These five knee systems have varying combinations of excellent initial fixation, low articular surface constraint, and precise preparation of the upper tibial surface.

A study of 10-year results with cemented and cementless technique with the use of the AGC (Biomet) knee implant revealed no difference in loosening, pain, and knee scores with the two fixation methods. It is important to note in this study that the most difficult patients—young, active male patients—all underwent cementless technique.[2] The PFC knee design was evaluated in a randomized, prospective study comparing cemented and cementless fixation.[26] Clinical performances were virtually identical, but radiolucent lines were found to be significantly more likely to occur in cemented components. The status of cementless total knee arthroplasty is now at the same point as was cemented total knee arthroplasty 10 to 15 years after its introduction. The design characteristics that consistently lead to success are now well known, and the surgical procedure is effective when performed by surgeons who are expert in its use.

Cemented total knee replacement is fairly consistently successful but has not yet become standardized. Some authors recommend superficial penetration of cement into the surface of the bone,[17] whereas others recommend deep penetration. Some authors recommend cementing only the tibial component,[21] whereas others recommend that all components be cemented.[17] Although many reports of excellent long-term results with cemented all-polyethylene tibial components are available in the literature, efforts to design an all-polyethylene tibial component that is reliable with full cement technique have been fraught with fixation problems. One clinical review reported that 18% of patients had to undergo revision or experienced gross loosening 1 year after surgery.[10] Although this finding may be related to the articular surface design and to the flatness of the femoral component surface, the reasons have not been fully established, and there may be other subtle features of cemented total knee replacement design that make it less than completely reliable.

Close evaluation of published long-term results indicate a rapid fall in prosthetic survival rate after 10 years in service.[31, 34] This is especially true in heavy, active patients, who begin to show radiographic evidence of failure as early as 4 years after surgery.[34] One group reported a good 10-year survival rate (approximately 94%) when revision for loosening was considered the endpoint, but when the endpoint represented moderate pain, loosening, or revision, the survival rate dropped to 84% at 10 years.[31] Worsening results in their series over the 10-year period were caused by progressively increasing pain, instability, and deformity. This suggests that the implants gradually loosen, move, and migrate. This explanation was supported in a report on motion of the tibial component of radiographically intact cemented total condylar knee arthroplasties.[36] In this study, 27 cemented knee arthroplasties were evaluated for motion between the tibial component and bone during varus-valgus stress testing. The least amount of motion was 0.2 mm, and the greatest was 2.1 mm. All knees had detectable motion between the cement and bone.

Because the bone-cement interface is subject to progressive osteolytic attack, and because this attack is especially rapid in cement interfaces with cancellous bone, as is the case with the acetabular component in total hip arthroplasty,[39] it is not unlikely that the bone-cement interface in total knee arthroplasty is undermined during the first few years and develops a fibrous tissue interface without surrounding sclerotic margin. Early studies comparing migration of cemented implants to that of cementless ones implanted by means of the radiostereophotogrammetry technique revealed less migration in cemented components. But as these studies progress and as the more effective cementless tibial component techniques are evaluated, it appears that progressive migration is minimized as reliably with cementless technique when stem and screws are used.[37] Reports comparing current cementless technique to cemented fixation of the tibial component showed progressive migration of the cemented components over the 5-year observation period, whereas the cementless implants ceased to migrate during the first year.[32]

CEMENTLESS REVISION AND BONE RECONSTRUCTION IN TOTAL KNEE REPLACEMENT

Of the few modern-design cementless implants that require revision, few require major bone grafting or cementing to restore bone stock and achieve stability.[56] The bone-implant interface has been remarkably benign, even in cases with severe patellar wear and massive contamination of the joint by metal and particulate polyethylene debris.

In patients who have massive bone loss, cementless

technique has been used successfully in revision arthroplasty of previously cemented or noncemented knees.[38, 50, 51, 56] Bone deficit has been managed with block and morselized grafting techniques in combination with various implant systems. Although larger defects are commonly thought to require a block allograft and a specially designed prosthesis,[41] a high rate of success has been reported with morselized graft and a regular prosthesis.[38, 50, 51, 56]

Although it seems that bone loss around the knee joint would cause irreversible laxity and chronic instability, it is possible to restore the joint surface in relation to the ligament attachments. However, injury and chronic deformity usually do cause adaptive changes of the fibrous tissue structures about the knee so that reconstruction of the femur and tibia to their original lengths may not be possible. As in knees with prolonged flexion contracture, permanent shortening of the posterior capsular structures occurs in a failing joint to accommodate the sinking implants; therefore, restoration of the joint surfaces to their original lengths requires in situ reconstruction.

When total knee arthroplasty fails, the cancellous bone in the distal femur and proximal tibia has usually been damaged severely or destroyed completely, leaving a sclerotic shell with large peripheral deficits. In most cases, however, enough diaphyseal cortical structure remains intact above and below the knee that implants with long stems can be used to engage this bone. Articular surfaces then can be augmented to rest on the rim of the deficient femoral and tibial metaphyses. The capsular ligaments can be tensioned so that constrained implants seldom are necessary.

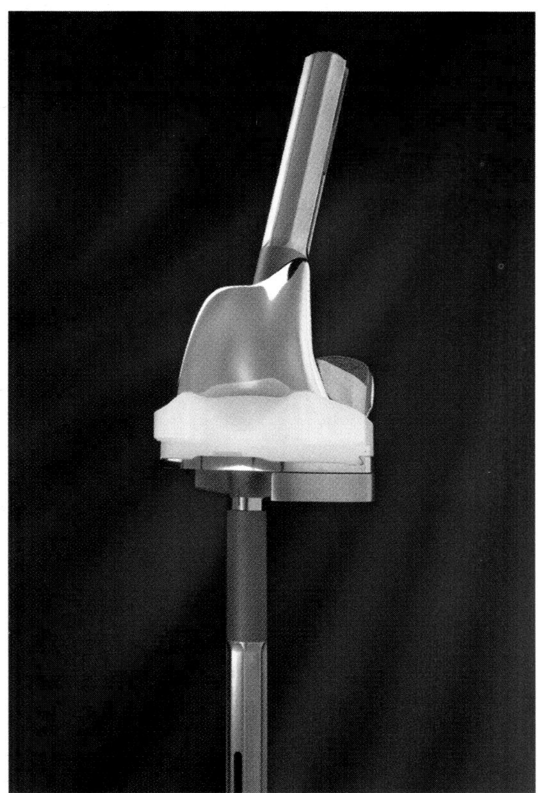

FIGURE 79.9 ➢ The Profix revision total knee replacement system (Smith and Nephew, Inc., Memphis, TN) features femoral and tibial components with a long stem for stability, posterodistal and distal-only wedges on the femoral component for severe structural bone loss, and conforming polyethylene with anterior build-up for anteroposterior stability.

Operative Procedure

The operative procedure includes complete removal of the implant and cement, débridement of the reactive membrane, and curettage to expose viable bone at all accessible surfaces. The medullary canals of the femur and tibia are reamed to accept an implant with a stem length of at least 150 mm and are fit tightly into the diaphyseal isthmus over a 2- to 4-cm length. The metaphyseal bone surface is prepared to accept seating of the femoral and tibial components over at least 25% of the rim circumference, and an effort is made to seat the femoral component posteriorly against substantial bone structure. Three thicknesses of femoral component are generally available for each size of implant in modern revision total knee arthroplasty systems, as are tibial thicknesses from 10 to 35 mm (Fig. 79.9). Posteriorly thickened femoral components make it possible to seat the implant posteriorly on bone so that linked hinges or highly constrained systems are not necessary to achieve stability.

Bone Grafting Procedure

Fresh-frozen allograft with morsels measuring 0.5 to 1 cm in diameter is soaked for 5 to 10 minutes in normal saline with a concentration of polymyxin, 500,000 U; bacitracin, 50,000 U; and cefazolin, 1 g/L. Ten milliliters of powdered demineralized cancellous bone are added to each 30 mL of fresh frozen cancellous allograft. The bone defects are packed with this mixture, and the implants are impacted to seat on the remnant of viable bone while the morselized bone graft is compacted.

Clinical Results

In a clinical review of 62 patients using this operative and bone grafting treatment program, all patients except one had a significant improvement in postoperative pain scores in comparison with preoperative scores, and 82.6% of patients were pain free at the 1-year postoperative follow-up visit (Figs. 79.10 to 79.12). Although the complication rate was high (22.5% of patients required repeated surgical treatment), only two patients required repeated revision for implant loosening. Pain was eliminated in one patient and was reduced to mild in the other.[56]

Rationale

Cancellous and cortical bone loss after failure of total knee arthroplasty necessitates replacement with allo-

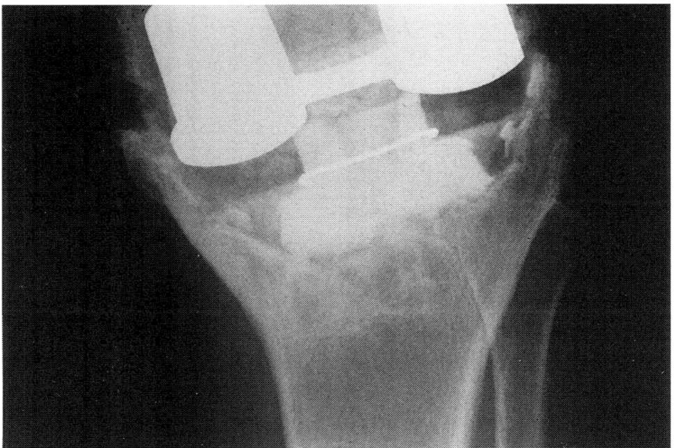

FIGURE 79.10 ➢ Preoperative radiograph of a left knee with a failed cemented component. Massive central and peripheral bone loss has occurred. (From Whiteside LA, Bicalho PS: Radiologic and histologic analysis of morselized allograft in revision total knee replacement. Clin Orthop 357:152, 1998.)

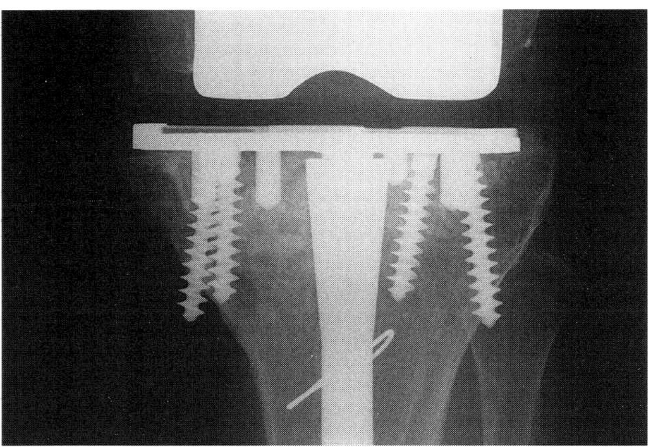

FIGURE 79.12 ➢ Radiograph, 7 years after surgery, of the knee shown in Figure 79.10. The graft has ossified, and trabecular bone is evident along the medial side of the tibia. (From Whiteside LA, Bicalho PS: Radiologic and histologic analysis of morselized allograft in revision total knee replacement. Clin Orthop 357:152, 1998.)

graft, and although block allografts have been advocated for such large deficits, the described morselized grafting technique obviates the more expensive, prolonged, and complicated block operation. Use of morselized allograft was developed in conjunction with stem-stabilized augmented implants that allowed rigid fixation and adjustment of joint surface position, and it was found that revision for loosening was seldom needed.[50, 51] The ready availability of morselized allograft and its history of clinical success led to its use for reconstruction of bone defects. Granulated allograft bone that is smaller than the 0.5- to 1-cm pieces advocated is often resorbed and removed by the inflammatory process.[11] Pieces larger than those advocated are much more difficult to construct, slower to ossify, and slower to incorporate.[9] Rapid healing and ossification occurred in the reported series, probably because the implants were stable and the allograft was surrounded by viable bone[56] (Figs. 79.13 to 79.16).

Although morselized cancellous allograft is osteoconductive rather than osteoinductive, it can serve as a scaffolding for new bone formation. The demineralized bone added to the morselized allograft provides the osteoinductive stimulus and probably augments healing of failed hinge cases in which massive defects are encountered. Bone formation appears to begin early and progresses slowly through the first 18 months to 2 years. Findings from the biopsy specimens taken from patients undergoing this treatment program suggest that the graft is fully mature by 3 years after surgery.[56]

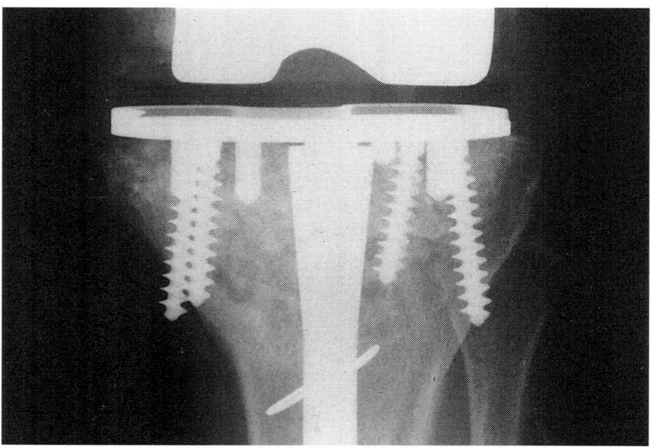

FIGURE 79.11 ➢ Radiograph, 1 month after surgery, of the knee shown in Figure 79.10. Tibial grafting with morselized allograft fills the defect. The lateral edge of the tibial tray is resting on bone. The stem prevents the medial edge from sinking into the allograft. (From Whiteside LA, Bicalho PS: Radiologic and histologic analysis of morselized allograft in revision total knee replacement. Clin Orthop 357:152, 1998.)

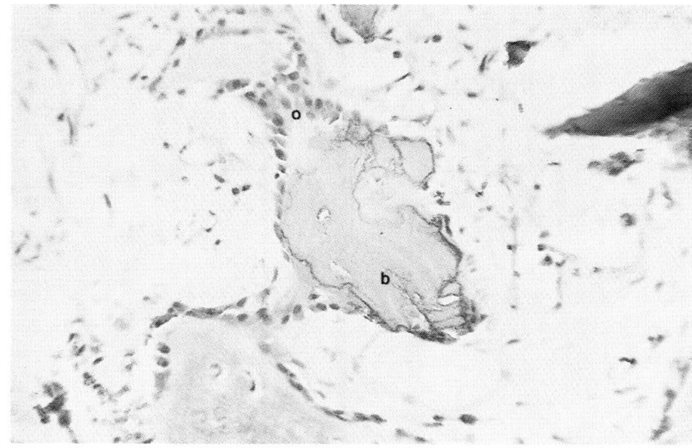

FIGURE 79.13 ➢ Photograph of histological section from a 3-week postoperative biopsy specimen. Granules of demineralized bone (b) are visible surrounded by plump osteoblasts (o) and new osteoid. Vascular stroma is present throughout the allografted area. There is no histological evidence of bone resorption. (Stain, hematoxylin and eosin; original magnification ×160.) (From Whiteside LA: Results: Cementless. In Rorabeck CH, Engh GA, eds: Revision Total Knee Arthroplasty. Baltimore, Williams & Wilkins, 1997, p 456.)

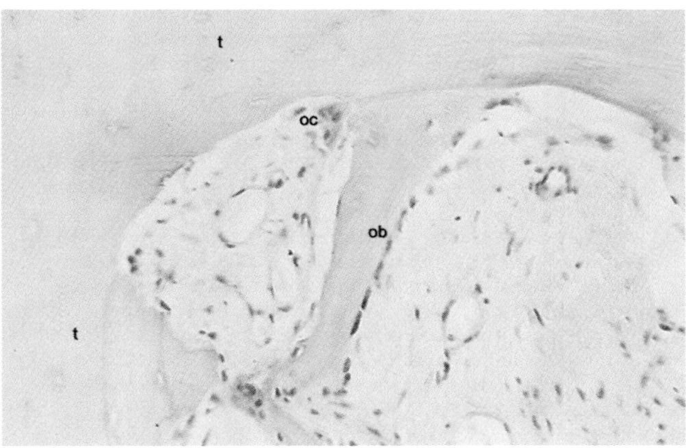

FIGURE 79.14 ➢ Photograph of histological section from a 3-month biopsy specimen. Dead trabeculae (t) are still abundant. Osteoclasts (oc) and new osteoid with osteoblasts (ob) are evident adjacent to the allograft. The allografted area contains multiple sites of bone resorption. New osteoid is often found on one surface of a trabecula, and osteoclastic resorption is found on the opposite surface. Osteoblasts at this interval are flatter and less numerous than in the 3-week biopsy specimen. (Stain, hematoxylin and eosin; original magnification ×160.) (From Whiteside LA: Results: Cementless. In Rorabeck CH, Engh GA, eds: Revision Total Knee Arthroplasty. Baltimore, Williams & Wilkins, 1997, p 456.)

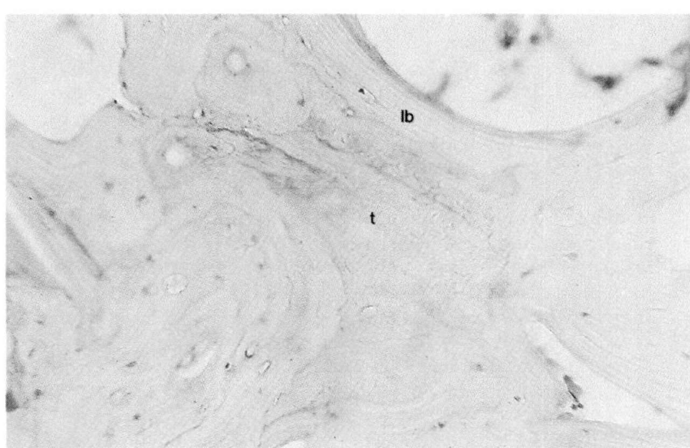

FIGURE 79.16 ➢ Photograph of histological section from a 37-month biopsy specimen. Entombed trabeculae (t) are present throughout the allograft. The visible allograft is encased completely by mature lamellar bone (lb). Bone remodeling continues at normal levels. Few osteoclasts are found, and there is minimal evidence of osteoblastic activity. (Stain, hematoxylin and eosin; original magnification ×100.) (From Whiteside LA: Results: Cementless. In Rorabeck CH, Engh GA, eds: Revision Total Knee Arthroplasty. Baltimore, Williams & Wilkins, 1997, p 457.)

Most of the bone visible in the grafted areas is a combination of entombed allograft trabeculae and new lamellar bone. This information indicates that bone graft healing and maturation of morselized cancellous allograft fortified with demineralized bone powder is similar to the mechanism of fracture callus formation. Structurally reliable bone is produced to support the implant and can be relied upon in the event that a revision operation is required.

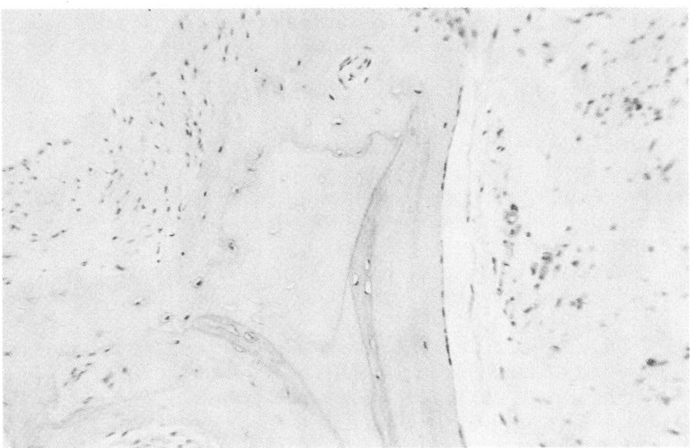

FIGURE 79.15 ➢ Photograph of histological section from a 21-month biopsy specimen. Mature lamellar bone and disorganized woven bone surround the allograft. The bone remodeling rate in the allografted area has decreased significantly. Trabeculae now are entombed completely by mature or woven bone. Bone remodeling has decreased, and osteoblastic or osteoclastic activity is directed toward new bone, not toward the allograft. (Stain, hematoxylin and eosin; original magnification ×100.) (From Whiteside LA: Results: Cementless. In Rorabeck CH, Engh GA, eds: Revision Total Knee Arthroplasty. Baltimore, Williams & Wilkins, 1997, p 457.)

SUMMARY

After 20 years of clinical experience with cementless total knee replacement, it can be recommended without reservation. A cementless total knee replacement operation can be performed quickly and effectively, the results are reliable and durable, and complications are relatively easy to handle. In cases of revision total knee arthroplasty, cementless technique can be used if certain issues are addressed. Adequate rigidity of fixation must be achieved with long-stemmed implants seated on structurally reliable bone and placed atop bone graft material with osteoinductive properties. Massive cementing is not necessary even in the presence of severe metaphyseal bone loss in the femur and tibia, provided that a rigidly fixed diaphyseal stem is used.

References

1. Bartel DL, Burstein AH, Santavirta EA, et al: Performance of the tibial component in total knee replacement. J Bone Joint Surg Am 64:1026, 1982.
2. Bassett RW: Results of 1000 Performance knees: Cementless versus cemented fixation. J Arthroplasty 13:409, 1998.
3. Bloebaum RD, Nelson K, Dorr LD, et al: Investigation of early surface delamination observed in retrieved heat-pressed tibial inserts. Clin Orthop 269:120, 1991.
4. Blunn GW, Walker PS, Joshi A, et al: The dominance of cyclic sliding in producing wear in total knee replacements. Clin Orthop 273:253, 1991.
5. Bobyn JD, Jacobs JJ, Tanzer M, et al: The susceptibility of smooth implant surfaces to peri-implant fibrosis and migration of polyethylene wear debris. Clin Orthop 311:21, 1995.
6. Buechel FF, Rosa RA, Pappas MJ: A metal-backed, rotating-bearing patellar prosthesis to lower contact stress. Clin Orthop 248: 34, 1989.
7. Emoto G, DeWeese FT, Arizono T, et al: Comparison of intraarticular pressure in normal and retrieved specimens and its effect

on effusion volume and flexion angle. Proc Am Acad Orthop Surgeons 1:249, 1999.
8. Engh GA, Dwyer KA, Hanes CK: Polyethylene wear of metal-backed tibial components in total and unicompartmental knee prostheses. J Bone Joint Surg Br 74:9, 1992.
9. Enneking WF, Mindell ER: Observations on massive retrieved human allografts. J Bone Joint Surg Am 7:1123, 1991.
10. Faris PM, Ritter MA, Meding JB, et al: Minimum two year clinical evaluation and finite element evaluation of a flat all polyethylene tibial component. Orthop Trans 19:387, 1995.
11. Friedlander GE: Current concepts review: Bone grafts. J Bone Joint Surg Am 69:786, 1987.
12. Haddad RJ, Cook SD, Thomas KA, et al: Histologic and microradiographic analysis of noncemented retrieved PCA knee components. Presented at the 53rd Annual Meeting of the American Academy of Orthopaedic Surgeons, New Orleans, LA, Feb. 20–25, 1986.
13. Harrington IJ: A bioengineering analysis of force actions at the knee in normal and pathological gait. Biomed Eng 11:167, 1976.
14. Hofmann AA, Murdock LE, Wyatt RWB, et al: Total knee arthroplasty. Two- to four-year experience using an asymmetric tibial tray and a deep trochlear-grooved femoral component. Clin Orthop 269:78, 1991.
15. Hungerford DS, Kenna RV: Preliminary experiences with a total knee prosthesis with porous coating used without cement. Clin Orthop 176:95, 1983.
16. Hvid I, Hansen SL: Trabecular bone strength patterns at the proximal tibial epiphysis. J Orthop Res 3:462, 1985.
17. Insall JN, Tria AJ, Scott WN: The total condylar knee prosthesis: The first 5 years. Clin Orthop 145:68, 1979.
18. Johnson JA, Krug WH, Nahon D, et al: An evaluation of the load bearing capability of the cancellous proximal tibia with special interest in the design of knee implants. Trans Orthop Res Soc 8: 403, 1983.
19. Kagan A: Mechanical causes of loosening in knee joint replacement. J Biomech 10:387, 1977.
20. Kenna RV, Hedley AK, Hungerford DS, et al: The PCA total hip system (Technical Monograph). Harrington Arthritis Research Foundation, 1984.
21. Kobs JK, Lachiewicz PF: Hybrid total knee arthroplasty. Two- to five-year results using the Miller-Galante prosthesis. Clin Orthop 286:78, 1993.
22. Kostuik JP, Schmidt O, Harris WR, et al: A study of weight transmission through the knee joint with applied varus and valgus loads. Clin Orthop 108:95, 1975.
23. Lewis JL, Askew MJ, Jaycox DP: A comparative evaluation of tibial component designs of total knee prosthesis. J Bone Joint Surg Am 64:129, 1982.
24. Maloney WJ, Jasty M, Harris WH, et al: Endosteal erosion in association with stable uncemented femoral components. J Bone Joint Surg Am 72:1025, 1990.
25. Martin JW, Whiteside LA: Osteolysis associated with mobile polyethylene components in total hip and total knee arthroplasty. Orthop Trans 21; 243. 1997;
26. McCaskie AW, Deehan DJ, Green TP, et al: Randomised, prospective study comparing cemented and cementless total knee replacement. J Bone Joint Surg Br 80:971, 1998.
27. Minns RJ: Forces at the knee joint: Anatomical considerations. J Biomech 14:633, 1980.
28. Miura H, Whiteside LA, Easley JC, et al: Effects of screws and a sleeve on initial fixation in uncemented total knee tibial components. Clin Orthop 259:160, 1990.
29. Morrison JB: The mechanics of the knee joint in relation to normal walking. J Biomech 3:51, 1970.
30. Murase K, Crowninshield RD, Pedersen DR, et al: An analysis of tibial component design in total knee arthroplasty. J Biomech 16:13, 1982.
31. Nelissen RGHH, Brand R, Rozing PM: Survivorship analysis in total condylar knee arthroplasty. J Bone Joint Surg Am 74:383, 1992.
32. Nilsson KG, Karrholm J: Increased varus-valgus tilting of screw-fixated knee prostheses: Stereoradiographic study of uncemented versus cemented tibial components. J Arthroplasty 8: 529, 1993.
33. Oishi CS, Walker RH, Colwell CW Jr: The femoral component in total hip arthroplasty. J Bone Joint Surg Am 76:1130, 1994.
34. Ranawat CS, Flynn WF, Saddler S, et al: Long-term results of the total condylar knee arthroplasty: A 15-year survivorship study. Clin Orthop 286:94, 1993.
35. Rosenqvist R, Bylander B, Knutson K, et al: Loosening of the porous coating of bicompartmental prostheses in patients with rheumatoid arthritis. J Bone Joint Surg Am 68:538, 1986.
36. Ryd L, Lindstrand A, Rosenquist R, et al: Micromotion of conventionally cemented all-polyethylene tibial components in total knee replacements. Arch Orthop Trauma Surg 106:82, 1987.
37. Ryd L: The role of roentgen stereophotogrammetric analysis (RSA) in knee surgery. Am J Knee Surg 5:44, 1992.
38. Samuelson K: Bone grafting and noncemented revision arthroplasty of the knee. Clin Orthop 226:93, 1988.
39. Schmalzried TP, Kwong LM, Jasty M, et al: The mechanism of loosening of cemented acetabular components in total hip arthroplasty. Clin Orthop 274:60, 1992.
40. Tanner MG, Whiteside LA, White SE: Effect of polyethylene quality on wear in total knee arthroplasty. Clin Orthop 317:83, 1995.
41. Tsahakis PJ, Beaver WB, Brick GW: Technique and results of allograft reconstruction in revision total knee arthroplasty. Clin Orthop 303:86, 1994.
42. Volz RG, Nisbet J, Lee R, et al: The mechanical stability of various noncemented tibial components. Clin Orthop 226:38, 1988.
43. Walker PS, Soudry M, Ewald FC, et al: Control of cement penetration in total knee arthroplasty. Clin Orthop 185:155, 1984.
44. Walker PS, Granholm J, Lowrey R: The fixation of femoral components of condylar knee prostheses. Eng Med 11:135, 1982.
45. Walker PS, Greene D, Reilly D, et al: Fixation of tibial components of knee prostheses. J Bone Joint Surg Am 63:258, 1981.
46. Walker PS, Hajek JV: The load bearing area in the knee joint. J Biomech 5:581, 1972.
47. Ward WG, Johnson KS, Dorey FJ, et al: Extramedullary porous coating to prevent diaphyseal osteolysis and radiolucent lines around proximal tibial replacements. J Bone Joint Surg Am 75: 976, 1993.
48. White SE, Tanner MG, Whiteside LA: Effects of sterilization on wear in total knee arthroplasty. Clin Orthop 331:164, 1996.
49. Whiteside LA, Summers RG: Anatomical landmarks for an intramedullary alignment system for total knee replacement. Orthop Trans 7:546, 1983.
50. Whiteside LA: Cementless reconstruction of massive tibial bone loss in revision total knee arthroplasty. Clin Orthop 248:80, 1989.
51. Whiteside LA: Cementless revision total knee arthroplasty. Clin Orthop 286:160, 1993.
52. Whiteside LA: Clinical results of cementless total knee replacement at 12–15 year followup. Orthop Trans 21:220, 1997.
53. Whiteside LA: Effect of porous-coating configuration on tibial osteolysis after total knee arthroplasty. Clin Orthop 321:92, 1995.
54. Whiteside LA, Fosco DR, Brooks JG Jr: Fracture of the femoral component in cementless total knee arthroplasty. Clin Orthop 286:71, 1993.
55. Whiteside LA, Pafford J: Load transfer characteristics of a noncemented total knee arthroplasty. Clin Orthop 239:168, 1989.
56. Whiteside LA, Bicalho PS: Radiologic and histologic analysis of morselized allograft in revision total knee replacement. Clin Orthop 357:149, 1998.
57. Woolson ST, Maloney WJ: Cementless total hip arthroplasty using a porous-coated prosthesis for bone ingrowth fixation. J Arthroplasty 7:381, 1992.

80 Meniscal-Bearing Knee Replacement

JOHN N. INSALL • PAOLO AGLIETTI • A. BALDINI • MARK E. EASLEY

INTRODUCTION

The natural menisci provide conformity and mobility. While conforming to the femoral condyles, the menisci are able to rotate, to some degree, on the tibial plateau. This combination of conformity and mobility allows for stability and load distribution not only in the neutral position but also when the femur is rotated in relation to the tibia.

Standard fixed-bearing total knee arthroplasty (TKA) has proved successful in long-term outcome studies, with 95% good-to-excellent results 10 to 15 years after surgery.[25] These results, however, apply almost exclusively to TKAs performed in elderly patients with low activity levels, who rarely test the durability of the prosthesis. Select reports suggest that nonconstrained fixed-bearing TKA may be equally successful in a younger, more active patient population.[26] Despite this success, the greater demands placed on these prostheses by younger patients will in all likelihood limit their durability.

The fixed-bearing TKA cannot simulate the kinematics of the natural knee. Conformity of the menisci and femoral condyles can be matched by increasing the conformity of the articulating surfaces but not without introducing excessive constraint. Because of its inherent lack of physiological rotation of the menisci, the fixed-bearing TKA remains a compromise between conformity and mobility.

Until both conformity and mobility are optimized, component loosening and polyethylene wear may limit the long-term success of fixed-bearing TKA in younger patients. Component loosening occurs with excessive conformity (and hence excessive constraint) as stresses are transmitted to the bone-prosthesis (or bone-cement) interface. Polyethylene wear can result from either too little or too much conformity. Limited conformity fails to permit diffusion of load, resulting in limited contact area and greater contact stresses; this situation may introduce increased articular surface polyethylene wear.

On the other hand, excessive conformity transfers stresses not only to the bone-prosthesis interface but also to the baseplate-polyethylene interface. Investigations have revealed that a significant amount of wear debris is generated at the undersurface of polyethylene inserts in conventional TKA.[32] Until an optimal locking mechanism is devised, micromotion between the plastic and unpolished tibial tray of modular fixed-bearing prostheses will continue to generate polyethylene undersurface wear.[75]

The mobile- (or meniscal-) bearing knee prosthesis was designed in an effort to reproduce natural knee function. Goodfellow and O'Connor developed the first mobile-bearing knee in 1976. The second, Buechel's Low Contact Stress (LCS) knee, has remained the most widely used meniscal-bearing design since its introduction in 1977. With the rotating mobile bearing, maximal conformity between the articulating components is possible with minimum constraint; optimal stability is thus present at any degree of rotation while diminishing the risks of loosening and wear. Load is distributed over a large surface regardless of the rotational position of the femur in relation to the tibia. The bicondylar contact area of a mobile-bearing knee may exceed 1000 mm^2, which is approximately five times the contact area of a standard, partially conforming, fixed-bearing design. Accordingly, the decrease in contact stress is approximately 25 MPa (fixed bearing) to less than 5 MPa (mobile bearing).[47]

The mobile bearing need not be limited to rotation; anterior-posterior (AP) translation is a feature of several meniscal-bearing designs. In fact, a combination of rotation and AP translation may mimic physiological meniscal function most closely. AP sliding also improves flexion. As full flexion becomes more desirable in TKA, AP translation, with or without rotation on the tibial platform, facilitates even load distribution in flexion by adjusting for the posterior shift in contact points. Furthermore, if AP translation and rotation on the tibial baseplate are used in combination with a femoral component in which the sagittal radius diminishes with flexion, physiological "high flexion" may be possible without excessive posterior contact stress or impingement.

The mobile-bearing TKA has limitations and will probably never duplicate physiological knee function. The composition and arrangement of collagen fibers on the meniscal and articular surfaces, combined with the knee's natural lubrication system, create virtually frictionless motion. Although highly polished tibial baseplates are available, the interface with the mobile polyethylene undersurface will approach but not match the gliding characteristics of the natural knee. Even though the rotational platform allows greater conformity of the articular surfaces to reduce contact stresses, the artificial materials cannot recreate the complex properties of shock absorption of the viscoelastic meniscus. Finally, failure and dislocation of the bearing remain concerns. Currently, however, meniscal-bearing designs most closely simulate normal knee function. As the mobile-bearing knee continues to evolve, long-term follow-up will determine whether its design characteristics improve the durability for TKA in younger, more active patients.

This chapter reviews the most commonly used mobile-bearing designs, including their most salient features. The emphasis, however, is on our meniscal-bearing prosthesis, the Mobile Bearing Knee with its medially biased kinematics (MBK). We present the principles of the MBK design and surgical technique, most of which are applicable to meniscal-bearing prostheses in general. We also provide our experience with the MBK prosthesis, including preliminary clinical outcome and in vitro testing performed in collaboration with several investigators around the world.

MOBILE-BEARING KNEES

Mobile-bearing prostheses are categorized on the basis of the degree of articular surface conformity: either partially or fully conforming. A third category has been introduced: the posterior stabilized meniscal-bearing prostheses. Several mobile-bearing prostheses are available, each with design modifications that provide theoretical advantages. We have summarized the salient features of the most popular mobile-bearing designs and categorized them as partially conforming, fully conforming, or posterior stabilized.

Partially Conforming

Low Contact Stress Total Knee System

The Low Contact Stress (LCS) total knee system (Depuy, Inc., Warsaw, IN), with either the rotating platform or the anatomically separated two-meniscal-bearing design, remains the most widely used mobile-bearing design since Buechel and Pappas developed it in the late 1970s. Buechel and Pappas' original version comprised two independent plastic bearings situated in curved tracks on the tibial tray and preserved both cruciate ligaments. The second version features a single plastic bearing that freely rotates about its post, seated within a hole in the tibial tray. Although not physiological, the reciprocal motion of the medial and lateral aspects of the tray is simple and functional. In extension, this design is highly congruent in both the coronal and sagittal planes, providing a large contact area with low contact stress that affords anteroposterior stability despite sacrificing the posterior cruciate ligament (PCL). The sagittal conformity is diminished in flexion. The patellar component also features a rotating bearing, designed to maintain a spherical contact area on both the medial and lateral facets with the femoral trochlea throughout flexion.[17] Originally, the prostheses were cemented[13]; in 1981, noncemented designs were introduced with sintered-bead porous coating (Fig. 80.1).

Reports conclude that the cemented and uncemented unicompartmental meniscal knee replacements have 91% and 98% rates of survival, respectively, at 10 years.[16, 19] The cemented bicruciate-retaining meniscal-bearing design has a 90% reported rate of survival at 10 years; for the cementless device, the survival rate is 95%. Failure with these devices was observed in cases of previous high tibial osteotomy or tibial plateau fracture (Hamelynck, personal communication). The authors surmised that such conditions appear to alter blood flow, limiting osteointegration in cementless bicruciate-retaining knees. A second cause of failure with these implants was a deficient anterior cruciate ligament (ACL). In fact, in these cases, early or late ACL rupture renders arthroplasty function equal to that of an ACL-deficient knee.[18, 21] The cemented and cementless rotating platform designs have a reported survival rate of 97.5% at 10 years' follow-up.[14, 20] In an analysis of a series of 665 consecutive cementless rotating platform prostheses implanted by a single surgeon, the survival rate at 11 years was 94.7%; the revision rate was 2%.[87]

Mechanical complications have been identified for meniscal bearings, rotating platforms, and rotating-bearing patellar replacements,[22] including bearing dislocation, fracture, patella bearing "spin out," wear,

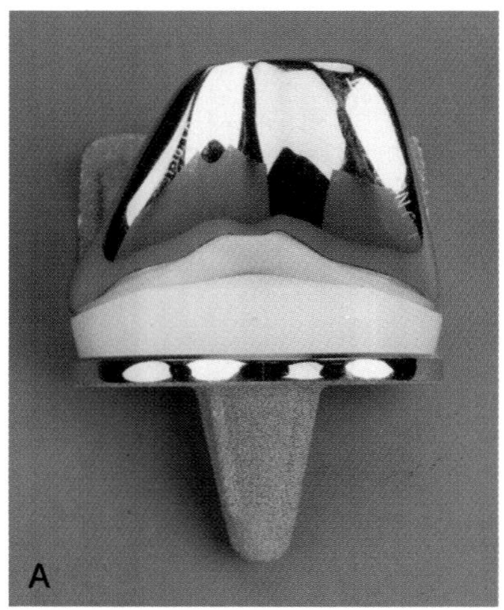

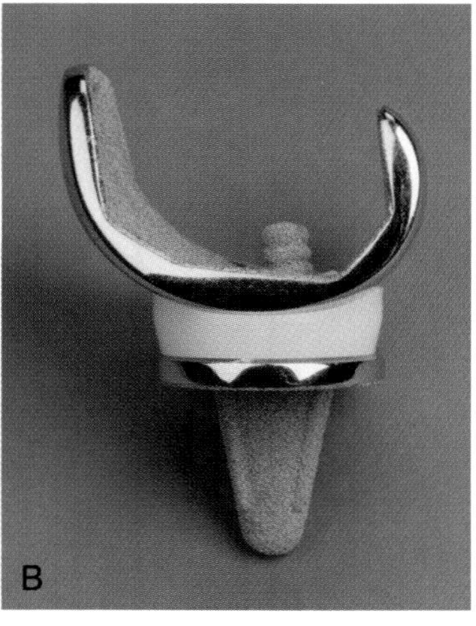

FIGURE 80.1 ➢ Cruciate-retaining, porous-coated Low Contact Stress (LCS) prosthesis. *A*, Coronal view. *B*, Sagittal view.

aseptic loosening, and osteolysis. Meniscal-bearing dislocation was observed by Buechel et al in 1.1% of primary TKAs during U.S. Food and Drug Administration clinical trials and was associated with tibial component malrotation and flexion-extension gap imbalance. Similarly, fracture of the meniscal bearing occurred in 1.1% of primary TKAs and was associated with malrotation of the tibial component, a thin flexible lip on the bearing, poorly manufactured polyethylene, and gamma irradiation in air sterilization. Severe wear prompted bearing exchange or revision in 1% of the cases at between 8 and 19 years of follow-up. Rotating platform dislocation was observed in fewer than 0.5% of primary TKAs or TKAs in multiply operated knees and in 5% of revision TKAs over a 12-year period.[15] Bert reported a dislocation rate of 9.3% with PCL-retaining, rotating-platform LCS knee replacements.[10] In 473 cementless cruciate-retaining, meniscal-bearing LCS TKAs that were monitored for an average of 5 years, Jordan et al reported a 3.6% rate of mechanical failure, including 12 polyethylene fractures or dislocations and five tibial subluxations secondary to ligamentous instability.[48] The authors suggested that high dislocation rates may be caused by failure to achieve proper intraoperative flexion-extension balance.[17] Rotating-bearing patellar replacements dislocated, dissociated, fractured, or exhibited catastrophic wear in fewer than 1% of all cases over a 20-year period, and patellar component "spin out" occurred in less than 0.05%.[22]

Stiehl et al, using fluoroscopy and image-matching techniques, conducted in vivo kinematic analysis in 10 normal patients and 10 patients with PCL-retaining bimeniscal-bearing LCS knee prostheses. In extension, the initial tibiofemoral contact point of the LCS knee is more posterior than in the normal knee, and beyond 60 degrees of flexion, anterior femoral translation is common. Kinematic patterns in more than 60 degrees of flexion are variable and do not simulate normal knee function. Five of the knees with meniscal bearings exhibited anterior sliding of the bearings with flexion; the five other bearings remained stationary in relation to the tibial tray.[98]

Self Aligning Mobile-Bearing Knee

The Self Aligning (SAL) Mobile Bearing Knee (Sulzer Orthopaedics, Baar, Switzerland) was designed by Bourne and Rorabeck in 1987. An oval recess in the posterior aspect of the polyethylene allows unlimited rotation and limited AP translation about a tibial tray peg. The femoral component is relatively flat in the coronal plane but maintains full sagittal conformity throughout the first 70 to 75 degrees of flexion; the posterior condyles are only partially conforming. The trochlear groove is deep and extended. Right and left femoral components are available. Whereas the original tibial component was made of titanium, the current tibial tray is constructed from stiff, polished cobalt-chromium-molybdenum (CoCrMo) with a single peg on the upper surface and two fixation pegs and a central stem (25 or 50 mm) on the undersurface. The patella (25 or 30 mm) is a single-pegged, symmetric dome design that is sensitive to position because of its central eminence (9 mm thick). Component fixation is either cemented (authors' preference) or cementless.

A polyethylene wear study was conducted with three-dimensional measurements in relation to markers in the polyethylene. Wear was not observed on either the articular surface or the undersurface of the polyethylene. The first 10 SAL knees were implanted in 1988. In a multicenter European clinical trial started in 1993, 234 SAL-I knee replacements were evaluated at 2 and 5 years' follow-up. The preoperative diagnosis was osteoarthritis in 172 patients. The average Knee Society rating score increased from 35 points preoperatively to 84 points at 2 years and 90 points at 5 years. Patellar lateral release was performed in 24 (10%) knees. The PCL was retained in approximately 85% of cases, recessed in 10% of cases, and sacrificed in approximately 5% of cases. The revision rate was 5.1%. Three revisions were for femoral component loosening and two were for vertical patellar fractures (Rorabeck, personal communication).

Total Articulating Cementless Knee

The Total Articulating Cementless Knee (TACK) (Waldemar Link, Hamburg, Germany) has been used since 1990. The total condylar femoral components are available for right and left knees that articulate with a rotating polyethylene platform. The tibial tray has two semicircular guides that engage circular tracks on both sides of the platform, permitting free rotational movement. PCL retention is accommodated by a posterior recess in the platform and tibial tray. The three-dimensional grid on the back surfaces of the tibial and femoral components is available with a hydroxyapatite coating to improve cementless fixation. Clinical outcomes are not yet available.

Interax Integrated Secure Asymmetric

The Interax Integrated Secure Asymmetric (ISA) (Howmedica International, Rutherford, NJ) prosthesis has nearly full conformity between the spherical distal condyles of the asymmetric femoral component (available for left and right knees) and the tibial meniscal bearing in extension; the conformity gradually decreases in flexion. The tibial baseplate is symmetric and has two central posts designed with a circular mushroom cap that engages a curved, T-shaped guide track within the meniscal bearing; the curved track determines right and left configurations. This design confers medially biased knee kinematics. The mechanism allows 36 degrees of internal and external rotation of the bearing, pivoting around a point in the medial compartment. From extension to flexion, 14 to 24 mm of AP translation occurs.[61] Fixation options include a unique Cast-Mesh ingrowth surface or Cast-Mesh with hydroxyapatite for cementless designs and a "Diamond" macro-textured surface for cemented prostheses.

An ongoing prospective clinical study is being conducted at four European centers. One hundred fifty-three patients entered into the trial from November 1995 to April 1997. Observations during a mean follow-up period of 2 years were available for 57 of these patients. The average age was 68 years (range, 32 to 86) and 79% were female. Eighty-four percent of patients had osteoarthritis. All prostheses were noncemented, and approximately two thirds of the patellae were not resurfaced. Patellar retinacular lateral release was performed in 12% of the cases. The PCL was retained in the majority of cases (97.4%). The Knee Society score improved from 42.3 preoperatively (n = 153) to 91.5 at 2-year follow-up (n = 57); the function score improved from 44.5 (n = 153) to a maximum of 85.3 at 2 years (n = 57). Range of motion improved from 98.2 degrees (n = 153) to 110.4 degrees at 2 years (n = 57) (M. Marcacci, personal communication).

Total Rotating Knee

Professor F. Ghilsellini, who designed the Total Rotating Knee (TRK) (Cremascoli, Milan, Italy), has implanted approximately 500 of these prostheses since 1992. The TRK comprises a total condylar-type femoral component and a metal tibial tray with a central post projecting from the center of the plate, both made of cobalt-chromium alloy for use with or without cement. The patella is an all-polyethylene, single-pegged dome. The two types of plastic bearings are available in five sizes and four thicknesses. The first ("R," for rotating) has a rounded hole in the undersurface that fits the post of the tibial tray to allow freedom of rotation, intended to be used when the PCL is excised. The second type ("RS," for rotating and sliding), with a slot allowing 10 mm of AP sliding and freedom of rotation, is indicated when the PCL is retained. Dr. Ghisellini's preliminary results (F. Ghisellini, personal communication) are encouraging, and wear testing, performed with a knee joint simulator in cadaveric specimens, demonstrates only minor abrasive and adhesive wear without signs of fatigue wear after 4 million cycles.

Minns Meniscal Knee Prosthesis

The Minns meniscal knee prosthesis (Zimmer UK, Swindon, UK) has a total condylar femoral component and a tibial platform with dovetail AP slots that engage two separate polyethylene "menisci," permitting rolling and sliding movements during flexion. Because the slots are straight and parallel, rotation is limited by a single sliding plateau design that engages both slots. The two-independent-menisci design allows 59 degrees of rotation (both internal and external), and the sliding single-plateau prosthesis has torque-rotation characteristics comparable with those of the total condylar design. The tibial tray has a central recess to accommodate both cruciate ligaments.

Forty patients with a Minns meniscal knee prosthesis were studied by means of fluoroscopy to obtain lateral spot films taken at four different angles of flexion. In six patients, the menisci did not appear to move. Meniscal starting position in relation to the tibial tray was variable. In most of the cases, the menisci moved forward during the first 20 to 30 degrees of flexion and then backward. In some patients, the medial meniscus moved more than the lateral meniscus, whereas in others, the opposite was noted.

The authors performed wear testing using a knee simulator in cadaver knees to a maximum of one million cycles at 3000 N of load. They studied contact area every 100,000 cycles with Fuji contact films. After the first 100,000 cycles they observed a minimal amount of wear; with further cycling wear was negligible, as the contact area increased.[67]

In a review of the first 165 implants at a maximal follow-up period of 5 years, the implants were rated good to excellent in 88% of the cases. Bearing dislocations and fractures occurred in the first series.[67] The investigators concluded that posterior tibial component placement was responsible for fracture of the bearing because of the high loading on the anterior aspect of the polyethylene that was overhanging from the tibial plate. The tibial surface cutting guide was modified to include a curved viewing slot that improves referencing to avoid posterior tibial positioning. The surgeons solved problems with bearing dislocation by substituting the meniscal bearing (at surgery or as a revision procedure) with the single sliding plateau.[65-67]

Fully Conforming

The Oxford Unicompartmental Knee Replacement

The Oxford unicompartmental knee replacement (Biomet Ltd, Bridgend, South Wales, Australia) was the first mobile-bearing design to be introduced by Goodfellow and O'Connor (1976).[35] Their cruciate-retaining design has independent femoral and tibial bearing surfaces that can be implanted in the medial or lateral compartment for unicompartmental arthritis or in both compartments for bicompartmental disease. The femoral component has a spherical articular surface with a 24-mm radius. Free meniscal bearings that are spherical on the articular surface and flat on the undersurface are positioned between the curved femoral component (available in only a single size) and the flat tibial component (available in five sizes). The position of the meniscal bearings is maintained by their geometry and ligamentous tension.[39] The meniscal bearings are available in several thicknesses, ranging from 3.5 mm to 11.5 mm. The surfaces are congruent throughout the range of motion, affording a contact area of 600 mm^2 per condyle in all joint positions.[36] Retrieval studies of prostheses implanted from 1 to 9 years demonstrated low penetration wear rates (0.026 to 0.043 mm per year) of the meniscal bearings.[4]

The success of the Oxford unicompartmental prosthesis is dependent on ACL function. In an evaluation of 125 unicompartmental prostheses implanted bicompartmentally, Goodfellow et al reported a failure rate of 8.8% in patients with ACL insufficiency, as opposed to 4.8% in knees with intact ACL function, after an average follow-up period of 6 years.[33] In a subsequent review of 301 knee replacements with the same prostheses, the cumulative 60-year survival rates of the Oxford prostheses with and without intact ACL function were 95% and 81%, respectively.[38] The results were similar in 103 prostheses implanted for unicompartmental arthritis: A 16.2% failure rate was observed in the 37 knees with a damaged ACL, and a 4.8% failure rate was observed in 63 knees with intact ACL function.[37] A success rate of 99.1% at 7 years was observed in 121 knees with medial compartment replacement that met these criteria: (1) functional ACL, (2) intact cartilage in the lateral compartment of the knee, and (3) anteromedial osteoarthritis with varus deformity passively correctable to neutral.[48]

Rotaglide Total Knee System

The Rotaglide total knee system (Cozim Medical, Cirencester, UK) designed in 1986 by Polyzoides and Tsakonas has a femoral component that maintains the same intercondylar distance and radius of curvature in all sizes. This feature is represented also on the articular surface of the one-piece polyethylene meniscal component, providing a contact area of 600 mm^2 per condyle that is maintained essentially from full extension to maximum flexion, with complete matching of all femoral and tibial sizes. The flat undersurface of the polyethylene platform glides 5 mm in an AP direction and rotates 12.5 degrees toward each side on the polished tibial tray. The tibial plateau has an anterior bollard that prevents anterior dislocation while restricting the rotation of the platform and another bollard in the middle of the tray that resists posterior dislocation. In both the femoral and tibial components, a single stem is used for fixation; tibial component fixation is augmented by two broach pegs. Cement fixation is typically favored.

Between 1988 and 1998, 1600 patients have undergone TKA with the Rotaglide prosthesis at two institutions. Preoperative diagnoses included degenerative and inflammatory arthritis. The follow-up period ranged from 6 to 10 years. According to the British Orthopaedic Association Chart,[1] patient satisfaction was 96%; relief of pain was experienced by 97.8%. All TKAs were stable, and flexion averaged 115 degrees. In the osteoarthritic population, the average walking distance was 3 km per day. The authors observed patellar problems in 3.3% of rheumatoid patients and in 1.2% of osteoarthritic patients. No radiological evidence of polyethylene wear or osteolysis was present, and no tibial component loosening was observed. The 0.9% revision rate among these 1600 knees reflects infection, patellar problems, and femoral component loosening.[78]

Medially Biased Kinematics Knee

The Medially Biased Kinematics (MBK) knee (Zimmer, Warsaw, IN) was developed in 1992 by John Insall, Paolo Aglietti, and Peter Walker (see Fig. 80.1). The design concept of this prosthesis is complete conformity between the femoral component and the polyethylene insert at any degree of flexion and during rotation and AP translation of the polyethylene insert on the tibial tray.[62] The details of this prosthesis are presented later in this chapter.

Posterior Stabilized

Two Radii Area Contact Mobile-Bearing Total Knee Replacement

The Two Radii Area Contact (TRAC) mobile-bearing total knee replacement (Biomet, Warsaw, IN), designed by Draganich and Pottenger, was introduced in 1997. This prosthesis features two different areas of tibiofemoral contact created by separating the femoral condylar surfaces into two radii of curvature. The femoral condyles have a greater radius of curvature on their larger distal aspect than on the smaller posterior aspect. From approximately 5 degrees of hyperextension through 8 degrees of flexion, the larger femoral curvature fully conforms with a more centrally located inner track of the meniscal bearing. When the cam engages the post to induce rollback at 8 degrees of flexion, tibiofemoral contact occurs between the smaller femoral curvature and the more peripherally located outer track of the meniscal bearing. The surface area of tibiofemoral contact diminishes from 1077 mm^2 in extension to 674 mm^2 in flexion.

The preliminary results of the first 86 TRAC prostheses reported by the designers showed an average Hospital for Special Surgery clinical score of 85 points at one year follow-up (Pottenger, personal communication).

Other PS Designs

Other TKAs in this category of PS-Mobile-Bearing Knees include the Rotaglide-PS (Cozim Medical, Cirencester, UK), the Low Contact Stress-PS (DePuy, Inc., Warsaw, IN), and the Noiles-PS (Johnson & Johnson Orthopaedics, Berkshire, UK). These designs are based on the "cam and post" mechanism on a rotating polyethylene platform. The common feature is the cam situated between the posterior femoral condyles that engages a post projecting from the mobile polyethylene platform.

MBK PRINCIPLES AND DESIGN

Principles

Rotation occurs at the knee during most activities, including walking. Three-dimensional gait analysis demonstrates that the tibia briefly rotates internally during stance phase (i.e., with load applied) and rotates externally 10 degrees during the swing phase (i.e., without load applied).[56] It has been estimated that modern knee prostheses require a minimum of 12 degrees of rotation to accommodate most non-weightbearing activities of daily living.

Restrained by the PCL, the femur translates posteriorly on the tibia with flexion. Because of the greater inherent stability of the medial joint compartment in relation to the lateral side, femoral rollback results in internal tibial torsion about its long axis.[6, 23, 83, 94] Through the 0- to 120-degree flexion range, the femorotibial contact points move posteriorly an average of 8 mm, particularly laterally. Fluoroscopic analysis of TKAs demonstrates that these knee kinematics occur only when the PCL is appropriately tensioned.[92]

Although femoral anatomy was traditionally described as having a decreasing radius for the posterior condyles, more recent studies have shown that a constant posterior condylar radius is approximately 21 to 23 mm for the medial femoral condyle.[29, 43] Therefore, a femoral component with a constant sagittal radius appears to be the most desirable in TKA.

Some researchers have postulated that the knee flexes about an axis closely approximating the femoral epicondyles. This axis passes through the centers of the posterior femoral condyles[43] and is perpendicular to the tibial axis at all degrees of flexion. A second rotational axis that is essentially parallel to the tibial long axis and medial to the joint center has also been identified.[53]

Using 10 fresh autopsy specimens and a photographic method, Trent and Walker observed that the center of transverse tibial rotation was located on the medial aspect of the tibial spine.[95] Their findings imply that there are two distinct components of knee motion: (1) flexion-extension about the transepicondylar axis and (2) internal-external rotation about a medially biased tibial axis. This "compound hinge model" was proved, through three-dimensional kinematic analysis by Churchill et al, in 15 cadaveric knees tested in simulated squatting.[23] These biomechanical principles of physiological knee kinematics have been applied to the design of the MBK (medially biased kinematics) knee prosthesis.

Design

The MBK prosthesis was designed to improve durability and function in TKA. On the basis of the aforementioned principles, the features of the MBK prosthesis design are as follows:

1. Reduced wear.
2. Smooth patellar tracking.
3. Medial kinematics.
4. Freedom of rotation.
5. Limitation of translation.
6. Plastic bearing stability.
7. Interchangeability.
8. Baseplate strength.
9. Physiological flexion and extension.

Reduced Wear

Wear limits durability in total knee replacement[52] and is associated with high contact stresses, excessive tibiofemoral sliding, undersurface shear stresses, and gradual oxidation of materials. Wear occurs by three mechanisms: adhesion, abrasion (superficial wear), and fatigue (pitting and delamination/deep wear).

Typically, wear is multifactorial. Multiple studies have associated wear damage with clinical, material, and design factors. Retrieval studies have demonstrated correlations between wear damage and weight, activity level, and the length of time that the component was implanted.[44]

Polyethylene's strength and deformation properties are determined by fusion defects, molecular weight, and molecule cross-linking.[58] Polyethylene is cross-linked through radiation at high temperatures. Because cross-linked polyethylene has been shown to resist adhesive wear, it has been used in several new total hip arthroplasty designs. Although the high stiffness created by cross-linking is not ideal for fixed-bearing knee prostheses, it may be acceptable for mobile-bearing prostheses. Cross-linking may also offset the effects of oxidative degradation, including reduced molecular weight, stiffness, and wear resistance.[54, 80, 82]

Clinical and mechanical factors under the surgeon's control, including component size and position, knee alignment, and ligament balance, may lead to wear, especially when unconstrained tibial components are used. Design factors influencing wear are polyethylene thickness and conformity. In an analytic study of the Insall-Burstein total condylar design, Bartel et al showed that stresses increased significantly for polyethylene insert thickness less than 8 mm.[6-8] Prosthetic articular surface conformity and contact stresses generated in the weightbearing area also influence wear characteristics.[9]

The MBK prosthesis has complete femorotibial conformity throughout motion because of the fixed radius of the posterior femoral condyles. The radius ratio is 1:1 in both the sagittal and coronal planes (Fig. 80.2). Contact stresses increase significantly when the ratio between the radii of the prosthetic design surfaces becomes larger. An increasing potential for polyethylene compromise is observed with increasing contact

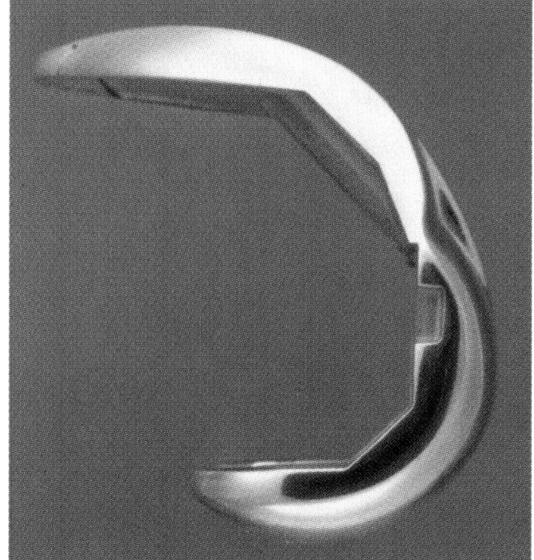

FIGURE 80.2 ➢ Side view of the Mobile-Bearing Knee with its medially biased kinematics femoral component, showing the fixed radius of the posterior femoral condyles.

stresses[10]; several investigations have demonstrated that contact stresses exceeding 5 to 10 MPa damage the polyethylene inserts.[17, 45, 73] For a 4000-N load, equivalent to approximately 5½ times body weight, a surface of at least 400 mm² is necessary to limit contact stresses to 10 MPa. Per condyle, the standard fixed-bearing prosthesis has a contact area of 100 to 150 mm² per condyle; the LCS knee, approximately 225 mm²; the Rotaglide and the Oxford prostheses, almost 600 mm²; and the MBK, 535 mm². With a 4000-N load, the MBK prosthesis has contact stresses of 3.6 MPa when contact is symmetric in both condyles and 7.0 MPa when errors in alignment force loading of only one condyle.

A three-dimensional finite-element study conducted by Greenwald et al analyzed articular and undersurface stresses of mobile-bearing tibial inserts from various knee systems, including the MBK, using an applied load of 2500 N (3½ times body weight) in full extension. With regard to the MBK, the bicondylar articular surface and total undersurface contact areas were 530 mm² and 293 mm², respectively.[69] All of the mobile-bearing tibial inserts studied demonstrated lower-than-expected contact areas and greater-than-expected undersurface perimeter contact. The finite-element method used in this investigation may have been limited by excessive artifact introduced by mobile-bearing prostheses. Another study of the MBK prosthesis by Walsh and Harris (Walsh, personal communication), who used a computerized contact area and pressure measurement system (Tekscan Inc., South Boston, MA), demonstrated different results in the MBK 14-mm polyethylene insert. The K-Scan 4000 system comprises a plastic laminated, thin (0.1-mm) film, electronic pressure transducer (a sensor with 4576 sensing elements); hardware and software for an IBM-compatible personal computer; and a coupler to connect the computer to the transducer. Tests were performed by applying loads of 3600 N, 3240 N, and 2880 N (equal to 5, 4.5, and 4 times ideal body weight) at flexion angles of 0, 30, 60, 90, and 110 degrees. Average contact stresses were 4 MPa for all loads and degrees of flexion, except for 110 degrees of flexion, for which 7.5 MPa was observed. Peak contact stresses in compression were below the failure stress of polyethylene for all combinations of load and flexion, except for 110 degrees of flexion, at which the peak stress was 22 MPa. The MBK articulating surface total contact area approximated 800 mm² at 0, 30, and 60 degrees of flexion; 700 mm² at 90 degrees; and 380 mm² at 110 degrees. The nonarticulating surface total contact area analyzed with ultra super low (USL) Fuji film (Fuji Photo Film Co., Tokyo, Japan) was about 1200 mm² for all tested degrees of flexion.

Smooth Patellar Tracking

The femoral component has separate femoropatellar and femorotibial surfaces. The femorotibial surfaces and the posterior femoral condyles are separated from the patellar flange by two condylotrochlear grooves

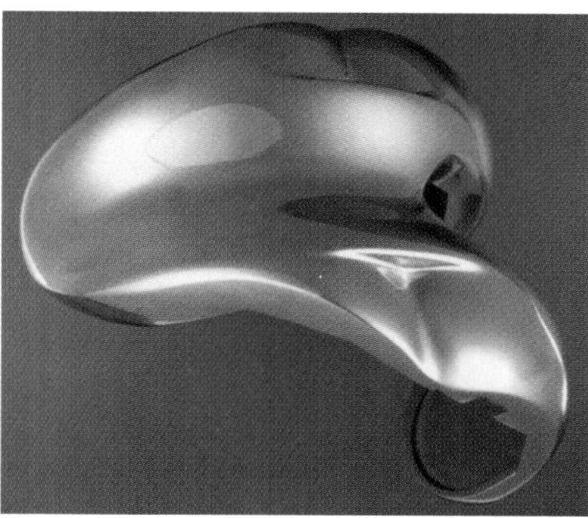

FIGURE 80.3 ➢ The femoral component has a deep and elongated trochlea. Two condylotrochlear grooves separate the femorotibial surface and the posterior femoral condyles.

(Fig. 80.3). The femoral condyles have a constant radius of curvature; this radius changes in proportion to prosthetic size. The patellar sulcus is deep, extends distally, and is displaced slightly laterally to improve patellar tracking in flexion. It can accommodate the natural patella. Right and left femoral components are available.

The patellar component can be either dome- or sombrero-shaped; the sombrero shape more closely simulates that of the natural patella. The sombrero design provides the greatest contact with the MBK femoral trochlea, but concerns about patellar alignment have prompted us to routinely use the dome-shaped design, which is more tolerant of tilting. Although the dome patella design affords only point-line contact with the femoral trochlea, plastic deformation of the polyethylene surface after implantation creates a larger contact area in the positions under high contact stress.[25] This behavior of the polyethylene imparts biological-like properties to the material ("bio-poly").

Medial Kinematics

Despite the symmetric design of the tibial component, the prosthesis design features medially biased kinematics, guided by the natural knee's stronger medial structures and greater lateral mobility. In essence, natural properties of the knee obviate the need for artificial devices that guide knee kinematics about a medial compartment center.

Freedom of Rotation

The polyethylene insert has approximately 20 degrees of both internal and external rotation on the tibial baseplate (Fig. 80.4). The degree of rotation is limited by soft tissues. Rotational freedom affords the potential advantage of tolerance of up to 15 degrees of tibial tray rotational malpositioning. The fully conforming articular surface forces the tibia to rotate into a position dictated by the femoral component, especially when the knee is fully extended. However, with noncon-

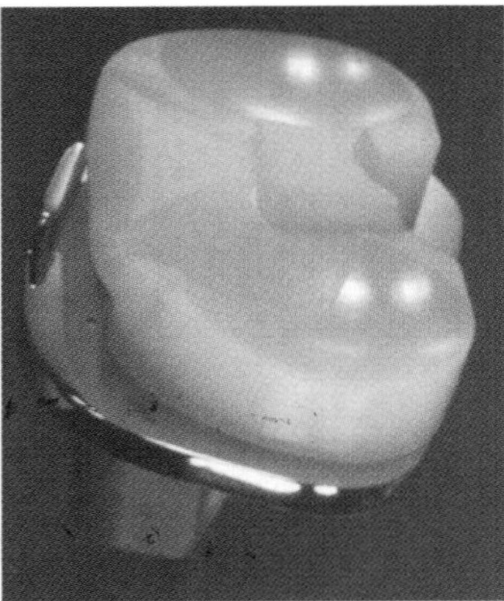

FIGURE 80.4 ➢ The polyethylene insert of the MBK can rotate 20 degrees internally and externally on the tibial tray.

forming articulations, tibial rotational position is determined by ligament tension rather than by component position. In a cadaveric study, Nagamine and Whiteside analyzed patellar tracking before and after TKR. They compared semiconstrained and unconstrained articular surfaces with the tibial tray in neutral position, in 15 degrees of internal rotation, and in 15 degrees of external rotation. In all three positions, only minimal tibial rotation was acceptable for the semiconstrained prosthesis; 15 degrees of malrotation of the unconstrained tray did not affect patellar tracking.[72]

Limitation of Translation

The plastic bearing translates 4.5 mm in an AP direction on the tibial tray (Fig. 80.5). An anterior stop prevents the plastic bearing from sliding off the tibial

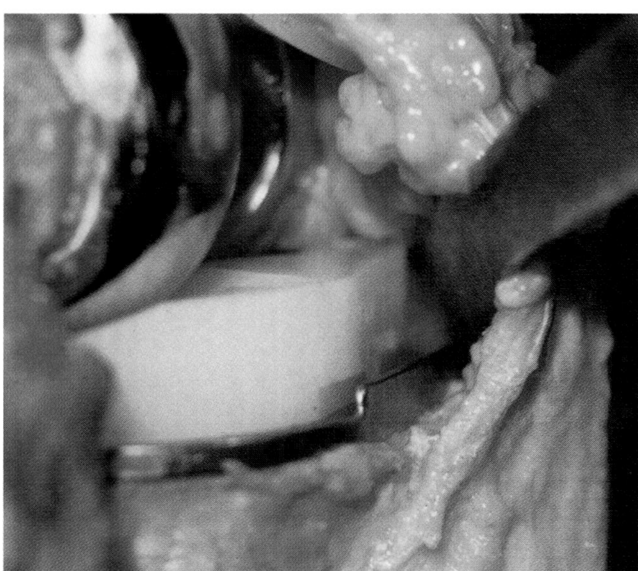

FIGURE 80.5 ➢ Implanted MBK showing posterior sliding of the polyethylene insert with knee flexion.

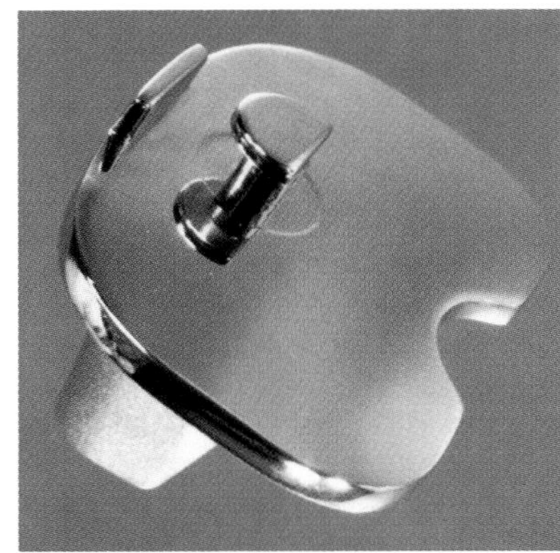

FIGURE 80.6 ➢ The tibial tray of the MBK.

tray and limits rotation in extension (Fig. 80.6). The anterior lip of the plastic bearing supplements the PCL in its function of providing posterior knee stability (Fig. 80.7). With posterior tibial stress, anterior translation of the mobile bearing is restricted by the tibial tray's metal rail and posterior aspect of the mushroom-shaped post; with anteriorly directed tibial stress posterior polyethylene displacement is blocked by the anterior aspect of the post (Fig. 80.8).

Medial-lateral translation is prevented by an asymmetric intercondylar "saddle" (Fig. 80.9). The medial aspect of the saddle conforms to the femoral condyle during single condyle loading (in varus position).

Stability of Plastic Bearing

A D-shaped "mushroom" on the tibial tray guides the mobile polyethylene. The mushroom snaps into a polyethylene undersurface slot, preventing liftoff of the plastic from the tibial tray (Fig. 80.10). The polyethyl-

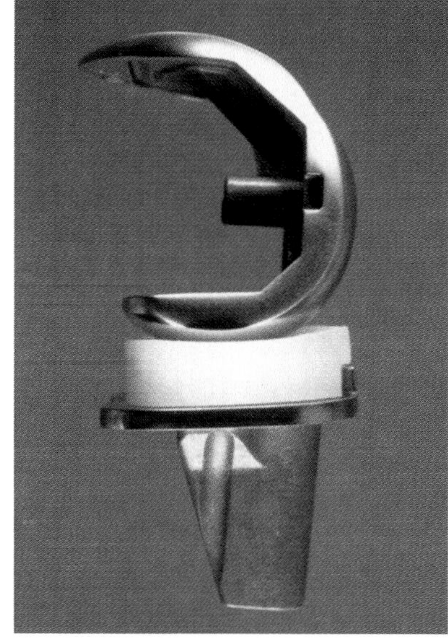

FIGURE 80.7 ➢ Side view of the MBK.

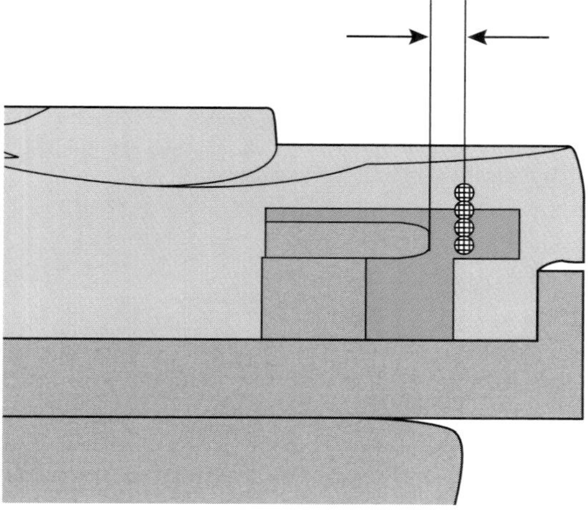

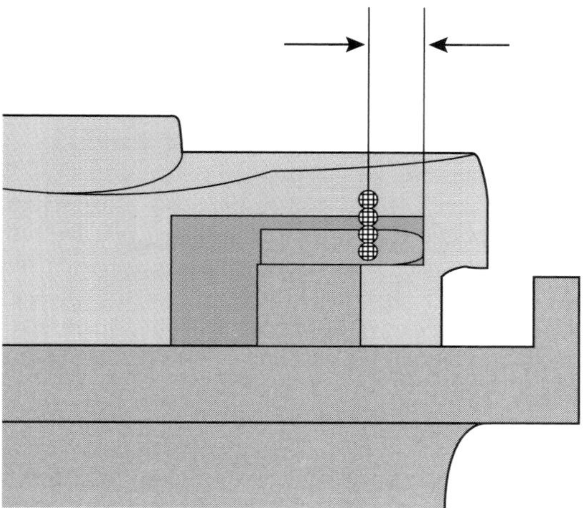

FIGURE 80.8 ➢ Section view of the polyethylene insert at the mushroom-shaped post. Multiple contact points between the mobile-bearing and the rail and post diffuse anteriorly or posteriorly directed tibial stresses.

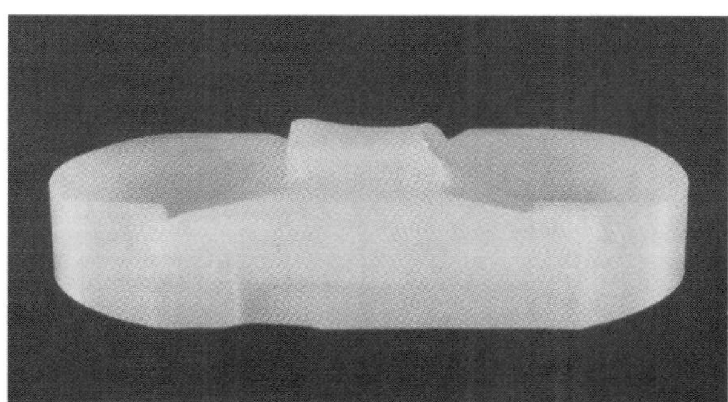

FIGURE 80.9 ➢ Front view of the polyethylene insert, showing the asymmetrically shaped intercondylar "saddle."

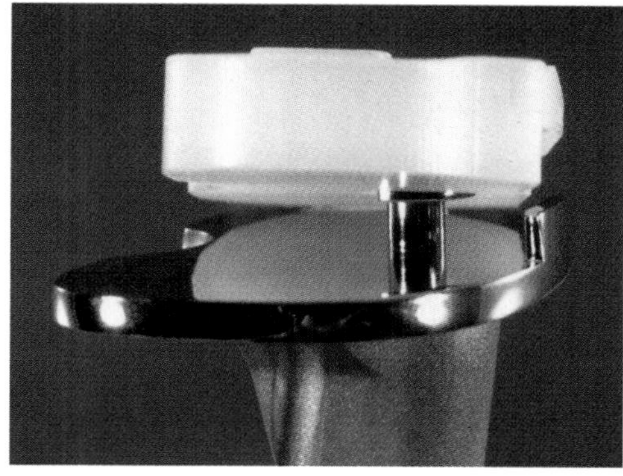

FIGURE 80.10 ➢ The D-shaped "mushroom" snaps into the polyethylene undersurface slot.

ene insert is secured to the baseplate in 20 degrees of internal rotation, to facilitate insertion or change of the insert during surgery. A specially designed instrument is used to change the insert; it wedges between the tray's anterior rail and the mobile insert while maintaining the insert in the proper rotation to allow for its extraction.

Interchangeability

The articular surface of the polyethylene bearings matches the corresponding femoral components exactly, and each femoral component is compatible with three tibial tray sizes (Fig. 80.11). This permits the surgeon to select the tibial component that optimizes cortical loading while maintaining correct matching with the femoral component.

Baseplate Strength

The tibial component's fluted design improves tibial tray stiffness. The nonporous tibial tray is made of

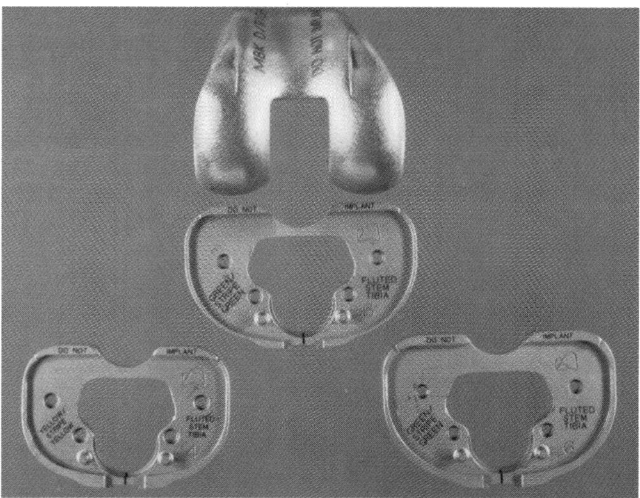

FIGURE 80.11 ➢ Interchangeability is afforded by the fact that each femoral component is compatible with three tibial tray sizes.

CoCrMo and is 4 mm thick. The polished tibial plate finishing has a low tolerance in the order of 0.1 μ (Fig. 80.12). Investigators at Zimmer have compared plate stiffness of several Zimmer tibial tray designs by measuring the tray deflection at 300 lb of load (data on file). The stiffest tibial baseplate was the nonporous, fluted MBK tibial tray designed with short and thick lateral flutes. Observed average deflections were 0.003 inch for the MBK (0.004 for mediolateral deflection and 0.0025 for posterior deflection), 0.006 inch for the Nexgen, and 0.010 inch for the IB-II. We believe that optimal stiffness of the tray reduces radiolucent lines and enhances tibial fixation.

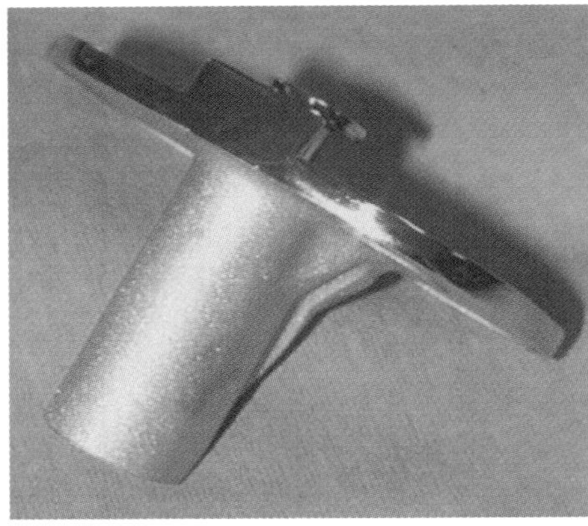

FIGURE 80.12 ➢ The fluted tibial tray design of the MBK.

Flexion and Extension Properties

Fully conforming knee prostheses inevitably lead to posterior polyethylene protrusion beyond 90 degrees of flexion. Despite this, the MBK prosthesis should afford approximately 120 degrees of flexion, provided that the posterior recesses are clear of impingement from osteophytes and soft tissue (Fig. 80.13). Furthermore, having a free posterior recess is important because posterior translation of tibiofemoral contact with progressive flexion inherent in the MBK design leads to earlier impingement with posterior structures. We routinely clear the medial and lateral posterior recesses with a curved osteotome and/or an elevator (see section on technique).

The MBK prosthetic design allows 12 degrees of hyperextension. Implantation of the tibial component with 7 degrees of posterior slope and of the femoral component in 3 degrees of flexion necessitates a prosthesis with 10 degrees of hyperextension just for the knee to achieve full extension.

SURGICAL TECHNIQUE

The patient, under epidural anesthesia, is placed in the supine position, and a tourniquet is applied to the proximal thigh.

Our preferred surgical approach involves a straight, longitudinal, midline anterior skin incision. With the extensor mechanism exposed, a longitudinal anteromedial parapatellar capsulotomy is made, beginning at the apex of the quadriceps tendon. The capsulotomy is extended distally, elevating the tendon from the medial border of the patella. The capsulotomy is continued parallel to the medial patellar tendon and completed on the anteromedial tibia 1 cm from the tuberosity. The distal extension of the incision on the anteromedial tibia is continued through the periosteum 1 cm medial to the tibial tubercle. In this approach, some periosteum remains attached to the tubercle; it can be used to improve the distal wound closure.

The patella is everted after forward translation and external rotation of the tibia, facilitated by transection of the ACL and release of the meniscotibial ligaments and deep medial collateral ligament (MCL) from the proximal tibia. Further external rotation requires elevation of the semimembranosus and pes anserinus tendons from the tibia. The superficial MCL fibers are elevated distally. Less medial dissection is required in valgus knees.

The operative sequence includes (1) distal femoral cut, (2) selection of the correct femoral rotational alignment, (3) anterior and posterior femoral cuts, (4) proximal tibial cut, (5) check of extension and flexion gaps with spacer blocks and possibly more extensive medial or lateral collateral ligament release (by the multiple puncture technique), (6) insertion of trial components, (7) possible PCL complete release from the tibia, (8) check of posterior stability in flexion, and (9) patellar resurfacing and assessment of patellar tracking.

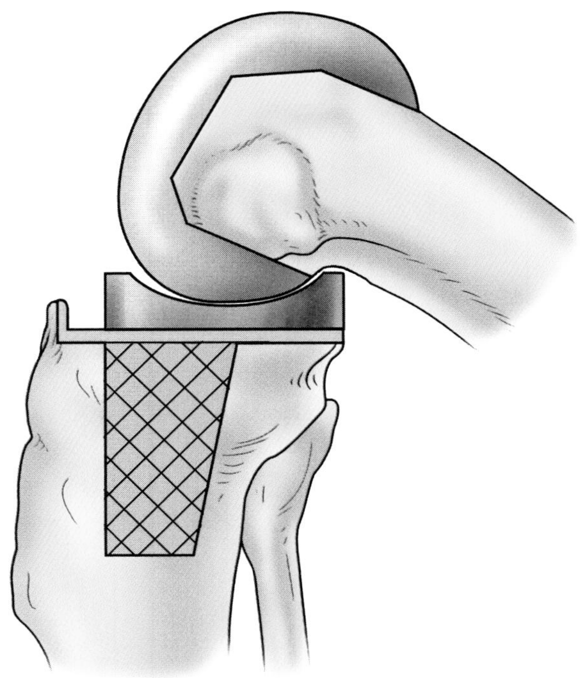

FIGURE 80.13 ➢ Flexion characteristics of the MBK design.

Distal Femoral Cut

Although this is not essential, we typically initiate the bone cuts on the femoral side. Before cutting the distal femur, we drill a 12-mm hole centered over the distal intramedullary canal approximately 1 cm anterior to the PCL insertion for the 8-mm femoral intramedullary guide. Creating a 12-mm hole for the 8-mm intramedullary rod allows an exit for bone marrow and fat, to reduce intramedullary pressure.

Correct valgus alignment for the distal femoral cut is established through the use of an intramedullary guide; we routinely confirm the position with an extramedullary rod aligned with the hip center, approximated by a point two fingerbreadths medial to the anterior superior iliac spine palpated through the drapes. Eight to 10 mm of distal femur is removed (referenced from the least affected condyle) with the distal femoral cutting block set in 6 to 7 degrees of valgus position in relation to the anatomic femoral axis. Usually a 2-mm distal femoral under-resection is performed when there is no preoperative flexion contracture. The MBK instrumentation imparts 3 degrees of flexion to the distal femoral cut in relation to the distal femoral axis; flexion at the distal femur reduces the risk of anterior notching, particularly when in-between sizing dictates use of the smaller femoral component.

Femoral Rotational Alignment

The preparation of the distal femur continues with exposure of the epicondyles that serve as landmarks for determining femoral component rotation.[9, 55, 71, 86] We aim for a few (3 to 4) degrees of external rotation in relation to the posterior condylar line, in order to improve patellar tracking and to compensate for physiological lateral collateral laxity.[51] The MBK instrumentation that we use is termed the "epicondylar" system; in fact, the epicondylar instrumentation system was originally developed in conjunction with the MBK prosthesis.

Excessive external rotation (≥10 degrees) is avoided because it may cause notching of the anterolateral femoral cortex or lead to component undersizing.[57] Furthermore, excessive external rotation can paradoxically increase patellar subluxations in flexion, because the anterior sulcus is rotated externally but the posterior aspect of the MBK condylofemoral sulcus is directed medially. Finally, excessive external rotation may produce medial joint laxity and a rotational mismatch of the flexion and extension gaps.[71]

There are several methods of establishing proper femoral rotation. The traditional method of referencing from the posterior condylar line[46] is limited by posterior condylar erosion or dysplasia. In valgus deformities, erosion of the posterior lateral condyle may lead to internal rotation of the femoral component, whereas erosion of the posterior medial condyle (in varus knees) may lead to excessive external rotation of the femoral component.

The second method of establishing proper femoral component rotation involves cutting the tibial first, tensing the collateral ligaments in flexion, and resecting the posterior condyles parallel to the tibial cut (parallel flexion gap method).[90, 97] Laminar spreaders or other specialized devices (tensors) may be used to adjust the ligament balance before femoral rotation is set.

The third method is to measure bone resections from the distal and posterior cuts, equalizing their amounts to establish appropriate rotation (G. A. Engh, personal communication). In our experience with this method, proper femoral rotation is rarely achieved because of variations in condylar bone deficiency.

The fourth method requires using the trochlear AP line (Whiteside's line), which is usually perpendicular to the epicondylar line. This method has been found to be particularly useful in the valgus knee.[5] Although the trochlear AP line is generally reliable, it may be distorted by a shallow sulcus or lateral femoral condylar dysplasia. In our opinion, the AP line shows too much variability in comparison with the epicondylar axis.

The method that we prefer requires identification of the epicondyles.[76] By referencing off the transepicondylar line, we routinely establish proper external rotation of a few degrees (average 4 degrees; range, 1 to 7 degrees) in relation to the posterior condylar line. The degree of external rotation varies according to the type of deformity; in a cadaveric study, the transepicondylar axis averaged 3.5 degrees in varus knees and 4.4 degrees in the valgus knees.[76]

The relationship of the epicondyles to other distal femoral landmarks was defined by Griffin et al, who used magnetic resonance imaging in 104 nonarthritic knees.[36, 37] The authors demonstrated that the distance between the distal joint line and the medial epicondylar sulcus averaged 27.4 ± 2.9 mm, with a statistically significant difference between genders (in females, average was 26.3 mm; in males, 29.2 mm). The distance from the posterior joint line to the medial sulcus averaged 29.0 ± 2.7 mm, again with a statistically significant difference between females (average, 27.8 mm) and males (average, 30.8 mm). The distance from the distal joint line to the lateral epicondyle was 24.3 ± 2.6 mm on average (in females, average was 23.4 mm; in males, 25.6 mm), and the distance from the posterior joint line to the lateral epicondyle averaged 25.0 ± 2.6 mm (in females, average was 23.9 mm; in males, 26.7 mm).

The angle between the surgical epicondylar axis (medial epicondylar sulcus to lateral epicondyle) and the tangent to the posterior condyles (posterior condylar angle) averaged 3.11 ± 1.75 degrees.[41] Griffin et al measured this angle in another study of 107 osteoarthritic knees by using a posterior reference/rotation guide. Varus knees measured 3.3 ± 1.9 degrees on average, whereas valgus knees measured 5.4 ± 2.3 degrees on average as a result of the deficient lateral posterior condyle.[36, 37]

The epicondyles are exposed by carefully removing the overlying synovium and dividing the lateral patellofemoral ligament. The lateral epicondyle is more easily identified because it tapers to a prominence, whereas

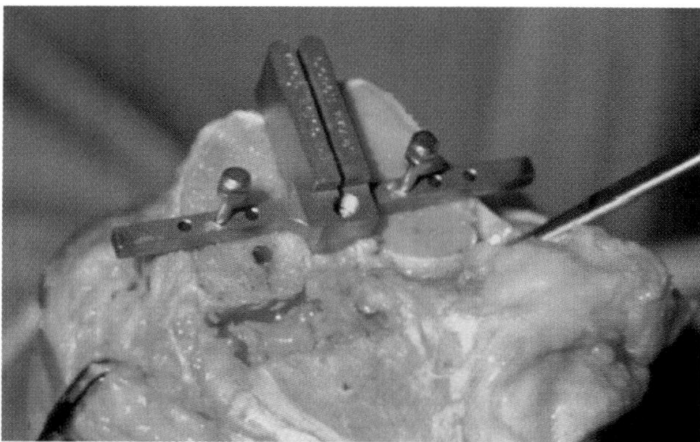

FIGURE 80.14 ➢ Slotted guide aligned with the epicondylar axis.

the less prominent fan-shaped medial epicondyle requires careful identification of landmarks to locate its center. We use a combination of the bull's-eye technique (defining the epicondylar ridge and marking its center) and the sulcus technique (locating the depression between the separate insertion ridges of the superficial and deep MCL).[10] Although a small vessel is often present at the superficial ridge, we have found that the location of this vessel is not consistent. The epicondylar line is marked on the resected distal femur with methylene blue, and a specially designed slotted instrument is aligned with the epicondylar line (Fig. 80.14). Through the use of the guide, a bony slot is created with the saw perpendicular to the epicondylar line. The slot serves to align the AP cutting block in appropriate femoral rotation; it is only 5 mm deep and does not compromise the PCL.

AP Femoral Cuts

The femoral (AP) sizing guide is inserted in the femur and referenced off the anterior lateral cortex (or middle aspect of the anterior cortex) and posterior condyles of the femur. The component size is read directly from the guide (letters A, B, C, and so forth). If the indicator is in between available sizes, the smaller component size is typically used.

The appropriate AP cutting block is engaged in the previously created slot with correct rotation. The cutting block is appropriately placed in the AP plane, referencing from both the anterior femoral cortex and the posterior condyles; an anterior "boom" and posterior reference/rotation guide determine the AP resection. The anterior boom should contact the middle to lateral anterior femoral cortex. Posteriorly, the runners of the guide are placed flush with the posterior condyles; with proper AP positioning of the cutting block, the guide should indicate a zero setting, which determines a posterior condylar resection of 9 to 10 mm to avoid potential imbalance of the flexion and extension gaps (Fig. 80.15). Because a few degrees of external rotation are desired, resection of the posterior condyles is usually more than 10 mm medially and less than 10 mm laterally. When a smaller femoral size is used (because of being between available sizes), additional bone must be removed either anteriorly or posteriorly. Additional posterior resection enlarges the flexion gap, introducing a potential for instability, whereas additional anterior resection increases the risk of notching the femur. "In-between" placement of the cutting block minimizes both of these effects. By moving the anterior boom of the AP cutting block medially, the guide can be translated more posteriorly to resect several additional millimeters of anterior bone.

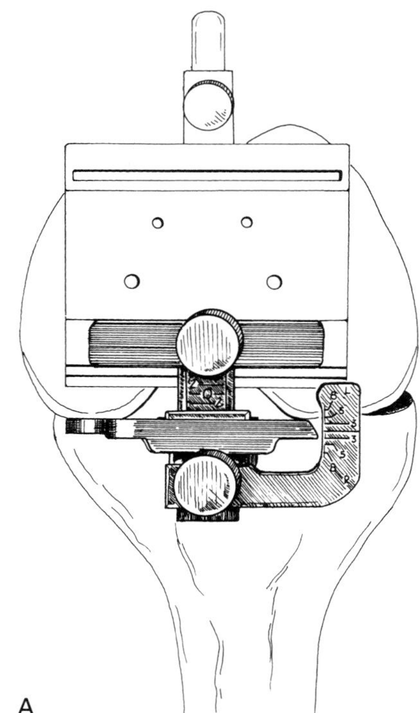

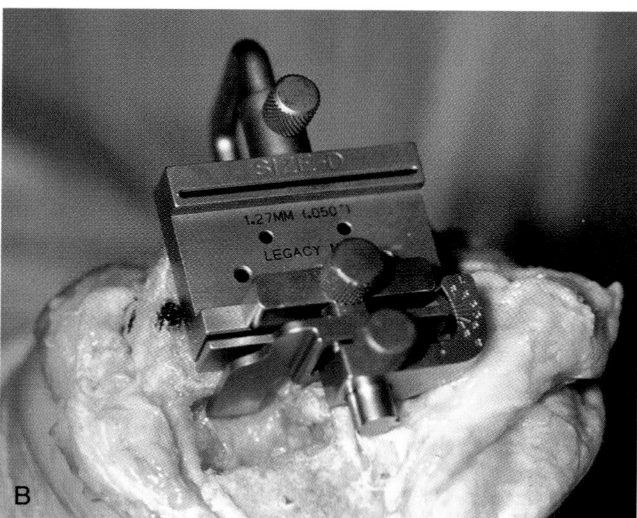

FIGURE 80.15 ➢ *A*, Anteroposterior (AP) cutting block connected to the posterior reference/rotation guide (which helps with proper AP and rotational positioning of the femoral component). *B*, Intraoperative photograph.

The 3 degrees of flexion in the distal femoral cut protect against potential anterior notching. The posterior reference/rotation guide helps to determine "in-between" placement. The guide indicates deviation from the standard bone resection. For example, the 2-mm line below the zero setting indicates that 2 mm of additional posterior condyle bone should be resected. If the posterior resection, as determined by the guide, is not within the 2-mm markings, the femoral size should be reevaluated.

Proximal Tibial Cut

The proximal tibial cut is aligned in accordance with an extramedullary guide. This guide references off the malleoli of the ankle. The true center of the ankle is about 5 to 10 mm medial to the midpoint between the medial and lateral malleoli.[68] Proximally, the alignment of the cut is perpendicular to the tibial axis in the coronal plane and with a 3- to 5-degree posterior slope. We typically remove 10 mm of bone from the least involved tibial plateau to maintain adequate stiffness of the underlying bone.

Harada et al suggested that the proximal tibia weakens below a depth of 5 mm,[38] prompting many surgeons to resect as little bone as possible. Because this requires use of thinner polyethylene inserts, the potential risk of stress-related wear is introduced. However, we have little reservation resecting an average of 10 mm of proximal tibia, because Goldstein et al demonstrated that significantly weaker bone is observed only beyond a depth of 20 mm.[30]

After the tibial cut, we use laminar spreaders for exposure to remove any remnants of the menisci. While we protect the PCL, we carefully remove posterior and notch osteophytes, using thin curved and straight osteotomes; detached tissues are removed with a hernia forceps (Fig. 80.16). This posterior débridement improves postoperative flexion.

Assessment of Extension and Flexion Gaps

The flexion and extension gaps are sized with spacer blocks.[51] Simultaneously, mediolateral stability and overall limb alignment are evaluated with the knee fully extended. If necessary, a medial or lateral ligament release is performed in a graduated manner. Medial release is performed by a distal release of the

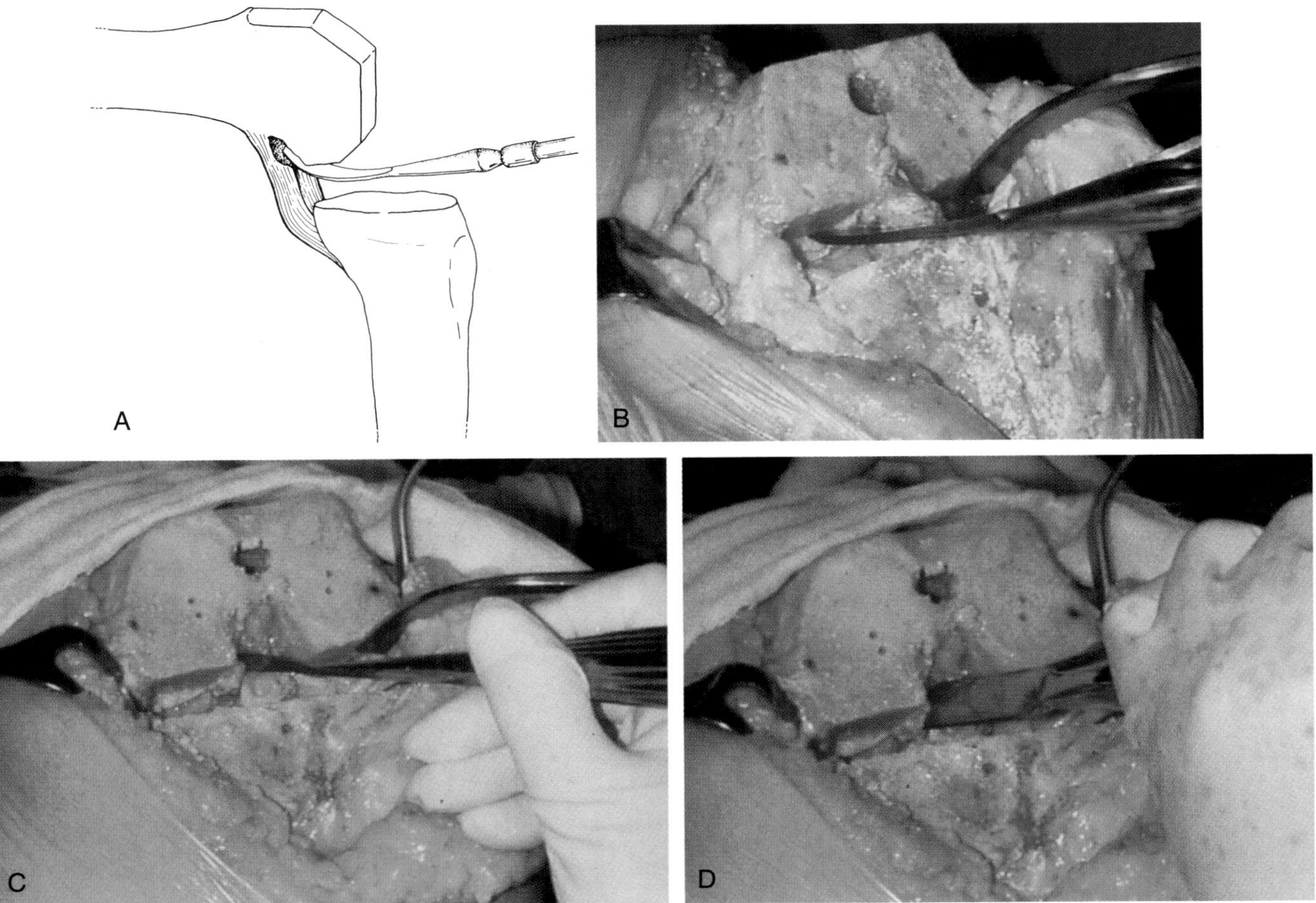

FIGURE 80.16 ➢ *A*, Posterior work with a curved osteotome to clean posterior recesses from the osteophytes. *B*, Intraoperative photograph. *C* and *D*, Removal of notch osteophytes while preserving the PCL.

superficial collateral ligament from the tibia; a lateral release is performed by the multiple puncture technique in extension.

PCL Management and Check of Stability in Flexion

The PCL is protected while the femoral and tibial bone cuts are made. During the proximal tibial cut, we prefer to insert a thin osteotome in front of the posterior spine to protect the PCL tibial insertion (Fig. 80.17).[6] After the proximal tibial cut, the residual spine is resected to the level of the tibial cut while the PCL is protected with an elevator (Fig. 80.18*A, B*). Alternatively, the surgeon may choose to cut across the proximal tibia initially to obtain a partial PCL release at the level of the proximal tibial cut. After insertion of the trial components, the knee is taken through a range of motion while PCL tension is assessed. In our experience with the MBK, PCL tension is frequently too tight, resulting in limited flexion, excessive femoral sliding back, and/or polyethylene insert anterior liftoff. The liftoff is exaggerated if the patella is everted and therefore should be assessed with the patella reduced. In the case of excessive tension, the PCL is released.[49, 81, 85] This can be done off the femur by selectively cutting the anterior fibers or (as we prefer) from the tibia by releasing the insertion with a small knife and periosteal elevator (Fig. 80.19). We release the PCL from the tibia because the ligament fibers remain attached to the posterior capsule, maintaining some tension and potential for healing back to the tibia at a new resting tension (Fig. 80.20). We feel that PCL recession from the tibia helps preserve the ligament's fundamental function of resisting posterior tibial subluxation.

Stability of the knee must be obtained in both extension and flexion. In flexion, we check stability with the spacer block and again with the trial components, performing AP drawer testing with the knee flexed to 90 degrees (Fig. 80.21). A thicker polyethylene insert is chosen if posterior stability is inadequate.

Flexion instability is an underdiagnosed cause of knee symptoms after TKA. Possible surgical causes of flexion instability include (1) femoral component undersizing with over-resection of the posterior femoral condyles; (2) femoral component malrotation with an asymmetric, trapezoidal flexion gap and a loose collateral ligament; (3) extensive lateral release in valgus knees; (4) flexion contracture corrected by the selection of a thinner plastic insert to bring the knee into extension; and (5) PCL insufficiency resulting from improper balancing, failure to recognize PCL incompetence (as in rheumatoid arthritis), or a partial release that becomes complete in the postoperative period. We prefer to reference the femoral AP cuts posteriorly to minimize the risk of flexion instability.

Next, the femoral Chamfer guide is placed flush with the anterior and distal surfaces of the femur. We center the box on the PCL, but we favor a slightly lateral position when possible. The fixation holes for the two femoral pegs are created. Then the anterior and posterior Chamfers and trochlear recesses are cut through the slots without compromising the PCL.

The tibia is finished before trial reduction. We select the tibial sizing plate that provides a good platform coverage[12] and rotate it toward the medial half of the tibial tubercle.[70] The space for the tibial stem is then prepared with a 15-mm drill, followed by a broach impactor.

Patellar Resurfacing

We routinely resurface the patella except in cases when the patellar surface is intact and tracks normally. The patellar osteotomy is performed with a saw or a specialized reaming device that produces congruent resection at a thickness sufficient to anchor the patellar prosthesis. Caliper measurements of patellar thickness before and after resurfacing are important.[79] The

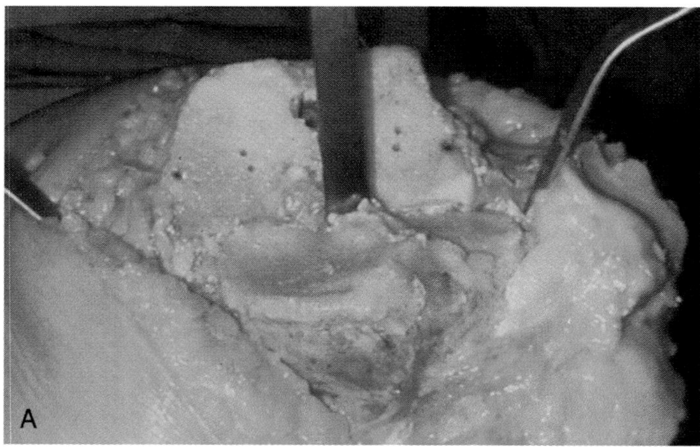

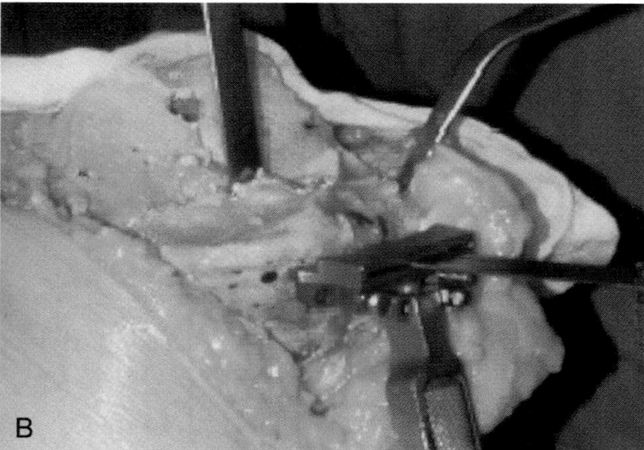

FIGURE 80.17 ➢ *A,* Thin osteotome inserted in front of the posterior spine to protect the PCL. *B,* Proximal tibial cut.

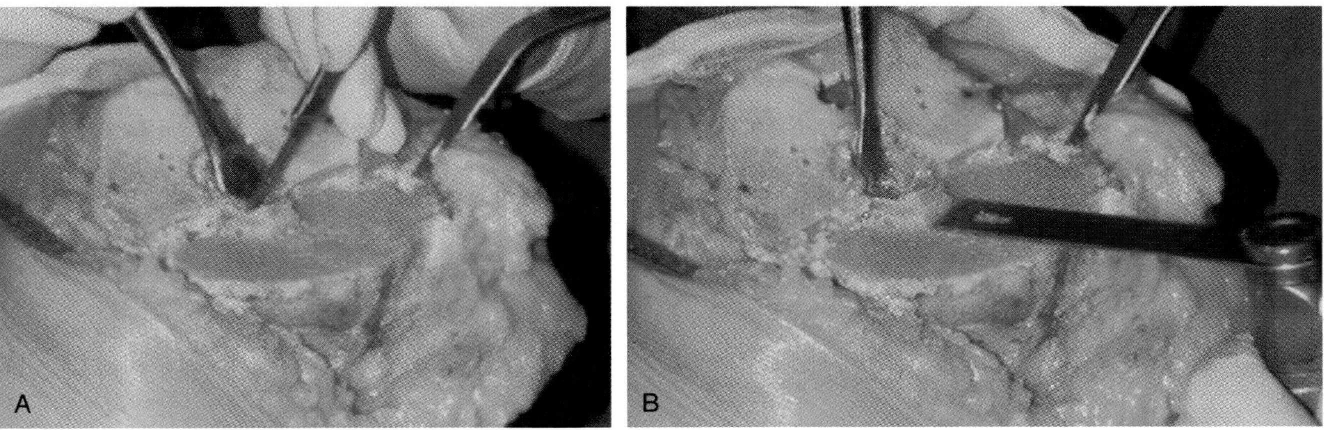

FIGURE 80.18 ➢ *A,* Careful release of the PCL from the residual spine. *B,* Resection of the residual spine while the PCL is protected with an elevator.

patellar thickness with the trial should be equal to or slightly less than the original thickness of the patella. Three fixation holes are reamed into the resected patellar surface, while the implant is slightly medialized.[96] The trial patellar button is inserted to observe patellar tracking during trial reduction. The "no thumb" test[31] is used to assess patellar tracking. The medial border of the patella should remain in contact with the femoral component throughout the range of motion without the lateral pressure of the surgeon's thumb. We remove slack from the quadriceps tendon during the assessment of patellar tracking by applying longitudinal tension to the rectus with a clamp (Fig. 80.22). If necessary, a lateral retinacular release is performed by means of the oblique cut technique or the multiple puncture technique; attention is given to save the superolateral geniculate vessels.[61, 64]

Proper limb alignment is confirmed by external (proximal and distal) landmarks, and flexion (see Fig. 80.21) and extension stability are reassessed. After careful bone cleaning by pulsatile lavage, the final components are cemented. The patellar and femoral

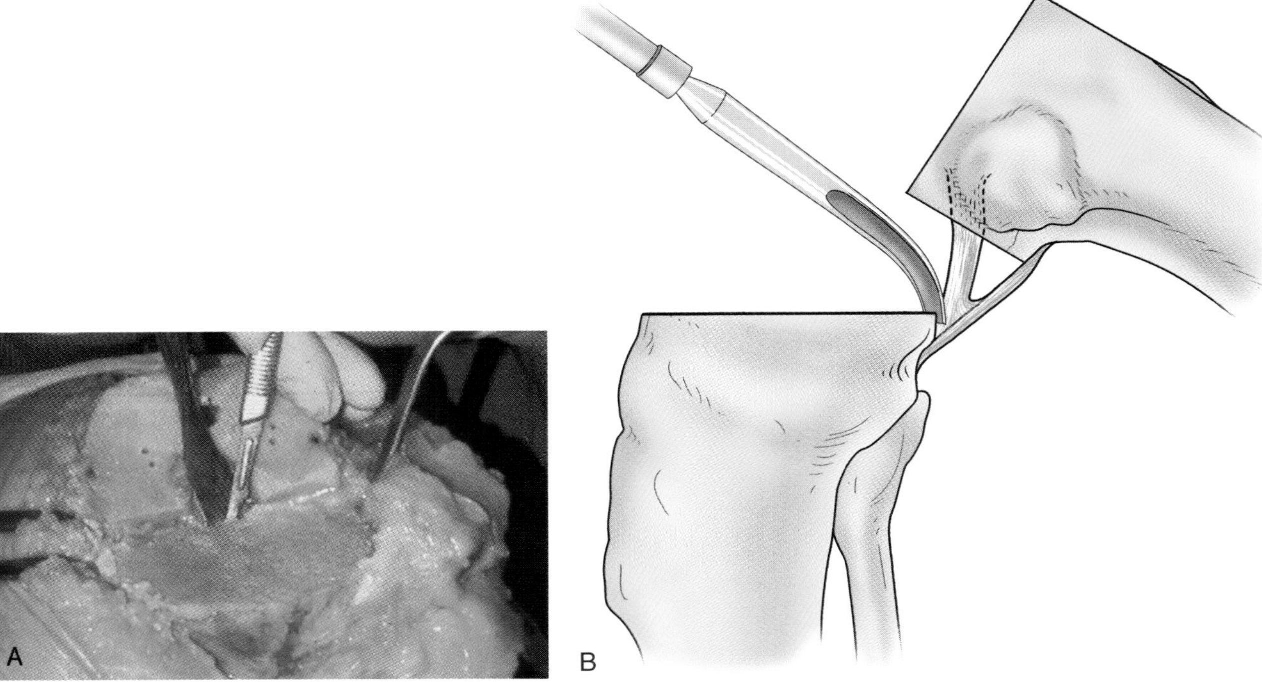

FIGURE 80.19 ➢ *A,* Subperiosteal PCL recession from the back of the tibia is performed with the use of a small knife and an elevator. *B,* Subperiosteal PCL recession, leaving the PCL attached to the posterior capsule.

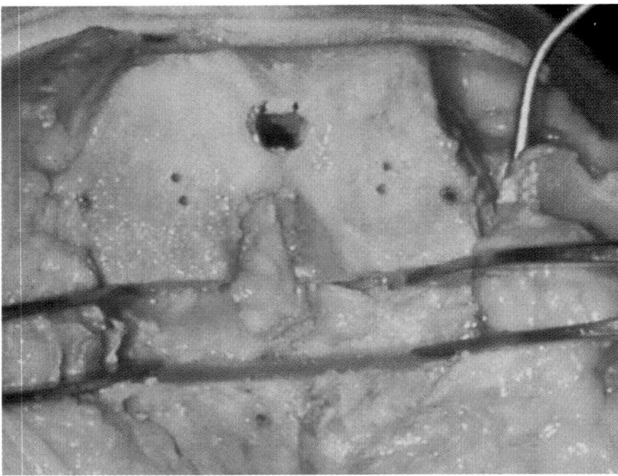

FIGURE 80.20 ➢ Recessed PCL that remains attached to the posterior capsule.

components are cemented before the tibial component is placed. The polyethylene is attached to the tibial baseplate. Excess cement must be completely removed to prevent cement particles from becoming entrapped under the mobile platform. After fixation of the components, appropriate knee stability, intraoperative motion, and patellar tracking are confirmed.

The arthrotomy is closed with interrupted sutures after the drain is placed. Adequate closure of the arthrotomy is verified with knee flexion. The skin is reapproximated, and a sterile dressing is applied. Radiographs are obtained in the recovery room.

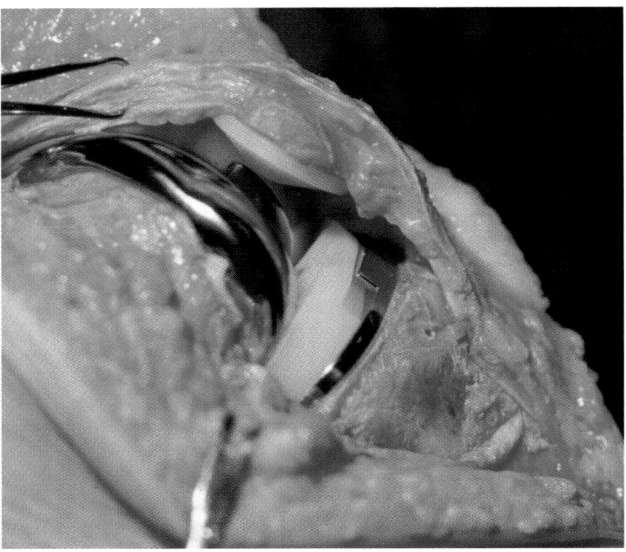

FIGURE 80.22 ➢ Assessment of patellar tracking while the slack is removed from the quadriceps tendon with a clamp.

REHABILITATION

Patients begin using a continuous passive motion machine in the immediate postoperative period. Range of motion is advanced from an initial setting of 60 degrees as tolerated, with the objective being flexion of at least 90 degrees by postoperative day 4 or 5.

We encourage the patient to stand on the first postoperative day and to take a few steps with a walker by the second day. Progress is variable and age depen-

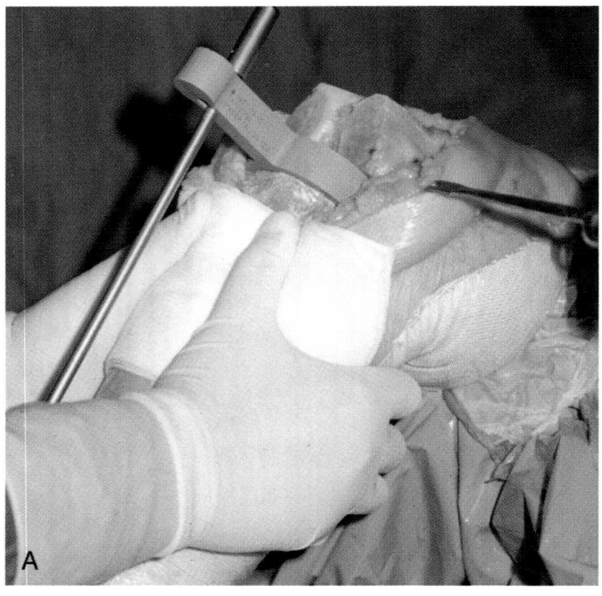

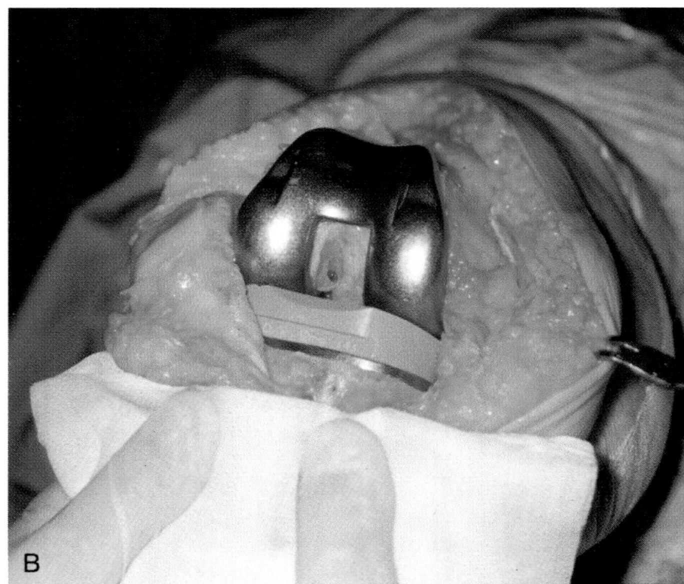

FIGURE 80.21 ➢ Assessment of knee stability in flexion with the spacer block *(A)* and with the trial components *(B)*.

dent. Ambulation is initiated with a walker until the patient is steady enough to use a single cane. Full weightbearing without a cane is permitted only when the patient demonstrates adequate stability and confidence.

Muscle strengthening exercises begin in the immediate postoperative period and include active plantar and dorsiflexion of the feet (to limit venous stasis) and isometric exercises for the for quadriceps and gluteus muscles. Straight-leg raising is started as soon as possible. Stationary bicycle exercises are initiated once the patient demonstrates adequate flexion.

Patients are typically discharged from the hospital after 5 to 7 days, provided that they can walk unassisted, flex to at least 90 degrees, and climb several steps while using an handrail. Physical therapy with emphasis on bicycling, range of motion, and isometric quadriceps exercises is continued under supervision of a physical therapist.

MBK STUDIES

In Vitro Studies of Wear

Several in vitro investigations to determine the wear characteristics of the MBK polyethylene are currently being conducted. These studies are assessing wear of the articular surface, the rotating surface, the undersurface "mushroom" slot, and the anterior rail slot. Although the mobile-bearing design should exhibit minimal wear at the articular surface with its large contact area and minimal constraint, some researchers are concerned about wear at other sites of contact between the polyethylene and tibial baseplate.

Using a simulator of natural knee function and motion, Peter Walker is comparing wear characteristics of the MBK to the IBII. At 10 million cycles (approximately equal to average weightbearing over 7 to 8 years) the MBK exhibits less penetration wear but approximately 30% greater volumetric wear than does the IBII. Differential analysis of the articulating and nonarticulating surfaces demonstrates that the MBK produces negligible wear from its articulating surface (only minor burnishing) but substantial undersurface wear, primarily by adhesive and abrasive mechanisms. Delamination of the polyethylene was not observed.

A limitation of this in vitro study is that lubrication between the polyethylene and baseplate does not simulate the natural knee lubrication mechanisms. Perhaps wear would be reduced if the bovine serum used in experimentation were redistributed to the rotating surface more frequently than every 150,000 cycles, during which time the load remains constant. Furthermore, the baseplate finish may have to be improved to a lower tolerance than 0.1 μ to further limit adhesive and abrasive wear.

The debris particles produced from this in vitro experimentation are studied by P. Campbell at the University of California, Los Angeles (P. Campbell, personal communication). This limb of the investigation quantifies the amounts of various wear particle sizes: (1) granules (<1 mm), (2) fibrils (3 mm), and (3) flakes (5 to 10 mm). In comparison with the IBII, fewer small particles are observed with the MBK polyethylene wear. From investigations of osteolysis after total hip arthroplasty,[84] it has been demonstrated that these smaller particles are the most active in stimulating the biological responses responsible for osteolysis, implying that the MBK prosthesis may diminish the risk of failure caused by osteolysis.

Other areas of stress concentration that may induce wear are the undersurface mushroom slot and anterior rail. In a separate laboratory experiment, no plastic deformation was observed at the undersurface slot with 1.5 million cycles of 400-N to 800-N shear stress applied (Zimmer, Inc.). With posterior tibial translation, the plastic contacts the anterior rail stop. Because these forces are distributed over a large area, no plastic deformation has been observed in this location. With anterior tibial translation (a rare occurrence in TKA), the mushroom head and peg contact the relatively thin plastic at the undersurface slot. During laboratory testing, no plastic deformation occurred at this site of potential wear.

Gait Analysis

Using a previously described method of gait analysis[1] combined with limb electromyography, Catani and colleagues compared the MBK and IBII prostheses in gait analysis and stair climbing (Catani, personal communication). While maintaining an adequate flexion moment, the MBK group demonstrated a reduction in the extension moment, which suggests better quadriceps function than in the IBII group. The adduction moment was significantly less in the MBK group, resulting in more symmetric loading (and therefore less medial compartment loading) during the late stance phase of gait. The advantage of symmetric loading may be attributed to external rotation of the polyethylene in the late stance phase. Unique to the MBK group was some irregularity of the flexion moment during late stance phase, as opposed to the fluid flexion moment observed in the IBII group. These irregularities are probably secondary to sliding of the polyethylene on the tibial baseplate.

Muscle activity during stair ascent in both groups demonstrated prolonged activity of the rectus femoris and of the anterior tibialis throughout the late stance phase. Increased activation of the hamstrings was observed in the MBK group, probably as a response to the AP sliding movements of the bearing. Physiological knee function was observed in both groups during stair descent.

Kinematics

Barrett and Walker performed video fluoroscopic analysis of the MBK prosthesis during stair climbing, applying techniques described by Stiehl et al. They analyzed the fluoroscopic videos by using an inverse perspective method that requires image matching and created digital libraries containing three-dimensional computer-assisted design drawings. At each increment of flexion, the two-dimensional fluoroscopic images were replaced by the library's closest matching three-dimensional computer-assisted design drawing. Despite considerable variation, several trends were observed. During stair climbing, the femoral component initially translated posteriorly on the tibia as the knee progressed from flexion to extension. With greater extension, however, the femur translated anteriorly in relation to the tibia. Finally, at terminal extension, the femur again translated posteriorly on the tibia.

Variability was also observed with regard to internal and external rotation, ranging from 6 to 8 degrees. However, terminal tibial external rotation was similar to that occurring in physiological knee function. In contrast to previous reports, lateral condylar liftoff was not observed. Stiehl et al, using a three-dimensional interactive modeling analysis of 20 LCS cruciate-sacrificing, mobile-bearing knees, estimated the lateral liftoff rate during heel strike at approximately 50%.[93] The average AP displacement of 3.1 mm was not fluid but instead occurred in bursts, which suggests that frictional forces (approximately 150 N) resist shear forces generated during stair climbing.

Clinical Outcomes

Our series of TKAs with the cruciate-sparing MBK design includes three versions of the prosthesis. The original model (Mark I) was implanted in 24 patients between October 1993 and June 1994. The second version (Mark II) was implanted in 24 patients between December 1994 and June 1996. The current design (Mark III) was implanted in 21 patients between December 1996 and April 1997. The evolution of the prosthesis from Mark I and Mark II involved design modifications to improve knee extension, whereas the changes from Mark II to the Mark III were made to avoid component translocation. In the Mark III, the femoral component condylotrochlear junction was shifted more anteriorly and proximally and the polyethylene anterior lip was reduced, thereby affording 12 degrees of hyperextension. As noted earlier, given the 6 to 7 degrees of posterior slope of the tibia and 3 degrees of flexion of the femoral component, this results in only approximately 2 to 3 degrees of actual hyperextension. The Mark III features a polyethylene "saddle" that prevents component translocation observed intraoperatively in several cases in which the previous models were used, particularly after lateral ligament release in valgus knees.

The average age of the 69 patients was 67.5 years (range, 58 to 80 years). There were 10 males and 59 females. The diagnosis was osteoarthritis in 64, rheumatoid arthritis in 4, and osteonecrosis in 1 patient.

Preoperative deformities included varus position (range, 1 to 27 degrees) in 56% of the cases, valgus position (range, 1 to 14 degrees) in 16%, and fixed flexion (greater than 15 degrees) in 14% (Fig. 80.23*A*, *B*). Fourteen percent of patients did not have preoperative knee deformities. Previous surgical procedures included high tibial osteotomy (7 patients), synovectomy (6 patients), and open reduction/internal fixation of a tibial plateau fracture (1 patient). The PCL was spared in all patients and was left at its resting tension in 23 cases (33%), was partially recessed from the tibia in 14 cases (20%), and was fully recessed in 32 (47%).

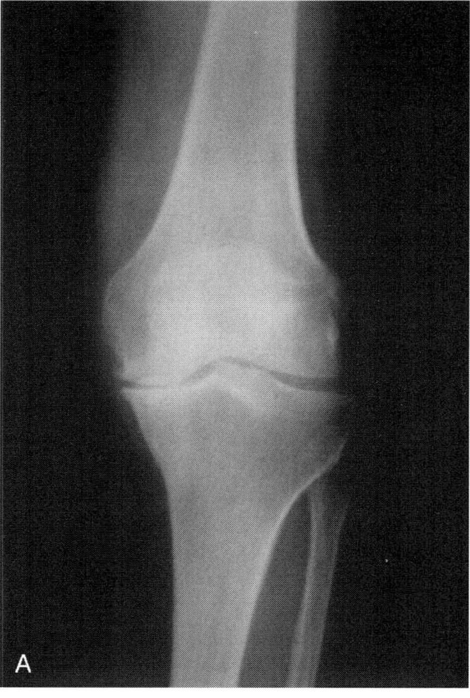

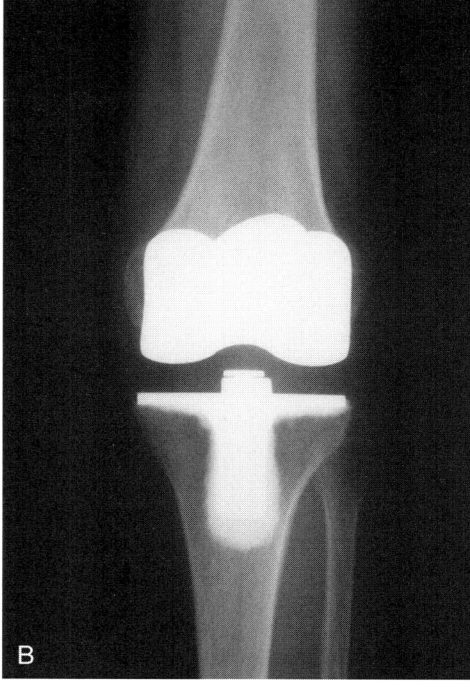

FIGURE 80.23 ➢ *A,* Preoperative radiograph of an osteoarthritic left knee with varus deformity. *B,* Postoperative radiograph at 1 year of follow-up of a Mark III MBK knee replacement.

We performed a lateral retinacular release in 18 cases (29%). The patella was resurfaced in all knees with a cemented all-polyethylene dome design.

Clinical and radiographic follow-up data were available for 61 of the original 69 patients (52 females and 9 males). The mean follow-up period was 2.5 years (range, 1.5 to 5.0). At follow-up, 5 patients had died of unrelated causes, 2 were bedridden, and 1 could not be located. The average knee score according to the Knee Society rating system[50] increased from 37.5 points preoperatively to 89 points at follow-up. The results were excellent in 35 knees (57%), good in 23 (38%), fair in 2 (3%), and poor in 1 (2%) (Fig. 80.24). Mean postoperative active flexion was 110 degrees (range, 90 to 130 degrees); 4 patients had an extension lag averaging 7 degrees.

The Knee Society functional score at follow-up was excellent in 32 patients (52%), good in 14 (23%), fair in 10 (17%), and poor in 5 (8%) (see Fig. 80.24). Anterior drawer testing was within 5 mm of the contralateral knee in 71% of the knees, between 5 to 10 mm in 24%, and greater than 10 mm in 5%. (The inherent AP translation of the prosthesis is 4.5 mm.) Only one patient had excessive AP laxity documented by radiological stress testing (Fig. 80.25). We attribute the excessive translation in this patient to undersizing of the femoral component and resultant flexion instability from over-resection of the posterior condyles. Postoperative coronal alignment was within 5 mm of physiological valgus position in 48 patients (79%), between 5 and 10 mm in 9 (15%), and greater than 10 mm in 4 (6%). All patients were able to adequately transfer from a chair. In accordance with Charnley's system, 81.5% of the patients in category A (only one knee involved) and 75% of the patients in category B (both knees replaced) were able to perform stair climbing.

Forty-eight patients had no pain at follow-up, 9 had mild pain, 3 had moderate pain, and 1 had severe pain. Seven patients (11.5%) noted a subjective "click" in the knee. The clicks seem attributable to contact of the polyethylene with the stopping mechanisms. In one very active patient, an audible extension "snap" occurred during the swing phase of gait, probably as a result of the same mechanism.

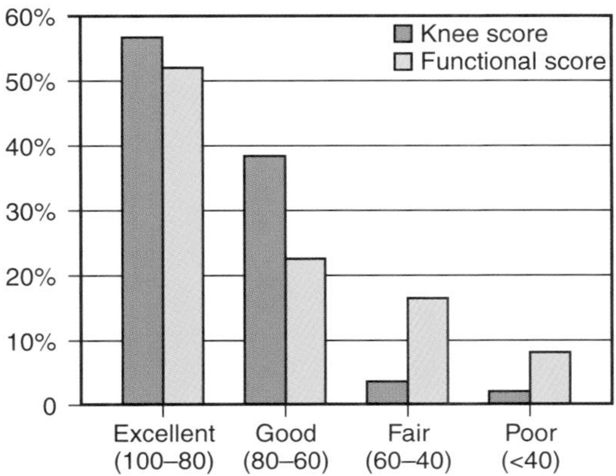

FIGURE 80.24 ➢ Postoperative Knee Society score and function score.

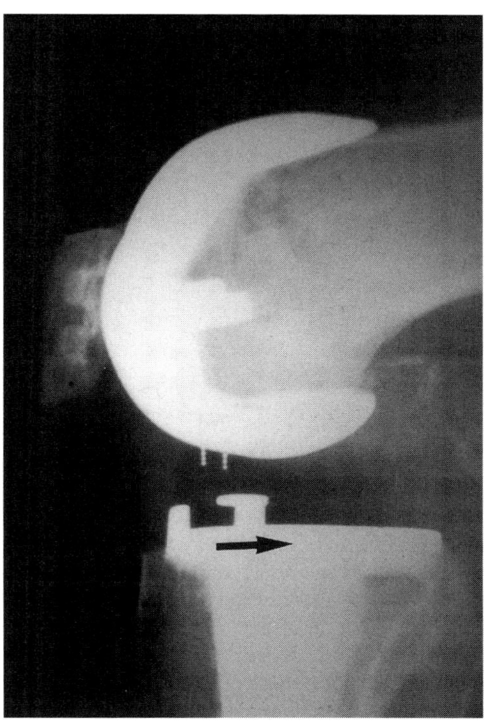

FIGURE 80.25 ➢ Radiological stress test demonstrating posterior subluxation of a Mark I knee replacement.

Asymptomatic painless patellar crepitus was present in 10 knees, and one patient had a patellar "clunk." On Merchant's views,[63] the patella was tilted medially in 7% of cases, tilted laterally in 24% of cases, and subluxated laterally in 12% of cases (Fig. 80.26). Two patients (3%) had radiographic evidence of an asymptomatic type I patellar stress fracture.[33] According to lateral radiographs, seven patients (11.5%) had patella baja; the majority of these cases were in patients after high tibial osteotomy.

We evaluated the radiographs according to the Knee Society Roentgenographic Evaluation System.[30] We used preoperative and postoperative long standing roentgenograms of the knee to determine overall limb alignment and fluoroscopic positioning in AP and lateral views to identify radiolucent lines.

Radiographic analysis with long standing films showed satisfactory good alignment over the mechanical axis (0 ± 5 degrees) in all patients, with 41 knees (67%) within 2 degrees of physiological alignment. In the coronal plane, the tibial component was at 90 ± 2 degrees in 97% of cases; the femoral component in the coronal plane was at 90 ± 5 degrees of valgus position in all the patients and at 90 ± 2 degrees in 52 cases.

Radiolucent lines were present on the medial side (zones 1 to 2) in 19% of tibial components and in 13% of femoral components (zone 4); no radiolucent lines

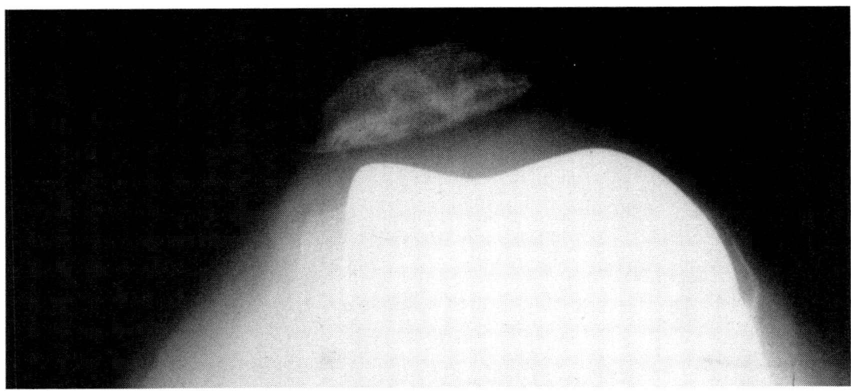

FIGURE 80.26 ➢ Merchant's view showing lateral patellar subluxation.

occurred laterally. One Mark I femoral component subsided into excessive valgus position at 5 years (the first-generation femoral component lacked the two fixation pegs). Minor osteolytic areas developed under one tibial component and two femoral components. We observed no evidence of polyethylene wear according to established radiological methods.[25]

One patient underwent revision (Mark I) for loosening of the femoral component 5 years after surgery. At reoperation there was no wear detectable in the plastic insert.

The University of Dundee (UK) is leading an ongoing multicenter European clinical trial of 249 MBK Mark III prostheses implanted in 170 females and 79 males. Data from a minimal follow-up period of 1 year are available for 41 of these patients. The diagnosis was osteoarthritis in 90.8%. Mean age was 68 years (range, 31 to 86). In 35% of the cases the "epicondylar" instrumentation was used. In 38 cases (15%) the patella was not resurfaced. A lateral patellar retinacular release was performed in 33%.

The average Knee Society score increased from 32 points preoperatively to 81 points at follow-up, and the average function score increased from 56 points to 80 points. Mean active flexion at follow-up was 103 degrees (range, 60 to 125 degrees), and the passive extension lag averaged 0.92 degree (range, 0 to 15 degrees). Eighty-five percent of the patients were able to walk half a mile 1 year after surgery. Eighty-five percent of the patients had no pain at rest, and 63% had no pain climbing stairs. Whereas 85% of patients had experienced patellofemoral pain preoperatively, only 15% reported anterior knee pain at follow-up. No patient had to undergo revision or was scheduled for revision at the 1-year follow-up interval.

COMMENTS

The concept of the mobile-bearing knee is intellectually attractive; such prostheses can potentially reduce problems of polyethylene wear while improving kinematics and function.

We believe that the conventional fixed-bearing knee prosthesis will maintain its place in the field of total knee replacement, with standard technique and reliable long-term results.[25, 86, 89] However, we think that there is a place for the more sophisticated mobile-bearing knee prosthesis, possibly to be used for younger, more active patients with increased demands. This implant should improve performance and exhibit reduced polyethylene wear. The preliminary results of the MBK series are promising, but long-term evaluation is required. The MBK design offers the advantages of full conformity throughout flexion and the option of preserving the PCL. The prosthesis can be used in most cases of osteoarthritis.

In summary, the theoretical advantages of reducing wear and providing better knee function with more physiological knee kinematics still need a longer term evaluation. Potential disadvantages include the design's mechanical complexity and its higher cost in relation to simpler knee systems.

Fixed-bearing knee design has reached its ultimate expression; occasionally, this stage of development indicates impending obsolescence. The mobile-bearing knee offers an attractive avenue for future developments.[47]

References

1. Aichroth P, Freeman MAR, Smillie IS, et al: A knee function assessment chart. J Bone Joint Surg Br 60:308-309, 1978.
1a. Andriacchi TP, Galante JO, Fermier RW: The influence of total knee replacement design on walking and stair climbing. J Bone Joint Surg Am 64:1328-1335, 1982.
2. Anouchi YS, Whiteside LA, Kaiser AD, et al: The effects of axial rotational alignment of the femoral component on instability and patellar tracking in total knee arthroplasty demonstrated on autopsy specimens. Clin Orthop 287:170-177, 1993.
3. Argenson JN, O'Connor JJ: Polyethylene wear in meniscal knee replacement: A 1-9 year retrieval analysis of the Oxford Knee. J Bone Joint Surg Br 74:228-232, 1992.
4. Arima J, Whiteside LA, McCarty DS, et al: Femoral rotational alignment, based on the antero-posterior axis, in total knee arthroplasty in a valgus knee. J Bone Joint Surg Am 77:1331-1334, 1995.
5. Barnes CL, Sledge CB: Total knee arthroplasty with posterior cruciate ligament retention designs. In Insall JN, ed: Surgery of the Knee, 2nd ed. New York, Churchill Livingstone, 1993, pp 815-827.
6. Bartel DL, Bicknell VL, Wright TM: The effect of conformity, thickness, and material on stresses in ultra-high molecular weight components for total joint replacement. J Bone Joint Surg Am 68:1041-1051, 1986.

7. Bartel DL, Burnstein AH, Santavicca EA, et al: Performance of the tibial component in total knee replacement. Conventional and revision design. J Bone Joint Surg Am 64:26-33, 1982.
8. Bartel DL, Bicknell VL, Wright TM: The effect of conformity, thickness, and material on stress in UHMWPE components for joint replacement. J Bone Joint Surg Am 68:1041-1051, 1986.
9. Berger RA, Rubash HE, Seel MJ, et al: Determining the rotational alignment of the femoral component in total knee arthroplasty using the epicondylar axis. Clin Orthop 286:40-47, 1993.
10. Bert JM: Dislocation/subluxation of meniscal bearing elements after New Jersey Low-Contact Stress total knee arthroplasty. Clin Orthop 254:211, 1990.
11. Bloebaum RD, Bachus KN, Mitchell W, et al: Analysis of the bone surface area in resected tibia: Implications in tibial component subsidence and fixation. Clin Orthop 309:2-10, 1994.
12. Buechel FF, Pappas MJ: The New Jersey Low Contact Stress Knee replacement system: Biomechanical rationale and review of the first 123 cemented cases. Arch Orthop Trauma Surg 105: 197-204, 1986.
13. Buechel FF, Pappas MJ: Long-term survivorship analysis of the cruciate-sparing versus cruciate sacrificing knee prostheses using meniscal bearings. Clin Orthop 260:162-169, 1990.
14. Buechel FF: Cemented and cementless revision arthroplasty using rotating platform total knee implants: A 12 year experience. Orthop Rev Suppl 71, 1990.
15. Buechel FF: New Jersey LCS unicompartmental knee replacement: Clinical, radiographic, statistical and survivorship analyses of 106 cementless cases performed by 7 surgeons. Food and Drug Administration Panel Presentation, Rockville, MD, August 16, 1991.
16. Buechel FF, Pappas MJ, Greenwald AS: Evaluation of contact stresses in metal-baked patellar replacements: A predictor of survivorship. Clin Orthop 273:190-197, 1991.
17. Buechel FF: Cementless mobile bearing TKR: Concepts and 10 year evaluation. Presented at the 7th Annual Joint Replacement Symposium, Palm Beach, FL, October 23, 1992.
18. Buechel FF, Keblish PA, Lee JM, et al: Low contact stress meniscal bearing unicompartmental knee replacement: Long-term evaluation of cemented and cementless results. J Orthop Rheum 7:31-41, 1994.
19. Buechel FF: Meniscal bearing knee replacement: Development, long-term results, and future technology. In Scott NW, ed: The Knee. New York, Mosby, 1994, pp 1157-1177.
20. Buechel FF: Low-Contact-Stress, meniscal bearing knee replacement: Design concepts, failure mechanisms and long term survivorship. In Insall JN, Scott WN, Scuderi GR, eds: Current Concepts in Primary and Revision Total Knee Arthroplasty. Philadelphia, Lippincott-Raven, 1996, pp 47-64.
21. Buechel FF: Evolving clinical use of mobile bearing knee design concepts. The complications of long experience. Presented at the 14th Annual Current Concepts in Joint Replacements Symposium, Orlando, FL, December 11, 1998.
22. Chao EY, Laughman RK, Schneider E, et al: Normative data of knee joint motion and ground reaction forces in adult level walking. J Biomech 16:219, 1983.
23. Churchill DL, Incavo SJ, Johnson CC, et al: The transepicondylar axis approximates the optimal flexion axis of the knee. Clin Orthop 356:111-118, 1998.
24. Colizza WA, Insall JN, Scuderi GR: The Posterior Stabilized total knee prosthesis. Assessment of polyethylene damage and osteolysis after a ten-year minimum follow-up. J Bone Joint Surg Am 77:1713-1720, 1995.
24a. Diduch DR, Insall JN, Scott WN, et al: Total knee replacement in young, active patients: Long-term follow-up and functional outcome. J Bone Joint Surg Am 79:575-582, 1997.
24b. Duffy GP, Trousdale RT, Stuart MJ: Total knee arthroplasty in patients 55 years old or younger. Clin Orthop 356:22-27, 1998.
25. Elbert K, Bartel D, Wright TM: The effect of conformity on stresses in dome-shaped polyethylene patellar components. Clin Orthop 317:71-75, 1995.
26. Elias SG, Freeman MAR, Gockay EI: A correlative study and anatomy of the distal femur. Clin Orthop 260:98-103, 1990.
27. Ewald FC: The Knee Society total knee arthroplasty roentgenographic evaluation and scoring system. Clin Orthop 248:9-12, 1989.
28. Ewald FC: Leg-lift technique for simultaneous femoral, tibial and patellar prosthetic cementing: "Rule of no thumb" for patellar tracking and steel rod rule for ligament tension. Tech Orthop 6: 44-46, 1991.
28a. Gabriel SM, Dennis DA, Honey MJ, et al: Polyethylene wear on the distal tibial insert surface in total knee arthroplasty. Knee 5: 221-228, 1998.
29. Goldberg VM, Figgie HE, Inglis AE, et al: Patellar fracture type and prognosis in condylar total knee arthroplasty. Clin Orthop 236:115-122, 1988.
30. Goldstein SA, Wilson DL, Sostengard DA, et al: The mechanical properties of human tibial trabecular bone as a function of metaphyseal location. J Biomech 16:965-969, 1983.
31. Goodfellow JW, O'Connor JJ: The mechanics of the knee and prosthetic design. J Bone Joint Surg Br 60:369-385, 1978.
32. Goodfellow JW, O'Connor JJ: Clinical results of the Oxford knee. Clin Orthop 205:21-42, 1986.
33. Goodfellow JW: The Oxford Knee for unicompartmental osteoarthritis. J Bone Joint Surg Br 70:692-701, 1988.
34. Goodfellow JW, O'Connor JJ: The anterior cruciate ligament in knee arthroplasty: A risk factor with unconstrained meniscal prostheses. Clin Orthop 276:245-252, 1992.
35. Goodfellow JW, O'Connor JJ: The role of congruent meniscal bearings in knee arthroplasty. In Scott NW, ed: The Knee. New York, Mosby, 1994, pp 1143-1156.
36. Griffin FM, Math KM, Scuderi GR, et al: Anatomy of the epicondyles of the distal femur: MRI analysis of normal knees. In press.
37. Griffin FM, Insall JN, Scuderi GR: The posterior condylar angle in osteoarthritic knees. J Arthroplasty 13:812-815, 1998.
38. Harada Y, Wevers HW, Cooke TDV: Distribution of bone strength in the proximal tibia. J Arthroplasty 3:167-175, 1988.
39. Hollister AM, Jatana S, Singh AK, et al: The axes of rotation of the knee. Clin Orthop 290:259-268, 1993.
40. Hood RW, Wright TM, Burnstein AH: Retrieval analysis of total knee prostheses: A method and its application to forty-eight total condylar prostheses. J Biomed Mater Res 17:829-842, 1983.
41. Hostalen GUR: Hoechst Aktiengellschaft. Frankfurt, Germany, 1982, p 22.
42. Hungerford DS, Kenna RV: Preliminary experience with a total knee prosthesis with porous coating used without cement. Clin Orthop 226:49, 1988.
43. Incavo SJ, Johnson CC, Beynnon BD, et al: Posterior cruciate ligament strain biomechanics in total knee arthroplasty. Clin Orthop 309:88-93, 1994.
44. Insall JN, Dorr LD, Scott RD, et al: Rationale of the Knee Society clinical rating system. Clin Orthop 248:13-14, 1989.
45. Insall JN: Surgical techniques and instrumentation in total knee arthroplasty. In Insall JN, ed: Surgery of the Knee, 2nd ed. New York, Churchill Livingstone, 1993.
46. Insall JN: Adventures in mobile-bearing knee design: A mid-life crisis. Orthopedics 21:1021-1023, 1998.
47. Jahan MS, Wang C, Schwartz G, et al: Combined chemical and mechanical effects on free radicals in UHMWPE joints during implantation. J Biomed Mater Res 24:1005-1017, 1991.
48. Jordan LR, Olivo JL, Voorhost PE: Survivorship analysis of cementless meniscal bearing total knee arthroplasty. Clin Orthop 338:119-123, 1997.
49. Keyes GW: Oxford meniscal prosthesis for anteromedial osteoarthritis of the knee and intact ACL. J Bone Joint Surg Br 73:140, 1991.
50. Kilgus DJ, Moreland JR, Finerman GA, et al: Catastrophic wear of tibial polyethylene insert. Clin Orthop 273:223-231, 1991.
51. Kurosawa H, Walker PS, Abe S: Geometry and motion of the knee for implant and orthotic design. J Biomech 18:487-499, 1985.
52. La Fortune MA, Cavanagh PR, Sommer MS, et al: Three dimensional kinematics of the human knee during walking. J Biomech 25:347-357, 1992.
53. Laskin RS: Flexion space configuration in total knee arthroplasty. J Arthroplasty 10:657-660, 1995.
54. Li S, Howard EG: Characterization and description of an enhanced ultra high molecular weight polyethylene for orthopaedic bearing surfaces. Trans Soc Biomater 13:190, 1990.
55. Mantas JP, Bloebaum RD, Skedros JG, et al: Implications of reference axes used for rotational alignment of the femoral component in primary and revision total knee arthroplasty. J Arthroplasty 7:531, 1992.

56. Martelli S, Ellis RE, Marcacci M, et al: Total knee arthroplasty kinematics. Computer simulation and intraoperative evaluation. J Arthroplasty 13:145-155, 1998.
57. McMahon MS, Scuderi GR, Glasgow JL, et al: Scintigraphic determination of patellar viability after excision of infrapatellar fat pad and/or lateral retinacular release in total arthroplasty. Clin Orthop 260:10-16, 1990.
58. Menchetti PPM, Walker PS: Mechanical evaluation of mobile bearing knees. Am J Knee Surg 10(2):73-82, 1997.
59. Merchant AC, Mercher RL, Jacobsen RH, et al: Roentgenographic analysis of patello-femoral congruence. J Bone Joint Surg Am 56: 1391-1396, 1974.
60. Merkow RL, Soudry M, Insall JN: Patellar dislocation following total knee replacement. J Bone Joint Surg Am 67:1321-1327, 1985.
61. Minns RJ, Eng B, Campbell J: The meniscal testing of a sliding meniscus knee prosthesis. Clin Orthop 137:268-275, 1978.
62. Minns RJ: The Minns meniscal knee prosthesis: Biomechanical aspects of the surgical procedure and a review of the first 165 cases. Arch Orthop Trauma Surg 108:231-235, 1989.
63. Minns RJ, Blamey JM, Blunn GW, et al: The polyethylene wear of meniscal bearings in the early Minns meniscal knee replacement. Knee 1:57-64, 1994.
64. Moreland JR, Basset LW, Hanker GJ: Radiographic analysis of the axial alignment of the lower extremity. J Bone Joint Surg Am 69: 745-749, 1987.
65. Morra EA, Postak PD, Greenwald AS: The influence of mobile bearing knee geometry on the wear of UHMWPE tibial inserts: A finite model element study. Presented at the 65th Annual Meeting of the American Academy of Orthopaedic Surgeons, New Orleans, March 1998.
66. Nagamine R, Whiteside LA: The effect of tibial tray malrotation on patellar tracking in total knee arthroplasty. J Arthroplasty 10: 265-270, 1995.
67. Nagamine R, White SE, Whiteside LA: The effect of rotational malposition of the femoral component on knee stability characteristics after total knee arthroplasty. Presented at the 60th Annual Meeting of the American Academy of Orthopaedic Surgeons, San Francisco, February 1993.
68. Nagamine R, Whiteside LA, White SE, et al: Patellar tracking after total knee arthroplasty. The effect of tibial tray malrotation and articular surface configuration. Clin Orthop 304:263-271, 1994.
69. Pappas MJ, Makris J, Buechel FF: Biomaterials for hard tissue applications. In Pizzoferrato PG, ed: Biomaterials and Clinical Applications: Evaluation of Contact Stresses in Metal-Plastic Knee Replacements. Amsterdam, Elsevier, 1987, pp 259-264.
70. Pappas MJ, Buechel FF: On the use of constant radius femoral component in meniscal bearing knee replacement. J Orthop Rheum 7:27-29, 1994.
70a. Parks NL, Engh GA, Topoleski LDT, et al: Modular tibial insert micromotion: A concern with contemporary knee implants. Clin Orthop 356:10-15, 1998.
71. Poilvache PL, Insall JN, Scuderi GR, et al: Rotational landmarks and sizing of the distal femur in total knee arthroplasty. Clin Orthop 331:35-46, 1996.
72. Polyzoides AJ, Dendrinos GK, Tsakonas H: The Rotaglide total knee arthroplasty. Prosthesis design and early results. J Arthroplasty 11:453-459, 1996.
73. Polyzoides AJ, Brooks S, Tsakonas A, et al: Design characteristics, experimental work and 10 year clinical experience with a fully conforming mobile bearing knee prosthesis. Presented at the International Conference on Knee Replacement 1974-2024, ImechE Headquarters, London, April 22-24, 1999.
74. Rand JA: Patellar resurfacing in total knee arthroplasty. Clin Orthop 260:110-117, 1990.
75. Rimnac CM, Burnstein AH, Carr JM, et al: Chemical and mechanical degradations of UHMWPE. J Applied Biomater 5:17-22, 1994.
76. Ritter MA, Faris PM, Keating EM, et al: Posterior cruciate ligament balancing during total knee arthroplasty. J Arthropl 3:323-326, 1988.
77. Roe RJ, Grood ES, Shastri R, et al: Effect of radiation sterilization and aging on ultrahigh molecular weight polyethylene. J Biomed Mater Res 15:209-230, 1981.
78. Rovick JS, Reuben JD, Schrager RJ, et al: Relation between knee motion and ligament length patterns. Clin Biomech 6(4):213-220, 1991.
79. Schmalzried TS, Jasty M, Harris WH: Periprosthetic bone loss in total hip arthroplasty. Polyethylene wear debris and the concept of the effective joint space. J Bone Joint Surg Am 74:849-863, 1992.
80. Scott RD, Thornhill TS: Posterior cruciate supplementing total knee replacement using conforming inserts and cruciate recession. Effect on range of motion and radiolucent lines. Clin Orthop 309:146-149, 1994.
81. Scuderi GR, Insall JN, Windsor RE, et al: Survivorship of cemented knee replacement. J Bone Joint Surg Br 71:778-803, 1989.
82. Sorrells RB: The rotating platform mobile bearing TKA. Orthopedics 19:793-796, 1996.
83. Soudry M, Walker PS, Reilly D, et al: Effects of total knee replacement design on femoro-tibial conditions. J Arthroplasty 1: 35, 1986.
84. Stern SH, Bowen MK, Insall JN, et al: Cemented total knee arthroplasty for gonarthrosis in patients 55 years old or younger. Clin Orthop 260:124-129, 1990.
85. Stiehl JB, Abbot BD: Femoral component rotational alignment using the extramedullary tibial shaft axis: A technical note. J Orthop Rheum 8:23, 1995.
86. Stiehl JB, Abbot BD: Morphology of the transepicondylar axis and its applications in primary and revision total knee arthroplasty. J Arthroplasty 10:785, 1995.
87. Stiehl JB, Komistek RD, Dennis DA, et al: Fluoroscopic analysis of the kinematics after posterior cruciate retaining knee arthroplasty. J Bone Joint Surg Br 77:884-889, 1995.
88. Stiehl JB, Cherveny PM: Femoral rotational alignment using the tibial shaft axis in total knee arthroplasty. Clin Orthop 331:47-55, 1996.
89. Stiehl JB, Dennis DA, Komistek RD, et al: In vivo kinematic analysis of a mobile bearing total knee prosthesis. Clin Orthop 345:60-66, 1997.
90. Stiehl JB, Dennis DA, Komistek RD, et al: In vivo determination of condylar lift off and screw home in a mobile bearing total knee arthroplasty. Presented at the 65th Annual Meeting of the American Academy of Orthopaedic Surgeons, New Orleans, March 1998.
91. Thompson WO, Thaete FL, Fu FH, et al: Tibial meniscal dynamics using three-dimensional reconstruction of magnetic resonance images. Am J Sports Med 19:210-216, 1991.
92. Trent PS, Walker PS, Wolf B: Ligament length patterns, strength, and rotational axes of the knee joint. Clin Orthop 117:263-270, 1976.
93. Walker PS: Design of total knee arthroplasty. In Insall JN, ed: Surgery of the Knee, 2nd ed. New York, Churchill Livingstone, 1993, pp 723-738.
93a. Wasielewski RC, Parks NL, Williams I, et al: The tibial insert undersurface as a contributing source of polyethylene wear debris. Clin Orthop 345:53-59, 1997.
94. Wasielewski RC, Galante JO, Leighty RM: Wear patterns on retrieved polyethylene tibial inserts and their relationship to technical considerations during total knee arthroplasty. Clin Orthop 299:31-43, 1994.
95. Wright TM, Bartel DL: The problem of surface damage in polyethylene total knee components. Clin Orthop 205:67-74, 1986.
96. Wright TM: Polyethylene failure. In Insall JN, Scott WN, Scuderi GR, eds: Current Concepts in Primary and Revision Total Knee Arthroplasty. Philadelphia, Lippincott-Raven, 1996, pp 123-130.
97. Yoshii I, Whiteside LA, Anouchi YS: The effect of patellar button placement and femoral component design on patellar tracking in total knee arthroplasty. Clin Orthop 275:211-219, 1992.
98. Yoshioka Y, Siu D, Cooke DV: The anatomy and functional axes of the femur. J Bone Joint Surg Am 69:873, 1987.

81 Patellar Replacement in Total Knee Arthroplasty

BERTRAND P. KAPER • ROBERT B. BOURNE

INTRODUCTION

Total knee arthroplasty (TKA) offers reliable relief of pain, improved function, and excellent durability for the arthritic knee. Despite excellent long-term results, considerable controversy still exists regarding the management of the patella during primary TKA. The addition of patellofemoral resurfacing fulfills the definition of a "total" knee arthroplasty yet concurrently introduces a new array of potential complications to this procedure (Fig. 81.1). There are numerous proponents both for and against routine patellar resurfacing. Essentially, there are three strategies that can be employed when dealing with the patella in TKA: always resurface the patella; never resurface the patella; or resurface the patella in only selected patients (e.g., those with rheumatoid arthritis or severe patellofemoral arthritis).

Historically, the first knee replacement systems did not feature patellofemoral replacement (Fig. 81.2). Early studies, examining patients in whom the patellofemoral joint was ignored, reported the prevalence rate of anterior knee pain up to 58%.[18, 22, 38, 39, 56, 76, 80] Whereas several implant systems made no attempt to resurface either side of the patellofemoral joint, femoral or patellar, other early designs featured a medial-to-lateral bar extending across the patellofemoral articulation, a factor that probably aggravated patellofemoral pain. Studies evaluating the results of such arthroplasty designs can, therefore, not be used as reference in the analysis of contemporary total knee replacement systems. The total condylar knee developed at the Hospital for Special Surgery was one of the first condylar implants that incorporated routine resurfacing of the anterior femoral articular surface and the patella. Reviews of this system and subsequent design improvements reflect what must be viewed as the representative function of contemporary implants. Historical data, reflecting older prosthetic designs, are limited in their usefulness when deciding whether the patellar should be resurfaced during primary knee replacement.

PATELLAR RESURFACING

Since the introduction of patellofemoral resurfacing, numerous studies have attempted to address the issue of patellar management in primary arthroplasties. The first reports reviewing TKAs incorporating patellofemoral resurfacing noted a relatively high rate of complications and of revision surgery for reasons related to the patella.[18, 83] Although retention of the articular surface of the patella is not without complications, the addition of patellofemoral resurfacing has the potential to produce a new set of complications if more recently established principles are not followed. These complications include patellofemoral instability, patellar fracture, component failure or loosening, patellar clunk, avascular necrosis, and tendon rupture. Before improvements in patellar resurfacing techniques were established, such complications were reported to occur in up to 12% of all TKAs[9, 13, 15, 18, 51, 57] and accounted for up to 50% of the indications for all TKA revision procedures.[13, 32, 83] Even with the use of current condylar designs, extensor mechanism complications remain a common failure mechanism.[28] These problems have prompted re-evaluation of the indications for patellar resurfacing in primary TKA.

The decision to resurface or retain the patella in primary knee arthroplasty should, ideally, be made on the basis of prospective, randomized, controlled double-blind study results. As suggested by Chalmers et al,[16] the use of such studies, with adequate follow-up, remains the most reliable method of ascertaining the effectiveness of a specific intervention. As related to the issue of patellar resurfacing, only a handful of such prospective studies exist in the literature.[3, 8, 21, 23, 44, 75, 79] A majority of the published reports are based on retrospective clinical analyses. Most of these studies are nonrandomized and have significant selection bias, often assessing only one technique, e.g., only resurfacing or only not resurfacing of the patella. The limitations of such studies, as noted by Chalmers et al, should be kept in mind when assessing results and conclusions.

Retrospective Studies

The consequences of patellar retention or resurfacing in primary TKA can be assessed via subjective and functional analyses.[1, 3, 8, 10, 21, 23, 44, 48, 49, 75, 80, 86] Conflicting data have been reported in this group of primarily retrospective analyses. Subjective results, with respect to anterior knee pain and Knee Society scores, have reported the following: diminished pain with resurfacing, when compared with not resurfacing the patella[3, 21, 48, 75]; decreased pain if the patella is not resurfaced[8]; and no difference between the two approaches.[1, 44, 79] From a functional perspective results vary widely from no functional differences,[1, 10, 44, 79] to enhanced stairclimbing ability or improved flexor torques without resurfacing.[8, 23, 80] Further complicat-

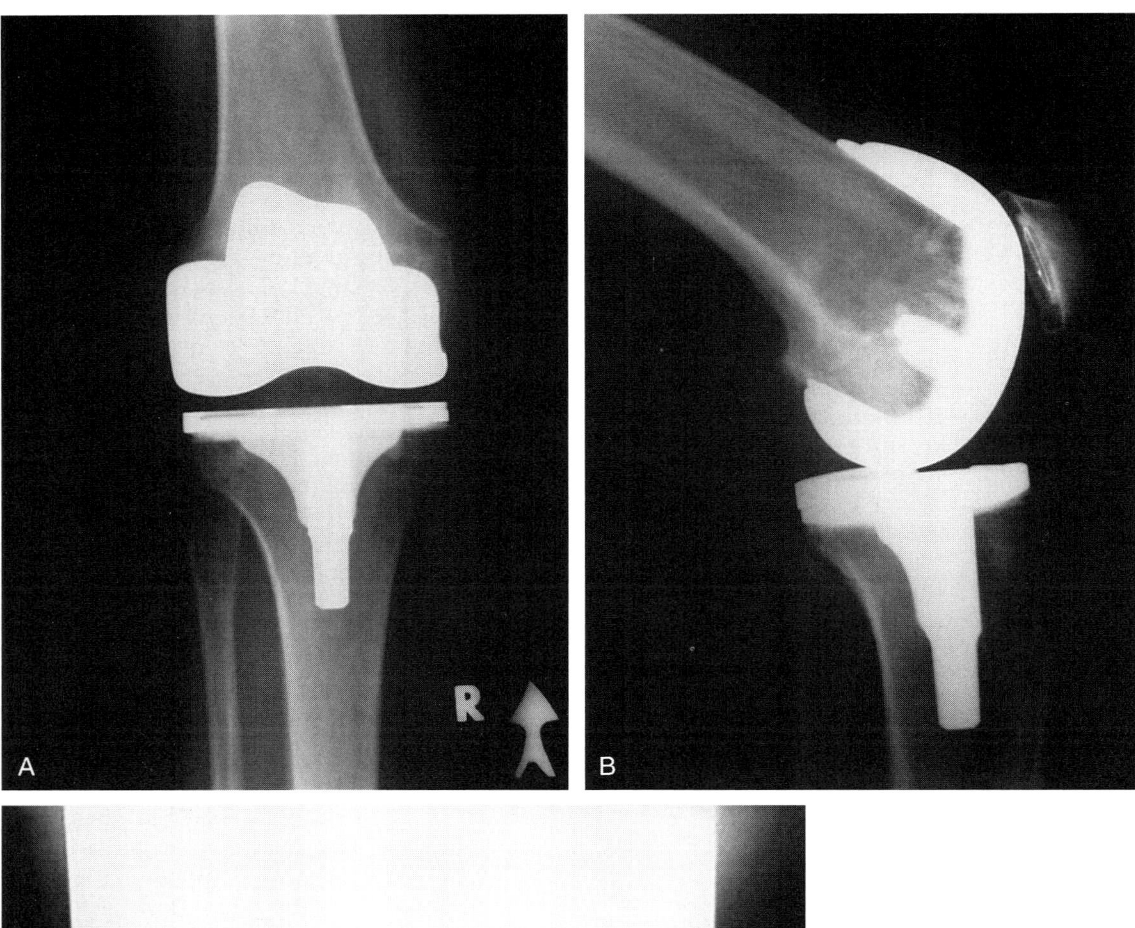

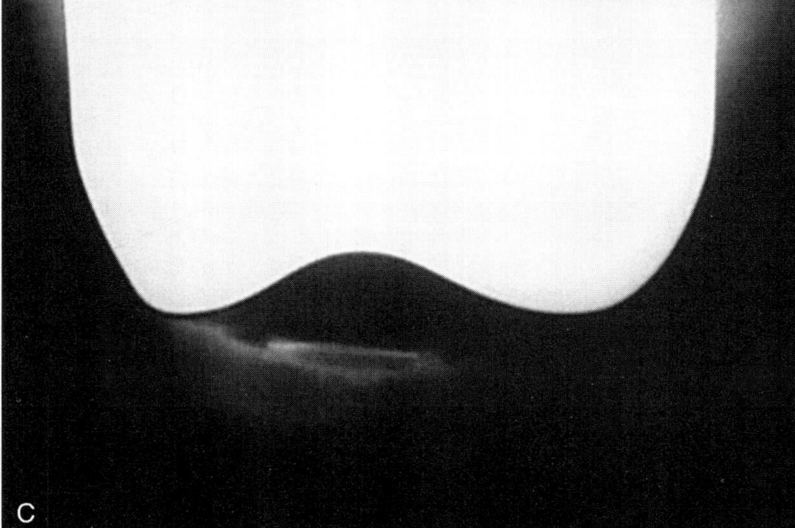

FIGURE 81.1 ➢ Anteroposterior (*A*), lateral (*B*), and skyline (*C*) radiographs, 2 years postoperative, of a contemporary TKA in a patient with no pain, good function, and 0 to 120 degrees range of motion. (Genesis II, Smith and Nephew, Memphis, TN.)

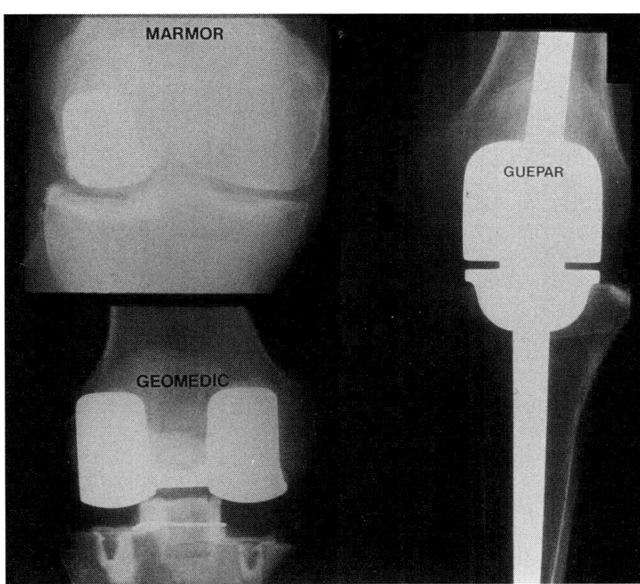

FIGURE 81.2 ➢ Examples of early total knee replacements where the patellofemoral joint was largely ignored.

ing the decision-making process are concerns related to the development of potential complications involving the extensor mechanism.[9, 63]

In a retrospective review of cases in which careful attention was paid to the surgical technique of resurfacing, Rand[62] reported no short- or long-term complications or anterior knee pain. In a much larger study, Boyd et al[9] retrospectively reviewed 891 TKAs in 684 patients to identify the prevalence of patellofemoral complications. A selective determination for resurfacing was made intraoperatively, based on loss of cartilage, exposed bone, gross surface irregularities, or tracking abnormalities. Complications, reported in the resurfacing group, were noted in 3.8% of knees, including five cases of patellar loosening, four cases of patellar subluxation, three patellar fractures, and three patellar tendon ruptures. In the unresurfaced group, patellar subluxation occurred in five knees, and rupture of the patellar tendon occurred in two knees—a 1.4% complication rate. Significant chronic peripatellar pain was reported in 51 patients without resurfacing (10.3%) yet in only 1 patient with resurfacing of the patella (0.2%).

In one of the most commonly cited references, Rhoads et al[69] attempted to identify criteria to be applied in the selective use of patellar resurfacing. One hundred TKAs were performed using a total condylar knee prosthesis, without patellar resurfacing, regardless of the intraoperative condition of the patellar cartilage. By means of retrospective analysis, a 29% prevalence rate of patellofemoral pain was reported at an average follow-up of 4.5 years (range 2 to 7 years). Of the 29 knees with postoperative pain, 7 had class III and the remaining 22 had class IV changes of the patellar cartilage, as described by Outerbridge.[58] A strong correlation between preoperative patellofemoral symptoms, class IV patellar surface changes, and postoperative patellofemoral pain was noted. Additionally, patient height, weight, and preoperative diagnosis were thought to influence postoperative results. The authors recommended routine patellar resurfacing in all patients with rheumatoid arthritis. Selective resurfacing was recommended in osteoarthritic patients with preoperative patellofemoral pain, height greater than 160 cm, weight greater than 60 kg, or advanced changes (class IV) of the patella noted intraoperatively.

Prospective Randomized Clinical Trials

The strengths of the available prospective, randomized studies in the literature merit specific attention. Barrack et al[3] performed a prospective, randomized double-blind study to compare resurfacing of the patella with retention of the patella. A group of 118 knees with a preoperative diagnosis of osteoarthritis underwent TKA with a nonanatomic designed implant. A 13% prevalence rate of anterior knee pain was noted in the nonresurfaced group, versus 7% in the resurfaced group. These numbers did not reach statistical significance. Ten percent of the unresurfaced patellae, however, subsequently underwent patellar resurfacing for persistent anterior knee pain. Postoperative clinical knee scores, postoperative anterior knee pain, and the need for subsequent resurfacing could not be predicted on the basis of preoperative anterior knee pain, obesity, or the grade of chondromalacia.

Bourne et al[8] prospectively randomized 100 patients undergoing TKA for osteoarthritis into two groups: patellar resurfacing versus nonresurfacing. With a minimum 2-year follow-up, disease-specific and functional capacity outcome measures were performed, following a double-blind protocol. Two knees (4%) in the unresurfaced group required reoperation for anterior knee pain (Fig. 81.3). However, the remaining patients in whom the patella was not resurfaced demonstrated significantly less pain and better knee flexor torques than did the resurfaced group. At 5 years, four knees (8%) of the unresurfaced group required resurfacing, compared with no reoperations in the resurfaced group. In the remaining patients, no significant differences were apparent at 5 years, with regards to Knee Society clinical ratings, pain scores, 30-second stair-climbing, and knee flexor/extensor torques.

Schroeder-Boersch et al[75] prospectively randomized 40 patients: 20 undergoing patellar resurfacing and 20 in whom the patella was left unresurfaced. Postoperative evaluation with Knee Society scores was performed in a nonblinded manner. At a minimum follow-up of 2 years, superior results were noted with patellar resurfacing. Superior functional results were noted in the setting of advanced osteoarthritis, leading the authors to conclude that regular resurfacing in this setting is indicated.

Keblish et al[44] prospectively performed patellar resurfacing to only one side of 52 pairs of bilateral mobile-bearing TKAs, with an anatomic implant design. Thirty patients were available for subjective, objective, and radiographic analysis, at a mean of 5.2 years. No

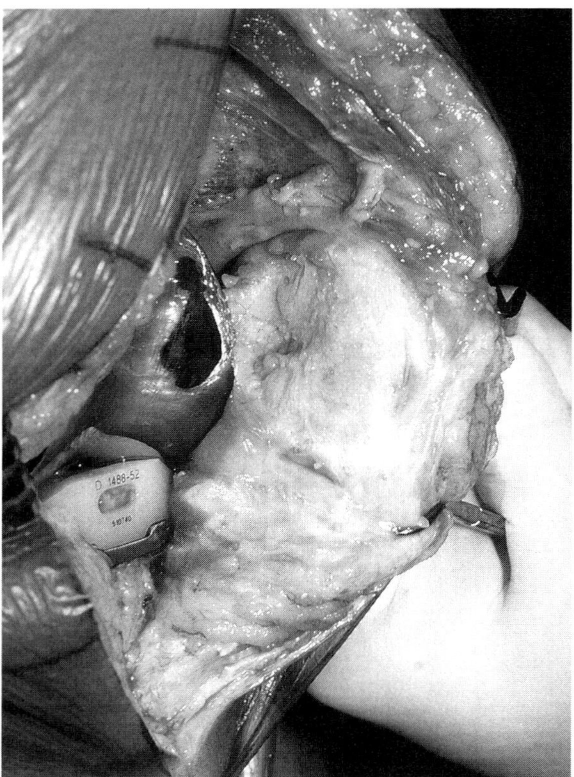

FIGURE 81.3 ➢ An intraoperative photograph of a patient in whom the patella was not resurfaced initially and revision resurfacing was necessary to relieve severe anterior knee pain. Note the disorganization of the patellar articular surface.

differences were noted with respect to subjective preference, stair-climbing ability, or anterior knee pain incidence. The authors concluded that retention of the patellar surface is an acceptable option if specific indications and criteria are followed. The loss of 22 pairs (42%) to follow-up weakens the observations of this study.

Shoji et al[79] randomly assigned 35 patients, with the selective preoperative diagnosis of rheumatoid arthritis undergoing bilateral TKA, to receive patellar replacement on one side but not on the other. At a minimum 2-year follow-up, relief of pain, functional improvement, range of motion, and muscle strength were equivocal in the two groups. The authors concluded that routine patellar replacement in rheumatoid patients with little or no deformity was not necessary.

Feller et al[23] selectively randomized 40 patients undergoing TKA, in whom the patella was not severely deformed, to either retention or resurfacing of the articular surface of the patella. Knee scores and a specifically designed patellar score reported no differences between the two groups. However, stair-climbing was noted to be significantly better in the unresurfaced group. There were no complications related to patellar resurfacing. The authors concluded that routine resurfacing of the patella, if it was not severely deformed, was not warranted.

In a prospective study of 25 patients with advanced

TABLE 81.1 **Clinical Factors for Determining Patellar Resurfacing in Primary TKA**

Factor	Patellar Not Resurfaced	Patellar Resurfacing
Preoperative diagnosis	Osteoarthritis	Inflammatory arthritis
Intraoperative appearance	Outerbridge I & II	Outerbridge III & IV
Implant design	Anatomic	Nonanatomic
Patellofemoral tracking	Satisfactory	Unsatisfactory
Age	<65 years	>65 years

patellofemoral arthritis receiving bilateral TKA, Enis et al[21] selectively performed patellar resurfacing in the right knee only. They found improved subjective and objective outcomes, with respect to pain relief and strength, in the resurfaced knee compared with the nonresurfaced knee. Routine resurfacing was, therefore, favored in knees with advanced patellofemoral disease.

Summary of the Literature

Proponents for and against patellar resurfacing can, therefore, cite any number of studies corroborating their viewpoint. The results of prospective studies, although few in number, have often not overcome previous suggestions made on the basis of retrospective analyses, which demonstrated weaknesses of sample size, length of follow-up, and methodological flaws. On balance, the majority of randomized clinical trials do support patellar resurfacing, at least in selective cases.

The use of modern TKAs, with an anatomic patellofemoral resurfacing design, boasts excellent results, with complication rates as low as 1.4% and reoperation rates as low as 0.56%.[31] Indications for selective resurfacing include inflammatory arthritis, such as rheumatoid arthritis; severe patellofemoral arthritis, as assessed pre- or intraoperatively; cystic changes within the patella; maltracking of the patella following femoral and tibial resurfacing; and incongruence between the patella and the trochlear design of the femoral prosthesis.[1, 9, 10, 41, 49, 59, 62, 76, 80] Patient height, weight, and age have also been suggested as decision-influencing variables.[59, 62, 76, 80] Inadequate bone stock constitutes the only relative contraindication to patellar resurfacing, as a minimum thickness is required to obtain fixation and avoid undue strain on the anterior patella. Clinical factors important in selective patellar resurfacing are summarized in Table 81.1 and the clinical algorithm, which we utilize, is depicted in Figure 81.4.

SURGICAL TECHNIQUE

Successful patellar resurfacing in the setting of a primary TKA requires the maintenance of an efficient extensor mechanism, with a stable and well-aligned

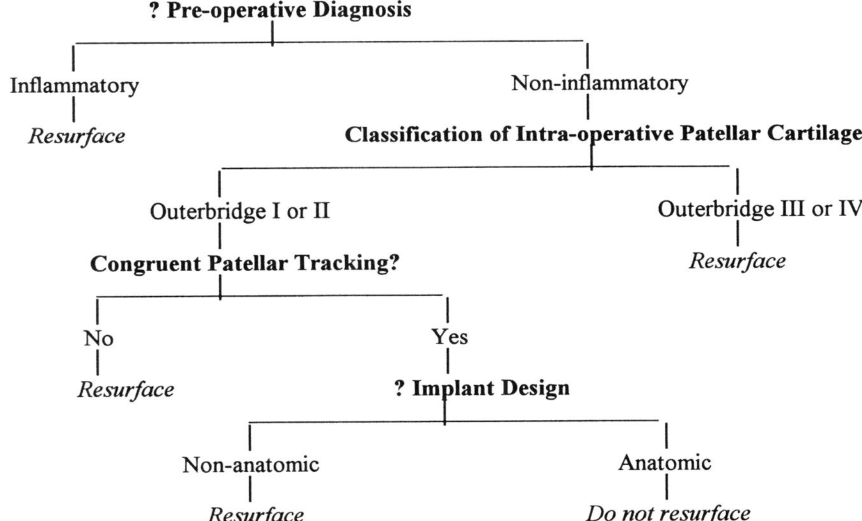

FIGURE 81.4 ➢ Clinical algorithm for patellar resurfacing decision-making in primary total knee arthroplasty.

patellar component. Attainment of these goals is dictated by (1) preservation of patellar vascularity; (2) achievement of appropriate patellar tracking, via restoration of patellar thickness and maintenance of patellar height; and (3) preservation of the quadriceps tendon and patellar tendon[65] (Fig. 81.5). Failure to attain these goals will typically preclude the achievement of satisfactory and reliable results and will predispose an additional array of complications. Complications specific to the patellofemoral articulation may include instability, fracture, component failure or loosening, patellar clunk, avascular necrosis, and tendon rupture. Successful patellofemoral resurfacing will, therefore, require attention dedicated to the prevention of such complications.

PATELLAR VASCULARITY

The arterial supply of the patella was well defined by Scapinelli.[74] The patella receives an extra- and intraosseous arterial inflow.[2, 74] A peripatellar anastomotic ring, from the supreme, superior medial, superior lateral, inferior medial, and inferior lateral geniculate arteries, constitutes the extraosseous blood supply. The intraosseous vascularity arises from a midpatellar, an apical, and a quadriceps tendon vessel. Portions of the extra- and intraosseous supply to the patella are routinely disrupted during a TKA, and other specific surgical maneuvers will risk the loss of the remaining vascularity. Knee arthrotomy, lateral release, menisectomy, and denervation procedures have the potential to compromise the extraosseous supply, whereas fat-pad excision and arthrotomy placement threaten the intraosseous supply. The clinical consequences of patellar devascularization have been demonstrated with an increased incidence of patellar stress fractures, fragmentation, and loosening (Fig. 81.6).[61, 62]

A medial peripatellar arthrotomy routinely divides the superior medial, inferior medial, and supreme geniculate arteries. Placement of the arthrotomy, whether medial or lateral, will risk disruption of a significant portion of the anastomotic ring. As demonstrated by cadaveric dye injections,[42] arthrotomies placed within 1 cm of the medial or lateral patellar border will interrupt the intraosseous vessels. Complete lateral menisectomy may result in division of the inferior lateral geniculate artery, thereby leaving the superior lateral vessel as the sole extraosseous blood supply to the patella. Débridement of the infrapatellar fat pad will further endanger patellar vascularity by means of disruption of the radial intraosseous vessels.[42] If a lateral release is required, preservation of the superior lateral geniculate artery is therefore mandatory. This vessel can be isolated in the subsynovial layer 1 to 2 cm distal to the inferior border of the vastus lateralis muscle. Knees with a significant preoperative valgus deformity (typically >20 degrees), in which a lateral release can be anticipated, deserve consideration of a lateral arthrotomy for exposure.[43] This approach will ensure preservation of the superior medial, inferior medial, and supreme geniculate vessels in such clinical scenarios.

Technetium 99m bone scanning has been employed to assess postoperative patellar vascularity. Wetzner et al[87] examined 41 consecutive TKAs to assess the potential development of postoperative avascular necrosis of the patella. Four patellae were noted to have decreased uptake, suggesting increased risk for the development of avascular necrosis. Prophylactic activity restrictions were recommended in this setting. Scuderi et al[77] compared the clinical effect of lateral release on patellar viability following TKA. The addition of a lateral release increased the incidence of vascular compromise from 15% to 56.4%. Only one of the knees requiring a lateral release, however, suffered a postoperative complication: a patellar fracture not requiring surgical intervention. McMahon et al[53] further investigated the effect of lateral release in conjunction with infrapatellar fat-pad excision. In 70 knees undergoing TKA, excision of the infrapatellar fat pad was not iden-

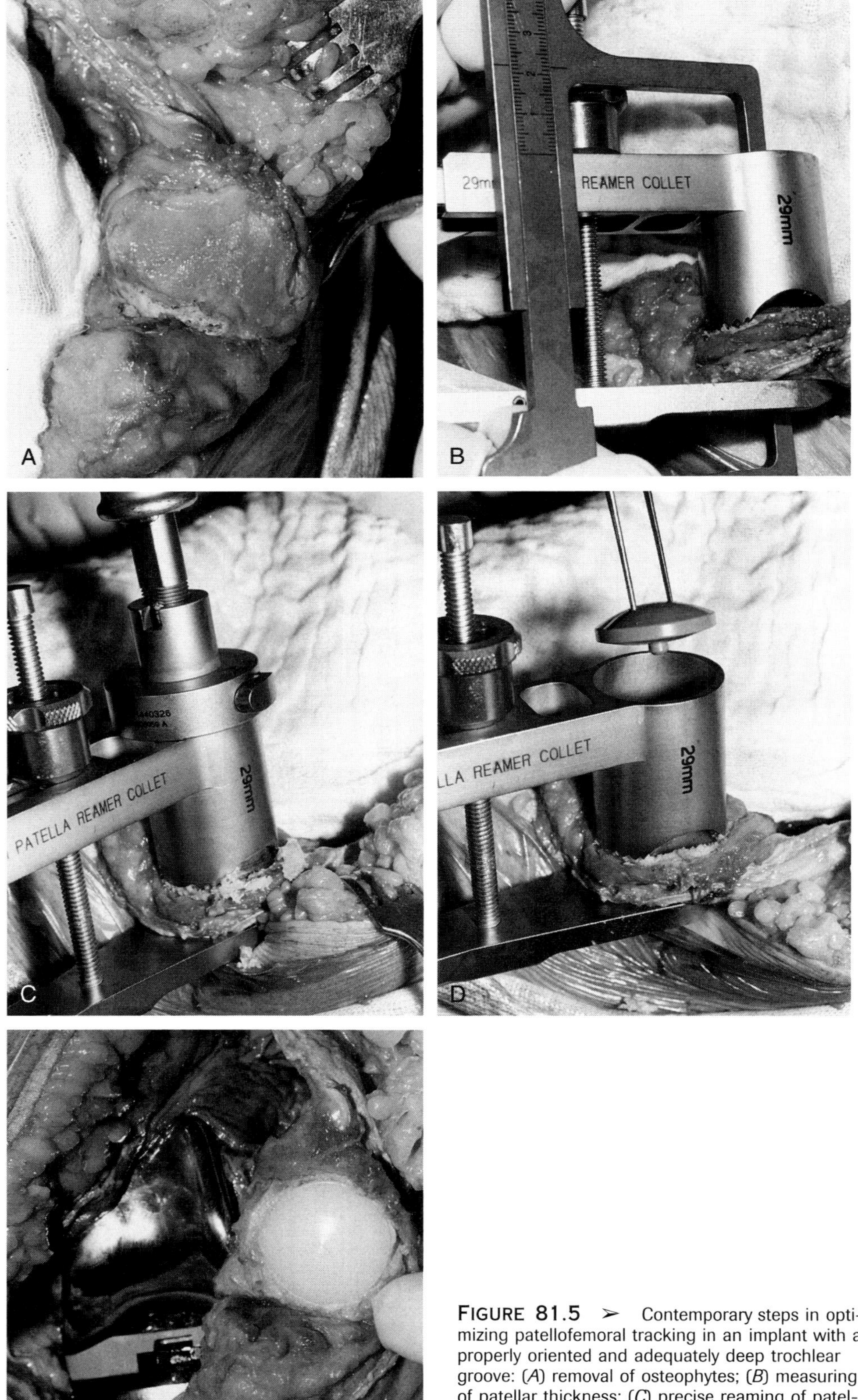

FIGURE 81.5 ➢ Contemporary steps in optimizing patellofemoral tracking in an implant with a properly oriented and adequately deep trochlear groove: (*A*) removal of osteophytes; (*B*) measuring of patellar thickness; (*C*) precise reaming of patellar implant bed; (*D*) measuring for patellar thickness with trial implant in place; and (*E*) cement fixation of the patellar prosthesis (note medialized position).

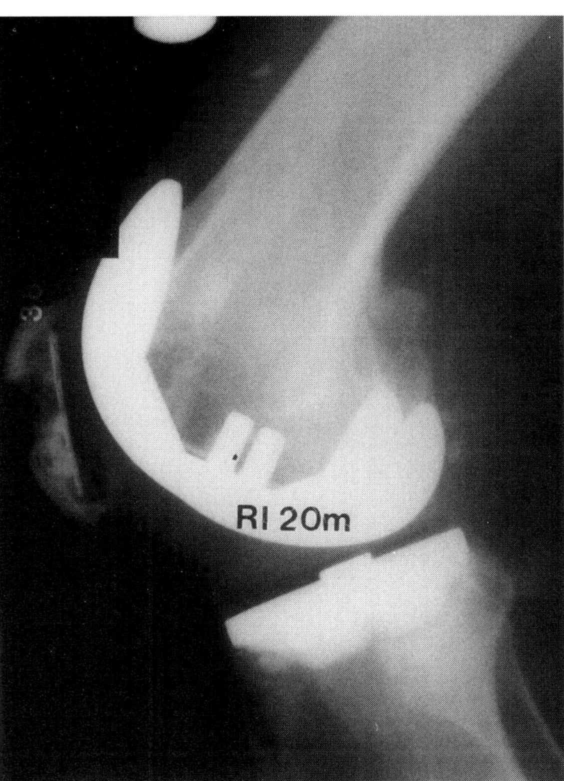

FIGURE 81.6 ➢ An example of an avascular patella 20 months following a total knee arthroplasty in which both a medial arthrotomy and a lateral retinacular release were performed. Note the subsequent patellar fragmentation and fracture, resulting in implant fixation compromise.

tified as an independent variable for compromise of patellar vascularity.

Ritter and Campbell[70] and Ritter et al[71] examined the consequences of lateral release in TKA. Forty-eight patients underwent simultaneous bilateral procedures in which one knee had a lateral release and the other did not. The knees were compared on the basis of clinical scores, roentgenographic findings, and technetium bone scans. No differences were noted between the two groups. No patellae developed signs of osteonecrosis. Similarly, a comparison of 84 knees requiring lateral release and 471 without lateral release showed no increase in prevalence of avascular necrosis, patellar component loosening, or fracture.

PATELLOFEMORAL STABILITY

The maintenance of an efficient extensor mechanism, with a stable and well-aligned patella, is obviously critical in the process of TKA. Difficulties with postoperative tilting, subluxation, and dislocation can occur in the setting of patellar resurfacing or retention.[13] Whereas the incidence rate of patellar subluxation following resurfacing has been reported as high as 31%,[7] reports on the incidence rate of clinically symptomatic patellar instability are typically less than 1%.[12, 28, 62] Intraoperative attention to technique and assessment of patellar tracking is, therefore, mandatory to minimize this potential complication. The cause of instability may be ascribed to several inter-related variables: component malposition, soft-tissue imbalance, and malalignment of the limb. Figure 81.5 highlights the contemporary steps in preventing postoperative patellar tilting, subluxation, and dislocation.

Proper selection and positioning of the femoral, tibial, and patellar implants, as dictated by preoperative radiographs and intraoperative assessment, is essential. Overstuffing of the knee joint in the anteroposterior plane will predispose to instability. This is seen clinically when a femoral implant too large in the anteroposterior dimension is used or the thickness of the patella-patellar implant composite, secondary to inadequate resection of patellar bone, is increased.[11, 28, 56, 62] The femoral and tibial components must be positioned to avoid medial shift and internal rotation, as both these orientations will predispose toward patellar subluxation or tilting.[33, 69] Five degrees of external femoral component rotation, versus a neutral or five-degree internally rotated position, has been demonstrated to provide superior patellar tracking and knee stability.[2] Newer prosthesis designs incorporate a slight degree of external rotation into the femoral component in the attempt to match the external rotation motion noted with knee extension and thereby facilitate enhanced patellar tracking and decrease the need to additional soft-tissue balancing.[33] For similar reasons, positioning of the patellar component is biased medially, avoiding lateral placement.[27, 88] The choice of patellar prosthesis also affects the risk of postoperative patellar tilt, subluxation, and the need for lateral release. Inset and resurfacing implants are available. Rand and Gustilo[64] noted that an inset patellar implant provided better radiographic alignment with statistically superior results with respect to tilt, subluxation, and the need for lateral release, when compared with a resurfacing component. The inset components were, however, noted to have a slightly higher incidence of complete patellar radiolucent lines.

Also inherent in patellar stability is the appropriate restoration of patellar thickness.[30, 36, 47, 54, 68] The premorbid anatomy of the patella may vary considerably, with a typical thickness between 22 and 25 mm. The use of calipers to accurately assess pre- and postresurfacing thickness is recommended.[54] When appropriate thickness is restored, the incidence of associated lateral release, performed for intraoperative instability, has been reported to decrease from 55% to 12.4%.[30]

The "no-thumbs" technique may be employed for accurate intraoperative dynamic tracking assessment. It is advisable to hold the lower leg in internal rotation when performing this maneuver. If tilting or subluxation of the patella is noted (ideally assessed after tourniquet deflation to release the capture of the quadriceps proximally) it can be addressed by means of lateral release. With contemporary techniques (see Fig. 81.5), lateral retinacular release should be necessary in less than 10% of cases. Postoperatively, a 45-degree Merchant view is recommended to assess patellar position and fixation. An average of nearly 5 degrees of postoperative patellar tilting has been noted in midflexion with three modern knee designs, despite a satisfactory assessment of intraoperative tracking.[17] Similarly, the incidence of radiographic patellar tilting has been reported as high as 31%, with a 14% incidence of subluxation or lateral displacement.[7] Preoperative tilting may in fact predispose to postoperative tilting, irrespective of the intraoperative management of the peripatellar soft tissues.

Surgical approach to the knee does not seem to significantly affect patellofemoral stability. Clinically equivalent results, with respect stability, have been demonstrated with both a mid- and subvastus approach when compared with a routine medial parapatellar approach.[20]

Treatment of symptomatic lateral patellar instability is performed by a proximal realignment with or without component revision. Distal realignment, using a modification of the Trillat procedure, has been employed successfully to treat recurrent patellar dislocation.[45] The combination of proximal and distal realignment is not recommended because of the significant risk of subsequent patellar tendon rupture.[28]

PATELLAR FRACTURE

Fractures of the patella following TKA are uncommon.[25, 29, 34, 72, 85] Varying causes have been proposed for these fractures: vascular compromise, component malposition, patellar subluxation, poor component design, trauma, thermal necrosis, and increased knee flexion. Prevalence reports dealing with modern arthroplasty designs range from 0% to 6.3%.[26, 29, 85]

Compromise of patellar vascularity has been recognized as a significant predisposing factor for subsequent patellar fracture. Disruption of a significant portion of the blood supply to the patella occurs after routine medial peripatellar arthrotomy. Fat-pad excision or lateral release represents an additional insult to the vascularity. In 18 cases of postoperative patellar fracture, Tria et al[85] identified a statistically significant correlation between lateral release and subsequent fracture.

Excessive patellar resection, resulting in less than 15 mm of remaining bone, will substantially weaken the host bone and increase anterior patellar strain.[68] Asymmetric patellar resection will lead to eccentric loading of the patellar component and of the underlying host bone. Inadequate bony resection will result in a thicker patella-patellar implant composite. Increased patellofemoral joint reactive forces and enhanced quadriceps tension will subsequently occur, increasing the strain on the component and anterior host bone.[81] Anterior translation or flexion of the femoral component, or a component too large in the anteroposterior dimensions, will similarly cause increased patellofemoral joint reaction forces.

Limb malalignment can predispose to fracture due to abnormal patellar tracking with increased contact forces. Figgie et al[24] reported a significant correlation between type of fracture and limb alignment. Minor deviation of limb alignment resulted in less severe fractures and better overall results. Major discrepancies in alignment resulted in more severe fractures with less satisfactory outcomes. Deviation from standard positioning of the patellar component will also increase the fracture risk, as this will predispose to abnormal patellar tracking or patellar component impingement on the tibial insert, typically seen in knees with a large flexion arc.

Thermal necrosis secondary to polymethylmethacrylate fixation has also been implicated in patellar fractures.

Treatment is dictated by extensor mechanism competence, fixation of the patellar implant, and anatomic location.[24, 26, 29, 34, 72] The natural history of patellar fractures following condylar TKA was reviewed in detail by Goldberg et al.[26] Four fracture configurations were identified: type I fractures occur through the midbody or superior pole, not involving the implant, cement, or quadriceps mechanism; type II disrupt the quadriceps mechanism or implant/bone/cement composite; type IIIA involve the inferior pole with disruption of the patellar tendon; type IIIB are nondisplaced through the inferior pole. Knees with implant loosening, patellar dislocation, or complete quadriceps disruption (types II and IIIA) require operative intervention. The remaining fractures, types I and IIIB, were noted to be better treated nonoperatively. Hozack et al[34] reviewed 21 fractures after TKA. Nondisplaced fractures and displaced fractures without an extensor lag demonstrated satisfactory results with nonoperative management. Recommendations for displaced fractures with an extensor lag was to proceed with operative intervention, although satisfactory results were reported for only 31% of these cases. Displaced distal pole fractures are treated with fracture fragment excision. Patellectomy is reserved for failures of all other treatments, as it will typically result in diminished quadriceps strength and extensor lag.

PATELLAR COMPONENT LOOSENING

The majority of modern patellofemoral resurfacing is accomplished with cement fixation of an all-polyethylene patellar component. Loosening is an uncommon complication, with an incidence rate ranging from 0.6% to 1.3%.[9, 13, 19, 55] Poor cementing technique, insults to the patellar vascularity, deficient host bone, component malposition, trauma, patellar fracture, and inadequate patellar preparation have all been implicated in patellar component loosening. Component design has also been suggested to influence loosening rates.

Whereas the incidence rate of patellar component loosening is low, the rate of complications related to isolated patellar revision is high. Berry and Rand[6] reported 14 significant complications in 42 knees (34%) undergoing patellar revision. There were five fractures, three cases of patellar instability, two peroneal nerve palsies, two cases of polyethylene wear, one deep infection, and one knee with an extensor lag. Similarly,

Lynch et al[52] noted a 24% complication rate in 37 isolated patellar revisions. Maintenance of an intact extensor mechanism dictates treatment. Options include observation, component revision, component removal and patellar débridement, and patellectomy. Overall satisfactory results have been obtained in 83% of knees.[6]

PATELLAR COMPONENT FAILURE

A large percentage of component failures in the setting of patellar resurfacing has occurred with the use of metal-backed implants.[4, 46, 50, 60, 73, 80] The initial design of the metal-backed patella was deemed desirable because of the uniform load transmission to the underlying patellar bone. Furthermore, the metal backing decreases the tendency of the polyethylene to deform under stress. The important considerations in the design of these implants, however, had to take into account: the total thickness of the implants; the thickness of the polyethylene; the modulus of elasticity of the polyethylene; the means of fixation of the polyethylene to the metal; the proportion of the polyethylene that is backed by metal; and the thickness and strength of the metal plate.[82] The basic mode of failure has either been wear or fracture of the polyethylene, or dissociation of the polyethylene from the base plate or fixation pegs. These failures result in significant particle debris generation, a metal-on-metal articulation, and a metal-induced proliferative synovitis.

Revision rates for TKA designs employing a metal-backed patella have been reported at 8.4% within 2 years and 33.3% at 6 years, with a 10-year revision rate estimated to be greater than 50%.[60] Good results, however, have been reported with the use of a metal-backed patella.[25, 46] Laskin and Bucknell[46] noted no implant failures in 451 knees. The design of the metal-backed patellar component used in this series employed maximum polyethylene thickness with inset of the metal-backing below the superficial surface of the host patellar bone. Similarly, Buechel et al[14] implanted 515 congruent-contact, metal-backed, rotating-bearing patellar components. Of 331 knees monitored for at least 2 years (mean 7.3 years), there were only 3 fractures and 1 dislocation. No polyethylene wear-through, separation from the metal base-plate, or implant failure was noted. Increased conformity of the patellar component onto the femoral flange improves the clinical situation by increasing contact area and maximizing polyethylene thickness.[37] The general use of metal-backed patellar components for patellar resurfacing, however, should be done with caution.

Factors implicated in the failure of all-polyethylene components have been related to the demands specific to the patellofemoral articulation. Enhanced postoperative flexion, typically greater than 115 degrees; increased patellofemoral loads; eccentric tracking with increased contact pressures; and excessive body weight have been reported to influence polyethylene wear.

PATELLAR "CLUNK" SYNDROME

The patellar "clunk" syndrome, as described by Hozack et al[35] in 1989, may be implicated as a cause of anterior knee pain following certain posterior-stabilized TKAs. A prominent, hyperplastic fibrous nodule forms at the posterior junction of the proximal patellar pole and the quadriceps tendon. This nodule lodges into the intercondylar notch of the femoral component during flexion and displaces with an audible catch or "clunk" as the quadriceps tendon and patella migrate proximally with extension of the knee. The presence of this "clunk" is especially noted in knees that have achieved a large flexion arc of motion. Impingement of the quadriceps tendon against the anterosuperior edge of the femoral intercondylar notch can lead to fibrous proliferation and nodule formation. Failure to sufficiently elevate the quadriceps tendon away from the femoral component through the use of a relatively thin patellar component or failure to reconstitute the height of the patella has been implicated. Superior placement of the patellar component beyond the proximal border of the patella may also predispose to fibrous nodule formation.

The majority of knees in which a "clunk" develops may be asymptomatic initially, but they will usually not remain so. Treatment is indicated for those knees in which symptoms persist. Although arthroscopic débridement of the nodule offers a minimally invasive means of treatment, Beight et al[5] reported 4 recurrences in 11 cases. Recurrence following open arthrotomy with or without patellar component revision has not been reported. While reports of the patellar clunk syndrome are limited to certain posterior-stabilized prosthetic designs, Shoji and Shimozaki[78] reported 11 cases of intraoperative patellar clunk syndrome. In these cases, catching was noted with the use of a cruciate-retaining design before patellar resurfacing. The catching was eliminated by patellar resurfacing in four knees and by shaving of the superior pole of the patella in the remaining seven cases.

The development of intra-articular fibrous bands following TKA has also been noted.[84] Similar to the patellar "clunk" syndrome, fibrous hyperplasia occurs, resulting either in tethering the patella laterally or inferiorly or displacing the patella from the sulcus of the femoral component. Arthroscopic débridement resulted in successful resolution of symptoms in all patients.

TENDON RUPTURE

Rupture of either the quadriceps or patellar tendon is an infrequent complication following TKA. Reports of incidence vary between 0.17% and 2.5%.[51, 55, 66, 67] Lynch et al[51] reported 3 quadriceps ruptures and 4 patellar tendon ruptures in 281 consecutive TKAs performed with patellar resurfacing. The use of an extensive lateral release may predispose to quadriceps tendon rupture, typically secondary to compromise of tendon vascularity. Patellar tendon rupture or avulsion may be seen in knees with significant preoperative limitations of flexion or previous surgeries. Postoperative manipulation under anesthesia to address arthrofibrosis presents an additional risk for failure of the extensor mechanism.

Treatment of patellar tendon ruptures is fraught with difficulties. Residual extensor lag, quadriceps weakness, increased risk of rerupture, and limited flexion have all been reported following attempts at repair of such ruptures. Numerous methods of repair and/or augmentation have been reported.[67] Operative repair techniques have been described with staples, screws, autograft, allograft, and synthetic ligament augment reconstruction. The use of a medial gastrocnemius flap to provide tissue for repair and vascular ingrowth has been described.[40] Given the marginal results with either operative or nonoperative approaches, careful attention to surgical technique to avoid these complications remains paramount.

CONCLUSIONS

Management of the patella in primary TKA remains controversial. Resurfacing of the patella at least in selected circumstances is indicated (see Table 81.1). Whether or not routine resurfacing is warranted has yet to be proven conclusively, with respect to improved long-term results and outcomes. The use of contemporary total knee implant systems, with improved instrumentation and operative techniques, has greatly improved the rate of satisfactory outcomes, which had previously been unacceptable. The risk of extensor mechanism complications exists in both the setting of resurfacing and not resurfacing of the patellar articular surface, and these problems still account for one of the most frequent reasons for reoperation following TKA. As with any operative procedure, attention to proper patient selection and surgical principles will result in optimization of the clinical results. At this time, our assessment of quality assurance and continuous improvement has led us to resurface 90% of patellae during primary TKA.

References

1. Abraham W, Buchanan JR, Dauber H, et al: Should the patella be resurfaced in total knee arthoplasty? Efficacy of patellar resurfacing. Clin Orthop 236:128, 1988.
2. Anouchi YS, Whiteside LA, Kaiser AD, et al: The effects of axial rotational alignment of the femoral component on knee stability and patellar tracking in total knee arthroplasty demonstrated on autopsy specimens. Clin Orthop 287:170, 1993.
3. Barrack RB, Wolfe MW, Waldman DA, et al: Resurfacing of the patella in total knee arthroplasty. J Bone Joint Surg Am 79:1121, 1997.
4. Bayley JC, Scott RD, Ewald FC, et al: Failure of the metal-backed patellar component after total knee replacement. J Bone Joint Surg Am 70:668, 1988.
5. Beight JL, Yao B, Hozack WJ, et al: The patellar "clunk" syndrome after posterior stabilized total knee arthoplasty. Clin Orthop 299:139, 1994.
6. Berry DJ, Rand JA: Isolated patellar component revision of total knee arthroplasty. Clin Orthop 286:110, 1993.
7. Bindelglass DF, Cohen JL, Dorr LD: Patellar tilt and subluxation in total knee arthroplasty: Relationship to pain, fixation, and design. Clin Orthop 286:103, 1993.
8. Bourne RB, Rorabeck CR, Vaz M, et al: Resurfacing versus not resurfacing of the patella during total knee replacement. Clin Orthop 321:156, 1995.
9. Boyd AD, Ewald FC, Thomas WH, et al: Long-term complications after total knee arthoplasty with or without resurfacing of the patella. J Bone Joint Surg Am 75:674, 1993.
10. Braakman M, Verburg AD, Bronsema G, et al: The outcome of three methods of patellar resurfacing in total knee arthroplasty. Int Orthop 19:7, 1995.
11. Briard JL, Hungerford DS: Patellofemoral instability in total knee arthroplasty. J Arthroplasty 4 (suppl):87, 1989.
12. Brick GW, Scott RD: Blood supply to the patella: Significance in total knee arthroplasty. J Arthroplasty 4 (suppl):75, 1989.
13. Brick GW, Scott RD: The patellofemoral component of total knee arthoplasty. Clin Orthop 231:163, 1988.
14. Buechel FF, Rosa RA, Pappas MJ: A metal-backed, rotating-bearing patellar prosthesis to lower contact stress: An 11-year clinical study. Clin Orthop 248:34, 1989.
15. Cameron HU, Fedorkow DM: The patella in total knee arthoplasty. Clin Orthop 165:197, 1982.
16. Chalmers TC, Celano P, Sacks HS, et al: Bias in treatment assignment in controlled clinical trials. N Engl J Med 309:1358, 1983.
17. Chew JT, Stewart NJ, Hanssen AD, et al: Differences in patellar tracking and knee kinematics among three different total knee designs. Clin Orthop 345:87, 1997.
18. Clayton ML, Thirupathi R: Patellar complications after total condylar arthroplasty. Clin Orthop 170:152, 1982.
19. Dennis DA: Patellofemoral complications in total knee arthoplasty: A literature review. Am J Knee Surg 5:156, 1992.
20. Engh GA, Holt BT, Parks NL: A midvastus muscle-splitting approach for total knee arthroplasty. J Arthroplasty 12:322, 1997.
21. Enis JE, Gardner R, Robledo MA, et al: Comparison of patellar resurfacing versus nonresurfacing in bilateral total knee arthroplasty. Clin Orthop 260:38, 1990.
22. Ewald FC, Thomas WH, Poss R, et al: Duo-patella total knee arthroplasty in rheumatoid arthritis. Orthop Trans 2:202, 1978.
23. Feller JA, Bartlett RJ, Lang DM: Patellar resurfacing versus retention in total knee arthroplasty. J Bone Joint Surg Br 78:226, 1996.
24. Figgie HE III, Goldberg VM, Figgie MP, et al: The effect of alignment of the implant on fractures of the patella after condylar total knee arthroplasty. J Bone Joint Surg, Am 71:1031, 1989.
25. Firestone TP, Teeny SM, Krackow KA, et al: The clinical and roentgenographic results of cementless porous-coated patellar fixation. Clin Orthop 273:184, 1991.
26. Goldberg VM, Figgie HE III, Inglis AE, et al: Patellar fracture type and prognosis in condylar total knee arthroplasty. Clin Orthop 236:115, 1988.
27. Gomes LSM, Bechtold JE, Gustilo RB: Patellar prosthesis positioning in total knee arthroplasty: A roentgenographic study. Clin Orthop 236:72, 1988.
28. Grace JN, Rand JA: Patellar instability after total knee arthoplasty. Clin Orthop 237:184, 1988.
29. Grace JN, Sim FH: Fracture of the patella after total knee arthroplasty. Clin Orthop 230:168, 1988.
30. Greenfield MA, Insall JN, Case GC, et al: Instrumentation of the patellar osteotomy in total knee arthroplasty: The relationship of patellar thickness and lateral retinacular release. Am J Knee Surg 9:129, 1996.
31. Harwin SF: Patellofemoral complications in symmetrical total knee arthoplasty. J Arthroplasty 13:753, 1998.
32. Hofmann GO, Hagena FW: Pathomechanics of the femoropatellar joint following total knee arthoplasty. Clin Orthop 224:251, 1987.
33. Hollister AM, Jatana S, Singh AK, et al: The axes of rotation of the knee. Clin Orthop 290:259, 1993.
34. Hozack WJ, Goll SR, Lotke PA, et al: The treatment of patellar fractures after total knee arthoplasty. Clin Orthop 236:123, 1988.
35. Hozack WJ, Rothman RH, Booth RE Jr, et al: The patellar clunk syndrome: A complication of posterior stabilized total knee arthoplasty. Clin Orthop 241:203, 1989.
36. Hsu HC, Luo ZP, Rand JA, et al: Influence of patellar thickness on patellar tracking and patellofemoral contact characteristics after total knee arthoplasty. J Arthroplasty 11:69, 1996.

37. Hsu HP, Walker PS: Wear and deformation of patellar components in total knee arthoplasty. Clin Orthop 246:260, 1989.
38. Insall JN, Ranawat CS, Aglietti P, et al: A comparison of four models of total knee replacement prostheses. J Bone Joint Surg Am 58:754, 1976.
39. Insall JN, Scott WN, Ranawat CS: The total condylar knee prosthesis. J Bone Joint Surg Am 61:173, 1979.
40. Jaureguito JW, Dubois CM, Smith SR, et al: Medial gastrocnemius transposition flap for the treatment of disruption of the extensor mechanism after total knee arthroplasty. J Bone Joint Surg Am 79:866, 1997.
41. Kawakubo M, Matsumoto H, Otani T, et al: Radiographic changes in the patella after total knee arthroplasty without resurfacing of the patella: Comparison of osteoarthritis and rheumatoid arthritis. Bull Hosp Jt Dis 56:237, 1997.
42. Kayler DE, Lyttle D: Surgical interruption of patellar blood supply by total knee arthroplasty. Clin Orthop 229:221, 1988.
43. Keblish P: Valgus deformity in total knee replacement (TKR): The lateral retinacular approach. Orthop Trans 9:28, 1985.
44. Keblish PA, Varma AK, Greenwald AS: Patellar resurfacing or retention in total knee arthoplasty: A prospective study of patients with bilateral replacements. J Bone Joint Surg Br 76:930, 1994.
45. Kirk P, Rorabeck CH, Bourne RB, et al: Management of recurrent dislocation of the patella following total knee arthroplasty. J Arthroplasty 7:229, 1992.
46. Laskin RS, Bucknell A: The use of metal-backed patellar prosthesis in total knee arthroplasty. Clin Orthop 260:52, 1990.
47. Lee TQ, Kim WC: Anatomically based patellar resection criteria in total knee arthroplasty. Am J Knee Surg 11:161, 1998.
48. Levai JP, McLeod HC, Freeman MAR: Why not resurface the patella? J Bone Joint Surg Br 65:448, 1983.
49. Levitsky KA, Harris WJ, McManus J, et al: Total knee arthoplasty without patellar resurfacing. Clin Orthop 286:116, 1993.
50. Lombardi AV, Engh GA, Volz RG, et al: Fracture/dissociation of the polyethylene in metal-backed patellar components in total knee arthoplasty. J Bone Joint Surg Am 70:675, 1988.
51. Lynch AF, Rorabeck CR, Bourne RB: Extensor mechanism complications following total knee arthoplasty. J Arthroplasty 2:135, 1987.
52. Lynch JA, Baker PL, Lepse PS, et al: Solitary patellar component revision following total knee arthroplasty. Presented at the Annual Meeting of the American Academy of Orthopaedic Surgeons, San Francisco, CA, Feb 20, 1993.
53. McMahon MS, Scuderi GR, Glashow JL, et al: Scintigraphic determination of patellar viability after excision of infrapatellar fat pad and/or lateral retinacular release in total knee arthroplasty. Clin Orthop 260:10, 1990.
54. Marmor L: Technique for patellar resurfacing in total knee arthroplasty. Clin Orthop 230:166, 1988.
55. Mason MD, Brick GW, Scott RD, et al: Three pegged all-polyethylene patella: 2-6-year results. Orthop Trans 17:991, 1994.
56. Merkow RL, Soudry M, Insall JN: Patellar dislocation following total knee arthroplasty. J Bone Joint Surg Am 67:1321, 1985.
57. Mochizuki RM, Schurman DJ: Patellar complications following total knee arthroplasty. J Bone Joint Surg Am 61:879, 1979.
58. Outerbridge RE: The etiology of chondromalacia patellae. J Bone Joint Surg Br 43:752, 1961.
59. Picetti GD III, McGann WA, Welch RB: The patellofemoral joint after total knee arthoplasty without patellar resurfacing. J Bone Joint Surg Am 72:1379, 1990.
60. Rader CP, Lohr J, Wittmann R, et al: Results of total knee arthoplasty with a metal-backed patellar component. J Arthroplasty 11:923, 1996.
61. Ranawat CS: The patellofemoral joint in total condylar knee arthroplasty: Pros and cons based on five-to-ten-year follow-up observations. Clin Orthop 205:93, 1986.
62. Rand JA: The patellofemoral joint in total knee arthoplasty. J Bone Joint Surg Am 76:612, 1994.
63. Rand JA: Patellar resurfacing in total knee arthroplasty. Clin Orthop 260:110, 1990.
64. Rand JA, Gustilo RB: Comparison of inset and resurfacing patellar prostheses in total knee arthroplasty. Acta Orthop Belg 62(suppl):154, 1996.
65. Rand JA, Gustilo RB: Technique of patellar resurfacing in total knee arthroplasty. Tech Orthop 3:57, 1988.
66. Rand JA, Morrey BF, Bryan RS: Patellar tendon rupture after total knee arthroplasty. Clin Orthop 244:233, 1989.
67. Rand JA, Morrey BF, Bryan RS: Patellar tendon rupture following total knee arthroplasty. Tech Orthop 3:45, 1988.
68. Reuben JD, McDonald CL, Woodard PL, et al: Effect of patella thickness on patella strain following total knee arthroplasty. J Arthroplasty 6:251, 1991.
69. Rhoads DD, Noble PC, Reuben JD, et al: The effect of femoral component position on patellar tracking after total knee arthroplasty. Clin Orthop 260:43, 1990.
70. Ritter MA, Campbell ED: Postoperative patellar complications with or without lateral release during total knee arthroplasty. Clin Orthop 219:163, 1987.
71. Ritter MA, Keating EM, Faris PM: Clinical, roentgenographic and scintigraphic results after interruption of the superior lateral genicular artery during total knee arthroplasty. Clin Orthop 248: 145, 1989.
72. Roffman M, Hirsh DM, Mendes DG: Fracture of the resurfaced patella in total knee replacement. Clin Orthop 148:112, 1980.
73. Rosenberg AG, Andriacchi TP, Barden R, et al: Patellar component failure in cementless total knee arthoplasty. Clin Orthop 236:106, 1988.
74. Scapinelli R: Blood supply to human patella. J Bone Joint Surg Br 49:563, 1967.
75. Schroeder-Boersch H, Scheller G, Fischer J, et al: Advantages of patellar resurfacing in total knee arthroplasty: Two-year results of a prospective randomized study. Arch Orthop Trauma Surg 117:73, 1998.
76. Scott RD: Prosthetic replacement of the patellofemoral joint. Orthop Clin North Am 10:129, 1979.
77. Scuderi G, Scharf SC, Meltzer LP, et al: The relationship of lateral releases to patellar viability in total knee arthroplasty. J Arthroplasy 2:209, 1987.
78. Shoji H, Shimozaki E: Patellar clunk syndrome in total knee arthroplasty without patellar resurfacing. J Arthroplasty 11:198, 1996.
79. Shoji H, Yoshino S, Kajino A: Patellar replacement in bilateral total knee arthroplasty: A study of patients who had rheumatoid arthritis and no gross deformity of the patella. J Bone Joint Surg Am 71:853, 1989.
80. Soudry M, Mestriner LA, Binazzi R, et al: Total knee arthoplasty without patellar resurfacing. Clin Orthop 205:166, 1986.
81. Star MJ, Kaufman KR, Irby Se, et al: The effects of patellar thickness on patellofemoral forces after resurfacing. Clin Orthop 322:279, 1996.
82. Stulberg SD, Stulberg BN, Hamati Y, et al: Failure mechanisms of metal-backed patellar components. Clin Orthop 236:88, 1988.
83. Thomas WH, Ewald FC, Poss R: Duopatellar total knee arthroplasty. Orthop Trans 4:329, 1980.
84. Thorpe CD, Bocell JR, Tullos HS: Intra-articular fibrous bands: Patellar complications after total knee arthroplasty. J Bone Joint Surg Am 72:811, 1990.
85. Tria AJ, Harwood DA, Alicea JA, et al: Patellar fractures in posterior stabilized knee arthroplasties. Clin Orthop 299:131, 1994.
86. Vince KG, McPherson EJ: The patella in total knee arthoplasty. Orthop Clin North Am 23:675, 1992.
87. Wetzner SM, Bezreh JS, Scott RD, et al: Bone scanning in the assessment of patellar viability following knee replacement. Clin Orthop 199:215, 1985.
88. Yoshi I, Whiteside LA, Anouchi YS: The effect of patellar button placement and femoral component design on patellar tracking in total knee arthroplasty. Clin Orthop 275:211, 1992.

82 Transfusion Considerations in Total Knee Arthroplasty

PHILIP M. FARIS • E. MICHAEL KEATING

Total knee arthroplasty has enjoyed a relatively long and successful reign as a beneficial adjunct in the treatment of various maladies of the painful knee. Complication rates have been relatively low, consisting predominantly of mechanical, infectious, and thromboembolic phenomena. However, as concerns over viral disease transmission through blood and blood product transfusion mount, more clinical and basic science research is being directed toward controlling and preventing disease transfer. Extensive investigation has begun not only into the identification and treatment of these viruses, which is beyond the scope of this chapter, but also, more practically, into methods of preventing their transmission. Three perioperative time periods should be considered, as the need for the use of blood products may be determined preoperatively, intraoperatively, and postoperatively. This chapter considers each of these perioperative periods and attempts to elucidate hematologic changes that occur and how these can affect blood usage during total knee arthroplasty.

PREOPERATIVE PERIOD

Patient factors are important in determining the necessity for postoperative blood usage. Primarily, the patient's coagulation status should be assessed. Bleeding time is the best general test for coagulation status but probably is not a necessary study in the mature patient with no medical history of a bleeding diathesis. Any patient or family history of coagulation defect should be evaluated. Anticoagulants such as warfarin (Coumadin) should be discontinued, if possible, prior to surgery. Since the half-life of warfarin is 2½ days, the drug should be discontinued at least 3 days prior to surgery. Some residual effect may be seen for 4 to 5 days; however, this effect is negligible and the drug can usually be resumed the evening before surgery for thromboembolic prophylaxis. Serum prothrombin time should be determined prior to surgery to verify adequate coagulability, and vitamin K may aid in reversing the warfarin effect.

Nonsteroidal anti-inflammatory drugs inhibit platelet aggregation and may prolong bleeding times.[1] The effect of these agents is dependent on their half-lives. Drugs with longer half-lives, e.g., piroxicam with a mean half-life of 50 hours, should be discontinued at least 5 days prior to surgery. Drugs with shorter half-lives, such as indomethacin, may be continued until 2 days prior to surgery. Because aspirin has a more direct and profound effect on platelet function, it should be discontinued 10 days prior to surgery, if possible.

The remainder of the preoperative patient preparation is devoted to preparing the patient for the expected blood loss of surgery. This is achieved currently by autologous self-donation and or with the use of recombinant human erythropoietin. Viral contamination and transfusion-related reactions and complications remain the major reasons to avoid the use of allogeneic blood. Viral contamination by the human immunodeficiency virus (HIV) stimulated public concern over transfusion-related problems. However; cytomegalovirus (CMV); hepatitis viruses A, B, and C; and other non-A, non-B viruses are also transmitted via the allogeneic transfusions. Particularly, the non-A, non-B forms have high rates of chronic sequelae such as chronic active hepatitis and cirrhosis that may result in the need for liver transplantation.[8, 14, 16, 26, 62] Complications from allogeneic transfusions may also result from mismatching, patient misidentification, transportation, storage mistakes, and unexpected transfusion reactions. Between 60 and 230 patients die each year of fatal hemolytic reactions.

Screening tests of allogeneic blood for viral contamination continue to be modified and developed and have decreased the windows in which undetected contamination occurs.[18, 49] Consequently, the blood pool is continually improving; however, risks continue and viral evolution will undoubtedly continue to put the donor pool at risk.[8, 14, 23, 62, 63]

Preoperative diligence must continue in identifying patients at risk for transfusion and the procedures that have high blood loss potential (Fig. 82.1). Then we can create environments that decrease the need for allogeneic blood. Our techniques for creating allogeneic blood free environments continue to improve. The gold standard for blood conservation remains preoperative autologous donation. However; it is also important to try to identify those patients who are at highest risk for allogeneic exposure in the postoperative period. With this in mind, at our institution and others, attempts are being made to identify the patients who are at the greatest risk for allogeneic usage and to counsel our patient populations as to their

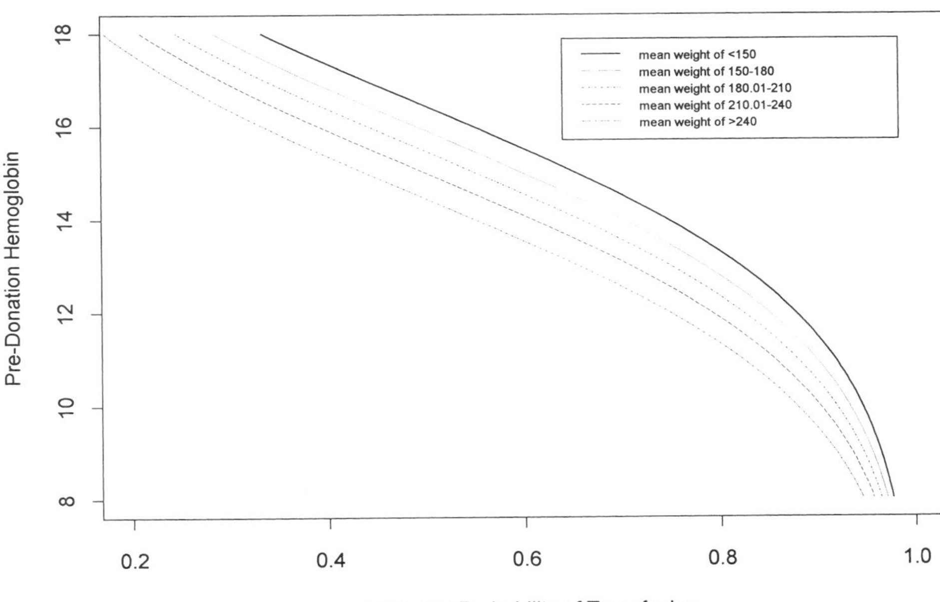

FIGURE 82.1 ➢ Bilateral total knee replacement transfusion risk with predonation hemoglobin and weight.

optimum modes of blood usage. This may evolve into the use of a blood algorithm. As Cohen suggested, autologous donation is a form of chronic hemodilution, which leads to lower postoperative hemoglobins, resulting in transfusions, which may not have been required had the preoperative donation not been performed.[12] Kickler and Spivak noted that the degree of anemia created by the preoperative donation is often not adequate to stimulate an erythropoietic response.[37] Consequently, patients are commonly coming to surgery with iatrogenic anemia. On the other hand, approximately 50% of preoperatively donated blood is unused and is discarded. This percentage may be as high as 70%. This reduces the cost effectiveness of preoperative autologous donation programs. In an attempt to identify the best preoperative strategies for blood management, we recently retrospectively reviewed the records of 279 primary unilateral total knee replacement patients and 200 primary bilateral total knee replacement patients. We determined that the estimated blood loss in the unilateral group was 3.85 g of hemoglobin and in the bilateral group 5.42 g of hemoglobin. In the unilateral group, if the preoperative hemoglobin was greater than 13 g/dL, 78% of the autologous blood was wasted; in those whose hemoglobin was between 10 and 13 g/dL, 56% of the autologous blood was wasted. These patients had preoperatively donated 1 unit of autologous blood.

In the bilateral total knee replacement group, if predonation hemoglobin was between 10 and 14, 32.3% used supplementary allogeneic blood in addition to the two units of autologous blood that they had preoperatively donated. If the predonation hemoglobin was greater than 13, only 6% received supplementary allogeneic blood. Hospital stays were statistically longer in both groups if allogeneic blood was transfused. Utilizing logistic regression analysis, predonated hemoglobin, age, weight, and blood volume were strong predictors of allogeneic transfusion. Nomograms (Fig. 82.2) were developed for both unilateral and bilateral total knee replacement groups and reveal the importance of treating preoperative anemia prior to both preoperative autologous donations and surgery. We also suggest an algorithm for decision making in total knee blood management (Fig. 82.3). Preoperative anemia may be treated with recombinant human erythropoietin. Several studies have elucidated the safety and efficacy of this therapy. Further evaluation of dosage regimens have outlined the safest, most efficacious, and most patient friendly regimen to be 600 international units per kg given on a one day per week basis beginning 3 weeks before surgery. A final fourth dose is given on the evening of surgery. This regimen has been quite efficacious and beneficial in decreasing allogeneic blood usage in the postoperative period.[18, 20]

Patients should be offered the opportunity to predonate. Some patients, however, will be at high risk for phlebotomy. As a predonation has become more prominent, blood bank personnel acceptance of higher-risk and more elderly patients has increased. Spiess et al.[61] categorize high-risk patients as having one or more of the following: a history of angina, myocardial infarction, cardiac dysrhythmia, hypertension requiring two or more medications for control, congestive heart failure, valvular heart disease, congenital heart disease, seizure disorder, previous cerebrovascular accident, or cerebrovascular insufficiency. They exclude from predonation those patients with unstable angina, aortic stenosis, and those who have suffered a myocardial infarction in the last 6 months. Using hemodynamic monitoring, they noted systolic blood pressure drops of 20% or more in 49 of 123 high-risk patients. Although this does not preclude predonation by this

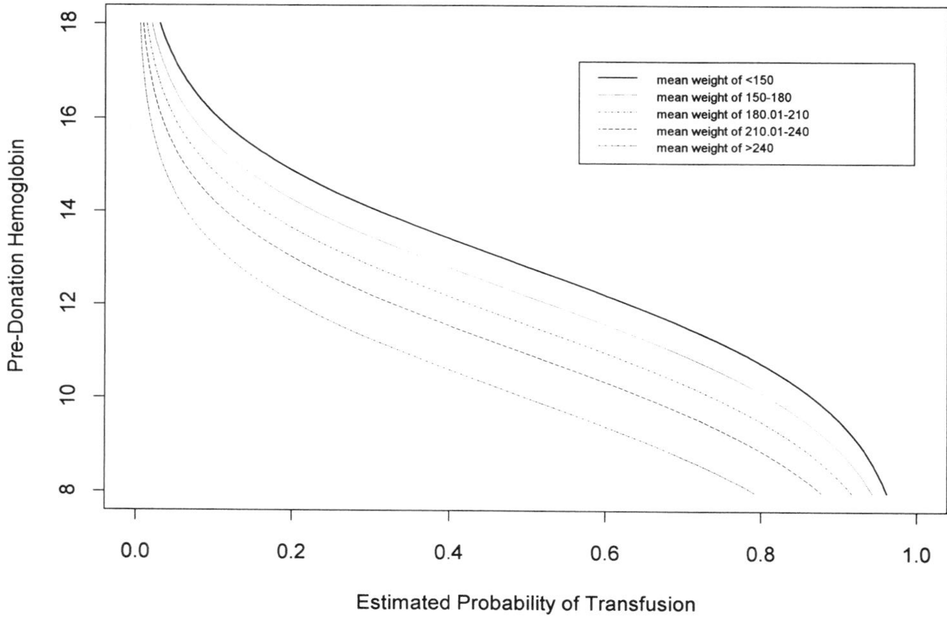

FIGURE 82.2 ➢ Unilateral total knee replacement transfusion risk with predonation hemoglobin and weight.

group of patients, it does point out the importance of monitoring these patients during phlebotomy.[52]

Spacing of preoperative donations in the normal knee replacement patient population is generally 10 to 14 days. This conservatively spaced period is allowable because of the elective nature of the procedure and the normal physiology of the hematopoietic response. Without the use of oral iron replacement, reticulcytosis peaks at approximately 9 days post phlebotomy and 1 unit of red blood cells can be replaced in 3 to 4 weeks. Red blood cell synthesis can be maximized with routine oral doses (i.e., 150 mg two to three times a day) of iron, which can result in the replacement of 1 unit of red cells in 3 to 5 days. With oral iron replacement, significant responses can be attained even in iron-deficient patients. Oral iron supplementation should be initiated 2 to 3 days prior to phlebotomy. Through maximization techniques, autologous donations may be procured every fourth day and surgery should be delayed until the fourth day after the last donation.[22–24, 52, 60]

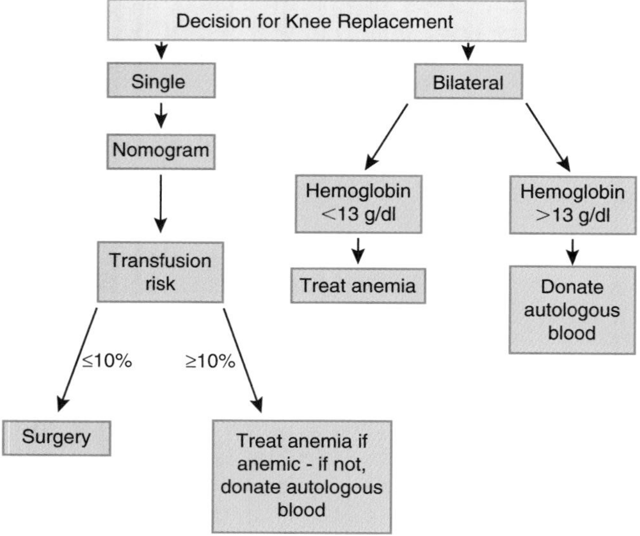

FIGURE 82.3 ➢ Algorithm for blood management for total knee replacement.

THE INTRAOPERATIVE PERIOD

Unlike orthopaedic procedures performed above the thigh, total knee arthroplasty is amenable to the use of a tourniquet. Tourniquet use allows a clean, dry surgical field and prevents significant blood loss during the procedure. Intraoperative techniques for blood loss prevention, then, are mainly to prevent postoperative drainage losses. Careful hemostasis during the procedure should be obtained, but it is not necessary to release the tourniquet prior to wound closure. In separate articles by Lotke et al,[39] Newman et al,[48] Erskin et al,[17] and Gannon et al,[19] tourniquet release prior to wound closure had no effect on total blood loss. Other techniques, such as the smearing of fibrin on the bone and soft tissue surfaces, have likewise had no effect on measurable postoperative blood loss; however, inapparent patient blood loss, which may amount to 31% of the postoperative loss, may be reduced by this method.[41, 49] The superior lateral genicular artery should be sought during lateral retinacular release and either preserved or coagulated because substantial blood loss and tense hematomas may result from its laceration.

The only significant factor in intraoperative blood loss appears to be the use of polymethyl metharcrylate for prosthetic fixation. Whether polymethyl methacrylate decreases blood loss via simple tamponade, as suggested by Charnley; increased venous pressure, which blocks sinusoids, as suggested by Tronzo; protein coagulation by monomer, as described by Jeffries; or heat cauterization of vessels caused by the exothermic curing reaction, cement decreases significantly the blood loss associated with total knee replacement.[13, 17, 44]

Other topically or locally active techniques under investigation to reduceinapparent postoperative loss include the pharmacological products known as antifibrinolytics. These include aprotinin and sigma-aminocaproic acid. These compounds are administered intraoperatively or postoperatively and are variably effective.[4–6, 28, 29, 31, 34, 44, 58, 64] There appear to be no consistent data as to whether these significantly decreased the actual blood loss involved in total knee replacement.

The postoperative dressing should be a soft compressive dressing made of burn gauze and elastic bandages. The dressing is designed to improve patient comfort and to allow some knee motion. Various forms of ice application have been designed that may improve patient comfort; however, good prospective, randomized studies are lacking relating to blood loss prevention, pain control, and economic justification that would allow us to recommend them for routine use.

POSTOPERATIVE PERIOD

The postoperative period in total knee replacement continues to hold promise for salvage and preservation of blood and blood products. Prior to discussing these techniques, note should be made of the effects of tourniquet use and surgery in general on the coagulation system. During surgical procedures, activation of both the fibrinolytic and coagulation systems occurs. This appears to be a general response and is noted after all surgical cases. An in-depth discussion of the multitude of factors involved in these cascades is beyond the scope of this chapter. In general, elevation of fibrinogen and fibrin degradation products occurs along with a decrease in platelet count. Stimulation of the system begins with tissue trauma, whether it be soft tissue or bone, and is mediated by a variety of kinins.[3, 10, 15, 35, 63, 69] Of interest in total knee surgery is the enhanced effect on this system by the hypoxia of tourniquet use.[15, 30, 35, 50] A study on dogs using tourniquet application for 4 hours in three separate groups demonstrated increased bleeding from the anterior tibial muscle, and prolongation of the bleeding time just prior to tourniquet release, maximizing at 5 minutes after release, and normalizing at 15 minutes after release. Blood platelet counts increased slightly throughout the study, and capillary permeability increased in the ischemic muscle. Venous occlusion without arterial occlusion can, of itself, increase fibrinolytic activity in the occluded extremity. These concepts, when combined with the tissue trauma occurring during knee arthroplasty, would seem to portend significant hematologic postoperative changes.[46]

Stern et al[63] studied platelet counts, fibrinogen, and fibrin degradation products in unilateral and bilateral total knee arthroplasties. Overall blood platelets decreased from a mean of 314/nL to a postoperative mean of 173/nL, fibrinogen increased from 304 mg/dL to 647 mg/dL, and variable elevations of fibrin degradation products occurred. All of these changes were enhanced by the performance of bilateral procedures; however, only platelet counts were statistically lower. They suggest that evaluation of preoperative platelet counts are important, especially in patients undergoing bilateral procedures in whom platelet counts decreased by an average of 60%. Stern et al did not give guidelines for maintenance of platelet counts; we prefer to maintain counts of above 25/nL and will transfuse platelets preoperatively to ensure that these levels are maintained in the postoperative period.

Since most blood loss in total knee replacement occurs in the postoperative period, techniques for postoperative salvage of shed blood have been developed. These techniques derive from techniques previously used for intraoperative blood salvage. Washed and centrifuged red blood cells for reinfusion have been used successfully and safely since the introduction of the Cell Saver (Haemonetics, Braintree, MA) in the mid-1970s. This device has been safely and efficaciously adapted to postoperative red blood cell salvage after total knee replacement. However, unless the device is used intraoperatively, the expense of using it in the postoperative period is prohibitive since it requires a technician for operation and the machine is extremely expensive.[2, 9, 25, 32, 36, 40–42, 51, 56, 57, 65, 67, 69]

A second method of postoperative shed blood salvage is through the use of unwashed shed red blood cells. This is accomplished via collection through a sterile drainage and filtration system,[18, 19, 54] e.g., Solcotrans (Solco Basle, Billingham, MA). Ansell et al[2] demonstrated comparable survival rates of red blood cells between these two different techniques of shed blood collection and preparation. Direct reinfusion of the shed, unwashed, filtered red blood cells and blood products can be accomplished. We have demonstrated in detail the hematologic properties of the shed blood and also the safety of the product when it is used properly.[18] The only major side effect was febrile reactions occurring in 2% of patients in whom shed blood collection lasted less than 6 hours at the time of reinfusion. Our study, however, failed to document efficacy. Reduction of postoperative transfusions using this system was documented by Groh et al.[27] in 1990 and by Majkowski et al[41] in 1991. These studies, however, were retrospective, and the factors that led to transfusion are not documented. In a recent prospective study using a triggering hematocrit of 27%, we found no significant difference in transfusion requirements, postoperative drainage, wound problems, or retardation of physical therapy progress regardless of whether a drainage system was used.[55] Consequently, we currently do not use any form of postoperative wound evacuation system after unilateral or bilateral total knee replacement.

Continuous passive motion machines have not been associated with increased blood loss or wound problems in the postoperative period; however, controversy exists as to their benefits in improving postoperative range of motion in knee replacement patients.[21, 39, 47, 56, 65] At this time, based on the current literature, we do not think the expense justifies their use.

SUMMARY

Total knee replacement surgery has proved to be a highly successful form of management of the painful, arthritic knee. Methods of preoperative, intraoperative, and postoperative management of blood loss, blood preservation, and hematopoietic stimulation can reduce the amount of homologous blood usage. However, sorting out of these techniques as to their efficacy and economic feasibility requires closely controlled prospective studies, and predonation of autologous blood, along with the use of recombinant human erythropoietin, remains the mainstay of blood loss management in total knee replacement patients.

REFERENCES

1. Anderson SK, Shaikh A: Dicolofenac in combination with opiate infusion after joint replacement surgery. Anaesth Intensive Care 19:535, 1991.
2. Ansell J: Survival of autotransfused red blood cells recovered from the surgical field during cardiovascular operations. J Thorac Cardiovascular Surg 84:387, 1982.
3. Aranda A, Paramo JA, Rocha E: Fibrinolytic activity in plasma after gynecological and urological surgery. Haemostasis 18:129, 1988.
4. Benoni G, Fredin H: Fibrinolytic inhibition with tranexamic acid reduces blood loss and blood transfusion after knee arthroplasty. A prospective, randomised, double-blind study of 86 patients. J Bone Joint Surg Br 78B(3):434, 1996.
5. Benoni G, Lethagen S, Fredin H: The effect of tranexamic acid on local plasma fibrinolytic during total knee arthroplasty. Thromb Res 85:195, 1997.
6. Benoni G, Carlsson A, Petersson C, Fredin H: Does tranexamic acid reduce blood loss in knee arthroplasty? Am J Knee Surg 8: 88, 1995.
7. Blaise G, Jackmusth R: Preoperative autotransfusion for total hip prostheses. Acta Anaesthesiol Belg 3:175, 1979.
8. Bove J: Transfusion transmitted diseases: Current problems and challenges. Prog Hematol 14:123, 1986.
9. Bovill DF: The efficacy of intraoperative autologous transfusion in major orthopedic surgery: A regression analysis. Orthopedics 9:1403, 1986.
10. Bredbacka S: Activation of cascade systems in hip arthroplasty. Acta Anaesthesiol Scand 58:231, 1987.
11. Chambers LA: Directed donor programs may adversely affect autologous donor participation. Transfusion 30:246, 1990.
12. Cohen JA, Brecher ME: Preoperative autologous blood donation: Benefit or detriment? A mathematical analysis. Transfusion 35: 640, 1995.
13. Cushner FD, Friedman RJ: Blood loss in total knee arthroplasty. Clin Orthop 269:98, 1991.
14. Dodd RY: Transfusion and AIDS. Int Ophthalmol Clin 29:83, 1989.
15. Donadoni R: Coagulation and fibrinolytic parameters in patients undergoing total hip replacement: Influence of the anaesthesia technique. Acta Anaesthesiol Scand 33:588, 1989.
16. Editorial. Am J Clin Pathol 29:78, 1992.
17. Erskin JG: Blood loss with knee joint replacement. J R Coll Surg Edin 26:295, 1981.
18. Faris PM: Unwashed filtered shed blood collected after knee and hip arthroplasties. J Bone Joint Surg Am 73:1169, 1991.
19. Gannon DM: An evaluation of the efficacy of postoperative blood salvage after total joint arthroplasty. J Arthroplasty 1:109, 1991.
20. Golberg MA, McCutchen JW, Jove M, et al: A safety and efficacy comparison study of two dosing regimens of epoetin alfa in patients undergoing major orthopedic surgery. Am J Orthop 25: 544, 1996.
21. Goletz TH, Henry JH: Continuous passive motion after total knee arthroplasty. South Med J 79:1116, 1986.
22. Goodnough LT, Brittenham GM: Limitations of the erythropoietic response to serial phlebotomy: Implications for autologous blood donor programs. J Lab Clin Med 115:28, 1990.
23. Goodnough LT, Shuck JM: Risk, options, and informed consent for blood transfusion in elective surgery. Am J Surg 159:602, 1990.
24. Goodnough LT: Limitations to donating adequate autologous blood prior to elective surgery. Arch Surg 124:494, 1989.
25. Goodnough LT: Increased preoperative collection of autologous blood with recombinant human erythropoietin therapy. N Engl J Med 321:1163, 1989.
26. Goulet JA: Intraoperative autologous transfusion in orthopaedic patients. J Bone Joint Surg Am 71:3, 1989.
27. Groh GI, Buchert PK, Allen WC: A comparison of transfusion requirements after total knee arthroplasty using the Solcotrans Autotransfusion System. J Arthroplasty 3:281, 1990.
28. Hayes A, Murphy DB, McCarroll M: The efficacy of single-dose aprotinin 2 million KIU in reducing blood loss and its impact on the incidence of deep venous thrombosis in patients undergoing total hip replacement surgery. J Clin Anesth 8:357, 1996.
29. Hiippala ST, Strid LJ, Wennerstrand MI, et al: Tranexamic acid radically decreases blood loss and transfusions associated with total knee arthroplasty. Anesth Analg 84:839, 1997.
30. Holemans R: Increase in fibrinolytic activity by venous occlusion. J Appl Physiol 18:1123.
31. Howes JP, Sharma V, Cohen AT: Tranexamic acid reduces blood loss after knee arthroplasty. J Bone Joint Surg Br 78(6):995, 1996.
32. Isbister JP: Autotransfusion: An impossible dream? Anaesth Intensive Care 12:236, 1984.
33. Isbister JP: Strategies for avoiding or minimizing homologous blood transfusion: A sequel to the AIDS scare. Med J Aust 142: 596, 1985.
34. Janssens M, Joris J, David JL: High-dose aprotinin reduces blood loss in patients undergoing total hip replacement surgery. Anesthesiology 80:23, 1994.
35. Kambayashi J: Activation of coagulation and fibrinolysis during surgery, analysed by molecular markers. Thromb Res 60:157, 1990.
36. Keeling MM: Intraoperative autotransfusion experience in 725 consecutive cases. Ann Surg 197:536, 1982.
37. Kickler TS, Spivak JL: Effect of repeated whole blood donations on serum immunoreactive erythropoietin levels in autologous donors. JAMA 260:65, 1988.
38. Levin EA: Increasing autologous blood donation with recombinant human erythropoietin. Surgery 88:327, 1991.
39. Lotke PA: Blood loss after total knee replacement. Effects of tourniquet release and continuous passive motion. J Bone Joint Surg Am 73:1937, 1991.
40. Mayer ED: Reduction of postoperative donor blood requirement by use of the cell separator. Scand J Thorac Cardiovasc Surg 19: 165, 1985.
41. Majkowski RS, Currie IC, Newman JH: Postoperative collection and reinfusion of autologous blood in total knee arthroplasty. Ann R Coll Surg Engl 73:381, 1991.
42. Marmor L, Avoy DR, McCabe A: Effect of fibrinogen concentrates on blood loss in total knee arthroplasty. Clin Orthop 273: 136, 1991.
43. McCarthy PM: Effect of blood conservation efforts in cardiac operations at the Mayo Clinic. Mayo Clin Proc 63:225, 1988.
44. Murkin JM, Shannon NA, Bourne RB, et al: Aprotinin decreases blood loss in patients undergoing revision or bilateral total hip arthroplasty. Anesth Analg 80:343, 1995.
45. Mylod AG: Perioperative blood loss associated with total knee arthroplasty. J Bone Joint Surg Am 72:1010, 1990.
46. Nakahara M, Sakahashi H: Effect of application of a tourniquet on bleeding factors in dogs. J Bone Joint Surg Am 49:1345, 1967.
47. Nielsen PT, Rechnagel K, Nielsen SE: No effect of continuous passive motion after arthroplasty of the knee. Acta Orthop Scand 59:580, 1988.

48. Newman JH, Jackson JP, Waugh W: Timing of tourniquet removal after knee replacment. J R Soc Med 72:492, 1979.
49. Page HP, Shepherd BD, Harrison JM: Reduction of blood loss in knee arthroplasty. Aust N Z J Surg 54:141, 1984.
50. Petaja J: Fibrinolysis after application of a pneumatic tourniquet. Acta Chir Scand 153:647, 1987.
51. Popovsky MA, Devine PA: Intraoperataive autologous transfusion. Mayo Clin Proc 60:125, 1985.
52. Preoperative autologous blood donations by hish-risk patients (editorial). Transfusion 32:1, 1992.
53. Rebulla P: Autologous blood predeposit for elective surgery: A program for better use and conservation of blood. Surgery 97: 463, 1984.
54. Reilly TJ: The use of postoperative suction drainage in total knee arthroplasty. Clin Orthop 208:238, 1986.
55. Ritter MA, Keating EM, Faris PM: Closed wound drainage: A prospective randomized study. Unpublished manuscript.
56. Romness DW, Rand JA: The role of continuous passive motion following total knee arthroplasty. Clin Orthop 226:34, 1988.
57. Ronai AK, Glass JJ, Shapiro AS: Improving autologous blood harvest: Recovery of red cells from sponges and suction. Anaesth Intensive Care 15:421, 1987.
58. Schott U, Sollen C, Axelsson K, et al: Desmopressin in acetate does not reduce blood loss during total hip replacement in patients receiving dextran. Acta Anaesthesiol Scand 39:593, 1995.
59. Semkiw LE: Postoperative blood salvage using the cell saver after total joint arthroplasty. J Bone Joint Surg Am 71:823, 1989.
60. Special communication. The use of autologous blood. The National Blood Resource Education Program Expert Panel. JAMA 263:414, 1990.
61. Spiess BD: Autologous blood donation: Hemodynamics in a high-risk patient population. Transfusion 32(1):17, 1992.
62. Starkey JM: Markers for transfusion-transmitted disease in different groups of blood donors. JAMA 262:3452, 1989.
63. Stern SH, Insall JN: Hematological effects of total knee arthroplasty: A prospective evaluation. Annual Meeting of the American Orthopaedic Surgery, 1992.
64. Theroux MC, Corddry DH, Tietz AE, et al: A Study of desmopressin and blood loss during spinal fusion for neuromuscular scoliosis: A randomized, controlled, doubleblinded study. Anesthesiology 87:260, 1997.
65. Thompson JD: Prior deposition of autologous blood in elective orthopaedic surgery. J Bone Joint Surg Am 69:325, 1987.
66. Vince KG: Continuous passive motion after total knee arthroplasty. J Arthroplasty 2:281, 1987.
67. Wasman J, Goodnough LT: Autologous blood donation for elective surgery. JAMA 258:3135, 1987.
68. Williamson KR, Taswell HF: Intraoperative blood salvage: A review. Transfusion 31, 1991.
69. Wilson J: Coagulation and fibronolysis during hip surgery. Hip Surg 51:439, 1988.
70. Wilson WJ: Intraoperatiave autologous transfusion in revision total hip arthroplasty. J Bone Joint Surg Am 71:8, 1989.
71. Woodson ST, Marsh JS, Tanner JB: Transfusion of previously deposited autologous blood for patients undergoing hip-replacement surgery. J Bone Joint Surg 69:320, 1987.
72. Young JN: Autologous blood retrieval in thoracic cardiovascular, and orthopedic surgery. Am J Surg 144:48, 1982.

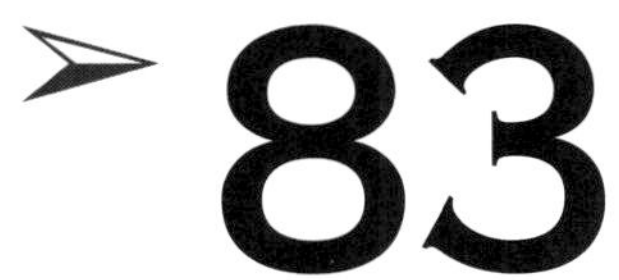

Thrombophlebitis in Knee Arthroplasty

CLIFFORD W. COLWELL • MARY E. HARDWICK

INTRODUCTION

Thromboembolic disease management remains one of the most controversial subjects in knee arthroplasty after decades of studies and debates. Without prophylaxis, venous thromboembolism has been reported in 40% to 84% of patients having total knee arthroplasty. In 9% to 20% of the knee arthroplasty cases, venous thromboembolism occurs proximally. Pulmonary embolism is reported to occur in 1.8% to 7% of patients having lower extremity orthopedic surgery, with fatal events occurring in 0.7% of cases.[8]

Venous thrombi contain fibrin and red blood cells with variable platelet and leukocyte components. Virchow, in 1846, first revealed that clinically important pulmonary embolisms nearly always begin as venous thrombi, typically in the large deep veins of the pelvis and thigh.[61] Virchow's triad describes the formation of thrombus as a result of a combination of vascular injury, activation of blood coagulation, and venous stasis.

The period of risk for postoperative development of venous thromboembolism begins at the time of knee arthroplasty. Thrombi of clinically significant proportions may be present beginning 24 to 48 hours postoperatively, peaking at 5 to 10 days, and continuing for up to several weeks.[5] The true prevalence of venous thromboembolism is uncertain largely because of the nonspecific nature of clinical signs and symptoms that may or may not indicate that a patient has venous thromboembolism. Classic clinical findings, such as leg pain and swelling, shortness of breath, and chest pain, are absent in more than half of all individuals who have venous thromboembolism, including a majority of those who die of pulmonary embolism. Furthermore, more than half of all individuals who present with typical signs and symptoms of venous thromboembolism do not have the disease.

Early diagnostic tests for venous thromboembolism included ^{125}I-fibrinogen scanning and impedance plethysmography. The most common tests for diagnosing venous thromboembolism in present-day management are venography and Doppler flow/duplex ultrasonography.

The idea of providing some form of venous thromboembolism prophylaxis during the overall risk period (from days to weeks postoperatively, depending on individual risk factors) after knee arthroplasty is generally accepted and should prevent the majority of clinically important pulmonary embolisms.[8, 11, 20] Accepted prophylaxis includes mechanical methods, such as sequential compression devices or intermittent compression boots, and pharmacological methods, such as warfarin or low-molecular-weight heparin. Duration of prophylaxis remains controversial; programs vary from 7 to 10 days up to 6 months.

DIAGNOSIS AND SURVEILLANCE TECHNIQUES

Pulmonary embolism is frequently the first clinical presentation of venous thromboembolism; 50% of deaths from pulmonary embolism occur within the first hour after embolization. This has led some surgeons to advocate for routine surveillance with noninvasive techniques as well as testing when clinical signs and symptoms are present.

Diagnostic Tests for Venous Thrombosis

The early diagnostic tests of impedance plethysmography (IPG) and ^{125}I-fibrinogen scanning may still be used in some settings. IPG measures changes in blood volume produced by deliberate temporary venous obstruction, so it can be thought of as a stress test of the venous system. An unobstructed venous system responds to the increasing volume challenge of IPG with a proportionately greater outflow rate; if there is a thrombus, the outflow rate decreases. IPG's advantages are that it is noninvasive and can detect thrombi in the groin and pelvis better than other models.

Because interpretations are based on nonstandardized measurements of venous outflow, the borderline between normal and abnormal is wide. Another limitation of IPG is its low sensitivity in the calf (17%), where false-negative readings can occur due to collateral blood flow. In addition, IPG has less than 13% sensitivity for proximal deep venous thrombosis (DVT) in high-risk asymptomatic patients[47]; it is much more sensitive in symptomatic patients, who unfortunately are far outnumbered by their asymptomatic counterparts.

In ^{125}I-fibrinogen scanning, circulating iodine-labeled fibrinogen is incorporated into a thrombus present in a lower extremity to create an overlying area of surface radioactivity measurable by an isotope detector. This test is positive for DVT if there is a 220% increase in the radioactive reading compared with readings taken over adjacent points in the same leg or similar points in the opposite leg. In addition to being a good test for screening high-risk patients for whom DVT prophylaxis is otherwise contraindicated, ^{125}I-fibrinogen scanning may also be used as an adjunct to IPG or ultrasonography. It may be diagnostic in patients with clinically suspected acute recurrence of DVT.

Although it is highly sensitive for calf DVT and relatively sensitive for mid- and lower-thigh DVT, ^{125}I-fibrinogen scanning has limited accuracy in the proximal thigh (possibly because surgical wounds and other tissue anomalies produce high readings) and is insensitive to DVT in the pelvis. ^{125}I-fibrinogen scanning should never be used as the sole diagnostic test for DVT because it fails to detect many proximal thrombi.[34] In addition, the radioactive fibrinogen injection, although generally acceptable, is prepared from pooled human serum donors and, therefore, theoretically poses the risk of hepatitis or AIDS. Following 100 U Ci of ^{125}I-fibrinogen injection, approximately 200 mrem is delivered to the blood, 70 mrem to soft tissues, and 5 mrem to the kidneys. This is less than the recommended 500 mrem annual total-body absorbed radiation dose.[36] Finally, a scan may not be positive for hours or even days after injection.

For lower-extremity venous thrombosis, venography remains the gold standard for diagnosis, providing good visualization of thrombi in the calf and thigh and up to 70% accuracy in diagnosis of thrombi in the iliac veins. Interpretation can be difficult, however, not only because the venogram is a two-dimensional representation of the three-dimensional venous system but also because it is a static rather than a dynamic image, and phasic blood flow cannot be visualized.

Other factors that limit venography include its high cost (up to $1500 for a single extremity); it is invasive and uncomfortable and, therefore, often unrepeatable; about 5% of patients have difficult venous access; improper dye/blood mixing; misinterpretation due to previously occluded veins; occasional contrast hypersensitivity; and a 1% or lower incidence of postvenography phlebitis.

For many clinicians, today's diagnostic standard for DVT is *duplex* ultrasonography. The term duplex refers to simultaneously viewing the vein in three dimensions and listening to the blood flow. A direct compression test in the area of a suspected thrombus can indicate whether a thrombus is present. Duplex ultrasonography has been shown in most studies to be nearly 100% specific, sensitive, and accurate for proximal DVT.[1, 4, 12, 13, 18, 34, 50, 51, 54, 65] The accuracy of duplex ultrasonography remains controversial, however. Some recent studies have reported a much lower sensitivity, especially for detection of distal DVT.[7, 19] Its main disadvantage is that it is highly operator-dependent; with a less skilled ultrasonographer, sensitivity to distal DVT drops markedly. There may also be problems with obese patients or with limb edema. It is incumbent upon every orthopedist using duplex ultrasonography to confirm the accuracy of this modality as compared with venography.[42, 52]

Surveillance for Deep Venous Thrombosis

Duplex ultrasonography, used by many orthopedic surgeons as a diagnostic test, can also be used routinely to examine patients after total knee arthroplasty for venous thromboembolism.[21, 46] Surveillance with duplex ultrasonography has advantages for detection of DVT: it is portable, painless, and noninvasive; has no side effects; and is less expensive than venography. In some institutions, it is as reliable as venography in both proximal and distal clots.[37, 52] In other institutions, the sensitivity, especially in the calf, is low.[7] It can be an excellent tool for screening and surveillance of DVT in patients who have had total knee arthroplasty in institutions where sensitivity, specificity, and accuracy have proved to be excellent.

Grady-Benson et al[21] reported that, in a study of 100 total knee arthroplasty patients managed with pneumatic compression devices and aspirin for prophylaxis, 7% had proximal DVT and 22% had distal DVT on the 4th postoperative day. None of these patients were symptomatic. Oishi et al[46] reported an overall rate of DVT of 23% when screening patients on postoperative day 4. Serial duplex ultrasonography on postoperative days 7 and 14 indicated that 18% (5/27) of the distal clots had propagated. Routine duplex ultrasonography screening in all patients is not recommended[6, 8, 53] in total knee arthroplasty because of the low yield in the proximal, more dangerous, clots.

VENOUS THROMBOEMBOLISM PROPHYLAXIS

Most orthopedic surgeons agree that an ideal prophylactic agent should (1) be effective, (2) be easy to administer and monitor, 3) have a low complication rate, and (4) have a reasonable cost. A number of different modalities are available for venous thromboembolism prophylaxis, but none meet all four criteria.

Mechanical Prophylaxis

Mechanical prophylaxis for venous thromboembolism after total knee arthroplasty has the advantage of not increasing the risk of bleeding associated with pharmacological methods of prophylaxis. Intermittent pneumatic compression (IPC) devices are thought to prevent thrombi by increasing venous blood flow and enhancing fibrinolytic activity.[2, 28, 32, 48] Two forms of IPC devices are available: sequential leg compression devices, which cover the lower leg and thigh, providing sequential compression from the ankle to the groin; and pulsatile pneumatic plantar compression devices, which cover the foot, providing pulsatile compression in the plantar plexus of the foot.

The prevalence of proximal clots ranges from 14% to 17% when intermittent pneumatic leg compression devices are started in the postanesthesia recovery unit as the only prophylactic agent.[32, 48, 66] Woolson and Watt[66] reported a proximal thrombosis rate of 12% with pneumatic leg compression devices alone when started preoperatively. There is some concern, however, that the leg compression devices do not adequately compress the proximal thigh, limiting the effectiveness in preventing formation of proximal thrombi. Paiement et al[48a] and Bailey et al[5a] noted a trend toward an increased rate of proximal thrombi with use of leg compression devices compared with patients receiving low-dose warfarin. Francis et al[15] demonstrated overall rate of DVT formation was the same in patients treated with two-step warfarin (31%) as with leg compression devices (27%). However, warfarin was significantly more effective than compression devices in reducing proximal clot formation (3% versus 15%).[16] Although leg compression devices reduce distal thrombus formation, their efficacy in reducing proximal thrombus formation is questionable and requires further investigation, particularly in total knee arthroplasty; most studies have been done in total hip arthroplasty.

Pulsatile pneumatic plantar compression devices (foot pumps) simulate weightbearing in nonambulatory patients to prevent venous stasis. A small study of 28 patients using the foot pump reported a 17.8% prevalence of proximal thrombi.[64] Westrich et al[63] reported an overall prevalence of DVT of 27% and proximal prevalence of 10% in 81 knee arthroplasty patients using foot pumps prophylactically after surgery. A study using foot pump and aspirin for prophylaxis reported a prevalence of 22% in 36 patients with unilateral knee arthroplasty and 48% of 25 patients with bilateral knee arthroplasty.[23] One study in hip arthroplasty compared use of the foot pump with use of enoxaparin, showing an overall prevalence of DVT of 18% (18/136) for the foot pump and 13% (18/138) for enoxaparin.[62] Similar studies with larger numbers of knee arthroplasty patients comparing warfarin or low-molecular-weight heparin with the foot pump would increase the confidence in prophylactic use of foot pumps.

A compilation of four studies using intermittent compression devices reported an 11% prevalence of DVT in 366 knee replacement patients.[8] Utility of IPC devices is limited by nonuse during physical therapy, patient intolerance, and the inability to continue prophylaxis after hospital discharge. These IPC devices are reasonable prophylaxis for patients who may be intolerable of pharmacological prophylaxis.

Influence of various types of anesthesia, such as general, spinal, or epidural, on venous thrombosis formation is receiving increasing attention in orthopedic literature. Though many of these studies have been done in total hip arthroplasty, knee arthroplasty data also suggest that use of hypotensive epidural anesthesia may play a significant role in decreasing thrombus rates.[35, 56] The overall effect of hypotensive epidural anesthesia is enhancement of lower extremity blood flow and more normal coagulation profile than is usually associated with general anesthesia. Although hypotensive epidural anesthesia appears to be safe in high-risk patients, it does require additional anesthetic expertise and monitoring that may not be available in all centers.

Pharmacological Prophylaxis

Dextran was put on trial as a prophylactic agent because of its ability to decrease platelet aggregation and blood viscosity and to stabilize endothelium. However, dextran was associated with problems related to intravenous access, fluid overload, and anaphylaxis that have limited its use for prophylaxis.[16, 25, 55]

Aspirin was thought to be an ideal prophylactic agent for DVT because of its antiplatelet action and its inhibition of cyclooxygenase, but several randomized trials could not demonstrate any reduction in venous thromboembolic rate with its use.[22, 24–27] In general, aspirin should not be used in the primary prophylaxis after total knee arthroplasty.

Warfarin has been in use as an anticoagulant agent in hip surgery for close to 40 years. Warfarin, a vitamin K antagonist, exerts its anticoagulant effect by inhibiting vitamin K epoxide and possibly vitamin K reductase. This leads to limited carboxylation of vitamin K-dependent proteins (prothrombin, factor VII, factor IX, and factor X). In addition, warfarin limits the carboxylation of proteins C and S by impairing their natural anticoagulant effect.

The observed anticoagulant effect is delayed 24 to 36 hours, representing the time necessary for replacement of the normal clotting factors with the newer decarboxylated factors. Because factor VII has the shortest half-life (6 to 7 hours), the initial anticoagulant effect is caused by the turnover of this factor. The full anticoagulant effect is not realized until 72 to 96 hours, when complete replacement of the other vitamin K-dependent factors occurs. Suppression of the natural anticoagulant protein C takes place early because of its short half-life, which may lead to a prothrombic phase at approximately the time of factor VII inhibition. This may explain both the lack of early anticoagulation induced by factor VII inhibition and the need for heparinization early in warfarin therapy.[30]

Warfarin prophylaxis is administered at a dose sufficient to prolong the International Normalized Ratio to between 2.0 and 3.0. The most appropriate time to administer the initial warfarin dose is uncertain because of the delay in reaching full anticoagulant effect. The initial dose may be given the day before surgery or started immediately after surgery. Even with this dosing schedule, therapeutic range of the International Normalized Ratio is not reached until the 2nd or 3rd postoperative day.

Warfarin has been used as a control in several recent studies. DVT ranged from 41% to 59%, with proximal DVT ranging from 10% to 13% in total knee arthroplasty patients (Table 83.1).

A compilation of six studies using warfarin with a combined enrollment of 1108 knee arthroplasty patients indicated a 49% prevalence of venous thromboembolism.[8] Based on postoperative venography in clinical trials, DVT rates with warfarin prophylaxis remain substantial, ranging from 38% to 59% in total knee arthroplasty patients.

Unfractionated heparin has been evaluated extensively in patients having surgery associated with moderate to high incidence of postoperative venous thromboembolic disease complications[9, 17, 43] and has been shown to be an effective prophylactic agent. A meta-analysis of large numbers of clinical trials using unfrac-

TABLE 83.1 CONTROLLED LOW-MOLECULAR-WEIGHT HEPARIN STUDIES IN ELECTIVE TOTAL KNEE ARTHROPLASTY

Author	Low-Molecular-Weight Heparin	Deep Venous Thrombosis	Deep Venous Thrombosis Proximal	Operative Site Hemorrhage	Major Hemorrhage	Control	Deep Venous Thrombosis	Deep Venous Thrombosis Proximal	Operative Site Hemorrhage	Major Hemorrhage
Hull et al[31]	Tinzaparin	116/258 (45%)	20/258 (18%)	28/317 (9%)	9/317 (3%)	Warfarin	152/227 (55%)	34/227 (12%)	19/324 (6%)	3/324 (1%)
RD Heparin Group[59]	Ardeparin	41/149 (28%)	7/149 (5%)	N/A	N/A	Warfarin	60/147 (41%)	15/147 (10%)	N/A	N/A
Leclerc et al[39]	Enoxaparin	8/41 (19%)	0/41 (0%)	2/66 (3%)	0/66 (0%)	Placebo	35/54 (65%)	11/54 (20%)	1/65 (2%)	1/65 (2%)
Leclerc et al[38]	Enoxaparin	79/206 (37%)	24/206 (12%)	18/336 (5%)	7/336 (2%)	Warfarin	109/211 (52%)	22/211 (10%)	18/334 (5%)	6/334 (2%)
Spiro et al[58]	Enoxaparin	41/108 (38%)	3/108 (3%)	12/173 (7%)	9/173 (5%)	Warfarin	72/122 (59%)	16/122 (13%)	6/176 (13%)	4/176 (2%)
Fauno et al[14]	Enoxaparin	29/92 (23%)	3/92 (3%)	8/92 (9%)	N/A	Heparin	25/93 (27%)	5/93 (5%)	5/93 (5%)	N/A
Colwell et al[10]	Enoxaparin	54/145 (37%)	4/145 (2%)	9/228 (4%)	3/228 (1%)	Heparin	74/143 (52%)	22/143 (15%)	22/143 (15%)	3/225 (1%)
Heit et al[29]	Ardeparin	62/232 (27%)	15/232 (6%)	13/277 (5%)	9/277 (3%)	Warfarin	85/222 (38%)	15/222 (7%)	10/275 (4%)	1/275 (0.3%)

tionated heparin has shown significant risk reduction in patients having general surgery and urologic surgery.[9] For patients having orthopedic surgery, the incidence of treatment failure was 24% in those receiving unfractionated heparin, compared with 47% in those receiving placebo.[9] Two studies using low-dose heparin (5000 IU every 8 hours) that included 386 patients indicated a venous thrombosis prevalence of 42% in knee arthroplasty patients.[8, 10]

Standard unfractionated heparin is a naturally occurring mucopolysaccharide, with a mean molecular weight of 12,000 to 15,000 daltons. It is usually obtained from either bovine or porcine intestinal mucosa. Unfractionated heparin acts by binding to antithrombin III, a natural inhibitor of the coagulation cascade, thereby forming a complex that inhibits a number of clotting factors, particularly factors IIa and Xa. The ratio of anti-Xa activity to anti-IIa activity for unfractionated heparin is 1:1. The increased activity of antithrombin III can be monitored by following the activated partial thromboplastin time because of the significant effects of unfractionated heparin on antithrombin IIa.

Unfractionated heparin has poor bioavailability (approximately 30%), a short half-life (1 hour), and poor clearance mechanisms, necessitating subcutaneous administration up to three times a day. Frequent monitoring of the activated partial thromboplastin time is therefore required in order to achieve optimal therapeutic effects while avoiding dangerously elevated concentrations. Because reversible thrombocytopenia occurs in about 10% of the patients taking the drug, frequent monitoring of the platelet count is necessary as well. Low-dose heparin is not any more effective than other agents, and most surgeons consider adjusted-dose heparin prophylaxis to be impractical for routine use.

Low-molecular-weight heparins, the most recent agents added to the list of prophylaxis, are derived from unfractionated heparin. Low-molecular-weight heparins are formed by individual depolymerization procedures. The molecular weights of these compounds are between 3000 and 10,000 daltons, compared with 12,000 to 15,000 daltons for unfractionated heparin.[41] The most investigated and utilized low-molecular-weight heparins are enoxaparin, ardeparin, dalteparin, tinzaparin, and nadroparin.

The pharmacological properties of low-molecular-weight heparins are entirely different from those of unfractionated heparin.[41] The molecular weight of a heparin constituent is inversely proportional to its anti-Xa-anti-thrombin (factor IIa) ratio. The highly predictable pharmacokinetic properties and high bioavailability, as well as the lower associated incidence of thrombocytopenia and ability to target factor Xa while affecting factor IIa to a lesser extent, make the low-molecular-weight heparins particularly appealing as prophylactic agents.

The pharmacokinetic properties of low-molecular-weight heparins are highly predictable after subcutaneous administration. The bioavailability in terms of anti-Xa activity is over 90%, which is approximately three times that of unfractionated heparin. The half-life of low-molecular-weight heparins can vary between 3 and 8 hours, depending on the specific agent used, compared with 1 hour for unfractionated heparin. The primary route of excretion appears to be renal. Whereas unfractionated heparin has saturable mechanism in its routes of excretion, low-molecular-weight heparins appear to have an advantage of dose-independent elimination. The favorable pharmacokinetics of low-molecular-weight heparins allow them to be administered subcutaneously once or twice daily with no requirement to follow drug levels or activity.[41] Levels of low-molecular-weight heparin cannot be measured directly. Anti-Xa activity can be monitored in international units with a clot-based test, but this is used mostly for research purposes and has little clinical application.

In recent studies with low-molecular-weight heparin, DVT ranged from 19% to 45%, with proximal DVT ranging from 0% to 18% in total knee arthroplasty patients (see Table 83.1). Eight studies consisting of 1499 knee arthroplasty patients reported a prevalence of venous thrombosis of 31%.[8] Low-molecular-weight heparins have been studied extensively and are safe and effective for prophylaxis after total knee arthroplasty surgery. The venographic prevalence of DVT, however, remains appreciable at 19% to 45% among knee arthroplasty patients.

SUMMARY

With the occurrence of venous thromboembolism in knee arthroplasty patients without prophylaxis as high as 84%, some type of prophylaxis is mandatory. Specific diagnostic test, prophylaxis treatment, and length of prophylaxis for venous thromboembolism remain a subject of debate.

Most common diagnostic tests are venography and duplex ultrasonography, both of which have advantages and disadvantages. Though cost and convenience may affect the selection of diagnostic test, the test used should be based on clinical presentation of symptoms and the accuracy of these tests at the specific institution. Presently, prehospital discharge routine screening is not recommended as an alternative to prophylaxis.

Total knee arthroplasty patients are especially recalcitrant to prophylaxis as noted in a number of studies.[31, 58, 59] Current recommendations for pharmacological prophylaxis after knee arthroplasty are either low-molecular-weight heparin or adjusted-dose warfarin.[8] Both pharmacological methods have advantages and disadvantages, as outlined here. Although intermittent pneumatic compression is recommended for knee arthroplasty, the results of IPC studies are smaller in number than those of pharmacology studies and lack comparison with warfarin and low-molecular-weight heparin for knee arthroplasty.

In this climate of cost containment and managed care, cost is also a consideration. Studies are divided as to cost-effectiveness of these two drugs.[31, 33, 45] The choice of low-molecular-weight heparin or warfarin prophylaxis is best tailored to the individual patient, based on the clinical assessment of postoperative thrombosis and bleeding risk as well as the specific cost and convenience of the prophylaxis.

The optimal duration of prophylaxis after knee arthroplasty is uncertain, although prophylaxis for 7 to 10 days has been shown to be extremely effective and is the recommendation of the American College of Chest Physicians.[8] With the current duration of hospitalization often 5 days or less, the duration of hospital prophylaxis may be inadequate. Several hip replacement studies suggest that the risk for DVT may persist for up to 2 months after surgery.[44, 57, 60] However, other studies of knee arthroplasty with 9 days of prophylaxis with either low-molecular-weight heparin or warfarin reported a symptomatic venous thrombosis occurrence of 3% (35/1099) during a 90-day follow-up.[3, 40] Studies detecting thrombosis by venography usually have a higher occurrence rate than those using a symptomatic endpoint because of the silent nature of venous thrombosis.

Genetic risk factors are being more clearly defined,[49, 67] and clinical tests to determine these risk factors are being put on trial. Genetic risk factors include polymorphism in coagulation factor V, which is manifested by resistance to activated protein C. With heterozygote carriers, the occurrence of thrombosis is 8 times greater, whereas with homozygote carriers, the occurrence of thrombosis is 80 times greater than in the normal population.

The future has new diagnostic and surveillance tests as well as new types of prophylaxis on the horizon. A diagnostic and surveillance technique now being researched is radioisotope labeling, which is specific for venous clots either peripheral or lung in nature. Specificity and sensitivity of the isotype is under investigation.

On the prophylactic side, new pharmacological tools are becoming available. A synthetic pentasaccharide is in clinical trials and shows promise. The synthetic pentasaccharide is a pure anti-Xa compound obtained by chemical synthesis that is devoid of antithrombin activity and does not potentiate adenosine diphosphate or collage-induced platelet aggregation. Also under development are oral preparations that would eliminate the inconvenience of subcutaneous injections. Recombinant hirudin, which is a direct thrombin inhibitor, also appears to be a possibility in future prophylaxis.

With the continued prevalence of venous thrombosis by venography in mechanical or pharmacological prophylaxed knee arthroplasty patients from 31% to 49%, there are still new modalities to be tested and many exciting research possibilities.

References

1. Aitken AGF, Godden DJ: Real-time ultrasound diagnosis of deep vein thrombosis: A comparison with venography. Clin Radiol 38: 309, 1987.
2. Allenby F, Pflug JJ, Boardman L, et al: Effects of external pneumatic intermittent compression on fibrinolysis in man. Lancet 12:1412, 1973.
3. Anderson DR, Gross M, Robinson KS, et al: Ultrasonographic screening for deep vein thrombosis following arthroplasty fails to reduce posthospital thromboembolic complications: The Postarthroplasty Screening Study (PASS). Chest 114:119S, 1998.
4. Appelman PT, De Jong TE, Lampmann LE: Deep venous thrombosis of the leg: US findings. Radiology 163:743, 1987.
5. Arcelus JI, Caprini JA: Prevention after hospital discharge. In Goldhaber SZ, ed: Prevention of Venous Thromboembolism, New York, Marcel Dekker, Inc., 1993, p 497.

5a. Bailey JP, Kruger MP, Solano FX, et al: Prospective randomized trial of sequential compression devices vs low-dose warfarin for deep venous thrombosis prophylaxis in total hip arthroplasty. J Arthroplasty 6:29, 1991.

6. Brothers TE, Frank CE, Frank B, et al: Is duplex venous surveillance worthwhile after arthroplasty? J Surg Res 67:72, 1997.
7. Ciccone WJ II, Fox PS, Neumyer M, et al: Ultrasound surveillance for asymptomatic deep venous thrombosis after total joint replacement. J Bone Joint Surg Am 80:1167, 1998.
8. Clagett GP, Anderson FA Jr, Geerts W, et al: Prevention of venous thromboembolism. Chest 114:531S, 1998.
9. Collins R, Scrimgour A, Vusul S, et al: Reduction in fatal pulmonary embolism and venous thrombosis by perioperative administration of subcutaneous heparin. N Engl J Med 318:1162, 1988.
10. Colwell CW Jr, Spiro TE, Trowbridge AA, et al: Efficacy and safety of enoxaparin versus unfractionated heparin for prevention of deep venous thrombosis after elective knee arthroplasty. Clin Orthop 321:19, 1995.
11. Consensus Conference: Prevention of venous thrombosis and pulmonary embolism. JAMA 256:744, 1986.
12. Cronan JJ, Dorfman GS, Grusmark J: Lower-extremity deep venous thrombosis: Further experience with and refinements of US assessment. Radiology 168:101, 1988.
13. Dauzat MM, Laroche J-P, Charras C, et al: Real-time B-mode ultrasonography for better specificity in the noninvasive diagnosis of deep venous thrombosis. J Ultrasound Med 5:625, 1986.
14. Fauno P, Soumalainen O, Rehnberg V, et al: Prophylaxis for the prevention of venous thromboembolism after total knee arthroplasty. J Bone Joint Surg Am 76:1814, 1994.
15. Francis CW, Pellegrini VD Jr, Marder VJ, et al: Comparison of warfarin and external pneumatic compression in prevention of venous thrombosis after total hip replacement. JAMA 267:2911, 1992.
16. Francis CW, Pellegrini VD Jr, Marder VJ, et al: Prevention of venous thrombosis after total hip arthroplasty: Antithrombin III and low-dose heparin compared with dextran 40. J Bone Joint Surg Am 71:327, 1989.
17. Francis CW, Pellegrini VD Jr, Stulberg BN, et al: Prevention of venous thrombosis after total knee arthroplasty: Comparison of antithrombin III and low-dose heparin with dextran. J Bone Joint Surg Am 72:976, 1990.
18. Froehlich JA, Dorfman GS, Cronan JJ, et al: Compression ultrasonography for the detection of deep venous thrombosis in patients who have a fracture of the hip. J Bone Joint Surg Am 71: 249, 1989.
19. Garino JP, Lotke PA, Kitziger KJ, et al: Deep venous thrombosis after total joint arthroplasty: The role of compression ultrasonography and the importance of the experience of the technician. J Bone Joint Surg Am 78:1359, 1996.
20. Goldhaber SZ, Hennekens CH, Evans DA, et al: Factors associated with correct antemortem diagnosis of major pulmonary embolism. Am J Med 73:822, 1982.
21. Grady-Benson JC, Oishi CS, Hanson PB, et al: Postoperative surveillance for deep vein thrombosis with duplex ultrasonography after total knee arthroplasty. J Bone Joint Surg Am 76:1649, 1994.
22. Guyer RD, Booth RE Jr, Rothman RH: The detection and prevention of pulmonary embolism in total hip replacement: A study comparing aspirin and low-dose warfarin. J Bone Joint Surg Am 64:1040, 1982.
23. Haas SB, Insall JN, Scuderi GR, et al: Pneumatic sequential-compression boots compared with aspirin prophylaxis of deep-vein thrombosis after total knee arthroplasty. J Bone Joint Surg Am 72:27, 1990.
24. Harris WH, Athanasoulis CA, Waltman AC, et al: High and low-dose aspirin prophylaxis against venous thromboembolic disease in total hip replacement. J Bone Joint Surg Am 64:63, 1982.

25. Harris WH, Athanasoulis CA, Waltman AC, et al: Prophylaxis of deep-vein thrombosis after total hip replacement: Dextran and external pneumatic compression compared with 1.2 or 0.3 gram of aspirin daily. J Bone Joint Surg Am 67:57, 1985.
26. Harris WH, Salzman EW, Athanasoulis CA, et al: Aspirin prophylaxis of venous thromboembolism after total hip replacement. N Engl J Med 297:1246, 1977.
27. Harris WH, Salzman EW, Athanasoulis CA, et al: Comparison of warfarin, low-molecular-weight dextran, aspirin, and subcutaneous heparin in prevention of venous thromboembolism following total hip replacement. J Bone Joint Surg Am 56:1552, 1974.
28. Hartman JT, Pugh JL, Smith RD, et al: Cyclic sequential compression of the lower limb in prevention of deep venous thrombosis. J Bone Joint Surg Am 64:1059, 1982.
29. Heit JA, Berkowitz SD, Bona R, et al: Efficacy and safety of low molecular weight heparin (ardeparin sodium) compared to warfarin for the prevention of venous thromboembolism after total knee replacement surgery: A double-blind, dose-ranging study. Thromb Haemost 77(1):32, 1997.
30. Hirsch J, Dalen JE, Deykin D, et al: Oral anticoagulants: Mechanism of action, clinical effectiveness, and optimal therapeutic range. Chest 102:312S, 1992.
31. Hull R, Raskob G, Pineo G, et al: A comparison of subcutaneous low-molecular weight heparin with warfarin sodium for prophylaxis against deep vein thrombosis after hip or knee implantation. N Engl J Med 329:1370, 1993.
32. Hull RD, Raskob GE, Gent M: Effectiveness of intermittent pneumatic leg compression for preventing deep vein thrombosis after total hip replacement. JAMA 263:2313, 1990.
33. Hull RD, Raskob GE, Pineo GF, et al: Subcutaneous low-molecular-weight heparin vs warfarin for prophylaxis of deep vein thrombosis after hip or knee implantation: An economic perspective. Arch Intern Med 157:298, 1997.
34. Hull RD, Secker-Walker RH, Hirsh J: Diagnosis of deep-vein thrombosis. In Coleman RW, Hirsh J, Marder V, et al, eds: Hemostasis and Thrombosis. Philadelphia, Lippincott, 1987, p 1220.
35. Jorgensen LN, Rasmussen LS, Nielsen PT, et al: Antithrombotic efficacy of continuous extradural analgesia after knee replacement. Br J Anaesth 66:8, 1991.
36. Kakkar VV: Fibrinogen uptake test for detection of deep vein thrombosis: A review of current practice. Semin Nucl Med 7: 229, 1977.
37. Kraay MJ, Goldberg VM, Herbener TE: Vascular ultrasonography for deep venous thrombosis after total knee arthroplasty. Clin Orthop 286:18, 1993.
38. Leclerc JR, Geerts WH, Desjardins L, et al: Prevention of venous thromboembolism (VTE) after knee arthroplasty: A randomized double-blind trial comparing a low molecular weight heparin fragment (enoxaparin) to warfarin. Blood 10:246, 1994..
39. Leclerc JR, Geerts WH, Desjardins L, et al: Prevention of deep vein thrombosis after major knee surgery: A randomized, double-blind trial comparing a low molecular weight heparin fragment (enoxaparin) to placebo. Thromb Haemost 67:417, 1992.
40. Leclerc JR, Gent M, Hirsh J, et al: The incidence of symptomatic venous thromboembolism during and after prophylaxis with enoxaparin: A multi-institutional cohort study of patients who underwent hip or knee arthroplasty. Arch Intern Med 158:873, 1998.
41. Leizorovicz A, Haugh MC, Chapuis FR: Low molecular weight heparin in prevention of perioperative thrombosis. Br Med J 305:913, 1992.
42. Leutz DW, Stauffer ES: Color duplex Doppler ultrasound scanning for detection of deep venous thrombosis in total knee and hip arthroplasty patients: Incidence, location, and diagnostic accuracy compared with ascending venography. J Arthroplasty 9: 543, 1994.
43. Leyvraz PF, Richard J, Bachmann F, et al: Adjusted versus fixed dose subcutaneous heparin in the prevention of deep vein thrombosis after total hip replacement. N Engl J Med 309:954, 1983.
44. Lotke PA, Steinberg ME, Ecker ML: Significance of deep venous thrombosis in the lower extremity after total joint arthroplasty. Clin Orthop 299:25, 1994.
45. O'Brien BJ, Anderson DR, Goeree R: Cost-effectiveness of enoxaparin versus warfarin prophylaxis against deep-vein thrombosis after total hip replacement. Canadian Med Assoc J 150:1083, 1994.
46. Oishi CS, Grady-Benson JC, Otis SM, et al: The clinical course of distal deep venous thrombosis after total hip and total knee arthroplasty as determined with duplex ultrasonography. J Bone Joint Surg Am 76:1658, 1994.
47. Paiement G, Wessinger SJ, Waltman AC, et al: Surveillance of deep vein thrombosis in asymptomatic total hip replacement patients: Impedance phlebography and fibrinogen scanning versus roentgenographic phlebography. Am J Surg 155:400, 1988.
48. Paiement GD, Bell D, Wessinger SJ, et al: New advances in the prevention, diagnosis, and cost effectiveness of venous thromboembolic diseases in patients with total hip replacement. In Hip Society Proceedings: Fourteenth Open Scientific Meeting of the Hip Society. St. Louis, C.V. Mosby, 1986, p 94.
48a. Paiement G, Wessinger SJ, Waltman AC, et al: Low-dose warfarin versus external pneumatic compression for prophylaxis against thromboembolism following total hip replacement. J Arthroplasty 2:23, 1987.
49. Patäjä J, Fernández JA, Gruber A, et al: Anticoagulant synergism of heparin and activated protein C in vitro: Role of a novel anticoagulant mechanism of heparin; enhancement of inactivation of factor V by activated protein C. J Clin Invest 99:2655, 1997.
50. Persson AV, Jones C, Zide R, et al: Use of the triplex scanner in diagnosis of deep venous thrombosis. Arch Surg 124:593, 1989.
51. Raghavendra BN, Horii SC, Hilton S, et al: Deep venous thrombosis: Detection by probe compression of veins. J Ultrasound Med 5:89, 1986.
52. Robinson KS, Anderson DR, Gross M, et al: Accuracy of screening compression ultrasonography and clinical examination for the diagnosis of deep vein thrombosis after total hip or knee arthroplasty. Can J Surg 41:368, 1998.
53. Robinson KS, Anderson DR, Gross M, et al: Ultrasonographic screening before hospital discharge for deep venous thrombosis after arthroplasty: The post-arthroplasty screening study—a randomized, controlled trial. Arch Intern Med 127:439, 1997.
54. Rollins DL, Semrow CM, Friedell ML, et al: Progress in the diagnosis of deep venous thrombosis: The efficacy of real-time B-mode ultrasonic imaging. J Vasc Surg 7:638, 1988.
55. Salvati EA, Lachiewicz P: Thromboembolism following total hip replacement arthroplasty: The efficacy of dextran-aspirin and dextran-warfarin in prophylaxis. J Bone Joint Surg Am 58:921, 1976.
56. Sharrock NE, Haas SB, Hargett MJ, et al: Effects of epidural anesthesia on the incidence of deep-vein thrombosis after total knee arthroplasty. J Bone Joint Surg Am 73:502, 1991.
57. Sikorski JM, Hampson WG, Staddon GE: The natural history and aetiology of deep vein thrombosis after total hip replacement. J Bone Joint Surg Br 63:171, 1981.
58. Spiro TE, Fitzgerald RH, Trowbridge AA, et al: Enoxaparin: A low molecular weight heparin and warfarin for the prevention of venous thromboembolic disease after elective knee replacement surgery. Blood 10:246, 1994.
59. RD Heparin Arthroplasty Group: RD heparin compared with warfarin for prevention of venous thromboembolic disease following total hip or knee arthroplasty. J Bone Joint Surg Am 76: 1174, 1994.
60. Trowbridge A, Boese CK, Woodruff B, et al: Incidence of posthospitalization proximal deep venous thrombosis after total hip arthroplasty: A pilot study. Clin Orthop 299:203, 1994.
61. Warren R: Behavior of venous thrombosis and pulmonary embolism. Arch Surg 115:1151, 1980.
62. Warwick D, Harrison J, Glew D, et al: Comparison of the use of a foot pump with the use of low-molecular-weight heparin for the prevention of deep-vein thrombosis after total hip replacement: A prospective, randomized trial. J Bone Joint Surg Am 80: 1158, 1998.
63. Westrich GH, Sculco TP: Prophylaxis against deep venous thrombosis after total knee arthroplasty: Pneumatic plantar compression and aspirin compared with aspirin alone. J Bone Joint Surg Am 78:826, 1996.
64. Wilson NV, Das SK, Kakkar VV, et al: Thromboembolic prophylaxis in total knee replacement: Evaluation of the A-V impulse system. J Bone Joint Surg Br 74:50, 1992.

65. Woolson ST, McCrory DW, Walter JF, et al: B-mode ultrasound scanning in the detection of proximal venous thrombosis after total hip replacement. J Bone Joint Surg Am 72:983, 1990.
66. Woolson ST, Watt JM: Intermittent pneumatic compression to prevent proximal deep venous thrombosis during and after total hip replacement: A prospective, randomized study of compression alone, compression and aspirin, and compression and low-dose warfarin. J Bone Joint Surg Am 73:507, 1991.
67. Zivelin A, Griffin JH, Xu X, et al: A single genetic origin for a common Caucasian risk factor for venous thrombosis. Blood 89: 397, 1997.

84 Mechanical Compression Treatment for the Prevention of Thrombophlebitis

GEOFFREY H. WESTRICH

INTRODUCTION

One of the most serious postoperative developments after total knee surgery is the development of thromboembolic disease, specifically, deep-vein thrombosis leading to pulmonary embolus. Deep-vein thrombosis after total knee arthroplasty (TKA), occurs most commonly in the calf and is more frequent after bilateral arthroplasty than unilateral knee arthroplasty. Isolated proximal vein thromboses are less frequent after TKA when compared with total hip arthroplasty. It is well documented that the proximal propagation of calf thrombi to the popliteal and femoral venous system occurs. This is the causative factor for the majority of fatal pulmonary embolisms after total knee replacement surgery.[1, 11, 13, 15, 20–22]

The incidence of deep-vein thrombosis after total knee replacement has been reported to be between 50% and 88%.[20, 67, 97] Although the majority of the thrombi occur in the calf, up to 24% propagate to the proximal veins.[67] Between 1% and 10% of patients will develop a proximal thrombus within 1 week of a total knee replacement.

Because of the mrobidity associated with these complications, it is essential to provide prophylaxis for deep-vein thrombosis as well as pulmonary embolism.[1–86] There are many different modalities available to the clinician, with both chemical and mechanical treatments. However, the pharmaceutical methods are not without their associated side effects and costs.[37, 38] Newer pharmacological treatments such as low-molecular-weight heparin have shown reduction in the risk of thromboembolic disease after orthopedic surgery, yet there is a growing concern due to the associated morbidity such as potential hemorrhagic complications, increasing cost, need for dosing by injection, and in rare occasions, the development of thrombocytopenia. In addition, low-molecular-weight heparin is contraindicated with epidural anesthesia/analgesia and has been associated with epidural hematomas and paralysis.[37, 38] Mechanical methods of prophylaxis have the advantages of being safe and inexpensive and have proved their efficacy in multiple surgical subspecialties.[2–31]

Many clinicians have advocated the use of early mobilization, continuous passive motion machines, and graded compression stockings for the prophylaxis of deep-vein thrombosis after a variety of surgical procedures and traumas. Recent studies for mechanical compression devices have shown that they reduce venous stasis and subsequently reduce the rate of deep-vein thrombosis after total joint arthroplasty.[1–31] There are a great number of devices on the market, with differences including length and location of sleeve and bladder, frequency and duration of activation, rate of pressure rise, maximum pressure achieved, and simultaneous versus sequential compression. These devices are further categorized as foot pumps, foot-calf pumps, calf pumps, and calf-thigh pumps, of which some are single chamber whereas others provide sequential chambers with a number of compartments. This chapter discusses the specifications of the mechanical devices in relation to their clinical efficacy as well as the effects on venous hemodynamics and physiology.

EFFECT OF PNEUMATIC COMPRESSION ON THE VENOUS SYSTEM

There are many types of pneumatic compression devices available, but the optimal contribution of augmented venous velocity and volume necessary to provide adequate deep-vein thrombosis prophylaxis in the lower extremity has not been elucidated. Newer mechanical devices that produce pulsatile venous pumping as opposed to a slow rise in venous return have recently been developed. Whereas the theoretical benefit of such devices, namely a reduction in the formation of thrombosis, is appreciated, the true flow and volume profiles of these devices in a patient population indicated for thromboembolic disease prophylaxis are unclear.

The formation of deep-vein thrombosis was best described by Virchow in 1856.[29] Virchow's triad includes hypercoagulability, endothelial injury, and venous stasis in the pathogenesis of deep-vein thrombosis. In the human vascular system there is a delicate balance between thrombosis and fibrinolysis and total knee replacement affects all three aspects of Virchow's triad. Risk factors such as advanced age (more than 40 years), female sex, obesity, immobilization, oral contraceptive use, superficial thrombophlebitis, a history of thromboembolic disease, and a history of cardiac disease will also result in an elevated risk for developing deep-vein thrombosis.

It has been proposed that these pumps are effective by two mechanisms: decreased stasis (accelerated venous emptying) and increased fibrinolysis.[1–18, 21–32] However, the relative contribution of these two mechanisms is unknown. Rapid compression devices are thought to produce an increase in peak venous velocity as compared with gradual compression, explaining their rise in usage. However, it has still not been proved what the optimal contribution of increased venous velocity or increased venous volume is necessary to provide adequate deep-vein thrombosis prophylaxis in the lower extremity.[1–18, 21–32] In addition, the fibrinolytic effect of such rapid compression devices has not been fully elucidated.

Intermittent pneumatic devices include polyvinyl boots or sleeves, stockings with inflatable bladders, multicompartment vinyl sleeves, and foot pumps.[85, 87] Generally, pressures reach 35 to 55 mm Hg and inflate in cycles of 20 to 90 seconds. The devices are intended to decrease stasis by augmenting venous flow in the lower extremities. In addition, studies have shown stimulation of the fibrinolytic system with the intermittent compression.[22, 85]

The boot or stockings can be applied to the nonoperative leg preoperatively and then postoperatively begun on the operative exterernity during TKA. The pneumatic devices are continued until the patient is ambulating independently. In addition, these devices can be used in conjunction with continuous passive motion.

Static venous blood accumulates in valve pockets during immobilization, as shown by cadaveric studies, and is a well-known risk factor for the formation of deep-vein thrombosis.[22,29] In theory, a pneumatic compression device with the greatest ability to augment venous velocity would not only increase turbulence behind valve pockets but also endothelial shear stresses, which has been shown to produce a reflex vasodilatation. Mechanical devices that produce rapid compression, as opposed to a slow rise in venous return, have recently been popularized and follow the above theory.

PNEUMATIC FOOT COMPRESSION

In 1959, Lovgren and Rastgeldi[94] first evaluated intermittent pneumatic pedal compression. Research continued in the 1960s with Henry and Winsor.[95] In the 1970s, Gaskell and Parrott[96] used a pneumatic foot pump to increase blood flow to the foot in patients with compromised vasculature. In 1983, Gardner and Fox described a physiological venous foot pump in the sole of the foot involving the venae comitans of the lateral plantar artery.[8] This "pump" has a 20-mL stroke volume that empties only through the deep venous system, and is activated solely upon weightbearing.[8]

Pneumatic compression devices that compress the plantar plexus are starting to gain appeal in that the range of applicability is increased and is not influenced by any postoperative dressing or external immobilization. The compliance from both the nursing and patient sides has seemingly improved because of the simplicity and comfort of the devices. The stroke volume of these devices is relatively small, approximately 30 mL, and the increase in peak venous velocity in the common femoral vein was considerably less than devices that pump the calf, specifically the soleal sinus. However, the foot pumps are capable of generating a 250% increase in peak venous velocity in the popliteal vein, and this may explain the efficacy of pneumatic foot compression.

A pneumatic plantar compression device was developed to activate this pump in patients who are nonambulatory. In addition to increasing venous return, it is hypothesized that foot compression may prevent deep-vein thrombosis by several other factors.[6–9] First, high flow states create increased turbulence around venous valve pockets, thus decreasing thrombus formation. Second, hemodynamic studies have confirmed increased blood flow and tissue perfusion with the release of endothelial derived relaxing factor (EDRF) and prostacyclin. Third, Allenby and colleagues documented enhancement of fibrinolysis using external pneumatic compression,[32] and fibrinolytic activity with foot compression is thought to exist as with other pneumatic devices.[9]

VENOUS HEMODYNAMICS

The hemodynamic effects of several types of mechanical devices vary in rate, method, and force of compression applied,[18, 72, 74, 75] whereas the formation of thrombosis may not directly correlate with the changes in venous blood flow resulting from the application of a pneumatic compression device. Mechanical devices have been developed to compress the foot, calf, and thigh, yet the difference in venous enhancement from the location of compression has not been evaluated. Furthermore, the number of compartments as well as the type of pressure applied (i.e., single or sequential wavelike pulsations) is also variable, but only limited studies exist as to the efficacy of these parameters.[71, 74, 75]

Nicolaides and coworkers[71] demonstrated increased venous flow in the common femoral vein with intermittent calf compression and accelerated flow with sequential compression. Roberts and associates[74] established that the rate of inflation was directly proportional to the increase in femoral vein velocity, and that devices with a greater rate of inflation produced improved flow augmentation as compared with devices with a slower rate of inflation. However, Salzman and colleagues[75] compared a graded-sequential filling device, a uniform multicompartment device, and a uniform pressure single-chamber device in a cohort of neurosurgical patients and found a similar incidence of deep-vein thrombosis. Although they noted that a larger study, with increased statistical power, might show graded sequential filling to be superior, they

TABLE 84.1 TOTAL KNEE ARTHROPLASTY: PEAK VELOCITY AUGMENTATION BELOW SAPHENOUS COMMON FEMORAL VEIN JUNCTION

Device	% Increase ± SD	Range	
		Minimum	*Maximum*
AV Impulse System	29 ± 39	0	100
PlexiPulse Foot	65 ± 76	0	252
PlexiPulse Foot-Calf	221 ± 75	150	348
VenaFlow	302 ± 125	125	454
Flowtron DVT	87 ± 69	6	206
SCD System	116 ± 53	42	217
Jobst Athrombic Pump	263 ± 245	71	890
Dorsiplantar Flexion	175 ± 116	25	377

concluded that the cost-to-benefit ratio of the more complex system might not justify its use.[75] With the increased popularization of rapid-compression devices, the above discussion may be superfluous, since impressive venous velocity augmentation can be achieved with only a foot-calf or calf-only mechanical compression device.

The true effect of venous volume augmentation for prophylaxis of deep-vein thrombosis is unknown. Measurements of peak venous velocity are much more accurate and reproducible than determinations of volume, especially in the venous system.[49, 73] Veins are elastic and distensible, which makes volume calculations less accurate.[49, 73] In addition, the measurement of turbulent flow, generated by rapid-flow compression devices, is more difficult and less predictable than laminar flow.[73] Sources of error in quantitative blood flow Doppler measurements may occur, and the reduction of these errors depends on the exact measurements of the vessel diameter and time-average velocity.[73] This may be difficult in that blood flow measurements are obtained with a handheld transducer, and alignment of the ultrasonic beam with the longitudinal axis of the vessel is imperative.[49, 73] In addition, the exact positioning of the sample volume in the center of the vessel is difficult to obtain reproducibly.[73]

VARIANCE OF PNEUMATIC COMPRESSION DEVICES

Postoperatively, patients have a marked decrease in pulsatile blood flow due to loss of normal physiologic muscular contraction in the lower extremities. Active dorsiplantar flexion is a normal physiological mechanism that increases venous return and should be the standard with which all pneumatic compression devices are compared. Unfortunately, continuous and forceful active dorsiplantar flexion is not possible postoperatively, and it is in this capacity that pneumatic compression devices, which are capable of reversing venous stasis, are able to prevent deep-vein thrombosis. All the pneumatic compression devices studied in this chapter augment both peak venous velocity and venous volume. The greatest effect of these devices is observed below the junction of the greater saphenous vein and the common femoral vein, namely in the deep-venous system. Pulsatile calf compression with a rapid inflation time produces the greatest increase in peak venous velocity, and sequential compression of the calf and thigh demonstates the greatest increase in venous volume.

At the author's Hospital for Special Surgery, a hemodynamic study was carried out, evaluating the efficacy of various intermittent pneumatic compression devices and active dorsiplantar flexion in terms of femoral venous velocity and venous flow following TKA.[90] The pneumatic devices evaluated included two foot pumps, the AV Impulse (Kendall, Mansfield, MA) and the PlexiPulse (NuTech, San Antonio, TX); a foot-calf pump, PlexiPulse; a calf pump, VenaFlow (Aircast, Summit, NJ); and three calf-thigh pumps, Flowtron AC500/DVT (NHE Healthcare, Manalapin, NJ), Sequential Compression Device (SCD) System 5325 (Kendall, Mansfield, MA), and Jobst Athrombic Pump System 2500 (NuTech, San Antonio, TX).

Below the greater saphenous - common femoral vein junction, the increase in peak venous velocity (over the baseline) assessed by the Acuson 128XP/10 duplex ultrasound unit with a 5-MHz linear array probe for each test condition was significant (see Table 84.1). Pulsatile calf compression with a rapid inflation time produced the greatest increase in peak venous velocity, whereas compression of the calf and thigh demonstrated the greatest overall increase in venous volume.

To critically compare the relative efficacy of the devices, one must understand that the increases in peak venous velocity or venous volume that were observed in this study only presume a reduction in thromboembolic disease. However, based on the results of this study in the deep-venous system, newer pulsatile devices such as the PlexiPulse foot-calf device and the VenaFlow device appear to significantly augment peak venous velocity. The Jobst Athrombic Pump had a much greater increase in peak venous velocity than the other two calf-thigh devices tested, namely the Flowtron DVT and the SCD System. Because patient and nursing compliance is so essential to the success of mechanical prophylaxis for thromboembolic disease, the more simple yet efficacious devices appear to have a greater likelihood of success. Because the recently popularized pulsatile devices that pump the calf alone or foot and calf together produce a marked increase in peak venous velocity greater than active dorsiplantar flexion, one has to question the necessity of more bulky calf-thigh compression sleeves, which may reduce patient and nursing compliance.

CLINICAL TRIALS

The incidence of deep-vein thrombosis with the use of calf- and thigh-length devices has been reported to be between 7.5% and 33% after unilateral TKA.[17, 47] Haas and associates evaluated the efficacy of a multichamber thigh-length pneumatic compression device compared with aspirin in a randomized prospective study in unilateral TKA and found that the incidence of deep-vein thrombosis was reduced to 22% with pneumatic stockings compared with 47% with aspirin.[11] The greatest reduction was seen in large thrombi (greater than 6 cm), which were reduced from 31% with aspirin to 6% with the pneumatic stockings. Patients undergoing simultaneous bilateral TKA have an even higher risk for development of deep-vein thrombosis. Despite the use of pneumatic compression stockings, 48% of the bilateral total knee replacement patients in Haas' study developed a deep-vein thrombosis compared with 68% with aspirin alone ($p < .20$).

Woolson and coworkers conducted a prospective study of the prevalence of proximal deep-vein thrombosis in total knee replacement patients who had prophylaxis for thrombosis with a combination of low-dose warfarin and intermittent pneumatic compression[91]; 297 patients who underwent 377 consecutive total knee replacements were studied. All patients were treated with low-dose warfarin and intermittent pneumatic compression using thigh-high sleeves. Surveillance for proximal thrombosis was done by duplex ultrasonography. Proximal thrombosis was detected in 19 patients, for a prevalence of 5%. There were 3 patients who had a major bleeding complication, for a prevalence of .9% for the 337 procedures performed. Although there was no concurrent control group of patients treated with another means of prophylaxis to compare with these patients, the low prevalence of proximal thrombosis and the low risk of major bleeding complications indicate the safety and efficacy of intermittent pneumatic compression with low-dose warfarin.

Grady-Benson and colleagues studied 100 patients who had had a TKA and had been managed with pneumatic compression stockings and aspirin for prophylaxis against deep-vein thrombosis. These patients had screening of both lower extremities with duplex ultrasonography on the fourth postoperative day.[51] Duplex ultrasonography demonstrated proximal deep-vein thrombosis in 7 patients (7%) and distal deep-vein thrombosis in 22 patients (22%); all 29 patients were asymptomatic. The patients who had distal deep-vein thrombosis had surveillance with serial duplex ultrasonography on the 7th and 14th postoperative days; 5 of these patients were found to have had propagation of the thrombosis to the proximal deep veins.

More recently, there has been increased interest in the use of foot pump devices. These devices increase venous circulation by applying a rapid increase in pressure to the plantar plexus and collateral veins in the foot. Studies have shown that these devices can lead to a significant increase in venous flow in the lower extremity.[89] Two studies have evaluated foot pumps in knee replacement. Westrich and Sculco evaluated the efficacy of the PlexiPulse foot pump device combined with aspirin compared with aspirin alone.[30] The authors found a significant reduction in deep-vein thrombosis with the use of the PlexiPulse; 27% of patients using the PlexiPulse developed a deep-vein thrombosis compared with 59% with aspirin alone. The incidence of major calf thrombi was only 9.9%. Although no patient using PlexiPulse developed proximal thrombosis, 14% of the patients using aspirin alone were found to have a proximal thrombosis. Westrich and Sculco also evaluated compliance and found a relationship between deep-vein thrombosis and the duration for which the device was used. Wilson and associates also evaluated the efficacy of foot compression after TKA.[87] They found a significant reduction in proximal thrombi; 19% in the control group compared with 0% with foot pumps, in a small series of 60 patients.

Pneumatic devices on the feet and the legs have been shown in numerous studies to lower the incidence of both proximal and distal thromboses after total joint replacement. Additionally, these devices have been associated with an extremely low rate of complications. Generally, however, leg-compression devices are recommended to be used on patients who do not have severe peripheral vascular disease. All of the devices are relatively inexpensive but compliance problems have been noted by some. Comerota and colleagues noted only a 33% patient compliance rate with the Kendall SCD calf device.[40] The foot pump devices appear to be well tolerated and we are now using them routinely on our knee replacement patients at the Hospital for Special Surgery. The efficacy of the pneumatic compression system is extremely dependent on patient and nursing compliance. The PlexiPulse foot pump system appears to have increased compliance compared with other calf- and thigh-length devices.

DATA FROM A META-ANALYSIS STUDY

We reviewed all published studies in the English literature in which TKA was performed on patients who were postoperatively assessed for deep-vein thrombosis. A meta-analysis was performed at the Hospital for Special Surgery to assess the efficacy of four common modalities of thromboembolic prophylaxis after TKA: intermittent pneumatic compression, warfarin, aspirin, and low-molecular-weight heparin. Only papers that used routine venography to assess deep-vein thrombosis and perfusion lung scan, ventilation-perfusion lung scan, or angiography to assess pulmonary embolism were included; 122 articles and abstracts

TABLE 84.2 RATES OF DEEP-VEIN THROMBOSIS

Deep-Vein Thrombosis	No. of Patients	Rates of DVT
Prophylaxis Type		
Aspirin	3235	53.4%
Warfarin	1201	43.8%
Low-molecular-weight heparin	1115	29.6%
Intermittent pneumatic compression device	509	17.5%

From Westrich GH, Hass SB, Mosca P, et al: Meta-analysis of thromboembolic prophylaxis after TKA. Br J Bone Jt Surg (in press).

TABLE 84.3 RATES OF PULMONARY EMBOLISM

Pulmonary Embolism	No. of Patients	% Asymptomatic PE
Prophylaxis Type		
Aspirin	2351	10.7%
Warfarin	1229	8.2%
Low-molecular-weight heparin	N/A	N/A
Intermittent pneumatic compression device	378	6.3%

From Westrich GH, Hass SB, Mosca P, et al: Meta-analysis of thromboemboic prophylaxis after TKA. Br J Bone Jt Surg (in press).-

were identified and reviewed. A total of 25 studies (6060 patients) were included in the analysis.

In assessing deep-vein thrombosis and pulmonary embolism, the results can be seen in Tables 84.2 and 84.3. Intermittent pneumatic compression devices and low-molecular-weight heparin were significantly better than warfarin ($p < .0001$) or aspirin ($p < .0001$) in preventing deep-vein thrombosis. Warfarin was significantly better than aspirin ($p < .0001$) in preventing deep-vein thrombosis. There was no statistically significant difference between low-molecular-weight heparin and intermittent pneumatic compression. In assessing asymptomatic pulmonary emboli, the rate for aspirin was 10.7%, warfarin, 8.2%, and intermittent pneumatic compression devices, 6.3%. The rate for aspirin was significantly higher than the rates for warfarin and pneumatic compression ($p < .05$). The rate for warfarin use was not statistically significant when compared with the rate for an intermittent pneumatic compression device ($p = 1$). In assessing symptomatic pulmonary embolism, the rate for an intermittent pneumatic compression device 0% was better than that of aspirin, 1.2% warfarin, 0.5%, or low-molecular-weight heparin, 0.3%, but there was no statistical significance.

CONTINUOUS PASSIVE MOTION

There are few studies that assess whether the use of continuous passive motion (CPM) after TKA is effective in reducing deep-vein thrombosis. However, a few studies confirm that it is advantageous to use CPM after total joint arthroplasty to improve postoperative function and range of motion. The use of CPM after TKA still remains controversial.

Yashar and coworkers evaluated a new approach, starting CPM at 70 to 100 degrees flexion in the recovery room (group 1).[92] A randomized, prospective study of 210 consecutive TKAs was performed at two institutions. The control population (group 2) started CPM at zero to 30 degrees, and progressed toward 100 degrees flexion. Flexion at postoperative day 3 was significantly different (Table 84.4). However, there was no significant difference between the groups at 4 weeks (see Table 84.4). In group 1, wound necrosis developed in one patient, which required a gastrocnemius flap. This major complication was caused by a tight dressing, and was not necessarily due to the accelerated flexion CPM. Although routine screening for deep-vein thrombosis or pulmonary embolism was not performed, no patient in either group developed a clinically symptomatic deep-vein thrombosis or pulmonary embolism.

Lynch and colleagues evaluated 150 consecutive patients who underwent TKA[93]; 75 had routine physiotherapy and 75 had CPM of the lower limb that had been operated on as well as routine physiotherapy. A pulmonary embolus did not develop in any patient, but about 40% had thrombosis in the veins of the calf, whether passive motion had been administered or not. Radiographically, the deep-vein thrombosis was seen to extend into or proximal to the popliteal vessel in 5% of the patients in each group. Sex, age, obesity, or a history of hypertension or diabetes did not influence the incidence of venous thrombosis.

CONCLUSION

Because newer pharmacological forms of prophylaxis are constantly being developed and studied, innovations with mechanical prophylaxis warrant the same evaluation. Mechanical prophylaxis offers several advantages over pharmacological prophylaxis in that it is safe, efficacious, and may be more cost effective. According to the literature, intermittent pneumatic compression devices are the most effective modality in preventing the occurrence of deep-vein thrombosis after TKA. Both intermittent pneumatic compression devices and warfarin may be better than aspirin in reducing the incidence of pulmonary embolism. Large, prospective randomized trials are needed to identify the benefit of combining prophylactic regimens. Because nursing and patient compliance are essential to the success of mechanical prophylaxis, the more sim-

TABLE 84.4 CONTINUOUS PASSIVE MOTION DATA

	Group 1 *Degrees of Flexion*	Group 2 *Degrees of Flexion*
Postop day 3	82.5	72.8
Day of discharge	89.1	84.3
Week 4	5.-104.1	5.6-102
Week 6	2.3-104.8	2.7-103.6
Week 12	1.7-107.7	4.7-108.2
Week 52	.5-113.2	1.8-110.5

ple devices seem to have a higher possibility for performing well.

References

1. Borow M, Goldson HJ: Prevention of postoperative deep venous thrombosis and pulmonary emboli with combined modalities. Am Surg 49:599, 1983.
2. Bradley JG, Krugener GH, Horst JJ: The effectiveness of intermittent plantar venous compression in prevention of deep venous thrombosis after total hip arthroplasty. J Arthroplasty 8:57, 1993.
3. Fordyce MJF, Ling RSM: A venous foot pump reduces thrombosis after total hip replacement. J Bone Joint Surg Br 74:45, 1992.
4. Francis CW, Pellegrini VD, Marder VJ, et al: Comparison of warfarin and external pneumatic compression in prevention of venous thrombosis after total hip replacement. JAMA 267:2911, 1992.
5. Gardner AMN, Fox RH: The return of blood to the heart against the force of gravity. In Negus D, Janet G, eds: Phlebology 1985, London: Libby, 1986, pp 68-71.
6. Gardner AMN, Fox RH: The return of blood to the heart: Venous pumps in health and disease. London, John Libbey and Co, 1989.
7. Gardner AMN, Fox RH: The venous footpump: Influence on tissue perfusion and prevention of venous thrombosis. Ann Rheum Dis 51:1173, 1992.
8. Gardner AMN, Fox RH: The venous pump of the human foot—Preliminary report. Bristol Med Chir J 98:109, 1983.
9. Gardner AMN, Fox RH, MacEachern AG, et al: Reduction of post-traumatic swelling and compartment pressure by impulse compression of the foot. J Bone Joint Surg Br 72:810, 1990.
10. Grossman RS: Changing patterns of prophylaxis for deep venous thrombosis following elective hip replacement. Orthopaedics 16: 19, 1993.
11. Haas SB, Insall JN, Scuderi GR, et al: Pneumatic sequential-compression boots compared to aspirin prophylaxis of deep venous thrombosis after total knee arthroplasty. J Bone Joint Surg 72:27, 1990.
12. Hartman JT, Pugh JL, Smith RD, et al: Cyclic sequential compression of the lower limb in prevention of deep venous thrombosis. J Bone Joint Surg Am 64:1059, 1982.
13. Hull R, Delmore TJ, Hirsh J, et al: Effectiveness of intermittent pulsatile elastic stockings for the prevention of calf and thigh vein thrombosis in patients undergoing elective knee surgery. Thromb Res 16:37, 1979.
14. Hull RD, Raskob GE: Current concepts review. Prophylaxis of venous thromboembolic disease following hip and knee surgery. J Bone Joint Surg Am 68:146, 1986.
15. Hull RD, Raskob GE, Gent M, et al: Effectiveness of intermittent pneumatic leg compression for preventing deep vein thrombosis after total hip replacement. JAMA 263:2313, 1990.
16. Janssen H, Trevino C, Williams D: Hemodynamic alterations in venous blood flow produced by external pneumatic compression. J Cardiovasc Surg 34:441, 1993.
17. Kaempffe FA, Lifeso RM, Meinking C: Intermittent pneumatic compression versus Coumadin. Clin Orthop 269:89, 1991.
18. Kamm R, Butcher R, Froelich J, et al: Optimization of indices of external pneumatic compression for prophylaxis against deep vein thrombosis: Radionuclide gated imaging studies. Cardiovasc Res 20:588, 1986.
19. Lieberman JR, Huo MM, Hanway J, et al: The prevalence of deep venous thrombosis after total hip arthroplasty with hypotensive epidural anesthesia. J Bone Joint Surg Am 76:341, 1994.
20. Lotke PA, Ecker ML, Alavi A, et al: Indications of the treatment of deep venous thrombosis following total knee replacement. J Bone Joint Surg Am 66:202, 1984.
21. McKenna R, Galante J, Bachmann F, et al: Prevention of venous thromboembolism after total knee replacement by high-dose aspirin or intermittent calf and thigh compression. British Med J 280:514, 1980.
22. McLachlin AD, McLachlin JA, Jory TA, et al: Venous stasis in the lower extremities. Ann Surg 152:678, 1960.
23. Moser KM, LeMoine JR: Is embolic risk conditioned by location of deep venous thrombosis? Ann Int Med 94:439, 1981.
24. Myerson MS, Henderson MR: Clinical applications of a pneumatic intermittent impulse compression device after trauma and major surgery to the foot and ankle. Foot Ankle 14:198, 1993.
25. Paiement GD, Beisaw N, Lotke P, et al: Advances in the prevention of venous thromboembolic disease after hip and knee surgery. Orthop Rev 18:1, 1989.
26. Paiement GD, Wessinger SJ, Waltman AC, et al: Low-dose warfarin versus extenal pneumatic compression for prophylaxis against venous thromboembolism following total hip replacement. J Arthroplasty 2:23, 1987.
27. Roberts TS, Nelson CL, Barnes LL, et al: Low dose dextran 40 in reconstructive hip surgery patients. Orthopedics 12:797, 1989.
28. Stannard JP, Harris RM, Bucknell AL, et al: Prophylaxis of deep venous thrombosis after total hip arthroplasty by using intermittent compression of the plantar venous plexus. Amer J Orthop 2:127, 1996.
29. Virchow R: Neuer fall von todlicher emboli der lungenarterie. Arch Path Anat 10:225, 1856.
30. Westrich GH, Sculco TP: Prophylaxis for deep venous thrombosis after total knee arthroplasty: Pneumatic plantar compression compared with aspirin. J Bone Joint Surg 78(6):826-834, 1996.
31. Wille-Jorgensen P, Winter CS, Bjerg-Nielsen A, et al: Prevention of thromboembolism following elective hip surgery. The value of regional anesthesia and graded compression stockings. Clin Orthop 247:163, 1989.
32. Allenby F, Pflug JJ, Boardman L, et al: Effects of external pneumatic compression on fibrinolysis in man. Lancet 2:1412, 1973.
33. Bromage PR: Epidural Analgesia. Philadelphia, WB Saunders, 1978.
34. Antiplatelet Trialists' Collaboration: Collaborative overview of randomized trials of antiplatelet therapy—III: Reduction in venous thrombosis and pulmonary embolism by antiplatelet prophylaxis among surgical and medical patients. Brit J Med 308: 235, 1994.
35. Barnes CL, Nelson CL, Nix ML, et al: Duplex scanning versus venography as a screening examination in total hip arthroplasty patients. Clin Orthop 271:180, 1991.
36. Clagett GP: Prevention of postoperative venous thromboembolism: An update. Am J Surg 168:515, 1994.
37. Cohen SJ, Ehrlich GE, Kauffman MS, et al: Thrombophlebitis following knee surgery. J Bone Joint Surg Am 55:106, 1973.
38. Colwell CW Jr, Spiro TE: Efficacy and safety of enoxaparin to prevent deep vein thrombosis after hip arthroplasty. Clin Orthop 319:215, 1995.
39. Colwell CW Jr, Spiro TE, Trowbridge AA, et al: Efficacy and safety of enoxaparin versus unfractionated heparin for prevention of deep venous thrombosis after elective knee arthroplasty. Clin Orthop 321:19, 1995.
40. Comerota AJ, Katz ML, White JV: Why does prophylaxis with external pneumatic compression for deep venous thrombosis prophylaxis fail? Am J Surg 164, 265, 1992.
41. Coventry MB, Nolan DR, Beckenbaugh RD: "Delayed" prophylactic anticoagulation: A study of results and complications in 2,012 total hip arthroplasties. J Bone Joint Surg Am 55:1487, 1973.
42. DeLee JC, Rockwood CA Jr: Current concepts review: The use of aspirin in thromboembolic disease. J Bone and Joint Surg Am 62:149, 1980.
43. Doouss TW: The clinical significance of venous thrombosis of the calf. Brit J Surg 63:377, 1976.
44. Evarts CM, Feil EJ: Prevention of thromboembolic disease after elective surgery of the hip. J Bone Joint Surg Am 53:1271, 1971.
45. Evarts CM: Prevention of venous thromboembolism. Clin Orthop 222:98, 1987.
46. Fitzgerald RH Jr, Spiro TE, Trowbridge AA, et al: A randomized and prospective comparision of enoxaparin and warfarin in the prevention of thromboembolic disease following total knee arthroplasty. Orthop Trans 1995.
47. Geerts WH, Code KI, Jay RM, et al: A prospective study of venous thromboembolism after major trauma. N Eng J Med 331: 1601, 1994.
48. Giachino A: Relationship between deep vein thrombosis in the calf and fatal pulmonary embolism. Can J Surg 31:129, 1988.
49. Gill RW: Measurement of blood flow by ultrasound: Accuracy and sources of error. Ultrasound Med Biol 11:625, 1985.
50. Gold EW: Prophylaxis of deep venous thromboembolism. Orthopedics 11:1197, 1988.

51. Grady-Benson JC, Oishi CS, Hannson PB, et al: Postoperative surveillance for deep venous thrombosis with duplex ultrasound after total knee arthroplasty. J Bone Joint Surg Am 76:1649, 1994.
52. Guyer RD, Booth RE, Rothman RH: The detection and prevention of pulmonary embolism in total hip replacement. J Bone Joint Surg Am 64:1040, 1982.
53. Haake DA, Berkman SA: Venous thromboembolic disease after hip surgery. Clin Orthop 242:212, 1989.
54. Harris WH, Salzman EW, Athanasoulis C, et al: Comparison of warfarin, low-molecular-weight dextran, aspirin, and subcutaneous heparin in prevention of venous thromboembolism following total hip replacement. J Bone Joint Surg Am 56:1552, 1974.
55. Harris WH, Athanasoulis C, Waltman AC, et al: Cuff-impedance phlebography and 125I fibrinogen scanning versus roentgenographic phlebography for diagnosis of thrombophlebitis following hip surgery. J Bone Joint Surg Am 58:939, 1976.
56. Harris WH, Athanasoulis C, Waltman AC, et al: High- and low-dose aspirin prophylaxis against venous thromboembolic disease in total hip replacement. J Bone Joint Surg Am 64:63, 1982.
57. Harris WH, McKusick K, Athanasoulis CA, et al: Detection of pulmonary emboli after total hip replacement. J Bone Joint Surg Am 66:1388, 1984.
58. Harris WH, Athanasoulis C, Waltman AC, et al: Prophylaxis of deep-vein thrombosis after total hip replacement. J Bone Joint Surg Am 67:57, 1985.
59. Hartman JT, Altner PC, Freeark RJ: The effect of limb elevation in preventing venous thrombosis. J Bone Joint Surg Am 52:1618, 1970.
60. Insall JI, Haas SB: Complications of total knee arthroplasty. In Insall JI, ed: Surgery of the Knee, 2 ed: New York, Churchill Livingstone, 1993, pp 891–899.
61. Johnson R, Green JR, Charnley J: Pulmonary embolism and its prophylaxis following the Charnley total hip replacement. Clin Orthop 127:123, 1977.
62. Kakkar VV, Howe CT, Flanc C, et al: Natural history of postoperative deep vein thrombosis. Lancet 2:230, 1969.
63. Lotke PA: Asymptomatic pulmonary embolism after total knee replacement. Orthop Trans 10:490, 1986.
64. Lotke PA: Thromboembolic disease: A critical review. Bull Am Acad Orthop Surg 37:20, 1989.
65. Lotke PA: Aspirin prophylaxis for thromboembolic disease. In Instructional Course Lectures, The American Academy of Orthopedic Surgeons, vol 44, St. Louis, CV Mosby, 1995.
66. McCardel BR, Lachiewich PF, Jones K: Aspirin prophylaxis and surveillance of pulmonary embolism and deep vein thrombosis in total hip arthroplasty. J Arthroplasty 5:181, 1990.
67. McKenna R, Bachmann F, Kaushal SP, et al: Thromboembolic disease in patients undergoing total knee replacement. J Bone Joint Surg Am 58:928, 1976.
68. McNally MA, Mollan RA: Total hip replacement, lower limb blood flow and venous thrombogenesis. J Bone Joint Surg Br 75: 640, 1993.
69. Modig J, Borg T, Karlstrom G, et al: Thromboembolism after total hip replacement: Role of epidural and general anesthesia. Anesth Analg 62:174, 1983.
70. Morrey BF, Adams RA, Ilstrup DM, et al: Complications and mortality associated with bilateral or unilateral total knee arthroplasty. J Bone Jont Surg Am 69:484, 1987.
71. Nicolaides AN, Fernandes JF, Pollock AV: Intermittent sequential pneumatic compression of the legs in the prevention of venous stasis and postoperative deep venous thrombosis. J Surgery 87: 69, 1980.
72. Paiement GD, Beisaw N, Harris W, et al: Advances in prevention of venous thromboembolic disease after elective hip surgery. In Instructional Course Lectures, The American Academy of Orthopedic Surgeons. 39:413, 1990.
73. Ranke C, Hendrickx P, Roth U, et al: Color and conventional image-directed doppler ultrasonography: Accuracy and sources of error in quantitative blood flow measurements. J Clin Ultrasound 20:187, 1992.
74. Roberts VC, Sabri S, Beeley AH, et al: The effect of intermittently applied external pressure on the hemodynamics of the lower limb in man. Br J Surg 59:223, 1972.
75. Salzman EW, McManama GP, Shapiro AH, et al: Effects of optimization of hemodynamics on fibrinolytic activity and antithrombotic efficacy of external pneumatic calf compression. Ann Surg 206:636, 1987.
76. Sandler DA, Martin JF: Autopsy proven pulmonary embolism in hospital patients: Are we detecting enough deep venous thrombosis? Royal Soc Med 82:203, 1989.
77. Santori FS, Vitullo A, Stopponi M, et al: Prophylaxis against deep-vein thrombosis in total hip replacement. Comparison of heparin and foot impulse pump. J Bone Joint Surg Br 76:579, 1994.
78. Sharrock NE, Brien WW, Salvati EA, et al: The effect of intravenous fixed-dose heparin during total hip arthroplasty on the incidence of deep-vein thrombosis. J Bone Joint Surg Am 72: 1456, 1990.
79. Sharrock NE, Haas SB, Hargett MJ, et al: Effects of epidural anesthesia on the incidence of deep venous thrombosis after total knee arthroplasty. J Bone Joint Surg 73:502, 1991.
80. Siegel RS: The use of indium-111 labeled platelet scanning for the detection of asymptomatic deep venous thrombosis in a high risk population. Orthop 12:1439, 1989.
81. Sikorski JM, Hampson WG, Staddon GE: The natural history and etiology of deep vein thrombosis after total hip replacement. J Bone Joint Surg Br 63:171, 1981.
82. Stranks GJ, McKenzie NA, Grover MI, et al: The A-V impulse system reduces deep vein thrombosis and swelling after hemiarthroplasty for hip fractures. J Bone Joint Surg Br 74:775, 1992.
83. Stringer MD, Steadman CA, Hedges AR, et al: Deep vein thrombosis after elective knee surgery. An incidence study in 312 patients. J Bone Joint Surg Br 71:492, 1989.
84. Stulberg BN, Dorr LD, Ranawat CS, et al: Aspirin prophylaxis for pulmonary embolism following total hip arthroplasty. Clin Orthop 168:119, 1982.
85. Tarnay TJ, et al: Pneumatic calf compression, fibrinolysis and the prevention of the deep vein thrombosis. Surgery 88:489, 1986.
86. Vaughn BK, Knezevich S, Lombardi A, et al: Use of the Greenfield filter to prevent fatal pulmonary embolism associated with total hip and knee arthroplasty. J Bone Joint Surg Am 71:1542, 1989.
87. Wilson NV, Das SK, Kakkar VV, et al: Thrombo-embolic prophylaxis in total knee replacement: Evaluation of the A-V impulse system. J Bone Joint Surg Br 74:50, 1992.
88. Woolson ST, Watt JM: Intermittent pneumatic compression to prevent proximal deep venous thrombosis during and after total hip replacement. J Bone Joint Surg Am 73:507, 1991.
89. Friedel HA, Balfour JA: Tinzaparin: A review of its pharmacology and clinical potential in the prevention and treatment of thromboembolic disorders. Drugs 48:638, 1994.
90. Westrich GW, Specht LM, Sharrock NE, et al: Venous haemodynamics after total knee arthroplasty. J Bone Joint Surg Br 80:6, 1998.
91. Woolson ST, Robinson RK, Khan NQ, et al: Deep venous thrombosis prophylaxis for knee replacement: Warfarin and pneumatic compression. Am J Orthop 27:4, 1998.
92. Yashar AA, Venn Watson E, Welsh T, et al: Continuous passive motion with accelerated flexion after total knee arthroplasty. Clin Orthop 345:38, 1997.
93. Lynch JA, Lynch AF, Bourne RB, et al: Deep-vein thrombosis and continuous passive motion after total knee arthroplasty. J Bone Joint Surg 70:1, 1988.
94. Lovgren O, Rastgeldi S: Treatment of rheumatoid arthritis by local application of intermittent pressure. Acta Rheum Scand 5: 240, 1959.
95. Henry JP, Winsor T: Compensation of arterial insufficiency by augmenting the circulation with intermittent compression of the limbs. Am Heart J 70:79, 1965.
96. Gaskell P, Parrott JCW: The effect of a mechanical venous pump on the circulation of the feet in the presence of arterial obstruction. Surg Gynecol Obstet 146:583, 1978.
97. Stulberg BN, Insall JN, Williams GW, et al: Deep vein thrombosis following total knee replacement. J Bone Joint Surg Am 66:194, 1984.

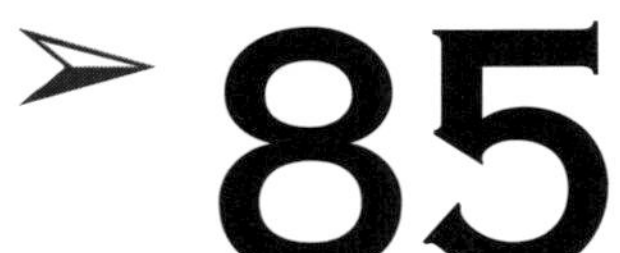

Partial Denervation for the Treatment of Painful Neuromata Complicating Total Knee Replacement

A. Lee Dellon • Michael A. Mont • David S. Hungerford

INTRODUCTION

Successful management of knee pain is critical to the practice of most orthopedic surgeons. Nonoperative treatment of knee pain of musculoskeletal origin is within the daily activity of most orthopedic surgeons. Operative approaches to the treatment of knee pain have been described extensively, and range from relatively less invasive procedures like arthroscopy and the correction of patellofemoral tracking to high tibial osteotomies, Maquet's procedure, and total knee replacement. Management of persistent knee pain after the above approaches have given a less than satisfactory approach remains perplexing, time consuming, and usually frustrating for the orthopedic surgeon. It is the goal of this chapter to provide an algorithm for the care of patients with persistent knee pain.

For a patient to perceive pain, there must be a neural pathway for transmission of the impulses generated from the injured tissues. This concept is easily accepted for the skin, where a direct injury may disrupt, crush, or stretch a nerve that innervates a piece of skin. Although the mechanisms to be discussed have been introduced for upper-extremity pain over the past two decades, their application to knee pain was begun just 5 years ago. An analogy will be helpful to provide the theoretical framework for the lower-extremity application.

If, after an injury to the dorsoradial aspect of the distal forearm, a patient complained of pain in that region, and physical examination suggested that the musculoskeletal system was intact, and radiographic imaging demonstrated no abnormalities, then a neuroma or compression of the radial sensory nerve would be the likely source of pain. If the anatomic variations of that region of skin were considered carefully, the differential diagnosis would be expanded to consider an injury to the lateral antebrachial cutaneous nerve, which overlaps with the radial sensory nerve in 75% of people.[37] Similarly, if a ganglion were removed from the dorsal aspect of the wrist, and the postoperative incision were painful, and remained painful, it would raise the possibility of a neuroma of a branch of these same two cutaneous nerves. However, if the patient's pain after ganglion removal were deeper, and became worse with wrist flexion and extension, then a nerve pathway that involved the dorsal wrist capsule would need to be considered in the cause of the pain. It is known that the terminal branch of the posterior interosseous nerve innervates the dorsal wrist capsule, and in particular the scapholunate ligament.[17] Therefore, a neuroma of this nerve may have resulted when the ganglion was excised from a portion of this ligament. If the patient's pain did not resolve with therapy, steroid massage, or steroid injection, and if pain limited hand function, successful treatment can be achieved by appropriate treatment of the involved nerve. Which is the involved nerve? Nerve blocks would be used to identify the source of pain as coming from either one or both cutaneous nerves and/or the nerve that innervates the wrist joint. For the cutaneous neuroma, the treatment must include resection of the neuroma or at least interruption of its neural pathway, as the neuroma can be a pain-generating source.[44] For the dorsoradial aspect of the hand, the appropriate treatment is to transfer the proximal end(s) of the cutaneous nerve(s) into a proximal large muscle, such as the brachioradialis.[39] For the dorsal wrist, a partial (dorsal) wrist denervation is indicated.[6]

Why has it taken so long for this approach, proven successful for management of upper-extremity pain, to be applied to the lower extremity? Almost certainly, the reason is related to continuing misconceptions about neuroma formation and treatment, and to lack of information about innervation of joints and ligaments. For the knee in particular, there was until recently an absence of any accepted anatomic basis about innervation of the knee joint. Before describing the neuroanatomy of the knee region, however, a review of the pathophysiology of neuroma formation and of the treatment of the painful neuroms is in order.

PATHOPHYSIOLOGY OF NEUROMA FORMATION

In the peripheral nervous system, the response to division of a peripheral nerve has been well documented. That response involves degeneration of the distal axons, survival of the distal Schwann's cells, sprouting of the proximal nerve fibers (because this is the physiologic response of the cell bodies located in the dorsal root ganglion), and production of nerve growth factor by the distal (denervated) Schwann's cells. This results in the proximal axon sprouts regenerating distally toward the chemotactic gradient of nerve growth factor. These sprouts track along the basement, whose fibronectin, type I collagen, and laminen also attract the sprouts.[8, 40] There is currently no available biological tool to prevent this cascade of events. Without destruction of the dorsal root ganglion, neuroma formation will always occur.

One of the most common misconceptions about management of the painful neuroma is that resection of the neuroma always results in another painful neuroma. From the above neurophysiology, it is clear that resection of a painful neuroma will always result in an attempt by the nerve to regenerate. A recurrent painful neuroma will result if that regeneration is allowed to occur into an area of movement, frequent contact or trauma, or into scar. A recurrent painful neuroma will not occur if the proximal end is allowed to regenerate into a peaceful area, e.g., innervated muscle away from an area of contact or trauma. Another suitable area into which to put the proximal end of the nerve after neuroma resection is a large area containing fat, which is also away from contact points. A common example of this is when the sural nerve is harvested for nerve grafting, and the proximal end of the nerve is allowed to lie in the popliteal fossa. A recurrent painful neuroma will not occur if the proximal end of the nerve is permitted to regenerate into a appropriate end-organ. An example of this is the type of regeneration that occurs when a nerve is divided and then reconstructed either with a nerve repair or a nerve graft; the nerve regenerates into its own distal territory.

TREATMENT OF A PAINFUL NEUROMA

Management of the painful neuroma can be done successfully if the following three steps are followed:

1. Identify the correct peripheral nerve that is the source of the pain; this requires careful clinical evaluation, understanding of anomalous innervation, and diagnostic nerve blocks.[37, 38]
2. Resect the end-bulb neuroma, as it is the source of spontaneous C-fiber and A-delta fiber activity that signals pain, and it is mechano- and chemosensitive.[44]
3. Relocate the proximal nerve into a site that is away from joint movement, away from nerve growth factor stimulation, and away from usual physical contact points; intramuscular placement has proven a successful strategy.[12, 14]

Studies in monkeys have demonstrated that when the proximal nerve sprouts into an environment of innervated muscle, and when that muscle is chosen to have minimal excursion, classic end-bulb neuromas do not form.[41] Clinically, this approach has proven successful for both the upper and lower extremities, for example, the radial sensory and lateral antebrachial cutaneous nerves into the brachioradialis muscle,[39] the palmar cutaneous branch of the median nerve into the pronator quadratus muscle,[20] the plantar digital nerves into the foot intrinsic muscles,[7] and the superficial and deep peroneal nerves into the anterolateral compartment muscles.[9] For neuromas related to nerves that innervate joints, resection of the neuroma or the peripheral nerve in an area proximal to the joint usually allows the resected proximal end of the nerve to lie in an internervous plane, and direct muscle implantation is therefore not needed. Examples of this are the anterior and posterior interosseous nerves in the forearm.[6, 8, 11]

HISTORY OF PARTIAL JOINT DENERVATION IN THE EXTREMITIES

In 1966, Wilhelm[53] published, in German, his approach to the treatment of persistent wrist joint pain. This concept became available to non-German-reading surgeons in 1977, when Buck-Gramcko[3] reviewed the German-speaking people's experience with 313 patients. With an 80% follow-up that exceeded 2 years, their results included excellent results in 69% of 195 patients. This was a complex review, including results from many surgeons, with as many as 10 separate nerves being resected circumferentially about the wrist during a total wrist denervation. Many patients had "incomplete" or partial denervations done based upon local anesthetic blocks. The patient population included patients who had persistent pain after forearm or wrist fractures, advanced arthritis, carpal instability, and severe sprains. Poorest results were in those with unstable wrists, who later required fusions.

In 1978, Dellon and Seif[17] published a description of the innervation of the dorsal wrist capsule by the terminal branch of the posterior interosseous nerve. This nerve could be identified easily over the distal dorsal forearm, proximal to the wrist. This implied that if wrist pain, regardless of its cause, could be isolated to neural transmission along this nerve pathway, then that pathway alone could be interrupted, eliminating wrist pain: a partial, rather than a total, approach to wrist denervation. This hypothesis was tested in a group of 29 patients studied between July 1981 and June 1984.[6] The cause of their pain was wrist fracture (8), carpal instability (4), arthritis (3), severe wrist sprain (10), and dorsal ganglionectomy (4). Range of wrist motion and grip strength were measured, an anesthetic block of the posterior interosseous nerve was done, and the range of motion and grip strength were then repeated (Fig. 85.1). There had to be pain relief, increased range of motion, and increased grip strength for the patient to be considered a surgical candidate. The results were that 90% of the patients achieved pain relief and improved wrist function; 83% returned to work. Failure occurred in three of the four patients with carpal instability, who required a subsequent wrist fusion. Three patients had reflex sympathetic dystrophy (RSD) after their wrist fracture; two of these

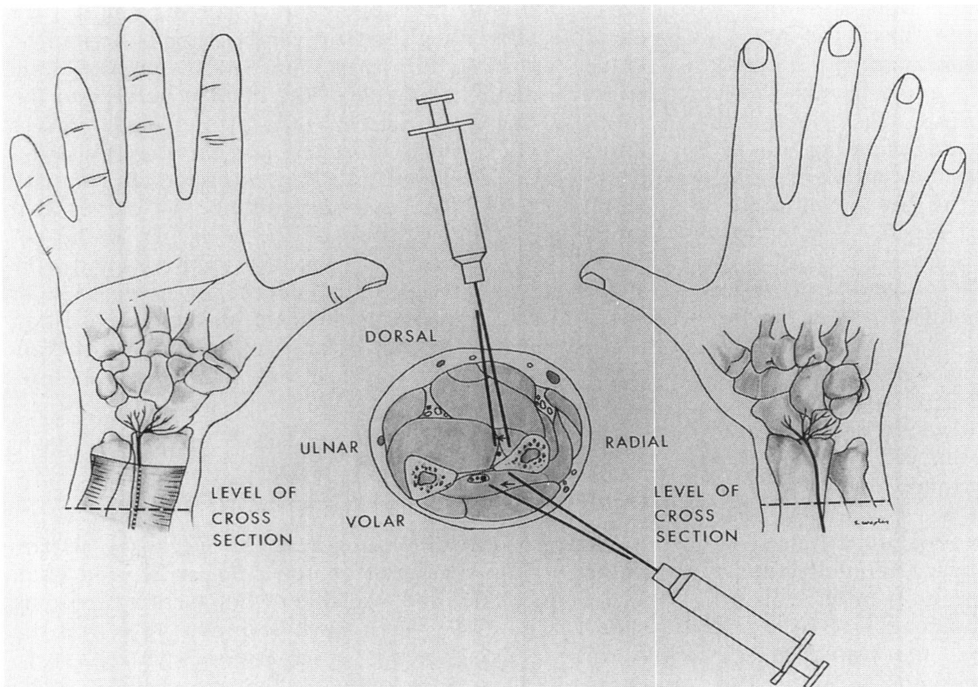

FIGURE 85.1 ➢ Local anesthetic nerve block. In order to identify the nerve that is the neural transmission route for the pain signal, it is essential to block a specific nerve with a local anesthetic. Relief of pain with either a regional or an intra-articular block is not sufficient to identify the individual nerves that may be rejected in a partial joint denervation. This type of block is illustrated here for the wrist, where either the anterior or the posterior interosseous nerves can be blocked. In the wrist, there are many patients who have either a dorsal or a volar injury, and a single nerve may be the source of pain. For some problems, like a triangular fibrocartilage tear, it may be necessary to block both of these nerves to obtain pain relief. This same approach must be used in the knee to identify individual components of pain arising from either the medial or lateral retinacular nerve, or both.

patients had previously had Darrach's procedures, and two had had a carpal tunnel decompression. Two of the RSD patients had subjective improvement after partial dorsal wrist denervation, had improved range of motion, but none of the three returned to work. The conclusion was that partial joint denervation was effective in pain relief and improving function in selected patients, that total joint denervation was not necessary, and that structural instability was a contraindication to joint denervation.

Logically, there would be a group of patients for whom anterior wrist pain could be treated by a partial volar wrist denervation procedure. In 1984, Dellon et al,[11] after basic anatomic dissections to identify the terminal branch of the anterior interosseous nerve distal to the pronator quadratus muscle, attempted partial volar wrist denervation in a small group of patients. From April 1982 through March 1984, there were 11 patients with persistent volar wrist pain; 9 of whom had work-related injuries, and 2 involved in motor vehicle accidents. Each had good relief of pain, increased wrist range of motion, and increased grip strength after a block of the anterior interosseous nerve (see Fig. 85.1). At a mean follow-up of 12.8 months (range 4 to 24 months) these patients each had good to excellent relief of their pain; 4 had returned to their regular job, 3 returned to "light duty" jobs, and 4 were in vocational rehabilitation. The conclusion was that partial joint denervation was effective in pain relief and improving function in selected patients, and that total joint denervation was not necessary.

In 1993, Dellon's experience in 51 patients treated for wrist pain with partial denervation was reviewed.[10] Overall, there was a 98% improvement for pain, with the visual analog scale level decreasing in all patients between 6 and 8 points out of 10. Improved range of motion occurred in 60% of the whole group. No patients with carpal instability were included in this more recent group.

Currently, partial wrist denervation is an accepted procedure for patients (1) whose wrist pain persists after at least 6 months of nonoperative management, (2) who have no carpal instability, and (3) who respond appropriately with decreased pain and increased motion after specific local anesthetic blocks of selected, identifiable, peripheral nerves.

Before the lessons learned in upper extremity joint denervation can be applied to the lower extremity, it is essential to identify the specific nerves that mediate pain from the knee region.

CUTANEOUS INNERVATION OF THE KNEE REGION

Virtually all anatomy books agree on the presence of the saphenous nerve innervating the infrapatellar region. It must be remembered that the saphenous nerve originates medially, from the femoral nerve, and descends in the medial thigh through the adductor canal to emerge around the sartorius muscle or through the sartorius muscle. The infrapatellar branch divides from the femoral nerve variably: in the proximal third of the thigh (17.6%), in the middle third of the thigh (58.8%), and in the distal third of the thigh (23.5%).[26] In 86% of the people, there are two saphenous nerve branches in Hunter's canal.[26] In this situation, the more anterior of the two branches will become the intrapatellar branch of the saphenous nerve, which when it enters the medial knee region is about 3 to 4 mm in width and begins to branch as it ap-

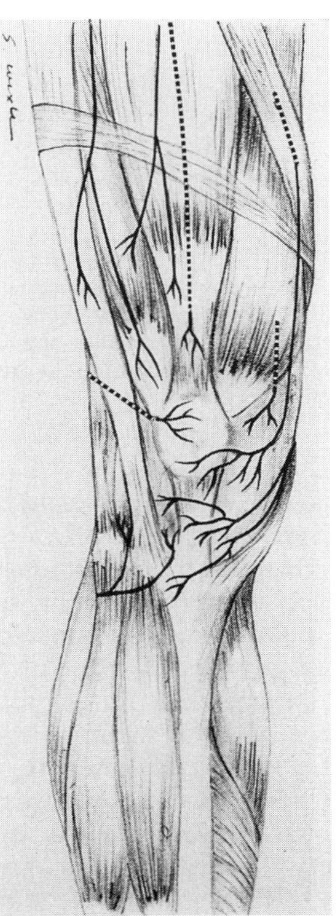

FIGURE 85.2 ➢ Innervation of the knee region; anterior view. Medial cutaneous nerve of the thigh. Medial retinacular nerve. Infrapatellar branch of the saphenous nerve. Lateral retinacular nerve. Lateral femoral cutaneous nerve. Anterior femoral cutaneous nerve. Innervation of the prepatellar bursal structures. Innervation of the proximal tibiofibular joint. The dotted lines are innervation of the knee joint.

proaches the anterior midline. It always crosses the leg below the patella, and usually has branches from below the patella to below the tibial tuberosity. The infrapatellar branch of the saphenous nerve innervates the anterior midline of the region below the patella and the lateral region below the patella. It does not innervate the skin covering the patella (Figs. 85.2, 85.3). It may send branches into the distal anterior knee joint capsule.[26]

The skin covering the patella is innervated by the medial cutaneous nerve of the thigh. This is a better name for this nerve than the anterior or medial femoral cutaneous nerve, because this nerve almost always branches from the saphenous nerve and travels as a separate branch, superficial to (39.1%), through (30.4), or deep to (30.5%) the sartorius, to emerge in the region of the femoral condyle, lying in the superficial subcutaneous plane.[26] This nerve may range in size from 0.6 to 1.1 mm, and there may be more than one branch. Its branches often lie directly over the medial retinacular nerve, and therefore a local anesthetic block in this region will block both nerves (see Figs. 85.2, 85.3).

It remains unclear as to whether the obturator nerve contributes branches to one or both of the branches of the saphenous nerve. The obturator nerve's sensory branches enter into the complex of nerves within the adductor canal, and do not emerge as a single identifiable branch in this distal thigh or knee region. Branches of the obturator nerve do participate in the innervation of the posterior knee capsule (Fig. 85.4).

The distal saphenous nerve theoretically begins distal to the infrapatellar branch of the saphenous nerve. Usually it has a separate branch in the thigh or it may be the continuation of the saphenous nerve after the infrapatellar branch. Most often, regardless of its origin, in the region distal to the tibial tuberosity, the distal saphenous nerve gives off one or more transverse branches that may become a source of pain from long anterior or medial incisions. The terminal skin innervated by the distal saphenous nerve includes the medial dorsum of the foot, and a region posterior to the medial malleous (see Figs. 85.2, 85.3).

The anterior femoral cutaneous nerve originates from the femoral nerve in the groin region and terminates at the patellar region. It has many small (<1 mm) branches in this region, and therefore there is usually not an identifiable neuroma of this nerve (see Fig. 85.2).

The medial femoral cutaneous nerve probably does not exist as such. The territories shown for it are best considered from a surgical anatomy point of view as being supplied by either the anterior femoral cutaneous nerve or by the medial cutaneous nerve of the thigh.

The lateral femoral cutaneous nerve begins at the hip region as a continuation of the L1 and L2 nerve roots. It has a branch that innervates the lateral buttock and a branch that innervates the lateral thigh skin extending to the level of the lateral knee. At the level of the inguinal ligament, the lateral femoral cutaneous nerve is 3 to 7 mm in size. At the lateral knee region, it has just terminal branches, which are usually too small to identify. Although pain can be referred to the knee from compression of the lateral femoral cutaneous nerve at the hip, direct injury to the knee or surgery in the knee region almost never causes a neuroma of this nerve. Lateral knee skin pain is almost always due to a neuroma of the medial cutaneous nerve of the thigh or the infrapatellar branch of the saphenous nerve (see Fig. 85.2).

INNERVATION OF THE KNEE JOINT

The innervation of the human knee joint has been described by Ruedinger (1857),[50] Druner (1927),[18] Jeletsky (1931),[30] Gardner (1948),[24] Wilhelm (1958),[52] Kennedy and coworkers (1982),[33] and Wojtys and associates. (1990).[54] None of these descriptions were from a large number of fresh human cadavers, and none provided detailed anatomic drawings sufficient to permit surgical approaches to these nerves. Furthermore, clarification of nomenclature was required. Such a study was reported in 1994 by Horner and Dellon[26] and serves as the basis for the following description and nomenclature. In that study, 45 fresh cadaver adult knees were dissected using loupe magnification.

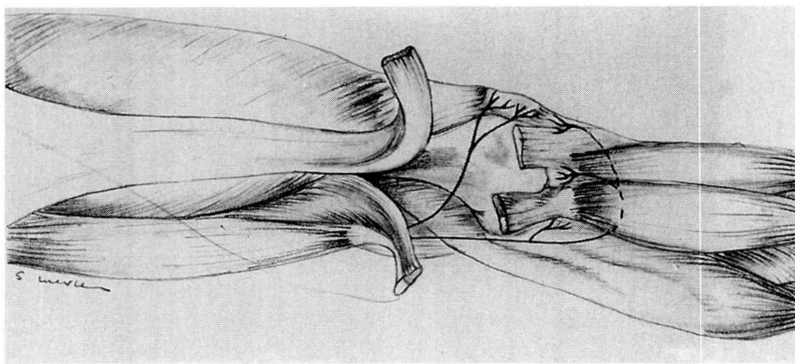

FIGURE 85.3 ➢ Innervation of the knee region: lateral view. The biceps femoris and the iliotibial tract have been divided and reflected. The lateral retinacular nerve innervating the lateral knee joint structures after arising from the sciatic nerve. The innervation of the proximal tibiofibular joint, from the common peroneal nerve.

The following description is based upon that study, and supplemented by clinical and operative experience over the past 4 years.

The lateral retinacular nerve is consistently present. It arises directly from the sciatic nerve, proximal to the popliteal fossa, and continues laterally to go beneath the biceps femoris tendon to reach the lateral retinacular structures. The lateral retinacular nerve lies beneath the lateral retinaculum. At this level, it exists as two or three, 1-mm branches, entering into the deeper structures of the knee joint. It is always accompanied by the recurrent lateral geniculate vessel and is always just distal to the vastus lateralis muscle. It is immediately superficial to the synovial structures of the knee joint (Figs. 85.2, 85.4, 85.5)

The medial retinacular nerve is consistently present. It arises from the branch of the femoral nerve that innervates the vastus medialis muscle. It exits from beneath the distal posterior aspect of the vastus medialis and travels anteriorly to innervate the medial retinacular structures in 90%, while in the other 10%, it exits through the muscle to innervate the medial retinacular structures.[26] The medial retinacular nerve lies beneath the medial retinaculum and at this level exists as two or three, 1-mm branches, entering into the deeper structures of the knee joint. It is always accompanied by the recurrent medial geniculate vessels, and is always just distal to the vastus medialis muscle. It is

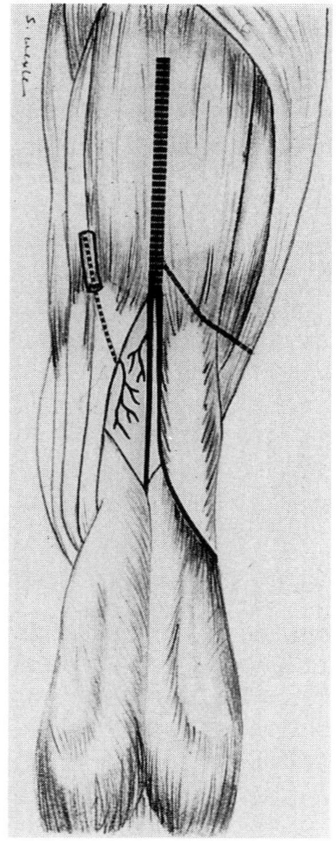

FIGURE 85.4 ➢ Innervation of the knee joint: posterior view. *A*, Lateral retinacular nerve arising from the sciatic nerve. The posterior knee capsule is innervated from branches of the obturator nerve coming through the adductor canal and from branches of the sciatic nerve.

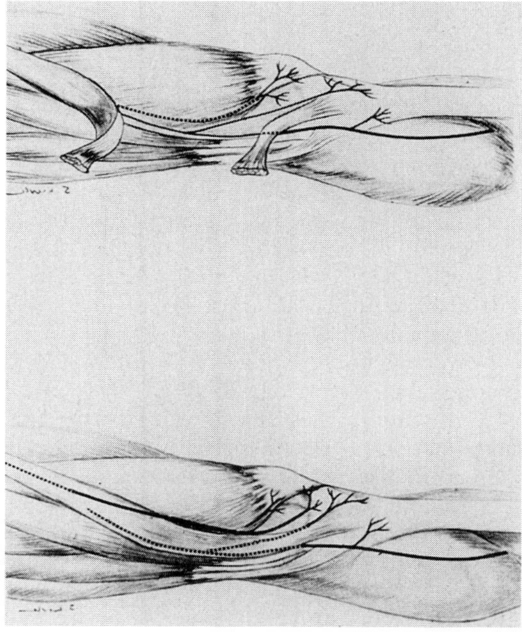

FIGURE 85.5 ➢ Innervation of the knee region: medial view. The sartorius muscle (top) has been divided and reflected. (bottom), The medial retinacular nerve continues distally after innervating the vastus medialis, to enter the medial knee joint structures. The saphenous nerve and its branches are unlabeled.

immediately superficial to the synovial structures of the knee joint (see Figs. 85.2, 85.3).

Nerves to the prepatellar bursal structures arise from the terminal branches of femoral nerves that innervate the vastus intermedius muscle. These continue distal to the muscle, lying on the anteromedial side of the distal femur, to enter into the prepatellar bursa and its surrounding structures. There is no unique name given to these nerve branches, which are approximately 1 mm each in diameter (see Fig. 85.2).

Nerves to the posterior knee capsule arise from the sciatic nerve over a 2-cm distance and widely innervate the posterior knee structures. There is no unique name given to these nerve branches, which are about <1 mm each in diameter (see Fig. 85.4) Druner[18] observed in 1927 that the posterior knee capsule received branches from the obturator nerve through Hunter's canal. The confluence of these branches with those from the sciatic nerve has been named by Ruedinger in 1931 as the popliteal plexus.[50]

INNERVATION OF THE PROXIMAL TIBIOFIBULAR JOINT

Although it is clear that the proximal tibiofibular joint is not part of the true knee joint, pain from the proximal tibiofibular joint may accompany knee pain in a patient's complaints. It is critical to be able to discern the difference between these two joints, and appreciate the separate source of innervation of the proximal tibiofibular joint from the true knee joint.

The common peroneal branch of the sciatic nerve gives the branches that innervate the proximal tibiofibular joint. These branches do not have a unique name. There is one branch that arises proximal to the fibular head and one or two that arise just distal to the fibular head. These branches are quite small, generally <1 mm in diameter, and require loupe magnification to identify. They travel into the structures between the fibular head and Gerdy's tubercle of the tibia (Figs. 85.2, 85.4, 85.5).

Immediately adjacent to these two small nerves are motor branches that innervate the tibialis anterior muscle. They cannot be distinguished morphologically. It is critical to use intraoperative electrical stimulation to identify the motor branches of the tibial nerve. To be most correct, it is critical to stimulate the nerve fiber believed to innervate this joint, and ensure that it is not a motor nerve by demonstrating that it does not cause a muscle contraction before it is cut.

RATIONALE FOR DENERVATION FOR PERSISTENT PAIN AFTER TOTAL KNEE ARTHROPLASTY

Nerve injury has been associated with virtually all orthopedic lower-extremity procedures, from relatively "simple" procedures like arthroscopy or arthrotomy,[1, 5, 27, 35, 51, 55] to total joint replacement.[25, 26] These reports, however, have described injury to well-known peripheral nerves like the sciatic, common peroneal, femoral, saphenous, and posterior tibial. The treatment of these nerve injuries varies from the conservative "observation," when nerve compression is thought to be the cause, to resection of individual small cutaneous nerves when they can be identified, to indwelling spinal cathethers or lumbar sympathetic blocks for the treatment of major pain, such as reflex sympathetic dystrophy.[21, 31, 32, 48, 49]

TABLE 85.1 INDICATIONS FOR KNEE DENERVATION

1. Persistent pain for at least 6 months after a knee procedure or an injury that was not relieved by nonsteroidal anti-inflammatory medications
2. Absence of active synovitis, knee joint effusion, or infection
3. Absence of radiographic evidence of bony or implant problems
4. Absence of mechanical reasons that could account for the pain, e.g., ligamentous instability (laxity in the mediolateral or anteroposterior plane greater than .5 cm)

Pain following total knee replacement may have a structural or biomechanical cause, such as malalignment or loosening, or may have a medical cause, such as infection. Once these possibilities have been carefully evaluated by traditional orthopedic approaches, it is plausible that the persistent pain may be of neural origin (Table 85.1). As with any incision anywhere on the body, a cutaneous nerve may become entrapped in the scar or have been divided during the surgery. Clearly, a cutaneous neuroma should be treated according to the rationale given above for a peripheral nerve in the upper extremity. The rationale of treating pain arising from the knee joint itself after a total knee arthroplasty (TKA) may seem to involve a contradiction: how can a joint that has been surgically removed be a source of pain?

Once it is accepted that there are identifiable nerves to the knee joint structures, just as there are to the wrist joint, then it becomes clear that some of these nerves must be transected in every TKA during the process of removing the necessary bone. What happens to the proximal end of these normal nerves after the surgery? Most probably, related to the degree of traction that occurs during the procedure, they retract into proximal tissues and form their neuromas in a quiet region, i.e., they form a nonpainful neuroma. This is most likely the explanation for the excellent results that occur in greater than 97% of patients having total knee replacement.[22] It is hypothesized that the cause of the deep knee pain in 1% to 3% of TKA patients who have persistent pain is the nerves supplying the knee joint. These nerves, i.e., the medial and lateral retinacular nerves, are most likely transected during the procedure and become adherent to the capsule that forms around the implant. If this is true, then postoperative range of motion of the knee stimulates these nerves through stretch/traction, eliciting a neural response that the brain interprets as a painful knee.[15] In one of the first denervation operations, the lateral retinacular nerve was followed down to the

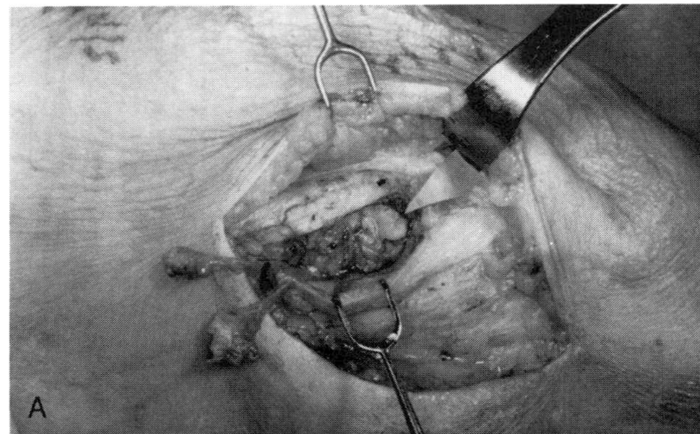

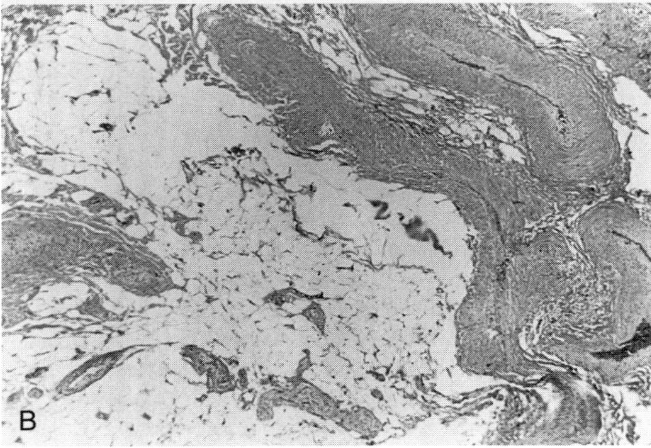

FIGURE 85.6 ➢ Neuroma formation on the lateral retinacular nerve after total knee replacement. *A*, The intraoperative appearance of the neuromas on branches of the lateral retinacular nerve in a patient with persistent pain after a total knee replacement. *B*, The histologic appearance of the specimen, which demonstrates a true neuroma. (H&E stain, 1 × 25.)

capsule, and resected with a portion of the capsule. The pathology report demonstrated a true neuroma (Fig. 85.6). As described below, this approach is *not* recommended, because a synovial leak developed in this patient, requiring reoperation. Nevertheless, the specimen obtained at that time supported this rationale.

DIAGNOSIS OF KNEE PAIN OF NEURAL ORIGIN

In general, each patient must have every musculoskeletal problem treated to the highest level. Denervating a joint cannot restore structural integrity. Conversely, restoring structural integrity will not always relieve pain. Although modern radiographic imaging can identify small defects in ligaments, menisci, and cartilage, they cannot identify the small nerves that innervate the knee joints and the surrounding skin.

Knee pain, in the presence of a relatively normal physical examination of the musculoskeletal system, in the presence of normal x-rays and a normal MRI, and even in the presence of a relatively normal or "negative" arthroscopy, should be considered of neural origin. The diagnosis must be made based upon nerve blocks.

The first step in deciding which nerves to block is to listen to the patient's complaints. Try to decide whether the complaints are just related to the knee joint or also involve the skin. Critical historical points include learning whether there was any direct injury to the knee itself, i.e., a fall during which the knee hit the floor or an object. A previous surgery, like a knee replacement procedure, will satisfy this historical point, as will a previous arthroscopy. Any previous surgery in the knee region may have resulted in a neuroma of one of its cutaneous nerves. The patient may indicate that the bedclothes or clothing is painful or disturbing when it touches the knee. These historical points implicate a cutaneous nerve. At the same time, complaints related to knee function, i.e., kneeling, walking, and climbing steps, suggest that nerves innervating the knee structures are implicated in the pain mechanism. The patient should be asked to give a numerical value to the level of the pain, using a rating scale from zero (no pain) to ten (the worst pain they ever had). If possible, a formal visual analog scale should be used. In general, to be considered a candidate for surgery, the pain level should be five or higher.

The physical examination must attempt to locate the source of the trigger zones that will identify the site of the involved nerve and the site for the nerve block. First, locate areas of decreased sensation to a moving-touch stimulus at the patellar and infrapatellar areas by touching these areas bilaterally. Then begin distally over the pretibial region and work toward the tibial tuberosity, pressing deeply to identify sites where cutaneous nerves may be sending impulses from a neuroma. Even if no incision touches this area, in an operation requiring as much retraction and dissection as a total knee replacement, it is conceivable that cutaneous nerves may have become scarred at these relatively remote sites. Sites of cutaneous neuromas are most commonly noted near a transverse distal saphenous nerve branch, at the infrapatellar branch of the saphenous nerve just medial to the tibial tuberosity, and at the medial cutaneous nerve of the thigh just medial to the patella (Fig. 85.7). The final area for a painful cutaneous neuroma is in the anterior scar proximal to the patella. Often the scar will be depressed where the skin is adherent to the quadriceps tendon.

Identifying involvement of the joint afferents in the pain syndrome can be done during the physical examination. Deep pressure just distal to the femoral condyles and posterior to the patella will reveal these nerves, which are sufficiently thickened from scar tissue that they become palpable.

Pain related to the innervation of the proximal tibiofibular joint can be identified by pressure just anterior to the fibular head. Historically, these patients have usually had either a high tibial osteotomy, a Maquet procedure, or a fibular fracture. There may be an associated compression of the common peroneal nerve at the fibular head. This can be found during the physical examination by gentle pressure of this nerve

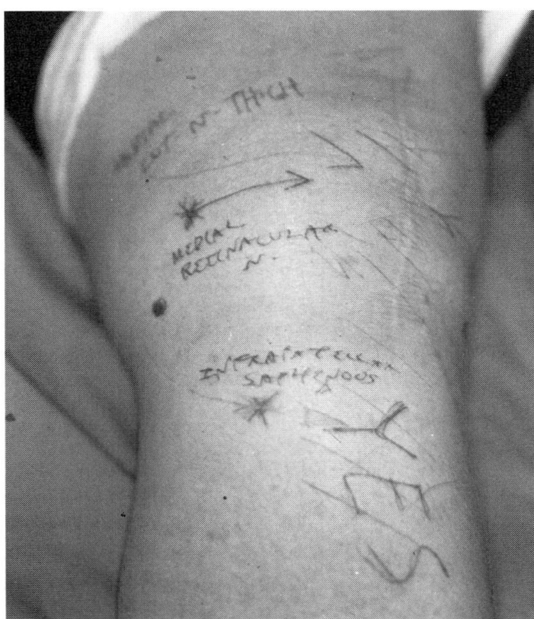

FIGURE 85.7 ➢ Clinical evaluation of the knee preoperatively. Note that abnormal areas of skin sensibility have been roughly estimated by crosshatched lines on the skin. These territories suggest that both the medial cutaneous nerve of the thigh as well as the intrapatellar branch of the saphenous nerve are involved in the pain mechanism, directing the examination to find the Tinel's sign locations or trigger spots for the neuromas. These are denoted by inked asterisks on the skin, to help with intraoperative localization.

against the fibular head (this is not usually painful), by identifying weakness in the muscles innervated by this nerve (weakness of the extensor hallucies longus often is the first to be detected), and by observing abnormal sensibility in the distribution of the superficial or deep peroneal nerves.

The physical examination has not been useful in identifying problems with innervation of the posterior knee joint capsule.

A diagnostic nerve block is not an intra-articular block. Clearly, anesthetic injected into the knee joint will diffuse to many different areas. It is unclear from an intra-articular anesthetic injection which nerve has been blocked.

Based upon the anatomic descriptions given above, it is possible to block specifically the individual nerves that may be the source of pain. The only overlap of these nerves is in the intersection in a superficial and deep plane of the medial cutaneous nerve of the thigh and the medial retinacular nerve. It is clear that if the skin of the patellar region is either reduced, dysesthetic, or actually painful, then in addition to the complaints of deep medial joint pain related to the medial retinacular nerve, there must be a cutaneous nerve involved as well. Most commonly, both of these nerves are involved in the painful knee.

The block should be done using aseptic technique. An iodine-containing skin preparation is preferred. The authors use 1% lidocaine and 0.5% bupivacaine, each without epinephrine; 5 mL of a 1:1 mixture of these two anesthetics is used. Each of the identified cutaneous and joint afferents is blocked, usually all at the same time. If for some reason it is difficult to identify the contributing sites, the medial side can be blocked, and then later during the same office visit or at a second office visit, the lateral side can be blocked. This may be needed especially if the patient's complaints are localized to the distal anterior knee joint region or to the "whole knee." Another example of the patient who may require more than one period of anesthetic administration is the one who has a "reflex sympathetic dystrophy" of the knee. If the nerve to the proximal tibiofibular joint is to be blocked, do not block the common peroneal nerve, which will interfere with the patient's ambulation. In order to block the nerve to the proximal tibiofibular joint, inject a local anesthetic adjacent to the anterior region of the fibular head.

After the anesthetic block, the patient must have knee function stressed. At about 15 minutes after the block, the patient should be asked to climb a flight of steps, walk in the hall, or kneel on a padded chair. During this time, he or she should be accompanied by a relative or a member of the office staff. Observations should be recorded for the office chart. The patient should again give a numerical assessment of the pain level, preferably on a visual analogue scale. If there is residual pain, its location should be identified, and, if necessary another nerve block done, with the knee function and pain score being repeated.

Operative Technique

The patient is interviewed and examined in the induction area, prior to surgery. The surgery is done on an outpatient basis, but, depending upon the medical situation, an overnight stay in the hospital may be justified. The exact sites of pain are marked with indelible ink, to aid in the incision making in the operating room. Typically, there will be a 3- to 5-cm incision over the medial knee (to approach the medial cutaneous nerve of the thigh and the medial retinacular nerves), a similar one over the lateral knee (to approach the lateral retinacular nerve), and a third incision about 3 cm distal to the medial incision, which is used to identify the infrapatellar branch of the saphenous nerve. When one long medial incision is made, there seems to be higher postoperative incidence of bruising or hematoma formation. A neuroma is not resected, but rather a segment of nerve, which may pathologically demonstrate fibrosis, is resected. This is technically a denervation rather than a neuroma resection. If the pathology report indicates that a normal nerve has been removed, this is acceptable. The patient receives 1 g of a cephalosporin drug intravenously in the induction area (another drug is used if there is a penicillin allergy history).

Knee denervation surgery should be considered peripheral nerve surgery and, as such, employ bipolar coagulation and loupe magnification. A microscope is not needed. The patient is placed supine on the operating table. The surgery should be done in a bloodless

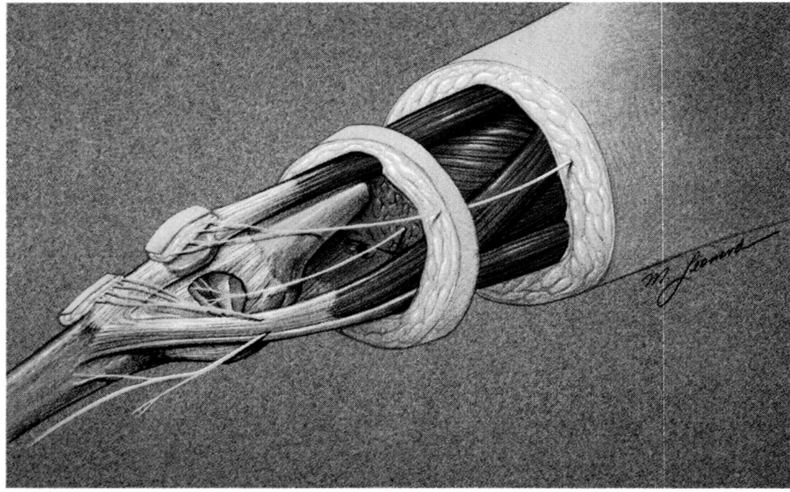

FIGURE 85.8 ➢ Anatomy of the innervation of the medial knee: three-dimensional view. Note the differing relationships of the medial nerves to the skin of the patellar and infrapatellar regions at the knee level and at the level below the knee. Note also the medial retinacular nerve traveling through the muscle of the vastus medialis to enter the knee joint structures beneath the medial retinaculum, in a location that places it immediately below the medial cutaneous nerve of the thigh.

field; a pneumatic tourniquet should be used. The patient is placed under spinal or general anesthesia. Unless just one nerve is to be resected, local anesthesia is not sufficient to remove the discomfort of the upper thigh tourniquet plus anesthetize the incision site. Depending on the patient's size and systolic pressure, the tourniquet is inflated to either 300 or 350 mm Hg after removing most of the blood from the leg with an Ace bandage. Since a guide to identifying the nerves is the blood in the vessels that accompany the nerve, it is suggested that the leg not be exsanguinated completely. It is our preference to cauterize extensively during the surgery, close each incision, dress the leg with a dressing that includes a tightly applied Ace bandage, and then let down the tourniquet. The Ace bandage is removed after half an hour in the recovery room, prior to the patient being discharged. Alternatively, the tourniquet can be let down at the completion of the procedure, hemostasis obtained, local anesthetic instilled, and the wounds closed.

During the medial dissection about the knee, the leg is externally rotated at the hip with the knee flexed, "frog-legged." During the lateral dissection, the knee is flexed and the leg is internally rotated, and the hip is flexed, bringing the knee up off the operating table.

Medially, the incision is deepened into the subcutaneous tissue, looking for the medial cutaneous nerve of the thigh over the site of the marking where the medial retinacular nerve is expected to be found. In the superficial subcutaneous plane, search for any small blood vessels going from posterior to anterior, not from proximal to distal. The soft tissues are spread with the scissors, which will cause the nerve to be identified by its relatively stable position. When the structure suspected to be the medial cutaneous nerve of the thigh is identified, it is dissected proximally. If the structure is the nerve and not connective tissue, it will be able to be followed proximally. One centimeter of the nerve is resected distally as it approaches the longitudinal incision that was used for the knee replacement, and it is submitted to the pathology department. Note that a true neuroma is not resected but rather a segment of the nerve is. The proximal end is turned, a widow created in the fascia of the vastus medialis, and the nerve implanted loose for a 2-cm length into the muscle. A suture is not needed. Bupivacaine is instilled into the implantation site at this time (Figs. 85.8–85.10).

Medially, the medial retinacular nerve is identified through the same incision used for the medial cutaneous nerve of the thigh by incising the fascia transversely just distal to the vastus medialis muscle. In this area, the recurrent medial geniculate vessel should be present. The nerve accompanies this vessel, and at this

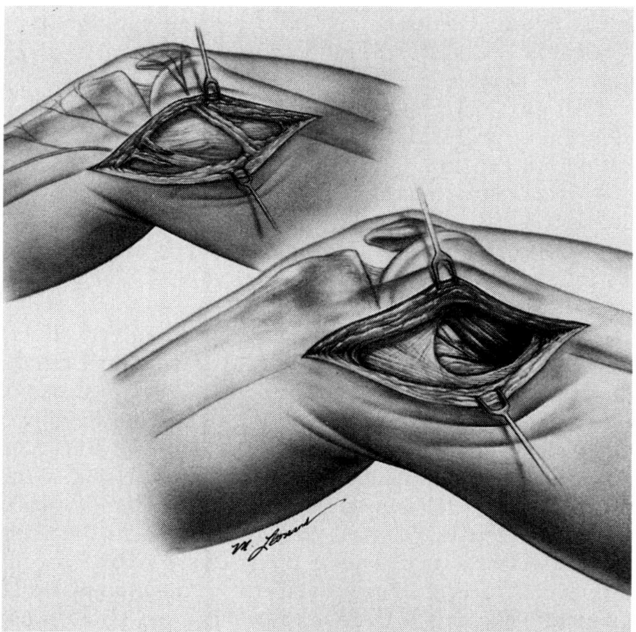

FIGURE 85.9 ➢ Operative approach to medial knee denervation. An incision is made medially at the knee, the medial retinaculum is approached, and the medial retinacular nerve is identified at this level. A segment is rejected, with the proximal level of resection lying beneath or within the vastus medialis muscle.

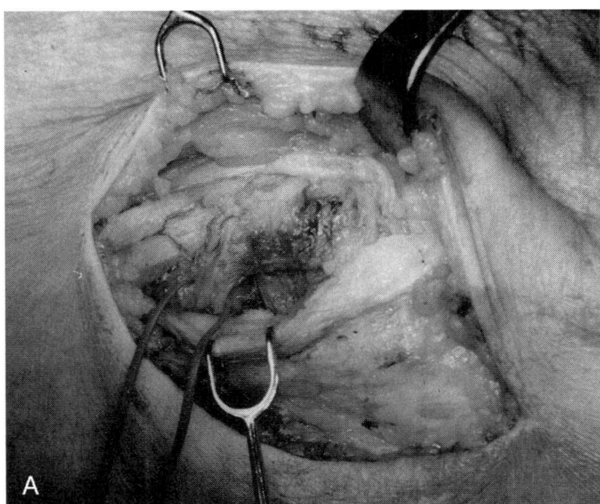

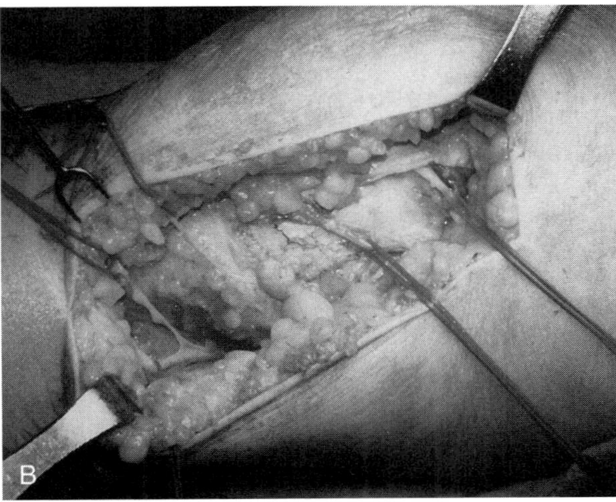

FIGURE 85.10 ➢ Intraoperative view during knee denervation. *A*, The lateral retinacular nerve. *B*, The medial retinacular nerve.

level the nerve has already branched. The bipolar coagulator is used to both dissect and cauterize anteriorly and distally until all the structures accompanying these vessels can be dissected proximally toward their origin from beneath the vastus medialis muscle. There may be significant scarring in this region from the previous joint replacement surgery. The proximal end is followed, and it will be noted that a clear neurovascular pedicle is identified. This is cauterized at the level at which it lies completely beneath the muscle, and the distal segment is submitted to pathology. Note that a true neuroma is not resected, the joint capsule around the implant is not identified, and the implant is not exposed during the dissection. The synovium is not biopsied. The medial retinaculum is closed with a figure-of-8, No. 4-0 absorbable polyglycolic acid sutures. Bupivacaine is instilled, and the wound is closed with No. 4-0 absorbable suture in the dermis and interrupted and continuous No. 5-0 nylon in the skin (see Figs. 85.8 - 85.10).

A new incision is made to identify the infrapatellar branch of the saphenous nerve. This nerve is deep to the subcutaneous tissue, lying on the deep fascia, and accompanied by a vein. The nerve may be pulled on to reveal dimpling of the skin in the region of the painful incision from the knee replacement. The nerve is dissected far proximally, where it will extend along a tunnel to have a relationship with the sartorius muscle. The distal 2 cm of the nerve is resected and submitted to the pathology department. Note that a neuroma is not resected. A long curved clamp facilitates the dissection that will create a tunnel into the sartorius muscle. The proximal end of the nerve is turned and implanted into the sartorius muscle tunnel for a length of about 2 cm. The nerve does not need to be sutured into the muscle. Bupivacaine is instilled into the wound, and it is then closed as above (see Figs. 85.8 - 85.10).

If there is a more distal pain trigger zone medially, and it cannot be reached through the same incision as one used to resect the infrapatellar branch of the saphenous nerve, a third incision should be made to identify the transverse, distal branch of the saphenous nerve. This is located in the deep subcutaneous tissue, often on the periosteum. There will be an accompanying small vessel. The proximal dissection leads to the saphenous vein and terminal branch of the saphenous nerve. These are left intact.

Laterally, the lateral retinacular nerve is identified through a 3- to 5-cm incision made laterally at the knee centered over the tender point marked preoperatively. The incision is deepened down to the lateral retinaculum. The iliotibial band is incised longitudinally with a scalpel beginning just over the distal end of the vastus lateralis and extended distally until just past the recurrent geniculate vessels, which will be apparent in the underlying tissues. The nerve accompanies this vessel; at this level the nerve has already branched. If a previous lateral release has been done during the knee replacement surgery, this area may be extensively scarred. The small nerve branches may not be seen. The bipolar coagulator is used to both dissect and cauterize anteriorly and distally until all the structures accompanying the geniculate vessels have been dissected proximally toward their origin from beneath the iliotibial band and the biceps tendon. This is facilitated by placing a double hook into the iliotibial band and retracting laterally. The proximal end is followed, and it will be noted that a clear neurovascular pedicle is identified originating from the popliteal fossa. This is cauterized at the level at which it lies completely deep to the iliotibial band and where the proximal end can be cauterized adequately. The distal segment is resected and submitted to Pathology. Note that a true neuroma is not resected, the joint capsule around the implant is not identified, and the implant is not exposed during the dissection. The synovium also is not biopsied. The lateral retinaculum is closed with three figure-of-8, No. 4-0 absorbable polyglycolic acid sutures. Bupivacaine is instilled and the wound closed with 4-0 absorbable suture in the dermis and interrupted with continuous No. 5-0 nylon in the skin (Figs. 85.10 - 85.12).

The innervation of the proximal tibiofibular joint is

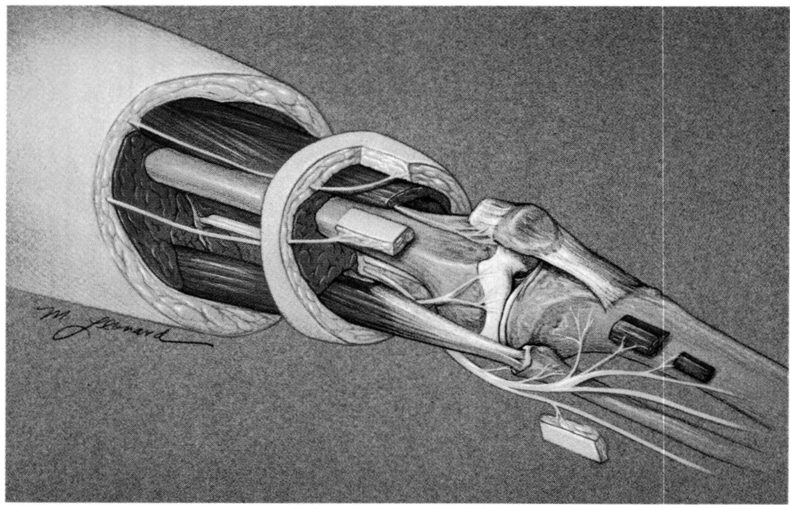

FIGURE 85.11 ➢ Anatomy of the innervation of the lateral knee: three-dimensional view. Note the lateral retinacular nerve arising posteriorly from the sciatic nerve and entering the region from beneath the biceps femoris. This nerve enters the lateral knee structures deep to the lateral retinaculum. Note the innervation of the proximal tibiofibular joint arising from the common peroneal nerve.

identified through an approach that requires a formal neurolysis of the common peroneal nerve at the fibular head. A 6-cm incision is made over the fibular head, obliquely, deepened into the subcutaneous tissue, and the lateral cutaneous nerve of the calf, if present, is preserved. The common peroneal nerve is palpated, the deep fascia covering is opened, and the common peroneal nerve is identified. It is followed anteriorly toward the fascia overlying the peroneus longus muscle. This fascia is slit transversely anteriorly, proximally, and distally. The muscle is elevated, and any deep bands are divided. The common peroneal nerve is then gently separated from all surrounding tissues, and using microsurgical dissecting instruments, the branches in and around the fibular head are separated from the fat, doing a fascicular dissection. At times, in order to identify these branches, an intrafascicular dissection is required. A disposable nerve stimulator is set on the lowest setting, and the gastrocnemius or peroneus muscle is stimulated as a positive control. Then the individual fascicles are stimulated to identify those to the tibialis anterior. The one to three small fascicles (<1 mm) that do not stimulate a muscle contraction are presumed to be those that innervate the proximal tibiofibular joint. These are resected and submitted to Pathology. In order for intraoperative electrical stimulation to work oxygen must be present in the nerve. Therefore, this portion of the procedure should be done first, before the tourniquet time has exceeded one-half hour. Bupivacaine is instilled just into the skin edges so that peroneal motor function will not be lost in the recovery room. The deep fascial structures are not sutured, in order to prevent peroneal nerve entrapment. The skin is closed as above (Figs. 85.11–85.13).

If the anterior femoral cutaneous nerve or the nerve that innervates the prepatellar bursa must be approached, the existing scar is opened and the dissection carried out. The superficial cutaneous nerve will be small, and may not be directly identified. Rather, the deep scarred tissue down to the quadriceps tendon is rejected as a block of tissue and dissected proximally; at that point a small nerve twig may be identified. The entire scar is submitted to Pathology. In this instance of a small nerve twig, it is rejected back into the fat in this region. If a clearly identifiable nerve is present, it should be turned and implanted into the adjacent quadriceps muscle. If necessary, the dissection can be carried deeper with a muscle-splitting incision down to the femur. In the fat at this level, and accompanied by a vessel, will be one or more small nerves going distally into the bursal region. These

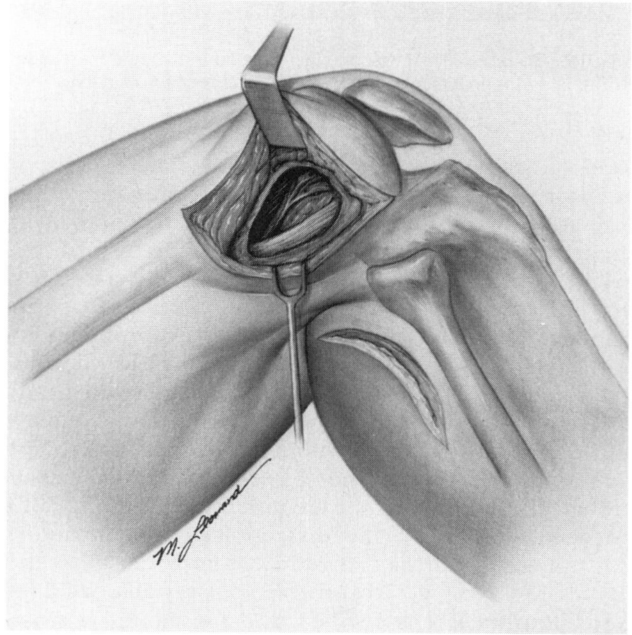

FIGURE 85.12 ➢ Operative approach to lateral knee denervation. An incision is made laterally at the knee; the iliotibial band is approached and incised just distal to the vastus lateralis. The lateral retinacular nerve is identified at this level. A segment is rejected, with the proximal level of resection lying in the popliteal fossa.

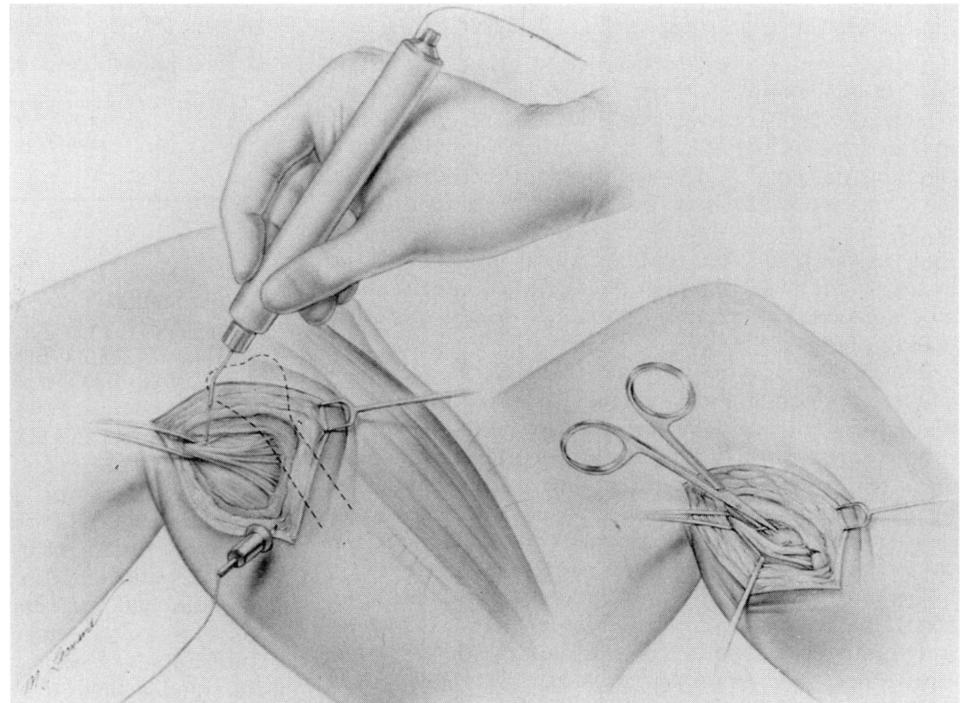

FIGURE 85.13 ➢ Intraoperative electrical stimulation to identify the innervation of the proximal tibiofibular joint. The common peroneal nerve is exposed and decompressed beneath the peroneus longus muscle. After a microdissection of the deep peroneal nerve, electric stimulation identifies small fascicles that cause muscle twitches. The first two or three small fascicles that do not cause a muscle contraction are the innervation of the proximal tibiofibular joint, and these are rejected.

nerves are rejected and submitted to Pathology, allowing their proximal ends to lie within the quadriceps muscles. Bupivacaine is instilled, and the skin is closed, usually with a separate set of sutures to pull some fat between the skin closure and quadriceps.

Postoperative Care

An excellent postoperative strategy is to encourage water walking in a heated pool for the second through the fourth weeks.

Beginning about the third postoperative week, a steroid cream is prescribed to massage into each scar. A 0.1% form of betamethasone is effective. This loosens the scar from the surrounding tissues, and helps to desensitive the skin that has been denervated. For some patients, the denervated skin territory presents a problem as the adjacent intact normal nerves regenerate (collateral sprouting), restoring sensation to these areas.

Most patients know that their original pain is either gone or different by the time of their first office visit, and are very happy with their result even at three weeks. It takes, however, 6 weeks for some patients to recover from the firmness and pain of the postoperative chemical inflammation from the fat oils, especially in the obese medial thigh area. Most patients resume full activity by 3 months after surgery.

Complications

The most common complication is postoperative bruising, with some swelling about the knee. This is present in about 40% of patients. It is treated with topical moist heat three times a day. It resolves during the first 2 weeks.

A chemical inflammation related to the oil from the fat cells causes a postoperative appearance similar to a cellulitis in about 10% of the patients. These patients are given an extra week of oral antibiotics; they apply warm compresses to the region three times a day and, if they are not intolerant of nonsteroidals, are given an anti-inflammatory medication.

Two patients have had to be taken back to surgery to drain a hematoma during the second week postoperatively, and one to have a local infection drained. This was done by their own orthopedic surgeon once the patients had returned to their own geographic area. No patient has had to be taken back acutely for bleeding.

Postoperative stiffness or limited range of motion of the knee that was present prior to the knee denervation was not considered a postoperative complication. Preoperative stiffness usually represented arthrofibrosis related to the initial injury or surgery and was not anticipated to be improved. Patients must be made aware, preoperatively, that denervation usually does not change knee range of motion.

A frequent postoperative problem associated with resection of cutaneous nerves is the hypersensitivity that results due to collateral sprouting from adjacent normal nerves. This is a normal process by which the uninjured adjacent nerve responds to the nerve growth factor released by the Schwann cells in the distal degenerated nerve fibers. The sprouting normal axons generate neural impulses that often are interpreted as recurrent pain. This is an area in which preoperative discussion with patients is critical to helping them understand postoperatively that this is expected, and is not recurrence of the preexisting pain. It is self-limited. Over 3 to 6 weeks, gentle desensitization will resolve the problem. Water walking or a hot tub is helpful, as is wearing long pants and touching the area. A neuropathic pain medication like Elavil or Neurontin may be helpful. A narcotic pain medication is certainly indicated during this period of time, as well as the topical application of steroid cream to the scars. Frequent office visits and reassurance are critical elements to success during this early healing phase.

One patient had to be taken back to surgery at 3 weeks after denervation in order to have draining synovial fluid corrected by oversewing the joint capsule. This was the only patient in whom there was an attempt to resect the neuroma where the retinacular nerve entered the joint capsule (see Fig. 85.6). This approach therefore is not recommended, i.e., a denervation not a neuroma resection is done at surgery.

The most disturbing complication is persistent knee pain. This is almost never the same pain that existed preoperatively, but rather pain in an area that was not approached. For example, a patient who has just a medial approach, may have lateral pain, or a patient who has both a medial and a lateral approach to the knee joint may have pain persist in the proximal tibiofibular joint. This problem occurred in almost 10% of the patients in the early series, requiring a second operation to remove another nerve. This problem is now reduced to about 5% of patients. There will be some patients who will require a second operation due to anatomic variations.

No patient has developed a Charcot joint after this operation. Since a TKA creates a totally denervated joint anyway, it is not logical to be concerned that this partial knee denervation will create one. But even when partial knee denervation is done for persistent knee pain in a patient who has had knee surgery but still retains his or her own knee, a Charcot joint will not result because this is a partial knee denervation. Nevertheless, this is a frequently asked question about a potential postoperative complication. It is supportive of this position for the knee to note that in up to 13 years of postoperative follow-up after wrist denervation, a Charcot joint was not observed.[3]

RESULTS OF PARTIAL KNEE DENERVATION

In 1993, the results of treatment of pain of neural origin after total knee replacement were presented to the American Academy of Orthopaedic Surgeons and later published. That initial experience comprised just 15 patients.[15] Each patient had had pain for at least 6 months after the arthroplasty. All patients were subjectively improved after selective denervation at a mean follow-up of 15 months (range 9 to 19 months). Knee Society objective scores improved from a mean of 55 points (range 30 to 60 points) to a mean of 90 points (range 80 to 100 points).

The first 70 patients having a knee denervation with this approach were reported in 1995.[16] The indications for knee denervation are given in Table 85.1. There were 46 men and 24 women. Mean age was 57 years, range 23 to 78 years. They had previously had a mean of 3.1 surgical procedures upon their painful knee (range, zero to 11 procedures). The number of nerves resected varied with the individual patient's pain pattern; 1 patient had six different nerves resected, and 5 patients had just one nerve rejected. Twenty-six patients had three nerves rejected, and 22 patients had four nerves resected. Twenty-eight patients had just the medial side denervated, 5 patients had just the lateral side denervated, and 37 patients had both medial and lateral knee denervations. The most commonly resected nerve was the infrapatellar branch of the saphenous nerve.[62] Open resected nerves included the medial retinacular nerve,[54] the medial cutaneous nerve of the thigh,[38] and the lateral retinacular nerve.[32] The proximal tibiofibular joint was denervated 13 times. Follow-up after the knee denervation procedure was a minimum of 12 months (range, 12 to 36 months). Of the 70 patients, 31 had a total knee replacement, 32 had previous knee injury, and 7 patients had a previous high tibial osteotomy or Maquet' procedure. All candidates were referred for knee denervation only after all traditional approaches for treatment had been exhausted. Each patient in the series had at least a 5-point reduction in their pain level after a local anesthetic block of specific nerve(s). The results demonstrated that 86% of patients were satisfied with the denervation as judged by direct questioning and a reduction in their preoperative pain visual analog score of 5 or more points. The average Knee Society score improved from 51 points (range, 40 to 62 points) to 82 points (range, 50 to 100 points), $p < .01$. Of 26 patients followed for a minimum of 24 months, 85%

TABLE 85.2 PARTIAL KNEE DENERVATION: 1993–1998

Indications	
Total knee arthroplasty	255
Knee injury	89
Total patients	344

TABLE 85.3 PARTIAL KNEE DENERVATION: 1993–1998

Results	
Excellent	70%
Good	20%
Improved	5%
No change (poor)	5%
Worse	0%

TABLE 85.4 PARTIAL KNEE DENERVATION: 1993–1998

Number of Nerves Removed		
One nerve	(0 patients)	0%
Two nerves	(66 patients)	19%
Three nerves	(44 patients)	13%
Four nerves	(89 patients)	26%
Five nerves	(37 patients)	11%
Six nerves	(108 patients)	31%
Total	344 patients	100%

had 5-point pain score reductions and 77% had Knee Society objective scores greater than 80 points, $p < .01$. In general, the patient's results at 6 months mirrored the results at 2 years. In 1998, a group of 15 knee denervations were reported by members of this group[36] with similar results.

The total experience of knee denervation from our records was recently reviewed and presented to the Western Pacific Orthopedic Association meeting in Japan in November 1998. There are now more than 300 patients who have had a denervation after total knee replacement (Table 85.2). The results, with many follow-ups of 4 or more years, continue to support our enthusiasm for partial knee denervation for the treatment of pain persisting after total knee replacement. It also supports treatment of pain persisting after knee injury or after other surgical approaches to the knee (Table 85.3). In general, the present trend is to be able to identify more nerves contributing to the overall painful knee than before, enabling more involved nerves to be resected at the initial knee denervation (Table 85.4). There is still a small group requiring a second denervation, and a rare individual who will require a third as more nerves or anomalous innervation to the knee joint is identified. Causes for poor results are in Table 85.5.

CONCLUSION

Partial knee denervation is more than a surgical procedure. It is an approach to the patient with knee pain that should be used increasingly in the orthopedic community. When knee pain can be understood as and persisting as a neural origin after the musculoskeletal system has been adequately treated, then a new dimension will open to patients previously thought to be beyond our reach.

TABLE 85.5 PARTIAL KNEE DENERVATION: 1993–1998

Causes for Poor Results (17 Patients)	
Alzheimer's disease	5 patients (29%)
Drug abuse (addiction)	3 patients (18%)
Workmen's compensation	9 patients (53%)

References

1. Abram LJ, Froimson AI: Saphenous nerve injury: An unusual arthropscopic complication. Am J Sports Med 18:41, 1991.
2. Aszman OC, Dellon AL, Birely B, et al: Innervation of the human shoulder joint and its implication for surgery. Clin Orthop Rel Res 330:202, 1996.
3. Buck-Gramcko D: Denervation of the wrist joint. J Hand Surg 2: 54, 1977.
4. Bosley RC: Total acromionectomy. A twenty-year review. J Bone Joint Surg Am 73:961, 1991.
5. Chambers GH: The prepatellar nerve: A cause of suboptimal results in knee arthrotomy. Clin Orthop 182:157, 1977.
6. Dellon AL: Partial dorsal wrist denervation: Resection of distal posterior interosseous nerve. J Hand Surg 10:527, 1985.
7. Dellon AL: Treatment of recurrent metatarsalgia by neuroma resection and muscle implantation: Case report and algorithm for management of Morton's "neuroma." Microsurg 10:256, 1989.
8. Dellon AL: Somatosensory Testing and Rehabilitation. Amer Occup Ther Assocn, Bethesda, MD, 1997, Chapter 14.
9. Dellon AL, Aszmann OC: Treatment of dorsal foot neuromas by translocation of nerves into the anterolateral compartment. Foot Ankle 19:700, 1998.
10. Dellon AL, Horner G: Partial wrist denervation. In Marsh J ed: Current Therapy in Plastic Surgery: The Wrist. Philadelphia, JB Lippincott, 1993, pp 252–261.
11. Dellon AL, Mackinnon SE, Daneshvar A: Terminal branch of anterior interosseous nerve as source of wrist pain. J Hand Surg 9:316, 1984.
12. Dellon AL, Mackinnon SE: Treatment of the painful neuroma by neuroma resection and muscle implantation. Plast Reconstr Surg 77:427, 1986.
13. Dellon AL, Mackinnon SE: Human ulnar neuropathy at the elbow: Clinical, electrical and morphometric correlation. J Reconstr Microsurg 4:179, 1988.
14. Dellon AL, Mackinon SE, Pestronk A: Implantation of sensory nerve into muscle: Preliminary clinical and experimental observation on neuroma formation. Ann Plast Surg 12:30, 1984.
15. Dellon AL, Mont MA, Hungerford DS: Partial denervation for treatment of persistent pain after total knee arthroplasty. Clin Orthop Rel Res 316:145, 1995.
16. Dellon AL, Mont MA, Mullick T, et al: Partial denervation for persistent neuroma pain around the knee. Clin Orthop Rel Res 329:216, 1966.
17. Dellon AL, Seif SS: Neuroma of the posterior interosseous nerve simulating a recurrent ganglion: Case report and anatomical dissection relating the posterior interosseous nerve to the carpus andetiology of dorsal ganglion pain. J Hand Surg 3:326, 1978.
18. Druner L: Ueber die Beteiligung des nervus obtutatorius an der Innervation des Knieglenks. AF Anat U Entwick 82:388, 1927.
19. Ellman H: Arthroscopic subacromial decompression for chronic impingement: Two to five year results. J Bone Joint Surg Br 73: 395, 1991.
20. Evans GRD, Dellon AL: Implantation of the palmar cutaneous branch of the median nerve into the pronator quadratus for treatment of painful neuroma. J Hand Surg 19:203, 1994.
21. Finterbush A: Reflex sympathetic dystrophy of the patellofemoral joint. Orthop Rev 20:877, 1991.
22. Fulkerson JP, Tennant R, Javin JS, et al: Histological evidence of retinacular nerve injury associated with patellofemoral malalignment. Clin Orthop 197:196, 1985.
23. Fulkerson JP, Gossling HR: Anatomy of the knee joint lateral retinaculum. Clin Orthop 153:183, 1980.
24. Gardner E: The innervation of the knee joint. Anat Rec 101:109, 1948.
25. Gardner E: The innervation of the shoulder joint. Anat Rec 102: 1, 1948.
26. Horner G, Dellon AL: Innervation of the human knee joint and implication for surgery. Clin Orthop Rel Res 301:221, 1994.
27. Huckle JR: Meniscectomy: A benign procedure? A long-term follow-up. Can J Surg 8:254, 1965.
28. Hungerford DS, Krackow KA, Kenna RV: Clinical experience with the PCA prosthesis with and without cement. In Hungerford DS, Krackow KA, Denna RV, eds. Total Knee Arthroplasty:

A Comprehensive Approach. Williams & Wilkins, Baltimore, 1984, pp 127–130.
29. Insall JN, Dorr LD, Scott RS, et al: Rationale of the Knee Society clinical rating system. Clinic Orthop 248:13, 1989.
30. Jeletsky AG: On the innervation of the capsule and epiphysis of the knee joint. Vestn Khir, 22:74, 1931.
31. Katz MM, Hungerford DS: Reflex sympathetic dystrophy affecting the knee. J Bone Joint Surg Br 69:797, 1987.
32. Katz MM, Hungerford DS, Krackow KA, et al: Reflex sympathetic dystrophy as a cause of poor results following total knee arthroplasty. J Arthros 1:117, 1986.
33. Kennedy JC, Alexander IJ, Hayes KC: Nerve supply to the human knee and its functional importance. Amer J Sports Med 10: 329, 1982.
34. Krackow KA, Maar DC, Mont MA, et al: Surgical decompression for peroneal nerve palsy after total knee arthroplasty. Clin Orthop 292:223, 1993.
35. Krompinger WJ, Fulkerson JP: Lateral retinacular release for intractable lateral pain. Clin Orthop 179:191, 1983.
36. Lewallen DG: Neurovascular injury associated with hip arthroplasty. J Bone Joint Surg Am 79:1870, 1997.
37. Mackinnon SE, Dellon AL: Overlap of lateral antebrachial cutaneous nerve and superficial sensory branch of the radial nerve. J Hand Surg 10:522, 1985.
38. Mackinnon SE, Dellon AL: Experimental study of chronic nerve compression: Clinical implications. Clin Hand Surg, 2:639, 1986.
39. Mackinnon SE, Dellon AL: Results of treatment of recurrent dorsoradial wrist neuromas. Ann Plast Surg 19:54, 1987.
40. Mackinnon SE, Dellon AL: Surgery of the Peripheral Nerve, New York, Thieme, 1988, Chapter 16.
41. Mackinnon SE, Dellon AL, Hudson AR, et al: Alteration of neuroma by manipulation of neural microenvironment. Plast Reconstr Surg 76:345, 1985.
42. Mackinnon SE, Dellon AL, Hudson AR, et al: A primate model for chronic nerve compression. J Reconstr Microsurg 1:185, 1985.
43. Mackinnon SE, Dellon AL, Hudson AR, et al: Histopathology of compression of the superficial radial nerve in the forearm. J Hand Surg 11:206, 1986.
44. Meyer RA, Raja SN, Campbell JN, et al: Neural activity originating from a neuroma in the baboon. Brain Res 325:255, 1985.
45. Mont MA, Dellon AL, Chen F, et al: Operative treatment of peroneal nerve palsy. J Bone Joint Surg Am 78:863, 1996.
46. Mori Y, Fujimoto A, Okumo H, et al: Lateral retinacular release in adolescent patellofemoral disorders: Its relationship to peripheral nerve injury in the lateral retinaculum. Bull Hosp Joint Dis Orthop Inst 51:218, 1981.
47. Nahabedian MY, Mont MA, Hungerford DS: Selective denervation of the knee. Amer J Knee Surg 11:175, 1998.
48. Ogilvie-Harris DJ, Marin R: Reflex sympathetic dystrophy of the knee. J Bone Joint Surg Br 69:804, 1987.
49. Poehling GG, Pollock FE, Jr, Koman LA: Reflex sympathetic dystrophy of the knee after sensory nerve injury. Arthroscopy 4: 31, 1988.
50. Ruedinger N: Die Gelenknerven des Mennschlichen Koerpers. Erlangen, Ferdinand Inke, 1857.
51. Swanson AJG: The incidence of prepatellar neuropathy following medial meniscectomy. Clin Orthop 181:151, 1983.
52. Wilhelm A: Zur Innervation der Gelenke der Oberen Extremitaet. Z. Anat und Entwicklungsgesch 120:331, 1958.
53. Wilhelm A: Die Gelenksdenervation und ihre anatomischen Grundlagen: Ein neues Behandlungsprinzip in der Handcirurgie. Hefte Unfallheilk 86:100, 1966.
54. Wojtys EM, Beaman DN, Glover RA, et al: Innervation of the human knee joint by substance P fibers. Arthoscopy 6:254, 1990.
55. Worth RM, Kettelkamp DB, Defalque RJ, et al: Saphenous nerve entrapment: A cause of medial knee pain. Am J Sports Med 12: 80, 1984.
56. Wrete M: The innervation of the shoulder joint in man. Acta Anat (Basel), 7:173, 1949.

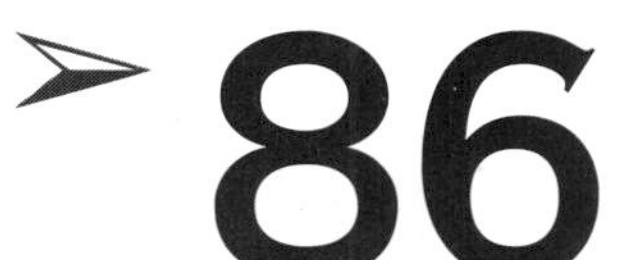

86 Bone Graft, Wedges, and Augments in Total Knee Arthroplasty

Mark W. Pagnano

The management of bone loss in total knee arthroplasty is directed by the extent and location of the bone deficiency. In primary total knee arthroplasty, the most frequently encountered form of bone loss is a posteromedial tibial plateau defect associated with marked varus angular deformity of the limb (Fig. 86.1). On the femoral side, marked bone loss is rare in the primary setting. An exception would be the severe valgus limb in which the lateral femoral condyle may have a combination of both distal and posterior bone loss (Fig. 86.2). In revision total knee arthroplasty, marked bone loss is encountered often, and the degree of bone loss typically exceeds that predicted by the preoperative radiographs. Osteolytic defects secondary to wear debris and iatrogenic bone loss at the time of component removal are major causes of large bony defects (Fig. 86.3). During revision total knee arthroplasty, bone loss from the distal and posterior femur must be routinely addressed (Fig. 86.4). Multiple options exist to fill those bony defects and include cement, autograft bone, allograft bone, and modular metal wedges and blocks.

The purpose of this chapter is to review the indications, limitations, detailed surgical techniques, and published clinical results for each of those methods of filling bone defects in total knee arthroplasty. An appropriate understanding of the benefits and limitations of each technique will allow the surgeon to deal efficiently and effectively with bone deficiency in total knee arthroplasty. Techniques to address bony defects must not compromise the basic principles of total knee replacement, which include the following: correct limb alignment, correct implant position, balance of the flexion and extension spaces, restoration of the joint line, central tracking of the patella, and adequate range of motion. A bony defect elegantly reconstructed with bone graft, metal wedges, and stems is still doomed to failure if the surgeon fails to obtain appropriate limb alignment, component position, and component fixation.

ASSESSMENT OF BONE LOSS

Assessment of bone deficiency in primary total knee arthroplasty is best done after making the standard bone cuts. Many defects that initially appear to require some type of augmentation are eliminated by the standard bony resection. This is often true with moderate-size posteromedial defects of the tibia in varus knees. Resection of an additional 1 to 2 mm of tibial bone

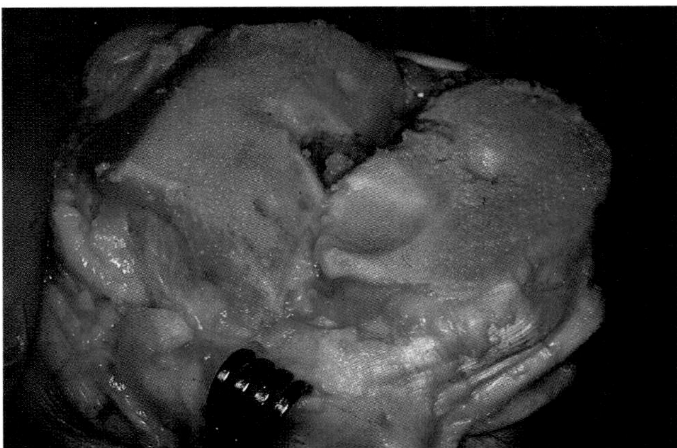

FIGURE 86.1 ➢ The most common bony defect in primary total knee arthroplasty is a posteromedial defect in a varus knee.

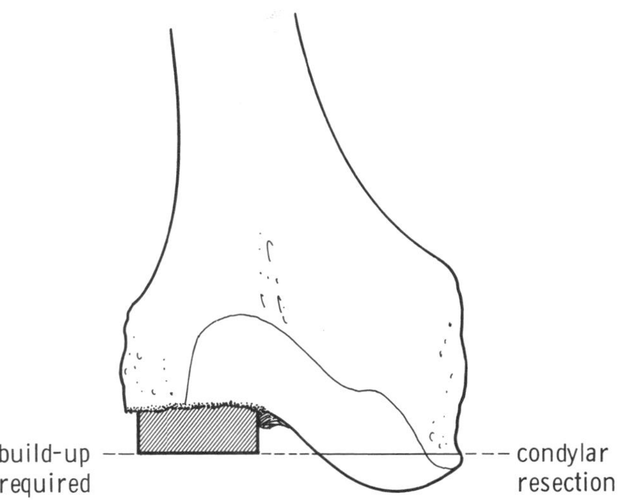

FIGURE 86.2 ➢ The valgus knee may have a lateral condyle that is deficient both distally and posteriorly. Often only a minimal amount of distal femoral bone is removed from the lateral condyle in the valgus knee. In some valgus knees, the level of resection may pass distal to the lateral condyle and require augmentation.

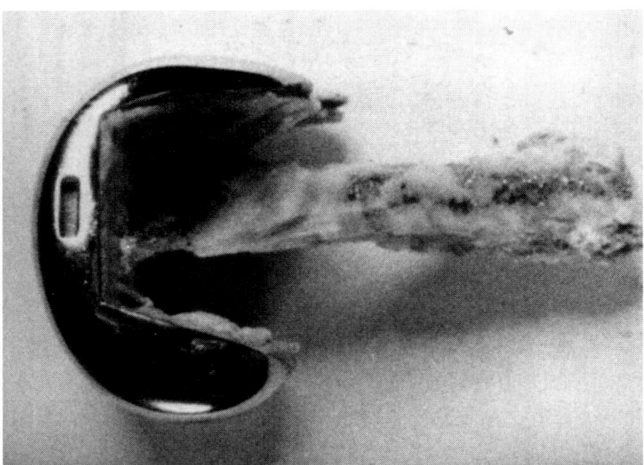

FIGURE 86.3 ➢ Care must be taken with the removal of components during revision total knee arthroplasty, or substantial bone may be lost inadvertently. All exposed prosthetic interfaces must be dissected free before the use of extraction devices.

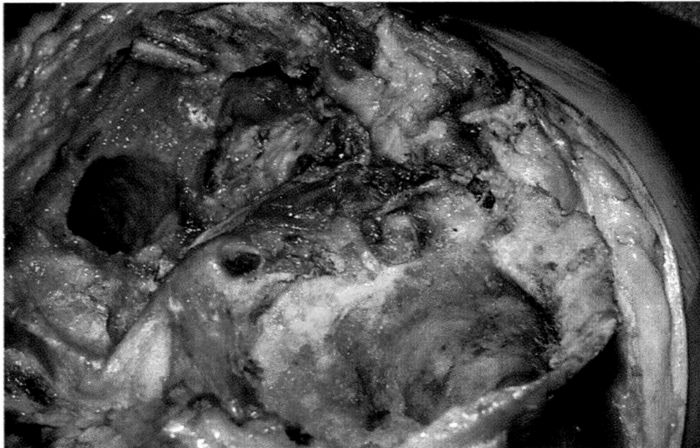

FIGURE 86.5 ➢ After careful removal of the components, the knee should be thoroughly débrided to remove any fibrous tissue associated with areas of osteolysis. At that point, the true extent of bone loss may be accurately assessed.

can eliminate some defects entirely, and such additional resection is appropriate if the initial resection was only 8 or 9 mm. Numerous biomechanical studies have demonstrated that trabecular bone strength in the proximal tibia decreases with greater distance from the joint surface.[22, 23, 40] Those studies have led many to caution against taking a larger proximal tibial resection. No study to date, however, has shown a clinically important relationship between tibial component survival and depth of tibial resection.

Assessment of bone deficiency during revision total knee arthroplasty is best done after removal of the components and débridement of all osteolytic regions (Fig. 86.5). A number of classification schemes exist to grade the extent of bone loss.[10, 11, 12] Most of these schemes distinguish between contained or cavitary defects (those with an intact peripheral cortex) and noncontained or segmental defects (those without a peripheral rim of bone). Although contained defects can often be filled adequately with morselized bone, segmental defects usually require structural graft, metal augments, or custom components.

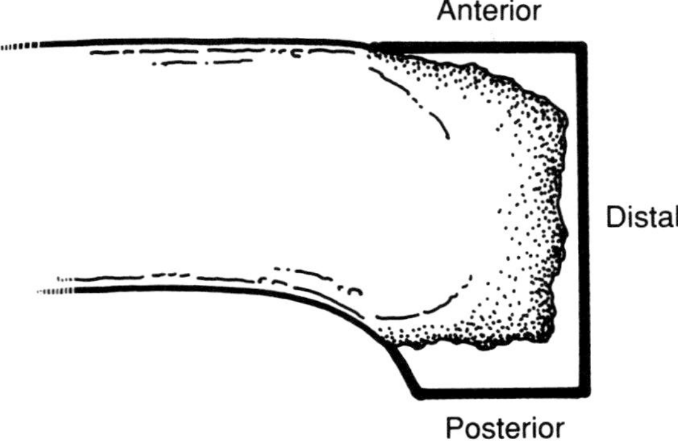

FIGURE 86.4 ➢ Distal and posterior femoral bone stock frequently must be augmented at the time of revision total knee arthroplasty.

BONE CEMENT

Indications: Small bony defects up to 5 mm in depth, preferably contained, in older patients

Limitations: The relatively poor biomechanical properties of cement that preclude its use in larger or segmental defects, particularly in younger patients

Bone cement is a useful means to fill small areas of bone deficiency. It is inexpensive, readily fills a defect, and does not require any major alteration in the performance of total knee arthroplasty. Cement has, however, relatively poor biomechanical properties. The modulus of elasticity of cement is lower than that of bone, and cement performs poorly when subjected to shear stresses. Brooks et al demonstrated that, when subject to axial loads, a simulated peripheral tibial defect filled with cement performed poorly in vitro.[5] Chen and Krackow have shown that it is biomechanically advantageous to convert defects into a step configuration when cement is used (Fig. 86.6).[8] The conversion of a wedge-shaped defect to a step-shaped construct minimizes shear force on the cement. Those authors' laboratory data suggested that a 20-degree wedge-shaped defect in the tibia could be converted to a step-shaped construct and filled with cement. In that setting, cement filling of the defect was as strong as a metal augmentation wedge. For larger defects, however, a metal wedge or metal augmentation block was recommended. Other authors have suggested that cement reinforced with bone screws can be used to fill larger defects.[14, 35, 36] In vitro biomechanical data suggest that use of screw reinforcement may result in a slight improvement over use of bone cement alone when filling defects.

Cement, however, does not restore bone stock, and

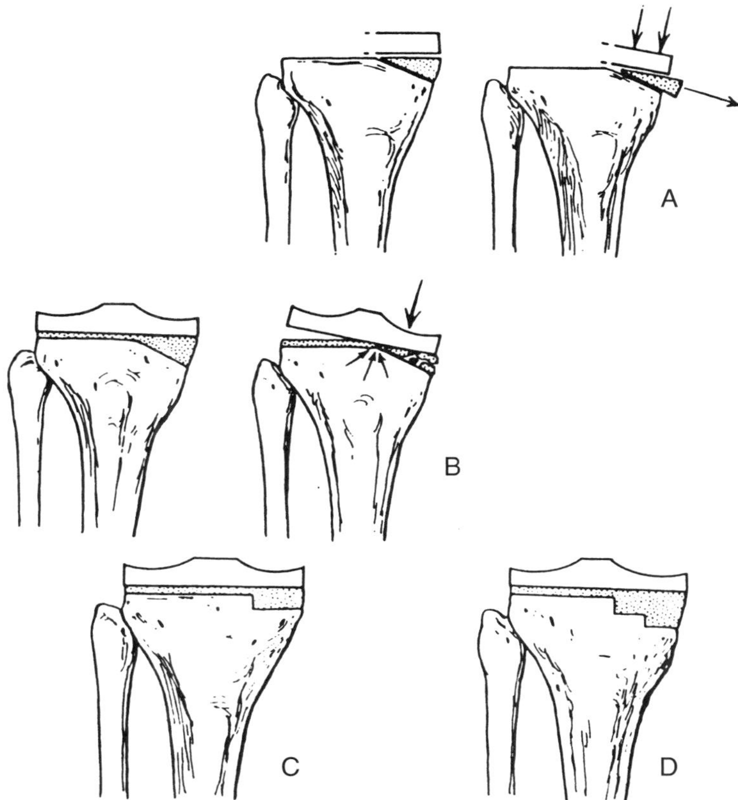

FIGURE 86.6 ➢ It is biomechanically advantageous to convert wedge-shaped bony defects to step-shaped defects if cement is used to fill the defect. *A,* Shear force may weaken the support of the overlying tibial component. *B,* Cement at the periphery of a wedge defect may be exposed to excessive stress. *C, D,* A step or terraced configuration will reduce the forces and lower the stresses on the cement. (From Chen F, Krackow K: Management of tibial defects in total knee arthroplasty. Clin Orthop 305:249, 1994.)

that may be important in younger patients who face the possibility of revision in the future. The young patient undergoing primary total knee replacement likely is better served by filling bony defects with autogenous bone rather than with cement. In that setting, the bone is readily available, reliably incorporates, and restores bone stock should the arthroplasty subsequently fail.

Clinical Results

At early and midterm follow-up, the results of use of cement and cement reinforced with screws to fill tibial defects in total knee arthroplasty have been satisfactory. Ritter et al reported on 47 patients with a minimum of 3 years' follow-up and an average of 6.1 years' follow-up after total knee arthroplasty with cement and screw filling of tibial defects.[35, 36] Those defects were defined as large with a depth of 9 ± 5 mm. Although nonprogressive radiolucent lines were common (27% of cases), there were no signs of cement failure or any loose prostheses. Those authors stated that cement and screw filling of tibial defects has proven to be satisfactory clinically. They further suggested that the presence of radiolucent lines adjacent to the cement-filled areas may be technique related. After adopting a technique to remove sclerotic bone, expose the underlying cancellous bone, and allow cement interdigitation, those authors found no early radiolucencies. Eleven knees were prepared in that manner, and no radiolucencies had developed in that group at 2 years' follow-up. Freeman reported good results with the use of cement reinforced with screws for tibial defects.[14] At early follow-up (mean, 32 months), many radiolucent lines were present, but none were progressive.

Surgical Technique

The tibia is prepared for a standard tibial tray in the typical fashion. The defect is assessed after the initial bone resection. The sclerotic base of the defect is débrided with a high speed bur, and multiple small drill holes are placed to encourage cement interdigitation. If the defect is wedge shaped, it is then converted into a step-shaped or terraced defect in an effort to minimize the shear forces on the cement construct. The bone is then thoroughly irrigated with a pulsatile lavage and dried. For larger defects, the cement can be reinforced with screws. Self-tapping cancellous bone screws are placed in the defect and advanced until the head of the screw will be below the level of the prosthesis. Because most tibial baseplates are titanium, titanium screws are favored to limit galvanic corrosion caused by dissimilar metals. The trial component is placed, and the screw depth is fine-tuned so that the screw heads do not directly contact the baseplate. The cement is mixed and introduced into the tibia when in a doughy state. Gentle pressurization of the cement into the base of the defect by finger packing is appropriate. Doughy cement is placed over the screw heads and on the underside of the baseplate to ensure that the prosthesis does not directly contact the screws. The tibial component is then inserted, excess cement is removed from the edge of the defect, and the cement is allowed to cure. Stem extensions on the tibial component are not required when small bony defects are filled with cement but should be used in the presence of larger defects or when the bone is markedly osteopenic.

AUTOGENOUS BONE GRAFT

Indications: Defects greater than 5 mm in depth or involving more than 50% of a tibial hemiplateau, particularly in a younger patient

Limitations: Limited availability of autogenous bone

Autogenous bone is an excellent material to fill defects at the time of total knee arthroplasty. Autogenous bone is readily incorporated, reliably heals, and appears to be durable when used to fill bony defects. Bone can be readily contoured to fit and fill segmental defects, or it can be morselized to fill contained defects. In primary total knee arthroplasty, adequate autogenous bone is often available from the distal femoral resection or the intercondylar resection. In revision total knee arthroplasty, autogenous bone is typically in short supply because of the marked bone loss and the limited need for resection of more bone. An exception would be the trapezoidal bone that is removed from the intercondylar region when converting from a cruciate retaining primary knee to a posterior stabilized revision implant. That autogenous bone can be used to fill small defects in the revision setting.

Clinical Results

Scuderi et al have reported good results in 26 total knee arthroplasties for which autogenous grafting was used.[38] Ninety-six percent good and excellent results were found, and the grafts were all incorporated by 1 year postoperatively. A nonprogressive radiolucency developed in two knees and in one of those cases was the result of graft collapse. Aglietti et al and Altcheck et al have had similar good results at comparable periods of follow-up.[1, 2] Dorr et al reported on 24 knees treated with autogenous graft to fill tibial defects.[10] All those patients were followed for a minimum of 3 years. Bone incorporation was seen in 22 of the cases. One graft failed because of collapse. That failure was linked to postoperative varus limb alignment.

Laskin has reported less satisfactory results with autogenous grafting of tibial defects.[26] Four knees in that series demonstrated graft collapse within 1 year postoperatively. Nine knees were biopsied more than 1 year after surgery, and fewer than half of the grafts were found to be living. Of interest is the choice of posterior femoral bone as the autogenous graft material in that series. The author has speculated that the large proportion of cortical and subchondral bone in those graft specimens may have contributed to the poor rate of incorporation and the high rate of failure. The overall success rate in that series was 67% at relatively early follow-up.

To date there are no studies that report the results for autogenous grafting of femoral bony defects.

Surgical Technique

Sculco has popularized the use of autogenous bone from the distal femoral resection (Fig. 86.7).[39] In that technique, the standard tibial resection is carried out. The sclerotic base of the tibial defect is then cut away to expose the underlying cancellous bone. Any underlying cystic regions in the tibia are curetted and filled with morselized cancellous autograft. To ensure that graft fixation is not compromised by the keel or stem of the tibial component, the tibia is prepared for the trial component. Next, the flat surfaces of the defect and the bone from the distal femoral resection are opposed and held in place with pins. Typically, the bone from the distal medial femur is more substantial and thus a better graft source than bone from the lateral side. The graft is appropriately shaped and then rigidly fixed with screws. The graft-host junction should be free of any gaps. Small defects can be packed with morselized cancellous graft. The graft-host junction is then protected against cement intrusion by caulking the interface. That caulking can be done with Gelfoam or with a small amount of cement itself if the femoral component is cemented separately. The tibial component is then cemented over the graft in the standard fashion. For femoral defects, a similar technique can be employed. The sclerotic bone on the deficient side is removed, exposing the underlying cancellous bone. Bone from the opposite condyle is then fixed into place and trimmed appropriately. The femoral component can then be cemented into place.

Windsor et al have suggested an alternative technique for autogenous grafting.[48] That method involves a so-called self-locking dowel technique. The proximal tibial resection is carried out, and the tibia is prepared for the trial tibial component. The defect is then converted into a trapezoidal shape, and the sclerotic base of the defect is removed with a high-speed bur. A matching trapezoid is made from the autogenous bone graft and is impacted into place. The press fit of the graft is temporarily supplemented with Kirschner wire fixation. The tibia is then cemented in the standard fashion.

ALLOGRAFT BONE

Indications: Large contained or segmental defects for which autogenous bone is not available or is insufficient to fill the defect

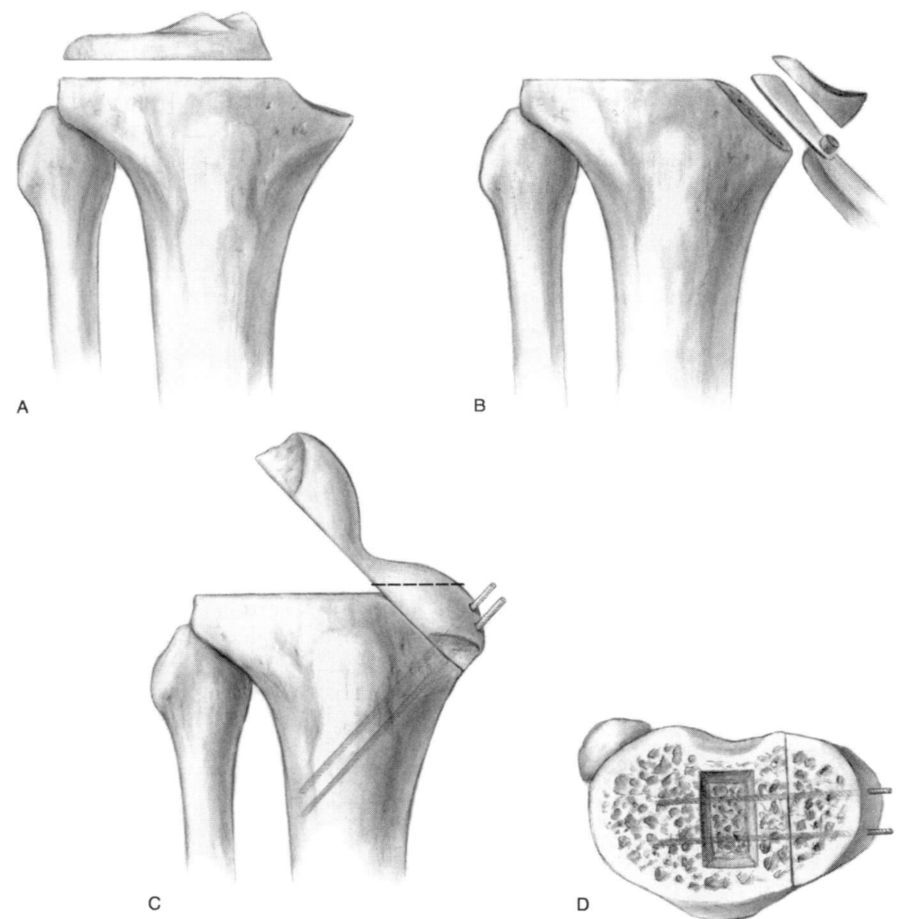

FIGURE 86.7 ➢ The proximal tibial resection (*A*) is carried out, and then the sclerotic base of the defect is removed (*B*) with an oscillating saw. The distal femoral graft (*C*) is fixed rigidly in place with bone screws. *D*, The construct as viewed from above, with the graft trimmed and prepared for the tibial component. (From Sculco TP: Bone grafting. In Lotke PA, ed: Master Techniques in Orthopedic Surgery, Knee Arthroplasty. New York, Raven Press, 1995.)

Limitations: Union of allograft to host required for long-term success; possibility that large grafts may fail late because they lack the ability to remodel in response to stress

Allograft bone is widely used in both revision total knee arthroplasty and revision total hip arthroplasty. The use of morselized cancellous allograft to fill contained defects appears to be both a reliable and a durable method. Impacted morselized allograft has been well studied in the hip and has been successfully used to fill large cavitary defects in both the femur and the acetabulum.[18, 19, 30] From a biological standpoint, morselized cancellous allograft lacks osteogenic properties but does possess osteoconductive properties and seems to incorporate much like a cancellous autograft, although at a slower rate. A well-vascularized recipient bed seems to facilitate incorporation of morselized allograft. There is, however, a paucity of scientific data on the use of such techniques in revision total knee arthroplasty.[44]

Large structural allografts are most often used to fill segmental defects at the time of revision total knee replacement.[17, 21, 25, 27, 41, 43, 47] Some reports of large structural allografts, however, have also detailed their use in filling extensive metaphyseal cavitary defects.[41] Allograft bone offers the chance to restore bone stock but requires that the graft unite to the underlying host bone.[15] Allograft bone is widely available, and the type of bone used can be tailored to the clinical situation (e.g., femoral head, proximal tibia, distal femur). Allograft bone can provide greater intraoperative flexibility at a lower cost than a custom implant. Disease transmission is a disadvantage in the use of allograft bone.[7] The risk of disease transmission is low and has been estimated at one in a million when strict donor selection criteria and thorough screening methods are employed.[6]

Complications with large structural allografts are not uncommon. The long-term success of a structural allograft requires union between the graft and the host. Typically, this occurs through a process of external callous formation and then revascularization followed by creeping substitution and remodeling.[15] If this process occurs too slowly, then a nonunion may ensue. If the process occurs too rapidly, then allograft integrity can be compromised and fracture or collapse may follow. Once the allograft has solidly united to the host, it has a very limited ability to remodel, and it essentially acts like an inert implant. Over long periods, that inability to remodel can lead to stress fracture and failure of the allograft construct. For that reason, structural allografts in total knee arthroplasty should be protected by an intramedullary stem that completely bypasses the graft.

Clinical Results

Several sets of authors have reported the results of morselized allograft in revision total knee arthroplasty.[37, 44, 46] Samuelson used morselized allograft to fill large tibial defects in 22 knees. Uncemented tibial components with intramedullary stems were used in all cases. At a minimum of 2 years' follow-up, one third of the implants had migrated but were felt to have reached a stable position. None of those implants were considered clinical failures. Whiteside reported 56 knees with either contained or segmental tibial defects that were filled with morselized allograft. The tibial components were all of an uncemented design with an extended intramedullary stem. Fixation was further augmented with screws placed through the tibial baseplate. At a minimum 2-year follow-up, nine knees had moderate or severe pain, one tibial component had migrated, three knees were unstable, three patellar dislocations had occurred, and one patellar tendon had ruptured. All grafts showed radiographic evidence of remodeling. Ullmark and Hovelius have reported on three patients treated with an impaction allografting technique similar to that described in the literature on hip arthroplasty. At 18 to 28 months' follow-up, all the patients were doing well clinically. Radiographs revealed incorporation of the allograft bone in two of the three patients.

Mow and Weidel used structural allografting in 15 total knees in which large segmental, cavitary, or combined deficiencies were present.[28] Both femoral and tibial defects were addressed. The allograft-host junction was bypassed with an intramedullary stem in all cases. Follow-up averaged 47 months. The Hospital for Special Surgery (HHS) knee scores improved from 47 prerevision to 86 at follow-up. One case failed because of tibial component loosening, and one case failed because of progressive lysis. There were no cases of infection. Mnaymneh et al reported the results with 14 structural allografts used to fill large distal femoral or proximal tibial defects.[27] Graft-host union occurred in 12 of those cases. Complications were common in this group, which had been followed for a mean of 3.3 years. Nonunion occurred in two cases, tibial loosening in two cases, dislocation in one case, and deep prosthetic infection in one case. Tsahakis et al used 48 bulk allografts in 30 revision total knee arthroplasties.[43] Excellent or good results were reported in 90% of those cases at a mean follow-up of 3.2 years. Those authors cemented the prostheses and used intramedullary stems to bypass the allograft in each case. Union was reliably obtained. Complications did occur in three cases as component failure, loosening, and ligamentous instability. Harris et al used structural allografts in 14 revision total knee arthroplasties with segmental defects.[21] Six whole tibial allografts, three medial tibial condyles, five whole femurs, and five medial femoral condyles were used. Intramedullary stems were used to bypass the allograft in 11 of the cases. At a mean follow-up of 43 months, 13 of the allografts had united and 11 of the 14 knees were considered clinical successes. Ghazavi et al have reported the use of structural allografts in 30 knee revisions.[17] These allografts were used to fill uncontained defects at least 3 cm in depth. A structural allograft was used on the femoral side alone in 16 cases, on the tibial side alone in 10 cases, and on both the femoral and the tibial sides in 4 cases. All allografts were bypassed with an intramedullary stem. There were three deep infections, two cases of tibial loosening, one graft fracture, one graft nonunion, one patellar tendon tear, and one wound necrosis. Twenty-three of the 30 knees (77%) were judged to be clinically successful. Wilde et al reported the results of bulk allografts used in 12 knees of 10 patients.[47] The allograft was used to fill a segmental defect in seven knees and a contained defect in five knees. Intramedullary stems were used in all cases, and supplemental fixation with a plate or screws was used for each case with a segmental defect. Nonunion occurred in one case. At a mean follow-up of 32 months, radiolucent lines beneath the tibial components were common but were not progressive. Two knees required revision for deep prosthetic infection.

Surgical Technique

Morselized Allograft. For contained defects, morselized cancellous or corticocancellous allograft can be efficiently used to restore bone stock. The host bone should be thoroughly débrided of any residual fibrous tissue to create a favorable environment for graft incorporation. For larger metaphyseal defects, the tibial or femoral canal should first be prepared to accept an appropriately sized intramedullary stem. The trial stem should be left in place, and the morselized cancellous allograft can be tightly packed around the stem. For large defects, several femoral heads may be needed. Preparation of the bone is facilitated by the use of a bone mill. To allow efficient packing, the bone should be processed through the bone mill several times to obtain suitably morselized bone. Alternatively, prepackaged morselized corticocancellous allograft can be obtained from several commercial sources. Once the defect has been tightly packed, the trial stem can be removed and the prosthesis and stem can be cemented in the standard fashion.

Structural Allograft. The host bone is débrided back to healthy bleeding bone to facilitate graft incorporation. When possible, the distal femoral and proxi-

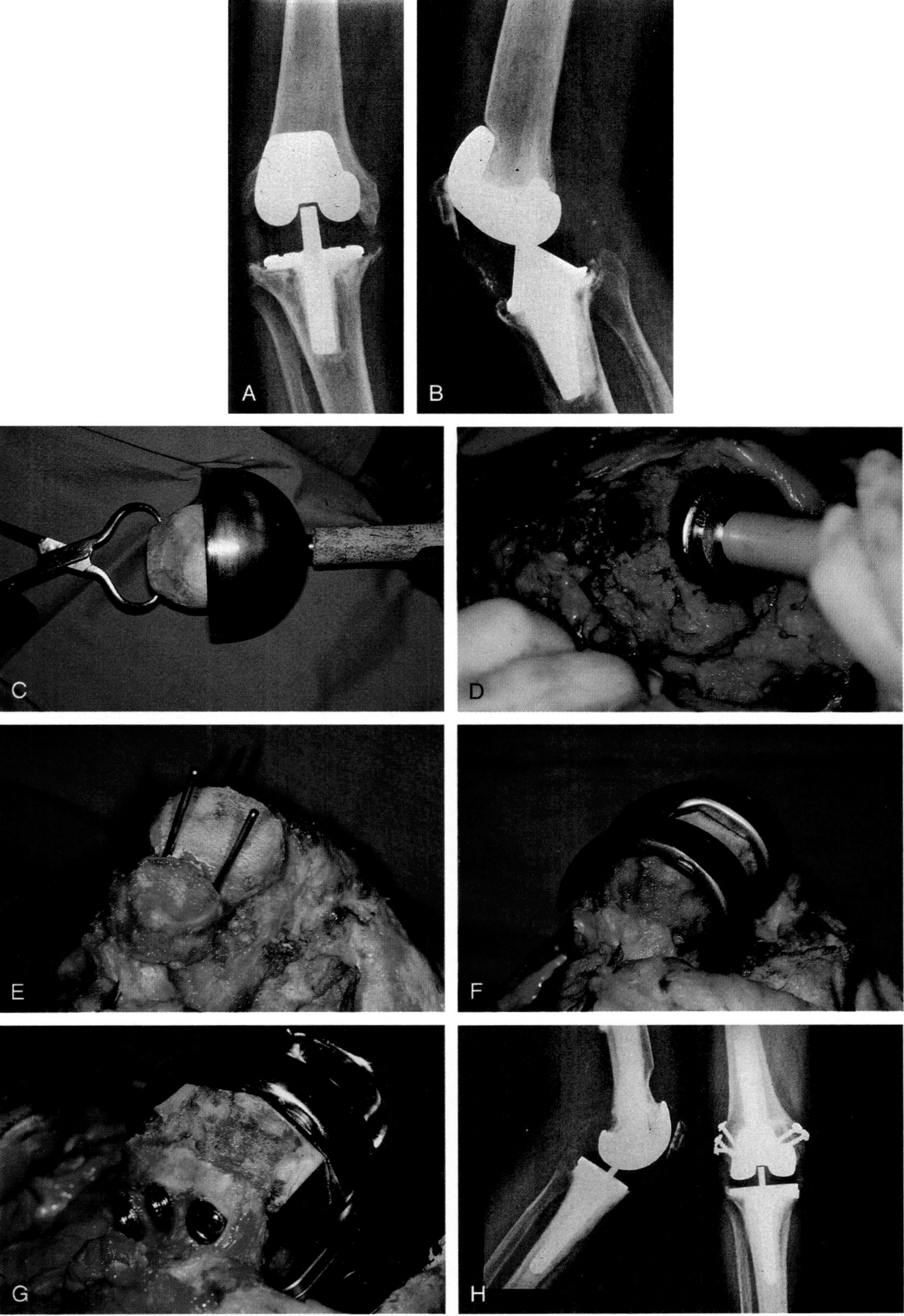

FIGURE 86.8 ➢ Anteroposterior (*A*) and lateral (*B*) views of a loose total knee arthroplasty with marked femoral and tibial bone loss. Femoral head allografts (*C*) are prepared using female resurfacing reamers. The host femur is prepared (*D*) with corresponding small acetabular reamers to allow intimate contact with the allograft femoral heads. Temporary graft fixation (*E*) is performed with Steinmann pins. The distal femur is prepared for the femoral component (*F*). *G,* Final graft fixation with cancellous bone screws and cementation of the femoral component with a long intramedullary stem are done. *H,* Postoperative anteroposterior and lateral views of the construct.

mal tibial resections are freshened by removing 1 to 2 mm of bone. That resection leaves a flat surface on which to seat the prosthesis and maximizes host bone contact with the implant while minimizing further bone sacrifice. The structural allograft is then contoured to fill the defect. In some cases, the host and the allograft bone can be fashioned into corresponding trapezoidal shapes to maximize fit and intrinsic stability. When a femoral head allograft has been chosen, the host bone may be prepared with an appropriately sized acetabular reamer (Fig. 86.8). Host cortical bone should not be sacrificed. Kirschner wires are used to supplement the mechanical fit between graft and host bone. Final shaping of the condylar surface of the allograft can be done with the standard knee-cutting guides. If the intrinsic mechanical fit of the graft to the host is poor, then supplemental fixation with cancellous bone screws is appropriate. In those cases where an entire distal femur or proximal tibia is required, the graft-host junction can be step-cut to enhance intrinsic stability. Strut allografts and cables can be used to enhance stability at the host-allograft junction. Alternatively, a so-called bone-within-bone approach has been described for the proximal tibia. In those cases, the allograft proximal tibia was invaginated into the remaining host tibia (Fig. 86.9). In all cases, an intramedullary stem is used to bypass the graft and to obtain fixation in the diaphyseal region. The prosthesis and stem should be cemented to the condylar surface and to the allograft because bone ingrowth from an avascular allograft to a porous

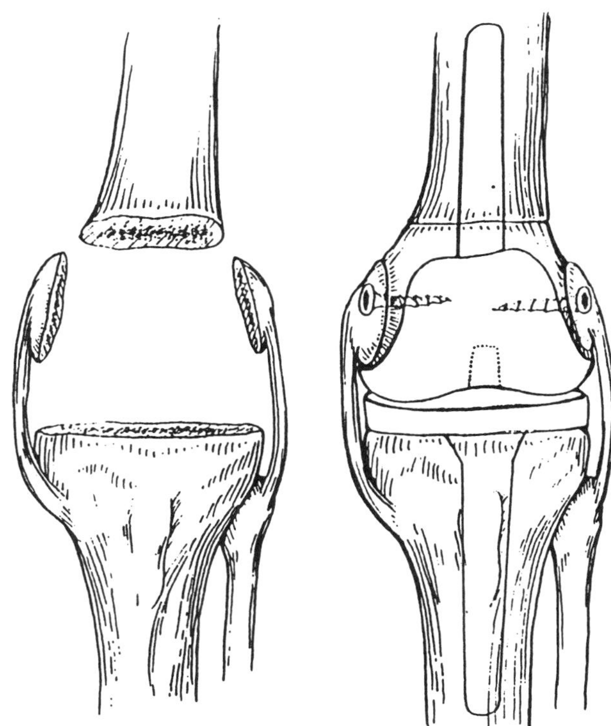

FIGURE 86.10 ➢ When a whole distal femoral allograft is needed, care should be taken to preserve the host bone at the epicondyles. The collateral ligaments can then be secured to the allograft with screws. (From Dennis DA: Structural allografting in revision total knee arthroplasty. In Insall JN, Scott WN, Scuderi GR, eds: Current Concepts in Primary and Revision Total Knee Arthroplasty. Philadelphia, Lippincott-Raven, 1996.)

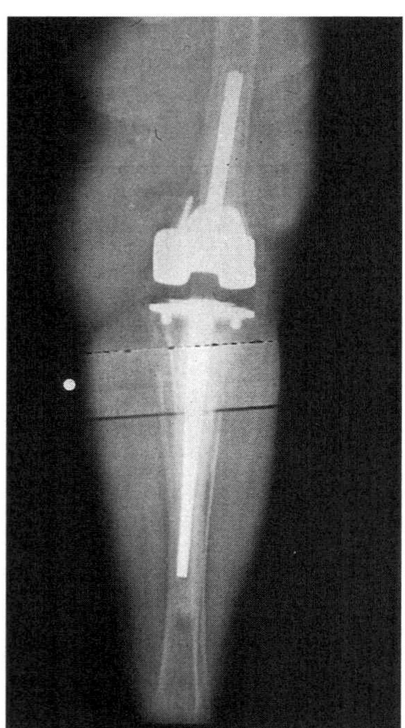

FIGURE 86.9 ➢ A bone-within-bone construct has been employed on the tibial side. The proximal tibial allograft was prepared for the tibial prosthesis and then invaginated within the remaining host tibia.

coated component is unlikely. The intramedullary stem itself either may be inserted in a press-fit fashion with diaphyseal cortical contact or may be cemented in place. Collateral ligament reattachment can be problematic if allograft reconstruction of the entire distal femur or proximal tibia has been done. In those cases, it is most appropriate to preserve the host ligament with a portion of bone attached. The ligament and attached host bone can then be fixed to the allograft with a bone screw. (Fig. 86.10). Host bone to allograft bone reattachment of the ligament appears to be the most reliable and durable way to restore appropriate collateral ligament function. Although soft-tissue reattachment to allograft can occur, obtaining appropriate ligament tension has proven problematic. In those cases requiring collateral ligament reattachment, it may be prudent to choose a prosthesis designed to provide some inherent medial-lateral constraint (e.g., constrained condylar knee). The postoperative management of the patient with a large allograft typically includes protected weightbearing for an extended period of time, particularly if the prosthesis is largely supported by allograft bone. In those cases, full weightbearing should be delayed until there is radiographic evidence of allograft incorporation.

METAL WEDGES AND AUGMENTS

Indications: Modular metal wedges and augments are particularly useful for moderate-size bony defects, particularly in older patients, and in revision knee surgery.

Limitations: Metal wedges and augments do not restore bone stock, which may be important in younger patients.

Modular metal wedges and block augments allow the intraoperative fabrication of a near-custom implant (Fig. 86.11). By selectively filling defects of the distal femur, posterior femur, and proximal tibia, the surgeon can maximize prosthetic contact with host bone. Metal wedges and blocks are not subject to the problems with incorporation, revascularization, or collapse that can occur with bone graft.[15] Laboratory data have demonstrated that modular wedges perform almost as well as custom implants in transmitting load across tibial defects.[5, 13] Modular implants are less expensive than custom implants and allow more intraoperative flexibility than do custom implants. Templating for a custom implant, particularly estimating the extent of bone loss, is fraught with difficulties. Inappropriate templating can result in the distressing intraoperative situation in which an expensive custom implant does not fit the patient.

Restoration of the joint line, balance of the flexion and extension gaps, and proper femoral rotational alignment can all be facilitated with the use of modular femoral wedges. Distal femoral wedges can compensate for distal femoral bone loss and thus allow the prosthetic joint line to be accurately restored. Reproducing the joint line both improves collateral ligament kinematic function and limits patellar impingement on the tibial component. To obtain equal flexion and extension spaces, it is often necessary to choose a femoral component with an anteroposterior dimension that is greater than the remaining host bone. Modular augmentation of the posterior femur can fill the gap between the prosthesis and the bone and allow the use of an appropriately sized femoral component. Femoral component rotation should be set parallel to the line that connects the medial and lateral epicondyles. Often, selectively augmenting the distal lateral femur slightly more than the distal medial femur aids in positioning the femoral component parallel to the transepicondylar axis. Care must be taken to avoid internal rotation of the femoral component relative to the transepidondylar axis because patellofemoral kinematics will be affected adversely.

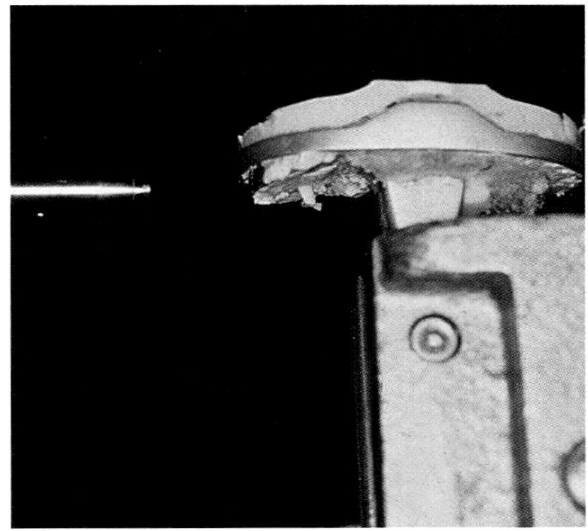

FIGURE 86.12 ➢ One cemented modular tibial wedge was retrieved after 6 years in vivo. The cement-wedge interface maintained 77% of its shear strength when compared with a freshly cemented wedge.

On the tibial side, in vitro data have been gathered that compare the use of metal wedges with the use of blocks in association with press-fit stems.[13] In that study, augmentation blocks performed slightly better than metal wedges, but the difference was small. Those authors concluded that in clinical practice the augment that best fills the bone defect should be chosen.

Clinical Results

Early and midterm results with the use of modular metal augments have been favorable.[4, 13, 31, 32] Long-term results are not available. The durability of the interface between the modular augments and the prosthesis has been questioned, but major problems have not emerged. One clinical retrieval of a cemented metal wedge showed that after 6 years in vivo the interface had maintained 77% of its shear strength as compared with a freshly cemented wedge (Fig. 86.12).[34] The study of Pagnano et al addressed modu-

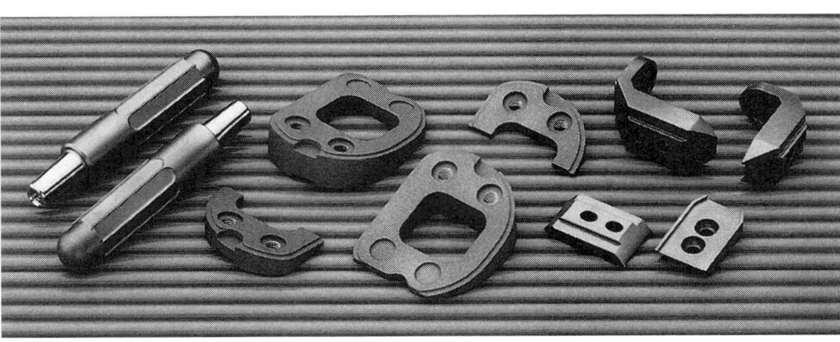

FIGURE 86.11 ➢ Modular metal wedges and blocks come in a variety of sizes and allow the intraoperative fabrication of a near-custom implant.

lar tibial augments in primary total knee arthroplasty and reviewed 25 knees in 21 patients.[31] At a mean follow-up of 4.8 years, excellent and good results were achieved in 96% of the patients. Although radiolucent lines were seen beneath the tibial component in 13 knees, none of those lucencies were progressive (Fig. 86.13).

Several studies have addressed the use of modular metal augments in revision total knee arthroplasty. Haas et al reviewed 76 revision knees with modular augments supplemented with press-fit intramedullary stems.[20] The intramedullary rods in that series were sized to obtain a so-called clinical press-fit but were not reamed to achieve intimate cortical contact in the diaphysis. At a mean follow-up of 3 years, excellent or good results were found in 84%. Survivorship of the implants was 83% at 8 years. Those authors felt that modular augmentation with press-fit rods was a reliable and durable procedure. Vince and Long reviewed 44 revisions with modular augmentations and press-fit intramedullary rods.[45] In 31 cases a posterior stabilized implant was used, and in 13 cases a constrained condylar implant was used. At follow-up of 2 to 6 years, 3 of the 13 constrained condylar knees had loosened, in contrast to none of the 31 posterior stabilized knees. Those authors initially suggested that press-fit rods may be inappropriate when coupled with a constrained condylar implant. Subsequent analysis has sug-

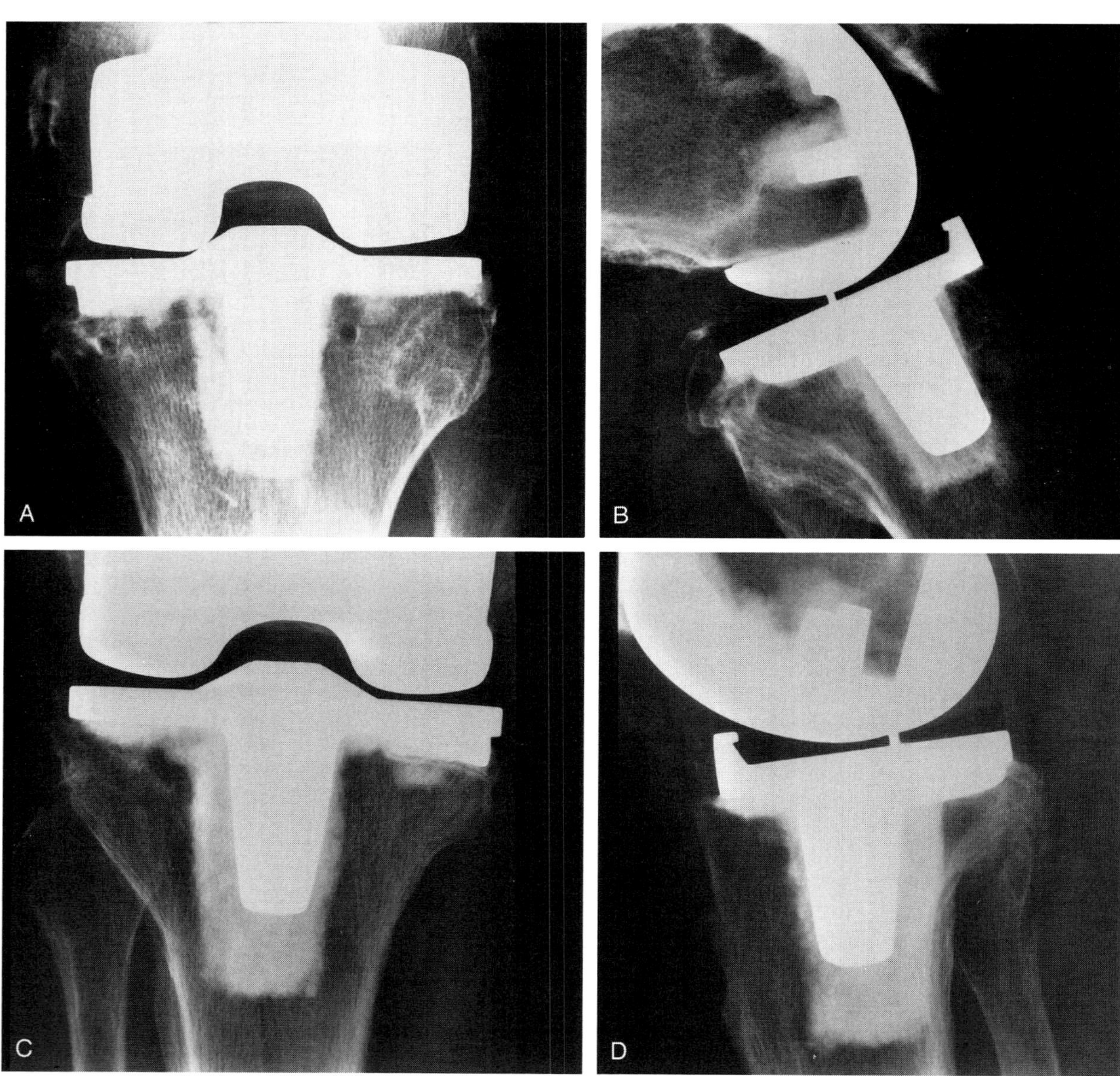

FIGURE 86.13 ➢ Anteroposterior (AP) (*A*) and lateral (*B*) views of a cemented modular metal wedge at 5 years demonstrate no radiolucency. AP (*C*) and lateral (*D*) views of a cemented modular wedge at 9 years show a nonprogressive radiolucent line beneath the wedge. The line was present in the early postoperative radiographs and showed no progression over 9 years.

gested that the mechanism of failure in those cases may have been related to suboptimal component alignment in part dictated by the intramedullary stem position. When press-fit stems dictate inappropriate component position, the surgeon must switch either to an off-set stem or to a smaller cemented stem to avoid component malposition (Fig. 86.14). Rand has studied 41 revision knees in which modular augmentation was used.[33] Modular augments were used for the distal femur alone in 2 knees, for the posterior femur alone in 16 knees, and for both the distal and the posterior femurs in 12 knees. Tibial augments were used medially in six knees, both medially and laterally in four knees, and as a custom augmentation in three knees. Intramedullary stems were used in all cases and included press-fit stems in 17 femurs and 16 tibias and cemented stems in 14 femurs and 13 tibias. At a mean of 3 years' follow-up, excellent and good results were found in 98% of the 41 revisions. There were no cases of loosening. Takahashi and Gustilo used the same implant system and reported satisfactory results in 39 cases at a mean of 20 months' follow-up.[42]

Surgical Technique

Tibial defects can be addressed with either metal wedges or metal blocks depending on the extent and location of the bony defect. Large metal wedges are also available that extend from one tibial condyle to the other. Most modular total knee systems have instrumentation that is designed to prepare the host tibia to accept a metal wedge or block. An intramedullary cutting guide can be useful because it will reproduce the component position that will be dictated by a press-fit intramedullary stem. Care must be taken to ensure that the tibial component is positioned perpendicular to the long axis of the tibia. If use of a press-fit stem will result in excessive varus or valgus positioning of the tibial component, then either a smaller-diameter cemented stem or an off-set tibial stem must be used. The surgeon must understand the design limits of the modular knee system he has chosen. In particular, he or she should realize that some intramedullary stems are not designed to be inserted with cement. Once proper axial alignment has been verified, the proximal tibia can be cut. In the revision situation, this is done as a freshening cut that removes 1 to 2 mm of bone from the more prominent side to provide a flat surface for the tibial baseplate. The tibial bone loss is surveyed, and an appropriately sized wedge or block is selected. A cutting guide for the block or wedge can then be assembled and a matching bone resection carried out. Care must be taken to set the tibial component rotation before the resection for the wedge or block. That step ensures that the real component, with its modular metal wedge, will sit flush with the resection and be appropriately aligned and rotated relative to the femoral component. The trial tibial component with the wedge or block and the intramedullary stem is assembled and trialed. If any questions about limb alignment or component position exist, then an intraoperative x-ray is obtained. The real components should be assembled and then inspected by the surgeon before cementing. Care must be taken to ensure that the appropriate-size component and stem have been assembled and that the augment positions are correct. If an off-set stem has been selected, verify that it is off-set in the proper direction. The real prosthesis can then be cemented into place.

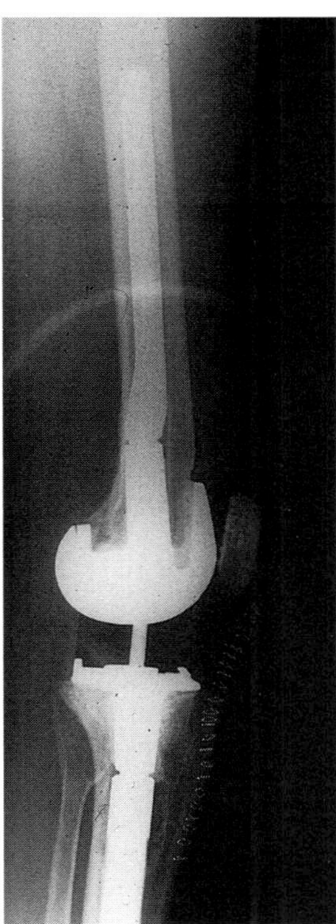

FIGURE 86.14 ➢ Off-set intramedullary stems are useful on both the femoral and the tibial sides. Here, an off-set femoral stem brings the femoral component more posteriorly and allows it to sit flush with the anterior cortex of the distal femur.

Femoral augmentation blocks are used to restore the joint line, fill the flexion space, and ensure femoral rotational alignment parallel to the transepicondylar axis. An intramedullary cutting guide is assembled, and the distal femoral cut should be freshened to provide a flat surface off which the revision prosthesis is assembled. Many revision systems will have rod-and-sleeve guides that allow the cuts to be made relative to the position dictated by a press-fit intramedullary rod. The first task is to choose the appropriate femoral component. Preoperative templating of the opposite knee can be useful in determining the proper femoral component size. In many failed total knees, there is a marked loss of posterior femoral bone, and the surgeon must avoid the temptation to downsize the femoral component to match the existing bone stock. A smaller femoral component may inadequately fill the flexion gap and could result in flexion instability. Once the proper size component has been selected, then the joint line must be reestablished. The most appropriate means in the revision setting is to identify the epicondyles and then measure distally from them. Typically, the joint line is 2.5 cm distal to the medial epicondyle. Distal augmentation blocks are then added to the femoral prosthesis to restore the joint line position. Femoral component rotation should be established by drawing a line across the distal femur that connects the medial and lateral epicondyles. The intercondylar box-cutting guide should then be rotated parallel to that line. When distal femoral augmentation is being used, the box-cutting guide should be moved distally a corresponding amount. That maneuver will preserve host bone in the intercondylar region. Finally, posterior femoral wedges are used to fill the gap between the posterior femoral runners and the posterior femur. Care is taken to avoid overstuffing the posterior medial side because this would tend to cause a compensatory internal rotation of the femoral component. The real component is then assembled and carefully inspected by the surgeon before cementing.

STEMS

Most revision total knee arthroplasties are cemented, at least at the condylar surface. Controversy still exists regarding cemented or press-fit fixation of intramedullary stems.[49] A common approach is to apply cement to the condylar surface and around the proximal portion of the stem-prosthesis housing but to press-fit the stem itself.[20] Care is taken with that approach to avoid cement at the junction between the stem and the baseplate because that cement can markedly interfere with component removal should revision be needed. Good results have been reported with the technique of cemented revision with press-fit intramedullary rods. Other authors have had good results with fully cemented rods (Fig. 86.15). Murray et al used cemented long stems in 40 revision total knee arthroplasties and found no cases of loosening at an average of 5 years' follow-up.[29] Rand has suggested that the choice of a cemented or press-fit intramedullary stem should be based on the bone quality and the effect of the rod on implant alignment.[33] A press-fit stem is preferred in most situations because it facilitates susequent revision. However, a press-fit rod may not be appropriate in the face of markedly osteopenic bone, with marked metaphyseal deformity, or in cases where the press-fit rod would result in limb malalignment or component malposition. Typically, one should not cement an intramedullary rod that has been designed for insertion in a press-fit fashion (Fig. 86.16). Most rods designed for

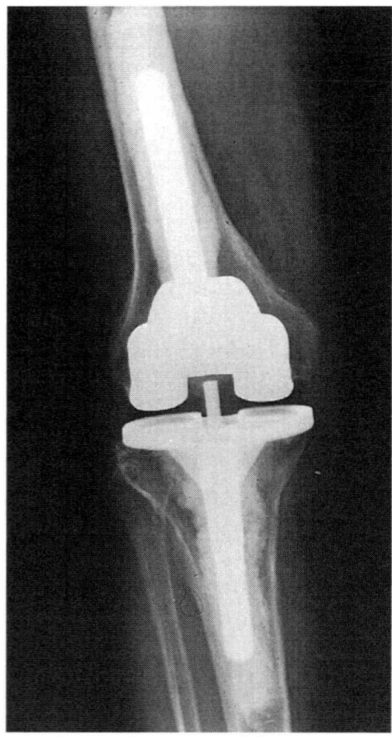

FIGURE 86.15 ➢ Fully cemented femoral and tibial rods after revision total knee arthroplasty.

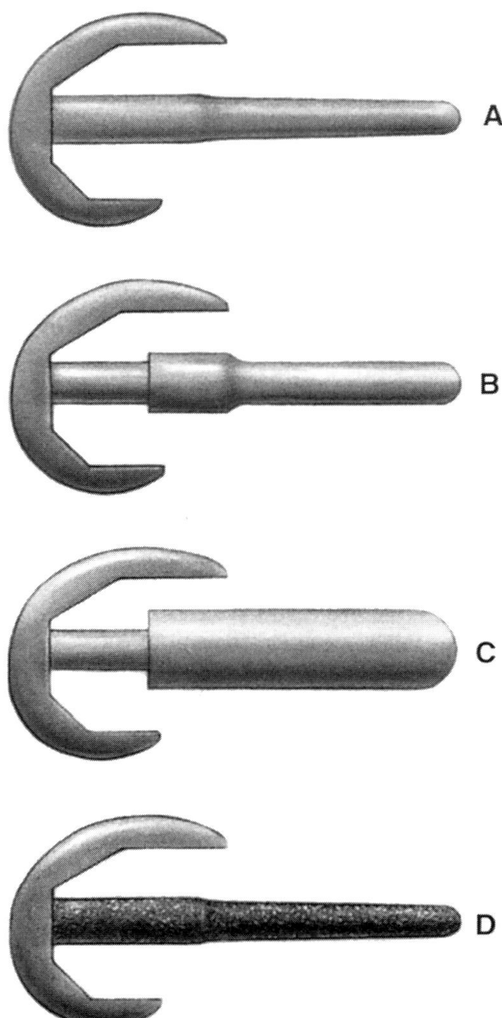

FIGURE 86.16 ➢ Smooth, tapered stems (*A*) are designed for insertion with bone cement. Stems with complex geometries (*B, C*) or with porous coating (*D*) should not be inserted with cement around the stem itself. (From Garino JP, Lotke PA: Fixation techniques in revision total knee surgery. In Lotke PA, Garino JP, eds: Revision Total Knee Arthroplasty. Philadelphia, Lippincott-Raven, 1999.)

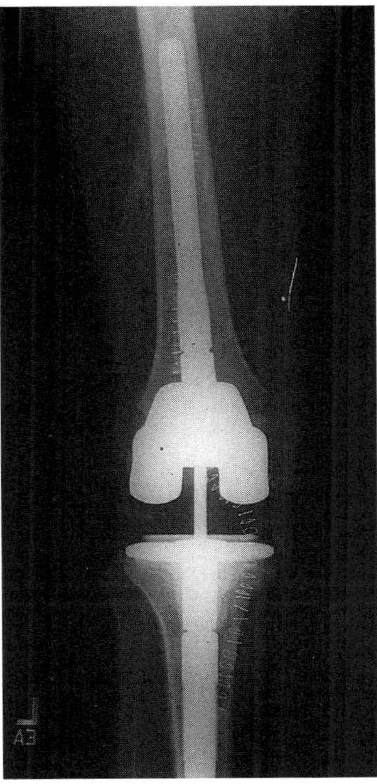

FIGURE 86.17 ➢ Press-fit rods are often fluted. Those rods should not be inserted with cement because the sharp flutes create an unfavorable cement-prosthesis interface.

insertion with cement have gently rounded surfaces to minimize stresses on the cement-prosthesis interface. In contrast, most press-fit rods are fluted. Those flutes cause high stresses at the bone-cement interface that could lead to cement mantle fracture (Fig. 86.17).

SUMMARY

Successfully reconstructing the knee with marked bone deficiency requires careful preoperative planning to ensure that the appropriate prosthetic components and allograft bone are available. Small defects localized to one condyle can be successfully addressed using autograft or allograft bone or with a modular metal wedge or block. Alternatively, small defects can be contoured into a step configuration and filled with bone cement. Larger tibial defects can be reconstituted with large modular wedges or blocks and a thicker polyethylene insert (Fig. 86.18). Structural allograft reconstruction of the tibia is typically required when the degree of bone loss results in a flexion-extension gap that exceeds 40 mm. At that point, the thickest modular augments and thickest polyethylene inserts of most modular revision knee systems will fail to fill the gaps adequately. On the femoral side, 12-mm augmentation blocks are commonly available, but defects of greater size will require structural grafts. Any reconstruction that requires extensive bone grafting or modular augmentation is best protected by an intramedullary stem that bypasses the defect. The choice of press-fit or cemented intramedullary stem fixation is dictated by the quality of the metaphyseal bone, the extent of bone loss, and the effect of the rod on implant and limb alignment.

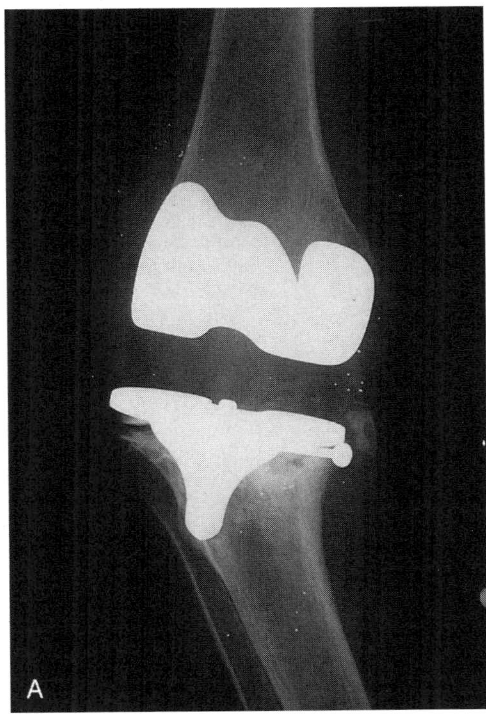

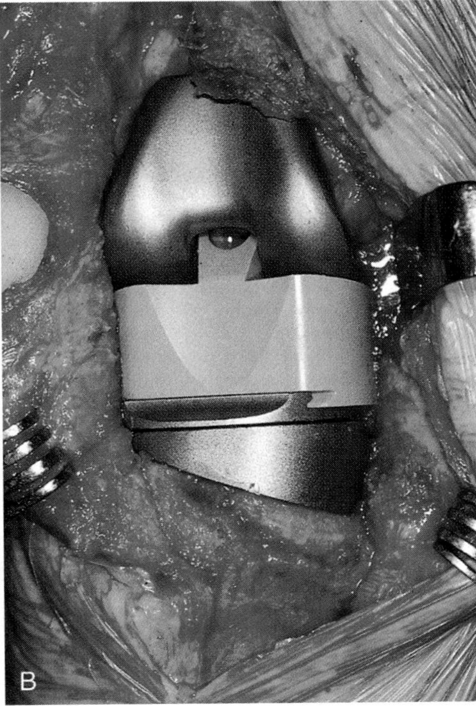

FIGURE 86.18 ➢ Marked medial tibial bone loss is seen on the preoperative radiograph (*A*). That defect is adequately filled with a full metal wedge and a thick tibial insert (*B*).

References

1. Aglietti P, Buzzi R, Scrobe F: Autologous bone grafting for medial defects in total knee arthroplasty. J Arthroplasty 6(4):287, 1991.
2. Altchek D, Sculco TP, Rawlins B: Autogenous bone grafting for severe angular deformity in total knee arthroplasty. J Arthroplasty 4(2):151, 1989.
3. Bourne RB, Finlay JB: The influence of tibial component intramedullary stems and implant-cortex contact on the strain distribution of the proximal tibia following total knee arthroplasty. Clin Orthop 208:95, 1986.
4. Brand MG, Daley RJ, Ewald FC, et al: Tibial tray augmentation with modular metal wedges for tibial bone stock deficiency. Clin Orthop 248:71, 1989.
5. Brooks P, Walker P, Scott R: Tibial component fixation in deficient tibial bone stock. Clin Orthop 184:302, 1984.
6. Buck BE, Malinin TI, Brown MD: Bone transplantation and human immunodeficiency virus: An estimate of acquired immunodeficiency virus syndrome (AIDS). Clin Orthop 240:129, 1989.
7. Campbell DG, Li P, Stephenson AJ, et al: Sterilization of HIV by gamma irradiation: A bone allograft model. Int Orthop 18:172, 1994.
8. Chen F, Krackow K: Management of tibial defects in total knee arthroplasty. Clin Orthop 305:249, 1994.
9. Dennis, DA: Structural allografting in revision total knee arthroplasty. In Insall JN, Scott WN, Scuderi GR, eds: Current Concepts in Primary and Revision Total Knee Arthroplasty. Philadelphia, Lippincott-Raven, 1996.
10. Dorr LD, Ranawat CS, Sculco TA, et al: Bone graft for tibial defects in total knee arthroplasty. Clin Orthop 205:153, 1986.
11. Elia E, Lotke PA: Results of revision total knee arthroplasty associated with significant bone loss. Clin Orthop 271:114, 1991.
12. Engh G, Parks NL: The classification and treatment options for bone defects in revision knee surgery [abstract]. Presented at the American Academy of Orthopedic Surgeons, February 24–28, 1994.
13. Fehring T, Peindl R, Humble R, et al: Modular tibial augmentation in total knee arthroplasty. Clin Orthop 327:207, 1996.
14. Freeman MAR, Bradley GW, Revell PA: Observations upon the interface between bone and polymethylmethacrylate cement. J Bone Joint Surg Br 64:489, 1982.
15. Garbuz DS, Masri BA, Czitrom AA: Biology of allografting. Orthop Clin North Am 29:199, 1998.
16. Garino JP, Lotke PA: Fixation techniques in revision total knee surgery. In Lotke PA, Garino JP, eds: Revision Total Knee Arthroplasty. Philadelphia, Lippincott-Raven, 1999.
17. Ghazavi MT, Stockley I, Yee G, et al: Reconstruction of massive bone defects with allograft in revision total knee arthroplasty. J Bone Joint Surg Am 79:17, 1997.
18. Gie GA, Linder L, Ling RS, et al: Contained morsellised allograft in revision total hip arthroplasty: Surgical technique. Orthop Clin North Am 24:717, 1993.
19. Gie GA, Linder L, Ling RSM, et al: Impacted cancellous allografts and cement for revision total hip arthroplasty. J Bone Joint Surg Br 75:14, 1993.
20. Haas S, Insall J, Montgomery W, et al: Revision total knee arthroplasty with use of modular components with stems inserted without cement. J Bone Joint Surg Am 77:1700, 1995.
21. Harris AL, Poddar S, Gitelis S, et al: Arthroplasty with a composite of an allograft and a prosthesis for knees with severe deficiency of bone. J Bone Joint Surg Am 77:373, 1995.
22. Harada Y, Wevers HW, Ir I, et al: Distribution of bone strength in the proximal tibia. J Arthroplasty 3(2):167, 1988.
23. Hvid I: Trabecular bone strength at the knee. Clin Orthop 227: 210, 1988.
24. Insall JN: Revision of aseptic failed total knee arthroplasty. In Insall JN, ed: Surgery of the Knee, 2nd ed. New York, Churchill-Livingstone, 1993.
25. Kraay MJ, Goldberg VM, Figgie MP, et al: Distal femoral replacement with allograft/prosthetic reconstruction for treatment of supracondylar fractures in patients with total knee arthroplasty. J Arthroplasty 7(1):7, 1992.
26. Laskin RS: Total knee arthroplasty in the presence of large bony defects of the tibia and marked knee instability. Clin Orthop 248:66, 1989.
27. Mnaymneh W, Emerson RH, Borja F, et al: Massive allografts in salvage revision of failed total knee arthroplasty. Clin Orthop 260:144, 1990.
28. Mow CS, Weidel JD: Structural allografting in revision total knee arthroplasty. J Arthroplasty 11:235, 1996.
29. Murray PB, Rand JA, Hanssen AD: Cemented long stem revision total knee arthroplasty. Clin Orthop 309:116, 1994.
30. Nielssen RG, Bauer TW, Weidenhelm LR, et al: Revision hip arthroplasty with the use of cement and impaction grafting: Histological analysis of four cases. J Bone Joint Surg Am 77:412, 1995.
31. Pagnano MW, Trousdale RT, Rand JA: Tibial wedge augmentation for bone deficiency in total knee arthroplasty—a followup study. Clin Orthop 321:151, 1995.
32. Rand JA: Bone deficiency in total knee arthroplasty: Use of metal wedge augmentation. Clin Orthop 271:63, 1991.
33. Rand J: Modularity in total knee arthroplasty. Acta Orthop Belg 62:180, 1996.
34. Rand J: Augmentation of a total knee arthroplasty with a modular metal wedge. J Bone Joint Surg Am 77:266, 1995.
35. Ritter MA: Screw and cement fixation of large defects in total knee arthroplasty. J Arthroplasty 1:125, 1986.
36. Ritter MA, Keating EM, Faris PM: Screw and cement fixation of large defects in total knee arthroplasty. A sequel. J Arthroplasty 8:63, 1993.
37. Samuelson KM: Bone grafting and noncemented revision arthroplasty of the knee. Clin Orthop 226:93, 1988.
38. Scuderi GR, Insall JH, Haas SB, et al: Inlay autogenic bone grafting of tibial defects in primary total knee arthroplasty. Clin Orthop 248:93, 1989.
39. Sculco TP: Bone grafting. In Lotke PA, ed: Master Techniques in Orthopedic Surgery, Knee Arthroplasty. New York, Raven Press, 1995.
40. Sneppen D, Christensen P, Larsen H, et al: Mechanical testing of trabecular bone in total knee replacement. Development of an osteopenetrometer. Int Orthop 5:251, 1981.
41. Stockley I, McAuley JP, Gross AE: Allograft reconstruction in total knee arthroplasty. J Bone Joint Surg Br 74:393, 1992.
42. Takahashi Y, Gustilo R: Nonconstrained implants in revision total knee arthroplasty. Clin Orthop 309:156, 1994.
43. Tsahakis PJ, Beaver WB, Brick GW: Technique and results of allograft reconstruction in revision total knee arthroplasty. Clin Orthop 303:86, 1994.
44. Ullmark G, Hovelius L: Impacted morselized allograft and cement for revision total knee arthroplasty: A preliminary report of 3 cases. Acta Orthop Scand 67:10, 1996.
45. Vince KG, Long W: Revision knee arthroplasty: The limits of press fit medullary fixation. Clin Orthop 317:172, 1995.
46. Whiteside LA: Cementless revision total knee arthroplasty. Clin Orthop 286:160, 1993.
47. Wilde AW, Schickendantz MS, Stulberg BN, et al: The incorporation of tibial allografts in total knee arthroplasty J Bone Joint Surg Am 72:815, 1990.
48. Windsor RE, Insall JN, Sculco TP: Bone grafting of tibial defects in primary and revision total knee arthroplasty. Clin Orthop 205: 132, 1986.
49. Winemaker M, Beingessner D, Rorabeck CH: Revision total knee arthroplasty: Should tibial stems be cemented or uncemented. In The Knee, in press.

87 Complications of Total Knee Arthroplasty

MARC F. BRASSARD • JOHN N. INSALL • GILES R. SCUDERI

GENERAL COMPLICATIONS

Despite the advanced age of most patients and the frequency of associated medical conditions such as arteriosclerotic heart disease, hypertension, diabetes, and chronic pulmonary disorders, the general complications of knee arthroplasty are relatively few. As with any substantial surgery, the major complications include cerebrovascular accidents, myocardial infarctions, and pulmonary embolism. In the postoperative period, patients are at risk for urinary retention and infections as well as deep vein thrombosis (DVT). However, considering that total knee arthroplasty (TKA) is a major surgical event, it is surprising that the operation can be performed so safely, especially when bilateral simultaneous procedures are done.[26, 197, 229] Several authors studied this aspect and failed to demonstrate increased risk with the bilateral procedures. The risk of a catastrophic medical event is, therefore, rare in a patient who is carefully monitored. Careful preoperative evaluation is essential, and the patient must be in the best possible medical health. The type of anesthesia is probably not critical, although we prefer epidural anesthesia. Intraoperative monitoring includes the use of a Swan-Ganz catheter in selected unilateral and most bilateral cases.

SYSTEMIC COMPLICATIONS

Thromboembolism

The importance of thromboembolic disease after TKA is controversial.[40, 67, 68, 83, 84, 100, 110, 118, 129, 173, 176, 178] It is undeniable and widely accepted that DVT occurs in approximately 50% of unilateral cases and in as many as 75% of bilateral cases when no prophylaxis is used. Although DVT occurs mainly in the calf veins (Fig. 87.1), life-threatening emboli do not arise from this region. Unlike the situation after total hip arthroplasty (THA), isolated proximal vein thrombosis does not seem to occur after knee surgery despite the possible trauma of a pneumatic tourniquet.

Some authors argued that distal thrombosis can be ignored, provided the patient convalesces normally and is not confined to bed for a lengthy period. We believe this view is too optimistic, although we concede that the risk of a fatal thromboembolus is small and is certainly lower than after THA. However, fatal emboli do occur, and 3 patients died of this cause in the first 400 arthroplasties performed at the Hospital for Special Surgery. No specific prophylaxis was used at that time; the cause of death was confirmed by autopsy in all cases. We believe that the incidence of fatal pulmonary emboli is underestimated. It is recognized that a certain proportion of calf clots propagate proximally to form the more dangerous clots in the popliteal and femoral veins. However, this process takes time; therefore, the major risk period for a fatal pulmonary embolism after TKA may be in the 3rd and 4th week after surgery (unlike the case after THA, in which a clot in the proximal veins may be found in one-fifth of cases after the 1st week). Because most total knee patients are now discharged after hospitalization of 4 to 7 days, sudden death at home in a patient having no clinical evidence of vein thrombosis may be attributed to myocardial infarction. It is also unlikely that an autopsy will be obtained.

Calf clots may not in themselves be important, but should be regarded as a harbinger of more proximal clotting. Haas et al[100] studied 1329 patients with 1697 TKAs. Thrombosis was found in 808 patients (61%): 53% had thrombosis of the calf vein and 8% had thrombosis of the proximal veins. The lung scans of 60 patients (4.5%) were positive, and symptomatic pulmonary emboli occurred in 14 patients (1.1%). All of these patients received aspirin as prophylaxis. Venography was performed between the 4th and 6th postoperative days. A perfusion lung scan obtained on the 5th to 7th day was compared with a preoperative baseline perfusion lung scan. Thrombosis of the calf vein was treated with warfarin (Coumadin); the dosage was adjusted to maintain a prothrombin time at approximately 1.5 times control. Only patients with symptomatic proximal thrombi or symptomatic pulmonary emboli were fully anticoagulated with intravenous heparin.

Although the natural history of thromboembolic disease was altered by prophylaxis and treatment, 6.5% of the patients with calf thrombi had a positive lung scan and 1.6% had symptomatic pulmonary emboli. This was compared with the patients who had no venographic evidence of DVT, of whom 1.9% had a positive lung scan and 0.2% had symptomatic pulmonary emboli. Statistical significance for the difference in lung scan and pulmonary embolus (PE) results were $p = .001$ and $p = .034$, respectively. Patients with calf or proximal thrombi were found to have similar rates of positive lung scans and symptomatic pulmonary emboli.

Kakkar et al[142] used venography and serial fibrinogen imaging to evaluate the progress of calf thrombi in

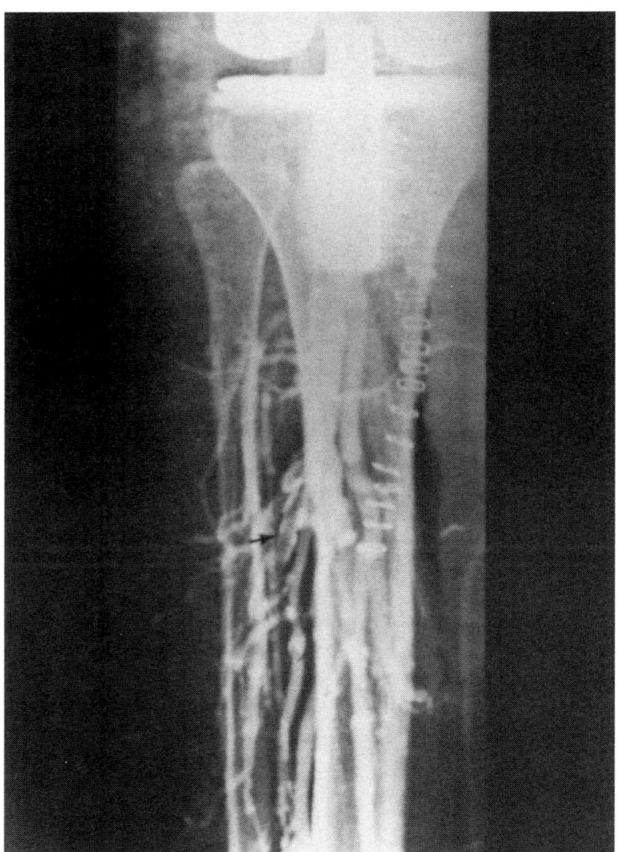

FIGURE 87.1 ➢ Venogram showing clots in the calf veins.

a group of postoperative patients. They found that 23% of calf thrombi propagated to the proximal veins. Doouss[58] performed a similar study and found a 5.6% propagation rate.

Detection of DVT

Many studies showed that clinical detection of DVT is unreliable. Both false-positive and false-negative results abound. The current trend in detection of DVT is the use of Doppler ultrasound.[155, 292] The sensitivity and specificity of ultrasound are approaching those of the gold standard in detection: contrast venography. The sensitivity of ultrasound is reported between 89% and 100%, the specificity between 95% and 100%, and the accuracy between 97% and 99%. However, these numbers apply to thigh clots only between the inguinal ligament and the popliteal vein. Another potential disadvantage of Doppler ultrasound is that the accuracy of the test may vary because it is technician/operator dependent. The distinct advantage of ultrasound over venography is that it is noninvasive and causes minimal discomfort for the patient, thus allowing for serial exams after surgery. Another advantage is that it will localize and quantitate the clot, which enables documentation of any changes in size and propagation. Other reliable objective diagnostic methods include iodine 125 fibrinogen scanning, impedance plethysmography, and ascending venography (see Fig. 87.1) for the diagnosis of venous thrombosis and ventilation-perfusion lung scanning and pulmonary angiography for pulmonary embolism. Iodine 125 fibrinogen scanning provides confusing data after knee surgery, and impedance plethysmography is logistically demanding. Currently, we use Doppler ultrasound on postoperative day 3 and 3 weeks postoperatively. Because we continue to have an interest in the natural history of DVT, we obtain a preoperative lung scan and a follow-up scan on postoperative day 3. This protocol may not be necessary as part of the routine screening.

The incidence of DVT after a TKA without prophylaxis is between 50% to 84% in the ipsilateral extremity. In the contralateral extremity, it is 3% to 5%.[171] Some confusion arises when discussing DVT based on the location of the thrombus. Most authors agree that thrombi below the popliteal vein are common and probably of little consequence, but they can propagate and become larger thrombi with more serious consequences. Larcom et al[161] determined that proximal DVT occurs in only 5% to 8% of TKA and THA. Many authors[100, 118, 166, 184] agree that isolated proximal venous thrombosis is infrequent after TKA, especially compared with THA.

Newer technology for the detection of DVT is being developed. One of the newer diagnostic modalities is magnetic resonance venography (MRV).[161] The major advantages of MRV over traditional contrast venography is that it is noninvasive. Its major advantage over venography and Doppler ultrasound is its ability to detect clots in the pelvis, for which both of the other techniques have extremely limited detection capability. Autopsy results from fatal pulmonary embolism show very large thrombi that seem to originate in the large veins of the thigh and pelvis immediately before their dislodgement.[161] This finding demonstrates the importance of detecting pelvic DVT. Larcom et al[161] performed a study comparing MRV with standard contrast venography. They found only a 45% sensitivity of MRV when interpreted by a dedicated magnetic resonance angiographer. This study demonstrates the need for further development of this technique. However, with improved equipment and more experience in interpretation, MRV could become the preferred technique.

Prophylaxis

DVT prophylaxis after TKA is still a prudent decision to make. With DVT rate as high as 80% after TKA with no prophylaxis, it is mandatory that the patient receive some form of prophylaxis. There is no clear-cut favorite for the one best form of prophylaxis. Those most commonly used include aspirin, low-molecular-weight heparin (LMWH), warfarin, heparin, and compression devices. Other methods that have lost popularity include low-molecular-weight dextran, antithrombin III, and elastic stockings. We review the more commonly used agents.

Warfarin has been in use for almost 50 years. Debates are still waged over its advantages versus disadvantages. Because warfarin is an oral agent, patient compliance is improved. There is low potential for excessive bleeding if careful control is maintained.[161] However, this characteristic is also a drawback because monitoring the prothrombin time requires weekly phlebotomy, which many patients find inconvenient as well as painful. This vigilant monitoring is essential to prevent excessive bleeding complications in the knee and other locations. Another important disadvantage is that the patient cannot take any aspirin or nonsteroidal anti-inflammatory medications (NSAIDs).[171]

Aspirin for the prevention of DVT is another controversial method. Most of the literature published on aspirin is from THA literature. As with warfarin, aspirin is an oral agent, making it is easy to take on discharge from the hospital. Another advantage of aspirin is its low dose and high patient tolerance. Because it is such a small pill, patients have an easier time swallowing it. Also its relatively low cost and over-the-counter availability make it an easier medication to obtain. The major disadvantage of aspirin is gastrointestinal (GI) intolerance, ranging from GI upset to ulcers. In addition, patients are reluctant to accept this common medication as an effective preventive measure for such a serious complication.[171]

LMWH has gained in popularity. In comparison to heparin, LMWH is a smaller and more homogenous molecule, which accounts for its more favorable binding affinity to activated factors X and II. This mechanism of action results in an antithrombotic effect that is exerted earlier in the clotting cascade and theoretically decreases the risk of concurrent bleeding complications compared with the risk with unfractionated heparin.[10] An advantage of fractionated heparin (LMWH) is that coagulation times do not need to be monitored. Also there is a decrease in side effects (i.e., thrombocytopenia) compared with heparin, and LMWH half-life is prolonged, which reduces its dosage requirements. Outpatient compliance may be limited because LMWH requires subcutaneous injection. Another limitation may be its restricted use with epidural anesthesia. There have been reports of epidural hematomas forming after the epidural was removed with patients on LMWH. Overall, some authors indicated there is an increase in bleeding complications, both at the operative wound and at the injection site with the use of LMWH.

Mechanical compression is basically one of two types: plantar compression or calf/thigh compression. Plantar compression (foot pumps) (Fig. 87.2) has been gaining in popularity in recent years. The foot pumps work by producing a forceful ejection of blood from the foot into the calf with a pressure of greater than 100 mm Hg (versus traditional calf compression devices providing a pressure of 20 to 30 mm Hg). The pulse wave originates in the plantar venous plexus and flows proximally into the popliteal and femoral veins, which can be demonstrated with both venography and Doppler ultrasound.[280] The foot pumps prevent DVT by (1) increasing the venous return, (2) inducing high-flow states, which increase turbulence around venous valves thus decrease the formation of thrombi, (3) increasing blood flow and tissue perfusion with the release of endothelial-derived relaxing factor and prostacyclin,[87] and (4) enhancing fibrinolysis with use of external pneumatic compression.[6] The advantages of compression devices as a whole include no medications to administer and no monitoring. Additional benefits of the foot pumps themselves include decreased postoperative thigh circumference and decreased wound drainage.[280] The disadvantages of external compression devices include patient compliance and the cost of the machines. There has been one report of a peroneal nerve palsy associated with the use of pneumatic compression device.[212]

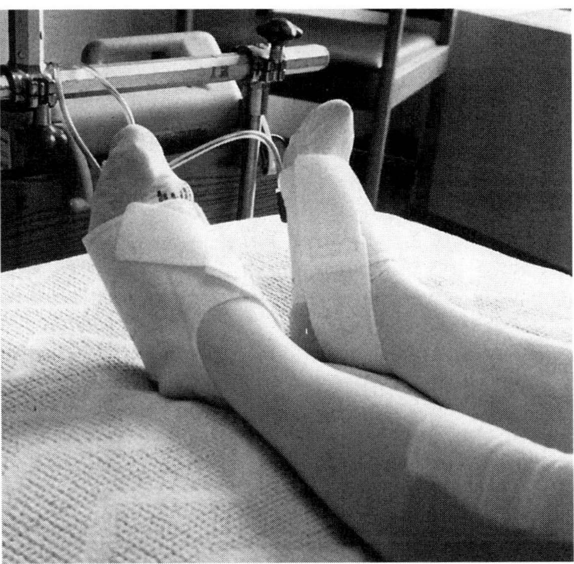

FIGURE 87.2 ➢ An example of a foot compression device. It provides intermittent, pulsatile plantar compression.

The standard external compression devices that compress either the calf or thigh have similar advantages to the plantar compression devices. Additional advantages of the calf-high sleeves are keeping pressure off the operative site and reducing the prevalence of thrombosis in the calf veins after a TKA.[100] The disadvantage of the thigh-high compression sleeves is that it covers the wound and could compress the operative site.

The question of which mode of DVT prophylaxis should be used has been debated for many years. There have been many conflicting studies, and there is no ideal method for DVT prophylaxis. Warfarin remains one of the most popular methods used today. Most studies demonstrate that when warfarin is used alone, it will decrease the rate of DVT. Laflamme et al[159] used warfarin in TKA patients and found a DVT incidence of 21% and no PE. They also had a 0.9% incidence of major bleeding and minor bleeding but no wound problems. Kaempffe et al[141] compared warfarin and pneumatic compression in THA and TKA patients. In TKA patients, warfarin was more effective than compression (19% versus 32%), but after THA compression was more effective than warfarin (16% versus 24%). The sampling size was small in this study, so the conclusion is somewhat limited. Hodge[107] compared warfarin to pneumatic calf compression after TKA. Again the sample size was small. In the warfarin patients, he found a DVT incidence of 30% with 6% in the thigh. In the compression group, he found a DVT incidence of 31% also with 6% in the thigh. The warfarin group had an increase in expenses of 50% compared with the compression group. Therefore, the author concluded that both forms are safe and effective, but compression devices are more economical.

In a study by Stulberg et al[258] of 517 patients with 638 total knee arthroplasties, 84% of 49 patients who did not receive prophylaxis experienced ipsilateral DVT. All the patients in this study had postoperative venograms performed for the detection of DVT. The incidence of thrombosis was 57% in the 468 patients who received some form of prophylaxis (aspirin, low-dose heparin, supplemented low-dose aspirin, or warfarin). In 11% there was evidence of thrombosis in the thigh or popliteal veins or both. Of the patients with bilateral TKA, 74% had evidence of thrombosis. No isolated popliteal or femoral clots were encountered.

Other studies compared the other forms of DVT prophylaxis. Haas et al[100] compared compression devices with aspirin after unilateral and bilateral TKA. In the unilateral group, the incidence of DVT in the compression group was 22% versus 47% in the aspirin group. In the bilateral group, the incidence of DVT in the compression group was 48% versus 68% in the aspirin group. The authors recommended the use of compression devices in unilateral TKA. Wilson et al[288] compared plantar compression devices with no prophylaxis. In a small sampling size, they found 0% DVT in the plantar compression group versus 19% in the no prophylaxis group. Westrich and Sculco[280] compared plantar compression and aspirin with aspirin alone. Overall, in unilateral and bilateral TKA, the compression plus aspirin group had a DVT rate of 27% compared with 59% in the aspirin alone group. Significantly, with the proximal thrombi being considered the most likely to embolize, they found no proximal thrombi in the compression group and 14% incidence in the aspirin alone group. Another key point in this study is the patient compliance factor and the amount of time the compression devices were worn. In the group that experienced DVT, the patients wore the devices an average of 13.4 h/day. Meanwhile, the group that did not experience DVT wore them 19.2 hours/day.

Many studies have examined the efficacy of LMWH. Colwell et al[43] compared LMWH with heparin. The incidence of DVT in the LMWH group was 24.6% and 34.2% in the heparin group. Fitzgerald et al[81] compared LMWH with low-dose heparin after TKA. They found that LMWH had a DVT incidence of 25% versus 45% for low-dose heparin. Levine et al[166] compared LMWH with compression stockings. They reported a DVT incidence of 29.8% in the LMWH group and 58.3% in the compression group. Also of interest in this study was that the incidence of bleeding events were similar between the two groups: 2.5% in the LMWH group and 2.4% in the compression group. Leclerc et al[163] compared LMWH with warfarin and found a 36.9% incidence of DVT in the LMWH group compared with 51.7% in the warfarin group. A similar incidence of bleeding events was also discovered. Spiro et al[253] examined LMWH and warfarin after TKA. LMWH had a lower incidence of DVT at 25.4% compared with warfarin at 45.4%. Proximal clots were also lower in the LMWH group, 1.7%, versus 11.4% in the warfarin group. They did find an increased incidence of hemorrhagic complications in the LMWH group, 6.9% compared with 3.4% in the warfarin group.

Currently, no one form of DVT prophylaxis enjoys wide-ranging acceptance because of the side effects, complications, or conflicting data on DVT incidence. The ideal prophylaxis method would be effective immediately postoperatively and last for at least 6 weeks. Currently, this profile of coverage requires two simultaneous methods. For example, warfarin has been shown to be an effective agent, but it requires several days to become effective. Maynard et al[184] demonstrated that a majority of thromboses form in the intraoperative or immediate postoperative period. Therefore, warfarin is not effective in preventing these clots. Maynard et al[184] also demonstrated that all thromboses propagated into or above the popliteal vein despite warfarin therapy initiated at the time of initial positive venogram. On the basis of this information, the ideal prophylaxis would be effective immediately in the recovery room, like compression devices. Then the ideal prophylaxis would remain effective for at least 6 weeks, until the patient resumes normal independent motion and the native muscles provide the necessary compressive forces.

We are examining a study protocol that evaluates warfarin alone, foot pumps alone, and both methods together. Ten milligrams of warfarin is given the night of surgery, and then no warfarin is given on postoperative day 1. Starting on postoperative day 2, it is given according to the daily prothrombin time. The goal is maintenance of a prothrombin time of 1.3 to 1.5 times the control (2 to 2.5 times the international normalized ratio). The warfarin is continued on discharge home; the patient has weekly monitoring of prothrombin times. We obtain a Doppler ultrasound and lung scan on postoperative day 3 and 3 weeks postoperatively. If the ultrasound at 3 weeks is negative, the warfarin is discontinued. If the ultrasound is positive, then the warfarin is continued for a total of 6 weeks. All of the patients wear thigh-high compression stockings from the recovery room to 6 weeks postoperatively.

Protocol for Patients With Documented Thromboembolic Disease

Positive Venography or Ultrasound

Patients with calf, popliteal, or femoral thrombi are treated with warfarin for a period of 6 weeks. Asymptomatic pulmonary emboli are treated in the same manner.

Symptomatic proximal thrombi and symptomatic pulmonary emboli[275] are treated with heparin until the effect of warfarin is established. Based on the discretion of the individual medical consultant, heparin treatment intravenously may be continued for as long as 1 week.

Intravenous heparin carries an extreme risk of local bleeding complications, and, in our opinion, should be used only in potentially life-threatening situations. This policy may sometimes cause conflict among medical advisors, who often may wish to use heparin in less threatening circumstances. We recommend that orthopedic surgeons plan their own policy and guidelines within their own institution.

Greenfield Filter

When warfarin prophylaxis fails to prevent a PE, when warfarin is contraindicated in a high-risk patient, or when complications develop as a result of anticoagulation, a Greenfield filter should be considered. Vaughn et al[270] reported on its use in 66 patients and found the technique to be safe, easy, and effective. They inserted the filter preoperatively in 42 patients who were considered at high risk for PE (group I) and postoperatively in 24 patients (group II). The preferred site of insertion was by way of the right internal jugular vein, and the implantations were done by a vascular surgeon. One patient in group II died of a massive pulmonary embolism 3 days after implantation. At follow-up, none of the remaining patients experienced migration of the filter, nor was there any evidence of postphlebitic syndrome or chronic symptomatic edema of the lower extremity.

Fat Embolism Syndrome

The diagnosis of fat embolism can be elusive,[17, 31, 60, 71, 194] and we suspect the condition may often pass unrecognized as the cause of transient confusional states after surgery. The syndrome results from the embolization of fat from the femur or tibia and travels mostly to the lungs. The initial effects in the lungs are mechanical, with an increase in perfusion pressure, engorgement of the vessels in the lungs, and secondary right-sided heart strain. In the presence of hypovolemic shock, the patient may die from acute right-sided heart failure. The delayed effects of fat embolism occur after 48 to 72 hours because of the chemical effects of fat. The pulmonary tissue secretes lipase, which hydrolyzes fat into free fatty acids and glycerol. These free fatty acids increase capillary permeability, cause destruction of alveolar architecture, and damage lung surfactant. The end result of all these changes is hypoxia.[214]

Clinical findings of fat embolism syndrome include tachypnea, dyspnea, profuse tracheobronchial secretions, apprehension, anxiety, delirium, confusion, unconsciousness, and petechial hemorrhage. Laboratory findings are hypoxemia on arterial blood gas and thrombocytopenia below 150,000 mm^3. Treatment is supportive. Mechanical ventilation may be required in advanced cases. Corticosteroids may be of benefit in diminishing the inflammatory response from the chemical effects of fat emboli.[209]

Monto et al,[194] in a review of the literature, reported 19 cases with 9 deaths, 15 of which were associated with long-stem cemented prostheses such as the Guepar hinge. Four cases were associated with total condylar arthroplasty. These authors reported one case associated with intramedullary instrumentation. Fahmy et al[71] showed human intramedullary femoral canal pressures between 500 and 1000 mm Hg generated by using standard alignment rod techniques. Venting the canal did not lower the canal pressure significantly. Only by overdrilling the femoral canal and gently placing the guide rod were intramedullary pressures maintained within normal limits. The use of a pneumatic tourniquet does not protect against fat embolism, and with the popularity of intramedullary guidance systems for femoral and tibial components, an increase in the incidence of fat embolism syndrome may be expected.

Blood Loss

There is little blood loss during the operation of TKA; most occurs postoperatively through suction drainage.[95, 202] Reinfusion drains are useful, but nonetheless one must be prepared for additional blood transfusion, particularly in bilateral cases. Given the current anxiety about receiving blood products, autologous transfusion is the choice of most patients for elective surgery. We recommend obtaining 1 unit of blood for each knee arthroplasty to ensure that homologous blood will not be needed. Although retransfusion of the blood may not be strictly necessary, we believe avoidance of postoperative anemia is helpful in promoting more rapid recovery, especially considering the advanced age and myriad medical problems with which our arthroplasty patients present.

LOCAL COMPLICATIONS

Wound Drainage and Delayed Wound Healing

In a series of 220 total condylar arthroplasties studied some years ago, 49 knees did not have primary wound healing[88] or had some wound drainage. Cultures were taken of 41 knees, of which 35 were negative. The most frequently isolated organism was *Staphylococcus epidermidis.* One case with skin necrosis became secondarily infected (mixed organisms) and eventually developed a deep wound infection. With this exception, early wound drainage was not related to periprosthetic infection.

Altering the skin incision from midline to slightly curved medial parapatella[134, 136] and improved techniques in tissue management have greatly increased the incidence of primary wound healing in more recent cases. Continuous passive motion (CPM), in routine use for at least the last decade, begun immediately postoperatively has not adversely affected wound healing.[273] Johnson[133] recommended that 40 degrees of flexion not be exceeded in the first few days, but we routinely start CPM in the recovery room at 60 degrees of motion, and we have not seen any increased incidence of wound problems.

Excessive bleeding will contribute to postoperative wound drainage and should be controlled. Although Lotke (personal communication, 1999) demonstrated in his own cases that there was no advantage in releasing the tourniquet before wound closure, we recommend that this be done. Not infrequently, rapid hemorrhage from one of the genicular vessels does occur when the tourniquet is released, and occasionally patients have been returned to the operating room for control of bleeding when the tourniquet was not released (Fig. 87.3). We have found two areas of particular concern: the posterior lateral corner at the level of the tibia, which is supplied by the lateral inferior geniculate artery, and the area near the insertion of the posterior cruciate ligament (PCL) on the tibia. Both these areas tend to bleed profusely if not properly coagulated. Aneurysm of the medial genicular artery[55, 254] secondary to injury during surgery has also been reported. Tourniquet release is recommended after insertion of the components when cement has cured.

Management of Wound Drainage

Serosanguineous drainage from the incision is not uncommon and is only a cause for concern when the drainage is profuse and persistent. If there is no purulence or erythema, initial management should be a compression dressing, immobilization, and observation. Wound healing takes precedence over motion. When there is drainage, antibiotic therapy is controversial because it may mask a deep infection, thus making it difficult to identify the causative organism. We recommend consulting with an infectious diseases specialist and administering intravenous antibiotics in selected cases. Clearly, this is a matter of clinical judgment, but we do not consider antibiotics in these circumstances necessarily wrong. Prolonged and persistent serosanguineous drainage raises the issue of a capsular defect that should be surgically repaired. Some authors advocated that if drainage does not stop after 5 days of appropriate treatment, then an open débridement should be performed.

Hematoma

Naturally, a certain amount of bleeding into the knee is normal, and on occasion a profuse amount may exit through the suction drain. In the latter event, we recommend removal of the drain, application of compression dressing, and observation. We also advocate stopping the CPM and range of motion (ROM) with therapy. If bleeding continues, as evidenced by tense and painful swelling, the knee must be reopened and the source of the bleeding identified (an argument for intraoperative tourniquet release). Later development of a hematoma is usually secondary to anticoagulant therapy. A period of immobilization and observation is permissible, and many hematomas subside spontaneously. However, when leakage through the incision occurs, it is best to evacuate the hematoma surgically. Another indication to evaluate a hematoma surgically is in the case of impending skin necrosis secondary to excessive soft tissue extension. The hematoma may be localized to the subcutaneous tissues, but if it is deep there is risk of prosthetic contamination. Probing and squeezing the wound to evacuate a hematoma are not recommended and may lead to retrograde contamination.

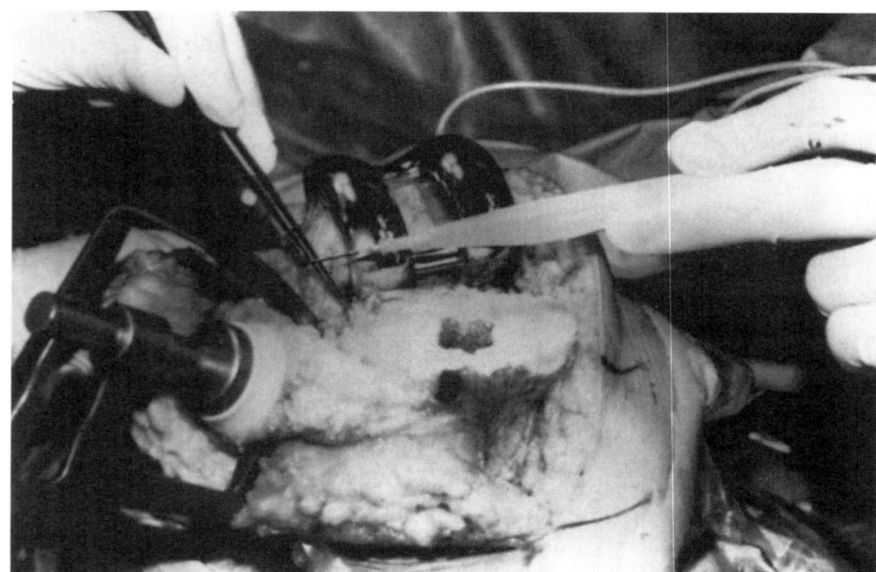

FIGURE 87.3 ➢ Photograph showing cautery of the lateral genicular artery. Unless this artery is clearly seen, it is advisable to release the tourniquet before closure so that the vessel can be clearly identified. It is the major source of dangerous postoperative bleeding.

SKIN NECROSIS

In the total condylar knee series, seven had skin necrosis or wound separation, three required secondary closure, and two required skin grafts. Skin necrosis (Fig. 87.4) is particularly likely in previously operated knees, especially when midmedial or midlateral incisions are already present. The use of such previous incisions involves raising a substantial skin flap, to which making a new incision seems preferable. When there are multiple scars, the most lateral scar should be used. This is done to avoid a large lateral skin flap with multiple scars in it and concern over its viability. Johnson[134] demonstrated a reduction in oxygenation of the skin in the lateral region after skin incisions about the knee through measurement of transcutaneous oxygen. When the surgeon is faced with ill-placed scars, it may be better to make a "sham" incision 10 to 14 days before the projected arthroplasty or to consider soft tissue expanders. Transverse incisions, such as are made in high tibial osteotomy, can be crossed with impunity. Sometimes part of a previous incision (such as incisions used for the fixation of tibial plateau fractures) can be reopened.

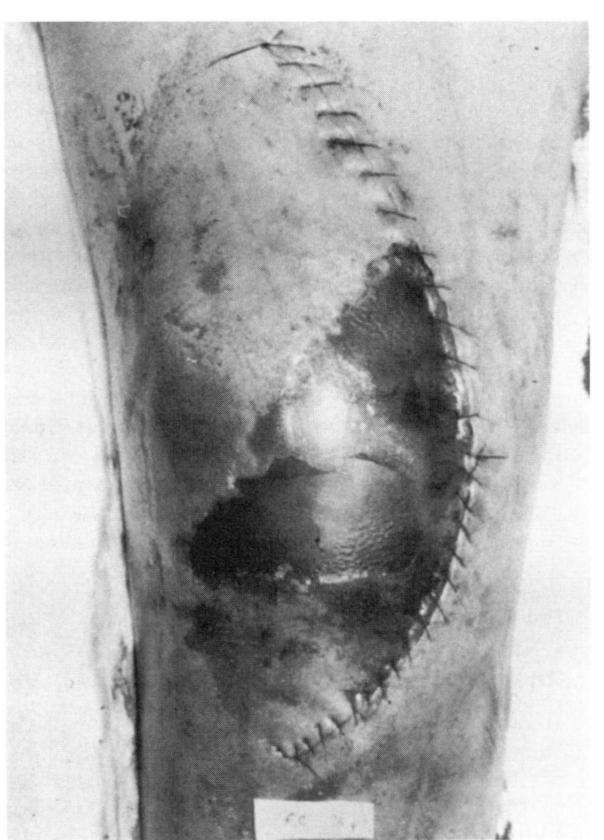

FIGURE 87.4 ➢ Because of its subcutaneous position, skin necrosis is a particular hazard in knee joint replacement. Overaggressive débridement can lead to deep infection. When necrosis occurs, the knee should be immobilized until the eschar separates.

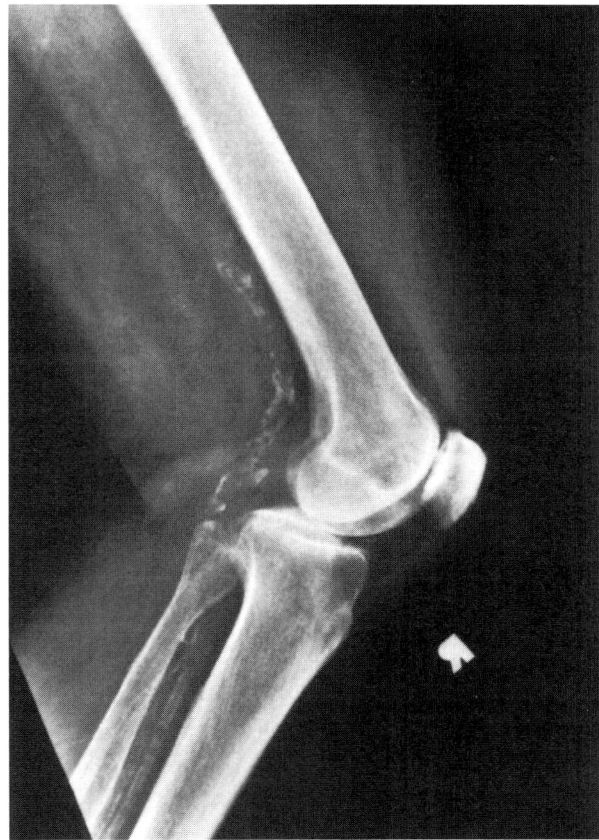

FIGURE 87.5 ➢ Lateral radiograph showing extensive calcification in the femoral, popliteal, posterotibial posterior tibial, and peroneal arteries. Although this patient had palpable peripheral pulses, knee surgery may result in arterial occlusion by a dislodged clot. Some investigators recommended avoidance of a tourniquet. The patient should be watched closely after surgery for evidence of arterial insufficiency.

VASCULAR COMPLICATIONS

Arterial complications are, fortunately, rare,[158, 216] and the preoperative absence of peripheral pulses has not been regarded as a contraindication to surgery, provided that the capillary circulation was adequate. In a large Mayo Clinic series, Rand[216] found the incidence of arterial insufficiency to be only 0.03% in 9022 TKA performed between 1971 to 1986. Rush et al[237] reported on arterial complications of TKA in Australia. By means of a questionnaire sent to Fellows of the Australian Orthopaedic Association, a total of 13 cases were reported: 4 with injury to the popliteal artery, 1 with arterial venous fistula involving the lateral genicular artery, and 8 with acute ischemia resulting from superficial femoral or popliteal artery thrombosis. The authors suggested that thrombosis was due to local pressure from the tourniquet and recommended that, in the presence of extensive calcification of the proximal arteries (Fig. 87.5) and poor peripheral pulses, a tourniquet not be used.

Absolute vascular contraindications for performing a

TKA include the presence of verified vascular claudication with minimal or no activity, active skin ulcerations secondary to arterial insufficiency or venous stasis, and ischemia or frank necrosis in the toes. If there are any questions or doubts, a vascular surgeon should be consulted. Others cautioned against the use of a tourniquet after previous bypass surgery. In our own experience, there have been seven instances of arterial compromise in more than 5000 arthroplasties; three resulted in amputation.

When there is concern about the circulation, we recommend a preoperative evaluation by a vascular surgeon. The operation should be scheduled at a time of day when consultant advice will be available postoperatively, so that prompt investigation with arteriography can be done if the state of the circulation is in doubt. Prompt embolectomy will usually restore the circulation. In one of our eventual amputations, embolectomy was delayed beyond the point at which it would have been useful. The other two amputations would not have been prevented by avoidance of a tourniquet.

Prolonged observation of postoperative vascular insufficiency is justified only in a setting of extreme vigilance and under the guidance of a vascular surgeon.

NERVE PALSY/NEUROLOGICAL COMPLICATIONS

Anatomy of the Peroneal Nerve

Although we have encountered two cases of transient paralysis of the popliteal nerve after correction of a severe flexion contracture, most nerve palsies involve the peroneal nerve.[9, 51, 56, 104, 105, 175, 233] This nerve is composed of fibers from the dorsal portion of the L4 and L5 and S1 and S2 nerves. As the nerve courses down from the thigh, it curves laterally behind the head of the fibula to reach the two heads of the peroneus longus. The nerve flattens as it passes between these two heads, separating the bundles and exposing unprotected nutrient vessels. Then the nerve curves around the neck of the fibula and divides into deep and superficial branches.

The deep peroneal nerve continues under the extensor digitorum longus along the anterior aspect of the intraosseous membrane. It sends motor branches to the tibialis anterior, extensor digitorum longus, extensor hallucis longus, and peroneus tertius. The nerve continues distally, ending in the medial and lateral terminal branches, which, among other functions, supply sensation to the first web space of the foot.

The superficial peroneal nerve passes distally between the peronei and extensor digitorum longus. Motor branches are given off to both the peroneus longus and peroneus brevis. In the lower one-third of the leg, the nerve branches into the medial and intermediate dorsal cutaneous nerves. These terminal branches complete the sensory innervation of the feet.

Postoperative Clinical Findings

Peroneal nerve palsy is an infrequent but worrisome complication after TKA. The incidence is higher in revision cases than primary TKA.[9] They are most commonly seen after correction of severe flexion and valgus deformities or combination of the two. Factors that have not been found to be associated with peroneal nerve palsy include age, gender, type of arthritis, and duration of tourniquet. It is most commonly diagnosed within 2 days after the TKA.

The prevalence of peroneal nerve palsy has been reported many times in the literature. Mont et al[191] reviewed the literature and found the cumulative prevalence to be 0.58% (74/12,784). Asp and Rand[9] reported an incidence of 0.3% in 8754 TKAs performed at the Mayo Clinic. A total of 2626 TKAs were performed at the Hospital for Special Surgery from January 1974 to December 1980. During that time, there were 23 peroneal nerve palsies in 22 patients.[233] One patient experienced a peroneal nerve palsy after both TKAs, which were done 5 months apart. The preoperative deformities were varus in 5 knees, neutral alignment in 7 knees, and valgus in 11 knees. In addition, some degree of flexion contracture was found in 14 patients, being severe in 9. Five patients underwent exploration and release of the peroneal nerve, and a nerve palsy developed despite this precaution. These explorations were done in knees with severe flexion contractures (30 degrees and 80 degrees) and in severe valgus deformities (27 degrees, 35 degrees, and 40 degrees).

The time of presentation of the problem was variable, ranging from discovery in the recovery room to the 6th postoperative day. Most cases were noted early; eight were found in the recovery room and another eight were discovered during the 1st postoperative day. Then three were noted on postoperative day 2, two on postoperative day 3, and two on postoperative day 6. The motor fibers of the tibialis anterior and extensor hallucis longus muscles were affected in all cases; a sensory deficit was noticed in 20 cases (87%). The peroneus longus muscle was affected in nine cases (39%). During the early postoperative period, six patients underwent electromyographic evaluation; a diffuse motor neuropathy was found in the mild cases and denervation potentials in muscles supplied by the deep branch of the common peroneal nerve in the more severely involved cases.

Treatment and Results

The treatment rendered on discovery of these findings varied according to the discretion of the surgeon involved. The most frequent therapeutic measure was to loosen the Robert Jones dressing and place the knee in a more flexed position. In two cases, this maneuver brought immediate improvement of both motor and sensory deficits.

The time interval between discovery and the beginning of the return of function ranged from immediately in the two cases mentioned to 6 months. Motor improvement occurred first, with sensory return lagging behind.

In 13 cases, traction secondary to correction of a valgus or flexion deformity or both was the cause of the palsy. In three cases, the palsy was caused by the medial and lateral splints used to hold the knee in full extension with "tight" components and the consequent traction on the nerve by this stretching mechanism. In four cases, the dressing containing the medial and lateral plaster splints was too tight or improperly padded, causing direct pressure on the peroneal nerve. In three cases no explanation could be determined.

Of the 23 peroneal palsies, 17 were extensive enough to require a drop-foot brace. The remaining six cases were mild and did not need any dorsiflexion assist. At follow-up examination, a residual deficit was found in all 18 patients in whom a sensory deficit had been present. Motor power was clinically normal in 6 of the patients (26%), the remaining 17 patients had motor power clinically assessed in the poor to good range. Only two patients, neither of whom had a sensory deficit initially, achieved full clinical recovery, both within 6 months. Four additional patients had complete motor recovery but with a residual sensory deficit.

The following factors contribute to the development of peroneal nerve palsy:

1. Stretching of the nerve in valgus and flexion contractures.
2. Fascial compression of the nerve and its vascular supply.
3. Direct pressure from the dressing.
4. Rare idiopathic cases in which none of the mechanisms just listed seems to apply.

Idusuyi and Morrey[123] examined a series of TKA patients seen at Mayo Clinic between 1979 through 1992. There were 10,321 TKAs performed with 32 postoperative peroneal nerve palsies. The following factors were associated with peroneal nerve palsy: epidural anesthesia for postoperative pain control, previous laminectomy, and preoperative valgus deformity. The relative risk for patients who had previous proximal tibial osteotomy was doubled but not statistically significant. Asp and Rand[9] described a similar Mayo Clinic experience with peroneal nerve palsy. Among 8998 arthroplasties, there were 26 nerve palsies. The circumstances in which they occurred were similar to our own, but recovery was generally better. Complete recovery was more likely when the palsy was initially incomplete. Removal of dressing and flexion of the knee on diagnosis did not always help.

The treatment of chronic peroneal nerve palsy usually consists of an ankle-foot orthosis for a foot drop and passive ankle ROM to prevent an equinus deformity. Complete recovery of a peroneal palsy is rare. The recovery seen is usually partial, with sensory deficits that may be permanent; residual motor deficits are not usually of clinical significance. Occasional marked weakness, especially of the great toe extensor, may be seen. Asp and Rand[9] studied 26 postoperative peroneal palsies. Palsies were complete in 18 and incomplete in 8. Twenty-three of the patients had both motor and sensory deficits, 3 had only motor deficits. At 5-year follow-up, recovery was complete for 13 palsies and partial for 12. Complete recovery was more likely in those palsies that were incomplete initially. Although most investigators support nonoperative treatment of this complication, others disagree. Krackow et al[156] treated five patients with operative exploration and decompression of the peroneal nerve for a postoperative palsy. The procedure was performed 5 to 45 months after the index TKA. All patients demonstrated improved nerve function. Four of five patients had full peroneal nerve recovery. All patients were able to discontinue their ankle-foot orthosis.

It is apparent that patients with excessive total deformities are prone to experience peroneal nerve palsies. The large soft tissue dissections required to balance the more severe deformities may be responsible for increased traction or vascular compromise in this area. The alternative method of bone sacrifice to correct large deformities, although appealing because of the elimination of the need for obtaining soft tissue balance, does not entirely avoid peroneal nerve palsy. The bone-sacrificing method also leaves a residual leg length discrepancy that is permanent and may be associated with an extensor lag because of relative lengthening of the quadriceps mechanism. When ligament balance is not attempted, a constrained prosthesis is needed. In younger patients this may lead to eventual loosening, although, with the constrained condylar prosthesis, this has not happened at the time of writing. In elderly patients at high risk for peroneal nerve palsy, the use of the constrained condylar knee is a suitable alternative. These patients recover much more rapidly than after major release procedures, and because of their age the risk of ultimate loosening is low.

We have also encountered two cases of transient paralysis of the popliteal nerve after correction of severe flexion contractures. In one of these there was complete recovery, but in the other the recognition of the palsy was delayed because a continued epidural anesthetic interfered with the clinical examination. Although it is sometimes necessary to splint the knee in extension after correction of a severe flexion contracture, evidence of nerve palsy demands immediate removal of the splints and flexion of the knee. If this is done promptly, complete recovery can be expected. In the case of valgus deformities, splinting is not necessary, and the intermittent flexion and relaxation that occurs with immediate continuous passive motion has greatly lessened the occurrence of peroneal nerve palsies. Tight dressings that might press directly on the peroneal nerve should also be avoided.

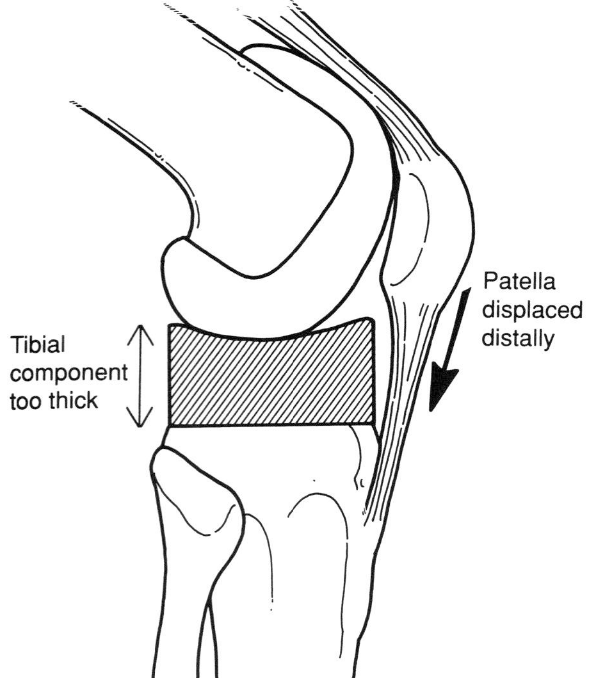

FIGURE 87.6 ➢ If an extra thick tibial component is needed to stabilize the knee, the patella is displaced distally, causing a patella infera. Undersizing of the femoral component in the sagittal plane or anterior malpositioning are possible causes. Excessive distal resection of the femur moving the joint line proximally is another cause.

MECHANICAL COMPLICATIONS

Instability

Instability after knee arthroplasty can be subdivided into three types: extension instability, flexion instability, and genu recurvatum.

Extension Instability

Instability in extension can be either symmetric or asymmetric. Either type is accentuated when there is malposition of the components or overall malalignment of the extremity. Conversely, the effects of extension instability are lessened and sometimes masked altogether when position and alignment are correct.

Symmetric Instability

Symmetric instability is caused whenever the thickness of the components is less than the extension gap between the bone ends. It can be caused by removal of excessive bone from the distal femur either because of miscalculation or because the collateral ligaments were not tensioned properly.

Over-resection of tibial bone is compensated for by use of a thicker tibial component, which makes up for the extra bone removed. The only adverse consequence is the seating of the prosthesis on more distal and potentially weaker tibial bone. Over-resection of the distal femur has more serious consequences and requires augmentation of the femoral component by blocks attached to the distal femur, which are available in many revision systems. Over-resection is less probable with tensor systems but is also unlikely to happen when a measured osteotomy (calculated to replace bone with prosthesis) is performed. When it is not due to excessive bone resection, extension instability may be the consequence of abnormal ligament length (i.e., in genu recurvatum and after extensive ligament releases). Although one remedy is to stabilize the knee by using a thicker tibial component, this will alter the joint mechanics by moving the joint axis proximally, an action that has secondary effects on ligament tension and stability[182] as well as patellar function (Fig. 87.6) by creating a low-lying patella. When preoperative and intraoperative assessment of the knee suggests this might happen, the femur should be deliberately under-resected by the initial osteotomy (Fig. 87.7). Later in the procedure, if either spacer blocks or the trial components suggest that further resection is necessary, it can be done by recutting the distal femur. Alternatively, if the osteotomy has already been made, augmentation of the distal femur as described previously can be tried as an alternative to a thicker tibial component.

Asymmetric Instability

Asymmetric instability is the most frequent variant (Fig. 87.8). Most arthritic knees possess some degree of ligament asymmetry, and if the bone cuts are made without regard to this fundamental anomaly, the arthroplasty will be unstable on one side. One of the

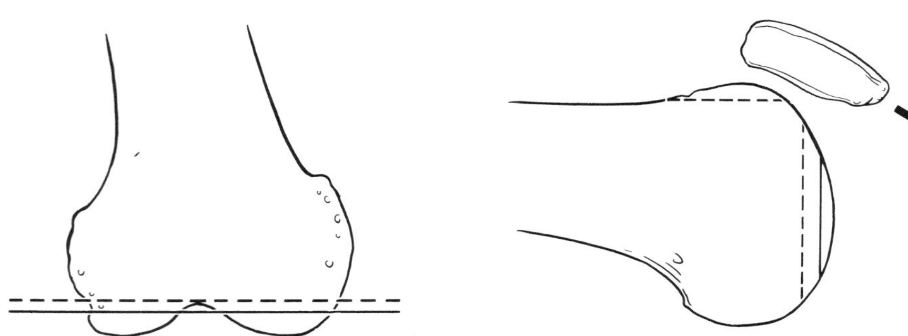

FIGURE 87.7 ➢ In cases with considerable ligamentous laxity, an under-resection of the distal femur may be preferable. The standard femoral resection will necessitate a thicker tibial component to take up the slack in the soft tissues and may cause distal migration of the patella. By under-resecting the femur, desirable patellar position is maintained.

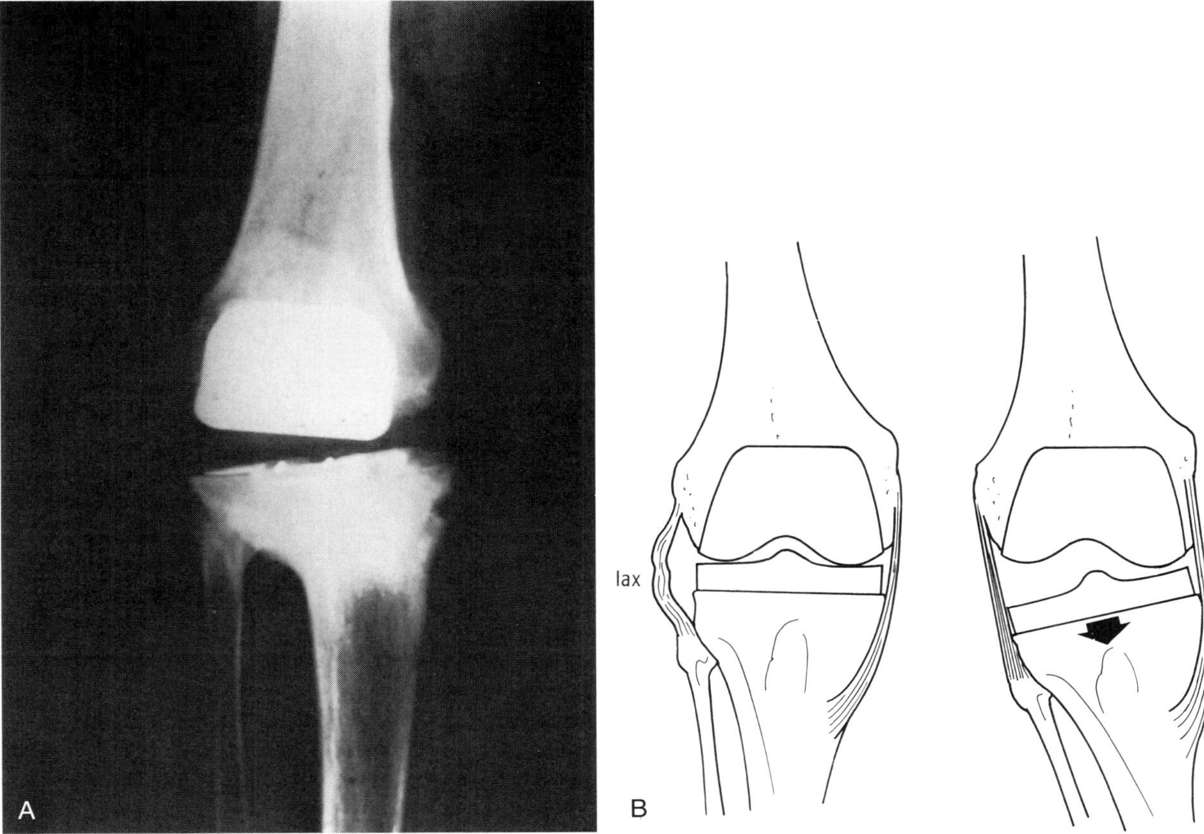

FIGURE 87.8 ➢ *A,* This arthroplasty is unstable, but not because of a ligament deficiency. *B,* The medial ligament was not released; hence, an asymmetric instability remains.

most common mistakes in technique is to release a tight ligament inadequately because of a natural fear of causing instability. How much instability can be accepted? Here a matter of surgical judgment is involved because, as discussed in Chapter 88, some degree of tightening laterally may be expected, provided the alignment of the components is satisfactory. As a rule of thumb, we accept very little medial laxity after correction of valgus (because there is little potential for spontaneous tightening), and we accept lateral laxity after varus correction providing the knee cannot be brought back to neutral with the components inserted. Further medial release should be done if this is possible. We have seen many knees that remained unstable because of insufficient medial release but few that have been over-released. Laskin and Schob[162] described 4 knees with instability of 68 severe varus deformities requiring medial capsular resection. All of these knees had appeared stable at the time of the operation. One knee had stability improved by inserting a thicker tibial component, and in one a probable neuropathic joint may have contributed to the instability. One knee was unsuccessfully revised by a ligament reconstruction, and the fourth knee required revision to a more constrained prosthesis. In our own practice, we have also seen occasional cases of instability after medial release. The first patient, who underwent bilateral TKR with varus release, experienced postoperative instability on one side. She responded to 6 weeks of postoperative bracing with an orthosis, and now, 3 years later, the result is highly successful, with no difference in laxity discernible between the two knees. The second patient, who also underwent bilateral TKR with corrective soft-tissue release, had a possible neuropathic joint on one side. The laxity was not noticed in the hospital, but 1 month later it became obvious that the knee was developing a progressive valgus. An orthosis was not successful in this case, perhaps because it was poorly tolerated by the patient. However, significant improvement occurred over the next year. She now has good stability on walking but notices a medial thrust on stairs. Another iatrogenic cause of asymmetric instability is damage of the medial collateral ligament during surgery (Fig. 87.9). This can occur when cutting the proximal tibia or posterior femur. If noticed during surgery, it should be treated by using a constrained condylar prosthesis because operative repair of the ligament is unlikely to be successful.

Apart from such iatrogenic causes, asymmetric instability is very rarely due to complete absence of ligaments. This situation might be expected in post-traumatic cases, but even then the torn ligaments normally heal, so that the end result is elongation rather than absence. It is often believed that the ligaments in rheumatoid knees are incompetent or sometimes damaged by synovitis, but if so, it must be most unusual. It is true that in loose rheumatoid knees some degree of postoperative stretching can occur, so that a tight fit is desirable.

Bone loss accompanying severe instability and deformity is not in itself an indication for a constrained prosthesis. It is a technical mistake to cut back excessively on either the tibia or the femur to produce a flat bone surface. On the tibial side large asymmetric defects, usually medial, are often found. Resection at the bottom level of the defect removes a large amount of tibial bone; the remaining cancellous bone is weak, and often the cross-sectional area of the tibia is reduced. It is preferable to resect the tibia at the usual level as if no defect existed and then build up the uneven surface on one side with a bone graft. Alternatively, the defect can be filled by using an asymmetric tibial component, and several wedge-shaped augments are now available (Fig. 87.10).

Femoral defects are usually lateral. It may be that the indicated level of resection removes bone from the medial femoral condyle but passes distal to the lateral condyle. The same solution applies; a distal augment laterally on the femoral component is the preferred solution (Fig. 87.11).

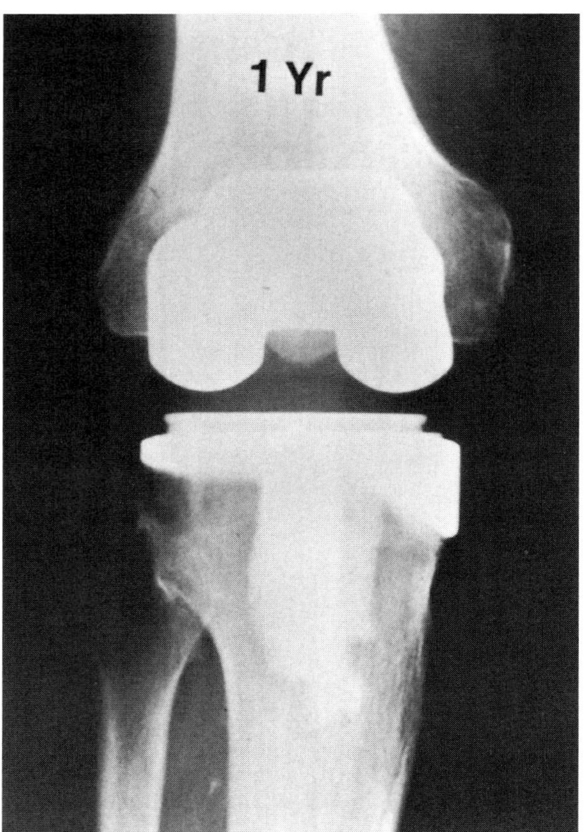

FIGURE 87.10 ➢ A large medial tibial bone deficiency has been compensated by the use of a medial wedge tibial component. The articular surface of the prosthesis is standard total condylar and is not constrained.

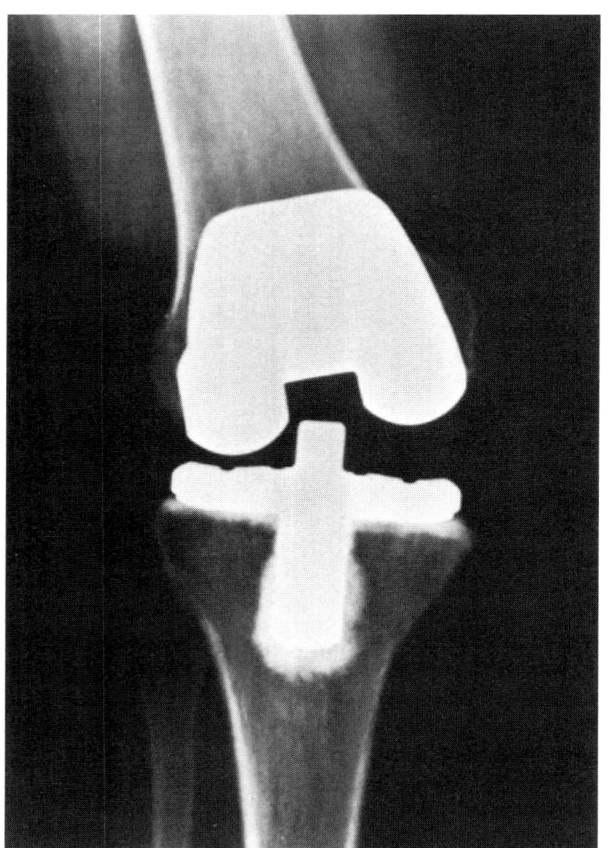

FIGURE 87.9 ➢ Radiograph showing the instability that results from a transected medial collateral ligament. This is not the result of an overzealous medial release.

Although stems are a means of gaining extra fixation to the bone, use of a stem should not be confused with constraint in the prosthetic joint itself, although most constrained or hinged prostheses do have long intramedullary stems. Particularly in revision operations, constrained prostheses are often used unnecessarily, not because the instability cannot be managed by other means but because the stabilizing prostheses have a stem.

Flexion Instability

The knee is stable in extension but not in flexion. The underlying problem is that the flexion space is relatively too large for the thickness of the tibial component (Fig. 87.12). This situation can arise in a number of ways. First, the femoral component is undersized anteroposteriorly. The remedy is to use a larger femoral component with posterior augments. Second, the knee has a flexion contracture with the trial components. Instead of dealing with the problem by troublesome additional distal femoral resection or posterior capsulotomy, the surgeon may choose to achieve extension by using a thinner tibial component or by

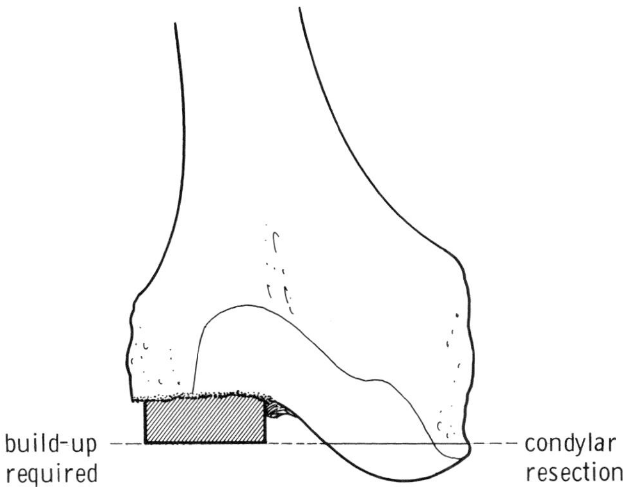

FIGURE 87.11 ➢ In some valgus knees, the level of femoral resection may pass distal to the lateral femoral condyle. Lateral augmentation of the femoral component is required.

additional tibial resection. Third, lateral release from the distal femur impairs the lateral ligamentous support, which has been the cause of several dislocations of the posterior stabilized knee that we have encountered (Fig. 87.13); it has been reported by Galinat et al[86] with the posterior stabilized knee and Gebhard and Kilgus[89] with the Kinematic stabilizer. This possibility may not be recognized intraoperatively, but if it is seen the remedy is either a thicker tibial component or revision to a constrained condylar prosthesis. Fourth, related to that just discussed is the rotational position of the femoral component. After lateral release, lateral laxity should be compensated for by externally rotating the femoral component.[28] A similar type of lateral laxity is created when a transverse tibial osteotomy is done, combined with an anatomic rotational placement of the femoral component (that is referenced from the posterior femoral condyle). Although the normal tibia is described as having a 3-degree medial slope,[144] there is considerable natural variation with an angle of 6.5 degrees recorded in one normal male volunteer.[196] A knee with this anatomy cut in the manner just described will have a discrepancy of ligament tensions in flexion. We believe the epicondylar axis is the best landmark for determining femoral component rotation. The anteroposterior axis of the femur, tibial shaft, and ligament tension are also methods of confirming rotational position of the femoral component.

Flexion instability will be manifest according to the design of the prosthesis. Posterior stabilized designs (see Fig. 87.13) may have episodes of posterior dislocation, which, when reduced, allows the knee to function normally again. Often the dislocation is caused by certain activities, such as crossing one leg over the other to put on a shoe or a sock. It is most likely to happen in patients who had a valgus deformity and in those who rapidly regained flexion probably because the speed of rehabilitation interfered with healing of the lateral structures. Early dislocations should be managed by a period of bracing, avoiding those activities known to cause dislocation. Otherwise, recurrent dislocation is treated by inserting a thicker polyethylene tibial component or revision to a constrained condylar prosthesis.

When the prosthesis is a cruciate-retaining model, the remedy may be exchange of the tibial component for a thicker one, but if this is not judged successful intraoperatively, revision of the components to a posterior stabilized or a constrained condylar design should be considered. Manifestation of this instability depends on the constraint in the original tibial component. One study[206] examined 25 patients with flexion instability with a cruciate-retaining device. Twenty-two of the knee replacements were revised to posterior stabilized implants, and 3 underwent tibial polyethylene liner exchange only. Nineteen of the 22 patients who had a revision to a posterior stabilized implant were improved markedly after the revision surgery. Only one of three patients who had a polyethylene exchange improved. The Knee Society knee scores improved from 45 to 90 points and function scores improved from 42 to 75 points. We recommend that revision surgery in these cases focus on balancing the

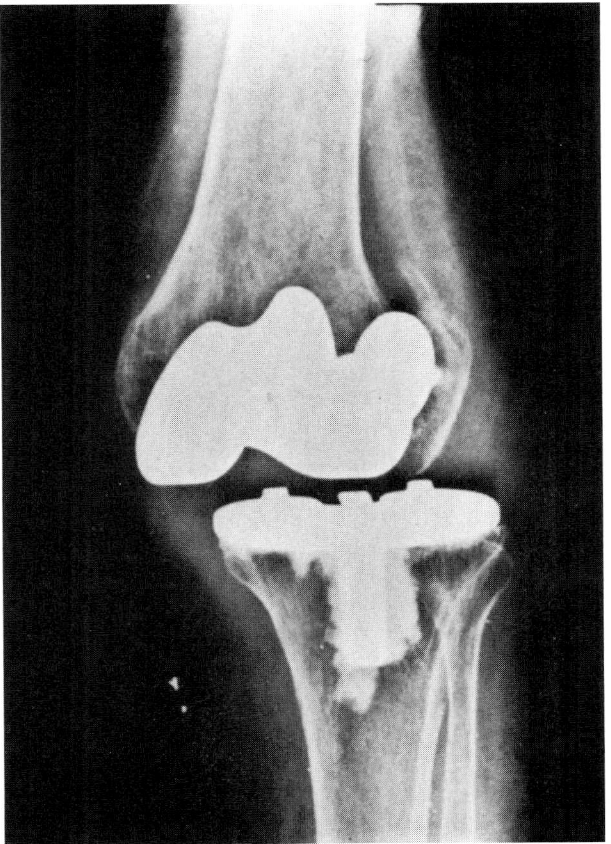

FIGURE 87.12 ➢ Anteroposterior radiograph of a knee with flexion instability. With the knee in flexion, a posterolateral dislocation is observed. This is caused by inequality between the flexion and extension gaps, and the posterior cruciate ligament is not sufficient to provide stability, particularly when the prosthesis is unconstrained.

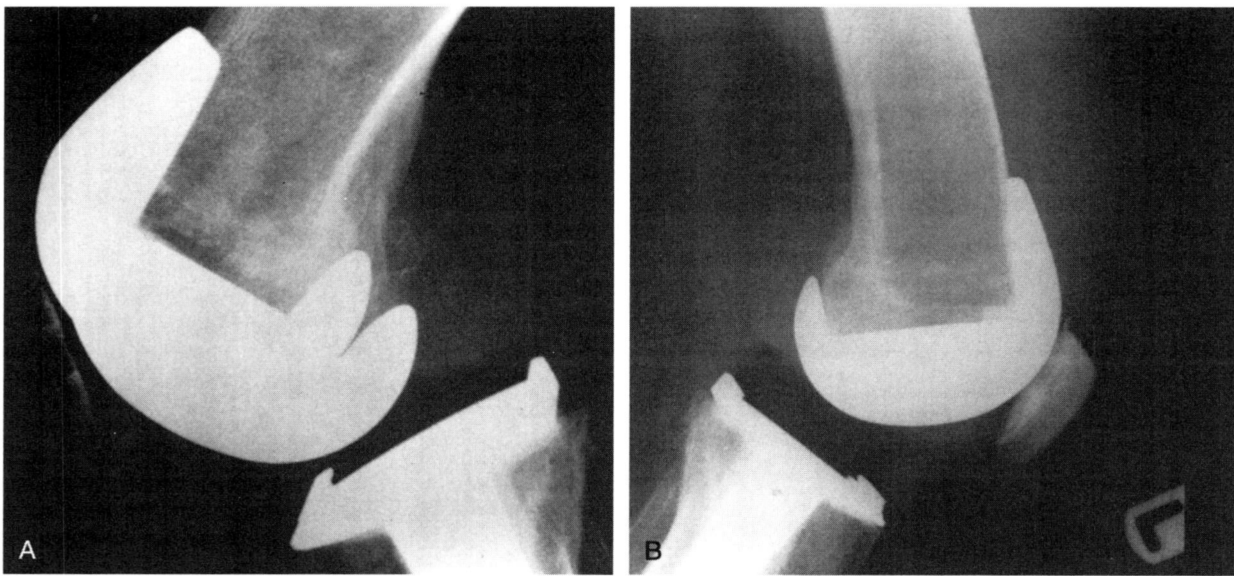

FIGURE 87.13 ➢ *A,* Posterior dislocation of a posterior stabilized prosthesis. *B,* After reduction.

flexion and extension spaces and convert to a posterior stabilized design. Similar results were reported by Waslewski et al[279]; in this study six of six patients who underwent conversion to posterior stabilized design improved.

Genu Recurvatum

The condition of genu recurvatum occurs almost exclusively in patients with rheumatoid arthritis and with muscle paralysis. Recurvatum and anterior subluxation of the tibia have been reported after polycentric arthroplasty in rheumatoid arthritis. Although it is generally true that a knee that does not hyperextend at the conclusion of surgery will not develop recurvatum later, an exception is in those patients who lack muscle control. Patients with long-standing weakness from poliomyelitis may experience osteoarthritis and often also have recurvatum. An arthroplasty should not be undertaken unless there is good power in the quadriceps muscle, but sometimes a functioning quadriceps is present in an otherwise almost flail extremity. These knees should be approached with great caution because, in the absence of hamstring and calf musculature, a slowly developing recurvatum is likely with any kind of surface replacement. Probably if these knees are to be replaced at all there is an indication for a constrained prosthesis with an extension stop, but, of course, the increased risk of loosening with such a device must be carefully weighed before making a decision. In patients with neuromuscular disorders and some collagen vascular disorders (i.e., Ehlers-Danlos syndrome), we will under-resect the distal femur by 1 to 2 mm. This may leave the patient with a slight flexion contracture, but eventually they will return toward full extension.

Krackow and Weiss[157] described a technique in which the origins of the collateral ligaments are transferred proximally and posteriorly, whereby the cam action of the prosthesis will prevent recurvatum.

INADEQUATE MOTION

The ROM obtained after arthroplasty is dependent on several factors, including body habitus, patient motivation, adequacy of physical therapy, and prosthetic design. However, probably the most important determinant is the ROM that existed before the arthroplasty. A knee that is very stiff to begin with is difficult to mobilize satisfactorily because of quadriceps contracture and capsular fibrosis. Even if an adequate ROM is achieved in the operating theater, this may not be realized postoperatively. For this reason, very stiff or ankylosed knees[2, 21, 109, 204] should be approached with caution and with the expectation that 45 to 60 degrees of flexion is the likely end result. Arthrodesed knees in which more extensive damage to the extensor mechanism might be expected, and in which the ligaments were probably divided, should not be considered for arthroplasty at all. Two studies have had conflicting results for TKA in ankylosed or arthrodesed knees. Montgomery et al[193] examined 71 patients with 82 TKA; all had preoperative arc of motion of ≤50 degrees. The average preoperative knee score was 38, average preoperative arc of motion was 36 degrees, average flexion contracture of 22 degrees, and average maximum flexion of 58 degrees. Postoperatively, the average knee score was 80, average postoperative arc of motion was 93 degrees, and average maximum flexion was 94 degrees. Postoperatively, no knee had a flexion contracture greater than 10 degrees. They concluded that TKA in ankylosed knees can lead to significant improvement in ROM and pain. In contrast to Montgomery et al's findings, Naranja et al[203] studied 37 knees that were either surgically fused or ankylosed and had a TKA performed. The results included an average 7 degrees lack of extension and 62 degrees flexion. The total complication rate was 57%. A satisfactory outcome (no pain and an unlimited ambulation distance) was obtained in only 10 patients (27%). They concluded that the lack of consistent adequate motion and the complication rate may suggest that the surgeon reconsider the risks and benefits of this difficult procedure. A linked design is more successful in improving motion than a surface replacement because the ligaments and capsule are not required for stability and can be excised. The difficulty in exposing a very stiff knee has been alluded to, and a quadriceps snip is recommended. A partial quadricepsplasty can be achieved if only the vastus medialis and rectus femoris components of the quadriceps are resutured, leaving the vastus intermedius and vastus lateralis completely or partially unattached.

Knee stiffness or decrease ROM after a TKA is disturbing to the patient and the surgeon. The stiff knee can be painful and lead to decrease use and disability. Reoperation on a stiff knee is no guarantee of success because the success depends on the cause of stiffness. If the stiffness is caused by component malposition, then revision of components can be successful. If stiffness is caused by excessive scarring or patella baja, then reoperation is limited in its results.[61] Nicholls and Dorr[204] found revision was successful in relieving pain in 12 of 13 knees. There was no significant improvement in ROM except in knees that had incorrect component position. ROM was not improved in knees that had stiffness from scarring, such as the "stiffening" type of rheumatoid arthritis or in knees that had patella baja.

It has been our policy to manipulate knees postoperatively if motion is not rapidly regained, and usually this is done during the 6th to 12th postoperative week when flexion is not 75 degrees or more by this time. Full muscular relaxation is needed because if tone remains in the quadriceps muscle the increased resistance may damage the extensor mechanism or possibly cause a fracture adjoining the prosthesis. Epidural anesthesia is convenient but does not always give the required degree of relaxation: spinal and general anesthesia are better in this respect. The purpose of the manipulation is to overcome intra-articular adhesions, and this can be done with less force when quadriceps resistance is eliminated. We have manipulated approximately 400 knees in this manner. Only two complications have been recorded: one was a supracondylar femoral fracture in a knee that was ankylosed before the arthroplasty, and the other a patellar ligament avulsion also occurring in a previously stiff knee. Both of these complications appeared early in our experience when the value of muscle-relaxing agents was not appreciated and might have been avoided had the quadriceps been paralyzed.

Some of our patients may not have needed a manipulation and might have regained motion if left alone to continue physical therapy. Fox and Poss[82] studied 343 total knee replacements performed in a 12-month period, of which 81 (23%) were manipulated, the indication being the failure to achieve 90 degrees of comfortable, active flexion by the end of the 2nd postoperative week. Manipulation did not increase the ultimate flexion of the knee when compared with the larger group of knees that were not manipulated at all. However, their study did not address the critical question of whether the knees chosen for manipulation would have done just as well without. Some patients do not easily regain flexion of the knee after arthroplasty, and in some patients restriction of motion may be permanent. We have seen examples of this in patients who were not manipulated either because a second anesthetic was prevented by a medical problem or because the surgeon involved did not consider manipulation desirable. A selective manipulation is done for the following reasons: (1) it improves the immediate course by allowing more normal function and by making the continued physical therapy easier and less painful; and (2) it prevents permanent restriction of motion in certain patients who are not easily identified until it is too late for manipulation to be effective.

We believe that prediction of the postoperative ROM is more certain for cruciate-sacrificing designs. Accurate tensioning is required with cruciate retention to prevent the PCL from acting as a check rein; this happens when the geometry of the prosthesis is of different curvature than the preexisting anatomic surfaces, causing the posterior cruciate to tighten with flexion.

Other intra-articular causes of loss of flexion are an oversized or malrotated femoral component (which may require component revision) and adhesive capsulitis. The latter is likely to follow a hematoma or other wound-healing problem that results in a long delay in physical therapy. Even so, most patients gradually regain motion, given sufficient time. When a lateral retinacular release has not been done, tightening of the lateral capsule makes flexion difficult; in particularly resistant cases, a lateral retinacular release followed by a manipulation will sometimes successfully regain motion. In addition, a tight PCL in a cruciate-retaining knee design can be a cause of loss of flexion.

Sympathetic dystrophy is an extreme example of adhesive capsulitis in which the whole joint is chronically swollen and the capsule greatly increased in thickness. Usually the other signs associated with a sympathetic dystrophy are present, and the patients invariably complain of excessive pain. The diagnosis of sympathetic dystrophy should be especially entertained if the pain is out of proportion to examination findings.

A persistent flexion contracture is usually the result of incorrect bone cuts at surgery or failure to strip and divide the posterior capsule. The latter maneuver is necessary when there is a severe (greater than 30-degree) preoperative flexion contracture and is in practice mostly limited to rheumatoid knees. Very rarely does this degree of contracture develop in gonarthrosis. With this exception, a postoperative flexion contracture is due to removal of an inadequate amount of bone from the distal femur, and normally this should be noticed when inserting the appropriate spacer in extension. If the components have already

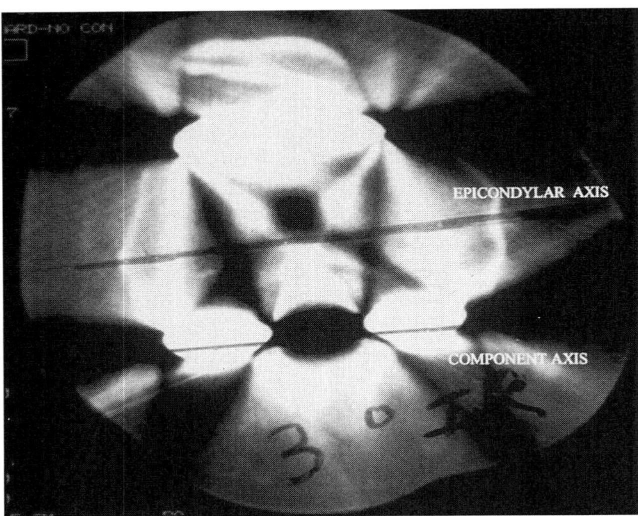

FIGURE 87.14 ➢ Computed tomography scan demonstrating 3 degrees of internal rotation of the femoral component compared with reference line through the epicondylar axis.

been fitted, it is tempting to overcome the flexion contracture by excising more bone from the upper tibia; to recut the distal femur requires more reshaping and is a more complicated and troublesome process. However, if the flexion contracture is relieved by removing extra tibial bone, the flexion gap will also be enlarged: the result will be a posterior sag with PCL-retaining prosthesis or possible dislocation with cruciate-sacrificing or posterior stabilized devices.[86, 89] Therefore, the distal femur should be recut; only then will the correct flexion balance be retained.

Knee prostheses in current use allow potential motion of 120 degrees or more, whether they be cruciate retaining or cruciate substituting. Clinical studies show an average motion of 110 degrees for the cruciate-retaining Kinematic design[293] and 115 degrees for the posterior stabilized cruciate-substituting design.[126] For various reasons and, most importantly, the preoperative ROM, many knees do not achieve the motion intended by the prosthetic designers, and knee arthroplasty for the purpose of increasing motion alone is generally disappointing.

In knees that do not obtain or regain the expected ROM, component malposition or malrotation, particularly internal rotation of the femoral component, should be considered. Femoral malrotation can be determined with precision by a computed tomography (CT) scan, which identifies the femoral epicondyles (Fig. 87.14).

LOOSENING

Component loosening, usually of the tibial component, was the most frequent cause of failure with hinged prosthesis and early surface replacements. The results of hinges often appear deceptively good when the follow-up time is short, because loosening is a time-related phenomenon and usually heralded by the development of a complete radiolucency at the bone-cement interface (Fig. 87.15). In contrast, with the surface replacements, most component loosening occurs within the first 2 years and is technique related, although the incidence of loosening does increase slowly thereafter (Fig. 87.16). Therefore, a 2-year follow-up examination of a surface replacement model serves as some indication of the security of fixation, whereas similar data for a constrained prosthesis may be misleading. For example, Deburge and Guepar,[53] using the Guepar prosthesis, reported a 2% loosening rate before 2 years; at 5 years a total of 15% of the prostheses had aseptic loosening. More sophisticated constrained designs also seem to share this characteristic, albeit to a lesser degree. Kaufer and Matthews,[146] using the spherocentric prosthesis, reported a 7.7% loosening after an average follow-up of 34 months. In addition, 10% of the femoral components and 14% of the tibial components showed a progressive radiolucency, indicating further incipient loosening.

There is reason to believe that the high failure rate caused by tibial component loosening (Fig. 87.17) represents a design problem that is now on the way to solution (Fig. 87.18). High rates of loosening have been reported with polycentric, geometric, and early Freeman-Swanson designs. In addition to loosening, plastic deformation and cold flow were reported with the original UCI prosthesis, indicating that the rigidity

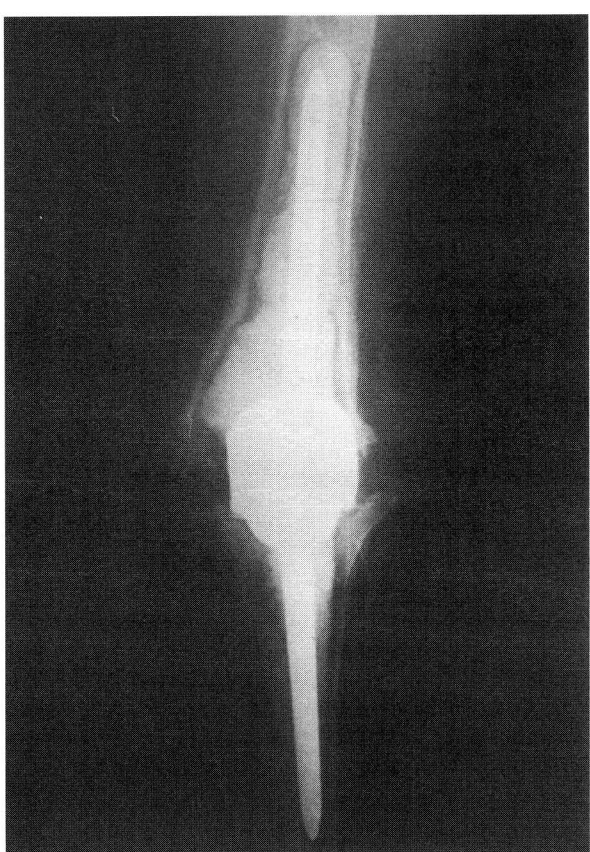

FIGURE 87.15 ➢ With hinge designs, loosening is time related.

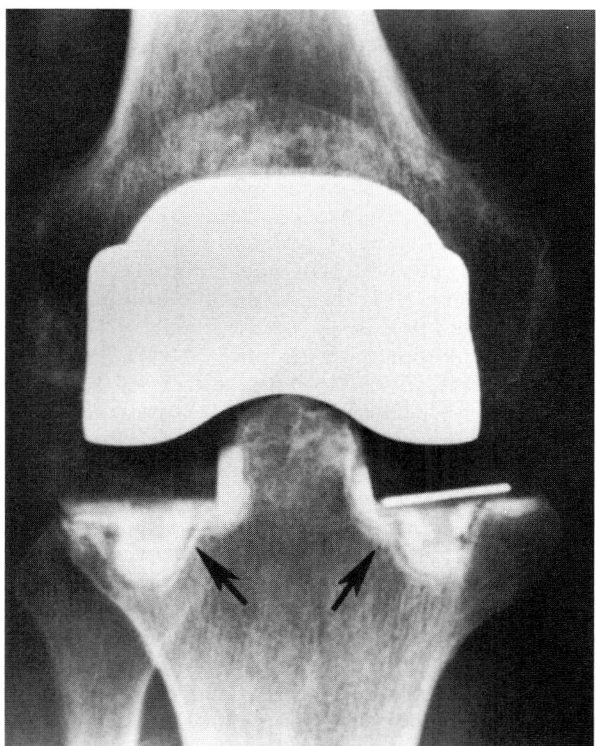

FIGURE 87.16 ➢ Complete radiolucent lines are frequently seen around two-piece polyethylene tibial components.

of polyethylene can be compromised by excessively thin components and generous cruciate cutouts. Modifications to the tibial components have been made in subsequent designs. The total condylar prosthesis, for example, has a one-piece tibial component and a central fixation peg, and no component loosening was seen in 220 knees monitored from 3 to 5 years. Reports from the Brigham and Women's Hospital in Boston on the PCL-retaining, but otherwise similar, Kinematic prosthesis[293] also showed aseptic loosening to be negligible.

We reported the 10- to 12-year follow-up of the same total condylar prosthesis.[272] All had a one-piece polyethylene tibia with a 3.5-cm central peg, and all were cemented. We observed three tibial loosenings and one femoral loosening. All of the tibial component loosenings were positioned in varus (Fig. 87.19). This confirmed our belief that the mechanism of loosening of the tibial component was one of progressive sinkage and migration into the medial tibia, producing an overall varus position. Hsu and Walker[116] showed experimentally that the ideal position for the Kinematic prosthesis is 7 degrees of femorotibial valgus with the tibia positioned at 90 degrees to the long axis of the tibia. In this situation, the component is loaded with a 51% to 49% distribution between medial and lateral plateaus, at least in a static position.[137] These authors conceded that adduction and abduction motions occurring during the gait cycle would, in reality, produce different loading patterns in the patient. It seems self-

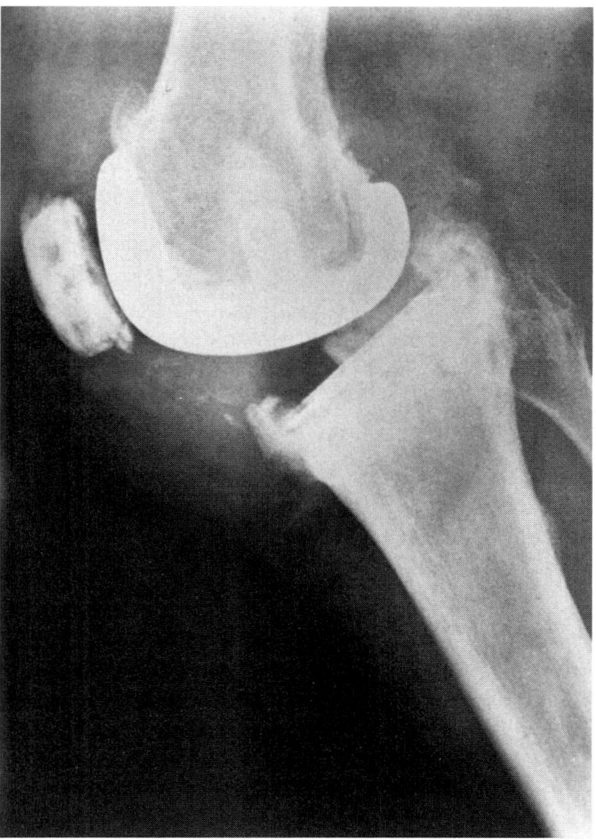

FIGURE 87.17 ➢ Flat tibial components, although one piece, are inadequately supported by the cancellous bone of the upper tibia and are susceptible to sinkage usually in anterior or medial directions.

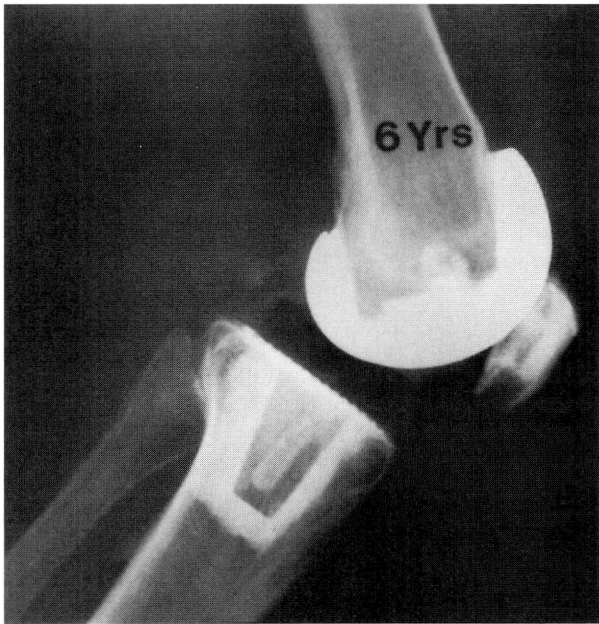

FIGURE 87.18 ➢ The addition of a central fixation peg to the tibial component virtually eliminates tibial component loosening.

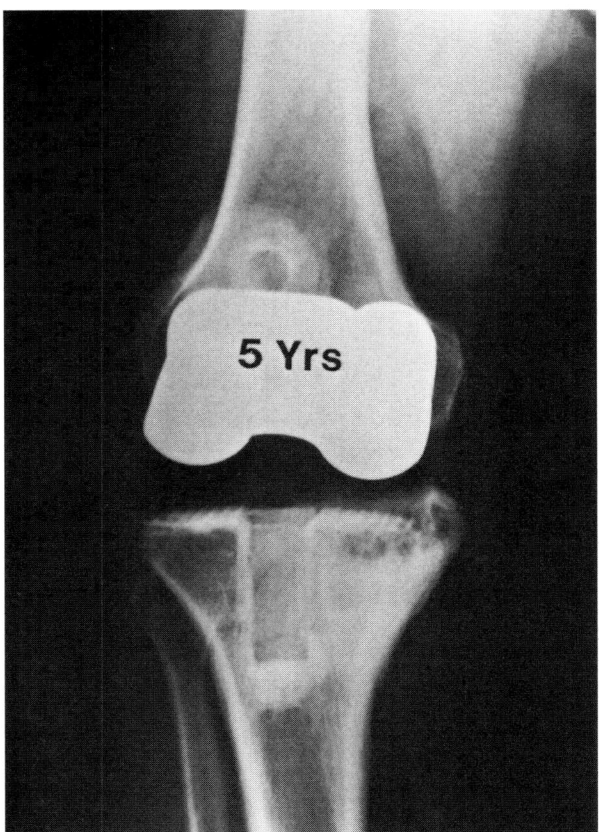

FIGURE 87.19 ➢ The importance of axial alignment. This total condylar knee prosthesis was positioned at surgery in slight varus, which gradually increased over a 5-year period. Collapse of the medial bone support with distortion of the polyethylene can be seen.

evident that malalignment and malposition should be related to mechanical loosening and perhaps are the main cause of it (Fig. 87.20). There is certainly some evidence for this. Lotke and Ecker[172] showed correlation between malalignment and radiolucent lines. These findings were confirmed by Hvid and Neilson.[122] Dorr and Boiardo[59] stated that "prosthetic alignment is the most important factor influencing postoperative loosening and instability." However, Hsu and Hsu[115, 117] were unable to show an association between varus positioning and component loosening, and Smith et al,[252] using a cemented total condylar prosthesis, could find no relationship between either radiolucent lines or loosening and component position. However, Cornell et al,[48] also using the total condylar prosthesis, did find a correlation between radiolucency (although not loosening) and varus positioning. Tew and Waugh[264] found the association between positioning and loosening inconclusive. There are possible explanations for these discrepancies. Loosening rates for modern prostheses are very low, and most certainly not all protheses positioned in varus will loosen. The identification and interpretation of radiolucent lines are confusing to the point that their analysis is probably meaningless (Fig. 87.21), unless the radiolucency is complete and progressive, a circumstance usually accompanied by clinical symptoms (Fig. 87.22). Our own belief is that a lack of statistical correlation between position and loosening is not established, but this is not a reason for carelessness about component positioning. Undeniably, when tibial components fail, they do so into varus, seldom into valgus, and the characteristic bone loss is medial, not lateral. These anecdotal observations, coupled with biomechanical analysis, strongly suggest that positioning remains of critical importance.

The use of metal-backed tibial components has further reduced the incidence of tibial loosening, presumably by distributing stress more evenly. The earliest version of the posterior stabilized knee had an all-polyethylene tibial component, and at 9- to 12-year follow-up a 3% tibial loosening rate was recorded.[255] More recently, a minimum 10-year study[41] of the same prosthesis with a metal-backed tibial component showed no tibial loosenings and no complete radiolucent lines. Also of interest, partial radiolucent lines were seen in 50% of the all-polyethylene components compared with 10% of the metal-backed components.

The mechanism of loosening is also of interest. Miller[188] believed that the process was initiated by micromotion between component and bone, postulating that micromotion could be reduced or eliminated by improving the interlock between cement and cancellous bone. This argument, like others in the field of

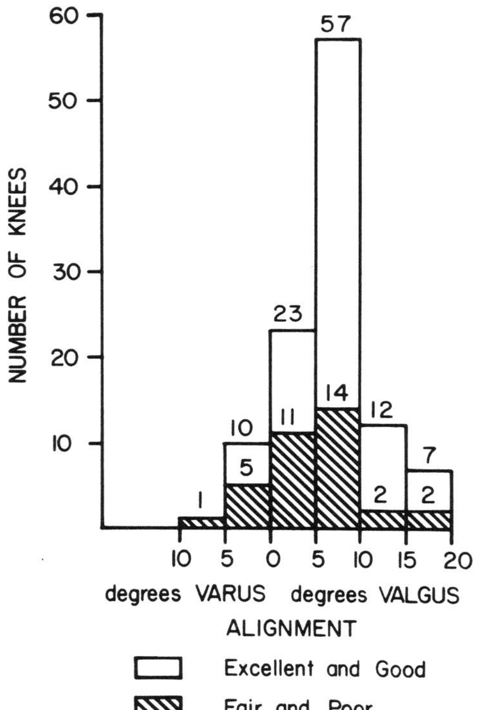

FIGURE 87.20 ➢ Bar graph showing the relationship between postoperative alignment and the clinical rating. The best results were obtained in knees aligned between 5 and 15 degrees of valgus. However, the relationship between alignment and the clinical result is by no means absolute. (From Insall J, Hood RW, Vanni M: The correction of knee alignment in 225 consecutive total condylar knee replacements. Clin Orthop 160:94, 1981.)

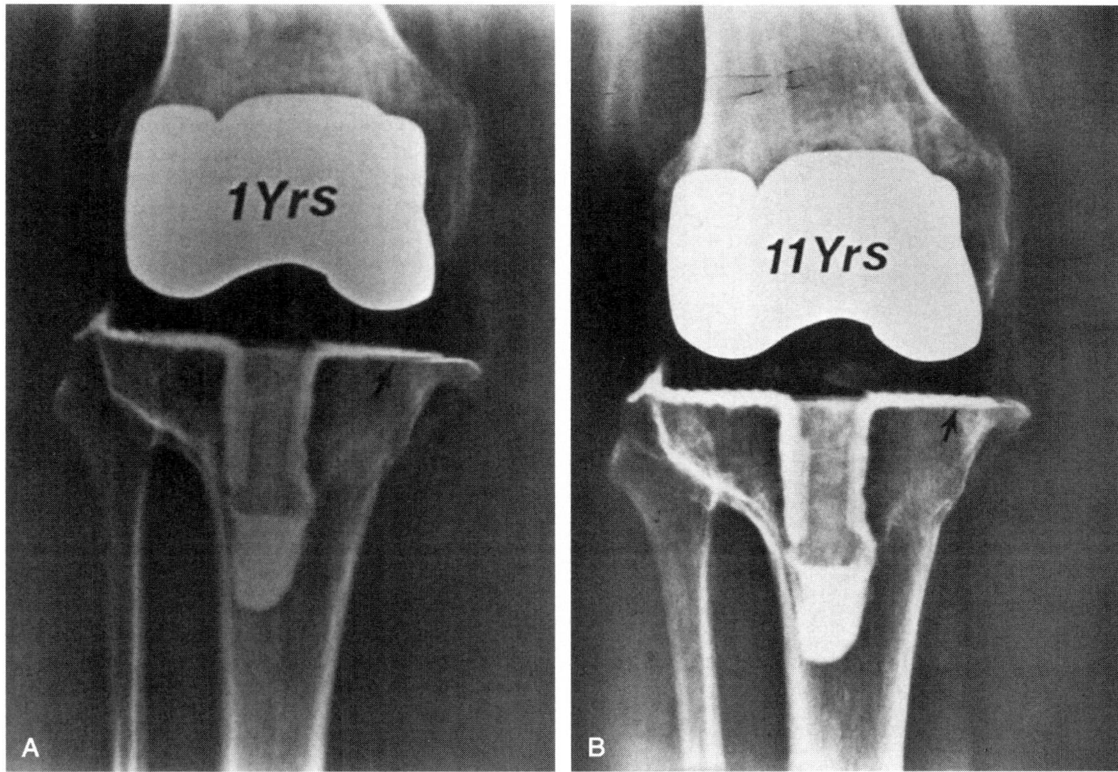

FIGURE 87.21 ➢ *A,* Small partial radiolucency beneath the medial tibial plateau. *B,* Ten years later the radiolucency is barely perceptible (probably because of a slight difference in projection).

joint arthroplasty, may well apply more to hip prostheses than to knee arthroplasty.

Another possible mechanism of loosening is that the components sink or subside into the bone. Seitz et al,[250] using CT, showed a loss of bone density for several months after knee arthroplasty, coupled with a tendency for the implant to migrate in a mediolateral direction.

Periprosthetic osteolysis is another cause of component loosening. The tibia is the more common site, but there have been documented cases in the literature involving both femoral and tibial components. Osteolysis is discussed in more detail in the next section.

Ryd et al[238–241, 267] extensively studied fixation of knee prostheses in vivo using roentgenstereophotogrammetric analysis (RSA). This technique was developed in Lund by Selvik in 1974 and applied to various orthopedic problems such as spinal fusion stability, healing of tibial osteotomy, and skeletal growth patterns. It has also been used for assessing hip joint prosthetic loosening. In the knee, three or more tantalum balls of 0.8-mm diameter are implanted into the tibial metaphysis, using a special instrument with needle and piston. Markers are also introduced about 3 mm into the polyethylene tibial component from underneath, using holes made with a dentist's drill. The postoperative reference examination, using a biplanar radiographic technique (Fig. 87.23), is administered to the supine patient before the operated leg has become weightbearing. The follow-up examination is carried out with the patient standing on the operated leg only. Rotations about the transverse and sagittal axes were the only movements determined. The initial study was performed on Marmor unicondylar replacements, all of which were clinically successful. The study showed that none of the prostheses were rigidly fixed to the skeleton, and a degree of micromotion and migration occurred. There was some pattern to migration. Of the six patients studied, five showed posterior and downward migration, and four showed medial tilting away from the central axis of the knee. Subsequent studies have been performed with both cemented and uncemented prostheses, with very similar results. Migration was greatest in the 1st year, after which it tended to stabilize; the direction tended to be medial, posterior, and downward. The mode of fixation was important, and migration was greater for uncemented prostheses. The magnitude was about 1 mm for a cemented total condylar prosthesis and 2.6 mm for an uncemented PCA prosthesis. In another study the same authors examined 26 patients randomized in the cemented or cementless TKA.[267] Using a similar study design, they found the migration between the two groups to be similar. At 1 year, the cemented tibial migration was 1.0 $\pm$0.2 mm compared with 1.4 $\pm$0.22 mm for the cementless. Ryd and Linder[240] published a description of the bone-cement interface in three well-functioning unicondylar replacements that

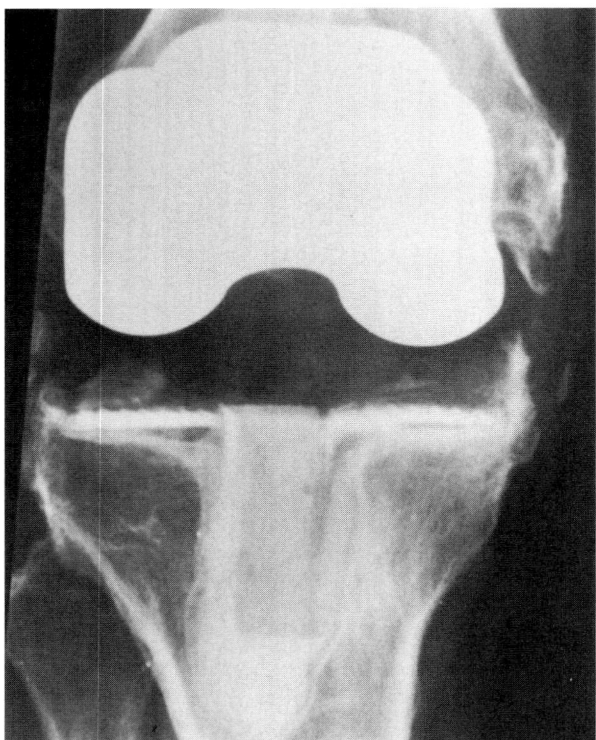

FIGURE 87.22 ➢ With the total condylar prosthesis, a complete radiolucency is attributed to low-grade infection until proved otherwise.

had initially been shown to migrate by RSA. The three prostheses were removed for reasons other than fixation. The tibial components were solidly fixed to the bone. The three interfaces had a similar distribution of fibrous tissue and fibrocartilage. The peripheral 5 to 10 mm consisted of fibrous tissue, whereas the remainder of the supporting tissue was fibrocartilage. This layer of cartilage always rested on bone sometimes with a seam of osteoid "sandwiched" between the bone and the cartilage. The bone underneath the cartilage was vital. There was a total absence of any cellular reaction in the fibrocartilage.

Ryd et al's[238–241, 267] studies showed that there is no such thing as rigid fixation between prosthesis and bone and that the normal situation allows some degree of micromotion. Prostheses move or migrate a certain amount early on and then, in most cases, stabilize into a state of equilibrium, which is compatible with satisfactory long-term function. The normal interface between cement and bone consists of fibrocartilage and fibrous tissue with little cellular reaction. This interface probably corresponds with thin, stable radiolucencies that can be identified in long-term studies of well-functioning knee arthroplasties. Hvid[120, 121] concluded that bone strength may be critical from the point of view of fatigue. From this information it can be argued that excessive penetration of cement into the cancellous bone of the knee may, in fact, be undesirable. It is unlikely that bone trabeculae enclosed within a massive amount of cement remain viable; thus, although the initial mechanical interlock may be improved, the long-term effect may be to transfer the interface to a more distal area of the tibia and into an area in which the strength of the bone is weaker. If one believes this argument, cement penetration should be minimal: 2 to 3 mm is ideal.[277] The theoretical argument coincides with clinical observations. Long-term studies of prostheses, using "old-fashioned" cement techniques that gave very little bone penetration, have shown extremely good survival. For about 2 years, roughly encompassing 1984 and 1985, we sought greater cement penetration, using low-viscosity cement[188]; however, after realizing that our earlier patients continued to function very well, we returned to the earlier cement techniques. Thus, the majority of our metal-backed tibial components have been fixed, using a thin layer of cement with very little attempt to penetrate the cancellous bone.

For bone ingrowth prostheses, close bony apposition, rigid initial fixation,[22, 54, 259, 260, 274] and avoidance of early weightbearing to minimize fixation stresses that could prejudice bone ingrowth have been recommended. In fact, bone ingrowth does not usually extensively attach to tibial components, and such bone that does attach to the prosthesis is limited to small areas, usually around fixation lugs.[46] Tibial fixation is thus mainly by fibrous tissue,[45] although this does seem compatible with good clinical function. Possibly the use of compression screws into the upper tibia will improve the amount of bone ingrowth.[285] The addition of an uncemented central stem has been shown to reduce tilting and sinkage of a proximally cemented tibia, and RSA has shown the least amount of migration with this type of design.[4, 5] Evolution of

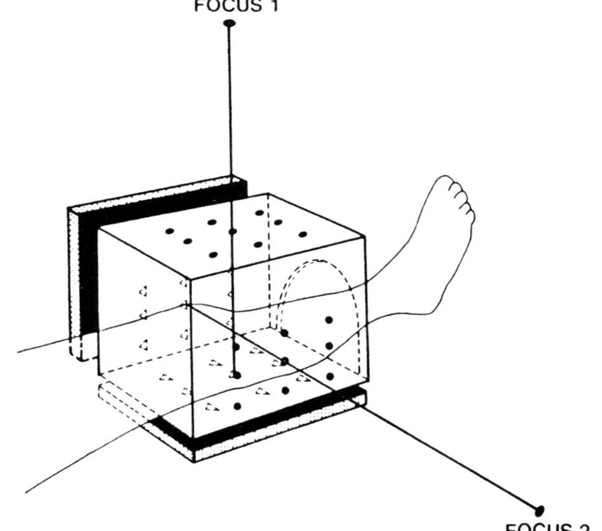

FIGURE 87.23 ➢ Biplanar radiographic setup for roentgenstereophotogrammetric analysis of the knee joint. (From Ryd L, Boegard T, Egund N, et al: Migration of the tibial component in successful unicompartmental knee arthroplasty: A clinical, radiographic, and roentgenstereophotogrammetric study. Acta Orthop Scand 54:408, 1983.)

prosthetic design is perhaps toward a central stem with screws in uncemented prostheses to protect against initial rotational stresses. Both cemented and uncemented prostheses migrate and then reach a stage of equilibrium, after which a certain degree of "normal" micromotion occurs without further sinkage or gross movement. The interface in both types of fixation is predominantly of fibrous tissue. Whiteside and Ohl[284] observed the development of bone hypertrophy underneath a stemmed, uncemented tibial component during the 1st year. Anterolateral sinking was noted in 6 of the first 46 patients, but was not seen again in the series after a design change was made to fix the stem in the bone of the upper tibia more rigidly. Sinkage in these patients was estimated from routine radiographs. Hypertrophy of the bone of the distal femur was also observed around the uncemented femoral components, more posteriorly than anteriorly, and once bone hypertrophy was presented, it did not regress.

Alignment is more critical in cementless knees because cement fixation is not present to help protect against excessive point loading, which may occur with malalignment. With cement fixation, load is more evenly distributed across the tibia, even when malalignment is present. Without cement fixation, this even distribution of load is not present and a point-load situation is created, which will certainly cause necrosis of bone under the overloaded tibial component. Also, without the protective effect of cement fixation, failure of fixation at the opposite condyle occurs from excessive tension at the interface.[61]

Loosening of femoral components is uncommon whether cemented or uncemented. When it does occur, however, it follows a particular pattern in which the bone resorbs posteriorly, allowing the femur to migrate anteriorly and rotate into flexion (Fig. 87.24). King and Scott[149] described a series of 15 loose, cemented duopatellar femoral prostheses. The incidence of femoral loosening is not stated, but in one series at the Hospital for Special Surgery there were 6 femoral loosenings in 430 cemented arthroplasties (1.4%) over a 15-year follow-up period. The mechanism of loosening was similar to that described by King and Scott,[149] who believed that lack of posterior femoral support as a result of either to osteoporotic bone or poor technique was the cause. It was in this region that cancellous bone hypertrophy was reported by Whiteside and Pafford,[285] and it is this region of the femur that is most likely to be highly stressed.

Loosening of the patellar component is most often associated with patellar fractures or with dissociation of polyethylene and metal-back components. Loosening of cemented all-polyethylene patellas in other circumstances is infrequent. The incidence of patella component loosening is about 1% but has been reported as high as 3%.[293] Loosening of the patella was more common with the small central lug, but more recently the tripod configuration of three small peripheral lugs has become popular. Mason et al[183] reported no loose patella components among 577 tripod configuration patellas at an average of 3 years.

Firestone et al[80] found loosening rates of 0.6% to 11.1% in several cementless patella component designs. Factors associated with loosening include insertion of the prosthesis with cement into worn or sclerotic bone, malpositioning of the patellar component, subluxation, fracture or avascular necrosis of the patella, osteoporosis, asymmetric resection, loosening of other prosthetic components, and lack of osseous growth into the porous coating.[24, 221] Reduction in the rate of loosening of the patella component requires improved bone preparation and cementing techniques, proper patella resection, avoidance of asymmetric or excessive bone removal, and central patella tracking.[10]

OSTEOLYSIS

Osteolysis after a TKA is a relatively recently observed phenomenon (Fig. 87.25). Although it is well documented in THA literature in response to particulate debris, it has only recently been discussed in total knee literature. The cause of the osteolysis in the knee is the same as the hip: inflammatory response to particulate debris. The first reported series of osteolysis as a complication was in 1992[210]; the authors reported a 16% incidence in 174 consecutive cementless TKAs, using tibial fixation with bone screws. Since then, there have been reports of osteolysis after both cemented and cementless TKA.[66, 69, 210, 230, 281]

The presentation of a patient with osteolysis is variable. Most patients with well-fixed components are asymptomatic. Other patients present with symptoms of boggy synovitis.[210] There can be mild or moderate diffuse pain with activity, especially in patients in whom the tibial component is not stable.[210] The radiographic criteria for diagnosis of osteolysis as proposed by Peters et al[210] are a lytic osseous defect that extends beyond the limits of that potentially caused by loosening of the implant alone, absence of cancellous bone trabeculae, and geographic demarcation by a shell of bone.

There has been an increased recognition of osteolysis after a TKA in recent literature. Meanwhile, osteolysis involving a THA has been discussed in the literature for approximately 20 years. This is of interest because TKA actually produces greater wear of the polyethylene surface than THA. Engh et al[66] described four factors that could explain this phenomenon. First is the size of the particles produced, which is related to the type of wear (i.e., delamination and abrasion in TKA). This releases large fragments of polyethylene, rarely seen in THA. Large particles produced in the TKA are relatively bioinert. Second, the synovial cavity of the knee is the most extensive of any synovial joint in the body and has greater capacity to engulf and digest wear debris (i.e., greater resistance to osteolysis). Third, the fixation interface with polymethylmethacrylate (PMMA) is a better seal to potential debris than PMMA in a THA. Fourth, the shear and tensile stresses on PMMA may be less at the knee than at the hip. The modulus of elasticity of PMMA is relatively close to that of the cancellous bone of the upper tibia and the tibial component. The decreased amount of

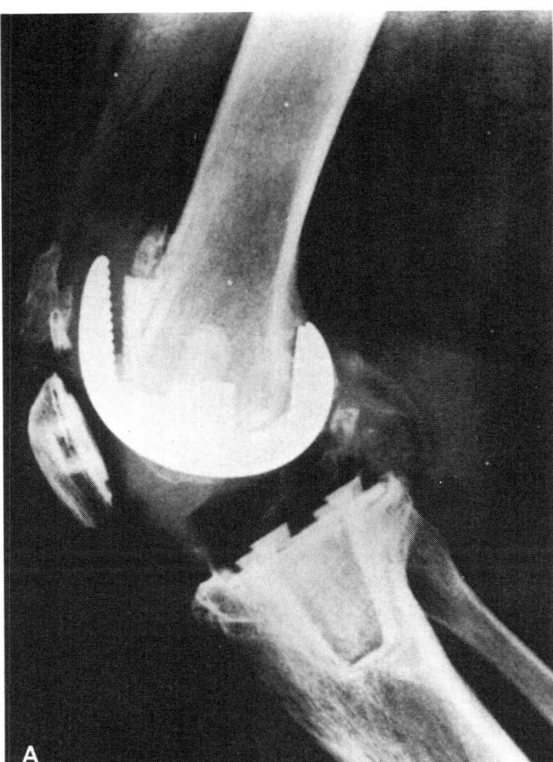

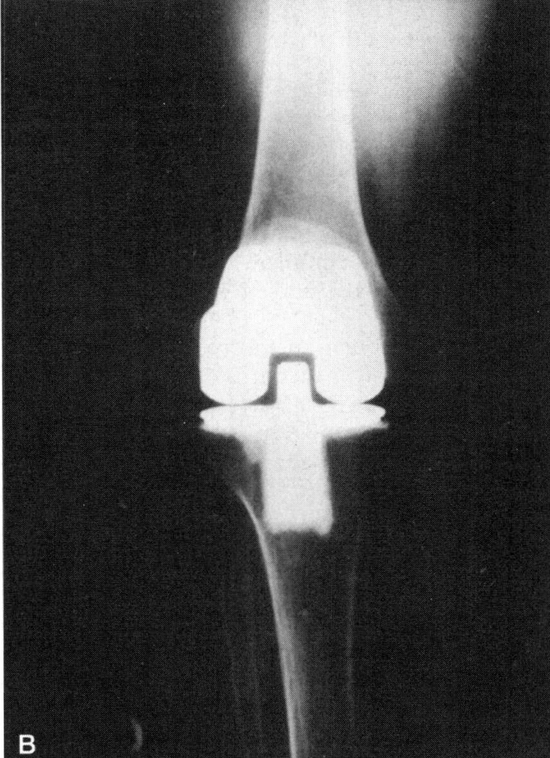

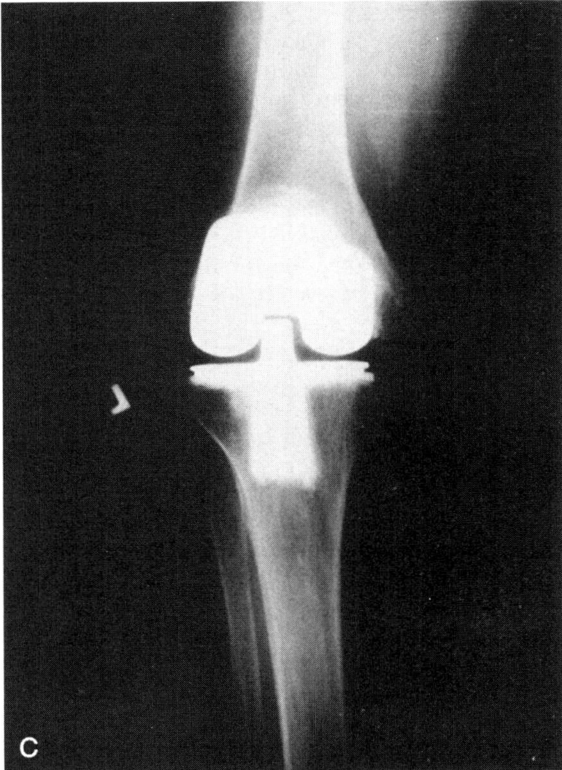

FIGURE 87.24 ➢ *A,* A radiograph showing a typical example of femoral loosening. In the lateral view, the femur has migrated anteriorly and moved into a flexed position as a result of resorption of posterior bone. *B* and *C,* The diagnosis of femoral loosening in the anteroposterior view is not always easy to make. The femur tends to migrate proximally so that there is the appearance of bone overgrowth either medially or laterally. In this case, the diagnosis of loosening was made because a change in position into varus was noted and was confirmed by overlapping the radiographs.

stress and fatigue means decreased fracture of the cement mantle, which leads to decreased access for debris to bone-cement interface.

When osteolysis does appear in the knee after a TKA, it usually appears on the tibial side. This occurrence is probably a multifactorial event. Peters et al[210] offered three possible factors for this occurrence. First, gravity and weightbearing through the medial side of

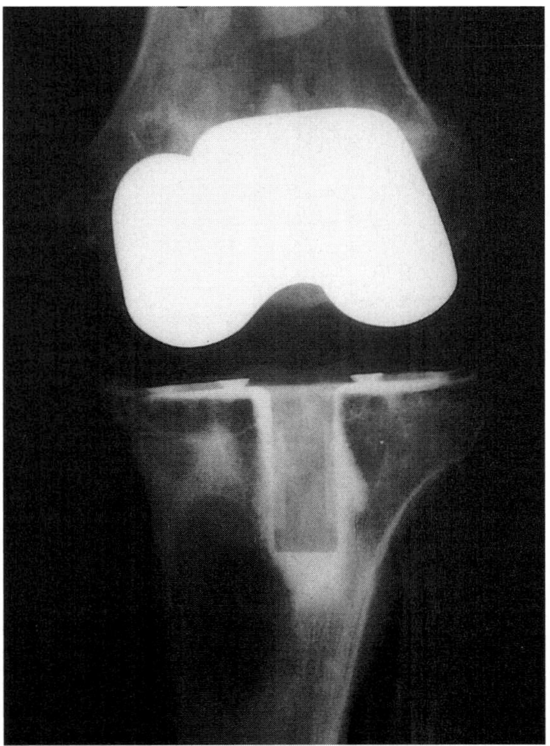

FIGURE 87.25 ➢ Radiograph demonstrating an example of osteolysis involving a prosthesis.

the knee tend to localize the particulate polyethylene on the tibial side. Second, on the femoral side, if the osteolytic process is initiated along the implant bone interface, the flanges of the femoral implant tend to obscure a radiographic diagnosis. Last, the addition of screws to the tibial implant provides avenues for the migration of debris into metaphyseal bone.

The incidence of osteolysis around a knee replacement is difficult to assess for many reasons. First and foremost is obtaining an accurate radiographic assessment at the interface. For example, if there is tibial osteolysis below the tray and the x-ray angle is from slightly above the joint, this lysis may be missed on x-ray film. In addition, Engh et al[66] indicated that femoral lesions are not well recognized as quickly secondary to being hidden by the femoral component on anteroposterior (AP) radiograph. Another reason for the difficulty in assessing the incidence of osteolysis is the length of follow-up. Ezzet et al[69] reported a strong correlation between length of follow-up and the prevalence of osteolysis. Before 24 months, no cases of osteolysis were identified; between 24 and 60 months, the incidence was 15%; and follow-up greater than 60 months had a 39% prevalence of osteolysis.

The reported incidence of osteolysis after a TKA is wide ranging. Whiteside[281] reported a 0% incidence using the Ortholoc II (Dow Corning Wright, Arlington, TN) components in which the tibial component is completely covered with porous coating. On the other end of the spectrum, Ezzet et al[69] reported an incidence of 30% in which the tibial component was fixed with cement and screws and the femoral component was cemented. The actual incidence probably lies between these two reported rates.

Factors in advancement of osteolysis include tibia components that use screws in cemented and cementless designs. The screw acts as a conduit for debris into the cancellous bone. Ezzet et al[69] recommended that screws not be used at all. Another factor is the design of the components and its coating. Whiteside[281] compared two types of cementless components, Ortholoc II and Ortholoc modular, to study osteolysis rates. The only difference between the two components is that Ortholoc II is completely porous coated, whereas the Ortholoc modular is only partially porous coated with smooth metal bridges connecting the four screw holes. They found a 0% rate of osteolysis with the Ortholoc II component and a 20% rate with the Ortholoc modular. Ezzet et al concluded that the smooth metal tracks conduct debris from the joint cavity to the area surrounding the stem. Whiteside attributed the low osteolysis rate of the Ortholoc II to the full porous coating. He believed there is a gasket effect that prevents polyethylene debris from traveling down the stem. Also there is protection of the implant bone interface by the fibrous tissue mantle that permeates the porous coating, preventing polyethylene debris from penetrating. Ezzet et al[69] indicated that a press fit femoral component may contribute to an increased incidence of osteolysis. Whiteside[281] did not believe that large amounts of polyethylene debris are needed to cause osteolysis as long as free access is available to the medullary canal of the tibia. Once the debris enters the medullary canal of the bone, there is no mechanism to remove it from the vicinity, and the macrophage build-up and subsequent osteolysis can become clinically significant.

Histological analysis of synovial tissue and osteolytic tissue has been performed. The synovial tissue of knees associated with osteolysis demonstrates subsynovial infiltrates consisting of histiocyte and giant cells.[210] Both polyethylene and metal particulate debris has been found in specimens. The size and type of material are important. Polyethylene less that 3 μm are usually engulfed by giant cells. Polyethylene particles greater that 3 μm are found in the cytoplasm of histiocytes and occasionally within giant cells. Larger particles of metal, greater than 5 μm, usually elicit little cellular response.[210] Histological examinations of osteolytic tissue revealed a hypercellular membrane consisting of sheets of histiocytes and occasional giant cells. There is no necrosis and little associated vascularity.

The treatment of osteolysis around a TKA is controversial. If the implant is stable and the patient is asymptomatic, one can observe the patient with serial x-ray films on a yearly basis. If the patient is symptomatic or the prosthesis is obviously loose, there are several different options. For patients who are symptomatic and prosthesis is not loose but excessive polyethylene wear is seen, one can remove the defects with a curet, pack with morselized bone graft, and replace the polyethylene. Engh et al[66] either changed out the polyethylene or performed removal of screws, curettage, and polyethylene exchange. In this series, they reported good results with no tibial defects progressing and no development of new lesions. If the components are grossly loose, then revision of components is in order. Because the defects are always larger in situ than they appear on x-ray film, a full armamentarium of revision instruments should be ready. In most of these situations, allograft and the full complement of modular augments should be available. In Engh et al's series,[66] in which the components were revised and structural allograft was used, four of five patients had excellent fixation interfaces at 2 years. There were no lucencies and no graft resorption. One rheumatoid patient had 1- to 2-mm radiolucency beneath the tibial plateau without change in component alignment. The patient was pain free at 6 years. Robinson et al[230] reported on 17 revisions they performed for osteolysis. The original method of component fixation was a mixture of hybrid fixation and cemented and cementless implants. The average time interval from the index surgery to radiographic evidence of osteolysis was 56 months. The prostheses used in the treatment of these 17 revisions were posterior stabilized implants in 65% of cases and a constrained implant in 30%. Osteolytic defects were reconstructed with cement only in 47%, allograft in 30%, and metallic wedges in 35%. No follow-up or outcome data were available from this series.

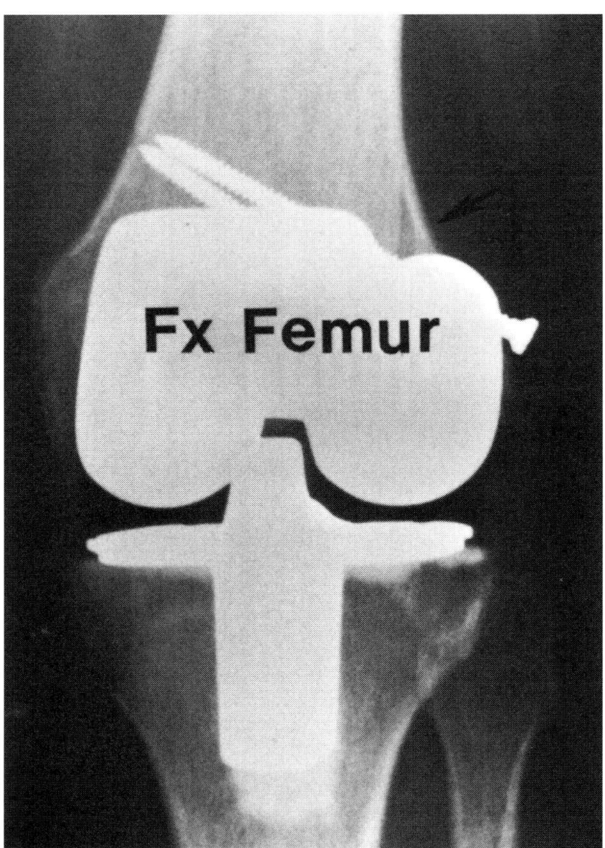

FIGURE 87.26 ➢ An intraoperative fracture of the lateral femoral condyle occurred in this case. After fixation with two screws, the aftercare was uneventful, and weightbearing as usual was permitted.

FRACTURES

Three types of fractures occur around the prosthesis: (1) intraoperative, (2) stress or fatigue related, and (3) postoperative.

Intraoperative Fractures

Intraoperative fractures can occur on either the tibial plateau or the femoral condyles. They are most likely to occur when bone is brittle and when the prosthesis is driven hard onto the bone. Tibial fractures can occur with central stem models when the stem hole is undersized; these are seldom of consequence and require no special treatment. Femoral condyle fractures may occur when the bone is very soft, as in rheumatoid arthritis, and the component is driven into the bone more than intended, resulting in a malposition. In posterior stabilizing designs with a central box, insertion of the femoral condyles may split the femur vertically (Fig. 87.26) when the bone cuts for the box are not exactly parallel. If the fracture is stable, no fixation is required, although screws may be needed (see Fig. 87.26). The addition of a stem to the femoral component may also be considered.

Intraoperative fractures are usually nondisplaced with minimal or no comminution. These fractures seldom require any special postoperative management, except perhaps a crutch assist for a longer time. Motion does not need to be delayed.

Intraoperative patella fractures are most commonly seen in the revision setting, with removal of the stable component. There are generally two types: horizontal and vertical. Horizontal fractures are more difficult to deal with, mainly secondary to concern over the integrity of the extensor mechanism. Usually a tension band technique is required to stabilize the patella and allow for some early motion. If the tension band is successful, then the patella component is not replaced. If the fragments cannot be satisfactorily repaired, other options include patellectomy or, in rare circumstances, an extensor mechanism allograft.

Intraoperative femoral fracture usually involves splitting or fracturing one of the condyles. Another observed fracture is perforation or fracture of the anterior cortex with the alignment rod. The condyles are usually handled with cancellous screws across the condyles or, in situations with greater comminution, a long-stemmed femoral component. The breach of the anterior cortex is treated also with a long-stemmed femoral component.

Intraoperative tibia fractures are usually of the vertical variety. They are caused by impingement of the stem or impaction during surgery. These fractures usually heal very well with little intervention. They are best treated with partial weightbearing and full ROM in the early postoperative period.

Stress or Fatigue Fractures

Stress fractures[220] adjoining the components usually occur in the patella (see later discussion) but also occur in the femur (Fig. 87.27) and tibia. These have been seen after a stripping of the lateral femoral condyle for the correction of fixed valgus deformity apparently caused by avascularity of the bone. Stress fracture of the tibia with medial sinkage and displacement of the tibial component has also been seen in a rheumatoid patient. Stress fractures involving femoral and tibial components usually require revision with the addition of appropriate augments and stems.

Stress fractures of the hip[79] may occur in patients who, before surgery, were unable to walk. This has occurred in two of our patients, and we have also seen fractures of the pubic rami. These complications might be avoided by prolonged use of crutches or a walker, but, unfortunately, in patients at risk it may not be practical.

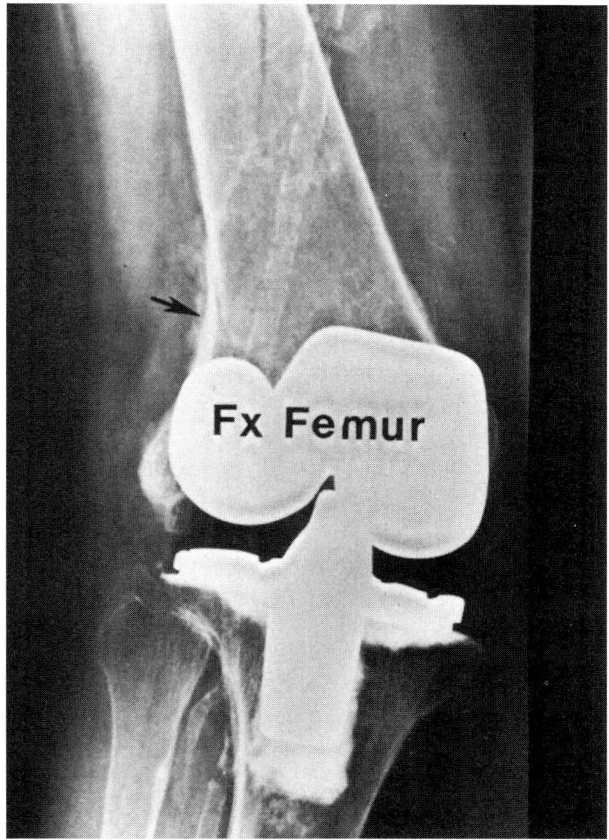

FIGURE 87.27 ➢ In this rheumatoid patient, a lateral soft tissue release was done to correct a severe valgus deformity. Two months after operation, pain and a recurrent valgus deformity developed. A stress fracture of the lateral femoral condyle was observed that healed in a position of deformity. The femoral component in this case is apparently not loose, and the knee is painless.

Postoperative Fractures

Postoperative periprosthetic fractures are somewhat more difficult to treat than intraoperative fractures. Patella and femoral fractures are more common than tibia fractures. The overall incidence is reported to be 0.3% to 2%.[38] The cause of these fractures include trauma, anterior notching of femoral cortex, osteoporosis, prolonged steroid use, preexisting neurological condition, stress shielding caused by rigid implants, pharmacological causes, hormonal influences, rheumatoid arthritis, and arthrofibrosis.[10, 36, 38] The goal of treatment is to restore the prefracture functional status by achieving fracture union and maintaining proper limb alignment and ROM with preservation of prosthetic component if stable.

Preoperative assessment and planning are extremely important in this situation. In particular, emphasis on the physical examination evaluating active ROM, stability of components, presence of extensor lag, palpation for obvious defect in the extensor mechanism, and quadriceps strength is crucial. Radiographs with a minimum of AP, lateral, and Merchant views should be obtained. Assessment of the fracture for size and displacement is also essential, as is assessment of the components for obvious signs of loosening. Finally, scrutinize the patient for any type of osseous defects, whether from comminution or osteolysis. If surgery is contemplated, then a medical consult is advised secondary to the older age and multiple medical problems.

Many classification systems have been proposed for these types of fractures. We use a system where type I is a nondisplaced fracture with stable components. Type IIA is a displaced fracture with no comminution and stable components. Type IIB is a displaced fracture with comminution and stable components. Type III is either a nondisplaced or displaced fracture with loose components. In general, type I fractures are treated nonoperatively, type II fractures usually require some type of manipulation and or fixation with retention of components, and type III fractures require revision arthroplasty.

Postoperative patella fractures are often asymptomatic. Occasionally patients will report a sudden onset of pain with knee flexion or difficulty climbing stairs. The causes of patella fractures have been attributed to certain design features of the femoral implant or to patella maltracking, both causing excessive concentrations of patella stress. The integrity of the bone and its capacity for repair of microtrauma may also be compromised by devascularization of the patella during lateral release resection of the fat pad or aggressive stripping of soft tissue around the patella.[131, 147] Tria et al[268] found an increased rate of patella fracture associated with lateral release in which the lateral superior genicular artery was not preserved. Patellar fractures after TKA can occur with and without patellar resurfacing, although they are more common when a patellar implant has been used.[25, 76, 97, 113, 140, 225, 227, 290] Treatment is dependent on three factors: integrity of extensor mechanism, displacement of the fracture, and prosthetic fixation. A nondisplaced fracture or mini-

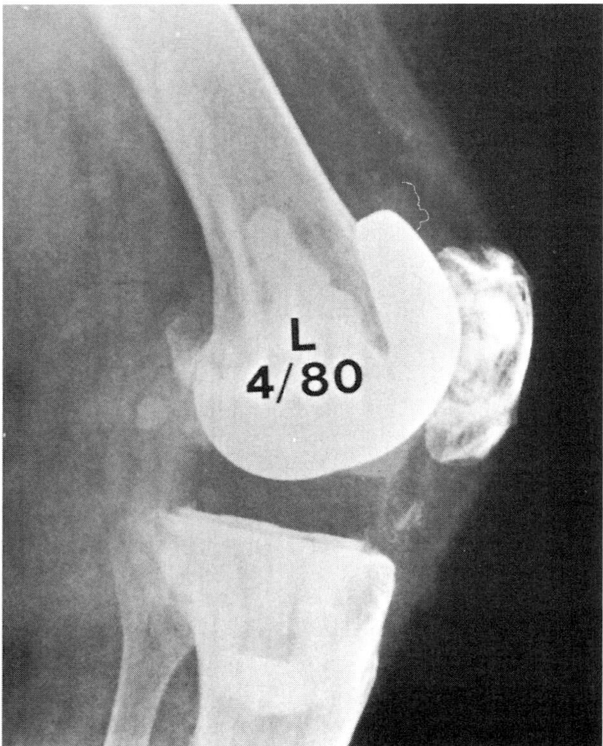

FIGURE 87.28 ➢ A healed fracture of the lower pole of the patella. This patient has an excellent result and no quadriceps weakness.

mally displaced fracture (<3 mm) may be treated in a knee immobilizer or cylinder cast for 3 to 4 weeks (Fig. 87.28). Surgery is reserved for displaced fractures, disruption of extensor mechanism, and prosthetic loosening. The main goal of treatment is fracture healing, even if that means removing a well-fixed component or not replacing a loose one. Tension band wiring technique can be used with excision of any loose or comminuted pieces of bone that cannot be properly incorporated into the repair. Patellectomy is a last resort.

Postoperative femoral fractures can be very difficult to treat. Most fractures that result from a fall or other injury occur in the lower femur adjoining the prosthesis and may be comminuted and displaced.[1, 32, 47, 50, 77, 106, 186, 232, 251] Fractures seem more likely to occur in this region if the femur was breached at operation by notching of the anterior femoral cortex (Fig. 87.29). Ritter et al[226] do not believe that femoral notching predisposes to fracture, but others consider it is a contributing factor. Notching was more likely before a complete range of femoral sizes became available. Size mismatch creates the need to fit a relatively small prosthesis onto a larger bone (Fig. 87.30). Techniques that size the femoral component from the posterior femoral condyles may also predispose the femur to notching because the adjustment cut in between sizes will be made anteriorly. Techniques that reference the anterior femoral cortex should be immune from this risk.

Supracondylar fractures are often comminuted with displacement of the femoral component posteriorly and laterally (Fig. 87.31). Operative fixation is complicated by the presence of the femoral component, which interferes with fixation of the distal fragment. Periprosthetic fractures have a higher rate of nonunion than other supracondylar femoral fractures in the elderly. This finding has been attributed to premorbid alterations in vascularity at the fracture site as a result of previous surgery, the presence of a metal implant and intramedullary PMMA, or long-term oral corticosteroid administration.

A type I fracture that is nondisplaced with the component well fixed is best treated nonoperatively. The treatment is with a brace or cast brace, allowing for ROM. In some situations, a long-leg cast may be applied for 3 weeks followed by a brace until healed. Traction (Fig. 87.32) with a tibial or os calcis pin has lost most of its popularity secondary to concerns with DVT, PE, pressure sores, and pulmonary infections in this elderly population. The key to nonoperative treatment is close monitoring to ensure there is no displacement of the fracture or alignment changes in the

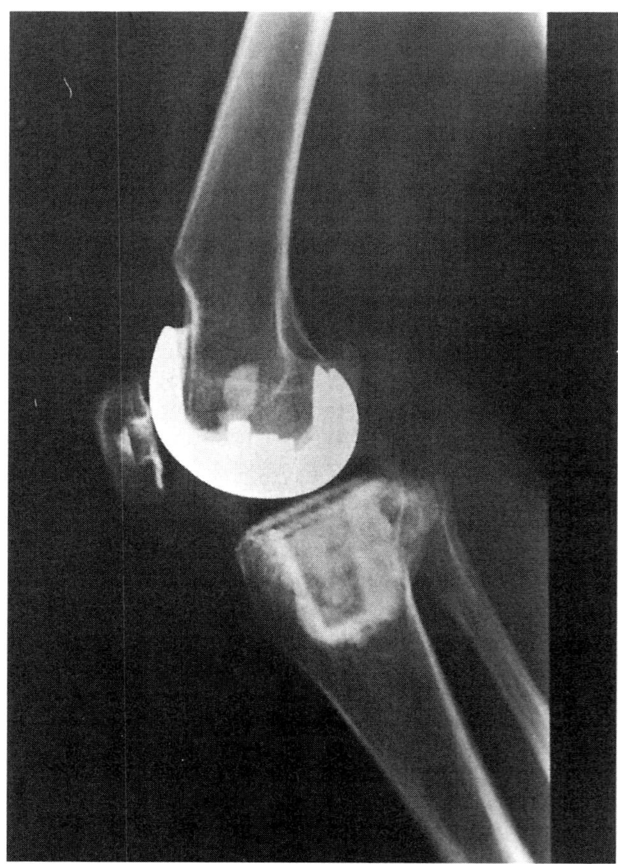

FIGURE 87.29 ➢ A lateral radiograph showing a notch in the femur caused by miscutting the anterior surface. Notching of the femur predisposes to supracondylar fracture.

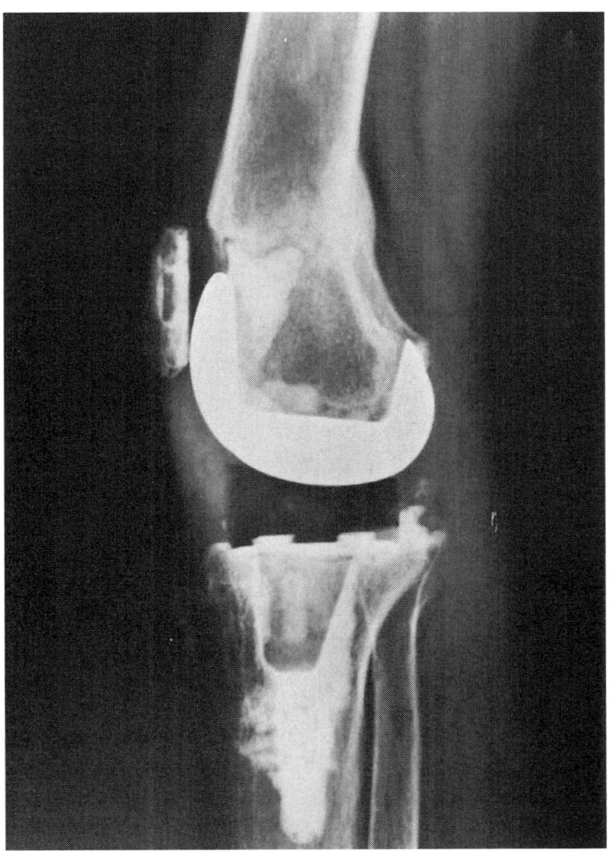

FIGURE 87.30 ➢ The saw has violated the anterior cortex of the femur. The weakened bone makes it susceptible to fracture.

extremity. Operative intervention is necessary for displacement of fracture, for malalignment, and in patients who are not able to tolerate the brace or have difficulty with the restricted weightbearing. Surgical options include retrograde nail, blade plate (Fig. 87.33), condylar buttress plate, condylar screw, Rush rods, or Zickel supracondylar rods. All have inherent advantages and disadvantages. The intramedullary devices like the retrograde nail, Rush rod, and Zickel rod do not disrupt the fracture site. Retrograde nails cannot be used if the patient has a posterior stabilized femoral component with closed housing or a long-stemmed component. The buttress plate, blade plate, and condylar screw have the disadvantage of requiring a long lateral scar and disruption of the fracture site.

A type II fracture with displacement but stable components usually requires operative intervention. In the appropriate situation, a trial of closed reduction with subsequent bracing or casting may be attempted. This treatment is seldom successful and requires a surgical procedure. There are many devices to choose from, but there are some important factors to consider when choosing this device: type of implant, comminution, displacement, and angulation of the fracture, bone quality, and extremity alignment. The selection of devices is similar to those used for the type I fracture. The buttress plate may be difficult to use in this elderly population secondary to poor bone quality and comminution. If the retrograde nail is to be used, then the intercondylar space needs to be ascertained. This is done by knowledge of the prosthesis or measurement on a notch or sunrise radiograph. A minimum of 12 mm is needed.

A type III fracture with loosening of the component is usually treated with a revision. This can be accomplished in one of two ways. First, the fracture may be treated first, allowed to heal, and then a revision performed. Alternatively, one may elect to perform the revision as part of the fracture stabilization. We prefer to perform the revision as part of the fracture stabilization, the underlying rationale being early mobilization of the patient. Most of the patients are elderly with multiple medical problems, and early mobilization decreases the incidence of medical complications, muscle atrophy, and so on. If the fracture is treated first, it could take 4 to 6 months to heal. Then after the revision it could be another 4 to 6 months for the patient to be independent again. If the revision and stabilization are performed simultaneously, the total recovery time is usually 4 to 6 months. There are two main advantages to delaying a revision procedure and treating the fracture first: (1) revision of a knee that has an anatomically healed supracondylar fracture is far easier than revision of one that has an unstable condylar fragments; (2) a standard revision implant can be used rather than a tumor replacement, a custom-made implant, or a large structural allograft. During the revision, a long-stemmed femoral component should be used. If the condyles are too comminuted or there is large amount of bone loss, then one must be prepared with alternatives to replace the deficiencies. Options include allograft,[35] implants made to replace distal femur, allograft-implant composites, and tumor prosthesis. For these cases, it may be necessary to cement the femoral stem extension.

Postoperative periprosthetic tibial fractures are more rare than femoral or patella fractures. The largest published series to date is by Felix et al,[74] with 83 fractures occurring in the postoperative period. Before that series, the largest series was 15 reported by Rand.[216] The classification system proposed by Felix et al[74] is the most commonly used system. There are four types, subclassified as A (prosthesis radiographically well fixed), B (loose), and C (intraoperative). Type I involves the tibial plateau; in type II the fracture is adjacent to the prosthetic stem; type III fracture is distal to the stem; and in type IV the fracture involves the tibial tubercle.

Treatment of a type IA fracture is nonoperative with a brace or cast, along with protected weightbearing. Type IB, which is more common, is best treated with revision of components and treatment of the depression with bone graft or metal wedges. Type IIA and IIIA fractures, if nondisplaced, can be treated with brace or cast, along with protected weightbearing. If displaced, then an attempt at closed reduction and casting is made. If unsuccessful, then open reduction

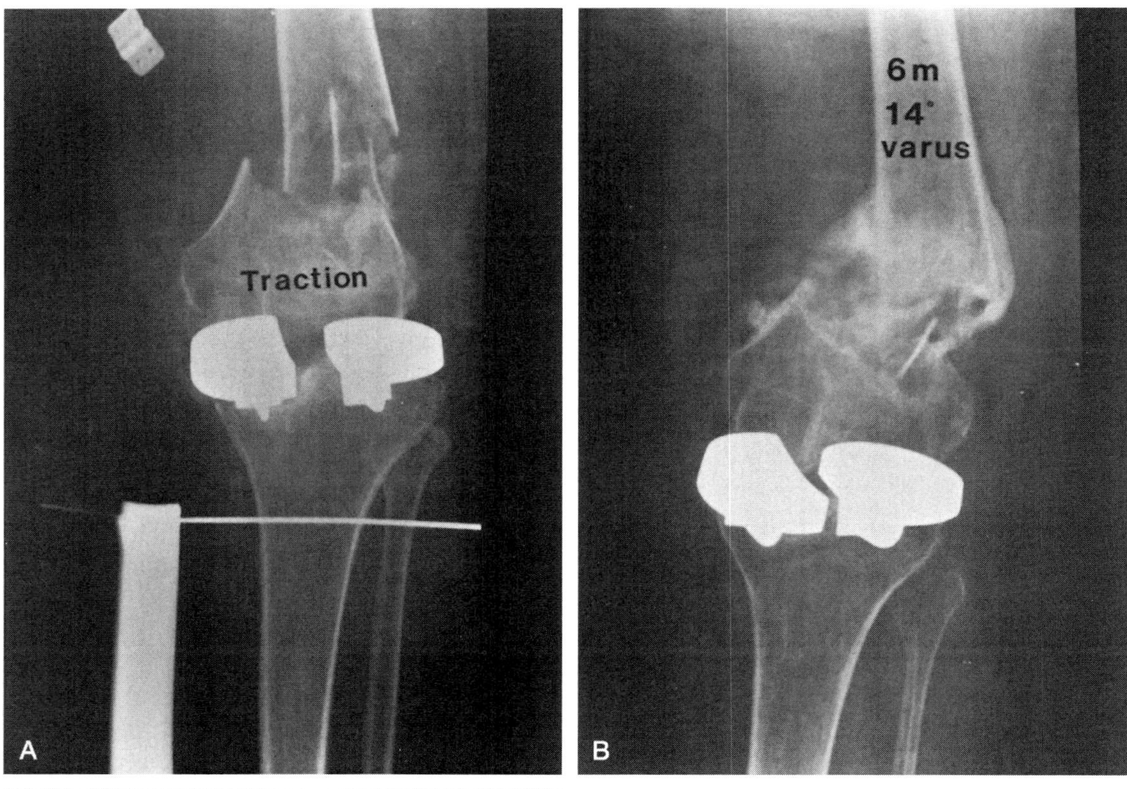

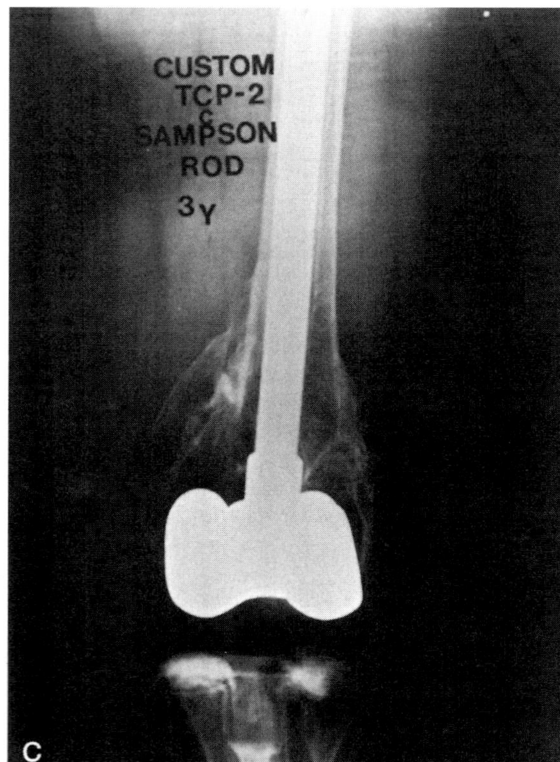

FIGURE 87.31 ➢ *A,* Radiograph of a supracondylar fracture of the femur adjacent to McKeever prostheses. *B,* Nonunion of the fracture after traction. *C,* Replacement of the knee with a prosthesis, which has a custom Sampson rod attached to the femoral component and used for internal fixation of the fracture, which united.

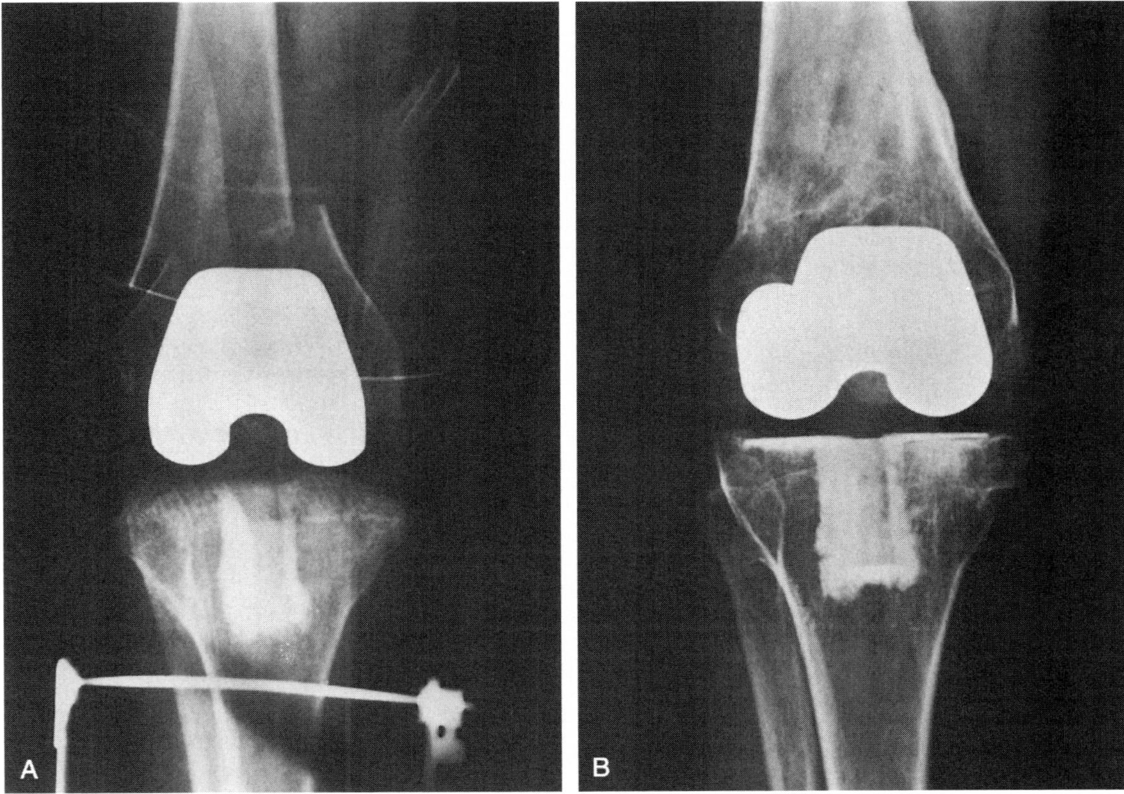

FIGURE 87.32 ➢ *A,* Supracondylar fracture of the femur treated by traction. *B,* Result after the fracture healed; good alignment and good function were preserved. (From Sisto DJ, Lachiewicz PR, Insall JN: Treatment of supracondylar fractures following prosthetic arthroplasty of the knee. Clin Orthop 196:265, 1985.)

and internal fixation (ORIF) is performed. Type IIB and IIIB fractures require revision arthroplasty with long-stemmed components. Nondisplaced type IV fractures are treated in extension with cast or knee immobilizer. Displaced type IV fractures are treated with ORIF.[74]

Results

The results of intraoperative fracture treatment are sparse for a number of reasons. First, it is rare. Second, it is largely unreported. Lombardi et al[170] reported on 41 intercondylar distal femoral fractures; 6 were identified intraoperatively and treated with a long-stemmed femoral component, screw fixation, or both. All six went on to heal without modification of postoperative regimen. The other 35 fractures were incidental findings on postoperative radiographs. All healed with the standard physical therapy protocol. Felix et al[74] reported on 19 intraoperative tibia fractures. Eleven were type IC fractures. Nine were fixed intraoperatively, and two were found postoperatively and treated with either a cast or activity modification. Nine of 11 (81%) had no pain or mild occasional pain. One patient had pain with weightbearing and was unable to walk five blocks. The last patient underwent revision for component loosening. Seven were type IIC fractures. Four were seen intraoperatively. Two required no treatment, and two required bone grafting. Three fractures were seen on postoperative radiographs; all were treated with a brace or a weightbearing restrictions. Six of seven patients had no knee pain at mean follow-up of 50 months. One patient had a type IIIC fracture that was treated with casting and non-weightbearing for 7 weeks. The patient had multiple medical problems and died 8 months after surgery.

More results are available for treatment of postoperative patella fractures. For type I fractures that are non- or minimally displaced and treated nonoperatively, the results were universally good.[25, 91, 113, 265] The results of operative treatment of displaced patellar fractures, especially with an extensor lag, have been poor.[25, 91, 113, 265] A representative study of treatment of patella fractures was one done at the Hospital for Special Surgery.[265] Of 18 patella fractures occurring after a TKA, 4 were treated operatively and 14 nonoperatively. The results of the four treated operatively were rated good in three and fair in one. Of the 14 nonoperatively treated knees, results in 10 were rated excellent and in 4 good. None of this group had demonstrable quadriceps weakness or an extension lag.

The results of nonoperative treatment for nondisplaced femoral fractures are very good.[36, 186, 195] The outcome of treatment of displaced femoral fractures is a little more variable because of the varied treatment

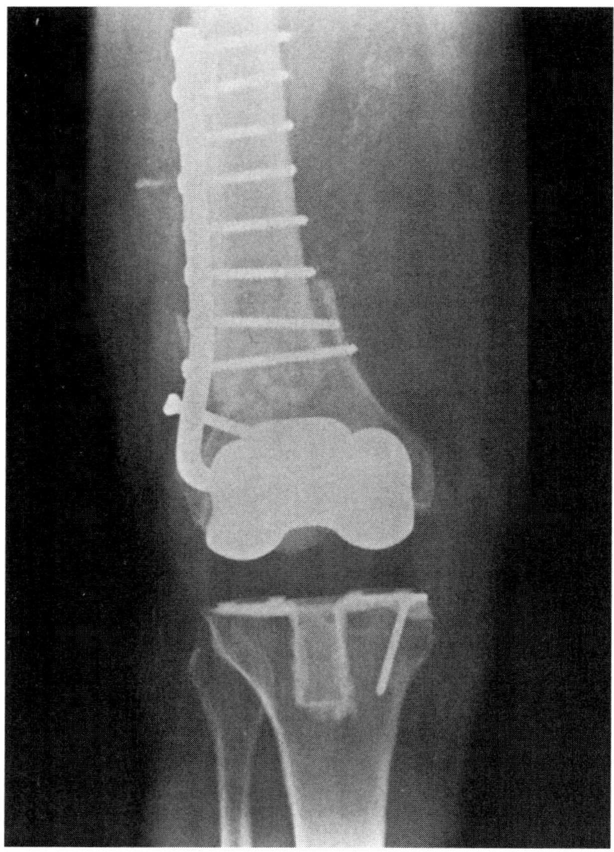

FIGURE 87.33 ➢ Fixation of a supracondylar fracture with a blade plate and screws. A low-grade infection subsequently developed requiring removal of the hardware and the knee implant.

options. One study that examined the use of Rush rods in 22 fractures found that all healed in 3 to 4 months. Two of the fractures healed in 15 degrees of valgus because of technical error. The patients recovered an average of 108 degrees of knee flexion. [228] The results of treatment with plates and screws is, for the most part, encouraging. Healy et al[103] found that 18 of 20 fractures healed after treatment with blade plate, a condylar screw, or a buttress plate. Bone graft was used in 15 of the patients. The postoperative Knee Society scores were equivalent to the prefracture scores. Culp et al[50] reported that 17 of 20 fractures healed after treatment with a compression plate. There have been reports of poor results with treatment with plates and screws.[47, 77, 205] Most of the failures and poor outcomes using plates and screws may be attributed to angulation of the fracture (malunion), migration of the condylar screw or plate, nonunion, poor knee motion, and infection.[64] The clinical results of the use of retrograde intramedullary rods is encouraging, but the numbers in most studies are small.[128, 185, 201, 231] Complications of this method of treatment include migration of the rod into the knee joint, femoral shortening, nonunion, loss of motion, and infection.

For type III fractures of the femur that include loosening of the component, requiring use of a revision component, the results are good. Cordeiro et al[47] reported on five fractures treated with a revision stem; all five healed with good results. Kraay et al[154] used a combination long-stemmed prosthesis and allograft in seven patients, all of whom had a satisfactory outcome. McLaren et al[185] treated 25 knees, most of which received a long-stemmed revision; 24 had a satisfactory outcome.

Overall clinical results of management of femoral fractures after TKA was reviewed by Chen et al.[36] The review incorporated 195 fractures in 12 published studies. Satisfactory results were achieved in 83% of the patients with nondisplaced fractures that were treated without surgery. In the patients with displaced fractures, 64% had satisfactory results with and without surgery. There was no statistically significant difference in satisfactory outcomes between nonoperative and operative treatments (67% versus 61%).

There are very few reports of treatment results of postoperative tibia fractures after TKA. Rand and Coventry[220] reported on 15 type IB fractures with loose prostheses. All were treated with revision surgery, and all did well. All the knees with tibia fractures had axial malalignment with increased varus compared with the control group. Lotke and Ecker[172] reported on five fractures of the medial tibial plateau; four of the five tibial components were aligned in varus. Cordeiro et al[47] reported on one tibial fracture that occurred below the prosthesis with loose components (type IIIB) that was treated by a long-stemmed revision. This fracture went on to heal without incident.

COMPONENT BREAKAGE

Breakage of components is rare[33, 98, 198] and usually restricted to hinges and linked designs.[200] Breakage is manifest by instability, pain, and deformity, but does not necessarily call for immediate revision. One of our patients had a fracture of the femoral stem associated with an episode of transient pain 3 years after the arthroplasty. Although some instability was present, this patient functioned at a high level with little or no pain for another 5 years before revision became necessary for an increasing varus deformity.

Mechanical failure in surface replacement is very rare. We have encountered three fractured femoral components in the early version of the uni- and duocondylar prostheses. In these, the femoral runner was made of considerably thinner metal than that used on subsequent designs, and it is not expected that similar fatigue failure will be seen in current models. Fracture of unicondylar metal components has also been reported.[33] Whiteside et al[282] examined fracture of femoral components in cementless TKA. They compared 6172 Ortholoc II femoral components with double-bead layers with 16,230 Ortholoc II femoral components with single-bead layers for fracture of components. They found 32 fractured femoral components in all, 31 of which were in the double-bead layers. The overall minimum rate of failure for the double-bead layers was 0.42%, whereas for the single-bead layer it was 0.006%. They found that all the failures occurred at the junction between one of the level surfaces and the distal surface of the implant.

Fracture of the metallic tibial tray has been reported on isolated occasions.[98, 248] Subsequently, in these designs, the metal tray was strengthened, particularly in the region of the posterior cruciate cutout. We have not seen a metal tray fracture in a cruciate-substituting design.

COMPONENT WEAR

Retrieval analysis of removed total joint implants has consistently revealed polyethylene particles in the synovium.[29, 93, 94, 190] In addition, acrylic debris and occasionally metallic particles have also been seen. Inspection of the removed components often reveals embedded cement particles in the polyethylene component with scratching, pitting, and burnishing of the articular surface. Distortion of the polyethylene and gross deformation of the component as a result of cold flow (Fig. 87.34) may also occur and is particularly likely when the tibial polyethylene component is thin. Some of the earlier designs possessed a component that was deliberately made thin to minimize bone removal and, in addition, often had a cruciate cutout. This combination led, in some instances, to gross distortion and deformation, which contributed to loosening of the component. (The early UCI design was prone to this type of failure.) It is now considered that, unless the component is reinforced with a metal tray, a minimum thickness of 8 mm is desirable.

Metal femoral components may be observed to have scratches in the highly polished articular surface in more than one-half of the retrieved specimens.

It is believed that some of the debris is generated from free cement particles that have become entrapped between the articular surfaces. Careful surgical technique can lessen cement entrapment; however, even in the absence of evidence of cement or body wear, polyethylene failure at the articular surface may be observed. This is manifested by pitting, scratching, burnishing, and abrasion of the surface. The amount of surface failure is highly correlated with the level of patient activity, body weight, and length of implantation, and seems to be of a greater degree than noted in retrieval analysis of total hip implants.[111]

The type of motion occurring in the articulation is also of importance. Sliding as opposed to rolling movements cause much greater wear, especially of the delamination type. Thus, the kinematic conditions in the joint seem to be of great importance.[18] Uncomforming flat surfaces, together with lax ligaments, predispose to various sliding motions.

The durability of a spherically convex polyethylene patellar implant may be questioned in that this shape theoretically causes more wear. Retrieval analysis at the Hospital for Special Surgery of 20 patellar buttons[112] did not indicate that the rate of wear is greater than that of the tibial plateau. There is, however, some deformation of the polyethylene, usually with elongation in the long axis and some flattening of the convex shape where it articulates with the femoral component. Figgie et al[78] examined all polyethylene dome patellar components and found a positive correlation between the amount of polyethylene damage and the ROM achieved postoperatively.

Metal backing of patellar components has not improved the wear performance characteristics but rather has led to the increase in wear-related complications.[11, 12, 170, 234, 261]

Hsu and Walker[116] more recently studied wear patterns in patellar components. They found that wear occurred regardless of the design shape, although wear was most rapid in dome patellas with metal inlays. A dome patella is only in line contact with the femur until approximately 70 degrees of flexion, after which the patella contacts peripherally with the condylar runners. Contouring the shape of the patella (central convexity and peripheral concavity) greatly improved the wear characteristics, which was better still when the component was metal backed. However, even with optimal shape and metal backing,

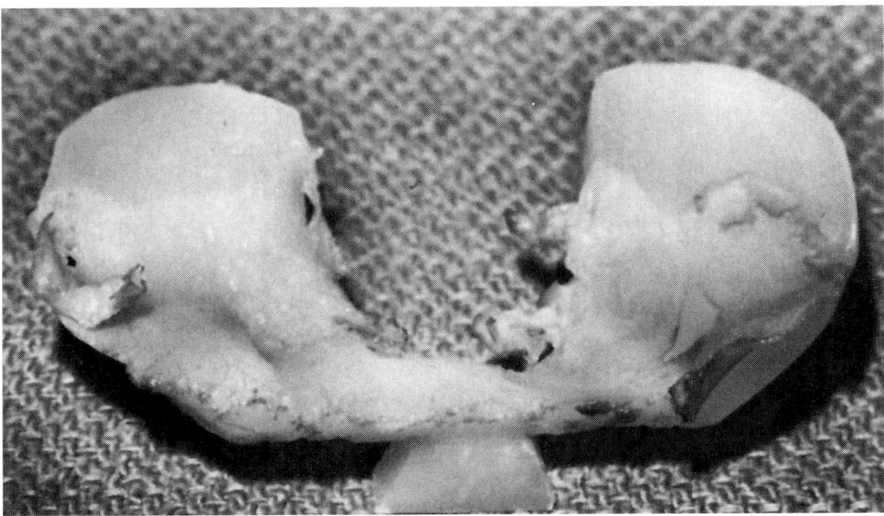

FIGURE 87.34 ➢ A retrieved geometric tibial component showing severe wear.

wear-through was ultimately predicted because of design constraints on the thickness of the polyethylene (approximately 3 mm). They concluded that currently onset patellar replacements with metal backing should not be used. Inlaying the patellar component allows a thicker layer of plastic, which may be an improvement from the wear point of view, but does not allow polyethylene resurfacing at the margins of the patella, the regions that will be subject to the greatest contact pressures when the knee is flexed. There has been a general return to cemented all-polyethylene patellar components, although agreement on this point is not uniform.[44]

Tibial polyethylene wear has emerged as a major clinical problem,[42, 65, 92, 138, 148, 189] particularly with designs having flat tibial surfaces and thin polyethylene.[37] Isolated cases of wear-through initially were reported for the porous-coated anatomic prosthesis[63] and the variable axis prosthesis. In the described cases, the medial polyethylene wore through to the metal base plate (see Fig. 87.35). The original thickness of the components was about 5 mm. These were treated by replacing the polyethylene insert with a thicker one. Posterior wear-through to metal has been seen on the Robert Brigham unicondylar design on 6-mm components[152, 153] and also on the posterior polyethylene of

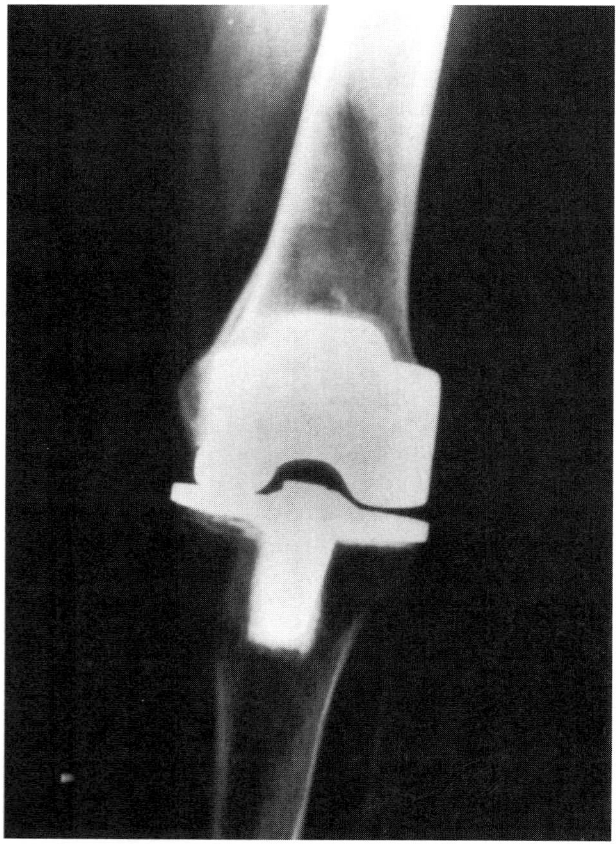

FIGURE 87.35 ➢ Radiograph of a Kinematic prosthesis 5 years postoperatively showing wear-through of the medial tibia.

Kinematic components, in which it was judged that excessive femoral rollback had occurred.

Wear damage to polyethylene is influenced by both clinical and design factors.[224] Studies performed on tibial components of a single design showed significant correlation between the amount of polyethylene damage to the articulating surface and both patient weight and the length of implantation of the component.[294] There has also been found to be greater wear damage in patients who achieved better ambulatory status postoperatively.

It seems likely that thinner components will also wear through, particularly in younger, more active people. The minimum thickness of polyethylene is, at this time, thought to be about 8 mm. Increasing conformity between the components (Fig. 87.36) will improve the wear characteristics, which, on current evidence, is a greater priority than reducing fixation stresses. Even relatively constrained articular shapes have negligible loosening,[249] and it is encouraging that the long-term study of the total condylar prosthesis did not reveal measurable polyethylene wear in any case.[272]

With the increased modularity afforded by metal tibial trays, a new problem has arisen: undersurface wear.[208] This is caused by micromotion between the polyethylene insert and the tray (usually made of titanium), causing particulate polyethylene debris to accumulate. In uncemented trays, the debris can filter down the screw holes, initiating osteolysis. Studies documented that, under physiological loading, modular designs have motion between the tray and the polyethylene insert regardless of the locking mechanism.[207] Wasielewski et al[278] examined 67 polyethylene tibial inserts from cementless TKA retrieved at autopsy or revision surgery. The mean implantation time was 62.8 months. Polyethylene cold flow and abrasive wear on the monoarticulating insert surface (undersurface) was assigned a wear severity score (grade 0 to 4). They found that severe grade 4 wear of the tibial insert undersurface was associated with tibial metaphyseal osteolysis or osteolysis around fixation screws. Time in situ was statistically related to grade 4 undersurface wear and tibial metaphyseal osteolysis.

Meniscal-bearing designs such as the Oxford and LCS (low contact stress) are theoretically the least liable to wear, but the possibility of dislocation of the bearings offsets the advantage to some extent.[16]

Lessons learned from the polished undersurface of the mobile bearing designs may be applied to fixed platform designs. Retrieval analysis of mobile bearing designs have not shown excessive wear of the back insert surface or tibial metaphyseal osteolysis.[27] With studies demonstrating that micromotion occurs between the insert and the tray regardless of locking mechanism, the next step is to polish the trays and analyze wear pattern and debris generation.

Landy and Walker[160] examined 90 retrieved knee prostheses with implant times of up to 10 years. Polyethylene wear was much greater than seen in wear studies of acetabular components in total hip prostheses. Abrasion, burnishing, and deformation was seen in

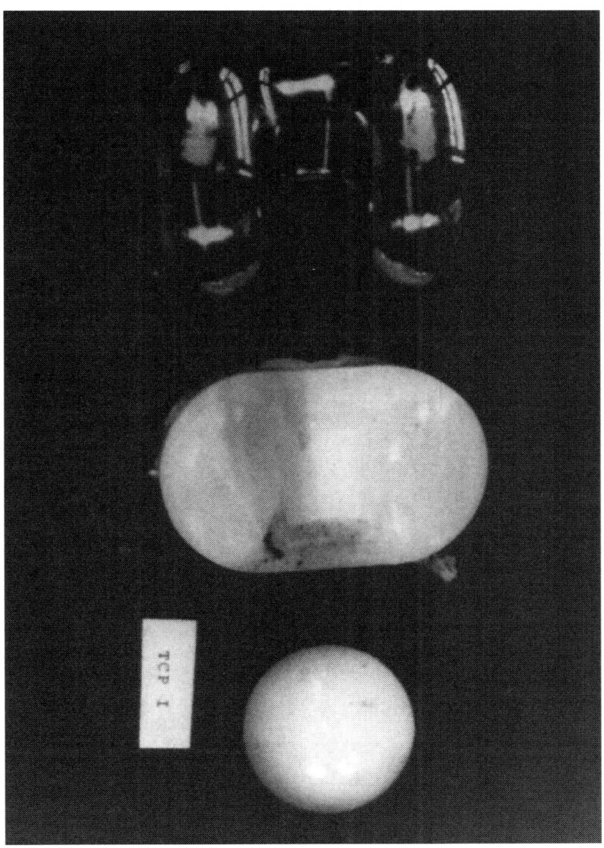

FIGURE 87.36 ➢ Retrieved total condylar prosthesis removed because of infection having been implanted for 7 years in an active patient. The appearance of the tibial component shows some burnishing and a few small pits. The patellar component shows slight flattening in one area. There is no other evidence of cold flow, delamination, or cracking of the polyethylene.

approximately 90% of the components. Cement particles embedded in the surface were found in about one-half. Delamination, the most severe form of polyethylene degradation, was found in 37%. Eight flat unicondylar components, which had the longest mean implant times (7.8 years), showed the most severe delamination. Twelve dished unicondylar components (6.3-year implant time) demonstrated less delamination. Six one-piece tibial components, with a mean wear time of 4.3 years, showed much less delamination, almost entirely restricted to the central margin.

There was considerable variation in the range of molecular weights between manufacturers and even between different components from the same manufacturer: the wear score for compression-molded components was higher than for other components.

The authors concluded that ultra-high-molecular-weight polyethylene is a questionable material for total knee components. However, currently, a suitable alternative is not available. The widespread adoption of metal-backed tibial components reduces deformation (Fig. 87.37), but the extra thickness of the metal is obtained either at the expense of greater tibial resection or thinner polyethylene. Apel et al[7] found that thicker (greater than 10 mm) all-polyethylene components behaved similarly to metal-backed components. For this reason as well as economic ones, we believe there may be some interest in returning to all-polyethylene components or monoblock metal back tibial augments.[164]

EXTENSOR MECHANISM AND PATELLAR-FEMORAL COMPLICATIONS

A number of complications involving the extensor mechanism can occur concomitant with TKA.[177]

Tibial Tubercle Avulsion

Avulsion of the tibial tubercle (Fig. 87.38) is an intraoperative complication that should be avoided rather than treated. Exposure can be difficult in knees that are tight or stiff, and, with the patella dislocated laterally, considerable traction is exerted on insertion of the patellar ligament. Avulsion of the tubercle during intraoperative maneuvers can easily happen, and if the periosteum tears across, an adequate reconstruction is very difficult. Three preventive measures are possible.

First, one can make the vertical capsular incision onto the tibia 1 cm medial to the tibial tubercle, so that a cuff of periosteum is reflected in continuity with the ligamentum patellae. If the insertion then begins to peel away from the tibial tubercle, the periosteal cuff is taken with the patellar ligament, thereby preserving distal soft tissue integrity.

Second, one can convert the exposure to a quadriceps snip by cutting obliquely at a 45-degree angle across the quadriceps tendon from its apex into the vastus lateralis until the quadriceps tendon and the patella can be turned distally and laterally. The quadriceps snip modification has been described earlier.

Third, one can osteotomize the tibial tubercle.[284]

An additional step intraoperatively to avoid tibia tubercle avulsion is to place a towel clip or Steinmann pin into the tibia tubercle. This will provide an extra point of fixation/stabilization. If a Steinmann pin or large Kirschner wire is used, it should be smooth rather than threaded to prevent damage to the tendon. During the procedure, it is wise to occasionally assess the amount of tension on the patellar tendon and tubercle. An assistant can unwittingly be placing tension on this area with a retractor.

Avulsion can also occur as a result of a manipulation or a fall. It has also been reported as occurring spontaneously during postoperative physical therapy, but probably this is more in the nature of a spontaneous detachment of an insertion already weakened by the operative exposure. A manipulative avulsion is avoidable, provided that the quadriceps muscle is paralyzed by a muscle relaxant before the manipulation is performed.

Once established, we know of no satisfactory method of repairing an avulsed tibial tubercle. Avulsion is most likely when the tibial bone is osteoporotic, and this factor complicates the repair. Open repair by suture, screw, or staple can be done, but all

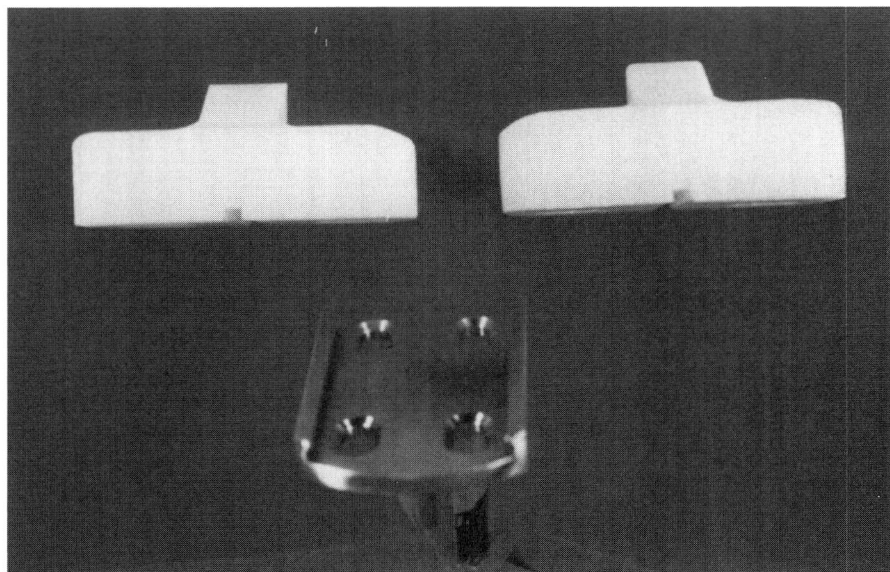

FIGURE 87.37 ➢ Metal tray support of the polyethylene prevents deformation.

too often rerupture occurs even after 6 to 8 weeks of immobilization. If the avulsion fracture is nondisplaced and the component is well fixed, a period of immobilization in extension is the best option. If the component is well fixed but the fracture is displaced, then ORIF with screw fixation should be attempted. If the fracture is displaced or nondisplaced but the component is loose, then a revision of the tibia component plus ORIF of the fracture is the best treatment.

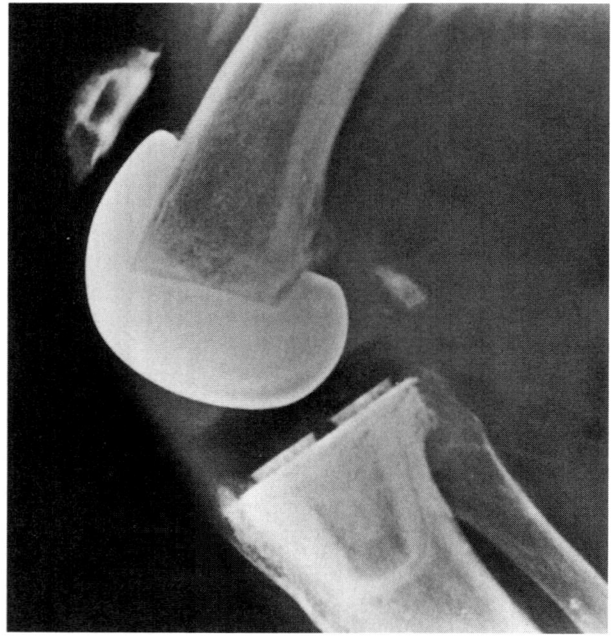

FIGURE 87.38 ➢ The patellar ligament has been avulsed from the tibial tubercle, and the patella is very high riding. There is a 40-degree extension lag.

Patellar Ligament or Quadriceps Tendon Rupture

Rupture of the patellar ligament[222] or quadriceps tendon can also happen. The incidence has been reported to range from 0.17% (14/8288)[222] to 2.5% (7/281).[172] There is an increased incidence in patients who have had a lateral release, secondary to devascularization, previous knee surgery, excision of fat pad, too deep a patellar osteotomy, closed manipulation of the knee, or osteotomy of the tibial tubercle for realignment of the extensor mechanism. The tissues are often of poor quality, making repair difficult. Many treatment options are available, including fixation with wires, staples, screws, or sutures; immobilization; ligament augmentation; and reconstruction with an allograft. None of these techniques have yielded consistently good results. Rand et al[222] cited persistent rupture after treatment in 11 of 18 knees. Cadambi and Engh[30] reported some success in treating this problem. They reported the successful clinical results in seven knees treated with autologous semitendinous tendon graft. This repair was followed by 6 weeks of immobilization in a cast. Only three of seven patients achieved more than 90 degrees of flexion. Emerson et al[62] reported their results using an allograft for a late reconstruction of a rupture of the patellar ligament. In their follow-up, only 3 of 10 allografts failed. With mostly dismal reports on treatment of this problem, prevention is the best treatment.

Patellar Complications

Subluxation and Dislocation

Various technical and design factors may contribute to subluxation and dislocation of the patella (Fig. 87.39).[15, 23, 96, 150, 169, 187, 215]

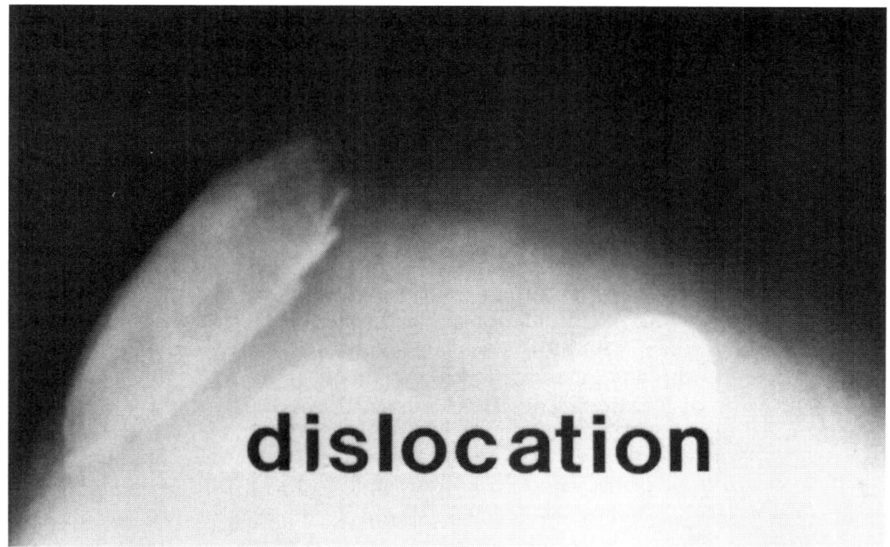

FIGURE 87.39 ➢ Gross rotary malposition of the tibial component leads to patellar dislocation.

Depth of the Femoral Trochlea. The design of the femoral sulcus is a compromise. A shallow sulcus predisposes the patella to instability, but an overly deep sulcus offers excessive constraint to the patella, which may lead to patellar component loosening and patellar fracture.

Position of the Femoral Component. Placement of the femoral component in internal rotation increases the lateral soft tissue tension as the knee is flexed.[223] As discussed elsewhere, some degree of external rotation is preferred (Fig. 87.40). We use the epicondylar axis to set the femoral rotation.

Malrotation of the Tibial Component. Internal rotation of the tibial component gives an external placement of the tibial tubercle, increasing the quadriceps angle and contributing to patellar instability. Malrotation of the tibial component is often the result of inadequate exposure. Sufficient dissection around the tibia to displace the tibial surface anteriorly gives the

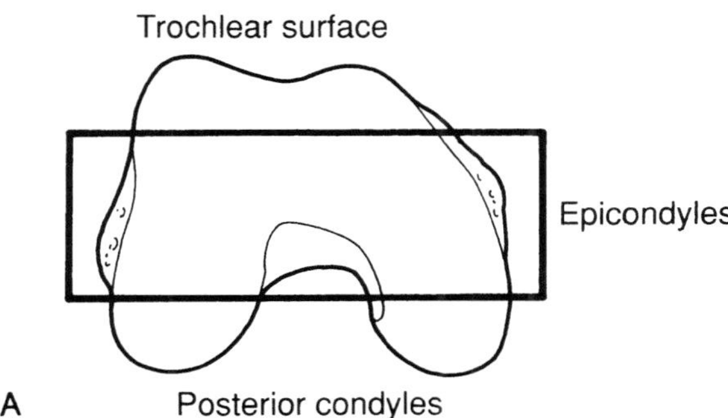

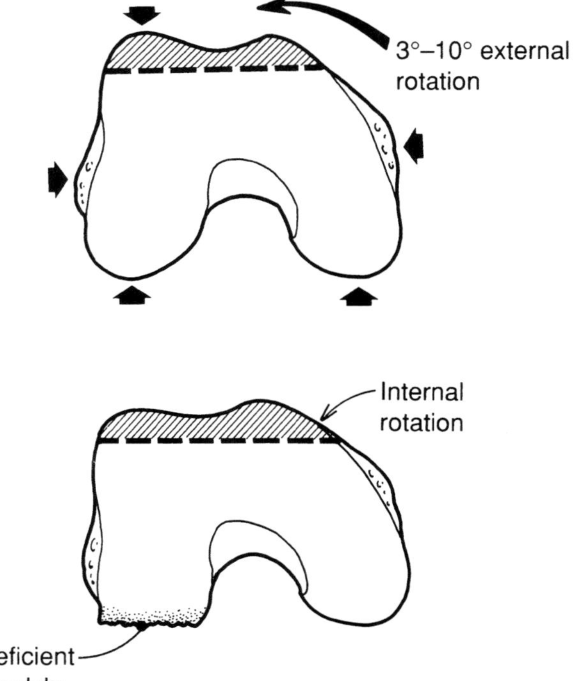

FIGURE 87.40 ➢ Internal rotation of the femoral component is a cause of patellar dislocation. The component should always be in slight *external* rotation.

best visualization of the various landmarks for tibial component placement (Fig. 87.41).

Overall Valgus Alignment. Excessive valgus position increases the quadriceps angle. Reports suggested that often patellar instability occurs in knees that were originally valgus.

Tight Lateral Retinaculum. A tight lateral retinaculum can contribute to patellar dislocation.

Patellar tracking problems after TKA have been reported to occur with an incidence as high as 29%.[131] Subluxation is more common than dislocation.[25] Patients usually complain of anterior knee pain or gross subluxation or dislocation. The treatment of this complication is dependent on its cause. A patient with mild subluxation and a weak vastus medialis would benefit from intense physical therapy. The components could be malpositioned or malaligned, which could be determined preoperatively with a CT scan (see Fig. 87.14). If this is the cause, then a revision would be appropriate. In most of the cases, the treatment is a lateral retinaculum release, sometimes in conjunction with a proximal realignment. We do not recommend a tibial tubercle transposition because of its high complication rate.

Results of surgical treatment for patella instability are good for combined lateral release and proximal realignment procedures. Grace and Rand[96] studied 25 knees with symptomatic lateral patellar instability after TKA. The knees were treated by one of three methods: proximal realignment, combined proximal and distal realignment, or component revision. At 50 months follow-up, 20 knees had normal patellar tracking, and 5 had recurrent instability. Two of nine patients who had a combined realignment had patellar tendon rupture. The authors recommended proximal realignment alone in the absence of component malposition. If the component is malpositioned, then component revision should be performed.

Merkow et al[187] reported the experience at the Hospital for Special Surgery. Between 1974 and 1982 12 dislocations occurred in 11 patients. Trauma was the cause of dislocation in three knees, incorrect tracking of the patella in six, and malrotation of the tibial component in three. Many of the knees were in valgus preoperatively. Dislocations occurred in four different prosthetic designs, suggesting that, in this series, design was not a factor. Unrestrained tibial rotation has been described as predisposing to patellar dislocation by others. Whiteside et al[283] maintained that the degree of tibial rotation is determined by the ligaments, provided they are correctly tensioned during surgery. They believe that rotational constraint in the prosthesis is unnecessary and may predispose to loosening. However, we believe that knees with initial external rotation deformities of the tibia are more easily managed by a design with rotational constraint, and this feature is also useful in managing a patellar dislocation that has already occurred. Altering the rotational position of the tibial component in a design with some constraint is the equivalent of transferring the tibial tubercle.

In Merkow's series,[187] the patellar dislocation was managed by proximal realignment in 10 cases, lateral release in 1, and proximal realignment and revision of the tibial component into a more desirable externally rotated position in 1. None of the dislocations recurred, and in none was transposition of the tibial tubercle required. We agree with Rand and Bryan[218] that tibial tubercle transposition is inadvisable after TKA because the bone quality is often poor and the proportion of complications high. Wolff et al[291] and Whiteside and Ohl[284] claimed that tibial tubercle transposition is effective with good technique. They recommended taking a relatively large fragment of the tibial tubercle so that secure fixation with screws is attainable.

Soft-Tissue Impingement

In 1982 we described a case in which a fibrous nodule was excised from the suprapatellar region of the quadriceps tendon. This nodule gave rise to what has become known as the patellar clunk syndrome (Fig. 87.42).[13, 114, 266, 271] It is most commonly associated with use of a posterior stabilized prosthesis.

The clinical manifestation is postoperative grating and catching on active extension of the knee, signs that usually appear 6 to 12 months after arthroplasty. The radiographs appear entirely normal, and no evidence of patellar subluxation is found. The cause is soft tissue impingement between the peripatellar synovium and the femoral component. Most often this in-

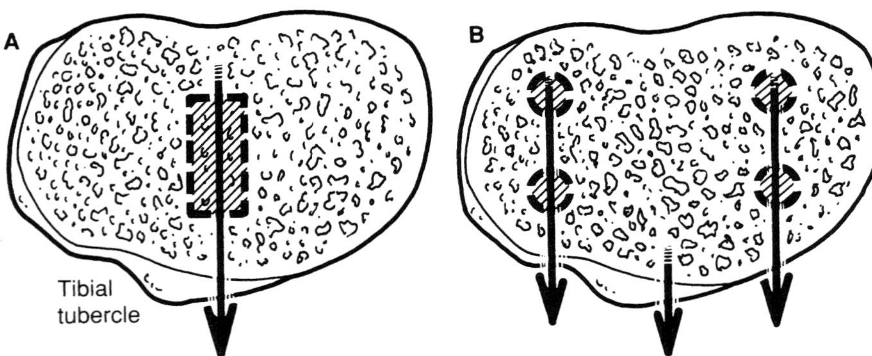

FIGURE 87.41 ➢ Alignment of the tibial component is projected at a point slightly medial to the tibial tubercle. Alignment of a symmetrical component with the posterior margin of the tibial plateau will usually result in some internal rotation of the tibial component. One should err on the side of external rotation.

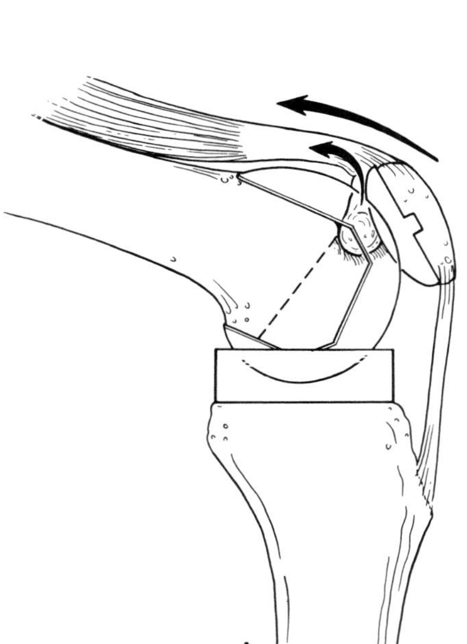

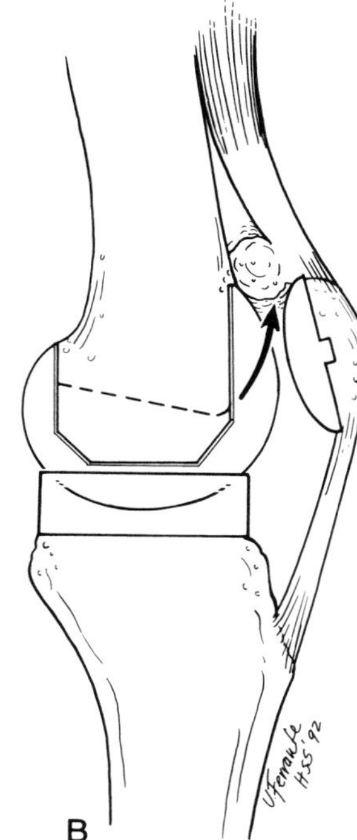

FIGURE 87.42 ➢ The patellar clunk syndrome. The cause of this peculiar symptom is a suprapatellar mass of synovium and fibrous tissue that forms a nodule, which is caught between the patella and the femoral component. This typically occurs at between 60 and 45 degrees of flexion and can result in locking of the knee in this position. As the knee is brought into terminal extension, the patella can be seen to pop and the nodule releases from its entrapped position. The symptom can be cured by arthroscopic removal of the fibrous nodule.

volves a portion of the suprapatellar synovium, which becomes irritated, inflamed, and swollen. Occasionally, a sizable mass can result, which catches within the anterior lip of the intercondylar recess of the femoral component. Because specific implant designs with a short femoral flange has been implicated, it is preferable to select an implant with a long deep femoral sulcus and a smooth transition into the intercondylar recess. These designs have greatly reduced the incidence of patellar crepitus and virtually eliminated the patellar clunk syndrome.

Soft tissue impingement and patellar clunk syndrome can be cured by the removal of the excess tissue and the "patellar meniscus" that forms around the patellar prosthetic margins. Initially, this was done by arthrotomy but more recently by arthroscopy.[271] The advantages of using arthroscopy over open arthrotomy are simplicity, decreased recurrence, decreased risk of infection, and quicker postoperative rehabilitation. Indications for open arthrotomy and excision of nodule are failure of arthroscopic débridement, malpositioned patella component, which can be a cause requiring revision of the component along with excision of nodule, and patella clunk with a loose prosthetic component. With a sharp decline in the incidence of patella clunk secondary to prosthetic design modifications, there are only a few reports of treatment outcomes. Diduch et al[57] had a success rate of 82% (14 of 17 knees) with a follow-up of 19.9 months after arthroscopic treatment of patella clunk.

UNEXPLAINED PAIN

A certain proportion of patients continue to complain of pain for which there is no obvious explanation. Sometimes the arthroplasty will objectively be functioning well and have a good ROM. The pain may be present continuously or mainly at rest. One of our patients was able to walk considerable distances and climb stairs normally without difficulty. He complained of severe pain when sitting, and, because his occupation involved frequent flying, this was a considerable problem for him. On other occasions, complaints of pain may be associated with lack of motion or flexion contracture, although the components appeared to be well seated and well positioned. We estimate the incidence of these cases to be approximately 1 in 300 arthroplasties. The cause is usually difficult to demonstrate. There is an overlap with reflex sympathetic dystrophy,[145] particularly in patients who have restricted motion. It may seem, in retrospect, that the preoperative symptoms were worse than the pathological condition of the knee. Some kind of material allergy has been suspected but never proven, although in one of our patients with a loose metal-on-metal hinge prosthesis we were able to demonstrate a skin allergy to cobalt chloride. Low-grade infection is always a possibility.

In the management of these patients, infection must be excluded as much as possible. Aspiration should be attempted, and if sufficient fluid is obtained cultures can be quite reliable; 90% of our infected knees have been diagnosed by culture of the aspirate. Bone scintigraphy[108, 143, 213] may also be useful, although technetium 99m scanning after total knee replacement gives highly variable results,[244] in that asymptomatic knees may continue to have abnormal scans indefinitely. Indium scanning[217] was found to be 85% reliable in 18 infected knees. However, in a group of 20 knees with aseptic loosening, the scan results were not given.

When reflex sympathetic dystrophy is suspected, sympathetic block should be tried. If the response is good, a lumbar sympathectomy should be considered. Nicholls and Dorr[204] reported success in surgical revision of stiff and painful knees with improvement of both motion and pain. This has not been our experience, and in most cases the results have been disappointing.

A 1996 study[192] examined the role of exploratory surgery in unexplained pain in TKA. Twenty-seven patients underwent exploration of their TKA secondary to severe debilitating pain of an unknown origin. They were divided into two groups: those with ROM less than 80 degrees and those with ROM greater than 80 degrees. At final follow-up, there were 11 excellent and good results (41%) and 16 fair or poor results (59%). Of the 15 patients with decreased ROM, 9 (60%) had good or excellent results. The ROM arc improved from a preoperative 43-degree average to an 81-degree average. For the pain only group, there were only two excellent or good results (17%). If a problem was identified at surgery, only 3 of 12 knees (25%) had successful outcomes. This study highlights the frustration of performing surgery on patients for unexplained pain. Even when the authors identified a problem at the time of surgery and corrected it, they only had a 25% success rate.

If the work-up of a painful TKA is negative, then one must consider obtaining fluoroscopically assisted radiographs. In this way, near-perfect perpendicular radiographs can be obtained to evaluate any radiolucencies, especially under the tibial tray. In one study[73] that examined painful TKA without explanation, the authors used fluoroscopic evaluation to study the knees. They had 20 patients referred to them for pain and disability after TKA with normal-appearing radiographs. All 20 patients had fluoroscopic radiographs obtained. In 14 of the 20 patients, the diagnosis of aseptic loosening was made with the new radiographs. Each of the patients thought to have a loose component at fluoroscopy did, in fact, have a loose component at revision. Each patient improved after revision with an increase in the Hospital for Special Surgery score of 26 points.

Great caution is recommended when deciding to revise a knee without good explanation of the pain, and in most cases the condition of the patient will be either unimproved or worse after revision unless a convincing intraoperative cause is found. Sometimes overgrown soft tissues or an interposed meniscal fragment will be found. Because these conditions can be managed without arthrotomy, an arthroscopic examination is recommended before revision is attempted.

INFECTION

Infection is one of the most serious complications.[3, 8, 14, 19, 20, 34, 39, 49, 52, 72, 85, 90, 99, 102] Infection is usually classified as acute (less than 3 months) or chronic (greater than 3 months). The treatment of acute infections is somewhat debatable. If the organism is of low virulence, then one may attempt an open irrigation and débridement with exchange of polyethylene. This procedure is followed by 6 weeks of intravenous antibiotics and close observation.[14, 199, 246, 263] The most appropriate treatment for a chronic infection is removal of components, débridement, and placement of a cement spacer followed by 6 weeks of intravenous antibiotics. At 6 weeks, the new components may be reimplanted if intraoperative Gram's stain and frozen sections are negative.[14, 19, 39, 199, 263, 286, 287, 289] The importance of the prevention and management of infection warrants a full-chapter discussion.

The treatment options for infection are as follows:

1. Antibiotic suppression.
2. Débridement with prosthesis in situ.
3. Removal of prosthesis.
   a. One-stage reimplantation.
   b. Two-stage reimplantation.
   c. Pseudarthrosis.
   d. "Beef-burger" operation.[139]
   e. Arthrodesis.[70, 75, 101, 132, 135, 151, 168, 180, 269, 276]

References

1. Aaron RK, Scott R: Supracondylar fracture of the femur after total knee arthroplasty. Clin Orthop 219:136, 1987.
2. Aglietti P, Windsor RE, Buzzi R, et al: Arthroplasty for the stiff or ankylosed knee. J Arthroplasty 4:1, 1989.
3. Ainscow DAP, Denham RA: The risk of haematogenous infection in total joint replacements. J Bone Joint Surg Br 66:589, 1984.
4. Albrektsson BEJ, Herberts P: ICLH knee arthroplasty: A consecutive study of 108 knees with uncemented tibial component fixation. J Arthroplasty 3:145, 1988.
5. Albrektsson BEJ, Ryd L, Carlsson LV, et al: The effect of a stem on the tibial component of knee arthroplasty: A roentgen stereophotogrammetric study of uncemented tibial components in the Freeman-Samuelson knee arthroplasty. J Bone Joint Surg Br 72:252, 1990.
6. Allenby F, Boardman L, Pflug JJ, et al: Effects of interval pneumatic intermittent compression on fibrinolysis in man. Lancet 2:1412, 1973.
7. Apel DM, Tozzi JM, Dorr LD: Clinical comparison of all-polyethylene and metal-backed tibial components in total knee arthroplasty. Clin Orthop 273:243, 1991.
8. Artz TD, Macys J, Salvati EA, et al: Hematogenous infection of total hip replacements: A report of four cases. J Bone Joint Surg Am 57:1024, 1975.
9. Asp JPL, Rand JA: Peroneal nerve palsy after total knee arthroplasty. Clin Orthop 261:233, 1990.
10. Ayers DC, Dennis DA, Johanson NA, et al: Common complications of total knee arthroplasty. J Bone Joint Surg Am 79:278, 1997.
11. Bayley JC, Scott RD: Further observations on metal-backed patellar component failure. Clin Orthop 236:82, 1988.
12. Bayley JC, Scott RD, Ewald FC, et al: Failure of the metal-backed patellar component after total knee replacement. J Bone Joint Surg Am 70:668, 1988.
13. Beight JL, Yao B, Hozack WJ, et al: The patellar clunk syndrome after posterior stabilized total knee arthroplasty. Clin Orthop 299:139, 1994.
14. Bengtson S, Knutson K, Lindgren L: Treatment of infected knee arthroplasty. Clin Orthop 245:173, 1989.
15. Berger RA, Crossett LS, Jacobs JJ, et al: Malrotation causing patellofemoral complications after total knee arthroplasty. Clin Orthop 356:144, 1998.
16. Bert JM: Dislocation/subluxation of meniscal bearing elements after New Jersey low-contact stress total knee arthroplasty. Clin Orthop 254:211, 1990.
17. Bisla RS, Inglis AE, Lewis RJ: Fat embolism following bilateral total knee replacement with the Guepar prosthesis: A case report. Clin Orthop 115:195, 1976.

18. Blunn GW, Walker PS, Joshi A, et al: The dominance of cyclic sliding in producing wear in total knee replacements. Clin Orthop 273:253, 1991.
19. Booth RE Jr, Lotke PA: The results of spacer block technique in revision of infected total knee arthroplasty. Clin Orthop 248:57, 1989.
20. Borden LS, Gearen PF: Infected total knee arthroplasty: A protocol for management. J Arthroplasty 2:27, 1987.
21. Bradley GW, Freeman MAR, Albrektsson BEJ: Total prosthetic replacement of ankylosed knees. J Arthroplasty 2:179, 1987.
22. Branson PJ, Steege JW, Wixson RL, et al: Rigidity of initial fixation with uncemented tibial knee implants. J Arthroplasty 4: 21, 1989.
23. Briard J-L, Hungerford DS: Patellofemoral instability in total knee arthroplasty. J Arthroplasty 4:587, 1989.
24. Brick GW, Scott RD: Blood supply to the patella: Significance in total knee arthroplasty. J Arthroplasty 4:575, 1989.
25. Brick GW, Scott RD: The patellofemoral component of total knee arthroplasty. Clin Orthop 231:163, 1988.
26. Brotherton SL, Roberson JR, De Andrade JR, et al: Staged versus simultaneous bilateral total knee replacement. J Arthroplasty 1:221, 1986.
27. Buechel FF: Cementless meniscal bearing knee arthroplasty: 7-12 year outcome analysis. Orthopedics 17:833, 1994.
28. Buechel FF: A sequential three-step lateral release for correcting fixed valgus knee deformities during total knee arthroplasty. Clin Orthop 260:170, 1990.
29. Bullough PG, Insall JN, Ranawat CS, et al: Wear and tissue reaction in failed knee arthroplasty. J Bone Joint Surg Br 58: 366, 1976.
30. Cadambi A, Engh GA: Use of a semitendinous tendon autogenous graft for rupture of the patellar ligament after total knee arthroplasty: A report of seven cases. J Bone Joint Surg Am 74: 974, 1992.
31. Caillouette JT, Anzel SH: Fat embolism syndrome following the intramedullary alignment guide in total knee arthroplasty. Clin Orthop 251:198, 1990.
32. Cain PR, Rubash HE, Wissinger HA, et al: Periprosthetic femoral fractures following total knee arthroplasty. Clin Orthop 208: 205, 1986.
33. Cameron HU, Welsh RP: Fracture of the femoral component in unicompartmental total knee arthroplasty. J Arthroplasty 5:315, 1990.
34. Carlsson AS, Josefsson G, Lindberg L: Revision with gentamicin-impregnated cement for deep infections in total hip arthroplasties. J Bone Joint Surg Am 60:1059, 1978.
35. Chandler HP, Tigges RG: The role of allografts in the treatment of periprosthetic femoral fractures. J Bone Joint Surg Am 79: 1422, 1997.
36. Chen F, Mont MA, Bachner RS: Management of ipsilateral supracondylar femur fractures following total knee arthroplasty. J Arthroplasty 9:521, 1994.
37. Chillag KJ, Barth E: An analysis of polyethylene thickness in modular total knee components. Clin Orthop 273:261, 1991.
38. Chmell MJ, Moran MC, Scott RD: Periarticular fractures after total knee arthroplasty: Principles of management. J Am Acad Orthop Surg 4:109, 1996.
39. Cohen JC, Hozack WJ, Cuckler JM, et al: Two-stage reimplantation of septic total knee arthroplasty. J Arthroplasty 3:369, 1988.
40. Cohen SH, Ehrlich GE, Kauffman MS, et al: Thrombophlebitis following knee surgery. J Bone Joint Surg Am 55:106, 1973.
41. Colizza WA, Insall JN, Scuderi GR: The posterior stabilized total knee prosthesis: Assessment of polyethylene damage and osteolysis after a ten-year minimum follow-up. J Bone Joint Surg Am 77:1713, 1995.
42. Collier JP, Mayor MB, McNamara JL, et al: Analysis of the failure of 122 polyethylene inserts from uncemented tibial knee components. Clin Orthop 273:232, 1991.
43. Colwell CW, Spiro TE, Trowbridge AA, et al for The Enoxaparin Clinical Trial Group: Efficacy and safety of enoxaparin versus unfractionated heparin for prevention of deep venous thrombosis after elective knee arthroplasty. Clin Orthop 321: 19, 1995.
44. Convery FR, Minteer-Convery M, Malcom LL: The spherocentric knee: A re-evaluation and modification. J Bone Joint Surg Am 62:320, 1980.
45. Cook SD, Barrack RL, Thomas KA, et al: Quantitative histologic analysis of tissue growth into porous total knee components. J Arthroplasty 4:533, 1989.
46. Cook SD, Thomas KA, Haddad RJ Jr: Histologic analysis of retrieved human porous-coated total joint components. Clin Orthop 234:90, 1988.
47. Cordeiro EN, Costa RC, Carazzato JG, et al: Periprosthetic fractures in patients with total knee arthroplasties. Clin Orthop 252:182, 1990.
48. Cornell CN, Ranawat CS, Burstein AH: A clinical and radiographic analysis of loosening of total knee arthroplasty components using a bilateral model. J Arthroplasty 1:157, 1986.
49. Cruess RL, Bickel WS, Von Kessler KLC: Infections in total hips secondary to a primary source elsewhere. Clin Orthop 106:99, 1975.
50. Culp RW, Schmidt RG, Hanks G, et al: Supracondylar fracture of the femur following prosthetic knee arthroplasty. Clin Orthop 22:212, 1987.
51. Curley P, Eyres K, Brezinova V, et al: Common peroneal nerve dysfunction after high tibial osteotomy. J Bone Joint Surg Br 72:405, 1990.
52. D'Ambrosia RD, Shoji H, Heater R: Secondarily infected total joint replacements by hematogenous spread. J Bone Joint Surg Am 58:450, 1976.
53. Deburge A: Guepar hinge prosthesis: Complications and results with two years follow-up. Clin Orthop 120:47, 1976.
54. Dempsey AJ, Finlay JB, Bourne RB, et al: Stability and anchorage considerations for cementless tibial components. J Arthroplasty 4:223, 1989.
55. Dennis DA, Neumann RD, Toma P, et al: Arteriovenous fistula with false aneurysm of the inferior medial geniculate artery: A complication of total knee arthroplasty. Clin Orthop 222:255, 1987.
56. Denny-Brown D, Doherty MM: Effects of transient stretching of peripheral nerve. Arch Neurol Psychiatry 54:116, 1945.
57. Diduch DR, Scuderi GR, Scott WN, et al: The efficacy of arthroscopy following total knee replacement. Arthroscopy 13: 166, 1997.
58. Doouss TW: The clinical significance of venous thrombosis of the calf. Br J Surg 63:377, 1976.
59. Dorr LD, Boiardo RA: Technical considerations in total knee arthroplasty. Clin Orthop 205:5, 1986.
60. Dorr LD, Merkel C, Mellman MF, et al: Fat emboli in bilateral total knee arthroplasty: Predictive factors for neurologic manifestations. Clin Orthop 248:112, 1989.
61. Dorr LD, Serocki JH: Mechanism of failure of total knee arthroplasty. In Scott WN, ed: The Knee. St. Louis, MO, CV Mosby, 1994, pp 1239.
62. Emerson RH Jr, Head WC, Malinin TI: Reconstruction of patellar tendon rupture after total knee arthroplasty with an extensor mechanism allograft. Clin Orthop 260:154, 1990.
63. Engh GA: Failure of the polyethylene bearing surface of a total knee replacement within four years: A case report. J Bone Joint Surg Am 70:1093, 1988.
64. Engh GA, Ammeen DJ: Periprosthetic fractures adjacent to total knee implants. J Bone Joint Surg Am 79:1100, 1997.
65. Engh GA, Dwyer KA, Hanes CK: Polyethylene wear of metal-backed tibial components in total and unicompartmental knee prostheses. J Bone Joint Surg Br 74:9, 1992.
66. Engh GA, Parks NL, Ammeen DJ: Tibial osteolysis in cementless total knee arthroplasty. Clin Orthop 309:33, 1994.
67. Evarts CM: Thromboembolism. In Rockwood CA Jr, Green DP, eds: Fractures. Vol. 1: Complications. Philadelphia, JB Lippincott, 1975, p 174.
68. Evarts CM: Prevention of venous thromboembolism. Clin Orthop 222:98, 1987.
69. Ezzet KA, Garcia R, Barrack RL: Effect of component fixation method on osteolysis in total knee arthroplasty. Clin Orthop 321:86, 1995.
70. Fahmy NRM, Barnes KL, Noble J: A technique for difficult arthrodesis of the knee. J Bone Joint Surg Br 66:367, 1984.
71. Fahmy NRM, Chandler HP, Danylchuk K, et al: Blood-gas and circulatory changes during total knee replacement: Role of the

intramedullary alignment rod. J Bone Joint Surg Am 72:19, 1990.

72. Falahee MH, Matthews LS, Kaufer H: Resection arthroplasty as a salvage procedure for a knee with infection after a total arthroplasty. J Bone Joint Surg Am 69:1013, 1987.
73. Fehring TK, McAvoy G: Fluoroscopic evaluation of the painful total knee arthroplasty. Clin Orthop 331:226, 1996.
74. Felix NA, Stuart MJ, Hanssen AD: Periprosthetic fractures of the tibia associated with total knee arthroplasty. Clin Orthop 345: 113, 1997.
75. Figgie HE III, Brody GA, Inglis AE, et al: Knee arthrodesis following total knee arthroplasty in rheumatoid arthritis. Clin Orthop 224:237, 1987.
76. Figgie HE III, Goldberg VM, Figgie MP, et al: The effect of alignment of the implant on fractures of the patella after condylar total knee arthroplasty. J Bone Joint Surg Am 71:1031, 1989.
77. Figgie MP, Goldberg VM, Figgie HE III, et al: The results of treatment of supracondylar fracture above total knee arthroplasty. J Arthroplasty 5:267, 1990.
78. Figgie MP: Performance of dome shaped patellar components in total knee arthroplasty. Trans Orthop Res Soc 14:531, 1989.
79. Fipp G: Stress fractures of the femoral neck following total knee arthroplasty. J Arthroplasty 3:347, 1988.
80. Firestone TP, Teeny SM, Krackow KA, et al: The clinical and roentgenographic results of cementless porous coated patellar fixation. Clin Orthop 273:184, 1991.
81. Fitzgerald RH, Spiro TE, Trowbridge AA, et al: A randomized and prospective comparison of enoxaparin and warfarin in the prevention of thromboembolic disease following total knee arthroplasty. Orthop Trans 19:335, 1995.
82. Fox JL, Poss R: The role of manipulation following total knee replacement. J Bone Joint Surg Am 63:357, 1981.
83. Francis CW, Pellegrini VD Jr, Stulberg BN et al: Prevention of venous thrombosis after total knee arthroplasty: Comparison of antithrombin III and low-dose heparin with dextran. J Bone Joint Surg Am 72:976, 1990.
84. Francis CW, Ricotta JJ, Evarts CM, et al: Long-term clinical observations and venous functional abnormalities after asymptomatic venous thrombosis following total hip or knee arthroplasty. Clin Orthop 232:271, 1988.
85. Freeman MAR, Sudlow RA, Casewell MW, et al: The management of infected total knee replacements. J Bone Joint Surg Br 67:764, 1985.
86. Galinat BJ, Vernace JV, Booth RE Jr, et al: Dislocation of the posterior stabilized total knee arthroplasty: A report of two cases. J Arthroplasty 3:363, 1988.
87. Gardner AM, Fox RH: The venous footpump: Influence on tissue perfusion and prevention of venous thrombosis. Ann Rheum Dis 51:1173, 1992.
88. Garner RW, Mowat AC, Hazleman BL: Wound healing after operations on patients with rheumatoid arthritis. J Bone Joint Surg Br 55:134, 1973.
89. Gebhard JS, Kilgus DJ: Dislocation of a posterior stabilized total knee prosthesis: A report of two cases. Clin Orthop 254:225, 1990.
90. Glynn MK, Sheehan JM: The significance of asymptomatic bacteriuria in patients undergoing hip/knee arthroplasty. Clin Orthop 185:151, 1984.
91. Goldberg VM, Figgie HE III, Inglis AE, et al: Patellar fracture type and prognosis in condylar total knee arthroplasty. Clin Orthop 236:115, 1988.
92. Goodfellow J: Knee prostheses: One step forward, two steps back. [editorial]. J Bone Joint Surg Br 74:1, 1992.
93. Goodman SB, Fornasier VL, Kei J: The effects of bulk versus particulate polymethylmethacrylate on bone. Clin Orthop 232: 255, 1988.
94. Goodman SB, Fornasier VL, Kei J: The effects of bulk versus particulate ultra-high-molecular-weight polyethylene on bone. J Arthroplasty 4:541, 1988.
95. Goodnough LT, Shafron D, Marcus RE: Utilization and effectiveness of autologous blood donation for arthroplastic surgery. J Arthroplasty 5(suppl):S89, 1990.
96. Grace JN, Rand JA: Patellar instability after total knee arthroplasty. Clin Orthop 237:184, 1988.
97. Grace JN, Sim FH: Fracture of the patella after total knee arthroplasty. Clin Orthop 230:168, 1988.
98. Gradisar IA Jr, Hoffmann ML, Askew MJ: Fracture of a fenestrated metal backing of a tibial knee component: A case report. J Arthroplasty 4:27, 1989.
99. Grogan TJ, Dorey F, Rollins J, et al: Deep sepsis following total knee arthroplasty: Ten-year experience at the University of California at Los Angeles Medical Center. J Bone Joint Surg Am 68: 226, 1986.
100. Haas SB, Insall JN, Scuderi GR, et al: Pneumatic sequential-compression boots compared with aspirin prophylaxis of deep-vein thrombosis after total knee arthroplasty. J Bone Joint Surg Am 72:27, 1990,
101. Hagemann WF, Woods GW, Tullos HS: Arthrodesis in failed total knee replacement. J Bone Joint Surg Am 60:790, 1978.
102. Hall AJ: Late infection about a total knee prosthesis. J Bone Joint Surg Br 56:144, 1974.
103. Healy WL, Siliski JM, Incavo SJ: Operative treatment of distal femoral fractures proximal to total knee replacements. J Bone Joint Surg Am 75:27, 1993.
104. Highet WB, Holmes W: Traction injuries to the lateral popliteal nerve and traction injuries to peripheral nerves after suture. Br J Surg 30:212, 1943.
105. Highet WB, Sanders FK: The effects of stretching nerves after suture. Br J Surg 30:355, 1943.
106. Hirsh DM, Bhalla S, Roffman M: Supracondylar fracture of the femur following total knee replacement: Report of four cases. J Bone Joint Surg Am 63:162, 1981.
107. Hodge WA: Prevention of deep vein thrombosis after total knee arthroplasty. Clin Orthop 271:101, 1991.
108. Hofmann AA, Wyatt RWB, Daniels AU, et al: Bone scans after total knee arthroplasty in asymptomatic patients: Cemented versus cementless. Clin Orthop 251:183, 1990.
109. Holden DL, Jackson DW: Considerations in total knee arthroplasty following previous knee fusion. Clin Orthop 227:223, 1988.
110. Hood RW, Flawn LB, Insall JN: The use of pulsatile compression stockings in total knee replacement for prevention of venous thrombosis: A prospective study. Trans Orthop Res Soc 7: 297, 1982.
111. Hood RW, Wright TM, Burstein AH, et al: Retrieval analysis of 70 total condylar knee prostheses. Orthop Trans 5:319, 1981.
112. Hood RW, Wright TM, Burstein AH, et al: Retrieval analysis of twenty polyethylene patellar buttons. Orthop Trans 5:291, 1981.
113. Hozack WJ, Goll SR, Lotke PA, et al: The treatment of patellar fractures after total knee arthroplasty. Clin Orthop 236:123, 1988.
114. Hozack WJ, Rothman RH, Booth RE Jr, et al: The patellar clunk syndrome: A complication of posterior stabilized total knee arthroplasty. Clin Orthop 241:203, 1989.
115. Hsu H-P, Garg A, Walker PS, et al: Effect of knee component alignment on tibial load distribution with clinical correlation. Clin Orthop 248:135, 1989.
116. Hsu H-P, Walker PS: Wear and deformation of patellar components in total knee arthroplasty. Clin Orthop 246:260, 1989.
117. Hsu RWW, Himeno S, Coventry MB, et al: Normal axial alignment of the lower extremity and load-bearing distribution at the knee. Clin Orthop 255:215, 1990.
118. Hull RD, Raskob GE: Prophylaxis of venous thromboembolic disease following hip and knee surgery. J Bone Joint Surg Am 68:146, 1986.
119. Hunter GA, Dandy D: Diagnosis and natural history of the infected total hip replacement. In The Hip Society: The Hip. Proceedings of the Fifth Open Scientific Meeting of The Hip Society. St. Louis, CV Mosby, 1977.
120. Hvid I: Mechanical strength of trabecular bone. Thesis, University of Aarhus, Denmark, 1988.
121. Hvid I: Trabecular bone strength at the knee. Clin Orthop 227: 210, 1988.
122. Hvid I, Nielsen S: Total condylar knee arthroplasty: Prosthetic component positioning and radiolucent lines. Acta Orthop Scand 55:160, 1984.
123. Idusuyi OB, Morrey BF: Peroneal nerve palsy after total knee arthroplasty. J Bone Joint Surg Am 78:177-184, 1996.
124. Infection in rheumatoid disease [editorial]. BMJ 2:549, 1972.

125. Insall JN: Infection in total knee arthroplasty. Instr Course Lect 31:42, 1982.
126. Insall JN, Lachiewicz PF, Burstein AH: The posterior stabilized condylar prosthesis: A modification of the total condylar design: Two to four year clinical experience. J Bone Joint Surg Am 64:1317, 1982.
127. Insall JN, Thompson FM, Brause DB, et al: Two-stage reimplantation for the salvage of infected total knee arthroplasty. Orthop Trans 6:369, 1982.
128. Jabczenski FF, Crawford M: Retrograde intramedullary nailing of supracondylar femur fracture above total knee arthroplasty: A preliminary report of four cases. J Arthroplasty 10:95, 1995.
129. Jennings JJ, Harris WH, Sarmiento A: A clinical evaluation of aspirin prophylaxis of thromboembolic disease after total hip arthroplasty. J Bone Joint Surg Am 58:926, 1976.
130. Jerry GJ Jr, Rand JA, Ilstrup D: Old sepsis prior to total knee arthroplasty. Clin Orthop 236:135, 1988.
131. Johanson NA: Extensor mechanism failure: Treatment of patella fracture, dislocation, and ligament rupture. In Lotke PA, ed: Master Techniques in Orthopedic Surgery, Knee Arthroplasty. New York, Raven Press, 1995, pp 219-240.
132. Johnson DP: Antibiotic prophylaxis with cefuroxime in arthroplasty of the knee. J Bone Joint Surg Br 69:787, 1987.
133. Johnson DP: The effect of continuous passive motion on wound-healing and joint mobility after knee arthroplasty. J Bone Joint Surg Am 72:421, 1990.
134. Johnson DP: Midline or parapatellar incision for knee arthroplasty: A comparative study of wound viability. J Bone Joint Surg Br 70:656, 1988.
135. Johnson DP, Donell ST: Antibiotic prophylaxis during bilateral knee arthroplasty: Brief report. J Bone Joint Surg Br 70:666, 1988.
136. Johnson DP, Houghton TA, Radford P: Anterior midline or medial parapatellar incision for arthroplasty of the knee: A comparative study. J Bone Joint Surg Br 68:812, 1986.
137. Johnson F, Leitl S, Waugh W: The distribution of load across the knee. J Bone Joint Surg Br 62:346, 1980.
138. Jones SMG, Pinder IM, Moran CG, et al: Polyethylene wear in uncemented knee replacements. J Bone Joint Surg Br 74:18, 1992.
139. Jones WA, Wroblewski BM: Salvage of failed total knee arthroplasty: The "beefburger" procedure. J Bone Joint Surg Br 68: 812, 1986.
140. Josefchak RG, Finlay JB, Bourne RB, et al: Cancellous bone support for patellar resurfacing. Clin Orthop 220:192, 1987.
141. Kaempffe FA, Lifeso RM, Meinking C: Intermittent pneumatic compression versus Coumadin: Prevention of deep vein thrombosis in lower extremity total joint arthroplasty. Clin Orthop 269:89, 1991.
142. Kakkar VV, Howe CT, Flanc C, et al: Natural history of postoperative deep-vein thrombosis. Lancet 2:230, 1969.
143. Kantor SG, Schneider R, Insall JN, et al: Radionuclide imaging of asymptomatic versus symptomatic total knee arthroplasties. Clin Orthop 260:118, 1990.
144. Kapandji IA: The Physiology of the Joints. Vol. II: The Lower Limb. London, Churchill Livingstone, 1970, p 120.
145. Katz MM, Hungerford DS, Krackow KA, et al: Reflex sympathetic dystrophy as a cause of poor results after total knee arthroplasty. J Arthroplasty 1:117, 1986.
146. Kaufer H, Matthews LS: Spherocentric arthroplasty of the knee. J Bone Joint Surg Am 63:545, 1981.
147. Kayler DE, Lyttle D: Surgical interruption of patellar blood supply by total knee arthroplasty. Clin Orthop 229:221, 1988.
148. Kilgus DJ, Moreland JR, Finerman GAM, et al: Catastrophic wear of tibial polyethylene inserts. Clin Orthop 273:223, 1991.
149. King TV, Scott RD: Femoral component loosening in total knee arthroplasty. Clin Orthop 194:285, 1985.
150. Kirk P, Rorabeck CH, Bourne RB, et al: Management of recurrent dislocation of the patella following total knee arthroplasty. J Arthroplasty 7:229, 1992.
151. Knutson K, Hovelius L, Lindstrand A, et al: Arthrodesis after failed knee arthroplasty: A nationwide multicenter investigation of 91 cases. Clin Orthop 191:202, 1984.
152. Kozinn SC, Marx C, Scott RD: Unicompartmental knee arthroplasty: A 4.5-6-year follow-up study with a metal-backed tibial component. J Arthroplasty 4:1, 1989.
153. Kozinn SC, Scott R: Unicondylar knee arthroplasty. J Bone Joint Surg Am 71:145, 1989.
154. Kraay MJ, Goldberg VM, Figgie MP, et al: Distal femoral replacement with allograft/prosthetic reconstruction for treatment of supracondylar fractures in patients with total knee arthroplasty. J Arthroplasty 7:7, 1992.
155. Kraay MJ, Goldberg VM, Herbener TE: Vascular ultrasonography for deep venous thrombosis after total knee arthroplasty. Clin Orthop 286:18, 1993.
156. Krackow KA, Maar DC, Mont MA, et al: Surgical decompression for peroneal nerve palsy after total knee arthroplasty. Clin Orthop 292:223, 1993.
157. Krackow KA, Weiss A-PC: Recurvatum deformity complicating performance of total knee arthroplasty: A brief note. J Bone Joint Surg Am 72:268, 1990.
158. Kumar SN, Chapman JA, Rawlins I: Vascular injuries in total knee arthroplasty. J Arthroplasty 13:211, 1998.
159. Laflamme GH, Laflamme GE, Beaumont P: Effectiveness and safety of low dose warfarin prophylaxis in cemented total knee prosthesis. J Bone Joint Surg Br 73:112, 1991.
160. Landy MM, Walker PS: Wear of ultra-high molecular-weight polyethylene components of 90 retrieved knee prostheses. J Arthroplasty 3(suppl):S73, 1988.
161. Larcom PG, Lotke PA, Steinberg ME: Magnetic resonance venography versus contrast venography to diagnose thrombosis after joint surgery. Clin Orthop 331:209, 1996.
162. Laskin RS, Schob CJ: Medial capsular recession for severe varus deformities. J Arthroplasty 2:313, 1987.
163. Leclerc JR, Geerts WN, Desjardins L: Prevention of venous thromboembolism after knee arthroplasty: A randomized double blind trial comparing a low molecular weight heparin fragment (enoxaparin) to warfarin. Blood 246:84, 1994.
164. Lee JG, Keating EM, Ritter MA, et al: Review of the all-polyethylene tibial component in total knee arthroplasty: A minimum seven-year follow-up period. Clin Orthop 260:87, 1990.
165. Lettin AWF, Neil MJ, Citron ND, et al: Excision arthroplasty for infected constrained total knee replacements. J Bone Joint Surg Br 72:220, 1990.
166. Levine MN, Gent M, Hirsh J, et al: Ardeparin (low molecular weight heparin) versus graduated compression stockings for the prevention of venous thromboembolism: A randomized trial in patients undergoing knee surgery. Arch Intern Med 156:851, 1996.
167. Lidwell OM: Clean air at operation and subsequent sepsis in the joint. Clin Orthop 211:91, 1986.
168. Lidwell OM, Elson RA, Lowbury EJL, et al: Ultraclean air and antibiotics for prevention of postoperative infection: A multicenter study of 8,052 joint replacement operations. Acta Orthop Scand 58:4, 1987.
169. Lombardi AV, Engh GA, Volz RG, et al: Fracture/dissociation of the polyethylene in metal-backed patellar components in total knee arthroplasty. J Bone Joint Surg Am 70:675, 1988.
170. Lombardi AV, Mallory TH, Waterman RA, et al: Intercondylar distal femoral fracture. J Arthroplasty 10:643, 1995.
171. Lotke PA: Thrombophlebitis in knee arthroplasty. In Scott WN, ed: The Knee. St Louis, CV Mosby, 1994, pp 1217-1225.
172. Lotke PA, Ecker ML: Influence of positioning of prosthesis in total knee replacement. J Bone Joint Surg Am 59:77, 1977.
173. Lotke PA, Ecker ML, Alavi A, et al: Indications for the treatment of deep venous thrombosis following total knee replacement. J Bone Joint Surg Am 66:202, 1984.
174. Lotke PA, Steinberg ME, Ecker ML: Significance of deep venous thrombosis in the lower extremity after total joint arthroplasty. Clin Orthop 299:25, 1994.
175. Lundborg G, Rydevik B: Effects of stretching the tibial nerve of the rabbit: A preliminary study of the intraneural circulation and barrier function of the perineurium. J Bone Joint Surg Br 55:390, 1973.
176. Lynch AF, Bourne RB, Rorabeck CH, et al: Deep-vein thrombosis and continuous passive motion after total knee arthroplasty. J Bone Joint Surg Am 70:11, 1988.
177. Lynch AF, Rorabeck CH, Bourne RB: Extensor mechanism complications following total knee arthroplasty. J Arthroplasty 2: 135, 1987.
178. Lynch JA, Baker PL, Polly RE, et al: Mechanical measures in the

prophylaxis of postoperative thromboembolism in total knee arthroplasty. Clin Orthop 260:24, 1990.
179. Maderazo EG, Judson S, Pasternak H: Late infections of total joint prostheses: A review and recommendations for prevention. Clin Orthop 229:131, 1988.
180. Marks KE, Nelson CL, Lautenschlager EP: Antibiotic-impregnated acrylic bone cement. J Bone Joint Surg Am 58:358, 1976.
181. Marsh PK, Cotler JM: Management of an anaerobic infection in a prosthetic knee with long-term antibiotic alone: A case report. Clin Orthop 155:133, 1981.
182. Martin JW, Whiteside LA: The influence of joint line position on knee stability after condylar knee arthroplasty. Clin Orthop 259:146, 1990.
183. Mason MD, Brick GW, Scott RD, et al: Three pegged all polyethylene patellae: Two to six year results. Orthop Trans 17: 991, 1994.
184. Maynard MJ, Sculco TP, Ghelman B: Progression and regression of deep vein thrombosis after total knee arthroplasty. Clin Orthop 273:125, 1991.
185. McLaren AC, Dupont JA, Schroeber DC: Open reduction internal fixation of supracondylar fractures above total knee arthroplasties using the intramedullary supracondylar rod. Clin Orthop 302:194, 1994.
186. Merkel KD, Johnson EW Jr: Supracondylar fracture of the femur after total knee arthroplasty. J Bone Joint Surg Am 68:29, 1986.
187. Merkow RL, Soudry M, Insall JN: Patellar dislocation following total knee replacement. J Bone Joint Surg Am 67:1321, 1985.
188. Miller J: Improved Fixation in Total Hip Arthroplasty Using L.V.C. Surgical Technique Brochure. Warsaw, IN, Zimmer, 1980.
189. Mintz L, Tsao AK, McCrae CR, et al: The arthroscopic evaluation and characteristics of severe polyethylene wear in total knee arthroplasty. Clin Orthop 273:215, 1991.
190. Mirra JM, Marder RA, Amstutz HC: The pathology of failed total joint arthroplasty. 170:175, 1982.
191. Mont MA, Dellon AL, Chen F, et al: The operative treatment of peroneal nerve palsy. J Bone Joint Surg Am 78:863, 1996.
192. Mont MA, Serna FK, Krackow KA, et al: Exploration of radiographically normal total knee replacements for unexplained pain. Clin Orthop 331:216, 1996.
193. Montgomery WH, Insall JN, Haas SB, et al: Primary total knee arthroplasty in stiff and ankylosed knees. Am J Knee Surg 11: 20, 1998.
194. Monto RR, Garcia J, Callaghan JJ: Fatal fat embolism following total condylar knee arthroplasty. J Arthroplasty 5:291, 1990.
195. Moran MC, Brick, Sledge CB, et al: Supracondylar femoral fracture following total knee arthroplasty. Clin Orthop 324:196, 1996.
196. Moreland JR, Hanker GJ: Lower extremity axial alignment of normal males. In Dorr LD, ed: The Knee. Baltimore, MD, University Park Press, 1985, p 55.
197. Morrey BF, Adams RA, Ilstrup DM, et al: Complications and mortality associated with bilateral or unilateral total knee arthroplasty. J Bone Joint Surg Am 69:484, 1987.
198. Morrey BF, Chao EYS: Fracture of the porous-coated metal tray of a biologically fixed knee prosthesis: Report of a case. Clin Orthop 228:182, 1988.
199. Morrey BF, Westholm F, Schoifet S, et al: Long-term results of various treatment options for infected total knee arthroplasty. Clin Orthop 248:120, 1989.
200. Murray DG, Wilde AH, Werner F, et al: Herbert total knee prosthesis: Combined laboratory and clinical assessment. J Bone Joint Surg Am 59:1026, 1977.
201. Murrell GA, Nunley JA: Interlocked supracondylar intramedullary nails for supracondylar fractures after total knee arthroplasty: A new treatment method. J Arthroplasty 10:37, 1995.
202. Mylod AG Jr, France MP, Muser DE, et al: Perioperative blood loss associated with total knee arthroplasty: A comparison of procedures performed with and without cementing. J Bone Joint Surg Am 72:1010, 1990.
203. Naranja RJ, Lotke PA, Pagnano MW, et al: Total knee arthroplasty in a previously ankylosed or arthrodesed knee. Clin Orthop 331:234, 1996.
204. Nicholls DW, Dorr LD: Revision surgery for stiff total knee arthroplasty. J Arthroplasty 5:73, 1990.
205. Nielsen BF, Petersen VS, Vanmarken JE: Fracture of the femur after knee arthroplasty. Acta Orthop Scand 59:155, 1989.
206. Pagnano MW, Hanssen AD, Lewallen DG, et al: Flexion instability after primary posterior cruciate retaining total knee arthroplasty. Clin Orthop 356:39, 1998.
207. Parks NI, Engh GA, Dwyer KA, et al: Micromotion of modular tibial components in total knee arthroplasty. Orthop Trans 18: 611, 1994.
208. Parks NI, Engh GA, Topoleski T, et al: Modular tibial insert micromotion: A concern with contemporary knee implants. Clin Orthop 356:10, 1998.
209. Peltier LF: Fat embolism. Clin Orthop 232: 263, 1988.
210. Peters PC, Engh GA, Dwyer KA, et al: Osteolysis after total knee arthroplasty without cement. J Bone Joint Surg Am 74: 864, 1992.
211. Petty W, Bryan RS, Coventry M: Infection following total knee arthroplasty. J Bone Joint Surg Br 57:394, 1975.
212. Pittman GR: Peroneal nerve palsy following sequential pneumatic compression. JAMA 261:2201, 1989.
213. Pring DJ, Henderson RG, Rivett AG, et al: Autologous granulocyte scanning of painful prosthetic joints. J Bone Joint Surg Br 68:647, 1986.
214. Rand JA: Neurovascular complications of total knee arthroplasty. In Rand JA, ed: Total Knee Arthroplasty. New York, Raven Press, 1993, pp 417–422.
215. Rand JA: The patellofemoral joint in total knee arthroplasty. J Bone Joint Surg Am 76:612, 1994.
216. Rand JA: Vascular complications of total knee arthroplasty: Report of three cases. J Arthroplasty 2:89, 1987.
217. Rand JA, Brown ML: The value of indium 111 leukocyte scanning in the evaluation of painful or infected total knee arthroplasties. Clin Orthop 259:179, 1990.
218. Rand JA, Bryan RS: Results of revision total knee arthroplasties using condylar prostheses: A review of fifty knees. J Bone Joint Surg Am 70:738, 1988.
219. Rand JA, Bryan RS, Morrey BF, et al: Management of infected total knee arthroplasty. Clin Orthop 205:75, 1986.
220. Rand JA, Coventry MB: Stress fractures after total knee arthroplasty. J Bone Joint Surg Am 62:226, 1980.
221. Rand JA, Gustilo RB: Technique of patellar resurfacing in total knee arthroplasty. Tech Orthop 3:57, 1988.
222. Rand JA, Morrey BF, Bryan RS: Patellar tendon rupture after total knee arthroplasty. Clin Orthop 244:233, 1989.
223. Rhoads DD, Noble PC, Reuben JD, et al: The effect of femoral component position on patellar tracking after total knee arthroplasty. Clin Orthop 260:43, 1990.
224. Rimnac CM, Wright TM: Retrieval analysis of knee replacements. In Scott WN, ed: The Knee. St. Louis, CV Mosby, 1994, pp 1251–1260.
225. Ritter MA, Campbell ED: Postoperative patellar complications with or without lateral release during total knee arthroplasty. Clin Orthop 219:163, 1987.
226. Ritter MA, Faris PM, Keating EM: Anterior femoral notching and ipsilateral supracondylar femur fracture in total knee arthroplasty. J Arthroplasty 3:185, 1988.
227. Ritter MA, Keating EM, Faris PM: Clinical roentgenographic and scintigraphic results after interruption of the superior lateral genicular artery during total knee arthroplasty. Clin Orthop 248:145, 1989.
228. Ritter MA, Keating EM, Faris PM, et al: Rush rod fixation of supracondylar fractures above total knee arthroplasties. J Arthroplasty 10:213, 1995.
229. Ritter MA, Meding JB: Bilateral simultaneous total knee arthroplasty. J Arthroplasty 2:185, 1987.
230. Robinson EJ, Mulliken BD, Bourne RB, et al: Catastrophic osteolysis in total knee replacement. Clin Orthop 321:98, 1995.
231. Rolston LR, Christ DJ, Halpern A, et al: Treatment of supracondylar fractures of the femur proximal to a total knee arthroplasty: A report of four cases. J Bone Joint Surg Am 77:924, 1995.
232. Roscoe MW, Goodman SB, Schatzker J: Supracondylar fracture of the femur after Guepar total knee arthroplasty: A new treatment method. Clin Orthop 241:221, 1989.
233. Rose HA, Hood RW, Otis JC, et al: Peroneal-nerve palsy following total knee arthroplasty: A review of the Hospital for Special Surgery experience. J Bone Joint Surg Am 64:347, 1982.

234. Rosenberg AG, Andriacchi TP, Barden R, et al: Patellar component failure in cementless total knee arthroplasty. Clin Orthop 236:106, 1988.
235. Rosenberg AG, Haas B, Barden R, et al: Salvage of infected total knee arthroplasty. Clin Orthop 226:29, 1988.
236. Rubin R, Salvati EA: Infected total hip replacement after dental procedures. Oral Surg 41:18, 1976.
237. Rush JH, Vidovich JD, Johnson MA: Arterial complications of total knee replacement: The Australian experience. J Bone Joint Surg Br 69:400, 1987.
238. Ryd L, Albrektsson BEJ, Herberts P, et al: Micromotion of noncemented Freeman-Samuelson knee prostheses in gonarthrosis: A roentgenstereophotogrammetric analysis of eight successful cases. Clin Orthop 229:205, 1988.
239. Ryd L, Boegard T, Egund N, et al: Migration of the tibial component in successful unicompartmental knee arthroplasty: A clinical, radiographic and roentgenstereophotogrammetric study. Acta Orthop Scand 54:408, 1983.
240. Ryd L, Linder L: On the correlation between micromotion and histology of the bone-cement interface: Report of three cases of knee arthroplasty followed by roentgenstereophotogrammetric analysis. J Arthroplasty 4:303, 1989.
241. Ryd L, Lindstrand A, Stenstrom A, et al: Porous coated anatomic tricompartmental tibial components: The relationship between prosthetic position and micromotion. Clin Orthop 251: 189, 1990.
242. Salvati EA, Brause BD, Chekofsky KM, et al: Reimplantation in infected total joint arthroplasty. Orthop Trans 5:449, 1981.
243. Salvati EA, Insall JN: The management of sepsis in total knee replacement. In Savastano AA, ed: Total Knee Replacement. New York, Appleton & Lange, 1980, p 49.
244. Schneider R, Soudry M: Radiographic and scintigraphic evaluation of total knee arthroplasty. Clin Orthop 205:108, 1986.
245. Schoifet SD, Morrey BF: Persistent infection after successful arthrodesis for infected total knee arthroplasty: A report of two cases. J Arthroplasty 5:277, 1990.
246. Schoifet SD, Morrey BF: Treatment of infection after total knee arthroplasty by debridement with retention of the components. J Bone Joint Surg Am 72:1383, 1990.
247. Schurman DJ, Johnson BL Jr, Amstutz HC: Knee joint infections with *Staphylococcus aureus* and *Micrococcus* species: Influence of antibiotics, metal debris, bacteremia, blood, and steroids, in a rabbit model. J Bone Joint Surg Am 57:40, 1975.
248. Scott RD, Ewald FC, Walker PS: Fracture of the metallic tibial tray following total knee replacement: Report of two cases. J Bone Joint Surg Am 66:780, 1984.
249. Scuderi GR, Insall JN, Windsor RE, et al: Survivorship of cemented knee replacements. J Bone Joint Surg Br 71:798, 1989.
250. Seitz P, Ruegsegger P, Gschwend N, et al: Changes in local bone density after knee arthroplasty: The use of quantitative computed tomography. J Bone Joint Surg Br 69:407, 1987.
251. Sisto DJ, Lachiewicz PF, Insall JN: Treatment of supracondylar fractures following prosthetic arthroplasty of the knee. Clin Orthop 196:265, 1985.
252. Smith JL Jr, Tullos HS, Davidson JP: Alignment of total knee arthroplasty. J Arthroplasty 4:55, 1989.
253. Spiro TE, Fitzgerald RH, Trowbridge AA, et al: Enoxaparin: A low molecular weight heparin and warfarin for the prevention of venous thromboembolic disease after elective knee replacement surgery. Blood 246:84, 1994.
254. Stanley D, Cumberland DC, Elson RA: Embolization for aneurysm after knee replacement: Brief report. J Bone Joint Surg Br 71:138, 1989.
255. Stern S, Insall JN: Posterior stabilized prosthesis: Results after follow-up on nine to twelve years. J Bone Joint Surg Am 74: 980, 1992.
256. Stinchfield FE, Bigliani LU, Neu HC, et al: Late hematogenous infection of total joint replacement. J Bone Joint Surg Am 62: 1345, 1980.
257. Stringer MD, Steadman CA, Hedges AR, et al: Deep vein thrombosis after elective knee surgery: An incidence study in 312 patients. J Bone Joint Surg Br 71:492, 1989.
258. Stulberg BN, Insall JN, Williams GW, et al: Deep-vein thrombosis following total knee replacement: An analysis of six hundred and thirty-eight arthroplasties. J Bone Joint Surg Am 66: 194, 1984.
259. Stulberg BN, Watson JT, Stulberg SD, et al: A new model to assess tibial fixation in knee arthroplasty: I. Histologic and roentgenographic results. Clin Orthop 263:288, 1991.
260. Stulberg BN, Watson JT, Stulberg SD, et al: A new model to assess tibial fixation: II. Concurrent histologic and biomechanical observations. Clin Orthop 263:303, 1991.
261. Stulberg SD, Stulberg BN, Hamati Y, et al: Failure mechanisms of metal-backed patellar components. Clin Orthop 236:88, 1988.
262. Sutherland CJ, Schurman JR: Complications associated with warfarin prophylaxis in total knee arthroplasty. Clin Orthop 219:158, 1987.
263. Teeny SM, Dorr L, Murato G, et al: Treatment of infected total knee arthroplasty: Irrigation and debridement versus two-stage reimplantation. J Arthroplasty 5:35, 1990.
264. Tew M, Waugh W: Tibiofemoral alignment and the results of knee replacement. J Bone Joint Surg Br 67:551, 1985.
265. Thompson FM, Hood RW, Insall JN: Patellar fractures in total knee arthroplasty. Orthop Trans 5:490, 1981.
266. Thorpe CD, Bocell JR, Tullos HS: Intra-articular fibrous bands: Patellar complications after total knee replacement. J Bone Joint Surg Am 72:811, 1990.
267. Toksuig-Larsen S, Ryd L, Lindstrand A: Early inducible displacement of tibial components in total knee prosthesis inserted with and without cement. J Bone Joint Surg Am 80:83, 1998.
268. Tria AJ, Harwood DA, Alicea JA, et al: Patellar fractures in posterior stabilized knee arthroplasties. Clin Orthop 299:131, 1994.
269. Trippel SB: Antibiotic-impregnated cement in total joint arthroplasty. J Bone Joint Surg Am 68:1297, 1986.
270. Vaughn BK, Knezevich S, Lombardi AV Jr, et al: Use of the Greenfield filter to prevent fatal pulmonary embolism associated with total hip and knee arthroplasty. J Bone Joint Surg Am 71:1542, 1989.
271. Vernace JV, Rothman RH, Booth RE Jr, et al: Arthroscopic management of the patellar clunk syndrome following posterior stabilized total knee arthroplasty. J Arthroplasty 4:179, 1989.
272. Vince KG, Insall JN, Kelly MA: The total condylar prosthesis: 10- to 12-year results of a cemented knee replacement. J Bone Joint Surg Br 71:793, 1989.
273. Vince KG, Kelly MA, Beck J, et al: Continuous passive motion after total knee arthroplasty. J Arthroplasty 2:281, 1987.
274. Volz RG, Nisbet JK, Lee RW, et al: The mechanical stability of various noncemented tibial components. Clin Orthop 226:38, 1988.
275. Vresilovic EJ, Hozack WJ, Booth RE, et al: Incidence of pulmonary embolism after total knee arthroplasty with low dose Coumadin prophylaxis. Clin Orthop 286:27, 1993.
276. Wade PJF, Denham RA: Arthrodesis of the knee after failed knee replacement. J Bone Joint Surg Br 66:362, 1984.
277. Walker PS, Soudry M, Ewald FC, et al: Control of cement penetration in total knee arthroplasty. Clin Orthop 185:155, 1984.
278. Wasielewski RC, Parks N, Williams I, et al: Tibial insert undersurface as a contributing source of polyethylene wear debris. Clin Orthop 345:53, 1997.
279. Waslewski GL, Marson BM, Benjamin JB: Early, incapacitating instability of posterior cruciate ligament-retaining total knee arthroplasty. J Arthroplasty 13:763, 1998.
280. Westrich GH, Sculco TP: Prophylaxis against deep venous thrombosis after total knee arthroplasty. J Bone Joint Surg Am 78:826, 1996.
281. Whiteside LA: Effect of porous coating configuration on tibial osteolysis after total knee arthroplasty. Clin Orthop 321:92, 1995.
282. Whiteside LA, Fosco DR, Brooks JG: Fracture of the femoral components in cementless total knee arthroplasty. Clin Orthop 286:71, 1993.
283. Whiteside LA, Kasselt MR, Haynes DW: Varus-valgus and rotational stability in rotationally unconstrained total knee arthroplasty. Clin Orthop 219:147, 1987.
284. Whiteside LA, Ohl MD: Tibial tubercle osteotomy for exposure of the difficult total knee arthroplasty. Clin Orthop 260:6, 1990.
285. Whiteside LA, Pafford J: Load transfer characteristics of a noncemented total knee arthroplasty. Clin Orthop 239:168, 1989.

286. Wilde AH, Ruth JT: Two-stage reimplantation in infected total knee arthroplasty. Clin Orthop 236:23, 1988.
287. Wilson MG, Kelley K, Thornhill TS: Infection as a complication of total knee-replacement arthroplasty: Risk factors and treatment in sixty-seven cases. J Bone Joint Surg Am 72:878, 1990.
288. Wilson NV, Das SK, Kakkar, et al: Thrombo-embolic prophylaxis in total knee replacement. Evaluation of the A-V impulse system. J Bone Joint Surg Br 74:50, 1992.
289. Windsor RE, Insall JN, Urs WK, et al: Two-stage reimplantation for the salvage of total knee arthroplasty complicated by infection: Further follow-up and refinement of indications. J Bone Joint Surg Am 72:272, 1990.
290. Windsor RE, Scuderi GR, Insall JN: Patellar fractures in total knee arthroplasty. J Arthroplasty 4:63, 1989.
291. Wolff AM, Hungerford DS, Krackow KA, et al: Osteotomy of the tibial tubercle during total knee replacement: A report of twenty-six cases. J Bone Joint Surg Am 71:848, 1989.
292. Woolson ST, Pottorff G: Venous ultrasonography in the detection of proximal vein thrombosis after total knee arthroplasty. Clin Orthop 273:131, 1991.
293. Wright J, Ewald FC, Walker PS, et al: Total knee arthroplasty with the Kinematic prosthesis: Results after five to nine years: A follow-up note. J Bone Joint Surg Am 72:1003, 1990.
294. Wright TM, Hood RW, Burstein AH: Analysis of material failures. Symposium on Total Knee Arthroplasty. Orthop Clin North Am 13:33, 1982.

88 Revision of Aseptic Failed Total Knee Arthroplasty

MARC F. BRASSARD • JOHN N. INSALL • GILES R. SCUDERI

INDICATIONS FOR REVISION

The causes of mechanical failure of total knee arthroplasty (TKA) are femoral and tibial loosening, osteolysis, instability, subluxation, and dislocation; polyethylene wear; patellar loosening; and lack of motion and malposition of the components.[17, 31] The cause of the arthroplasty failure must be evident, as exploration without due reason is not helpful, and the original error, if it is that, must be corrected. One study examined this outcome in exploration of 27 knees for severe pain of unknown origin following a TKA. At final follow-up, there was only 41% good and excellent results. Even if the problem was identified at time of surgery, only 25% had successful outcomes.[16] Most mechanical failures are either design- or technique-related, and probably a new type of revision prosthesis will be required.

PREOPERATIVE ASSESSMENT

As a general principle, revision surgery should be performed as soon as failure is diagnosed. Once components are loose and have shifted in position, failure is inevitable, and procrastination only results in progressive bone destruction and the creation of larger defects. Likewise, if polyethylene wear-through of tibial or patellar components (Fig. 88.1) is diagnosed, delay will produce a more massive metallic synovitis. Ligament instability is seldom improved by conservative means. A more satisfactory revision operation is obtained by early intervention.

Preoperatively, all cases must be reviewed carefully, and thought must be given to the type of prosthesis that will be required for the revision. Any special components that may be needed must be ordered. The need for bone graft must also be anticipated. Aspiration is advisable whenever joint fluid is present. The aspirate should be examined for cells, organisms, and metallic and polyethylene debris as well as sent for aerobic, anaerobic, and fungal cultures. When infection is seriously considered, fluid should be sent for analysis of protein and glucose levels, and preoperative antibiotics should be avoided. In the preoperative period, reflex sympathetic dystrophy should be ruled out. This diagnosis should be considered especially in situations where there are no obvious signs of failure of the components and pain is out of proportion to the examination.

An important principle in revision knee surgery concerns the identification of the exact failure mode of the preceding arthroplasty. If the mode of failure is not clearly understood, the revision is not likely to succeed. Intraoperative surprises should be very infrequent.

The size of the original components should be estimated and confirmed whenever possible. If the patient had the previous arthroplasty performed by another surgeon, the operative report should be obtained to ascertain the correct sizes and other pertinent information. Templates for the selected revision components can be helpful. The amount of bone loss to be expected after the components are removed is assessed as well. New revision components of the correct sizes should preferably be modular to allow intraoperative attachment of augments, wedges, and stems. In our view, the revision proceeds more smoothly when the cruciate ligaments are excised, and both posterior stabilized and constrained polyethylene inserts should be available. The ligament stability and the integrity of the extensor mechanism are assessed. The position of previous incisions are noted, and if skin viability is in question, a plastic surgery consultation should be obtained.

SURGICAL TECHNIQUE

Exposure

In the exposure of a revision case, a previous incision should be used whenever possible. Recently, use of soft-tissue expanders preoperatively in the revision setting has been successful.[8] If the knee is stiff, a quadriceps snip may be anticipated and should be done early in the procedure to avoid damage to the tibial tubercle. A medial subperiosteal exposure that allows the tibia to be externally rotated and anteriorly subluxed is done as part of the exposure and may be incorporated into a medial release, if indicated. When eversion of the patella is difficult, the patella may at first be subluxed laterally without eversion while the femoral and tibial components are removed. When a quadriceps snip does not allow adequate exposure, a tibial tubercle osteotomy should be considered. If a tibial tubercle osteotomy is to be performed, then a long osteotomy as described by Whiteside and Ohl is the best option.[28] It is best to leave the lateral soft-tissue attachments to the osteomized bone and hinge the osteotomy open.

Fixed angular deformities are commonly encountered and should be addressed during the exposure. A fixed varus deformity is corrected by subperiosteal release of the deep and superficial portions of the me-

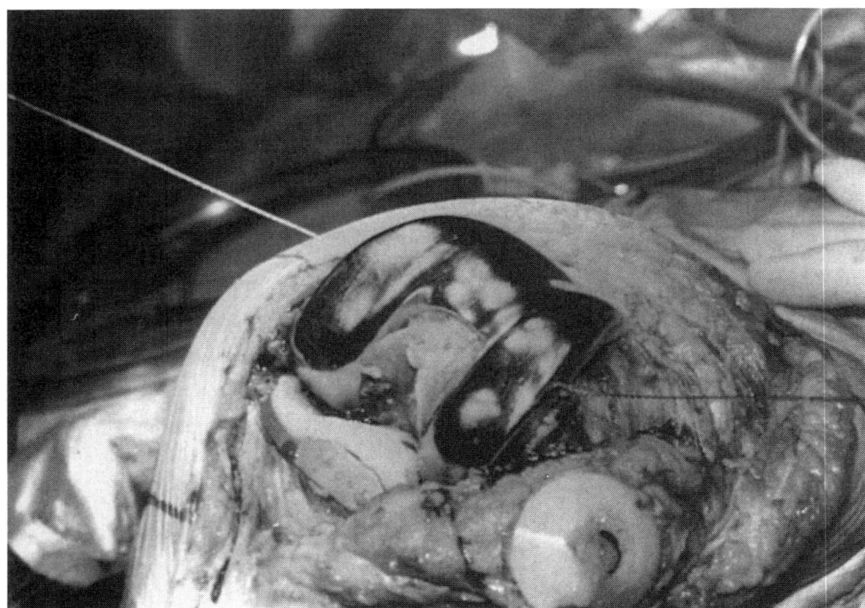

FIGURE 88.1 ➢ Photograph of a kinematic prosthesis showing central wear-through of a metal-backed patellar component.

dial collateral ligament and the pes anserine insertion in the metaphyseal region. The distal insertion of the superficial medial collateral ligament is elevated subperiosteally in an incremental fashion using a periosteal elevator or osteotome. Finally, the semimembranous and the posterior capsule are released, allowing full exposure of the proximal tibia. A fixed valgus deformity is unusual in the revision setting; however, if one is present, the most appropriate solution is to perform small, multiple horizontal incisions in the lateral structures (posterior capsule, lateral collateral ligament, and iliotibial band) in a "pie crusting" manner. The small incisions, approximately 1 to 2 cm in length, are performed both at the level of the joint and proximally. It is helpful to have some tension on the lateral structure during this procedure, which is accomplished either by placement of laminar spreaders between the femur and tibia or by manual distraction of the leg by an assistant. Severe fixed valgus deformities may require complete release of the lateral supporting structures from the femoral condyle. For cases with a rigid deformity and arthrofibrosis, it may be necessary to perform a femoral peel. Because this involves a complete release of the medial and lateral supporting structures, it will be necessary to revise the knee to a constrained design.

Débridement

A débridement of the supra- and parapatellar regions should be done routinely. Failed knees often produce considerable debris of polyethylene, polymethylmethacrylate, and bone fragments that can become incorporated into the synovium.

Removal of Components

When operative inspection reveals granulation tissue, necrotic tissue, or other evidence of infection, the components should be removed, a thorough débridement completed, and frozen-section tissue examined. Evidence of acute inflammation is a reason for aborting the procedure until microbacterial cultures are available. Closing the wound over an antibiotic impregnated polymethylmethacrylate spacer (Fig. 88.2) makes subsequent re-entry of the knee easier in the event that cultures prove negative.

Revision operations are increasingly performed for reasons other than loosening. Removal of well-fixed components can be a difficult task, particularly if they are porous-coated. Special instruments can facilitate removal, and we have found a large sliding hammer (Fig. 88.3) with various gripping devices invaluable for extraction. A Gigli saw, flexible osteotomes, and a high-speed, low-torque pneumatic drill are also useful. Recently, we have been using a microsagittal saw blade that is placed directly under the component and moved parallel to the component to avoid cutting into the bone (Fig. 88.4). This action will break down the adhesion between the cement and the component, leaving the bone mostly intact. If this technique is done appropriately, the cement is left behind, still attached to the bone. The cement is then removed by cracking it with a small osteotome in a mosaic pattern. The osteotome should be used lightly on the cement to just crack it and prevent any gouging or iatrogenic bone loss. A diamond-tip drill may sometimes be required to remove a well-fixed component piecemeal.[30] Shedding of beads can be expected when removing porous-coated implants. When the components are not loose, they must be removed with minimal loss of bone.

Working around the femoral component with a microsagittal saw should free the surfaces up to the fixation pegs or stems. Afterward, thin flexible osteotomes are used to further disrupt the cement-component interface. When the interface is completely severed, an

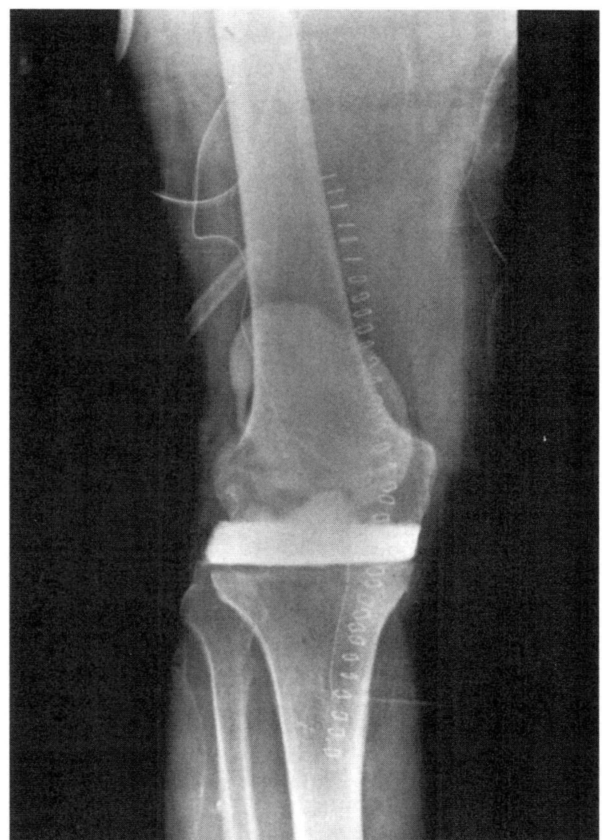

FIGURE 88.2 ➢ Radiograph showing antibiotic-impregnated cement spacers used after the removal of an infected implant. The use of spacers contributes to patient comfort and makes reimplantation technically easier.

extraction device may be utilized. This device locks onto the component; with the slap-hammer attachment, the component is carefully distracted from the bone.

An all-polyethylene tibial component can be separated from the tibial surface with a microsagittal saw, giving better access for removal of pegs or stems. For metal-backed components, the microsagittal saw blade can be passed just under the tray in a manner similar to that used for the femur. The key to using the saw blade is to remain parallel to the surface and avoid digging into the bone. Once the bond is broken between the cement and the component, stacked osteotomes may be used to gently lift the tray and central stem from the tibia. Again, with the remaining cement, use an osteotome to crack the cement gently in a mosaic pattern. Some models allow removal of the polyethylene tibial component to give access to intramedullary stems. Removal of the cemented porous-coated prosthesis can be a very difficult task, especially with stems designed for bone ingrowth. It may be necessary to disassemble the components to gain access to the stems (Fig. 88.5). In the present situation, with many of the tibial components being modular, it is usually helpful to remove the polyethylene as early as possible. This method will greatly enhance exposure of the tibia and the femur.

Polyethylene patellar components can be cut across with an oscillating saw. The removal of metal-backed components, especially cementless components, may be more difficult, and it may be necessary to use a high-speed diamond-edged saw.

With the components out, the bone surfaces are thoroughly cleaned of cement, debris, and granulation tissue. If a small area of cement is difficult to remove from bone, then the small oscillating saw blade may also be used. With the saw blade, the surgeon has more control over removing the cement and "freshening up" the bone ends. Use of an osteotome, rongeur, or curet to remove this small area of cement may cause further bone loss. In a revision setting, where infection has been ruled out, it is better to leave remaining well-fixed cement in the canal rather than risking excessive bone loss or perforating the canal trying to remove it. The soft tissues in the posterior compartment of the knee should also be débrided.

Reconstruction

After the removal of the components and thorough débridement is the time to rebuild the knee. The basic principle of revision arthroplasty involves creating a kinematically stable arthroplasty that is well fixed and well aligned. This involves the management of the residual bone and the soft tissue. The key to revision surgery is to create equal flexion and extension gaps; however, when this is not readily achieved, adjustments need to be made. Adjustments on the femoral side can affect the knee in either flexion or extension, whereas any adjustments on the tibial side will affect both.

When performing revisions, we prefer to use a three-step method. The three steps are recreating the femur, rebuilding the flexion space, and rebuilding the extension space. The femur is prepared first because of the availability of more reliable anatomical landmarks. In addition, this method is also the order in which primary TKAs are performed; familiarity with these steps will aid the surgeon.

Recreate the Femur

SIZE THE FEMUR

Choosing the correct size of components is an essential step. It is helpful preoperatively to procure the operative notes from the previous procedure. Another useful preoperative step is to template the opposite side in order to obtain a relative idea of the sizes. Look at the size of the femoral component that is being removed and determine if it is an appropriate size. The remaining bone should be templated in the anteroposterior plane. There is usually posterior bone loss, so templating intraoperatively runs the risk of undersizing the femoral component (Fig. 88.6). The epicondylar width of the femur can also be helpful in selecting the appropriate femoral size.

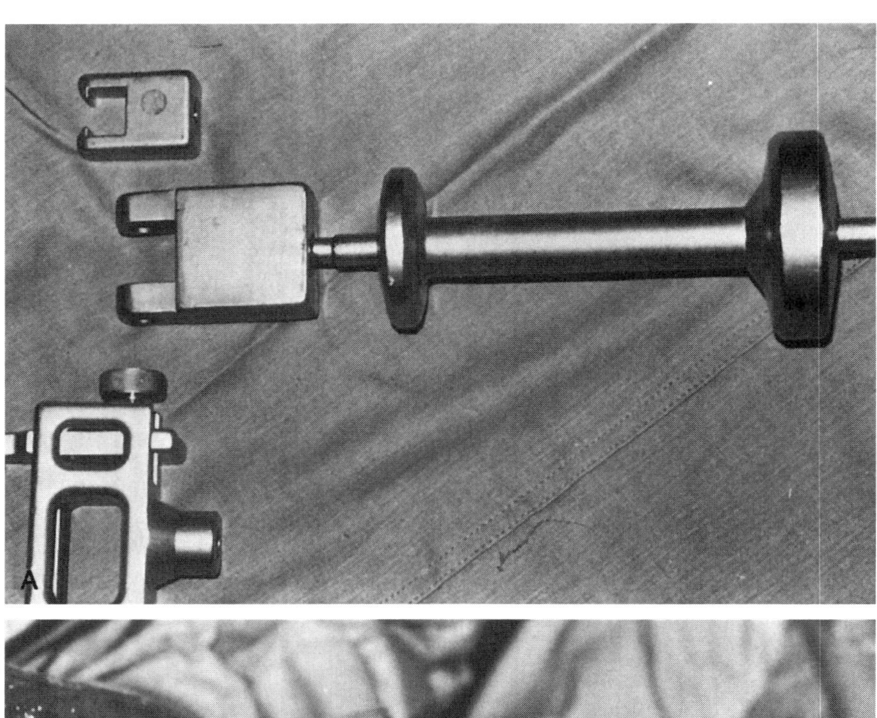

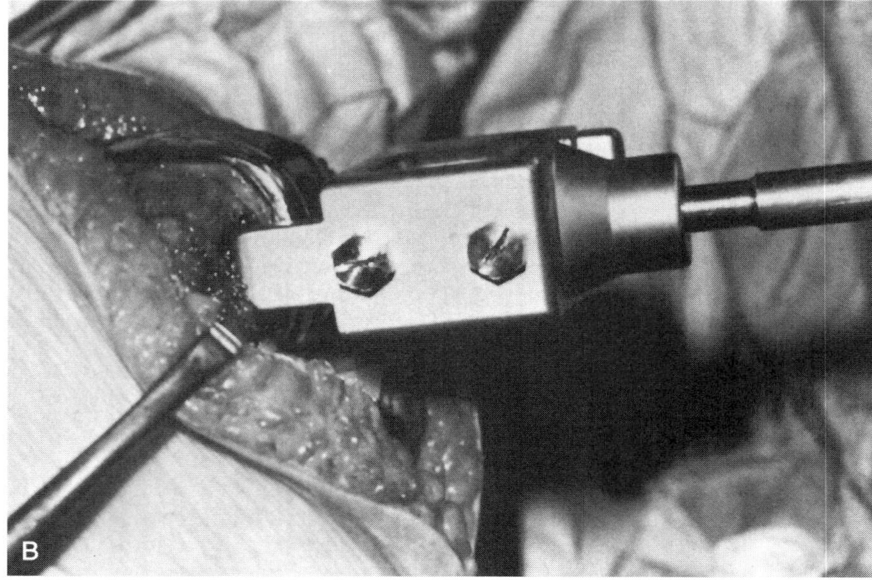

FIGURE 88.3 ➢ A sliding hammer with special attachments is very helpful for removing prosthetic components, especially those with stems.

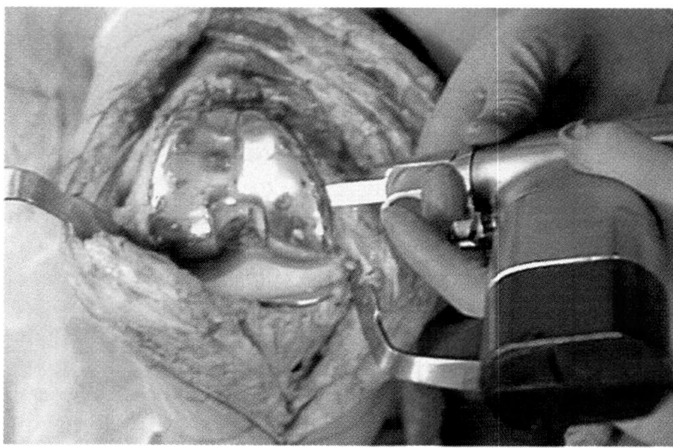

FIGURE 88.4 ➢ Photograph showing the use of a microsagittal saw blade around the femoral component.

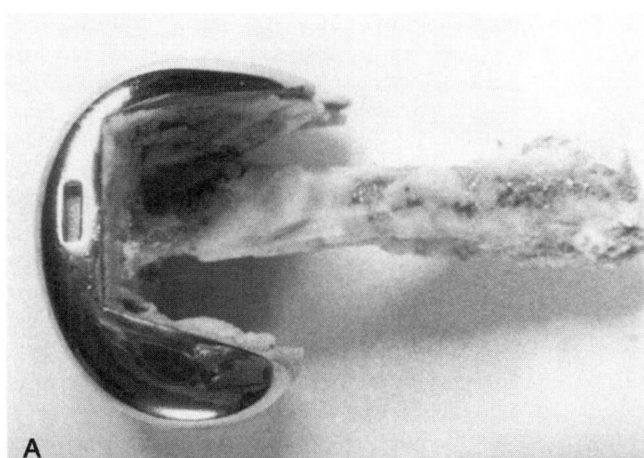

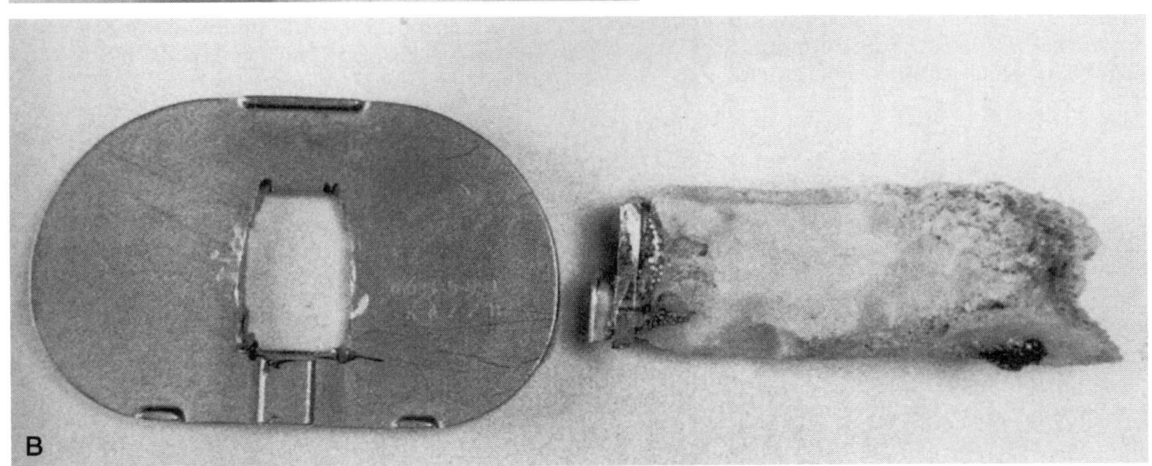

FIGURE 88.5 ➢ Photograph showing porous cemented components that were removed because of infection. This was a very difficult task and resulted in some bone loss, both on the posterior surface of the femur and on the posterior surface of the tibia. The tibial component could not be extracted until the central peg had been cut from the base plate with a diamond-tip saw.

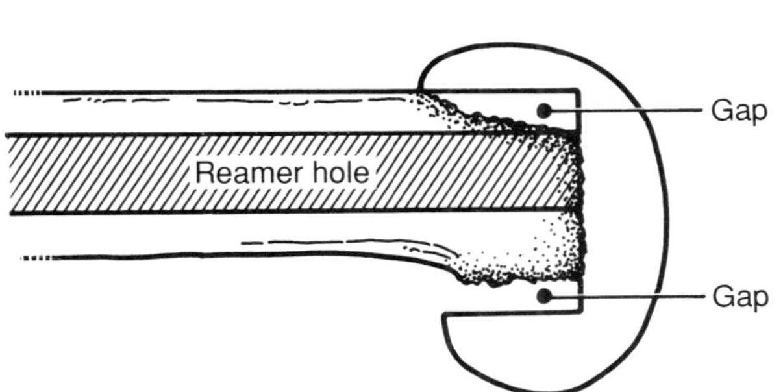

FIGURE 88.6 ➢ The revision femoral component must be sized from measurements of the opposite knee or estimated from the removed components. Typically, there will be gaps anteriorly and posteriorly.

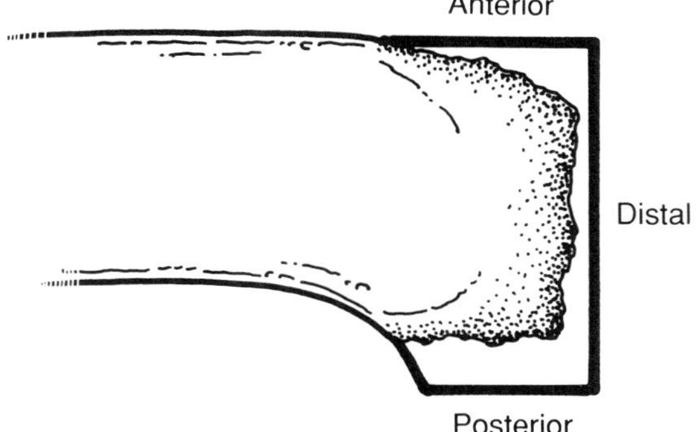

FIGURE 88.7 ➢ Typical bone loss after removal of a femoral component. There are bone deficiencies distally, anteriorly, and posteriorly.

The danger in selecting an excessively small femoral component is that it will compromise flexion stability. It is better to select a larger femoral component and augment the posterior condyles to restore the anteroposterior dimension. Bone loss is usually most significant in the posterior femoral condyle area, but anterior femoral bone loss can occur, influencing sizing, especially of the component in the sagittal position of the femoral component (Fig. 88.7).

FEMORAL COMPONENT ROTATION

The correct femoral component rotation is vital to knee kinematics and patella tracking. The best way to determine rotation is to identify the medial and lateral epicondyles and to establish the epicondylar axis. Rotational adjustments should be made to the residual distal femur, which usually require shaving bone from the anterolateral and posteromedial femur if the prior component was rotated internally. To ensure the correct rotation, the posterolateral condyle usually has to be augmented. If a posterior stabilized prosthesis or similar prosthesis is used, the intercondylar notch is prepared 90 degrees to the epicondylar axis (Fig. 88.8).

DISTAL FEMUR POSITION

The key to this step is restoring the distance from the joint line, distally and posteriorly. The epicondyles are a useful landmark to determine the joint line. The joint line on average is 25 mm from the lateral epicondyle and 30 mm from the medial epicondyle. Because the tibial cut is established at 90 degrees to the tibial shaft, the joint line of the prosthetic knee, of average size, is 30 mm from both epicondyles.

After determining the appropriate joint line, the femoral component can be set provisionally to reestablish the distal joint line. Provisional distal augmentation can be used at this time (Fig. 88.9), especially if there is asymmetric femoral bone loss. The distance from the epicondyles to the posterior joint line is similar to that of the distal joint line and is helpful in confirming the correct femoral component size.

Because this step is provisional, no bone should be resected to fit the augments until the final position and the size of the femoral component are determined. Additional adjustments to the position and the size of the femoral component may be needed as the flexion and extension gaps are balanced.

Rebuild the Flexion Space

CREATE A FLAT TIBIAL SURFACE

The key in selecting the correct size tibial component is to choose a size that will cover the entire proximal tibia without overhang. The tibial surface should be perpendicular to the tibial shaft. This should be accomplished with minimal bone resection; when necessary, appropriate wedge or block augmentation should be added (Fig. 88.10).

BALANCE THE FLEXION SPACE

This step requires choosing the correct tibial polyethylene articulation. The provisional femoral component needs to be in place. The size of the polyethylene chosen should fill the flexion space (Fig. 88.11).

Rebuild the Extension Space

To assess the extension space, retain the polyethylene used to create the flexion space, and bring the knee into full extension. If the gaps are equal and stable,

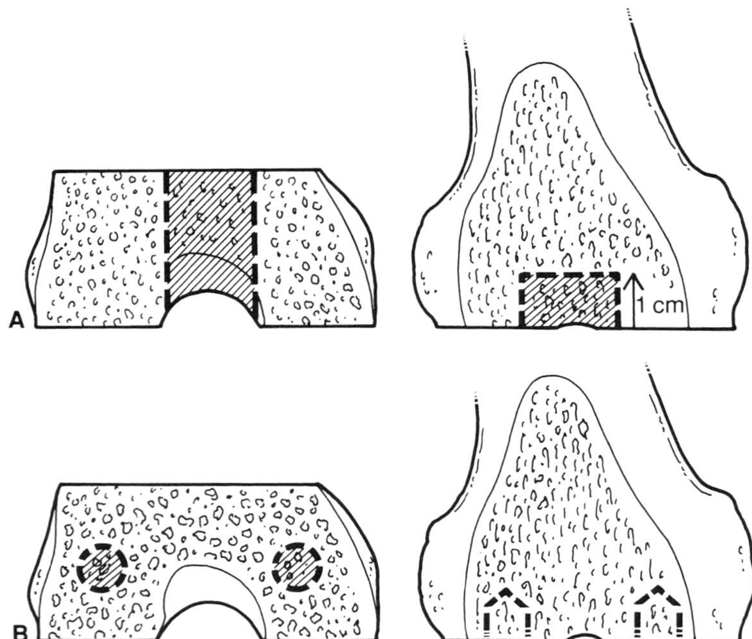

FIGURE 88.8 ➢ Femoral fixation can be enhanced by a central box *(A)* usually found with posterior stabilized designs or *(B)* medial and lateral fixation lugs.

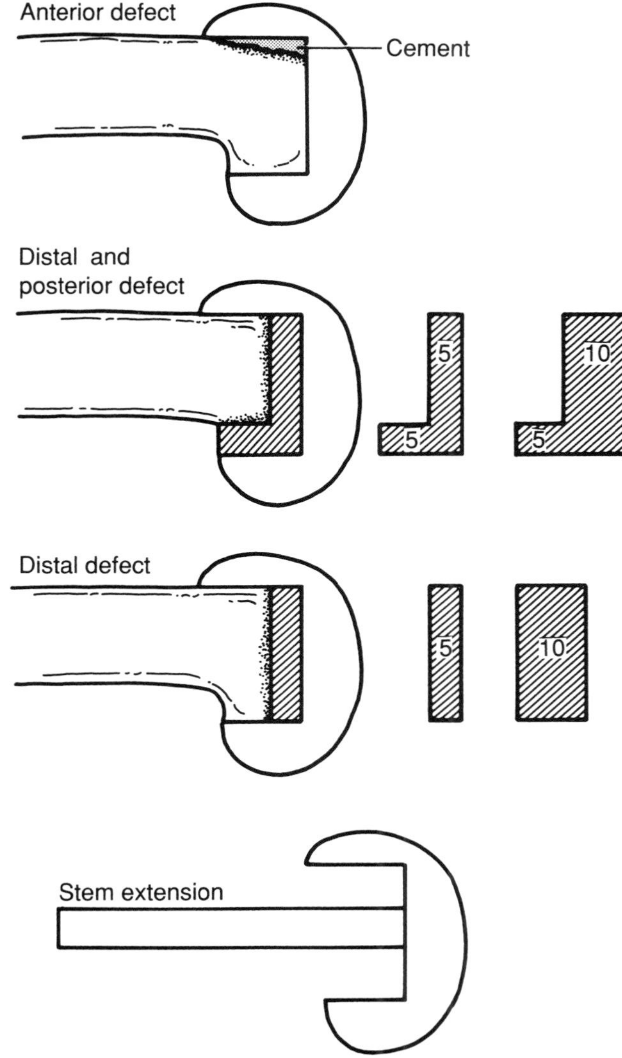

FIGURE 88.9 ➢ Augmentation of the distal femur. The revision femoral component should have a stem extension; usually, both distal and posterior augments are required, although the amount of augmentation at each site may differ. Thus, 5 mm may be sufficient posteriorly, although distal augmentation of 10 mm is required. This can be judged by considering the spacers needed in flexion and extension and the amount of distal augmentation needed to restore the joint line.

then the polyethylene is the correctly sized articulation, and the femoral augments are finalized. Minor adjustments to the tibial polyethylene thickness can be made to balance the gaps. If an imbalance is present after the minor adjustments are made, then refer to the following nine decision points:

1. If the knee is too tight in both flexion and extension, reducing the thickness of the tibial component may be sufficient to balance the knee.
2. If the knee is tight in flexion but acceptable in extension, there are two options:
   a. Check the sagittal position of the femoral component. If it is positioned too posteriorly, consider using an offset femoral stem extension. This will move the femoral component more anteriorly, but be careful not to overstuff the patellofemoral joint—this will adversely affect motion and patellofemoral tracking.
   b. Downsize the femoral component.
3. If the knee is tight in flexion and loose in extension, consider these options:
   a. Check the sagittal position of the femoral component as in point 2, and consider using a thicker tibial component.
   b. Downsize the femoral component, and use a thicker tibial component.
   c. If the femoral component is the correct size, increase the distal femoral augmentation until the extension gap is equal to the flexion gap. This may require a thinner tibial component to balance the knee. Be careful not to move the joint line too far distally because this will adversely affect patellar tracking.
4. If the knee is acceptable in flexion but tight in extension, there are two options:
   a. Either reduce distal femoral augmentation or resect more distal femoral bone. This will move the femoral component more proximally, increasing the extension space.
   b. If a preoperative flexion contracture is present, release the posterior capsule, preferably from the femur.
5. If both the flexion and extension gaps are equal, then no further adjustments are necessary.
6. If the knee is acceptable in flexion and loose in extension, the solution is to augment the distal femur so that the extension gap requires the same amount of tibial polyethylene as the flexion gap.
7. The most common problem is that the flexion space is larger than the extension space. If the knee is loose in flexion and tight in extension, then the solution is to go through a series of checks and adjustments.
   a. Check the sagittal position of the femoral component. If it is positioned too anteriorly, then consider using an offset femoral stem extension. This will move the femoral component more posteriorly and reduce the flexion space.
   b. Check the distal position of the femoral component. Consider reducing the distal augmentation or resecting more distal femoral bone.
   c. Check the femoral component size. If the size appears to be too small, consider choosing the next larger size, but be careful not to oversize the femur.
   d. If the prior maneuvers fail to balance the gaps, then there may be a need for a constrained condylar knee (CCK) articulation.
   e. Depending on the experience of the surgeon, collateral ligament advancement and reconstruction may be considered.

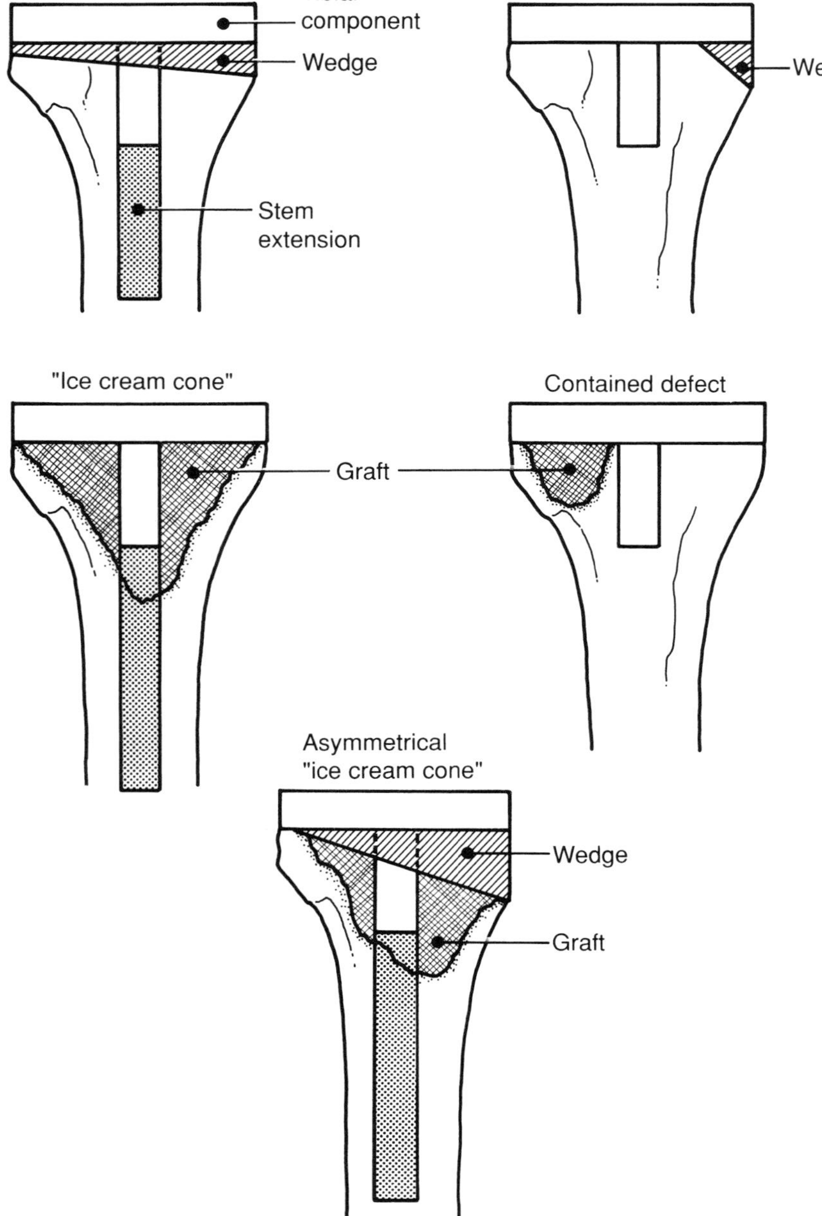

FIGURE 88.10 ➢ Reconstruction of tibial defects. Symmetric tibial deficiency can be compensated by a thicker tibial polyethylene. Stem extension is usually advisable.

8. If the knee is loose in flexion and acceptable in extension, moving the femoral component proximally and using a thicker tibial component may solve the problem. If this does not balance the knee, then the options in point 7 should be considered.
9. If the knee is symmetrically loose in flexion and extension, then a thicker tibial component will solve the problem.

Management of Bone Loss

Bone loss is common in the revision setting. Even unicompartmental replacements (Figs. 88.12 and 88.13) leave substantial asymmetric bony deficiencies.[20] The best way to be prepared for intraoperative surprises is to be well prepared preoperatively. At the time of revision, the surgeon should make sure all the materials for reconstruction are available. These include wedges, blocks, allografts, and special components.

Bone defects can be classified as contained, uncontained, or a combination (Figs. 88.14 and 88.15). A contained defect has an intact cortical rim. An uncontained defect has segmental bone loss with no remaining cortex. The treatment of bone defects depends on two factors: (1) whether the defect is contained or uncontained and (2) the size of the defect. A small (less than 5 mm) contained defect can be treated with cement or morseled bone graft. The cement can be

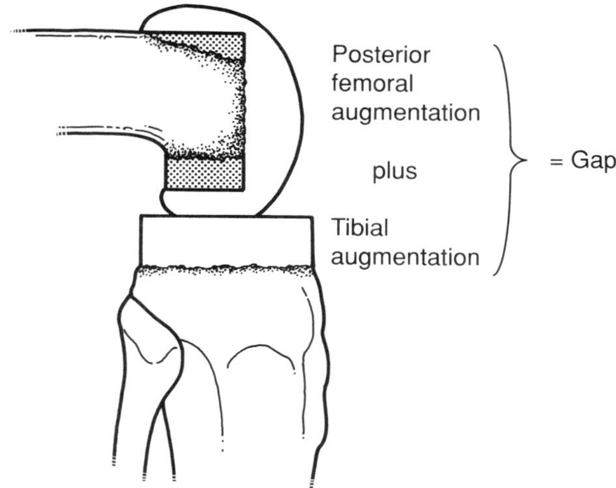

FIGURE 88.11 ➢ In the reconstruction, the flexion gap is restored by a combination of posterior femoral and tibial augmentation.

reinforced with screws and have good long-term results.[22] Large contained cavitary defects can be treated with autogenous or allograft bone. Small (less than 5 mm) uncontained defects can also be repaired with cement alone or cement and screws. Intermediate (5 to 10 mm) uncontained defects can be managed with modular wedges.[21] Large (greater than 10 mm) uncontained defects are best managed with modular augments or structural allografts.[4, 7, 15, 23, 29]

Use of allograft in managing bone defects has many advantages: bone stock restoration, biocompatibility, potential for ligamentous reattachment, versatility, and cost-effectiveness. Its disadvantages include donor availability, late resorption, nonunion, fracture, and risk of disease transmission. Absolute contraindication to allograft is a chronic infection. Relative contraindications include immunosuppression, metabolic bone disorders, neuropathic arthropathy, and inadequate extensor mechanism. The use of bone grafts in anatomically matching sites (e.g., proximal tibia allograft for metaphyseal tibia bone loss) allows for accurate orientation of trabeculae along the lines of force. This may lessen the likelihood of early mechanical failure.[24]

In revisions, severe and extensive bone loss can involve a large portion of the distal femoral metaphysis. This may include one or both condyles, along with the collateral ligaments. Epicondylar flaring sometimes occurs when a grossly loose femoral component subsides; along with significant femoral bone loss, the distal femur appears to be trumpet-shaped. In these situations, the reconstruction is complex and requires a knowledge of ligament reconstruction and bone-grafting techniques. The surgical options include a tumor-type prosthesis, which may be a constrained or hinged design or reconstruction with a structural allograft.

Structural allografting of the distal femur depends on the extent of the bone loss and the location of the lesion. If the loss is isolated to one entire condyle, then it may be possible to reestablish the distal femur

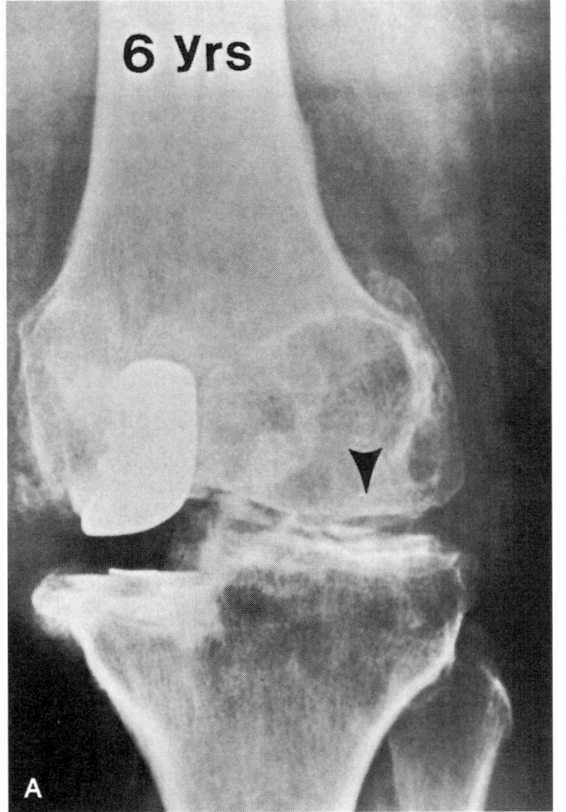

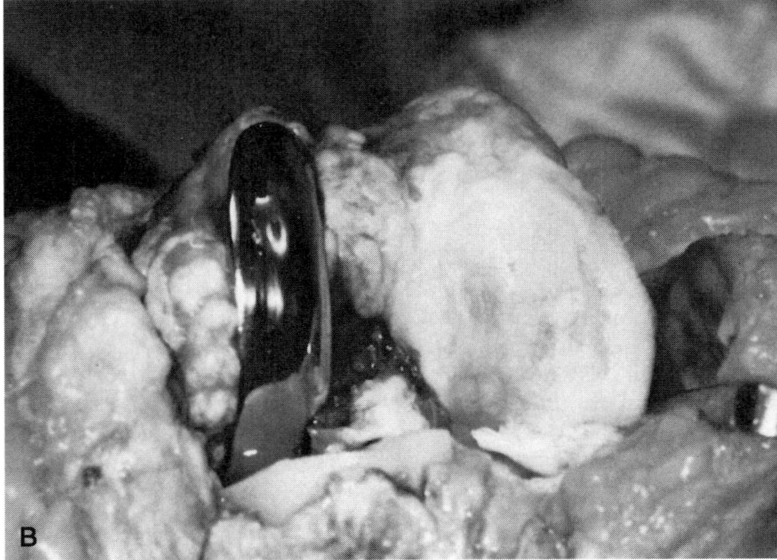

FIGURE 88.12 ➢ The most common reason for failure of unicondylar replacement is progressive arthritis of the unreplaced compartments of the knee. Free or embedded particles of acrylic cement are frequently found.

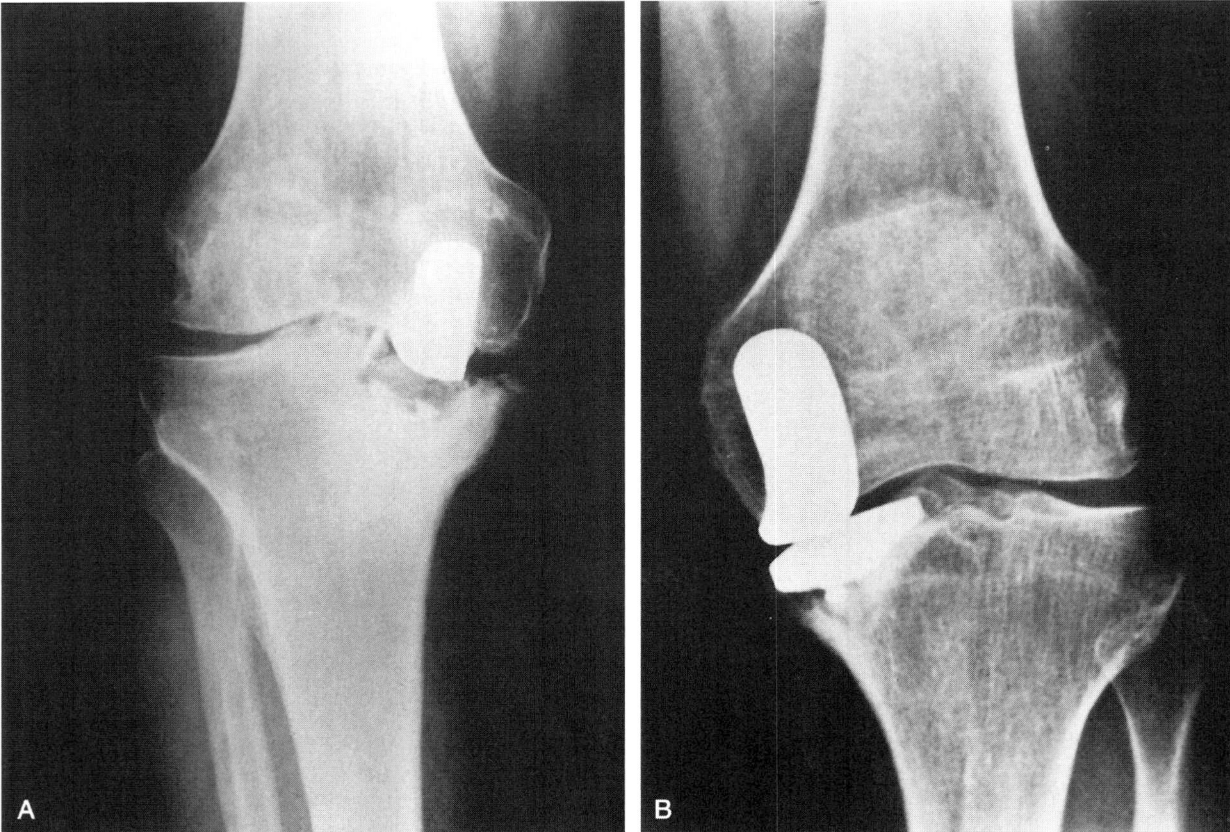

FIGURE 88.13 ➢ *A*, A failed unicompartmental arthroplasty showing the amount of medial bone loss to be anticipated in the tibia. This is an old design. *B*, Radiograph of a more modern type of unicondylar arthroplasty, which has also failed by tibial loosening. A similar degree of medial tibial bone loss can be anticipated.

with a femoral head allograft. In this case, the femoral head is contoured and matched to the distal femur. Engh et al[5] described a technique where the distal femoral defect is prepared with a reamer and the femoral head is prepared with a reversed-shaped reamer. This allows the allograft to mate to the defect. The graft is then secured provisionally to the host, and the construct is prepared to accept the implant. In these cases, it is necessary to utilize a canal-filling stem to secure the implant in place. More extreme cases, with loss of both condyles including the metaphysis, require either two femoral heads or a distal femoral allograft. Fixation of two femoral heads is similar to the method described above but can at times be cumbersome. In this situation, it may be easier to rebuild the metaphyseal bone loss with a distal femoral allograft that can be fitted onto the residual bone. A distal femoral allograft can also be fitted into the trumpet-shaped or "ice cream cone" defect of the femur that is seen with epicondylar flaring (Fig. 88.16). This apparent widening of the distal femur occurs when the component is grossly loose; along with osteolysis, it results in subsidence of the component. The amount of metaphyseal bone loss can be extensive.

Preparation of the allograft is a two-stage process. While one surgeon prepares the allograft to accept the femoral component, the other surgeon prepares the residual femur. If present, the epicondyles along with the collateral ligaments should be preserved for later attachment. Most likely a constrained implant will be necessary. When positioning the allograft, care must be taken to achieve the correct length and rotation. There are several ways to achieve fixation of the allograft to the residual bone. One technique is to secure the composite with a canal-filling stem and supplement the fixation with a plate. Another method requires cementing the stem extension in the femoral diaphysis, securing the construct with cerclage wires. Whereas this controls rotation, final fixation is achieved with a press-fit canal-filling stem. In using either method, a step cut can be made in the host femur and allograft to improve rotational stability. When the construct is secure, the epicondyles and collateral ligaments can be reattached to the allograft.

Structural allograft for proximal tibial metaphyseal bone loss is also an appealing option. The type of allograft is depends on the size and location of the bone loss. A trumpet-like proximal tibia, which is a contained defect, may easily accommodate one or two

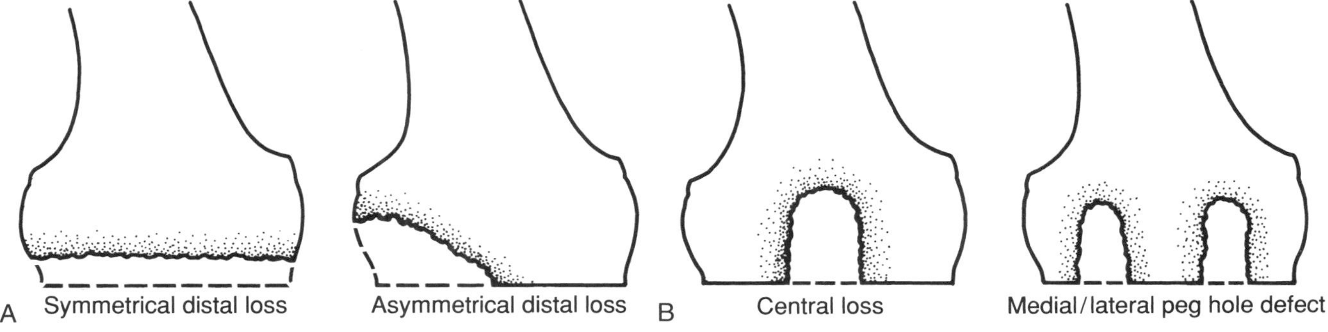

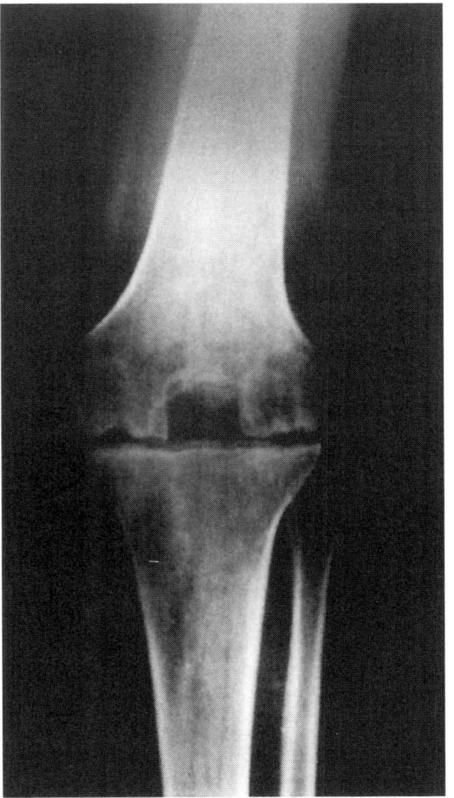

FIGURE 88.14 ➢ *A,* In the coronal plane, distal femoral bone loss may be symmetric or asymmetric. *B,* There may also be contained defects created by central or peripheral fixation lugs. *C,* Radiograph showing defects left after removal of the prosthesis, with a central box on the femur and a central stem on the tibia. Note good preservation of medial and lateral bone.

femoral heads. An asymmetric uncontained defect may accommodate a femoral head as described above for femoral bone loss. Larger defects, with loss of both the medial and lateral tibial plateaux, can be reconstructed with a proximal tibial allograft. Rotational stability and fixation are achieved by the techniques described above, with a step cut and press-fit canal-filling stem being the best option. If bone loss is so extensive that the tibial tubercle is involved, it will be necessary to have available a proximal tibia with the extensor mechanism still attached. Loss of the collateral ligament attachments necessitates implantation of a constrained knee.

MANAGEMENT OF THE PATELLA

When the components are inserted for a final check, patellar tracking is assessed by means of a lateral patellar release and balancing when necessary. If the augments have been chosen correctly, the patellar position will be in the "neutral zone." If it is not, altering the distribution of the augments between femur and tibia should be considered (Fig. 88.17); remember that some prerevision knees already have a patellar infera that, if due to actual shortening of the patellar ligament, must be accepted. In extreme situations, the patellar ligament may be so shortened that the patella actually articulates with the tibial polyethylene. Patellar lengthening and tibial tubercle advancement have been described; we believe there is too much risk of disruption or late failure of the patellar ligament to take this route. We prefer to reduce the size of the patellar bone and omit the patellar prosthesis.

The decision to use a patellar prosthetic component must depend not only on the patellar position but also on the amount of remaining bone stock. In most cases it is possible to reshape the patella and cement in a three-peg component. However, the patellar prosthesis

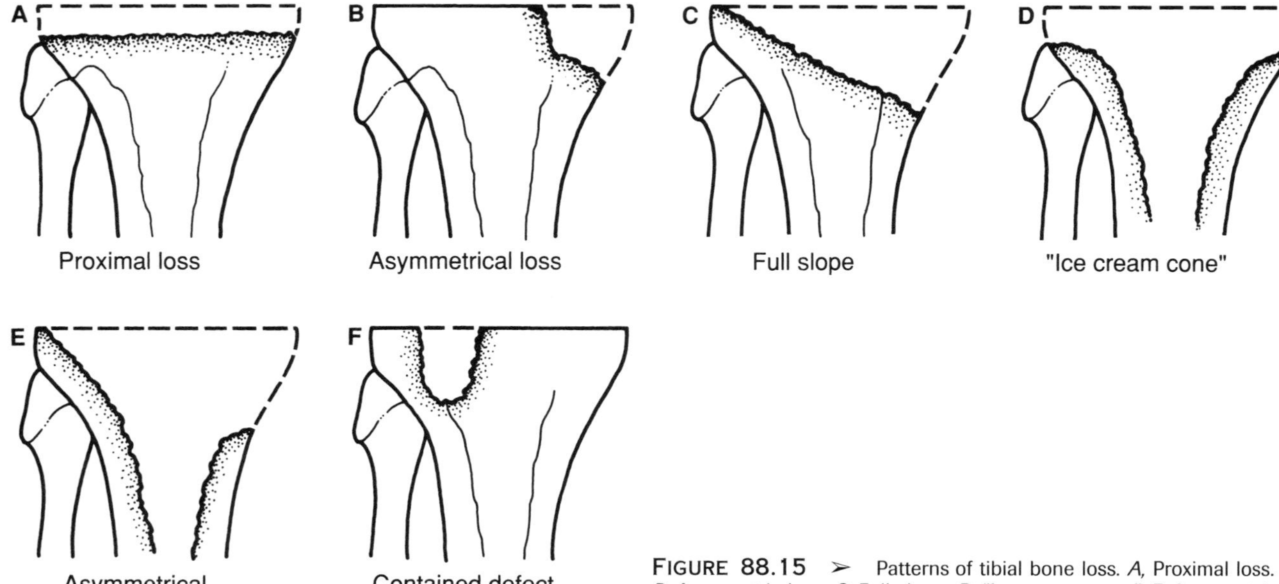

FIGURE 88.15 ➢ Patterns of tibial bone loss. *A,* Proximal loss. *B,* Asymmetric loss. *C,* Full slope. *D,* "Ice cream cone." *E,* Asymmetric "ice cream cone." *F,* Contained defect.

can be omitted when the bone stock is insufficient (less than 12 mm) or of very poor quality: the remaining patellar bone is then trimmed so that a reasonable fit in the femoral sulcus is obtained, commonly referred to as a "patelloplasty." At this point, the tourniquet is released, and major bleeding points are secured before reapplying the Esmarch bandage and reinflating the tourniquet.

Final Preparation

The bone surfaces are cleaned with pulsatile lavage. Note that in most revision cases, even with considerable bone loss, the margins of the defect will consist of sclerotic bone or irregular contours. This bone represents the strongest available, and it should not be removed or drilled, and no attempt should be made to obtain a cancellous surface. Even when this is possible, the quality of the bone may be poor and inadequate for providing proper prosthetic support.

The final components are assembled (Fig. 88.18),

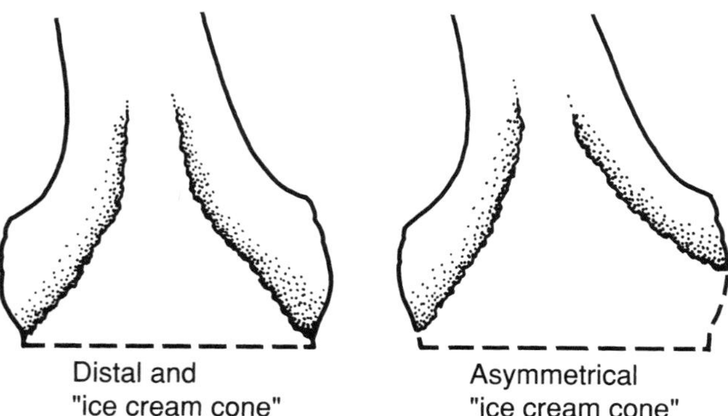

FIGURE 88.16 ➢ Cone defects in the distal femur are usually caused by removal of cemented stemmed components. This very extensive bone loss may be symmetric or asymmetric; bone grafting is often required in addition to augmentation.

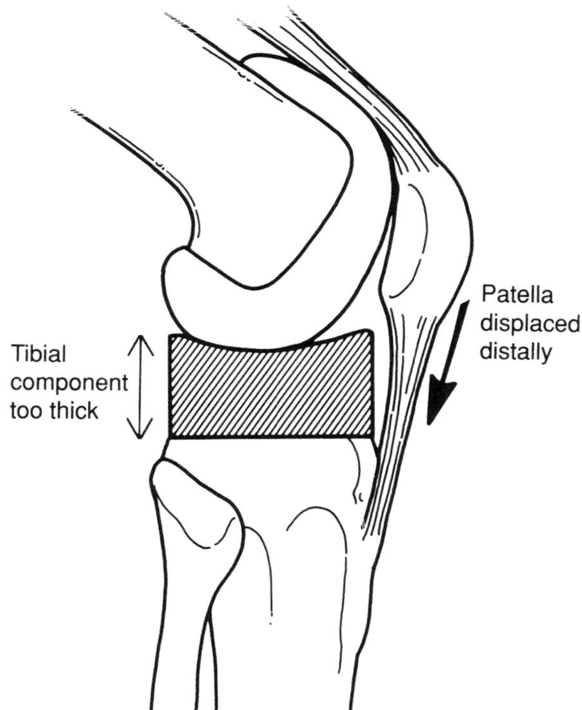

FIGURE 88.17 ➢ If an extra-thick tibial component is needed to stabilize the knee, the patella is displaced distally, causing a patella infera. Undersizing of the femoral component in the sagittal plane or anterior malpositioning are possible causes. Excessive distal resection of the femur moving the joint line proximally is another cause.

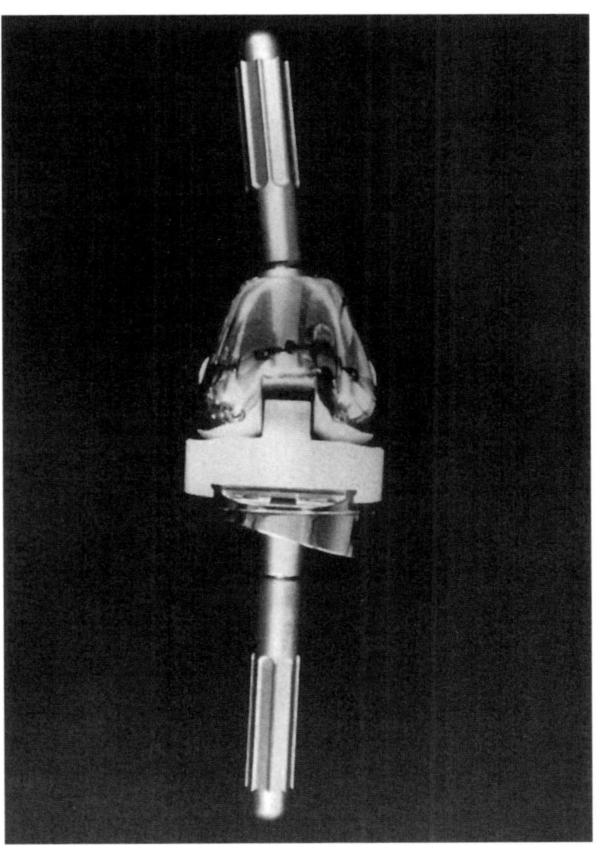

FIGURE 88.18 ➢ A modular IB II posterior stabilized prosthesis with stems and a full wedge augment to the tibia assembled in the operating room for implantation into a knee with a failed implant. There are also augments on the distal femur (not seen). Although this implant has a posterior stabilized articulation, by changing the polyethylene insert, it could be converted into a CCK (constrained condylar knee). The CCK metal components are compatible with both posterior stabilized and CCK tibial inserts.

the selected modular augments and wedges are fixed with screws or cement according to the designer's intention, and the intramedullary stems are attached. It is recommended that these stems be 1 mm larger than the stems used for the trial reduction to get the firmest possible fit.

Cementing

Although cementless reconstruction has its advocates,[18, 27] the use of cement has many attractions, and its use ensures that the new prosthesis fits perfectly on bone surfaces, which are inherently irregular. Bone resection that would otherwise be needed is avoided. Provided that cement is prevented from entering the intramedullary canals, later removal of the prosthesis (e.g., in the event of infection) is not difficult. The object of cement use is to level the bone ends and to give even loading beneath the prosthesis. Fixation itself is obtained by the component shape and the intramedullary stems (Fig. 88.19).

Two batches of cement are usually required for each component; they should contain an antibiotic powder. If gentamicin-impregnated cement is not available, 1 g of tobramycin powder for each bag of cement is used. The cement is used in the doughy stage and applied to the undersurface of the core femoral component. As intramedullary cement is to be avoided, care is taken not to allow cement to be pushed around the stem. The prosthesis is inserted and gradually impacted into the bone until it is firmly seated on the bony surface. The cement should be doughy because, if in a liquid phase, the cement will "leak" from under the prosthesis.

The patellar component, when it is used, can be cemented with the femur and held with a clamp until cured.

The cement for tibial fixation is then mixed. Once again it is applied to the underside of the core prosthesis in a doughy condition, and the prosthesis is inserted and gently impacted into the bone. When morseled graft has been used, insertion of the components must be done gently so as not to displace the graft into the intramedullary canal (Fig. 88.20).

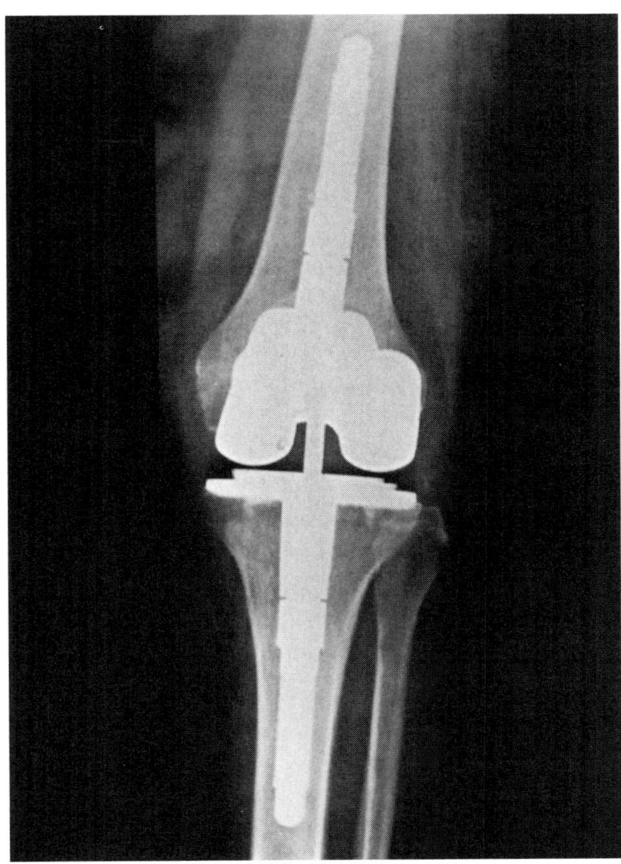

FIGURE 88.19 ➢ Prostheses that are fixed with bone cement as a grouting material at the interface with uncemented stem extensions have been shown by roentgen stereophotogrammetric analysis to have minimal micromotion. It is not necessary for the stems to contact the cortices.

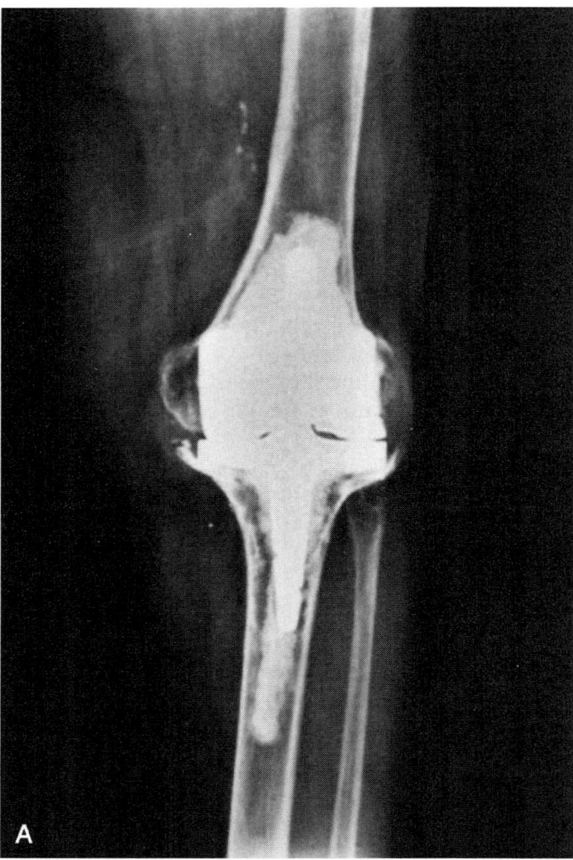

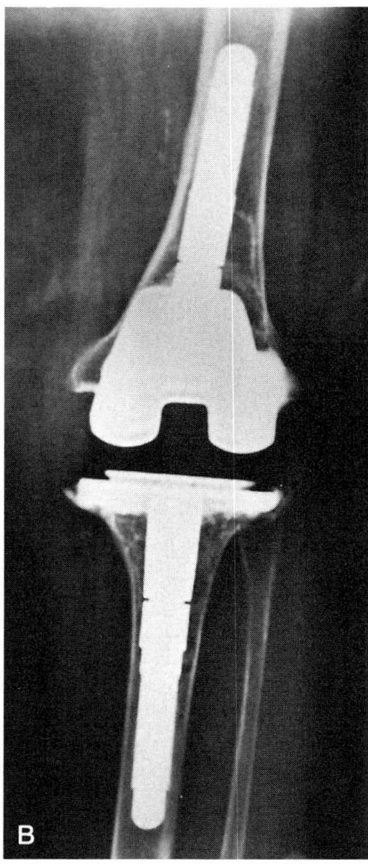

FIGURE 88.20 ➢ *A,* Radiograph showing a loose spherocentric prosthesis. From the distribution of the cement, extensive bone loss was anticipated. *B,* Radiograph taken after revision using constrained condylar knee metal implants with a posterior stabilized polyethylene insert. The contained defects have been packed with cancellous bone graft. Cement was used to level the bone ends, and the stems were uncemented.

Aftercare

Aftercare for revision surgery does not differ from that indicated for primary cases, unless there has been extensive bone grafting, which would require some protection in weightbearing. Even with the use of a "quadriceps snip" or a tibial tubercle osteotomy, we still progress with range-of-motion and strengthening exercises. If there is any question of the fixation of the tibial tubercle osteotomy, then motion and quadriceps exercises are limited for 6 to 8 weeks or until the osteotomy is healed.

RESULTS OF REVISION SURGERY

It is difficult to give meaningful results of revision surgery because, even more than for primary arthroplasty, techniques are continually evolving. Long-term results of revision surgery, therefore, describe cases using techniques not applicable today. Customized components, metal augments, wedges, stems, and allograft techniques are still being refined.

Bertin and colleagues[1] were the first to give revision results using noncemented stems (on the ICLH prosthesis), which were, if anything, better than those with primary arthroplasty. This experience led Freeman (personal communication) to use similar stems for all of his replacements.

The results obtained at The Hospital for Special Surgery with customized prostheses (Fig. 88.21) using augments, wedges, and stems were examined.[25] The infection rate was 5%, and mechanical loosening was 3%, all in cemented and short-stem components. None of the long-stem noncemented components loosened. Of the noncemented stems, 96% showed a sclerotic halo around the stem and, in most cases, cortical reaction at the distal tip of the stem. Problems of sizing and fit occurred with the custom prosthesis because it was difficult to estimate from preoperative radiographs the exact shape and location of bone defects and, in some cases, the optimal stem size; there were many component misfits, which led to the newer concept of modular design.

The results, although as durable as those of primary arthroplasty, were not equal in quality. In 1982 Insall and Dethmers[12] recorded an 89% good and excellent result in a series of cemented revisions. However, the period of follow-up was relatively short, and the incidence rate of radiolucent lines around the components was high. There were fewer excellent and more good results than in a primary arthroplasty series. Goldberg and colleagues[9] gave the results of 65 consecutive revision TKAs performed for mechanical failure. The types of implants used included total condylar, posterior stabilized, total condylar III, and a kinematic rotating hinge prosthesis. In this series 46% of the knees was considered excellent or good, and 42% was poor or failure. The infection rate was 4.5%, and multiple revisions did poorly. Jacobs et al[13] reviewed 24 patients

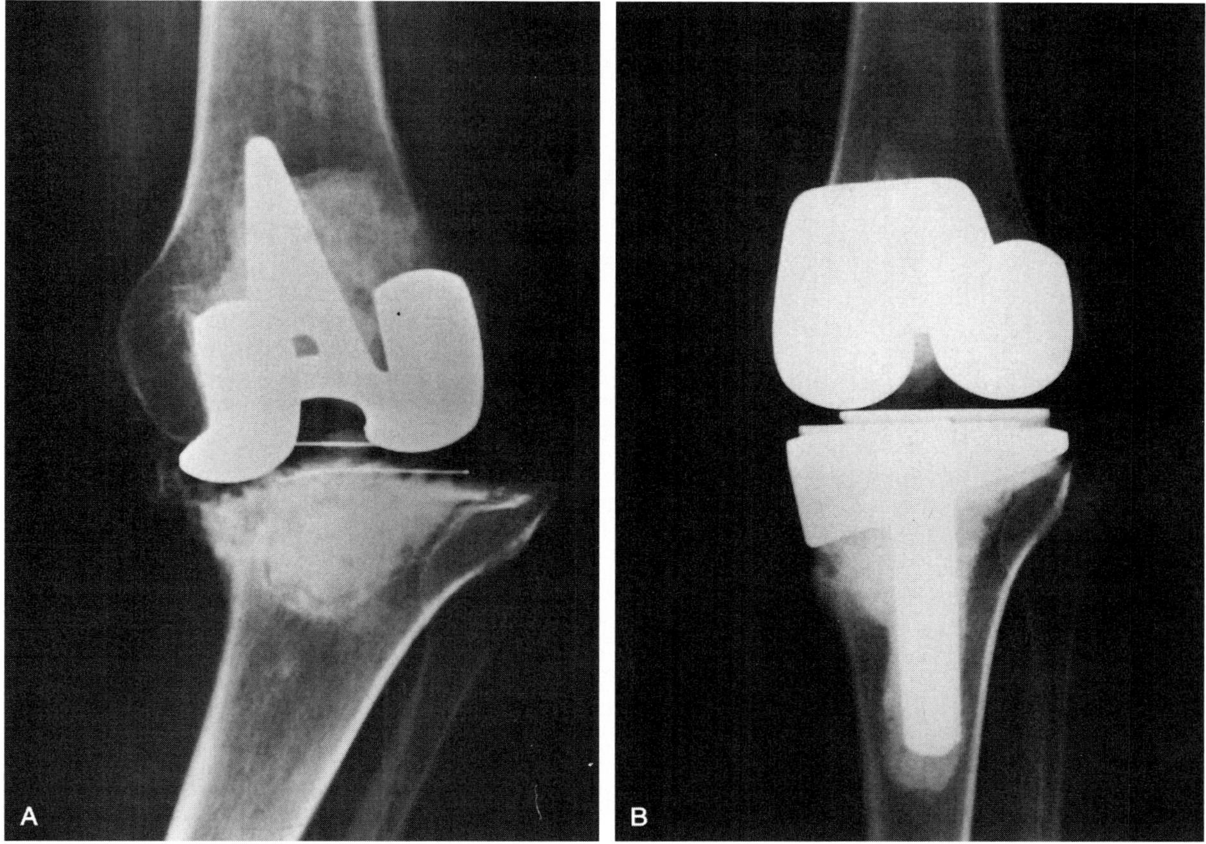

FIGURE 88.21 ➢ In the revision of this prosthesis with severe collapse of the medial tibia, a custom-made prosthesis with a full wedge was used. The articular surfaces of the revision prosthesis are standard posterior stabilized condylar design.

with 28 failed TKAs replaced with porous-coated anatomic components. Good and excellent results occurred in 68%, and there were three failures. Patients who had revision operations for severe pain or who had no clearly definable problem were not improved. Friedman and coworkers[6] gave results of 137 revision total knees at the Brigham and Women's Hospital in Boston. Function instability, motion, and pain, all improved after revision, but improvements were significantly less than those seen after primary total knee replacement. One-third of the patients still walked with crutches, a walker, or not at all. Loosening was the most common reason for failure. The clinical success rate was 63% for a single revision, and the failure rate at 5 years was 5.8%.

The results of using allograft to manage bony defects has had some encouraging results for small and large defects. Whiteside[26] used morseled allograft for localized areas of bone defects in 56 cementless revisions. All 56 knees demonstrated increase density in the grafted zone. For larger defects, Wilde et al[29] reported their results on 12 knees. Five of the knees had contained defects and seven knees had an uncontained defect; all were treated with structural allograft. Radiographs demonstrated complete incorporation of the graft in 11 of the 12 knees at an average of 23 months after operation. Single photon emission computed tomography scans showed uniform activity in the area of the graft in four of the five knees that were studied. Laskin[14] demonstrated poor results using autogenous bone graft for large bony defects. He examined 26 patients with severe tibial bone loss and secondary varus-valgus instability of greater than 20 degrees treated with TKA and autogenous bone graft. He found that four grafts demonstrated fragmentation and dissolution within the first year with implant subsidence. Needle biopsy in 9 other knees 1 year postoperatively revealed osteocytes in the lacunae in only 4 grafts. In four other knees there was a complete radiolucency between the graft and the tibial host bone. The overall success rate at 5 years was only 67%.

Other studies of allograft use in mostly uncontained defects demonstrated good results. Harris and colleagues[11] reported on 14 cases with a 43 month follow-up. Seven of the eight cases (87.5%) that involved the distal femur obtained good or excellent results. Tsahakis et al[24] reported even better results. In their study of 13 large uncontained femoral defects, at a mean follow-up of 2.1 years, all 13 cases had host-allograft union. In this study, all six proximal tibial

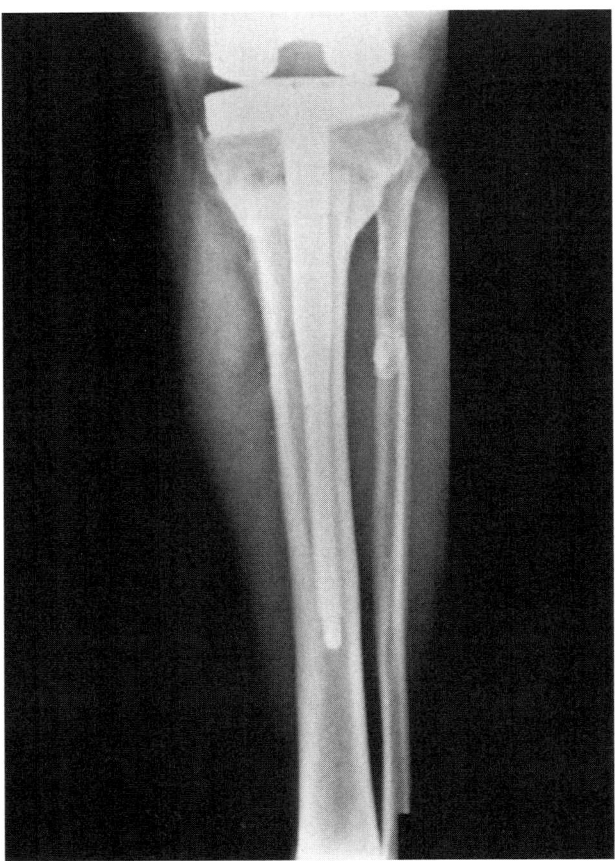

FIGURE 88.22 ➢ Radiograph showing a stem attachment to a tibial component for a nonunion of an upper tibial osteotomy. This method has proved very successful and predictable in obtaining healing of the fracture.

allografts also healed. Mow and Wiedel[19] also reported good results with uncemented component fixation. They used 15 allografts, including 10 for the proximal tibia. There was 1 failure (at 3 years) due to allograft failure. During the revision of the failure, they found the graft had incorporated, but the component lost support with subsequent implant fracture. They concluded that all 15 allografts had healed to host bone.

The use of metal augments in the form of wedges or blocks has overall good results in revision knee surgery. Brooks et al[3] compared five different techniques in the treatment of wedge-shaped proximal tibial defects. They concluded that a metal wedge was an acceptable alternative to a custom-made component in the reconstruction of tibial bone stock defects. Brand and colleagues[2] reported their good results in using a metal wedge for proximal tibial defects. In their series, 22 knees (20 patients) were monitored for an average of 37 months. No failures and no loosening of tibial components were reported. However, there was a 27% incidence of nonprogressive radiolucent lines. None of these patients required revision surgery, and all but one patient was pain-free.

The results of our own experience with CCK components and uncemented stems have been examined.[10] There were 68 revision operations, and follow-up was for 2 to 10 years. Excellent and good results were obtained in 56 knees, and there were 11 poor results. A further revision was performed on six knees, all because of infection. The posterior stabilized tibial insert was used in 49 knees, of which 43 (87%) were excellent and good, with 4 further revisions. The CCK tibial insert was needed to give greater stability in 18 knees, and there were 13 (82%) knees rated excellent and good, with 2 further revisions. The overall infection rate was high (9%), confirming the wisdom of avoiding intramedullary cement. Survivorship analysis of this group of patients was calculated as 80% at 10 years, a figure less satisfactory than a similar analysis performed on the total condylar and posterior stabilized prostheses (90% and 94%, respectively). Thus, even with so-called "modern" techniques, the results of revision surgery are understandably less satisfactory than primary arthroplasty. The point made by Jacobs and coworkers[13] about the poor results of revision surgery done for pain, without clear definition of the reason, is well taken and cannot be overemphasized. Our own experience confirms this, although we un-

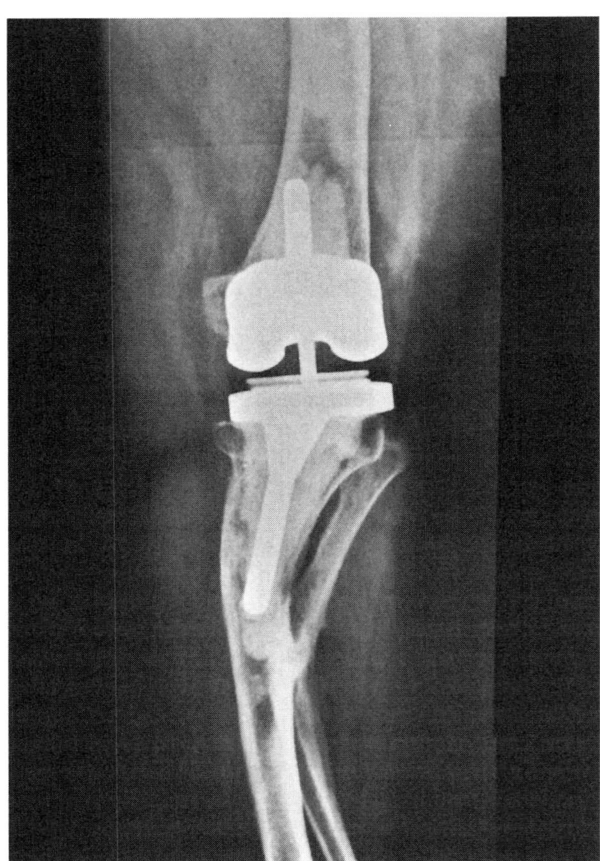

FIGURE 88.23 ➢ This bizarre prosthesis is a posterior stabilized design used for the revision of a hinged prosthesis. An angulated tibial stem was used because of bone deformity of the upper tibia.

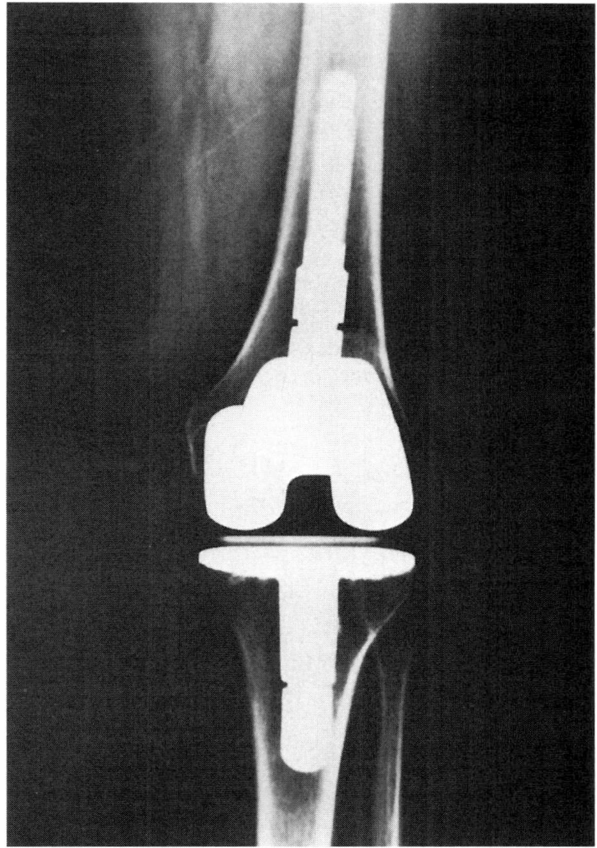

FIGURE 88.24 ➢ Radiograph of a "stubby" stem extension on the tibial component. The stubby stem impinges against the lateral cortex of the tibia. If a longer stem extension had been used, the tibial component would have tilted into the valgus. Alternatively, the whole component could be medialized, but this would cause medial overhang of the prosthesis. In this case, an offset stem is required.

derstand how difficult it is to manage a patient with a painful arthroplasty. The temptation to "give it a go" is sometimes irresistible, but the result will be failure.

CUSTOM COMPONENTS

Since the introduction of modularity, custom components have a limited role in revision knee arthroplasty. A custom prosthesis can be considered if one of the following conditions prevails:

1. The bone is so oversized or undersized that standard components will not fit.
2. Stems are needed to enhance fixation, but the bone shapes preclude the use of standard devices (for example, when there is a fracture malunion adjacent to the prosthesis [Fig. 88.22] or an offset stem is needed because of peculiarities in intramedullary alignment [Fig. 88.23]; shorter modular stem extensions and offset stems also provide a solution to this problem [Fig. 88.24]).
3. The size or location of bone loss cannot be accommodated by standard augments.

Otherwise, custom components should be avoided, for the following reasons:

1. There are no instruments designed for implanting custom components.
2. The use of a custom component does not provide for sizing options intraoperatively.

Generally, the high degree of modularity available with today's knee systems has replaced what little need there is for custom components.

SUMMARY

Revision knee surgery is not straightforward and is not always technically easy. Instruments are not as useful as they are for primary arthroplasty, although the use of stems is helpful in obtaining alignment. Above all, the surgeon should develop a good understanding of the principles of revision knee arthroplasty and perform the appropriate preoperative preparations.

References

1. Bertin KC, Freeman MAR, Samuelson KM, et al: Stemmed revision arthroplasty for aseptic loosening of total knee replacement. J Bone Joint Surg Br 67:242, 1985.
2. Brand MG, Daley RJ, Ewald FC, et al: Tibial tray augmentation with modular metal wedges for tibial bone stock deficiency. Clin Orthop 248:71, 1989.
3. Brooks PJ, Walker PS, Scott RD: Tibial component fixation in deficient tibial bone stock. Clin Orthop 184:302, 1984.
4. Chen F, Krackow KA: Management of tibial defects in total knee arthroplasty. Clin Orthop 305:249, 1994.
5. Engh GA, Herzwurm PJ, Parks NL: Treatment of major defects of bone with bulk allografts and stemmed components during total knee arthroplasty. J Bone Joint Surg Am 79:1030, 1997.
6. Friedman RJ, Hirst P, Poss R, et al: Results of revision total knee arthroplasty performed for aseptic loosening. Clin Orthop 255: 235, 1990.
7. Ghazavi MT, Stockley I, Yee G, et al: Reconstruction of massive bone defects with allograft in revision total knee arthroplasty. J Bone Joint Surg Am 79:17, 1997.
8. Gold DA, Scott WN, Scott SA: Soft tissue expanders prior to total knee replacement in the multioperated knee: A new method to prevent catastrophic skin problems. J Arthroplasty 11:512, 1996.
9. Goldberg VM, Figgie MP, Figgie HE III, et al: The results of revision total knee arthroplasty. Clin Orthop 226:86, 1988.
10. Haas SB, Insall JN, Montgomery W, et al: Revision total knee arthroplasty with use of modular components with stems inserted without cement. J Bone Joint Surg Am 77:1700, 1995.
11. Harris AI, Poddar S, Gitelis S, et al: Arthroplasty with a composite of an allograft and a prosthesis for knees with severe deficiency of bone. J Bone Joint Surg Am 77:373, 1995.
12. Insall JN, Dethmers DA: Revision of total knee arthroplasty. Clin Orthop 170:123, 1982.
13. Jacobs MA, Hungerford DS, Krackow KA, et al: Revision total knee arthroplasty for aseptic failure. Clin Orthop 226:78, 1988.
14. Laskin RS: Total knee arthroplasty in the presence of large bony defects of the tibia and marked knee instability. Clin Orthop 248:66, 1989.
15. Mnaymneh W, Emerson RH, Borja F, et al: Massive allografts in salvage revisions of failed total knee arthroplasties. Clin Orthop 260:144, 1990.
16. Mont MA, Serna FK, Krackow KA, et al: Exploration of radiographically normal total knee replacements for unexplained pain. Clin Orthop 331:216, 1996.
17. Moreland JR: Mechanisms of failure in total knee arthroplasty. Clin Orthop 226:49, 1988.

18. Mow CS, Wiedel JD: Noncemented revision total knee arthroplasty. Clin Orthop 309:110, 1994.
19. Mow CS, Wiedel JD: Structural allografting in revision total knee arthroplasty. J Arthroplasty 11:235, 1996.
20. Padgett DE, Stern SH, Insall JN: Revision total knee arthroplasty for failed unicompartmental replacement. J Bone Joint Surg Am 73:186, 1991.
21. Pagnano MW, Trousdale RT, Rand JA: Tibial wedge augmentation for bone deficiency in total knee arthroplasty. Clin Orthop 321:151, 1995.
22. Ritter MA, Keating M, Faris PM: Screw and cement fixation of large defects in total knee arthroplasty. J Arthroplasty 8:63, 1993.
23. Stockley I, McAuley JP, Gross AE: Allograft reconstruction in total knee arthroplasty. J Bone Joint Surg Br 74:393, 1992.
24. Tsahakis PJ, Beaver WB, Brick GW: Technique and results of allograft reconstruction in revision total knee arthroplasty. Clin Orthop 303:86, 1994.
25. Urs WK, Binazzi R, Insall JN, et al: Custom total knee arthroplasty. Orthop Trans 12:711, 1988.
26. Whiteside LA: Cementless reconstruction of massive tibial bone loss in revision total knee arthroplasty. Clin Orthop 248:80, 1989.
27. Whiteside LA: Cementless revision total knee arthroplasty. Clin Orthop 286:160, 1993.
28. Whiteside LA, Ohl MD: Tibial tubercle osteotomy for exposure of the difficult total knee arthroplasty. Clin Orthop 260:6, 1990.
29. Wilde AH, Schickendantz MS, Stulberg BN, et al: The incorporation of tibial allografts in total knee arthroplasty. J Bone Joint Surg Am 72:815, 1990.
30. Windsor RE, Scuderi GR, Insall JN: Revision of well-fixed cemented, porous total knee arthroplasty: Report of six cases. J Arthroplasty 3:87, 1988.
31. Windsor RE, Scuderi GR, Moran MC, et al: Mechanisms of failure of the femoral and tibial components in total knee arthroplasty. Clin Orthop 248:15, 1989.

Extensor Mechanism Disruption After Total Knee Arthroplasty

RAJ K. SINHA • LAWRENCE S. CROSSETT • HARRY E. RUBASH

Total knee arthroplasty (TKA) has developed into one of the most successful and reliable surgical treatment options for the debilitated knee. However, despite the favorable results for the vast majority of patients, complications of the patellofemoral joint continue to haunt surgeons and patients alike. Complications range from minor inconveniences to major catastrophes and may include such undesirable results as painless crepitus with range of motion, persistent anterior knee pain, patellar subluxation or dislocation, patellar clunk, patellar component loosening, patellar component wear, patella fracture, and patellar tendon rupture. This chapter discusses the rare but devastating complication of extensor mechanism disruption. Rorabeck et al[32] reviewed other patellofemoral complications listed, and many of these complications are discussed elsewhere in this book.

QUADRICEPS TENDON DISRUPTION

Rupture of the quadriceps tendon after TKA is exceedingly rare. As reported by Lynch et al,[26] quadriceps tendon rupture occurred in 3 of 281 (1.1%) TKAs. In addition, Fernandez-Baillo et al[11] reported a single case, and Grace and Sim[14] reported a single quadriceps tendon rupture after patellectomy for treatment of a patella fracture after TKA.

It is difficult to determine whether certain conditions predispose a TKA patient to quadriceps rupture, because the complication is rare. Rheumatoid arthritis (RA) was implicated by Fernandez-Baillo et al,[11] whereas technical errors such as over-resection of the patella with violation of the quadriceps tendon were suggested by Lynch et al[26] and Grace and Sim.[14] Additional possible causes include poor preoperative range of motion necessitating a rectus snip or V-Y turndown and subsequent incomplete healing, postoperative manipulation, or trauma.

Fernandez-Baillo et al[11] used Scuderi's technique of primary quadriceps tendon repair with proximal turndown over the repair with Dacron tape reinforcement followed by a long-leg cast with the knee in extension for 6 weeks. At the 1-year follow-up, the functional result was reported to be good. For quadriceps rupture, we have attempted primary repair and Achilles tendon allograft reconstruction. Both techniques are less than optimal, although a slightly better functional outcome results with allograft reconstruction.

Treatment of quadriceps rupture remains frustrating, and the condition may be prevented with meticulous surgical technique and careful attention to preservation of the blood supply during TKA.

PATELLA FRACTURE

Stress fracture or traumatic fracture of the patella after TKA has been reported in several series.[2, 3, 6, 14, 16, 19, 26, 30, 33, 37, 38] The incidence of patella fracture ranges from 0.3% to 5.4% (Table 89.1). Clayton and Thirupathi[6] reported six fractures in 111 total condylar TKAs at 2-year follow-up. All fractures occurred within 18 months of surgery, and five required further surgical intervention. Of the five surgical patients, only three patients had a satisfactory result. Similarly, four patella fractures at average 6.6-year follow-up were reported by Insall et al[19] from a study of 88 total condylar TKAs. Despite appropriate treatment, the TKA patients with the patella fractures had decreased ultimate results. Following duopatellar TKA, Scott et al[33] found the incidence of patella fracture to be 0.5% (6 of 1213). Three of the six patients were treated nonoperatively with good results. However, two of three patients treated surgically eventually required patellectomy. In a series by Grace and Sim,[14] 12 of 8249 (0.15%) TKAs were complicated by patella fracture. Eight patients had operative intervention, and three had significant complications including quadriceps rupture, sepsis, and refracture. Brick and Scott[3] identified 15 fractures in 2887 cases (0.52%), 9 of which required reoperation. Seven of these patients had significant complications after initial reoperation that resulted in a poorer outcome than initially existed after TKA. Thus, despite its low incidence, patella fracture adversely affects results following TKA.

Factors that may increase the likelihood of eventual patella fracture (Table 89.2) include resurfacing of the patella,[2, 14, 33] lateral release,[16, 32, 33] use of press-fit components,[16, 32] revision surgery,[14] malalignment of the arthroplasty,[12, 37] entire fat pad excision,[6] over-resection resulting in a thin patella,[6, 14, 32, 33] use of patellar clamps,[32] size or orientation of the fixation lugs,[32, 33] thermal necrosis from cement,[6, 14] osteoporosis,[3] osteo-

TABLE 89.1 REPORTED INCIDENCE OF EXTENSOR MECHANISM DISRUPTION

Quadriceps Tendon Ruptures		
Fernandez-Baillo et al (11)	1 case report	Repaired with Dacron tapes
Lynch et al (26)	3/281 (1.1%)	
Patella Fractures		
Scott et al (33)		Stress fractures; duopatellar prosthesis
Resurfaced	5/372 (1.3%)	
Unresurfaced	1/841 (0.12%)	
Clayton and Thirupathi (6)	6/111 (5.4%)	Total condylar knee
Lynch et al (26)	5/281 (1.8%)	
Webster and Murray (38)	1/366 (0.27%)	Variable axis TKA
Insall et al (19)	4/88 (5.4%)	Total condylar prosthesis
Ritter and Campbell (30)		Superior geniculate artery sacrificed
Lateral release	1/84 (1.2%)	
No lateral release	17/471 (3.6%)	
Brick and Scott (3)	15/2887 (0.52%)	
Grace and Sim (14)		
Resurfaced	9/2719 (0.33%)	
Unresurfaced	3/5530 (0.05%)	
Boyd et al (2)		Duopatellar prosthesis
Resurfaced	3/396 (0.76%)	
Unresurfaced	0/495	
Tria et al (37)	18/504 (3.6%)	All fractures after lateral release
Healy et al (16)	5/211 (2.4%)	Cementless fixation; lateral release correlated with fracture
Patellar Tendon Ruptures		
Wilson and Venteers (39)	3/54 (5.6%)	Walldius hinged knee
Deburge (8)	5/292 (1.7%)	Guepar hinged knee
Lettin et al (24)	2/100 (2.0%)	Stanmore hinged knee
Yamamoto (41)	1/170 (0.59%)	Kodama-Yamamoto prosthesis
Wilson et al (40)	1/62 (1.6%)	Walldius hinged knee
Hui and Fitzgerald (18)	2/77 (2.6%)	After revisions
Kaufer and Matthews (22)	1/82 (1.2%)	Spherocentric prosthesis
Lettin et al (25)	1/20 (5.0%)	Stanmore hinged knee
Oglesby and Wilson (27)	4/160 (2.5%)	All after Walldius TKA; none after total condylar or geometric TKA
Townley (36)	2/532 (0.38%)	Anatomic total knee
Webster and Murray (38)	1/366 (0.27%)	Associated with steroid use
Lynch et al (26)	4/281 (1.4%)	
Grace and Rand (15)	2/25 (8.0%)	Revisons for instability
Rand et al (28)	17/8288 (0.21%)	Multiple treatments
Boyd et al (2)		Duopatellar prosthesis
Resurfaced	3/396 (0.76%)	
Unresurfaced	2/495 (0.40%)	
Healy et al (16)	1/211 (0.47%)	

TKA = total knee arthroplasty.

arthritic cysts,[3] patella subluxation,[14] incorrect patellar component size,[14] postoperative manipulation,[33] previous patella fracture,[33] hinged TKA,[31] male gender,[32] excessive early range of motion,[20] posterior stabilized femoral components,[32] inset patellar components,[32] and increased patellofemoral strain from increased thickness of the patella or anterior displacement of the femoral component.[28]

Of the myriad predisposing causes of patella fracture, a few have been shown to be statistically significant. For example, Grace and Sim[14] showed that fractures occurred in 9 of 2719 (0.33%) resurfaced patellae but in only 3 of 5530 (0.05%) nonresurfaced patellae ($p < 0.05$). Similarly, Scott et al[33] reported that 5 of 372 (1.3%) resurfaced patellae fractured, whereas only 1 of 841 (0.12%) unresurfaced patellae fractured. In the series of Boyd et al,[2] 3 of 396 (0.76%) resurfaced patellae fractured, and 0 of 495 unresurfaced patellae fractured. Thus, fractures appear to be more common after resurfacing of the patella.

Another commonly cited cause of patella fracture is lateral retinacular release and subsequent devascularization of the patella.[34] Healy et al[16] reported that four of five fractures occurred after lateral release ($p < 0.04$); Scott et al[33] found the same incidence. Similarly, Tria et al[37] determined that of 18 patella fractures, all had previous lateral release, although 82% of all cases required lateral release. However, Ritter et al[30] specifically addressed the question of lateral release and patella fracture and found a higher incidence of fracture in knees not requiring lateral release (3.6%) than in those requiring lateral release (1.4%), even though no attempt was made to preserve the superior lateral geniculate artery. Despite these conflicting reports, most authors agree that the benefits of lateral release to balance the extensor mechanism and improve patello-

TABLE 89.2 ETIOLOGY OF EXTENSOR MECHANISM RUPTURES

Condition	References
Quadriceps Rupture	
Rheumatoid arthritis	11
Patella Fracture	
Technical issues	
Lateral release	16, 32, 33
Component malalignment	12, 37
Patella subluxation	14
Over-resection of patellar bone	6, 14, 32, 33
Overstuffing of anterior compartment	29
Total fat pad excision	6
Thermal necrosis from cement	6, 14
Patellar clamps	32
Inset patellar components	32
Implant choice	
Resurfacing	2, 14, 33
Cementless fixation	16, 32
Hinged TKA	31
Posterior stabilized components	32
Patient factors	
Revision TKA	14
Previous patella fracture	33
Manipulation	33
Excessive early ROM	20
Male gender	32
Osteoporosis	3
Subchondral cysts	3
Patellar Tendon Rupture	
Technical issues	
Revision surgery	26, 28
Devascularization	9, 10
Mechanical impingement	9, 10
Patellar instability	15
Resurfacing	2
Implant choice	
Hinged TKA	42
Patient factors	
Chronic steroid use	4, 38, 39
Rheumatoid arthritis	4
Collagen vascular diseases	4
Diabetes mellitus	4
Trauma	42
Infection	39, 40

ROM = range of motion; TKA = total knee arthroplasty.

femoral mechanics far outweigh the risk of devascularization, although the superior lateral geniculate artery should be preserved if possible.

An additional predisposing factor of patella fracture is revision surgery. Three of 495 (0.61%) revision TKAs were complicated by patella fracture, compared with 9 of 7754 (0.12%) primary TKAs ($p < 0.05$).[14] Similarly, four of five fractures were observed after cementless patellar component fixation, compared with one of five fractures after cemented component fixation.[13] Tria et al[37] showed that minor malalignment of the arthroplasty[12] was related to 17 of 18 patella fractures. In addition, minor malalignment has been related to an increased severity of patella fracture compared with neutral alignment.[12] The remainder of the suggested predisposing factors listed in Table 89.2 are based on individual investigators' experience but have not been shown statistically to increase the risk of patella fracture.

The poorer quality of RA bone compared with osteoarthritic (OA) bone suggests that patella fracture would occur more often in RA bone. However, Scott et al[33] found fractures in 2 of 286 (0.7%) RA patients and in 3 of 86 (3.5%) OA patients. In addition, Ritter et al,[30] Grace and Sim,[14] and Brick and Scott[3] found no increased incidence of fracture in patients with RA. This may be the result of lower demand on the TKA and decreased range of motion seen in RA patients.

Classification and Treatment. Goldberg et al[13] attempted to classify and determine the natural history of various types of periprosthetic patella fractures by reviewing their treatment results for 36 patients. They identified five categories: type I—fractures not involving the implant-cement composite or quadriceps mechanism, type II—fractures involving the implant-cement composite or quadriceps mechanism, type IIIA—inferior pole fractures with patellar ligament rupture, type IIIB—inferior pole fractures without patellar ligament rupture, and type IV—fracture-dislocations.

Fourteen type I fractures were treated nonoperatively and resulted in good or excellent functional scores without pain, locking, or mechanical symptoms. All six patients with type II midbody fractures underwent operation for revision of loose components and quadriceps tendon repair. Four knees were unsatisfactory. Two of two type IIIB fractures treated nonoperatively resulted in no superior migration and had satisfactory results. Eight type IIIA fractures were identified, and revision was recommended for all to repair the ruptured patellar ligament. Five of seven operated knees had poor outcomes, as did the knee of one patient who refused surgery. Nine patients had type IV fractures, and all underwent surgical treatment. Four patients had unsatisfactory results. Overall, 13 of 22 surgically treated knees had unsatisfactory results.

Hozack et al[17] treated 21 periprosthetic patella fractures and retrospectively reviewed the outcomes. A wide variety of treatments was rendered to this heterogeneous group of patients. Seven patients had nondisplaced fractures, five of which were comminuted. Four of these patients had patellectomy with subsequent good range of motion, no extensor lag, and good functional knee scores, but three of four had decreased quadriceps strength. Three of these patients were treated in a cylinder cast, and one patient had a poor result because of limited flexion after treatment. Fourteen patients had displaced fractures. Six patients were treated with a patellectomy, and only two of these had a satisfactory clinical outcome. The remainder of patient outcomes were complicated by decreased quadriceps strength and residual extensor lags. Two patients were treated with open reduction and internal fixation (ORIF) of their displaced inferior pole fractures, and both failed. Two patients were treated nonoperatively and had satisfactory results in terms of extensor lag, quadriceps strength, and range of motion. Of the four patients who were treated with fragment excision, two patients had favorable results and two had poor results. On the basis of these results, Hozack et al recommended the following treatment: Treat nondisplaced fractures and displaced fractures with no extensor lag nonoperatively with casting or bracing in extension. Displaced fractures with extensor lag have poor results despite operative treatment, and distal fragment excision should be considered. Reserve patellectomy for all failed interventions.

Authors' Preferred Treatment

On the basis of our experience, we have identified several criteria that determine treatment and outcome after periprosthetic patella fracture. These criteria include integrity of the extensor mechanism, displacement of the fracture, involvement of the patellar component (i.e., integrity of the prosthesis-bone interface), and vascularity of the patella. We have established a useful treatment algorithm based on these criteria (Fig. 89.1).

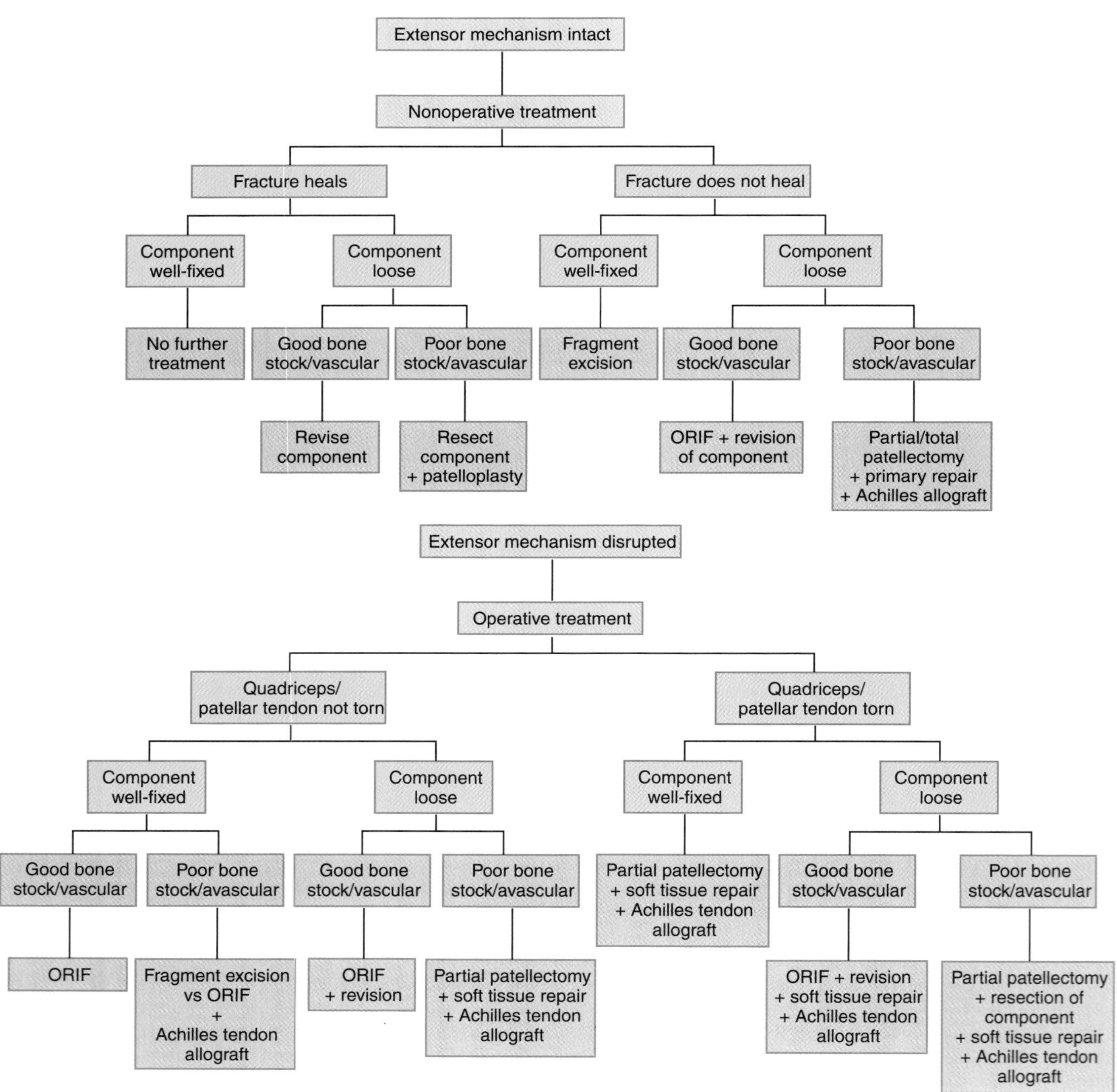

FIGURE 89.1 ➢ Algorithm for treatment of patella fractures after total knee arthroplasty.

When a patient presents with a patella fracture, we first assess the integrity of the extensor mechanism. If the patient is able to fully extend the limb against gravity or to do a straight-leg raise, then the extensor mechanism is intact. These patients generally have a nondisplaced fracture that does not involve the quadriceps or patellar ligament and can be treated very effectively and reliably with casting or bracing in extension for approximately 6 weeks or until the fracture heals. Once the fracture heals, the stability of the component is assessed. If the fracture does not involve the component-bone interface, no further treatment is needed. If the fracture heals but the component is loose (typically seen with comminuted fractures), the quality of the bone stock and the degree of vascularity determine whether revision or resection is appropriate. If the fracture does not heal, then component integrity determines the next step. Displaced fractures that do not involve the component-bone interface (typically vertical and marginal fractures; Fig. 89.2) may progress to nonunion and require late fragment excision. If the fracture involves the component-bone interface and the component is loose, depending on the quality of the remaining patellar bone and its vascularity, the component can be revised with ORIF or resected with primary soft-tissue repair and possible Achilles tendon allograft supplementation (technique described later).

Displaced transverse fractures typically involve the component-bone interface and disrupt the extensor mechanism (Fig. 89.3). These require operative intervention. If the component is well fixed and the remaining patellar bone is vascular and sufficiently thick, then ORIF is appropriate. If the component is loose, but bone stock and vascularity are sufficient, then ORIF with component revision is undertaken. If the patella is avascular or too thin or ectatic for resurfacing, or if the fracture disrupts the patellar or quadriceps tendon (Fig. 89.4), we favor partial or total patellectomy coupled with primary repair and Achilles tendon allograft supplementation. In addition, chronic fractures with displacement and loss of extensor mechanism function are put through the same algorithm and, in our practice, are generally supplemented with Achilles tendon allograft.

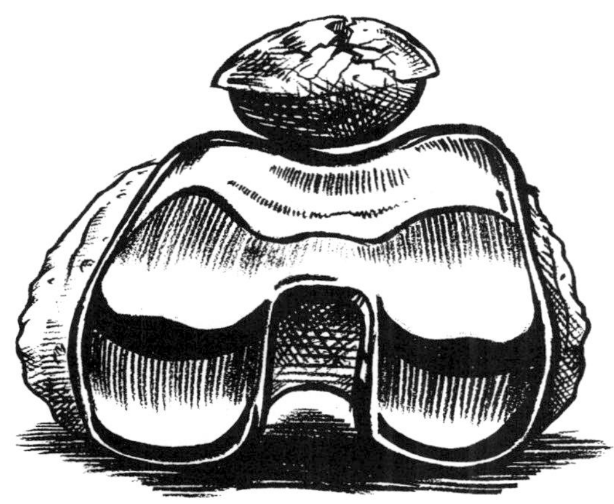

FIGURE 89.2 ➢ Schematic representation of marginal patella fracture after TKA. Note that the fracture does not extend into the prosthesis-bone interface.

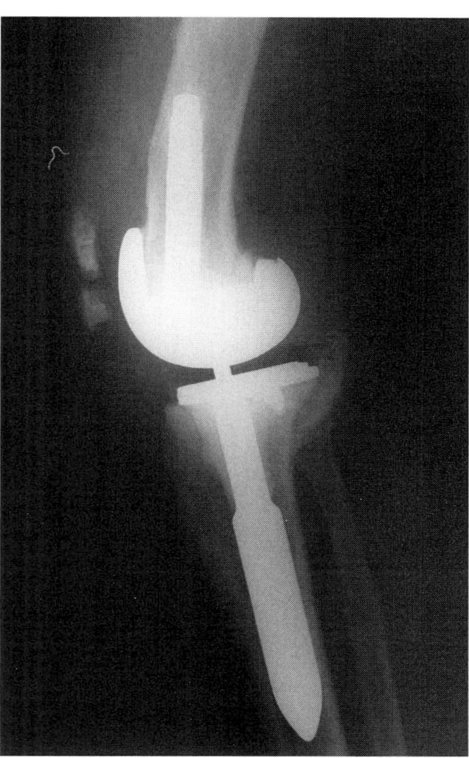

FIGURE 89.3 ➢ Radiograph depicting transverse patella fracture after revision total knee arthroplasty. The patient had a subsequent 40-degree extensor lag.

One caveat to remember when treating disrupted extensor mechanisms associated with patella fractures is that the patient may not be a candidate for further operative treatment. Elderly patients with minimal function, patients with poor skin that would threaten soft-tissue coverage, and patients with debilitating comorbidities, among others, may be better treated with bracing despite the resultant extensor lag.

Another important surgical issue to consider is component alignment and rotational orientation. When operative treatment is required, we routinely assess femoral and tibial component orientation and perform revision of one or more components as indicated. Failure to address component orientation may result in recurrent patella fracture or subluxation.

PATELLAR TENDON RUPTURE

Incidence. Like patella fracture, patellar tendon rupture after TKA is an uncommon but potentially devastating complication (Fig. 89.5). Despite its low incidence, most large series reporting on results of a wide variety of prosthesis types discuss patellar tendon ruptures (summarized in Table 89.1).

For example, a review of results with the Stanmore hinged prosthesis by Lettin et al[24] found two avulsions

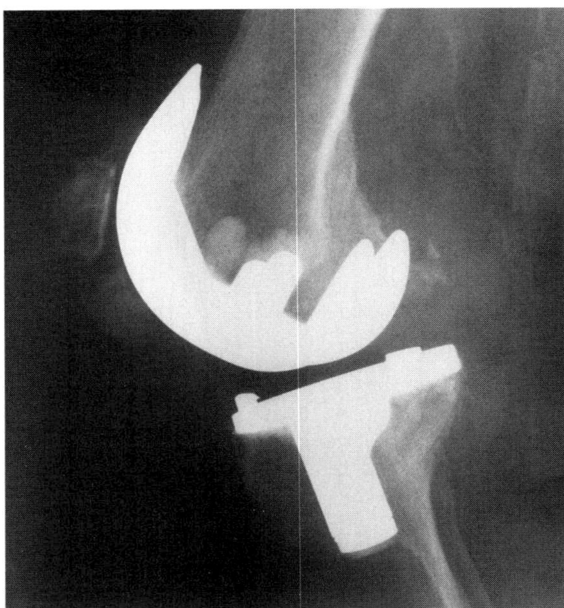

FIGURE 89.4 ➢ Radiograph depicting patella fracture after total knee arthroplasty that extended into the patellar tendon.

at the time of surgery and two subsequent ruptures (4% incidence). Both of the latter patients required supports for walking after the complication. The same group found an additional rupture in the 20 (5% incidence) patients who were followed up for more than 10 years.[25] A study detailing results with the Walldius hinged TKA found 3 of 54 (5.6%) patients with patellar tendon rupture.[39] Similarly, in a comparative study between the Walldius hinged and the geometric TKAs,[40] 1 of 62 (1.6%) patients sustained a patellar ligament rupture 4 months after hinged TKA. After repair, the patient went on to develop deep sepsis and eventually had a 35-degree extensor lag. Another comparative study of the Walldius, geometric, and total condylar TKAs[27] showed 5 of 160 (3.1%) patellar tendon ruptures, 4 of which occurred in the Walldius group. All four patellar tendon ruptures had primary repair but had resultant extensor lags of 10 to 35 degrees. Using another hinged TKA, the Guepar prosthesis, Deburge[8] reported that five tendon ruptures occurred during 292 TKAs (1.7%). Furthermore, another series of hinged Walldius and Guepar TKAs from the Mayo Clinic showed a 2.6% incidence (2 of 77) of patellar tendon rupture.[18]

Patellar tendon rupture has also occurred with other knee designs. Kaufer and Matthews[22] reported an incidence of 1 of 82 (1.2%) patellar tendon ruptures with the spherocentric knee. A 20-degree extensor lag resulted, but the patient did not undergo further surgery. Similarly, Yamamoto[41] found an incidence of 1 of 170 (0.59%) avulsions from the tibial tubercle during surgery; it was successfully reattached with a staple. With the Townley prosthesis, 2 of 532 (0.38%) TKAs were complicated by patellar tendon rupture or avulsion.[36] Lynch et al[26] demonstrated a 1.4% incidence (4 of 281), while Boyd et al[2] reported a 0.56% incidence (5 of 891) of patellar tendon ruptures. Similarly, Cadambi and Engh[4] noted a 0.55% incidence in their large series, while Healy et al[16] reported an incidence of 1 of 211 (0.5%), and Rand et al[28] reported a 0.17% incidence out of 8288 TKAs. Thus, the overall incidence of patellar tendon ruptures ranges from 0.17% to 5.6% after primary TKA.

Like quadriceps tendon ruptures, the relative infrequency of patellar tendon ruptures after TKA makes it difficult to draw definite conclusions regarding predisposing factors. However, several authors have pointed to potential causes (outlined in Table 89.2). For example, Rand et al[28] suggested that the most common cause is related to attempts to obtain exposure in the knee with limited range of motion. In addition, chronic steroid use has been implicated,[4, 38, 39] as well as trauma,[42] multiple surgeries,[26] devascularization,[9, 10] and mechanical impingement by the tibial or patellar components.[9, 10] Infection can clearly result in patellar tendon rupture.[39, 40] In the study of Cadambi and Engh,[4] five of seven patients suffered from systemic diseases such as diabetes mellitus and RA. These authors also suggested that collagen vascular diseases such as systemic lupus erythematosus may be a precipitating factor. In addition, Grace and Rand found that two patellar tendon ruptures occurred after 25 realignment procedures for patellar instability.[15] Also, hinged TKAs have been suggested to be more likely to result in patellar tendon rupture because of the increased constraint.[42] There may also be a slightly increased predisposition for rupture after patellar resurfacing (0.76% versus 0.40%).[2] Finally, dislocation of a TKA may result from a ruptured patellar tendon.[35]

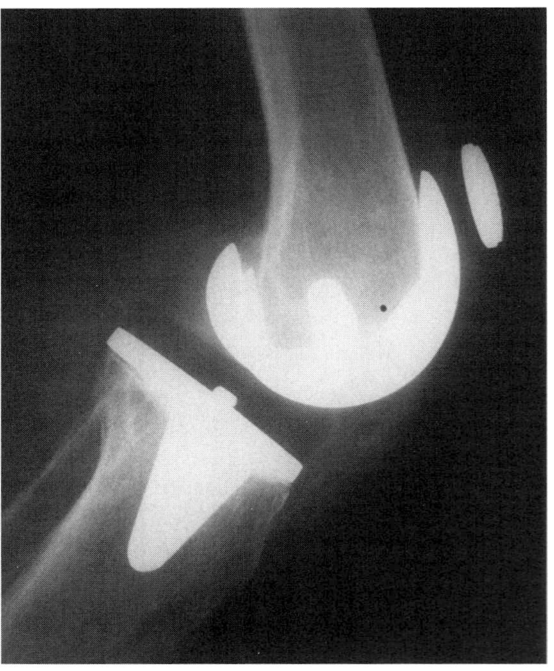

FIGURE 89.5 ➢ Radiograph of patellar tendon rupture after total knee arthroplasty. Note that patella alta exists.

Treatment and Results. As briefly discussed earlier, initial attempts at primary repair of patellar tendon ruptures were fraught with unpredictable results at best and catastrophic results at worst. One exception may be peeling off of the tendon at its insertion to the tibial tubercle at the time of surgery. In our experience, if the tendon peels off with the periosteal sleeve intact, it can be reattached primarily with a suture-anchor or through drill holes. Results of the TKA seem to be unaffected, even with no change in standard rehabilitation protocols. However, repair of later ruptures or avulsions presents an entirely different treatment dilemma.

In an early report, Wilson and Venteers[39] used the plantaris tendon to repair midsubstance patellar tendon ruptures. In both patients, full active extension was achieved, although details of the repair technique and of the postoperative protocol were not provided. More recently, Rand et al[28] reviewed their results after treating 18 tendon ruptures. Nine patients received primary suture repair, and in all nine cases, the repair failed, as defined by lack of full active extension. Four patients had staple fixation of tendon avulsions, and this was successful in two patients. One patient had a primary suture repair with semitendinosus tendon augmentation, and this treatment failed. An additional two knees had xenograft reconstruction, and both of these were successful. The final two patients had cast immobilization, and this treatment was unsuccessful. Thus, of 18 treated patellar tendon ruptures, the authors achieved successful outcomes in only four cases, and the mean flexion was only 81 degrees. It is important to note that three of these patients also had cast immobilization for 3 to 8 weeks postoperatively. This study further illustrates the difficulty in treating patellar tendon ruptures and the frustration that results for both patients and surgeons.

Emerson and associates first reported on an allografting technique in 1990[9] and later reported intermediate-term follow-up in 1994.[10] In their technique, the allograft consisted of quadriceps tendon, patella with cemented prosthesis, patellar tendon, and tibial tubercle. The tubercle of the allograft was keyed into the host tibia at its anatomic location and secured with screw or wire fixation. The patella was then placed on the anterior flange of the femoral prosthesis and tensioned, and the quadriceps tendon was attached to host tendon with nonabsorbable sutures to allow 60 degrees of flexion without undue tension. Postoperatively, the patient was allowed only limited flexion for several weeks, followed by gradual increase in range of motion. At an average follow-up of 23 months in 10 patients, the authors found two graft ruptures and one patella fracture, all of which led to failure of the construct. In the remaining patients, all tubercles healed and all quadriceps tendons healed. Nine patients were followed up for 4.1 years.[10] The average flexion was 106 degrees. Six patients had full active extension, but three had extensor lags ranging from 20 to 40 degrees. There were no additional graft ruptures, but two patellar prostheses had become loose and required revision. Thus, the authors questioned the need to resurface the patella. Overall, they felt that their technique was a viable option for extensor mechanism - deficient TKAs, especially in lower-demand patients, although durability was a concern.

Cadambi and Engh[4] used a different approach to reconstruct seven ruptured patellar tendons. They divided the semitendinosus tendon at its proximal muscle junction and maintained the distal insertion. The graft was routed along the medial border of the remnant patellar tendon through a quarter-inch drill hole in the distal pole of the patella and then resutured to itself at the distal insertion. The knee was flexed to 90 degrees to ensure that excessive tension was not placed on the graft. Immediate full weightbearing with a knee immobilizer was allowed for 6 weeks. After 6 weeks, limited flexion to 60 degrees for an additional 6 weeks was allowed with a knee immobilizer for walking. In this group of seven patients, the average extensor lag was 10 degrees, with average flexion of only 79 degrees. Four patients required a cane to ambulate. The authors concluded that use of autogenous graft was superior to primary repair or allograft and that it restored sufficient quadriceps strength and motion of the knee.

Jauregito and associates[21] used another type of autogenous graft to reconstruct six patellar tendon ruptures after TKA. A medial gastrocnemius muscle flap was mobilized and sutured transversely to the anterior muscle compartment at the level of the tibial tubercle. The patellar tendon stump was then sutured to the medial border of the gastrocnemius flap. Postoperatively, patients were held in an above-knee cast in full extension for 6 weeks, followed by a hinged knee brace for an additional 8 weeks, with progressive flexion dialed into the brace. At an average 26-month follow-up, the average range of motion was 100 degrees, with an average extensor lag of 24 degrees. The ambulation status of all patients improved, with two each requiring no aids, a cane, or a walker. There were two complications: One postoperative manipulation resulted in a 30-degree extensor lag, and one patient had a small area of skin necrosis that required skin grafting. The authors concluded that a medial gastrocnemius flap appeared to be a reliable option for reconstructing ruptured patellar tendons, with the added benefit of simultaneously improving soft-tissue coverage for these often multiply operated knees.

Several case reports elucidate other methods to treat ruptured patellar tendons after TKA. For example, Abril et al[1] performed Bunnell repairs with nonabsorbable suture placed through two drill holes in the tubercle for two patellar tendon avulsions. The repair was protected with a figure-eight wire placed superiorly through the quadriceps tendon and inferiorly around a screw in the tubercle. Both patients achieved full active extension and 85 or 95 degrees of flexion and were able to ambulate without walking aids. Similarly, Zanotti et al[42] used a bone - patellar tendon - bone allograft, which is similar to those used for anterior cruciate ligament reconstructions. Proximally, interference fit was used to secure the allograft to the patella, and, distally, the graft was secured with an interference screw. The patient was held in a cast at full extension for 12 weeks, followed by gradual increases in flexion. At 2 years, the patient had full active extension but intermittently required a knee-foot-ankle orthosis to control 5 to 10 degrees of chronic hyperextension. Flexion was not mentioned. Alternatively, Chiou et al[5] used an autogenous lateral gastrocnemius-Achilles tendon graft to reconstruct a patellar tendon rupture with overlying skin defect. The results were reported as satisfactory. Finally, Kempenaar and Cameron[23] reported a patellotibial fusion for a chronic patellar tendon rupture. This was accomplished by downsizing the tibial articular spacer. The patient achieved an active range of motion of −20 to 90 degrees. Although each of these techniques may be an option, additional experience with longer follow-up is necessary before definitive statements can be made.

Authors' Method for Achilles Tendon Allograft Reconstruction

On the basis of the experience of various authors, we have used a fresh-frozen Achilles tendon allograft with os calcis bone block to reconstruct patellar and quadriceps tendon ruptures, as well as to supplement patella fractures as outlined in Figure 89.1. This is based on several observations: (1) Primary repairs alone often result in residual extensor lag with dependence on ambulatory aids; (2) freeze-dried allografts are weaker than fresh-frozen allografts[9, 10]; (3) bony allografts appear to heal without difficulty if securely fixed to the tibia[9, 10]; (4) allograft tendon appears to heal reliably when sutured with nonabsorbable suture to the quadriceps myofascia and tendon[9, 10]; (5) autograft tendons are of unreliable length, thickness, strength, and integrity[4]; and (6) use of autogenous muscle-tendon autografts is technically very challenging and presents the likelihood of otherwise avoidable donor-site morbidities.[5, 21] There are several important points to remember when using this technique: (1) Fresh-frozen allograft is used rather than freeze-dried allograft; (2) autogenous tissue is not removed, and, if possible, primary repairs are performed; (3) the tendinous portion of the allograft is handled carefully, and no crushing instruments are used; (4) the bony portion of the allograft is maintained sufficiently thick so as not to weaken the allograft and thus predispose it to fracture; (5) atraumatic tapered needles should be used so as not to traumatize the tendon; (6) thick skin and subcutaneous flaps must be created, and they must be closed without undue tension; and (7) strict adherence to postoperative rehabilitation protocols is necessary. We have reported our preliminary results with this technique.[7] We are pleased with the improved early outcomes as compared with other techniques discussed previously.

Figure 89.6*A* shows a TKA complicated by patellar tendon rupture. At the time of surgery, there was a remnant patellar tendon with fibroplastic ends. After revision of the loose tibial tray, primary repair (Fig. 89.6*B*) was achieved and the patella was returned to its appropriate position. However, the repair was expectedly tenuous and supplemented in the following manner. On the back table, the allograft was prepared (Fig. 89.6*C*) so that the bony portion could be secured into a tibial defect by interference fit and then was further secured to the tibia with lag screw fixation. The medial collateral ligament was elevated subperiosteally along the medial border of the tibia. The location for the bony portion of the allograft was marked as close to the tubercle as possible on the medial side of the tibia. A defect was created in the host tibia with a high-speed bur (Fig. 89.6*D*, *E*). Care was taken to keep the allograft more than 15 mm thick and to not injure the tendon-bone junction. In addition, the allograft was gently impacted into the tibial defect to avoid fracture of the allograft (Fig. 89.6*F*) and then secured with a lag screw (Fig. 89.6*G*, *H*). With the knee in full extension (or slight hyperextension, if possible), the allograft tendon was placed over the patellar tendon, patella, and quadriceps myofascia. The tendon was secured to the underlying tissue with multiple no. 2 Ethibond simple sutures using a tapered, atraumatic needle (Fig. 89.6*I*). Importantly, no attempts were made to flex the knee at this point. The wound was closed without any tension on the skin. Also, if the components require revision, a posterior stabilized TKA is favored.

Postoperatively, the patient was maintained in a hinged knee brace locked at full extension with touch-down weightbearing. Isometric exercises were allowed. After 1 month, the patient was progressed to 50% weightbearing and the brace was set to allow 0 to 40 degrees of motion. Active and passive range-of-motion exercises coupled with quadriceps strengthening were instituted. After the second month, the brace was reset to allow 90 degrees of flexion. Weightbearing was continued at 50%. Strengthening exercises and active and passive range of motion were allowed. At the end of the third month, weightbearing was advanced to full (on the basis of evidence of radiographic union) and the brace was discontinued. Physical therapy was continued for an additional 6 to 12 weeks.

Results were reported on 11 patients.[7] Of the three failures, the first patient fell and acutely hyperflexed his knee and dislodged the bony block. This was resecured surgically, and the patient went on to have no extensor lag and 110 degrees of flexion. The second patient did not comply with the postoperative regimen and removed her brace at 1 month. She had a resultant 45-degree extensor lag and was excluded from further analysis. The third patient sustained a tibial shaft fracture at the allograft fixation site that occurred 14 months postoperatively. This patient was treated in a long-leg cast for 6 weeks but had a persistent nonunion. After revision of the tibial tray with a long stem that bypassed the nonunion site, the fracture united and the patient had no extensor lag with 110 degrees of flexion at 24 months after the initial allograft.

Thus, 10 patients at average 30-month follow-up were included. The average preoperative extensor lag was 40 degrees. Postoperatively, two patients had 5-

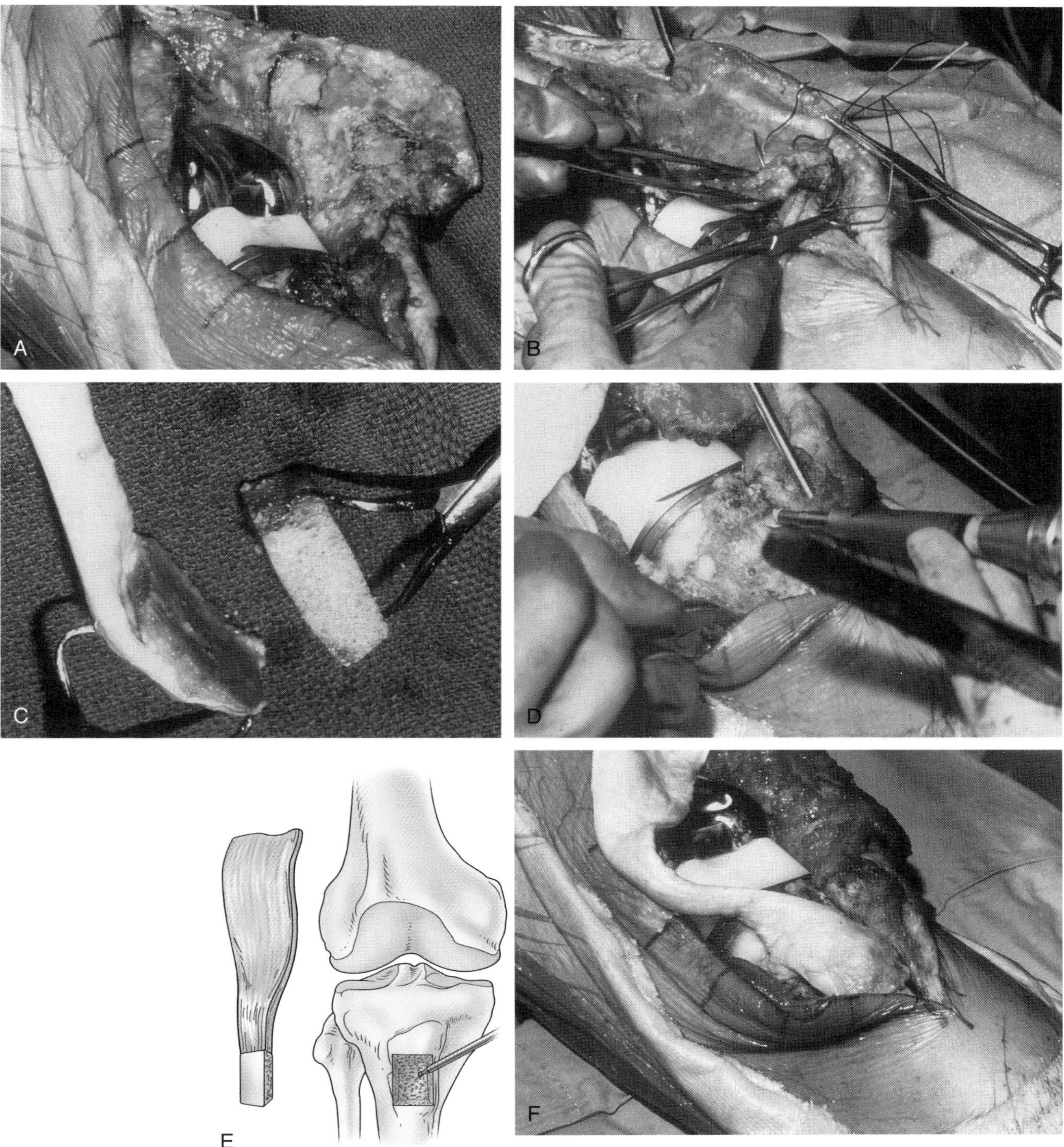

FIGURE 89.6 ➢ Technique of Achilles tendon allograft reconstruction. *A*, Intraoperative appearance of total knee arthroplasty with ruptured patellar tendon. *B*, Primary repair of patellar tendon with nonresorbable suture. This step returns the patella to its proper position. *C*, Appearance of thawed allograft after sectioning of the os calcis bone block. The remaining bone is a minimum of 15 mm thick. *D*, Preparation of the tibia using a high-speed bur for placement of the allograft bone block. The window in the tibia is located as close to the native tubercle as possible and is slightly undersized compared with the allograft bone block so as to achieve interference fit. *E*, Schematic representation of tibial bed prepared for os calcis bone block. *F*, Appearance of allograft bone block impacted into tibial bed and achieving interference fit.

Illustration continued on following page

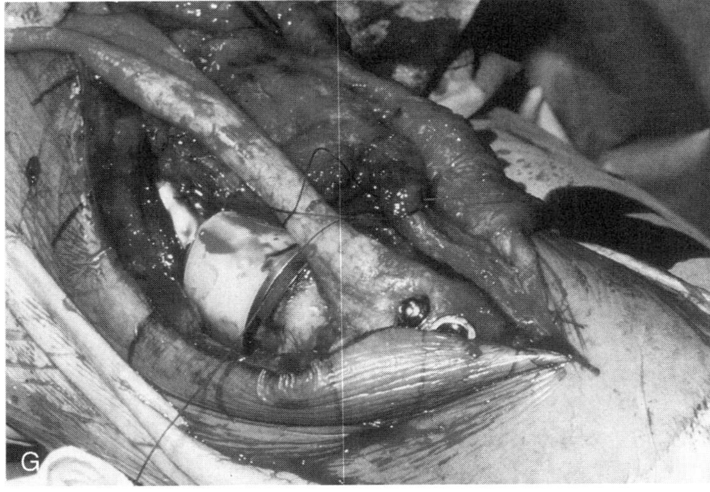

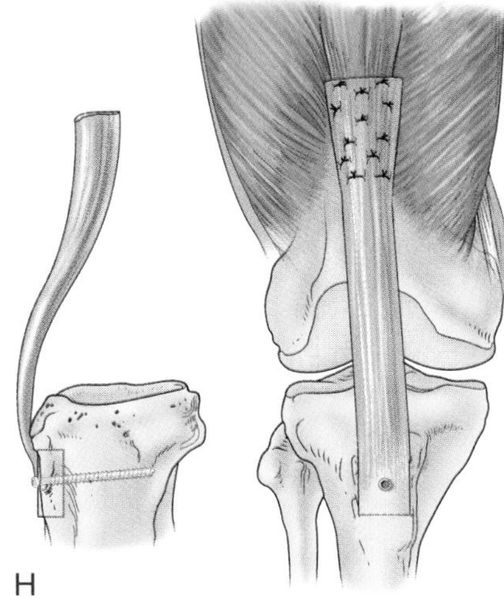

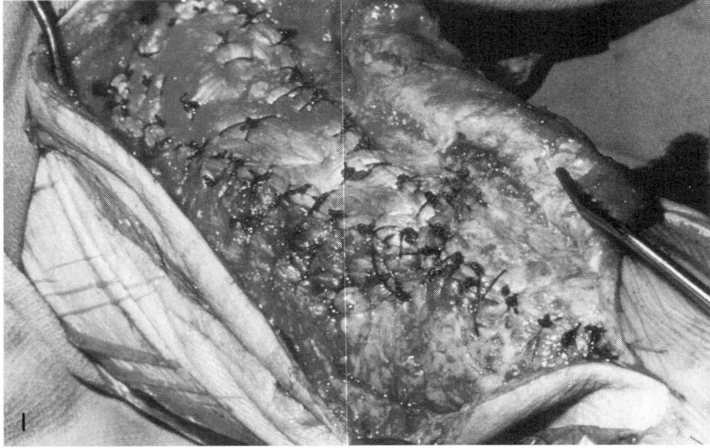

FIGURE 89.6 *Continued* ➢ *G,* Fixation of the allograft by two cortical lag screws. *H,* Schematic representation of fixation of the bone block. The lag screw must often be angled to avoid the tibial stem. *I,* Closure of the quadriceps tendon and capsule with nonresorbable suture. The tendinous portion of the allograft has also been secured with multiple sutures. Importantly, the construct should *not* be flexed to test tension.

degree extensor lags and, of note, eight patients had no extensor lag (Fig. 89.7). The average flexion was 101 degrees, which was improved from 89 degrees preoperatively. All patients improved their ambulation status. Seven patients required a cane, and three patients required a walker.

CONCLUSIONS

Ruptured extensor mechanisms after TKA are potentially devastating injuries. It is important to differentiate between these injuries in arthroplasty knees and in nonarthroplasty knees. In the absence of TKA, these injuries are much more straightforward to diagnose and treat. However, after TKA they can result in extreme disability. Therefore, a systematic approach to treatment is necessary. Experience since the 1980s suggests that surgery is not always indicated. However, when surgery is required, primary repair is usually insufficient. A grafting procedure is usually required to supplement the repair to improve outcomes. It is also important to note that TKA patients represent a difficult population in that they have multiple comorbidities and are frequently elderly. Thus, minor complica-

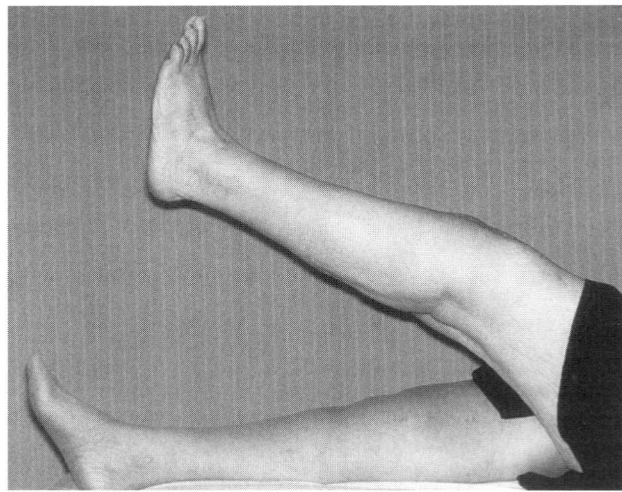

FIGURE 89.7 ➢ A patient with full active extension 3 months after Achilles tendon allograft reconstruction for a ruptured patellar tendon.

tions are fairly frequent, and treatment for each case must be based on its individual features. However, with the appropriate approach, good outcomes can be achieved consistently.

References

1. Abril JC, Alvarez L, Vallejo JC: Patellar tendon avulsion after total knee arthroplasty. J Arthroplasty 10:275, 1995.
2. Boyd AD, Ewald FC, Thomas WH, et al: Long-term complications after total knee arthroplasty with or without resurfacing of the patella. J Bone Joint Surg Am 75:674, 1993.
3. Brick GW, Scott RD: The patellofemoral component of total knee arthroplasty. Clin Orthop 231:163, 1988.
4. Cadambi A, Engh GA: Use of a semitendinosus tendon autogenous graft for rupture of the patellar ligament after total knee arthroplasty. J Bone Joint Surg Am 74:974, 1992.
5. Chiou HM, Chang MC, Lo WH: One-stage reconstruction of skin defect and patellar tendon rupture after total knee arthroplasty. J Arthroplasty 12:575, 1997.
6. Clayton ML, Thirupathi R: Patellar complications after total condylar arthroplasty. Clin Orthop 170:152, 1982.
7. Crossett LC, Zimmerman GW, Fada R, et al: Patellar Tendon Reconstruction Using Tendon Allograft Following Total Knee Arthroplasty [Final Program]. American Academy of Orthopaedic Surgeons, New Orleans, 65th Annual Meeting, 168, 1998.
8. Deburge A: Guepar hinge prosthesis. Clin Orthop 120:47, 1976.
9. Emerson RH, Head WC, Malinin TI: Reconstruction of patellar tendon rupture after total knee arthroplasty with an extensor mechanism allograft. Clin Orthop 260:154, 1990.
10. Emerson RH, Head WC, Malinin TI: Extensor mechanism reconstruction with an allograft after total knee arthroplasty. Clin Orthop 303:79, 1994.
11. Fernandez-Baillo N, Garay EG, Ordonez JM: Rupture of the quadriceps tendon after total knee arthroplasty. J Arthoplasty 8:331, 1993.
12. Figgie HE, Goldberg VM, Figgie MP, et al: The effect of alignment of the implant on fractures of the patella after condylar knee arthroplasty. J Bone Joint Surg Am 71:1031, 1989.
13. Goldberg VM, Figgie HE, Inglis AE, et al: Patellar fracture type and prognosis in condylar total knee arthroplasty. Clin Orthop 236:115, 1988.
14. Grace JN, Sim FH: Fracture of the patella after total knee arthroplasty. Clin Orthop 230:168, 1988.
15. Grace JN, Rand JA: Patellar instability after total knee arthroplasty. Clin Orthop 237:184, 1988.
16. Healy WL, Wasilewski SA, Takei R, et al: Patellofemoral complications following total knee arthroplasty. J Arthroplasty 10:197, 1995.
17. Hozack WJ, Goll SR, Lotke PA, et al: The treatment of patella fractures after total knee arthroplasty. Clin Orthop 236:123, 1988.
18. Hui FC, Fitzgerald RH: Hinged total knee arthroplasty. J Bone Joint Surg Am 62:513, 1980.
19. Insall JN, Hood RW, Flawn LB, et al: The total condylar knee prosthesis in gonarthrosis. J Bone Joint Surg Am 65:619, 1983.
20. Insall JN, Haas SB: Complications of total knee arthroplasty. In Insall JN, Windsor RE, Scott WN, et al, eds: Surgery of the Knee. New York, Churchill Livingstone, 1993, p 891.
21. Jauregito JW, Dubois CM, Smith SR, et al: Medial gastrocnemius transposition flap for the treatment of disruption of the extensor mechanism after total knee arthroplasty. J Bone Joint Surg Am 79:866, 1997.
22. Kaufer H, Matthews LS: Spherocentric arthroplasty of the knee. J Bone Joint Surg Am 63:545, 1981.
23. Kempenaar JW, Cameron JC: Patellotibial fusion for patellar tendon rupture after total knee arthroplasty. J Arthroplasty 14:115, 1999.
24. Lettin AWF, DeLiss LJ, Blackburne JS, et al: The Stanmore hinged knee arthroplasty. J Bone Joint Surg Br 60:327, 1978.
25. Lettin AWF, Kavanagh TG, Scales JT: The long-term results of Stanmore total knee replacement. J Bone Joint Surg Br 66:349, 1984.
26. Lynch AF, Rorabeck CH, Bourne RB: Extensor mechanism complications following total knee arthroplasty. J Arthroplasty 2:135, 1987.
27. Oglesby JW, Wilson FC: The evolution of knee arthroplasty. Clin Orthop 186:96, 1984.
28. Rand JA, Morrey BF, Bryan RS: Patellar tendon rupture after total knee arthroplasty. Clin Orthop 44:233, 1989.
29. Reuben JD, McDonald L, Woodard PL, et al: The effect of patella thickness on patella strain following total knee arthroplasty. J Arthroplasty 6:251, 1991.
30. Ritter MA, Campbell ED: Postoperative patellar complications with or without lateral release during total knee arthroplasty. Clin Orthop 219:163, 1987.
31. Roffman M, Hirsh DM, Mended DG: Fracture of the resurfaced patella in total knee replacement. Clin Orthop 148:112, 1980.
32. Rorabeck CH, Angliss RD, Lewis L: Fractures of the femur, tibia, and patella after total knee arthroplasty: Decision making and principles of management. In Dilworth Cannon W Jr, ed: Instructional Course Lectures, vol. 47. Rosemont, IL, American Academy of Orthopaedic Surgeons, 1998, p 449.
33. Scott RD, Turoff N, Ewald FC: Stress fracture of the patella following duopatellar knee arthroplasty with patellar resurfacing. Clin Orthop 170:147, 1982.
34. Scuderi G, Scharf SC, Meltzer LP: The relationship of lateral releases to patella viability in total knee arthroplasty. J Arthroplasty 2:209, 1987.
35. Sharkey PF, Hozack WJ, Booth RE, et al: Posterior dislocation of total knee arthroplasty. Clin Orthop 278:128, 1992.
36. Townley CO: The anatomic total knee resurfacing arthroplasty. Clin Orthop 192:82, 1985.
37. Tria AJ, Harwood DA, Alicea JA, et al: Patellar fractures in posterior stabilized knee arthroplasties. Clin Orthop 299:131, 1994.
38. Webster DA, Murray DG: Complications of variable axis total knee arthroplasty. Clin Orthop 193:162, 1985.
39. Wilson FC, Venteers GC: Results of knee replacement with the Walldius prosthesis. Clin Orthop 120:39, 1976.
40. Wilson FC, Fajgenbaum DM, Venteers GC: Results of knee replacement with Walldius and geometric prostheses. J Bone Joint Surg Am 62:497, 1980.
41. Yamamoto S: Total knee replacement with the Kodama-Yamamoto prosthesis. Clin Orthop 145:60, 1979.
42. Zanotti RM, Freiberg AA, Matthews LS: Use of patellar allograft to reconstruct a patellar tendon-deficient knee after total joint arthroplasty. J Arthroplasty 10:271, 1995.

Infected Total Knee Arthroplasty

THOMAS J. MULVEY • THOMAS S. THORNHILL

Infection is one of the most dreaded complications that can occur after total knee arthroplasty (TKA). It presents a formidable challenge to the orthopedic surgeon in that treatment is difficult and prolonged. For the patient who is expecting a significant improvement in pain relief and quality of life, infection is devastating, requiring additional surgical procedures, intravenous (IV) antibiotics, prolonged rehabilitation; in addition, a diminished functional outcome is possible.

It is estimated that in the United States alone more than 200,000 TKAs are performed annually. This number is expected to double by the end of the next decade. With a contemporary infection rate of 1% to 2%,[2, 10, 107] one can predict several thousand cases of infection per year. Moreover, the expanding use of TKA in the younger patient population with significant remaining life expectancy and the potential need for revision surgery creates an even greater problem given the increased risk of infection in the revision setting.

The economic impact of treating infected TKA is substantial. With the current infection rate and an approximate per case cost of $70,000,[5] a conservative estimate of the burden on the current health care system is 200 to 300 million dollars annually. It has been demonstrated that hospital resource utilization is increased three to four times for treatment of an infected TKA compared with primary TKA and twice that required for aseptic revision.[43] The increasing socioeconomic burden of this complication combined with diminishing payer reimbursement results in large losses for treating institutions.

To minimize the morbidity associated with this complication, a thorough understanding of the multiple issues surrounding infected TKA is necessary for those involved in the management. Maximization of our preventive measures, prompt diagnosis, and sound management along with continued refinement of our treatment protocols is essential. This chapter reviews the incidence, risk factors, microbiology, diagnosis, and current treatment protocols. It serves as a review and guide for the orthopedic surgeon who is confronted with the responsibility of treating an infected TKA.

INCIDENCE AND RISK FACTORS

With the advent of TKA, infection rates of up to 23% were reported.[54] A review of reports published throughout the 1970s disclosed an overall infection rate of 5%,[50] whereas several studies reported contemporary infection rates to be in the 1% to 2% range.[2, 7, 108] Higher incidences in early reports were noted before the routine use of prophylactic antibiotics, now considered the most important factor in limiting infection. Moreover, the routine use of implants with greater constraint, such as the Guepar hinge prosthesis[22] or Kinematic rotating hinge,[85] likely contributed to the higher infection rates as well. In fact, it has been demonstrated that infection rates of up to 16% can be seen with the use of constrained implants, even with modern prophylactic measures.[53] This is presumably due to the increased loosening and particulate debris formation that leads to hyperemia and a local environment conducive to bacterial seeding and growth.

Although advances in TKA have decreased the incidence of infection, the overall rates have remained relatively constant over the past 2 decades. As in any surgical procedure, infection is, and will continue to be, a potential complication that can never be completely eliminated. It has been proposed that there are inherent anatomic factors that contribute to this in addition to the multiple perioperative and surgical factors.[4] These include the joint's relatively superficial position, lack of vascularized muscle coverage, and a marginal vascular supply to the skin anteriorly, increasing the risk of wound complications.

A comprehensive list of risk factors associated with infection is found in Table 90.1. They can be broadly categorized as host factors and those related to the perioperative environment or surgical technique. Although many of the issues related to the host cannot be altered, appropriate intervention of the multiple other variables should be undertaken before surgery to minimize risk.

Immunocompromise has clearly been associated with infection, as seen in the rheumatoid population. The rate of infection in the rheumatoid population is reported as 2.6 times greater than in those with an underlying diagnosis of osteoarthritis.[78] Wilson et al[107] reviewed 4171 TKAs and found 67 cases of infection, 45 of which were associated with a primary diagnosis of rheumatoid arthritis compared with 16 with osteoarthritis. In the rheumatoid group corrected for gender bias, men were affected more than twice as frequently as women. Use of oral steroid medication has also been found to be associated with a higher rate of infection, particularly in the rheumatoid population. Patients with diabetes mellitus have been shown to have higher infection rates as well, ranging from 3%[75] to 7%[28] in reported series. Malnourished patients

TABLE 90.1 Factors Associated With Infection in Total Knee Arthroplasty

Host	Perioperative Environment	Surgical Technique
Immunocompromise	Operating room personnel	Implant factors
Rheumatoid arthritis	Number	Constraint
Steroids	Traffic	Tissue handling
Diabetes mellitus	Operative site preparation	Hematoma
Malignancy	Air flow systems	Wound dehiscence
Poor nutrition	Surgical team attire	Operative time
Obesity		Previous incisions
Skin ulceration		
Concurrent infection		
UTI		
Skin		
Soft tissue		
Previous surgery		
Previous infection		
Septic arthritis		
Osteomyelitis		
Psoriasis		
Organ transplantation		
Debilitation		
Advanced age		
Alcoholism		
Renal failure		
Prolonged preoperative hospitalization		

UTI = urinary tract infection.

should be assessed and supplemented to restore adequate albumin levels and total lymphocyte counts before elective TKA.

Obesity has also been associated with an increased incidence of infection.[107] A 1998 study evaluating TKA in 50 morbidly obese patients found that, at a mean follow-up of 5 years, there were five infections (10%).[110] Three of the cases were associated with wound complications, and all five occurred within the first 20 weeks after surgery. Although this patient population has been shown to benefit from TKA, awareness of the high risk of complications and wound healing issues is critical in risk analysis.

Previous surgery on the knee is a well-known risk factor for infection after TKA. The report of Wilson et al[107] showed an incidence of 1.4% in patients with osteoarthritis who had previous surgery compared with 0.3% in nonoperated knees. Rates of infection in the revision setting have also been reported to be higher. In a review of revision operations involving 2714 knees between 1969 and 1996, a 5.6% overall incidence of infection was found.[39] Repeated procedures increase the amount of poorly vascularized scar tissue and potential bacterial seeding of the joint. A subset of these revision cases also likely represents low-grade cryptogenic infection before revision that became clinically manifest after revision. Patients with previous infection have an even greater risk of subsequent infection; one study reported a 4% incidence in patients with a history of septic arthritis and 15% in those with a history of osteomyelitis.[52]

The greatest source of bacteria within the operating suite is the operating personnel. Minimizing the number of people as well as the amount of traffic within the room is beneficial in limiting bacterial contamination.[88] One study has shown that bacterial shedding ranging from 1000 to 10,000 organisms per minute per person occurs, a significant source of bacterial contamination.[86] Because skin preparation cannot remove bacteria in hair follicles or sebaceous glands, all surgical wounds are contaminated to some extent. A report using iodophor drapes, however, found lower wound bacteria counts and recommended that they be used.[87] The same study showed that, with laminar flow, antibiotics, and use of an iodophor drape, an infection rate of less than 0.5% in 649 TKAs was obtained. Adherence to meticulous operative technique should minimize the risk of intraoperative contamination, the main cause of early infection.

Additional perioperative factors that may impact on infection include clean air systems, ultraviolet light, and surgical attire. Air circulation using horizontal and vertical laminar flow has the benefit of decreasing bacterial counts and, therefore, lowering the risk of infection.[37] Some controversy exists in TKA, however, with the use of horizontal flow, as reported by Salvati et al.[91] They found a 3.9% incidence of infection with the use of horizontal laminar flow compared with 1.4% without it and explained that interposition of operating room personnel between the air source and patient increased bacterial shedding into the operative site. Possible solutions include the use of body exhaust suites or vertical flow systems. Ultraviolet light has been demonstrated to reduce the infection rate further by creating an ultra-clean air environment at a relatively low cost, as described by Berg et al.[8, 9] There is some evidence that closed air exhaust suits may reduce infection,[19, 61] although a 1996 report disputes these findings.[95] The results of the report suggested that no additional protection from airborne contamination was detected around the surgical field compared with appropriately used hoods and masks. A protocol of enclosed hoods, impermeable gowns, shoe covers, and double gloving with frequent change and for passing sharp instruments has been shown to help control contamination of the operative team in joint arthroplasty.[44]

As mentioned, decreasing the amount of constraint in the implant has favorable effects on infection rates. Meticulous surgical technique minimizing tissue devitalization and maintenance of adequate hemostasis limit wound complications and subsequent problems. Execution of a well-planned procedure in an expeditious manner is extremely important to minimize bacterial contamination further. It has been reported that as operative time increases, contamination of gloves, instruments, and suction tips increases.[88]

A 1997 study reported a series of joint arthroplasty infection in patients with kidney or liver transplantation.[98] They found an infection rate of 19% (5 of 27 joints) in those who had the procedure after organ transplantation compared with no infections in the group that first had an arthroplasty. Although these patients have been shown to benefit from arthroplasty, they stated that more intense immunosuppressive medication combined with the increasing use of organ transplants is alarming. There are contrasting reports in the literature regarding TKA in the HIV-infected hemophiliac population. One study demonstrated a 44% mortality rate,[56] whereas another showed no cases of infected TKA after an average follow-up of 4.4 years.[99] Other studies have been published to support the latter, and it appears that HIV seropositivity should not contraindicate elective orthopedic procedures unless the CD4 count is low, and great care is taken to minimize patient and surgical team contamination.

MICROBIOLOGY

The organisms most commonly involved in deep prosthetic infection are reviewed in Table 90.2. In a series of 76 infections, the infecting organism was gram-positive in 39 cases, gram-negative in 18, and mixed in 19.[102] Another study reviewing 64 infected cases involved a single gram-positive organism in 43 patients, a gram-negative organism in 13, and a mixed organism in 5.[39] In both series the predominant gram-positive organisms were *Staphylococcus aureus, S. epidermidis,* and streptococci, whereas gram-negative infections most commonly involved *Escherichia coli* and *Pseudomonas aeruginosa.* Some reports demonstrated the increasing prevalence of *S. epidermidis* as the predominant organism involved in implant-related infections.[7, 83] Specific infectious patterns at individual institutions will vary to some degree and should be frequently monitored as part of an infection control program.

Reports of bacterial resistance to standard antimicrobial agents have been a concern. Methicillin-resistant *S. aureus* (MRSA) and *S. epidermidis* (MRSE) have led to the increased use of vancomycin as standard prophylaxis in certain centers. Even more concerning are the rare but reported cases of vancomycin-resistant enterococci for which there is truly no effective treatment. Inappropriate use and overuse of vancomycin and other antibiotics should be avoided in the "postantibiotic era" in which no therapy will be available to treat these resistant organisms.[1] For these reasons, we recommend restricting the use of vancomycin to institutions in which frequent infections with MRSA or MRSE occur.

Fungal infections are unusual, and a review of the English literature found only 21 reported cases after TKA.[16, 100] The majority of these cases were caused by a *Candida* species. Tuberculosis has also been reported as an infectious agent in total hip and knee arthroplasty.[10, 58] Suspicion for these rare but potential causes of infection should be considered in the evaluation of infected joint arthroplasty and treatment determined on a case-by-case basis. Furthermore, patients with associated underlying diseases, such as the gastrointestinal tract, in whom infection develops around TKA should be specifically evaluated for organisms that are normally found in these organ systems.

An understanding of the pathophysiology of infection related to orthopedic implants is necessary for those involved in the management of infected TKA. Bacterial adhesion to polymers and metal via glycoproteins, pili, and binding forces increase resistance.[55] The production of a glycocalix or mucopolysaccharide "slime" by some bacteria, particularly *S. epidermidis,* increases its virulence by protection from antibiotics and host defenses.[2, 6] Physical properties of implants, their chemical composition, precoating, and surface tension interact in a variety of ways to impact the overall risk of infection.[18, 24] These factors make it difficult to eradicate infection using nonsurgical means and raise concerns with those treatment protocols that advocate prosthesis retention. Consultation with an infectious disease specialist familiar with these issues is helpful in formulating a treatment plan.

Antibiotic prophylaxis is the greatest single contribution to minimizing infection in total joint arthroplasty. Antibiotics chosen should cover the most likely contaminating organisms and be administered before surgery. It appears that the first dose is crucial and should be given 5 to 30 minutes before tourniquet inflation to provide maximum concentrations in bone and soft tissue during TKA.[35] Table 90.3 lists the recommended antibiotics for surgical prophylaxis. Cephalosporins have been recommended for prophylaxis based on their low toxicity, bone and soft tissue penetration, and cost.[59, 104] Cefazolin remains our antibiotic of choice. Vancomycin and clindamycin provide a reasonable alternative for patients with anaphylaxis to penicillin or allergic reaction to the cephalosporins. Twenty-four hours' duration of antibiotics is adequate for routine cases,[69] whereas 48 hours may be appropriate if bladder catheterization or postoperative wound drains are left in place until the 2nd postoperative day.

The use of prophylactic antibiotics in cement in routine TKA may be beneficial in certain cases and has been advocated by several authors.[36, 65] There appears to be a lack of consensus, however, with this method

TABLE 90.2 ORGANISMS MOST COMMONLY INVOLVED IN DEEP PROSTHETIC INFECTION

Predominant Organisms	Emerging Organisms	Other Organisms
Gram positive	Gram positive	Gram negative
Staphylococcus aureus (coagulase positive)	Methicillin-resistant *S. aureus*	*Escherichia coli*
Staphylococcus epidermidis (coagulase negative)	Methicillin-resistant *S. epidermidis*	*Pseudomonas aeruginosa*
Streptococci	Vancomycin-resistant *Enterococcus* species	*Proteus* species
		Serratia
		Klebsiella
		Enterobacter
		Anaerobic
		Peptostreptococcus
		Propionibacterium acnes
		Bacteroides fragilis
		Fungal
		Candida albicans
		Candida species
		Mycobacteria
		Mycobacterium tuberculosis
		M. fortuitum
		Brucella
		Mixed infection

because of potential concerns such as allergic reactions, organism resistance, and adverse effects on the structural properties of the cement. In fact, a 1995 survey of 1015 orthopedic surgeons regarding their use of antibiotics in cement showed wide variation in clinical practice patterns.[42] Only 56% of respondents used antibiotics in cement; the most common reason for doing so was septic revision surgery. Reasonable indications along with medications and recommended doses are listed in Table 90.4. It has been demonstrated that antibiotics used in these doses will not affect the strength or structural properties of the cement.[94, 111] Significantly higher doses can be used in staged procedures when cement or articulating spacers are used as antibiotic depots when one is not concerned about the long-term structural properties of the cement, as discussed later in this chapter. The antibiotic should be heat stable, have adequate elution properties from polymethylmethacrylate, and be in a powder form because liquid antibiotics have detrimental effects on the cement.[42] Several commercially available premixed products are also available for use.

The potential for late prosthetic seeding after dental manipulation has created controversy. Although the dental literature recommends that routine antibiotic prophylaxis is unnecessary in patients with prosthetic joints,[30] the risk of deep sepsis is disturbing. In fact, in a 1997 retrospective review of 3490 patients treated with TKA, 62 late infections were noted, 7 (11% of all infections or 0.2% of all TKAs) of which were strongly linked to a dental procedure.[101] In addition, 2 of 12 infected cases referred to their institution during that time were also believed to be related to dental work. They found that these patients had systemic risk factors for infection such as rheumatoid arthritis or diabetes mellitus and had extensive dental procedures. They cautioned that infections associated with dental work may be more common than suspected and that patients meeting these criteria should have prophylaxis. Interestingly, these authors also recommended the use of a first-generation cephalosporin as the drug of choice based on the organisms identified in their study

TABLE 90.3 SURGICAL ANTIBIOTIC PROPHYLAXIS

Standard Prophylaxis
Cefazolin, 1 g IV at surgery, then q8h for 24-48 h
Cefuroxime, 1.5 g IV at surgery, then 750 mg q8h for 24-48 h
Penicillin Allergic
Clindamycin, 600 mg at surgery, then q8h for 24-48 h
Vancomycin,* 1 g at surgery, then 500-1000 mg q12h for 24-48 h
Gram-Negative Organisms
Gentamicin, 2.0 mg/kg at surgery, then 1.0 mg/kg q8h for 24-48 h

* Avoid routine use to minimize organism resistance.

TABLE 90.4 INDICATIONS FOR ANTIBIOTICS IN CEMENT FOR PROSTHETIC REIMPLANTATION

Indications
Previous infection
Revision surgery
Immunocompromised host
Rheumatoid arthritis
Diabetes mellitus
Immunosuppressive medication
Systemic illness
Antibiotic/Dose*
Tobramycin, 600 mg
Cephamandole, 1 g
Vancomycin,† 1 g
Gentamicin, 500 mg to 1 g

* Per 40 g cement.
† Avoid routine use to minimize bacterial resistance.

TABLE 90.5 ANTIBIOTIC DENTAL, GASTROINTESTINAL, AND GENITOURINARY, PROPHYLAXIS

Antibiotic	Dose
No Penicillin Allergy	
Amoxicillin or	3 g po 1 h before procedure
cephalexin	2 g po 1 h before procedure
Penicillin Allergy	
Clindamycin	600 mg po 1 h before procedure

and that it be administered 1 hour before and 8 hours after dental manipulation, although they did not offer a specific dose. Current recommendations suggest a compromise in which all patients receive prophylaxis for the first 2 years postoperatively and subsequently in all patients determined to be at high risk. Table 90.5 reviews the current antibiotic recommendations.

DIAGNOSIS

Deep sepsis is evident when the infection extends subfascially and involves the prosthesis and bone interface, whereas superficial wound infections are limited to the skin and subcutaneous tissues. The differentiation between the two can often be difficult, especially in the early postoperative period. Most surgeons at some point are faced with the dilemma involving the patient with wound drainage, erythema, and increased pain in the early postsurgical course. Establishing a diagnosis of a noninfectious wound complication versus superficial or deep infection and the appropriate treatment can be problematic. Factors that should heighten the suspicion for infection in the acute period include changes in the intensity or character of pain, increasing medication requirements, and variation from the usual gradual improvement in the normal postoperative course. Increasing drainage and wound-healing problems are also findings that may be associated with an infectious cause. The differentiation is important in that superficial infection carries with it a much more favorable prognosis. Nonetheless, early accurate diagnosis of superficial infection should be managed aggressively with surgical débridement and hematoma evacuation followed by culture-guided antibiotic therapy.

An important factor that has significant implications for prognosis and treatment is the time of onset of the infection in relation to the index procedure and, perhaps more importantly, the duration of symptoms. As a general principle, early infections are usually due to perioperative contamination, whereas late infections are secondary to hematogenous seeding. Multiple classification schemes are described and vary with regard to the specific time periods for which they are defined. The value of these methods of classification lies in their ability to assist in determining cause and to serve as a guide in directing treatment.

Insall[48] described early infection as occurring within 3 months of surgery or late if it occurred after this time. Rand[81] described a three-tiered classification: early, within 2 months of surgery; intermediate, if the infection occurred 2 to 24 months afterward; and late, if the onset was after 2 years. Others described these periods to be as early as 6 weeks and as late as 6 months. The importance in the differentiation is that acute, or early, infection is more likely to be successfully treated with prosthesis-retaining procedures, whereas late infections are more appropriately treated with a staged procedure, including prosthetic removal.

Two studies demonstrated that symptom duration may actually be more important than the overall timing of the infection in relation to the index procedure. In one study of 76 infected TKAs treated between 1981 and 1990, patients were classified on the basis of symptom duration: acute, fewer than 2 weeks, or chronic, more than 2 weeks.[102] Prosthesis-retaining procedures were frequently used in the acute group. At a minimum 2-year follow-up, the initial treatment modality chosen was successful in eliminating infection in 69 of 76 patients (90%). The authors concluded that careful treatment selection based on symptom duration is predictably successful. Another prospective study evaluated the results of 24 infected TKAs treated with multiple irrigation and débridement with prosthetic retention.[72] Strict criteria for selection included symptom duration of less than 30 days. At an average follow-up of 48 months, infection was eliminated in 10 of 10 postsurgical infections (100%) and in 10 of 14 late hematogenously infected patients (71%). It appears that, although the timing of infection in relation to the index procedure is an important predictor of outcome, another important element that impacts surgical decision making and ultimate outcome is the duration of symptoms.

The complaint most consistent with deep infection is pain. Any patient who presents for evaluation of a painful TKA should be assumed to have an infection until proven otherwise. A differential diagnosis should include periprosthetic fracture, patellofemoral problems, aseptic loosening, soft tissue disruption, instability, reflex sympathetic dystrophy, heterotopic ossification, and arthrofibrosis. Rest pain or night pain is also more suspicious for an infectious cause compared with start-up or activity-related pain that is consistent with mechanical loosening or instability.

Typical physical examination findings consistent with infection may be seen, although there are occasions when minimal findings are present as a result of a subacute or chronic low-grade infection. Classic findings include the presence of an effusion, warmth, erythema, tenderness, an overall inflamed appearance, or skin breakdown, as demonstrated in Figure 90.1. Patients may show signs of change of activity related to their normal baseline level of function or have significantly limited range of motion. The presence of wound drainage or obvious purulence is highly suspicious for infection and chronic drainage, or a draining sinus tract essentially ensures subfascial involvement.

Standard hematological testing is usually performed early in the work-up because of the widespread availa-

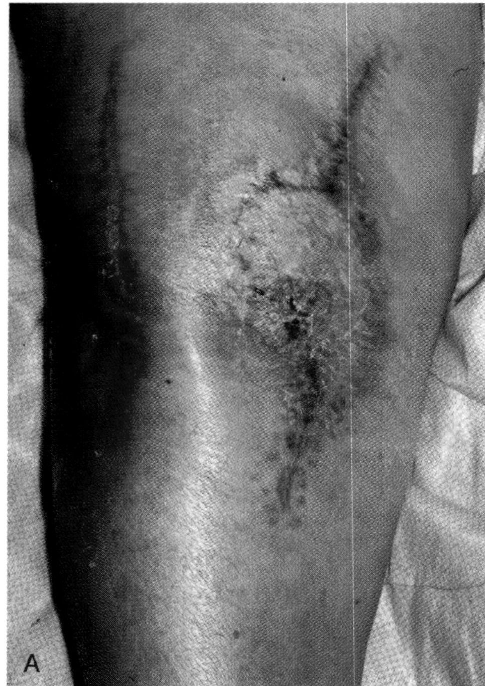

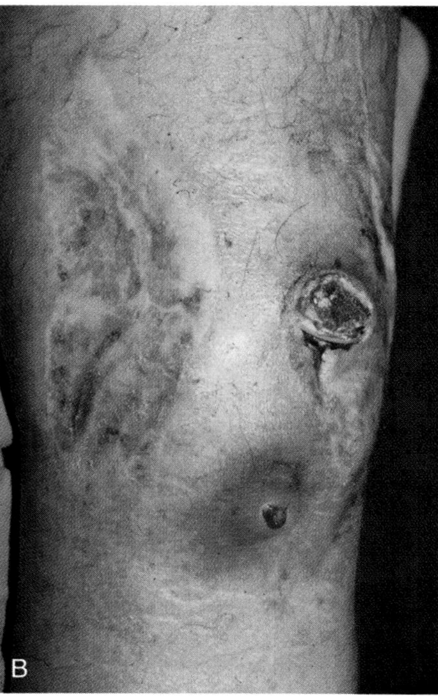

FIGURE 90.1 ➢ *A,* Photograph of a patient with an infected total knee arthroplasty demonstrating multiple previous incisions, erythema, and a swollen, inflamed appearance. *B,* This patient has obvious signs of deep infection, including a draining sinus tract inferiorly, along with skin necrosis, soft tissue loss, and exposure of prosthetic components. (From Scott WN: The Knee, vol 2. St. Louis, Mosby-Year Book, 1994, pp 1263, 1266.)

bility and the ease of performance. The most commonly ordered tests include peripheral leukocyte count, erythrocyte sedimentation rate (ESR), and C-reactive protein (CRP). Peripheral white cell counts have been shown repeatedly to be inconsistently elevated, and reliance on this test should be avoided.[40] The ESR has also been shown to be somewhat unreliable. A study of 52 patients treated for infected TKA revealed an average white cell count of 8300 (range = 5800 to 14,000) and an ESR of 63 (range = 4 to 125).[108] Levitsky et al[60] demonstrated that a preoperative ESR greater than 30 had a sensitivity of 60% and a specificity of only 65% in evaluating possible infection in painful prosthetic joints. The CRP may be more specific in that it tends to be elevated in cases of infection but remains normal when the cause is mechanical in nature.[96] Additionally, it tends to return to a normal level 3 weeks after surgery, whereas the ESR often remains elevated for a prolonged period.[73] Although these tests may be of some limited value in the preoperative evaluation of a possibly infected TKA and be included as part of a diagnostic scheme, they may be better used as a method of assessing response to treatment once the diagnosis is established.

Radiological imaging studies that can be obtained include plain films and bone scanning with the use of technetium 99, gallium 111, indium-labeled white cells, and labeled monoclonal or polyclonal antibodies. Plain radiographs will be negative in the early course of infection unless loosening or other findings were present before infection. Later findings include erosion, osteitis, marginal osseous resorption, and loosening.[4] Radiolucencies around the central tibial stem of a well-aligned knee should be considered as infection until proven otherwise. Furthermore, overall alignment, fracture, polyethylene wear, and other modes of failure can be assessed, and radiographs should, therefore, be obtained in every case.

A study reviewing the value of technetium 99 bone scanning in the evaluation of the painful prosthetic joint revealed a sensitivity of 33% and a specificity of 86%.[60] The authors stated that the low sensitivity and poor positive predictive value of 30% significantly limited the test's usefulness and concluded it was an unwarranted and expensive procedure. Gallium scanning used in the diagnosis of musculoskeletal infection has widely variable results; reports of sensitivity range from 22% to 100% and specificity from 0% to 100%.[103] Differential scanning with technetium and gallium has been attempted to improve the results, although this has been shown to be problematic.[71] Rand and Brown[82] reviewed the use of indium-labeled leukocyte scanning in 38 painful or infected TKAs and found a sensitivity of 83%, a specificity of 85%, and an accuracy of 84%. They concluded that, although indium scans may be useful in the evaluation of TKA, because of the possibility of false-positive or false-negative tests, the result must be considered along with the clinical evaluation of the patient.

Indium-labeled polyclonal antibody and technetium-labeled monoclonal antibody scans have been introduced and have been shown to be effective in the diagnosis of musculoskeletal infection. Preliminary reports are promising, and these tests may have a more widespread use in the future.[62, 74] At this time, we believe that nuclear medicine studies should not be considered first-line diagnostic tests and should be reserved for cases in which the diagnosis is unclear and further imaging is required, while remembering their associated limitations when they are used.

Although aspiration has been questioned by some because of false-negative results, it remains an essential component in the evaluation of the infected TKA. Windsor and Insall[109] stated that aspiration is the most important diagnostic test for conclusively determining deep joint infection. A 1996 study evaluating preoperative aspiration of the knee before revision arthroplasty in 64 patients had sensitivity, specificity, and accuracy of 100%.[26] The authors concluded that aspiration is the most helpful method for diagnosing infection in a prosthetic knee joint. Before aspiration, antibiotics should be discontinued for 10 to 14 days to avoid suppression of any sensitive organisms, and meticulous sterile technique must be used to prevent joint seeding or aspirate contamination with skin flora. In addition to aerobic and anaerobic cultures, a cell count should be routinely obtained. An elevated cell count should raise the suspicion of infection. The use of polymerase chain reaction (PCR) technology has been used to improve the diagnosis of infection in synovial aspirates in patients with TKA.[64] This method detects and amplifies the presence of bacterial DNA and has been reported to be accurate and rapid. Because of the limited reliability associated with standard microbiological synovial fluid assays, these authors stated that PCR should serve as an adjunctive diagnostic method or possibly even as an alternative in the future. The possibility of a high false-positive rate has been raised because of the detection of noninfectious or nonbacterial sequences, however.[39] As methods continue to be refined and future improvements with this technology are made, this will, it is hoped, become less of a problem.

In some cases in which the diagnosis remains uncertain, histological examination of tissue is necessary. Open biopsy has been recommended, and specimens of the bone-prosthesis interface and multiple synovial samples should be taken.[49, 81] Gram stains have a high false-negative rate, and although a positive stain is consistent with infection, a negative result does not rule out the possibility of an infection.[3] In an evaluation of 194 revision TKA/total hip arthroplasty in which 87% had an intraoperative Gram's stain, there were 32 infections and no positive Gram's stains for a sensitivity of 0%.[20] A 1995 study showed that frozen section is a reliable predictor of infection and should be performed at biopsy.[33] In a study using frozen sections to identify active infection in revision arthroplasty, using an index of 10 polymorphonuclear leukocytes (PMN) per high-power field (HPF) (these must be morphologically intact PMNs surrounding viable tissue from the most cellular areas), the authors obtained a sensitivity of 84%, a specificity of 99%, a positive predictive value of 89%, and a negative predictive value of 98%.[63] If there were fewer than 5 PMNs/HPF, infection was highly unlikely; if there were 5 to 10 PMNs/HPF, the surgeon needed other tests to differentiate. An experienced pathologist is required for interpretation of the biopsy material, and arrangements for this should be made preoperatively. Other authors also demonstrated intraoperative frozen section to be useful and reliable for the diagnosis of infection.[32]

It is important to remember that no single test can be used to diagnose infection accurately in all cases. A suspicion for the diagnosis combined with risk factor assessment, physical examination, various laboratory, radiographic studies, and aspiration should provide sufficient information to make an accurate diagnosis.

TREATMENT

Treatment options for managing an infected TKA are summarized in Table 90.6. They can be broadly categorized as prosthetic retaining, prosthetic exchange, or salvage procedures. Decision making requires a basic understanding of the complexity of each situation and the multiple factors involved, including host immunocompetence, infecting organism(s), symptom duration, and condition of the soft tissue. As a general rule, infected TKA involves surgical pathology requiring operative intervention, and although nonsurgical options often seem attractive in an attempt to eradicate infection, they frequently are found to be unsuccessful.

It is helpful to consult an infectious disease expert preoperatively once a diagnosis is established to assist with the selection of appropriate antibiotic therapy. Moreover, they are essential to ensure adequate dosing and drug concentrations and to monitor treatment duration. It may also be helpful to consult a plastic surgeon when there are significant areas of skin necrosis or wound breakdown, as seen in Figure 90.2, in which a gastrocnemius flap or vascularized muscle transfer may be required for wound closure.

Antibiotics/Aspiration

Because of the reportedly poor results with this method, it should be regarded more as a form of suppression rather than treatment. Multiple reports show poor long-term success rates that range between 21% and 38%.[45] In addition, significant potential downsides of prolonged antibiotic treatment include side effects, allergic reactions, toxicity, and the emergence of resistant organisms.[66] Other potential risks include the frequent failure of this method, with subsequent bone and soft tissue destruction compromising future definitive treatment options or the development of systemic infection.

Although this form of treatment cannot be consistently recommended, there are select circumstances in which it may be the only option. In patients who are severely debilitated or medically compromised and who cannot withstand the rigors of a surgical procedure, chronic antibiotic suppression as a means to minimize morbidity may be indicated. Patients who have more than one prosthetic joint should probably not be considered because of the risk of hematogenous seeding of the other joints. Additionally, the use of more than one antibiotic, such as rifampin com-

TABLE 90.6 TREATMENT OPTIONS FOR INFECTED TOTAL KNEE ARTHROPLASTY

Prosthesis Retention	Prosthesis Exchange	Salvage Procedures
Antibiotic suppression	Immediate exchange	Arthrodesis
Aspiration	Early exchange	Resection arthroplasty
Irrigation and débridement	Delayed exchange ± articulating spacer	Amputation
Arthroscopic		
Open arthrotomy		

bined with a fluoroquinolone for the treatment of *Staphylococcus*-infected implants, has been shown to potentially improve treatment outcomes and should be considered.[25, 51] If chosen, close routine clinical and laboratory follow-up should be performed to ensure a favorable clinical course.

Unlike in the patient with septic arthritis in the absence of a TKA, aspiration combined with antibiotics has not been shown to be an effective means of eradicating infection. Bengston and Knutson[7] reported a series of 357 infected TKAs; they demonstrated only a 15% success rate with aspiration and antibiotics alone. Success rates are low because of the inability of the antibiotics to penetrate bacteria embedded within a biofilm layer adherent to the implant and cement surfaces. Use of this method should be limited to cases in which an early diagnosis is made, usually less than 48 hours, before significant bacterial resistance has been established. The isolated organism should be a penicillin-sensitive streptococci, and there should be no signs of significant synovial reaction. Furthermore, one should see a rapid clinical response, including decreased effusion, decreased synovial white cells, and negative culture on repeat aspiration. If variation from such a course occurs, this method should be abandoned in favor of a more aggressive surgical approach. Using this method, Wilson et al[107] eradicated infection in 5 of 12 patients when these criteria were applied.[107]

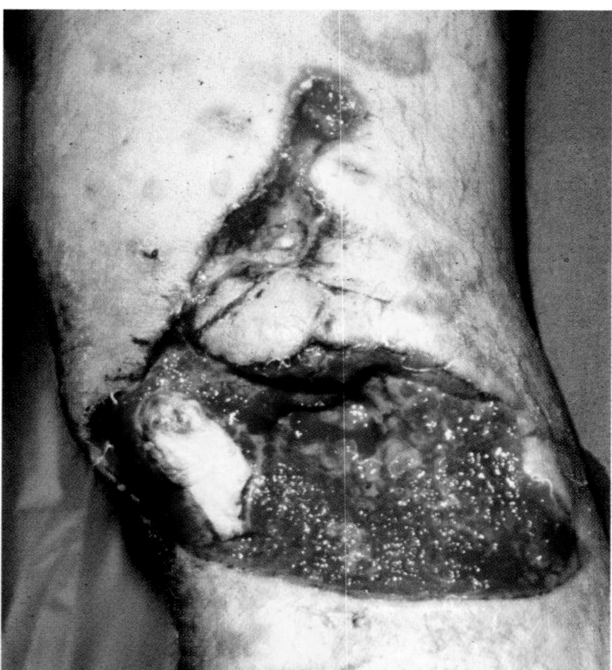

FIGURE 90.2 ➢ Infected total knee arthroplasty with significant loss of soft tissues, which required a gastrocnemius flap and skin graft to obtain wound coverage at the time of surgery.

Irrigation and Débridement

A review of earlier reports on the use of irrigation and débridement, antibiotic treatment, and retention of the components shows this method to be controversial. Multiple reports showed highly variable but overall dissatisfying results.[17, 93] A review of these studies shows success rates ranging from 18% to 52%. Rand[80] reviewed the literature and found elimination of infection in 110 of 377 cases, for an overall success rate of only 29% with attempted implant salvage.

In contrast, a review of the more recent literature has shown promising results with this method. In a retrospective study of 60 infected TKAs, Burger et al[17] recommended that implant salvage with aggressive débridement and antibiotics be strongly considered in certain cases. They found an increased chance of success in patients who had short symptom duration (<2 weeks), a susceptible gram-positive organism, absence of significant postoperative drainage or sinus tract formation, and a well-fixed implant. Although their success rate was only 17.9% overall, when their selection criteria was reapplied (only five knees met the criteria) all had a successful result. Another prospective study using strict entry criteria treated 24 cases with irrigation, débridement, and implant retention.[72] Selection criteria included onset of infection within 30 days of the index arthroplasty or symptom duration less than 30 days in the late hematogenous group without radiographic signs of component loosening. They were able to eliminate infection in 100% (10 of 10) of the early postsurgical group and in 71% (10 of 14) of late infections at average follow-up of 48 months. Patients did require repeated débridement (one to three procedures), which the authors believed was important in obtaining higher cure rates. They concluded that, in select cases, this method can provide adequate success and limited morbidity. Other reports confirmed these findings using these more rigid selection criteria.[70, 102]

A method of administration of long-term high concentration of antibiotics combined with soft tissue débridement has been reported in a small series of patients.[21] These authors used a subcutaneously implantable pump along with high-dose amikacin to treat 23 patients with arthroplasty infections. Selection criteria for inclusion were a susceptible organism, acute infection (0 to 3 months), and a stable component. The average treatment duration was 18 weeks (10 to 32 weeks), and the authors were able to eradicate infection in 17 of 20 patients with adequate follow-up. No significant adverse effects were seen, and the authors stated that one could still resort to other treatment regimens should this method fail.

Débridement may be performed arthroscopically or through an open arthrotomy. Although arthroscopy is appealing, significant scarring, adhesions, and fibrosis may prevent a thorough débridement, often rendering an synovectomy incomplete at best. Although one is able to potentially elevate a polyethylene liner and irrigate the undersurface, concerns over the adequacy of débridement exist. Furthermore, one is unable to exchange the modular insert, which is strongly recommended at the time of débridement. Moreover, all of the studies demonstrating improved success using this method were done through an open procedure, a fact that likely contributed to the better results.

We believe that candidates for open débridement include those patients who are not suitable for aspiration alone, have no evidence of loosening or osteolysis, have normal alignment, and are immunocompetent. Importantly, the duration of infection in either the early postoperative group or symptoms in the late hematogenously infected group was less than 2 weeks. The organism should be identified to be gram positive and be sensitive to penicillin. Multiple procedures may be necessary, and close follow-up, including repeated aspirations and clinical monitoring for improvement, is recommended. If this method fails, one should subsequently convert to a two-stage procedure. Prolonged delays in recognizing failure should be prevented to avoid compromise of further treatment. A diagnosis of *S. aureus* as the infecting organism is a predictor of a poor outcome and should be considered when this method of treatment is used. In Wilson et al's[107] study, irrigation and débridement with prosthesis retention in cases of *S. aureus* infection failed 50% of the time.

Immediate/Early Exchange

The indications for immediate or early exchange arthroplasty are somewhat unclear because most series involve limited numbers of patients. The Mayo Clinic reported on a series of 14 acutely infected TKAs in which six of seven low-virulence infections and two of seven high-virulence infections were salvaged, although only a 35% overall satisfactory functional result was obtained.[90] Borden and Gearen[12] reported a small series of three patients; all cases were successfully treated with immediate exchange. Freeman et al[34] reported on a series of 18 patients with septic TKA, all of whom were infected with gram-positive organisms and had loosening of the components. Their protocol included a one-stage revision with gentamicin-impregnated cement followed by 3 months of oral antibiotics; 17 of the 18 original infections were successfully treated. They used separate instruments for the débridement and implantation portions of the procedure and intraoperative redraping between procedures. Advantages of such a procedure include less surgery and improved soft tissue status and functional outcome at lower costs.

Currently, we believe that immediate exchange can be cautiously considered when there is a loose or maligned prosthesis that would otherwise fulfill the criteria for less aggressive surgical management. Criteria include an acute presentation of less than 2 weeks, isolation of a susceptible gram-positive organism, adequate soft tissue status, and an immunocompetent host. Antibiotics in cement at the time of reimplantation, careful surgical technique, and a course of antibiotics postoperatively should be used. If this method fails, the patient should be managed with prosthetic removal and delayed reimplantation.

Early exchange protocols, described as occurring within 2 weeks of prosthetic removal, have met with variable success. Various studies reported success rates of 30% to 80% depending on organism virulence and multiple other factors.[70, 77, 80] There is no doubt that more consistent results are obtained with delayed reimplantation. In our opinion, although certain patients may fulfill the criteria for a one-stage exchange, as noted previously, most infected TKAs should be treated with a staged procedure, delaying reimplantation until completion of a course of 6 weeks of IV antibiotics to maximize the likelihood of success.

As newer antibiotics and treatment regimens are developed, indications for prosthetic retention and immediate or early exchange protocols may increase. As mentioned, when used in appropriate circumstances, these methods can achieve high cure rates. There is concern that economic factors may influence treatment choice. With hospital reimbursement structured such that significant losses occur in the management of these cases, as well as the fear of institution colonization, some centers are considering limiting treatment to those patients whose index arthroplasty was performed at their hospital. It would be sad indeed if economic pressures rather than patient-driven factors influence triage. Moreover, if less costly immediate exchange can expect 80% success compared with the results obtained with delayed two-stage exchange, will a 10% to 15% improvement in results justify the increased expense?

Delayed Two-Stage Exchange Arthroplasty

Although certain cases of infection may be treated with other methods with a reasonable expectation of a successful result, the technique of prosthetic removal and débridement followed by a period of IV antibiotics and subsequent reimplantation remains the standard of care. This method continues to provide the greatest likelihood of successful eradication of infection when prosthetic retention is not recommended or when other treatment methods have failed. Table 90.7 provides a summary of the results of several studies using

TABLE 90.7 SUMMARY OF RESULTS USING DELAYED TWO-STAGE EXCHANGE ARTHROPLASTY

Study	No. Patients	Average Follow-Up	Success Rate*
Wasielewski et al[102]	50	57 months	92% (46/50)
Hirakawa et al[45]	55	61.9 months	87.2% (48/55)
Goldman et al[38]	64	7.5 years	97% (62/64)
Windsor and Insall[109]	38	4 years	97.4% (37/38)
Hannsen et al[41]	36	52 months	89% (32/36)
Hofmann et al[47]	26	30 months	100% (26/26)

* Eradication rates of original deep infection.

this method with significant follow-up. The data demonstrate success rates of 87.2% to 100%, higher than any other treatment option providing a well-functioning prosthetic knee.

Most protocols for delayed reimplantation include removal of the implant, thorough débridement of the bone and soft tissues, and complete removal of all cement. At the initial procedure, a local antibiotic depot or articulating spacer impregnated with high doses of antibiotics may be inserted. This is followed by several weeks of IV antibiotics and close clinical follow-up. Final reimplantation is performed when the knee is free of infection, usually determined by repeat aspiration and culture after completion of the antibiotic. Antibiotics in cement should be used at the time of reinsertion because they have been shown to improve cure rates.[13]

There has been some debate over the optimal duration for the period of IV antibiotic administration. Multiple reports using 6 weeks have shown this to be effective.[38, 50, 108] One study including 14 patients using a time period of 4 weeks until reimplantation was reported.[13] The authors found no significant adverse effects on the overall cure rate with this shortened time interval. At this time, however, because of consistently reproducible results using a 6-week protocol, it remains the gold standard. The drugs chosen should be the most effective against the isolated organism and be the least toxic to the host. It is important that close monitoring be performed to maintain serum levels in the therapeutic, but not the toxic, range.

Reimplantation success rates may be adversely affected by certain variables. A review of 66 infected TKAs treated with two-stage reimplantation demonstrated the negative effects of organism virulence, underlying diagnosis, and previous surgery on eradication rates.[45] The authors found 80% success with low-virulence organisms compared with 71.4% and 66.7% with polymicrobial infections and highly virulent organisms, respectively. Osteoarthritics had an overall treatment success of 82% compared with 54% in the rheumatoid population. Finally, infection was successfully treated 92% of the time if it occurred after a primary TKA but only 41% of the time if it occurred after multiple previous operations. They also noted that should infection occur, it was most likely to be seen in the first 24 months after surgery.

The use of an antibiotic spacer is an important aspect of a staged protocol. Cement beads or blocks able to deliver high-dose local antibiotic concentrations may increase the chance of curing the infection and have a favorable effect on the soft tissue envelope.[11, 12, 105] Advances have expanded this concept and demonstrated improved patient outcomes by providing a more functional spacer compared with the original crude block techniques. Hofmann et al[47] fashioned an articulating spacer using tobramycin-impregnated cement at a dose of 4.8 g/40 g along with the cleaned and autoclaved femoral component, new polyethylene tibial insert, and, on occasion, a patellar component with the pegs removed. A 6-week course of parenteral antibiotics followed by reimplantation led to no recurrences of infection at follow-up of 13 to 70 months with 92% good to excellent functional results. Benefits over a one-stage procedure include repeat débridement and the ability to add antibiotics to cement in high concentrations.

Another temporary functional spacer that has been used is the prosthesis of antibiotic-loaded acrylic cement, or PROSTALAC, system. It is constructed using high-dose antibiotic cement and a small amount of metal and plastic to form a smooth articulation that allows motion. The authors reviewed their series of 36 patents with 37 infections and found a recurrence in three cases for a cure rate of 92% at average follow-up of 3.1 years.[68] They also found a significantly greater level of pain relief postoperatively and improved motion when this system was used. Protocols that allow weightbearing, motion, and maintenance of soft tissue tension appear to have favorable effects on the overall functional outcome. Benefits over cement blocks include improved bone quality and a healthier soft tissue envelope, which facilitates reimplantation, wound healing, and improved motion.

The success of systems using local antibiotic depots requires maintenance of adequate intra-articular concentrations. This necessitates use of a cement with adequate elution properties and addition of appropriate amounts of antibiotics. Hofmann et al[47] used 4.8 g tobramycin per 40 g of Simplex P cement with good results. An in vitro study combining two drugs, vancomycin and tobramycin, improved elution of these medications and formed the basis of a clinical series.[76] A group of 49 patients using this drug combination and the PROSTALAC system demonstrated that 3.6 g of tobramycin and 1 g of vancomycin per 40 g of cement maintained local bactericidal levels ($p < .05$).[67] Lower doses were found to provide inadequate intra-articular bactericidal concentrations. Although these authors were unable to demonstrate a statistically significant difference in elution characteristics between Palacos-R and Simplex P cement, others have shown Palacos-R to be superior.[27, 46, 65] At this time, it appears either cement may be used with adequate success.

As noted, treatment protocols extend the use of an articulating spacer to include addition of a metal femoral component and a polyethylene tibial component. This, when combined with a high dose of antibiotic-impregnated cement, affords the patient the benefit of high-dose concentration of locally released antibiotics coupled with the benefits of a metal to plastic articulation. This intriguing treatment protocol of delayed reconstruction raises several possible benefits and concerns. The benefit of a high concentration of local antibiotics coupled with an interim articulating surface, allowing motion and function, has an obvious positive side. There are also several potential negative aspects. Will the addition of polyethylene and metal as well as methylmethacrylate facilitate the growth and protection of glycocalix-forming bacteria? Will the high-dose local antibiotic sufficiently improve the results compared with an immediate exchange procedure using antibiotic-impregnated cement in standard concentrations? It is true that any delayed exchange protocol is more time consuming and costly and is associated with a greater patient morbidity than an immediate exchange protocol. If the results are the same or nearly the same, is the added morbidity and expense justified? If the local high concentration of antibiotics is indeed beneficial, could we perform immediate exchange and local antibiotic delivery by some other mechanism? The answers to these questions can only be obtained from well-controlled prospective multicenter studies in which each of these variables is controlled in the data analysis.

A 1996 in vitro study evaluated bacterial growth on antibiotic-loaded acrylic cement and demonstrated that bone cement is a suitable substrate for bacterial growth, even in the presence of antibiotics.[55] This confirms our concerns regarding the ability to eradicate infection fully and perhaps challenges this method of treatment. At this time, however, based on the high cure rates achieved in multiple series, the use of high-dose antibiotic-loaded cement in combination with or without small amounts of plastic and metal to create a functional spacer appears to be beneficial in the clinical management of the infected TKA.

SURGICAL TECHNIQUE

The surgical technique for reconstructing an infected TKA is challenging and, in fact, more difficult than in most revision knee arthroplasties. The difficulty of exposure in the presence of infected tissues, the need for a thorough débridement, dealing with the bone loss associated with débridement of devitalized tissue, and the scarring that occurs present a challenge to the treating surgeon.

In cases of open débridement in which prosthesis retention is indicated, it is not always essential to evert the patella during exposure. The previous incision from the index arthroplasty should be used and the extensor mechanism may be moved laterally without eversion of the patella. A thorough synovectomy and débridement can then be performed. It is important to remove a modular tibial insert and thoroughly irrigate the tibial tray before inserting a new polyethylene. Before electing to retain the prosthesis, the surgeon should carefully débride the bone cement or the bone-prosthesis interface to check for undermining of the implant and local pockets of infection. If a purulent cavity is encountered, the surgeon should strongly consider removal of the prosthesis and a more aggressive treatment option. In open débridement, it is often necessary to reinsert a component at least 2 mm thicker because of the soft tissue instability that occurs during the débridement process.

In cases of prosthesis removal in either immediate or delayed exchange, it is important to débride all loose and clearly infected bone; however, it is not necessary to remove all bone that is not bleeding. This would result in excessive débridement, and in many cases hard, nonbleeding bone will remain viable and provide valuable support for the new implant. Figure 90.3 demonstrates the appearance of a knee after careful removal of an infected prosthesis and thorough débridement to remove all infected tissue while preserving as much bone stock as possible.

In cases of delayed exchange, it is necessary to evert the patella to flex the knee. Of great concern is

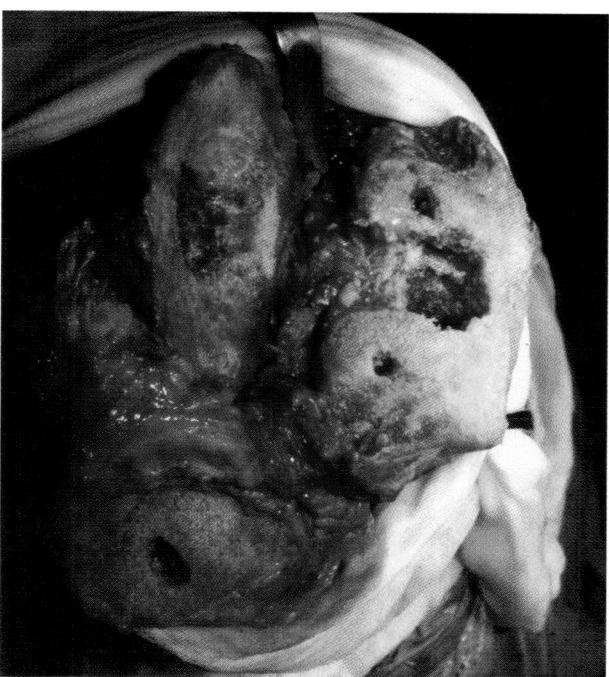

FIGURE 90.3 ➢ Intraoperative photograph demonstrating the appearance of bony surfaces after component removal and adequate débridement. Atraumatic removal of implants combined with judicious débridement has resulted in limiting bone loss to a small peripheral defect of the medial femoral condyle and a contained lesion of the proximal tibia.

the integrity of the infrapatellar tendon at the tibial tubercle. It is important for the surgeon to be patient and to go through a series of steps before everting the patella. The initial procedure is to perform a medial release and facilitate external rotation of the tibia. A lateral retinacular release combined with débridement of the lateral gutter may be performed. It is also helpful to fortify the tibial tubercle with either a towel clamp, a pin, or a strong suture to avoid avulsion throughout the procedure. If it is still difficult to evert the patella, the surgeon has a choice between either proximal or distal techniques. The proximal techniques include a rectus snip or a short quadriceps turn-down. The preferred distal technique is that of a tibial tubercle osteotomy. In our opinion, the best way to choose between these two techniques is to evert the patella and feel where the resistance occurs. If the resistance to eversion is along the free medial edge of the quadriceps mechanism, a quadriceps turn-down or rectus snip is preferable. If, as is frequently the case in reimplantation after delayed exchange, the entire quadriceps tendon is thick, it is preferable to proceed distally and perform a tibial tubercle osteotomy.

In fabricating a cement spacer or articulating spacer, it is important to consider the relative flexion and extension space. Although fashioning a large cement spacer in extension will facilitate stability, it may produce a discrepancy between the flexion and extension gaps and render revision arthroplasty more difficult. It is also important in fashioning a cement spacer to place a stem or fixation peg to prevent extrusion of the spacer and erosion of the extensor mechanism during the delayed exchange, as seen in Figure 90.4.

The specifics of exposure by suprapatellar and infrapatellar techniques as well as the principles of revision arthroplasty are beyond the scope of this chapter and are described elsewhere in this text.

SALVAGE PROCEDURES

Although the ultimate goal of providing the patient with a well-functioning knee prosthesis free of infection is often accomplished, alternative procedures are occasionally required. A poor soft tissue envelope, an extensor mechanism disruption, an immunocompromised host, or failure of other treatment methods may prohibit reimplantation. In these cases, salvage procedures are required to provide patients with a suitable limb to best meet their functional needs. Choices include resection arthroplasty, arthrodesis, and amputation. Thorough assessment of the individual, including age, level of disability, functional demands, and medical condition, is necessary to determine the optimal method of treatment.

Arthrodesis

Many different methods with varying success rates have been used to obtain solid arthrodesis, including internal and external fixation and intramedullary (IM) rods. Many complex problems must be addressed with the specific technique used that may not be seen when performed as a primary procedure. These problems include significant bone deficits, alignment deformity, soft tissue devitalization, and loss secondary to multiple previous operations.[106] Another major problem continues to be patient dissatisfaction with a stiff knee or with difficulty ambulating in multiply arthritic patients, especially in the rheumatoid population.[14] Nevertheless, arthrodesis is the most common salvage procedure used in failed TKA.

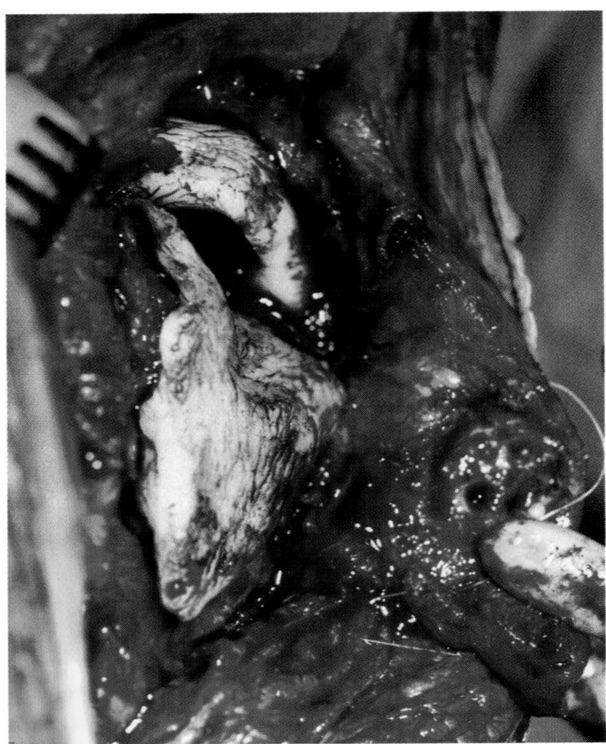

FIGURE 90.4 ➢ Antibiotic-laden cement spacer fashioned at the time of prosthetic removal and débridement. Proximal extension of the spacer into the suprapatellar region is important to minimize extensor mechanism adhesion and scarring.

Although consideration of multiple patient factors is important, it is also essential to adhere to general surgical principles if a favorable outcome is to be obtained. There is a general consensus that the most important factor that determines successful fusion is the ability to obtain and maintain rigid immobilization.[97] Unless the procedure is performed in a technically sound manner, fusion is unlikely to occur regardless of the specific technique chosen. Furthermore, long-term follow-up with periodic examination is recommended because successful fusion does not guarantee eradication of infection in all cases.[92]

Internal fixation with the use of one or more plates and screws can provide rigid immobilization. Potential downsides include the need for extensive soft tissue dissection to gain exposure for plate application, prolonged weightbearing restrictions, and the potential need for hardware removal. Moreover, as a result of stress shielding, there is a risk of fracture at the bone-plate junction.[97] This method of fixation is recommended when a prosthesis with long, large intramedullary stems is removed, leaving the remaining femur and tibia thin and relatively weak.

Success rates with external fixation have varied. A 1984 study evaluating a single-frame fixator showed poor results; fusion occurred in only one-third of cases, although a short application period and pin tract problems may have contributed to these failures.[57] The use of biplane external fixation may provide more rigid stability, as suggested by other authors.[15, 89] A 1987 study, however, using a new type of biplane external fixator had a success rate of 68% in 28 patients, results that are similar to those obtained with the use of other external fixators.[84] These authors concluded that other factors must also be important in providing union, because increasing frame rigidity did not show marked improvement in overall fusion rates. They believed the most important factor appeared to be the extent of bone loss; significant deficits minimized contact between the bone ends, resulting in an unstable situation unlikely to proceed to solid arthrodesis.

The results of fusion using external fixation after failed TKA are also dependent on the type of arthroplasty performed. Better results are seen after removal of a resurfacing prosthesis compared with more constrained implants. The Mayo Clinic reported success rates of 85% and 43% for resurfacing and hinged implants, respectively.[84] Maximal contact and compression of the two bone ends are limited when hollow tubes of cortical bone are present. Furthermore, pin tract infections, poor pin purchase, loosening, and fractures around the pins are well-known problems with these devices. Prolonged non-weightbearing and poor patient tolerance of the device are additional concerns. Therefore, the use of external fixation for arthrodesis, in our opinion, has limited application.

IM fixation appears to have the greatest success of fusion compared with other techniques, and it appears to be the procedure of choice for arthrodesis of the knee after failed TKA.[23] Caution should be taken when using IM fixation in cases of active infection as IM spread will increase the risk of systemic sepsis as well as chronic osteomyelitis. Wilde and Stearns[106] reviewed the literature and found the combined average fusion rate for cases of infected TKA treated with IM arthrodesis to be 84%. Donley et al[23] used IM fixation to obtain successful fusion in seven of eight infected cases, a success rate of 87.5%. The average time from prosthetic removal to fusion was 12 months (range = 5.5 to 36 months). They recommended a two-stage protocol with initial implant removal, with subsequent fusion only when infection was eliminated to improve effectiveness.

The advantages of IM fixation include ease of placement, creation of a stable situation in the presence of significant bone and soft tissue loss, and the ability to obtain solid fusion even when infection recurs. Weightbearing can be initiated early after the procedure, and external supports can often be avoided. Most important, this method can be used in cases of massive bone loss, when other methods have a significantly higher failure rate.[29] Patients with ipsilateral hip arthroplasty are not candidates for this method because of the presence of the femoral component in the medullary canal. Other drawbacks include long surgical times (average = 4.1 hours) and significant blood loss (average = 3.9 units) in one study.[23] Nevertheless, as a result of consistently reported high success rates, the use of an IM rod should be strongly considered when contemplating arthrodesis, especially in patients with significant bone loss.

Resection Arthroplasty

Removal of the components with thorough débridement and IV antibiotics followed by immobilization to allow soft tissue contracture and scarring for stability is a viable alternative in some select patients. Falahee et al[31] reviewed 28 infected TKAs in 26 patients between 1970 and 1983 who were treated with resection arthroplasty. They found that after resection alone 15 of the patients were able to walk independently, six required secondary arthrodesis, and three had spontaneous fusions in good alignment. Two patients were unable to walk, although both were unable to do so before the procedure. Systemic signs of infection were eliminated in all patients and local signs were eliminated in 89%. All patients required the use of a walking aid, and all but five patients required a knee brace for additional stability. They found that neither the type of prosthesis nor the underlying diagnosis was predictive of a successful outcome. The best indicator for a successful result was the level of patient disability. In general, those with the greatest disability were the most satisfied with the condition after the procedure, whereas those with little preoperative disability were more likely to be dissatisfied.

One of the difficulties with recommending arthrodesis is the poor acceptance of a stiff-leg gait and difficulty in positioning the extremity in a sitting position. The difficulty is determining whether patients will prefer this stiff, stable limb or perhaps a more flexible but relatively unstable joint. The benefits of resection include not only eradicating infection but also serving as a trial to determine which patients are more likely to be satisfied with a secondary arthrodesis on the basis of their previous experience with postoperative immobilization as part of the resection protocol.[31] Furthermore, the likelihood of successful fusion is increased in the absence of infection should this now be preferred.

We believe that resection arthroplasty should be selectively used as definitive treatment of infected TKA. Those who have reasonably good mobility before infection will most likely be unhappy with the pain and limitation in activity resulting from the inadequate stability obtained from resection alone. Nonambulators with multiarticular disease and limited functional demands are the most appropriate candidates. The lack of stability in these patients should not significantly further limit their activity, and a flexible knee will be beneficial for leg positioning, especially in sitting positions. Resection arthroplasty may also be considered as the salvage result in the patient with a failed arthrodesis.

Amputation

Amputation should be reserved as the last option in dealing with an infected TKA or in cases of life-threatening sepsis. Indications include evidence of systemic toxicity that cannot be controlled by local means, refractory infections with resistant or gas-forming organisms, and severe bone and soft tissue loss or intractable pain. Because of a combination of often associated medical comorbidities, the nature of the procedure, and the increased energy expenditure required for ambulation, a significant reduction in function is expected. A study reviewing mobility after amputation in 23 patients found that only 7 were able to ambulate, and 12 were confined to a wheelchair.[79] The authors concluded that amputation cannot be regarded as a satisfactory solution and that patients should be told they are likely to be wheelchair dependent.

REINFECTION AFTER REIMPLANTATION

Although rare, the recurrence of infection after successfully treated infected TKA presents a new set of challenges, even to the surgeon familiar with this complication. A retrospective study evaluating 24 such cases over a 16-year period demonstrated the overall poor outcome in this subset of patients.[41] The final outcome included 10 successful fusions, five persistent infections on oral suppression, four above-knee amputations, three cases of pseudarthrosis, one resection arthroplasty, and one uninfected TKA. The authors' experience led them to conclude that many of these patients will require multiple operations (average = 3.7) to obtain soft tissue coverage, wound closure, and eradication of infection. They stated that as experience and technology continue to grow there should be a more optimistic outlook for these patients, although they strongly recommended that alternative salvage procedures be considered, and performed earlier rather than later, to minimize the difficulty in performing them and enhance their overall success rate.

Another study involving a smaller number of patients evaluating the results of subsequent two-stage reimplantation for reinfection were reported at an average follow-up of 31 months.[5] The series included a total of 12 patients, nine of whom underwent a typical two-stage reimplantation protocol and three who had arthrodesis with an IM rod. On the basis of their early results, which evaluated recurrence of infection and overall knee function scores, they indicated that reimplantation is preferable to fusion and resection arthroplasty. They stated that certain criteria should be met before reimplantation, however: isolation of the infecting organism, IV antibiotics with a minimal bactericidal level of 1:8, host immune competence, adequate soft tissue coverage, and an intact extensor mechanism.

CONCLUSION

In summary, all cases of infection must be considered on an individual basis. A thorough evaluation of all involved variables is necessary so that the most reasonable treatment option may be selected. Through a cooperative effort among the surgeon, the infectious disease consultant, and an informed patient, a treatment regimen to eradicate infection and restore function can be selected. With improved antibiotics and antibiotic regimens, newer materials that will allow local antibiotic deliverance, and improved surgical technique, it is hoped that all total knee infections can be treated by a mechanism that will leave the patient with a functional arthroplasty.

Bibliography

1. American Academy Orthopaedic Surgeons: 1998 Annual Meeting Academy News, March 20, 1998.
2. Arizono T, Oga M, Sugioka Y: Increased resistance of bacteria after adherence to polymethylmethacrylate. Acta Orthop Scand 63:661, 1992.
3. Athanasou N, Pandey R, DeSteiger R, et al: Diagnosis of infection by frozen section during revision arthroplasty. J Bone Joint Surg Br 77:28, 1995.
4. Ayers D, Dennis D, Johanson N, et al: Common complications of total knee arthroplasty. J Bone Joint Surg Am 79:278, 1997.
5. Backe H, Wolff D, Windsor R: Total knee replacement infection after 2-stage reimplantation. Clin Orthop 331:125, 1996.
6. Bayston R, Rogers J: Production of extracellular slime by *Staphylococcus epidermidis* during stationary phase of growth. J Clin Pathol 43:866, 1990.
7. Bengston S, Knutson K: The infected knee arthroplasty. Acta Orthop Scand 62:301, 1991.
8. Berg M, Bergman B, Hoborn J: Ultraviolet air compared to ultraclean air exposure. Comparison of air bacteria counts in operating rooms. J Bone Joint Surg Br 73:811, 1991.
9. Berg-Prier M, Cederblad A, Persson U: Ultraviolet radiation and ultraclean air exposures in operating rooms. UV protection, economy and comfort. J Arthroplasty 7:457, 1992.
10. Besser M: Tuberculosis infection complicating total knee arthroplasty. J Bone Joint Surg 81:143, 1999.
11. Booth R, Lotke P: The results of spacer block technique in revision of infected total knee arthroplasty. Clin Orthop 248:57, 1989.
12. Borden L, Gearen P: Infected total knee arthroplasty. J Arthroplasty 2:27, 1987.
13. Bose W, Gearen P, Randall J, et al: Long term outcome of 42 knees with chronic infection after total knee arthroplasty. Clin Orthop 319:285, 1995.
14. Hakan A, Brattstrom M: Long term results in knee arthrodesis in rheumatoid arthritis. Acta Rheum Scand 17:86, 1971.
15. Brooker A, Hansen N: The biplane frame—Modified compression arthrodesis of the knee. Clin Orthop 160:163, 1981.
16. Brooks D, Pupparo F: Successful salvage of a primary total knee arthroplasty infected with candida parapsilosis. J Arthroplasty 13:707, 1998.
17. Burger R, Basch T, Hopson C: Implant salvage in infected total knee arthroplasty. Clin Orthop 273:105, 1991.
18. Chang C, Merritt K: Microbial adherence of polymethylmethacrylate surfaces. J Biomed Mater Res 26:197, 1992.
19. Charnley J, Eftekhar N: Postoperative infection in total prosthetic replacement arthroplasty of the hip joint and operating room bacterial counts. Br J Surg 56:641, 1969.
20. Chimento C, Finger S, Barrack R: Gram stain detection of infection during revision arthroplasty. J Bone Joint Surg Br 78:838, 1996.
21. Davenport K, Traina S, Perry C: Treatment of acutely infected arthroplasty with local antibiotics. J Arthroplasty 6:179, 1991.
22. Deburge A: Guepar hinge prosthesis—Complications

and results with two years' follow up. Clin Orthop 120:47, 1976.
23. Donley B, Matthews L, Kaufer H: Arthrodesis of the knee with an intramedullary nail. J Bone Joint Surg 73:907, 1991.
24. Dougherty S, Simmons R: Infections in bionic man—The pathobiology of infections in prosthetic devices. Curr Probl Surg 19:217, 1982.
25. Drancourt M, Stein A: Oral rifampin plus ofloxacin for treatment of staphylococcus infected orthopedic implants. Antimicrob Agents Chemother 37:1214, 1993.
26. Duff G, Lachiewicz P, Kelley S: Aspiration of the knee joint before revision arthroplasty. Clin Orthop 331:132, 1996.
27. Elson R, Jephcott A, et al: Antibiotic loaded acrylic cement. J Bone Joint Surg Br 59:197, 1977.
28. England S, Stern S, Insall J, et al: Total knee arthroplasty in diabetes mellitus. Clin Orthop 260:130, 1990.
29. Ennecking W, Shirley P: Resection arthrodesis for malignant and potentially malignant lesions about the knee using an intramedullary rod and local bone grafts. J Bone Joint Surg 59:223, 1977.
30. Eskinazi D: Is systemic antimicrobial prophylaxis justified in dental patients with prosthetic joints? Oral Surg Oral Med 66: 430, 1988.
31. Falahee M, Matthews L, Kaufer H: Resection arthroplasty as a salvage procedure for a knee with infection after a total arthroplasty. J Bone Joint Surg 69:1013, 1987.
32. Fehring T, McAlister J: Frozen histologic section as a guide to sepsis in revision joint arthroplasty. Clin Orthop 304:229, 1994.
33. Feldman D, Lonner J, Desai P, et al: The role of intraoperative frozen sections in revision total joint arthroplasty. J Bone Joint Surg 77:1807, 1995.
34. Freeman M, Sudlow R, Casewell M, et al: The management of infected total knee replacements. J Bone Joint Surg Br 67:764, 1985.
35. Friedman R, Friedrich L, White R, et al: Antibiotic prophylaxis and tourniquet inflation in total knee arthroplasty. Clin Orthop 260:17, 1990.
36. Garvin K, Salvati E, Brause B: Role of gentamicin impregnated cement in total joint arthroplasty. Orthop Clin North Am 19: 605, 1988.
37. Glynn M, Sheehan J: An analysis of the causes of deep infection after hip and knee arthroplasties. Clin Orthop 178:202, 1983.
38. Goldman R, Scuderi G, Insall J: Two stage reimplantation for infected total knee replacement. Clin Orthop 331:118, 1996.
39. Hanssen A, Rand J: Evaluation and treatment of infection at the site of total hip or knee arthroplasty. J Bone Joint Surg 80:910, 1998.
40. Hanssen A, Rand J, Osmon D: Treatment of the infected total knee arthroplasty with insertion of another prosthesis. The effect of antibiotic impregnated bone cement. Clin Orthop 309: 44, 1994.
41. Hanssen A, Trousdale R, Osmon D: Patient outcome with reinfection following reimplantation for the infected total knee arthroplasty. Clin Orthop 321:55, 1995.
42. Heck D, Rosenberg A, et al: Use of antibiotic impregnated cement during hip and knee arthroplasty in the United States. J Arthroplasty 10:470, 1995.
43. Herbert C, Williams R, Levy R, et al: Cost of treating an infected total knee replacement. Clin Orthop 331:140, 1996.
44. Hester R, Nelson C, Harrison S: Control of contamination of the operative team in total joint arthroplasty. J Arthroplasty 7: 267, 1992.
45. Hirakawa K, Stulberg B, Wilde A, et al: Results of two stage reimplantation for infected total knee arthroplasty. J Arthroplasty 13:22, 1998.
46. Hoff S, Fitzgerald R, Kelly P: The depot administration of penicillin-G and gentamicin in acrylic bone cement. J Bone Joint Surg 63:798, 1981.
47. Hofmann A, Kane K, Tkach T, et al: Treatment of infected total knee arthroplasty using an articulating spacer. Clin Orthop 321: 45, 1995.
48. Insall J: Infection in total knee arthroplasty. Instr Course Lect 31:42, 1982.
49. Insall J: Infection of total knee arthroplasty. Instr Course Lect 35:319, 1986.
50. Insall J, Thompson F, Brause B: Two stage reimplantation for the salvage of infected total knee arthroplasty. J Bone Joint Surg 65:1087, 1983.
51. Isiklar Z, Darouiche R, Landon G, et al: Efficacy of antibiotics alone for orthopaedic device related infections. Clin Orthop 332:184, 1996.
52. Jerry G, Rand J, Ilstrup D: Old sepsis prior to knee arthroplasty. Clin Orthop 236:135, 1988.
53. Johnson D, Bannister G: Outcome of infected arthroplasty of the knee. J Bone Joint Surg Br 68:289, 1986.
54. Jones E, Insall J, Inglis A, et al: Guepar knee arthroplasty and late complications. Clin Orthop 140:145, 1979.
55. Kendall R, Duncan C, Smith J, et al: Persistence of bacteria on antibiotic loaded acrylic depots. Clin Orthop 329:273, 1996.
56. Khaersgaard-Anderson P, Christiansen Singerslev J, et al: Total knee arthroplasty in classic hemophilia. Clin Orthop 256:137, 1990.
57. Knutson K, Hovelius L, Lindstrand A, et al: Arthrodesis after failed knee arthroplasty—A nationwide multicenter investigation of 91 cases. Clin Orthop 191:202, 1984.
58. Kreder H, Davey J: Total hip arthroplasty complicated by tuberculosis infection. J Arthroplasty 11:111, 1996.
59. Leigh D: Serum and bone concentrations of cefuroxime in patients undergoing knee arthroplasty. J Antimicrob Chemother 18:609, 1986.
60. Levitsky K, Hozack W, Balderson R, et al: Evaluation of the painful prosthetic joint. J Arthroplasty 6:237, 1991.
61. Lidwell O, Lowbury E, Whyte W, et al: Effect of ultraclean air in operating rooms on deep sepsis in the joint after total hip or knee replacement—A randomised study. BMJ 285:10, 1982.
62. Lind P, Langsteger W, Koltringer P, et al: Immunoscintigraphy of inflammatory processes with a technetium-99 labeled monoclonal antigranulocyte antibody. J Nucl Med 31:417, 1990.
63. Lonner J, Desai P, Dicesare P, et al: The reliability of analysis of intraoperative frozen sections for identifying active infection during revision hip or knee arthroplasty. J Bone Joint Surg 78: 1553, 1996.
65. Mariani B, Martin D, Levine M, et al: Polymerase chain reaction detection of bacterial infection in total knee arthroplasty. Clin Orthop 331:11, 1996.
64. Marks K, Nelson C, Lautenschlager E: Antibiotic impregnated acrylic bone cement. J Bone Joint Surg 58:358, 1976.
66. Masini M, Maguire J, Thornhill T: Infected total knee arthroplasty. In The Knee. St. Louis, MO, Mosby Year Book, 1261–1278, 1994.
67. Masri B, Duncan C, Beauchamp C: Long term elution of antibiotics from bone cement—An in vivo study using the prosthesis of antibiotic loaded acrylic cement system. J Arthroplasty 13: 331, 1998.
68. Masri B, Duncan C, Beauchamp C: The modified two stage exchange arthroplasty in treatment of infected total knee replacement. In Revision Total Knee Arthroplasty. Baltimore, MD, Williams & Wilkins, 1997, p 394.
69. Mauerhan D, Nelson C, Smith D, et al: Prophylaxis against infection in total joint arthroplasty. J Bone Joint Surg 76:39, 1994.
70. McLaren A, Spooner C: Salvage of infected total knee components. Clin Orthop 331:146, 1996.
71. Merkel K, Brown M, Dewanjee M, et al: Comparison of indium labeled leukocyte imaging with sequential technetium-gallium scanning in the diagnosis of low grade musculoskeletal sepsis. J Bone Joint Surg 67:465, 1985.
72. Mont M, Waldman B, Banerjee C, et al: Multiple irrigation, debridement, and retention of components in infected total knee arthroplasty. J Arthroplasty 12:426, 1997.
73. Niskanen R, Korkala O, Pammo H: Serum C-reactive protein levels after hip and knee arthroplasty. J Bone Joint Surg Br 78: 431, 1996.
74. Oyen W, vanHorn J, Claessens R, et al: Diagnosis of bone, joint and joint prosthetic infections with In-111 labeled nonspecific immunoglobulin G scintigraphy. Radiology 182:195, 1992.
75. Papagelopoulos P, Idusuyi O, Wallrichs S, et al: Long term outcome and survivorship analysis of primary knee arthroplasty in patients with diabetes mellitus. Clin Orthop 330:124, 1996.
76. Penner M, Masri B, Duncan C: Elution characteristics of vancomycin and tobramycin combined in acrylic bone cement. J Arthroplasty 11:939, 1996.

77. Petty W, Bryan R, Coventry M, et al: Infection after total knee arthroplasty. Orthop Clin North Am 6:1005, 1975.
78. Poss R, Thornhill T, Ewald F, et al: Factors influencing the incidence and outcome of infection following total joint arthroplasty. Clin Orthop 182:117, 1984.
79. Pring D, Marks L, Angel J: Mobility after amputation for failed knee replacement. J Bone Joint Surg Br 70:770, 1988.
80. Rand J: Alternatives to reimplantation for salvage of the total knee arthroplasty complicated by infection. J Bone Joint Surg 75:282, 1993.80. Rand J, Brown M: The value of indium 111 leukocyte scanning in the evaluation of painful or infected total knee arthroplasties. Clin Orthop 259:179, 1990.
81. Rand J: Sepsis following total knee arthroplasty. In Total Knee Arthroplasty. New York, Raven Press, 1993, pp 349-376.
82. Rand J, Brown M: The value of indium 111 leukocyte scanning in the evaluation of painful or infected total knee arthroplasties. Clin Orthop 259:179, 1990.
83. Rand J, Bryan R: Reimplantation for the salvage of an infected total knee arthroplasty. J Bone Joint Surg 65:1081, 1983.
84. Rand J, Bryan R, Chao E: Failed total knee arthroplasty treated by arthrodesis of the knee using the Ace-Fischer apparatus. J Bone Joint Surg 69:39, 1987.
85. Rand J, Chao E, Stauffer R: Kinematic rotating hinge total knee arthroplasty. J Bone Joint Surg 69:489, 1987.
86. Ritter M: Intraoperative controls for bacterial contamination during total knee replacement. Orthop Clin North Am 20:49, 1989.
87. Ritter M, Campbell E: Retrospective evaluation of an iodophor incorporated antimicrobial plastic adhesive wound drape. Clin Orthop 228:307, 1988.
88. Ritter M, Eitzen H, French M, et al: The effect that time, touch and environment have upon bacterial contamination of instruments during surgery. Ann Surg 184:642, 1976.
89. Rothacker G, Cabanela M: External fixation for arthrodesis of the knee and ankle. Clin Orthop 180:101, 1983.
90. Saliban A, Anzel S: Salvage of an infected knee prosthesis with medial and lateral gastrocnemius muscle flaps. J Bone Joint Surg 65:681, 1983.
91. Salvati E, Robinson R, Zeno S, et al: Infection rates after 3175 total hip and total knee replacements performed with and without a horizontal unidirectional filtered airflow system. J Bone Joint Surg 64:525, 1982.
92. Schoifet S, Morrey B: Persistent infection after successful arthrodesis for infected total knee arthroplasty—A report of two cases. J Arthroplasty 5:277, 1990.
93. Schoifet S, Morrey B: Treatment of infection after total knee arthroplasty by debridement with retention of the components. J Bone Joint Surg 72:1383, 1990.
94. Schurman D, Swenson L, Piiali R: Bone cement with and without antibiotics: A study of mechanical properties. In Proceedings of the 6th Meeting of the Hip Society. St. Louis, MO, CV Mosby, 1978, p 78.
95. Shaw J, Bordner M, Hamory B: Efficacy of the steri-shield filtered exhaust helmet in limiting bacterial counts in the operating room during total joint arthroplasty. J Arthroplasty 11:469, 1996.
96. Shih L, Wu J, Yang D: Erythrocyte sedimentation rates and C-reactive protein values in patients with total hip arthroplasty. Clin Orthop 225:238, 1987.
97. Stulberg S: Arthrodesis in failed total knee replacements. Orthop Clin North Am 13:213, 1982.
98. Tannenbaum D, Matthews L, Grady-Benson J: Infection around joint replacements in patients who have a renal or liver transplantation. J Bone Joint Surg 79:36, 1997.
99. Unger A, Kessler C, Lewis R: Total knee arthroplasty in human immunodeficiency virus infected hemophiliacs. J Arthroplasty 10:448, 1995.
100. Wada M, Baba H, Imura S: Prosthetic knee candida parapsilosis infection. J Arthroplasty 13:479, 1998.
101. Waldman B, Mont M, Hungerford D: Total knee arthroplasty infections associated with dental procedures. Clin Orthop 343:164, 1997.
102. Wasielewski R, Barden R, Rosenberg A: Results of different surgical procedures on total knee arthroplasty infections. J Arthroplasty 11:931, 1996.
103. Wegener W, Alavi A: Diagnostic imaging of musculoskeletal infection. Orthop Clin North Am 22:401, 1991.
104. Wiggins C, Nelson C, Clarke R, et al: Concentration of antibiotics in normal bone after intravenous injection. J Bone Joint Surg 60:93, 1978.
105. Wilde A, Ruth J: Two stage reimplantation in infected total knee arthroplasty. Clin Orthop 236:23, 1988.
106. Wilde A, Stearns K: Intramedullary fixation for arthrodesis of the knee after infected total knee arthroplasty. Clin Orthop 248:87, 1989.
107. Wilson M, Kelley K, Thornhill T: Infection as a complication of total knee replacement arthroplasty. J Bone Joint Surg 72:878, 1990.
108. Windsor R, Bono J: Infected total knee replacements. J Am Acad Orthop Surg 2:44, 1994.
109. Windsor R, Insall J: Management of the infected total knee arthroplasty. Surgery of the Knee, 2nd ed. New York, Churchill Livingstone, 1983, pp 959-974.
110. Winiarsky R, Barth P, Lotke P: Total knee arthroplasty in morbidly obese patients. J Bone Joint Surg 80:1770, 1998.
111. Wright T, Sullivan D, Arnoczky S: The effect of antibiotic additions on the fracture properties of bone cements. Acta Orthop Scand 55:414, 1984.

91 Cement Spacers in Knee Surgery

FARES S. HADDAD • BASSAM A. MASRI • CLIVE P. DUNCAN

Total knee arthroplasty has become one of the most common and most successful procedures performed in the field of joint reconstruction. In the United States, 50,000 total knee arthroplasties are performed each year.[15] Excellent long-term results have been reported in young as well as elderly patients.[38, 131, 136] However, in spite of rigorous prophylaxis, between 1.0% and 2.0% of total knee replacements are complicated by infection.[11, 12, 52, 132, 139] This leads to significant morbidity, is expensive and time consuming to treat,[8, 158] and usually results in an inferior functional outcome.

Sculco[142] reviewed the prevalence and economic impact of infected total hip and knee arthroplasty. In 1989, 80,647 total knee replacements were performed on Medicare patients in the United States. During the same year, 1795 implants were removed for infection, for an estimated prevalence of total knee sepsis of 2.23%. Sculco also estimated the cost of treatment of each infection at $50,000 to $60,000. The overall annual cost for the treatment of infected total knee replacements would, therefore, be between $90 million and $110 million per year.

Hebert et al[64] compared the cost of the treatment of 20 consecutive infected total knee replacements with that of 30 primary total knee arthroplasties and 30 aseptic revision knee arthroplasties during the same period. The surgical treatment of an infected total knee arthroplasty was twice as expensive as that of an aseptic revision and three to four times as expensive as a primary total knee replacement. The majority of the cost of treatment was related to the expense of the prolonged hospitalization that was often required. Any treatment method that allows earlier discharge from hospital not only would be desirable from the patient's viewpoint but would also have economic advantages.

In this chapter, we discuss the evolution and use of cement spacers and outline our preferred method of treating the infected total knee replacement. This method is a modification of the well-accepted two-stage exchange arthroplasty, in which the implant is removed and the knee is débrided at the first stage; after an interval period of several weeks, a permanent prosthesis is reimplanted. The modification of this method includes the insertion of an antibiotic-loaded facsimile of a total knee replacement prosthesis between stages (Fig. 91.1). In addition to the elution of high levels of antibiotics into the joint, this prosthesis allows ambulation and rehabilitation and earlier discharge from hospital between stages. It also facilitates the second-stage procedure by preserving knee motion and soft-tissue tension; this preserves soft-tissue planes and makes the exposure and reimplantation easier. The patient is readmitted for the second stage on an elective basis. This temporary functional spacer is now known as the *PROSThesis* of *Antibiotic-Loaded Acrylic Cement*, or simply PROSTALAC.[40–42, 79, 97]

PERIPROSTHETIC ENVIRONMENT

Of all the infections encountered in orthopedics, those involving implanted foreign material remain some of the most difficult to treat. Organisms usually considered nonpathogenic or exquisitely sensitive to antibiotics become resistant to all forms of treatment short of removal of the foreign material. This resistance to simple therapeutic measures is related to a number of interactions among the host, the prosthesis, and the infecting organism.

In the setting of a joint arthroplasty, the mechanical trauma of reaming and bone preparation and the thermal trauma of cement polymerization potentially create a bacterial culture medium of necrotic debris. Local trauma is also thought to increase fibronectin levels.[16, 130] This enhances the binding of *Staphylococcus aureus* to biomaterials by its attachment to the N-terminal portion of the fibronectin. Invasive forms of *S. aureus* have better adherence by this mechanism. Moreover, methyl methacrylate has been shown to have an inhibitory effect on macrophage function in vitro[60] and to increase the probability of infection in dogs.[125, 126] To the best of our knowledge, this has never been borne out in human studies but remains a theoretical consideration. The host defenses may be hampered further by the nature of the periprosthetic milieu, which has a relatively poor blood supply that insulates bacteria from the effects of systemic antibiotics.

Furthermore, in the presence of a prosthesis or an implant, bacterial adherence is enhanced by the formation of glycocalix, a polysaccharide layer that is produced around bacterial colonies and helps increase bacterial resistance to host defenses.[57–59, 61] This phenomenon has been observed with biomaterials when they become colonized with bacteria: they become coated with a biofilm consisting of both bacterial colonies and their glycocalix.[32, 57] The production of a biofilm allows the organism to adhere to and survive successfully on synthetic surfaces. Bacteria that exist within a biofilm are at least 500 times more resistant

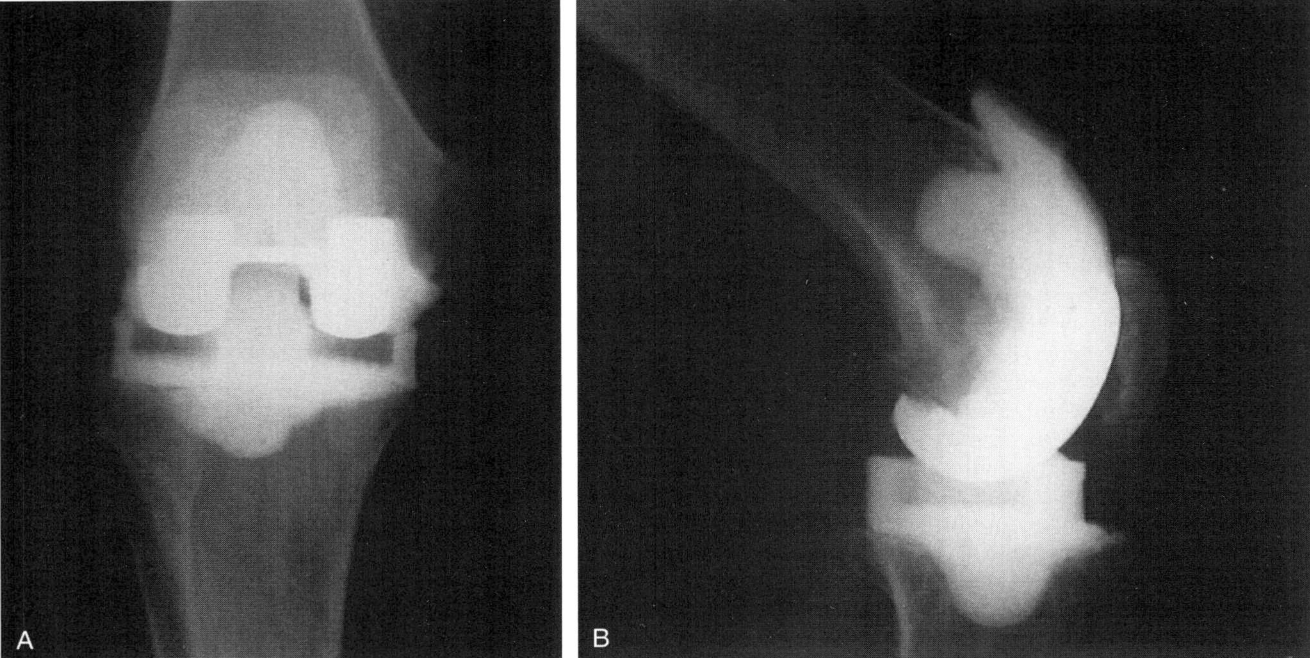

FIGURE 91.1 ➢ Anteroposterior *(A)* and lateral *(B)* radiographs of a PROSTALAC used in the treatment of an infected total knee arthroplasty.

to antibiotics than the planktonic forms.[33] In addition, they are also relatively resistant to complement activation and ingestion by neutrophils. The glycocalix not only isolates the infecting organism further from the host defenses, but may also make it difficult to detect such bacteria on joint aspiration.

Glycocalix production differs among bacteria, which may partly explain their very variable adherence properties. A number of tests are available to determine glycocalix/slime production in laboratory cultures. However, the correlation between glycocalix production by an organism and infection of a knee prosthesis is not sufficient for the test to have clear clinical relevance. In most reports of periprosthetic infection, *S. aureus* and *Staphylococcus epidermidis* are the most common infecting organisms, followed by a wide range of gram-positive and gram-negative bacteria. Many species of *S. aureus* and *S. epidermidis* are slime producers. Most gram-negative organisms are poor slime producers with the notable exception of the *Pseudomonas* species.

There is also evidence that the material from which a component is made and the surface finish of the component may influence the ease with which a prosthesis may become infected. Cordero et al[31] showed that chrome-cobalt surfaces are more easily infected with *S. aureus* than titanium surfaces and porous surfaces are more easily infected than polished surfaces in an animal model.[31] The better resistance of titanium surfaces to infection may be related to superior osseointegration properties, allowing the host tissues to adhere to the surface of the implant, before any microorganisms can adhere, elaborate glycocalix, and cause a clinical, yet indolent infection. This has been referred to as the "race for the surface."[61] The balance may be tipped in favor of infection when there is prosthetic motion or loosening. Petrie et al[120] showed a higher infection rate with the use of metal-backed patellas. They hypothesized that this was related to synovitis, effusions, and relative hyperemia of these knees in the presence of the particulate metal and polyethylene debris, which may increase the potential of bacterial seeding.

Host factors such as immunosuppression,[146] rheumatoid arthritis,[88, 128] diabetes mellitus,[46] advanced age, obesity, use of corticosteroids, malnutrition,[51, 56, 145] and preexisting or concurrent infection[108, 155] also contribute to an increased risk of sepsis in total knee replacements.

The interplay between all of these factors makes infection at the site of a total knee arthroplasty difficult to eradicate and necessitates a rapid and very aggressive response to any periprosthetic infection.

OPTIONS FOR THE INFECTED TOTAL KNEE REPLACEMENT

A number of strategies are available for the treatment of the infected arthroplasty.[132–135, 154, 155] These include suppressive antibiotic therapy, soft tissue débridement, and parenteral antibiotics with retention of the prosthesis, single-stage or two-stage exchange arthroplasty, arthrodesis, excision arthroplasty, and amputation.

Antibiotic Suppression

Antibiotics alone are very seldom a cure for an infected total knee replacement.[76, 134, 158] This is suppressive rather than curative therapy and is indicated only in those patients who are too frail or unwilling to undergo surgery.[92, 116] For it to be successful, the organism must be of low virulence and must be susceptible to the oral antibiotics used, and the patient must be able to tolerate the antibiotics without serious ill effects. Rand[132] combined the results of a number of series and concluded that antibiotic suppression was successful in 27% of cases.

Débridement

Débridement must be combined with the administration of appropriate antibiotics. These are usually delivered systemically but can also be delivered locally using infusion pumps[35] or antibiotic-loaded cement with retention of the total knee prosthesis.[99] This technique is most successful in acute hematogenous or early postoperative infections.[15, 102, 105, 107, 144] Débridement and suction irrigation along with long-term antibiotic therapy can salvage 50% to 60% of acutely infected total knee replacements.[102] Mont et al[105] reported the results of a prospective study of multiple irrigation and débridement, component retention, and at least 6 weeks of intravenous antibiotics, with a mean follow-up of 4 years and a minimum follow-up of 2 years. They treated early postsurgical and acute hematogenous infections presenting within 30 days. By adhering to strict inclusion criteria, including the absence of radiographic or intraoperative component loosening or evidence of osteolysis, and by carefully addressing all the possible sources of sepsis, they were able to retain the component in 10 of 10 knees with acute postsurgical infection and in 10 of 14 knees with acute hematogenous infection (71%). This approach fails for chronic infections.[13, 135, 158]

Resection Arthroplasty/Knee Arthrodesis

In most cases, resection arthroplasty and knee arthrodesis are unsatisfactory options in the treatment of infected total knee arthroplasties, controlling the infection at the price of a painful or poorly functioning limb.[43, 48, 107] Consideration should, however, be given to arthrodesis, particularly in young patients, when multiple attempts at prosthetic reimplantation may make later arthrodesis very difficult.[63]

Amputation

Amputation may be necessary when the alternative modalities fail to eradicate pain or sepsis,[77, 132] when there is massive bone loss, or when sepsis is life threatening. In contrast to the outcome after above-knee amputation for other reasons, the outcome in this setting seldom results in satisfactory function. Many of the patients do not return to an ambulatory status.[129]

One-Stage Exchange Arthroplasty

The successful reports of one-stage exchange arthroplasty for infection have not been replicated by many groups. Borden and Gearen[15] reported no recurrence of infection in three patients in whom a one-stage exchange arthroplasty was performed. This was, however, a very small number in whom infection was caused by gram-positive organisms. Freeman et al[48] were able to control the infection in all eight patients with septic loosening of total knee replacements, who were treated with a one-stage exchange protocol in which gentamicin-loaded Palacos R cement (Smith and Nephew Richards, Memphis, TN) was used for the fixation of the revision arthroplasty. A strict protocol was followed, with separate intraoperative preparation, draping, and instruments for the débridement and reimplantation portions of the procedure, the use of antiseptic solutions, and oral antibiotics for a minimum of 3 months after surgery. In this series, six knees were infected with *S. aureus,* and two knees yielded negative cultures because of prior antibiotic therapy. In a later series by Göksan and Freeman,[53] the original infection was controlled in 17 of 18 knees with gram-positive infections. One of these 17 knees subsequently became infected with a different organism, for an overall success rate of 16 of 18 knees (89%). These results may not apply to infections caused by gram-negative organisms or when the presence of draining sinuses, soft-tissue deficiency requiring flap coverage, or bony deficiency requiring bone grafting must be addressed.

Two-Stage Exchange Arthroplasty

Although some authors reported successful immediate reimplantation,[15, 48, 147] the best results were obtained when reimplantation was delayed by at least 6 weeks.[15, 76, 137, 156-158] Intravenous antibiotics are administered in the interim with or without the use of local antibiotic-loaded cement, and antibiotic-loaded cement is used for fixation of the new implant. The first report of a successful reimplantation of an infected knee replacement using a two-stage exchange technique with an antibiotic-loaded cement spacer was published in 1979.[73] The first series of reimplantation for salvage of infected total knee replacements were reported in 1983 by Rand and Bryan,[133] Insall et al,[76] and Woods et al.[158] These series showed good results with two-stage exchange arthroplasty with a delay of at least 6 weeks between stages. When the delay was less than 2 weeks, particularly with more virulent organisms, the results were not as encouraging. Since Rand and Bryan's and Insall's series, many others have been reported using two-stage exchange arthroplasty.[14, 15, 50, 54, 62, 69, 71, 137, 141, 147, 150, 153, 156, 157]

The currently used protocols for the treatment of infected total knee arthroplasties are modifications of the two-stage exchange arthroplasty described by Insall et al.[76] The technique of Insall et al is a two-stage exchange arthroplasty in which the infected implant, infected material, and retained cement are carefully removed at the first stage. Intravenous antibiotic therapy is then administered for a 6-week period. Serum bactericidal titers are measured using a serial two-fold tube-dilution technique, and bactericidal titers are maintained at a dilution level of 1:8 or greater. These serum titers are maintained for a full 6-week period, and any days during which the serum titers are not adequate do not count toward the 6-week period. A definitive resurfacing total knee arthroplasty is then reimplanted. All antibiotics are discontinued after reimplantation. Using this method, the authors reported no recurrence of the initial infection in a prospective series of 11 infected knee replacements with an average follow-up of 34 months.[76] There was one new infection, with a different organism, secondary to an infected bunion. It should be noted that the mean inpatient stay averaged 12 weeks.

In a series of 11 patients treated with a two-stage exchange technique, Borden and Gearen[15] reported control of the infection in 10. The one uncontrolled case involved an infected Guepar-hinged prosthesis. This was treated successfully with a knee arthrodesis. The authors used antibiotic-loaded bone cement for the reimplantation, and in eight of 11 cases antibiotic-loaded cement beads were used as a spacer between stages. During the interval period, bactericidal levels of antibiotics were given for 3 weeks, after which, if two separate aspirations revealed no growth of organisms, the second stage was performed.

Rosenberg et al[137] reported on 25 patients with 26 infected total knee replacements treated with a two-stage exchange arthroplasty, with 6 weeks of intravenous antibiotic therapy between stages. Antibiotic-loaded bone cement was used for reimplantation in all cases. There was no clinical recurrence of infection, but three patients had positive cultures at second stage, including one with a tuberculous infection that was treated with a long course of antituberculous medication. The other two patients were treated with oral antibiotics for 3 to 6 months after reimplantation.

In a subsequent report by the same group, Wasielewski et al[150] reviewed 76 consecutive infected total knee replacements with an average follow-up of 57 months. A two-stage procedure was successful in 100% (six of six) acute cases and in 91% (40 of 44) chronic infections.

Windsor et al[157] reported on the management of 38 infected total knee replacements (35 patients) using the technique first described by Insall et al at the Hospital for Special Surgery (HSS). Of these knees, eight had been previously reported by Insall et al.[76] At a mean follow-up of 4 years (range 2.5 to 10 years), infection recurred in one knee and reinfection with a different organism occurred in another two knees. If the successful eradication of infection is defined as the prevention of recurrent infection with the initial infecting organisms, the success rate is 97%. If all the reinfections are considered failures, the success rate is 89%.

Similarly, no recurrence of infection was reported by Teeny et al[147] in a series of seven knees that were treated using a two-stage exchange technique after failure of débridement and irrigation.

Whiteside[153] reported the results of two-stage exchange arthroplasty in 33 infected total knee replacements. Antibiotic-loaded bone cement beads were used between stages in addition to parenteral antibiotic therapy. In 28 knees, a single débridement was sufficient for control of infection. In four knees, one or two further débridements were required before reimplantation to control the infection. In one knee, infection could not be controlled, and the patient eventually underwent an above-knee amputation. In the 32 knees that were salvaged (97%), reimplantation was delayed by at least 6 weeks after the last débridement, and all revision prostheses were cementless and were implanted with antibiotic-loaded morselized allograft to fill bony defects.

Insall's group published their longer term results in 1996.[54] Sixty-four infected total knee replacements treated with the previously described two-stage protocol for reimplantation were reviewed at an average follow-up of 7.5 years (range 2 to 17 years). Six knees (9%) became reinfected, but only two with the same organism. The 10-year predicted survivorship of two-stage reimplantation for infection was 77.4%.

Backe et al,[5] in 1996, reported the results of two-stage reimplantation after previous two-stage excision arthroplasties. Twelve patients underwent salvage of reinfected total knee replacements. Nine of the patients underwent reimplantation surgery and three of the patients underwent arthrodesis. At an average 31 months follow-up, there was no evidence of reinfection. The three patients who did not undergo reimplantation surgery had solid fusions in good position but were less satisfied than those in whom a further prosthesis was inserted. The authors pointed out, however, that success is dependent on identifying the infecting organism, organizing effective antibiotic therapy, and ensuring that the patient is not immunosuppressed, has the potential for adequate soft-tissue cover, and has an intact extensor mechanism.

Role of Antibiotic-Loaded Bone Cement

Despite the excellent results obtained by Insall et al[76] and Windsor et al[157] in which two-stage exchange arthroplasty was performed without antibiotic-loaded bone cement, the current techniques of two-stage exchange arthroplasty include the use of antibiotic-loaded bone cement for fixation of the revision prosthesis at the second stage of the procedure. In a study of 89 infected total knee replacements,[62] the only factor that was found to correlate with a better result after two-stage exchange arthroplasty was the use of antibiotic-loaded bone cement for the fixation of the definitive prosthesis.

In a multicenter, randomized, prospective study

comparing gentamicin-loaded bead implantation to conventional parenteral antibiotic therapy in two-stage exchange arthroplasty for infected total hip and knee replacements, antibiotic-loaded bone cement beads seemed to have a protective effect compared with parenteral antibiotic therapy.[112] Infection recurred in fewer cases in the antibiotic-loaded cement bead group (2 of 15; 13%) than in the parenteral antibiotic group (4 of 13; 30%), but in view of the small numbers, this difference did not reach statistical significance.

Thus, removal of the infected hardware, along with adjunctive antibiotic therapy, both locally and systemically, appears to be the current gold standard initial treatment for the infected total knee arthroplasty. Reimplantation of a new total knee prosthesis, if technically feasible, is the most acceptable option after removal of the infected prosthesis.

ANTIBIOTICS IN BONE CEMENT

Up to 88% of physicians with an interest in adult joint reconstruction use antibiotic-loaded bone cement in their routine practice.[65] This reflects a rapid rise in the popularity of antibiotic-loaded cements in North America over the past decade.[47] A better understanding of the basic properties of antibiotic-loaded bone cement will allow the surgeon to use this material more effectively in the treatment of infected total knee replacements.

Elution

The elution properties of antibiotic bone cement have been thoroughly investigated over the past 2 decades. Both in vitro[2, 6, 9, 27, 28, 39, 44, 55, 68, 70, 80, 81, 85, 94] and in vivo[2, 6, 9, 17, 21, 27, 28, 44, 91, 93, 94, 138, 148, 149] studies showed that many commonly used antibiotics are released from bone cement in such a way that the local antibiotic levels vastly exceed the minimal inhibitory concentration of most susceptible pathogens. Moreover, these levels are much higher than those achieved with parenteral therapy.[17, 138] In general, most antibiotics elute rapidly, with maximum antibiotic release occurring during the first few days, followed by a rapid decrease in elution.[91, 148] The elution characteristics are influenced by the types and concentration of antibiotic used and by the type of bone cement,[91] any substances added to it,[81] its preparation,[4] its surface characteristics,[95] and its porosity.[6]

Of the bone cements in common use, Palacos R has the best in vitro elution characteristics.[44, 70, 91, 148] Each antibiotic has distinctive elution characteristics. For example, tobramycin elutes in much higher concentrations than vancomycin early on, but its in vitro elution also decays at a much faster rate than that of vancomycin.[94, 119] In combination, the two antibiotics appear to have a synergistic effect; the presence of tobramycin significantly improves the elution profile of vancomycin.[119] This has been termed “passive opportunism” and has been ascribed to the increased porosity of the cement with the presence and elution of one antibiotic improving the elution characteristics of the other.

Only a limited number of studies addressed the long-term elution of antibiotics from bone cement.[21, 27, 68, 93, 148] In an in vitro assay, clindamycin was found to elute for up to 56 days.[68] In rabbits, antibiotic-loaded cement pellets can elute antibiotics for up to 37 days.[27] In a series of 3 sheep with gentamicin-loaded bone cement within the femur, gentamicin levels in bone at 18 months after insertion of the antibiotic-loaded cement ranged from 7 to 36 mg/kg.[21]

The in vivo long-term elution of antibiotics in humans has been reported in two series.[93, 148] In 1 study, therapeutic levels of gentamicin were measured in the periprosthetic connective tissue, cancellous bone, or cortical bone in 17 patients several months after total hip arthroplasty with gentamicin-loaded bone cement.[148] In 1 patient, 5.75 years after surgery, gentamicin concentrations of 5.4 to 6.6 mg/kg of tissue (wet weight) and 6.6 mg/kg were measured from periprosthetic connective tissue and cancellous bone, respectively. In this study, the joint fluid was not assayed for gentamicin levels. The long-term antibiotic elution from the PROSTALAC hip[40, 79] and knee[97] systems was studied in 49 patients. The intra-articular antibiotic concentrations of tobramycin and vancomycin were measured at the removal of the PROSTALAC spacer.[93] This averaged 118 days from implantation. Tobramycin had superior and more reliable elution characteristics. Therapeutic tobramycin levels were maintained throughout the study period, particularly when 3.6 g per 40-g package of bone cement was used. The breakpoint sensitivity limit is defined as the antimicrobial level that marks the transition between bacterial susceptibility and the induction of bacterial resistance. The use of 3.6 g of tobramycin kept the elution above the breakpoint sensitivity limit throughout the study period. This study confirmed the in vivo passive opportunism of combining the two antibiotics. These findings also suggested that it was preferable to use vancomycin in combination with tobramycin in bone cement rather than using it as the only antibiotic.[93]

It should also be noted that even when antibiotics stop eluting from bone cement, there are still antibiotic stores that can be released if the cement surface is violated. This occurs at the time of revision surgery; samples should, therefore, be taken for culture before the cement is split.

Not only does antibiotic-loaded bone cement allow the elution of high levels of antibiotics into the periprosthetic milieu, but it has been shown that antibiotics within bone cement implanted within the medullary cavity of a cadaver femur are able to permeate through dead cortical bone.[45] This finding has obvious therapeutic advantages in the case of the severely infected total knee arthroplasty with osteomyelitis and devascularization.

The safety of this form of antibiotic depot has also been clearly established. In our own patients treated with antibiotic-loaded bone cement for infected hip and knee arthroplasties, we have never been able to measure tobramycin or vancomycin serum levels higher than 3 mg/L. This has also been shown by other investigators both in humans and in animal models.[1, 27, 44, 70, 91, 149] Care should be taken, however, if autotransfusion of drainage fluid is considered in such cases. This may add to the systemic antibiotic load and could potentially take blood levels over the toxic threshold.

Baker and Greenham,[6] through in vivo and in vitro studies with scanning electron microscopy, described the mechanism of elution of antibiotics from bone cement. The release of antibiotics occurs only from the surface through voids and cracks in the bone cement. They concluded that increasing the concentration of antibiotics within the bone cement would improve the elution characteristics of antibiotics. This was confirmed in human studies by Wahlig et al,[149] who showed that doubling the concentration of gentamicin from 0.5 g to 1.0 g per 40 g of cement doubled the concentration of gentamicin in wound secretions. Baker and Greenham[6] also concluded that bone cements with a higher porosity would be expected to allow higher antibiotic release than those with a lower porosity. Moreover, they hypothesized that methods of cement preparation that are designed to minimize porosity (such as vacuum mixing or centrifugation) could have a deleterious effect on antibiotic elution.

Biomechanics

The change in mechanical strength of antibiotic-loaded bone cement compared with plain cement has also been studied[7, 36, 83, 84, 106, 113, 159] both in static and dynamic/fatigue situations. The addition of small amounts of antibiotics in powder form does not seem to weaken bone cement significantly,[36, 83] whereas the addition of antibiotics in the liquid form causes significant weakening.[84] Other studies showed that the addition of any amount of antibiotic powder will cause some weakening of the antibiotic - bone cement composite.[7, 106] The degree of weakening depends on the proportional weight of antibiotics added to the bone cements.[83] Centrifugation may improve the fatigue properties of some antibiotic-loaded bone cements.[36] Lautenschlager et al[83] showed that mixing more than 4.5 g of gentamicin sulfate can significantly weaken bone cement to the point that its compressive strength is decreased to below the minimum acceptable standards. This was only when samples were tested in compression. Fatigue testing of the cement is difficult to perform because physiological cycling would require a very prolonged period of time, but there is some evidence that antibiotic-loaded cement weakens with time.[113] The present consensus in the literature suggests that a limit of about 2 g of antibiotic powder per 40 g of bone cement appears to be a safe estimate for the maximum allowable concentration of antibiotics in bone cement (5% of the mass), if the fatigue life of the acrylic is important. These limits do not necessarily apply when antibiotics are added to bone cement in temporary spacers, which are removed after a few weeks or months in a two-stage exchange arthroplasty.

Further Considerations

The role of bone cement in both encouraging or preventing infection has been debated. Petty and others expressed concern regarding the potential deleterious effects of bone cement on the immune system.[82, 118, 121-124, 140] Concerns have also been expressed regarding the ability of bacteria to survive on antibiotic-loaded cement.[3, 25-26, 78, 89, 111] This has, however, not been the case in human in vivo retrieval studies.[78] Kendall et al[78] examined antibiotic loaded cement and tissues obtained at the second stage of two-stage revisions for infection. No organisms were cultured from the surface of any of the specimens. These findings have been corroborated in animal studies.[45, 89]

Another possible advantage to the use of antibiotic-loaded bone cement is its potential role in decreasing bacterial adherence. In one study, the adherence of *S. epidermidis* was reduced when tobramycin was added to bone cement.[115] Another study showed that the use of clindamycin can inhibit glycocalix production in an experimental streptococcal endocarditis model.[34] Whether such an interaction is applicable in the case of orthopedic implant infections remains to be seen.

The antibiotics that are added to bone cement are chosen according to the sensitivity profile of the infecting organisms. The choice of antibiotic also depends on the criteria outlined by Murray.[109] These include antibiotic safety, thermostability, hypoallergenicity, water solubility, adequate bactericidal spectrum, and availability in a sterile powder form. In a minority of cases, in which the most appropriate antibiotic is available only in liquid form, the liquid may be lyophilized under sterile conditions, and a sterile powder may be obtained, on a customized basis. This, however, requires highly specialized facilities.

Some antibiotics should not be routinely mixed with bone cement. Penicillin and its derivatives may be inactivated by cement polymerization.[148-149] Lincomycin, chloramphenicol, and tetracycline are also inactivated by the polymerization process, and rifampicin produces a black tacky composite that does not harden for several days.[10, 86]

Clinical Studies

Antibiotic-loaded cement beads have been used in the management of open fractures and soft-tissue and bone infections.[66-67, 90, 127] A variety of organisms and infections have been addressed, including those caused by mycobacteria and methicillin-resistant *S. aureus*.[96, 117]

Since Buchholz et al[18-20] successfully demonstrated that antibiotics can elute from the surface of bone cement in concentrations sufficient to achieve local control of the infection in the periprosthetic space, it has become common practice to use antibiotic-loaded cement in the reimplantation phase after septic failure of a total joint replacement. Antibiotic-loaded cement beads have been used to occupy the medullary canal after removal of infected total hip prostheses.[42, 73] Likewise, antibiotic-loaded cement spacers have been used after removal of infected total knee implants.[15, 29, 102, 107, 156] These are discussed in the next section.

McLaren and Spooner reported the use of an antibiotic-loaded cement spacer with retention of the knee prosthesis.[99] The infected knee is thoroughly débrided, and all modular components are removed. The bone-cement-implant interface is then carefully assessed. If this is intact, the decision is made to retain the prosthesis. It is washed with 0.125% sodium hypochlorite to penetrate the biofilm. The remaining dead space is then filled with bone cement loaded with high doses of vancomycin (4 g per packet), tobramycin (3.6 g per packet), and cefoxitin (6 g per packet). Their preliminary data suggest that this leads to sufficient antibiotic concentrations to penetrate the biofilm. The knee is then redébrided at 3 weeks, followed by 6 weeks of parenteral antibiotics and then 6 weeks of oral antibiotics. The knee is then left for a minimum of 4 weeks before serological reinvestigation and aspiration. The modular parts are then reimplanted. The authors reported no evidence of reinfection at 18-month follow-up in four knees treated using this protocol. They also noted similar success with other infected joints, including some polymicrobial infections. Although this represents the short-term follow-up of a very small number of patients, this technique is worthy of further consideration for the well-fixed infected total knee replacement.

There is a negative side to the routine use of antibiotic-loaded cement. In a review of 246 infected total hip replacements between 1976 and 1987, Hope et al[72] reported that 91 cases were caused by coagulase-negative staphylococci. Twenty-seven of these were caused by two or more strains of this organism. It was found that in 30 of 34 (88%) patients whose primary arthroplasty contained gentamicin-loaded bone cement, at least one of the infecting strains of *Staphylococcus* was resistant to gentamicin. In contrast, only nine of 57 (16%) patients whose index arthroplasty did not contain gentamicin-loaded cement grew gentamicin-resistant coagulase-negative staphylococci. These findings are echoed in the current concern and debate over the emergence of vancomycin-resistant bacteria.[37, 49, 87, 98, 103, 104, 114, 151, 152] We no longer advocate the use of vancomycin alone, and are moving away from its inclusion in bone cement unless indicated by the sensitivities of the infecting organisms. Because of this tendency toward the emergence of resistant strains when antibiotic-loaded bone cement is used, the prophylactic use of antibiotic cement should be approached with caution, and it should only be used when the anticipated benefits outweigh the potential risks.

EVOLUTION OF TWO-STAGE EXCHANGE ARTHROPLASTY WITH A SPACER

The steadily improving results of reimplantation for the treatment of the infected total knee replacement have been achieved using two-stage exchange arthroplasty protocols. However, the efficacy of the two-stage exchange arthroplasty in the treatment of the infected total knee arthroplasty does not come without a price. In addition to having to perform two surgical procedures, the other disadvantages include

- The patient is uncomfortable, discouraged, and often confined to the hospital with limited mobility and activity during the interval between the two procedures.
- The delayed reimplantation procedures are technically more difficult because of scar formation, shortening, disuse osteoporosis, and distorted anatomy.
- It may be difficult to stabilize a limb between stages when a major bone deficit exists, and immobilization in a brace or cast may be necessary.

Almost 20% of Insall's patients had a less than optimal result directly or indirectly attributable to the delay between the two stages.[74, 76, 157] The knee between the two stages is flail and painful and is incapable of a normal range of motion and weightbearing. This contributes to joint contractures and muscle weakness, making postoperative rehabilitation after the second stage more difficult and possibly contributing to a worse functional result. The analgesic and nursing requirements are increased, and the mobilization of the patient is restricted, thus increasing the morbidity of the procedure. The exposure for the reimplantation procedure is generally difficult, and skeletization of the distal femur is often required. Because of tension on the extensor mechanism, a Coonse-Adams quadriceps turn-down,[30] or one of its modifications, or a tibial tubercle osteotomy may be required.[23] The scarring and shortening may ultimately necessitate flap soft-tissue cover or the use of soft-tissue expansion techniques.[110]

Several techniques can help preserve limb length and minimize soft-tissue contractures, including a variety of antibiotic-loaded bone cement spacer blocks and articulated spacers. In addition to their ability to elute high levels of antibiotics, these spacer blocks, in contrast to antibiotic-loaded cement beads, decrease the scarring within the joint space and facilitate reimplantation. The use of these spacers was first reported in 1988. Cohen et al[29] reported on three patients treated with this method. Infection was controlled in all three patients, and the authors were able to successfully implant a well-functioning total knee replacement as late as 6 months after removing the infected implants. Wilde and Ruth[156] reported a series of 21 infected total knee arthroplasties treated using a two-stage exchange technique, but only 15 cases had a follow-up longer than 1 year. A spacer block was used in 10 of these cases. The mean delay between stages

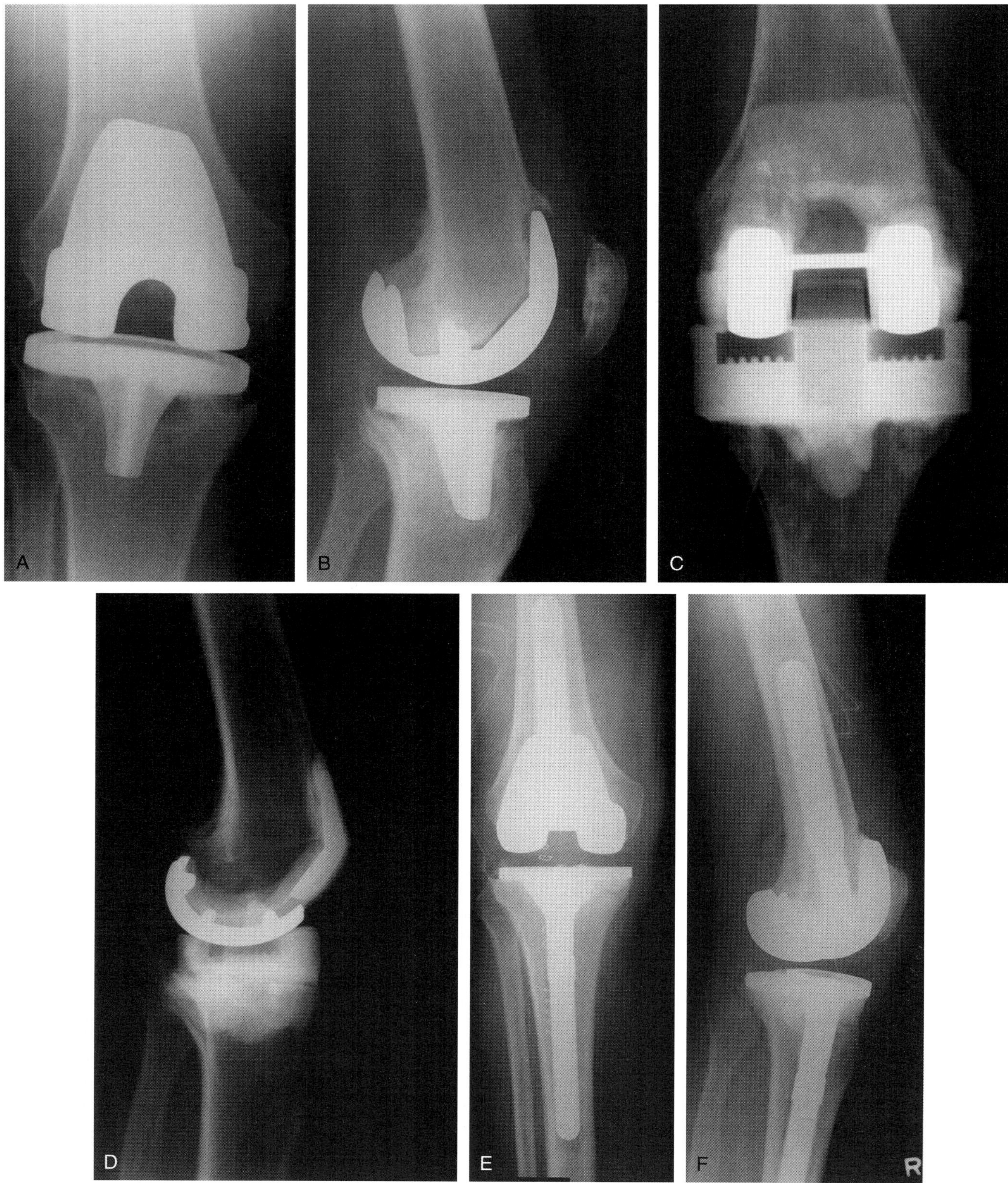

FIGURE 91.2 ➢ *A* and *B*, Preoperative radiographs of loose infected total knee arthroplasty. *C* and *D*, Radiographs of the PROSTALAC articulated spacer during the interval period. *E* and *F*, Radiographs of reconstruction performed after a 3-month interval period.

was 6 weeks, and the mean duration of intravenous antibiotic therapy was 4.2 weeks. Of the 10 patients with spacers, there were no definite infections, and one patient was presumed infected and underwent revision elsewhere, for an infection control rate of 90%. Although these numbers are small, the presence of a spacer did not seem to have a detrimental effect on infection control. In a larger series of infected knee replacements treated with two-stage exchange arthroplasty with an interim antibiotic-loaded cement spacer, Booth and Lotke[14] reported one failure among 25 cases, with a mean follow-up of 25 months. The delay between stages ranged from 3 weeks to 17 months, and even at 17 months, a successful arthroplasty was achieved with a range of motion of 0 to 105 degrees. The authors believed that the reimplantation was facilitated by the presence of the spacer and that the use of cement spacers enhanced bone quality.

These blocks are usually handmade in the operating room and are sized to fit the defect created by removal of the infected prosthesis. Ideally, a small cement stem should be fashioned and added to the spacer block to allow anchoring of the block to the tibia and prevent its migration. Moreover, a thin layer of cement between the femur and the patella may prevent the scarring of the extensor mechanism to the distal femur. In most cases, a minimum of two packs of bone cement are required. Despite these efforts, in our experience, the revision procedure is still difficult and scarring still substantial, particularly in the lateral and medial gutters. In our opinion, the patient should not be allowed to move the knee with the spacer in place, and full weightbearing should be discouraged because of the risk of bone erosion with a mobile one-piece spacer, especially in patients with weak bone. These spacers should not be used if further surgery is not possible, and excision arthroplasty will be the definitive method of treatment because of the risk of dislodgment as well as the risk of this spacer acting as a foreign body after elution of the antibiotics within the surface layer of the spacer. Calton et al[23] studied the bone loss during treatment of 25 knees with infected total knee replacements managed with débridement, component removal, and insertion of an antibiotic-loaded cement spacer block. During the interval period, the patients' knees were kept in a knee immobilizer, and they were not allowed to bear weight. Tibial bone loss was present in 10 (40%) cases and averaged 6.2 mm. Femoral bone loss was present in 11 (44%) cases and averaged 12.8 mm. Bone loss was more common when spacer blocks were undersized. None of the 15 spacer blocks that were made with a small intramedullary stem displaced. Three of the remaining 10 spacer blocks made without an intramedullary stem did displace with associated bone loss. They recommended the use of intramedullary extensions, while ensuring that the spacer rests on the cortical rim of the femur and tibia to minimize invagination into the soft cancellous bone. They also emphasized the importance of maintaining collateral ligament tension and the full extension gap to prevent varus-valgus instability.

ARTICULATED SPACERS IN TWO-STAGE EXCHANGE ARTHROPLASTY

As a corollary to the increased ease in reimplantation that Booth and Lotke[14] noted, and as a solution to some of the problems later noted by Calton et al,[23] the presence of a spacer that allows not only distraction of the joint space but also motion between stages would be expected to even further increase the ease of revision and potentially improve the final functional outcome. Articulated spacers allow the patient some function between stages, maintain the soft tissues out to length, and decrease scarring within the periprosthetic tissues (Fig. 91.2).

In addition to the PROSTALAC system, which was first reported in 1992,[41] several other articulated spacer systems have been described.[22, 71, 100, 101, 141] The advantages of such articulated spacers include continued mobility, ease of rehabilitation, and ease of reimplantation (Fig. 91.3). Moreover, a higher antibiotic dose can be added to the bone cement in a spacer than in a one-stage exchange or a definitive reimplantation when the antibiotic dose has to be limited because of the risk of weakening of the cement. The disadvantages amount to the increased cost of the prosthesis that is used as a spacer and later discarded.

In 1993, Scott et al[141] described a novel modification of two-stage exchange arthroplasty. In this technique, the infected implant and all cement are removed at first stage. After a thorough débridement and irrigation, antibiotic-loaded cement beads are threaded on a braided wire, and the beads are inserted within any open medullary canals and also within the joint space. A sterile prosthesis is then loosely cemented with antibiotic-loaded bone cement to act as a spacer and to allow motion. At 6 weeks, a definitive reimplantation using antibiotic-loaded bone cement is performed. The antibiotics that are added to bone cement are chosen based on the sensitivity profile of the infecting organisms. All seven knees treated using this modified two-stage exchange arthroplasty were free of infection at final review.

A similar articulated spacer technique was described by Hoffmann et al.[71] A two-stage exchange technique is used, with a 6-week interval between stages. After an adequate débridement at the first stage, the removed femoral component is flash sterilized and is reinserted with antibiotic-loaded bone cement at a late stage in cement polymerization to prevent thorough interdigitation between the cement and bone and facilitate the removal of the component at the second stage. On the tibial side, a new polyethylene liner of an adequate thickness is likewise fixed loosely with antibiotic-loaded bone cement. Tobramycin was used in bone cement, at a dosage level of 4.8 g of tobramycin per 40-g package of Simplex P (Howmedica, Rutherford, NJ) bone cement. After 6 weeks of intravenous antibiotic therapy, this temporary spacer is removed, and a knee replacement is reimplanted using antibiotic-impregnated bone cement. At a mean follow-up of 30 months, with a minimum follow-up of 13 months,

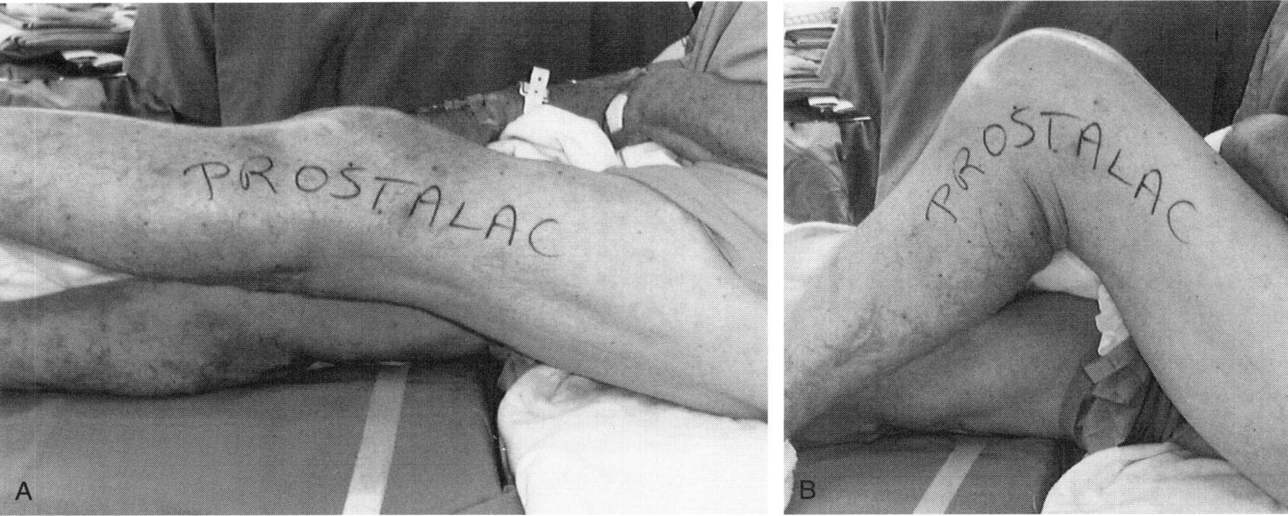

FIGURE 91.3 ➢ Typical range of motion with PROSTALAC articulated spacer. These photographs *(A,B)* were taken before reimplantation. The patient was able to move the knee actively through this range without significant discomfort.

there was no reinfection in 25 infected knee replacements.

Cadambi et al[22] described another similar technique for the treatment of infected knee and hip replacements. The surgical technique is similar to that described by Scott et al.[141] The only difference is that reimplantation was performed only 2 weeks after the first stage of the procedure, and parenteral antibiotic therapy was continued for 6 weeks after reimplantation. Eleven infected knee replacements were treated using this protocol. Infection was controlled in all but one knee. The only failure was in a 72-year-old diabetic with congestive heart failure and peripheral vascular disease. McPherson et al[101] reported on the use of a handmade facsimile of a knee replacement that is inserted between stages in a two-stage exchange protocol. This handmade facsimile is made of antibiotic-loaded bone cement. This allows motion and partial weightbearing between stages. Because of this crude design, stability was not well maintained, and a knee immobilizer was required for walking.

Notably, all of these articulated spacer protocols were developed independently over the past few years at a variety of centers. This reflects the difficulty encountered with reimplantation after a standard excision arthroplasty. It also potentially reflects the dissatisfaction of both the patient and the surgeon with the function between stages when the patient is left without a functional knee joint. Like others, we have also been dissatisfied with patients' function between stages, hence the development of PROSTALAC, beginning in 1987. This modified two-stage exchange protocol combines many of the features of the aforementioned articulated spacers. The difference is that it allows intraoperative flexibility regardless of the intraoperative findings, while using the least possible amount of metal and plastic within the joint.

PROSTALAC SYSTEM

The purpose of this system is to allow mobility and protected weightbearing between stages while maintaining adequate soft tissue tension and joint stability. It is also intended to simplify the reimplantation procedure. Because excellent function is maintained between stages, the patient may be discharged from hospital, thus greatly reducing costs.

System Design and Evolution

The PROSTALAC prototype was first implanted in 1987. This was a handmade facsimile of a total knee replacement prosthesis made entirely of antibiotic-loaded bone cement. Because of the difficulty in fashioning a smooth articular surface using a handmade technique, the first-generation PROSTALAC was introduced in early 1991. This was also a facsimile of a knee replacement with a cement on cement articulation. The articular surfaces on the femoral and tibial components, however, were smooth because of the introduction of a flexible polyethylene mold that allowed the creation of smooth articular surfaces. For the most part, motion was painless, and a range of flexion of at least 75 degrees was the norm. However, patients complained that motion was quite noisy because of the high friction, and painless crepitus was easily audible. The normal rhythm of gait was disrupted, and their movement appeared awkward. A further problem was both posterior and mediolateral knee instability. Because the molds were flexible, it was difficult to control the thickness of the femoral and tibial components adequately, and sufficient restoration of the level of joint line, as well as soft-tissue balancing, was difficult. The design also did not allow substitution of posterior cruciate ligament function, which is commonly absent in cases of infected total knee replacement. These problems have been addressed in the current design. The difficulty with the high-friction articulation was solved by the addition of small stainless-steel femoral runners and polyethylene tibial skids. To avoid the use of large amount of metal and plastic, the design of the tibial skid was quite flat because a conforming tibial skid would require much thicker polyethylene. The design was also changed to that of a posterior-stabilized prosthesis, with a cement post on the tibial component and a small metal bar connecting the two femoral runners so that a cam mechanism is created. Despite this modification, the amount of metal and plastic within this spacer is still small, and the majority of the exposed surface of the implant is made of antibiotic-loaded bone cement (Fig. 91.4). The flexible polyethylene molds have also been replaced with more rigid modular molds that allow the easy production of different component sizes and permit accurate determination of the distal thickness of the femoral component and the total thickness of the tibial component.

The thickness of the femoral and tibial components required is determined on the basis of intraoperative measurements using any revision total knee system. Specific trial components for the PROSTALAC system are now in production. In the meantime, trial implants from any revision knee system can be adapted and used. With the ability to manufacture the femoral and tibial components intraoperatively, the joint line can be accurately reproduced, and knee kinematics and stability are improved. When the collateral ligaments are absent and a constrained knee is required, a hinged knee brace could be used postoperatively so that knee stability is maintained. Motion and protected weightbearing are encouraged.

Surgical Technique

This is a modified two-stage exchange arthroplasty, as described by Insall et al.[76] At the first stage, the infected implants are removed with all the residual cement. It is our policy to remove all cement at the first stage, using a combination of hand and power instruments. In some cases, an intraoperative radiograph may help visualize any retained cement. A wide exposure is required to remove the components and perform a thorough débridement. In many of our cases a rectus "snip," as described by Insall,[75] or in some cases a modified Coonse-Adams turn-down may be required.[24, 30]

One or more components may be loose, or all implants may be rigidly fixed. The removal of a rigidly fixed cementless femoral component is greatly facilitated by the use of flexible osteotomes. A Gigli saw may also be passed at the prosthetic interface to facilitate the breakdown of the areas of bone ingrowth. Once the implant has been loosened, a variety of extraction devices may be used. For the rigidly cemented femoral component, similar techniques may be used; however, great care has to be taken to remain within the prosthetic-cement interface and not the bone-cement interface. As with any revision surgery, caution is necessary so as not to sacrifice bone stock unnecessarily. Similar techniques may be used for the removal of the tibial component, although the Gigli saw is more difficult to apply. Proximal skeletization of the tibia may be necessary but should be limited so as not to devitalize the bone.

Several specimens should be obtained for culture and sensitivity. We generally obtain samples from the capsule, the synovial lining, the membrane at the femoral, tibial, and patellar interfaces, as well as the medullary canals of the tibia and femur if applicable. Systemic antibiotics are withheld until adequate samples are obtained. These samples should be sent for aerobic, anaerobic, mycobacterial, and fungal cultures. A thorough synovectomy should then be performed. All devitalized tissue and all metal and polyethylene wear debris should be removed. The knee should then be copiously irrigated using several liters of an antibiotic-containing saline solution. At the end of the débridement and irrigation, the appearance of the knee joint should be not unlike that of a knee joint that is being revised for aseptic reasons.

After débridement, the knee is prepared for a revision knee replacement, and very modest preliminary bone cuts are made removing minimal bone. The flexion and extension spaces are then measured, and the position of the joint line is estimated. A decision is then made on the required thickness of the components of the PROSTALAC implants. Distal femoral deficiencies are made up by increasing the distal thickness of the PROSTALAC femoral component. The minimum thickness of the femoral component is 12.5 mm. This may be increased by 5, 10, or 15 mm if necessary. Posterior deficiencies are simply made up with bone cement when the final implant is inserted. Likewise, the desired thickness of the tibial component is determined. Each tibial size allows an implant thickness ranging from 12 mm to 34 mm (Fig. 91.5).

While the knee is being prepared for reimplantation, an assistant assembles the PROSTALAC molds and manufactures the required implants. Each PROSTALAC component is custom made in the operating room to suit the needs of the individual patient. The antibiotics are selected based on the sensitivity profile of the infecting organism. In most cases, however, a combination of tobramycin and vancomycin is adequate. Based on studies of the long-term antibiotic concentrations within the joint after insertion of PROSTALAC implants,[93] we currently recommend the use of 3.6 g of tobramycin and 1.0 g of vancomycin. We do not recommend the use of vancomycin alone because its elution properties, when used alone, are not as reliable as when used in combination with tobramycin. This has been demonstrated in both in vitro[119] and in vivo[93, 94] studies. We also recommend the use of Palacos R bone cement because of its more favorable antibiotic elution characteristics.

The femoral component is manufactured as shown in Figure 91.6. The femoral skids are placed within their respective cavities in mold no. 1 (Fig 91.6A and B). Antibiotic-loaded Palacos R cement is then poured

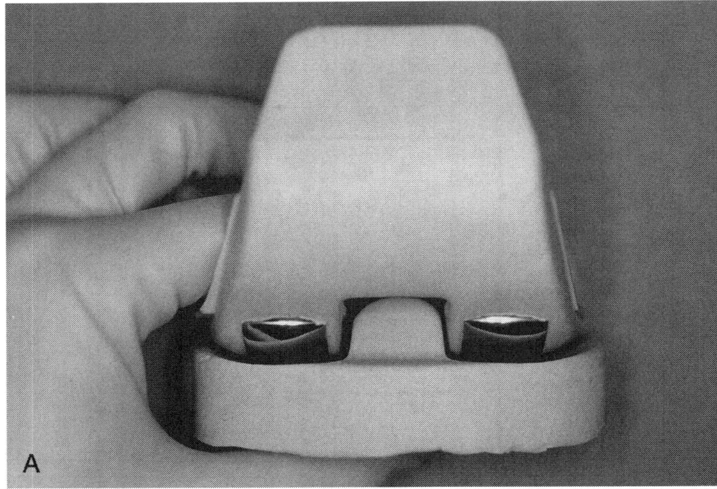

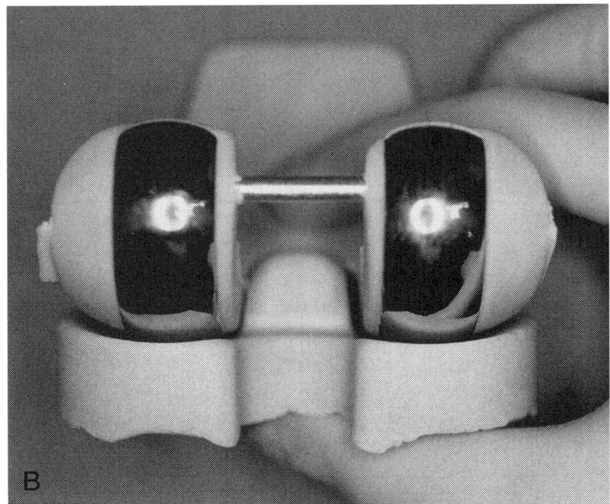

FIGURE 91.4 ➢ Anterior *(A)* and posterior *(B)* views of the PROSTALAC components. The cam mechanism prevents posterior dislocation of the tibia.

into the mold, and the appropriate size mold no. 2 is chosen to provide the required distal femoral thickness (Fig 91.6C). Mold no. 2 is inserted within mold no. 1, and its thickness determines the final distal thickness of the PROSTALAC component (Fig 91.6D).

The tibial component is manufactured in the operating room using a similar technique. The tibial skids are placed within their respective cavities within tibial mold no. 1 (Fig. 91.7A), and antibiotic-loaded Palacos R cement is then poured into the mold. Mold no. 2 is then used to obtain the appropriate thickness of the tibial component (Fig 91.7B and C).

Once the cement has hardened, the implants are removed from the molds (Fig. 91.8) and are cemented to the host bone (Fig. 91.9) at a late stage of antibiotic-cement polymerization. This is to allow some fixation but not such solid fixation that removal of the implants at the second stage will remove valuable bone stock. Excessive pressurization of the bone cement is avoided. Bone cement is used to fill any bone defects that are not filled by the PROSTALAC implant. The patella is not resurfaced, but great care is taken to ensure appropriate rotation of the femoral and tibial components, and a lateral retinacular release is performed if needed. This minimizes the risk of patellar instability, which was a problem early in our experience with this system.

Postoperatively, the knee is wrapped in a modified Robert Jones bandage for 24 to 48 hours. The patient is then allowed to walk with partial weightbearing.

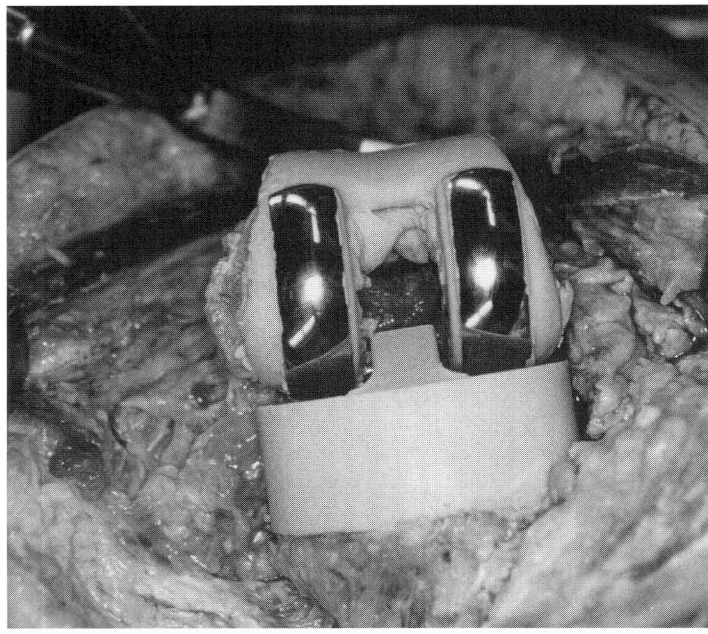

FIGURE 91.5 ➢ Intraoperative photograph of a PROSTALAC spacer for which a thick tibial component was required.

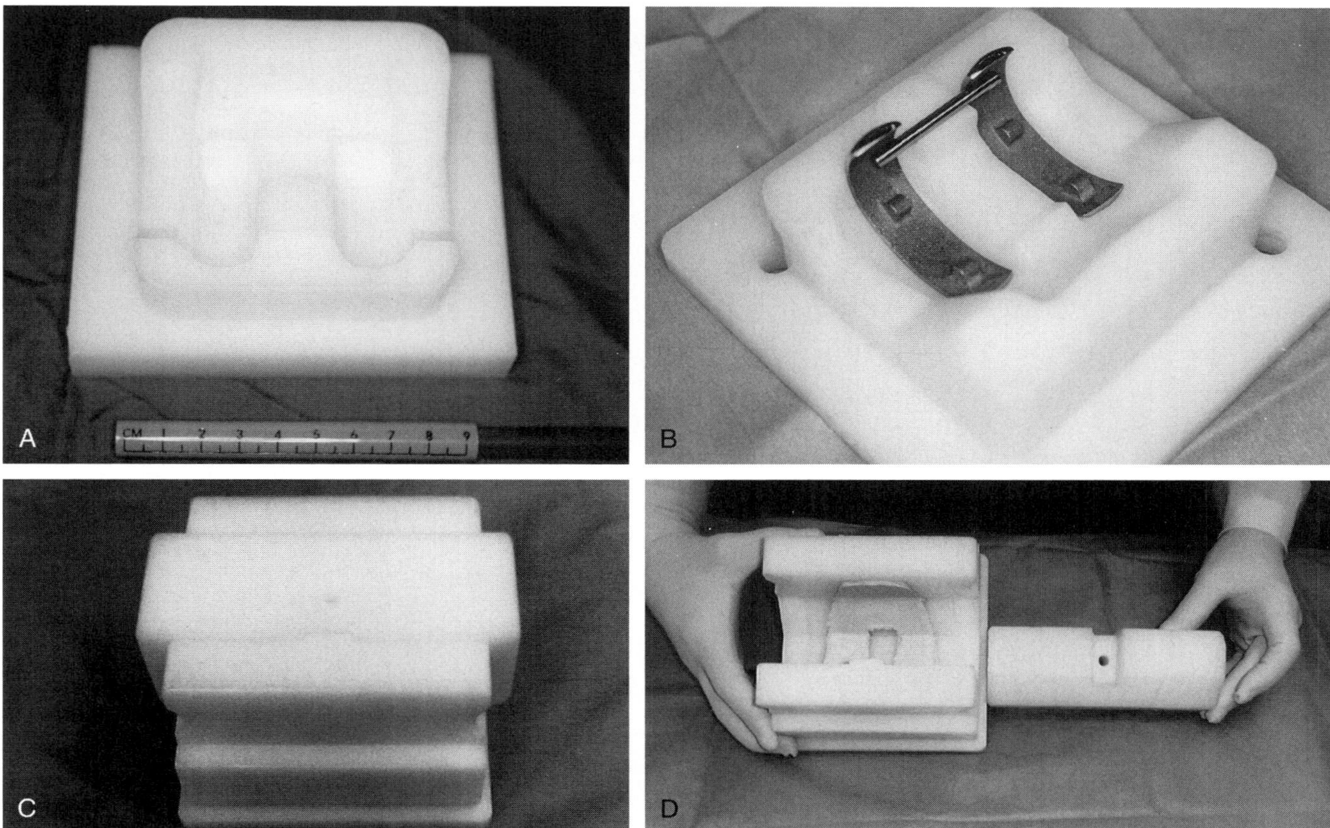

FIGURE 91.6 ➢ Intraoperative manufacture of the femoral component. The appropriate size femoral mold *(A)* and skids *(B)* are chosen. Antibiotic-loaded Palacos R cement is then poured into the mold, and the appropriate size mold no. 2 is chosen to provide the required distal femoral thickness *(C)*. Once the cement has cured *(D)*, mold no. 2 is removed and the femoral component extracted.

Free knee motion is encouraged without a brace, unless collateral insufficiency was detected intraoperatively. In such cases, a hinged knee brace is used, but the hinges are unlocked to allow free mobility. The patient is then treated at home or at an outside facility with a 3- to 6-week course of intravenous antibiotics. Four weeks after the discontinuation of antibiotics, a repeat aspiration biopsy is performed to confirm eradication of infection (Fig. 91.10). We do not routinely measure minimum bactericidal levels, as suggested by Insall et al[76] and Windsor et al.[157] Physiotherapy is continued between stages, with an emphasis on range of motion and muscle strengthening.

Three months after the first stage, the patient is readmitted to our hospital for reimplantation (Fig. 91.11). It is not always possible to follow this schedule precisely, and some leeway is allowed depending on the specific circumstances. In our experience, reimplantation is greatly facilitated by the presence of the PROSTALAC spacer. A rectus snip is nevertheless often required for exposure. A standard revision knee replacement is then performed. Intraoperative cultures are obtained and prophylactic antibiotics then administered. Removal of the PROSTALAC is easy and is accomplished in a few minutes. The cement is fractured with the use of an osteotome, and the fragmented components are then removed piecemeal. A thorough débridement and irrigation are performed, and the revision components are implanted. Antibiotic-loaded bone cement is used for the fixation of the components. If tobramycin is an appropriate antibiotic, we use 0.6 g of tobramycin per package of bone cement. If the infecting organism is not sensitive to tobramycin, another appropriate antibiotic is chosen. Regardless of the type of antibiotic, we prefer not to exceed 1 to 1.2 g of antibiotic per 40-g package of bone cement because of the risk of weakening the cement. Intravenous antibiotics are continued for 5 days postoperatively and are discontinued when the final results of intraoperative cultures are reported as negative.

Clinical Results

A total of 44 patients were treated for a diagnosis of an infected total knee arthroplasty between April 1987 and June 1994. Nine patients were excluded from this series for a variety of reasons that made reconstruction using the PROSTALAC system not feasible. Two patients underwent a two-stage exchange procedure using a block-and-bead antibiotic-loaded cement spacer between stages before the PROSTALAC system became our routine. One patient had bone and soft-tissue loss

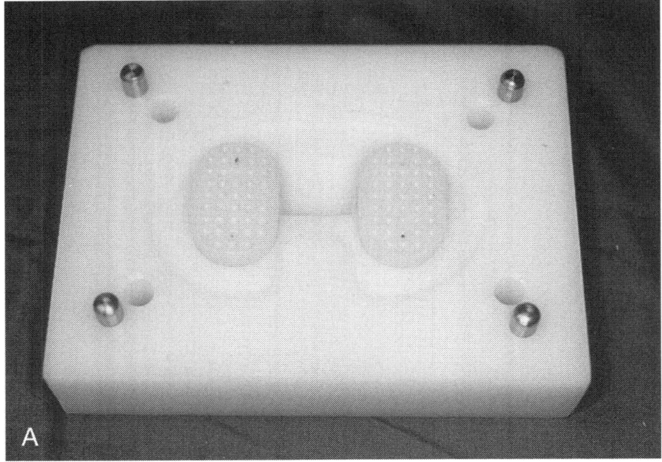

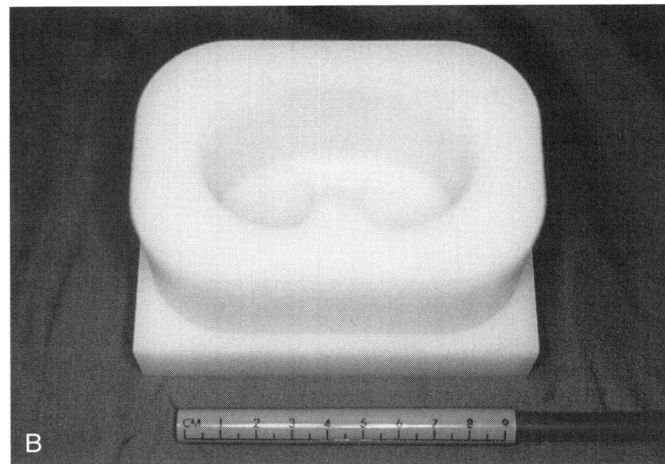

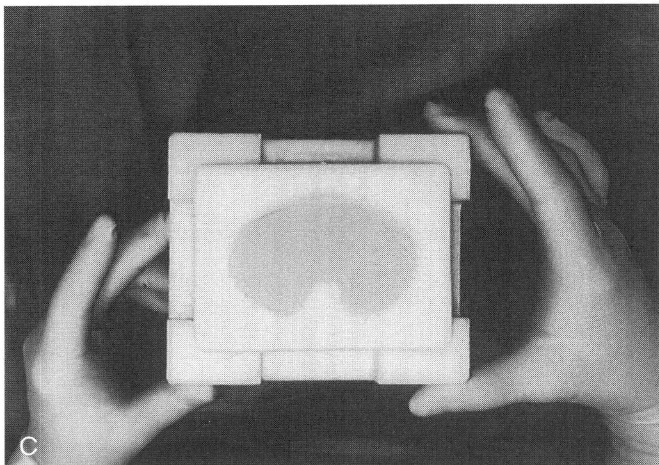

FIGURE 91.7 ➢ Intraoperative manufacture of the tibial component. The appropriate size of tibial mold and skids are chosen *(A)*. Antibiotic-loaded Palacos-R cement is then poured into the mold. Mold no. 2 *(B)* is then used to obtain the appropriate thickness of the PROSTALAC tibial component *(C)*.

that was so severe that reconstruction with the first-generation PROSTALAC implant was not possible. A block-and-bead antibiotic-loaded cement spacer was used between stages instead. This could now be reconstructed with the posterior-stabilized PROSTALAC, which was not available at that time. One patient underwent an above-knee amputation because of severe bone and soft-tissue loss, with loss of the extensor mechanism. A knee arthrodesis was performed in two patients in whom knee joint salvage was not technically feasible. Another patient underwent an uncomplicated first-stage replacement with the PROSTALAC prosthesis; however, while awaiting reimplantation, the patient died of unrelated causes and was, therefore, not included in the final analysis. A 26-year-old patient with severe juvenile rheumatoid arthritis had just undergone a revision knee arthroplasty using a custom long-stem femoral component. The femoral component was rigidly fixed, and removal of this prosthesis would have compromised bone stock. We elected to treat this patient with the unusual combination of débridement, retention of the femoral component, and removal of the tibial component and replacement with a highly antibiotic-loaded cement spacer with a thin polyethylene articular surface. This was subsequently revised as a preplanned second-stage procedure. Four years after surgery, there is no evidence of recurrent infection. The last patient who was not thought to be a candidate for two-stage exchange arthroplasty using the PROSTALAC system was 76 years old and had severe rheumatoid arthritis and a polyarticular deep infection affecting one knee, one hip, and one elbow. Because of frail health and polyarticular involvement, he was treated with débridement and irrigation and suppressive antibiotics. This patient died 2 years later from unrelated causes.

In addition to the remaining 35 patients with infected knee replacements, one patient with bilateral long-standing deep infections affecting both knee joints was included in this series. This 38-year-old patient had a history of chronic renal failure and previous renal transplantation. He had end-stage osteonecrosis of both femoral condyles and the right femoral head secondary to corticosteroids. He also had multifocal *Mycoplasma* septic arthritis affecting both knees and shoulders. In preparation for bilateral knee replacements, he was treated with the PROSTALAC knee system as if he had had an infected total knee arthroplasty because of the chronicity of the infection (more than 2 years) and because of end-stage degeneration.

A total of 36 patients (17 men and 19 women) with 37 infected knees, with a minimum 2-year follow-up,

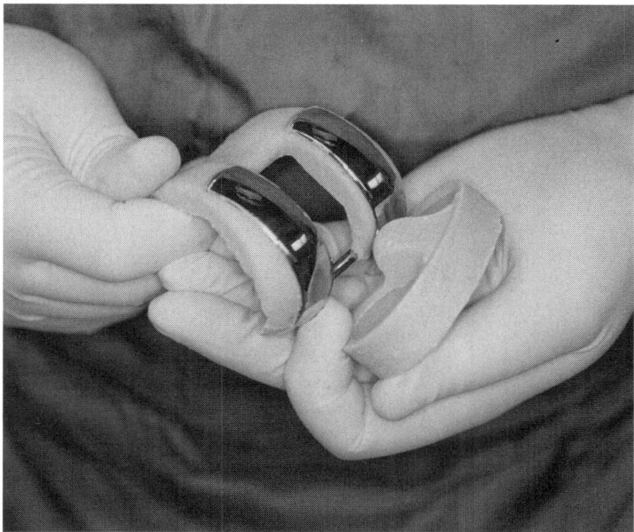

FIGURE 91.8 ➢ The PROSTALAC femoral and tibial components before insertion.

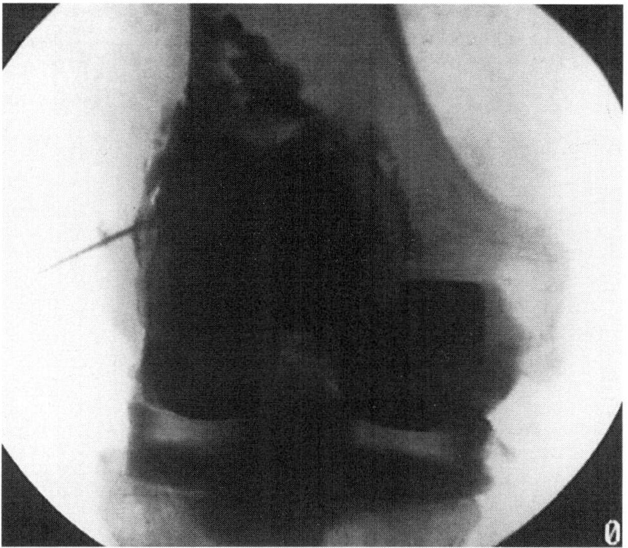

FIGURE 91.10 ➢ Aspiration biopsy 4 weeks after discontinuation of antibiotic therapy. The radiopaque dye was used to confirm the intra-articular location of the needle.

are, therefore, included in this series. The mean age was 66.2 years (range 26 to 83 years). The underlying diagnosis was osteoarthritis in 26, rheumatoid arthritis in four, post-traumatic arthritis in two, osteonecrosis in three, hemophilic arthropathy in one, and neuropathic arthropathy in one. Twelve patients (13 knees) were immunocompromised or at a high risk of infection. Four patients had rheumatoid arthritis, one of whom was still on corticosteroid therapy, one was treated with chemotherapy for chronic lymphocytic leukemia, one patient (two knees) was on chronic immunosuppressive therapy for a renal transplant, one patient was infected with HIV, three were diabetic, one had chronic lymphedema and recurrent cellulitis affecting the ipsilateral lower extremity, and one had renal calculi with recurrent urinary tract infections. The mean number of previous procedures was 2.4 (range 0 to 8). These procedures included nine patients who had already undergone a débridement and irrigation for infection without success. One of these patients had undergone two débridements without success. One patient had undergone excision ar-

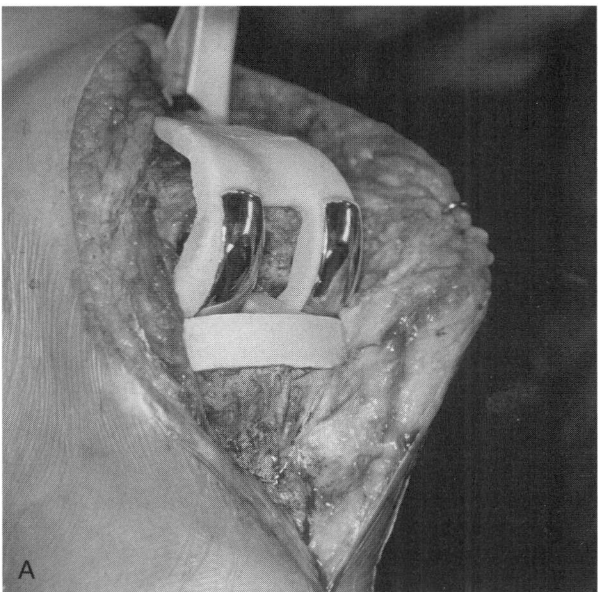

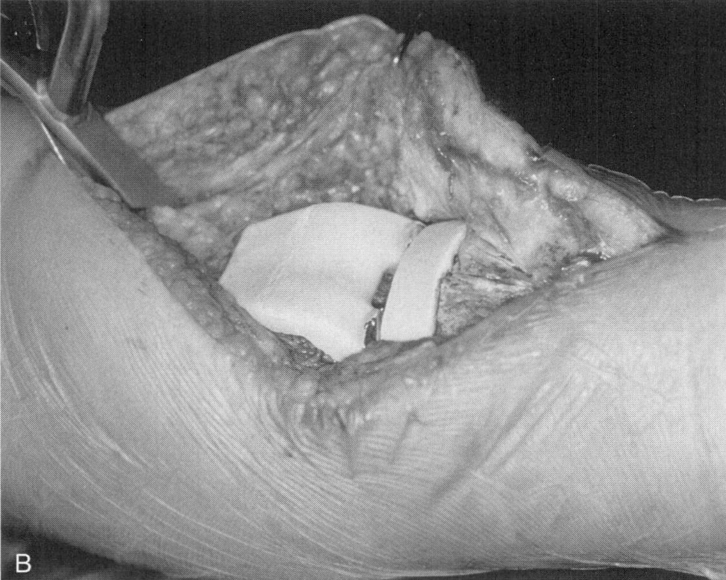

FIGURE 91.9 ➢ Intraoperative photographs in flexion *(A)* and extension *(B)* after insertion of the PROSTALAC spacer just before fixation with a single batch of antibiotic-loaded cement without pressurization.

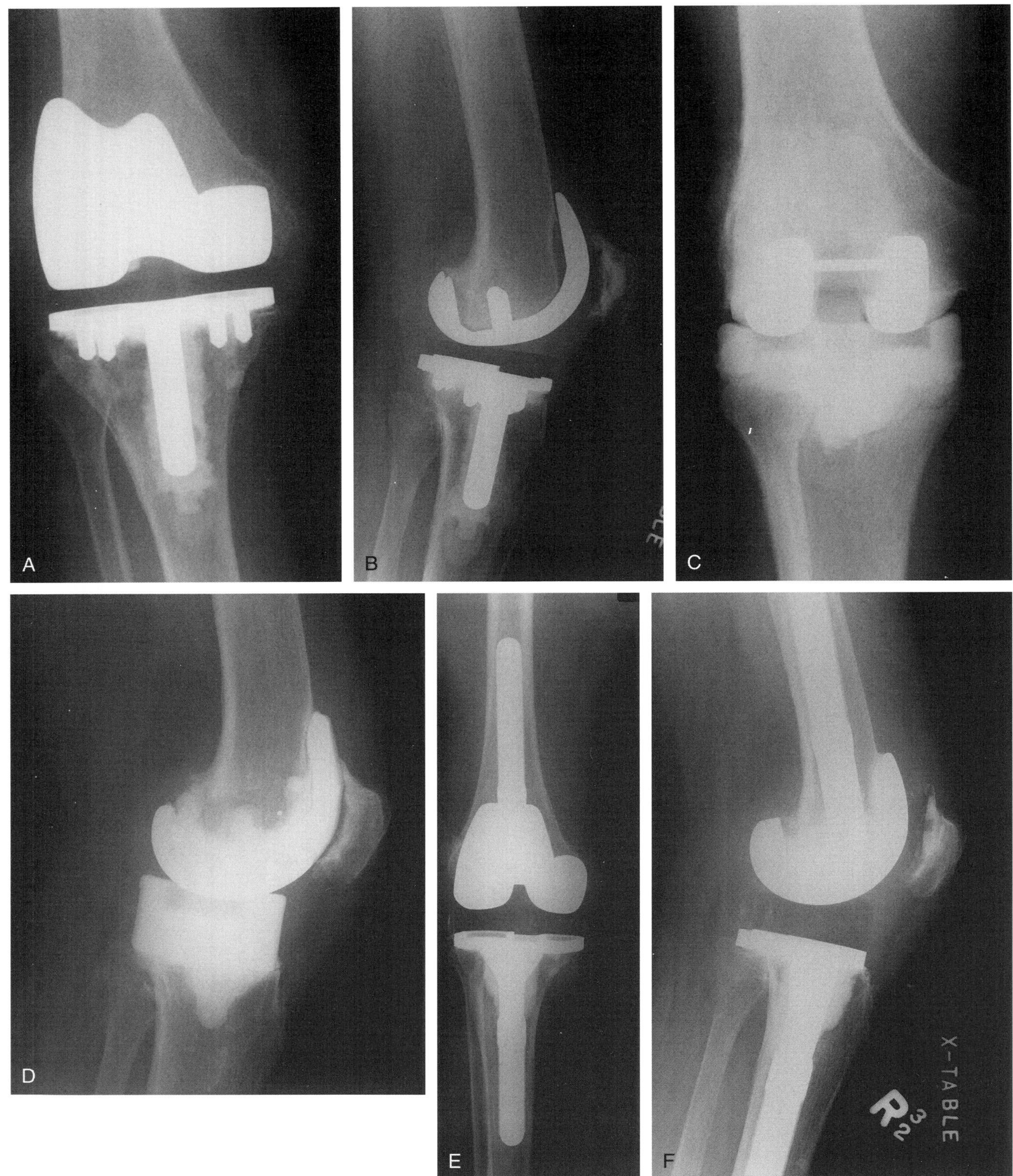

FIGURE 91.11 ➢ *A* and *B,* Preoperative radiographs of an infected total knee arthroplasty. *C* and *D,* Radiographs of the PROSTALAC articulated spacer during the interval period. A thick tibial component was necessary to maintain the appropriate soft tissue balance. *E* and *F,* Radiographs of reconstruction after a 12-week interval period.

throplasty and insertion of an antibiotic-loaded cement spacer without resolution of the infection.

The mean erythrocyte sedimentation rate (ESR) was 57 (range 1 to 126). Only two patients had an ESR less than 20. The infecting organisms were known in all but five cases (86%). In each of the five cases in which no organisms were cultured, the patient was on long-term oral antibiotics at presentation, and intraoperative findings on removal of the infected components revealed definite evidence of infection such as gross pus or a draining sinus. Fifteen patients presented with a draining sinus. There were four cases of mixed infection and 27 cases (26 patients) of isolated infection. In each of the cases of mixed infection, *S. epidermidis* was one of the infecting organisms. Overall, *S. epidermidis* was the most common organism and was isolated in 18 cultures. *S. aureus* was isolated in eight cases. *Mycoplasma, Peptostreptococcus,* and coagulase-negative *Staphylococcus* other than *S. epidermidis* were isolated from two knees each. *Bacillus, Streptococcus, Serratia, Enterococcus, Escherichia coli,* and *Mycobacterium tuberculosis* were isolated once each.

All of these patients completed a two-stage exchange knee arthroplasty protocol using the PROSTALAC knee prosthesis as a temporary antibiotic-loaded functional spacer. In seven knees, the PROSTALAC component was a handmade facsimile of a total knee prosthesis with a cement on cement articular surface. In three patients a first-generation cement-on-cement molded PROSTALAC implant was used. The second-generation low-friction PROSTALAC prosthesis was used in 14 patients. The third-generation posterior cruciate substituting PROSTALAC knee design was used in 13 patients in this series. The mean delay between the two stages was 94 days (range 25 to 234 days), after which reimplantation was performed. During the interval period, each patient was treated with a 3-week or longer course of intravenous antibiotics, followed by oral antibiotics for a minimum of another 3 weeks. Early in our experience, because of the lack of home intravenous antibiotic therapy programs, our routine was to switch from parenteral antibiotic to oral therapy, when appropriate, at 3 weeks. More recently, however, we have abandoned this practice and currently continue intravenous antibiotic therapy for 6 weeks. All the patients were discharged from our hospital before the second stage of the procedure. No deaths were directly related to the procedure; however, 2 patients (3 knees) died of unrelated causes between 2.5 and 7 years after surgery.

In each patient, the antibiotics used in the bone cement were customized based on the sensitivity profile of the infecting organisms. If no organism was isolated, a combination of tobramycin and vancomycin was used. Tobramycin and vancomycin were used in combination in 27 cases, and tobramycin in isolation was used in three. Vancomycin alone was used in four cases, although this is no longer our practice. Penicillin G was used in three cases but never in isolation. In two cases it was combined with tobramycin, and in one it was combined with both tobramycin and vancomycin. The amount of antibiotic added to each packet of cement varied between 2.4 and 4.8 g for tobramycin, 1.0 and 2.0 g for vancomycin and 5 and 10 million units for penicillin G. Early in our experience, we used Simplex P bone cement. In the latest nine cases in this series, we used Palacos R bone cement because of its better antibiotic elution profile.

The following additional procedures were required. At the first stage, a skin rotation flap and a medial gastrocnemius flap were required for soft-tissue coverage in one and two patients, respectively. Repair of a ruptured patellar tendon was required in one patient. At the second stage, proximal and distal extensor mechanism realignment was required in one patient and an extensive proximal extensor mechanism realignment in nine patients.

Pain Relief

The main advantage of this approach compared with a standard excision arthroplasty was the pain relief observed between stages. In the majority, there was complete pain relief after surgery. In the early cases, particularly those in which a low-friction-bearing surface was not used, there was mild to moderate residual pain in five of 10 knees. This pain was associated with a grating sensation and crepitus with knee movement. Only one of the patients who received the modified implant complained of persistent pain. This was in relation to severe heterotopic ossification in the anteromedial soft tissues.

Range of Motion

With the PROSTALAC prosthesis in situ, knee mobility was maintained in the majority of cases. There was no substantial change in range of motion after implantation of PROSTALAC implants compared with the preoperative range of motion. The mean range of motion was from 8 to 70 degrees before PROSTALAC compared with 8 to 72 degrees after the PROSTALAC procedure. Range of motion after the final reimplantation of a definitive total knee replacement prosthesis was improved, with a mean gain of 21 degrees in flexion and a 3-degree decrease in flexion deformity (average range of flexion = 5 to 91 degrees).

Knee Stability

Ligamentous laxity was a common finding in our patients at initial presentation. There was significant ligamentous laxity in 15 of 37 knees. This was due to either failure of the implant with subsequent bone deficiency or a previous excision arthroplasty. Two of these patients had instability so severe that immobilization in a cast was required while the patient was awaiting surgery. After excision arthroplasty and replacement with a PROSTALAC implant, ligamentous laxity was detected on physical examination in 14 patients; however, this was considered severe in only seven. Instability was marked in only one of the 13 patients who received a posterior-stabilized PROSTA-

LAC. Two of these patients required cast immobilization after implantation of the PROSTALAC prosthesis because of significant tibiofemoral instability. Another patient was immobilized in a cylinder cast prophylactically so that unprotected activity would not cause fragmentation and mechanical failure of the PROSTALAC implant. In this patient, the PROSTALAC implant was used simply as a spacer to maintain the soft tissues out to length and to facilitate revision arthroplasty at the second stage. Another patient required a knee brace between stages because of intraoperative rupture of the extensor mechanism and severe bone loss leading to significant instability. Because of severe bone loss, a hinged implant (Kinematic rotating hinge, Howmedica, Rutherford, NJ) was used for the final reconstruction at the second stage. Postoperatively, the patient was mobilized with a hinged knee brace. This is the only patient who was using a brace at final review. The only patient with a posterior-stabilized PROSTALAC who required bracing between stages had severe collateral ligament deficiency that could not be controlled with a posterior-stabilized design. A hinged knee brace was used between stages with good success.

Extensor Lag

The mean extensor lag at the time of presentation was 10 degrees (range = 0 to 35 degrees). After excision arthroplasty and replacement with the PROSTALAC prosthesis, the mean extensor lag was unchanged at a mean of 12 degrees (range = 0 to 35 degrees). At final review, the mean extensor lag was reduced to 4 degrees (range = 0 to 30 degrees), with only one patient with an extensor lag greater than 10 degrees. The one patient with a final extensor lag of 30 degrees was a 62-year-old man with severe rheumatoid arthritis who suffered a rupture of his extensor mechanism at the time of insertion of the PROSTALAC implant. This was the only complication involving disruption of the extensor mechanism. Despite this complication, his final extensor lag was no worse than his preoperative extensor lag of 35 degrees.

Patellar Instability

The majority of the complications in this series are related to the extensor mechanism. A thin patella that is difficult to resurface is at risk of subluxation and riding over the lateral femoral condyle. Maltracking of the patella was encountered in 13 knees in this series (35%). After insertion of the PROSTALAC prosthesis, there were two complete dislocations of the patella (8%). Patellar dislocation produced a significant decrease in the HSS knee score after insertion of the PROSTALAC implant (16 points and 18 points in these two patients). This decline in HSS knee score was due to anterior knee pain, quadriceps weakness, and extensor lag. At the second stage, one patient was treated with proximal extensor mechanism realignment and a final HSS knee score of 85 was obtained, and the other required a tibial tubercle osteotomy and proximal realignment, which resulted in a stable, pain-free patella with a final HSS knee score of 89.

There was persistent, yet asymptomatic lateral subluxation of the patella in 8 knees (22%) after insertion of the PROSTALAC implant. In all of these patients, the HSS score after implantation of the PROSTALAC prosthesis was improved compared with the preoperative HSS score. At final reconstruction, the patella was stable in all but one of these patients. Distal extensor mechanism realignment was not performed in any of these patients. The one patient with persistent subluxation had some anterior knee pain and an HSS knee score of 76. Patellar instability was not a problem in the patients in whom a posterior-stabilized PROSTALAC design was used.

Knee Score

All patients were evaluated using the HSS knee score at initial presentation, before removal of the PROSTALAC prosthesis, and at final follow-up. The mean HSS knee score at initial presentation was 41 (range = 11 to 76). After excision arthroplasty and replacement with the temporary PROSTALAC spacer, the mean HSS score increased to 55 (range = 18 to 87). At final review, the mean HSS knee score was improved to 81 (range = 46 to 95). After insertion of the PROSTALAC prosthesis, there was a significant decline in the HSS knee score in five patients. Two of these patients had a fixed dislocation of the patella. Another patient had an 8-point decline in his HSS score after insertion of the PROSTALAC implant. This was in relation to an avulsion of his extensor mechanism at the time of insertion of the PROSTALAC implant. In another patient, there was a 24-point decline in the HSS knee score as a result of severe heterotopic ossification on the anteromedial aspect of the knee, causing significant pain and stiffness. This patient was treated with radiation therapy (single dose of 700 rad) before the second stage of the procedure. At that time, a lateral parapatellar approach was required because of the severity of the heterotopic ossification within the medial soft tissues. At final review, the pain had resolved, and the patient achieved a range of motion of 0 to 85 degrees. His final HSS knee score has improved from 18 to 85. The last patient who had a decline in the HSS knee score after implantation of the PROSTALAC prosthesis had been immobilized in a cylinder cast prophylactically because of severe neuropathic arthropathy.

Summary of Complications

As discussed, the following complications were encountered:

- Persistent pain caused by the high-friction articular surface was noted in five patients. This problem was readily corrected by adding a low-friction-bearing surface.
- Tibiofemoral instability was seen in 14 patients.

This, however, was mild and caused no symptoms in the majority of patients (11/14). Symptomatic posterior subluxation of the tibia secondary to loss of the posterior cruciate ligament was encountered in two patients. This problem was addressed by modifying the PROSTALAC implant to a more constrained design with a tibial post and a femoral cam as a substitute for the deficient posterior cruciate ligament.

- Rupture of the patellar tendon was seen in one patient.
- Patellar instability was the most significant complication in this series. Two patients suffered from a fixed lateral dislocation of the patella that compromised the short-term outcome after insertion of the PROSTALAC implant, although it did not affect the final outcome. One of these patients has a stable patella at final review, whereas one had an asymptomatic yet chronically subluxated patella. Eight patients suffered from asymptomatic lateral subluxation of the patella after insertion of the PROSTALAC prosthesis. At final review, the patella was stable in all but one of these patients who had persistent, slightly symptomatic subluxation of the patella.
- The unusual complication of heterotopic ossification was encountered in two patients. In one patient, the outcome after insertion of the PROSTALAC was compromised because of pain and stiffness, but the final outcome was not compromised. This patient was treated with single-dose radiation therapy before the second stage.
- There was one intraoperative fracture of the femur during removal of the cement from the medullary canal of the femur during the first stage of the procedure. The fracture was unicortical and was stabilized using three 2.0-mm stainless-steel cables. The patient was mobilized postoperatively with minimal weightbearing. The fracture healed without any further complications.
- There was failure of the tibial component in one patient who received a rotating hinge constrained revision total knee replacement prosthesis. He presented 18 months after final reconstruction with dissociation of the tibial component. He underwent a second revision total knee arthroplasty without any complications. At the time of revision surgery, there was no evidence of infection, and all intraoperative cultures were negative.

Recurrent Infection

Infection recurred in four patients in this series, for an infection cure rate of 89% at a mean follow-up of 4.1 years. In all these cases the original infection was caused by *S. epidermidis.* One of these four patients was diabetic; the other three were not immune compromised. The post-PROSTALAC infection was caused by *Streptococcus agalactiae* in one case, by *S. aureus* in another, by a combination of *S. epidermidis* and *Enterococcus* species in the third, and by *S. epidermidis* in the fourth. These patients have not been treated with a repeat two-stage exchange arthroplasty. Assuming that the two patients with *S. epidermidis* reinfection had a recurrence of the original infection, the infection recurrence rate is 5.4% and the reinfection rate 5.4%, for an overall failure rate of 10.8%, which still compares favorably with the overall results of two-stage exchange arthroplasty in the literature.

ADVANTAGES OF THE PROSTALAC SYSTEM

One of the advantages of articulated spacers in general, and the PROSTALAC system in particular, is the ability to add large amounts of antibiotic powder to the bone cement without fear of weakening the cement, because structural integrity of the cement becomes less important when these spacers are used for only a short period of time. This, in theory, should increase the levels and duration of antibiotic elution.

With the use of the PROSTALAC system, a second débridement is possible at reimplantation, and the interval between stages and antibiotics used both locally and systemically at reconstruction may be modified in accordance with culture results.

The advantages of mobility between stages are clear. The patient is more functional, can be discharged from hospital, and generally has a better outlook than one treated without a mobile spacer between stages. The reimplantation is much easier because of the presence of the spacer that stabilizes the soft tissues and preserves the joint cavity.

One of the drawbacks of the PROSTALAC and other articulated spacer techniques is the retention of foreign material within the joint in the presence of infection. On the basis of the various reports of articulated spacers and on our experience, it is clear that as long as antibiotic-loaded bone cement is used with these articulated spacers there are no adverse effects associated with the presence of small amounts of metal and plastic in addition to antibiotic-loaded bone cement.

SUMMARY

The safest and most efficacious approach to the treatment of chronically infected knee replacement is two-stage exchange arthroplasty. Antibiotic-loaded cement is increasingly being used in this setting. There has been a natural evolution from the use of beads, to antibiotic-loaded cement spacers, and ultimately to articulated spacers. The PROSTALAC is an interim functional spacer that is manufactured primarily of antibiotic-loaded cement and that resembles a knee replacement. It is used between stages in the two-stage exchange arthroplasty protocol and combines the advantages of high concentrations of local antibiotics with excellent motion between stages and the preservation of limb length, limb alignment, and soft tissue planes. The addition of small amounts of metal and plastic, in addition to antibiotic-loaded bone cement in interim spacers, does not seem to have an adverse effect on infection cure rates and has the advantage of improved function between stages. This technique has considerable economic advantages as well as high patient satisfaction.

Acknowledgments

Fares S. Haddad was supported by the John Charnley and BOA/Wishbone trusts and by the Norman Capener Travelling Fellowship.

References

1. Abendschein W: Arthroplasty Rounds. Salvage of infected total hip replacement: Use of antibiotic/PMMA spacer. Orthopedics 15:228, 1992.
2. Adams KA, Couch L, Cierny G, et al: In vitro and in vivo evaluation of antibiotic diffusion from antibiotic-impregnated polymethyl methacrylate beads. Clin Orthop 278:244, 1992.
3. Arizono T, Oga M, Sugioka Y: Increased resistance of bacteria after adherence to polymethyl methacrylate: An in vitro study. Acta Orthop Scand 63:661, 1992.
4. Askew MJ, Kufel MF, Fleissner PR Jr, et al: Effect of vacuum mixing on the mechanical properties of antibiotic impregnated methylmethacrylate bone cement. J Biomed Biomater Res 24: 573, 1990.
5. Backe HA Jr, Wolff DA, Windsor RE: Total knee replacement infection after 2-stage reimplantation: Results of subsequent 2-stage reimplantation. Clin Orthop 331:125, 1996.
6. Baker AS, Greenham LW: Release of gentamicin from acrylic bone cement. J Bone Joint Surg Am 70:1551, 1988.
7. Bargar WL, Martin RB, deJesus R, et al: The addition of tobramycin to contrast bone cement. J Arthroplasty 1:165, 1986.
8. Barrack RL: Economics of the infected total knee replacement. Orthopedics 19(9):780 1996.
9. Bayston R, Milner RDG: The sustained release of antimicrobial drugs from bone cement. J Bone Joint Surg Br 64(4):460, 1982.
10. Beeching NJ, Thomas MG, Roberts S, et al: Comparative in-vitro activity of antibiotics incorporated in acrylic bone cement. J Antimicrob Chemother 17:173, 1986.
11. Bengtson S, Knutson K: The infected knee arthroplasty. Acta Orthop Scand 62:301, 1991.
12. Bengtson S, Knutson K, Lidgren L: Revision of infected knee arthroplasty. Acta Orthop Scand 57:489, 1986.
13. Bliss DG, McBride GG: Infected total knee arthroplasties. Clin Orthop 199:207, 1985.
14. Booth RE Jr, Lotke P: The results of spacer block technique in revision of infected total knee arthroplasty. Clin Orthop 248:57, 1989.
15. Borden LS, Gearen PF: Infected total knee arthroplasty, a protocol for management. J Arthroplasty 2:27, 1987.
16. Brause BD: Infections associated with prosthetic joints. Clin Rheum Dis 12:523, 1986.
17. Brien WW, Salvati EA, Klein R, et al: Antibiotic impregnated bone cement in total hip arthroplasty. An in vivo comparison of the elution properties of tobramycin and vancomycin. Clin Orthop 296:242, 1993.
18. Buchholz HW, Elson RA, Engelbrecht E, et al: Management of deep infection of total hip arthroplasty. J Bone Joint Surg Br 63:342, 1981.
19. Buchholz HW, Elson RA, Heinert K: Antibiotic-loaded acrylic cement: Current concepts. Clin Orthop 190:96, 1984.
20. Buchholz HW, Engelbrecht H: Über die Depotwirkung einiger Antibiotica bei Vermischung mit dem Kunstharz Palacos. Chirurg 41:511, 1970.
21. Bunetel L, Segui A, Langlais F, et al: Osseous concentrations of gentamicin after implantation of acrylic bone cement in sheep femora. Eur J Drug Metab Pharmacokinet 19:99, 1994.
22. Cadambi A, Jones RE, Maale GE: A protocol for staged revision of infected total hip and knee arthroplasties: The use of antibiotic-cement-implant composites. Int Orthop 3:133, 1995.
23. Calton TF, Fehring TK, Griffin WL: Bone loss associated with the use of spacer blocks in infected total knee arthroplasty. Clin Orthop 345:148, 1997.
24. Campbell DG, Masri BA, Garbuz DS, et al: Seven specialized exposures in revision hip and knee replacement. Orthop Clin North Am 29(2):229, 1998.
25. Chang CC, Merritt K: Effect of *Staphylococcus epidermidis* on adherence of *Pseudomonas aeruginosa* and *Proteus mirabilis* to polymethyl methacrylate (PMMA) and gentamicin containing PMMA. J Orthop Res 9:284, 1991.
26. Chang CC, Merritt K: Microbial adherence on polymethylmethacrylate (PMMA) surfaces. J Biomed Mater Res 26:197, 1992.
27. Chapman MW, Hadley WK: The effect of polymethylmethacrylate and antibiotic combinations on bacterial viability: An in vitro and preliminary in vivo study. J Bone Joint Surg Am 58: 76, 1976.
28. Chohfi M, Langlais F, Fourastier J, et al: Pharmacokinetics, uses, and limitations of vancomycin-loaded bone cement. Int Orthop 22(3):171, 1998.
29. Cohen JC, Hozack WJ, Cuckler JM, et al: Two-stage reimplantation of septic total knee arthroplasty: Report of three cases using an antibiotic-PMMA spacer block. J Arthroplasty 3:369, 1988.
30. Coonse K, Adams JD: A new operative approach to the knee joint. Surg Gynecol Obstet 77:344, 1943.
31. Cordero J, Munuera L, Folgueira MD: Influence of metal implants on infection. An experimental study in rabbits. J Bone Joint Surg Br 76:717, 1994.
32. Costerton JW, Geesey GG, Cheng K-J: How bacteria stick. Sci Am 238:86, 1978.
33. Costerton JW, Lewandowski Z, Caldwell DE, et al: Microbial biofilms. Annu Rev Microbiol 49:711, 1995.
34. Dall L, Keilhofner M, Herndon B, et al: Clindamycin effect on glycocalyx production in experimental viridans streptococcal endocarditis. J Infect Dis 161:1221, 1990.
35. Davenport K, Trajna S, Perry C: Treatment of acutely infected arthroplasty with local antibiotics. J Arthroplasty 6:179, 1991.
36. Davies JP, O'Connor DO, Burke DW, et al: Influence of antibiotic impregnation on the fatigue life of Simplex P and Palacos R acrylic bone cements, with and without centrifugation. J Biomed Mater Res 23:379, 1989.
37. Dennesen PJ, Bonten MJ, Weinstein RA: Multiresistant bacteria as a hospital epidemic problem. Ann Med 30(2):176, 1998.
38. Diduch DR, Insall JN, Scott WN, et al: Total knee replacement in young, active patients. Long-term follow-up and functional outcome. J Bone Joint Surg Am 79:575, 1997.
39. DiMaio FR, O'Halloran JJ, Quale JM: In vitro elution of ciprofloxacin from polymethylmethacrylate cement beads. J Orthop Res 12:79, 1994.
40. Duncan CP, Beauchamp CP: A temporary antibiotic-loaded joint replacement system for management of complex infections involving the hip. Orthop Clin North Am 24:751, 1993.
41. Duncan CP, Beauchamp CP, Masri B, et al: The antibiotic loaded joint replacement system: A novel approach to the management of the infected knee replacement. J Bone Joint Surg Br 74(suppl III):296, 1992.
42. Duncan CP, Masri BA: Antibiotic depots. J Bone Joint Surg Br 75(3):349, 1993.
43. Ellingsen DE, Rand JA: Intramedullary arthrodesis of the knee after failed total knee arthroplasty. J Bone Joint Surg Am 76(6): 870, 1994.
44. Elson RA, Jephcott AE, McGechie DB, et al: Antibiotic-loaded acrylic cement. J Bone Joint Surg Br 59:200, 1977.
45. Elson RA, Jephcott AE, McGechie DB, et al: Bacterial infection and acrylic cement in the rat. J Bone Joint Surg Br 59:452, 1977.
46. England SP, Stern SH, Insall JN, et al: Total knee arthroplasty in diabetes mellitus. Clin Orthop 260:130, 1990.
47. Fish DN, Hoffman HM, Danziger LH: Antibiotic-impregnated cement use in U.S. hospitals. Am J Hosp Pharm 49(10):2469, 1992.
48. Freeman MAR, Sudlow RA, Casewell MW, et al: The management of infected total knee replacements. J Bone Joint Surg Br 67(5):764, 1985.
49. French GL: Enterococci and vancomycin resistance. Clin Infect Dis 27(suppl 1):S75, 1998.

50. Gacon G, Laurencon M, Van de Velde D, et al: Two stages reimplantation for infection after knee arthroplasty. Apropos of a series of 29 cases. Rev Chir Orthop Reparatrice Appar Mot 83(4):313, 1997.
51. Gherini S, Vaughn BK, Lombardi AV Jr, et al: Delayed wound healing and nutritional deficiencies after total hip arthroplasty. Clin Orthop 293:188, 1993.
52. Gill GS, Mills DM: Long term follow-up evaluation of 1000 consecutive cemented total knee arthroplasties. Clin Orthop 273:66, 1991.
53. Göksan SB, Freeman MA: One-stage reimplantation for infected total knee arthroplasty. J Bone Joint Surg 74:78, 1992.
54. Goldman RT, Scuderi GR, Insall JN: Two-stage reimplantation for infected total knee replacement. Clin Orthop 331:118, 1996.
55. Goodell JA, Flick AB, Herbert JC, et al: Preparation and release characteristics of tobramycin-impregnated polymethylmethacrylate beads. Am J Hosp Pharm 43:1454, 1986.
56. Greene KA, Wilde AN, Stulberg BN: Preoperative nutritional status of total joint patients. J Arthroplasty 6:321, 1991.
57. Gristina AG: Biomaterial-centered infection: Microbial adhesion versus tissue integration. Science 237:1588, 1987.
58. Gristina AG, Costerton JW: Bacterial adherence and the glycocalyx and their role in musculoskeletal infection. Orthop Clin North Am 15:517, 1984.
59. Gristina AG, Costerton JW: Bacterial adherence to biomaterials and tissue. The significance of its role in clinical sepsis. J Bone Joint Surg Am 67:264, 1985.
60. Gristina AG, Kolkin J: Current concepts review: Total joint replacement and sepsis. J Bone Joint Surg Am 65:128, 1983.
61. Gristina AG, Shibata Y, Giridhar G, et al: The glycocalyx, biofilm, microbes, and resistant infection. Semin Arthroplasty 5: 160, 1994.
62. Hanssen AD, Rand JA, Osmon DR: Treatment of the infected total knee arthroplasty with insertion of another prosthesis: The effect of antibiotic-impregnated bone cement. Clin Orthop 309:44, 1994.
63. Hanssen AD, Trousdale RT, Osmon DR: Patient outcome with reinfection following reimplantation for the infected total knee arthroplasty. Clin Orthop 321:55, 1995.
64. Hebert CK, Williams RE, Levy RS, et al: Cost of treating an infected total knee replacement. Clin Orthop 331:140, 1996.
65. Heck DA, Melfi CA, Mamlin LA, et al: Revision rates after knee replacement in the United States. Med Care 36(5):661, 1998.
66. Hedstrom SA, Lidgren L, Torholm C, et al: Antibiotic containing cement beads in the treatment of deep muscle and skeletal infections. Acta Orthop Scand 51:863, 1980.
67. Henry SL, Seligson D, Mangino P, et al: Antibiotic impregnated beads. Part I: Bead implantation versus systemic therapy. Orthop Rev 20:242, 1991.
68. Hill J, Klenerman L, Trustey S, et al: Diffusion of antibiotics from acrylic bone-cement in vitro. J Bone Joint Surg Am 59: 197, 1977.
69. Hirakawa K, Stulberg BN, Wilde AH, et al: Results of 2-stage reimplantation for infected total knee arthroplasty. J Arthroplasty 13(1):22, 1998.
70. Hoff SF, Fitzgerald RH Jr, Kelly PJ: The depot administration of penicillin G and gentamicin in acrylic bone cement. J Bone Joint Surg Am 63(5):798, 1981.
71. Hoffmann A, Kane K, Tkach T, et al: Treatment of infected total knee replacement arthroplasty using an articulating spacer. Clin Orthop 321:45, 1995.
72. Hope PG, Kristinsson KG, Norman P, et al: Deep infection of cemented total hip arthroplasties caused by coagulase-negative staphylococci. J Bone Joint Surg Br 71:851, 1989.
73. Hovelius L, Josefsson G: An alternative method for exchange operation of infected arthroplasty. Acta Orthop Scand 50:93, 1979.
74. Insall JN: Infection of total knee arthroplasty. Instr Course Lect 35:319, 1986.
75. Insall JN: Surgical techniques and instrumentation in total knee arthroplasty. In Insall JN, Windsor RE, Scott WN, et al, eds: Surgery of the Knee, 2nd ed. New York, Churchill Livingstone, 1993, pp 739–804.
76. Insall JN, Thompson FM, Brause BD: Two-stage reimplantation for the salvage of infected total knee arthroplasty. J Bone Joint Surg Am 65(8):1087, 1983.
77. Isiklar ZU, Landon GC, Tullos HS: Amputation after failed total knee arthroplasty. Clin Orthop 299:173, 1994.
78. Kendall RW, Duncan CP, Beauchamp CP: Bacterial growth on antibiotic-loaded acrylic cement: A prospective in vivo retrieval study. J Arthroplasty 10:817, 1995.
79. Kendall RW, Masri BA, Duncan CP, et al: Temporary antibiotic loaded acrylic hip replacement: A novel method for management of the infected THA. Semin Arthroplasty 5:171, 1994.
80. Kirkpatrick DK, Trachenberg LS, Mangino PD, et al: In vitro characteristics of tobramycin-PMMA beads, compressive strength and leaching. Orthopedics 8:1130, 1985.
81. Kuechle DK, Landon GC, Musher DM, et al: Elution of vancomycin, daptomycin, and amikacin from acrylic bone cement. Clin Orthop 264:302, 1991.
82. Landon GC, Muscher D, Gounder S, et al: Susceptibility to infection: A comparison of cemented and cementless implants. Orthop Trans 14:408, 1990.
83. Lautenschlager EP, Jacobs JJ, Marshall GW, et al: Mechanical properties of bone cements containing large doses of antibiotic powder. J Biomed Mater Res 10:929, 1976.
84. Lautenschlager EP, Marshall GW, Marks KE, et al: Mechanical strength of acrylic bone cements impregnated with antibiotics. J Biomed Mater Res 10:837, 1976.
85. Lawson KJ, Marks KE, Brems J, et al: Vancomycin and tobramycin elution from polymethylmethacrylate: An in vitro study. Orthopedics 13:521, 1990.
86. Levin PD: The effectiveness of various antibiotics in methylmethacrylate. J Bone Joint Surg Br 57:234, 1975.
87. Linden PK: Clinical implications of nosocomial gram-positive bacteremia and superimposed antimicrobial resistance. Am J Med 104(5A):24S, 1998.
88. Luessenhop CP, Higgins LD, Brause BD, et al: Multiple prosthetic infections after total joint arthroplasty. Risk factor analysis. J Arthroplasty 11:862, 1996.
89. Lyons VO, Henri SL, Faghri M, et al: Bacterial adherence to plain and tobramycin laden polymethylmethacrylate beads. Clin Orthop 278:260, 1992.
90. Majid SA, Lindberg ST, Gutenberg B, et al: Gentamicin-PMMA beads in the treatment of chronic osteomyelitis. Acta Orthop Scand 56:265, 1985.
91. Marks KE, Nelson CL, Lautenschlager EP: Antibiotic-impregnated acrylic bone cement. J Bone Joint Surg Am 58:358, 1976.
92. Marsh PK, Cotler JM: Management of an anaerobic infection in a prosthetic knee with long term antibiotics alone. Clin Orthop 155:133, 1981.
93. Masri B, Duncan CP, Beauchamp CP: Long-term elution of antibiotics from bone cement: An in vivo study using the PROSTALAC system. J Arthroplasty 13:331, 1998.
94. Masri BA, Duncan CP, Beauchamp CP, et al: Tobramycin and vancomycin elution from bone cement. An in vitro and in vivo study. Orthop Trans 18:130, 1994.
95. Masri BA, Duncan CP, Beauchamp CP, et al: Effect of varying surface patterns on antibiotic elution from antibiotic-loaded bone cement. J Arthroplasty 10(4):453, 1995.
96. Masri B, Duncan CP, Jewesson P, et al: Streptomycin loaded bone cement in the treatment of tuberculous osteomyelitis: An adjunct to conventional therapy. Can J Surg 38:64, 1995.
97. Masri BA, Kendall RW, Duncan CP, et al: Two-stage exchange arthroplasty using a functional antibiotic-loaded spacer in the treatment of the infected knee replacement: The Vancouver experience. Semin Arthroplasty 5:122, 1994.
98. May J, Shannon K, King A, et al: Glycopeptide tolerance in *Staphylococcus aureus*. J Antimicrob Chemother 42(2):189, 1998.
99. McLaren AC, Spooner CE: Salvage of infected total knee components. Clin Orthop 331:146, 1996.
100. McMaster WC: Technique for intraoperative construction of PMMA spacer in total knee revision. Am J Orthop 24(2):178, 1995.
101. McPherson EJ, Lewonowski K, Dorr LD: Use of an articulated PMMA spacer in the infected total knee arthroplasty. J Arthroplasty 10:87, 1995.
102. Meislin R, Zuckerman JD: Management of an infected total knee arthroplasty. Bull Hosp Jt Dis 49(1):21, 1989.

103. Moellering RC Jr: The specter of glycopeptide resistance: Current trends and future considerations. Am J Med 104(5A):3S, 1998.
104. Moellering RC Jr, Linden PK: The specter of glycopeptide resistance: current trends and future considerations. Am J Med 104(5A):1S, 1998.
105. Mont MA, Waldman B, Banerjee C, et al: Multiple irrigation, debridement and retention of components in infected total knee arthroplasty. J Arthroplasty 12:426, 1997.
106. Moran JM, Greenwald SA, Matejczyk M-B: Effect of gentamicin on shear and interface strengths of bone cement. Clin Orthop 141:96, 1979.
107. Morrey BF, Westholm F, Schoifet S, et al: Long-term results of various treatment options for infected total knee arthroplasty. Clin Orthop 248:120, 1989.
108. Murray RP, Bourne MH, Fitzgerald RH: Metachronous infection in patients who have had more than one total joint arthroplasty. J Bone Joint Surg Am 75:1469, 1993.
109. Murray WR: Use of antibiotic-containing bone cement. Clin Orthop 190:89, 1984.
110. Namba RS, Diao E: Tissue expansion for staged reimplantation of infected total knee arthroplasty. J Arthroplasty 12(4):471, 1997.
111. Naylor PT, Myrvik QN, Gristina AG: Antibiotic resistance of biomaterial-adherent coagulase negative and coagulase positive staphylococci. Clin Orthop 261:126, 1990.
112. Nelson CL, Evans RP, Blaha JD, et al: A comparison of gentamicin-impregnated polymethylmethacrylate bead implantation to conventional parenteral antibiotic therapy in infected total hip and knee arthroplasty. Clin Orthop 295:96, 1993.
113. Nelson RC, Hoffman RO, Burton TA: The effect of antibiotic additions on the mechanical properties of acrylic cement. J Biomed Mater Res 12:473, 1978.
114. Nichols RL: Postoperative infections in the age of drug-resistant gram-positive bacteria. Am J Med 104(5A):11S, 1998.
115. Oga M, Arizono T, Sugioka Y: Inhibition of bacterial adhesion by tobramycin-impregnated PMMA bone cement. Acta Orthop Scand 63:301, 1992.
116. Orti A, Roig P, Alcala R, et al: Brucellar prosthetic arthritis in a total knee replacement. Eur J Clin Microbiol Infect Dis 16(11): 843, 1997.
117. Ozaki T, Yoshitaka T, Kunisada T, et al: Vancomycin-impregnated polymethylmethacrylate beads for methicillin-resistant *Staphylococcus aureus* (MRSA) infection: Report of two cases. J Orthop Sci 3(3):163, 1998.
118. Panush RS, Petty RW: Inhibition of human lymphocyte responses by methylmethacrylate. Clin Orthop 134:356, 1978.
119. Penner MJ, Masri BA, Duncan CP: Elution characteristics of vancomycin and tobramycin combined in acrylic bone cement. J Arthroplasty 11:939, 1996.
120. Petrie RS, Hanssen AD, Osmon DR, et al: Metal-backed patellar component failure in total knee arthroplasty: A possible risk for late infection. Am J Orthop 27(3):172, 1998.
121. Petty W: The effect of methylmethacrylate on the bacterial inhibiting properties of normal human serum. Clin Orthop 132: 266, 1978.
122. Petty W: The effect of methylmethacrylate on chemotaxis of polymorphonuclear leukocytes. J Bone Joint Surg Am 60:492, 1978.
123. Petty W: The effect of methylmethacrylate on bacterial phagocytosis and killing by human polymorphonuclear leukocytes. J Bone Joint Surg Am 60:752, 1978.
124. Petty W, Caldwell JR: The effect of methylmethacrylate on complement activity. Clin Orthop 128:354, 1977.
125. Petty W, Spanier S, Shuster JJ: Prevention of infection after total joint replacement. Experiments with a canine model. J Bone Joint Surg Am 70:536, 1988.
126. Petty W, Spanier S, Shuster JJ, et al: The influence of skeletal implants on incidence of infection. Experiments in a canine model. J Bone Joint Surg Am 67:1236, 1985.
127. Popham GJ, Mangino P, Seligson D, et al: Antibiotic impregnated beads. Part II: Factors in antibiotic selection. Orthop Rev 20:331, 1991.
128. Poss R, Thornhill TS, Ewald FC, et al: Factors influencing the incidence and outcome of infection following total joint arthroplasty. Clin Orthop 182:117, 1984.
129. Pring DJ, Marks L, Angel JC: Mobility after amputation for failed knee replacement. J Bone Joint Surg Br 70:770, 1988.
130. Proctor RA, Hamill RJ, Mosher DF, et al: Effects of subinhibitory concentrations of antibiotics on *Staphylococcus aureus* interactions with fibronectin. J Antimicrob Ther 12(suppl C): 85, 1983.
131. Ranawat CS, Flynn WF, Saddler S, et al: Long-term results of the total condylar knee arthroplasty. Clin Orthop 286:94, 1993.
132. Rand JA: Alternatives to reimplantation for salvage of the total knee arthroplasty complicated by infection. J Bone Joint Surg 75(2):282, 1993.
133. Rand JA, Bryan RS: Reimplantation for the salvage of an infected total knee arthroplasty. J Bone Joint Surg Am 65:1081, 1983.
134. Rand JA, Bryan RS, Morrey BF, et al: Management of infected total knee arthroplasty. Clin Orthop 205:75, 1986.
135. Rand JA, Fitzgerald RH: Diagnosis and management of the infected total knee arthroplasty. Orthop Clin North Am 20(2): 201, 1989.
136. Robertsson O, Knutson K, Lewold S, et al: Knee arthroplasty in rheumatoid arthritis. A report from the Swedish Knee Arthroplasty Register on 4,381 primary operations 1985-1995. Acta Orthop Scand 68(6):545, 1997.
137. Rosenberg AG, Haas B, Barden R, et al: Salvage of infected total knee arthroplasty. Clin Orthop 226:29, 1988.
138. Salvati EA, Callaghan JJ, Brause BD, et al: Reimplantation in infection: Elution of gentamicin from cement and beads. Clin Orthop 207:83, 1986.
139. Salvati EA, Robinson RP, Zeno SM, et al: Infection rates after 3175 total hip and total knee replacements performed with and without a horizontal unidirectional filtered air-flow system. J Bone Joint Surg Am 64:525, 1982.
140. Samuelson KM, Daniels AU, Rasmussen GL, et al: Evaluation of cemented versus finned peg cementless fixation and fixation in canine total joint arthroplasties. Orthop Trans 7:339, 1983.
141. Scott IR, Stockley I, Getty CJM: Exchange arthroplasty for infected knee replacements. A new method. J Bone Joint Surg Br 74:28, 1993.
142. Sculco TP: The economic impact of infected total joint arthroplasty. In Heckman JD, ed: American Academy of Orthopaedic Surgeons, Instructor Course Lectures, vol. 42. Rosemont, American Academy of Orthopaedic Surgeons, 1993, pp 349-351.
143. Seyral P, Zannier A, Argenson JN, et al: The release in vitro of vancomycin and tobramycin from acrylic bone cement. J Antimicrob Chemotherapy 33:337, 1994.
144. Simonian PT, Brause BD, Wickiewicz TL: *Candida* infection after total knee arthroplasty. Management without resection or amphotericin B. J Arthroplasty 12(7):825, 1997.
145. Smith TK: Nutrition: Its relationship to orthopaedic infections. Orthop Clin North Am 22:373, 1991.
146. Tannenbaum DA, Matthews LS, Grady-Benson JC: Infection around joint replacements in patients who have a renal or liver transplantation. J Bone Joint Surg Am 79:36, 1997.
147. Teeny SM, Dorr L, Murata G, et al: Treatment of infected total knee arthroplasty: Irrigation and debridement versus two-stage reimplantation. J Arthroplasty 5:35, 1990.
148. Wahlig H, Dingeldein E: Antibiotics and bone cement. Acta Orthop Scand 5:49, 1980.
149. Wahlig H, Dingeldein E, Buchholz HW, et al: Pharmacokinetic study of gentamicin-loaded cement in total hip replacements: Comparative effects of varying dosage. J Bone Joint Surg Br 66(2):175, 1984.
150. Wasielewski RC, Barden RM, Rosenberg AG: Results of different surgical procedures on total knee arthroplasty infections. J Arthroplasty 11:931, 1996.
151. Webb LX, Holman J, de Araujo B, et al: Antibiotic resistance in staphylococci adherent to cortical bone. J Orthop Trauma 8(1): 28, 1994.
152. Weinstein RA: Nosocomial infection update. Emerg Infect Dis 4(3):416, 1998.
153. Whiteside L: Treatment of infected total knee arthroplasty. Clin Orthop 299:169, 1994.
154. Wilde AH: Management of infected knee and hip prostheses. Curr Opin Rheumatol 6(2):172, 1994.
155. Wilde AH: Management of infected knee and hip prostheses. Curr Opin Rheumatol 5(3):317, 1993.

156. Wilde AH, Ruth JT: Two-stage reimplantation in infected total knee arthroplasty. Clin Orthop 236:23, 1988.
157. Windsor RE, Insall JN, Urs WR, et al: Two-stage reimplantation for the salvage of total knee arthroplasty complicated by infection: Further follow-up and refinement of indications. J Bone Joint Surg Am 72(2):272, 1990.
158. Woods GW, Lionberger DR, Tullos HS: Failed total knee arthroplasty: Revision and arthrodesis for infection and noninfectious complications. Clin Orthop 173:184, 1983.
159. Wright TM, Sullivan DJ, Arnoczky SP: The effect of antibiotic additions on the fracture properties of bone cements. Acta Orthop Scand 55:414, 1984.

92 Knee Arthrodesis and Resection Arthroplasty

JOHN J. CALLAGHAN • ARLEN D. HANSSEN

The improvement in results of total knee arthroplasty in general and in the treatment of the infected knee replacement specifically have diminished the need for arthrodesis and resection arthroplasty. As fewer arthrodeses are being performed and experience with the procedure is dwindling, the need to strictly follow the surgical principles of bone apposition, compressive force between bone ends, and rigid immobilization of the distal femur and proximal tibia is paramount in achieving successful fusion.[8, 14, 15, 17, 25, 41, 43] Since successful fusion occurs only in 80 to 90% of cases, techniques that optimize the fusion rate should be utilized. Resection arthroplasty, although performed less commonly than knee arthrodesis, should still be considered in the case of the infected total knee replacement where the host is compromised by many comorbidities that limit the patient's life expectancy.

INDICATIONS FOR ARTHRODESIS IN PATIENTS WITHOUT PREVIOUS ARTHROPLASTY

Over the years, the patients' and the surgeons' acceptance and enthusiasm for the arthrodesis procedure have markedly diminished. From the patients' perspective, they have heard about and seen the remarkable results of total knee replacement, and the concept of a stiff straight leg is not appealing. From the standpoint of the surgeon, he or she has gained more confidence in the total knee arthroplasty procedure and is always trying to broaden the indication for the procedure. There is a feeling of defeat if this cannot be accomplished for the individual patient. In addition, the surgeon understands that, unlike hip arthrodesis, which can be successfully converted to total hip replacement after many years of functional use, the knee arthrodesis is permanent, as the conversion of knee fusion to total knee replacement has had only very limited success. Indications for primary knee arthrodesis include (1) malignant and aggressive benign knee lesions; (2) unilateral posttraumatic arthritis in the young adult; (3) neuropathic joint; (4) the multiply operated knee; (5) paralytic conditions; and (6) painful ankylosis.

Cases of malignant and aggressive benign tumors of the knee remain one of the most important indications for knee arthrodesis today.[11, 44] Because no long term follow-up reports are available for total knee replacements with mechanically limited rotating hinge type modular devices and allograft surgery,[20, 33, 37, 38, 47, 48] fusion for lesions such as aggressive giant cell tumor, chondrosarcoma, osteosarcoma, and recurrent chondroblastoma is a reasonable option in combination with local resection.

Lexer first described local resection and arthrodesis for tumors about the knee in 1907.[30, 31] Enneking and Shirley[11] reported the treatment of local resection and arthrodesis using an intramedullary rod and autologous segmental cortical grafts for 20 malignant and aggressive benign lesions in the distal femur and proximal tibia. Only one local recurrence was reported. A customized bent fluted rod was used in most cases. More recently, Arroyo, Garvin, and Neff[1] reported the use of a titanium modular intramedullary nail that couples at the knee. Union occurred in all 16 cases where this device was used for tumors. No recurrence was noted.

Young patients with posttraumatic arthritis of the knee who plan to continue to perform manual labor should be offered a knee arthrodesis if nonoperative modalities including weight reduction, activity modification, braces, and medications do not relieve them of disabling pain. Before such recommendation, all other options including osteotomy and local allografts should be considered. In addition, the potential of vocational rehabilitation should be explored. Arthrodesis should be considered only for the most motivated individual who plans and needs to perform manual labor for a livelihood. Other young adults with disabling severe posttraumatic arthritis are probably better candidates for total knee replacement. As an example, a nonmotivated obese male or female is not the optimal candidate for knee arthrodesis.

A patient with arthrodesis of a Charcot knee that has failed to respond to bracing (i.e., progressive deformity and pain) has always been considered a candidate for knee fusion and contraindicated for knee replacement. However, successful fusion is limited and nonunion is high. Drennan and colleagues[10] reported better results when complete removal of the thick, boggy, and edematous synovium is performed in addition to débridement of all bone detritus. However, for the reasonable patient, and especially in bilateral cases, total knee replacement can be considered for at least one knee if not both. Bone defects should be reconstructed with metal augments rather than bone grafts, and long press-fit intramedullary stems should be considered. Permanent external bracing should be recommended, although compliance is difficult.[42]

The young patient with the multiply operated knee who has disabling pain, multiple incisions, and severe degenerative changes on radiographs may rarely be indicated for knee arthrodesis. However, nonoperative treatment with any pain relieving modality is the most appropriate treatment. Knee arthrodesis in this population, in the authors' experience, performs as poorly if not worse than total knee replacement in the workman's compensation group.

Fortunately, the sequela of poliomyelitis is rare in the United States today. The genu recurvatum and angular deformity that can occur are usually treated by bracing. When bracing fails, fusion can address the quadriceps weakness and deformity. However, the authors have also treated this problem with total knee replacement and bracing in the recent past.

The patient with a knee that is stiff and painful from previous sepsis including tuberculosis or from previous severe trauma and is basically ankylosed (no more than 10 to 20 degrees of motion) is an optimal candidate for formal knee arthrodesis. Many times the patient has an acceptable mindset for the procedure because he or she has lived with a stiff knee for many years. The surgeon also has an acceptable mindset because he or she realizes that arthroplasty performed in these circumstances produces suboptimal results. However, the surgeon should also recognize that in cases of anklylosis resulting from rheumatoid arthritis or uncomplicated osteoarthritis, successful knee replacement with limited knee flexion (usually less than 90 degrees) can be obtained by using quadriceps turndown techniques, employing skeletonization of the femur and tibia, and removing all scarred and contracted tissues from the medial and lateral gutters.[34, 35]

INDICATIONS FOR ARTHRODESIS IN PATIENTS WITH FAILED TOTAL KNEE ARTHROPLASTY

The main reason a surgeon considers knee arthrodesis today is for the failed total knee replacement, septic or aseptic. In the case of an infected total knee replacement, circumstances that warrant knee arthrodesis consideration include (1) persistent infection after multiple débridements with the end result a painful stiff knee with sinus tract formation and resistant bacteria; (2) infection with incompetent extensor mechanism; (3) infection with resistant organisms (i.e., methicillin-resistant *Staphylococcus* or vancomycin-resistant enterococcus) or infection requiring toxic antibiotic therapy (i.e., *Candida* or other fungal infections),[22, 27, 29, 45] especially in an immunocompromised patient (i.e., rheumatoid arthritis, diabetes, malignancy); (4) infection in the case of a failed two stage reimplantation; or (5) if this procedure is preferred by the patient (especially older debilitated patients, although these may be excellent candidates for resection arthroplasty). In the aseptic case, the patient with an incompetent extensor mechanism in whom reconstruction has failed is indicated for knee arthrodesis, especially if bracing fails or is unacceptable to the patient.

When considering the infected situation, the first scenario of the multiply débrided knee case should be avoided. If one débridement does not eradicate an infection, removal of the implant with radical débridement and two stage reimplantation should be an early

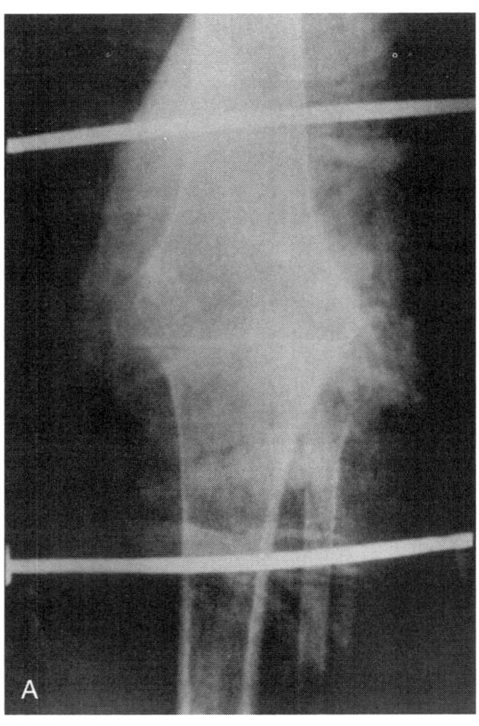

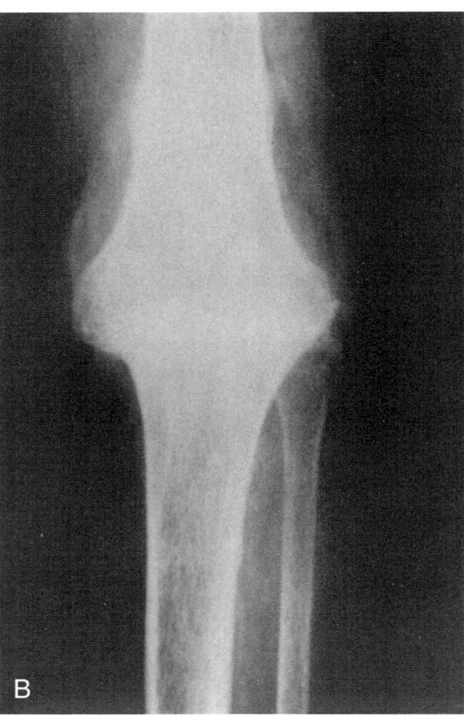

FIGURE 92.1 ➢ *A, B,* Compression arthrodesis using a Charnley clamp.

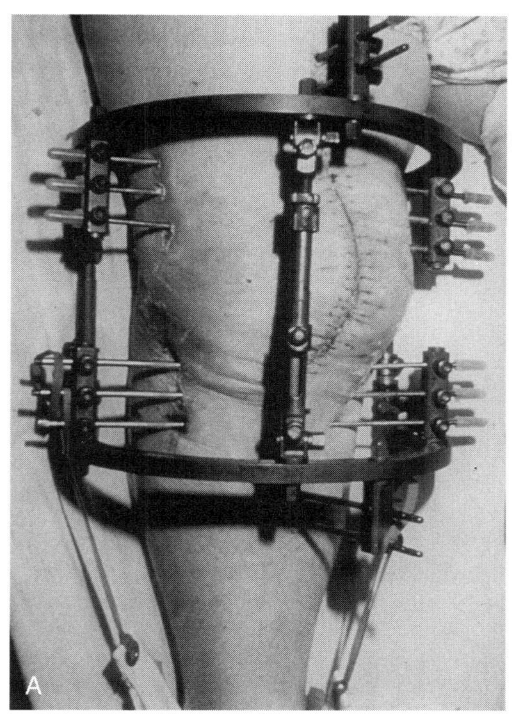

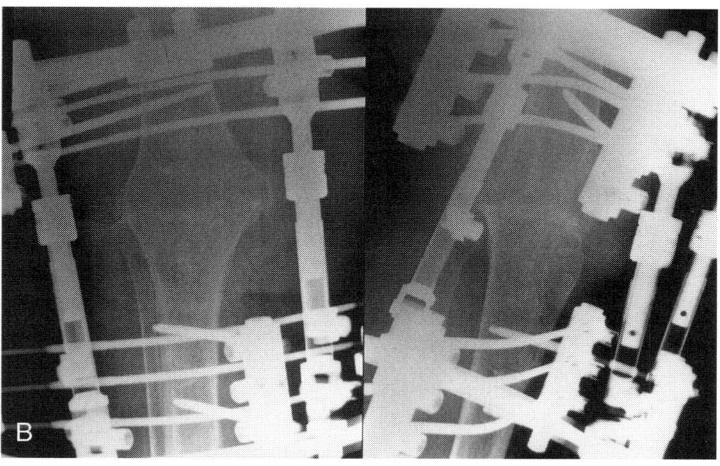

FIGURE 92.2 ➢ *A* and *B*, Ace Fischer device with multiple plane pins.

consideration. Most of these patients in whom the authors recommend the approach of arthrodesis have had 5 to 10 débridements and now have an extremely stiff knee. It is not uncommon to see extensor tendon avulsion in the same patient who has had multiple débridements. Because reconstruction of extensor tendon avulsion has limited success in a one-stage procedure, let alone in a two-stage procedure, the authors consider arthrodesis an option for these patients. If patients have resistant bacterial organisms infecting their replacement, the authors consider arthrodesis, especially in the immunocompromised patient, as their risk for recurrence is much higher than for infections with bacteria that are highly sensitive to antibiotic therapy. Although the authors do perform multiple two stage exchange procedures, when one such procedure has failed, the patient is always given the option of knee arthrodesis. However, a recent study demonstrates relatively poor results when fusion is performed following a failed two stage reimplantation.[18]

ARTHRODESIS TECHNIQUES

Surgical arthrodesis may be performed by one of three methods: (1) external fixation compression arthrodesis; (2) intramedullary rod fixation; and (3) plate and screws.

External Fixation Compression Arthrodesis

Compression, using a pin and frame technique, was described by Key[24] and by Charnley.[5, 6] Reasonable results with fusion rates as high as 85% can be achieved.[3] Fusion rates have been reported in only about 50% of cases when the procedure was performed for failure of hinged prostheses because of the large loss of bone in these cases. Most authors recommended application of the fixator for 3 months fol-

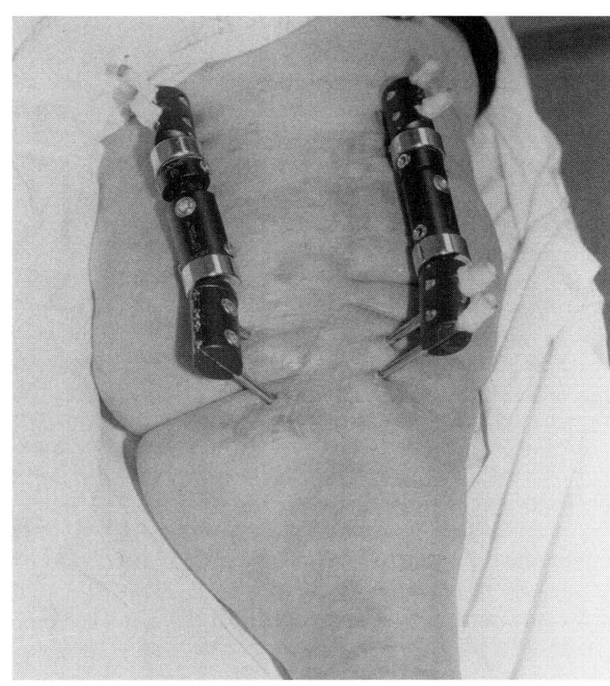

FIGURE 92.3 ➢ Medial and lateral monoblock EBI fixators in obese patient.

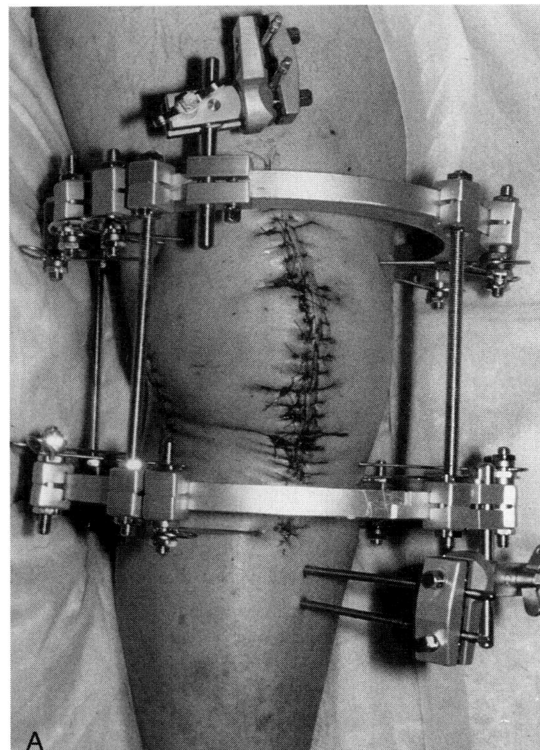

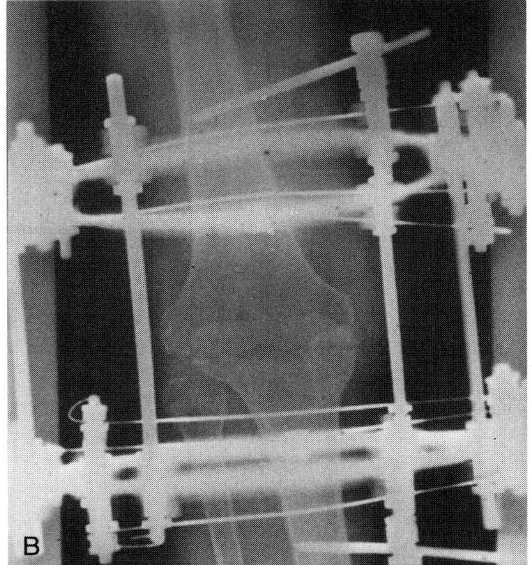

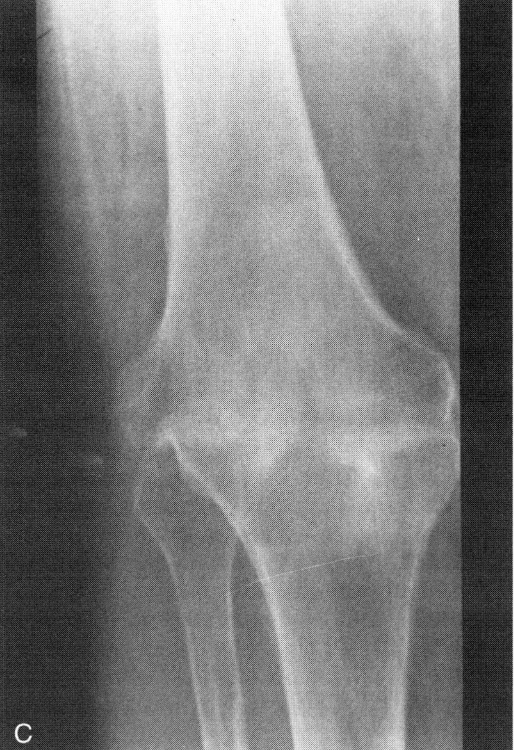

FIGURE 92.4 ➢ *A–C*, Ring fixator (Spinelli type, *A* and *B*) and final result (*C*).

lowed by cast immobilization until union occurs. The advantage of this technique is that it can be performed in one stage and the device can be easily removed leaving no remaining metal in place. Fixators can be placed in multiple planes, adding to the anterior posterior stability of the construct.[2, 26] The disadvantages of this technique include pin tract infections, poor patient compliance, and the need for casting following fixator application.

Surgical Procedure

For primary arthrodesis, the knee is approached through a midline incision and medial parapatellar approach. Total knee alignment jigs are used to resect approximately 1 or 2 cm of distal femur (using 5-degree valgus jig) and proximal tibia (with 5 to 10 degrees posterior slope) so that good cancellous bone is available for compression. The patella can be left alone, or the articular cartilage can be removed. Femo-

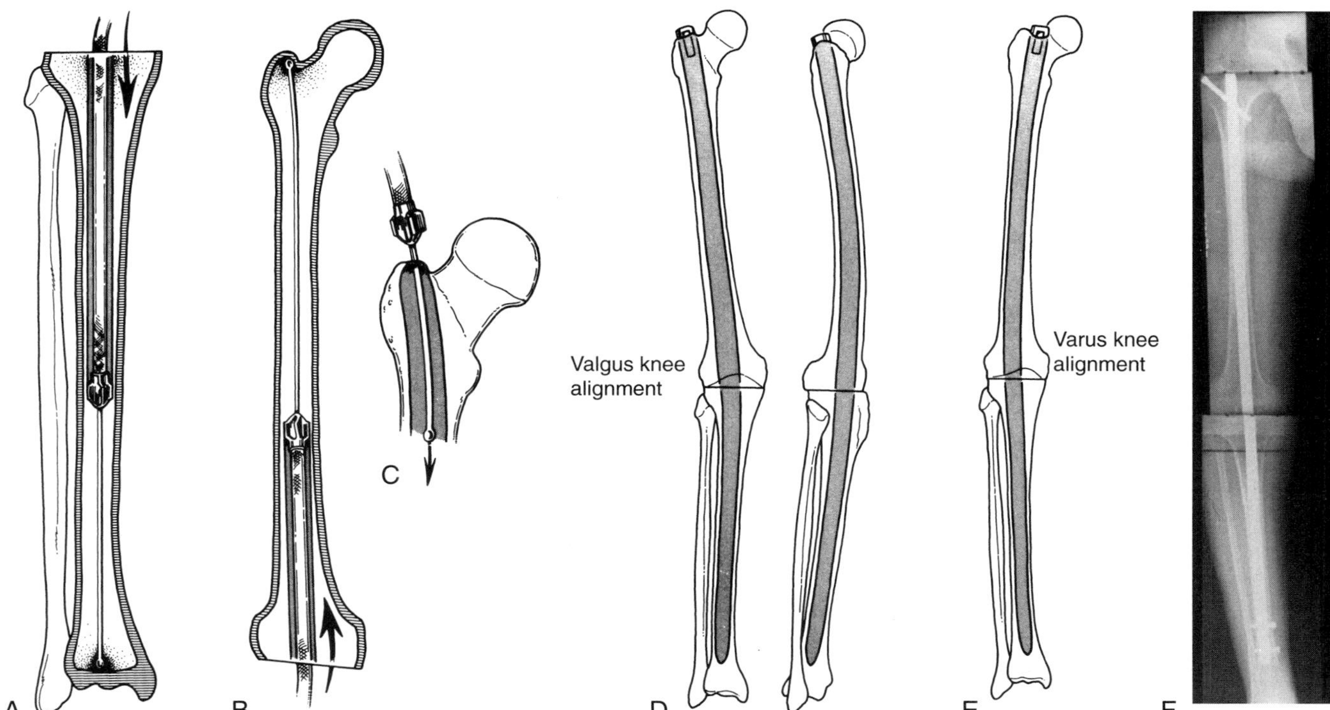

FIGURE 92.5 ➢ Technique of intramedullary arthrodesis. *A,* Tibial reaming to level of tibial plafond. The largest diameter to engage the tibial isthmus will be used for intramedullary nail diameter. *B,* Retrograde femoral reaming to inferior aspect of greater trochanter. Ream to diameter of the largest tibial reamer utilized. *C,* Antegrade reaming of the piriformis fossa to 1 mm greater than the nail diameter. *D,* Correct position of the nail convexity anteromedially to allow valgus and flexion of the arthrodesis site. *E,* Incorrect anterolateral positioning of the nail convexity, which drives the arthrodesis into a varus position. *F,* Case of intramedullary arthrodesis with proximal and distal interlock to avoid nail migration.

ral patella groove cartilage should also be resected if the patella articular cartilage is removed. The femur and tibia should be placed in contact with the desired alignment of 0 to 5 degrees of valgus and 10 to 15 degrees of flexion.

For cases of failed total knee arthroplasty, the remaining distal femur and proximal tibia should be interdigitated. No further bone resection should be performed. The patella can be used to fill any large bony defects. Today in addition to medial to lateral transfixion pins, anterior half pins are also placed for anterior-posterior stability. Illustrations demonstrate the use of Charnley compression clamp (Fig. 92.1); Ace Fischer device with a combination of transfixion and half pins (Fig. 92.2); multiple monoplane fixators (EBI, Warsaw, IN) (Fig. 92.3); and a ring fixator (Spinelli, Richards, Memphis, TN) (Fig. 92.4).

If stable, partial weightbearing is usually begun in the immediate postoperative period. Fixators are usually removed at 3 months or when pin tracts become a problem. A cast is applied until healing is complete.

Intramedullary Rod Fixation

Intramedullary rod fixation for knee arthrodesis has achieved fusion in 66 to 100% of reported cases.[9, 13, 16, 19, 23, 32, 46] The benefits of the intramedullary rod technique include immediate weightbearing and compression across the fusion bed, easier rehabilitation, the avoidance of pain tract problems, and the high fusion rate. Disadvantages include the need for a two stage procedure (in infection) and the difficulty of obtaining correct alignment.

Surgical Technique

Intramedullary arthrodesis has gained popularity for the salvage of severely infected total knee arthroplasties. Most authors recommend two stage procedures; however, Puranen[39] and colleagues have performed one stage procedures in cases with bacteria that are extremely sensitive to antibiotic agents. We usually perform the procedure after 4 weeks of antibiotic therapy or after the wound looks entirely benign.

The current technique utilizes the original longitudinal incision. The knee is widely exposed and débrided. The bone ends are prepared to allow maximum cancellous bone contact between the distal femur and proximal tibia. Using cannulated flexible reamers, the tibial shaft is reamed down to the tibial plafond (Fig. 92.5). The diameter of the largest reamer to engage the tibial isthmus is used for the size of the

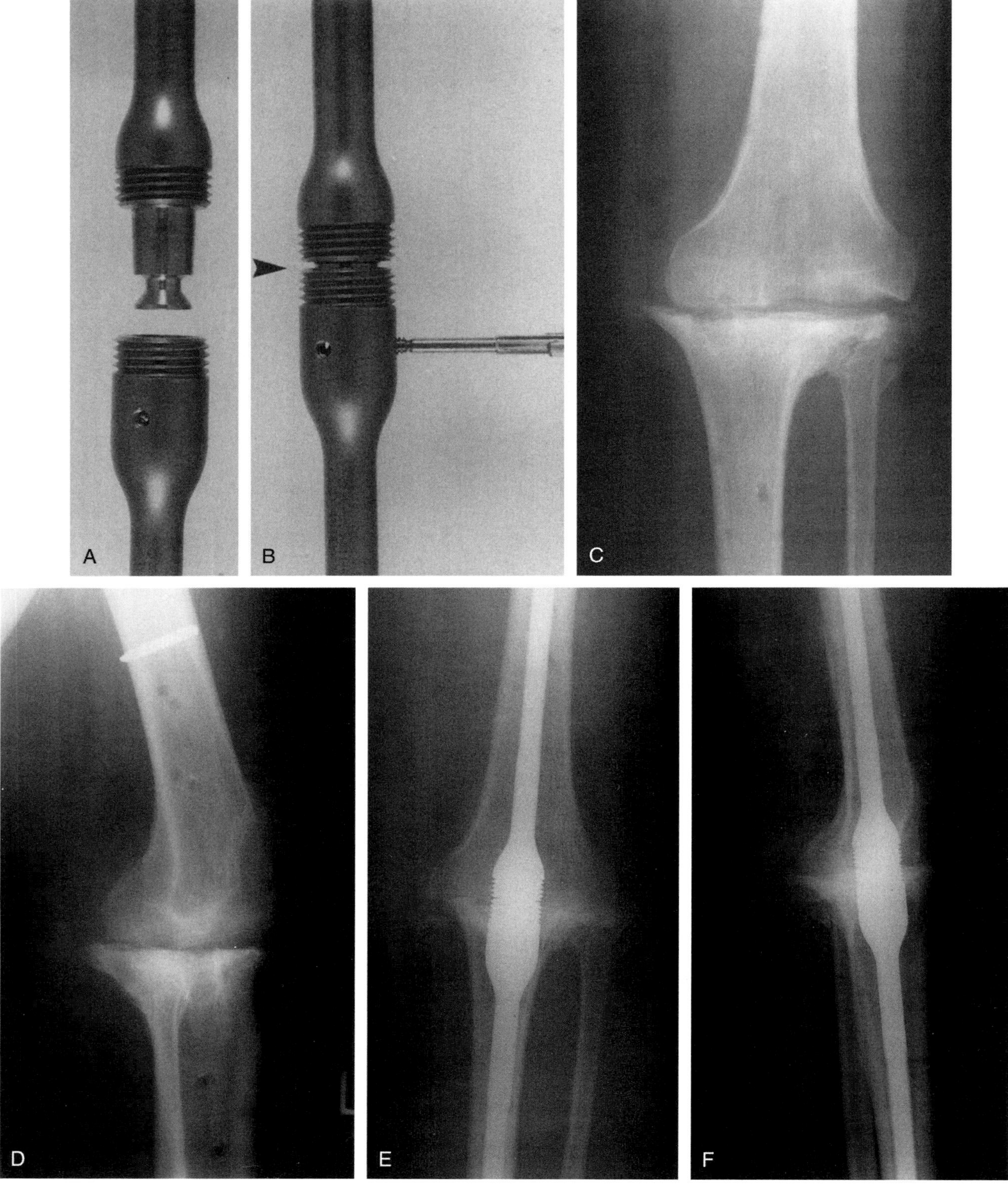

FIGURE 92.6 ➢ Modular intramedullary arthrodesis. Unlocked (*A*) and locked (*B*) modular connections of titanium modular intramedullary nail. Pre-fusion (*C, D*) and post-fusion (*E, F*) with a modular intramedullary nail performed for failed fusion following infected total knee replacement.

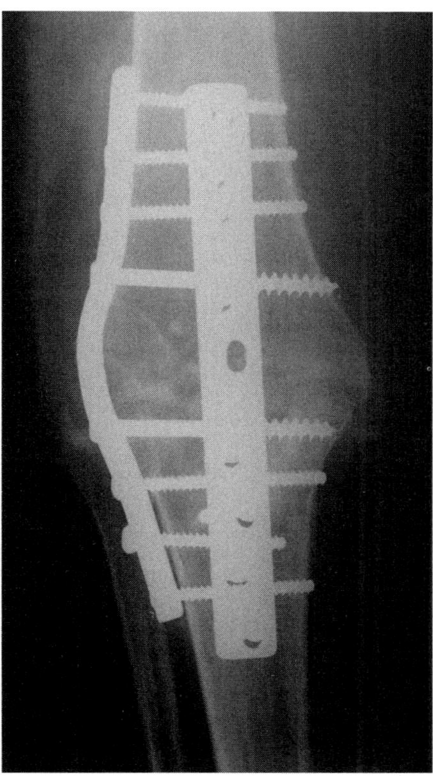

FIGURE 92.7 ➢ Knee arthrodesis performed with plate and screws. Plates are placed at right angles for stability.

rod. The desired tibial length of the rod is from the entrance into the tibia proximally to the tibial plafond. The guide wire is then inserted into the femoral canal to the inferior surface of the greater trochanter. The canal is reamed to the diameter of the previously reamed tibial isthmus. The femoral length is measured using the guide wire, and the length of the nail to be used is 1 cm shorter than the total femur and tibial length. The guide wire is then notched through the piriformis fossa with the thigh adducted. An incision is made over the subcutaneous tissue where the guide wire protrudes, and the incision is carried through the gluteus musculature to the piriformis recess. The recess is reamed to 1 mm greater than the diameter of the rod to be inserted. After reaming, a 90-cm curved Küntschner arthrodesis nail (Biomet, Inc., Warsaw, IN) is cut to the measured length (femoral plus tibial length minus 1 cm) using a high-speed diamond tip cutting tool (Midas Rex, Fort Worth, TX). In the technique of intramedullary arthrodesis, the rod is inserted with the curve positioned anteromedially down the femoral shaft. The rod will then come through the tibia in valgus alignment and in slight flexion. If the rod follows the anterolateral bow of the femur, it will enter the tibia in varus alignment with slight hyperextension. The anterior flare of the tibia can be forced forward by the rod, and the anterior tibial bone may need to be resected. It can be used for bone grafting. Some authors recommend wiring of the proximal position of the rod to prevent proximal migration. Some newer rods have a place for a proximal interlocking screw.

Recently, a modular titanium modular nail has been used for fusion (Fig. 92.6). Four of five cases in which the nail was used for failure of a total knee replacement healed; however, one of the cases required a second bone grafting procedure. The advantages of this approach are that the entire procedure can be performed through the knee incision, and in addition the tibia and femoral diameters can be independently sized. Concerns include the need to take down the fusion to retrieve the nail if late sepsis occurs around the nail. Also, the nail may be in the way of a future hip replacement, if it is required, because of the development of hip arthritis above the fusion. Attempts should be made to use a short femoral segment.[7, 28]

Arthrodesis With Plate and Screws

Some authors recommend internal fixation of the arthrodesis with plates and screws (Fig. 92.7). This can provide rigid fixation. Two plates perpendicular to each other have been recommended to provide a more steady construct. Concerns include potential wound closure problems because of proud plates. In addition, plates will need to be removed if sepsis recurs.

COMPLICATIONS OF ARTHRODESIS

The two major complications following knee arthrodesis are residual pain, which has been reported in up to 15% of cases; and nonunion, reported in 10 to 20% of all cases and in upwards of 50% of cases where a hinged prosthesis was utilized. In the case of residual pain, it must be explained preoperatively that 15% of patients may continue to have pain. Also, to avoid unrealistic expectations following surgery, placing the patient in a cylinder cast preoperatively for a time prior to surgery should help the patient understand the quality of life he or she can expect following fusion. The patient must understand that the procedure is a salvage operation and that it is permanent.

Nonunion can occur with any attempt at arthrodesis. When it occurs around an intramedullary nail, the nail can break. Breakage usually occurs at the knee, and arthrodesis may be repeated using a larger nail and bone grafting (Fig. 92.8). Vascularized fibular bone grafts have been successful in helping to achieve union in these cases.[40]

An additional complication is infection at pin tract sites or in cases of intramedullary nailing recurrent sepsis at the fusion site. These infected nails need to be removed with or without a later attempt at refusion. Such a case would require extensive bone destruction if a modular nail has been utilized. Especially if short nails are utilized, there is potential for fracture of the tibia at the end of the nail. For this reason, the nail should be seated well into the metaphysis of the distal tibia.

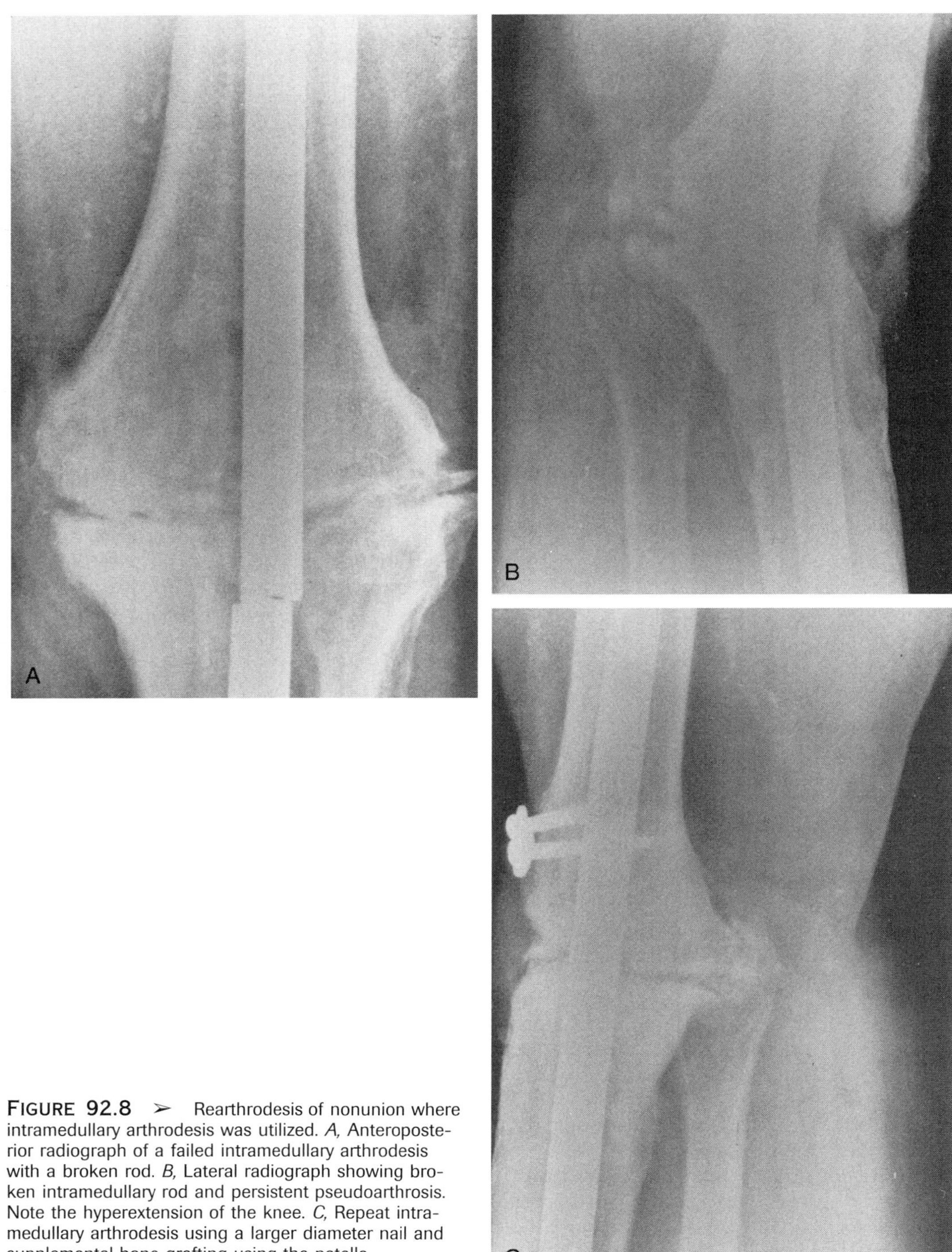

FIGURE 92.8 ➢ Rearthrodesis of nonunion where intramedullary arthrodesis was utilized. *A,* Anteroposterior radiograph of a failed intramedullary arthrodesis with a broken rod. *B,* Lateral radiograph showing broken intramedullary rod and persistent pseudoarthrosis. Note the hyperextension of the knee. *C,* Repeat intramedullary arthrodesis using a larger diameter nail and supplemental bone grafting using the patella.

CONVERSION OF ARTHRODESIS TO TOTAL KNEE REPLACEMENT

One should refrain from converting a fused knee to a total knee replacement (Fig. 92.9). A long-standing fusion results in permanent scarring and contracture of surrounding muscle, limiting acceptable knee flexion. Collateral ligament integrity is suspect. Muscle atrophy contributes to significant extensors lags. There is a high rate of recurrent sepsis.[4, 21, 36] There is no guarantee for a successful fusion if this operation fails. The best results are obtained if the knee is fused in excessive flexion. In addition, a knee fused in this position is one in which the arthrodesis limits activity.

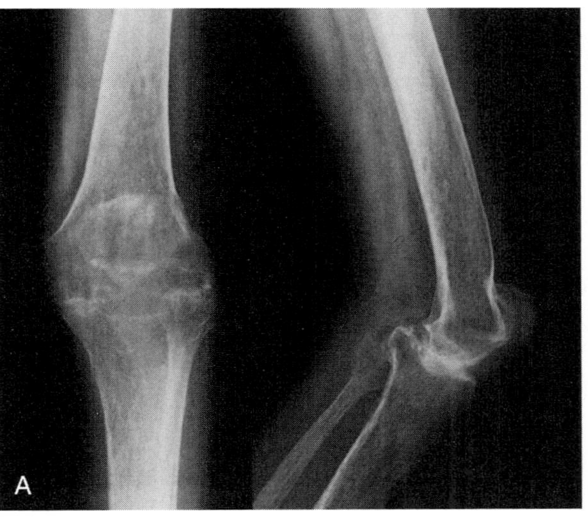

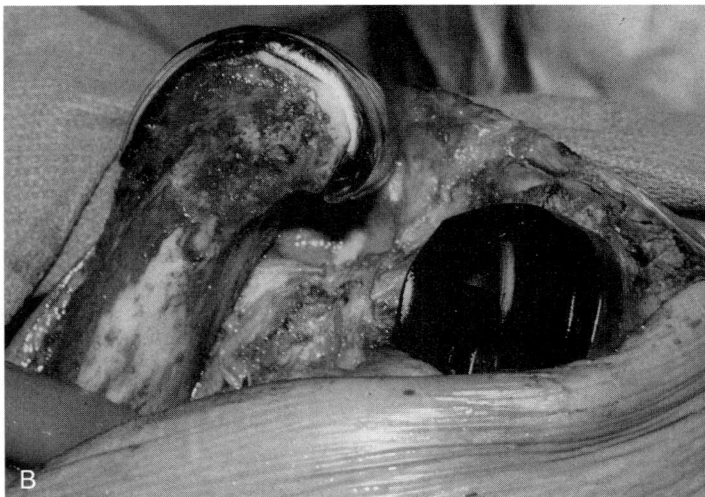

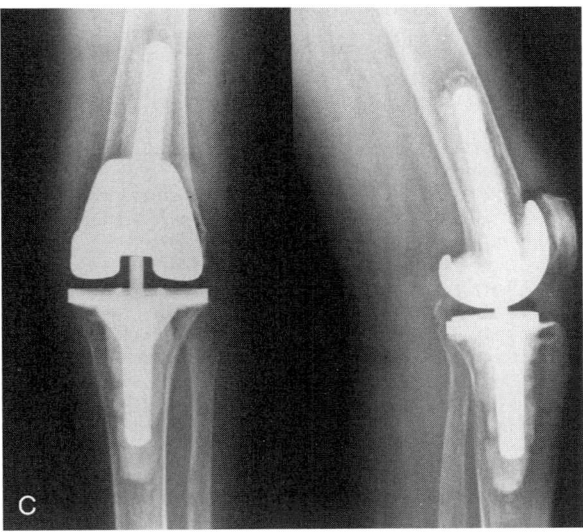

FIGURE 92.9 ➢ Arthrodesis conversion to total knee replacement; 54-year-old patient with rheumatoid arthritis and knee fusion following removal of septic knee. The knee was fused in 40 degrees of external rotation and 45 degrees of flexion (*A*) and was of no functional use to the patient. *B*, Intraoperative photograph demonstrates medial femoral peel. *C*, Patient postoperatively has 5 to 70 degrees of knee flexion.

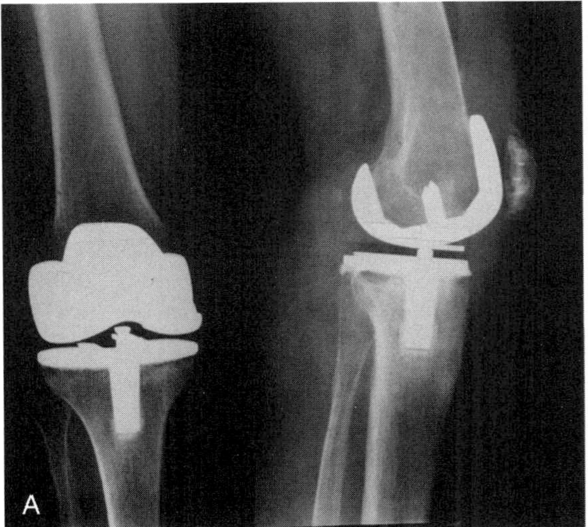

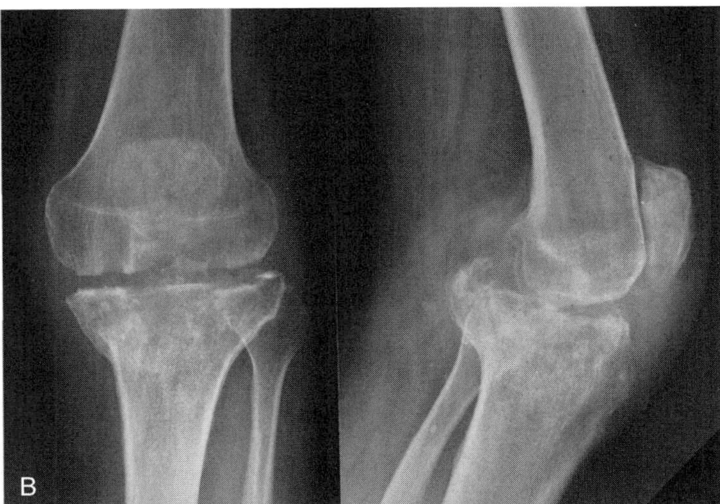

FIGURE 92.10 ➢ Immunocompromised male (88 years old) who minimally ambulated before surgery. He had a total knee replacement (*A*) infected with methicillin-resistant *Staphylococcus aureus* and *Pseudomonas* and was treated with resection arthroplasty (*B*).

RESECTION ARTHROPLASTY

For debilitated patients with low demands and high comorbidities, simple resection of an infected total knee replacement may be an excellent option (Fig. 92.10). Falahee et al[12] reviewed 28 knees with resection arthroplasty. Local infection was eliminated in 89 per cent of cases. The patients who had had the most severe disability before the total knee arthroplasty were most likely to be satisfied. We have also found that patients with better bone stock do better. One misconception is that this operation works best if the knee flexes more. After thorough débridement, we cast the patients or brace them in extension for 6 to 12 weeks with the intention that they will obtain 30 to 50 degrees of flexion but that the knee will be relatively stable in the medial lateral direction.

References

1. Arroyo JS, Garvin KL, Neff JF: Arthrodesis of the knee with a modular titanium intramedullary nail. J Bone Joint Surg Am 79: 26, 1997.
2. Briggs B, Chao EYS: The mechanical performance of the standard Hoffmann-Vidal external fixation apparatus. J Bone Joint Surg Am 64:566, 1982.
3. Brodersen MP, Fitzgerald RH Jr, Peterson LFA, et al: Arthrodesis of the knee following failed total knee arthroplasty. J Bone Joint Surg Am 61:181, 1979.
4. Cameron HU, Hu C: Results of total knee arthroplasty following takedown of femoral knee fusion. J Arthroplasty 11:732, 1996.
5. Charnley JC: Positive pressure in arthrodesis of the knee joint. J Bone Joint Surg Br 30:478, 1948.
6. Charnley J, Baker SL: Compression arthrodesis of the knee: A clinical and histological study. J Bone Joint Surg Br 34:187, 1952.
7. Cheng SL, Gross AE: Knee arthrodesis using a short locked intramedullary nail: A new technique. Am J Knee Surg 8:56, 1995.
8. Dee R: The case for arthrodesis of the knee. Orthop Clin North Am 10(1):249, 1979.
9. Donley BG, Matthews LS, Kaufer H: Arthrodesis of the knee with an intramedullary nail. J Bone Joint Surg Am 73:907, 1991.
10. Drennan DB, Fahey JJ, Maylahn DJ: Important factors in achieving arthrodesis of the Charcot knee. J Bone Joint Surg 73:907, 1991.
11. Enneking WF, Shirley PD: Resection-arthrodesis for malignant and potentially malignant lesions about the knee using an intramedullary rod and local bone grafts. J Bone Joint Surg Am 59: 223, 1977.
12. Falahee MH, Matthews LS, Kaufer H: Resection arthroplasty as a salvage procedure for a knee with infection after total arthroplasty. J Bone Joint Surg Am 69:1013, 1987.
13. Fern ED, Stewart HD, Newton G: Curved Küntscher nail arthrodesis after failure of knee replacement. J Bone Joint Surg Br 71: 588, 1989.
14. Figgie HE III, Brody GA, Inglis AE, et al: Knee arthrodesis following total knee arthroplasty in rheumatoid arthritis. Clin Orthop 224:237, 1987.
15. Green DP, Parkes JC II, Stinchfield FE: Arthrodesis of the knee: A follow-up study. J Bone Joint Surg Am 49:1065, 1967.
16. Griend RV: Arthrodesis of the knee with intramedullary fixation. Clin Orthop 181:146, 1983.
17. Hagemann WF,Woods GW, Tullos HS: Arthrodesis in failed total knee replacement. J Bone Joint Surg Am 60:790, 1978.
18. Hanssen AD, Trousdale RT, Osmon DR: Patient outcome with reinfection following reimplantation for the infected total knee arthroplasty. Clin Orthop 321:55, 1995.
19. Harris CM, Froehlich J: Knee fusion with intramedullary rods for failed total knee arthroplasty. Clin Orthop 197:209, 1985.
20. Higinbotham ML, Coley BL: The treatment of bone tumors by resection and replacement with massive grafts. Instr Course Lect 7:26, 1950.
21. Holden DL, Jackson DW: Considerations in total knee arthroplasty following previous knee fusion. Clin Orthop 227:223, 1988.
22. Iskander MK, Khan MA: *Candida albicans* infection of a prosthetic knee replacement [letter]. J Rheumatol 15(10):1594, 1988.
23. Kaufer H, Irvine G, Matthews LS: Intramedullary arthrodesis of the knee. Orthop Trans 7:547, 1983.
24. Key JA: Positive pressure in arthrodesis for tuberculosis of the knee joint. South Med J 25:909, 1932.
25. Knutson K, Hovelius L, Lindstrand A, Lidgren L: Arthrodesis after failed knee arthroplasty: A nationwide multicenter investigation of 91 cases. Clin Orthop 191:202, 1984.
26. Knutson K, Bodelind B, Lidgren L: Stability of external fixators used for knee arthrodesis after failed knee arthroplasty. J Bone Joint Surg Br 67:47, 1985.
27. Koch AE: *Candida albicans* infection of a prosthetic knee replacement: A report and review of the literature. J Rheumatol 15(2):362, 1988.
28. Lai K, Shen WJ, Yang CY: Arthrodesis with a short Huckstep nail as a salvage procedure for failed total knee arthroplasty. J Bone Joint Surg Am 80:380, 1988.
29. Levine M, Rehm SJ, Wilde AH: Infection with *Candida albicans* of a total knee arthroplasty: Case report and review of the literature. Clin Orthop 226:235, 1988.
30. Lexer E: Substitution of whole or half joints from freshly amputated extremities by free plastic operation. Surg Gynecol Obstet 6:501, 1908.
31. Lexer E: Joint transplantations and arthroplasty. Surg Gynecol Obstet 40:782, 1925.
32. Mazet R, Urist MR: Arthrodesis of the knee with intramedullary nail fixation. Clin Orthop 18:43, 1960.
33. Merle D'Aubigne R, Dejouany JP: Diaphyso-epiphyseal resection for bone tumor at the knee: With reports of nine cases. J Bone Joint Surg Br 40:385, 1958.
34. Montgomery WH III, Insall JN, Haas SB, et al: Primary total knee arthroplasty in stiff and ankylosed knees. Am J Knee Surg 11:20, 1998.
35. Montgomery WH, Becker MW, Windsor RE, Insall JN: Primary total knee arthroplasty in stiff and ankylosed knees. Orthop Trans 15:54, 1991.
36. Naranja RJ, Lotke PA, Pagnano MW, Hanssen AD: Total knee arthroplasty in a previously ankylosed or arthrodesed knee. Clin Orthop 331:234.
37. Parrish FF: Treatment of bone tumors by total excision and replacement with massive autologous and homologous grafts. J Bone Joint Surg Am 48:968, 1966.
38. Phemister DB: Rapid repair of defect of femur by massive bone grafts after resection for tumors. Surg Gynecol Obstet 80:120, 1945.
39. Puranen J, Kortelainen P, Jalovaara P: Arthrodesis of the knee with intramedullary nail fixation. J Bone Joint Surg 72:433, 1990.
40. Rasmussen MR, Bishop AT, Wood MB: Arthrodesis of the knee with a vascularized fibular rotatory graft. J Bone Joint Surg Am 77:751 1995.
41. Siller TN, Hadjipavlou A: Arthrodesis of the knee. In The American Academy of Orthopaedic Surgeons Symposium on Reconstructive Surgery of the Knee. St. Louis, CV Mosby, 1978, p 161.
42. Soudry M, Binazzi R, Johanson NA, et al: Total knee arthroplasty in Charcot and Charcot-like joints. Clin Orthop 208:199, 1986.
43. Stulberg SD: Arthrodesis in failed total knee replacements. Orthop Clin North Am 12(1):213, 1982.
44. Tuli SM: Bridging of bone defects by massive bone grafts in tumorous conditions and in osteomyelitis. Clin Orthop 87:60, 1972.
45. Wilde AH, Sweeney RS, Borden LS: Hematogenously acquired infection of a total knee arthroplasty by *Clostridium perfringens.* Clin Orthop 229:228, 1988.
46. Wilde AH, Stearns KL: Intramedullary fixation for arthrodesis of the knee after infected total knee arthroplasty. Clin Orthop 248: 86, 1989.
47. Wilson PD, Lance EM: Surgical reconstruction of the skeleton following segmental resection for bone tumors. J Bone Joint Surg Am 47:1629, 1965.
48. Wilson PD Jr: A clinical study of the biomechanical behavior of massive bone transplants used to reconstruct large bone defects. Clin Orthop 87:81, 1972.

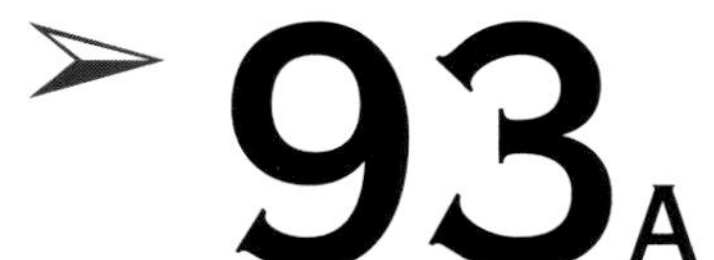

Revision Knee Arthroplasty: How I Do It

LAWRENCE D. DORR

PREOPERATIVE ASSESSMENT

Preoperatively, the most important clinical assessment is the determination of the range of motion of the knee and the ligamentous stability of the knee. If the patient has had multiple previous surgeries, the knowledge of all of the previous skin incisions about the knee is critical. Preoperative range of motion is important because in patients who do not have flexion to 90 degrees and have a stable knee, the release of the attachment of the superficial medial collateral ligament at the tibia is important during the approach so that this ligament does not tear during full flexion of the knee. Secondly, in patients who do not have 90 degrees of flexion, the surgeon should anticipate that some release of the extensor mechanism will be required to obtain good postoperative flexion. The choice is proximal with the extensor mechanism or distal with the tibial tubercle elevation. I always use proximal release. The presence of a flexion contracture beyond 15 degrees also requires special attention of the surgeon to the flexion space and most often will require the release of posterior capsule from the posterior femur and certainly the sacrifice of the posterior cruciate ligament.

Preoperative assessment of the radiograph is important for determination of bone loss. Bone loss of the distal femur most often can be replaced with augments. However, it is important to know that the use of augments is limited by the necessity to be sure that the posterior condyles of the femoral implant are hooked under posterior femoral bone. If not, there is not good rotational stability of the distal femoral component and it can become loose at the Morse taper fit to any stem that is used. Therefore, I am willing not to restore the joint line if it would compromise rotational stability of the distal femoral component. Bone graft for the distal femur can be anticipated if it is necessary to provide rotational stability of the femoral component.

For the tibia, the tibial condylar plate must also sit on some bone. The tibia cannot simply be fixed by a stem into a diaphyseal tube. This will result in rapid loosening of the tibia. The use of proximal tibial allograft can be anticipated when the entire tibial metaphysis is missing. This proximal tibial allograft will be necessary to provide tilt and rotational stability of the tibial component. Particulate graft can be used in the tibia only for filling of cavitary defects and not proximal segmental loss.

SKIN INCISION AND APPROACH

Prior to preparation and draping of the leg, we place a support for the foot that allows the leg to be stabilized in flexion without the foot slipping. We also use a support against the greater trochanter (often this is adjacent to the level of the tourniquet) to prevent the leg from falling sideways. With the leg supported in flexion and from falling sideways, the leg is stabilized, which frees the hands of the assistant from holding the leg.

In a patient with multiple scars on the knee, I will select the scar that is most anterior or most medial parapatellar. If a knee has only a long lateral parapatellar scar, I will use the lateral scar for the skin and subcutaneous incision and then undermine the subcutaneous tissue to the medial side of the patella and enter the knee through a medial parapatellar approach. I do not use a lateral approach, even with the presence of a lateral scar, because of the difficulty in everting the patella medially without a tubercle osteotomy and the difficulty in closing the lateral fascial incision. The skin incision extends a minimum of four fingerbreadths above the superior pole of the patella and two fingerbreaths below the tibial tubercle. If the skin incision is anterior or medial parapatellar, it is undermined subcutaneously across the top of the patella to expose the entire quadriceps tendon and the entire patella ligament. In a stiff knee that will require an extended rectus snip approach, the incision is carried even further proximally.

Approach

Once the quadriceps tendon, patella, and patella ligament have been exposed, the incision is made through the medial side of the quadriceps tendon as close to the vastus medialis obliquus muscle as possible (leaving a 2 to 3 mm cuff of tendon attached to the vastus medialis obliquus muscle). The incision is carried medially to the patella just enough to allow reattachment of the medial capsule to the patella and finally is carried through the scar tissue just medial to the patella ligament and its attachment to the tibial tubercle. Usu-

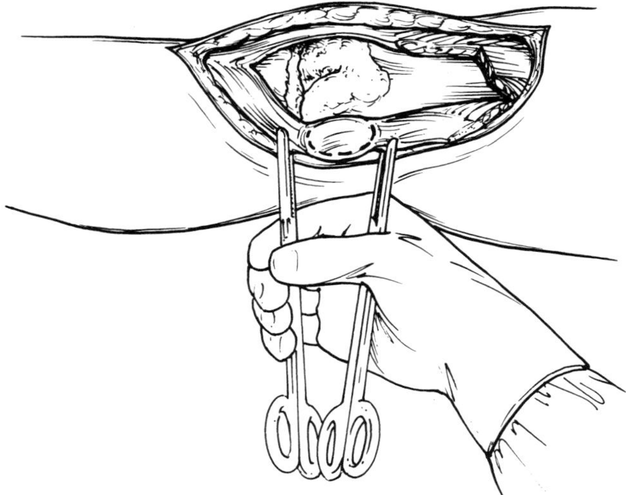

FIGURE 93–1 ➢ Rectus snip incision with proximal lateral extension of the incision across the quadriceps tendon and into the vastus lateralis muscle in line with its fibers allows eversion of the patella without tension on the patella ligament.

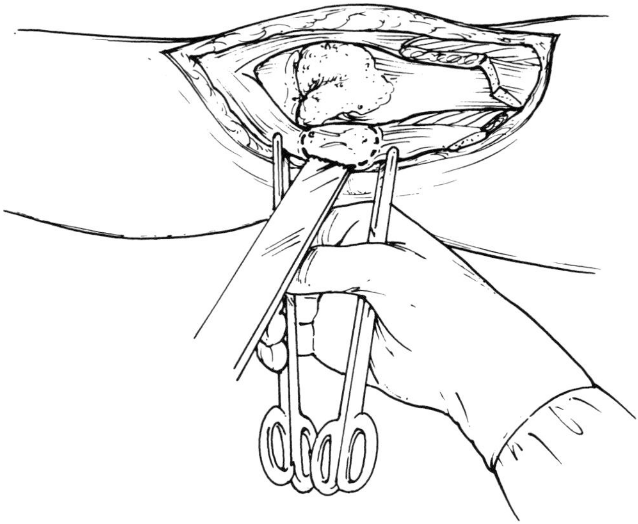

FIGURE 93–2 ➢ The patient cut is made with two Kochler clamps stabilizing the patella. One Kochler clamp (or towel clip clamp) is superior on the quadriceps tendon, and one is inferior to the patella on the patella ligament.

ally with revision surgery this tissue is thickened over the proximal tibia, which makes it easier to make a medial cuff of tissue for reattachment to the patella ligament.

In a patient with a stiff total knee, a rectus snip is always done and is extended proximally through the vastus lateralis muscle in an oblique fashion directed proximally (Fig. 93.1). Eversion of the patella is further facilitated by excision of any scar in the lateral recess and any lateral scar tissue in the suprapatellar pouch between the quadriceps mechanism or vastus lateralis muscle and the femur. Eversion of the patella should be performed sufficiently to allow the patella to be held superiorly and inferiorly to the patella with Kochler clamps for excision of scar tissue around the patella and removal of the patella component (Fig. 93.2). Eversion should also be sufficient to allow the patella to be retracted completely laterally of the tibial plateau when the knee is in full flexion (Fig. 93.3). We will elevate one third of the patella ligament attachment to the tibial tubercle to relieve any tension on the attachment of the tendon to the tubercle. The tendon can be also protected by one or two towel clips, which are placed through the tendon and into the tibial tubercle.

At the completion of the approach, the knee should be able to be fully mobilized from full extension to complete flexion with the patella everted laterally.

REMOVAL OF THE COMPONENTS

The first component removed by us is the modular tibial insert (if one is present). If the knee is stiff, this modular tibial component is removed even prior to full flexion of the knee to facilitate mobilization of the knee. The modular plastic is removed by using an osteotome between the plastic and the metal tray to loosen the locking mechanism so that the plastic can be lifted out of the metal tray.

Removal of the femoral component must be done without removal of bone. I prefer the use of a Gigli saw across the trochlea to the level of the housing of a PS knee or the pegs of a cruciate retaining knee. I will use a high-speed drill with a thin pointed bit to

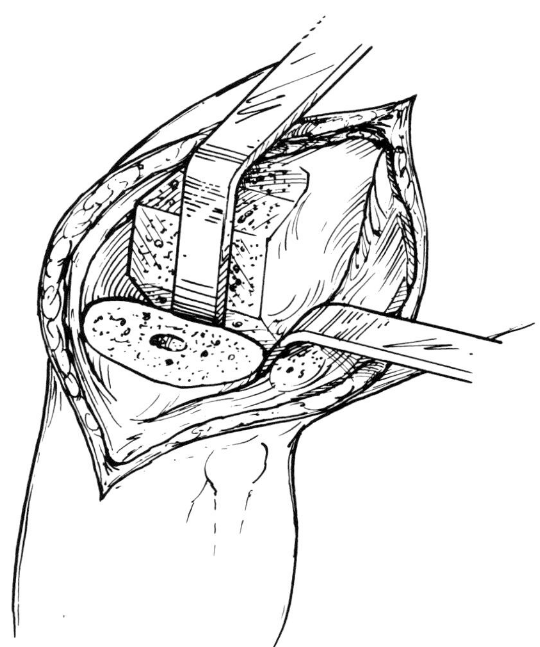

FIGURE 93–3 ➢ The tibia is retracted anterior to the femur and the patella is retracted lateral.

fragment the cement or the bone ingrowth fixation between the metal and the distal femoral condyles and the posterior condyles. Once the interface has been fragmented in this fashion, the femoral component can be removed from the femur by using a bone tamp and knocking it off in an axial direction. With careful attention to the fragmentation of the interface, the femoral component can always be removed without fracture of a condyle or removal of excessive distal femoral bone.

If the femoral component has a stem that is well fixed into the diaphysis with either bone ingrowth through a porous coated stem, or a fixed cemented stem to a roughened surface, the femoral component cannot be knocked out in an axial direction. In this situation, I remove a window of anterior femur bone to provide access to the interface between the metal stem and the fixation (Fig. 93.4) The pointed bit of the high-speed drill is again used to fragment the fixation of the stem, which then allows removal of the femoral component. The window is reattached with either cables or wires.

The tibial component is removed by using a saw to fragment the interface between the tibial component and the tibial bone. If there are screws into the tibial component, they are removed prior to the use of the saw. If there are pegs under the tibial tray, again the pointed bur of the high speed drill is used to reach those areas between the pegs that cannot be reached with a saw. Once the tibial condylar fixation is fragmented, a metal tray can be removed in an axial direction if there is a smooth metal stem. If there is an all polyethylene tibial component, the saw is used to cut across the tibial stem for removal of the tibial condylar plastic. The cemented polyethylene tibial stem is removed separately.

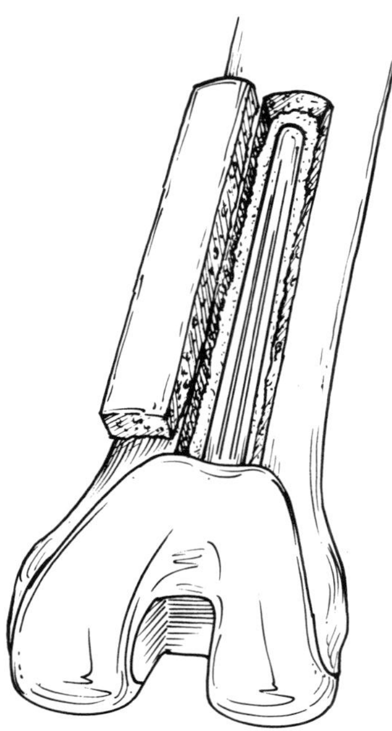

FIGURE 93–4 ➢ An anterior femoral bone window is removed to expose the stem and the fixation.

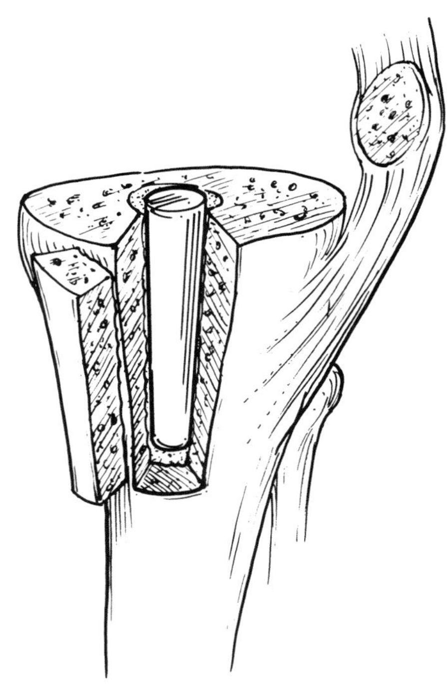

FIGURE 93–5 ➢ An anterior tibial window medial to the tibial tubercle is removed to expose stem and fixation.

If there is a fixed tibial stem into the diaphysis by either porous coating bone ingrowth fixation or cemented fixation to a roughened stem, a window is made in the tibia. This is done by removing the bone medial to the tibial tubercle so that the attachment of the patella ligament is not jeopardized (Fig. 93.5). The strip of bone that is removed can be whatever length is necessary to have access to the entire length of the stem. The stem fixation interface is again fragmented using the pointed burr of the high speed drill. The tibial window is reattached using either cables or wires.

Removal of the patella component should also be done if it is significantly worn, if it is metal-backed and worn at all, or if it has a shape that is specific to a trochlea that is different from the one being reimplanted. The patella component can be removed by gripping the quadriceps tendon superiorly and the patella ligament inferiorly with a Kochler clamp or (a towel clip). The patella is stabilized by the assistant holding the Kochler clamps with a knuckle of the index finger pushing up onto the surface of the patella bone (see Fig. 93.2). All soft tissue is excised from around the edge of the patella component so that the interface between the patella component and the bone is visible. A saw is used again to fragment the interface and if the patella is an all polyethylene patella, the saw can be used to divide the pegs from the patella implant substrate. The pegs can then be removed separately. If there is a metal-backed patella, again the pointed bit of the high-speed drill can be used to fragment the interface between the metal pegs to loosen the metal interface from the bone and allow removal of the component without fracture or destruction of the patella bone.

REVISION INSTRUMENTS

The principles for use of instruments for the femur is to provide the correct valgus and rotational orientation of the femoral component. The valgus of the femur will be determined by the stem if the stem is press fit. The stem of the Apollo revision knee (ACK, Sulzer Medica, Austin, TX) is 7 degrees. In a primary knee, I prefer 4 to 5 degrees of valgus; therefore, if I use a cemented stem, I will try to achieve 4 to 5 degrees of valgus (Fig. 93.6). It is important that the revision instruments allow the intercondylar notch cut for a posterior stabilized or constrained condylar revision knee to be oriented in the same external rotation as is desired for the femoral component.

For the tibia, the principle for instrumentation is that the varus/valgus alignment be as close to 0 degrees as possible. The posterior tilt for the ACK knee system requires 3 degrees posterior tilt. The intramedullary canal of the bony tibia is off-set 3 to 5 mm in most knees; therefore, if non-cemented stems are used centrally on the tibial tray, the tibial stem will cause overhang of the tibial tray. Therefore, the offset of the tibial intramedullary canal must be compensated by off-set of the stem on the tibial tray. The revision instruments must also provide for satisfactory preparation of the metaphyseal stem position. The flare of the metaphyseal stem must be aligned correctly for rotational control of the tibial component. Ninety-five percent of the time, this rotation will be correct when aligned over the medial third of the tibial tubercle.

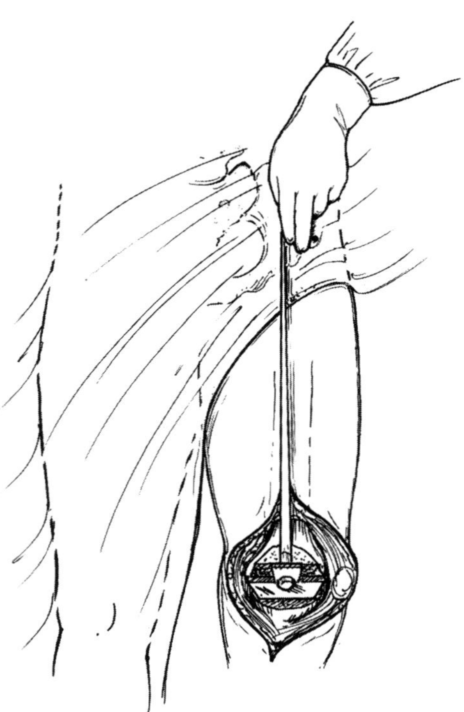

FIGURE 93–6 ➢ An anterior rod over the femur points to two fingerbreadths inside (medial to) the anterior superior spine of the pelvis. This position provides a distal femoral cut of approximately 5 degrees of valgus.

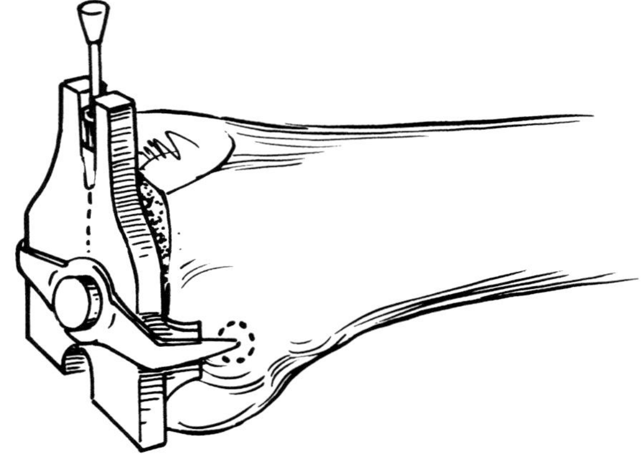

FIGURE 93–7 ➢ Rotation of the femur is determined by aligning the rotational tool with the lateral epicondyle that provides approximately 3 degrees of external rotation.

The only revision instruments for the patella for us are two Kocher clamps. A Kocher clamp is placed across the quadriceps tendon and across the patella ligament so that the patella can be stabilized for removal of the previous patella component and bone preparation for the new patella component. A drill guide is necessary to correctly position the drill holes for the pegs of the patella. Because the bone in the patella will be variable in a revision knee, the choice for three pegs or a single central peg should be available.

Femoral Tools

For preparation of the femur, the instrument that I favor the most for revision surgery is the femoral aligning tool. This tool has a plate that is angulated 6 degrees so that the distal end of the femur can be cut with a saw parallel to the plate and corrected to 5 to 7 degrees of valgus. The use of this tool provides a rapid accurate check of the distal femoral angle after removal of the previous component and allows this angle to be quickly prepared at the correct angulation. The second tool that is required is a distal femoral block that allows correct preparation of the rotation of the femur by the anterior and posterior cut. This block is set so that it is along the epicondylar axis. In practice, we simply align it with the apex of the lateral epicondyle and the block can then be fixed in this position so that the anterior and posterior cuts are then made with correct rotation (Fig. 93.7). The distal femoral block is attached onto a stem in the femoral

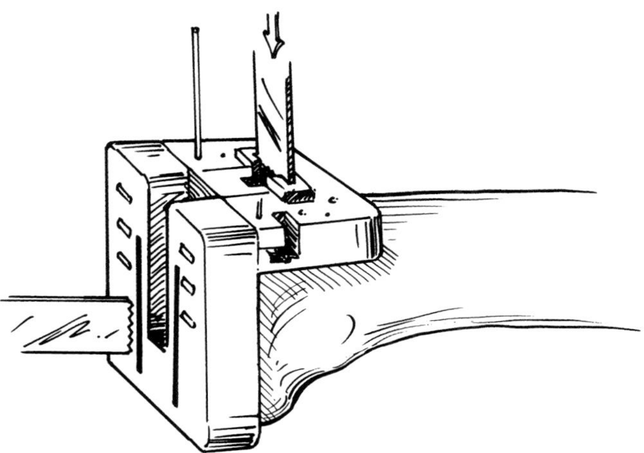

FIGURE 93–8 ➢ The intercondylar cut must be in external rotation that matches the rotational cut of the femur. The cutting tool provides this external rotation by resting on the anterior femoral cut. The osteotome placed proximally protects against the saw cutting through a condyle.

canal that gives stability to the block. The size stem for the medullary canal is determined by using hand reamers sequentially until there is a good mechanical grip of the reamer in the intramedullary canal, indicating the correct size.

The last step for femoral preparation is the intercondylar notch cut. The tool is set on the anterior cut of the femur so that the rotation will be correct. The depth and width of the cut are then made through the intercondylar notch cut guide (Fig. 93.8).

Tibial Tools

The most useful instrument for the tibia, again, is the aligner tool (Fig. 93.9). The tibial plate has a 7-degree posterior tilt, and therefore with an intramedullary rod the varus/valgus and posterior tilt position of the tibial cut can be evaluated. The varus/valgus position is preferred to be 90 degrees to the axis of the tibia, and the posterior tilt of the ACK is 3 degrees. With the aligning tool in the canal, a saw can be used to cut parallel to the surface of the plate to produce the varus/valgus cut. The posterior tilt would be somewhat less than is present in the metal plate of the aligner. If there is a significant medial or lateral defect, the tibial cutting jig is applied by attaching to the intramedullary stem. The hand-held reamer is again used to determine the size of the tibial intramedullary canal, and a tibial stem of that size is inserted. The cutting block is attached to this tibial stem. The cutting block will allow the varus/valgus cut to be made at 90 degrees and has slots to make a cut for the necessary augment to compensate for the defect (Fig. 93.10). The last step in preparation of the tibia is to punch the proximal tibia for the metaphyseal stem of the tibial component. This metaphyseal stem has medial and lateral fins that provide rotational stability.

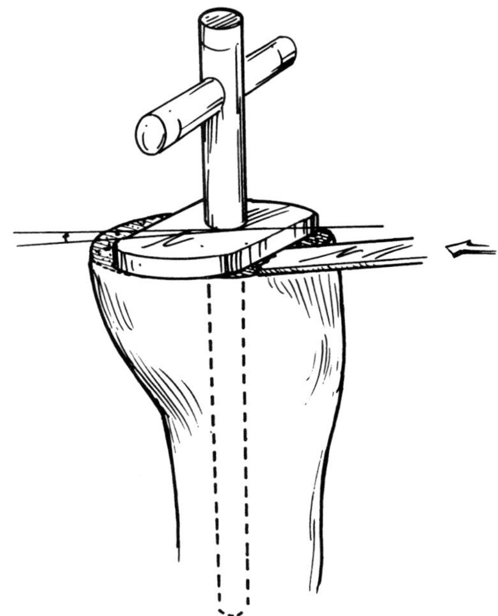

FIGURE 93–9 ➢ The tibial aligner tool can be used to recut the tibial surface so that it has a 90 degree varus/valgus angle with posterior slope.

Patella Tools

The patella tools are two Kocher clamps as previously described (see Fig. 93.2). The patella surface can be cut with a saw to ensure that it is flat and gives equal thickness medial and lateral. Previous cement that is present in peg holes does not need to be removed and should be left if the removal of this cement would significantly weaken the structure of the patella. Once the drill holes have been placed into the patella, the patella trial can be inserted to ensure that it has stabil-

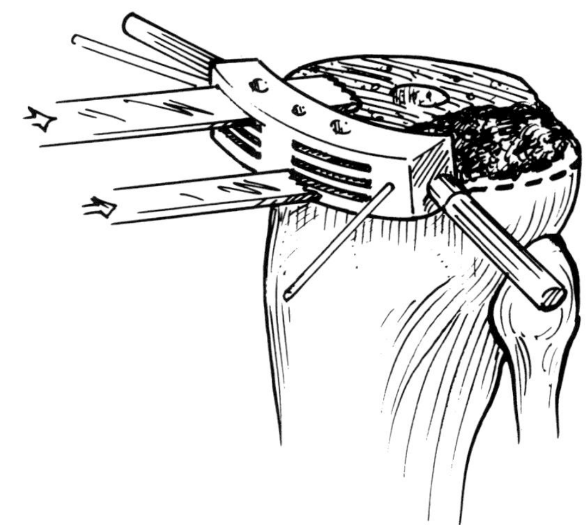

FIGURE 93–10 ➢ The tibial cutting tool permits the tibial cut to be made for use of an augment when needed for a defect either medially or laterally.

ity. It is important that the patella component have press-fit stability within the bone, if at all possible, with cement being used to simply secure the fixation. Sometimes in revision knees it is not possible to obtain a good press fit stability of the patella and the cement must be used to provide all of the stability for the patella. We still prefer to use a patella component, even in these circumstances, because the clinical results for the patient are better with a patella component rather than leaving the patella bone unresurfaced. The incidence of anterior knee pain is much higher in patients without a resurfaced patella component.[1]

STABILITY OF THE ARTHROPLASTY

Mediolateral and anteroposterior stability must be present throughout the range of motion of the revised knee. It is not satisfactory to have mediolateral stability just in full extension and to have a sloppy knee in mid-flexion. The anterior posterior stability should also be good throughout the range of motion and not just at 90 degrees of flexion. Therefore, it is important that the gap between the femur and the tibia be equal in flexion and extension if a posterior stabilized knee is to be used. Since I always sacrifice the posterior cruciate ligament at revision surgery, the choice is posterior stabilized or a constrained condylar design prosthesis. The posterior stabilized knee requires that the flexion and extension gaps be equal while the constrained condylar knee can have a flexion gap that is 5 to 6 mm bigger than the extension gap. Secondly, the Apollo constrained condylar knee is used when there is an intact medial collateral ligament but unequal stability between the medial and lateral ligamentous structures. The constrained condylar tibial post provides increased mediolateral stability when ligamentous imbalance is present and provides increased anteroposterior stability when the flexion gap is greater than the extension gap. The joint line does not need to be reestablished to use a constrained condylar design knee.

We use either a tissue balancer or spacer blocks to compare the thickness of the flexion and extension gaps (Fig. 93.11). Posterior structures can be released through the space of the tissue balancer to provide equality of tissue balance on the medial and lateral knee. If the flexion gap is greater than the extension gap, and there already is a significant loss of distal femoral bone, I choose to use a constrained condylar implant and I will not worry about returning the distal femur to the correct joint line for reasons listed above. If there is a significant amount of distal femoral bone and there is good and equal medial and lateral ligamentous stability, additional distal femoral bone can be removed to allow equality of the flexion and extension gaps and a posterior stabilized tibial insert can be used rather than the higher tibial post of the constrained condylar knee. Mostly, I use the constrained condylar knee because there is usually not equality of the ligamentous stability and not equality of the flexion and extension gaps. My experience has shown that there is

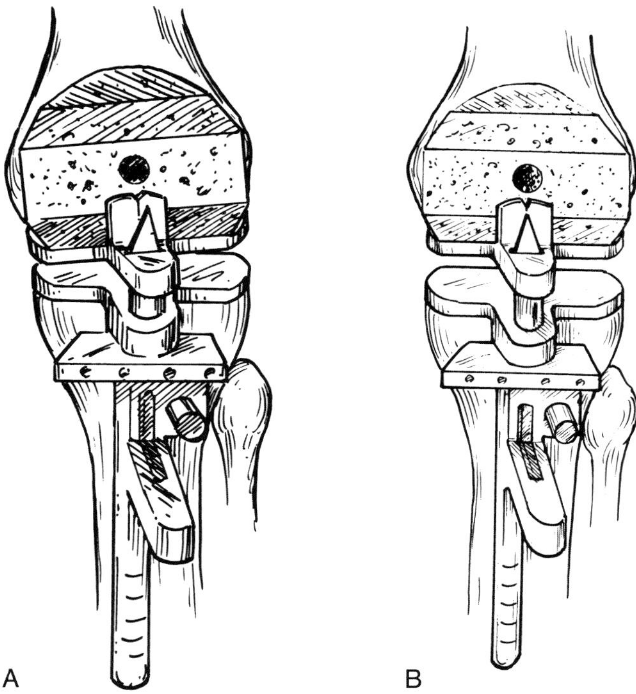

FIGURE 93–11 ➢ *A,* The tensioning device demonstrates the lack of equality of medial and lateral flexion gaps. Soft tissue release is necessary on the tight side to equalize gaps. *B,* After the appropriate soft tissue release, the tensioning device demonstrates that the medial and lateral gaps are equal. This device can also be used to demonstrate that flexion and extension gaps are equal.

good range of motion with this constrained condylar device no matter the joint line and that the durability of this design has been excellent, as evidenced by results of the constrained condylar knee reported in other chapters of this book.

Of greater difficulty in revision knees is the stability of the extensor mechanism. Often the revision is being performed because of problems with the extensor mechanism. Either the knee has been too stiff or the knee has been too unstable. For almost all knees, an extended rectus snip will allow satisfactory tracking of the patella. Often with stiff knees the release of the extensor mechanism must be extended along the lateral aspect of the patella. When we extend the release along the lateral aspect of the patella, even to the lateral aspect of the patella ligament, we leave the vastus lateralis fibers attached to the quadriceps tendon superiorly, which does provide blood supply to the tendon. Secondly, once the patella is balanced in the trochlear groove throughout the range of motion, we will close as much of the lateral defect as possible during the closure (as described below). This closure provides less lateral "pooch" for the patient and greater comfort.

We are most concerned with tracking of the patella during the first 30 degrees because it is during this range that clinical subluxation of the patella occurs. Even with the rectus snip, if there is tilt during the

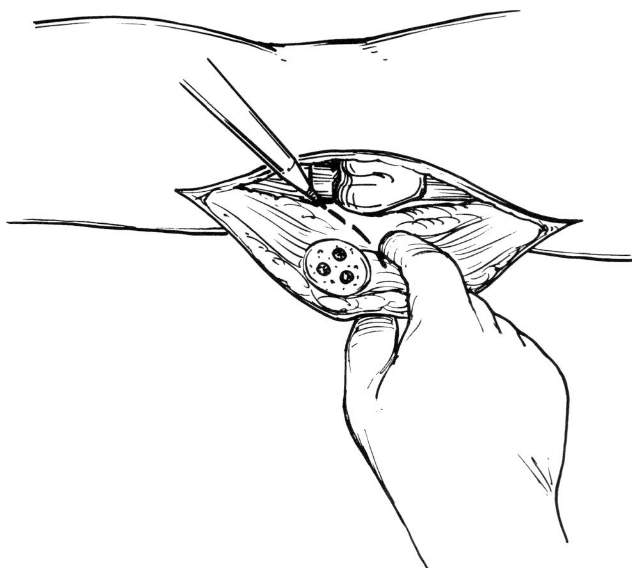

FIGURE 93–12 ➢ An oblique lateral release of the lateral retinaculum goes from the tibial surface to the superior edge of the patella (do not cut the tendon). The lateral superior geniculate artery is 3 mm proximal to the superior edge of the patella.

first 30 degrees, we will use an oblique release that extends from the tibia to the superior pole of the patella, and this almost always eradicates any tilt in the first 30 degrees (Fig. 93.12). This oblique release protects the superior geniculate artery, which runs approximately 3 mm above the superior pole of the patella. If an extended lateral release has been performed, as described above, the superior geniculate artery is sacrificed.

PROSTHETIC SELECTION

Some of the principles for prosthetic selection are discussed in the section on stability. A posterior stabilized knee can be used if the flexion and extension gaps are equalized. The femoral components should be stable both for tilt and rotation on the distal end of the femur without a stem. Augments or bone graft can be used for the distal femoral component to provide this stability. However, the posterior condyle of the implant must engage the posterior femur sufficiently that the femoral component has tilt and rotational stability. If this engagement of the posterior condyles on posterior femoral bone requires that the joint line be significantly elevated, a constrained condylar post should be used for the revision knee.

Either femoral or tibial stems should be added for stability of the components if there are defects of the condyles (Fig. 93.13). The stem can be non-cemented if good press-fit stability of the stem can be obtained and if the bone has sufficient cortical thickness to provide good stability for the stem. Significantly osteoporotic bone will not stabilize a non-cemented stem well, and rapid evidence of demarcation between the stem and the bone can be seen by the evidence of radiolucent lines. In this type of bone, the stem should be cemented. This is true for both the tibia and the femur. The cortical support for a stem is worse in the femur than the tibia because of the shape of the canal.

For the tibia, a stem should be used if there is not good stability of the tibial tray without the stem. This means stability for tilt in either the mediolateral or anteroposterior direction. If there is a significant defect (greater than 1 cm) of either the medial or the lateral condyle, a stem should be added to provide better support for the tibial tray. The stem can be non-cemented as long as a good press-fit can be obtained into cortical bone.

The patella component should always be used unless there is insufficient bone to obtain fixation. If this is so, the patella bone should be removed sufficiently to reduce the contact between the remaining patella bone and the metal trochlea. Only sufficient patella bone to maintain structural integrity of the extensor mechanism should be left. Our experience, and that reported by Pagnano et al.[1] and by Barrack et al.,[2] indicates that leaving the patella without a patella component in revision knees has a high incidence of anterior knee pain. The size of the patella should be sufficient to cover the extent of the patella bone. In primary arthroplasty, it has been recommended that the patella component be placed only on the medial two thirds of the patella,[3] but in a revision situation the patella should cover the entire bone.

If there is an absent medial collateral ligament, or global instability of the knee, a rotating hinged knee should be selected. Our experience with the use of the kinematic rotating hinge (Howmedica, Rutherford, NJ) has been very good for its limited use by us in the last 15 years. We have had less experience with the S-ROM rotating hinge knee (Johnson and Johnson, Raynham, MA).

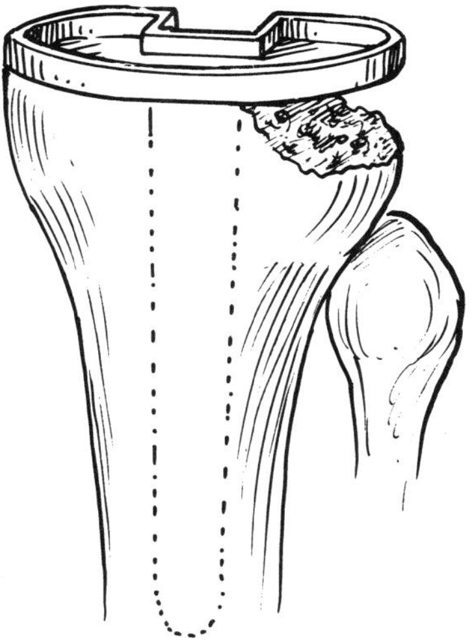

FIGURE 93–13 ➢ A tibial stem is needed when a defect includes 80% or more of an entire condyle. This same principle is true for the femur.

FIXATION

Although non-cemented stems are favored by most surgeons at this time, I still cement a majority of these stems with the use of the ACK constrained condylar knee. I have had outstanding success with cemented stems with the Total Condylar III knee (Johnson and Johnson, Raynhoun, MA) for 20 years. The technique used for the cementing of these stems has been the same technique used for cementing of a femoral stem. A plug is placed into the canal; cement is inserted into the femur with a gun and then manually pressurized. The cement is inserted in a doughy state so that when the stem is inserted into the canal further pressurization of the cement can occur. For the tibia the plug is also used in the intramedullary canal, but the cement is inserted manually because it can be pushed into the canal in a downward fashion. The cement is then manually pressurized. Further cement is put onto the stems, and as they are inserted into doughy cement, further pressurization of the cement can occur. The use of non-cemented stems for me is limited to those patients in whom there is good cortical bone for support of the non-cemented stem. Because these stems do not have any biological fixation, and therefore have only a mechanical grip in the bone, the cortical bone must be strong enough to sustain this mechanical grip against the difference in the stiffness of the stem versus the bone. The appearance of radiolucent lines around the stem in the femur or tibia suggests impending failure to me. This motion of the stem will translate into micromotion of the cemented fixation of deficient condylar bone, and I believe that the longevity of the arthroplasty will be compromised.

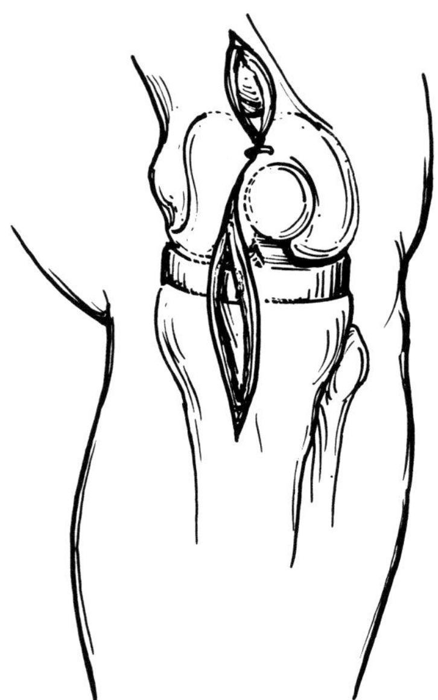

FIGURE 93–14 ➢ One suture is placed at the superior edge of the patella, and the knee is moved to full flexion. The suture should not break, which indicates the tension on the extensor mechanism is not excessive.

CLOSURE

Closure of the knee is initially performed with the knee in flexion. The knee is placed into nearly complete flexion with the foot resting against the foot plate. A suture is used to reattach the vastus medialis obliquus to the superior corner of the patella with the knee in extension (Fig. 93.14). The "single suture test" is then used as the knee is taken to full flexion to ensure that the knee mechanism is not too tight. If the single suture breaks, further release of the extensor mechanism is needed or the patient will have difficulty obtaining flexion. If the suture remains intact, the closure is performed in flexion until the edges of the distal wound are parallel (Fig. 93.15). The proximal wound is closed at the proximal end because this is easier to access in flexion. Two further sutures are placed just above the patella to close the distal end of the quadriceps tendon. The knee is then taken to extension and the remainder of the closure done with the knee in extension. A drain is most commonly used in revision surgery.

If a distal lateral extension of the rectus snip has been performed, this distal, lateral wound is also closed with the knee in flexion. These sutures may be placed only through the synovium if the wound is tight. Sometimes the sutures can be placed through the edges of the cut lateral retinaculum. After each two or three sutures, the knee is taken to extension and brought back to flexion to be sure that the patella tracks centrally and that the lateral sutures do not break. If the sutures break, they are not reattached

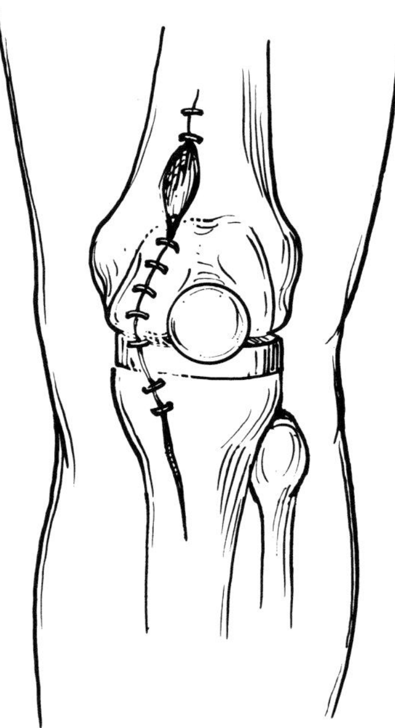

FIGURE 93–15 ➢ The wound is closed in extension once a suture is placed at the superior and inferior pole of the patella and the superior end of the wound in flexion. These first sutures should remove any tension on the wound, and the edges should then be parallel, which indicates this tension is in fact removed.

because this closure is tightening the lateral side too much. Sometimes the entire lateral wound can be closed. When closure of the wound can be obtained, there is more comfort for the patient because there is not a lateral defect that results in a pooched-out appearance of the lateral knee and thin tissue over the lateral side of the knee implants. Following complete closure, the patient is placed into a knee immobilizer.

POSTOPERATIVE REHABILITATION

Postoperatively, the patient is maintained with an epidural for 36 to 48 hours. Morphine can be given through the epidural, and this gives excellent pain relief. This allows the initiation of the postoperative rehabilitation with minimal pain on the first postoperative day. The patient is seated on the edge of the bed or in a chair, and the knee is flexed with active assisted motion.[4] Usually knee flexion of 90 degrees is obtained while the epidural is effective. Once the epidural is removed, this knee flexion will usually reduce to 60 to 70 degrees and the average discharge flexion is 80 degrees. The patients are allowed to bear weight fully unless there is a significant bone graft for the proximal tibia or distal femur. If there is a significant allograft (which is rare in our experience), the patient is maintained in a brace that keeps the knee at extension for 4 to 6 weeks before active rehabilitation is begun. No continuous passive motion (CPM) machines are used by us except for patients with a large allograft or patients with a significant lateral extension for release of the extensor mechanism. These two groups of patients will be placed onto a CPM for 1 week to allow motion that will inhibit suprapatellar pouch scarring. With the allograft, a cast is then placed for 1 month. With the modified V-Y release, active flexion is begun between 7 and 10 days postoperatively.

For patients who do not have either an allograft or a modified V-Y extensor release, the patient is allowed to be fully weightbearing on two crutches. When the leg strength allows this (even before discharge from the hospital if possible), the patient will be allowed to go to one crutch. One or two crutch support will be maintained for 6 weeks to allow healing of the bone and muscles from the surgery. The primary rehabilitation used for these patients is walking, and they are encouraged to go outdoors and gradually increase their walking distance up to 1 mile. Ninety percent of the patients do not require any formal physical therapy once they leave the hospital. I believe it is critical that the patient not become significantly painful postoperatively, and this is less likely to occur if they are controlling their own therapy and using a walking program. The patient is educated completely in regard to the significance of not allowing excessive pain to occur, and if it does, to cease any rehabilitation until the pain is controlled.

POSTOPERATIVE THROMBOEMBOLIC PROPHYLAXIS

I have used aspirin combined with mechanical compression as the only thromboembolic prophylaxis for 20 years. The record with this has been superb. We have not had a death from a pulmonary embolism since 1985. The advantage of aspirin with mechanical compression is the lower incidence of drainage and hematoma formation. The patients are also gotten out of bed the afternoon of the surgery or the next morning after the surgery. They continue to be gotten out of bed a minimum of two times a day during their hospitalization. I believe that a short surgery duration and early rapid mobilization of the patient are more important than the chemical prophylaxis used. Because our incidence of clinical thrombophlebitis in 2000 total hip and knee patients during the past 5 years is 0.6%, I continue to use aspirin and mechanical compression. The patients are discharged home with TED stockings and aspirin which is taken as 650 mg (2 adult aspirin) twice a day. This treatment is continued for 1 month, and then the aspirin and the stockings are discontinued.

References

1. Pagnano MW, Scuderi GR, Insall JN: Patellar component resection in revision and reimplantation total knee arthroplasty. Clin Orthop 356:34, 1998.
2. Barrack RL, Matzkin E, Ingraham R, Engh G, et al: Rorabeck C: Revision knee arthroplasty with patella replacement vs. bony shell. Clin Orthop 356:139, 1988.
3. Lewonowski K, Dorr LD, McPherson EJ, et al: Medialization of the patella in total knee arthroplasty. J Arthrop 2(2):151, 1997.
4. Kumar JP, McPherson EJ, Dorr LD, et al: Rehabilitation after total knee arthroplasty. Clin Orthop 331:93, 1996.

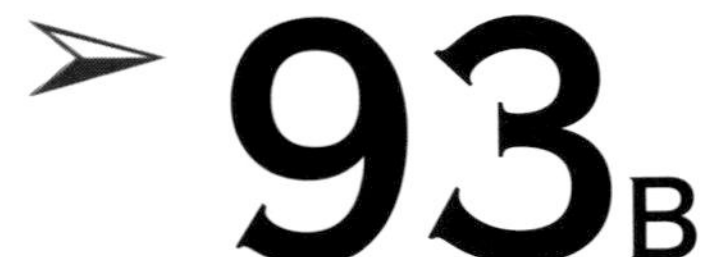

Revision Knee Arthroplasty: How I Do It

Douglas A. Dennis

PREOPERATIVE ASSESSMENT

Preoperative patient evaluation involves obtaining a thorough history and performing a clinical examination in addition to a laboratory assessment and a critical review of radiographs. The goals of the history are to determine if the patient's symptomatology is consistent with a failed total knee arthroplasty (TKA) and to rule out conditions in which revision TKA may be contraindicated such as infection, Charcot's arthropathy, neuromuscular disease, or adverse medical conditions. Analysis of previous surgical procedures, including review of previous operative reports, is necessary to assess the previous surgical approach used, soft-tissue releases performed, and size and type of present prosthetic components.

Clinical examination includes assessment of range of motion, ligamentous stability, lower-limb alignment, and patellofemoral tracking. The skin is carefully inspected to determine previous skin incisions, mobility of the anterior soft tissues of the knee, and presence of any preexisting ulcerations that would require treatment before proceeding with revision TKA. A neurological examination is performed to ensure adequate motor control of the operative lower extremity and to rule out neurological conditions in which revision TKA would be contraindicated, such as Charcot's arthropathy. If diminished pulses are observed on vascular examination noninvasive arterial studies are obtained, and a preoperative vascular surgery consultation is considered. Signs of venous insufficiency are evaluated with duplex color ultrasonography. Lastly, clinical examination must confirm that the patient's symptoms are truly secondary to a failed TKA by ruling out referred pain from adjacent areas, such as a diseased hip joint, or radicular pain from spinal nerve root impingement.

Laboratory blood tests customary for patients undergoing a major surgical procedure (e.g., complete blood count, electrolytes, urinalysis) are routinely performed. Prothrombin time and partial thromboplastin time are obtained as an initial assessment for preoperative coagulopathy and to provide guidance for perioperative anticoagulation. Further coagulation studies are indicated if the patient provides a history of excessive bleeding. An erythrocyte sedimentation rate or C-reactive protein is obtained as an initial screening to rule out infection. It is my preference to routinely aspirate the knee joint before all revision TKA procedures for Gram's stain and cultures. Although the problem of false-positive cultures exists, studies show the value of negative cultures in ruling out infection.[2, 8]

Routine radiographic evaluation includes a weightbearing anteroposterior view of both knees as well as lateral and Merchant's patellar[26] views. These views are used for implant sizing, bone stock assessment, present implant position, patellar height and coronal position, and diaphyseal deformities. Additionally, a full-length, weightbearing, anteroposterior radiograph of the entire operative extremity is obtained to determine the angle of distal femoral resection, the presence of diaphyseal deformities, and the status of the ipsilateral hip joint. If the patient's symptomatology exceeds clinical and routine radiographic findings, additional radiographs such as varus and valgus stress views and a 45-degree posteroanterior flexion weightbearing radiograph[37] are obtained. If the status of prosthetic fixation is in question, fluoroscopically guided radiographs[11] positioned exactly parallel to the implant interfaces and a technetium bone scan are considered. Cervical spine radiographs are obtained in patients with rheumatoid arthritis and history of atlantoaxial instability or in those with a history of difficult endotracheal intubation.

The goal at completion of preoperative assessment is to precisely determine the mechanism of failure and to not repeat mistakes that may have led to the initial TKA failure. The surgeon needs to determine what is deficient and, subsequently, what is necessary to reconstruct both the bone and the soft-tissue deficits. Revision TKA in cases of unexplained pain are often unsatisfactory, and one must carefully rule out conditions such as reflex sympathetic dystrophy, indolent infection, subtle instability, pes anserine bursitis, snapping popliteal tendon, or component loosening.

SKIN INCISION

Use of the same type of skin incision as used previously is generally recommended. Although it is usually safe to ignore previous short medial or lateral peripatellar skin incisions, one should be aware of wide scars with thin or absent subcutaneous tissue, because damage to the underlying dermal plexus is likely, increasing the risk of wound necrosis.[7, 21] Problems with placement of a longitudinal incision crossing a transverse incision previously used for patellectomy or high tibial osteotomy are uncommon.[9, 46]

If long parallel skin incisions exit, choice of the lateralmost incision is favorable to avoid a large lateral skin flap that has been previously compromised at the time of the initial skin incision. Transcutaneous oxygen measurements, both before and after skin incisions about the knee, have demonstrated reduced oxygenation of the lateral skin region.[19, 20]

In complex situations, such as knees with multiple skin incisions or previously burned or irradiated skin, consideration of plastic surgical consultation is wise, for the design of the upcoming skin incision as well as for consideration of preoperative muscle flap procedures if the risk of skin necrosis is substantial. In selected complex situations, wound problems can be reduced by using a staged technique. A "prerevision" skin incision to the depth of the capsular layer is made and then is closed. If this incision heals without difficulty, one can later proceed with a TKA through this incision with greater confidence.

Soft-tissue expansion techniques have been used successfully in cases of contracted soft tissues from previous skin incisions or exposure of the skin to radiation or burns.[1, 15, 22–24, 31, 34] These techniques involve implantation, usually subcutaneously, of an expandable reservoir, into which saline can be intermittently injected to expand the surface area of the skin. Studies have shown that this technique maintains epidermal thickness. Although some dermal thinning is encountered, actual dermal collagen synthesis is increased. Complications with soft-tissue expansion are minimal and include hematoma formation, reservoir deflation, infection, and skin necrosis from overly vigorous soft-tissue expansion.

Skin circulation of the anterior aspect of the knee is dependent on the dermal plexus, which originates directly from arterioles traveling within the subcutaneous fascia. Any surgical dissection performed superficial to this subcutaneous fascial layer disrupts the arterial supply to the skin and increases the possibility of skin necrosis. Elevation of skin flaps about the anterior aspect of the knee requires dissection deep to the subcutaneous fascia to preserve the perforating arteriolar network between the subcutaneous fascia and the dermal plexus.[7, 21]

APPROACH

After the skin incision has been made, I prefer a medial peripatellar arthrotomy because of its extensile capabilities to deal with challenges found at the time of revision TKA. To gain adequate exposure in cases with excessive preoperative stiffness, the medial arthrotomy is extended, and all intra-articular adhesions are released. An extensive peripheral release of the deep medial collateral ligament, including the posteromedial capsule, to the origin of the posterior cruciate ligament, allows external rotation of the tibia. This reduces tension on the extensor mechanism and facilitates eversion of the patella.

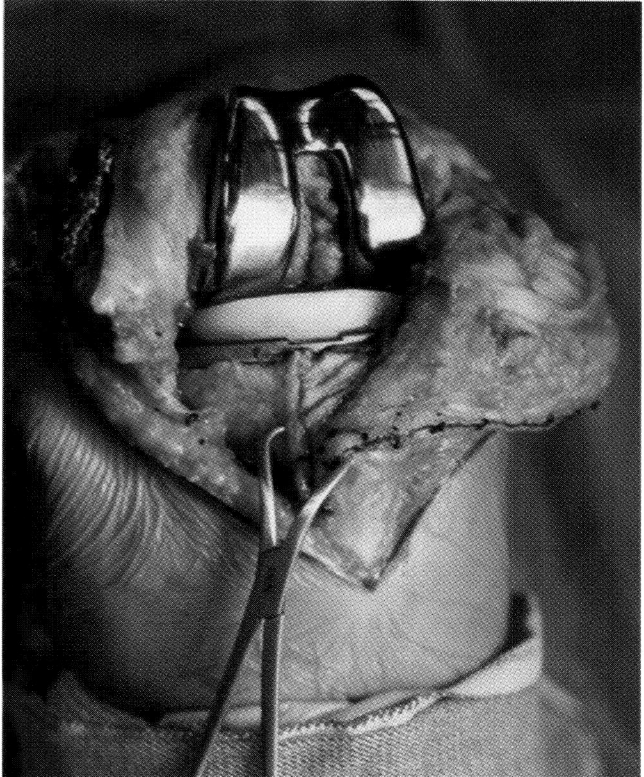

FIGURE 93.16 ➢ Intraoperative photograph demonstrating a small bone tenaculum anchored to the medial aspect of the patellar ligament and a hole drilled medial to the tibial tubercle to prevent inadvertent disruption of the patellar ligament.

With any surgical approach, it is critical to protect the patellar ligament attachment. A partial release of the patellar ligament is not performed because of an increased incidence of later patellar ligament rupture.[32] A small hole is drilled medial to the patellar ligament insertion. A bone tenaculum is then placed through the medial aspect of the patellar ligament at its insertion, as well as into the previously drilled hole to prevent inadvertent disruption of the patellar ligament while proceeding to gain better surgical exposure (Fig. 93.16).[3] A lateral retinacular release may be performed if difficulties with patellar eversion persist.

If the above surgical maneuvers have been completed and exposure remains inadequate, extensile exposure options, such as a rectus snip,[13] modified V-Y quadricepsplasty,[38, 41] or extended tibial tubercle osteotomy,[43, 44] are necessary. I favor use of a rectus snip because it provides satisfactory exposure for the most complex revision TKA cases with minimal complications. It also allows routine postoperative rehabilitation measures following revision TKA. The rectus tendon snip is performed 8 to 10 cm proximal to the superior pole of the patella to ensure good side-to-side repair of the extensor mechanism (Fig. 93.17). After adequate exposure has been obtained, preliminary soft-tissue releases are performed based on the type and degree of the preoperative deformity. One must determine if

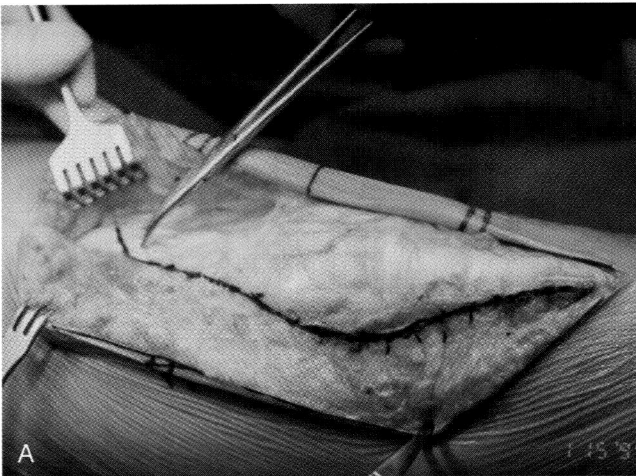
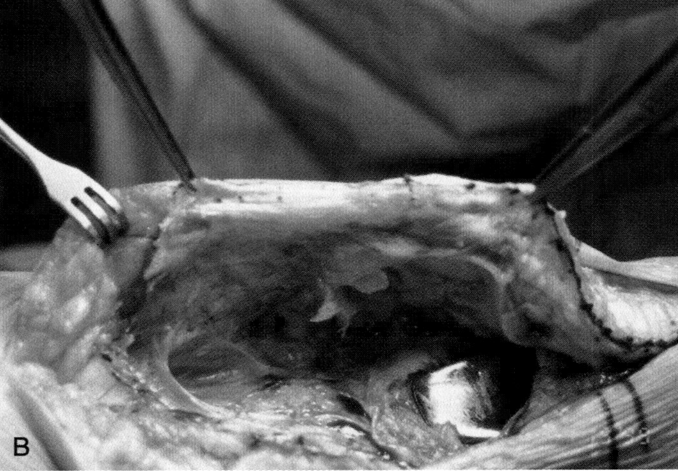

FIGURE 93.17 ➢ Intraoperative photograph outlining the medial arthrotomy (*A*) and rectus tendon transection (rectus snip). After completion of rectus snip, extensile exposure of the knee joint is provided (*B*).

preoperative deformities are fixed or flexible. If deformities are flexible and easily corrected passively, soft-tissue releases can often be minimized.

COMPONENT REMOVAL

Multiple instruments are available for component removal including osteotomes, power saws, Gigli's saw, disimpaction punches, and component-specific extraction devices. The component fixation interface is initially divided using a thin, oscillating saw blade and is completed with thin osteotomes. If cemented components are to be removed, division of the prosthesis-cement interface is initially pursued. After component removal, the bone cement can then be easily removed under direct vision. After division of the fixation interface is completed, the components are usually easily removed with a disimpaction punch (Fig. 93.18). In cases of difficult component removal, stacking osteotomes at the fixation interface is helpful to disengage components.

Occasionally, in cases of difficult component removal, metal sectioning with either a high-speed carbide drill or a diamond wheel saw is necessary. Component removal difficulty may be encountered in removal of metal-backed patellar components, particularly if good bone ingrowth has occurred into porous coated fixation pegs. In such cases, the metal peg-plate junction is divided using a high-speed diamond wheel saw and is then removed. This provides easy access to the well-fixed, porous ingrown pegs. These are then removed by a circumferential disruption of the fixation interface using a high-speed, side-cutting, pencil-tipped drill (Fig. 93.19).[6]

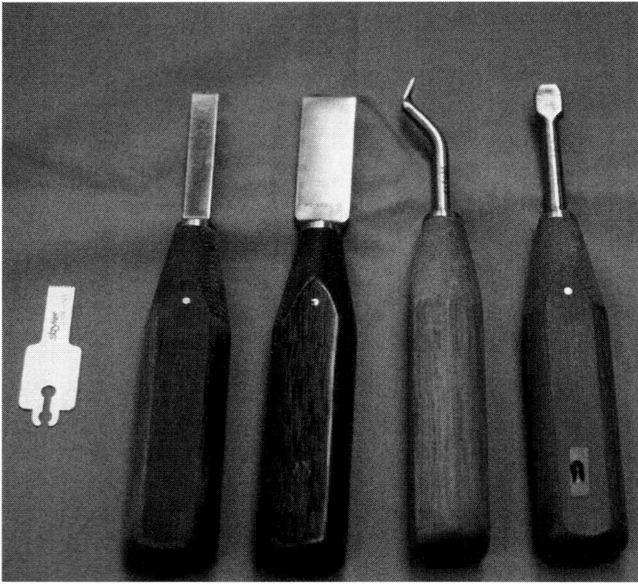

FIGURE 93.18 ➢ Surgical instruments commonly used for component removal, including a thin oscillating saw blade, thin osteotomes, and a disimpaction punch.

ASSESSING STABILITY

After component removal, spacer blocks are inserted into both the flexion and the extension gaps to assess the medial-lateral symmetry of each gap as well as the balance of the flexion gap versus the extension gap. The data obtained from this maneuver are valuable in determining later component sizing and positioning. It is common to find asymmetry, particularly of the flexion gap, with the lateral aspect having a greater dimension than the medial aspect because of previous femoral component internal rotation relative to the transepicondylar axis. Typically, this is corrected by derotation of the new femoral component, positioning of it parallel to the transepicondylar axis, and use of a posterior femoral augmentation placed laterally. It is also common to find the dimensions of the flexion gap larger than those of the extension gap. This is often

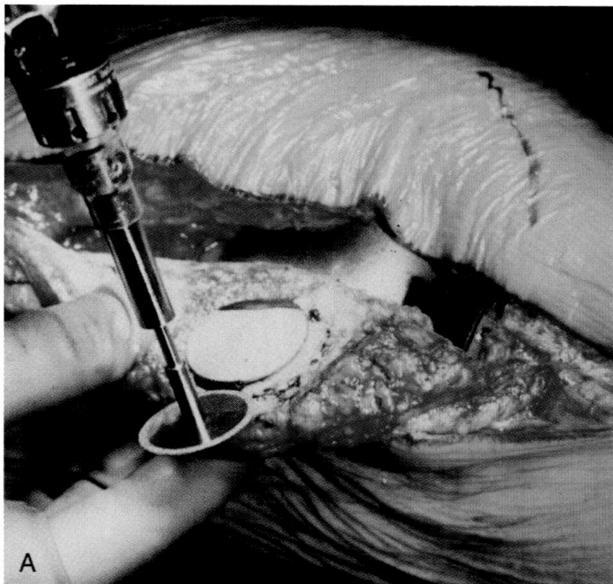

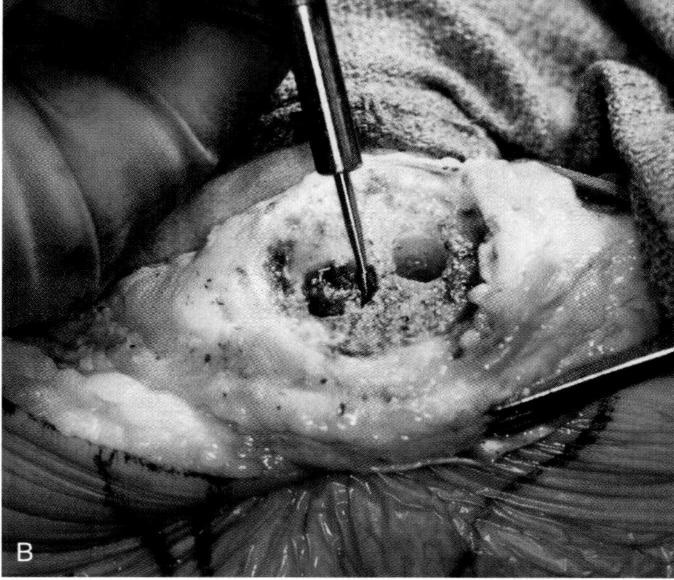

FIGURE 93.19 ➢ Intraoperative photographs displaying removal of a metal-backed patellar component with bone ingrown fixation lugs. Initially, a high-speed, diamond wheel saw is used to disrupt the metal plate-fixation lug interface (*A*). After metal plate removal, fixation lugs are removed by circumferential disruption of the fixation interface using a high-speed, side-cutting, pencil-tipped drill (*B*).

managed with use of a larger femoral component size and posterior augmentations placed medially and laterally on the femoral component. The surgeon must be aware of the multiple possible flexion-extension gap mismatches that may occur and of exactly what options are available to correct these variances (Table 93.1). A key to stable and successful revision TKA is good prosthetic alignment in the coronal, sagittal, and transverse planes as well as reestablishing symmetry and equality of the flexion and extension gaps.

BONE RESECTION SEQUENCE

A principle of revision TKA is to minimize additional bone resection, remembering that a substantial amount of bone has already been removed at the time of the previous TKA. Only 1 to 2 mm of bone are removed from the most prominent femoral or tibial condyle to provide a unicondylar platform onto which resection guides can be placed. Residual defects of the contralateral condyles are managed with bone graft or prosthetic augmentation.

I favor resection of the proximal tibia initially because this resection affects both the flexion and the extension gaps. The flexion gap is then established through proper resection of the anterior and posterior aspects of the distal femur and selection of the correct femoral component size. If the flexion gap is larger than the extension gap, a larger femoral component size is selected; a smaller femoral component is selected if the flexion gap is smaller than the extension gap. External rotation of the anteroposterior femoral cutting guide is usually required to obtain symmetry of the flexion gap. In revision TKA, the patellofemoral

TABLE 93.1 **FLEXION-EXTENSION GAP IMBALANCE: TREATMENT OPTIONS**

	Extension Adequate	Extension Loose	Extension Tight
Flexion Adequate	Make no changes.	Augment distal femur. Bone graft distal femur.	Resect distal femur. Perform posterior release. Resect posterior osteophytes.
Flexion Loose	Select larger femoral component with posterior augmentation.	Select thicker tibial component.	Select larger femoral component with posterior augmentation and resect distal femur.
Flexion Tight	Select smaller femoral component. Perform posteriorly angled tibial resection. Consider posterior cruciate ligament substitution.	Select smaller femoral component with distal augmentation. Consider posterior cruciate ligament substitution.	Select thinner tibial component. Resect tibia.

joint and the posterior femoral condyles have already been resected. Therefore, the anteroposterior and posterior condylar axes are of little value in determining proper femoral component rotation. The best remaining landmark to use is the transepicondylar axis.[25, 30, 47] As previously mentioned, it is common to resect no additional bone from the medial aspect of the anterior femur or the posterior aspect of the lateral femur because of previous placement of the femoral component internally rotated relative to the transepicondylar axis (Fig. 93.20).

The distal aspect of the femur is then resected perpendicular to the mechanical axis at a level appropriate to balance the extension gap to the previously determined flexion gap. A common error is to resect too much distal femur, which results in elevation of the joint line and subsequent patella intera. The chamfer cuts are performed last to complete the femoral resections.

Should prosthetic augmentation of the tibial component be required, augmentation resection is delayed until after trial reduction of components is completed to ensure proper rotational alignment of augmentation resection.

Removal of patellar components is not always required. If a dome patellar component design is present without malposition, loosening, or excessive polyethylene wear, it is usually safe to preserve the patellar component and allow it to articulate with the newly revised femoral component if a dome design trochlear flange is selected. My experience is that small geometric mismatches between the dome configuration of the retained patellar component and the new femoral component trochlear groove are well tolerated because of the development of a "patellar meniscus" around the periphery of the retained patellar component.[5]

BONE LOSS

Some degree of bone loss is present in all revision TKA. Most contained defects are managed with morselized local autograft or allograft. If massive contained defects are present, structural allograft is used with invagination of the graft into the contained cavity.

Numerous options are available for treating small, noncontained osseous defects, including cement and screws,[35, 36] prosthetic augmentation,[4, 29, 33] and structural allografting.[10, 14, 18, 27, 40, 42, 45] As a result of the highly successful midterm results of prosthetic augmentation, I will use these most commonly because of the absence of disease transmission, nonunion, malunion, or collapse, which may occur with bone grafting. Bone grafting is favored to reestablish bone stock in younger patients in whom additional revision TKA is probable. Cement and screws are occasionally used for small defects (5 to 10 mm) in elderly patients for economic reasons.

In large, noncontained defects, structural allografts are routinely used. In large defects, I often try to obtain anatomically matching structural allograft specimens and position them to orient the allograft trabeculae parallel to the axial loads normally placed across the deficient host defect. To prepare for structural allografting, the host defect must be cleared of any intervening soft tissue and hypersclerotic bone to provide a well-vascularized host bed of autogenous bone. Geometric shaping of the host defect (removing minimal bone) is sometimes required to maximize mechanical interlock of the structural allograft into the host defect. Meticulous shaping of the structural allograft to maximize surface area contact with host bone is paramount. Rigid fixation is imperative to enhance allograft-host union. Diaphyseal engaging stems, which maximize fixation into virgin host bone and offload the allograft during incorporation, are always used (Fig. 93.21). Occasionally, axially placed screws or cortical plates are used to further enhance fixation.

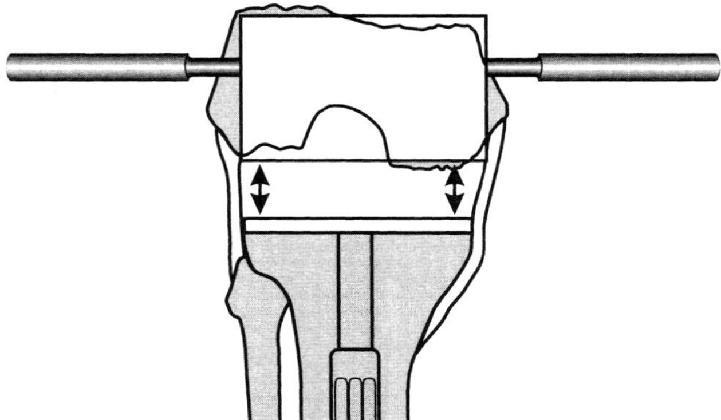

FIGURE 93.20 ➢ Schematic diagram demonstrating placement of anteroposterior resection guide parallel to the transepicondylar axis. Note that no bone is removed from the posterior aspect of the lateral femoral condyle because of internal rotation of the anterior and posterior resections (relative to the transepicondylar axis) at the time of the initial total knee arthroplasty.

JOINT LINE

Reestablishing the joint line at the true anatomic level is required for optimal stability and joint kinematics. If the posterior cruciate ligament is preserved, studies have shown that the joint line must be restored to within 3 mm of its original position to maximize stability and kinematic function.[16] If posterior cruciate substitution is selected, restoration of the joint line to within 8 mm is necessary to optimize function.[12] The joint line is adjusted by selection of the appropriate femoral component size and thickness of the tibial polyethylene insert. In revision TKA, it is often necessary to further adjust the joint line through the use of structural bone graft or prosthetic augmentation.

Landmarks to determine the anatomic joint line include the old meniscal scar, one finger width above the fibular head, and one finger width below the inferior pole of the patella. More detailed anatomic studies have determined the joint line to be positioned at a mean distance of 3.08 cm below the medial epicondyle and 2.53 cm below the lateral epicondyle.[39]

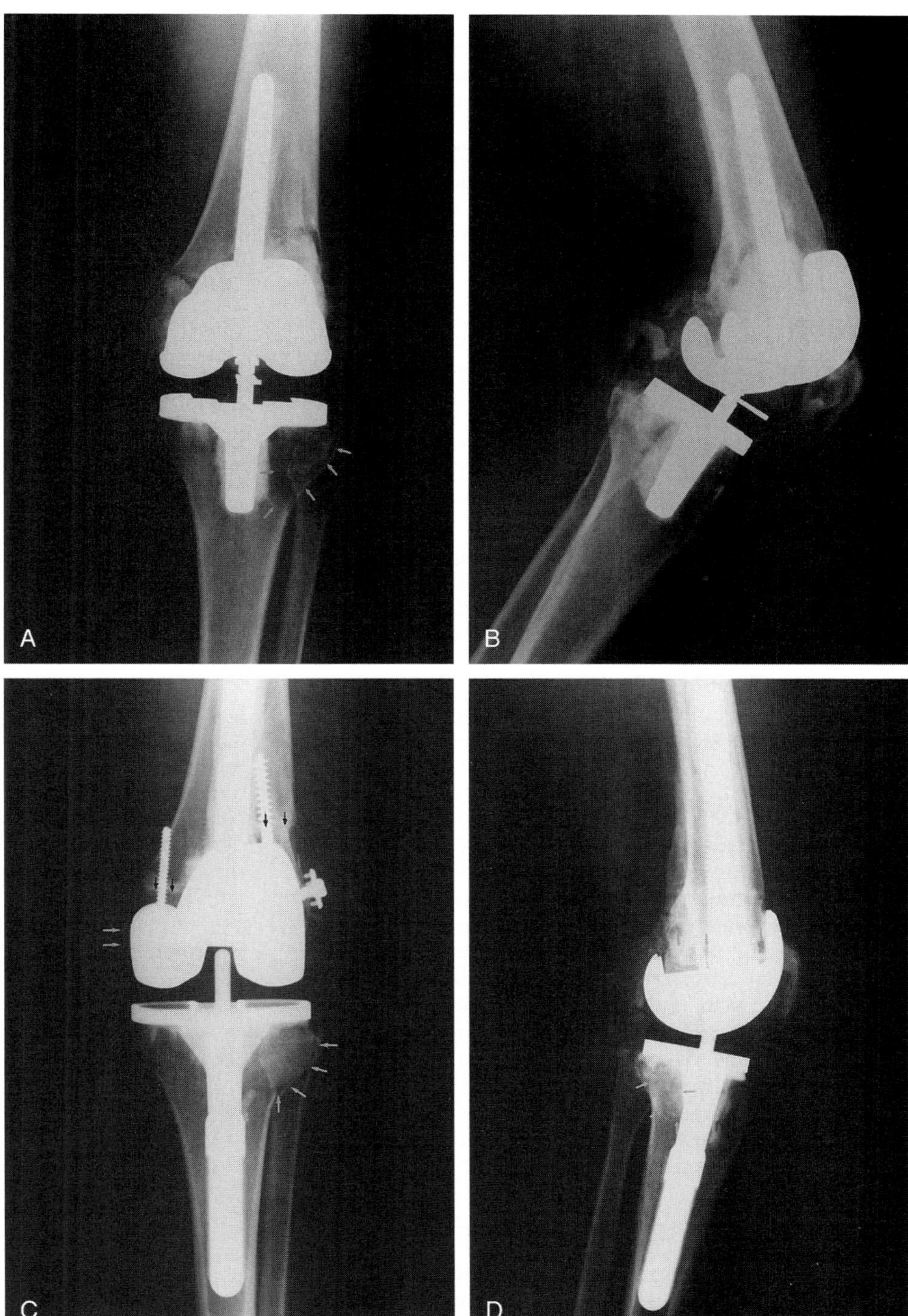

FIGURE 93.21 ➢ Preoperative anteroposterior (*A*) and lateral (*B*) radiographs of a failed revision total knee arthroplasty resulting from femoral component loosening and proximal tibial osteolysis (*arrows*). Postoperative anteroposterior (*C*) and lateral (*D*) radiographs following repeat revision total knee arthroplasty. Structural allografts have been used to reconstruct a large, noncontained osseous defect of the distal femur and a contained osseous defect of the proximal tibia (*arrows*).

PROSTHESIS SELECTION

To successfully address the myriad of problems faced in revision TKA, a prosthetic TKA system possessing multiple types of prosthetic components is required, including options of multiple levels of prosthetic constraint, femoral and tibial prosthetic augmentations, and diaphyseal engaging stems. One must realize that long-term durability of the prosthetic components, as well as fixation, is inversely proportional to prosthetic constraint. Therefore, selecting the least constrained prosthetic components that provide satisfactory stability is wise. In my experience with revision TKA, however, the posterior cruciate ligament is frequently damaged, and posterior cruciate ligament substitution is recommended.

Constrained condylar components are selected in cases of extreme collateral ligamentous injury or when a marked flexion-extension gap mismatch is present that cannot be managed by proper component selection and orientation, soft-tissue balancing, and joint line restoration. In my experience, linked constrained devices are rarely required and are reserved for cases of severe posterior capsular insufficiency and uncontrolled hyperextension.

Use of diaphyseal engaging stems is indicated whenever existing condylar bone support is compromised, which includes the majority of revision TKAs performed.

FIXATION

Although both cemented and cementless revision TKA components are available, I favor use of cement for condylar fixation of both the femoral and the tibial components. If diaphyseal engaging stems are required, review of the literature suggests that use of either press-fit[17] or cemented[28] stem designs provides similar success at midterm follow-up. I most commonly select a press-fit diaphyseal engaging stem because of the ease of extraction if additional revision TKA becomes necessary in the future. Cemented stems are considered in patients with advanced age (especially with advanced osteopenia) and in cases associated with anatomic abnormalities in which use of press-fit stems would distort proper condylar positioning of either the femoral or the tibial component.

WOUND CLOSURE

Before wound closure, the tourniquet is released both to assess patellar tracking and to obtain meticulous hemostasis. A drain is used in all cases to reduce the risk of postoperative hematoma. The wound is closed in layers, using a nonabsorbable suture for capsular closure and an absorbable suture for subcutaneous repair while the skin is reapproximated with skin clips. One must avoid excessive tension during wound closure because this risks later skin necrosis. Occasionally, excessive tightness is observed, particularly in the area of the proximal tibia. In such cases, soft-tissue transfer, typically using a rotational medial gastrocnemius myocutaneous flap, is required.

POSTOPERATIVE REHABILITATION

Rapid postoperative mobilization is helpful to minimize postoperative complications associated with inactivity such as thromboembolic disease, urinary retention, gastrointestinal ileus, and pneumonia. The patient is stood at the bedside on the evening of surgery, and protected ambulation with either a walker or bilateral crutches is initiated on the first postoperative day. Weightbearing status is individualized based on the quality of fixation and the strength of the remaining condylar and metaphyseal bone. In cases of extensive structural allografting, protected weightbearing is extended until union of the allograft is radiographically apparent, typically at 3 to 4 months after the operative procedure.

Active-assisted range-of-motion exercises, transfers, stair ambulation, and strengthening are initiated under the guidance of a physiotherapist on the first postoperative day. Continuous passive motion machines are not routinely used because benefits such as early range of motion are usually obtained with aggressive, early range-of-motion exercises initiated by the physiotherapist and the patient.

POSTOPERATIVE THROMBOEMBOLIC DISEASE PROPHYLAXIS

Unless it is medically contraindicated, all patients are treated with a combination of medicinal and mechanical measures. Warfarin is initiated the night before the operative procedure and continued for a period of 3 weeks postoperatively. Mechanical foot pumps are used both intraoperatively and postoperatively until hospital discharge. Thigh-high thromboembolic stockings are worn bilaterally for 1 month following the operative procedure. Following completion of warfarin, patients are placed on salicylates for an additional 3-week period.

SUMMARY

Successful revision TKA requires a thorough preoperative evaluation and proper patient selection. The exact mechanism of failure must be determined preoperatively, because results of revision TKA for unexplained pain are often poor. A surgical "game plan" is then developed and meticulously executed in the operating room theater to provide optimum results.

References

1. Argenta LC, Marks MW, Pasyk KA: Advances in tissue expansion. Clin Plast Surg 12:159, 1985.
2. Barrack RL, Jennings RW, Wolfe MW, et al: The Coventry award. The value of preoperative aspiration before total knee revision. Clin Orthop 345:8, 1997.
3. Booth RE Jr: Personal communication. Philadelphia, 1996.
4. Brand MG, Daley RJ, Ewald FC, et al: Tibial tray augmentation with modular metal wedges for tibial bone stock deficiency. Clin Orthop 248:71, 1989.
5. Cameron HU, Cameron GM: The patellar meniscus in total knee replacement. Orthop Rev 16:75, 1987.
6. Dennis DA: Removal of well fixed cementless metal-backed patellar components. J Arthroplasty 7:217, 1992.
7. Dennis DA: Wound complications in total knee arthroplasty. Instr Course Lect 46:165, 1997.
8. Duff GP, Lachiewicz PF, Kelley SS: Aspiration of the knee joint before revision arthroplasty. Clin Orthop 331:132, 1996.
9. Ecker ML, Lotke PA: Wound healing complications. In Rand JA, ed: Total Knee Arthroplasty. New York, Raven Press, 1993, pp 403–437.
10. Engh GA, Herzwurm PJ, Parks NL: Treatment of major defects of bone with bulk allografts and stemmed components during total knee arthroplasty. J Bone Joint Surg Am 79:1030, 1997.
11. Fehring TK, McAvoy G: Fluoroscopic evaluation of the painful total knee arthroplasty. Clin Orthop 331:226, 1996.
12. Figgie HE III, Goldberg VM, Heiple KG, et al: The influence of tibial-patellofemoral location on function of the knee in patients with the posterior stabilized condylar knee prosthesis. J Bone Joint Surg Am 68:1035, 1986.
13. Garvin KL, Scuderi G, Insall JN: Evolution of the quadriceps snip. Clin Orthop 321:131, 1995.

14. Ghazavi MT, Stockley I, Yee G, et al: Reconstruction of massive bone defects with allograft in revision total knee arthroplasty. J Bone Joint Surg Am 79:17, 1997.
15. Gold DA, Scott SC, Scott WN: Soft tissue expansion prior to arthroplasty in the multiply-operated knee. A new method of preventing catastrophic skin problems. J Arthroplasty 11:512, 1996.
16. Grady-Benson JC, Kaufman KR, Irby SE, et al: The influence of joint line location on tibiofemoral forces after total knee arthroplasty. Presented at the 38th Annual Meeting of the Orthopaedic Research Society, Washington, DC, February 17-20, 1992.
17. Haas SB, Insall JN, Montgomery W III, et al: Revision total knee arthroplasty with use of modular components with stems inserted without cement. J Bone Joint Surg Am 77:1700, 1995.
18. Harris AI, Poddar S, Gitelis S, et al: Arthroplasty with a composite of an allograft and a prosthesis for knees with severe deficiency of bone. J Bone Joint Surg Am 77:373, 1995.
19. Johnson DP, Houghton TA, Radford P: Anterior midline or medial parapatellar incision for arthroplasty of the knee. A comparative study. J Bone Joint Surg Br 68:812, 1986.
20. Johnson DP: Midline or parapatellar incision for knee arthroplasty. A comparative study of wound viability. J Bone Joint Surg Br 70:656, 1988.
21. Klein NE, Cox CV: Wound problems in total knee arthroplasty. In Fu FH, Harner CD, Vince K, et al, eds: Knee Surgery. Baltimore, Williams & Wilkins, 1994, pp 1539-1552.
22. Mahomed N, McKee N, Solomon P, et al: Soft-tissue expansion before total knee arthroplasty in arthrodesed joints: A report of two cases. J Bone Joint Surg Br 76:88, 1994.
23. Manders EK, Oaks TE, Au VK, et al: Soft-tissue expansion in the lower extremities. Plast Reconstr Surg 81:208, 1988.
24. Manders EK, Schenden MJ, Furrey JA, et al: Soft-tissue expansion: Concepts and complications. Plast Reconstr Surg 74:493, 1984.
25. Mantas JP, Bloebaum RD, Skedros JG, et al: Implications of reference axes used for rotational alignment of the femoral component in primary and revision knee arthroplasty. J Arthroplasty 7: 531, 1992.
26. Merchant AC, Mercer RL, Jacobsen RH, et al: Roentgenographic analysis of patellofemoral congruence. J Bone Joint Surg Am 56: 1391, 1974.
27. Mnaymneh W, Emerson RH, Borja F, et al: Massive allografts in salvage revisions of failed total knee arthroplasties. Clin Orthop 260:144, 1990.
28. Murray PB, Rand JA, Hanssen AD: Cemented long-stem revision total knee arthroplasty. Clin Orthop 309:116, 1994.
29. Pagnano MW, Trousdale RT, Rand JA: Tibial wedge augmentation for bone deficiency in total knee arthroplasty. A follow-up study. Clin Orthop 321:151, 1995.
30. Poilvache PL, Insall JN, Scuderi GR, et al: Rotational landmarks and sizing of the distal femur in total knee arthroplasty. Clin Orthop 331:35, 1996.
31. Radovan C: Tissue expansion in soft-tissue reconstruction. Plast Reconstr Surg 74:482, 1984.
32. Rand JA, Morrey BF, Bryan AS: Patellar tendon rupture after total knee arthroplasty. Clin Orthop 244:233, 1989.
33. Rand JA: Bone deficiency in total knee arthroplasty. Use of metal wedge augmentation. Clin Orthop 271:63, 1991.
34. Riederman R, Noyes FR: Soft tissue skin expansion of contracted tissues prior to knee surgery. Am J Knee Surg 4:195, 1991.
35. Ritter MA: Screw and cement fixation of large defects in total knee arthroplasty. J Arthroplasty 1:125, 1986.
36. Ritter MA, Keating EM, Faris PM: Screw and cement fixation of large defects in total knee arthroplasty. A sequel. J Arthroplasty 8:63, 1993.
37. Rosenberg TD, Paulos LE, Parker RD, et al: The forty-five-degree posterior flexion weight-bearing radiograph of the knee. J Bone Joint Surg Am 70:1479, 1988.
38. Scott RD, Siliski JM: The use of modified V-Y quadricepsplasty during total knee replacement to gain exposure and improve flexion in the ankylosed knee. Orthopedics 8:45, 1985.
39. Stiehl JB, Abbott BD: Morphology of the transepicondylar axis and its application in primary and revision total knee arthroplasty. J Arthroplasty 10:785, 1995.
40. Stockley I, McAuley JP, Gross AE: Allograft reconstruction in total knee arthroplasty. J Bone Joint Surg Br 74:393, 1992.
41. Trousdale RT, Hanssen AD, Rand JA, et al: V-Y quadricepsplasty in total knee arthroplasty. Clin Orthop 286:48, 1993.
42. Tsahakis PJ, Beaver WB, Brick GW: Technique and results of allograft reconstruction in revision total knee arthroplasty. Clin Orthop 303:86, 1994.
43. Whiteside LA, Ohl MD: Tibial tubercle osteotomy for exposure of the difficult total knee arthroplasty. Clin Orthop 260:6, 1990.
44. Whiteside LA: Surgical exposure in revision total knee arthroplasty. Instr Course Lect 46:221, 1997.
45. Wilde AH, Schickendantz MS, Stulberg BN, et al: The incorporation of tibial allografts in total knee arthroplasty. J Bone Joint Surg Am 72:815, 1990.
46. Windsor RE, Insall JN, Vince KG: Technical consideration of total knee arthroplasty after proximal tibial osteotomy. J Bone Joint Surg Am 70:547, 1988.
47. Yoshioka Y, Siu D, Cooke TD: The anatomy and functional axes of the femur. J Bone Joint Surg Am 69:873, 1987.

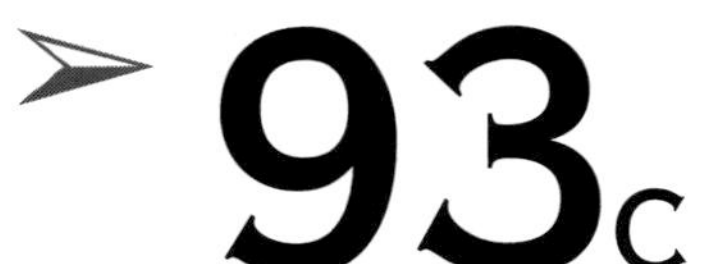

Revision Knee Arthroplasty: How I Do It

FERNANDO SANCHEZ • GERARD A. ENGH

The patient in the following case came to the Anderson Orthopaedic Clinic because of chronic pain 18 months after a total knee arthroplasty revision. His history, physical examination, and radiographic findings led to a presumptive diagnosis of a chronic, indolent, deep, periprosthetic infection with loosening of the tibial tray. We chose to summarize this case because it illustrated several concerns related to revisions. First, it showed that even with negative cultures, infections can be present. Second, this was a difficult revision, which required a unique surgical approach to gain exposure. Third, because sepsis was suspected, we determined whether to do a one-stage, early two-stage, or delayed two-stage reimplantation from information gained during implant removal. Fourth, this case exemplified our approach to managing bone loss through the use of large structural bulk allograft.

HISTORY

This 64-year-old man came to our clinic in 1998, 18 months after a total knee arthroplasty revision, because of constant pain in his revised knee. The patient had a primary right total knee arthroplasty in November 1995 and was free from pain until involved in a car accident 6 months following surgery. After the accident, he had constant discomfort in his right knee. Diagnosed with aseptic loosening secondary to the accident, he underwent a revision total knee arthroplasty in December 1996. During the revision, his tibial component was found to be grossly loose. No cultures were obtained during the revision. Afterward, he continued to have constant, sharp pain while walking and at rest. He required narcotics for pain relief and could walk only short distances with a cane and a hinged brace. He had recurrent swelling and decreased range of motion of his right knee, but no drainage, fever, chills, or associated constitutional symptoms.

PHYSICAL AND RADIOGRAPHIC EXAMINATION

During his physical examination at our clinic, the patient walked slowly, favoring his right knee. He wore a hinged brace and used a cane for support. His right knee had a midline scar with no sinus tracts, erythema, rubor, or cellulitis. On palpation of the knee, he had tenderness over the proximal tibia.

An assessment of stability showed a normal anterior translation of 5 mm, no posterior sag, a stable posterolateral corner, and approximately 7 mm of laxity medially with valgus stress. We detected a grade 1 effusion with a boggy synovium. His range of motion was 0 to 100 degrees with no extension lag and normal patellar tracking. His neurovascular status was normal.

We reviewed serial weightbearing anteroposterior (AP), supine AP, lateral, and sunrise radiographs of both knees. Radiographs of his primary knee arthroplasty (Johnson-Johnson P.F.C. primary system, Raynham, MA) showed an incomplete radiolucency around both the tibial and the femoral components. Radiographs of his revision knee arthroplasty (Johnson-Johnson P.F.C. revision knee system) taken at our clinic showed progressive and complete tibial radiolucencies with evidence of a varus shift of the tibial component (Fig. 93.22). A circumferential reactive line was present adjacent to the stem of the tibial component (Fig. 93.23).

PRELIMINARY DIAGNOSIS

Two different mechanisms could have caused implant loosening just 1 year after total knee arthroplasty revision. One possibility was septic loosening from wound contamination during surgery or from hematogenous seeding in the early postoperative interval. The other possibility was a technical mistake, such as poor soft-tissue balancing or inadequate placement and fixation of the prosthetic components. The patient's persistent pain, swelling, and decreased range of motion from the time of his revision and the extensive radiolucencies around the tibial stem led us to believe that septic loosening was the likely cause of failure.

The single most important test in determining the presence of deep periprosthetic infection is a culture of joint fluid. A positive culture establishes a diagnosis of sepsis. Single or multiple negative cultures reduce the likelihood of deep infection but do not rule it out. Blood tests provide additional valuable information: if the erythrocyte sedimentation rate (ESR) and C-reactive protein (CRP) are normal, an infection is unlikely.

We performed both joint fluid culture and blood tests on this patient. He was taken off all antibiotics

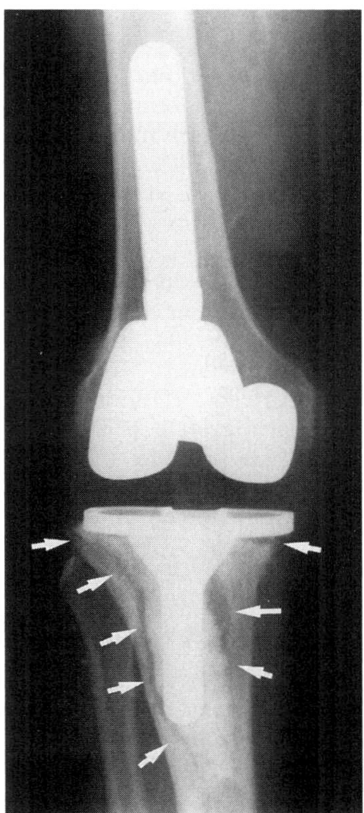

FIGURE 93.22 ➢ Radiographs of the revised knee (Johnson-Johnson P.F.C. revision knee system) taken 1 year after the revision showed circumferential demarcation at the tibial bone-cement interface. Our presumptive diagnosis was joint implant sepsis.

for 2 weeks before aspirating the joint fluid sample. As seen in Table 93.2, results from the synovial fluid tests showed an elevated white blood cell count with an abnormal differential. The blood tests showed elevated CRP and ESR, compatible with our diagnosis of prosthetic infection.

In general, we rarely use nuclear medicine scans to assess painful total knee replacements because of their relatively low sensitivity and specificity. This patient, however, underwent indium 111-labeled leukocyte scintigraphy at an outside institution before coming to our clinic. As is often the case, the scan showed no conclusive evidence of infection.

PRESUMPTIVE DIAGNOSIS

The laboratory tests supported our clinical impression of chronic, indolent, deep, periprosthetic infection (Gustilo type IV)[5] with septic loosening of the tibial tray. With this presumptive diagnosis, we considered three surgical options: a one-stage arthroplasty, an early two-stage (4 to 7 days) exchange arthroplasty, or a delayed two-stage exchange arthroplasty. We would determine the most appropriate procedure from intraoperative information and tests performed during the removal of the loose implants. Table 93.3 gives indications for each procedure.

TABLE 93.2 LABORATORY STUDIES

Blood Tests	Joint Aspiration
White blood count: 7.7 K	White blood count: 48 K with 82% PMNs
C-reactive protein: 2.5 (reference less than 0.5)	Gram's stain: negative
Erythrocyte sedimentation rate: 50 (reference 0–10)	Culture: negative

PMNs = polymorphonuclear white cells.

PREOPERATIVE PREPARATION

Preoperative planning for revision surgery begins with identifying the implant type and manufacturer from preoperative radiographs. Ascertaining the nuances of a component's removal or disassembly helps us anticipate potential difficulties involved with detaching the stem or disengaging the polyethylene insert. If surgeons are unfamiliar with a specific implant, they can obtain information from a manufacturing representative. Old operative notes also are useful in identifying implant specifications.

Expecting that this patient's femoral stem would be stable and difficult to extract, we planned to use Moreland Knee Revision instruments (DePuy, Warsaw, IN). These instruments enable extraction of well-fixed components without significant force. Because we also anticipated an infection, we notified the pathologist that a frozen section would be taken. The anesthesia team received instructions to institute antibiotics only after deep cultures were obtained.

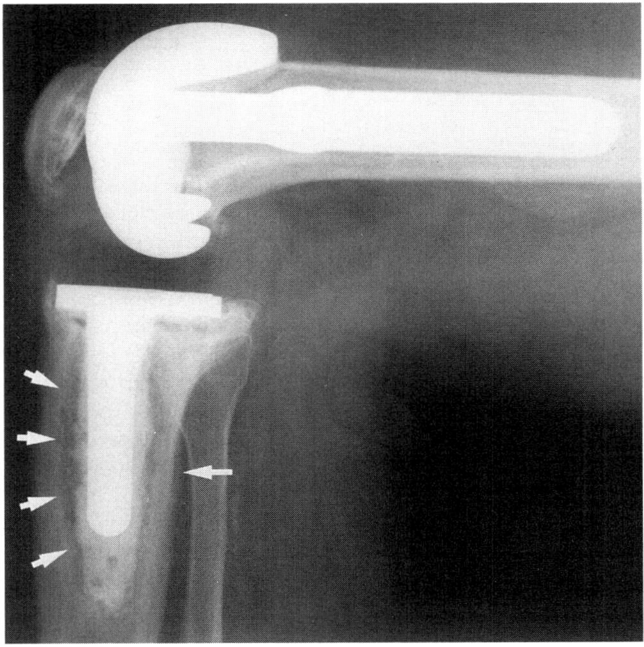

FIGURE 93.23 ➢ Extensive bone resorption at the tibial bone-cement interface on the revised knee is outlined. A thin reactive line of new bone formation is also seen on the posterior aspect of the tibia (*single arrow.*)

TABLE 93.3 THE SURGICAL OPTIONS FOR AN INFECTED TOTAL KNEE ARTHROPLASTY ARE DEPENDENT ON LABORATORY TESTS AND INTRAOPERATIVE EVALUATION

Prerequisites	Type of Revision
Acute onset (infection <48 hours)	One-stage reimplantation
Clear or turbid joint fluid Frozen sections <5 PMNs/HPF* Permanent sections <5 PMNs/HPF All cultures negative at 72 hours	Early two-stage reimplantation (4–7 days)
Purulent joint fluid Frozen sections >5 PMNs/HPF Positive Gram's stains Permanent sections >5 PMNs/HPF	Delayed two-stage reimplantation

* PMNs = Polymorphonuclear white cells per high-power field.

Before entering the operating room, we determined the surgical exposure. The patient had a midline scar that could be extended to give wide exposure of the distal femur and proximal tibia. Because the range of motion in his knee was 0 to 100 degrees, we did not envision difficulties in everting and dislocating the patella.

EXPOSURE

For fear of disseminating organisms into the patient's general circulation, we did not exsanguinate the knee. Flaps were developed superficial to the galea aponeurotica for retraction of skin and fatty tissue, thereby avoiding subcutaneous dissection that could have caused skin necrosis.

We achieved intra-articular access to the knee with a modification of a standard medial parapatellar arthrotomy. Incising the transition between the vastus medialis and the quadriceps tendon, we left just enough tendinous tissue attached to the vastus medialis for proper extensor mechanism repair. This technique reduced the risk of creating patellofemoral instability. The distal periosteal incision was made 1 cm medial to the tibial tubercle to preserve soft tissues in proximity with the patellar tendon. This extended sleeve of tissue protected the patellar tendon from inadvertent detachment and later would be used for suture repair.

After achieving access to the intra-articular space, we sent joint fluid for cultures, which included aerobic, anaerobic, fungus, and tuberculosis cultures. The joint fluid was turbid, but no purulence was obvious.

IMPLANT REMOVAL

The cemented tibial component in this patient was grossly loose, but, as suspected, the patellar and femoral components were well fixed. We obtained frozen and permanent histological sections from three sites, including the most suspicious areas. The frozen section result, which took about 20 minutes, showed greater than 10 polymorphonuclear white cells per high-power field (PMNs/HPF) in more than five fields, confirming our diagnosis of deep periprosthetic infection. We elected to perform a delayed two-stage reimplantation in this patient's knee. At this point, a first-generation cephalosporin was given.

We removed all components and cement with the Moreland Knee Revision instruments. To minimize bone loss, we were careful to free the implants at the prosthetic-cement interface. While protecting the collateral ligaments, we performed an extensive synovectomy-debridement. To expose the posterior capsule and excise the posterior synovium, we elevated the femur with an intramedullary femoral rod while displacing the proximal tibia posteriorly.

ARTICULATED SPACER PLACEMENT

In two-stage procedures, we use an articulated spacer of antibiotic-laden cement to maintain distraction of the joint space and permit limited knee motion in the interval before reimplantation. After irrigating this patient's knee with 3 L of normal saline, we made a McPherson articulated spacer[8] of antibiotic-loaded bone cement (Fig. 93.24), using 80 g of Palacos cement with 4.8 g of tobramycin and 2 g of vancomycin. At a late stage in cement polymerization, we deflated the tourniquet and inserted the spacer. This minimized interdigitation between the cement and the bone, thereby easing spacer removal without additional bone loss during reimplantation.

PATIENT REGIMEN FOLLOWING THE FIRST STAGE

A Hemovac was left in place for 1 day. Our patient's therapy involved weightbearing-as-tolerated ambulation, active range-of-motion and strengthening exercises, and terminal extension exercises. A polycentric-axis hinge brace provided stability during ambulation and physical therapy.

All final intraoperative cultures were negative. However, results from the frozen and permanent sections demonstrated greater than 10 PMNs/HPF, again substantiating a diagnosis of infection and our decision to perform delayed two-stage reimplantation. A central catheter line was introduced, and the antibiotic changed empirically from first-generation cephalosporin to vancomycin (1 g intravenously per day), an antibiotic more appropriate for organisms that commonly cause joint arthroplasty sepsis. We also requested an infectious disease consult.

After 4 weeks of intravenous antibiotics, the CRP level was less than 0.5, and the ESR was 5. A physical examination showed a well-healed scar with no obvious signs of active infection. The patient's range of motion was +12 to 90 degrees of flexion. At this

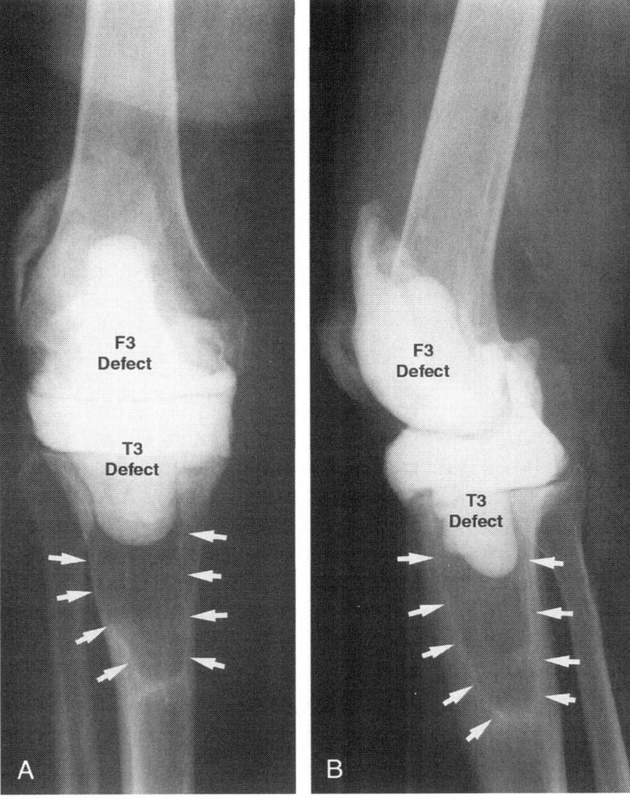

FIGURE 93.24 ➢ Anteroposterior and lateral radiographs showed the cement spacer filling the large bone loss from the femur and the tibia. The massive bone loss from the anterior and distal femur and the extensive cavitary defect in the central tibia (*arrows*) led this to be classified as F3-T3, "deficient bone."

point, his reimplantation was scheduled for 6 weeks after the component removal.

SECOND STAGE–REIMPLANTATION

Preoperative Planning

When planning for revision total knee arthroplasty or reimplantation, we use the Anderson Orthopaedic Research Institute (AORI) bone defect classification system that categorizes cases into groups of comparable difficulty by describing the extent and location of bone damage.[2] The severity of bone loss influences the type of prosthesis and the need for bone graft material or special equipment, such as Midas Rex instruments. The AORI bone defect classification is based on preoperative radiographs and intraoperative findings. We prepare for the worst-case scenario of bone loss and order the equipment necessary to perform the reconstruction efficaciously.

In this patient, we anticipated a type 3 defect (deficient metaphyseal segment) in both the distal femur and the proximal tibia (see Fig. 93.24). We planned to reconstruct the femoral condyles and tibial plateaus with structural allograft, augments, wedges, and cement. Although we rarely use hinged components, we had one available in case our planned options were unsuitable.

Exposure

We began the second stage by reopening our previous medial parapatellar incision. We then placed a 0.62-in Steinmann pin through the middle of the tibial tubercle to avoid tendon avulsion. The pin was directed so that intramedullary access to the proximal tibia was possible. To prevent injury during the procedure, we cut the pin short, bent it out of the way, and covered it with a plastic cap.

We encountered exuberant capsular fibrosis when reopening this patient's knee. We excised the thickened pseudocapsule, releasing adhesions between the extensor expansion and the femoral condyles. The capsular fibrosis also produced tension on the patellar tendon insertion into the tibial tubercle, making it impossible to evert the patella without a proximal or distal release of the extensor mechanism.

In most instances, we prefer a proximal extensor mechanism release to a tibial tubercle osteotomy.[1] Therefore, we performed the proximal releases of the extensor mechanism incrementally, starting with a lateral retinaculum release and following with a rectus snip. To preserve blood supply to the patella, we maintained a bridge of tissue consisting of the insertion of the vastus lateralis into the quadriceps tendon.[6]

To further enhance exposure of the patient's ankylosed knee, we performed a medial epicondylar osteotomy.[4] The medial epicondylar osteotomy was performed with the knee flexed 90 degrees and placed in a figure-four position. We directed a 1-in osteotome from the distal end of the femur proximally along the long axis of the femur. We then detached a wafer of bone 4 cm in diameter by 1 cm that included the medial epicondyle and the adductor tubercle. By hinging this wafer of bone posterior to the condyle, we exposed the posteromedial joint capsule. Fibers of the posterior oblique ligament and posteromedial joint capsule were then released from the posteromedial corner of the knee. The osteotomy relaxed the contracted structures on the medial side of the knee and destabilized the knee in flexion. The epicondylar osteotomy enabled us to angle the tibia into exaggerated valgus and external rotation, easing patellar dislocation.

After dislocating and everting the patella, we flexed the knee and removed the articulated spacer. Tissue from three sites was sent for frozen histological section analysis. The results showed no PMNs/HPF in more than five fields; we proceeded with the reimplantation.

Reconstruction of Large Bone Deficiencies Using Allograft

The use of allograft in a delayed two-stage reimplantation involving infection is controversial because of the potential for dead bone to serve as a nidus for reinfection. Although we recognized the potential for reinfection, we chose bulk allograft for this case because of the mechanical stability it would provide. Not only would host bone heal rapidly to allograft bone, but the allograft would also provide an optimum cancellous structure for bone-cement interdigitation. Two alternatives to a bone graft would have been a linked revision implant or filling the large bone defect with antibiotic-impregnated bone cement. The bone cement would not have bonded well to the damaged and sclerotic bone. With this patient's partially lost condyle and plateau, we preferred allografts because of the ease of machining the graft and the bone defect to matching shapes. The resulting interference fit would provide stability for the implant, as well as an increased surface area for rapid bone healing.

We obtained the allograft from the Red Cross bone bank. It had been routinely screened for hepatitis, cytomegalovirus, and human immunodefiency virus and had undergone cultures and biopsies to rule out infection and bone pathology. Harvested under sterile conditions and triple-wrapped in sterile material, the allograft was stored at −70°C until needed. (The allograft was delivered to the operating room in dry ice, which permitted us to return it without incurring the cost of the allograft if it proved unnecessary.)

We opened the allograft in a sterile fashion in the operating room and thawed it completely in saline, which took about 30 minutes. While waiting, we débrided tissue, detritus, remaining bone cement, and nonviable bone from the patient's knee.

The next step was preparing the graft.[7] We used an Allogrip device (Depuy, Warsaw, IN) to stabilize the graft. After drilling a hole in the femoral neck of the allograft, we inserted the threaded post of the Allogrip device into the femoral neck. We then mounted the graft on the Allogrip platform. With a female reamer about the diameter of the femoral head, we machined the graft until a hemispheric shape was obtained and cancellous bone was exposed. Flushing the graft with saline removed marrow elements and reduced potential immunogenicity of the graft.

This patient's distal femur had an irregularly shaped, deficient metaphyseal segment with a partially intact peripheral rim of bone (F3 defect). It would have been impossible to machine a graft to match this irregular bone defect. To achieve an interference-graft fit, we reamed the host bone with a male acetabular reamer that was 2 mm smaller than the prepared femoral head. By reaming, we created bleeding bone for rapid healing at the allograft-host junction and preserved the shell of bone and cortical rim that provided ligament stability. Treating the bone defect as if it were a delayed or nonunion fracture site, we reconstructed the cancellous structure of the lateral femoral condyle in this fashion.

We secured the graft to the host bone with two Kirschner wires. These wires were positioned to avoid impinging on the component's stem. We trimmed the protruding wires, leaving enough for their subsequent removal.

The proximal tibial metaphyseal deficit (T3 defect) also required femoral head allografting. This was performed following the same techniques described for the femoral side.

Revision Instruments

Bone deficiencies make it difficult to position and stabilize the cutting guides of the revision instrumentation. In the revision setting, the intramedullary canals of the tibia or femur are often the most reliable bone landmarks available for orienting the components. By fitting a stemmed cutting guide in the intramedullary canal, we determined the component's final position and secured guides for correct bone cuts. The protruding neck of each femoral head allograft was removed with preliminary rough cuts. We then attached the cutting blocks to the appropriate trial stem and placed the assembly into the intramedullary canal for completion of bone preparation.

Stability Assessment

A sequence of surgical steps was followed to acquire knee stability: restoring the tibial level joint, attaining flexion stability, assessing the extension gap, and determining the need for constrained implants.

Joint Line Restoration. Because tibial component height affects both the flexion and the extension gaps, we reconstructed the height of the tibia without sacrificing viable bone. The tibial tubercle and the fibular head provided easily visible references. To preserve as much tibial host bone as possible, we selected a tibial tray with a 5-degree medial wedge. We set component rotation by orienting the tibial cutting block to the medial aspect of the tibia tubercle.

Restoration of Flexion Stability. To restore flexion stability, we selected a component size larger than the host bone that would tense the collateral and capsular ligaments and maintain an adequate distance from the epicondyles to the back of the femoral condyles. We filled the bone deficiency with augments. To orient the femoral rotation and restore flexion stability, we used medial and lateral posterior augments of different widths.

Extension Gap Assessment. We used spacer blocks for gross assessment of the gap and trial implants for fine-tuning. A tibial insert thickness was selected that provided knee stability in flexion. However, on extension, the knee was unstable. To achieve extension stability, we added distal augments to move the femur distal toward the joint line. The distal femur augment tightened the gap in full extension, whereas the tibial insert provided adequate knee stability in flexion.

Use of Constrained Implants. Our goal was to achieve a stable knee with the least amount of implant constraint. Starting with a nonconstrained trial component, we assessed knee stability. After careful soft-tissue balancing, the patient had a stable knee in extension but an unstable knee in flexion. The instability was mainly because of extensive bone loss, the absence of the posterior cruciate ligament, the popliteal tendon, and weak capsular ligament. Therefore, we selected a varus-valgus constrained implant to render the knee stable.

Cementing or Not

The cancellous surface of resected bone provided an excellent bed for cement fixation. In essence, we captured the bone graft between the component and the host bone and secured the implant with cement to the reconstructed metaphyseal bone segments.

A long-stemmed component decreased the load at the allograft-host bone interface and the allograft-cement-implant interface. To permit easier implant removal if a re-revision were to become necessary, we did not cement the stem. The uncemented stem also permitted axial loading on the bone graft, thereby encouraging graft union such as in compression arthrodesis.

Once the final components were in place and the cement was cured, we removed the Kirschner wires securing the bone grafts.

Closure

The osteotomy of the medial femoral epicondyle was inherently stable except in flexion. The adductor tendon inserting into the bone fragment created proximal stability. Using heavy sutures to prevent posterior displacement, we reattached the osteotomized bone fragment to what we call the "cortical" bridge of the medial femoral condyle.[3] The patient's knee was then flexed to ensure that the repair eliminated motion at the osteotomy site.

POSTOPERATIVE REHABILITATION

The mobilization and weightbearing status of the patient after surgery depend on the extent of the reconstruction. In this case, we encouraged the patient to begin motion early in the postoperative period. A continuous passive motion machine helped the patient recover early motion without hindering wound healing. We instructed the patient to use a walker and to maintain a 50% weightbearing status. At the 6-week postoperative visit, the patient was advanced to full weightbearing with a cane. On his second visit, 4 months after surgery, the cane was discontinued.

Postoperative Thromboembolic Prophylaxis

The type and duration of anticoagulation therapy to minimize the incidence of deep vein thrombosis (DVT) should be tailored to each patient's individual risk factors. We do not use chemical prophylaxis unless the patient has a history of DVT, pulmonary embolism, or obvious clinical risk factors for DVT.

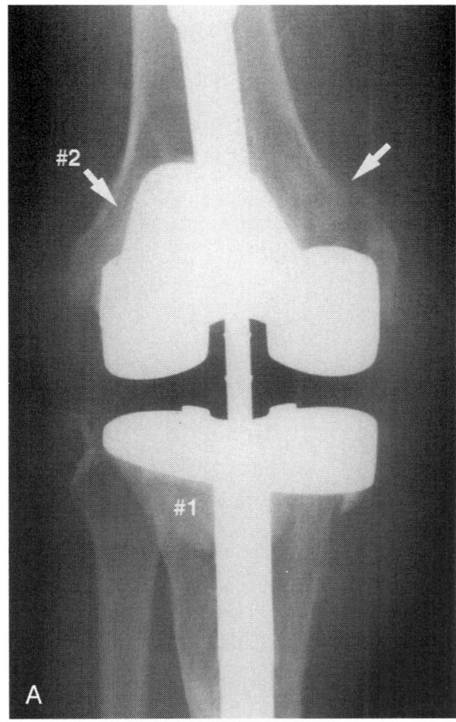

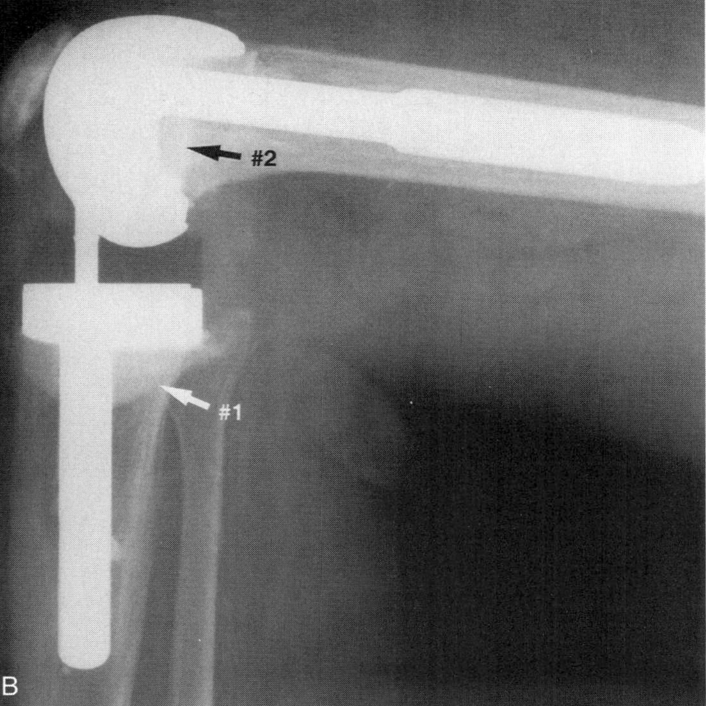

FIGURE 93.25 ➢ The large cavitary bone defects were repaired with femoral head allografts (*#1 and #2*). The unlabeled arrow identifies the healing medial epicondylar osteotomy.

We placed this patient on mechanical prophylaxis consisting of foot pumps and thigh-high thromboembolic disease (TED) hoses on both lower extremities. At his 6-week postoperative visit, we performed a color Doppler ultrasound and ruled out DVT. The TED hoses were discontinued at this time.

PATIENT OUTCOME

At our patient's last office visit, 4 months postoperatively he had no discomfort in his right knee, was walking without support, and was highly pleased with his results.

On physical examination, he had a mild limp favoring his right lower extremity. His scar was well healed with no signs of superficial infection. He had no instability in flexion or extension, and his range of motion was +10 to 114 degrees with 3 degrees of extension lag and normal patella tracking. He had no discomfort on range of motion or direct palpation. His clinical tibiofemoral alignment was 6 degrees of valgus, and there was no leg-length discrepancy.

His radiographs showed a well-fixed component in 5 degrees of valgus alignment. There were no changes associated with the allograft heads. Fibrous union of the epicondylar osteotomy site had occurred (Fig. 93.25).

References

1. Barrack PL, Smith P, Munn B, et al: Comparison of surgical approaches in total knee arthroplasty. Clin Orthop 356:16, 1998.
2. Engh GA: Bone defect classification. In Engh GA, Rorabeck CH: Revision Total Knee Arthroplasty. Baltimore, Williams & Wilkins, 1997, pp 63–120.
3. Engh GA, Ammeen D: The Clinical Results of Total Knee Arthroplasty with Medial Epicondyle to Correct Severe Genu Varum: Knee Society 1999. Clin Orthop 367:141, 1999.
4. Engh GA, McAuley JP: Joint line restoration and flexion-extension balance with revision total knee arthroplasty. In Engh GA, Rorabeck CH: Revision Total Knee Arthroplasty. Baltimore, Williams & Wilkins, 1997, pp 242–244.
5. Hanssen AD: Management of the infected total knee arthroplasty. In Engh GA, Rorabeck CH: Revision Total Knee Arthroplasty. Baltimore, Williams & Wilkins, 1997, p 373.
6. Insall JN: Surgical techniques and instrumentation in total knee arthroplasty. Insall JN, Windsor RE, Scott WN; Surgery of the Knee, 2nd ed. New York, Churchill Livingstone, 1993, pp 756–758.
7. McAuley JP, Engh GA: Allografts in revision total knee arthroplasty. In Engh GA, Rorabeck CH: Revision Total Knee Arthroplasty. Baltimore, Williams & Wilkins, 1997, pp 252–274.
8. McPherson EJ, Lewonowski K, Dorr LD. Use of an articulated PMMA spacer in the infected total knee arthroplasty. J Arthroplasty 10:87, 1995.

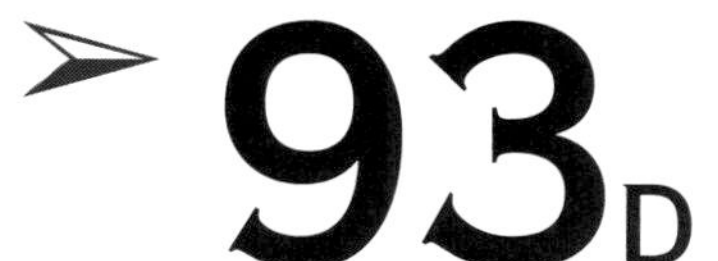

93D Revision Knee Arthroplasty: How I Do It

Cecil H. Rorabeck • James Taylor

The aim of revision total knee arthroplasty is to obtain a stable and durable construct in combination with a high level of patient satisfaction. The postoperative success of a patient undergoing revision total knee replacement depends on careful preoperative assessment.

PREOPERATIVE CLINICAL ASSESSMENT

From the preoperative clinical assessment, it is important for the surgeon to obtain an adequate history of all previous operations on the patient's knee and, of course, to rule out infection. Ideally, sequential x-rays should be present at the time of consultation, as should previous operative notes so that the operating surgeon can identify the prosthesis in place. From a historical standpoint, we find it helpful to assess the success of previous operations performed on the patient. For example, if the patient has had five or six previous operations on the same knee, none of which have been successful, then it is unlikely that the next operation that we are planning to do will be greeted with great enthusiasm by the patient. One needs to get to know the patient and get a sense of his or her expectations.

Preoperative clinical assessment of the knee centers around three major areas—namely, stability, integrity of the extensor mechanism, and possibility of sepsis. When we examine such a patient in the office, we try to determine the integrity of the patient's ligaments in an attempt to decide what type of reconstruction should be considered. For example, does the patient have varus-valgus instability as well as sagittal plane instability? Does the patient have a generalized global instability indicating dysfunction of all the supporting structures around the knee? If that is the case, one should be thinking of a hinged implant as opposed to a nonlinked hinged implant. It is relatively simple for the surgeon to assess varus-valgus stability in extension, but one should also look carefully for sagittal plane instability and, in particular, for a loose flexion gap. If the patient has a history of subluxation of the knee, she or he may well have incompetent lateral collateral ligament with midflexion instability, particularly when the limb is placed in a figure-four position. A patient with global instability, on the other hand, will have flexion and extension gaps with generalized laxity irrespective of the position of the limb. As part of the physical examination, we ask ourselves whether we will need to restore the stability of the knee at the time of revision. If the answer to that question is no, then we would probably plan to do a revision knee arthroplasty incorporating a posterior stabilized or varus, valgus-constrained liner. If the answer to the question is yes, then we would more likely think about a hinged component.

Careful assessment of the extensor mechanism is also made at this point. If the extensor mechanism is not intact and is nonreconstructable, then, of course, revision is contraindicated.

Radiographic Assessment

We obtain three x-rays, including standing 3-ft anteroposterior (AP) x-rays and a non-weightbearing lateral x-ray of the knee taken in 90 degrees, if possible. In addition, it is useful to take a sunrise view to assess the relationship of the patella to the femoral component. From these radiographs, we are able to determine the alignment of the knee. We are also able to assess the position of the implant, as well as the type, and possibly determine the mechanism of failure. It is important, when obtaining radiographs, that the opposite knee be included. The normal side is often a useful check for preoperative templating.

Although preoperative templating is not ordinarily done at the time of the first office visit, the radiographs taken at that time will form the basis for careful preoperative planning, which is carried out at our preoperative planning conference the week before the patient's surgery. From the radiographs, it is important to assess the bone loss. This can be done by carefully examining the radiographs in the AP and lateral plane and looking for defects, not only in the femur and tibia, but also in the patella. The identification of bone defects on the femoral side can be particularly troublesome because of the overlying femoral component. Often, the only clue the surgeon gets is an apparent area of osteopenia on the lateral x-ray. We look at these x-rays sequentially and carefully review them for *any* suggestion of osteolysis. Osteolysis on the tibial side is a little easier to see, but, once again, all radiographs need to be studied carefully (Fig. 93.26). It is usually not possible to classify bone defects preopera-

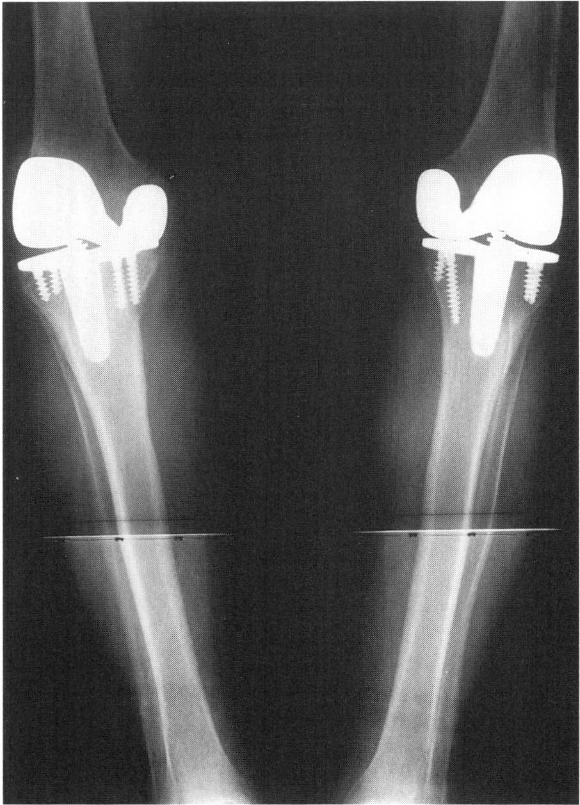

FIGURE 93.26 ➢ Osteolysis is clearly seen in the common site around the tibial screws.

tively with complete accuracy; however, it is possible to get a good idea as to what will be needed in the way of structural allograft. As a general rule, intraoperative bone defects are always *worse* than they appear on the radiographs.

As part of the radiographic evaluation, it is important, we believe, to assess the joint line and to determine where that joint line should be in the revised knee. Our experience with revision knee replacement would lead us to believe that most surgeons tend to elevate the joint line, often failing to recognize significant bone defects on the femoral side, which necessitates augments to distalize the femoral component. One should look for the fibular head on both projections and also identify the patella and its relationship to the femur to get an idea as to the desired joint line.

As we evaluate these x-rays, we ask ourselves, "How should these bone defects be managed? Are we going to be able to deal with cement, or will we need augments or allografts?" It is very important to consider these things preoperatively so that everything is available intraoperatively in the event that it is required.

Planning the Approach

At the time of our preoperative assessment of the patient, we look carefully at the patient's previous incisions, range of motion, and radiographs. It never hurts to ask the question, "What exposure will I use?" Revision total knee replacement can often be done through a simple medial parapatellar incision with proximal extension. Many patients, however, require a more extensile exposure, and it is important for the surgeon to have those exposures in her or his armamentarium so that, if necessary, they can be used to facilitate the surgery. A multiply operated knee is always a concern (Fig. 93.27). Generally, the most lateral incision should be used, but this is not always practical.

A careful analysis of the radiographs may assist the surgeon in defining the type of exposure to be used. For example, if the patient has a long cemented tibial stem and the cement appears to be solid and the implant firmly fixed, then we would advise a tibial tubercle osteotomy,[5] not only to facilitate the exposure but also for cement removal. Similarly, if a patient has a very limited arc of motion (<60 degrees), it is useful to consider an extensile exposure. We would normally start with the standard medial parapatellar, taking the incision proximally into the quadriceps tendon. At the upper end we often do a "rectus snip"[3] and combine that with a lateral release from outside in. A pin is placed in the patellar tendon, and an attempt is made to evert the patella. Our tolerance for doing a more extensile exposure in the event that the patella is difficult to evert is minimal. Our preference is to do a tibial tubercle osteotomy. The other option is a quadriceps turndown,[1, 4] which can be used; how-

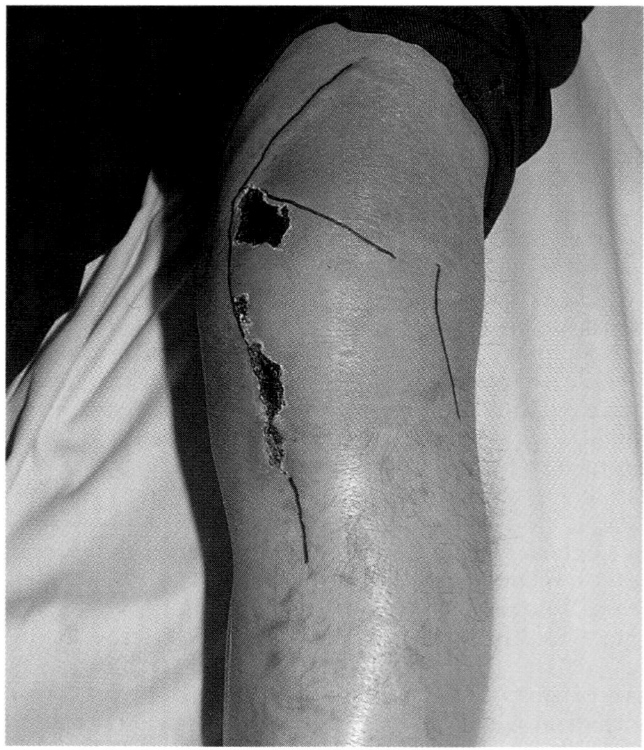

FIGURE 93.27 ➢ An example of the type of wound one tries to avoid with careful assessment and handling of the soft tissues.

ever, it is associated with a significant incidence of avascular necrosis of the patella, which may cause problems in the future (Fig. 93.28, 93.29, 93.30, and 93.31).

Component Selection

The selection of the component is perhaps the least important part of the proposed operation and is determined by the degree and severity of bone defects as well as the restoration of stability at the time of revision. If bone defects are likely, then stems are required. The length of the stem, to some extent, depends on the severity of the bone defect, but generally we prefer to use longer stems (140 mm) in the presence of significant bone defects. How much constraint will be required in the implant chosen? To some extent, this has to be assessed intraoperatively, but one can often get an idea preoperatively. For example, a patient with global instability of the knee with absent varus-valgus and sagittal plane stability may well require a hinge. Most patients, however, can be managed with a less constrained insert—either a posterior stabilized or a varus-valgus constrained. The difference between these inserts is the amount of stability offered to the knee in extension and in flexion. Posterior stabilized inserts provide considerably more rotation than do varus-valgus constrained inserts.

PREOPERATIVE CONFERENCE

Approximately 1100 total joint replacements are done each year in our institution. Every Thursday morning, a preoperative conference is held for each patient who will be operated on during the following week, and plans are discussed with the operating room nurses present. Thus, the preoperative planning is done at that time, and the operating room nurses are told what will be required in the way of implants, bone graft, and so on. Preoperative templating is done at this time (Fig. 93.32).

At the preoperative conference, the mechanism of failure is determined and each radiograph is carefully examined for bone defects. To describe the bone defects, we prefer the classification of Engh,[2] which is useful to guide treatment (Table 93.4).

THE OPERATION

A clinical case has been chosen to help illustrate the surgical technique (Fig. 93.33A). We do the surgery with the use of a tourniquet that exsanguinates the limb. The exposure that we use has been discussed previously, but in most cases it is a medial parapatellar incision with or without a lateral release and a rectus snip. Occasionally, more extensile approaches are required (tibial tubercle osteotomy or quadriceps turndown). Although it is sometimes obvious preoperatively that a tibial tubercle osteotomy (for example) will be required, most often the decision to use an extensile exposure is made intraoperatively. During exposure, we take great care to ensure that the patellar tendon will not be avulsed. To that end, a pin is often placed in the patellar tendon during the exposure, and it stays there for most of the case, if possible. To gain further exposure at the time of surgery, we usually get around well laterally and medially and, if necesssary, "skeletonize" the distal femur by releasing all scar tissue in the medial lateral gutters. With patience, one can usually get the desired exposure without having to violate the extensor mechanism.

We take cultures once the knee is open. We do not routinely send synovium for histological assessment unless we are concerned that there may be infection that we had not been aware of.

The component removal begins on the femoral side. If the implant being removed is cementless and is fully bony ingrown, then Gigli's saw is helpful (Fig. 93.33B). We also use fine osteotomes to get distal to the pegs. It is extremely important to run these instruments distally and posteriorly to loosen up the osseous-implant interface as much as possible. It is easy to loosen it up proximally and distally but more difficult distally and posteriorly. Once that has been done, Gigli's saw is used and the femoral component is gently tapped off using a reverse hook and a hammer. Ideally, little, if any, of the host bone should be removed with the cementless implant. If the implant to be removed is cemented, then we usually use osteotomes to break up the interface, although on occasion we use Gigli's saw. These are usually easier to remove, and one is less likely to damage the host bone. Once the femoral component has been removed, we measure the internal dimensions of it to get an idea as to the sizing of the femoral component, which we will be replacing (Fig. 93.33C). The removed component is then denuded of tissue and placed back onto the native femur to facilitate retraction and subluxation of the tibial component.

To loosen the interface between the tibial component and the bone, we generally use an oscillating saw with a narrow blade. One needs to be careful with this instrument because it is possible for the blade to "submarine," thereby resulting in removal of host bone. The small blade with the power saw allows us to get around the central post or the lateral pegs, as the case may be. Once the tibial surface has been loosened, it remains to be determined if the tibial component can be extracted simply. If the component is cemented and if the stem is smooth, then one can probably tap the tibial component out of the cement mantle relatively easily, or stacked osteotomes can be used (Fig. 93.33D). On the other hand, if the component is cemented, and if recessed areas are present on the stem, it can be extremely difficult and, frankly, dangerous to do that. In that situation, it is better to do a tibial tubercle osteotomy and come up from below, to loosen the cement mantle from the prosthesis. This can be determined preoperatively by knowledge of the implant to be removed, and, therefore, it should not pose an unexpected problem at the time of surgery. Fully ingrown cementless stems need to be removed using a tibial tubercle osteotomy. Once the interface has been loosened around the tibial compo-

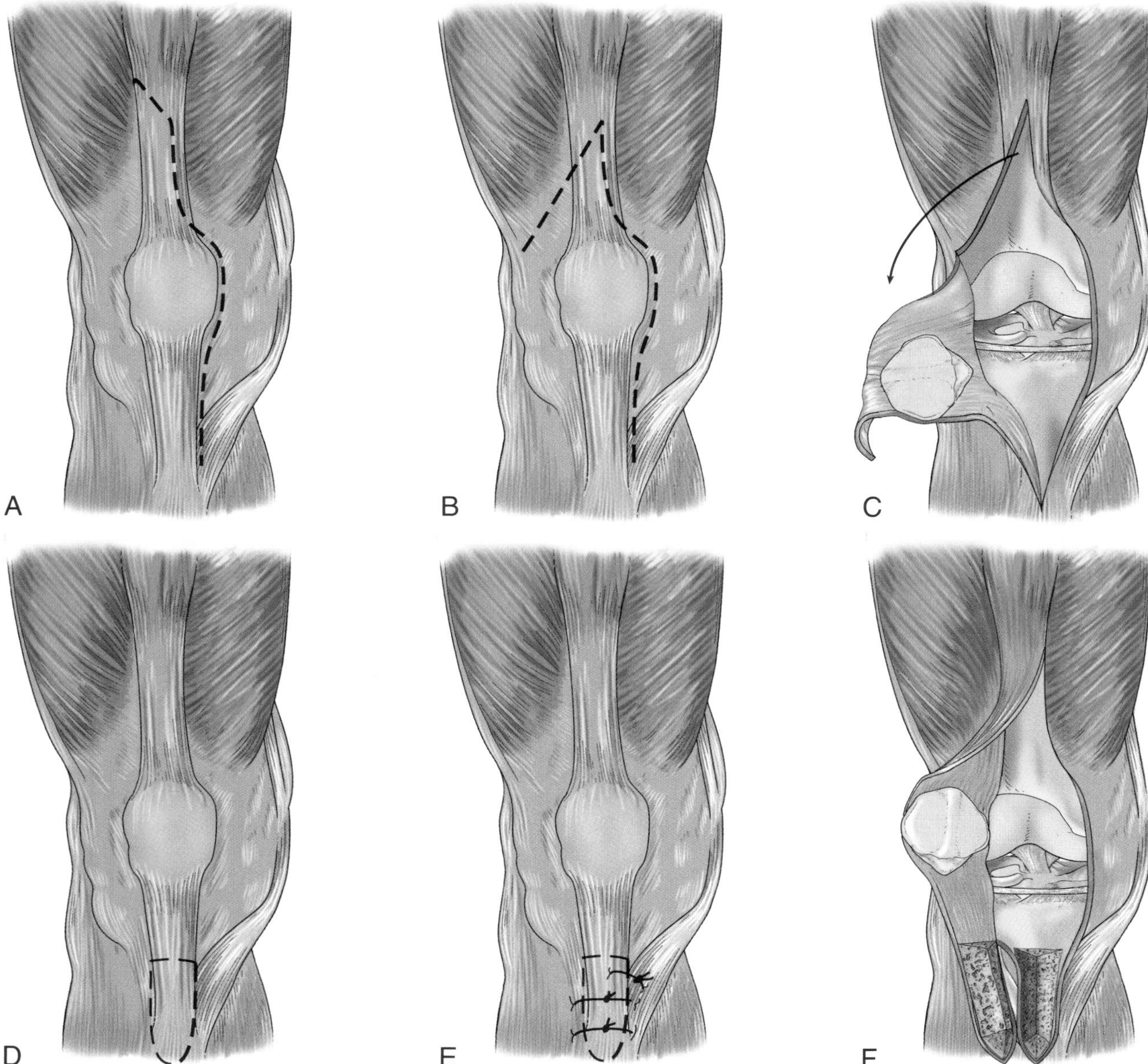

FIGURE 93.28 ➢ Diagrams depicting the alternative methods used to improve exposure. *A,* The incision used to perform a rectus snip. A medial parapatellar approach is used, and the incision is then directed across, laterally and proximally, at the proximal end. Note that the incision remains within the tendon throughout. *B and C,* A quadriceps turndown. It is preferable to restrict the lateral limb of the incision to preserve as much blood supply to the patella as possible, but the incision can be extended if required for exposure. *D, E and F,* A tibial tubercle osteotomy. Note that the osteotomy is cut from the medial side using an oscillating saw, leaving the soft tissues attached laterally. The osteotomy is rotated laterally to provide access to the knee. The osteotomy is reattached, usually using three wires. The most proximal wire is passed through the osteotomy and then out of the tibia medially. The distal wires are passed through the tibia and wrap around the osteotomy. The wires are passed before insertion of the prosthesis and tightened while the cement is setting.

nent, it could be tapped out using a hook and a hammer.

Once the tibial component has been removed, excess cement and debris are removed (Fig. 93.33E). We excise the remnants of the posterior cruciate ligament and make certain that the capsule at the back of the tibia is identified and that the tibial margins are carefully exposed (Fig. 93.33F). A blunt Hohman retractor is placed posteriorly, retracting against the replaced femoral component. It is distinctly unwise to use these

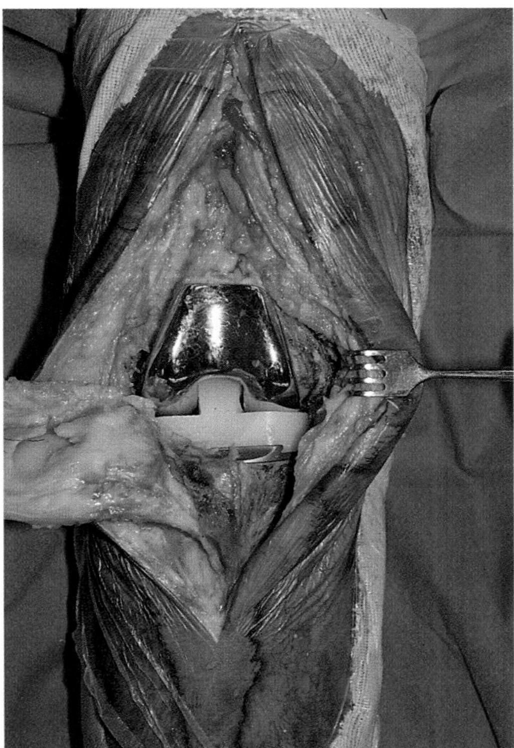

FIGURE 93.29 ➢ Quadriceps turndown providing excellent exposure of the knee.

retractors without the femoral component being in place.

Once the tibial and femoral components are removed, we examine the flexion and extension gaps in

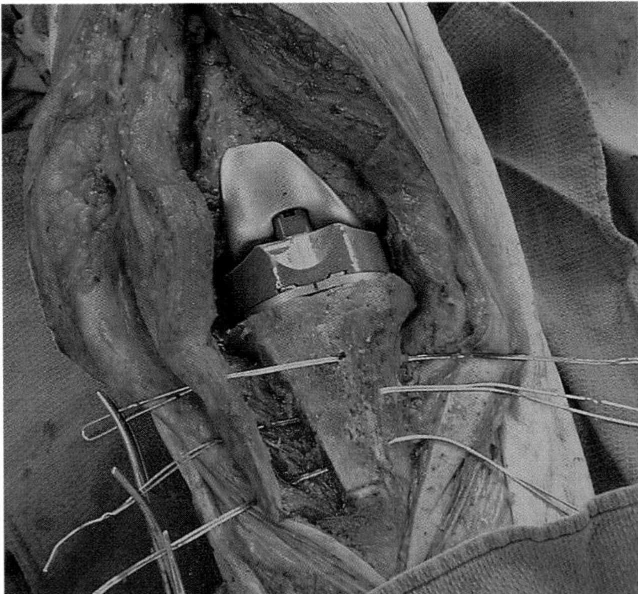

FIGURE 93.30 ➢ Tibial tubercle osteotomy with the wires in place clearly showing their positioning.

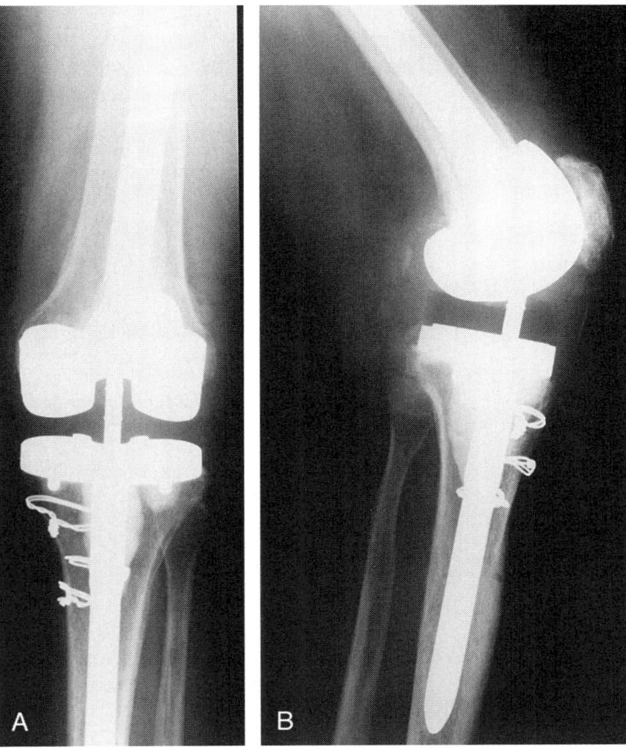

FIGURE 93.31 ➢ Postoperative anteroposterior and lateral radiographs showing a tibial tubercle osteotomy healed in position.

the knee and measure them with a ruler to get a rough idea as to how much bone may or may not have to be removed and whether augments will be required to center the joint line where we want it.

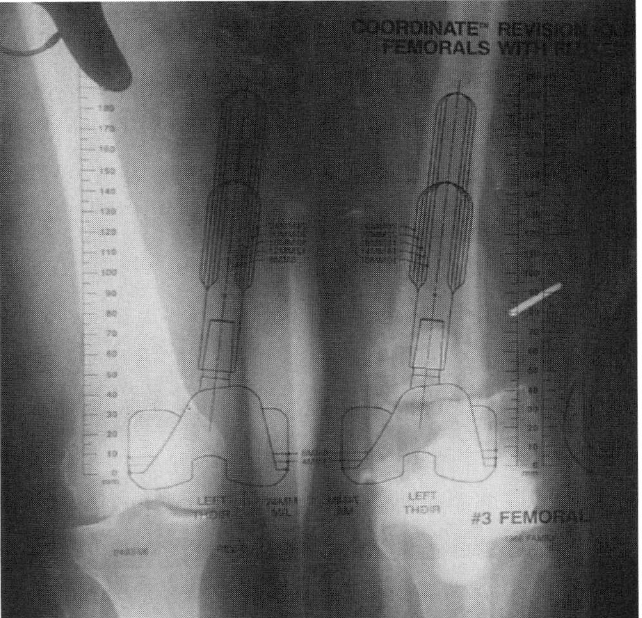

FIGURE 93.32 ➢ Preoperative templating is an essential part of the planning process.

TABLE 93.4 **ANDERSON ORTHOPAEDIC RESEARCH INSTITUTE CLASSIFICATION OF BONE DEFECTS IN FAILED TOTAL KNEE ARTHROPLASTY**

Classification	Bone Defects	Surgical Options
Type 1	Intact metaphyseal bone, minor bone defects, revision component expected to be stable	Small defects can be filled with cement or morselized bone graft.
Femur (F1)	Normal joint line, condyles intact	
Tibia (T1)	Component above fibular head and metaphysis intact	
Type 2 (2A - one condyle) (2B - both condyles)	Damaged metaphyseal bone, cancellous bone loss	Most defects are able to be reconstructed with an augmented component. Stems are required.
Femur (F2)	Joint line elevated and condyles damaged	
Tibia (T2)	Component at or below the tip of the fibular head and tibial width reduced	
Type 3	Deficient metaphyseal segment, major bone defect, collateral or patellar ligaments possibly detached	Reconstruction with structural bone graft or large augments, maximally constrained or hinged components may be required.
Femur (F3)	Implant migration or osteolysis to the level of the epicondyles	
Tibia (T3)	Component migration or osteolysis causing loss of the tibial flare	

This is a crude determination at this point, but it does allow us to be thinking about these things as we proceed with the operation.

A 6-mm intramedullary rod is passed down the shaft of the tibia once the cement has been removed. This rod is placed right to the ankle, and a cutting block (0 degrees) is then pinned into place (Fig. 93.33G). Generally speaking, a minimum amount of bone needs to be removed from the tibia, but, to some extent, this will be determined by the preoperative planning. It is important in most situations that this first cut be placed at 90 degrees to the sagittal and coronal plane so that when finished, it will be at right angles to the floor. However, depending on the presence of bone defects, angled cuts may sometimes need to be made (Fig. 93.33H). Once the block is pinned in position and the cut is made, the bone is then removed and the medullary canal of the tibia is reamed by hand, beginning with an 8-mm reamer and progressing until we have good cortical chatter. If (for example) this occurs at 12 mm, then a trial reduction with a 12-mm stem on an appropriately sized baseplate will be applied. The stem will be canal filling and will also allow us to determine the accuracy of the cut on the proximal tibia. Before seating the trial all the way, we use the undersurface of the tibial plate as a reference to trim and "fine-tune" the tibial cut. The tibial component trial is then seated in an appropriate degree of external rotation.

Attention is turned to the femur following completion of the tibia. The femoral canal is opened slightly medial to the posterior cruciate ligament attachment to allow appropriate centering of the prosthesis. The femur is reamed progressively, by hand, until cortical chatter is achieved and the distal femoral cutting block is applied (Fig. 93.33I). At this point, one has to determine the rotation of the femoral component. There are a number of "clues" as to the correct rotational orientation of the femoral component. The position of the removed implant is a help. Some of the older implants are often internally rotated, and one can note that at the time of removal. We also identify the epicondyles at this point, as well as the anterior surface of the femur. The epicondyles are not always easy to find; nevertheless, the exercise of identification is important because it does allow one to seat the femoral component parallel to the transepicondylar axis. We can now place the distal femoral cutting block in the same position with the correct rotation and check its position referable to the epicondyles and to the ante-

FIGURE 93.33 ➢ 77-year-old woman who required revision of a right total knee arthroplasty 4 years after the index operation. She developed increasing pain and a progressive varus deformity, with varus-valgus instability present on examination. An aspiration of the knee was negative on bacterial culture. *A,* Preoperative radiographs show that the tibial component has collapsed into varus and that the femoral component is in an excessive degree of valgus. *B,* Use of Gigli's saw to free the femoral component before disimpaction. *C,* The inside dimensions as well as the width of the removed femoral component are measured to help decide on the size of the revision femoral component. *D,* Stacked osteotomes are useful to remove the tibial component once it has been freed up. *E,* Débridement of the bone ends. *F,* To easily find the plane of dissection at the posterior aspect of the tibia, an oscillating saw is used to cut a wafer of bone that is then "greensticked" upward. This peels the soft tissue off the posterior cortex of the tibia at this point and allows for safe access for retractors. *G,* Extramedullary guide for the tibial cutting block. In this case, because of the medial bone defect, a wedged tibial component will be used, and so the cutting guide is angled. *H,* Minimal bone is removed from the proximal tibia.

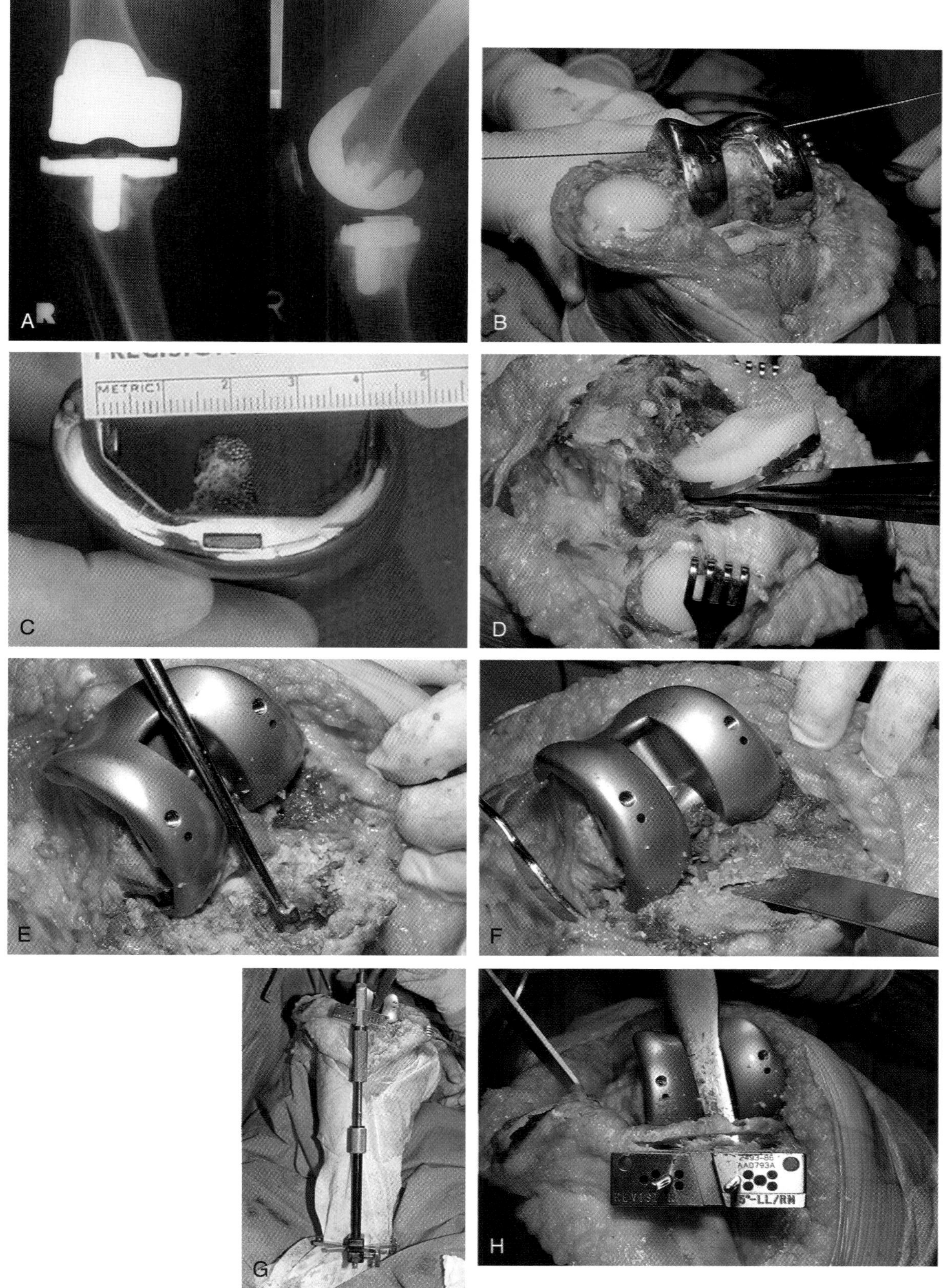

FIGURE 93.33 ➢ *See legend on opposite page.*

Illustration continued on following page

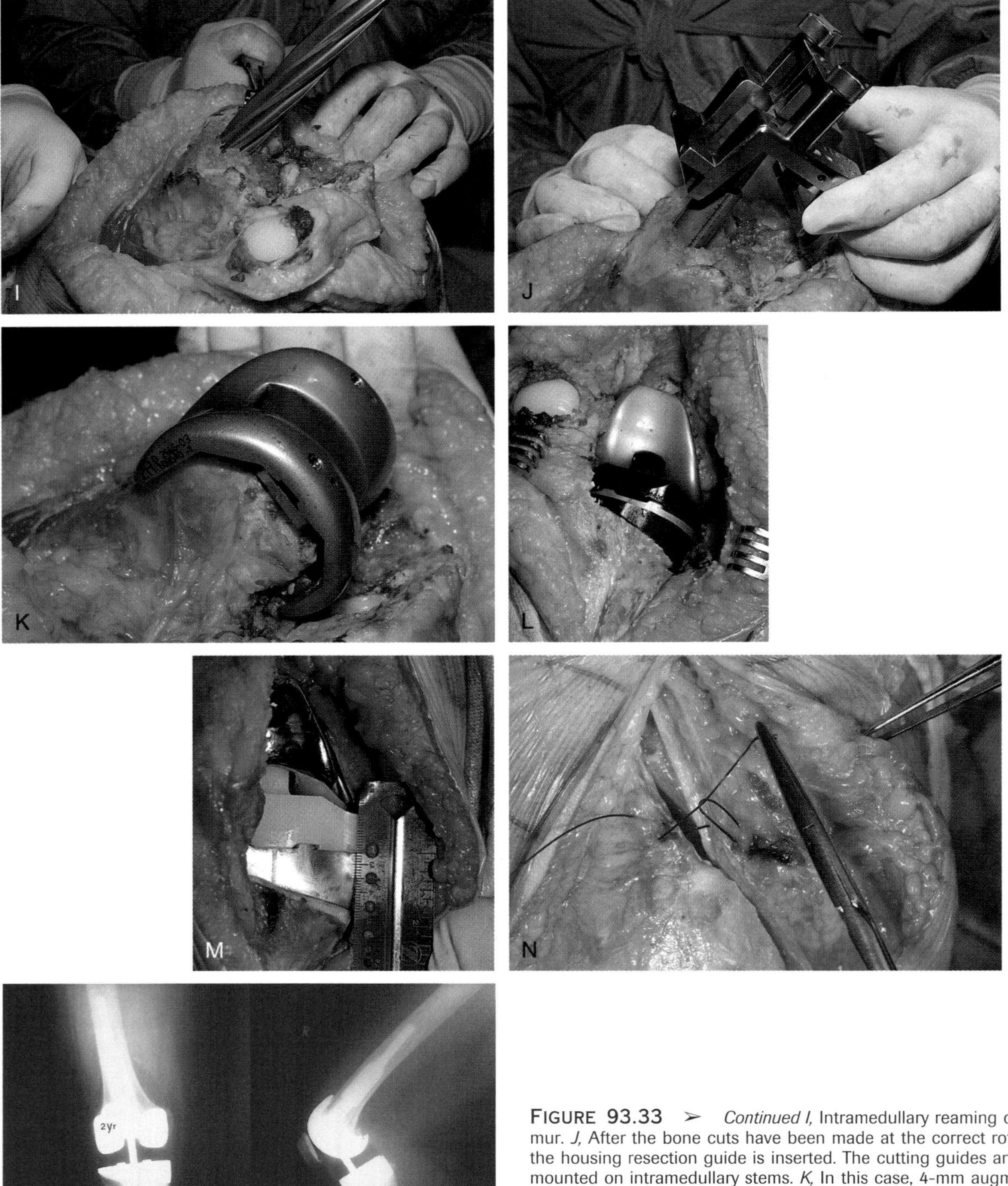

FIGURE 93.33 ➢ *Continued I,* Intramedullary reaming of the femur. *J,* After the bone cuts have been made at the correct rotation, the housing resection guide is inserted. The cutting guides are mounted on intramedullary stems. *K,* In this case, 4-mm augments were used distally and posteriorally on the lateral side, as seen on the trial femoral component. *L,* The trial components in place. *M,* The definitive components have been cemented in place. One can see the size of the defect that has been replaced. *N,* The locking stitch used in the extensor mechanism to ensure a sturdy repair. *O,* Radiographs taken 2 years postoperatively. The clinical result was excellent.

rior surface of the femur. Using canal referencing instruments, it is possible for the distal femoral cutting guide to "sag" posteriorly with the weight of gravity. Thus, we normally use a saw capture on the front of this guide and insert a crab-claw or an empty saw blade to reference the anterior cortex. The block is now pinned in position. This allows us to "shim" the distal femur at either 4 mm or 8 mm, depending on the degree of bone loss and the desired position of the femoral component (Fig. 93.33J). As has been indicated previously, there is a tendency by most surgeons to move the joint line proximally, and thus it is our practice to remove a *minimal* amount of bone from the distal femur.

AP and mediolateral sizing of the new femoral component will be done by measuring the internal dimensions of the removed femoral components and templating to the normal side. Thus, at this point, a size-3 (for example) housing resection guide will be inserted with the appropriate-sized stem and centered on the distal femur (Fig. 93.33K). Stem position is extremely important in determining the position of the housing resection guide. If the start point is too far lateral, one may have lateral overhang, which is undesirable. We make every effort to ensure that the housing resection guide is properly seated mediolaterally and in the AP plane. Depending on the bone defects on the femoral side, augments may be placed distally or posteriorly on the housing resection guide, medially or laterally, to recreate the normal dimensions of the host femur. With the housing resection guide firmly seated in position, the central piece of bone is removed. With the housing resection guide removed and the trial tibial component in place, flexion-extension gap measurement is carried out. The cuts are now fine-tuned to ensure symmetry. Using the appropriate-sized trial intramedullary stem, the chamfer cutter is now applied to the femur and the anterior and posterior chamfer is completed. A trial femoral component, with the appropriate trial augments, is inserted, and a tibial insert is chosen (Fig. 93.33 L) Stability at this point needs to be assessed carefully. In particular, one often sees flexion-space instability, and it is extremely important to check the integrity of the construct in varus and valgus as well as in a sagittal plane with the patella reduced. If one has done an extensile exposure (tibial tubercle osteotomy or quadriceps turndown), then, of course, the flexion space will be somewhat looser than it should be. To assess this, the extensor mechanism should be temporarily coapted.

We now turn our attention to the patella and make a decision as to whether we are going to leave the native patella in situ or are going to remove it. If the patella is a nonanatomic design (i.e., domed) and is not metal backed with minimal polywear, then we will leave it in situ. We do not believe it matters if it is not from the same manufacturer as the component being replaced. An anatomic patella, however, needs to be removed and a decision made at that time as to whether it will be replaced. We try, as much as possible, to replace *all* patellae with a cemented, all-polyethylene, domed button. If, however, the remaining bone is less than 8 mm, then the risk of fracturing it at the time of replacement is high, and then we prefer not to replace it.

The trial components are now removed, the surface is cleaned and dried, and a single mix of "warm" bone cement is used to attach the augments to the femoral or tibial components. While this is curing, three batches of cement are mixed (two at room temperature and one from the warming oven). The "real" femoral component with attached stem is cemented into position, cementing only the metaphysis and the housing, *not* the stem. We like to get a good press-fit of the stem. Our attention is now turned to the tibia, where the metaphyseal area of the tibia is cemented, following which the tibial component is hammered into place. Once again, we will have a good press fit of the tibial stem; therefore, the stem is not cemented. The knee is brought out into extension with the trial spacer, and the patellar component is cemented into place. Excess glue is removed, stability is assessed, and the appropriate-sized insert is applied (Fig. 93.33M). Once the cement is set, the tourniquet is generally released. If a tibial tubercle osteotomy has been performed, it is now wired back into position, and closure is carried out using a locking suture in the capsule over an ⅛-in drain (Fig. 93.33N). Once the capsule is closed, the knee is flexed to 90 degrees to ensure integrity of the suture line, and the closure is completed. Radiographs are taken in the postoperative recovery room to assess component position (Fig. 93.33O).

Postoperatively, continuous passive motion is started in the recovery room at 70 to 110 degrees as a routine and continues overnight. The patient is mobilized with weightbearing as tolerated from postoperative day 2 unless bone grafting has been performed, in which case the patient is kept to touch weightbearing. A brace is not usually required.

Intravenous antibiotics are continued until the results of cultures taken intraoperatively are available, which is usually in 5 days. All patients are placed on a warfarin (Coumadin) protocol to maintain the International Normalized Ratio in the therapeutic range (2.0) until discharge.

CONCLUSION

Revision knee arthroplasty is a challenging procedure with many potential complications. By adhering to these simple guidelines, and with attention to detail, it is possible to consistently achieve good results. Careful preoperative planning, as well as the ability to modify that plan intraoperatively if required, is essential.

References

1. Coonse K, Adams JD: A new operative approach to the knee joint. Surg Gynecol Obstet 77:344, 1943.
2. Engh GA: Bone defect classification. In Engh GA, Rorabeck CH, eds: Revision Total Knee Arthroplasty. Baltimore, Williams & Wilkins, 1997, p 63.
3. Garvin KL, Scuderi G, Insall JN: Evolution of the quadriceps snip. Clin Orthop 321:131, 1995.
4. Trousdale RT, Hanssen AD, Rand JA, et al: VY quadricepsplasty in total knee arthroplasty. Clin Orthop 286:48, 1993.
5. Whiteside LA, Ohl MD: Tibial tubercle osteotomy for exposure of the difficult total knee arthroplasty. Clin Orthop 260:6, 1990.

93E Revision Knee Arthroplasty: How I Do It

Kelly G. Vince

PREOPERATIVE ASSESSMENT

The case discussed in this chapter illustrates difficulties with a failed revision knee arthroplasty. Most failed primary total knee arthroplasties still leave the surgeon with adequate amounts of bone and intact ligament structures for a reasonably uncomplicated revision arthroplasty. Failure, however, to observe principles of revision surgery and failure to reconstruct missing bone as needed with allograft material often lead to failure of revision arthroplasty. The patient discussed in this chapter, a woman still gainfully employed at age 63 years, had a cemented cruciate retaining knee that failed secondary to loosening with probable angular and rotational malalignment of components (Fig. 93.34). Evaluation of this failed primary knee arthroplasty might have included a computed tomography (CT) scan, which is very useful in depicting the three-dimensional positioning of components. Despite scatter that is often observed in these studies, the epicondyles and the rotational position of the femoral component can usually be identified. Similarly, the tibial tubercle and the tibial component can be identified. This helps in planning the revision knee arthroplasty in terms of correcting malrotation.

Undoubtedly, this patient presented to the first revision surgeon with pain. An important distinction among patients with painful knee arthroplasties is whether there was ever pain relief after the primary arthroplasty. Patients suffering persistent pain that is similar to the pain that predated the knee arthroplasty may be suffering from referred symptoms that originate in spinal pathology or in an arthritic hip ipsilateral to the knee where the knee arthroplasty was performed. Careful history, physical examination, and a bone scan are helpful in avoiding revision knee arthroplasty for pain that originates in another location.

The second type of presentation is pain that has persisted from the time of the primary knee arthroplasty but that differs in quality. These patients may be suffering from sepsis, failure of bone ingrowth into a porous coated prosthesis, malrotation of components, or an overstuffed joint that leaves them feeling tight and painful. Most tight joints will flex poorly and may have a flexion contracture. Aspiration of the arthroplasty is essential to determine whether sepsis is present. The fluid should be sent, not only for culture and sensitivity, but also for cell count, including a differential of the white cells.

The third situation is the patient who enjoyed good function with excellent pain relief following the arthroplasty but who at a later date began to develop problems. This is a typical presentation for loosening of the components, breakage of the prosthesis, or new onset of sepsis. Individuals who may suffer fracture of the bone adjacent to the prosthesis are included in this group. Supracondylar femur fractures usually have a dramatic presentation with little doubt as to the diagnosis, but fractures of the patella may present insidiously with small amounts of pain and a radiograph that is initially normal. Repeat films and a bone scan are very helpful in diagnosing patellar fracture. At any rate, it is incumbent on the surgeon to establish the diagnosis and the cause of pain. I find it very useful to place the patient in one of the nine categories of failure that have been established in the literature (Table 93.5).

In an early paper, Hungerford and associates described the first four causes of revision knee arthroplasty. Causes five through eight were included in the review of failed total knee arthroplasties that I published, and I have since added a ninth cause—fracture. It should be noted that cause number four, "no diagnosis for the pain," represents a contraindication to revision knee arthroplasty. As I have gained more experience in evaluating painful knee replacements, this category, sometimes described as the "mystery knee," often turns out to be pain secondary to failed bone ingrowth or pain secondary to malrotation of components.[1]

The patient presented to me with a failed, painful revision knee arthroplasty (Fig. 93.35). The failed revision arthroplasty demonstrated several problems. The first was the use of the constrained implant when the failed primary radiograph indicated a high probability that collateral ligaments were intact. This should have allowed the surgeon to reestablish integrity of collateral ligaments and to avoid use of the constrained implant. The knee had been aligned in excess valgus. Valgus alignment combined with a constrained implant is likely to result in problems. The medial thrust imparted by the valgus alignment either breaks the components or rapidly results in loosening. This valgus

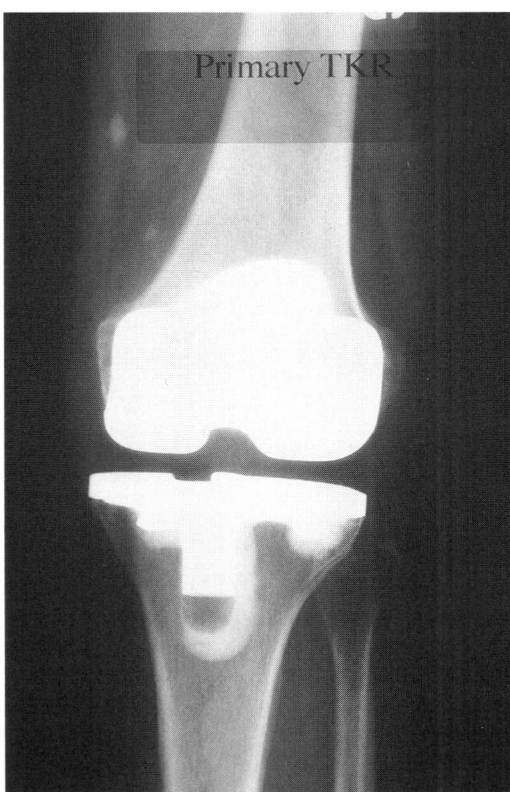

FIGURE 93.34 ➢ Original primary total knee arthroplasty with cemented cruciate retaining prosthesis. Note the relative anteroposterior radiograph of the femoral component in conjunction a malrotated tibial component. This implies that the tibia, the femoral component, or both suffered malalignment. This undoubtedly contributed to the failure of the prosthesis.

alignment had resulted from the positioning of the femoral component stem, a wide-diameter, uncemented component. Undoubtedly, the entry point was too far lateral; the surgeon, in this case, had become a "slave to the stem," positioning the component where the stem dictated. It would also seem that the lateral femoral condylar bone was inevitably deficient and, instead of being reconstructed with allograft or prosthesis, the component was simply seated on deficient bone, which contributed further to the valgus positioning.

The anteroposterior (AP) radiograph showed a relatively straight view of the femoral component but an asymmetric view of the tibia, implying that these revision components were malrotated. The third problem in this revision was the extent of bone loss that had been accepted by the surgeon as opposed to being reconstructed with allograft. I have noted how loss of lateral femoral bone contributed to unacceptable valgus alignment of the femoral component. In addition, there was considerable bone loss on the proximal tibia such that the fixation of the revision components could not be satisfactory and were particularly inadequate for a constrained component.

My evaluation indicated no sepsis, based on a benign cell count with benign differential and negative

TABLE 93.5 **NINE CAUSES OF FAILURE OF TOTAL KNEE ARTHROPLASTY**

	Indications for Revision TKR	
Type	***Diagnosis***	***% Good or Excellent***
1	Loosening and progression of arthritis in a unicompartmental replacement	76
2	Instability	100
3	Malrotation and patellar instability	100
4	Undiagnosed pain	0
5	Breakage	
6	Sepsis	
7	Extensor rupture	
8	Stiffness	
9	Fracture	

TKR = total knee replacement.

Data from: Jacobs MA, Hungerford DS, Krackow KA, et al: Revision total knee arthoplasty for aseptic failure. Clin Orthop 226:78, 1988. Vince KG, Long W: Revision knee arthroplasty. The limits of press-fit medullary fixation. Clin Orthop 317:172, 1995.

cultures. In addition, the history indicated no problems with wound healing or other symptoms suggestive of sepsis at the time of the primary arthroplasty or the first revision. The diagnosis was loosening of the femoral and tibial components with malalignment and additional patellar tracking problems.

A plan was made for revision knee arthroplasty surgery with preparations for allograft bone graft reconstruction of the distal femur and the proximal tibia. Special attention would be given to reestablishing correct valgus alignment and correct rotational positioning of components.

SKIN INCISION AND APPROACH

This patient had a well-placed skin incision from the primary knee arthroplasty that was appropriately reentered on the revision. The only improvement that could have been made in the positioning was the fact that the distal aspect of the incision lay over the tibial tubercle. This is a common shortcoming in approaches to the knee. Incisions placed over the tubercle can be uncomfortable, lying as they do on a bony prominence. In addition, if the surgeon continues the arthrotomy at the same point, she or he will inevitably elevate part of the patellar tendon on its medial side, and this predisposes patients to avulsion of the patellar tendon. The surgical approach is facilitated by an incision that angles laterally proximal to the knee. This follows the "Q-angle" of the knee, creates a smaller lateral skin flap to evert during surgery, and makes it easier to turn the extensor mechanism out of the way.

Had difficulties been encountered with the expo-

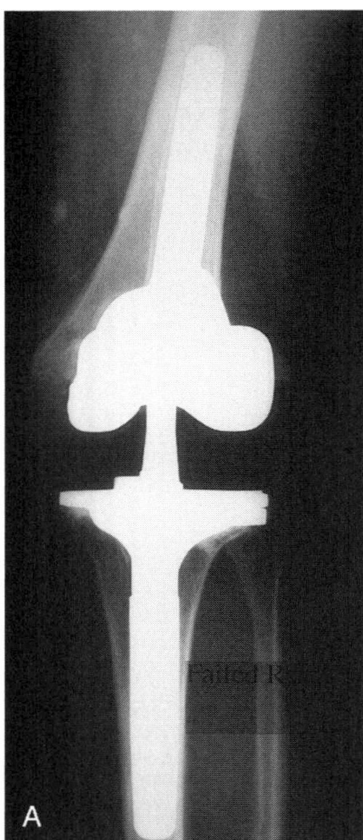

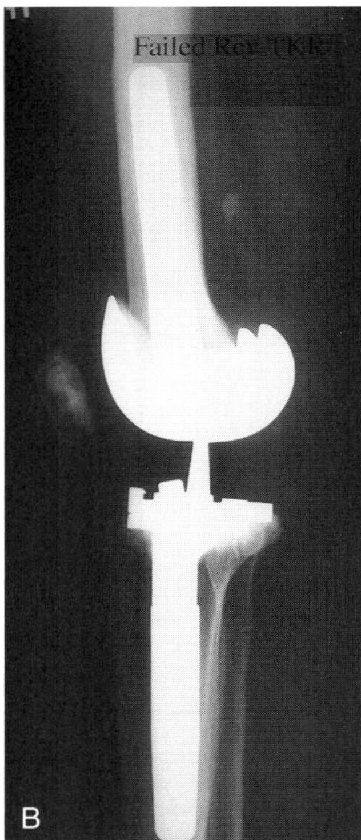

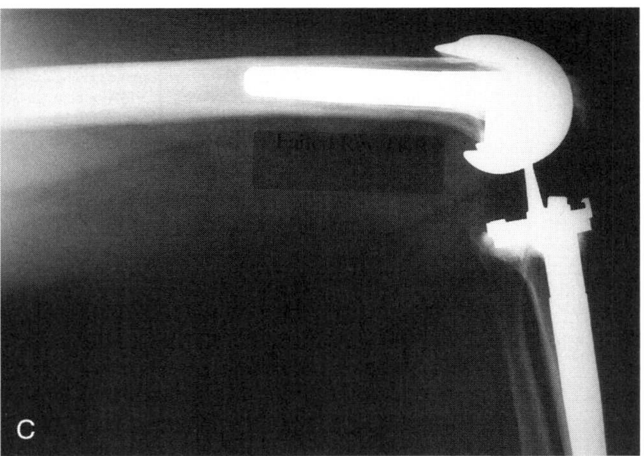

FIGURE 93.35A ➢ Painful revision arthroplasty. Was constraint essential? Note the excess valgus resulting from position of femoral component stem. Relative anteroposterior view of the femoral component is at odds with the rotated view of the tibia, suggesting component malrotation. Tibial component is placed very low on the tibia inferior to the tibiofibular head.

FIGURE 93.35B ➢ The lateral view of the failed revision knee arthroplasty demonstrates a relatively low position of the patella and a relatively high position of the joint line. Reflecting back to Figure 93.35A, the elevation of the joint line is apparent. Note that the femoral component size and its anteroposterior dimension appear to be satisfactory. This implies that the flexion gap will be tight. Consider that inordinately thick polyethylene was used to stabilize the knee in extension but that a normal-size femoral component was used, and we see that the extension gap was probably wider than the flexion gap. This also produced elevation of the joint line. Anterior position of patella indicates a chronic effusion.

FIGURE 93.35C ➢ Lateral radiograph in maximum flexion of failed revision knee arthroplasty. Flexion is limited to less than 90 degrees, which results from a failure to balance the flexion and extension gaps. This implies that the flexion gap is tight. This further indicates that of the two gap-type problems in this knee both gaps are unacceptably large because of failure to reconstruct distal bone and flexion of a too-small femoral component. However, it would seem that the extension gap is still considerably larger than the flexion gap, explaining why the knee flexes poorly. The solution is a larger femoral component and reconstruction of the distal femur with allograft.

sure, the first goal would be to pay attention to surgical details. Accordingly, the gutters on either side of the femur should be freed of scar. A lateral patellar retinacular release is often useful in facilitating eversion. An extensive synovectomy removing abundant scar tissue makes it easier to expose the knee. Given the undue valgus alignment in this arthroplasty, it would be undesirable to elevate extensive amounts of medial capsule and medial collateral ligament, which would have further compromised stability.

In the vast majority of revisions, attention to these details permits adequate exposure without jeopardy to the extensor mechanism. If eversion remains a problem, the quadriceps muscle can simply be split more proximally in line with the arthrotomy. It is only in rare cases that a "quadriceps snip" approach is necessary. It is my preference to avoid tubercle osteotomies because they compromise the integrity of the tibial bone and the tibial component fixation (Fig. 93.35B).

REMOVAL OF THE COMPONENTS

Numerous innovative methods have been suggested for removal of cemented and uncemented components. Having tried them all, I have found that the fastest, most efficient, and most bone-conserving method is to disrupt the interface with a sagittal saw. These narrow-bladed saws can be inserted between most of the appendages common to knee prostheses. They cut easily between the bone-cement interface or the cement-prosthetic interface or between a porous coated component and the bone. Once the interface

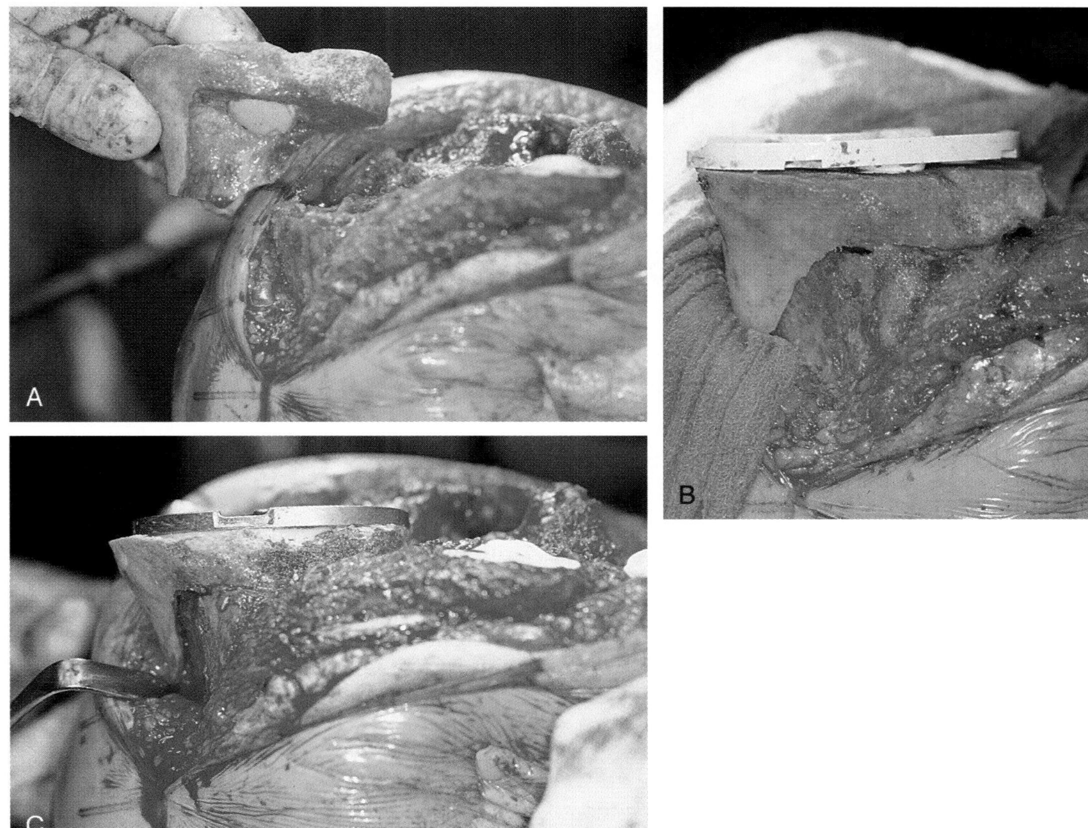

FIGURE 93.36A ➢ A proximal tibial allograft specimen is shaped to mate up with the host bone. The medial diaphyseal cortex has been retained to overlap the host and provide additional interface material as well as enhance rotational stability. There is always a difficulty in allograft reconstruction of accommodating the desired size of graft. Large defects soon seem too small for structural allograft. Reducing the size of the allograft compromises its strength.

FIGURE 93.36B ➢ Tibial allograft in place retained by a trial component and its intramedullary stem.

FIGURE 93.36C ➢ Tibial allograft in place retained by the implanted revision tibial component.

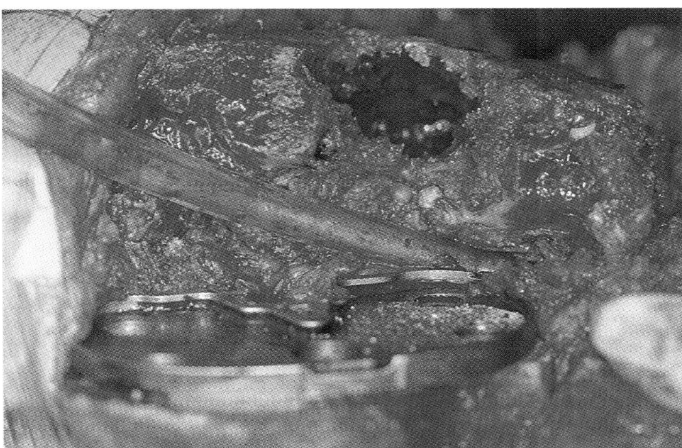

FIGURE 93.37 ➢ The distal femoral bone is compromised. The condyles are severely deficient, indicating that a prosthetic femoral component would not enjoy rotational stability on host bone.

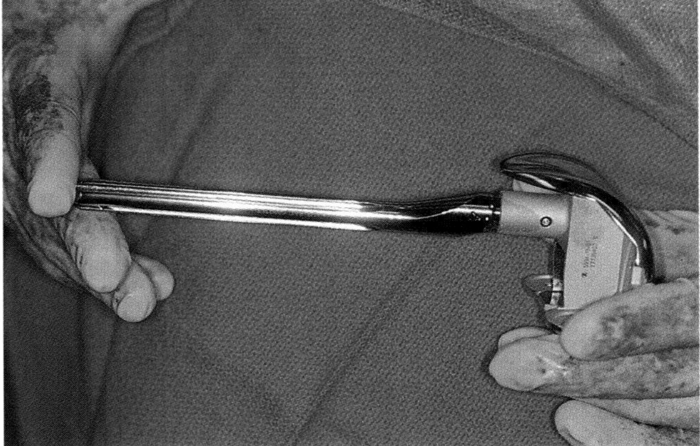

FIGURE 93.38 ➢ Side view of the prosthesis and modular offset stem showing the femoral component translated anteriorly, allowing the intramedullary stem to sit in the middle of the femoral canal.

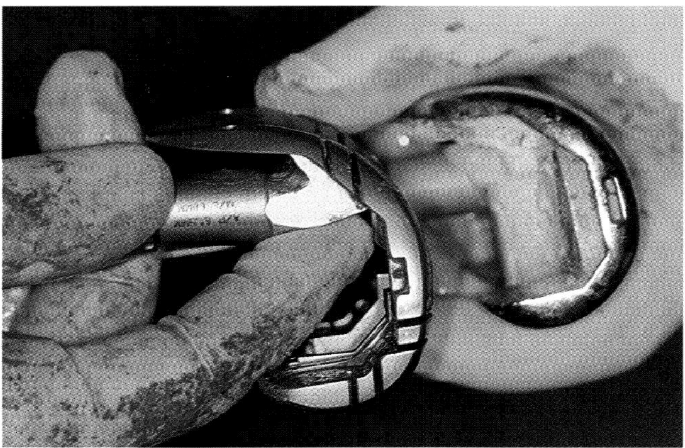

FIGURE 93.39 ➢ Comparison of the failed femoral component on the right with the new second revision component that will be implanted to stabilize the knee in flexion indicates that a larger size is required.

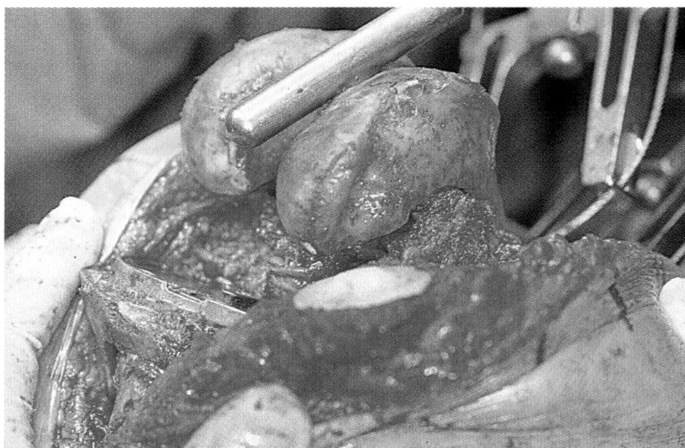

FIGURE 93.40 ➢ Femoral allograft positioned on distal femur.

has been disrupted maximally with the saw, osteotomes of about ¼ to ½-inch width can be inserted into the interface with a mallet to elevate the component and separate it from the bone. This is sometimes a slow process. Additional osteotomes may be stacked on top of the one that has been inserted. It is wise to avoid levering the osteotome because this will inevitably destroy some bone. The goal is to distribute the force on as broad a surface as possible using wider osteotomes when feasible. Axial slap hammer extractors have long been recommended for component removal, but I avoid them. They can be difficult to attach to modern asymmetric components, and, when attached, they easily apply unacceptably large amounts of force that can remove bone along with the prosthesis.

A small metal punch or bone tamp can be used to apply axial force to the components with a mallet and facilitate removal. With the component removed, there may be residual bone or adherent cement in some places. The conventional approach recommends fragmentation of the cement with an osteotome as a means of preserving bone. I find that this creates abundant debris and still leaves poor-quality bone, which must be resected to establish the solid osseous foundation. Accordingly, to conserve both bone and time, apply a sagittal saw to the bone, removing thin wafers along with the undesired cement and the component.

REVISION INSTRUMENTS

There are few specific instruments that are truly useful in revision knee arthroplasty surgery. The surgeon is best equipped who has a sound grasp of principles and a coherent plan for the reconstruction. Trial components function as instruments, and some prosthetic systems have adapted the trial components with cutting blocks to facilitate reimplantation.

REVISION KNEE ARTHROPLASTY

Since the 1980s, I have employed a three-step technique for revision knee arthroplasty.[2] This series of steps is useful for planning and execution of revision knee arthroplasty. Inherent in these steps is the importance of alignment, equalization of flexion and extension gaps, and reestablishment of the most appropriate joint line height.

Step 1: Proximal Tibia Platform. The word *platform* is consciously chosen here to discriminate between the steps in which the articular surface is determined. It is useful to begin the reconstruction by reestablishing a foundation on which the knee can be rebuilt. In this particular case, large amounts of proximal tibial bone had been lost from the primary as well as the failed revision arthroplasty surgery. A decision was made before surgery that allograft bone graft would be necessary.

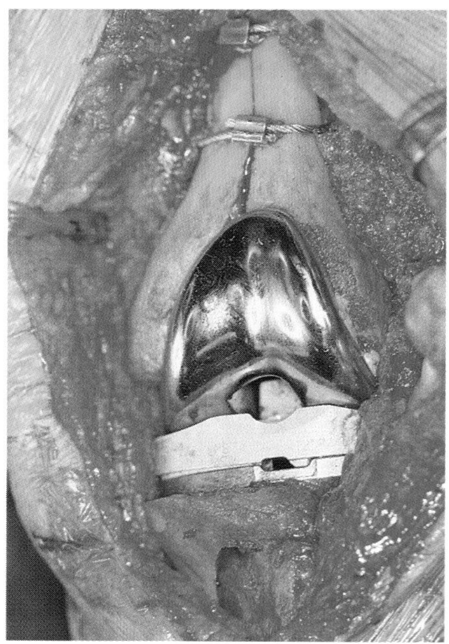

FIGURE 93.41 ➢ Second revision completed.

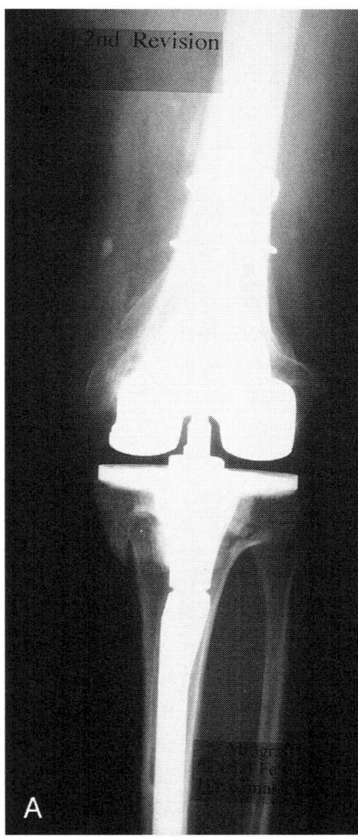

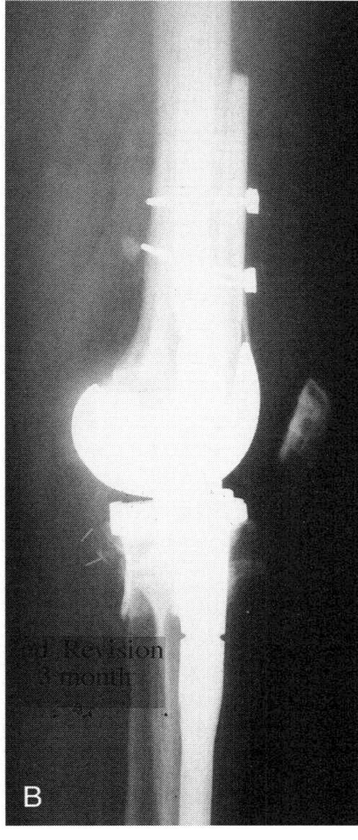

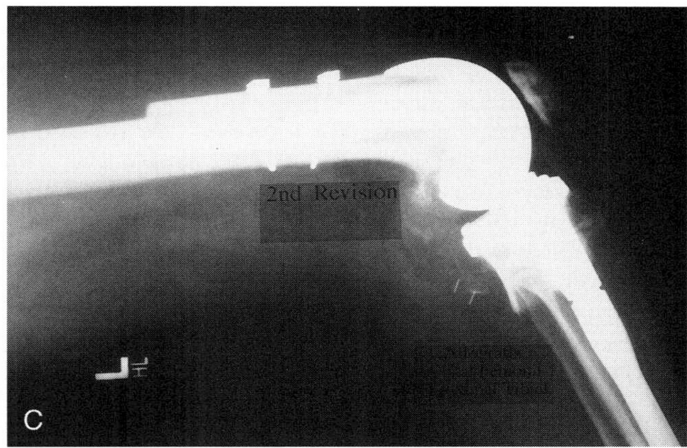

FIGURE 93.42 ➢ Post-second revision radiographs. *A,* The desired valgus alignment has been restored. Offset stems in the tibia allow large-diameter stems that seat well in the medullary canal, with a tibial component that is also seated centrally on the tibia. *B,* Lateral radiograph. The offset stem in the femur has allowed the anterior cortex of the graft to sit on the patient's own bone while the stem reaches posteriorly into the host canal. *C,* The flexed knee viewed laterally. Patellar height is maintained.

The first step in this case, as in other revision arthroplasty cases in which intramedullary fixation is required, was to open the medullary canal and insert an instrument that indicated the axis of the intramedullary canal as well as the inner dimensions. Reaming to enlarge or change the shape of the canal was inappropriate given the thin cortical bone available. Usually, the tibia is asymmetric and the center of the isthmus will not correspond to the center of the proximal tibial surface. Offset stems may be required. In the case under discussion, a cadaver allograft proximal tibia had been selected to reestablish bone stock. One of the problems in revision surgery when bone graft is required but not used is that the residual sclerotic patient host bone is not amenable to the use of methacrylate cement. The advantage of structural allograft is to provide "transitional interfaces." Specifically, cement intrusion into the allograft is excellent, providing solid union with the prosthesis. The second interface between allograft and host bone is biologically active in a way that methacrylate against host cannot be. We expect, at best, that there will be union at the interface between the host and the allograft without revascularization and inevitable destruction of the allograft.

The technique of structural allograft reconstruction necessarily involves retention of as much structural integrity of the allograft as possible and provision of maximal interface contact between the graft and the host for stability and biological union. In most revision surgeries, a trial tibial component is implanted provisionally in step 1 of the procedure. Once the balance of the knee has been reconstructed, the surgeon then implants the final components. When allograft reconstruction is employed, however, it is sometimes preferable to complete step 1 by fully cementing in the actual component as a means of protecting and preserving the allograft bone. It should be noted that the tibial platform is selected as the first phase because the tibial articular surface is always in contact with the femur from extension to full flexion. As such, the tibial component position relative to the tip of the fibular head, for example, has virtually no significance for kinematics or alterations of the flexion and extension gaps, assuming that it has not been reconstructed too high. It is only the distal position of the femoral component and the posterior position of its articular condyles that can lead to constructive manipulation of the flexion and extension gaps. The principle remains, however, that the surgeon should not accept large amounts of missing proximal tibial bone.

Step 2: Stabilization of the Knee in Flexion. Irrespective of deformity or bone loss, the femoral component position must be correct rotationally, usually with respect to the position of the epicondyles. Most of the osseous landmarks for accurate rotational positioning of the femoral component are compromised in revision surgery. The surgeon who practices identifying the location of the epicondyles during primary surgery will have an advantage in the most difficult revision situation. The femoral component is ideally situated with a rotation parallel to the transepicondylar axis. The only other reliable indicator of rotational positioning during revision is the amount of residual posterior bone on the posterior condyles that can be palpated but not observed. For example, examination of the failed knee arthroplasty at the time of revision will reveal a greater amount of palpable bone on the posterior femoral condyle on the medial side than on the lateral side if the component has been internally rotated. Preoperative CT scans are useful in this assessment. The solution to the problem is to apply a posterolateral augment to the revision component, forcing the prosthetic femur into the correct, relatively externally rotated position.

However, when large amounts of bone have been lost from the distal femur, allograft distal femur reconstruction may be necessary. My indication for the use of structural allograft on the femur is sufficient loss of bone such that there can be no rotational stability provided to the posterior femoral condyles of the component by the bone. A decision had been made on this patient preoperatively to reconstruct the distal femur with structural allograft. Again, the important principle in allograft reconstruction is to maintain the integrity of the allograft by not decreasing its size and by maximizing the surface contact area between the host and the allograft to enhance junctional union between the two. The technique that I have employed is to preserve an anterior strip of allograft femoral cortex that lies against the host bone. Fixation will be provided by cerclage wires and an extended intramedullary stem. The sculpting of the allograft provides rotational stability. Cerclage wires allow the allograft to be compacted proximally against the host bone. Offset stems are of particular use in this situation because the allograft femur is necessarily translated a little anteriorly to preserve the position of the anterior femoral cortex of the host bone.

Step 2a: Establishing Femoral Component Rotation. Distal femoral allografts are rarely required, but when they are, there is no substitute. Planning and then executing the distal femoral allograft must be incorporated into step 2a because allograft reconstruction poses huge challenges to establishing the correct rotational position of the femoral component. First, the allograft itself must be applied to the host bone in a reasonably correct rotation, and then the femoral component must be implanted with the correct rotational position not simply to the allograft, but more importantly to the host bone and host extensor mechanism.

When structural allografts were first employed in the 1980s, there was usually recourse only to fresh-frozen femoral heads. These did not fill all the gaps in the distal femur and were often implanted by first drilling a large hole through the femoral head through which passed the intramedullary stem of the femoral component. The use of actual distal femurs was later performed by making bone cuts on the back table such that the allograft fit the component precisely. This creates the problem, however, of sculpting the graft (now attached to the prosthesis) so that it can sit on the host bone well and permit the intramedullary stem extension to sit properly in the femur. I have preferred to apply the allograft to the host first, focusing on accurate sculpting and fit between host and graft bone. Once this has been secured with cerclage wires, the allograft can then be prepared very much like a primary arthroplasty with the standard cutting jigs and instruments. The final cuts must not be performed, however, until the end of Step 2.

Step 2b: Selection of Femoral Component Size. One of the most common errors in revision total knee arthroplasty is to select a femoral component so that it fits the residual bone on the failed arthroplasty. It will usually be too small. The AP dimension of the femoral component size should be selected with strict observance of what is required to restore ligament stability in flexion.

The situation is clearer when structural allograft is not required. A femoral component is selected and attached to an intramedullary stem if bone defects are present; the knee is flexed to 90 degrees and distracted. The space between the posterior articular condyles and the residual proximal tibia indicate the dimensions of the gap that will have to be filled with tibial baseplates and articular polyethylene. Radiographs of the knee before the primary arthroplasty or radiographs of the contralateral knee may be useful guidelines to the appropriate femoral component size. In addition, the size of the femoral component that was removed is a helpful indicator. When revision of knees that were unstable in flexion is performed, a larger femoral component may be indicated. When revisions for the knee that flexes poorly are performed, a smaller femoral component may be helpful to decrease the tension in flexion and enhance motion.

The patient described here had a smaller, somewhat undersized, femoral component used for the first revision. Accordingly, a larger second-revision component was selected.

The gaps that usually result after selecting the appropriate size of femoral component are necessarily filled with posterior augments on the femoral component. In my case, because of the technique employed for structural femoral allografting, the femoral component was shifted anteriorly. A somewhat larger component was required to balance the flexion gap with this translation. The largest dimension that can be employed will be limited by the medial to lateral dimension of the component and the patient's bone.

Step 2c: Joint Line Height. It is clear that the flexion gap of a knee arthroplasty can be balanced with more than one size of femoral component. A small femoral component may be coupled with thicker articular polyethylene to provide stability in flexion. Ultimately, a larger femoral component may be coupled with thinner polyethylene to provide the same stability. The difference between these two circumstances is the level of the joint line. The small femoral component necessarily drives the joint line proximally. This happens immediately in flexion and, when I create the extension gap, the femoral component has to be positioned more proximally to accommodate the thicker polyethylene. This is generally undesirable.

There are several ways to determine the desired

joint line height. In the majority of cases, it is important to remember that balancing the flexion and extension gaps, restoring alignment and stability to the knee, and securing adequate fixation are far more important goals than reestablishing the joint line. In the multiply revised knee or the reimplantation after infection, there will usually be so much damage to soft tissues that the concept of the normal joint line will not be as beneficial to the soft tissue as one might anticipate. The position of the extensor mechanism is also of consequence. When the patellar tendon remains a normal length and has suffered from neither stretching and elongation nor contracture and shortening, the inferior pole of the patella is best kept slightly above the level of the joint line. Quantitative guidelines have been established whereby the transepicondylar distance may be used as a ratio to determine precisely where the joint line should lie relative to the tip of the fibular head. In step 2c, a femoral component that has been placed on the distal femur is coupled with articular polyethylene that stabilizes the knee in flexion and provides a workable joint line height.

Step 3: Seating the Femoral Component and Creating a Stable Extension Gap. The femoral component can be seated either more proximally or more distally to balance the knee in extension. In most revision cases, the stem of the component can be slid inside the femoral canal to adjust its position. Additional distal femur will be removed only in rare cases, usually when a flexion contracture must be corrected. A surgeon who decides that additional distal femur must be removed to achieve full extension should re-evaluate the choice of femoral component size, specifically its AP dimension. If a thick polyethylene insert was required for flexion and it is hard to accommodate this insert in extension, chances are that the femoral component is too small.

More commonly, distal augments will be necessary to bring the femoral component down to the normal joint line and compensate for lost bone. In more extreme cases, such as the one described here, augments will be inadequate and structural allograft is necessary to stabilize the knee. Allograft reconstruction of the distal femur complicates the determination of femoral component position distally. Instruments are not yet available that provide a quantitative assessment of this position with subsequently adequate bone cuts. Much of the work is done freehand. The surgeon must reestablish stability in extension, eliminate recurvatum, and ensure full extension, yet not compromise integrity of the allograft by resecting too much bone. In this case, the distal femur was seated with cerclage wires holding the allograft in place. The intramedullary stem provided enhanced fixation. Full extension without recurvatum was established.

ASSESSING STABILITY

Assessment of stability in revision knee arthroplasty is basically deciding whether or not mechanical constraint will be required in the reconstruction. Linked constrained devices (hinges) are rarely, if ever, required, and nonlinked constrained devices (constrained condylar types) are seldom required. There are two specific indications for constraint:

1. Instability in extension to varus or valgus forces resulting from compromise of the collateral ligaments.
2. A flexion gap that exceeds the dimensions of the extension gap profoundly as a result of failure of soft tissues. This mismatch of flexion and extension gaps, which may result in posterior tibial dislocation, can be remedied with a constrained component.

Inappropriate use of constrained prostheses includes failure to perform necessary collateral ligament releases to correct deformity that was left uncorrected at the time of the arthroplasty that failed. In addition, it is inappropriate to select constrained devices when the instability results from pseudolaxity originating in deficient bone. In many revisions, stability will be restored when the bone stock has been restored and the soft tissues brought out to length.

PROSTHETIC SELECTION

The choices for prosthesis in revision knee arthroplasty need not be many. The system should be modular, allowing the surgeon to address problems of deficient bone, instability, and compromised fixation. As such, intramedullary stems will be required when bone quality is compromised or when defects are present that will be reconstructed with augments or grafts. These stems may, in some cases, be fully cemented with a technique resembling that of hip arthroplasty. Any surgeon who cements such a stem should be prepared to remove it in the event of infection. Small-diameter smooth stems are appropriate for this application. Longer, more slender stems that achieve a three-point fixation without cement may be employed, as may shorter, modular, larger-diameter stems that achieve a press fit. Stems with an offset design will enable a press fit without compromising alignment in the majority of cases. Fully porous coated stems for uncemented application are generally not used.

Fortunately, some revision arthroplasties will be straightforward and require neither modular augments nor stem extensions. If a revision presents the surgeon with bone stock very similar to what had been present at the time of the primary arthroplasty, then primary knee arthroplasty components may be considered for the revision.

The articular geometry of the implants should be, at a minimum, conforming, if not posterior stabilized. This implies that stability to varus-valgus stresses will be provided by collateral ligaments. The implant may contribute to posterior stability of the tibia but only as a function of intact ligaments. Elimination of recurvatum with fully constrained implants that feature an extension stop carries a very high risk of loosening.

Cementing or Not?

Revision knee arthroplasty has been practiced widely, with the use of methacrylate bone cement for fixation. The cement is applied to the cut bone surfaces and restricted from entry into the medullary canal. Uncemented fixation in revision knee arthroplasty has been performed in a limited number of centers. The knowledge and follow-up data of this technique are available but not extensive.

CLOSURE

Wound-closure techniques need not differ from what has been employed in primary knee arthroplasty. My preference has been absorbable suture material in the arthrotomy, subcutaneous, and subcuticular layers. The recommendation to perform a patellectomy because tissues are too tight to close should be regarded with extreme caution. This implies that the revision has been overstuffed, that there is such extensive scarring that a flap should have been required originally, or that simple steps such as a lateral patellar retinacular release have not been performed to facilitate closure. This situation is most likely to arise during the reimplantation after two-stage treatment for infection. It compromises the patient's functional capacity and, in the worst cases, may jeopardize the functional integrity of the extensor mechanism.

A sterile dressing is applied under a fishnet type of tubular gauze that eliminates adhesive tape contact with the skin and facilitates dressing changes. This also easily accommodates the swelling that occurs with revision surgery.

POSTOPERATIVE REHABILITATION

With rare exception, postoperative rehabilitation should proceed identical to the protocol of the primary knee arthroplasty. Exceptions may include reconstruction of the extensor mechanism, especially in the form of allograft implantation, that may require protection from full flexion in the early phase. This is one of the rare indications for a brace that would include dial-lock hinges and drop locks. Ligament advancements and reconstructions, which I have added to the techniques for revision knee arthroplasty surgery in my own practice, should be sufficiently well fixed to bone that bracing is not required. Cast immobilization is quite simply never indicated unless there is a plan to deal with the inevitable stiffness that will ensue.

TABLE 93.6 MANAGING BONE DEFECTS

1. Contained defect	Particulate bone graft or cement
2. Noncontained defect	Prosthetic modular augments
3. Massive bone loss	Structural allograft

TABLE 93.7 REVISION KNEE ARTHROPLASTY

Step 1: Tibial platform reconstruction	1. Establish a foundation for the knee.
Step 2: Stabilization of the knee in flexion	2. Establish flexion gap.
Step 2a: Femoral component rotation	
Step 2b: Selection of femoral component size	
Step 2c: Combination of femoral component and tibial polyethylene to establish joint line	
Step 3: Seating of femoral component to stabilize in extension	3. Create extension gap equal to flexion gap.

SUMMARY

The keys to successful revision knee arthroplasty, no matter how difficult the case, are included in the three tables presented here. Table 93.5, describing the nine causes of failure, focuses on the importance of a preoperative diagnosis and a specific mechanical plan that addresses the reason that the prior arthroplasty failed to begin with. Table 93.6 demonstrates an organized approach to managing bone defects. To simply ignore them or to try to compensate with the use of an inappropriate degree of constraint will necessarily lead to problems as is observed in the failed knee arthroplasty presented in this chapter. Table 93.7 describes an organized approach to the execution of the knee arthroplasty. Following these steps enables the surgeon to address each of the significant issues in revision knee arthroplasty: stability, bone defect reconstruction, fixation, and motion. These three steps can be used to plan the surgical technique. By following each one sequentially in a plan, the surgeon can better anticipate required materials and equipment.

Revision knee arthroplasty differs significantly from primary reconstruction of the arthritic joint. Success will come from this realization, with accurate planning and greater experience in the actual reconstructions themselves.

References

1. Kharazzi D, Spitzer A, Vince K: Femoral component malrotation as a cause of pain and stiffness in total knee arthroplasty. Presented at the Meeting of the Societé Internationale de Chirurgie Orthopedique et Traumatologique, Sydney, Australia, Jan. 1999.
2. Vince K, et al: Revision TKR with a Three Step Technique. Presented at the Meeting of the Combined Societies of the English Speaking World, Auckland, NZ, 1998.

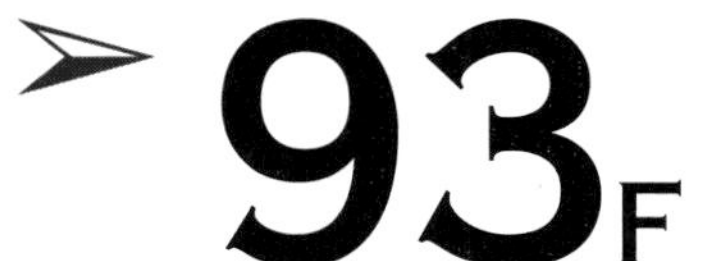

Revision Knee Arthroplasty: How I Do It

STEVEN F. HARWIN

I find it best to approach all surgery in general, and revision surgery in particular, in a systematic fashion so that a thorough and accurate work-up and diagnosis can be achieved. If we follow the same procedures each time, we are less likely to overlook important factors.

In order to perform successful revision surgery, we must first establish the cause of failure. Work-up will include a thorough history and physical examination, review of serial radiographs, aspiration of the knee, technetium and indium scans, complete blood count, sedimentation rate, and C-reactive protein. A computed tomography scan is done if rotational malalignment is suspected. Once infection has been ruled out and the reason for failure of the index procedure has been established, preparation for revision is addressed. The soft tissues are examined to ensure adequate coverage and quality of skin. Previous incisions are located, and a decision is made as to the approach to be used. Tissue expanders can be considered if skin is thin or deficient, or if difficulty with closure is anticipated.

Based on the radiographs and the physical examination, prosthetic options must be considered and chosen. At surgery, the knee should be exposed widely, with no tension on the skin and the patellar tendon. The failed implant should be removed, preserving as much bone as possible. Trial implants are positioned and stability and kinematics are checked. The final implant, with the proper level of constraint and appropriate augments, is chosen. The patella is then considered for replacement or patellaplasty. Postoperatively, proper wound healing must be ensured.

To illustrate this approach, I present the following typical case of revision for aseptic loosening and instability.

CASE PROFILE

The patient was a 66-year-old female who had had a history of osteoarthritis for more than 12 years. She had undergone bilateral total knee arthroplasties (TKAs) at another institution in 1995. She presented to me complaining of pain, instability, and loss of motion of both knees. She did have initial relief but after 2 years began to have pain, with a feeling of giving way and instability, with gradual loss of motion. The right knee was more symptomatic than the left; only the right knee is addressed here.

She denied any fever, chills, or any local inflammation of the wound, but she did report occasional swelling. Initial wound healing was normal. She described giving way especially when changing direction or going up and down stairs, with global pain about the knee.

Her presenting physical examination revealed a healthy-appearing female who walked with an antalgic gait. The knee appeared aligned in varus with moderate swelling anteriorly. There was a varus thrust when she walked. The wound was benign in appearance. The limb appeared normal regarding circulation, with no stasis changes. Results of examination of the spine, hip, ankle, and foot were within normal limits. No neurological deficit was noted.

The active range of motion (ROM) of the knee was from −30 degrees to 85 degrees. There was a moderate effusion, with some synovial thickening. Passive ROM was −25 degrees to 90 degrees with hard endpoints. In as much extension as possible, there was moderate valgus instability with laxity of about 15 to 20 mm. In 30 degrees to 40 degrees of flexion, there was more laxity, with 20 to 30 mm of opening. With passive flexion to 90 degrees, there was at least 10 mm of anterior laxity and 20 mm of posterior laxity. The tibial tray was easily displaced beyond the distal femoral condyles and the tibial tubercle had lost its normal prominence, consistent with subluxation. The patella was clinically located, but some decreased mobility was noted. Quadriceps tone and strength were normal.

The neurovascular status of the limb was intact. The skin was of normal turgor and temperature, with normal sensation, proprioception, and vibratory sense. The patient had difficulty arising from a chair, had to use the handrails, and had to go up and down stairs one at a time, using the railing for support.

Radiographs were taken in multiple projections, including anteroposterior, lateral, and Merchant's patella view. They revealed varus alignment of a condylar-type TKA that appeared to be a posterior cruciate ligament-retaining design (Fig. 93.43). Stress views confirmed incompetence of the medial collateral ligament (MCL) and the posterior collateral ligament (PCL). A standing leg-alignment radiograph with the hips,

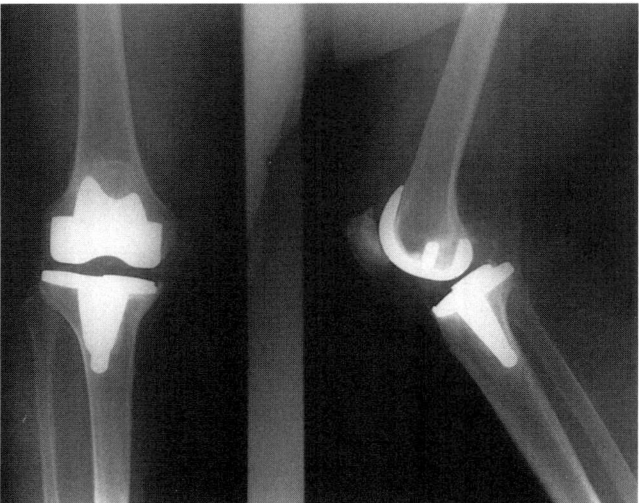

FIGURE 93.43 ➢ Condylar-type TKA with varus alignment and incompetence of MCL and PCL. Note upslope of tibial cut and thick patella.

knees, and ankles on the same plate was taken to assess the mechanical axis, which measured varus of 7 degrees. Some radiolucencies were seen beneath the tibial tray medially, and only a small amount of cement was apparent around the tray and stem. The tibial component was in varus and slightly posteriorly displaced in relation to the femur. The cut surface had a slight up-slope on sagittal view. The cemented patella was thick and asymmetrically resurfaced. The femoral component was in valgus with minimal visible cement. No radiographic evidence of loosening was noted, and there was no osteolysis. There was no cement beneath the anterior flange. The stress views revealed pathological laxity of the MCL and PCL.

Aspiration of the knee under sterile conditions revealed 20 mL of clear yellow fluid. Gram's stain revealed no organisms and few polymorpholeukocytes. Culture subsequently was negative. Blood studies revealed a normal CBC and C-reactive protein. The patient's sedimentation rate was 5. She was sent for a technetium bone scan which revealed some increased activity on the tibial side. An indium scan revealed no mismatch.

Review of the index operation report confirmed that a PCL-retaining device had seen implanted. No specific mention was made about patella thickness and ligament balancing of the MCL or PCL. Immediate postoperative radiographs of her index arthroplasty were reviewed and, when compared with the current films, confirmed some varus shift of the tibial component. Based on the history, physical examination and work-up, a diagnosis of failure of the TKA was made, given the instability of the MCL and PCL, with possible tibial loosening and stuffing of the patellofemoral joint. Infection would still have to be ruled out at surgery. In preparation for surgery, a complete medical evaluation was performed; the patient was found fit for surgery. One unit of blood was donated before the surgery.

The patient's wound was carefully examined for any healing defects or potential problems in coverage or healing, and no contraindications or significant concerns were found.

Implants necessary in preparation for revision were reviewed. The revision implant system chosen was the Kinemax Plus Modular TKA system, which includes a PCL-retaining primary implant, a posteriorly stabilized prosthesis, a modular revision stabilizer prosthesis to allow for distal or posterior augments to the femur as well as for stem extensions, a constrained prosthesis that will substitute for the MCL and lateral ligaments (Superstabilizer), and a rotating hinge prosthesis for salvage surgery. In this case, it will be likely that a constrained prosthesis will be necessary because of the instability. Given the adequate bone stock and only moderate instability, it is unlikely that a hinge prosthesis will be needed. Regardless of implant system chosen, a full system including augments and bone graft material is required in order to be prepared for all eventualities.

SURGICAL PROCEDURE

The patient arrived at the hospital on the day of surgery 2 hours before start time, having had nothing by mouth since midnight. She was interviewed by the anesthesiologist. There was also a discussion of the type of anesthesia. My preference is for epidural anesthesia so that the catheter may be left in postoperatively to allow for early maximal ROM with reduced pain. The patient agreed. Antibiotics were deferred until intraoperative cultures were taken. A frozen section with CBC was taken to rule out acute inflammation and likely infection.

The procedure is performed, in a vertical laminar flow operating room, under tourniquet control with a pressure of 350 mm Hg. The entire lower limb is prepared and draped free. An Esmarch bandage is used to exsanguinate after about 5 minutes of elevation. To achieve maximum length of the quadriceps mechanism, the knee is fully flexed before inflation.

The prior incision is used and extended proximally and distally, 12 cm above the superior pole of the patella and 4 cm below the tibial tubercle. There is much scarring in the soft tissues from the prior surgery. Care is taken to make the flaps as thick as possible. A medial parapatellar entry is made, leaving a cuff of tissue on the medial aspect of the patella for closure. The quadriceps incision is in the medial third of the tendon, allowing for options for improving exposure, such as a V-Y turndown or a quadriceps snip. (If necessary, a lateral retinacular release is performed early in the procedure, from outside in to allow for eversion of the patella. In this case, it was not necessary.)

The joint is opened, and clear yellow fluid is encountered. Cultures and frozen sections from multiple areas are taken. The joint does not appear to be infected. The soft tissues medially and laterally below the retinaculum are debulked. The patellofemoral ligament is released to aid in patellar mobilization. The Gram stain returns negative for organisms, and only 2 to 3 white blood cells per high-powered field are noted on frozen section. Based on these factors and the preoperative work-up, it is unlikely that infection is present. I then proceed with a one-stage revision. Antibiotics are now given (cefazolin, 2 g intravenously), to be continued (1 g intravenously every 6 hours) until the final culture returns. (If there were any question regarding the presence of infection—for example, if the fluid was cloudy, or if there were more than five to ten white blood cells per high-powered field on frozen section, then a two-stage procedure would be performed. An antibiotic impregnated cement spacer would be inserted, and reimplantation would be planned for a later date.)

Because of difficulty in mobilizing and everting the patella in this case, a quadriceps snip is used to improve exposure and to protect the insertion of the patella tendon. The medial quadriceps incision is extended proximally and laterally at 45 degrees into the vastus lateralis for a distance of about 4 cm. This allows a wide exposure and the patella to be everted with no tension on the patellar tendon. (If the insertion were at risk, a wire would be driven through the insertion to protect it. If this is not adequate for protection or the exposure is not satisfactory, then a tibial tubercle osteotomy would be performed. In my experience, this has rarely been necessary if a quadriceps snip is used.)

Before any extensive soft-tissue releases are performed, the knee is examined, and the instability due to incompetence of the MCL and PCL is confirmed. The medial side of the knee is released subperiosteally as is the posterior tibia to the midline to allow for complete external rotation of the tibia. In most cases, this will include the superficial and deep MCL as well as the insertion of the pes anserinus. The insertion of the semimembranosus is released to free the posteromedial corner. It is the external rotation maneuver, when combined with flexion of the knee and eversion of the patella, that will allow for adequate exposure. This should enable the tibia to be brought forward of the femur completely (Fig. 93.44). During the flexion-

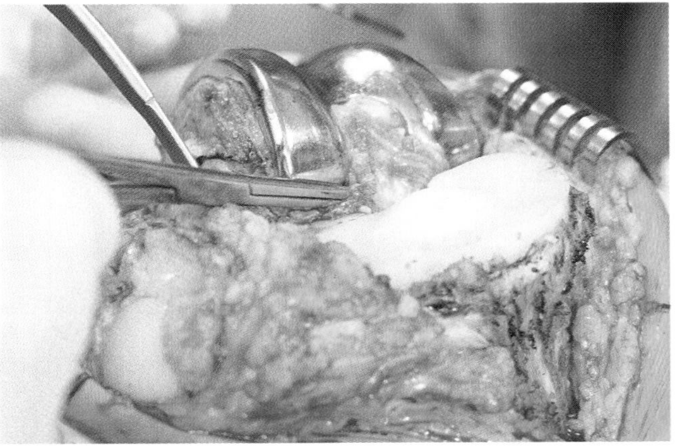

FIGURE 93.44 ➢ Wide exposure with tibia brought forward of the femur.

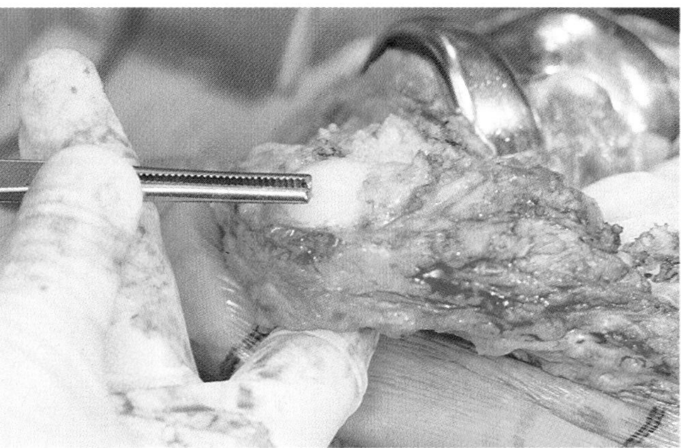

FIGURE 93.45 ➢ Small patellar dome with bone overgrowth laterally.

rotation maneuver, the insertion of the patellar tendon is observed for any evidence of tension or possible avulsion.

In this case, the MCL was lax, and it took up tension poorly. The PCL was incompetent as well with no well-defined structure present in the intercondylar notch. A PCL-retaining, relatively "flat-on-flat" implant was in place. At this point, the implant itself is examined. All components are checked for position, alignment, rotation, and loosening. The poly is worn posteriorly with some delamination and pitting present. The poly is now removed from the tibial tray to further expose the knee. The femoral component is found to have some scratches on the medial side. In this case, the femoral component was satisfactorily positioned and sized, and no malrotation was found. It was not grossly loose. The tibial component was in varus and grossly loose. Pressure on the baseplate produced movement and fluid from beneath the tray. The patellar thickness measured 30 mm, with poor coverage of only about 50% of the bony surface covered by the implant. The small dome rested almost entirely on the lateral facet, with bony overgrowth (Fig. 93.45). The preliminary diagnosis and cause of failure is confirmed: aseptic loosening and instability and stuffing of the patellofemoral joint.

The implant is now removed. The interface between the femoral prosthesis and the cement is located and developed to free the bond. Small rigid and flexible osteotomes are used as well as a short oscillating saw. Rarely, a Gigli saw may be used to disrupt a stubborn interface. Once the component is loosened, a slap-hammer extractor device is applied to remove it with several short, sharp blows. This prevents levering of the implant and potential fracture and bone loss. If the implant does not come off easily, check the interfaces to ensure that adequate preparation has been performed, especially about the femoral pegs if present. In this case, the implant comes off rather easily, although there is some unavoidable bone loss from the medial and lateral peg holes (Fig. 93.46). Some scant cement is found around the implant.

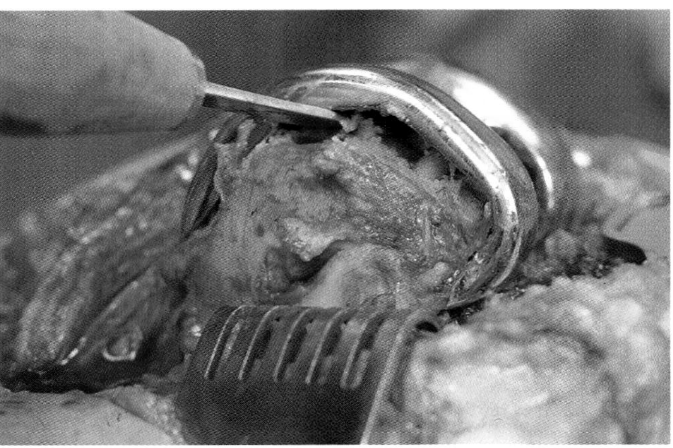

FIGURE 93.46 ➢ Femoral component removed with minimal bone loss. Osteotome develops prosthesis-cement interval.

Residual cement and fibrous tissue are removed from the femur, and cysts are curetted. Bone loss is assessed. Commonly, there is posterior and distal condylar loss, but in this case minimal loss was encountered. The joint line landmarks, including both epicondyles, are located and marked for reference.

The tibial component is now addressed. The same basic technique is used to remove the tibial tray. In this case, the tray exhibits gross motion. Osteotomes and an oscillating saw are used to further disrupt the tray-cement interface and to dislodge the central peg. A slap-hammer extractor is also helpful here. The tray is removed easily and residual cement and fibrous tissue are removed.

Now the bony defects left by implant removal are evaluated. The need for wedges and additional augments is determined. Combined incompetence of the PCL and MCL requires a constrained prosthesis; the Kinemax Plus Superstabilizer is used (Fig. 93.47). The femoral implant already has a 5-mm distal and posterior build-up, having been specifically designed for revision in which there is always some relative bone loss due to the bone resected for the prior implant. This feature accounts for less frequent use of add-on augments. Further augments of 5 and 10 mm distally and posteriorly are available if needed. Because they are cemented on the implant, either augment may be used individually. In this case, because of only minor bone loss, it appears that only a stem will be needed on the femoral side.

However, the tibia will most likely need a wedge on the medial side, rather than requiring more bone to be resected on the lateral side. In many situations, further resection of the lateral bone can be done, but in this case it would result in a level below the fibula head. Two factors influence the decision not to resect further: the quality of the bone is not as good, and the size of the residual bone is much smaller, possibly creating a bone-prosthesis mismatch. With conforming, constrained implants like the Superstabilizer, the tibial articular surface must match the femoral size, although the poly insert may be applied to any size baseplate. Either a half- or full-slope block wedge will be chosen. The large central defect from the tibial stem will be filled with the new stem and its extension and either bone graft or cement. Once the bone ends are cleaned and débrided, revision instrumentation is used to position the new implant and to establish the proper orientation and joint line position. Intramedullary rods and stabilizing pins are used to stabilize the jigs. In this case, for use of the Superstabilizer, the distal femur is cut at 7 degrees valgus and 0 degrees flexion; the tibia is cut at 90 degrees to the long axis of the tibia in both the coronal and sagittal plane. These cuts match the stem and central peg orientation on the implant. Little bone is removed with these cuts. The ends are merely "freshened" and made flat. Because stem extensions will be always used with a constrained implant, instrumentation for the Superstabilizer uses the medullary canal as a reference point for the cutting and positioning guides.

Intramedullary stems are used on the cutting jigs and the trial components to create stability and to allow proper mediolateral and anteroposterior positioning (Fig. 93.48). This eliminates any mismatch between the prosthesis position and that of the stem when the cuts are completed (the "slave-to-the-stem" phenomenon). Trial distal and posterior femoral augments and proximal tibial wedges and blocks are applied to the implant trials if necessary.

The femoral canal is opened; and reaming with blunt-end reamers begins. Reaming is started with power but may be completed by hand to obtain a "soft press-fit". If the reamer do not "toggle" in the canal, then the fit is correct, and the size and length are recorded (as this will be the size of the stem extension used). The distal femoral cutting jig is inserted and stabilized with medial and lateral pins, and the femur is cut at 7 degrees valgus. Subsequent cutting jigs are applied to the intramedullary stem, positioned, and stabilized, and finishing cuts, including anterior, posterior, and chamfer cuts, if necessary, are

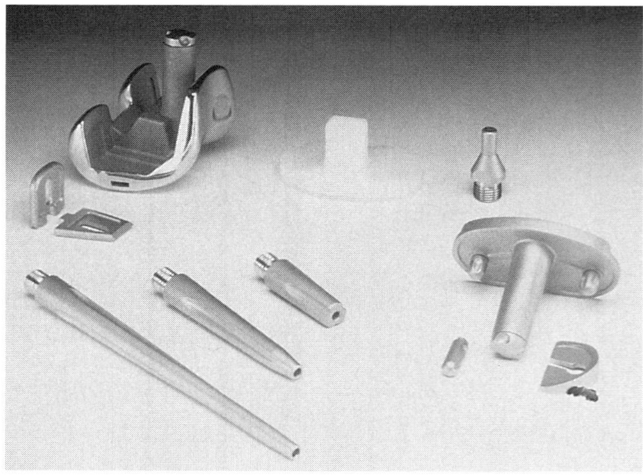

FIGURE 93.47 ➢ Modular revision prosthesis with metal tibial reinforcement post (Superstabilizer, Stryker-Howmedica Osteonics).

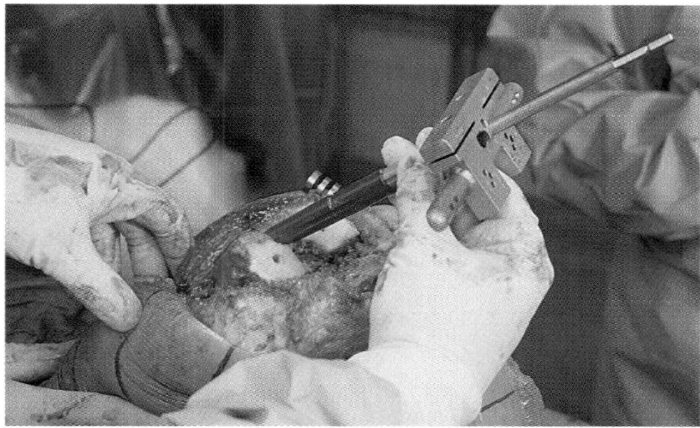

FIGURE 93.48 ➢ Intramedullary stem attached to cutting guide ensures proper positioning.

made. All jigs are referenced to the proper joint line and the epicondylar axis. Internal rotation must be avoided in all components. The femoral trial construct is then applied, and the relationship to the joint line and the epicondylar axis is confirmed. The need for bone graft or additional augments will be now readily apparent. In this case, because the chosen implant already has distal and posterior build-ups, no "add-on" augments will be needed. The proper joint line is restored, approximately 2 to 2.5 cm distal to the epicondyles. If these landmarks are absent or obscure, another useful guide will be to place the implant at a similar distance from the fibular head as that of the other knee and its axis parallel to the cut surface of the tibia. This will assure a relatively symmetrical and rectangular flexion and extension gap. In addition, if the tibia is cut at 90 degree to the long axis, this reference will provide relative external rotation to the femoral component and more favorable patellofemoral tracking.

The tibia is then addressed. I prefer a combination of intramedullary and extramedullary tibial cutting guides. Once the tibia is reamed to a soft press-fit, the combination intramedullary/extramedullary tibial cutting guide with its press-fit stem is applied. It is apparent that cutting the tibia at 90 degrees to the long axis by resecting bone laterally will end in a resection lower than the fibula head. While theoretically possible, this option is less than optimal for reasons discussed above. The standard jig is slipped off the fixation pins, and the full-slope wedge-cutting guide is applied (Fig. 93.49). After the tibia is cut, the proper size IM rod is left in place, and the appropriate size tibial baseplate template with the wedge trial is applied. The position is checked, ensuring the proper coronal, sagittal, and rotational alignment. Medial and lateral peg holes are drilled, and the trial construct, with the baseplate, full-slope wedge, and stem extension, is applied. The center of the baseplate should be directly behind, or slightly medial to, the tibial tubercle. If significant overhang of the baseplate is found, then an offset stem is used. Overhang on the medial side should be avoided if possible so as not to irritate the MCL or remaining soft tissues. This wedge has a tapered design, similar to that of the tibial metaphysis, to provide a low profile to the bone and collateral ligaments. In this case, an offset stem will not be needed. The trial reinforcement post is applied, then, trial reductions with various thicknesses of trial poly inserts assess the stability and kinematics.

Stability with any posteriorly stabilized implant is created with a stable flexion gap. Progressively thicker spacers are used until flexion stability is achieved. Once that is done, the extension gap is examined. If full extension cannot be achieved, then thought can be given to recutting the femur to allow for full extension. This must be in the context of possibly elevating the joint line, contributing to a patella baja and altered kinematics. Prior to doing that, a posterior release should be carried out. If full extension still cannot be achieved, one can consider accepting 5 to 10 degrees of fixed flexion, but this is less than optimal. The use of trial implants, spacer blocks, or a spacer-tensor device is helpful in this determination, as well as for fine-tuning the varus-valgus balancing.

The posterior recesses of the femur must also be recreated along with the posterior capsular space in order to allow for proper and adequate flexion. There must be no "booking" of the knee when it goes into flexion. This abnormal phenomenon is avoided by carefully using a curved osteotome to release the structures posteriorly and proximally on the femur and by electrocautery release at the joint line behind the tibia. Care must be taken to avoid the midline neurovascular structures during this step.

The final configuration of the implant and the level of constraint necessary must be determined. In this case, because of the incompetent MCL and PCL, a constrained Superstabilizer implant will be used with a full-slope medial wedge and femoral and tibial stem extensions. As a general principle, the surgeon should use the least constraint possible, yet stability must be ensured in all planes. The use of stem extensions with constrained implants of this type is recommended in all cases.

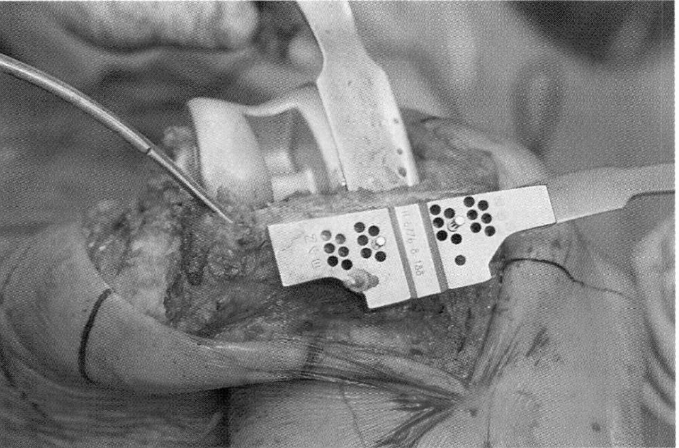

FIGURE 93.49 ➢ Full-slope tibial wedge-cutting guide in place. Minimal bone is removed.

Once this is done, the patella is addressed. The prosthetic-bone construct is measured with a caliper. In this case, it measures 30 mm, suggesting that the construct may have been overly thickened. A circumferential synovectomy is carried out to expose the insertion of the quadriceps and patella tendons. Bony overgrowth and osteophytes are trimmed.

The poly button is removed by using an oscillating saw and osteotomes, taking care not to lever the patella, which can create a fracture. It can be helpful to use "stacked" osteotomes to wedge the implant off. The residual cement and fibrous tissue are removed, and any cystic areas are débrided. The residual bony remnant is measured. In this case, it measures 20 mm. The resection guide is applied and another 6 mm is removed, leaving bone stock of 14 mm. Little bone is taken off the lateral side, and more is taken off the medial side to create a symmetrical patella. The Kinemax patellar component is a modified dome, with a 3-mm medial offset, to enhance tracking. It varies in superior-inferior and medial-lateral size and in thickness from 9 to 11 mm (small to large). In this case, I use a medium, which measures 10 mm in thickness. The remaining bone measures 14 mm, as planned, resulting in a new construct of 24 mm. The template is applied to the medial edge of the patella after osteotomy. Three peg holes are drilled, and the trial implant is applied. The medial-to-lateral orientation of the oval implant should be parallel to the new joint line.

If the residual bone stock were less than 10 to 12 mm, than a salvage resection arthroplasty would be considered. In that situation, the patella is trimmed and miniaturized, osteophytes are débrided, and then the patella is centralized in the femoral groove. Although I try to resurface the patella every time, I believe that a nonresurfaced patella is better than a poorly done or ill-advised resurfaced one. In some cases, especially in elderly or infirm patients, the previously placed patella can be left in situ if stable and relatively compatible with the revision implant. This option is even more attractive when removal of the implant might jeopardize the integrity of the extensor mechanism or possibly create a fracture of the patella.

The trial patella is applied, and tracking is assessed. The knee is reduced, the tibia is returned to its normal position, and patellar tracking is observed throughout the entire ROM. Although the "no thumb" technique must be used, it is acceptable to take the slack out of the quadriceps by applying proximal tension with a tenaculum. No medial vector is applied. If there is any question as to subluxation, tilt, or lift-off; then a lateral retinacular release should be performed or, if already done, extended. This assumes that the components have again been checked for position, alignment, and rotation. The patella is also examined for contact with the tibial poly as may occur with a patella baja. This phenomenon is not uncommon in revision surgery and may have to be accepted if not severe. Options to improve this include moving the component more proximally, osteotomizing the tibial tubercle, and trimming the tibial poly, but these measures are rarely needed. If the joint line has been elevated, this phenomenon is more frequent.

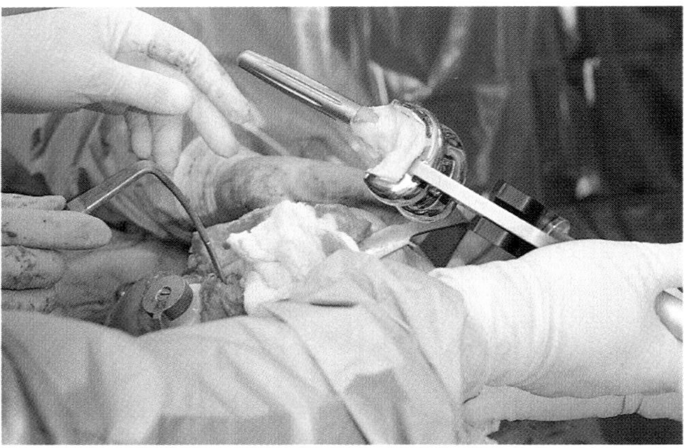

FIGURE 93.50 ➢ Femoral component prepared for insertion with cement. Stem is press-fit. Note build-up of distal and posterior femur inherent in Superstabilizer. Patella component has been cemented simultaneously.

Once these steps are completed, the final implant is cemented in place. For revision surgery, 1.2 g of tobramycin are added to each bag of cement used. The bone ends are prepared, using a pulsating lavage, dry sponges, hydrogen peroxide, and then dry sponges again, to produce a clean, dry, and bloodless surface for cementing. When using the Superstabilizer, the femoral component with its augments, if needed, is prepared first. Stem extensions are screwed into the central housing and tightened with a torque wrench to 80 inch-pounds to ensure proper security.

The choice whether to cement the stem is always left to the surgeon. I prefer a soft press-fit, which will be done in this case. (If it is decided to cement the stem, then typical preparation of the canal should be carried out as above, with a canal cement restrictor.) In the press-fit technique, cement is applied to the back of the implants and to the bone ends only. The femoral component is cemented simultaneously with the patella (Fig. 93.50).

The tibial component is now prepared with the full slope wedge and its stem extension. The surgeon can choose either to cement the wedge to the baseplate or to attach it with a screw-peg combination as was done in this case. Five-millimeter medial and lateral tibial pegs are standard on the implant. If longer pegs are needed, they may be changed for 20-mm pegs and may be removed completely if necessary, for example, to avoid hardware. The tibial component is cemented in place in a fashion similar to that for the femur. The knee is extended with the trial post and trial poly insert for pressurization (Fig. 93.51). After the cement has hardened, the patella tracking is again checked; if maltracking occurs, a lateral retinacular release, if not already done, may be performed. In rare cases, a medial muscle imbrication with proximal realignment and/or a tibial tubercle transfer may be necessary. Excess cement is trimmed away, and the back of the knee is examined for residual cement and overhanging

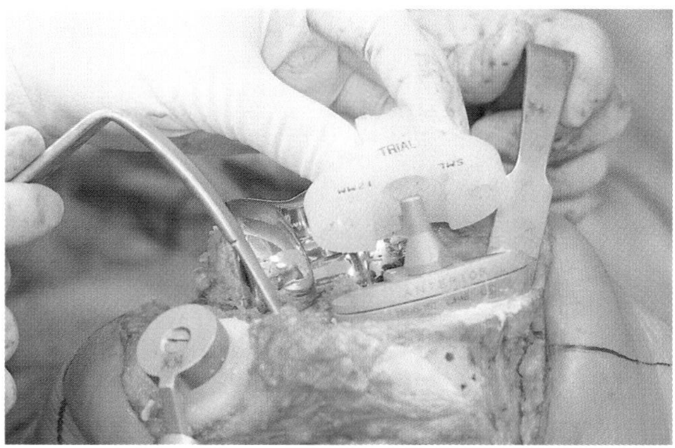
FIGURE 93.51 ➢ Tibial component with full slope wedge (and press fit stem) is cemented in place. Trial poly is placed over trial metal reinforcement post.

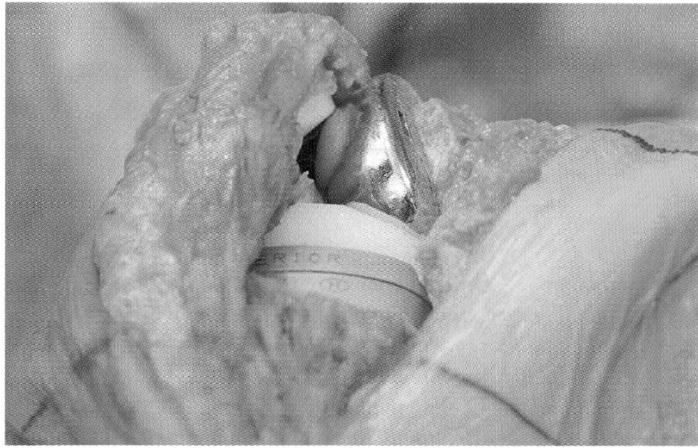
FIGURE 93.52 ➢ Patella relocated, demonstrating excellent tracking.

bone. After again checking stability, the final poly insert is chosen, but insertion is deferred until hemostasis is achieved in order to allow access to the back of the joint.

While in routine primary surgery, I deflate the tourniquet after the procedure is completed and the dressing is on. In revision or complex primary surgery, I deflate the tourniquet before closure to allow for hemostasis. This is especially important because the posterior recesses have been recreated and the posterior capsule and lateral retinaculum is often released. After hemostasis is achieved, the tibial reinforcement post is applied with a torque wrench, the real poly insert is applied, and the knee is again placed through an ROM to ensure stability, adequate kinematics, and patellar tracking (Fig. 93.52). The wound is now closed over a deep and superficial blood recovery drain. The quadriceps snip and tendon are routinely closed muscle to muscle and tendon to tendon using #1 Maxon suture or its equivalent. The repair is tested at maximal flexion to ensure ability to withstand early ROM. The subcutaneous tissue is closed in a double layer, with a 2-0 and 3-0 Vicryl or their equivalent. The skin is closed with staples; if any tension were to be encountered, individual AO mattress sutures with 3-0 nylon would be used.

POSTOPERATIVE

The postoperative regime is often overlooked as an important part of revision TKA surgery. I use a relatively light dressing, loosely applied, covered by a surgical support stocking, so that the knee will flex easily in the continuous passive motion machine and there is no undue pressure on the wound. I routinely flex to patient tolerance if an epidural catheter remains in place. If general anesthesia was used, then ROM begins at 0 to 60 degrees, increasing 10 degrees each day. Anteroposterior and lateral radiographs are taken in the recovery room to confirm proper position (Fig. 93.53).

Warfarin therapy for deep vein thrombosis prophylaxis is started the night of surgery, as long as there is no medical contraindication. The INR is kept at about 1.5, and therapy continues for 6 weeks. Antiembolism stockings are worn during that period. Continuous passive motion is not continued at home except under special circumstances. If the patient had formed heterotopic bone after the index operation, consideration is

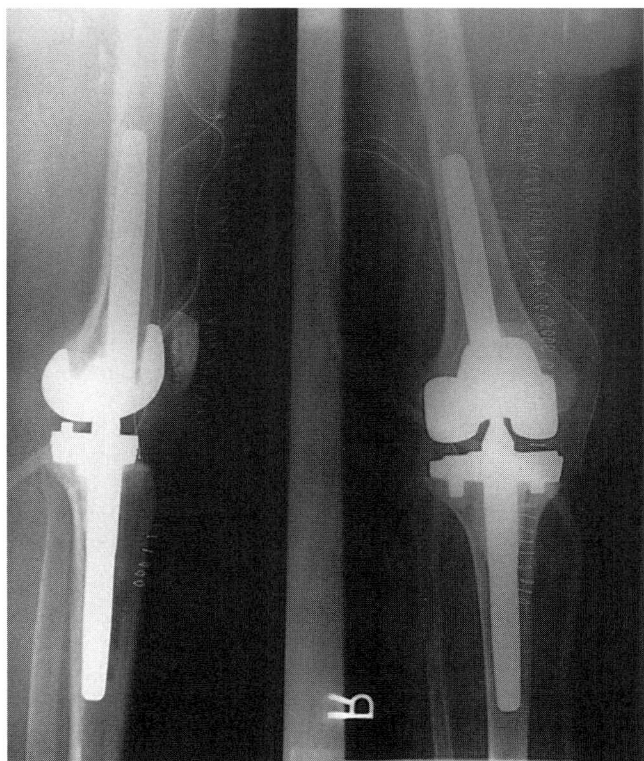
FIGURE 93.53 ➢ Postoperative radiograph showing excellent alignment with restoration of joint landmarks. Stem size is indicative of soft press-fit.

given to preoperative or postoperative radiotherapy in a single dose.

The dressing is changed the next day to reduce the bulk and to inspect the wound. The drains are usually removed at 24 hours but may be left longer if drainage is heavy. If the operative culture results are negative, the antibiotics are stopped.

Perhaps the most important principle in revision TKA (and arguably all joint replacement surgery) is that wound healing must be paramount. If wound drainage or necrosis occurs, I delay rehabilitation modalities, such as ambulation and ROM, until the wound demarcates and stabilizes. The wound must seal before I stress it with ROM and ambulation. No amount of elegant reconstructive surgery would be appreciated if a draining or infected wound is the end result.

In this case, the patient's wound was clean and dry with no significant drainage. The drain was removed at 24 hours, the culture results were negative, and the antibiotics were then stopped. If the operative culture returns positive, then an infectious disease specialist is consulted and the organism is studied as to whether it should be treated as a contaminant or a pathogen. If observed to be a pathogen, I would then most likely treat the patient with intravenous antibiotics via an implanted catheter for at least 6 to 8 weeks. This is done on an outpatient basis.

This patient was discharged on the 4th postoperative day, bearing full weight as tolerated with a walker, with an ROM from 0 to 90 degrees. Arrangements were made by social service specialists for a physiotherapist and a visiting nurse to see the patient three times a week at home. The rehabilitation protocol is not altered by the use of the quadriceps snip approach. Uncomplicated revisions are treated like a primary knee, they bear as much weight as possible and begin ROM exercises to tolerance.

The patient was seen in the office 2 weeks postoperative by a physician assistant who assessed the wound, removed the clips, and determined that the patient was making adequate progress regarding ROM. I saw the patient at 6 weeks. The wound was well healed, and the ROM was 0 to 100 degrees with no instability. Radiographs revealed satisfactory position of the implant with excellent patella tracking and no radiolucent lines. The patient complained only of incisional pain and walked with a simple cane for support. She will be seen at 3 months, 1 year, and yearly thereafter.

Using this type of systematic approach to revision surgery has resulted in satisfactory patient outcomes and few serious complications.

Selected Reading

1. Ahlberg A, Lunden A: Secondary operations after knee joint replacement. Clin Orthop 156:170, 1981.
2. Bertin KC, Freeman MAR, Samuelson KM, et al: Stemmed revision arthroplasty for aseptic loosening of total knee arthroplasty. J Bone Joint Surg 67:242, 1985.
3. Bryan RS, Rand JA: Revision total knee arthroplasty. Clin Orthop 170:116, 1982.
4. Cameron HU, Hunter GA: Failure in total knee arthroplasty: Mechanisms, revisions and results. Clin Orthop 170:141, 1982.
5. Chotivicht AL, Cracchiolo A, Chow GH, et al: Total knee arthroplasty using the Total Condylar III knee prosthesis. J Arthroplasty 16:341, 1991.
6. Donaldson WF, Sculco TP, Insall JN, et al: Total Condylar III knee prosthesis: Long-term follow-up study. Clin Orthop 226:21, 1988.
7. Goldberg VM, Figgie MP, Figgie HE, et al: The results of revision total knee arthroplasty. Clin Orthop 226:86, 1988.
8. Hanssen AD, Rand JA: A comparison of primary and revision total knee arthroplasty using the linematic stabilizer prosthesis. J Bone Joint Surg Am 70:491, 1988.
9. Harwin SF: Preoperative evaluation for TKA. In Scuderi GR, Tria AJ, eds: Surgical Techniques in Total Knee Arthroplasty. New York, Springer-Verlag. In press.
10. Insall JN, Dethmers DA: Revision of total knee arthroplasty. Clin Orthop 170:123, 1982.
11. Jacobs MA, Hungerford DS, Krachow KA, et al: Revision total knee arthroplasty for aseptic failure. Clin Orthop 226:78, 1988.
12. Lotke PA, Windsor R, Ecker ML, et al: Long-term results after total condylar knee replacement: Significance of radiolucent lines. Orthop Trans 8:398, 1984.
13. Peters CI, Hennessey R, Bardon RM, et al: Revision TKA with a cemented PS or constrained condylar prosthesis. J Arthroplasty 12:896, 1997.
14. Ranawat CS, Flynn WF, Deshmukh RG: Impact of modern technique on long-term results of total condylar knee arthroplasty. Clin Orthop 309:131, 1994.
15. Rand JA, Bryan RS: Results of revision total knee arthroplasties using condylar prostheses: A review of 50 knees. J Bone Joint Surg Am 70:738, 1988.
16. Ritter MS, Eizember LE, Fechtman RW, et al: Revision total knee arthroplasty: A survival analysis. J Arthroplasty 6:351, 1991.
17. Rosenberg AG, Yerner JJ, Galante JO: Clinical results of total knee revision using the Total Condylar III prosthesis. Clin Orthop 273:83, 1991.
18. Samuelson KM: Bone grafting and noncemented revision arthroplasty of the knee. Clin Orthop 226:93, 1988.
19. Scott RD: Revision total knee arthroplasty. Clin Orthop 226:65, 1988.
20. Stuart MJ, Larson JE, Morrey BE: Reoperation after condylar revision total knee arthroplasty. Clin Orthop 286:168, 1993.
21. Thornhill TS, Dalziel DW, Sledge CB: Alternatives to arthrodesis for the failed total knee arthroplasty: Clin Orthop 170:131, 1982.
22. Vince KG, Long W: Revision knee arthroplasty: The limits of press fit medullary fixation. Orthop Trans 8:76, 1994.
23. Whiteside LA: Cementless revision total knee arthoplasty. Clin Orthop 286:160, 1993.
24. Wilde AH, Schickendantz MS, Stulberg BN, et al: The incorporation of tibial allografts in total knee arthroplasty. J Bone Joint Surg Am 72:815, 1999.

SECTION XI

Tumors About the Knee

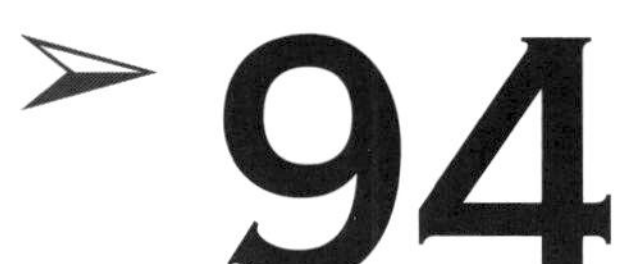

94 Bone Tumors and Tumor-Like Lesions of the Knee

VINCENT J. VIGORITA • BERNARD GHELMAN

Although bone tumors are relatively rare, the knee is the most common site.[37] In fact, one-third of bone tumors occur in the region of the knee, approximately half in the distal femur (Table 94.1). The proximal tibia is the next most common location for intraosseous bone tumors followed far less commonly by the proximal fibula. Less than 1% of reported bone tumors occur in the patella. Approximately half of the tumors that arise in the bony structures of the knee in general and distal femur in particular are malignant (Table 94.2). Bone tumors of the proximal tibia are more commonly benign (60% versus 40%). Most bone tumors arising in the proximal fibula and patella are benign.

Osteosarcoma is, by far, the most commonly reported primary knee tumor or tumor-like lesion, comprising 32% of all reported cases, followed by osteochondroma (19%), giant cell tumor (15%), nonossifying fibroma (7%), and fibrosarcoma (5%).* These tumors in the aggregate comprise more than 75% of all primary tumors and tumor-like conditions. At the distal femur, osteosarcoma accounts for approximately 36% of all tumors, followed by osteochondroma (20%), giant cell tumor (13%), nonossifying fibroma (7%), and fibrosarcoma. These tumors and tumor-like lesions account for more than 80% of all primary distal femur tumors. In the proximal tibia, the giant cell tumor follows the osteosarcoma (18% versus 28%); these tumors make up a smaller percentage than tumors at other knee bone sites.

In the proximal fibula, osteosarcoma accounts for 20% of all reported primary bone tumors, followed by osteochondroma (16%), nonossifying fibroma (14%), giant cell tumor (13%), and Ewing's sarcoma (7%); these five make up 75% of all primary proximal fibula tumors and tumor-like lesions. Fibrosarcoma is a less frequent diagnosis in this bone.

The large majority of tumors in the patella are benign; chondroblastoma is most frequently reported (32%), followed by giant cell tumor and osteoblastoma, each of which account for approximately 16% (Table 94.3). Kransdorf et al,[19] in 1989, reported on 42 proven primary patella tumors, 90% of which were benign: chondroblastoma accounted for 38%; giant cell tumor, 19%; and simple bone cyst, 14%.

DEVELOPMENTAL, HAMARTOMATOUS, AND TUMOR-LIKE LESIONS

Cystic Lesions of the Knee

The most common cystic-type replacement of bone tissue is that which ensues after remodeling of bone pursuant to degenerative joint disease. However, there are at least three well-defined primary cystic lesions of the skeleton that may involve bones around the knee.

Unicameral Bone Cyst

Unicameral or simple bone cyst is a benign replacement of cancellous bone by a serous fluid, the cause of which is unknown.[7] The lesion occurs most frequently in the proximal femur and proximal humerus. Initiating in the metaphysis, it may be progressively observed down the shaft as the proximal ends of the bone and distal ends of the bone grow away during endochondral ossification. Only 4% of unicameral bone

TABLE 94.1 TUMOR LOCATIONS AS PERCENTAGES OF TOTAL BONE TUMORS OF THE KNEE

Tumor Location	Percentage of All Bone Tumors	Percentage of Bone Tumors of the Knee
Knee	33.8	100
Distal femur	19.0	56.1
Proximal tibia	12.5	37.0
Proximal fibula	2.2	6.6
Patella	0.1	0.3

Modified from Vigorita VJ, Gatto C, Ghelman B: Tumors and tumor-like lesions of the knee. In Scott WN: The Knee, vol 2. Mosby-Year Book, St. Louis, 1994, pp 1421–1440.

*These figures represent reported cases in the literature, not the actual prevalence of these lesions.

TABLE 94.2 RATIO OF BENIGN VERSUS MALIGNANT BONE TUMORS IN BONES OF THE KNEE

Tumor Location	Benign Tumors (%)	Malignant Tumors (%)	Ratio
Knee	54	46	1.2 : 1
Distal femur	49	51	1 : 1
Proximal tibia	60	40	1.5 : 1
Proximal fibula	64	36	2 : 1
Patella	97	3	32 : 1

TABLE 94.3 PATELLA BONE TUMORS IN ORDER OF FREQUENCY (%)

Types of Bone Tumor	Total Reported Patella Tumors (%)
Chondroblastoma	32
Osteoblastoma	16
Giant cell tumor	16
Osteochondroma	10
Aneurysmal bone cyst	10
Osteoid osteoma	10
Osteosarcoma	3
Malignant fibrous histiocytoma	3

cysts occur at the knee. Unicameral bone cyst is the 16th most commonly reported primary osseous knee tumor or tumor-like lesion; its most common locations are the proximal tibia (56%), followed by the distal femur (32%), and the proximal fibula (12%). It has been rarely reported in the patella. More than 80% of unicameral bone cysts present between the ages of 5 and 20 years; the male-female ratio is generally 2.5:1. Roentgenographically, the lesion appears as a solitary metaphyseal radiolucency abutting but not involving the growth plate (Fig. 94.1). On magnetic resonance imaging, there is low signal intensity on T1-weighted images and very high intensity on T2-weighted images,

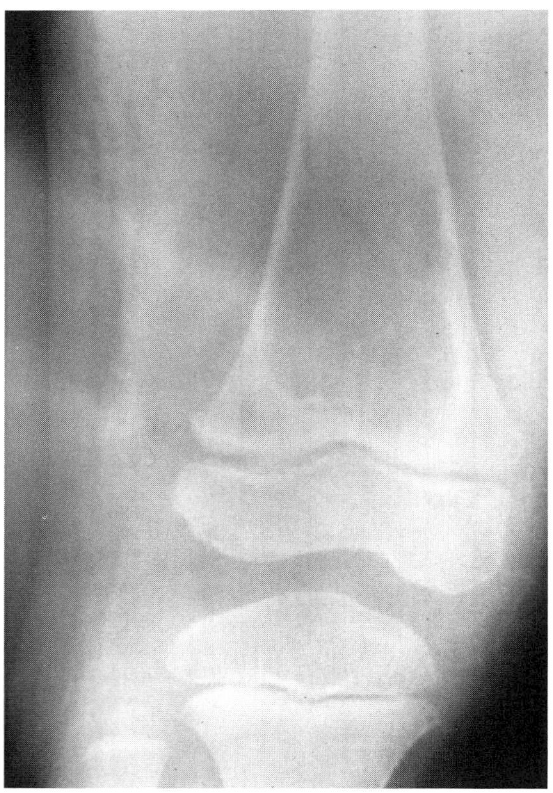

FIGURE 94.1 ➢ Unicameral bone cyst. Well-defined lucency is present in the distal metaphyses of the femur. The lesion extends to the growth plate but does not involve it or the adjacent epiphyses.

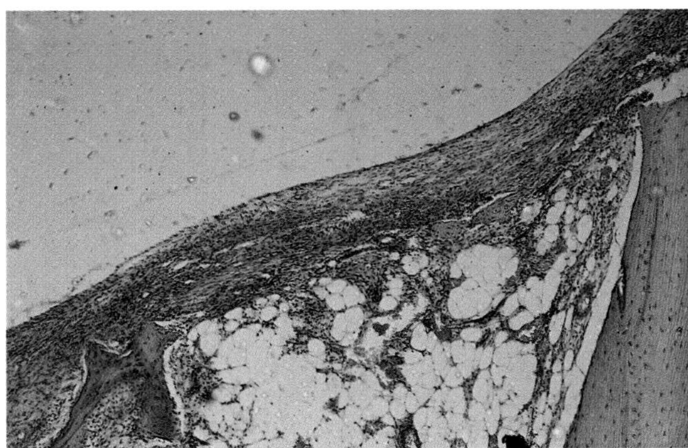

FIGURE 94.2 ➢ Unicameral bone cyst (histology). A bland, sparsely cellular fibrous membrane frames the cystic cavity. Underlying the membrane is host bone and fatty marrow.

reflecting high fluid content. Simple bone cysts may cause an expansion of the cortex on the roentgenogram because of the remodeling effect of cortical bone. This may result in fractures and thus pain, which is not an uncommon presentation of these lesions. Most simple bone cysts are asymptomatic and remain undetected. Microscopically, a thin lined fibrous membrane is seen, but secondary changes caused by fracture may lead to reactive bone, granulation tissue, hemosiderin, and cholesterol clefts (Fig. 94.2).

Aneurysmal Bone Cyst

The aneurysmal bone cyst (ABC) is a distinct, benign, pseudotumorous lesion of the bone that is usually differentiated from the simple bone cyst by both its roentgenographic and histopathological appearance.[36] Its exact cause is not known, but it may be the result of the secondary effects of bone remodeling pursuant to areas of intraosseous hemorrhage. Twenty-four percent of all ABCs occur at the knee. Classically, the ABC was described as an eccentric, trabeculated lesion in the skeleton, and it may occur at any osseous site. Studies showed that numerous bone lesions may be partly complicated by features of an ABC; therefore, the pathological diagnosis of ABC must be carefully correlated with the roentgenographic appearance to ensure adequate diagnostic accuracy. ABCs are the sixth most common primary osseous knee tumor, comprising 3% of all tumors and tumor-like lesions. Its most common location at the knee is the proximal tibia (48%), followed by the distal femur (38%), and the proximal fibula (14%). One percent of these tumors have been reported at the knee in the patella. It is usually metaphyseal in origin but may extend to the epiphysis in adults. The peak age of ABC occurrence is between 10 and 20 years; 75% of cases occur before 20 years of age. There is a more equal sex distribution for this lesion than for simple bone cyst.

The most common clinical finding is swelling at the lesion, which may or may not be painful. In one-third

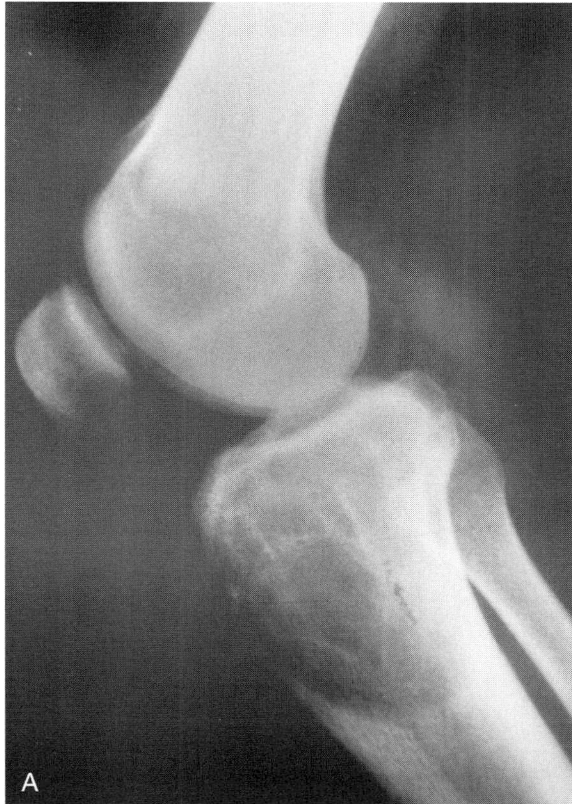

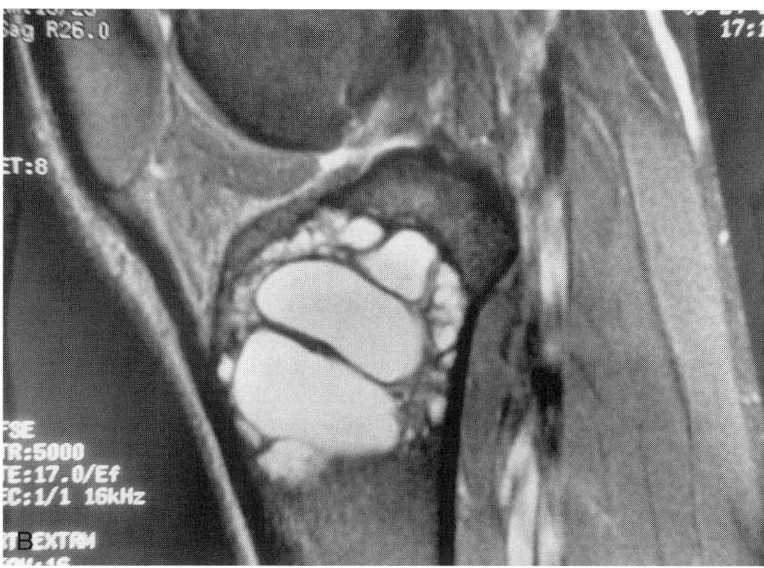

FIGURE 94.3 ➢ Aneurysmal bone cyst. *A,* Large lucency with well-defined margins is seen in the proximal end of the tibia in the lateral radiograph. *B,* T2-weighted sagittal magnetic resonance imaging (MRI) scan shows a multiloculated fluid-containing lesion in the proximal tibia. At times, the MRI scan of an aneurysmal bone cyst demonstrates fluid-fluid levels because of separation of blood into its heavier and lighter components.

of cases, the onset of symptoms may be related to trauma; pathological fracture may occur. Roentgenographically, there is a ballooning or expansile cystic change to the involved bone (Fig. 94.3). Computed tomography (CT) or MRI may be useful to evaluate the lesion; these show mostly a fluid appearance of its contents. The MRI pattern is a low signal on T1-weighted images and very high signal on T2-weighted images. Grossly, the periosteum is usually elevated and intact, enveloping a thin rim of reactive bone. The lesion proper may appear bluish because of acute and chronic bleeding; the cavity itself shows very hemorrhagic-appearing sponge-like cavities filled with blood and other fluid. Although not pulsatile, it is a vascular lesion. Bone tissue walls are thin, often with fibrous septa. The tissue itself is histologically different from that of a simple bone cyst, which has a bland membrane as its salient microscopic feature. In an ABC, there is a cellular cavity; often the membranes are filled with giant cells (Fig. 94.4). The clinical course of an ABC is variable but may show progression. Others may spontaneously cease and may slowly ossify, repairing themselves, as with simple bone cysts. ABCs may recur and, as mentioned, may be a complicating feature to a number of other neoplasms, such as giant cell tumor, chondroblastoma, chrondomyxoid fibroma, and other lesions. Although spontaneous remission of an ABC is well documented, growth is the rule. Recurrences are common and have been reported in one-fifth of cases, especially within 2 years.

The distinction from telangiectatic (hemorrhagic) osteosarcoma with its shared clinical, roentgenographic, and even histopathological similarities can be most difficult. However, microscopically, ABC is essentially a benign lesion. Telangiectatic osteosarcoma histologically displays conventional features of osteosarcoma within the ABC-like microscopic membranes.

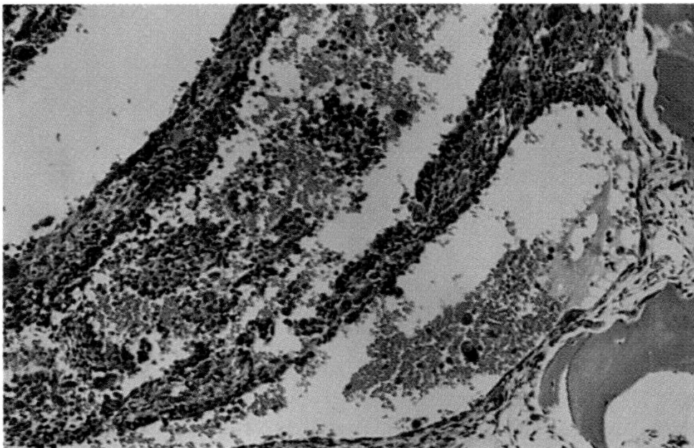

FIGURE 94.4 ➢ Photomicrograph of an aneurysmal bone cyst showing large vascular spaces filled with red blood cells. The underlying cancellous bone (lower right) is remodeling and is lined by a membrane composed of slender lining cells and multinucleated giant cells. Sinewy membrane extensions filled with mononuclear cells and giant cells course through the open vascular channels. (From Scott WN: The Knee, vol 2. St. Louis, Mosby-Year Book, 1994, p 1423.)

Ganglion Cysts

These rare benign cysts derive their name from the chemical and pathological similarity to their far more common soft tissue counterpart.[2] Characteristically, a clear, gelatinous, self-contained lesion is seen in juxtaposition to eroded para-articular bone.

Despite its proximity to a joint, the lesion rarely communicates with the joint. Two types have been described. Whereas a ganglion may be purely intraosseous, occasionally an overlying soft tissue ganglion is present, which may communicate with the intraosseous ganglion.

Roentgenographically, there is a well-circumscribed radiolucent lesion in the subchondral epiphyseal region of bone, which may extend into the metaphysis. As with other fluid-filled cystic lesions of bone, MRI signal is low on T1-weighted images and very high on T2-weighted images. Microscopically, the ganglion consists of clear gelatinous material with the bone cyst lined by a thin fibrous membrane.

Treated by curettage, recurrence is rare.

Fibrous Metaphyseal Defect

Fibrous metaphyseal defect (FMD) (nonossifying fibroma, fibrous cortical defect) is best considered a benign, hamartomatous, or developmental condition of the metaphyseal region of the bone in which there is a mixed fibroblastic, histiocytic, and foam cell proliferation, usually at the incorporation of tendinous or ligamentous insertions of the bone.[30] The anatomic occurrence at certain locations in the distal femur and proximal tibia support the diagnosis of it occurring as a developmental error, 55% of them at the knee. The nonossifying fibroma is the fourth most common reported tumor-like lesion of the knee, constituting approximately 7% of reported bone tumor cases. The most common location is the distal femur followed by the proximal tibia (54% versus 33%) and the proximal fibula (13%); no cases have been reported in the patella. This lesion occurs predominantly between the ages of 5 and 20 years; as many as one-third of all children age 4 to 10 years demonstrate such a lesion, usually a small, asymptomatic, regressing lesion.

Caffey,[8] in a roentgenographic survey of a pediatric population, showed that these lesions are quite common in the developmental group, with gradual disappearance as the skeleton reaches maturation. Lesions histologically identical to the nonossifying fibroma in an adult may be seen and are best regarded as a benign fibrous histiocytoma (Fig. 94.5).[11] Nonossifying fibromas are most commonly seen in males (1.5:1) and are most often completely asymptomatic. However, they may be large, causing mild pain and pathological fracture. Multiple nonossifying fibromas with associated pigmented skin lesions and congenital abnormalities have been reported in the literature. Roentgenographically, there is a characteristic lytic lesion located eccentrically involving the cortex with sclerotic borders. Appearance is oblong (i.e., along the longitudinal axis of the bone). These lesions have a gross appearance showing yellowish-brown tissue, which is usually solid. Histologically, it is composed of a mixture of cells, including giant cells, fibroblasts, histiocytes, and often foam cells. Hemosiderin may be present as well as areas of collagen production. The spindle-shaped fibroblasts proliferating in a swirling pattern may mimic a benign spindle cell tumor. However, small asymptomatic FMDs do not need to be treated. Large lesions with imminent fracture may require curettage and bone graft.

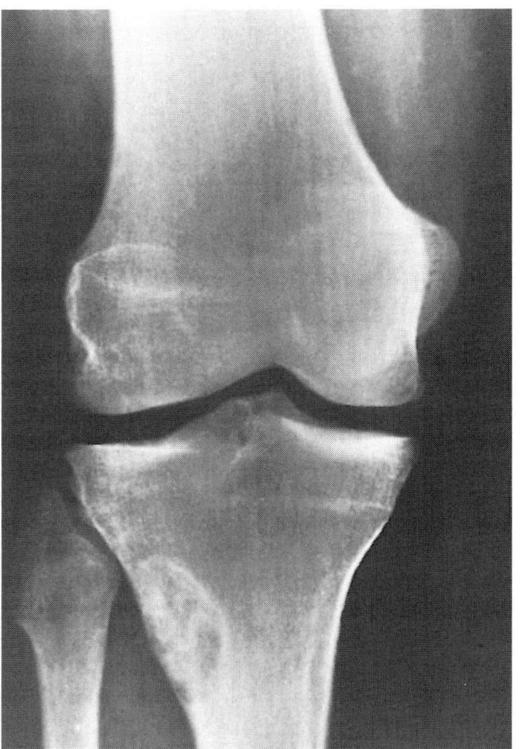

FIGURE 94.5 ➢ Benign fibrous histiocytoma. Frontal radiograph of a well-defined lucent lesion in the lateral border of the proximal tibial metaphysis. The lesion causes moderate thinning and mild bulging of the adjacent cortex. Areas of increased density are seen in the lesion. This is a healing benign fibrous histiocytoma. The same lesion in a younger patient would be interpreted as a nonossifying fibroma. (From Scott WN: The Knee, vol 2. St. Louis, MO, Mosby-Year Book, 1994, p 1424.)

Fibrous Dysplasia

Fibrous dysplasia is a slow-growing, developmental defect that replaces cancellous and eventually cortical bone with a fibro-osseous tissue.[32] Numerous types of fibrous dysplasia have been described, including monostotic and polyostotic variants, polyostotic variants with endocrinopathy and skin lesions (Albright's syndrome), and an unusual type involving the facial bones leading to the appearance of cherubism. Albright's syndrome occurs in less than 5% of fibrous dysplasia cases. In general, fibrous dysplasia in all its variants is seen in the knee in 23% of cases. It is the seventh most common reported tumor or tumor-like lesion of the knee, comprising approximately 3% of all cases. It occurs with almost equal distribution in the proximal tibia, distal femur, and proximal fibula and less frequently in the proximal fibula, with rare occurrences in the patella.

Fibrous dysplasia usually begins in childhood with a peak onset of symptoms between the ages of 5 and 20 years. The more extensive the case, the earlier is the onset of symptoms. There is an almost equal sex distribution. Symptoms, usually mild, are proportional to the extent of the lesion. With lesions involving the proximal fibula or tibia, there may be deformation as well as fractures. The radiographic appearance is very typical in advanced lesions, with replacement of predominantly cancellous, but also cortical, bone, by a fibrous and osseous stroma leading to relative radiolucency. There is often a fine granularity to the texture of the bone on x-ray film, giving the so-called ground-glass appearance. The cortex may be very thin with expansion of the overall diameter of the bone, often with cystic cavities. On gross examination the tumor has a compact, solid appearance; microscopic appearance shows a replacement of the cancellous tissue by benign-appearing, sparsely cellular fibrous tissue intermixed with irregular spicules of cellular or woven bone (Fig. 94.6). Rare foci of cartilage may occur, explaining the very rare complication of malignancy such as chondrosarcoma.

The course of fibrous dysplasia begins in childhood but is highly variable and dependent on the extent of the condition. Eventually maturation is seen in most cases. In general, patients younger than 18 years with lower extremity lesions need surgical intervention for optimal results.[34] Sarcomatous transformation is rare, occurring in less than 1% of cases.

Genetic findings in studies of Albright-McCune syndrome have shed light on the pathogenesis of fibrous dysplasia. Somatic mutations in the gene and coding of the G protein family (proteins that mediate transduction across cell membranes) lead to activation of adenylate cyclase and the proliferation and autonomous hyperfunction of hormonally responsive cells. Overproduction of cyclic adenosine monophosphate (cAMP) leads to endocrinopathies in endocrine tissues and dysregulation of osteogenic cells; the fibrous areas in fibrous dysplasia are probably manifestations of preosteogenic cells and abnormal fibroblasts. Increased expression of the *c-fos* proto-oncogene has also been described.[32]

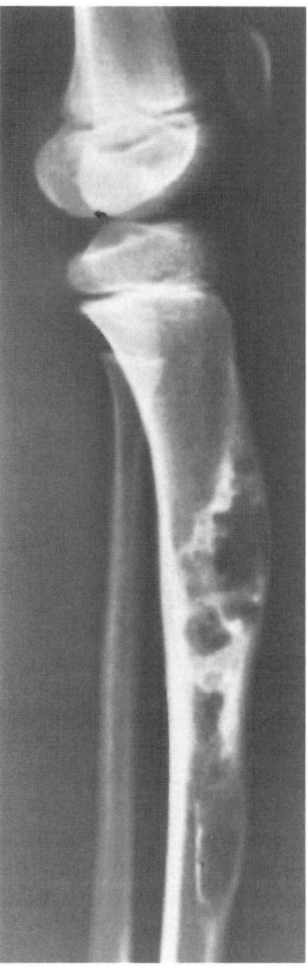

FIGURE 94.7 ➢ Osteofibrous dysplasia. Lateral radiograph of a well-defined lucent and partially sclerotic lesion involving the anterior cortex of the midtibial shaft. The lesion is located mainly in the diaphyses. There is mild anterior bowing of the tibia with a normal growth plate and epiphyses. (From Scott WN: The Knee, vol 2. St. Louis, MO, Mosby-Year Book, 1994, p 1425.)

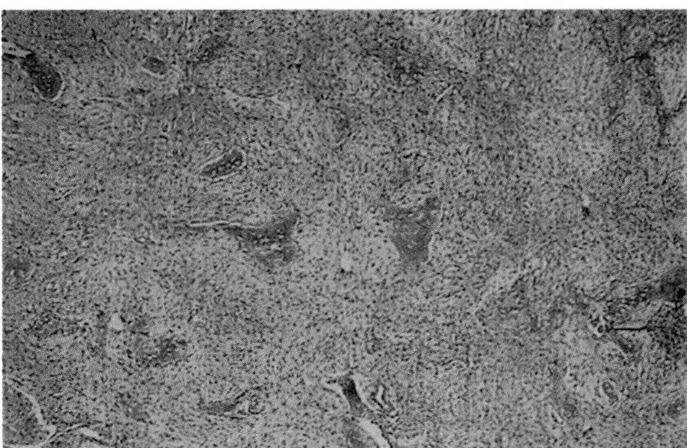

FIGURE 94.6 ➢ Fibrous dysplasia. Photomicrograph revealing irregularly shaped spicules of cellular woven bone enmeshed in a matrix of bland cellularity producing abundant collagenized matrix, the admixture of irregular woven bone spicules and bland fibrous tissue characteristic of fibrous dysplasia. (From Scott WN: The Knee, vol 2. St. Louis, MO, Mosby-Year Book, 1994, p 1424.)

Osteofibrous Dysplasia

A lesion of the skeleton predilected to the mandible and tibia and initially referred to as an ossifying fibroma because of prominent osteoblast rimming of bone spicules observed microscopically has been defined. Because it possibly represents a variant in a spectrum of fibro-osseous lesions of the skeleton, Campanacci popularized the term *osteofibrous dysplasia* for this lesion.[10] It is characterized by prominent cortical tibia involvement with anterior bowing (Fig. 94.7).

Desmoplastic Fibroma of Bone

Initially described by Cappell in 1935 in the fibula as an endosteal fibroma, Jaffe popularized the term *desmoplastic fibroma* a quarter of a century later for benign fibrous lesions arising within the bone with histological characteristics of the extraosseous desmoid tumors.[25] This rare, locally aggressive benign tumor may be extremely difficult to differentiate histologically from desmoids and low-grade fibrosarcomas and even fibrous histiocytoma, but combined characteristic pathological and roentgenographic features can distinguish this lesion. It tends to be diagnosed in the first 3 decades of life, with no sexual predilection. Thirty-two percent have been reported in the knee region, 15% in the distal femur, 5% in the proximal tibia, and 2% in the proximal fibula. Because of its insidious onset, the lesion is usually large at clinical diagnosis, with only slight occasional pain. Rarely, a pathological fracture may be the presenting symptom. Roentgenographically, these lesions are usually distinct expansile, lucent lesions with well-defined margins. Cortical erosion with pathological fracture may be seen. Computed tomographic (CT) scans may show evidence of soft tissue invasion where involved. Desmoplastic fibroma appears well defined on magnetic resonance imaging (MRI) revealing an intermediate signal intensity on T1-weighted images and a heterogeneous pattern on T2-weighted images. The clear separation of intraosseous tumor from normal bone marrow and extent of soft tissue involvement makes MRI extremely valuable in planning surgery. Histologically, the lesions are essentially identical to that of the desmoid tumor and are characterized by dense, collagenized tissue within which are uniform-appearing, benign fibroblasts (Fig. 94.8). Although cellularity may vary within the lesion, the cells are almost always small and regular with bland nuclei and little hyperchromasia and mitotic activity. There are no giant cells. The clinical course is local aggression, with recurrence in up to 72% after nonresection procedures, 17% with resections, and 0% when resected with a wide surgical margin. Therefore, recurrence may be avoided by a good surgical margin. Metastases have been reported after local recurrence in three of 184 cases (1.6%) reported in the literature.

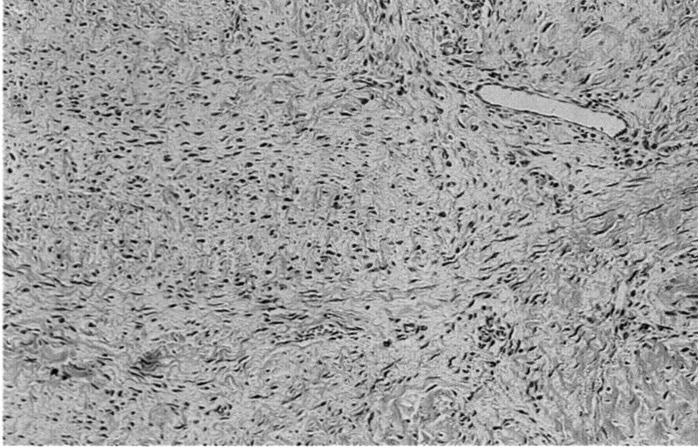

FIGURE 94.8 ➢ Desmoplastic fibroma (microscopic). Uniform benign fibroblasts in dense collagen stroma.

Osteochondroma (Exostosis)

Osteochondroma is a benign developmental tumor-like condition that represents an eccentric mass growing away from the joint space, most likely representing the independent growth of aberrant epiphyseal cartilage during early growth of the skeleton (Fig. 94.9). Best considered ectopic growth plates, these eccentric masses may be sessile or quite pedunculated in their appearance and usually present as a mass. They may or may not be symptomatic depending on pressure effects on nerves and fracture of the stalk. It is the second most common reported tumor or tumor-like lesion of the knee, making up approximately 19% of all reported cases. Its most common location is the distal femur (61%), followed by the proximal tibia (33%), proximal fibula (6%), and patella (less than 1%). Osteochondromas peak in the 10- to 18-year age range; growth is greatest during puberty. Osteochondromas usually cease growth after skeletal maturation. Any solitary osteochondroma that continues to grow after skeletal maturation, as well as those changing in size in multiple hereditary exostosis (MHE), should be considered carefully for the diagnosis of chondrosarcomatous transformation. There is a slight male predominance for osteochondroma. The gross pathology is that of a mature piece of bone capped by a thin cartilaginous cap. Histologically, one sees a band of periosteum covering a proliferating zone of organized columns of chondrocytes, which are undergoing endochondral ossification (Fig. 94.10). The cap may be variable in thickness, and fragments of the cap may separate after trauma, developing separate growths similar to osseocartilaginous loose bodies seen in synovial loose bodies.

As mentioned, the osteochondroma may be seen as multiple lesions in the condition known as hereditary exostosis,[26] which is 10 times less common than a solitary exostosis. In MHE there is often associated skeletal shortening of the involved limb or deformity and an increased incidence of malignant transformation, which most likely occurs in at least 1% to 10% of these cases.

Osteochondromatous-like proliferations may be seen in a wide range of settings, including after irradiation in a child, over the epiphysis associated with limb length inequality (dysplasia epiphysialis hemimelica), under the toenail (subungual exostosis), and on the surface of bone, so-called Nora's lesion or bizarre parosteal osteochondromatous proliferation of bone. A para-articular soft tissue osteochondroma has also been described.

Osteoid Osteoma

Pain, often severe at night, and relieved by aspirin, with a characteristic, hot, well-circumscribed lesion on bone scan is characteristic of osteoid osteoma, a small,

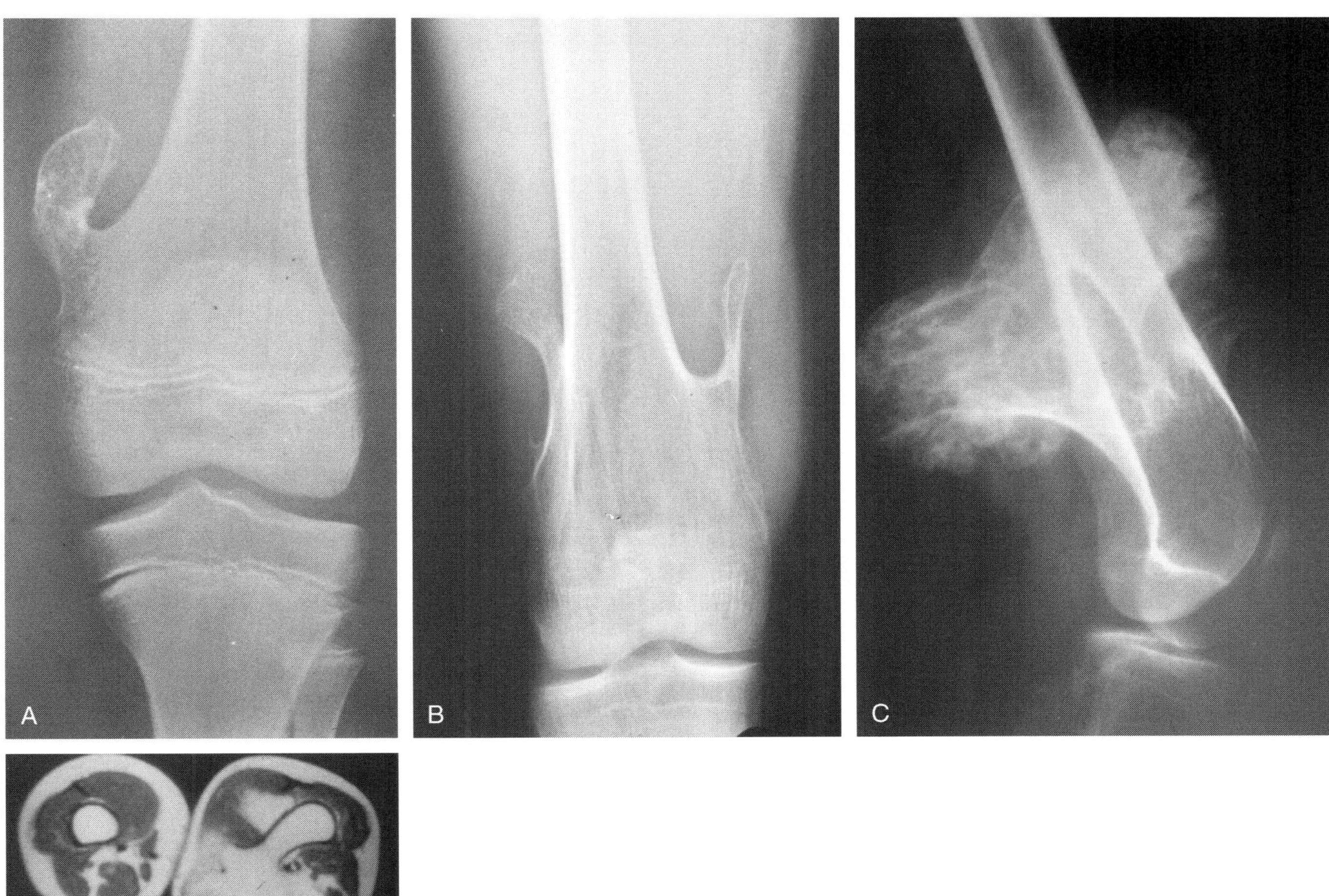

FIGURE 94.9 ➢ Frontal radiographs demonstrate (*A*) single and (*B*) multiple osteochondromas in the distal metaphyses of the femora. The lesions are pedunculated and point away from the knee joint. Notice the continuity of the cortex and marrow cavity of the bone into the osteochondromas. Lateral radiograph demonstrates large broad-based osteochondroma in the posterior surface of the distal femur (*C*). Magnetic resonance imaging scan demonstrates continuity of the cortical and marrow signal into the osteochondroma (*D*).

most likely reactive lesion of the skeleton. Osteoid osteoma most characteristically occurs as a well-defined nidus of remodeling spicules of cancellous-type bone within the cortex. Less commonly, it is seen in the cancellous marrow bone and even less frequently in a subarticular or juxta-articular location. It is the 11th most common tumor-like lesion in large series, composing approximately 2% of all reported cases but 13% of all cases occurring in the knee. The most common location in the knee is the cortical bone of the proximal tibia (61%), followed by the distal femur (33%), the proximal fibula (5%), and the patella (2%).

Osteoid osteoma has a classic roentgenographic appearance. It has a peak age of occurrence in the pediatric population: ages 11 to 20; 95% of cases occur between age 5 and 30 years. There is a 2.3:1 male predominance. The lesion is characteristically examined for its associated pain: roentgenography shows a zone of sclerosis. In many cases on the radiograph, and more sensitively on the CT scan, a centralized radiolucent nidus may be detected embedded within the sclerotic cortical bone (Fig. 94.11). These lesions may be difficult to localize surgically, but studies with bone-scanning agents have indicated that the central lucent nidus is the area of most intense radioactive uptake, a phenomenon that has formed the basis for

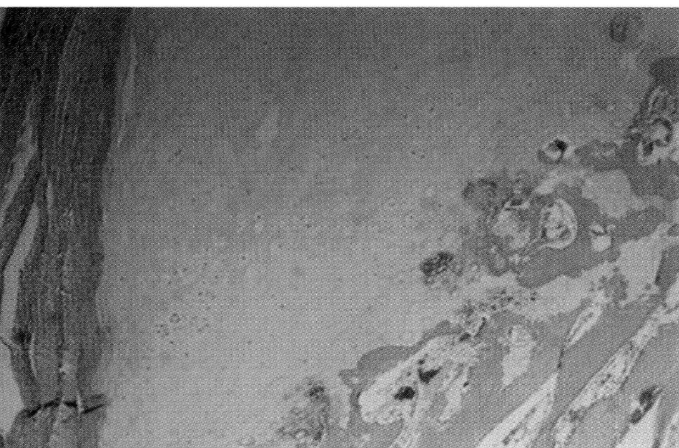

FIGURE 94.10 ➢ Osteochondroma. Photomicrograph revealing a cartilaginous cap lined by a fibrous periosteum (top). The cartilage cap consists of chondrocytes often lined up in columns that are undergoing endochondral ossification (central bottom), similar to that seen at an active epiphysis. The cartilage becomes calcified and then remodels into cancellous bone. (From Scott WN: The Knee, vol 2. St. Louis, MO, Mosby-Year Book, 1994, p 1425.)

radioisotope localization techniques to localize this lesion.[38] These lesions may be difficult to see grossly because they may be small, usually less than 1 cm (Fig. 94.12). Surgical removal is curative.

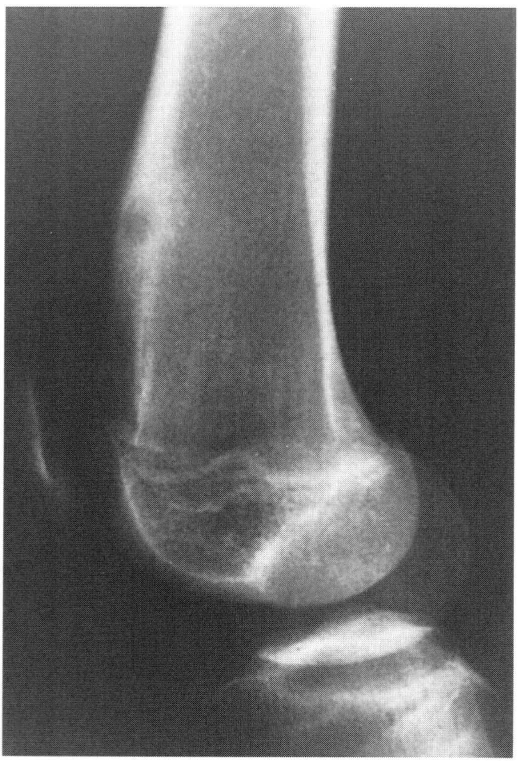

FIGURE 94.11 ➢ Osteoid osteoma. Lateral radiograph of a small central lucency (the nidus) surrounded by sclerosis in the anterior cortex of the distal femur. At times small central calcifications can be seen in the nidus of an osteoid osteoma. (From Scott WN: The Knee, vol 2. St. Louis, MO, Mosby-Year Book, 1994, p 1426.

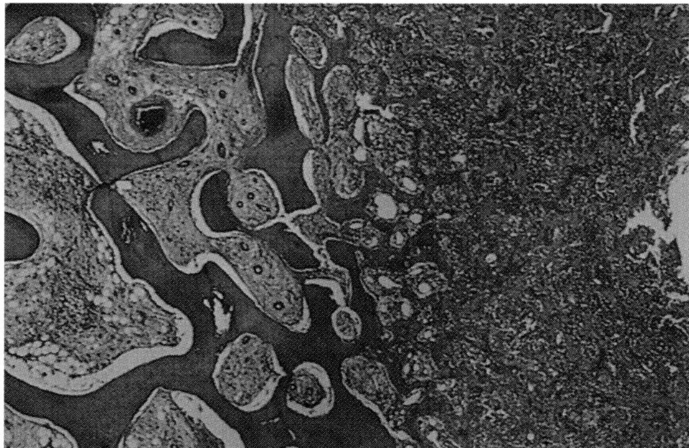

FIGURE 94.12 ➢ Osteoid osteoma. A well-circumscribed nidus (right) is seen in contradistinction to the surrounding remodeling bone (left) and is characterized by smaller, interweaving spicules of markedly remodeling bone, with osteoblasts forming abundant osteoid in a well-vascularized stroma. (From Scott WN: The Knee, vol 2. St. Louis, MO, Mosby-Year Book, 1994, p 1427.)

Grossly, osteoid osteoma may be difficult to identify because they are often small bone foci within sclerotic bone. Large lesions are reddish in color. The zonal architecture is characteristic.

The lesion is usually intracortical; a well-circumscribed round or oval nidus consists of interlacing spicules of cellular remodeling cancellous (trabecular) bone. The bone spicules are replete with bone-lining cells, including osteoclasts and numerous osteoblasts. Osteoid surfacing of the bone is abundant. Between spicules is a richly vascular loose fibrovascular tissue. Cartilage, bone marrow elements, and mitoses are usually not present. The nidus is characterized by more abundant mineralization centrally (a central sclerosis on x-ray film) and separation from host bone peripherally by a fibrovascular, sparsely mineralized perimeter.

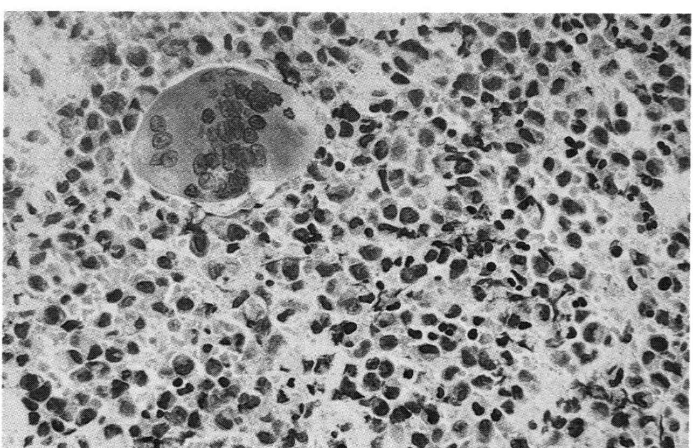

FIGURE 94.13 ➢ Langerhans' cell granulomatosis (eosinophilic granuloma) consists of a mixed population of eosinophils, giant cells, and large mononuclear cells, the latter the Langerhans' cells, which on electron microscopy, reveal the trilaminar Birbeck granules.

Langerhans' Cell Granulomatosis (Eosinophilic Granuloma)

Langerhans' cell granulomatosis (LCG) is a tumor-like proliferation of chronic inflammatory cells, eosinophils, histiocytes, and Langerhans' cells which may involve one or multiple bones, and in rare circumstances may be associated with diabetes insipidus and exophthalmos (Hand-Schüller-Christian disease) (Fig. 94.13). Most often, the clinical presentation of LCG to the orthopedic surgeon is that of a solitary lesion, which not uncommonly presents in the femur or tibia.[14] It often manifests with pain or swelling in the extremity of a child. The lesion may clinically and roentgenographically mimic osteomyelitis, fibrous dysplasia, Ewing's sarcoma, and in some instances even osteogenic sarcoma. A biopsy is necessary to confirm the diagnosis of LCG, which is a benign, usually nonprogressive osseous lesion of limited duration. Although lesions have been treated both surgically and with medical intervention, including chemotherapy, the solitary variant may follow a limited course and most likely represents a reactive or transient immunological abnormality. The diagnosis is confirmed by identifying the diagnostic Langerhans' giant cell, a cell that is present normally in numerous anatomic sites, including the skin, but proliferates in rare circumstances. The Langerhans' giant cell is identified by the characteristic Birbeck granules, peculiar pentalamellar structures identified by electron microscopy.[39] The Langerhans cells most probably are peripheral antigen-processing cells of bone marrow origin that process various antigens stimulating an immunological reaction.

Formerly, LCG was considered part of a spectrum of lesions termed histiocytosis X, which included the solitary eosinophilic granuloma, the Hand-Schüller-Christian disease and Letterer-Siwe disease. The last disorder, however, is a distinct clinicopathological entity that carries a poor prognosis and acts clinically more like a progressive lymphoproliferative disorder.

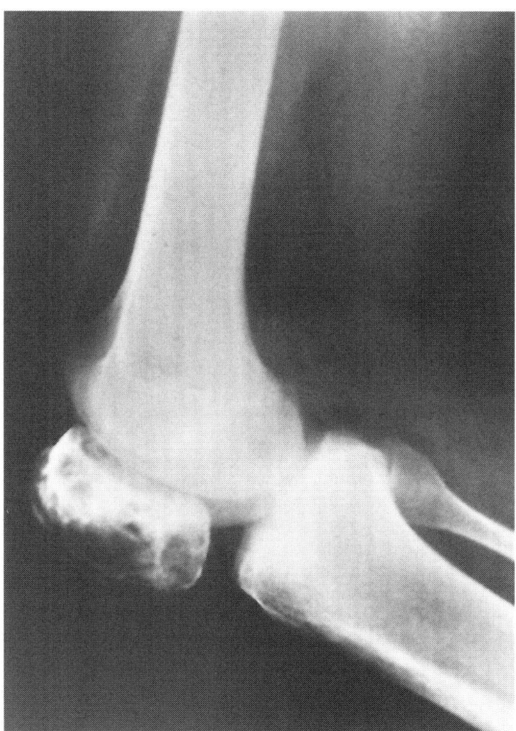

FIGURE 94.14 ➢ Chondroblastoma. Lateral radiograph of a large lucent and partially sclerotic lesion occupying most of the patella in this 17-year-old patient. Plain radiographs and computed tomography scan demonstrated the sclerosis mainly in the periphery of the lesion. There was no evidence for punctate calcifications in the lesion. This is an unusual location for chondroblastomas (Codman's tumor), most often found in the proximal humeral and femoral epiphyses. (From Scott WN: The Knee, vol 2. St. Louis, MO, Mosby-Year Book, 1994, p 1427.)

BENIGN TUMORS

Chondroblastoma

Chondroblastoma characteristically occurs as a slow-growing benign lytic lesion over the epiphysis in a skeletally immature person (Fig. 94.14).[33] Thirty-six percent of all chondroblastomas occur in the knee. It is the 12th most commonly reported primary osseous tumor of the knee and occurs with almost equal distribution between the proximal tibia (48%) and the distal femur (45%). Five percent of knee chondroblastomas occur in the patella; the fibula is the least common site (2%). The peak age of occurrence is between 10 and 20 years (85%), with a 1.8:1 male-female ratio. The lesion usually presents with pain and may rarely involve the articular cartilage, causing symptoms primarily associated with the joint. A fracture into the chondroblastoma may lead to loose bodies and may even mimic osteochondritis dissecans roentgenographically and clinically. The origins of chondroblastoma are not known, but ultrastructural studies suggested that the major cell in this tumor has some similarities to a primitive cartilaginous cell or chondroblast. Histologically, chondroblastoma is characterized by a polygonal cell population; focal areas of calcification are noted in approximately 50% of cases, the calcification often appearing in a linear fashion enveloping individual cells (Fig. 94.15). The lesion may be quite cellular and may be confused microscopically with a malignant tumor.

Enchondroma

Enchondromas are benign tumors of well-differentiated cartilage. Only 5% of all solitary enchondromas occur in the knee. Enchondromas may occur as a solitary lesion or as a more diffuse, developmental problem (enchondromatosis or Ollier's disease). Enchondromatosis may lead to marked deformities of the involved bone and is associated with the development of chondrosarcoma. Solitary enchondroma constitutes approximately 1% of all knee tumors. Its most common location at the knee is the distal femur (41%), followed by

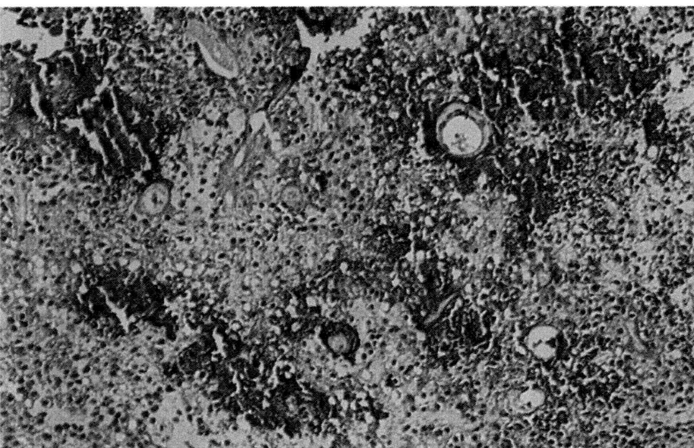

FIGURE 94.15 ➢ Chondroblastoma. These cellular lesions are characterized by proliferating mononuclear cells producing a grayish-blue chondroid matrix, which focally undergoes calcification, often surrounding individual chondrocytes in a punctate linear fashion. The cell population is polygonal with varying degrees of cytoplasm, chondroid matrix, and calcification. (From Scott WN: The Knee, vol 2. St. Louis, MO, Mosby-Year Book, 1994, p 1428.)

the proximal fibula (30%), proximal tibia (29%), and patella (1%). It is most commonly diagnosed in the knee during the first 20 years of life and has no sex predilection.

Enchondromas roentgenographically occur as purely lytic lesions or with a cluster of punctate calcifications. The latter may mimic a chondrosarcoma roentgenographically and histologically (Fig. 94.16). Histologically, enchondromas are characterized by well-differentiated cartilage with focal areas of calcification (Fig. 94.17). Unlike chondrosarcoma, these lesions are usually not pleomorphic and are usually enveloped by the normal surrounding lamella bone.

Periosteal (Juxtacortical) Chondroma

Periosteal or juxtacortical chondroma is a benign cartilage tumor usually arising on the surface of cortical bone in the diaphysis or metaphysis.[3] It is most common during adolescence or young adulthood and characteristically has an x-ray film appearance of a saucer-shaped indentation of the cortical bone. Because of increased cartilaginous cellularity, it may be misdiagnosed and overtreated. The most common presenting symptoms are pain and swelling. Marginal excision usually suffices.

Chondromyxoid Fibroma

Chondromyxoid fibroma is a benign tumor composed of fibrous tissue, myxoid connective tissue, and tissue differentiating toward cartilage.[41] It almost always arises in regions of fetal metaphyseal cartilage. Forty-five percent of all chondromyxoid fibromas reported in the literature occur in the knee; the proximal tibia accounts for 76%, the distal femur 15%, and the proximal fibula 10%. In general, more than 80% of cases

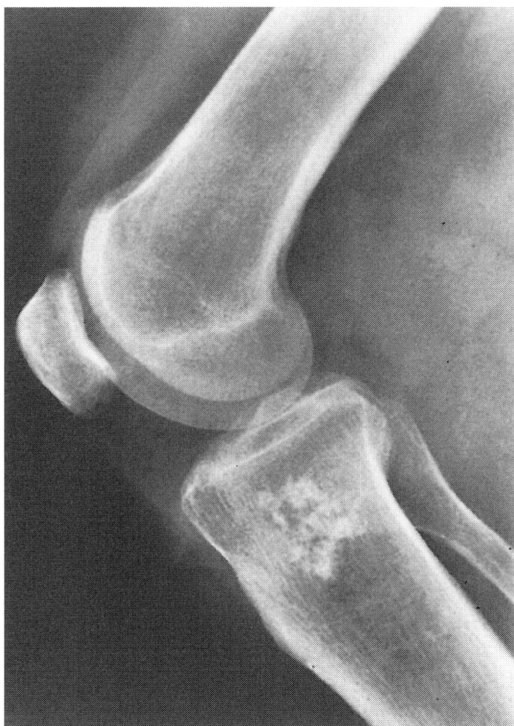

FIGURE 94.16 ➢ Enchondroma. Lateral radiograph showing punctate calcifications in the proximal metaphyses of the tibia, a lesion that can be confused with a bone infarction. (From Scott WN: The Knee, vol 2. St. Louis, MO, Mosby-Year Book, 1994, p 1428.)

occur between the ages of 5 and 30 years; there is a 1.5:1 male predominance.

Osteoma

Osteomas are benign slow-growing radiodense tumor-like lesions characterized pathologically by predomi-

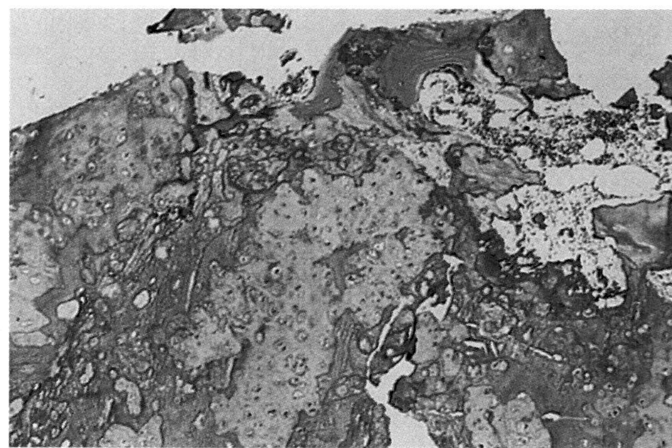

FIGURE 94.17 ➢ Enchondroma. Proliferative chondrocytes in a grayish-blue matrix are characteristic of enchondromas, which typically calcify (deep purple) and remodel into bone (pink) in interconnecting islands replacing the underlying normal marrow fat and bone (upper right). (From Scott WN: The Knee, vol 2. St. Louis, MO, Mosby-Year Book, 1994, p 1429.)

nantly mature lamellar bone. Osteomas may particularly affect the skull and facial bones, especially the mandible and frontal and ethmoid sinuses. Clinically, a painless mass is noted.

Parosteal osteomas (or long bone osteomas) are benign radiodense growths on the surface of bone composed of essentially cortical-type haversian bone.[5] Their importance rests in the distinction from parosteal osteosarcoma. They are usually reported in the lower extremity. Patients are usually in the 4th or 5th decade of life.

Roentgenographically, a dense or oval-shaped mass is noted contiguous with the cortical surface of the bone. There is no periosteal reaction, and there are no areas of radiolucency. The surface is smooth or smoothly lobulated. The underlying cortex of the host bone may be slightly thickened, and cross-sectional studies may show slight encroachment of medullary bone, but these changes are minimal if present.

Because of difficulty in distinguishing this lesion from osteosarcoma, some investigators recommend definitive surgical removal even when the diagnosis of osteoma is likely.

Osteomas of the mandible, calvarium, and even long bones are seen in association with colonic intestinal polyps in Gardner's syndrome, which is also characterized by odontomasa, supernumerary and unerupted teeth, and soft tissue tumors, including fibromas, retroperitoneal and mesenteric fibromatosis, and epidermal inclusion cysts. Gardner's syndrome is an autosomal-dominant genetic disorder of particular importance because of the associated malignant change seen in the adenomatous lesions of the intestine.

Osteomas usually consist of circumscribed foci of dense bone contiguous with host bone, primarily mature lamellar cortical-type haversian bone. Wide zones of either cortical or trabecular bone may be seen, and although usually mature lamellar bone predominates, immature woven bone may be noted. There are sparse interosseous spaces, which may be filled with vessels, fibrous tissue, fat, and even bone marrow. In general, the typical osteoma has a lobulated appearance on microscopy and consists of mature remodeling haversian bone, and it abuts rather than blends into the surrounding tissue. Active remodeling of bone in an osteoma showing numerous osteoblasts and osteoclasts may mimic an osteoblastoma, the so-called osteoblastoma-like osteoma.

Osteoblastoma

Osteoblastoma is a benign tumor characterized histologically by its similarity to osteoid osteoma, in which there is abundant osteoblast cellularity with production of osteoid and bone in an irregular organization.[18, 21] Only 10% of reported osteoblastomas occur in the knee, constituting less than 1% of primary bone tumors of the knee (proximal tibia, 64%; distal femur, 22%). The patella accounts for a surprising high percentage of knee cases (14%). Approximately 90% of these tumors occur between 5 and 30 years of age, with a 3:1 male predominance. These lesions are usually larger than 2 cm and have a roentgenographic appearance, which may vary from one of pure lysis to one in which there is detectable bone formation.

GIANT CELL TUMOR

Giant cell tumor, or osteoclastoma, occurs at the end of the bones as a well-circumscribed lytic lesion usually abutting the articular cartilage.[9, 20] It derives its name from a microscopic appearance in which there is a sea of multinucleated giant cells enmeshed in a noninflammatory mesodermal mononuclear cell matrix of uncertain histogenesis. Although most giant cell tumors are benign, the lesion may metastasize in less than 10% of cases. Giant cell tumors that are fully malignant from the start and act in a sarcomatous fashion are also well documented in the literature. This is the third most commonly reported primary osseous tumor of the knee, comprising 15% of all reported cases, and occurring with approximately equal distribution between the distal femur (48%) and the proximal tibia (46%); 6% of cases have been reported in the proximal fibula and less than 1% in the patella. The peak age of occurrence for giant cell tumor is the young adult; 80% of cases occur between 20 and 40 years of age. It is very rare before puberty. Thus, lytic lesions at the end of the bone before skeletal maturation favor the diagnosis of chondroblastoma and, after skeletal maturation, giant cell tumor. There is a slight female predilection in reported cases.

Clinically, the major symptom is pain, usually in the joint, with decreased range of motion often resulting from effusion or expansion of the bone. Although the tumor abuts the articular cartilage, it rarely extends into the joint space. There may be swelling, and pathological fracture is not uncommon. Characteristically, there is a well-defined radiolucent mass on the roentgenogram, with well-defined borders (Fig. 94.18). It is usually situated eccentrically at the metaphyseal-epiphyseal areas. Classification of giant cell tumors roentgenographically has been proposed and is reputed to be of prognostic value. In the Enneking staging system, stage I "quiescent" lesions appear small and slowly expand with an intact cortex and well-defined borders. Active lesions (stage II) usually show a thinned or missing cortex but have an intact periosteum. Borders are less clear. This is the most common form encountered. In stage III, or the aggressive giant cell tumor, the cortex is destroyed. The tumor is not confined by the periosteum. Here a large expansive lesion, possibly extending to articular cartilage, suggests rapid growth.

Grossly, giant cell tumors appear as usually solid lesions with a light brown to red color, uniform, without bone or calcification. There may be associated hyperemia and marked bleeding at incision. Histologically, the characteristic uniform and even distribution of giant cells is diagnostic (Fig. 94.19). However, the tumor is composed of two cell populations: the giant cells, osteoclast-like cells of probable monocyte-macrophage origin, and a second population of intervening mononuclear stromal cells, the cause of which is unclear. Histological study alone and even flow cytome-

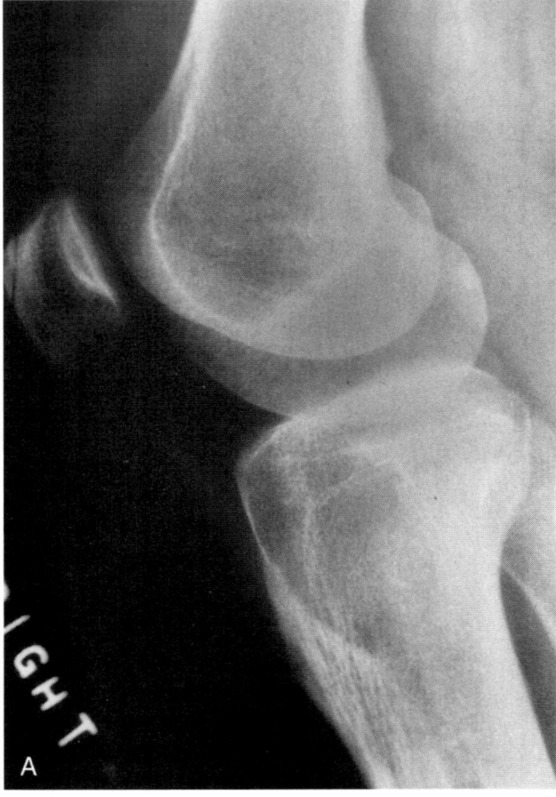

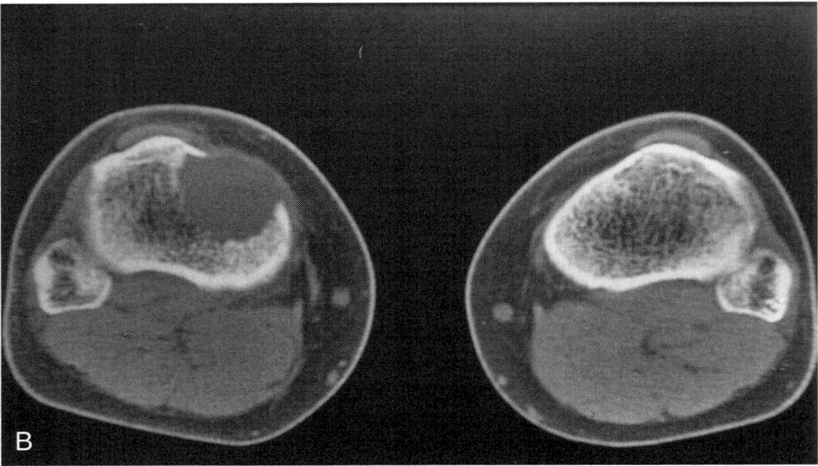

FIGURE 94.18 ➢ Giant cell tumor of bone. *A*, Lateral radiograph demonstrates well-defined lucent lesion in the proximal tibia extending into the subchondral surface of the bone. *B*, Computed tomography scan demonstrates well-marginated area of destruction of the bone trabeculae and cortex in the anteromedial surface of the tibia. Notice the absence of calcifications or of sclerosis surrounding the lesion.

try studies of the DNA content of the nuclei of cells from giant cell tumors are unable to predict those lesions that will metastasize.

The clinical course of giant cell tumors is highly variable, ranging from local growth over years to more rapid invasion in brief periods of time. Although malignant transformation has been reported in 5% of cases, one cannot exclude that these malignant giant cell tumors are not sarcomas from the beginning. Malignant giant cell tumors may have fibrosarcomatous, malignant fibrous histiocytomatous, or osteosarcomatous areas, raising the possibility of initial diagnostic accuracy. Radiation treatment is contraindicated because of the potential for sarcomatous stimulation. Local recurrence has been reported in less than 10% with appropriate surgical treatment and usually occurs within 3 years of surgery. Patients with pulmonary metastases have survived with surgical removal of pulmonary metastases and chemotherapy.

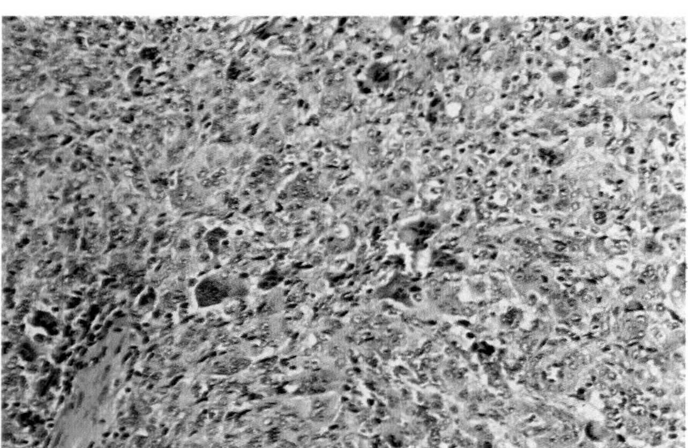

FIGURE 94.19 ➢ Giant cell tumor (histology). Cellular tumor composed of multinucleated giant cells evenly dispersed and admixed with stromal mononuclear cells of uncertain histogenesis.

MALIGNANT TUMORS OF THE KNEE

Osteosarcoma (Osteogenic Sarcoma)

Osteosarcoma, or osteogenic sarcoma, is a highly malignant tumor that, by definition, produces neoplastic osteoid or bone. It characteristically arises within the metaphysis of the long bones and grows circumferentially through the cortex into the soft tissue, raising the periosteum. It rarely invades the joint space. Fifty-six percent of all osteogenic sarcomas occur at the knee; thus, it is the most common primary osseous knee tumor reported in the literature (32%). Of osteogenic sarcomas of the knee, 64% occur in the distal femur, 32% in the proximal tibia, 4% in the proximal fibula, and less than 1% in the patella. Osteogenic sarcoma characteristically occurs at the adolescent growth spurt. The peak age of occurrence is between ages 10 and 20 years, 75% of all cases occur between 10 and 30 years of age. There is a male predominance of 1.5:1. In the immature skeleton with an intact growth plate, the epiphysis may act as a relative barrier to its growth. Osteogenic sarcoma typically presents with pain, which is often mild and intermittent initially but more continuous and exacerbated by deep palpation later. A mass or a swelling may be felt. Rarely, one encounters a pathological fracture. The laboratory hallmark of an osteogenic sarcoma is an elevated alkaline phosphatase, usually in excess of that noted during pediatric growth. The characteristic radiograph reveals a radiodense lesion over the metaphysis with indistinct borders and periosteal elevation (Fig. 94.20). The raised periosteum creates a triangle (referred to as Codman's triangle), the borders of which are the intact cortex, the tumor, and the periosteum proper. CT scans may be helpful in defining soft tissue or joint penetration: MRI defines involvement of cancellous and medullary bone.

Grossly, the osteogenic sarcoma is a hard, compact tumor (Fig. 94.21). The external layers tend to be softer and more suitable for biopsy. Histologically, osteogenic sarcoma is characterized by the presence of sarcomatous osteoblast cells producing a disorganized maze of calcified tissue, including osteoid and bone (Fig. 94.22). The lesion may vary from one that is very cellular with little osteoid or bone production to those that are sparsely cellular with abundant calcified matrix being produced. Osteogenic sarcoma, for which there is an animal model in the Great Dane, has a seeming predilection for areas of rapid growth. As mentioned, it occurs in the adolescent growth spurt and also is seen with increased incidence in bone

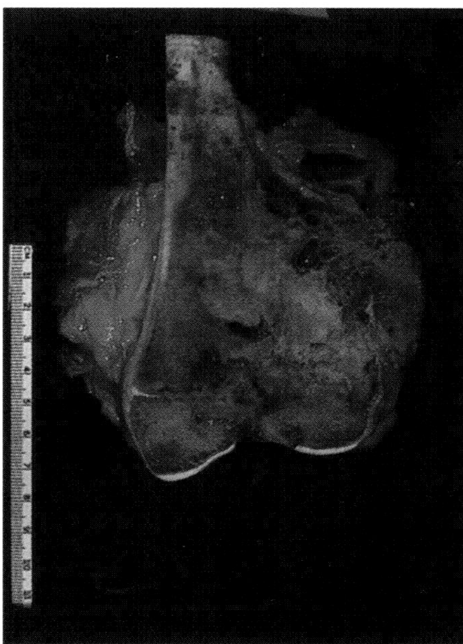

FIGURE 94.21 ➢ Gross photograph of osteogenic sarcoma at the distal metaphysis of the proximal femur showing a bone-forming lesion expanding into the surrounding soft tissue and lifting up the periosteum (top right). The marrow itself and surrounding soft tissue are replaced by a heterogeneous matrix destroying the bone; the epiphyseal growth plate acts as a relative barrier of spread with relative sparing of the epiphysis. (From Scott WN: The Knee, vol 2. St. Louis, MO, Mosby-Year Book, 1994, p 1431.)

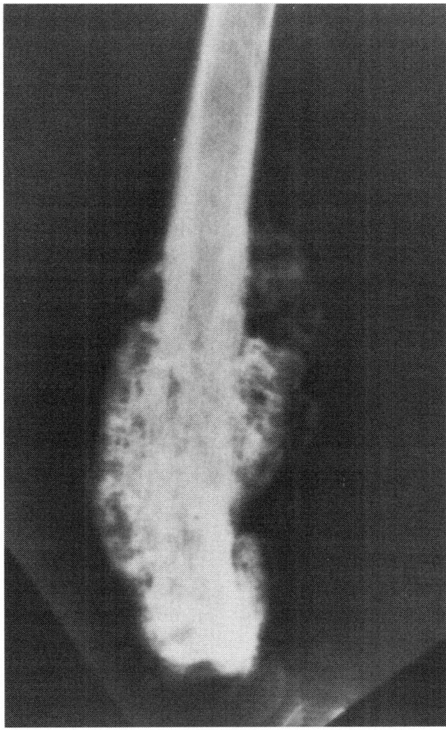

FIGURE 94.20 ➢ Osteogenic sarcoma. Lateral radiograph showing a large blastic lesion extending from the distal metaphyses to the diaphyses of the femur. Extensive periosteal and tumor bone formation surrounds the distal femur. Periosteal new bone formation tends to be better organized, with areas of density perpendicular or parallel to the involved bone. Tumor bone tends to be disorganized and is usually seen as patches of increased density. The differentiation between periosteal and tumor bone formation is difficult. In this case, the epiphyses of the distal femur is not involved by the tumor. (From Scott WN: The Knee, vol 2. St. Louis, MO, Mosby-Year Book, 1994, p 1430.)

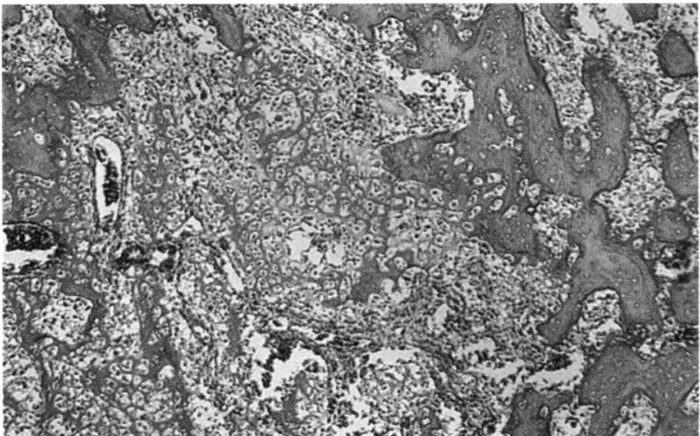

FIGURE 94.22 ➢ Photomicrograph of osteogenic sarcoma showing the underlying remodeling cancellous bone (lower left) being replaced by the juxtaposition of a highly irregular cellular population of cells, producing a highly disorganized bone matrix. The replacement of marrow fat and bone by irregular osteoid and bone production is characteristic of osteogenic sarcoma. (From Scott WN: The Knee, vol 2. St. Louis, MO, Mosby-Year Book, 1994, p 1431.)

affected by Paget's disease.[16, 31] Osteogenic sarcoma grows by relatively rapid local expansion and metastases to the lungs. With the advent of adjuvant therapy, including chemotherapy and surgical removal, the 5-year survival of children with osteogenic sarcoma without evidence of disseminated disease, is approximately 60% to 70%.[27] Of prognostic value is the response to preoperative chemotherapy; a favorable outlook is possible when 90% of the tumor is necrosed. Other prognostic indicators include the size and extent of cortical and soft tissue penetration.

Osteosarcoma Variants

Numerous variants of osteogenic sarcoma have been described, including a low-grade well-differentiated tumor, a hemorrhagic radiolucent lesion mimicking an aneurysmal bone cyst (telangiectatic osteogenic sarcoma)[28] (Fig. 94.23), and one confined to the cortex of bone (intracortical osteogenic sarcoma). Osteogenic sarcomas may also occur on the surface of the bone, and at least three variants have been described: a high-grade osteogenic sarcoma that mimics classic osteogenic sarcoma histologically; a periosteal osteogenic sarcoma that tends toward chondroblastic differentiation; and the most distinct of the group: the parosteal or juxtacortical osteogenic sarcoma, which is a lesion of fibroblastic differentiation with a predilection for the distal posterior aspect of the distal femur.[29] In addition to the anatomic variants, there are numerous histological variants, most notably the small cell osteogenic sarcoma, which is highly malignant and mimicks an undifferentiated small cell tumor such as Ewing's sarcoma.[22]

Parosteal or juxtacortical osteogenic sarcoma is generally slow growing. It is the 10th most common primary osseous tumor reported in the literature, accounting for approximately 2% of cases. Sixty-nine percent of all parosteal osteogenic sarcomas occur at the knee, a higher prevalence than classic osteogenic sarcoma. The distal femur is the most common location (86%), occurring posteriorly with growth or swelling into the popliteal space. Ten percent occur in the proximal tibia and 4% in the proximal fibula, with no cases reported in the patella. Parosteal or juxtacortical osteogenic sarcoma occurs in an older age group than classic osteogenic sarcoma; 95% of all cases occur between the ages of 15 and 40 years. In contradistinction to classic osteogenic sarcoma, there is a 1.4:1 female predilection. The tumor is characterized by pain and swelling late in the course of the disease with a decreased range of motion.

Roentgenographically, there is a mass at the surface of the bone, which is often radiodense. CT scans and MRI may be useful in ascertaining cortical invasion, a factor that has prognostic significance because the classic juxtacortical surface tumor carries a better prognosis than one involving the medullary cavity. On gross examination, the tumor is hard with a pseudocapsule; the tumor itself envelopes the bone. It may be adherent to the soft tissue or the cortex. The clinical course is a slow progression. Metastases by hematogenous spread may occur more than 5 years after excision. With a wide margin, recurrence is rare but

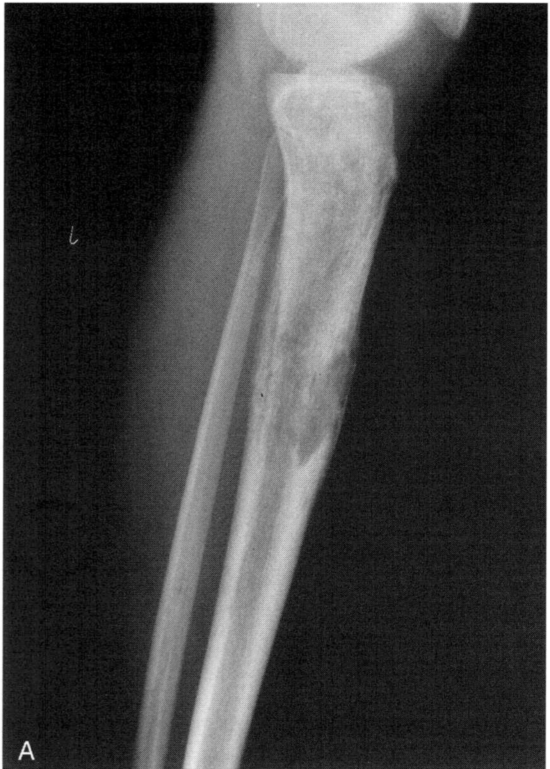

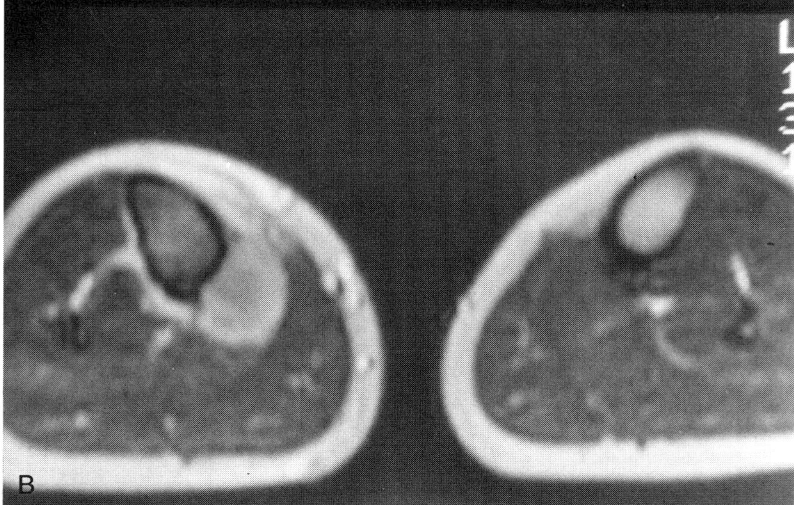

FIGURE 94.23 ➢ Lytic osteosarcoma (telangiectatic osteosarcoma). *A,* Lateral radiograph of the tibia demonstrates lucent lesion with cortical destruction and periosteal reaction at the junction of the proximal and middle one-third of the bone. *B,* T2-weighted magnetic resonance image at the junction of the proximal and middle one-third of the tibia demonstrate destruction of the posteromedial cortex of the bone with an adjacent soft tissue mass. Note the abnormal signal in the marrow cavity of the bone and soft tissue caused by replacement by tumor.

may occur as much as a decade after surgery. Overall, survival is approximately 80%.

Chondrosarcoma

Chondrosarcoma occurs as a malignant lesion within the medullary cavity in a skeletally mature individual.[13] Although the classic chondrosarcoma is one that arises de novo in essentially normal bone, chondrosarcoma may develop in preexisting lesions, including multiple hereditary exostoses and Ollier's disease. As with osteogenic sarcoma, there are several anatomic and microscopic variants of this tumor. Anatomically, chondrosarcomas may arise either on the surface of the bone — the periosteal chondrosarcoma — or in the soft tissue. They may also complicate, in rare circumstances, benign conditions such as synovial chondromatosis[13] and fibrous dysplasia. Well-described microscopic variants include those that mimic a small cell tumor (mesenchymal chondrosarcoma),[17] those that have a purely lyric appearance and mimic metastatic renal cell carcinoma (clear cell chondrosarcoma),[6] and one in which there is a highly malignant-appearing spindle cell tumor (dedifferentiated chondrosarcoma).[23]

Twelve percent of the classic cases of medullary chondrosarcomas occur at the knee. It is the 9th most commonly reported primary bone tumor, constituting approximately 2% of all bone tumors. Its most common location in the knee is the proximal tibia (54%), followed by the distal femur (40%) and the proximal fibula (6%). In adults, in whom it is most commonly reported, the chondrosarcoma frequently invades the epiphysis and may even involve the joint. Most cases occur between the ages of 30 and 70 years, with rare occurrences before 20 years of age. There is a 1.6:1 male-female ratio. Chondrosarcomas classically show a slow growth, often with a nonspecific clinical history, but vague, mild intermittent pain may occur. Epiphyseal involvement, which is common, can cause effusions. Pathological fractures are rare.

Roentgenographically, there is a slow-growing lytic lesion, usually calcified, eroding the inner aspect of the cortical bone, leaving a scalloped appearance. It is somewhat eccentric at the metaphyseal area and, unlike osteogenic sarcoma, preferentially grows down the medullary cavity. In general, the cortex is thinned and even perforated. Grossly, chondrosarcoma has a bluish-gray appearance with calcifications apparent. There is usually a finely gritty texture. Microscopically, the tumor is characterized by neoplastic pleomorphic cartilage cells; the degree of differentiation toward cartilage is variable (Fig. 94.24). In low-grade lesions, there may be only slight cytological abnormalities, making the differential diagnosis from benign enchondromas quite difficult. However, most cases exhibit a degree of variation from cell to cell and crowding of cells and abnormal mitotic figures, making the diagnosis less difficult. Obviously, large pleomorphic tumors carry a worse prognosis.

In general, the clinical course is more indolent than that of osteogenic sarcoma. The tumor spreads by the hematogenous route; therefore, pulmonary metastases may be encountered.

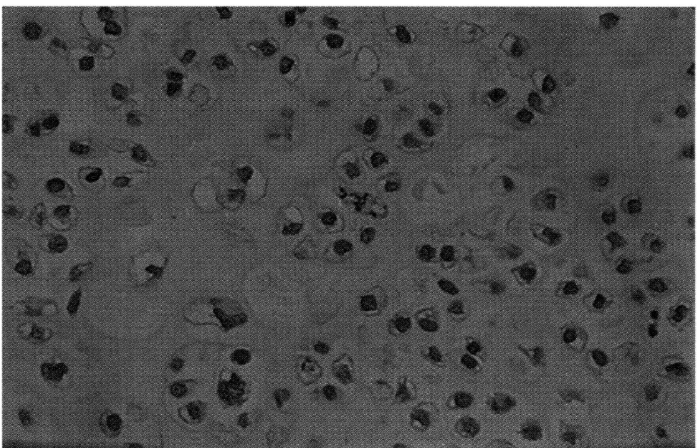

FIGURE 94.24 ➢ Photomicrograph of chondrosarcoma revealing pleomorphic chondrocytes with atypical mitoses (center) enmeshed in a chondroid matrix. The variation from cell to cell, the highly irregular nuclear configurations, the atypical mitoses, and the often binuclear chondrocytes are typical of a malignant cartilage tumor. (From Scott WN: The Knee, vol 2. St. Louis, MO, Mosby-Year Book, 1994, p 1432.)

Dedifferentiated Chondrosarcoma

The dedifferentiated chondrosarcoma is a highly malignant sarcomatous tumor originating in preexisting chondrosarcoma.[23] It is characterized by the juxtaposition of classic chondrosarcomatous areas with a fully malignant, spindle cell tumor, usually a fibrosarcoma or malignant fibrous histiocytoma. Some believe this tumor to be a pluripotential malignant tumor from its onset. However, the classic roentgenographic appearance showing a typical calcified cartilaginous tumor adjacent to a purely lytic permeative lesion supports a change in an underlying chondrosarcoma. Eighteen percent of all reported dedifferentiated chondrosarcomas occur in the knee; this tumor accounts for less than 1% of reported knee tumors. The most common location in the knee is the distal femur (76%), followed by the proximal tibia (24%); there are no reported cases in the proximal fibula and patella. Its more frequent occurrence in the knee than classic chondrosarcoma suggests a predilection for this unusual malignancy for this site. The tumor usually occurs after age 50 years, with a peak between 60 and 70 years. There is a slight male predominance. Dedifferentiated chondrosarcoma is a highly malignant tumor with a poor prognosis.

Mesenchymal Chondrosarcoma

Mesenchymal chondrosarcoma is a rare form of chondrosarcoma characterized by a population of undifferentiated, mononuclear malignant cells mimicking other small cell malignant tumors such as Ewing's sarcoma and lymphoma.[17] However, admixed with the poorly differentiated small cell population are areas of recognizable chondrosarcoma. The prognosis is poor. Only 8% of cases have been reported in the knee. This rare tumor may occur in the distal femur (50%), proximal fibula (30%), and proximal tibia (20%).

Malignant Fibrous Histiocytoma and Fibrosarcoma

Two predominantly fibroblastic malignancies of the knee are the fibrosarcoma and the malignant fibrous histiocytoma.[24] These highly malignant tumors are more frequently reported in soft tissue but may occur de novo in bone. They are distinguished by their microscopic appearance; the fibrosarcoma is composed predominantly of spindle cell pleomorphic fibroblasts, often arranged in a herringbone pattern, as opposed to the malignant fibrous histiocytoma (MFH), a tumor of heterogeneous cellularity that may include fibroblasts, macrophages or histiocytes, as well as inflammatory cells. In the MFH the disorganized growth pattern is striking; tumor cells proliferate in a swirling or storiform pattern. Forty-four percent of fibrosarcomas reported in the literature occur at the knee; fibrosarcoma represents the 5th most common primary osseous tumor, constituting 5% of all reported tumor cases. Its most common location in the knee is the distal femur (61%), followed by the proximal tibia (34%) and the proximal fibula (5%). Very rare before puberty, it is most diffusely distributed between the ages of 15 and 60 years and affects both sexes relatively equally. Pain is the most common feature; there is a frequent occurrence of pathologic fracture. Roentgenographically, the tumor is purely osteolytic, characteristic of most benign and malignant tumors of fibrous origin. The tumor is more indolent than osteogenic sarcoma, particularly those that have a low-grade histologically. However, high-grade tumors may spread hematogeneously; pulmonary and bone metastases are frequent.

Malignant fibrous histiocytoma has been reported with less frequency than fibrosarcoma (Fig. 94.25). Its roentgenographic appearance, clinical symptoms, age, and sex distribution mimic those of fibrosarcoma. Spindle cell tumors, such as fibrosarcoma and MFH, have been reported as complications of both radiotherapy and bone infarction.

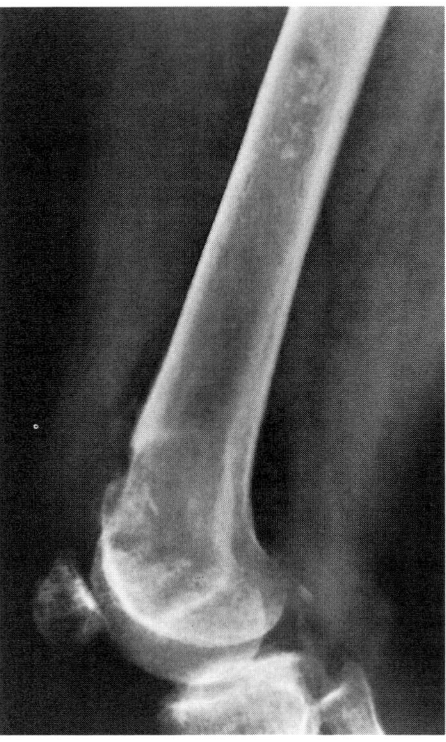

FIGURE 94.25 ➢ Malignant fibrous histiocytoma. Lateral radiograph demonstrating a poorly defined lucent lesion in the distal metaphyses of the femur. There is destruction of the adjacent cortex in the anterior surface of the distal femur. Faint calcifications are seen in the tumor as well as in the midportion of the femoral shaft. This is a case of bone infarctions with superimposed degeneration into a malignant fibrous histiocytoma. (From Scott WN: The Knee, vol 2. St. Louis, MO, Mosby-Year Book, 1994, p 1433.)

Ewing's Sarcoma

The classic Ewing's sarcoma is a permeating, destructive lesion of the diaphysis of a long bone in a child; laboratory, clinical, and roentgenographic symptoms often mimic those of osteomyelitis.[1] There may be fever, anemia, elevated sedimentation rate, and leukocytosis. The diagnosis is made by the histological identification of a population of undifferentiated round cells, which characteristically have abundant glycogen and express the MIC_2 antigen, a 30- to 32-kd cell surface glycoprotein. A chromosome translocation t(11;22)(q24;q12) has been shown to be characteristic of Ewing's sarcoma. Numerous small or round cell tumors may affect the skeleton either in a primary or secondary fashion, and laboratory expertise is required in differentiating them. These round cell tumors include lymphomas, acute leukemias, and other more rare entities. Thirteen percent of all reported cases of Ewing's sarcoma occur at the knee. It is the 8th most commonly reported primary osseous knee tumor, constituting approximately 3% of all cases. The most common location in the knee is the distal femur (46%), followed by the proximal tibia (35%) and the proximal fibula (19%). Approximately 90% of all cases occur between the ages of 5 and 25 years, with a 1.5:1 male-female ratio.

In general, Ewing's sarcoma presents with pain, which may be mild and intermittent but progressively severe. Swelling occurs early and associated symptoms include weight loss, low-grade fever, anemia, leukocytosis, and increased sedimentation rate. These symptoms may parallel progression of the tumor and indicate a poor prognosis. Radiographic features are variable, but the classic Ewing's sarcoma shows a permeative destructive lesion that anatomically invades the cortex and elevates the periosteum, causing a layering or onion-skin appearance to the periosteal tissue (Fig. 94.26). The spread of Ewing's sarcoma is more

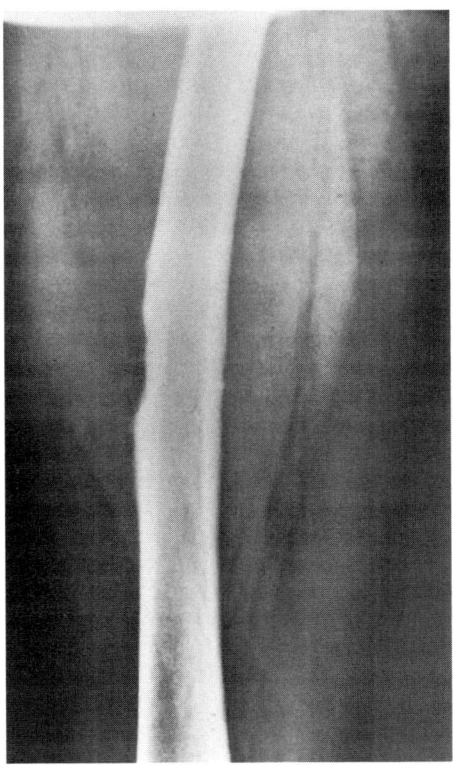

FIGURE 94.26 ➢ Ewing's sarcoma. Frontal radiographs of the femur showing shallow defect in the anteromedial cortex of the shaft of the bone. Faint periosteal reaction surrounds this defect. On biopsy, this proved to be a Ewing's sarcoma. These neoplasms arise from the marrow cavity of the bone and grow by invasion of the cortex and displacement of periosteum. Multilayered periosteal reaction ("onion skin" appearance) is typical for Ewing's sarcoma. At times, as in this case, the growth of the neoplasm is not circumferential and results in localized invasion of the cortex and localized periosteal reaction. The shallow defect (saucer sign) is seen at times in these lesions. The cortical defect is apparently due to pressure by the tumor on the outer surface of the bone. (From Scott WN: The Knee, vol 2. St. Louis, MO, Mosby-Year Book, 1994, p 1434.)

extensive than can be demonstrated by roentgenographic studies. In this regard, CT scans, bone scans, and MRI scans may be helpful.

On gross appearance, Ewing's sarcoma is a soft, grayish-white tumor with abundant areas of necrosis. The inflammation that accrues with necrosis may lead to misinterpretation of diagnosis. However, in an adequate sample, the diffuse population of homogeneous, small round cells with scant cytoplasm confirms the presence of a malignant tumor (Fig. 94.27). The histogenesis of Ewing's sarcoma is unknown. The usual clinical course is one of fairly rapid growth; if left untreated, it will disseminate quickly to other parts of the skeleton and hematogeneously throughout the body, including through lymphatic channels. The prognosis for Ewing's sarcoma has dramatically improved with the advent of adjuvant therapies. Treatment with a combination of surgery, chemotherapy, and radiation has improved the 5-year survival in the range of 50%. In long-term survivors of modern protocols, post-treatment malignancies, including osteosarcoma, have evolved.

Lymphoma

Both Hodgkin's and non-Hodgkin's lymphomas can arise de novo in the skeleton, although most lymphomas involve the skeleton in a secondary fashion after spread from lymph organs. Most patients with terminal lymphomas from lymph node origin have skeletal involvement at the time of death. However, lymphomas may arise within the skeleton as a primary process. Hodgkin's lymphoma is identified by the recognition histologically of a heterogeneous cell population, including eosinophils and plasma cells, but most importantly by the identification of the Reed-Sternberg cell, a cell characterized by its large mirror-image clear nucleus and red nucleolus. With regard to non-Hodgkin's lymphomas, studies using techniques applied to lymphomas arising within lymph nodes have shown that the histological type, stage, and presence and degree of soft tissue invasion are important indicators of survival potential in non-Hodgkin's lymphoma of the skeleton.[12]

Non-Hodgkin's lymphomas of the skeleton can be classified by the microscopic features of the predominant cell type; the most common reported non-Hodgkin's lymphoma of bone is a diffusely infiltrative large cell tumor. Those with cleaved nuclei have shown a better prognosis than those that have a noncleaved or immunoblastic appearance. Less commonly described variants of lymphoma include the undifferentiated or Burkitt's type as well as the well-differentiated or small lymphocytic type lymphomas. Long-term survivorship is far more likely in patients who present with osseous

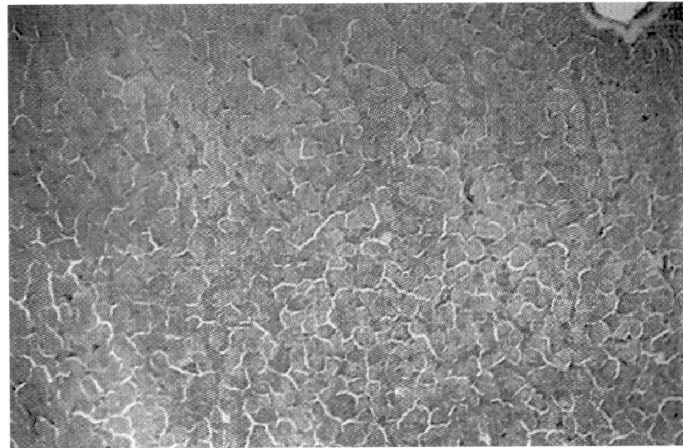

FIGURE 94.27 ➢ Photomicrograph of Ewing's sarcoma reveals a homogeneous cell population characterized by cells with sparse cytoplasm and bland nuclear detail characteristic of this malignant, small cell tumor. The pink cytoplasmic glycogen characteristic of Ewing's sarcoma is demonstrated here using a periodic-acid Schiff stain. Special studies such as genetic alterations and cytoplasmic markers are required for the specific classification of small cell tumors. (From Scott WN: The Knee, vol 2. St. Louis, MO, Mosby-Year Book, 1994, p 1434.)

lymphomas localized to one bone than those in which the tumor has disseminated in the skeleton. Lymphomas present with a lytic pattern but may have a mixed or primary sclerotic appearance in the skeleton.

Multiple Myeloma

Multiple myeloma is a malignant tumor of plasma cells associated with widespread intraosseous proliferation of plasma cells with ensuing destruction and lysis of bone. Clinically, multiple myeloma is usually associated clinically with severe bone pain. Lytic lesions occur throughout the skeleton, including the extremities, often leading to fracture. The laboratory abnormalities associated with multiple myeloma include hypercalcemia and hypergammaglobulinemia. The plasma cells produce a monoclonal gammopathy, which is identified by serum or urine immunoelectrophoresis. In screening for multiple myeloma, the hypergammaglobulinemia may be verified by performing serum protein electrophoresis in which a broad band is detected in the gamma globulin range. However, to detect a monoclonal gammopathy, a characteristic of plasma cell malignancies, the diagnostic tests are serum and urine immunoelectrophoresis, which detects the monoclonal production of one heavy chain (immunoglobulin [Ig]M, IgG, IgA, or others) or one light chain (kappa or lambda) or both.

Plasma cell aggregates filling at least one-half of a high-power microscopic field or obliterating one fatty marrow interspace have been estimated to identify myeloma correctly in 84% of cases.[35]

Efforts at further quantifying tumorous plasmacytosis have been elusive. Although plasmacytosis greater than 10% is considered worrisome, this can be seen in 15% of controls, and 40% of myeloma patients have had less than 10% plasmacytosis on presentation.[35] Nonetheless, notwithstanding important clinical staging parameters, packing of marrow by plasma cells and more than five mitoses per high-power field have been associated with a poor prognosis.

Other findings include amyloid production in fewer than 10% of cases; the amyloid may focally calcify superficially to create an appearance resembling that of osteosarcoma.

Myeloma cells produce bone-resorbing factors (cytokines such as interleukin-1β [IL-1β]) and tumor necrosis factor β [TNF-β]), which explains its destructive lysis of the skeleton. Roentgenographic abnormalities are typical. Classically, discrete, punched-out lytic lesions prevail, but diffuse osteoporosis (osteopenia) with vertebral compression fractures may prevail. The skull is involved in 20% of cases, and the findings are usually multiple lytic lesions.

The most common roentgenographic features of myeloma are demineralization and lytic bone lesions, which may be assessed by routine roentgenograms, CT, and MRI, the latter of which is the most sensitive. Bone densitometry techniques have been applied to myeloma patients. Unlike other modalities, dual-energy x-ray absorptiometry has demonstrated sensitivity in revealing new bone after treatment, which indicates a role for it in assessment of therapy.

Although sclerosis may occur, myeloma is almost always lytic, explaining the lack of uptake on bone scanning, because positive scanning requires either hypervascularity or increased mineralization activity or both. Hot myeloma scans usually indicate fracture. Affected bones may show remodeling expansion or soft tissue extension, but sclerosis and periosteal reactions are rare. Skeletal surveys remain negative in up to 20% of cases.

In rare circumstances, myeloma may be associated with bone production, a sclerotic variant or the POEMS syndrome (Polyneuropathy, Osteosclerotic bone lesions, Endocrinopathy, *M* protein, and Skin changes).

The natural history of multiple myeloma is progressive, and although there is currently no prospect for cure, realistic goals of achieving partial or complete remission sustained over time are achievable. Anemia, weakness, bone pain, fatigue, and fractures give way to renal failure, bleeding, recurrent infections, and death. Chemotherapy is the mainstay of treatment, both initially and after relapse. Intermittent courses of melphalan and prednisone have been standard; remissions are generally defined as a 75% reduction in serum myeloma protein, a 95% reduction in Bence Jones proteinuria, and fewer than 5% bone marrow plasma cells.

Thrombocytopenia, low hemoglobin and elevated creatinine levels, extensive lytic lesions, and a large tumor burden are considered poor prognostic indicators.

Metastatic Carcinoma

Metastatic cancer to the skeleton is the most common malignant tumor affecting bone. The bone is the third most common site of metastasis; bone metastasis is revealed in 60% of cancer patients at autopsy. The most frequently seen tumor affecting the skeleton in patients dying of metastatic cancer are those of the breast, prostate, lung, thyroid, and kidney. Metastatic cancer has a predilection for the marrow space of bone, but in rare circumstances it may affect cortical bone. This is usually due to metastatic lung cancer. The most commonly affected parts of the skeleton are the spine. The lumbar vertebrae are more commonly involved than thoracic, cervical, and sacral vertebrae. The exception is prostate cancer, which has a predilection for metastasis to the lumbar and sacral vertebral bodies, and breast and lung cancers, which prefer thoracic vertebrae. In order of decreasing frequency, after the spine, metastatic cancer occurs in the ribs, pelvis, proximal ends of the bones, sternum, and skull. Factors associated with metastatic spread have, for the most part, been elusive to investigators, but more than likely involve anatomic aspects of the vasculature, perhaps explaining the predilection of prostate cancer for vertebral bodies via Batson's plexus, variability in the susceptibility of different organs, and different properties of tumor cells themselves.

Metastatic cancer usually causes lysis or destruction; the most common features of metastatic cancer are radiolucencies and eventual fractures. Thyroid, kidney, lung, and gastrointestinal tumors most commonly cause lysis of the skeleton. Prostate most often causes bone formation and osteoblastic metastases. Breast cancer often gives a mixed picture.

More specifically in the skeleton, it has been estimated that 30% of metastatic osseous lesions are located in the femur; one-third of these occur below the subtrochanteric region in the shaft or in the supracondylar region.[40] Metastatic lesions may be suspected when a symptomatic lesion is seen on plain films or abnormal areas are found on bone scan, with either increased or decreased uptake. It should be pointed out, when contemplating biopsy to establish the diagnosis, that metastatic renal and thyroid tumors may have a significant increase in vascularity with even palpable pulses or bruits.

The tibia is a relatively infrequent site of involvement by metastatic cancer, and usually tibial metastases occur late in the development of metastatic disease.[4] It should be noted that metastatic bone disease may be the presenting complaint in patients with metastatic cancer; the primary site is not immediately appreciated. In fact, cases in which a primary cancer may be indeterminate after extensive clinical and roentgenographical work-up are well known. Even after autopsies in some studies, approximately 1% of patients presenting with metastatic cancer may have an undetectable primary site. More than likely, however, tumors uncovered after a careful search are common tumors, such as those of the breast, lung, thyroid, and kidney; an increased number of pancreatic cancers are evident in this group, requiring evaluation.

The reasons for bone-associated changes in metastatic cancer are not clear but may include a number of factors. Some tumors such as multiple myeloma secrete cytokine-resorbing factors such as IL-1β and TNF-β. Others secrete parathyroid-like hormones, which activate the remodeling cycle, in particular osteoclastic resorption. Tumors are well known to be associated with both marrow and bone necrosis, processes that may cause definable bone scan and plain film changes. The release of other local bone-mediating factors, as well as the possibility of direct mechanical or pressure effects, may also play a role.

SECONDARY MALIGNANCIES

Malignant bone tumors may occur in rare circumstances as a complication of benign tumors and tumor-like lesions of the skeleton as well as after infarction and iatrogenic intervention. Chondrosarcomas, for example, may complicate benign cartilaginous conditions, such as multiple hereditary exostosis (MHE) and Ollier's disease (enchondromatosis). The incidence varies considerably, but is probably less than 10% in MHE, but as high as 100% in Maffucci's syndrome, a variant of Ollier's disease. Solitary osteochondromas and solitary enchondromas are an extremely rare setting for the development of a malignant cartilaginous tumor. Chondrosarcomas have also been described as complicating cases of fibrous dysplasia and synovial chondromatosis, albeit rare phenomena.

Paget's disease, a metabolic disturbance of the skeleton in which there is an increased remodeling with marked increase in osteoblast and osteoclast remodeling of the skeleton, may be a monofocal or multifocal condition. The latter is associated with the development over time of malignant neoplasms, which include osteogenic sarcomas, chondrosarcomas, lymphomas, and even giant cell lesions (Avellino's tumor).[16]

Radioactivity may lead to the development of tumors, including leukemias; the classic description is their development in radium dial workers after oral ingestion of the radioactive dyes. Postirradiation sarcomas of the skeleton are now well described and, in fact, may be predicted in a small percentage of patients treated for a various number of tumors, including lymphomas.

Bone infarction may also be the setting for the development of malignancy in the skeleton, including leukemias. Interest has been generated in a number of reports showing an association between the implantation of orthopedic devices and the subsequent development of sarcomas at that site.[15] However, even though certain metal components are carcinogenic in laboratory animals, the sporadic and sparse reports of such associations in humans more than likely represent a coincidental occurrence, albeit one of potential serious concern.

In general, malignant transformation may occur in a broad range of lesions. Squamous cell carcinoma may arise in draining sinuses over many years' duration in chronic osteomyelitis. Infarction, of whatever cause, may lead to the development of malignancies, particularly MFH, osteogenic sarcomas, and even, most recently, angiosarcomas. Interestingly, malignancies reported as complications of underlying skeletal disorders are often composed of malignant spindle cell sarcomas, such as malignant fibrous histiocytoma. These spindle cell sarcomas have been reported complicating chrondromatosis, fibrous dysplasia, radiation disorders, Paget's disease, bone infarction, and even in association with metallic implants. In general, sarcomas developing in the setting of underlying bone disease are highly malignant and carry a poor prognosis.

Acknowledgment

We acknowledge Dr. Charles A. Gatto for his contribution to an earlier edition of this chapter.

References

1. Bacci G, Toni A, Avella M, et al: Long-term results in 144 localized Ewing's sarcoma patients treated with combined therapy. Cancer 63:1477, 1989.
2. Bauer TW, Dorfman HD: Intraosseous ganglion: A clinicopathologic study of 11 cases. Am J Surg Pathol 6:207, 1982.
3. Bauer TW, Dorfman HD, Lathan JT Jr: Periosteal chondroma: A clinicopathologic study of 23 cases. Am J Surg Pathol 6:631, 1982.

4. Beauchamp CP, Sim FH: Lesions of the tibia. In Sim FH, ed: Diagnosis and Treatment of Metastatic Bone Disease: A Multidisciplinary Approach to Management. New York, Raven Press, 1987.
5. Bertoni R, Unni K, Beabout JW, et al: Parosteal osteoma of bones other than of the skull and face. Cancer 75:2466, 1995.
6. Bjornsson J, Unni KK, Dahlin DC, et al: Clear cell chondrosarcoma of bone: Observations in 47 cases. Am J Surg Pathol 8:223, 1984.
7. Boseker EH, Bickel WH, Dahlin DC: A clinicopathologic study of simple unicameral bone cysts. Surg Gynecol Obstet 127:550, 1968.
8. Caffey J: On fibrous defects in cortical walls of growing tubular bones: Their radiologic appearance, structure, prevalence, natural course, and diagnostic significance. Adv Pediatr 7:13, 1955.
9. Campanacci M, Baldini N, Boriani S, et al: Giant-cell tumor of bone. J Bone Joint Surg Am 69(1):106, 1987.
10. Campanacci M, Laus M: Osteofibrous dysplasia of the tibia and fibula. J Bone Joint Surg Am 63:367, 1981.
11. Clarke BE, Xipell JM, Thomas DP: Benign fibrous histiocytoma of bone. Am J Surg Pathol 9(1):806, 1985.
12. Clayton F, Butler JJ, Ayala AG, et al: Non-Hodgkin's lymphoma in bone: Pathologic and radiologic features with clinical correlates. Cancer 60:2494, 1987.
13. Gitelis S, Bertoni F, Picci P, et al: Chondrosarcoma of bone: The experience at the Instituto Ortopedico Rizzoli. J Bone Joint Surg Am 63:1248, 1981.
14. Greis PE, Hankin FM: Eosinophiliac granuloma: The management of solitary lesions of bone. Clin Orthop 257:204, 1990.
15. Hamblen DL, Carter RL: Sarcoma and joint replacement [editorial]. J Bone Joint Surg Br 66(5):625, 1984.
16. Healey JH, Buss D: Radiation and pagetic osteosarcoma. Clin Orthop 270:128, 1991.
17. Huvos AG, Rosen G, Dabaka M, et al: Mesenchymal chondrosarcoma: A clinicopathologic analysis of 35 patients with emphasis on treatment. Cancer 51:1230, 1983.
18. Jackson RP, Reckling FW, Mantz FA: Osteoid osteoma and osteoblastoma: Similar histologic lesions with different natural histories. Clin Orthop 128:303, 1977.
19. Kransdorf MJ, Moser RP, Vinh TN, et al: Primary tumors of the patella. A review of 42 cases. Skeletal Radiol 128:303, 1989.
20. Larsson SE, Lorentzon R, Boquist L: Giant-cell tumor of bone: A demographic, clinical and histopathological study of all cases recorded in the Swedish Cancer Registry for years 1958 through 1968. J Bone Joint Surg Am 57:167, 1975.
21. Lucas DR, Unni K, McLeod RA, et al: Osteoblastoma. Clinicopathologic study of 306 cases. Hum Pathol 25:117, 1994.
22. Martin SE, Dwyer A, Kissane JM, et al: Small-cell osteosarcoma. Cancer 50:990, 1982.
23. McCarthy EF, Dorfman HD: Chondrosarcoma of bone with dedifferentiation: A study of eighteen cases. Hum Patrol 13:36, 1982.
24. Nishida J, Sim FH, Wenger DE, et al: Malignant fibrous histiocytoma of bone. A clinicopathologic study of 81 patients. Cancer 79:482, 1997.
25. Nishida J, Tajima K, Abe M, et al: Desmoplastic fibroma. Aggressive curettage as a surgical alternative to treatment. Clin Orthop 320:142, 1995.
26. Peterson HA: Multiple hereditary osteochondromata. Clin Orthop 239:222, 1989.
27. Petrilli AS, Gentil FC, Epelman S, et al: Increased survival, limb preservation, and prognostic factors for osteosarcoma. Cancer 68:733, 1991.
28. Pignatti G, Bacci G, Picci P, et al: Telangiectatic osteogenic sarcoma of the extremities: Results in 17 patients treated with neoadjuvant chemotherapy. Clin Orthop 270:99, 1991.
29. Raymond AK: Surface osteosarcoma. Clin Orthop 270:140, 1991.
30. Ritschl P, Karnel F, Hajek P: Fibrous metaphyseal defects—Determination of their origin and natural history using a radiomorphological study. Skeletal Radiol 17(15):8, 1988.
31. Schajowicz F: Tumors and Tumorlike Lesions of Bone and Joints. New York, Springer-Verlag, 1981.
32. Singer FR: Fibrous dysplasia of bone. The bone lesion unmasked. Am J Clin Pathol 151(6):1511, 1997.
33. Springfield DS, Capanna R, Gherlinzoni F, et al: Chondroblastoma: A review of seventy cases. J Bone Joint Surg Am 67:748, 1985.
34. Stephenson RB, Londen MD, Hankin FM, et al: Fibrous dysplasia: An analysis of options for treatment. J Bone Joint Surg Am 69(3): 400, 1987.
35. Sukpanichnant S, Cousar JB, Leelasiri A, et al: Diagnostic criteria and histologic grading in multiple myeloma: Histologic and immunohistologic analysis of 176 cases with clinical correlation. Hum Pathol 25:308, 1994.
36. Vergel DeDios AM, Bond JR, Shives TC, et al: Aneurysmal bone cyst: A clinicopathologic study of 238 cases. Cancer 69(12): 2921, 1992.
37. Vigorita VJ: Orthopaedic Pathology. Philadelphia, Lippincott-Williams-Wilkins, 1999.
38. Vigorita VJ, Ghelman B: Localization of osteoid osteomas —Use of radionuclide scanning and autoimaging in identifying the nidus. Am J Clin Pathol 79(2):223, 1983.
39. Wester SM, Beabout JW, Unni KK, et al: Langerhans' cell granulomatosis (histiocytosis X) of bone in adults. Am J Surg Pathol 6: 413, 1982.
40. Wilkins RM, Sim FH: Lesions of the femur. In Diagnosis and Treatment of Metastatic Bone Disease: A Multidisciplinary Approach to Management. New York, Raven Press, 1987.
41. Wu CT, Inwards CY, O'Laughlin S, et al: Chondromyxoid fibroma of bone. A clinicopathologic review of 278 cases. Hum Pathol 29:438, 1998.

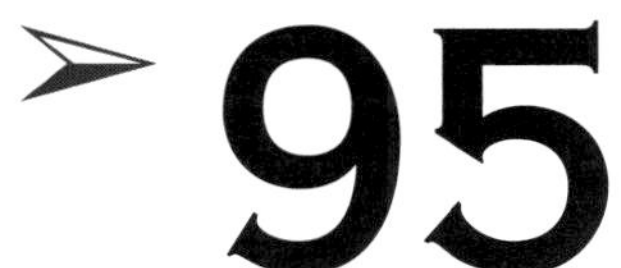

Bone and Soft-Tissue Tumors Around the Knee

JOHN H. HEALEY

Tumors about the knee are relatively common and should be considered routinely when evaluating a patient with knee pain or a mass. The entire spectrum of benign and malignant bone and soft-tissue lesions occur frequently in this location. Metastatic lesions may also present in this site, although less often than in the hip. Tumors must be recognized and treated promptly to optimize oncological and functional results. General orthopedists, sports medicine physicians, and knee specialists encounter many lesions in this region. They must recognize the clinical features, know the appropriate diagnostic tests to order, and be familiar with the therapeutic options for the common diagnostic entities.

This chapter presents clinical, epidemiological, and imaging information about bone and soft-tissue tumors that occur about the knee. It discusses general concepts of staging, biopsy, and treatment that are pertinent for all knee surgeons. The current data on the function and durability of reconstructions used after tumor excisions are reviewed. This information is of particular interest to tumor surgeons and adult reconstructive knee surgeons contending with increasingly complex primary and revision problems in nononcological practice.

BONE TUMORS

General Concepts

The two critical questions to answer in diagnosing bone tumors are (1) who needs a biopsy and (2) who should perform the biopsy.

Who needs a biopsy? Any person with a lesion that defies clinical and radiographic diagnosis or with a lesion that requires treatment. If the history, examination, and imaging studies cannot be reconciled, a tissue diagnosis is needed. A preliminary clinical diagnosis is reached from a careful history, a physical examination, and a knowledge of the epidemiology of tumors. This defines the "pretest probability" of diagnosing each of the lesions that can be found around the knee. Coupled with discriminating evaluation of the plain radiographs (still the most specific imaging study for bone tumors), these tools can determine which lesions need biopsy sampling.[25] If you are in doubt, get another opinion. Orthopedic oncological and imaging expertise is available in most medical centers.

Who should perform the biopsy? Generally, if you are not comfortable treating the diseases that could potentially be diagnosed from a biopsy of a lesion, it is better to refer the patient to a specialist. Whoever is going to treat the tumor should have the opportunity to biopsy it and analyze the clinical, radiographic, gross, and microscopic features of the tumor. This principle is crucial to correctly diagnose tumors and avoid tragedies.[95, 141] If the biopsy results, radiographs, and other clinical elements are inconsistent, further analysis is needed. This may be another test, biopsy, or clinical follow-up. Understanding tumor epidemiology and behavior is fundamental to this process.

Clinical Features

Pain is usually the first symptom. Bone pain is either lesional or mechanical. Lesional pain comes from increased pressure within the bone compartment or periosteal extension of the tumor and is highly correlated with growth rate. It may be worse at night. Malignant and aggressive benign bone tumors are almost always painful. Slowly growing tumors such as low-grade chondrosarcomas may be pain-free in as many as one-third of patients. A mechanical component is often present as well. Pain that is exacerbated by weight-bearing reflects structural insufficiency and may herald a fracture. Rarely, the presenting symptom is a pathological fracture.

The medical history can be diagnostic. It helps to exclude infection and congenital conditions. Primary tumors lack distinguishing histories in most cases. Focused examination may reveal the source of metastatic cancers. The family history is occasionally diagnostic. Notable examples include the Li-Fraumeni syndrome of multiple cancers that originate from a defect in the *p53* tumor suppressor gene. It often includes osteogenic sarcoma (OGS) or soft-tissue sarcoma. The most common benign familial condition is osteochondromatosis.

Coincidental findings are common. Thirty percent of patients report that they sustained trauma to the area. Usually, the injury brings a previously unsuspected lesion to the patient's attention. Patellar pain is ubiquitous, particularly after muscle atrophy and gait abnormalities develop from favoring of the affected extremity. The physician must exhibit great restraint to avoid diagnosing the obvious comorbid condition and miss the offending primary lesion or tumor. Therefore, even when a soft-tissue injury, malalignment syndrome, or benign intra-articular derangement is suspected, there may be an underlying tumor. If symptoms do not resolve predictably, patients should undergo radiographic examination. If surgery is planned, even arthroscopy alone, proper imaging should be obtained to exclude occult pathology.

Physical examination findings are nonspecific. A palpable mass, a painful or restricted joint motion, and an effusion may be detected. Tenderness is variable and most common in patients with tumors causing periosteal reactions. Vascular and neurological findings are uncommon but may reflect compression or invasion of popliteal structures. Examination of the hip is important because this may be the source of referred knee pain. Lymphoma is the only primary bone tumor that involves lymph nodes regularly. Lymphadenopathy from spindle cell and round cell sarcomas occurs in 1% to 2% of cases.[49] General examination of the chest, abdomen, and pelvic organs may reveal the site of the primary cancer in cases of metastatic disease.

As many as 43% of normal children have a developmental or neoplastic bony defect during growth as reported by Caffey.[20] Among these abnormalities, fibrous cortical defects or metaphyseal conversion defects are the most common (Fig. 95.1). It is estimated that 30% of children experience a defect in the metaphysis of the distal femur or proximal tibia sometime during growth. This lesion is usually found incidentally and is asymptomatic.

The importance of this lesion is to distinguish it from a true neoplasm that requires intervention. Most resolve spontaneously but require mechanical protection of the bone if they are large. If the lesion is painful, biopsy sampling and treatment are needed because pain indicates that either a microfracture is developing or the radiographic diagnosis is wrong. Although histologically indistinguishable from fibrous cortical defects, nonossifying fibromas differ clinically. They are larger, are corticated, and persist after skeletal maturity. They warrant excision and bone grafting.

The most common benign bone tumor (12% of all tumors and 50% of benign bone tumors) is the solitary osteochondroma (Fig. 95.2). Nearly one-half of these develop about the knee. They cause a variable amount of pain. Symptomatic osteochondromas and those growing after skeletal maturity warrant excisional biopsy if the diagnosis is ensured. The perichondrium and as much overlying bursae as is practical should be excised to prevent recurrence. Be careful when ascribing knee pain to the radiographically obvious osteochondroma. The lesion has been there for a long time, yet the symptoms only developed recently. Rule out other causes for the pain. A common error is to ascribe anterior knee pain to an osteochondroma of the medial femoral metaphysis.

Because the disease process is developmental and there is uniformly some distortion of the distal femur, patellofemoral malalignment and poor tracking occur routinely. Patellar pain syndromes may be exacerbated by surgery that weakens the vastus medialis while an osteochondroma is removed. Excision may need to be coupled with lateral retinacular release in such patients, one of the few occasions in which it is appropriate to perform incidental reconstructive surgery in tandem with tumor resection. Incisional biopsy and staged resection are reserved for osteochondromas with large cartilaginous caps (i.e., 1.5 cm or more) as seen on magnetic resonance imaging (MRI). Such lesions could have converted to chondrosarcomas, and a staged diagnostic and therapeutic approach is pre-

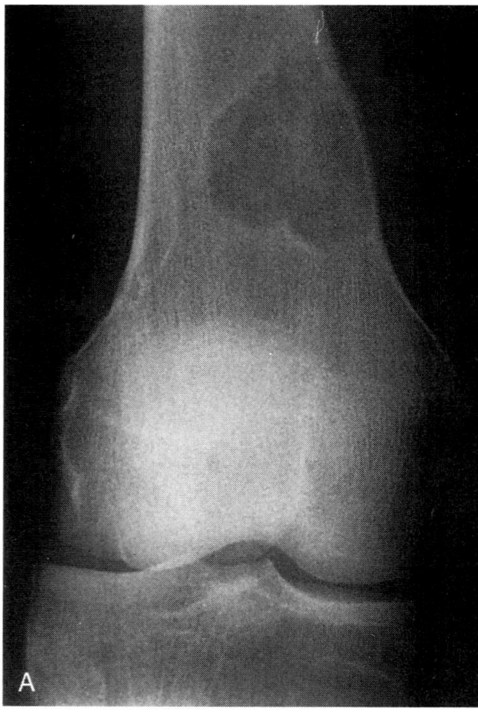

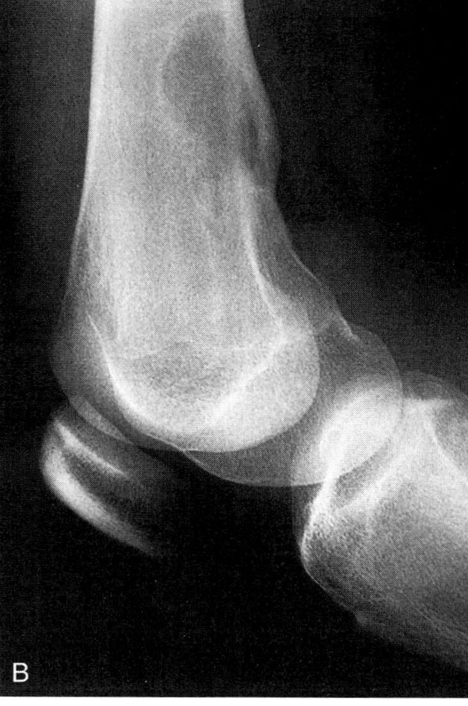

FIGURE 95.1 ➢ AP (*A*) and lateral (*B*) radiographs of a distal femoral nonossifying fibroma. Before closure of the growth plate, the lesion appears similar to incomplete ossification of the periosteal surface.

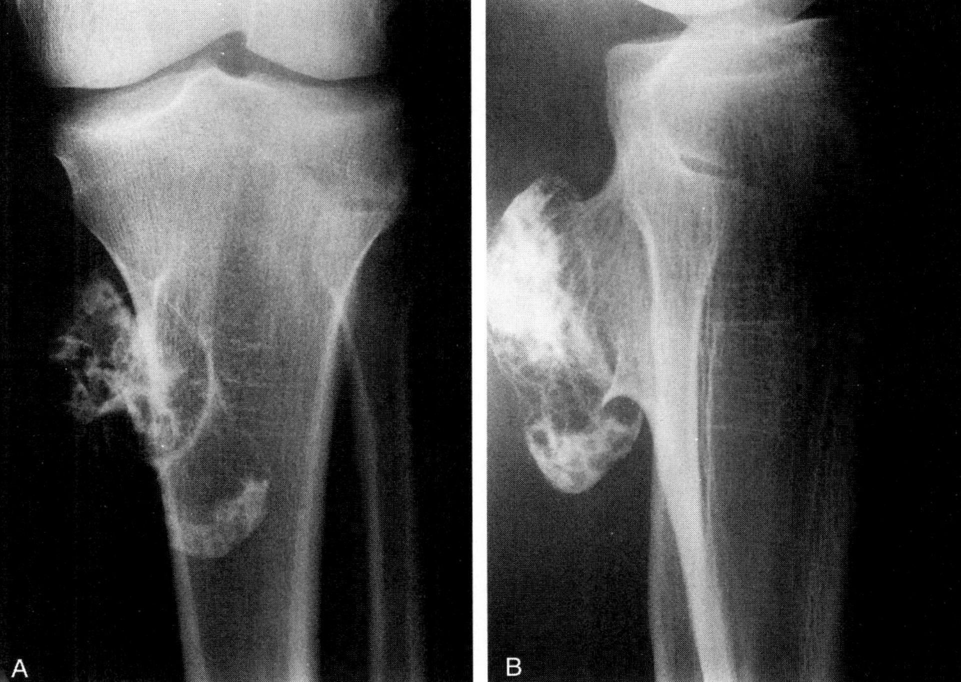

FIGURE 95.2 ➢ AP (*A*) and lateral (*B*) radiographs of a proximal tibial osteochondroma. Note the continuity of the cortex and cancellous bone between the lesion and the tibia. The entire surface is covered by a continuous ossification line, typically associated with a small benign cartilaginous cap.

ferred because the resection margin for a cancer would typically be larger (Fig. 95.3). Prophylactic excision of osteochondromas is rarely indicated because the surgical risks exceed the risk of sarcomatous degeneration (estimated at 0.1%). One should not operate simply because a lesion exists.

Giant cell tumors (GCTs) are lytic epiphyseal tumors that frequently (65%) occur in the distal femur or proximal tibia in young adults.[27, 40, 91, 102, 104, 111, 165] They lack reactive bone formation. When such a tumor is present, either a superimposed aneurysmal bone cyst is there or another diagnosis should be entertained.[97, 101, 116, 161] For example, chondroblastomas or calcifying epiphyseal GCTs usually have a rim of reactive bone. They share the same epiphyseal distribution as GCTs, one-third of cases are around the knee, and they characteristically occur in skeletally immature patients. The tibial spines, even involving the cruciate ligaments,[35] and femoral intercondylar notch are typical haunts for this tumor.[97, 101, 116, 161]

Chondromyxoid fibromas are very rare, but 45% occur in the proximal tibia or fibula.[112, 160] They may also occur at the osteocartilaginous junction of the anterior distal femur and cause considerable patellofemoral pain. These are a few of the benign tumors that have a nonrandom anatomic distribution or distinctive clinical presentation about the knee.

Malignant tumors are less common than benign bone tumors and significantly rarer than the developmental lesions that mimic bone tumors. Conventional OGS is the most common primary bone malignancy.[38] Approximately one-half of these high-grade cancers, an estimated 300 per year in the United States, occur about the knee.[67] The metaphyseal femur or tibia is the typical site (Fig. 95.4).[3, 13, 67, 114, 138] Low-grade surface variants of OGS have distinctive genetic profiles from classic OGS. Huvos reported that over 40% were on the posterior aspect of the femur (Fig. 95.5).[67] Periosteal variants are more cartilaginous and may develop in more diaphyseal locations.[12] Treatment for OGS is detailed later in this chapter and serves as the paradigm for the management of all bone sarcomas. In brief, patients with high-grade tumors need to receive chemotherapy and all tumors should be excised with a margin of normal tissue.

Chondrosarcomas, malignant fibrous histiocytomas, and fibrosarcomas are other malignant spindle cell, mesenchymal tumors that occur regularly about the knee. Their incidence is approximately one-half to two-thirds that of OGSs. These tumors all occur in a somewhat older population. Wide excision is the cornerstone of treatment for these sarcomas. Chemotherapy for these entities is controversial. Its record in chondrosarcoma is poor, but it is worthy of consideration in the highest-grade variants such as dedifferentiated chondrosarcoma because the prognosis is so discouraging.[147] Malignant fibrous histiocytoma is more responsive to chemotherapy and should probably be treated in a fashion similar to that for OGS.[7, 43, 58, 123]

Ewing's sarcoma is classically a diaphyseal cancer of youth. Even so, nearly 50% of them occur in nondiaphyseal locations, and about 20% may occur in young to middle-aged adults. Ewing's sarcoma is particularly common in the femur and is the most common malignancy of the fibula. It serves as the prototype for treatment of round cell tumors and is dealt with in detail later.

Lymphoma (mixed and histiocytic types) may de-

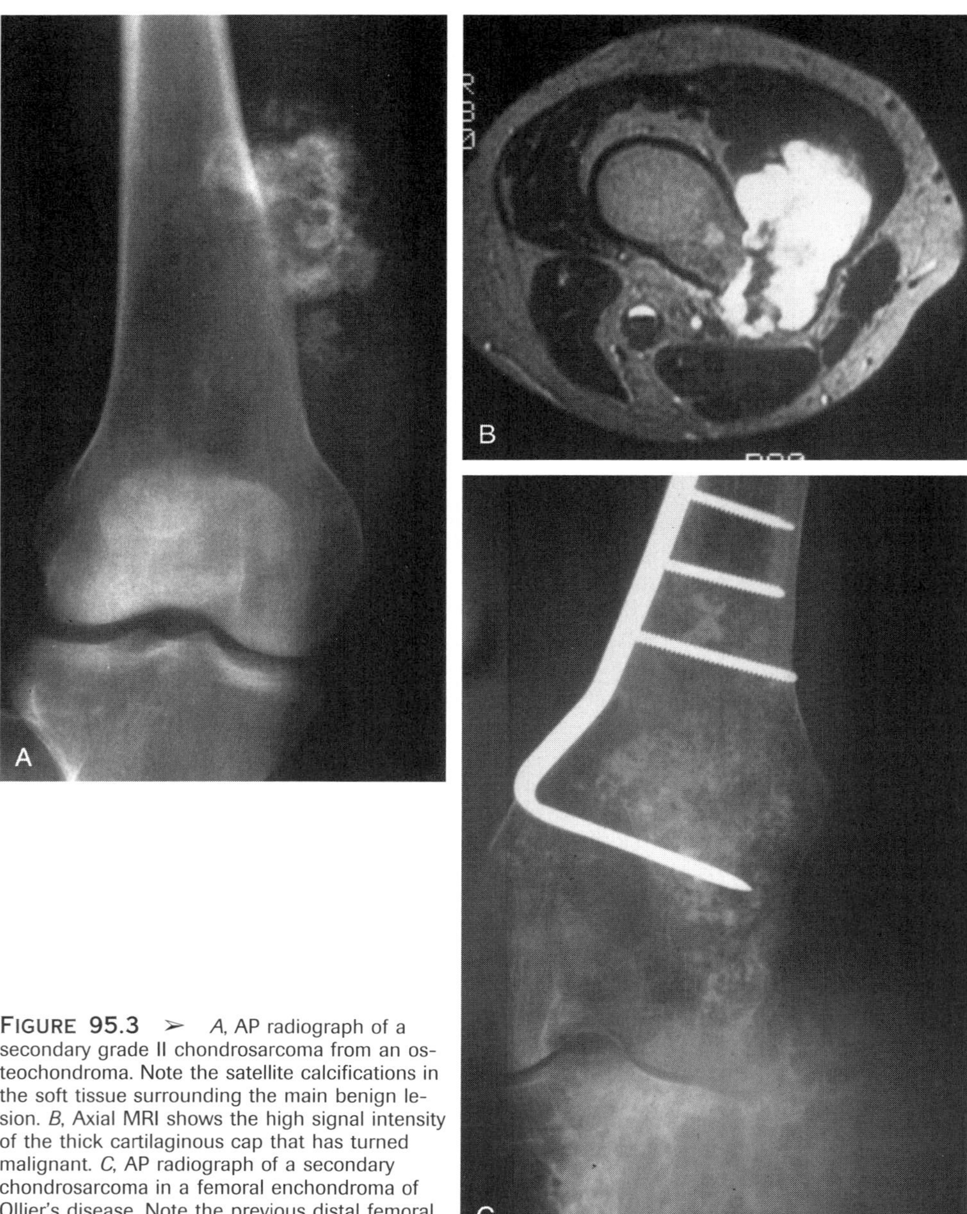

FIGURE 95.3 ➢ *A*, AP radiograph of a secondary grade II chondrosarcoma from an osteochondroma. Note the satellite calcifications in the soft tissue surrounding the main benign lesion. *B*, Axial MRI shows the high signal intensity of the thick cartilaginous cap that has turned malignant. *C*, AP radiograph of a secondary chondrosarcoma in a femoral enchondroma of Ollier's disease. Note the previous distal femoral osteotomy fixation.

velop as a primary bone tumor and seems to have a predilection for the femur in children or adults. Biopsy is usually the only surgery required. Ample tissue should be taken to permit the many special diagnostic studies such as cytogenetics and lymphoma markers.[88]

Multiple myeloma and metastatic lesions are the most common neoplastic knee region lesions in older adults. Breast, renal, and lung cancer are the usual suspects. Biopsy samples should be taken if the lesions are the first site of presumed disseminated disease. Otherwise, treatment should be for mechanical stabilization of diseased bone. Tumor resection and joint reconstruction, similar to that for primary bone tumors, should be reserved for patients with unresponsive tumors and long projected life expectancies.

Diagnostic Imaging Studies

Conventional biplane radiographs are the most useful and specific diagnostic tests.[25, 136, 140] They focus the differential diagnosis and suggest whether the tumor is benign or malignant. Benign lesions have sharp margins, a narrow zone of transition, and well-developed reactive bone surrounding them. They may expand the cortical bone but usually do not destroy it or extend into the soft tissue. Malignant lesions lack a sharp margin, have a wide zone of transition, and elicit a primitive host response such as elevating the periosteum. They often permeate through cortical and cancellous bone and extend into soft tissue. The matrix within the lesion can be diagnostic of specific bone

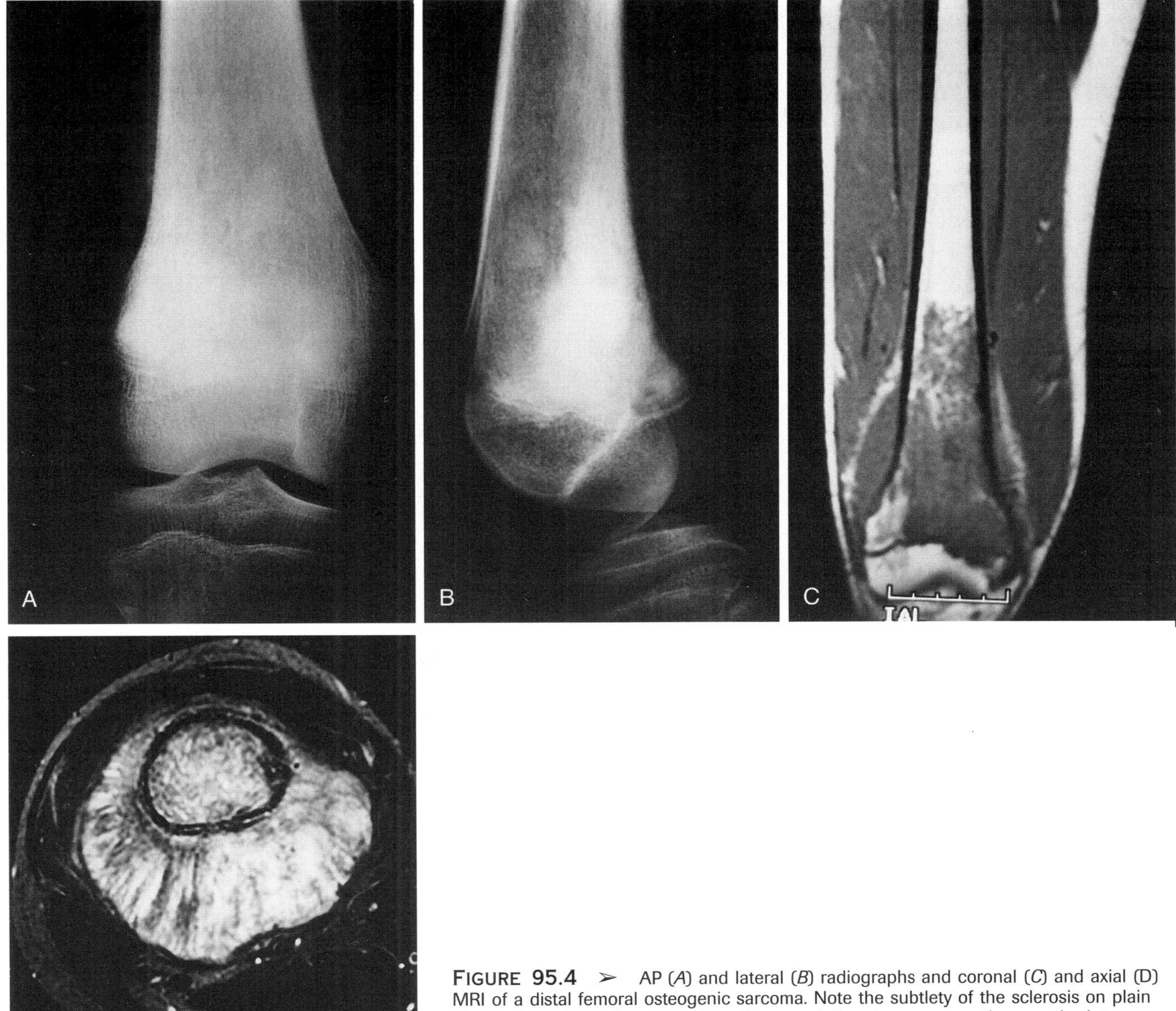

FIGURE 95.4 ➢ AP (*A*) and lateral (*B*) radiographs and coronal (*C*) and axial (D) MRI of a distal femoral osteogenic sarcoma. Note the subtlety of the sclerosis on plain film, periosteal reaction, extension of intramedullary tumor across the growth plate scar and onto the collateral ligament, and the large popliteal mass.

tumors. For example, OGS characteristically produces a white cloud of bony matrix.

Osteochondromas and fibrous cortical defects are radiographic diagnoses.[41, 118] Biopsy samples do not need to be taken unless they grow or become symptomatic. Biopsy samples should be taken from most other lesions.

Serum tests rarely are specific, so they should be ordered selectively. The erythrocyte sedimentation rate is mildly elevated in most malignant tumors, so it does not distinguish them from infections. Multiple myeloma causes significant elevations of the erythrocyte sedimentation rate as well as anemia, azotemia, and even hypercalcemia in widespread disease. The alkaline phosphatase level is elevated in 85% of OGSs and in most patients with Paget's disease of bone. Serum lactate dehydrogenase (LDH) is typically elevated in round cell tumors such as Ewing's sarcoma and lymphoma, with values correlating with tumor burden. Both LDH and alkaline phosphatase have prognostic significance. Patients presenting with elevated levels experience lower long-term survival than patients presenting with normal levels.[105] Serum calcium and parathyroid hormone levels are elevated in brown tumors of hyperparathyroidism, and these laboratory studies should be checked in all patients with multifocal or atypical GCTs because they may be impossible to differentiate histologically from brown tumors.

Pseudotumors of hemophilia should be suspected if there is an appropriate history of coagulopathy. Crystal

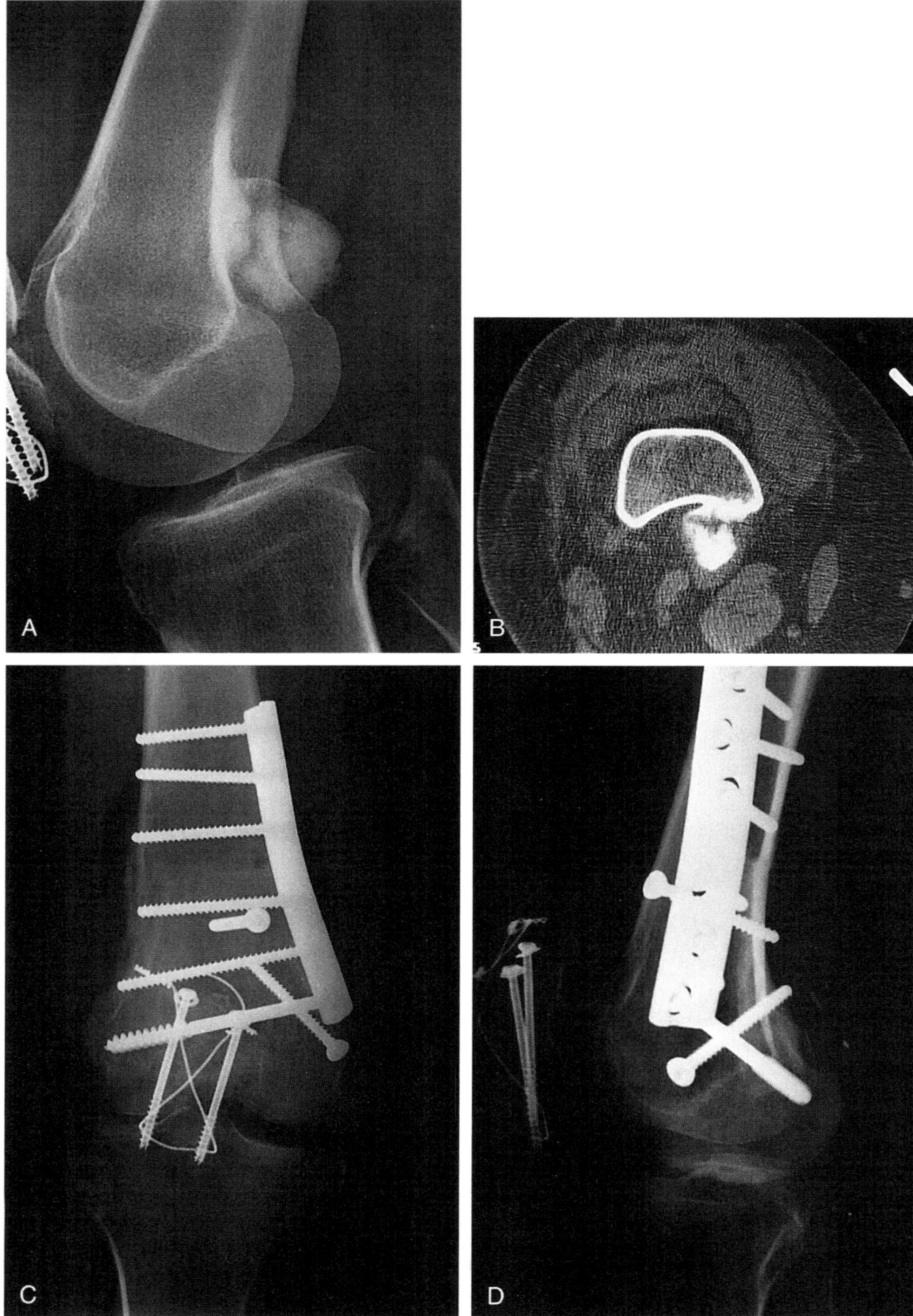

FIGURE 95.5 ➢ *A*, Lateral radiograph of a parosteal, juxtacortical osteogenic sarcoma of the distal femur. *B*, CT scan. AP (*C*) and lateral (*D*) radiographs of an allograft reconstruction that replaced the distal femur, posterior capsule, and posterior cruciate ligament. The articular surface could be spared. The patellar fracture brought the patient to medical attention, and the sarcoma was an incidental finding.

deposition disease may produce a mass that demonstrates the diagnostic uric acid or calcium pyrophosphate crystals.[31, 47, 52, 100, 166] In patients with chondrosarcoma (70%), glucose tolerance test results are abnormal.[98] Biochemical studies should be ordered when a metabolic disease or high-grade malignancy is suspected.

When a lesion displays benign and latent characteristics, no further imaging is warranted and the biopsy should be performed next. Conversely, if the diagnosis is unclear or if a more aggressive or possibly malignant lesion is suspected, further imaging will aid the diagnosis and treatment.

MRI provides valuable diagnostic information about both benign and malignant lesions yet still lacks diagnostic precision. The technique excels at defining normal and pathological anatomy, particularly defining soft-tissue, vascular, neural, and marrow space involvement by tumor.[25, 34] Imaging of only the affected limb maximizes the resolution of the test. It may even be too sensitive in identifying reactive and edematous tissue. This may suggest more extensive tumor involvement than actually exists. For example, Shima reported that joint involvement seen on MRI was frequently not corroborated histopathologically.

MRI scans that are narrowly focused on the joint or are taken with only one spin-echo sequence to evaluate intra-articular lesions (meniscal tears) can easily miss extra-articular soft-tissue and metaphyseal bone tumors. Therefore, the knee MRI protocol should include, at a minimum, a Tl-weighted coronal image, a T2-weighted sagittal image, and a gradient echo-weighted axial image to pick up the unsuspected lesion in the distal femur, proximal tibia, or soft tissues. The formal evaluation of a tumor requires at least axial T1 and T2 imaging in addition to the described sequences. Fat-suppressed images are increasingly helpful.

Computed tomography (CT) is the best tool to assess cortical bone and endosteal cortical erosions caused by tumors such as low-grade chondrosarcomas that frequent the distal femur and proximal tibia. CT can also detect cortical breakthrough and is sensitive in identifying soft-tissue calcification, such as that visible in synovial sarcoma.

A whole-body technetium-99m pyrophosphate bone scan is part of bone tumor staging. Repeat the whole-body study if only a localized bone scan has been performed (e.g., for the evaluation of tibial plateau or femoral condyle osteonecrosis). The bone scan is particularly important when metastatic disease is suspected because it may identify an alternative site to biopsy. Gallium scans are useful for round cell tumors.[142] Pulmonary metastatic or mediastinal nodal involvement can be ruled out by means of a chest film and CT. Chest CT detects a pulmonary metastasis missed on the plain film and is more sensitive than plain tomography. Table 95.1 summarizes the diagnostic studies used at Memorial Sloan-Kettering Cancer Center.

TABLE 95.1 RECOMMENDED DIAGNOSTIC STUDIES OF BONE TUMORS

Before biopsy	Physical examination Radiograph (biplanar) of primary site Chest radiograph Three-dimensional imaging of primary site (MRI or CT) Whole-body three-phase bone scan Biochemical profile (lactic dehydrogenase, alkaline phosphatase) Hematologic profile (complete blood count, erythrocyte sedimentation rate)
Post biopsy	Chest CT (high-grade and low-grade tumors) Gallium scan (round cell tumors) Bone marrow biopsy (round cell tumors)
Optional	Thallium scan

Staging

Benign and malignant tumors should be staged. This organizes the diagnostic process, predicts outcome, and suggests appropriate treatment.

Benign tumors are staged by one of two methods. The Enneking method is more comprehensive but cumbersome.[61] The Campanacci system, developed to classify aneurysmal bone cysts, is based solely on the radiograph.[23] Latent lesions (stage A) are contained within bone, without affecting the surrounding cortex. Active lesions (stage B) are also within bone but evoke a cortical reaction. Aggressive lesions (stage C) traverse the cortex and extend into the surrounding soft tissue. Benign tumor staging is valuable because it defines the extent and behavior of the tumor. It thereby helps in formulating proper tumor ablation and requisite skeletal reconstruction.

Malignant bone tumor staging is more standardized and prognostically accurate. In the Enneking system, bone cancers are graded as either low grade or high grade based on histological criteria and metastatic potential. Stage I tumors are low-grade lesions, and stage II tumors are high-grade lesions. Substage A denotes that the tumor is confined within the bony compartment, whereas substage B signifies that the tumor extends beyond the compartment into the surrounding joint or soft tissue. Stage III identifies all metastatic tumors, whether high or low grade. Most malignant tumors (both bone and soft-tissue) are high grade and extracompartmental (i.e., stage IIB lesions). A slightly different system is used to stage round cell tumors such as Ewing's sarcoma.

Prognosis has been shown to correlate with these stages. Refinements may account for the lesion's size and anatomic site. The popliteal space poses significant treatment problems that are not fully reflected in the staging system.[164] Because the area behind the knee is extracompartmental and not bounded by fascial planes, tumors in this location are stage IB or IIB. Soft-tissue malignancies can be classified by this same system but are better handled by the American Joint Committee on Cancer system, described later.[1] Molecular staging based on the tumor's genetic profile, invasiveness, and metastatic potential is rapidly coming on the heels of advances in tumor and cell biology.

Biopsy Technique

Various methods are available, and the most appropriate choice is determined by practical considerations such as the experience and preferences of your pathologist or the availability of operating room space. In general, lesions that have a virtually diagnostic radiographic appearance are good candidates for a needle biopsy, whereas lesions with atypical radiographic presentations are suitable for an open biopsy. Finally, fresh tissue is increasingly in demand for genetic testing of primary bone tumors; thus, an open biopsy is required to obtain adequate tissue for these tests. This concern will be eliminated in the near future with advances in fluorescent in situ hybridization that will allow a genetic profile to be obtained from as little as one tumor cell.

When the risk of local recurrence is low and treatment is similar for the lesions that could be potentially diagnosed, a biopsy that excises the entire lesion is suitable. For example, osteoid osteomas should be excised first and diagnosed afterward. The excision may be performed with narrow margins of normal tissue; intralesional treatment may be best for difficult locations. The diagnostic alternative is Brodie's abscess, appropriately treated in the same fashion, based on the location.

Most commonly, biopsy precedes treatment. The incisional procedure entails excising only a small portion of the tumor for diagnosis. Proper technique minimizes the possible complications associated with this procedure. Strive to follow the procedure outlined in Table 95.2.

Antibiotics should not be administered before the biopsy so that microorganisms may be recovered. Remember, when you biopsy it, culture it, and when you culture it, biopsy it.[72] A tourniquet is desirable to minimize bleeding. There is no evidence that a tourniquet alters the risk of tumor dissemination. However, avoid using a compression bandage to exsanguinate the limb because this embolizes tumor. Use gravity and patience instead.

The placement of the biopsy incision is crucial because it opens all tissue exposed to potential tumor contamination. At the time of surgical resection, this tissue must be excised in continuity with the tumor mass. Biopsy incisions about the knee should be over the tumor and linear. They should be extensile and facilitate exposures that will be used to perform the resection. Most incisions are placed anteromedially or anterolaterally to avoid contaminating the joint and minimize unnecessary extracompartmental contamination. It is difficult to avoid the neurovascular popliteal structures with a posterior incision. Transverse biopsy scars compromise the extensile exposure of the knee needed for en bloc limb-sparing resection. Make the incisions small to minimize tumor contamination. Large incisions must be widely excised and lead to substantial soft-tissue defects over the knee joint that would make wound closure impossible. Muscle flaps have improved the options for limb salvage by covering even large soft-tissue defects created by inappropriate biopsies. Nevertheless, proper biopsy technique can obviate the need for morbid muscle flap procedures.

TABLE 95.2 BONE BIOPSY TECHNIQUE

Needle biopsy if radiograph diagnostic
Open biopsy otherwise
- No preoperative antibiotics
- Exsanguinate by gravity, not compression bandage
- +/− tourniquet
- Small, extensile incision
- X-ray localization if necessary
- Soft-tissue biopsy if possible
- Round bone hole
- Frozen-section for adequacy
- Fresh tissue for special studies (genetics)
- Culture (fungus, tuberculosis, bacteriology)
- Absolute hemostasis
- Plug hole
- Drain in line with definitive incision (if necessary)
- Protect weight bearing

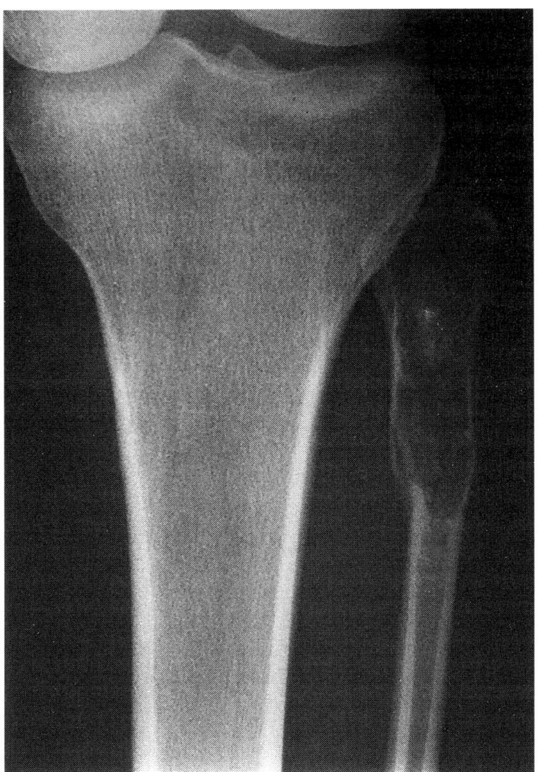

FIGURE 95.6 ➢ AP radiograph of a proximal fibular grade I chondrosarcoma with extension through the cortex. It fractured with minimal trauma and was treated with wide local excision and repair of the collateral ligament.

Biopsy samples of fibular lesions present a particular problem. A longitudinal incision over the anterolateral aspect of the bone is best, avoiding the peroneal nerve. It should not be isolated; otherwise, it may have to be sacrificed when a cancer is excised. Primary wide excision of the fibular head is useful in selected circumstances, as is discussed later. Intraosseous cartilaginous lesions, suspicious for chondrosarcoma, are amenable to primary excision of the proximal fibula (Fig. 95.6).

Bone biopsies should remove as little tissue as possible but as much as necessary. If possible, limit the biopsy to the soft-tissue component of the tumor to preserve remaining strength in the bone. If it is necessary to violate the bone, preserve the architectural relationship between the host bone and the lesion. A circular or oval hole minimizes the risk of postbiopsy fracture. A frozen-section analysis confirms sufficiency of the biopsy sample. The intraoperative examination may suggest the need for special studies that require fresh tissue. When appropriate, fungal, mycobacterial, aerobic, and anaerobic cultures should be obtained because infections may mimic tumors, and tumors rarely can also be secondarily infected. Contamination of surrounding tissue should be minimized by avoiding spillage of tumor and achieving meticulous hemostasis. Absorbable gelatin sponge (Gelfoam) and thrombin work well. On occasion, it is necessary to cement the cortical window in the bone to prevent postoperative hemorrhage. If a drain is used, it should be small and placed in line with the incision so that the tract of the drain is easily excised in continuity with the biopsy incision at the time of definitive tumor resection.

The patient must avoid unprotected weightbearing to prevent fracturing the pathological bone. A pathological fracture does not preclude limb salvage, but it disseminates tumor and makes it more difficult to obtain a wide margin of tumor resection, even if amputation is needed.

Treatment

A four-part staging system stratifies procedures, specifies the nature of any tumor excision, and defines the surgical margin that was attained.[61] An *intralesional margin* occurs when an incision passes through the tumor. For example, curettage is an intralesional procedure. Intralesional excisions are only suitable for benign lesions. A *marginal margin* is achieved when the excision courses through the layer of reactive, inflammatory tissue around a cancer. A common example is an excisional biopsy around the tumor pseudocapsule. It almost always leaves microscopic disease behind and is routinely associated with recurrence of malignant tumors. Re-excision of the tumor and surgical bed with a wide margin is recommended after marginal excision of a malignant bone or soft-tissue tumor. A *wide excision* removes the tumor and some amount of surrounding normal tissue. Most limb-sparing en bloc excisions for sarcomas obtain a wide surgical margin. A *radical margin* is obtained by removing not only the tumor but the entire soft-tissue and bone compartments that contain the tumor. This means, for example, removing the entire femur for a lesion of the distal femur or the entire quadriceps for a lesion in the distal vastus medialis.

Benign Bone Tumors

Benign bone tumors that have indisputable radiological features and are asymptomatic, such as osteochondromas or metaphyseal cortical defects, do not need to be treated or subjected to biopsy sampling. If the diagnosis is in doubt or known lesions become symptomatic, biopsy and treatment are appropriate. Latent lesions can be treated with curettage and bone grafting. Occasionally, it may be reasonable to closely follow small latent lesions. Active and aggressive lesions should always be excised and may require the addition of an adjuvant such as cryosurgery, phenol, bone cement, or even a limited en bloc excision. GCT treatment embodies the methods and common technical variations that are used for other benign tumors of similar virulence, such as aneurysmal bone cysts, chondroblastomas, and chondromyxoid fibromas.

GIANT CELL TUMOR

Treatment for GCT follows the principles previously articulated for benign bone tumors as modified to address the peculiar subchondral location and aggressiveness of this tumor. Most GCTs occur in the epiphyseal distal femur or proximal tibia and often extend to the subchondral surface (Fig. 95.7). Modern treatment that addresses tumor aggressiveness has reduced the historically high recurrence rate to less than 10% without sacrificing joint function.[14, 165] Many strategies have been advocated. The simplest, curettage and bone grafting, has an approximately 50% recurrence rate. At the other extreme, wide excision cures most cases, but this treatment has more morbidity and reconstructive difficulty and does not eliminate the possibility of metastatic disease.

Intralesional surgery has the best balance between risk of recurrence and risk of functional disruption. Fully exteriorize the tumor through a cortical bone window large enough to allow direct vision into all areas of the tumor. Curette the lesion aggressively and use a high-speed burr to eradicate fingers of tumor that extend though cancellous bone. The subchondral area can be treated with great precision and avoid disrupting the articular cartilage. Pay particular attention to the diaphyseal side of the tumor because, ironically, most recurrences happen in this region.

Despite careful, expert technique, recurrence still abounds. An important study from the Massachusetts General Hospital reported recurrence in 7 of 25 tibial and 3 of 23 distal femoral GCTs treated by curettage, burring, cement, and phenol in selected cases.[113] The improvement in local control that can be achieved by modern mechanical treatment with curetting-burring and bone grafting alone was shown by Blackley et al.[15] Recurrence was found in 7 of 59 cases, although it should be noted that 41% of cases were treated by en bloc excision, and careful case selection was used. These disappointing results highlight the need for aggressive treatment and suggest that surgical adjuvants warrant consideration.

Chemical and physical modalities extend the margin of tumor excision and improve tumor control. Acrylic cement produces heat and necroses a small rim of surrounding bone. This not only kills tumor but mechanically supports the defect, allowing early weightbearing. Long-term follow-up has shown that the cement functions well and that it need not be replaced electively with bone grafts.[14, 113] Supplemental cryosurgery can dramatically extend the volume of bone sterilized, potentially reducing the recurrence rate further.[91, 99] Cryosurgery theoretically can reduce bone healing and contribute to fatigue fractures. Prophylactic internal fixation preempts most of these problems. Malawar reported a local recurrence rate of 2% for

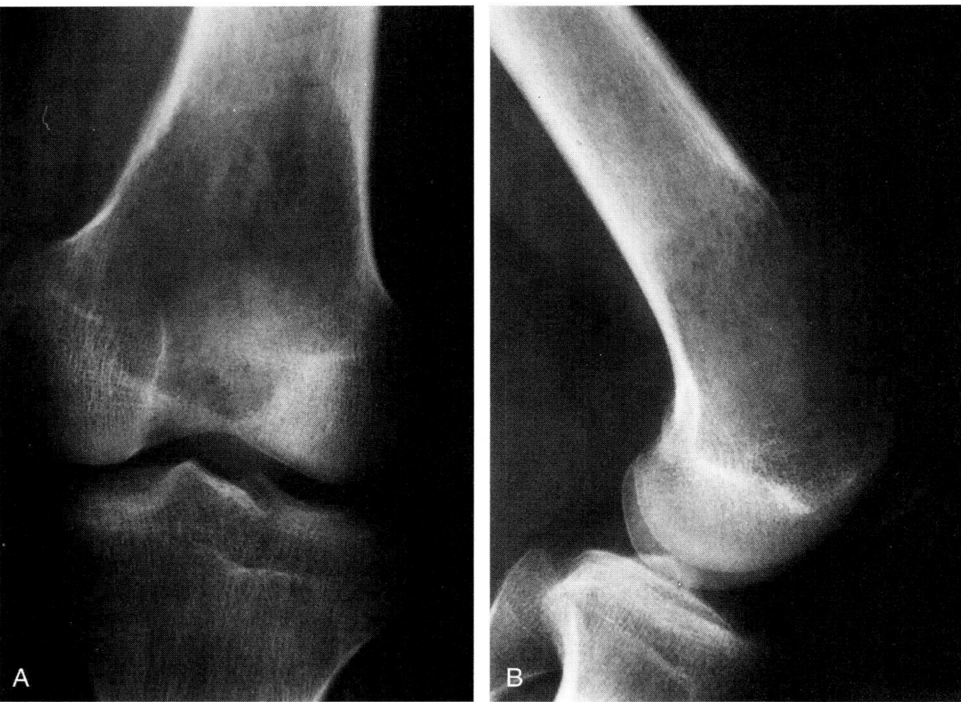

FIGURE 95.7 ➢ AP (*A*) and lateral (*B*) radiographs of a large lytic giant cell tumor of the distal femoral epiphysis. Note the destruction of the anterior femoral cortex.

primary tumors and 8% for recurrent tumors treated with cryosurgery. The fracture rate was 6%. Treatments such as phenol application and laser therapy affect the surface, do not extend the excision margin, and have no proven value to reduce recurrence rates.[129] Cement is an inexpensive filler, especially suitable after a local adjuvant has been used to create a layer of devitalized bone in the tumor cavity. Occasionally, it is necessary to bone graft the subchondral surface if it is very thin or fractured. Despite poor local vascularity, this bone graft has been reported to heal and function well.[3]

Pathological fracture (9% of cases) may be treated with closed reduction and casting, followed by treatment after the fracture heals, if the lesion is typical. If there is a clinical or radiographic concern about malignancy, a preliminary biopsy sample is needed. This is best done immediately, before early fracture healing produces osteoid that could be confused with OGS. Seeding of the synovium is uncommon but does occur, so synovectomy may be used selectively to remove contaminated areas. GCT extends into the adjacent joint in 5% of cases, particularly the tibial-fibular joint.[22] Excision of the involved tissue is necessary.

Intra-articular fracture or recurrence may disrupt the knee joint. Endoprosthetic knee replacement or allografts can salvage many such cases. Large eccentric tumors may destroy one tibial plateau or femoral condyle. Wide excision and replacement of a single condyle (or plateau) with an allograft is an excellent solution.[10, 111] (Fig. 95.8). This type of "hemi-joint" replacement preserves joint alignment, stability, and structure, and it has a high success rate. Range of motion is often restricted because of differences in condylar size and arc of curvature. The grafts heal rapidly because of the large cancellous appositional surfaces. Complete osteochondral allografts are occasionally necessary. Complication rates are higher and results poorer than for the hemi-joint replacements. Tibial osteoarticular allografts failed in 7 of 16 cases reported by Clohisy and Mankin,[32] and similar failure rates apply to distal femoral grafts.[167] Long-term follow-up of grafts reveal 19% fracture and 10% infection rates.[94] Instability is particularly common after femoral allografting, and degenerative arthritis is ubiquitous but usually painless. Fortunately, en bloc excision and complex reconstruction is rarely needed, and the intralesional technique effectively eradicates aggressive tumors such as GCT.

Rare tumors pose specialized problems when they occur around the knee. For example, chondroblastoma has a predilection for the subchondral bone in the intercondylar notch and the tibial spine, epiphyseal locations that are not easily visible by conventional radiographic imaging (Fig. 95.9). The deep central location limits direct access by conventional routes such as an extra-articular medial or lateral exposure. Intra-articular exposure is sometimes acceptable in order to limit the amount of normal bone that has to be removed, particularly when the lesion has already broken into the joint. Because these locations are nonweightbearing, the transarticular approach does not disrupt joint function. Nevertheless, it is critical to protect the uninvolved joint from tumor implantation. Isolation of the tumor bed with sponges and vigorous lavage of the joint after tumor removal effectively protects the remaining joint when approaching a tumor in this fashion. Tibial chondroblastomas often extend

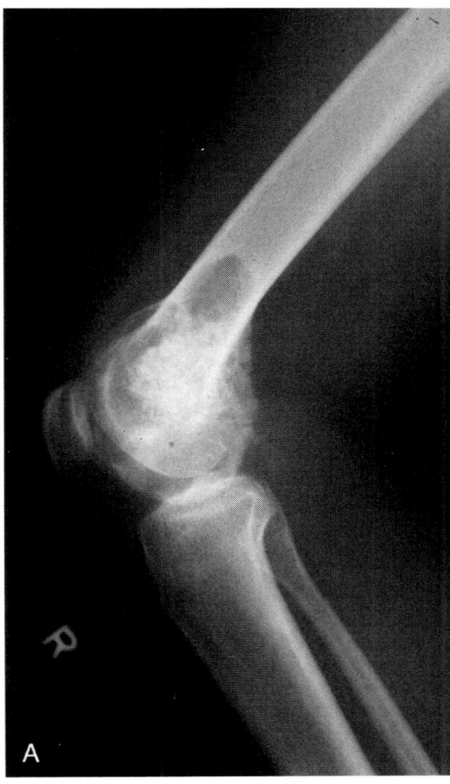

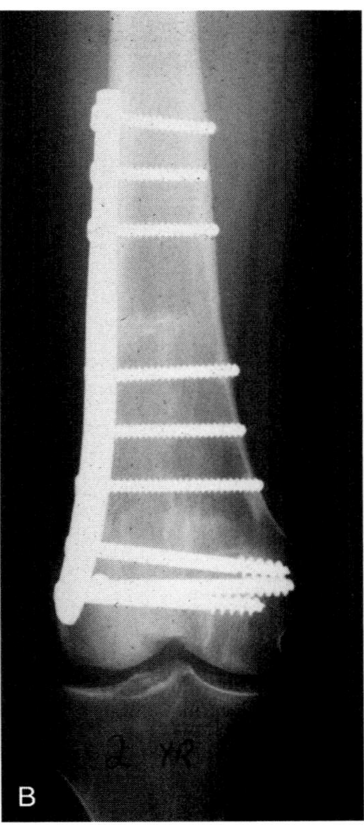

FIGURE 95.8 ➢ *A*, Lateral radiograph of a recurrent giant cell tumor of the distal femur. It had been treated with curettage, high-speed burring, and cement. Note the lucency around the cement in the distal femoral epiphysis and in the diaphyseal area. *B*, Treatment was with resection of the lateral femur and replacement with an allograft of the lateral femoral condyle. AP radiograph was taken 8 years after surgery.

along the growth plate and affect the tibial tubercle. Coronal and sagittal MRI helps to define tibial tubercle involvement. The shell of cortical bone remaining after tumor removal is susceptible to avulsion fracture. Reinforcement of the tubercle with a heavy nonabsorbable suture, or with screw and washer, should be considered. The postoperative rehabilitation program should be adjusted if the tubercle is unstable.

Malignant Bone Tumors

When an *effective* adjuvant is available, the current standard of practice for a bone or soft-tissue sarcoma is a wide local excision. The following two points should be emphasized:

- Because not all adjuvants are effective, the response to adjuvant therapy must be considered. For example, if the cancer does not respond to chemotherapy, it is prudent to obtain a wider surgical resection margin with limb preservation or amputation.
- Amputation is always an option when treating a sarcoma. It is difficult to argue against an option that is effective and potentially curative. However, not all amputations are equal, oncologically or functionally. Oncologically, amputations are not necessarily radical. For example, resection of the entire adductor compartment would be more radical treatment for a sarcoma of the distal gracilis than an above-knee amputation that cut through the adductor compartment. Functional differences are also important. For example, an excellent long above-knee amputation for a tibial cancer achieves dramatically better function than does a high above-knee amputation for a distal femoral lesion.

OSTEOGENIC SARCOMA

A long-term, multi-institutional follow-up study of patients treated for distal femoral OGS substantiated that limb preservation achieved similar survival rates as did amputation and hip disarticulation. Nevertheless, there was a difference in the local recurrence rate among the procedures: limb salvage, 11%; above-knee amputation, 8%; hip disarticulation, 0%. Even though few patients who suffer local recurrence are cured, this report curiously seemed to show that local recurrence does not reduce the cure rate. This paradox is thought to be due to the fact that patients who suffer from a recurrence have biologically aggressive disease and a high probability of dying of metastatic disease anyway.

Although associated with a bad prognosis, recurrence is not usually the cause of systemic failure. These results show that in the era of modern chemotherapy, treating resectable lesions with limb-sparing surgery causes no statistically adverse impact on survival. It should be noted that the studies published to date are highly selected case series that have a low power — only 10% (large beta error) — to rule out an important difference in survival between above-knee amputation and limb salvage. Consequently, limb salvage may have a small oncological risk that has not been adequately defined. This is of great importance when treating an individual patient. For example, a

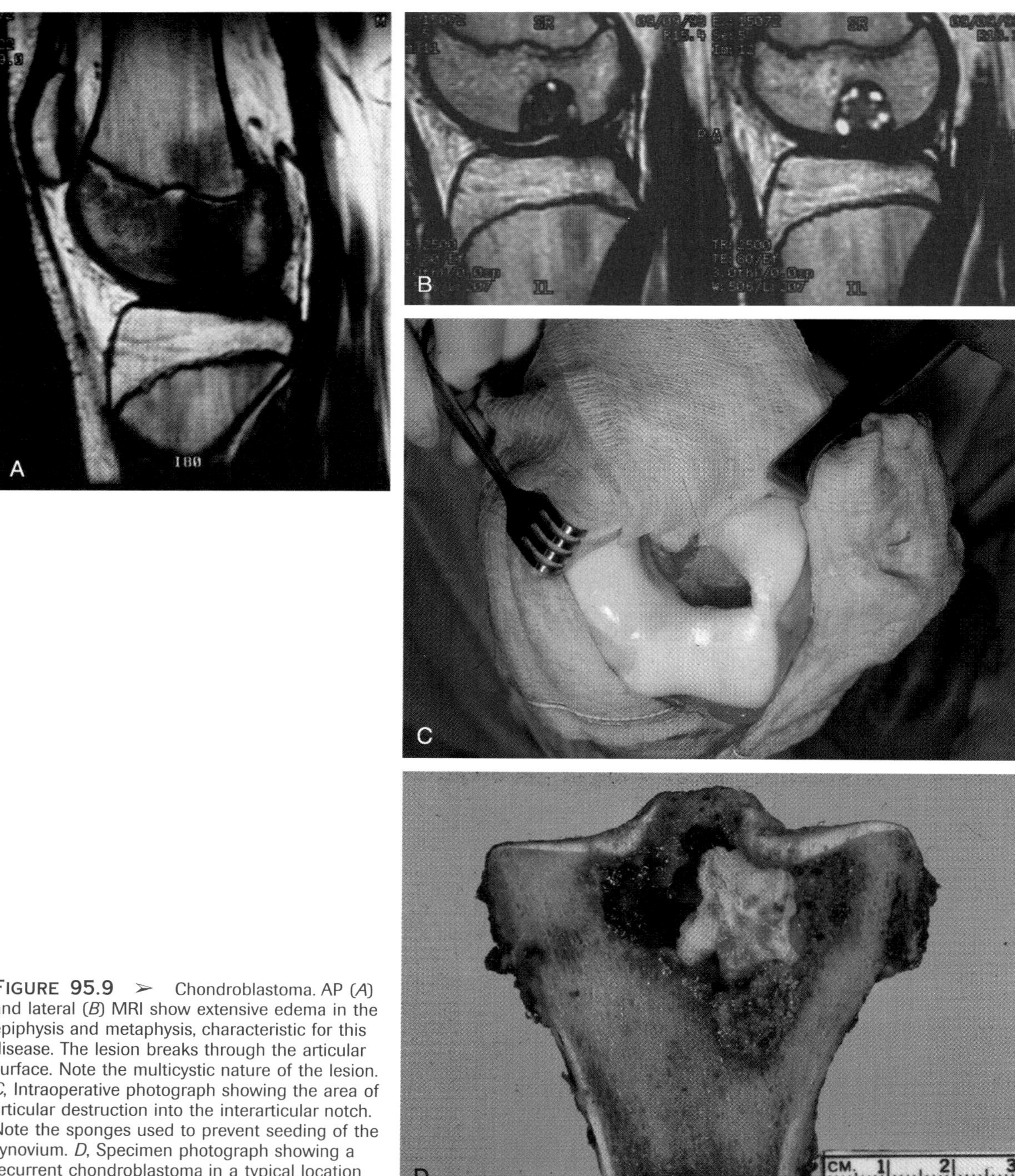

FIGURE 95.9 ➢ Chondroblastoma. AP (*A*) and lateral (*B*) MRI show extensive edema in the epiphysis and metaphysis, characteristic for this disease. The lesion breaks through the articular surface. Note the multicystic nature of the lesion. *C*, Intraoperative photograph showing the area of articular destruction into the interarticular notch. Note the sponges used to prevent seeding of the synovium. *D*, Specimen photograph showing a recurrent chondroblastoma in a typical location into the tibial spine.

large tumor that has responded poorly to chemotherapy is at a greater risk for local failure.[124] Consequently, a standard limb-preserving operation with a wide surgical margin exposes the patient to a higher risk of recurrence and possibly death. Limb salvage should not be automatic. Radical resection should be considered the most curative treatment.[6]

Survival rates of 80% can be expected for stage IIB lower-limb lesions, 90% for stage IIA lesions. In the Memorial Sloan-Kettering experience, disease-free survivals have been durable.[107] Differentiation of high- from low-risk cases is one of the major current challenges. They can be distinguished by intrinsic and treatment variables. The tumor site is important oncologically and functionally. Tibial lesions have a significantly better survival than distal femoral tumors,[107] yet limb salvage for tibial tumors is less predictable, function is not as good, and the reconstructions are less durable.[71, 75] Metastasis is a bad prognostic factor. Only 15% of patients with distant metastases can be cured. More radical surgery is inappropriate for patients with stage III disease.[8, 105, 155] Limb salvage is the humane and oncologically sound option to treat the local disease. Amputation is appropriate for stage III disease only if there is a pathological fracture or uncontrolled symptoms from the primary tumor. The response to chemotherapy is the strongest predictive factor of disease-free survival. Unfortunately, it has not been proved that in cases of poor response to preoperative chemotherapy, limbs can be salvaged by changing drugs postoperatively. Improvement in our ability to resolve high-risk cases is sorely needed.

Stage I, low-grade OGSs occur about one-tenth as often as the conventional OGSs. Most are surface, juxtacortical tumors, or they are rarely in the intramedullary space.[3, 26, 114, 135, 138] They develop in a slightly older population, involve different genetic changes than typical OGSs (ring chromosomes amplifying segments of the 12th chromosome), and a unique anatomic distribution.[11, 145] Surface tumors come in two varieties: parosteal and periosteal. Both have a predilection for the distal femur but also occur in the proximal tibia. Parosteal tumors typically grow in the popliteal space, just above the posterior knee capsular origin.

Periosteal tumors tend to be more diaphyseal. Despite their name, they invade the marrow space in up to 20% of cases. Furthermore, they may harbor high-grade elements in 15% to 20% of cases. Occasionally, long-standing parosteal OGSs may undergo dedifferentiation to very-high-grade sarcoma. Just because a tumor is predominantly on the bone surface, it still must be staged carefully and a biopsy is needed to direct treatment. If the tumor is high grade, chemotherapy is necessary, but chemotherapy should not be used for low-grade tumors. Wide local excision is the preferred treatment, and amputation is only needed for massive or recurrent tumors involving the neurovascular structures.

Resection is based on tumor extent and anatomy. The articular surface can often be preserved. Intercalary or, if necessary, osteoarticular allografts are attractive options because (1) the other side of the joint is uninvolved, so total-knee arthroplasty is not needed and (2) bone healing is better than it would be if chemotherapy were required for a high-grade tumor (see Fig. 95.5). Careful reconstruction of the posterior capsule and posterior cruciate ligament is needed in these cases, and the tissue that comes with the frozen allografts helps to augment the deficiencies of host tissue.

Adjuvant Chemotherapy

OGSs and Ewing's sarcomas are the paradigms of the current approach to high-grade malignant tumors. Adjuvant multiagent chemotherapy is standard treatment for high-grade malignant bone tumors. In OGS, chemotherapy has increased disease-free survival from less than 20% when treatment was radical surgery alone to approximately 70% to 80% for chemotherapy and wide excision. The data are incontrovertible for OGS and Ewing's sarcoma.[89]

Other histological tumor types may not be as responsive to existing chemotherapy. Chondrosarcomas have not been shown to be sensitive to chemotherapy, and most express the multidrug-resistance gene. There is much debate regarding routine adjuvant chemotherapy for high-grade soft-tissue sarcoma. Meta-analysis of published randomized studies suggests that there is an advantage to doxorubicin-based chemotherapy, reducing local failure by 6% and systemic failure by 10% after 10 years.[2] Data about new ifosfamide regimens are sparse but suggest that high-dose therapy may improve disease control significantly, especially for synovial sarcoma.

Because of the low incidence of bone sarcomas, there are not enough cases to test all potential chemotherapy combinations to establish which is the best option. It is difficult to demonstrate a statistically significant improvement beyond the current 70% to 80% cure rates for OGSs in the 3- to 5-year accrual window used to test new regimens. Furthermore, it is difficult for individual surgeons and medical centers to develop expertise in managing these rare diseases. To support a multispecialty treatment team, it is important that all cases of OGS and other rare cancers be treated in a comprehensive cancer center. This approach optimizes care, centralizes tissue banking for genetic studies, and allows enough cases to accrue improved chemotherapy regimens.

Most patients already have metastatic disease when an OGS is diagnosed. Fifteen percent have one or more lesions identified by chest CT scan, and 65% have only subclinical, microscopic foci of disease. Surgical resection is needed for identifiable metastases and systemic treatment for micrometastases.

Preoperative chemotherapy followed by resection of the tumor and consolidation postoperative chemotherapy is the paradigm to treat osteogenic and Ewing's sarcoma. The advantages of preoperative chemotherapy include the following:

- Early treatment of the life-threatening microscopic metastatic disease.
- Shrinkage of the primary tumor and sterilization of the reactive zone surrounding the sarcoma.
- Time to manufacture a custom prosthesis or obtain a suitable allograft.
- Time to establish a relationship with the patient and their family.

This interval allows careful consideration of the surgical options, and it provides a glimpse of how effective the chemotherapy will be in shrinking the local tumor. Occasionally, an unresectable tumor becomes resectable after a profound response to chemotherapy. Ewing's sarcoma lacks a rigid supportive matrix, so dramatic tumor shrinkage can occur, and the distinction between tumor and surrounding edema becomes clearer. This allows less tissue to be removed when resecting the sarcoma and increases the rate at which limbs can be saved. However, around the knee, the popliteal extension of tumor is usually the limiting distance that determines tumor resectability. Disappointingly, despite an overall reduction in volume, tumor shrinkage does not always occur in the most favorable sites. The relationship between displaced popliteal vessels and tumor may not change appreciably during chemotherapy. It should be kept in mind that despite the theoretic advantages, there has never been a proven survival advantage to starting chemotherapy before surgery.[55] Consequently, definitive surgery followed by the early introduction of intensive chemotherapy is an appropriate option for certain patients. Primary surgery is a useful strategy in patients for whom the diagnosis, or tumor grade, is uncertain. Evaluation of the entire specimen eliminates doubt and guides the decision for postoperative chemotherapy.

The extent of necrosis in the resected OGS and Ewing's sarcoma specimens predicts long-term disease-free survival.[106, 162] Necrosis, in tandem with assessment of the surgical margin, also predicts the likelihood of local tumor recurrence. Unfortunately, the idea that postoperative chemotherapy can be tailored according to the histological response to preoperative chemotherapy has not worked. New regimens based on ifosfamide and cisplatinum may induce greater necrosis in the primary tumor than occurs historically, but long-term follow-up is needed to determine whether the predictive value of tumor necrosis obtained with one type of chemotherapy can be extrapolated to new chemotherapy protocols.

Exciting new biological agents may enhance survival of human patients with OGS, as they have done in dogs with naturally occurring disease. A national trial of muramyl tripeptide phosphoethanolamine, a modulator of macrophage function, in 714 patients with OGS will be reported imminently.[79] These results may change the approach to sarcoma management.

Combination chemotherapy is the cornerstone of treatment for small cell malignancies such as Ewing's sarcoma. Nevertheless, sterilization of the primary tumor site is required. Radiation usually succeeds but has high short- and long-term complication rates. As many as 28% of patients irradiated for Ewing's sarcoma may experience local recurrence. About the knee, radiation of the growth plates predictably produces severe limb-length inequality and knee joint contractures.[54, 87, 109] Pathological fracture and delayed union or nonunion are common sequelae of the high doses of radiation used (>50 Gy). Finally, a startling rate (1% per year) of radiation-associated cancers has been reported in patients who have received radiation and modern high doses of alkylating agents.[42, 81] Therefore, most oncologists now recommend resection of the primary bone as the best way to achieve local control and avoid long-term complications. When the bone is "dispensable," such as the fibula, there is little controversy. When the femur is the primary site, however, the best method for local control is not always clear.[146] I recommend wide local excision and prosthetic replacement of the knee or diaphyseal replacement of the femur as dictated by the tumor location. Supplemental radiation is still occasionally needed if a wide margin is not obtained.

Surgical Technique for Malignant Bone Tumors

Decision-Making

Surgical decision making for malignant lesions about the knee is complex. It depends on many factors. Decision analysis of amputation versus limb salvage has been modeled and favors limb salvage for tumors about the knee. Accurate surgical staging and pathological diagnosis are of major importance. Imaging studies after preliminary chemotherapy should be repeated before making a final decision about which surgical procedure to recommend. The extent of bone, joint, soft-tissue, and neurovascular involvement are evaluated as well. The chemotherapeutic response based on tumor shrinkage, pain relief, biochemical changes (decreased alkaline phosphatase and LDH), and improvement in the imaging characteristics are assessed. If all of the test results are favorable, limb sparing is proper. If there is no improvement, amputation may be safer. Oncological principles must not be compromised just to preserve a limb because local recurrence and death will be the outcome.

The patient's age plays a major role in determining the type of surgical procedure that should be employed. Major limb-length inequality occurs in young children who lose their distal femoral and proximal tibial physes. The expandable prostheses touted for these patients are too small and biomechanically inadequate for the demands placed on the knee joint[33, 44, 78, 153] (Fig. 95.10). Furthermore, they must be expanded every 6 months to keep pace with growth. Children recovering from cancer and chemotherapy should be subjected to the minimum number of additional surgeries. If the femoral transaction level is within 7 cm of the lesser trochanter, stump-extending alternatives such as turnplasty or rotationplasty may be considered[21, 80] (Fig. 95.11). If a longer stump is feasible and the patient does not want rotationplasty, amputation remains the most suitable surgical option.

MRI provides accurate documentation of the proximal and distal margins of tumor, particularly the extent of intramedullary involvement. The presence of "skip" metastases is excluded by MRI and bone scan. Whether limb salvage or amputation is chosen, the bone is transected approximately 2 to 3 cm away from the bony limit of disease, although even these margins may be difficult to obtain in small children. Narrower margins have been elected increasingly in children to preserve the growth plate and/or articular surface. Improvements in chemotherapy and imaging allow these courageous efforts to improve function without significantly compromising the curative potential of the surgery.

En Bloc Excision of the Knee

Limb-sparing wide excision of the knee joint is usually an oncologically sound option to amputation. The surgical techniques of resection and reconstruction continue to evolve. These procedures should be performed in centers with extensive experience in the

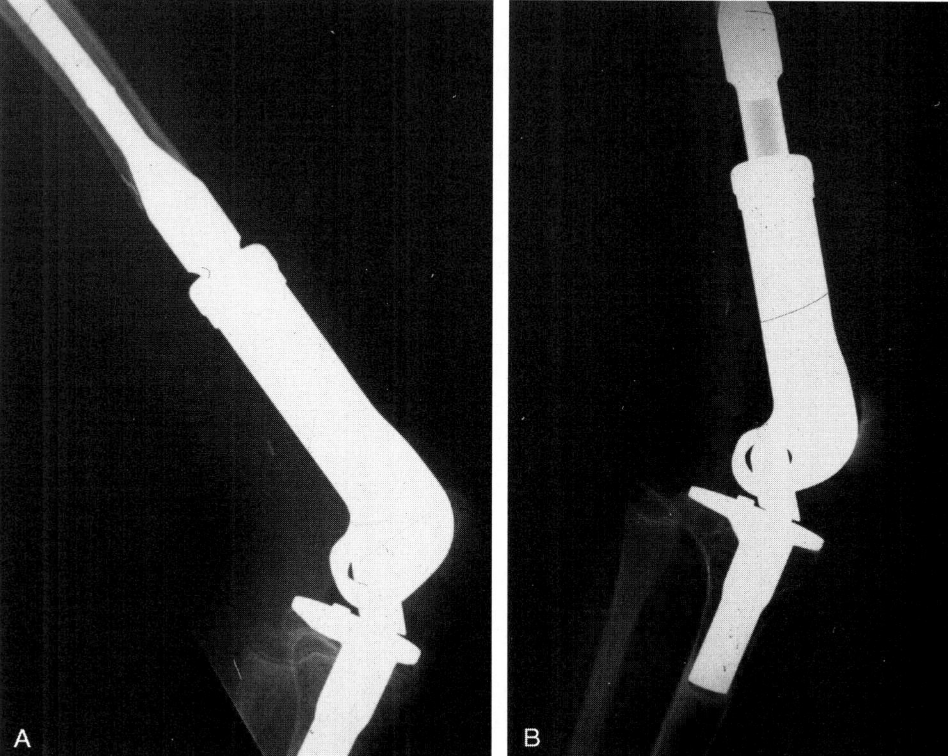

FIGURE 95.10 ➢ Lateral radiographs of an expandable Finn total knee replacement taken after the original implantation (*A*) and after having been expanded 6 cm in 1.5-cm increments (*B*). Note the radiolucency in the distal segment and narrowness of the proximal segment shaft.

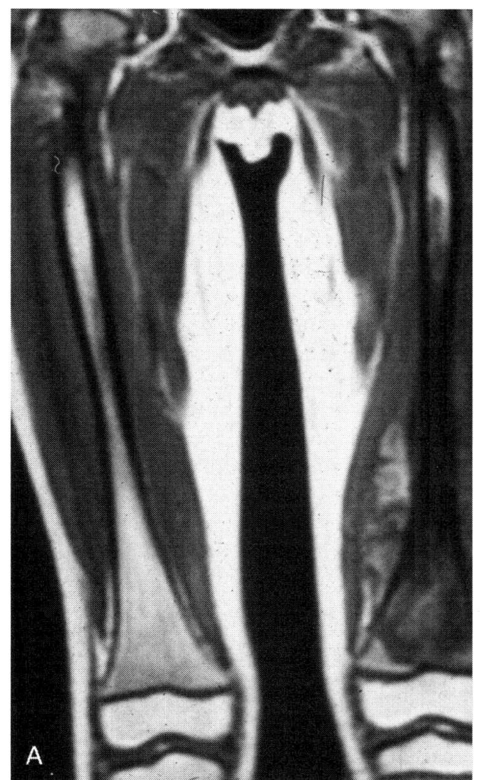

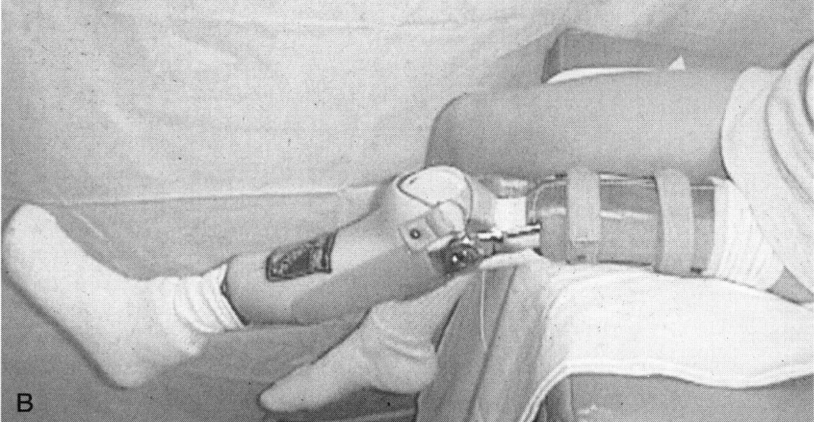

FIGURE 95.11 ➢ *A*, Coronal MRI of an osteogenic sarcoma of the entire diaphysis and distal metaphysis in a 7-year-old. The femur was resected from the subtrochanteric area to the knee joint. The leg was externally rotated 180 degrees and the tibia plated to the proximal femur. *B*, Clinical photograph of the alignment of the knee joints and the prosthesis with a thigh cuff. The patient plays baseball and basketball for his junior high school team.

methods of and access to multidisciplinary oncological care for these patients.

A tourniquet is applied to obtain a dry field during cementation of an endoprosthesis or if bleeding is a problem. The incision is placed longitudinally as dictated by the medial or lateral biopsy scar, with care taken not to compromise a potential site of proximal amputation with unnecessary incisions. The "no touch" technique is adhered to assiduously. The saphenous vein and nerve are preserved if possible. Flaps are created either above the fascia or below the fascia, as required. Retaining the fascia facilitates wound closure and improves healing but should not be done at the expense of obtaining a wide margin.

The semimembranosus, pes, and medial gastrocnemius are detached as necessary to allow exposure of the popliteal vessels. The popliteal areolar tissue is retained with the tumor. The vascular adventitia is split, and the artery and vein are shelled out separately, ligating all branches. The vessels are mobilized distally past the popliteal trifurcation. The vastus muscles and short head of the biceps are incised at the predetermined level down to the femur. The femur is transected, and the retained resection margin of proximal host bone and soft tissue are analyzed by frozen-section histology.

Tumor location and invasiveness determine the required extent of resection. Intra-articular excisions conserve one side of the joint and are technically easier to perform. More reconstructive options exist after intra-articular excisions (e.g., osteoarticular allografts), and functional results are theoretically superior to extra-articular excision. Improvements in preoperative imaging and adjuvant therapies foster this more conservative surgical approach. Performed selectively, intra-articular excision may be appropriate for approximately 85% of patients treated by limb-sparing surgical resection without compromising local recurrence or survival rates.[77]

Traditionally, distal femoral and proximal tibial sarcomas should be excised widely by removing the entire joint. About 15% of current procedures require extra-articular excision to address tumors invading the joint (anterior lesions associated with an effusion) or tracking along the capsule (posterior tumors involving the posterior cruciate ligament). Persistence of an effusion after chemotherapy is a relative indication for extra-articular excision. When performing extra-articular excision, it is difficult to preserve any extensor mechanism. In some cases, a useful extensor mechanism can be maintained by staying out of the joint, preserving the anterior portion of the quadriceps tendon and the patella (making a coronal cut in the patella and leaving the articular cartilage, subchondral bone, and synovium with the resected knee joint) (Fig. 95.12).

A modified extra-articular excision is applicable to most cases. The tibial-femoral joint is resected with the entire synovium and capsule en bloc. Arthrotomy is performed, and the capsular structures are dissected away from the patella, rectus femoris, and any vasti

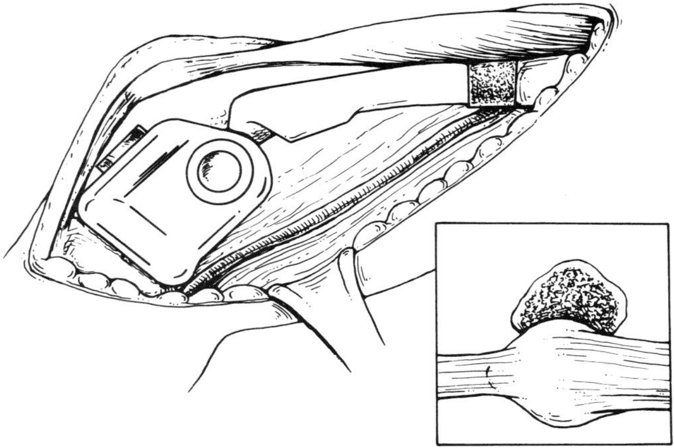

FIGURE 95.12 ➢ Illustration of the quadriceps-sparing, extra-articular resection. The patella is cut in situ with a coronal cut, analogous to that used in standard knee replacement surgery. The distal rectus femoris tendon is slightly thinned to stay out of the suprapatellar pouch. Reconstruction, including patellar resurfacing, can then be performed.

that can be retained. The remaining portion of the procedure is identical to the extra-articular excision.

If the extra-articular technique is chosen, the popliteal trifurcation vessels behind the tibia are protected. The tibia is cut 10 to 15 mm below the joint line, keeping the popliteus in continuity with the joint and tumor mass. If the intra-articular technique is chosen, the ligaments are cut well away from the tumor, ideally at their tibial insertions.

The technique for proximal tibial resection is similar.[32, 63, 66, 71] Most cases require, and are certainly made easier by, ligating the anterior tibial vessels on each side of the interosseous membrane. Commonly, it is necessary to excise the proximal tibial-fibular joint to obtain a wide margin. Small tumors may permit retention of the anterior tibial vessels and the joint. The tibial tubercle and patellar tendon usually must be sacrificed, so all cases need reconstruction of the extensor mechanism, described later.[121] Care must be taken to preserve vascularity to local structures such as the medial gastrocnemius that may be needed for the soft-tissue reconstruction. Because soft-tissue coverage is particularly problematic after tibial resections, plans are made for not only local muscle flap coverage and skin graft but for possible free tissue transfers such as latissimus dorsi microvascular transfers.[65, 68, 76, 83, 93, 103, 121]

Reconstruction

Reconstructive options about the knee include prosthetic arthroplasty, arthrodesis, and osteoarticular allografts. Each alternative must be adapted to the nature of the tumor resection and the magnitude and quality of the structural defect. Although intimately related, the resection must be performed independently of the reconstruction to avoid compromising the oncological success of the procedure. Remember, no tumor was ever cured by an allograft or prosthesis.

Endoprostheses

Prosthetic knee replacement is the preferred method of reconstruction in patients who undergo resection of high-grade malignancies and those in whom both sides of the joint were removed. The potentially short life expectancy of the patient, the need to resume chemotherapy promptly, and the compromise of bone healing during chemotherapy make segmental joint replacement the logical choice. Because soft tissues and ligamentous supports are lacking, a constrained prosthesis is needed. In our series, segmental defects averaging 24 cm of femur or 20 cm of tibia require replacement of the bone shaft coupled with the joint replacement. It is difficult to make the level of resection exactly at the predetermined level because exposure of the bony shaft is limited. Resection lengths are typically off by 1 cm or more. Custom prostheses do not allow for the clinical reality of variable resection lengths. Modular systems provide greater flexibility, and currently available models have interchangeable segments every 2 to 3 cm in length. The long lever arms on constrained prostheses create huge forces on the components, bone, and interface that may lead to early implant failure.

Efforts to reduce mechanical failure have centered around improving prosthetic design, metallurgy, and prosthetic fixation. Prosthetic designs have varied to reduce and dampen loads applied to the prosthesis (cement)-bone interface.

The most commonly used components employ a rotating-hinge design and reconstruct an anatomic joint line. The Kinematic (Howmedica, Rutherford, NJ),[58, 92] Kotz KMFTR (Howmedica),[28] Stanmore (Royal National Orthopaedic Hospital, England),[152] and Finn (Biomet, Warsaw, IN)[75] designs are most popular. They are well adapted to situations wherein a significant amount of the extensor mechanism is preserved. When the extensors are absent, as after classic extra-articular excision, a novel ball-and-socket design is appropriate. The Burstein-Lane prosthesis allows 3.5 degrees of knee hyperextension and 2.5 degrees of internal-external rotation, and it operates through a "sloppy hinge" mechanism.[77] There has also been interest in reducing the prosthetic constraint needed by combining the joint replacement with a segmental allograft. Gitelis and Piasecki refer to these reconstructions as "alloprostheses."[53] About the knee, an alloprosthesis can provide ligamentous and capsular tissue as well as replace the deficient segment. Arguably, one could then use a partially constrained component, resurfacing the articular surface of the allograft and repairing the allograft soft tissues to the remaining host structures (Fig. 95.13).

Most prostheses are made of titanium to reduce weight and maximize strength. Particulate debris is a significant problem with all existing designs, especially in light of the young age of so many tumor patients. Differences in long-term effects of titanium, cobalt-

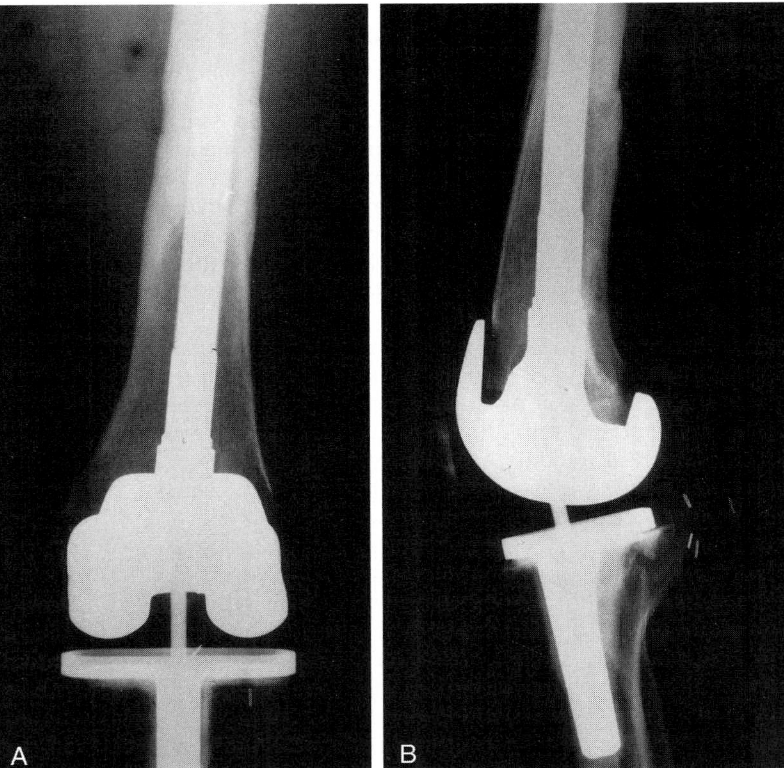

FIGURE 95.13 ➢ AP (*A*) and lateral (*B*) 8-year follow up radiographs of an allograft-prosthetic composite. An Insall-Burstein III knee was used rather than a more constrained, rotating hinge implant.

chromium, and stainless steel will no doubt influence the selection of prostheses in the future. These issues are particularly important in devices that have metal-on-metal gear mechanisms like the existing expandable prostheses. The worst metal wear problems we have encountered have been in such prostheses.[16] Polyethylene wear has not been reported to be a problem in oncological reconstructions. Now that more patients and limbs are being saved, this problem will undoubtedly surface in the near future.

Interface problems have been addressed by moving away from cementation of prostheses. Various uncemented fixation strategies are popular.[28] It is prudent to remember, however, that cement may be the best solution for very ill patients on chemotherapy in whom the integration of bone into prosthesis may be undependable. The role of biological fixation remains to be defined in tumor reconstructive surgery, and comparative studies are needed to evaluate the relative merits of the techniques. Uncemented implants rely on intramedullary press fit, intramedullary porous ingrowth, extramedullary fixation, or a combination of all three (Fig. 95.14). Press-fit fluted stems give excellent cortical bone purchase and rotatory control. However, it is difficult to match the host bone. Short, straight stems are easy to prepare and insert but provide inferior fixation. Longer curved stems are theoretically better, but the radius of prosthetic curvature rarely matches that of the host bone, instrumentation is limited, and precise preparation of the bone is impossible. It is not surprising then that insertion of such prostheses are apt to be loose or too tight.

Intramedullary porous ingrowth is an attractive concept with which most reconstructive surgeons are familiar. Data on the effectiveness and durability of such prostheses are limited. Chao and colleagues[56, 139] and others[154] advocated extramedullary porous fixation to take advantage of the periosteal-periprosthetic sleeve of bone that reliably forms at the junction of bone and component. Animal models support the use of this fixation method, and early clinical results from several centers have been favorable. Unfortunately, the large cuff of bone that develops during the first postoperative year seems to attenuate over time as stresses bypass the newly formed bone.

The Kotz prosthesis couples uncemented fixation with an extramedullary plate and interlocking screws, securing the stem and plate to the bone. They provide excellent torsional stability and may facilitate porous ingrowth. Unfortunately, they are very rigid and contribute to extensive bone loss attributed to the stress bypass effect, and these prostheses may be subject to greater metal debris problems. The original designs had a fixed hinge and suffered significant failure rates for the polyethylene bushings. New versions utilize a rotating hinge articulation. Only careful clinical and radiographic evaluation will determine which prostheses produce the most functional and long-lived reconstructions.

A final issue is the uncertain role of custom prostheses. Satisfactory options exist using standard modular components for distal femoral reconstructions. Unusual anatomic situations in the femur may require unique, customized solutions. For example, when long resections leave too little of the femoral isthmus to secure a stem, interlocking screws matching the intrinsic femoral neck anteversion give excellent fixation (Fig. 95.15). This custom design feature allows limb salvage and hip joint preservation. Low-frequency procedures such as proximal tibial replacements or long, multijoint reconstructions that would entail multiple couplings in a modular reconstruction system (e.g., total femur) are candidates for custom-designed prostheses.

Segmental knee replacement yields good to excellent results in most cases.[75] Pain-free, unassisted, and unlimited ambulation is the usual outcome. Function is inversely proportional to the magnitude of the bone and soft-tissue resection required to remove the tumors.[29, 74, 76, 148] Functionally, cancer patients undergoing knee replacement have better velocity, endurance, and oxygen utilization than amputees. Endoprosthetic reconstruction is chosen most often by patients and surgeons alike.

Complications are routine both early and late after major joint resection and reconstruction.[132] Acutely, the most frequent complication is marginal wound necrosis, which occurs in as many as 25% of cases of large femoral tumor and in most tibial resections. Wound healing problems are treated aggressively because they can delay the resumption of chemotherapy and compromise patient survival. Local muscle (gastrocnemius) or free tissue transfers (latissimus dorsi) are required to achieve tension-free closure with muscle coverage over all prostheses and allografts. If a wound slough still occurs, prompt wound revision and muscle coverage saves most limbs. Aseptic loosening occurs in as many as 25% of patients at 5 years of follow-up. Revision surgery successfully salvages most cases of prosthetic failure from aseptic loosening.[151, 158] Wound healing problems and infection plague attempted revisions, and careful soft-tissue management is critical. Tibial replacement failures are often converted to above-knee amputations because reasonable function can be achieved by a low above-knee amputation.[64] Femoral lesions warrant more aggressive attempts at revision because even a poor salvage is usually better than a high above-knee amputation or hip disarticulation.

Good results require proper postoperative management. Suction drains are kept in place until drainage is minimal. Antibiotic prophylaxis is used until the wound healing is secure. Physical therapy and continuous passive motion of the knee begin when the wound is dry and healing well. Knee flexors are often stronger than the residual knee extensors. Knee flexion contractures are avoided by splinting the knee in extension at night. This is critical in patients with absent quadriceps because a flexion contracture prevents them from keeping their weightbearing axis anterior to the knee flexion axis and precludes a stable stance phase during gait.

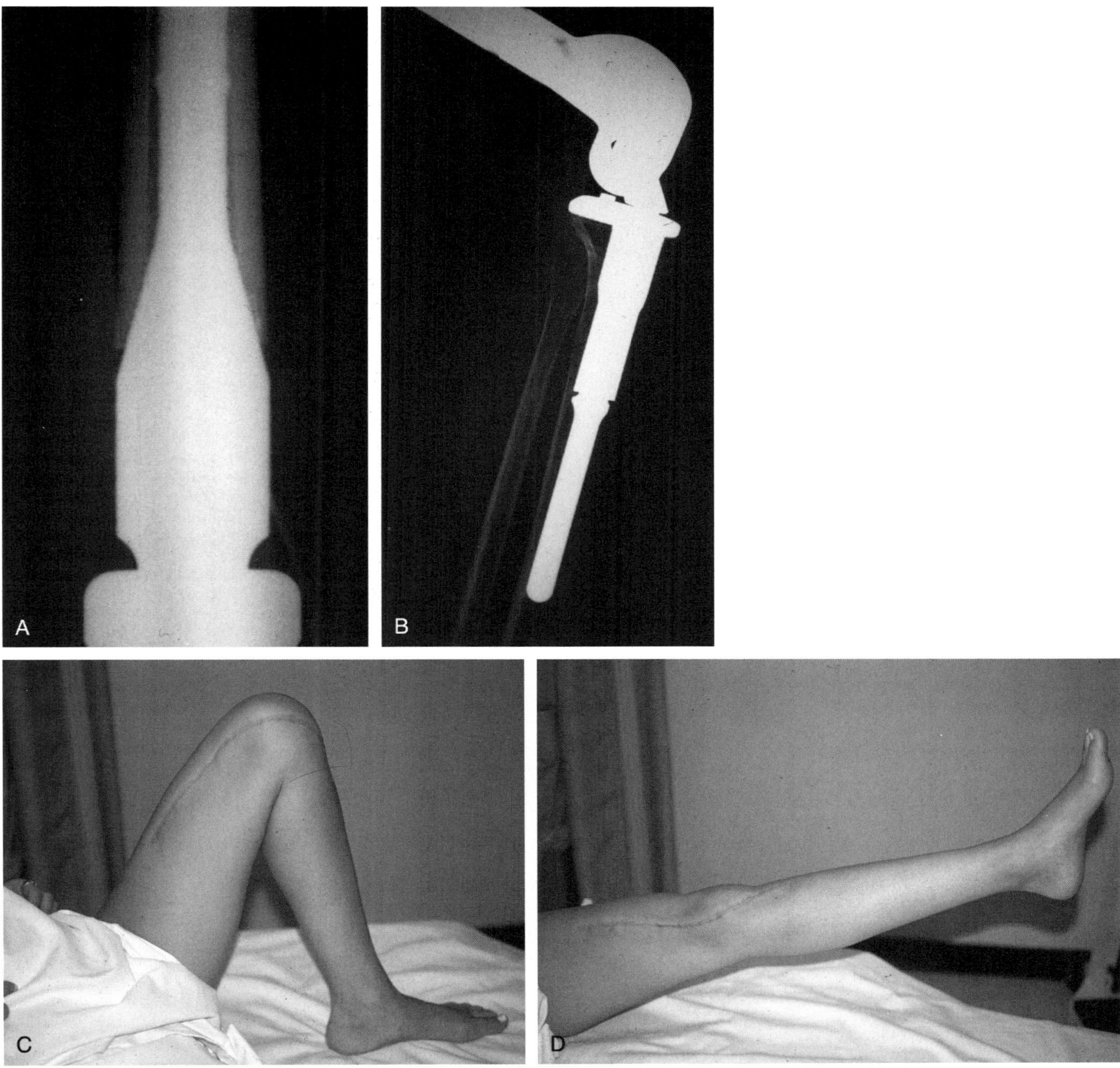

FIGURE 95.14 ➢ Finn uncemented rotating hinge knee replacement. *A*, AP radiograph of the press-fit, porous interface. *B*, Lateral radiograph of the joint and the intramedullary stem that is sometimes necessary to enhance fixation in the tibia. Note the increased anteroposterior dimension of the distal femur. This enhances the extensor mechanism torque generation, enhancing function. *C* and *D* Illustrate the typical motion achieved when the quadriceps can be preserved.

Arthrodesis

Arthrodesis is an alternative to endoprosthesis after resecting a malignant or recurrent benign tumor about the knee.[155, 156, 159] Various combinations of autologous or allogeneic grafts and intramedullary devices span the skeletal defect. Many surgeons prefer arthrodesis whenever the entire extensor mechanism is absent. Campanacci and Costa[24] use an anterior hemicylindrical graft taken from either the tibia or femur, whereas Enneking and Shirley[46] use a hemidiaphyseal graft sagittally turned down (up) from the remaining unaffected host bone. The method usually uses an intramedullary rod inserted antegrade from the greater trochanter-femoral neck.

Because the diameter of the femur and tibia rarely match, Neff modifies the technique. He joins a larger-diameter femoral rod inserted retrograde to an appropriately sized tibial fluted rod that is inserted in an

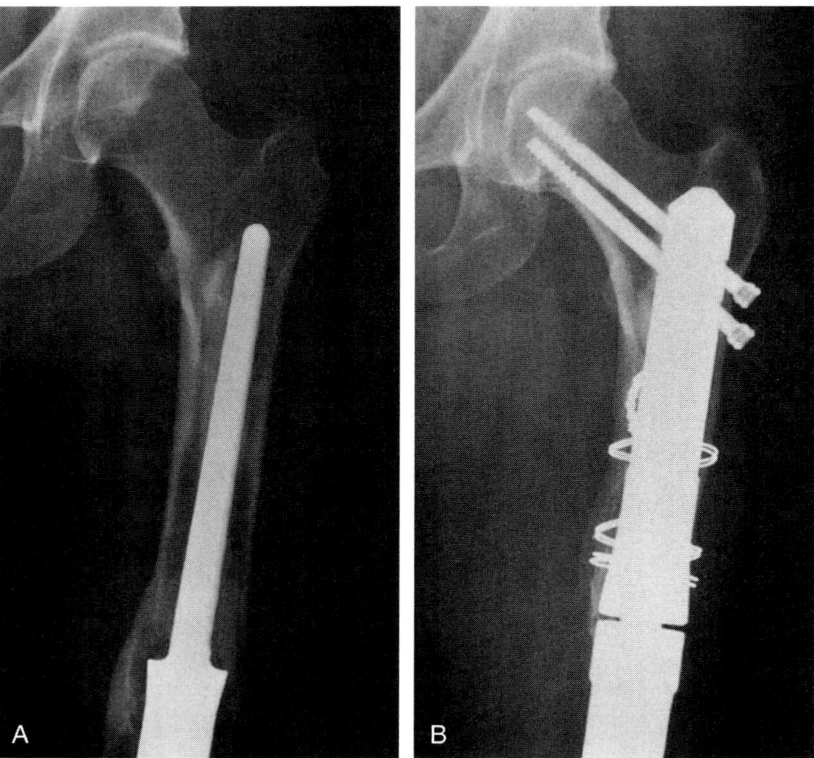

FIGURE 95.15 ➢ *A*, AP radiograph of a failed Guepar prosthesis with osteolysis, fracture, and fragmentation of the residual femoral shaft from radiation necrosis after 11,000 rads. *B*, AP radiograph of an uncemented revision implant. The proximal rotational fixation was provided by the interlocking reconstruction screws. Nine years later, the prosthesis is secure with excellent radiographic intramedullary and extramedullary ingrowth and stress-related changes with mild thinning of the distal cortex.

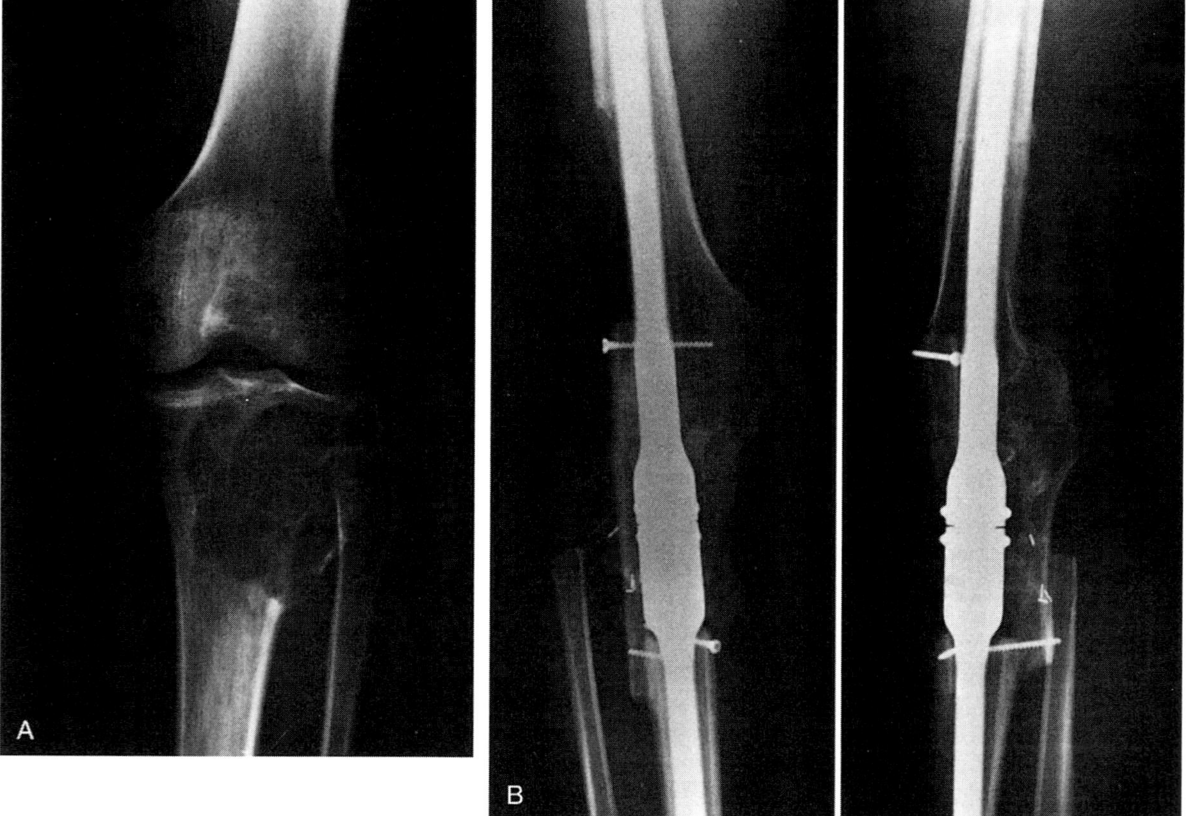

FIGURE 95.16 ➢ *A*, AP radiograph of a giant cell tumor of the proximal tibia that extended into the joint in a laborer. *B*, Knee arthrodesis using articulating-locking femoral and tibial rods was performed. A femoral turndown and fibular graft promoted union.

antegrade manner. The rods lock at the knee and supplemental grafts are placed around the rods (Fig. 95.16). Improved fixation results and avoids a second incision at the hip, but this technique can lead to insurmountable difficulty in extracting the rods if necessitated by infection or other complication. Campanacci and Costa achieved union in 92% of cases eventually, using repeated bone grafting in 15% of cases.[24] Full weightbearing was regained within 2 years in all patients with solid fusions. Infection occurred in 19% of cases, half of which were salvageable, half of which contributed to nonunion. These problems are serious and often prompt patients to request secondary amputation.

Harris et al compared the functional outcome and gait performance of patients with successful knee fusions, arthroplasty, and amputation after tumor resections.[59] There was no difference between the three groups. Some contend that the durability of the fusion makes it the preferred reconstruction. The slow healing and difficulty with sitting may be a worthwhile long-term tradeoff for patients who survive their cancer and would have faced multiple prosthetic revisions, but these limitations come at a high cost to patients who still succumb to their disease.

Intercalary defects in the femoral or tibial shafts behave similarly owing to the defect length, deficient soft tissue, and presence of two osteosynthesis sites. Vascularized[59] and nonvascularized fibular grafts have been used to span arthrodeses and diaphyseal defects. Enneking and Shirley noted that the likelihood of graft fracture increases dramatically whenever the graft length exceeds 12 cm.[46] Vascularized fibulae seem to heal faster and hypertrophy faster than nonvascularized fibular grafts. Unfortunately, the fibula substitutes poorly for the mechanical properties of a normal femur. Fractures typically occur during the time it takes the fibula to hypertrophy sufficiently. The fibular strengthening process takes 2 or more years.

Allografts solve the mechanical problem dependably but leave a biological problem of being slow to unite to host bone. Furthermore, although allografts have been used successfully to span arthrodesis defects, approximately 25% do not unite at one junction and require secondary bone grafting. This encourages the search for a mechanically sound alternative method that promotes bone healing. Some surgeons now combine allografts for structural support and vascularized fibulae for enhanced healing potential.[117]

Allografts—Autografts

Selected patients are candidates for allograft reconstructions. Diaphyseal defects are best reconstructed by intercalary allografts. Surgeons continue to narrow surgical margins and preserve the joint articular surface and ligaments, leaving a problem that can be solved by an intercalary graft. Allografts, vascularized autografts, or a combination can be used (Fig. 95.17). Bone transport has been used to solve intercalary defects, particularly in children. Infrequently, even the growth plate can be retained. Fixation of the small articular fragment is difficult and requires innovative solutions.

If an adequate articular fragment cannot be saved safely, an osteoarticular allograft with attached ligaments can effectively solve the reconstructive dilemma. The surgical technique is exacting. The bone cuts must be exact to align the joint. A step-cut may be considered to increase surface area for healing and reduce nonunions, but it is challenging to match the sizes of host and allograft bone. Generally, the ligaments and capsule should be repaired before the bone is fixed. This allows circumferential exposure of the joint and accurate placement of heavy nonresorbable sutures. The posterior capsular repair is most important and can be done in a vest-over-pants fashion, using both the transplanted and host tissues. Balancing the collateral ligaments is difficult because of the inevitable variation in the radius of curvature of the allograft compared with the host and problems identifying the true instant center of joint rotation. A balance must be achieved with a tight capsular repair that allows maximal knee motion. The cruciate ligaments, particularly the posterior ligament, are usually repaired as well in an end-to-end fashion.

It is important to avoid making extra drill holes or tunnels through the allograft bone because they lead to bone resorption and fracture of the allografts. Internal fixation of the bone graft is then performed. Increasingly, antibiotic cement is being used to fill the canal of the allograft. This may reduce the incidence of graft fracture and infection. It has not been proved, however, and the cement may make it difficult to place fixation screws or to resurface the articular surface if degenerative arthritis develops later. If the fascia cannot be closed primarily over the graft, a muscle flap should be used. I routinely use a gastrocnemius rotation flap to cover tibial allografts and reinforce the reconstruction of the tibial tendon. Motion can be started as soon as wound healing is satisfactory, and an extension stop at −10 degrees has helped to avoid late instability. I recommend a derotation brace for 3 months. Bone healing may take 12 to 18 months and is retarded by the postoperative chemotherapy needed to treat malignant tumors. Weightbearing should be protected until there is bone union. Unfortunately, this prolongs the recuperative period for all patients, and 25% to 50% of patients who experience metastatic disease will never have the opportunity to enjoy any of the potential benefits of their biological allograft reconstruction.

When used in patients requiring chemotherapy, allografts have unacceptably high infection, fracture, and nonunion rates. These complications seem to be less salvageable than similar problems encountered in prostheses. The strongest indication for allograft reconstruction is for tibial osteoarticular grafts in children with open distal femoral physes. Preservation of their major growth potential minimizes the predictable limb-length inequality. Allograft-prosthetic composites of the tibia should also be considered because repair of the transplanted patellar tendon is an excellent way to reconstruct the extensor mechanism. Whichever re-

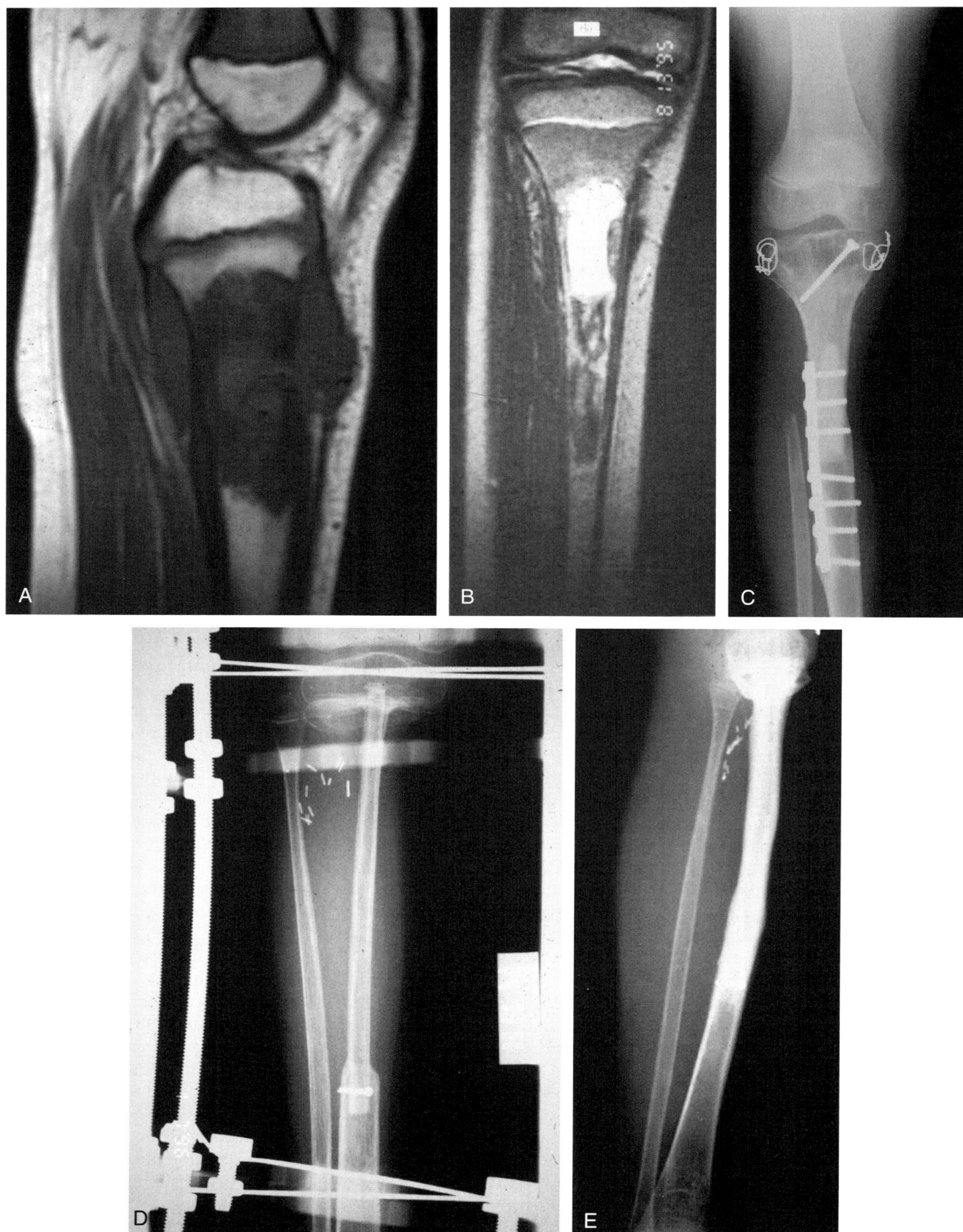

FIGURE 95.17 ➢ Intercalary defects treated by allograft (*A* and *B*) or vascularized fibular autograft (*C*, *D*, and *E*). A, Sagittal MRI of a proximal tibial osteogenic sarcoma in a 12-year-old. *B*, AP radiograph of the reconstruction that spared the upper 1 cm of tibia and used intra-articular screws under the menisci to transfix the junction site. *C*, Coronal MRI showing the tibial Ewing sarcoma, which was resected in an epiphysis-sparing fashion. *D*, An Ilizarov frame was used while a vascularized fibular graft was healing. *E*, Hypertrophy of the graft and preservation of the open growth plate is visible 2 years later.

construction option is chosen, patients should be selected carefully and educated before and after limb preservation.

As demonstrated, there are many options for reconstruction after limb salvage, and the treatment should be individualized. It is most functional and compassionate to keep all patients functioning, walking, and bending their knees during their remaining lifetime. Most patients are best served by endoprosthetic reconstruction.

All of these reconstructive alternatives restrict patient function. Altered muscle balance, stability, and proprioception affect function of salvaged limbs and may contribute to falls. These problems are compounded in patients who suffer peripheral neuropathies from chemotherapy (e.g., cisplatinum, vincristine). Patients should be counseled that despite undergoing limb salvage surgery, they will be permanently disabled and athletic activities should be modified accordingly.

Fibular Resection

Fibular lesions encompass a broad spectrum of diagnoses. Benign conditions include a disproportionate prevalence of aneurysmal bone cysts, enchondromas, unicameral bone cysts, and GCTs. Malignant lesions include Ewing's sarcoma (the most common cancer of the fibula), chondrosarcoma, and rare spindle cell sarcomas. Benign lesions are approached through a longitudinal lateral incision, with care taken to isolate the peroneal nerve. Primary resection[90, 96] or excisional biopsy is the most suitable technique for benign-aggressive and questionably malignant lesions. This solves the diagnostic and therapeutic problems expeditiously. It also minimizes the risk of peroneal nerve neuropraxia or tumor recurrence that is inherent in staged biopsy-excision procedures.

There is a limited role for surgical adjuvants in treating benign-aggressive or low-grade malignant tumors of the fibula. Tumors that are probably high-grade sarcomas, suitable for chemotherapy, should undergo incisional biopsy rather than primary resection. Because peroneal nerve sacrifice is usually essential to obtain a satisfactory margin around a proximal fibular malignancy, biopsy contamination does not compromise the ability to save the nerve at the time of definitive tumor resection. Appropriate systemic therapy is needed, as for other long bone cancers. Fibular sarcomas frequently extend across the tibial fibular joint or involve the popliteal artery trifurcation, precluding safe limb salvage. When at least one major artery can be saved, en bloc wide excision may be considered. Arteriography is helpful in preoperatively planning resection of the proximal fibula. Amputation still has a role in fibular sarcomas when the popliteal artery trifurcation is encased by tumor. Extra-articular excision of the proximal tibial-fibular joint is usually appropriate. The lateral collateral ligament insertion is lost from fibular excision. It can be reinserted into the proximal tibia with suture anchors to re-establish lateral stability, but residual instability is common.[39] Consider rotating the lateral gastrocnemius anteriorly to address the unsightly contour defect that accompanies large resections.

METASTATIC TUMORS ABOUT THE KNEE

Metastatic lesions about the knee cause pain, swelling, and pathological fracture. They are usually identified because of symptoms in a patient with a known cancer, but they can be the initial manifestation of a cancer. Breast cancer, kidney cancer, prostate cancer, and multiple myeloma are the most common cancers. Typically, there is widespread bone involvement.

The entire femur must be evaluated to exclude the presence of a significant lesion in the proximal femur causing referred knee pain or that may influence the reconstructive options. Small deposits that are mechanically stable should be treated with protected weightbearing and radiotherapy. If pain does not relent promptly, surgery is needed. Some poor surgical candidates with less than 3 months to live may get relief from a cast brace that allows weightbearing. Most patients have bone tenderness, a soft-tissue mass, or peripheral edema that precludes use of a cast brace. Pathological fracture of the supracondylar femur requires surgery in most instances. Good to excellent results are obtained in 70% of patients after fixing the fracture with a 95-degree blade plate or retrograde nail reinforced with polymethylmethacrylate.[60] Rigid fixation palliates symptoms and improves the quality of life. Postoperative radiotherapy is usually indicated to stop tumor progression.

Destructive epiphyseal disease of the proximal tibia or distal femur is best treated by local resection and total knee replacement (Fig. 95.18). When the joint is involved or a stable construct can not be achieved with internal fixation, resection arthroplasty and knee replacement meet the goal of palliation. Tissue such as the extensor mechanism is preserved whenever possible. In these circumstances, function is a priority. A constrained prosthesis is necessary because tumors progress and destabilize the components. Palliative amputation may be the fastest, most dependable treatment for uncontrollable lesions.

SOFT-TISSUE TUMORS

General Concepts

Soft-tissue tumors are approximately 10 times more common than bone tumors. This applies to both benign and malignant tumors. The tumors are generally painless masses, although pain may be present. Rapid growth is often reported in cases that turn out to be malignancies. It reflects not only the cell proliferation rate but hemorrhage and necrosis within the tumor. Physical examination is fundamental to identify the relationship of the tumor to the knee joint and important neurovascular structures. Transillumination is a useful technique to evaluate superficial lesions. Meniscal or ganglion cysts often transmit light because of their fluid-filled nature. These simple tests can obviate the need for formal biopsy of trivial lesions as well as

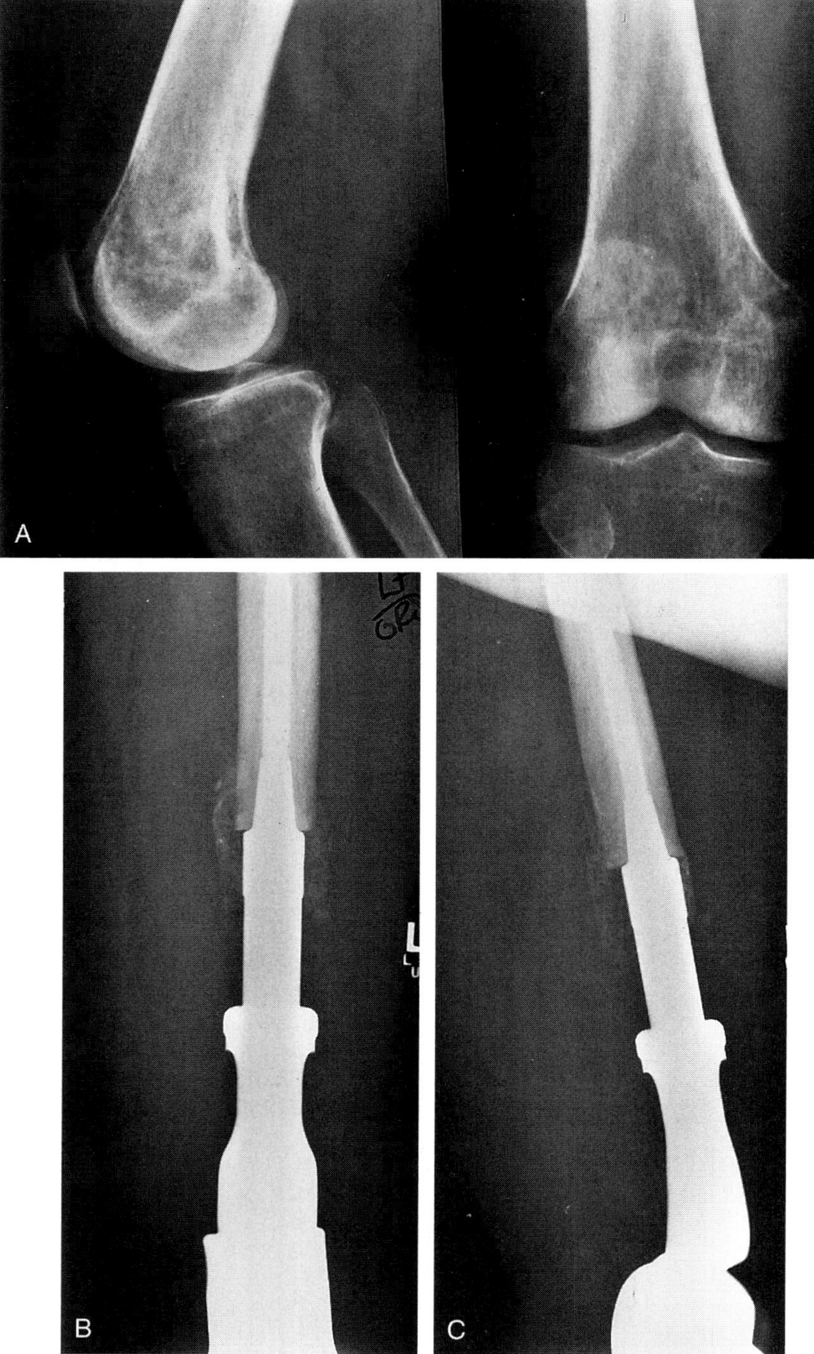

FIGURE 95.18 ➢ *A*, AP and lateral radiographs of metastatic disease permeating the distal femur. AP (*B*) and lateral (*C*) radiographs of the distal femoral reconstruction. Note the extramedullary bone formation on the porous ingrowth surface that augmented fixation.

highlight tumors that must be subject to biopsy sampling.

The diagnostic imaging work-up should be focused. Plain films and MRI or CT with contrast are the only relevant tests. Other studies waste time and resources and rarely provide information that alters diagnosis or treatment. Exceptions are arthrography (with or without CT), used to best demonstrate extension of a mass into or out of the joint, and sonography, which helps to define cystic lesions. These studies are warranted to distinguish tumors from popliteal or meniscal cysts when the clinical picture is not clear.[133, 150] Complete staging studies, including chest CT, should be performed selectively in patients who have an established malignant tumor.

Biopsy is the definitive diagnostic test. As for bone tumors, the physician must make a determination at this time if the local experience and facilities are suitable to treat the most involved tumor that is within the differential diagnosis. If not, the patient should be referred to a specialty center. Biopsy technique varies with the clinical situation, tumor size, and location.

Although surgery is the treatment of choice for all soft-tissue tumors, the magnitude of the resection, extent of surgical margins, possibility of preoperative radiation therapy or investigational chemotherapy or of intraoperative placement of brachytherapy catheters, and appropriate patient counseling justify a discrete biopsy procedure.

The simplest, least-expensive procedure is needle aspiration. This office procedure gives immediate diagnostic information about cystic lesions. If typical joint or ganglion fluid is not obtained, more expensive imaging or more invasive diagnostic tests should be undertaken. Aspiration biopsy cytology can be diagnostic.[110] Prior to any major tumor resection, the diagnosis should usually be established histologically. Needle biopsy is often adequate for this task.[140] The needle track must be marked for excision with the primary specimen. Avoid the common errors of plunging through the tumor and transporting the sarcoma to the underlying bone or into a new fascial compartment.

When the diagnosis is fairly certain, superficial small (<3 cm) lesions can be excised marginally, staying above the fascia. This approach is most suitable for lipomas. Because fatty tumors are notoriously difficult to evaluate by frozen-section histological analysis, primary excision is particularly appropriate. Biopsy samples of superficial large lesions should be taken first because removal of greater amounts of normal tissue is recommended if the lesion is found to be malignant.[120]

Deep lesions are much more often malignant than superficial lesions, although most are still benign. Biopsy samples of deep large tumors should be taken. Deep small tumors are uncommon and present an unusual set of clinical compromises for the surgeon. There is a rationale for incisional biopsy, excisional biopsy, and primary wide excision in dealing with deep small lesions. The final decision depends on the extent of additional disability that would be anticipated if a potential secondary wide excision were needed. If the extra disability is projected to be minimal, a preliminary biopsy procedure is warranted. Conversely, if important anatomic structures would have to be sacrificed if contaminated by the biopsy, the best opportunity to obtain a wide surgical margin without causing undue disability is at the time of the initial procedure. Under these unusual circumstances, a primary wide excision should be chosen.

Benign Soft-Tissue Tumors

Most benign lesions are simply excised and have low recurrence rates. Lipomas are among the most common of all lesions. Most are superficial and do not require treatment. Deeper, intramuscular lipomas are common, particularly in the distal thigh. When deep, painful, or demonstrably growing, suspected lipomas require further investigation. MRI can be virtually diagnostic, distinguishing benign from malignant fatty tumors, particularly when fat saturation sequences are used. Lipomas are removed by marginal excision. Atypical lipomas have a propensity to grow and recur and are common in the deep intramuscular tissue. Excision of atypical lipomas should be en bloc, removing a narrow muscle margin when possible. Follow-up must be sustained.

Popliteal cysts may be primary or secondary and are the most common soft-tissue masses found behind the knee. If the presumed cyst is not in the typical location adjacent to the semimembranosus or medial gastrocnemius, or if fluid cannot be aspirated, further work-up is needed because soft-tissue sarcomas may simulate popliteal cysts. Clinical examination should usually be supplemented with MRI, CT, or ultrasonography to confirm the cystic nature of the mass and help identify intra-articular pathology that may have contributed to the development of the cyst.[108, 134] A solid tumor is suspected if the arthrogram does not show communication between the joint and the lesion or if the sonogram shows echogenic solid areas. Biopsy should be performed when diagnosis is uncertain. Care must be taken to avoid contaminating popliteal neurovascular structures with tumor to maximize the potential to cure a possible malignancy with less than an amputation. Needle biopsy of the mass is often the prudent approach. Symptomatic cysts refractory to conservative treatment are excised. Popliteal cysts in children are usually painless, and most regress spontaneously.[36]

Extra-abdominal desmoid tumors are aggressive, infiltrating tumors that may develop after trauma. They recur frequently, grow invasively, and may develop in multiple sites within the extremity. Imaging these tumors is extremely difficult, particularly with CT, because the density of the tumor mimics that of the surrounding tissue. Therefore, contrast-enhanced MRI should be used.[45] Surgery is the only definitive treatment. Wide excision is preferred.[57, 62, 128] Trauma is implicated in many cases, and surgery may paradoxically trigger recurrent disease.

Adjuvant radiotherapy may reduce local recurrence but compromises follow-up examination of the radiated tissue and may cause extra morbidity such as neuropathy, edema, or even sarcomatous degeneration.[137] We use radiation selectively for recurrent cases or when recurrence has both a high probability and a significant consequence if it does occur. Favorable reports of chemotherapy,[119, 130, 144, 157] hormonal therapy,[69, 131, 149] or anti-inflammatory therapy[37, 82, 122] for desmoid tumors abound, but no controlled trials exist and response rates do not justify routine chemotherapy.

Synovial chondromatosis is an uncommon cause of painful knee swelling and effusion. Diagnostic metaplastic foci of cartilage develop in the synovium. Calcified or even ossified foci are usually visible radiographically (Fig. 95.19). They may detach and appear as loose bodies in the joint but usually remain fixed in the joint capsule or synovium. Double-contrast arthrography demonstrates these deposits particularly well. Histologically, the tissue appears very active or even pseudomalignant. Complete synovectomy and removal of the loose bodies are the indicated treatments. Arthroscopic treatment is sometimes sufficient, but large

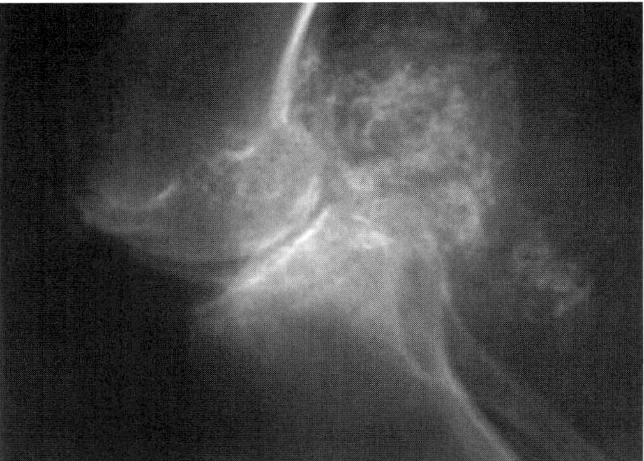

FIGURE 95.19 ➢ MRI of synovial chondromatosis with masses anterior and posterior to the knee joint and an associated popliteal cyst.

masses may develop in the posterior capsule that are amenable only to open surgical excision. Isolated loose bodies rarely recur, whereas extensive multifocal synovial involvement is difficult to eradicate.

Pigmented villonodular synovitis is a form of monoarthritis most common around the knee. It occurs in young and middle-aged adults. Similar to synovial chondromatosis, it is an inflammatory condition and is associated with a substantial amount of joint pain and sensitivity and recurrent hemarthrosis. Radiographs usually show only nonspecific synovitis, but erosions on both sides of the joint may result. Various inflammatory arthropathies and chronic infections such as tuberculosis can have this same appearance, both clinically and radiographically. Asymmetric cysts on one side of the joint have been mistaken for GCTs and malignant neoplasms. Pigmented villonodular synovitis must be distinguished histologically from nonspecific synovitis with focal hemorrhage and rheumatoid arthritis. Mild diffuse synovial disease can be treated by arthroscopic synovectomy. Extensive, erosive, and recurrent synovial disease is best treated by open total synovectomy. This may require two incisions, anticipating the future likelihood of total knee arthroplasty (Fig. 95.20). Localized nodular disease requires wide local excision to eradicate the tumor. Recurrent disease may require en bloc excision of the joint or even amputation.

Periarticular muscle is the most common site for intramuscular hemangiomas. The distal vastus muscles and the knee capsule are the commonest sites for this developmental, neoplastic condition (Fig. 95.21). Symptomatic masses usually arise in the third and fourth decades of life. They typically cause a dull aching pain that becomes severe and throbbing after exercise. Adolescents seem to be particularly prone to this activity-related pain from hemangiomas.

Smaller lesions may be exquisitely sensitive to percussion despite lacking tenderness to deep palpation.

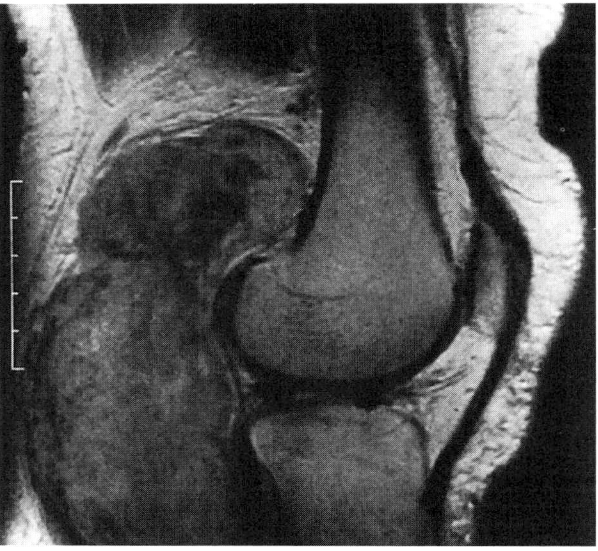

FIGURE 95.20 ➢ Lateral MRI of pigmented villonodular synovitis that demonstrates the typical mixed, low-signal-intensity mass in the popliteal space, enveloping the popliteal vessels.

Intramuscular hemangiomas are multifocal in at least 25% of cases. Therefore, although excision may be effective in eliminating pain, recurrence is frequent. Excision must be judicious to remove all the identifiable tumor yet preserve important joint and muscle tissue. Inadequate tumor excision merely spreads the disease in the periarticular tissue,[19] contributes to tumor recurrence, and is associated with chronic pain and disability in many instances. Experimental techniques, such as interferon-α administration[30] and intravascular sclerosis by embolization or injection, hold promise for improved treatment of this disorder. Keep

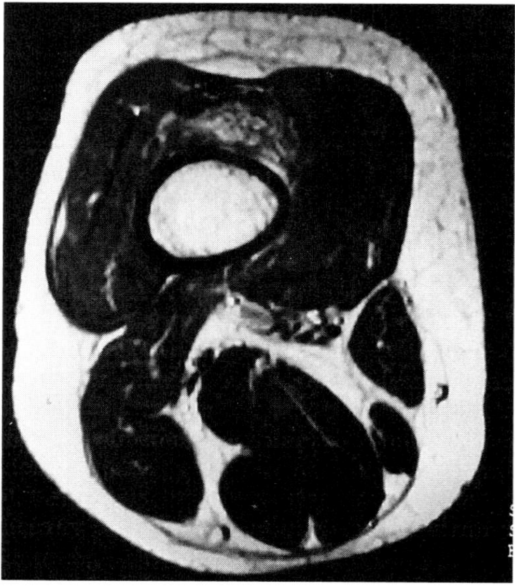

FIGURE 95.21 ➢ Axial MRI of the distal thigh, demonstrating the high-signal hemangioma in the vastus intermedius.

a tourniquet in abeyance, but avoid exsanguination of the limb before attempting excision because it deflates the dilated tumor vessels and it becomes difficult to define the extent of the lesion.

Soft-Tissue Sarcomas

Epidemiology and Clinical Features

Approximately one-third of soft-tissue sarcomas occur in the thigh or knee region. Malignant fibrous histiocytoma and liposarcoma are the most common. Around the knee, synovial sarcoma is also common, particularly in young adults. "Bone" malignancies such as mesenchymal and myxoid chondrosarcoma have a predilection for the popliteal area, despite their overall rarity. Perhaps the tumors that are most important to distinguish are embryonal rhabdomyosarcomas in children and young adults because chemotherapy plays an important role in their cure. Malignant peripheral nerve sheath tumors are among the most difficult to image accurately because of common intraneural spread, and they are refractory to adjuvant therapies. Some authors question whether these facts preclude successful limb salvage surgery for such tumors. Subclassification of soft-tissue sarcomas has not been proved to be of diagnostic or therapeutic value. Some investigators report that there may be some value because synovial sarcoma is particularly sensitive to high-dose ifosfamide and leiomyosarcoma is not very responsive to this agent.

There are no reliable historical or physical examination features that distinguish between benign and malignant soft-tissue lesions. For example, benign tumors and soft-tissue sarcomas are usually asymptomatic. Biopsy is usually required. Biopsy samples of persistent, painful, or growing deep masses should be taken. Biopsy samples of tumors fixed to skin or deep structures also must be taken. Lymphadenopathy may indicate neoplastic spread. Enlarged regional lymph nodes mandate biopsy sampling. However, most sarcomas metastasize via the hematogenous route, and lymphatic involvement is uncommon (1% to 5%).[49] Several sarcomas such as epithelioid sarcoma, embryonal rhabdomyosarcoma, clear cell sarcoma and, to a lesser extent, synovial sarcoma have a propensity to spread via the lymphatic system.

As noted previously, one should be parsimonious in ordering tests. Plain films are very important for identifying soft-tissue calcifications. Calcification can occur in any soft-tissue sarcoma, most commonly the ectopic "bone" tumors, synovial sarcoma, and leiomyosarcoma. MRI or contrast-enhanced CT is needed for three-dimensional imaging of the lesion. They may show important diagnostic information such as central necrosis or fluid-fluid levels but are nonspecific diagnostically. Bone scans have poor accuracy and poor positive predictive value in soft-tissue sarcomas. Gallium scans may be helpful for certain round cell tumors such as Ewing's sarcoma but are insensitive for mesenchymal tumors, failing to image primary and recurrent lesions under 5 cm reliably. Important staging studies such as chest CT can be performed if a malignancy is confirmed histologically.

Staging and Prognostic Factors

The most important early prognostic factor in patients with soft-tissue sarcomas is the histological grade of the tumor. Survival is inversely proportional to grade. Broder I and II, well-differentiated, Musculoskeletal Tumor Society (MSTS) stage I tumors have the best prognosis. Broder III and IV, poorly differentiated, MSTS stage II tumors have the worst prognosis. The Hadju system, which is based on tumor grade, size, and depth relative to the deep fascia, is more predictive of survival and local control than the MSTS staging system. The factors are independently predictive of outcome in multivariate analysis.[18, 49, 85, 125] Compartmentalization of soft-tissue sarcomas, significant by univariate analysis, ceases to be important in multivariate analysis. The importance of tumor size increases and tumor grade decreases over time.

These observations have led to the adoption of the American Joint Committee on Cancer Staging System, 5th edition, in 1997 (Table 95.3). This prognostic

TABLE 95.3 **AMERICAN JOINT COMMITTEE ON CANCER (AJCC) STAGING SYSTEM FOR SOFT TISSUE SARCOMA, 5TH ED**

Stage	Substage	Grade	Size	Depth
I	A	Low	Small	Superficial
	—	Low	Small	Deep
	B	Low	Large	Superficial
II	A	Low	Large	Deep
	B	High	Small	Superficial
	—	High	Small	Deep
	C	High	Large	Superficial
III	—	High	Large	Deep
IV	—	Metastases		

From Fleming ID, Cooper JS, Henson DE, et al: Soft tissue sarcoma. In Fleming DI, Cooper JS, Henson DE, et al, eds: AJCC Cancer Staging Manual, 5th ed. Philadelphia, Lippincott-Raven, 1997, pp 149–156.

value of this system is better than for the Enneking Musculoskeletal Tumor Society System. Disease-free survival (5-year) correlates with stage: I = 78%, II = 64%, III = 36%. Invasiveness may be an important additional factor. Karakousis et al found the lowest survival rates in patients with nerve, artery, or bone involvement.[73] Several investigators have reported independent prognostic value for tumor DNA ploidy (diploid, good prognosis; aneuploid, bad prognosis).[9] New biological markers are being investigated to identify tumors with the highest probability of metastasis and patients with the greatest need for effective systemic chemotherapy.[84] Recurrent sarcomas are more likely to recur again and to metastasize. Local recurrence is probably a marker for biologically aggressive disease. Occasionally, it may contribute to subsequent metastasis.[17, 86]

Surgery

Limb-sparing treatment is as effective as amputation in curing soft-tissue sarcoma, as shown by a randomized National Cancer Institute trial. Because of the locally invasive nature of these lesions, local recurrence rates of up to 30% occur with local excision of large high-grade sarcomas (stage IIC or III) unless an effective adjuvant is used. Radical compartment resection or wide excision plus radiation therapy (60 Gy) reduces local recurrence rates to less than 10%.[163] Preoperative radiotherapy followed by marginal excision works as effectively in selected cases.[127]

Patients who have undergone "total removal" of a mass that was later discovered to have been a soft-tissue sarcoma make up a mixed population. Generally, they should undergo repeat excision with a wide margin (Fig. 95.22). In such cases, gross tumor remains in one-third of patients, microscopic tumor remains in one-third, and most of the others have undetectable cancer that would inevitably recur without the re-excision. Despite successful re-excision, results may not be as good as would have been achieved if the tumor were adequately excised the first time.

The role of adjuvant radiation therapy in the treatment of large, low-grade sarcomas remains to be deter-

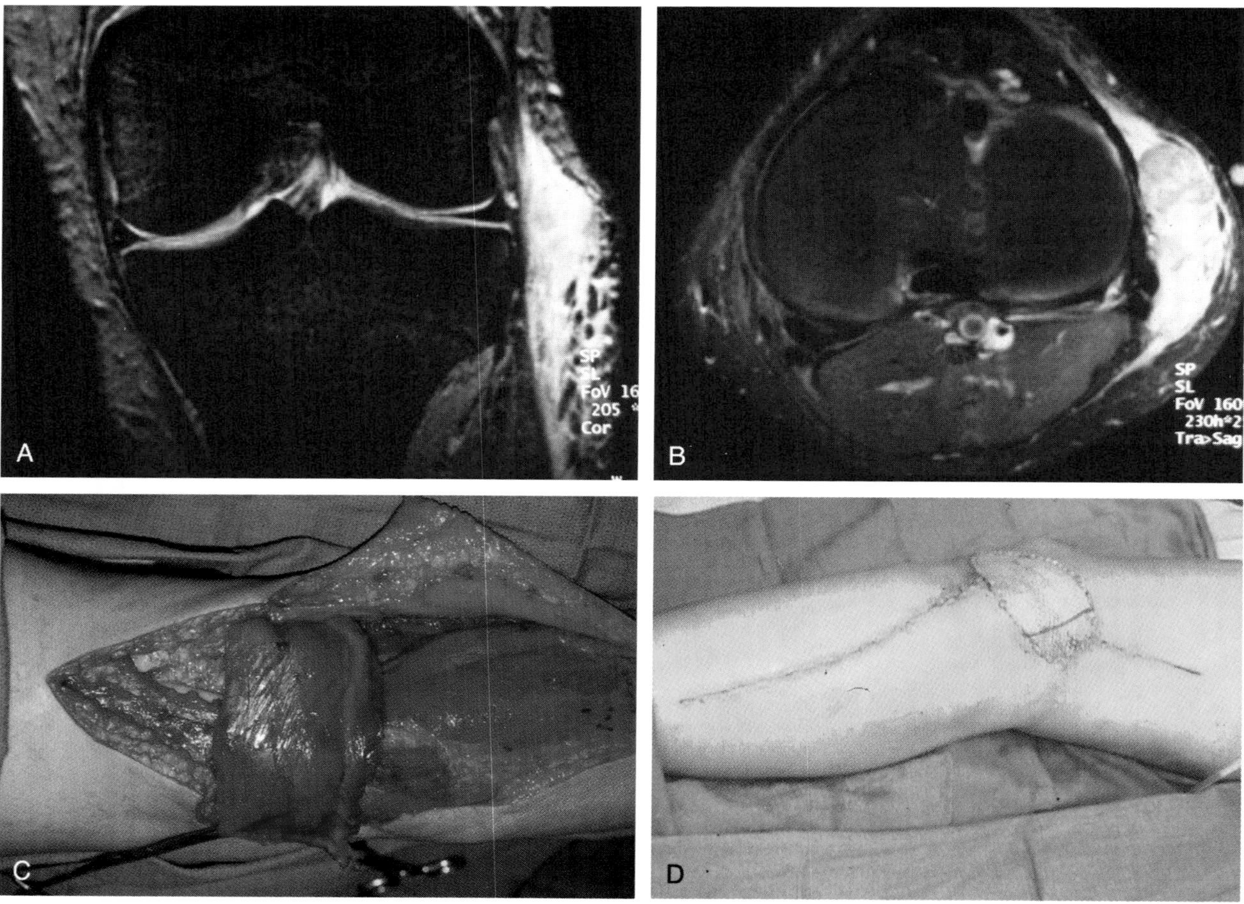

FIGURE 95.22 ➢ *A* and *B*, MRI of a soft tissue mass penetrating the deep fascia. It was enucleated at the same time the knee underwent arthroscopy for suspected intra-articular pathology. Malignant fibrous histiocytoma was found with positive margins. *C*, Intraoperative picture of the lateral gastrocnemius flap used to cover the large soft-tissue defect. *D*, Postoperative picture showing the skin-grafted site. Supplemental radiation was also given.

mined. Brachytherapy does not improve the results, but external beam radiation may. Small sarcomas (<5 cm), whether low (stage IA) or high grade, superficial or deep (stage IIA or B), can be treated with excision alone and no radiation therapy. The local recurrence rate with this technique is 10%, the 5-year survival rate is 94%, and neither outcome is improved with chemotherapy or radiation therapy.[51] Primary amputation continues to have a role for bulky, invasive tumors wherein vascular, bone or joint, and soft-tissue reconstruction cannot restore reasonable function in the extremity. Amputation for extensive recurrent disease remains the procedure of choice.

Radiation

Radiation oncologists use various methods to deliver adjuvant radiotherapy. At Sloan-Kettering, brachytherapy is used whenever possible to administer the equivalent of at least 60 Gy via iridium or iodine beads.[126] Empty catheters are placed intraoperatively. When the wound is healed adequately (about 5 days postoperatively), the radiation seeds are loaded into the catheters. When treatment is completed after 4 days of radiation, the catheters are removed. Total treatment time is shortened from the 6 weeks required for conventional cobalt external beam radiotherapy. Several centers are experimenting with intraoperative radiotherapy in combination with either preoperative or postoperative radiotherapy. Early results have shown this to be an effective technique, although at the expense of toxicity to neural structures.[143]

Chemotherapy

Because there is a 40% to 80% mortality rate with high-grade soft-tissue sarcoma, the need for effective systemic therapy is obvious. Adjuvant chemotherapy remains a tantalizing prospect to improve the outcome in patients with soft-tissue sarcoma with poor prognostic factors (large, high-grade, deep tumors). Doxorubicin-containing protocols appear to be the most effective for metastatic disease and have been tried as adjuvant therapies. However, promising reports of single-agent and multiagent chemotherapy regimens have not been corroborated in most randomized trials of adjuvant treatment. A meta-analysis of 14 randomized trials suggests that adjuvant doxorubicin-based chemotherapy significantly improves local recurrence-free survival by 6% and disease-free survival by 10% at 10 years. Overall survival was improved insignificantly (relative risk of failure, 0.89).[70] Chemotherapy is undependable for shrinking local soft-tissue sarcoma. Chemotherapy is being used with increasing frequency for localized soft-tissue sarcomas but should be used judiciously.

Soft-tissue tumors are within the orthopedist's purview. Careful work-up, staging, limb-sparing surgery, and adjuvant radiation therapy for large high-grade sarcomas are the standards of care. Patients should be referred for consideration of chemotherapy when the tumor is large, high grade, and deep. The orthopedist should remain involved as the best person to reconstruct the patient's limb, optimize functional results, and evaluate for recurrent disease.

REFERENCES

1. Aboulafia AJ, Rosenbaum DH, Sicard-Rosenbaum L, et al: Treatment of large subchondral tumors of the knee with cryosurgery and composite reconstruction. Clin Orthop 307:189, 1994.
2. Adjuvant chemotherapy for localized resectable soft-tissue sarcoma of adults: Meta-analysis of individual data. Sarcoma Meta-Analysis Collaboration. Lancet 350:1647, 1997.
3. Ahuja SC, Villacin AB, Smith J, et al: Juxtacortical (parosteal) osteogenic sarcoma: Histological grading and prognosis. J Bone Joint Surg Am 59:632, 1977.
4. AJCC Cancer Staging Manual, 5th ed. Philadelphia, Lippincott-Raven, 1997.
5. Arroyo JS, Garvin KL, Neff JR: Arthrodesis of the knee with a modular titanium intramedullary nail. J Bone Joint Surg Am 79: 26, 1997.
6. Bacci G, Ferrari S, Mercuri M, et al: Predictive factors for local recurrence in osteosarcoma: 540 patients with extremity tumors followed for minimum 2.5 years after neoadjuvant chemotherapy. Acta Orthop Scand 69:230, 1998.
7. Bacci G, Picci P, Mercuri M, et al: Neoadjuvant chemotherapy for high grade malignant fibrous histiocytoma of bone. Clin Orthop 178:346 1998.
8. Bacci G, Ruggieri P, Picci P, et al: Changing pattern of relapse in osteosarcoma of the extremities treated with adjuvant and neoadjuvant chemotherapy. J Chemother 7:230, 1995.
9. Bauer HCF, Kreicbergs A, Tribukait B: DNA content prognostic in soft-tissue sarcoma. Acta Orthop Scand 62:187, 1991.
10. Bell RS, Davis A, Allan DG, et al: Fresh osteochondral allografts for advanced giant cell tumors at the knee. J Arthroplasty 9: 603, 1994.
11. Bertoni F, Bacchini P, Fabbri N, et al: Osteosarcoma: Low-grade intraosseous-type osteosarcoma, histologicalally resembling parosteal osteosarcoma, fibrous dysplasia, and desmoplastic fibroma. Cancer 71:338, 1993.
12. Bertoni F, Boriani S, Laus M, et al: Periosteal chondrosarcoma and periosteal osteosarcoma: Two distinct entities. J Bone Joint Surg Br 64:370, 1982.
13. Bertoni F, Unni KK, Beabout JW, et al: Parosteal osteoma of bones other than of the skull and face. Cancer 75:2466, 1995.
14. Bini SA, Gill K, Johnston JO: Giant cell tumor of bone: Curettage and cement reconstruction. Clin Orthop 245:321, 1995.
15. Blackley HR, Wunder JS, Davis AM, et al: Treatment of giant-cell tumors of long bones with curettage and bone-grafting. J Bone Joint Surg Am 81:811, 1999.
16. Blunn GW, Wait ME, Lilley P, et al: The reactions of tissues to titanium wear generated from massive segmental bone defect prostheses. In Brown KLB, ed: Complications of Limb Salvage. Montreal, ISOLS, 1991, p 429.
17. Brennan MF: The enigma of local recurrence: The Society of Surgical Oncology. Ann Surg Oncol 4:1, 1997.
18. Brennan MF: Staging of soft-tissue sarcomas [editorial]. Ann Surg Oncol 6:8, 1999.
19. Bruns J, Eggers-Stroeder G, von Torklus D: Synovial hemangioma—a rare benign synovial tumor: Report of four cases. Knee Surg Sports Traumatol Arthrosc 2:186, 1994.
20. Caffey J: On fibrous defects in cortical walls of growing tubular bones: Their radiologic appearance, structure, prevalence, natural course, and diagnostic significance. Adv Pediatr 7:13, 1955.
21. Cammisa FP Jr, Glasser DB, Otis JC, et al: The Van Nes tibial rotationplasty: A functionally viable reconstructive procedure in children who have a tumor of the distal end of the femur. J Bone Joint Surg Am 72:1541, 1990.
22. Campanacci M, Baldini N, Boriani S, et al: Giant-cell tumor of bone. J Bone Joint Surg Am 69:106, 1987.
23. Campanacci M, Capanna R, Picci P: Unicameral and aneurysmal bone cysts. Clin Orthop 25:204, 1986.
24. Campanacci M, Costa P: Total resection of distal femur or proximal tibia for bone tumours: Autogenous bone grafts and arthrodesis in twenty-six cases. J Bone Joint Surg Br 61:455, 1979.

25. Campanacci M, Mercuri M, Gasbarrini A, et al: The value of imaging in the diagnosis and treatment of bone tumors. Eur J Radiol 27:116, 1998.
26. Campanacci M, Picci P, Gherlinzoni F, et al: Parosteal osteosarcoma. J Bone Joint Surg Br 66:313, 1984.
27. Capanna R, Fabbri N, Bettelli G: Curettage of giant cell tumor of bone: The effect of surgical technique and adjuvants on local recurrence rate. Chir Organi Mov 75:206, 1990.
28. Capanna R, Morris HG, Campanacci D, et al: Modular uncemented prosthetic reconstruction after resection of tumours of the distal femur. J Bone Joint Surg Br 76:178, 1994.
29. Capanna R, Ruggieri P, Biagini R, et al: The effect of quadriceps excision on functional results after distal femoral resection and prosthetic replacement of bone tumors. Clin Orthop 186: 267, 1991.
30. Chang E, Boyd A, Nelson CC, et al: Successful treatment of infantile hemangiomas with interferon-alpha-2b. J Pediatr Hematol Oncol 19:237, 1997.
31. Chen CK, Yeh LR, Pan HB, et al: Intra-articular gouty tophi of the knee: CT and MR imaging in 12 patients. Skeletal Radiol 28:75, 1999.
32. Clohisy DR, Mankin HJ: Osteoarticular allografts for reconstruction after resection of a musculoskeletal tumor in the proximal end of the tibia. J Bone Joint Surg Am 76:549, 1994.
33. Cool WP, Carter SR, Grimer RJ, et al: Growth after extendible endoprosthetic replacement of the distal femur. J Bone Joint Surg Br 79:938, 1997.
34. Dalinka MK, Zlatkin MB, Chao P, et al: The use of magnetic resonance imaging in the evaluation of bone and soft-tissue tumors. Rad Clin North Am 28:461, 1990.
35. De Boeck H, Aerts P, Casteleyn PP: Chondroblastoma of the upper end of the tibia, invading the attachment of the posterior cruciate ligament. Acta Orthop Belg 55:129, 1989.
36. Dinham JM: Popliteal cysts in children: The case against surgery. J Bone Joint Surg Br 57:69, 1975.
37. Dominguez-Malagon HR, Alfeiran-Ruiz A, Chavarria-Xicotencatl P, et al: Clinical and cellular effects of colchicine in fibromatosis. Cancer 69:2478, 1992.
38. Dorfman HD, Czerniak B: Bone cancers. Cancer 75:203, 1995.
39. Draganich LF, Nicholas RW, Shuster JK, et al: The effects of resection of the proximal part of the fibula on stability of the knee and on gait. J Bone Joint Surg Am 73:575, 1991.
40. Dreinhofer KE, Rydholm A, Bauer HC, et al: Giant-cell tumours with fracture at diagnosis: Curettage and acrylic cementing in ten cases. J Bone Joint Surg Br 77:189, 1995.
41. Dunham WK, Marcus NW, Enneking WF, et al: Developmental defects of the distal femoral metaphysis. J Bone Joint Surg Am 62:801, 1980.
42. Dunst J, Sauer R, Burgers JM, et al: Radiation therapy as local treatment in Ewing's sarcoma: Results of the Cooperative Ewing's Sarcoma Studies CESS 81 and CESS 86. Cancer 67:2818, 1993.
43. Earl HM, Pringle J, Kemp H, et al: Chemotherapy of malignant fibrous histiocytoma of bone. Ann Oncol 4:409, 1993.
44. Eckardt JJ, Safran MR, Eilber FR, et al: Expandable endoprosthetic reconstruction of the skeletally immature after malignant bone tumor resection. Clin Orthop 188:297, 1993.
45. Eich GF, Hoeffel JC, Tschappeler H, et al: Fibrous tumours in children: Imaging features of a heterogeneous group of disorders. Pediatr Radiol 28:500, 1998.
46. Enneking WF, Shirley PD: Resection-arthrodesis for malignant and potentially malignant lesions about the knee using an intramedullary rod and local bone grafts. J Bone Joint Surg Am 59: 223, 1977.
47. Fam AG: Calcium pyrophosphate crystal deposition disease and other crystal deposition diseases. Curr Opin Rheumatol 4:574, 1992.
48. Fleming ID, Cooper JS, Henson DE, et al: Soft Tissue Sarcoma. In: Fleming DI, Cooper JS, Henson DE, et al, eds: AJCC Cancer Staging Manual, 5th ed. Philadelphia, Lippincott-Raven, 1997, p 149.
49. Fong Y, Coit DG, Woodruff JM, et al: Lymph node metastasis from soft-tissue sarcoma in adults: Analysis of data from a prospective database of 1772 sarcoma patients. Ann Surg 217:72, 1993.
50. Freedman EL, Eckardt JJ: A modular endoprosthetic system for tumor and non-tumor reconstruction: Preliminary experience. Orthopedics 20:27, 1997.
51. Geer RJ, Woodruff J, Casper ES, et al: Management of small soft-tissue sarcoma of the extremity in adults [see comments]. Arch Surg 127:1285, 1992.
52. Gerster JC, Landry M, Duvoisin B, et al: Computed tomography of the knee joint as an indicator of intra-articular tophi in gout. Arthritis Rheum 39:1406, 1996.
53. Gitelis S, Piasecki P: Allograft prosthetic composite arthroplasty for osteosarcoma and other aggressive bone tumors. Clin Orthop 270:197, 1992.
54. Gonzalez-Herranz P, Burgos-Flores J, Ocete-Guzman JG, et al: The management of limb-length discrepancies in children after treatment of osteosarcoma and Ewing's sarcoma. J Pediatr Orthop 15:561, 1995.
55. Goorin A, Baker A, Gieser P, et al: No evidence for improved event free survival (EFS) with presurgical chemotherapy (PRE) for non-metastatic extremity osteogenic sarcoma (OGS): Preliminary results of randomized pediatric oncology group (POG) trial 8651 (Meeting abstract). Proceedings of the Annual Meeting of the Am Soc Clin Oncol 14:1420, 1995.
56. Gottsauner-Wolf F, Rock MG, Pritchard D, et al: Extracortical bone bridging for endoprosthetic shaft anchorage in segmental bone/joint defect replacement. In Brown KLB, ed: Complications of Limb Salvage. Montreal, ISOLS, 1991, p 439.
57. Goy BW, Lee SP, Fu YS, et al: Treatment results of unresected or partially resected desmoid tumors. Am J Clin Oncol 21:584, 1998.
58. Ham SJ, Hoekstra HJ, van der Graaf WT, et al: The value of high-dose methotrexate-based neoadjuvant chemotherapy in malignant fibrous histiocytoma of bone. J Clin Oncol 14:490, 1996.
59. Harris IE, Leff AR, Gitelis S, et al: Function after amputation, arthrodesis, or arthroplasty for tumors about the knee. J Bone Joint Surg Am 72:1477, 1990.
60. Healey JH, Lane JM: Treatment of pathological fractures of the distal femur with the Zickel supracondylar nail. Clin Orthop 250:216, 1990.
61. Heare TC, Enneking WF, Heare MM: Staging techniques and biopsy of bone tumors. Orthop Clin North Am 20:273, 1989.
62. Higaki S, Tateishi A, Ohno T, et al: Surgical treatment of extra-abdominal desmoid tumours (aggressive fibromatoses). Int Orthop 19:383, 1995.
63. Hornicek FJ Jr, Mnaymneh W, Lackman RD, et al: Limb salvage with osteoarticular allografts after resection of proximal tibia bone tumors. Clin Orthop 352:179, 1998.
64. Horowitz SM, Glasser DB, Lane JM, et al: Prosthetic and extremity survivorship after limb salvage for sarcoma: How long do the reconstructions last? Clin Orthop 280, 1993.
65. Horowitz SM, Lane JM, Healey JH: Soft-tissue management with prosthetic replacement for sarcomas around the knee. Clin Orthop 226, 1992.
66. Horowitz SM, Lane JM, Otis JC, et al: Prosthetic arthroplasty of the knee after resection of a sarcoma in the proximal end of the tibia: A report of sixteen cases. J Bone Joint Surg Am 73: 286, 1991.
67. Huvos AG: Osteogenic sarcoma. In Anonymous, ed: Bone Tumors: Diagnosis, Treatment, and Prognosis, 2nd ed. Philadelphia, WB Saunders, 1991, p 85.
68. Ikeda K, Tsuchiya H, Shimozaki E, et al: Use of latissimus dorsi flap for reconstruction with prostheses after tumor resection. Microsurgery 15:73, 1994.
69. Izes JK, Zinman LN, Larsen CR: Regression of large pelvic desmoid tumor by tamoxifen and sulindac. Urology 47:756, 1996.
70. Jaeger HJ, Kruegener GH, Donovan AG: Patellar metastasis from a malignant melanoma. Int Orthop 16:282, 1992.
71. Jeon DG, Kawai A, Boland P, et al: Algorithm for the surgical treatment of malignant lesions of the proximal tibia. Clin Orthop 15, 1999.
72. Juhn A, Healey JH, Ghelman B, et al: Subacute osteomyelitis presenting as bone tumors. Orthopedics 12:245, 1989.

73. Karakousis CP, Kontzoglou K, Driscoll D: Sarcomas near extremity joints in adults. J Surg Oncol 67:164, 1998.
74. Kawai A, Backus SI, Otis JC, et al: Interrelationships of clinical outcome, length of resection, and energy cost of walking after prosthetic knee replacement following resection of a malignant tumor of the distal aspect of the femur. J Bone Joint Surg Am 80:822, 1998.
75. Kawai A, Healey JH, Boland PJ, et al: A rotating-hinge knee replacement for malignant tumors of the femur and tibia. J Arthroplasty 14:187, 1999.
76. Kawai A, Lin PP, Boland PJ, et al: Relationship between magnitude of resection, complication, and prosthetic survival after prosthetic knee reconstructions for distal femoral tumors. J Surg Oncol 70:109, 1999.
77. Kawai A, Muschler GF, Lane JM, et al: Prosthetic knee replacement after resection of a malignant tumor of the distal part of the femur: Medium to long-term results. J Bone Joint Surg Am 80:636, 1998.
78. Kenan S, DeSimone DP, Lewis MM: Limb sparing for skeletally immature patients with osteosarcoma: The expandable prosthesis. Cancer Treat Res 62:205, 1993.
79. Kleinerman ES, Gano JB, Johnston DA, et al: Efficacy of liposomal muramyl tripeptide (CGP 19835A) in the treatment of relapsed osteosarcoma. Am J Clin Oncol 18:93, 1995.
80. Kotz R: Rotationplasty. Semin Surg Oncol 13:34, 1997.
81. Kuttesch JF Jr, Wexler LH, Marcus RB, et al: Second malignancies after Ewing's sarcoma: Radiation dose-dependency of secondary sarcomas. J Clin Oncol 14:2818, 1996.
82. Lackner H, Urban C, Kerbl R, et al: Noncytotoxic drug therapy in children with unresectable desmoid tumors. Cancer 80:334, 1997.
83. Lesavoy MA, Dubrow TJ, Wackym PA, Eckardt JJ: Muscle-flap coverage of exposed endoprostheses. Plast Reconstr Surg 83: 90, 1989.
84. Levine EA, Holzmayer T, Bacus S, et al: Evaluation of newer prognostic markers for adult soft-tissue sarcomas. J Clin Oncol 15:3249, 1997.
85. Lewis JJ, Leung D, Casper ES, et al: Multifactorial analysis of long-term follow-up (more than 5 years) of primary extremity sarcoma. Arch Surg 134:190, 1999.
86. Lewis JJ, Leung D, Heslin M, et al: Association of local recurrence with subsequent survival in extremity soft-tissue sarcoma. J Clin Oncol 15:646, 1997.
87. Lewis RJ, Marcove RC, Rosen G: Ewing's sarcoma—functional effects of radiation therapy. J Bone Joint Surg Am 59:325, 1977.
88. Lewis SJ, Bell RS, Fernandes BJ, et al: Malignant lymphoma of bone. Can J Surg 37:43, 1994.
89. Link MP, Goorin AM, Horowitz M, et al: Adjuvant chemotherapy of high-grade osteosarcoma of the extremity: Updated results of the Multi-Institutional Osteosarcoma Study. Clin Orthop 8, 1991.
90. Malawer MM: Surgical management of aggressive and malignant tumors of the proximal fibula. Clin Orthop 172, 1984.
91. Malawer MM, Bickels J, Meller I, et al: Cryosurgery in the treatment of giant cell tumor: A long term followup study. Clin Orthop Rel Res 359:176, 1999.
92. Malawer MM, Chou LB: Prosthetic survival and clinical results with use of large-segment replacements in the treatment of high-grade bone sarcomas. J Bone Joint Surg Am 77:1154, 1995.
93. Malawer MM, Price WM: Gastrocnemius transposition flap in conjunction with limb-sparing surgery for primary bone sarcomas around the knee. Plast Reconstr Surg 73:741, 1984.
94. Mankin HJ, Gebhardt MC, Jennings LC, et al: Long-term results of allograft replacement in the management of bone tumors. Clin Orthop 324:86, 1996.
95. Mankin HJ, Mankin CJ, Simon MA: The hazards of the biopsy, revisited: Members of the Musculoskeletal Tumor Society [see comments]. J Bone Joint Surg Am 78:656, 1996.
96. Marcove RC, Jensen MJ: Radical resection for osteogenic sarcoma of fibula with preservation of limb. Clin Orthop 125:173, 1977.
97. Marcove RC, Sheth DS, Takemoto S, et al: The treatment of aneurysmal bone cyst. Clin Orthop 157, 1995.
98. Marcove RC, Shoji H, Arlen M: Altered carbohydrate metabolism in cartilagenous tumors. Contemp Surg 5:53, 1974.
99. Marcove RC, Weis, Vaghaiwalla MR: Cryosurgery in the treatment of giant cell tumors of bone: A report of 52 consecutive cases. Cancer 41:957, 1978.
100. Marcove RC, Wolfe SW, Healey JH, et al: Massive solitary tophus containing calcium pyrophosphate dihydrate crystals at the acromioclavicular joint. Clin Orthop 227:305, 1988.
101. Martinez V, Sissons HA: Aneurysmal bone cyst: A review of 123 cases including primary lesions and those secondary to other bone pathology. Cancer 61:2291, 1988.
102. McDonald DJ, Sim FH, McLeod RA, et al: Giant cell tumor of bone. J Bone Joint Surg Am 68:235, 1986.
103. Meller I, Ariche A, Sagi A: The role of the gastrocnemius muscle flap in limb-sparing surgery for bone sarcomas of the distal femur: A proposed classification of muscle transfers. Plast Reconstr Surg 99:751, 1997.
104. Menendez LR, Murata GT, Cahill EL, et al: Polymethylmethacrylation in the treatment of giant cell tumors. In Langlais F, Tomeno B, eds: Limb Salvage—Major Reconstructions in Oncologic and Nontumoral Conditions. Berlin, Springer-Verlag, 1991, p 147.
105. Meyers PA, Heller G, Healey JH, et al: Osteogenic sarcoma with clinically detectable metastasis at initial presentation. J Clin Oncol 11:449, 1993.
106. Meyers PA, Heller G, Healey JH, et al: Chemotherapy for nonmetastatic osteogenic sarcoma: The Memorial Sloan-Kettering experience. J Clin Oncol 10:5, 1992.
107. Meyers PA, Heller G, Vlamis V: Osteosarcoma of the extremities: Chemotherapy experience at Memorial Sloan-Kettering. Cancer Treat Res 62:309, 1993.
108. Miller TT, Staron RB, Koenigsberg T, et al: MR imaging of Baker cysts: Association with internal derangement, effusion, and degenerative arthropathy [see comments]. Radiology 201: 247, 1996.
109. Moseley CF: Management of leg-length disparities after tumor surgery [editorial]. J Pediatr Orthop 15:559, 1995.
110. Muddu BN, Barrie JL, Morris MA: Aspiration and injection for meniscal cysts [see comments]. J Bone Joint Surg Br 74:627, 1992.
111. Muscolo DL, Ayerza MA, Calabrese ME, et al: The use of a bone allograft for reconstruction after resection of giant-cell tumor close to the knee. J Bone Joint Surg Am 75:1656, 1993.
112. Nimityongskul P, Anderson LD, Dowling EA: Chondromyxoid fibroma. Orthop Rev 21:863, 1992.
113. O'Donnell RJ, Springfield DS, Motwani HK, et al: Recurrence of giant-cell tumors of the long bones after curettage and packing with cement. J Bone Joint Surg Am 76:1827, 1994.
114. Okada K, Frassica FJ, Sim FH, et al: Periosteal osteosarcoma: A clinicopathological study. J Bone Joint Surg Am 76:366, 1994.
115. Otis JC, Lane JM, Krol MA: Energy cost during gait in osteosarcoma patients after resection and knee replacement and after above the knee amputation. J Bone Joint Surg Am 67:606, 1985.
116. Ozaki T, Hillmann A, Lindner N, Winkelmann W, et al: Cementation of primary aneurysmal bone cysts. Clin Orthop 240, 1997.
117. Ozaki T, Hillmann A, Wuisman P, et al: Reconstruction of tibia by ipsilateral vascularized fibula and allograft: 12 cases with malignant bone tumors. Acta Orthop Scand 68:298, 1997.
118. Ozaki T, Kawai A, Sugihara S, et al: Multiple osteocartilaginous exostosis: A follow-up study. Arch Orthop Trauma Surg 115: 255, 1996.
119. Patel SR, Evans HL, Benjamin RS: Combination chemotherapy in adult desmoid tumors. Cancer 72:3244, 1993.
120. Peabody TD, Monson D, Montag A, et al: A comparison of the prognoses for deep and subcutaneous sarcomas of the extremities. J Bone Joint Surg Am 76:1167, 1994.
121. Petschnig R, Baron R, Kotz R, et al: Muscle function after endoprosthetic replacement of the proximal tibia: Different techniques for extensor reconstruction in 17 tumor patients. Acta Orthop Scand 66:266, 1995.
122. Picariello L, Brandi ML, Formigli L, et al: Apoptosis induced by sulindac sulfide in epithelial and mesenchymal cells from human abdominal neoplasms. Eur J Pharmacol 360:105, 1998.

123. Picci P, Bacci G, Ferrari S, et al: Neoadjuvant chemotherapy in malignant fibrous histiocytoma of bone and in osteosarcoma located in the extremities: Analogies and differences between the two tumors. Ann Oncol 8:1107, 1997.
124. Picci P, Sangiorgi L, Bahamonde L, et al: Risk factors for local recurrences after limb-salvage surgery for high-grade osteosarcoma of the extremities. Ann Oncol 8:899, 1997.
125. Pisters PW, Harrison LB, Leung DH, et al: Long-term results of a prospective randomized trial of adjuvant brachytherapy in soft-tissue sarcoma. J Clin Oncol 14:859, 1996.
126. Pisters PW, Harrison LB, Woodruff JM, et al: A prospective randomized trial of adjuvant brachytherapy in the management of low-grade soft-tissue sarcomas of the extremity and superficial trunk. J Clin Oncol 12:1150, 1994.
127. Pollack A, Zagars GK, Goswitz MS, et al: Preoperative vs. postoperative radiotherapy in the treatment of soft-tissue sarcomas: A matter of presentation. Int J Radiat Oncol Biol Phys 42:563, 1998.
128. Pritchard DJ, Nascimento AG, Petersen IA: Local control of extra-abdominal desmoid tumors. J Bone Joint Surg Am 78:848, 1996.
129. Quint U, Muller RT, Muller G: Characteristics of phenol: Instillation in intralesional tumor excision of chondroblastoma, osteoclastoma and enchondroma. Arch Orthop Trauma Surg 117: 43, 1998.
130. Reich S, Overberg-Schmidt US, Buhrer C, et al: Low-dose chemotherapy with vinblastine and methotrexate in childhood desmoid tumors [letter]. J Clin Oncol 17:1086, 1999.
131. Reitamo JJ, Scheinin TM, Hayry P: The desmoid syndrome: New aspects in the cause, pathogenesis and treatment of the desmoid tumor. Am J Surg 151:230, 1986.
132. Ruggieri P, De Cristofaro R, Picci P, et al: Complications and surgical indications in 144 cases of nonmetastatic osteosarcoma of the extremities treated with neoadjuvant chemotherapy. Clin Orthop 226, 1993.
133. Rutten MJ, Collins JM, van Kampen A, et al: Meniscal cysts: Detection with high-resolution sonography. AJR Am J Roentgenol 171:491, 1998.
134. Sansone V, de Ponti A, Paluello GM, et al: Popliteal cysts and associated disorders of the knee: Critical review with MR imaging. Int Orthop 19:275, 1995.
135. Schajowicz F, McGuire MH, Santini Araujo E, et al: Osteosarcomas arising on the surfaces of long bones. J Bone Joint Surg Am 70:555, 1988.
136. Seeger LL, Dungan DH, Eckardt JJ, et al: Nonspecific findings on MR imaging: The importance of correlative studies and clinical information. Clin Orthop 306, 1991.
137. Sherman NE, Romsdahl M, Evans H, et al: Desmoid tumors: A 20-year radiotherapy experience. Int J Radiat Oncol Biol Phys 19:37, 1990.
138. Sheth DS, Yasko AW, Raymond AK, et al: Conventional and dedifferentiated parosteal osteosarcoma: Diagnosis, treatment, and outcome. Cancer 78:2136, 1996.
139. Sim FH, Beauchamp CP, Chao EYS: Reconstruction of musculoskeletal defects about the knee for tumors. Clin Orthop Rel Res 221:188, 1987.
140. Simon MA, Finn HA: Diagnostic strategy for bone and soft-tissue tumors. J Bone Joint Surg Am 75:622, 1993.
141. Simon MA, Finn HA: Diagnostic strategy for bone and soft-tissue tumors. Instr Course Lect 43:527, 1994.
142. Simon MA, Kirchner PT: Scintigraphic evaluation of primary bone tumors: Comparison of technetium-99m phosphonate and gallium citrate imaging. J Bone Joint Surg Am 62:758, 1980.
143. Sindelar WF, Kinsella TJ, Chen PW, et al: Intraoperative radiotherapy in retroperitoneal sarcomas: Final results of a prospective, randomized, clinical trial. Arch Surg 128:402, 1993.
144. Skapek SX, Hawk BJ, Hoffer FA, et al: Combination chemotherapy using vinblastine and methotrexate for the treatment of progressive desmoid tumor in children. J Clin Oncol 16:3021, 1998.
145. Szymanska J, Mandahl N, Mertens F, et al: Ring chromosomes in parosteal osteosarcoma contain sequences from 12q13-15: A combined cytogenetic and comparative genomic hybridization study. Genes Chromosomes Cancer 16:31, 1996.
146. Terek RM, Brien EW, Marcove RC, et al: Treatment of femoral Ewing's sarcoma. Cancer 78:70, 1996.
147. Terek RM, Schwartz GK, Devaney K, et al: Chemotherapy and P-glycoprotein expression in chondrosarcoma. J Orthop Res 16: 585, 1998.
148. Tsuboyama T, Windhager R, Dock W, et al: Knee function after operation for malignancy of the distal femur: Quadriceps muscle mass and knee extension strength in 21 patients with hinged endoprostheses. Acta Orthop Scand 64:673, 1993.
149. Tsukada K, Church JM, Jagelman DG, et al: Noncytotoxic drug therapy for intra-abdominal desmoid tumor in patients with familial adenomatous polyposis. Dis Colon Rectum 35:29, 1992.
150. Tyson LL, Daughters TC Jr, Ryu RK, et al: MRI appearance of meniscal cysts. Skeletal Radiol 24:421, 1995.
151. Unwin PS, Blunn GW, Cobb JP, et al: How successful are revisions of massive prostheses? In Brown KLB, ed: Complications of Limb Salvage. Montreal, ISOLS, 1991, p 183.
152. Unwin PS, Cannon SR, Grimer RJ, et al: Aseptic loosening in cemented custom-made prosthetic replacements for bone tumours of the lower limb. J Bone Joint Surg Br 78:5, 1996.
153. Unwin PS, Walker PS: Extendible endoprostheses for the skeletally immature. Clin Orthop 322:179, 1996.
154. Ward WG, Johnston KS, Dorey FJ, et al: Extramedullary porous coating to prevent diaphyseal osteolysis and radiolucent lines around proximal tibial replacements: A preliminary report. J Bone Joint Surg Am 75:976, 1993.
155. Ward WG, Mikaelian K, Dorey F, et al: Pulmonary metastases of stage IIB extremity osteosarcoma and subsequent pulmonary metastases. J Clin Oncol 12:1849, 1994.
156. Weiner SD, Scarborough M, Vander Griend RA: Resection arthrodesis of the knee with an intercalary allograft. J Bone Joint Surg Am 78:185, 1996.
157. Weiss AJ, Horowitz S, Lackmen RD: Therapy of desmoid tumors and fibromatosis using vinorelbine. Am J Clin Oncol 22: 193, 1999.
158. Wirganowicz PZ, Eckardt JJ, Dorey FJ, et al: Etiology and results of tumor endoprosthesis revision surgery in 64 patients. Clin Orthop 64, 1999.
159. Wolf RE, Scarborough MT, Enneking WF: Long-term followup of patients with autogenous resection arthrodesis of the knee. Clin Orthop 358:36, 1999.
160. Wu CT, Inwards CY, O'Laughlin S, et al: Chondromyxoid fibroma of bone: A clinicopathological review of 278 cases. Hum Pathol 29:438, 1998.
161. Wubben RC: Aneurysmal bone cyst arising after anterior cruciate ligament rupture. Am J Orthop 26:695, 1997.
162. Wunder JS, Paulian G, Huvos AG, et al: The histological response to chemotherapy as a predictor of the oncological outcome of operative treatment of Ewing's sarcoma. J Bone Joint Surg Am 80:1020, 1998.
163. Yang JC, Chang AE, Baker AR, et al: Randomized prospective study of the benefit of adjuvant radiation therapy in the treatment of soft-tissue sarcomas of the extremity. J Clin Oncol 16: 197, 1998.
164. Yang RS, Lane JM, Eilber FR, et al: High grade soft-tissue sarcoma of the flexor fossae: Size rather than compartmental status determine prognosis. Cancer 76:1398, 1995.
165. Yip KM, Leung PC, Kumta SM: Giant cell tumor of bone. Clin Orthop :60, 1996.
166. Yu JS, Chung C, Recht M, et al: MR imaging of tophaceous gout. AJR Am J Roentgenol 168:523, 1997.
167. Zatsepin ST, Burdygin VN: Replacement of the distal femur and proximal tibia with frozen allografts. Clin Orthop 303:95, 1994.

➢ Index

Note: Page numbers in *italics* refer to illustrations; page numbers followed by t refer to tables.